GASTROINTESTINAL PATHOLOGY

An Atlas and Text

THIRD EDITION

GASTROINTESTINAL PATHOLOGY
An Atlas and Text

THIRD EDITION

CECILIA M. FENOGLIO-PREISER, MD

Director of Gastrointestinal Pathology
AmeriPath Arizona
Phoenix, Arizona

AMY E. NOFFSINGER, MD

Associate Professor
University of Chicago
Chicago, Illinois

GRANT N. STEMMERMANN, MD

Professor of Pathology
University of Cincinnati College of Medicine
Cincinnati, Ohio

PATRICK E. LANTZ, MD

Associate Professor of Pathology
Wake Forest University Health Sciences
Winston-Salem, North Carolina

PETER G. ISAACSON, DM, DSc, FRCPath

Emeritus Professor
Department of Pathology
Royal Free and University College Medical School
London, United Kingdom

Wolters Kluwer | Lippincott Williams & Wilkins
Health
Philadelphia • Baltimore • New York • London
Buenos Aires • Hong Kong • Sydney • Tokyo

Acquisitions Editor: Jonathan Pine
Managing Editor: Jean McGough
Project Manager: Rosanne Hallowell
Manufacturing Manager: Kathleen Brown
Marketing Manager: Angela Panetta
Cover Designer/Design Coordinator: Stephen Druding
Production Services: Aptara, Inc.

Third Edition
© 2008 by Lippincott Williams & Wilkins, a Wolters Kluwer business
530 Walnut Street
Philadelphia, PA 19106
LWW.com

Second Edition © 1997 by Lippincott Williams & Wilkins
First Edition © 1989 by Raven Press

Printed in China.

Library of Congress Cataloging-in-Publication Data

Gastrointestinal pathology : an atlas and text / Cecilia M. Fenoglio-Preiser ... [et al.]. — 3rd ed.
       p. ; cm.
    Includes bibliographical references and index.
    ISBN-13: 978-0-7817-7146-7
    ISBN-10: 0-7817-7146-3
    1. Gastrointestinal system—Diseases.   2. Gastrointestinal system—Histopathology.
3. Gastrointestinal system—Diseases—Atlases.   4. Gastrointestinal system—Histopathology—
Atlases.   I. Fenoglio-Preiser, Cecilia M., 1943–
    [DNLM: 1. Gastrointestinal Diseases—pathology—Atlases.   2. Gastrointestinal Diseases—
pathology.   3. Digestive System—anatomy & histology—Atlases.   4. Digestive System—anatomy
& histology. WI 140 G2589 2008]
    RC802.9.G368 2008
    616.3'3071—dc22

                                                                                        2007033389

                                                                10 9 8 7 6 5 4 3

CCS0209

To Wolf, Rich, Nell, and Kreiter

CONTENTS

PREFACE

The third edition of this book has been a long time coming because it has been markedly expanded from the second edition. This expansion is the result of suggestions made by you, our readers. It is also the result of an explosion in our understanding of the pathophysiology of many disorders due to the use of animal models of disease and genetic investigations. Animal models have greatly enhanced our understanding of inflammatory bowel disease and motility disorders. Genetic studies have also contributed to our knowledge of predispositions to many types of neoplasms as well as serving as potential prognostic or therapeutic markers. The last decade has also seen an explosion in imaging and endoscopic diagnostic and therapeutic techniques, which is now generating novel types of specimens, including endomucosal resection specimens and increasing numbers of cytologic samples. During this time our understanding of many diseases has expanded, controversies have arisen, and new entities have emerged.

Because of the expansion in our knowledge, the size of this book would have been unmanageable (and the cost prohibitive) without some alterations from the previous edition. Therefore, some chapters have been eliminated such as the AIDS and cytology chapters as well as the separate chapter on the normal anatomy and histology of each site. This material has been integrated into other chapters. We have also eliminated many radiographs to provide space for additional histologic images or diagrams. One new chapter has been added on endocrine lesions to avoid duplication of material and give us more room to add new material. Some chapters have been exhaustively revised, particularly those dealing with gastrointestinal stromal tumors, gastrointestinal hematologic diseases, and motility disorders. We have also added in material that was on the CD that went with the second edition but was not in the printed version of the book.

We intend for this work to be comprehensive and helpful for those dealing with biopsies as well as cytology and resection specimens of all gastrointestinal sites, and it therefore contains information about benign and neoplastic gastrointestinal diseases that is not found in other textbooks. We have tried to arrange the material in a way that meets the reading or perusing needs of many of you. Because we believe that "a picture is worth a thousand words," the book is replete with illustrations, diagrams, and tables. As in previous editions, we have attempted to incorporate information concerning normal anatomy and histology, epidemiology, clinical features, and, of course, pathologic and prognostic features. We have added abundant new genetic information in many areas about both benign and malignant gastrointestinal diseases. The diseases covered include those affecting both children and adults.

Each of the "benign organ" chapters is arranged in a similar way. Each begins with a discussion of the normal anatomy and histology followed by discussions of congenital and acquired lesions, infectious diseases, drug-related diseases, and diseases resulting from altered blood flow, as well as many other entities. These chapters also contain basic information on the interpretation of mucosal biopsies. We hope that the third edition meets the needs of those both in academic centers and in other practice settings. We expect that our readers will continue to find this text helpful in eliminating the need to run to multiple sources to gain a clear understanding of gastrointestinal diseases. We hope that the reader finds the abundant illustrations and tables educational. We also hope that this book is practical for use by both the "generalist" and those practicing gastrointestinal pathology. We believe that this book will be useful to pathologists, gastroenterologists, radiologists, internists, and surgeons interested in gastrointestinal diseases, whether they be clinicians, clinician educators, or researchers.

Cecilia M. Fenoglio-Preiser, MD
Amy E. Noffsinger, MD
Grant N. Stemmermann, MD
Patrick E. Lantz, MD
Peter G. Isaacson, DM, DSc, FRCPath

PREFACE TO THE FIRST EDITION

his book originally started as an atlas of gastrointestinal diseases. As it developed, however, it became clear that there was no one book of gastrointestinal pathology that incorporates information concerning anatomy, infectious diseases, clinical manifestations, radiology, and pathologic analysis into a single convenient source. For this reason, it has gradually evolved into a comprehensively illustrated textbook of gastrointestinal pathology, with gross and microscopic photographs, line drawings, radiographs, and electron micrographs. We have tried to discuss and to illustrate the spectrum of changes that may be present throughout the entire gastrointestinal tract, drawing on the wealth of literature that is dispersed throughout scientific texts and journals.

The book is organized such that each anatomical section (esophagus, stomach, small bowel, large intestine, and anus) is divided into three chapters, i.e., normal anatomy, nonneoplastic conditions, and neoplasms involving that site. A single chapter is devoted to the appendix, since it shares features of both the small and large intestine and is affected by some unique entities. In addition, there are chapters devoted to inflammatory bowel disease, polyposis syndromes, endocrine cells, mesenchymal tumors, lymphoproliferative lesions, and cytological features since the discussions involve disorders affecting multiple anatomic sites. The nonneoplastic chapters are arranged similarly with discussion of the embryological (congenital) disorders followed by a discussion of inflammations and miscellaneous disorders.

We have not concentrated on the mucosal biopsy as many current texts of gastrointestinal pathology do; our intention has been to cover aspects of gastrointestinal diseases as seen through resection specimens, mucosal biopsy specimens, and cytology specimens. We expect the reader will find our discussion of various aspects of gastrointestinal disease helpful in eliminating the need to run to multiple sources to get a clear understanding of the disease processes. We also expect that the reader will find the illustrative material educational.

We believe this book will be useful to pathologists, gastroenterologists, radiologists, internists, and surgeons interested in the diseases of the gastrointestinal tract, particularly for those who teach in these areas.

Cecilia M. Fenoglio-Preiser, MD
Patrick E. Lantz, MD
Margaret B. Listrom, MD
Michael Davis, MD
Franco O. Rilke, MD

ACKNOWLEDGMENTS

Many pathologists contributed the illustrations provided in the text. We are reusing some illustrations previously acknowledged in the first and second editions. The authors would like to thank those residents at the University of New Mexico School of Medicine, Department of Pathology, during the preparation of the First Edition and residents at the University of Cincinnati during the preparation of the second and third editions who brought interesting gastrointestinal cases to our attention. We also would like to thank all of those who provided additional illustrative material. They are specifically acknowledged in the figure legends accompanying the individual figures.

Finally, we would like to thank our families for providing continual moral support and patience in the many years it took to revise this text. The third edition would not be a reality without the special contributions of all of these people.

GASTROINTESTINAL PATHOLOGY

An Atlas and Text

THIRD EDITION

CHAPTER 1

General Features of the Gastrointestinal Tract and Evaluation of Specimens Derived from It

GENERAL COMMENTS

In many ways the gastrointestinal (GI) tract is a remarkable organ. The embryonic endoderm will give rise to the future GI tract. The GI tract will acquire multiple cell types that will be dispersed into two planes: A vertical plane that allows one to recognize different layers of the bowel wall and a horizontal plane that develops into the esophagus, stomach, small intestine, colon, and anus. Although these cell types will resemble one another, important histologic differences allow specific physiologic functions to be carried out in each anatomic region. Interactions between cell populations regulate subsequent patterns of gene expression and organ development (1).

The physiology of the GI tract is also impressive. It serves as the digestive organ of the body, taking in everything that is swallowed and turning it into useful nutrients or discarding what is left over as waste. These processes begin in the mouth and terminate at the anus. While digesting everything to which it is exposed and breaking it down into smaller, absorbable, chemical substances, the gut is itself able to withstand these processes and avoid autodigestion. Complex neuromuscular interactions allow the GI tract to move food and liquids from one section of the gut to the next while at the same time controlling the passage of food in such a way that maximum digestion and absorption occurs in each of the appropriate spots. Even in a single organ, such as the small intestine, a differentiation gradient exists such that different substances are preferentially absorbed at different intestinal sites and through different parts of the cell. Not everything taken into the mouth and swallowed is healthy for the patient. Therefore, the GI tract serves as a major interface between the outside world and the rest of the body. The gut is continuously exposed to toxins and infectious organisms, yet it is often capable of eliminating these agents without causing any harm to itself. Not surprisingly, breakdown in these defense processes often results in disease. This generally occurs when the integrity of the bowel wall becomes compromised. The gut also serves as a major immune organ. It is the major site of the generation of mucosal immunity, hence the utility of oral vaccines. These immunologic processes largely take place in the small bowel. Finally, the GI tract is a major endocrine organ.

In humans, the gut is divided into four major organs: Esophagus, stomach, small intestine, and large intestine. These are separated by sphincters that control the passage of contents from one organ to the next. The junctions between organs are identifiable by an abrupt change in the mucosal nature and by the presence of the sphincters.

EMBRYOLOGY

Multiple interactions occur during development between and within the three germ layers (endoderm, mesoderm, and ectoderm). Each of these layers may reciprocally induce development of other layers. The endoderm induces the mesoderm (2). It also confers a dorsal-ventral pattern on it (2). The endoderm and ectoderm contact one another in the 2- to 4-week embryo. The endoderm, which forms the roof of the yolk sac, gives rise to the future gut, creating the majority of the epithelial lining of the GI tract, biliary passages, liver, and pancreas. The primitive gut temporarily consists of foregut, midgut, and hindgut. The splanchnic mesoderm surrounding the primitive gut forms the muscular and connective tissue layers. Embryologic development takes place with a large number of inducers that share overlapping expression patterns and redundant functions. The core of this system consists of a set of structurally similar genes known as homeobox genes. The embryology of each region is discussed in detail in the relevant chapters.

Multipotential neural progenitors give rise to various derivatives, including neurons, glia, and ganglia, as the result of local environmental signals. These progenitors differentiate based on specific molecules they encounter either during their migration or within the organ in which they terminally differentiate as discussed in detail in Chapter 10.

Abundant endocrine cells are present by 8 weeks' gestation. The diversity of the GI endocrine cell component is established early. There is a higher density of endocrine cells in both the proximal duodenum and distal colon/rectum compared with other areas. Endocrine cell numbers increase with age, roughly paralleling the growth of the gut. The full adult profile is attained by the second trimester. The endocrine system is discussed in detail in Chapter 17.

Peripheral lymph nodes develop by the second month of gestation. Mononuclear cell aggregates are also identified in the fetal intestine in proximity to the endodermal epithelium.

CELL PROLIFERATION

The GI tract undergoes continuous development and proliferation. Its mucosa varies from the esophagus to the colon and it contains multiple cell types. New cells form from stem cells within the basal layers of the anal and esophageal squamous epithelium, in the mucous neck region of the stomach, or from the bases of the crypts in the intestines (Fig. 1.1). Cells then migrate out of the proliferative zone and differentiate into multiple cell lineages. The differentiation pattern of the gut epithelium is influenced by other cells in its environment (3). Eventually the cells are shed into the lumen or undergo apoptosis. Cellular life span is 5 to 7 days in the duodenum and jejunum, 4 to 5 days in the ileum, and 4 to 6 days in the large intestine. Specific details of cell proliferation in the esophagus, stomach, small intestine, and colon are discussed in the relevant chapters.

The intestine alters its rates of cellular renewal and adapts to surgical, nutritional, and other toxic stimuli, as well as to physiologic and disease states. Stem cells show three general features: (a) the capacity to undergo asymmetric division, producing one daughter that remains a stem cell and another that undergoes a seemingly irreversible commitment to enter a differentiation pathway; (b) proliferative potential; and (c) the ability to retain a position in a particular environmental niche (4,5). Some stem cells are unipotential, giving rise to a single differentiated phenotype, whereas others are multipotential, giving rise to multiple cell types.

Of interest is the fact that not all stem cells that give rise to gastrointestinal epithelia are gastrointestinal stem cells. It now appears that bone marrow stem cells may be recruited to sites of injury and give rise to a host of cell lineages, including cells with mixed gastrointestinal phenotypes. This phenomenon is best exemplified in the development of gastric cancer following *Helicobacter pylori* infections as discussed in Chapter 5.

GASTROINTESTINAL STRUCTURE

In general, the gut consists of four concentric layers as one progresses outward from the lumen: The mucosa, submucosa, muscularis propria, and serosa or adventitia (Fig. 1.2). These layers are easily visualized histologically and can also be imaged using ultrasound. The high correlation that exists between the ultrasound image and the histologic features allows one to use ultrasound to provide diagnostic information about the status of the GI tract.

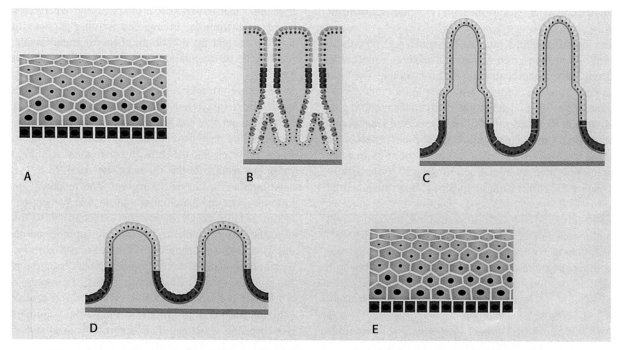

FIG. 1.1. Diagrammatic representation of the proliferative zones (*green*) in the various regions of the gastrointestinal tract. **A:** The proliferative zone of the esophagus is restricted to the basal cell layer of the stratified squamous epithelium. **B:** In the stomach, proliferation occurs in the neck region of the glands, and cells migrate in two directions to populate the pits and the bases of the glands. **C:** Proliferation in the small intestine occurs in the basal one third of the crypts. **D:** In the colon, proliferation is restricted to the basal one third to one half of the crypt. **E:** Like the esophagus, proliferation in the anus occurs in the basal zone of the epithelium.

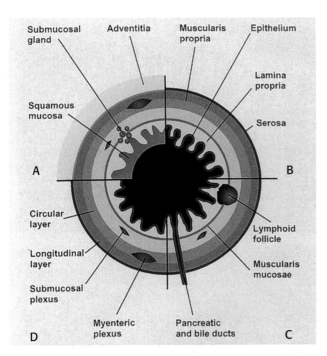

FIG. 1.2. Although the basic architecture is similar in all regions of the gastrointestinal tract, functional and histologic differences do exist. The four quadrants of the diagram compare the **(A)** esophagus, **(B)** stomach, **(C)** small intestine, and **(D)** large intestine.

Mucosa

The mucosa consists of an epithelial lining, a lamina propria that contains loose connective tissue rich in immunocompetent cells, and the muscularis mucosae. The lamina propria is most visible in the stomach, large and small intestines, and appendix, and is least visible in the esophagus and anus. The smooth muscle cells in the muscularis mucosae are predominantly arranged in a circular orientation, although some longitudinal muscle fibers are also present.

The epithelium may invaginate to form glands that extend into the (a) lamina propria (i.e., mucosal glands in the stomach) (Fig. 1.2), (b) submucosa (i.e., submucosal glands in the esophagus [Fig. 1.2] or Brunner glands in the duodenum), or (c) ducts that extend to organs outside the gut, such as to the pancreas or the liver. The mucosa and submucosa may also project into the GI lumen as folds (plicae or rugae) (Fig. 1.2). Additionally, villi may be present (Fig. 1.2).

GI epithelium differs substantially in various organs. Squamous epithelium lines the mucosa of the esophagus and anus (Fig. 1.3). In the stomach, the epithelium is divided into surface epithelium, pits, and glands (Fig. 1.3). In the small intestine, the mucosa consists of crypts and villi containing a population of intestinal epithelial cells. The colon contains similar cells but it lacks villi. The squamous lining of the esophagus protects it from the passage of undigested food over its surface. Likewise, in the anus, the squamous epithelium protects the mucosa from the damaging effects of the passage of solid waste. In the stomach, the mucosa facilitates digestion by secreting acid.

The epithelial lining of the small intestine is uniquely suited to the further digestion and absorption of nutrients along a gradient from the duodenum to the ileum. The colon predominantly resorbs water. The specific features of the various portions of the gut are discussed in their appropriate chapters.

The lamina propria forms the mucosal interglandular tissues. It appears as a delicate, loose, connective tissue containing lymphocytes, plasma cells (Fig. 1.4), eosinophils, rare neutrophils, and mast cells. The majority of the cells are plasma cells and lymphocytes, with the majority of plasma cells secreting IgA; however, IgM-, IgG-, and IgE-secreting cells are also present. The lamina propria also contains large numbers of macrophages, which play important roles in mucosal immunity, antigen presentation, elimination of exogenous pathologic antigens or organisms, immunoglobulin production, and immunoregulation (6).

The gut-associated lymphoid tissue (GALT) primarily lies within the lamina propria. It is distributed diffusely or appears as solitary (Fig. 1.5) or aggregated nodules, which in the ileum and appendix are called Peyer patches. Larger aggregates contain germinal centers. Peyer patches are present on the antimesenteric border of the intestine. These lymphoid nodules often span the muscularis mucosae (Fig. 1.5), breaking through into the superficial submucosa and creating gaps in the muscularis mucosae. Solitary nodules occur in the esophagus, in the gastric pylorus, and along the small and large intestines. Both blood and lymphatic capillaries form a plexus around the lymphoid follicles (7). The majority of the cells within the follicles are lymphocytes, macrophages, and plasma cells. The basement membrane overlying the Peyer patches is more porous than that of the adjacent epithelial areas, facilitating the bidirectional passage of lymphocytes during antigenic stimulation (8). The lamina propria also contains vessels and unmyelinated nerve fibers.

Mast cells comprise an important, but heterogeneous, component of the lamina propria and submucosa. Specialized contacts exist between mast cells and other cell types; these contacts facilitate intercellular communication. Mast cells often lie adjacent to blood vessels or lymphatics, near or within nerves, and beneath epithelial surfaces, particularly those of the GI tract where they are exposed to environmental antigens (9,10). Numerous cells respond to mast cell mediators, as exemplified by the presence of histamine receptors on their surfaces. Cells with surface histamine receptors include lymphocytes, macrophages, neutrophils, basophils, eosinophils, smooth muscle cells, and parietal cells. Neuropeptides and hormones influence mast cells, inducing them to release their mediators.

Mast cells initiate acute inflammation and propagate chronic inflammatory changes. These cells may also be antigen-presenting cells. In some IgE-dependent inflammatory responses, mast cells are the sole or primary initiator of the reaction, and in others they may influence pre-existing inflammation. By virtue of their location and number, mast cells participate in a wide variety of GI diseases. The most important include food allergies, eosinophilia, immunodeficiency

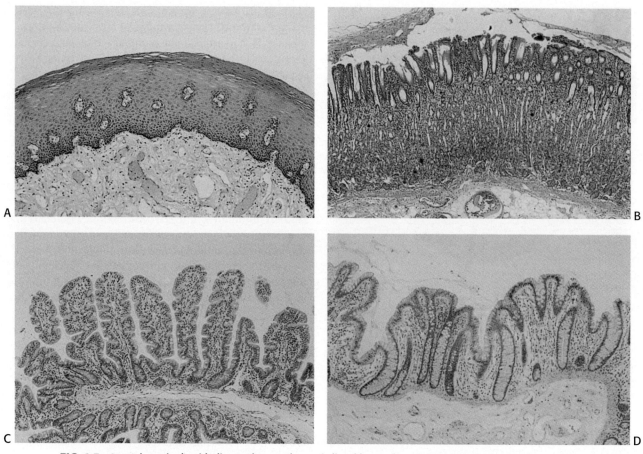

FIG. 1.3. Gastrointestinal epithelia. **A:** The esophagus is lined by nonkeratinizing stratified squamous epithelium. **B:** The epithelium of the stomach is arranged into pits and glands. The pits are lined by foveolar cells and have a similar appearance in all regions of the stomach. The glands contain numerous cell types that differ from one region of the stomach to another. **C:** The small intestinal mucosa consists of crypts and villi. **D:** The colon lacks villi and consists of rows of parallel crypts lined by columnar absorptive cells, goblet cells, and endocrine cells.

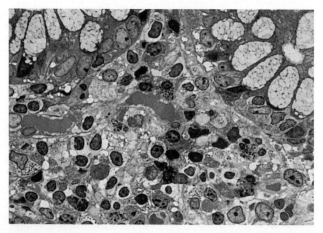

FIG. 1.4. Thick section from a portion of small bowel showing the lamina propria that contains large numbers of lymphocytes, plasma cells, and macrophages.

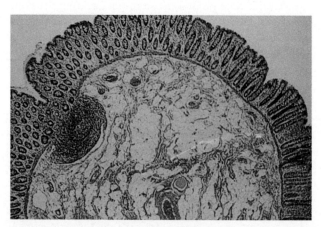

FIG. 1.5. The colonic mucosa is separated from the submucosa by the muscularis mucosae, which is punctuated only by the lymphoid follicle. Collagen bundles and large vessels are prominent in the submucosa.

syndromes, immediate hypersensitivity reactions, host responses to parasites and neoplasms, immunologically non-specific inflammatory and fibrotic conditions, and tissue remodeling. Mast cells are also important in angiogenesis, wound healing, peptic ulcer disease, and other chronic inflammatory conditions, including graft versus host disease and inflammatory bowel disease.

Eosinophils might also be present within the lamina propria. Eosinophils are most abundant in tissues with an epithelial interface, such as the GI tract. Their intracellular granules cause their tinctorial features. Eosinophils express receptors for IgG, IgE, and IgA on their external membranes (11). Eosinophils also have receptors for complement components and cytokines. They themselves produce and release numerous mediators in response to activation (11). Eosinophils have both beneficial and detrimental roles in the host. They function in host defense, including the phagocytosis and killing of bacteria and other microbes, but they also mediate allergic reactions, and the oxidative products of eosinophils can damage cells. The eosinophilic products that are most damaging are the cationic proteins (11).

Submucosa

The submucosa is a more densely collagenous, less cellular layer than the mucosa. However, in some areas it may have a loose organization. Major blood vessels, lymphatics, nerves, ganglia, and occasionally lymphoid collections are located here. It also contains fat.

Muscularis Propria

The muscularis propria is a continuous structure composed of two smooth muscle layers that extend from the upper esophagus to the anal canal (Fig. 1.6). The only exception to this occurs in the stomach, where three layers are present. At the junctions between adjacent organs, the muscular coat

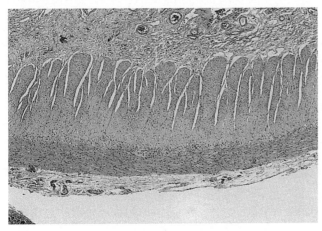

FIG. 1.6. Hematoxylin and eosin–stained section demonstrating the circular and longitudinal smooth muscle layers of the muscularis propria.

rearranges to form sphincters including the pharyngoesophageal, esophagogastric, pyloric, ileocecal, and anal sphincters. The function of these sphincters is based on physiologic and pharmacologic characteristics of the musculature and on their innervation. The muscle fibers are usually arranged in a concentric circular fashion in the inner muscular layer (the circular layer), whereas the outer muscle fibers are arranged longitudinally (the longitudinal layer). In the cecum and in parts of the colon, the longitudinal muscle is extremely attenuated except in the regions where it forms thick cords (i.e., the taeniae coli).

Circular muscle, from the esophagus to the internal anal sphincter, behaves as an electrical syncytium. The syncytial properties result from nexuses between the plasma membranes of contiguous muscle fibers. These nexuses function as intracellular pathways for conduction of excitation between adjacent cells. Even in the absence of neural influences, these syncytial properties allow for three-dimensional spread of excitation (12). Smooth muscle cells also contain gap junctions or nexuses that electrically couple adjacent cells (12).

The musculature also contains the interstitial cells of Cajal (ICCs). ICCs have three major functions: (a) they act as pacemakers for the GI muscle (13), (b) they facilitate active propagation of electrical events, and (c) they mediate neurotransmission. They may also act as mechanoreceptors (13). These cells may be abnormal in motility disorders as discussed in Chapter 10 and they give rise to the group of tumors known as GI stromal tumors (GISTs) as discussed in Chapter 19.

The cells of the muscularis propria contain numerous receptors, allowing them to respond to neural signals as well as other stimulatory and inhibitory signals during the digestive process. Contraction of the circular layer constricts the lumen; contraction of the longitudinal layer shortens the digestive tube. When the bowel becomes obstructed or the intestinal lumen distends on a persistent basis, the muscle increases in volume through both hypertrophy and hyperplasia. Smooth muscle hyperplasia also follows myenteric ablation. Obstruction results in a number of changes to both the muscular and neural layers.

Adventitia or Serosa

The adventitia consists of loose connective tissue containing fat, collagen, and elastic tissues (Fig. 1.7). If it is covered by mesothelium, it is called a serosa. A serosa is present on the stomach, those parts of the small intestine that are not retroperitoneal, the appendix, and the large intestine above the peritoneal reflection.

Blood Vessels

Both blood vessels and lymphatics enter the gut from the surrounding tissues. The largest arteries pass through the GI wall and are arranged longitudinally in a submucosal plexus.

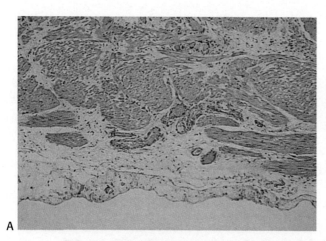

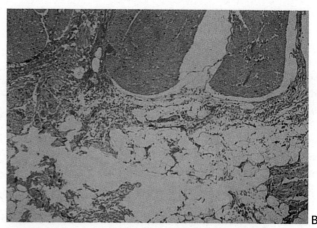

A   B

FIG. 1.7. Well-delineated serosal surface of the intestine **(A)** covered with mesothelium contrasts sharply with the irregular loose tissue of the adventitia of the esophagus **(B).**

The submucosal plexus sends arterioles and capillaries into the mucosa, muscularis, and adventitia or serosa. The mucosa contains an irregular capillary plexus, often with its most terminal branches underlying the luminal surface epithelium (Fig. 1.8). Within the muscular layer the vessels lie parallel to the muscle fibers. Veins arising in the mucosa anastomose in the submucosa and course with the arteries out of the intestine. Valves are present in veins in the adventitia or serosa. The vascular anatomy of each region of the GI tract is described in the relevant chapters.

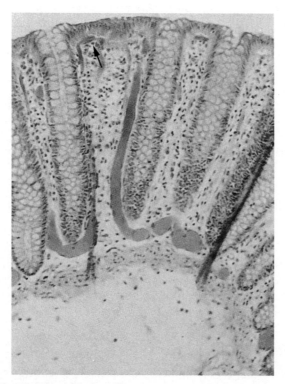

FIG. 1.8. Blood-filled capillary penetrates to the surface epithelium, where a rich capillary network is located (*arrow*).

The intestinal mucosa receives the highest vascular perfusion of any peripheral organ (14), a feature critical to the absorption of nutrients from this site. Vascular contractility is controlled by submucosal neurons whose excitation leads to vasodilation of the submucosal arterioles. This increases mucosal blood flow (15). Intestinal blood flow is determined by three mechanisms: intrinsic (myogenic and local metabolic), extrinsic (sympathetic nervous), and circulating vasoactive agents (14).

Nitric oxide (NO) is continuously released from the arterial and arteriolar endothelium (Fig. 1.9) (16). Vessels, particularly arteries, also contain large amounts of superoxide dismutase (SOD). This enzyme modulates NO activity. NO acts as an important intracellular signal causing smooth muscle relaxation, including the smooth muscle of the vascular system (17). NO also contributes to thromboresistance of vessel walls.

Lymphatics

The gut is richly supplied with lymphatics, but their distribution, particularly in the mucosa, varies with the location in the gut. The richest lymphatic distribution occurs in the small intestine, where the lymphatics are intimately involved in nutrient absorption. Larger submucosal lymphatics branch freely and contain numerous valves. Smaller mucosal and submucosal lymphatics may be difficult to detect because they are often collapsed and blend in with the surrounding connective tissue. They are also sometimes difficult to distinguish from small blood capillaries. However, each vessel type has distinctive features. The lymphatics from the submucosa pass through the gastrointestinal wall and eventually drain into the regional lymph nodes.

Innervation

The enteric nervous system (ENS) is the most complex portion of the peripheral nervous system. It is discussed in detail in Chapter 10.

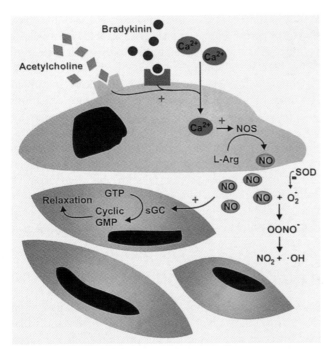

FIG. 1.9. Nitric oxide (NO) mediates vascular relaxation. NO is produced in endothelial cells by the action of calcium-dependent nitric oxide synthase (NOS). Mediators such as acetylcholine and bradykinin stimulate its production. NO acts on smooth muscle cells through a process involving conversion of guanosine triphosphate (GTP) to cyclic guanosine monophosphate (GMP), affecting relaxation. NO released into the interstitium may produce damaging free radicals after interacting with superoxide molecules. This process is inhibited by the action of superoxide dismutase (SOD) on superoxide.

Endocrine Cells

The gastrointestinal tract is the largest endocrine "organ" in the body and contains a large number and type of endocrine/paracrine cells. It is the second richest source of regulatory peptides outside of the brain. Some endocrine cell types found in the gut also occur in the pancreas, and thus the entire population is also sometimes referred to as the gastroenteropancreatic system. This system is discussed in detail in Chapter 17.

TYPES OF GASTROINTESTINAL SPECIMENS

GI pathology specimens fall into three major categories: Biopsy specimens, resection specimens, and cytology specimens. GI specimen interpretation is facilitated by a familiarity by the pathologist of clinical gastroenterology and the nature of the procedures used to obtain the specimens. Endoscopy, diagnostic imaging, and therapeutic instrumentation are currently generating biopsy or small resection specimens from sites that were previously inaccessible without a major resection. As a result, gastroenterologists, surgeons, endoscopists, and radiologists currently provide specimens to

the pathology laboratory. It is important that these individuals understand the information different types of specimens can provide and what the limitations of different types of specimens are.

Biopsies are taken to establish a specific diagnosis or to follow the evolution of a particular lesion or disease. They are also taken to determine disease extent as in inflammatory bowel disease or to judge its severity, to determine response to therapy, and to detect cancers or their premalignant stages. Biopsies may also be taken to acquire tissues for other specific purposes, including microbial culture, biochemical examination, ultrastructural examination, or evaluation by molecular markers. Specimen interpretation is always enhanced by an effective dialogue between the pathologist and the clinician, usually via pertinent information provided on the requisition form or through routine clinical-pathologic correlation conferences.

It is important that the clinician indicate the exact site of origin of a biopsy since this provides critical information for specimens from some locations. For example, the presence of gastritis in the proximal stomach versus the antrum has different clinical implications and etiologies. The significance of intestinal metaplasia in the esophagus differs from that in the stomach. Inflammation in the distal colon may have different implications than inflammation in the proximal colon. Thus, it is important that the clinician not submit samples from multiple locations in the stomach or colon in the same specimen bottle, as critical information can be lost when this occurs. This is especially true in the colon, where the distribution of a colitis provides important diagnostic information. It is also helpful to know whether the areas biopsied appeared endoscopically normal or abnormal.

Incisional biopsies (such as biopsies of cancer) represent only part of a lesion, and these are purely diagnostic biopsies. In contrast, excisional biopsies (such as a polypectomy) can be therapeutic as well as diagnostic. The decision of the clinician to perform an incisional or an excisional biopsy depends on the size of the lesion and, in some cases, its growth pattern.

Ideally, once biopsies are obtained, they should be oriented to avoid tangentially cutting when the specimen is processed and to facilitate the assessment of certain measurements such as a crypt:villus ratio in the small bowel or an evaluation of the length of the papillae in the esophagus. However, even if the specimens are received unoriented, the presence of multiple biopsies examined at several levels usually provides sufficient information that one can interpret the biopsies without special care having been taken to the orientation.

Some GI lesions will be sampled cytologically, although in the United States exfoliative cytology does not play the same role that gastrointestinal biopsy interpretation does, except possibly in the diagnosis of esophageal infections. However, cytologic examination can be an important adjunctive technology in the diagnosis of malignancies. Cytologic samples are particularly helpful in portions of the GI tract that are stenotic and therefore difficult to biopsy. Cytologic preparations can also be used in areas where a gross lesion is present because large areas of the surface can be sampled with a cytology brush. Cytologic examination can help confirm the presence of neoplasia. This approach has been used much more extensively for screening for cancer of the esophagus or stomach in places such as China and Japan. It is much less commonly used to diagnose colonic and rectal lesions.

Resections are performed to surgically treat cancer or precancerous lesions, life-threatening ischemia, severe ulcerating diseases, obstructions, and pseudo-obstructions, as well as various other conditions. Resection specimens received in the fresh state should be examined as soon as possible to determine whether or not the specimen requires special handling for procedures such as microbial cultures, ultrastructural examination, histochemical stains requiring frozen sections or special fixatives, biochemical analysis, imprints, cytogenetic studies, or molecular studies prior to fixation. The pathologist should be able to examine the entire specimen. It is a common practice to remove a fresh piece of tumor (or other disease) and normal mucosa for future research if this does not interfere with the pathology assessment. This should be done under the supervision of a pathologist and in compliance with Health Insurance Portability and Accountability Act (HIPAA) regulations. Removal of any tissue before a pathologist has examined the specimen often results in loss of critical material that is needed to properly interpret the specimen.

SPECIMEN FIXATION

Biopsies should be placed in an adequate amount of fixative, which for biopsies should be at least five times the volume of the specimens. Ten percent buffered formalin is the most commonly used fixative in histology laboratories because it is stable and allows staining with most currently used histochemical and immunohistochemical stains. It does, however, induce substantial tissue shrinkage. In some circumstances where a more accurate rendering of the cytologic features is required, additional fixatives can be used that contain heavy metals, such as Bouin, B5, or Hollende solution. These fixatives cause less tissue shrinkage and permit analysis of nuclei that appear less distorted. However, the latter fixatives interfere with the ability to isolate high-quality nucleic acids from the biopsy specimens should this be intended later. Additionally, these fixatives are often not routinely available.

In some cases it is important that the samples be presented in an unfixed state so that they can be handled in a special way. For example, in suspected lymphomas, fresh tissue should be obtained for flow cytometry, freezing, and other special studies. In patients with motility disorders such as Hirschsprung disease, submission of fresh tissue allows the use of enzyme histochemistry to evaluate the neural structures. Fresh tissue is also required to demonstrate fat within the tissues as in some lipid storage diseases. Finally,

rapidly acquired fresh tissue may be necessary for some genetic or chromosomal studies. There should be a duplicate sample that is fixed in formalin if all of the fresh tissue is to be used for special studies.

Glutaraldehyde is the fixative of choice for specimens that may require ultrastructural examinations. Situations where this might be necessary may include a search for microsporidia, an evaluation of storage diseases, or a mitochondrial myopathy. Ultrastructural examination may also be useful in the identification of certain tumors, although this is becoming less common with the wide array of immunohistochemical and more recently genetic markers that is available. A duplicate formalin-fixed specimen should also be submitted in these situations.

HANDLING RESECTION SPECIMENS

Resection specimens should be opened longitudinally and cleansed to remove blood, stool, and other substances that may interfere with obtaining information from the specimen. The prosector should describe all lesions, including tumors, ulcers, or other abnormal areas. Attention should be given to documenting the size, appearance, and anatomic relationship of any lesions. The distance of a tumor from the proximal, distal, and radial margins should be measured. The depth of invasion should be estimated and extension beyond the organ should be documented, if present. Specimen palpation helps delineate full tumor extent. Painting the margins with India ink can be useful in making these determinations. A comment should be as to whether or not the nodes appear to be grossly involved. If the resection specimen is a resection for ischemia, a search for thrombi should be made in the mesenteric vessels.

The specimen should be photographed if it contains an obvious lesion. These photographs are invaluable for presentations at tumor boards and other clinical care conferences. They also serve as invaluable teaching resources. They allow physicians to recognize the gross aspects of the diseases that are encountered on a daily basis. They also facilitate correlation with endoscopic and/or radiologic appearances. Carcinomas should be photographed from both the surface and the cut section to show the extent of tumor invasion. Vascular lesions can be enhanced by intravascular ingestion of ink or other compounds. When the specimen is photographed, it should be properly oriented and should include some normal tissue for orientation. The photographic table should be clean.

The resection specimen should be placed in 10% neutral buffered formalin with a fixative volume that is at least ten times that of the tissue. Bowel specimens should be pinned out to optimize flat, well-oriented lesions. If a specimen is pinned to a corkboard, gauze or paper towels can be placed beneath the specimen to serve as a wick for the fixative. Tissues should be adequately fixed prior to sectioning. Blocks should be obtained to evaluate the nature and extent of all lesions. If the patient has received preoperative radiation and/or chemotherapy, residual cancer may not be obvious and one may need to block an entire suspicious area in order to find remnants of tumor. This is especially true in esophageal, gastric and rectal resection specimens from patients undergoing neoadjuvant therapies. It is important that when sections are submitted, the origins of each section be noted in the gross description.

Sometimes vital staining is used in the evaluation of gross specimens, although this is most commonly done in research settings. Examples include Lugol staining of esophagectomy specimens with squamous cell lesions, alkaline phosphatase staining of gastric resections to map areas of intestinal metaplasia (see Chapter 4), or vital staining to identify aberrant crypt foci.

Endoscopic mucosal resection (EMR) specimens require special handling in order to determine whether the resection margins are microscopically complete (18). The specimen should be stretched and pinned to a block. Deep and lateral margins should be marked with India ink. The specimen should be sectioned longitudinally at 2-mm intervals after fixation for 24 hours in formaldehyde. A resection may be classified as complete for neoplasia if the deep and lateral margins are negative and complete for Barrett esophagus if the margins are composed of nonmetaplastic mucosa.

Patients with invasive duodenal adenocarcinomas are often treated with a pancreaticoduodenectomy (i.e., Whipple resection: A resection of the distal stomach, duodenum, distal biliary tree, and head of pancreas), and they require special handling. The stomach and duodenum should first be placed in a fixative, preferably formalin, to allow for deep fixation. Inserting a probe from the cut surface of the common bile duct through the biliary tree and into the duodenal lumen is not recommended. Metal probes damage and distort the lining cells of these ducts and subsequent sections will often show complete loss of the epithelial lining. Neoplasms involving the ampulla and distal bile ducts should be blocked in their entirety. Sections should be taken parallel to the long axis of the bile duct and pancreatic ducts as they enter the ampullary area. In this manner, the entire distal duct system can be followed and reconstructed, as the ducts will appear on more than one slide. In addition, the entire mucosal surface surrounding the ampulla should be examined. In many cases, residual adenomatous epithelium can be found involving the adjacent duodenal mucosa, the ampulla, or the biliary and/or pancreatic ducts.

If, on gross examination, a tumor grossly involves the serosal surface or the adjacent pancreas, sections should be taken in these areas to document the extent of local invasion. Sections should be taken of the pancreas, including the surgical line of resection, to examine the pancreatic ductal system. Carcinomas arising in the duodenum and ampulla will infrequently be associated with atypical changes within pancreatic ducts away from the ampulla, and usually not at the line of resection. Similarly, one should examine the resected end of the common bile duct to look for atypia of the lining cells. Again, as for the pancreatic ducts, one usually will not find dysplastic or neoplastic changes in the lining cells of the common bile duct at the line of resection when the tumor originates in the duodenum. However, an invasive carcinoma that has extended from a primary site may be found in the wall of the bile duct. The connective tissue between the duodenum and pancreas should be examined carefully for lymph nodes. Adenocarcinomas arising in the duodenum or ampulla metastasize first to these pancreaticoduodenal nodes and then more distantly.

Invasive carcinomas arising in longstanding Crohn disease or ulcerative colitis may produce grossly apparent lesions that resemble other small bowel carcinomas. However, the carcinomas may also produce stenotic areas or diffuse thickening of the bowel wall, mimicking the gross appearance of the underlying inflammatory bowel disease. Since these carcinomas may be difficult to identify by gross examination, we recommend that many sections be obtained of the resection specimen. Ideally, sections should be taken along the entire length of the grossly abnormal bowel, but this may not be practical, especially when long segments of bowel are involved. At least one section should be taken for every 5 cm of inflamed bowel.

Section Orientation

Sections, whether from biopsy or resection specimens, should be taken with the proper orientation, which usually involves a section perpendicular to the mucosa. This allows one to evaluate mucosal height and its component parts. In some circumstances, however, one may wish to produce an en face section. Unicryptal adenomas or aberrant crypt foci are identified in this way because it allows for evaluation of a greater number of crypts per slide. Sections should not be taken until the specimen is well fixed. Specimens submitted for histology should not be more than 3 mm thick because they do not fit appropriately into the cassettes and they fail to become adequately infiltrated.

Lymph Node Dissection

Although all pathologists agree that pathologic stage and grade are among the most important tumor prognosticators, sufficient care is often not taken to carefully dissect the lymph nodes. Optimally in the GI tract, the fatty tissue should be dissected from the muscularis propria while the specimen is fresh. Most lymph nodes lie closely apposed to the muscularis propria, so that the dissection should be done in such a way that the fat is cleaned off the muscle completely and then dissected to find the lymph nodes. It is often helpful to follow vasculature because many of the lymph nodes lie along the vessels. Examination of the fat at a distance from the specimen is usually not very productive and examination of the omentum is useless because lymph nodes are not present here. Fixation of the removed fatty tissues in Bouin, a clearing solution, or Carnoy solution helps highlight the lymph nodes.

If an entire colectomy is performed in a patient with multiple cancers or with dysplasia in ulcerative colitis, it is helpful to divide the bowel and its lymph nodes into four sections extending from the proximal to the distal bowel, keeping the lymph nodes from each section separate. This allows accurate staging of each cancer, should multiple cancers be present. It is also important to obtain as many lymph nodes as possible since the staging system for some tumors is based on the number of positive nodes that are present, as in gastric cancer (see Chapter 5). If insufficient lymph nodes are removed, understaging of a tumor may occur.

Detailed guidelines for handling and reporting gastrointestinal specimens are provided by the Collage of American Pathology in its guidelines (19–21).

REFERENCES

1. Ettensohn CA: The regulation of primary mesenchyme cell patterning. *Dev Biol* 1990;140:261.
2. Nieuwkoop PD: Short historical survey of pattern formation in the endo-mesoderm and the neural anlage in the vertebrates: the role of vertical and planar inductive actions. *Cell Mol Life Sci* 1997;53:305.
3. Simon-Assmann P, Bouziges F, Arnold C, et al: Epithelial-mesenchymal interactions in the production of basement membrane components in the gut. *Development* 1988;102:339.
4. Gordon JI: Understanding gastrointestinal epithelial cell biology: lessons from mice with help from worms and flies. *Gastroenterology* 1993; 104:315.
5. Potten CS, Loeffler M: Stem cells: attributes, cycles, spirals, pitfalls, and uncertainties—lessons for and from the crypt. *Development* 1990; 110:1001.
6. Bland PW, Kambarage DM: Antigen handling by the epithelium and lamina propria macrophages. *Gastroenterol Clin North Am* 1991;20:577.
7. Bhalla DK, Murakami T, Owen RL: Microcirculation of intestinal lymphoid follicles in rat Peyer's patches. *Gastroenterology* 1981;81:481.
8. McClugage SG, Low FN, Zimny ML: Porosity of the basement membrane overlying Peyer's patches in rats and monkeys. *Gastroenterology* 1986;91:1128.
9. Galli SJ, Dvorak AM, Dvorak HF: Basophils and mast cells: morphologic insights into their biology, secretory patterns, and function. *Prog Allergy* 1984;34:1.
10. Metcalfe DD, Kaliner M, Donlon MA: The mast cell. *CRC Crit Rev Immunol* 1981;2:23.
11. Weller PF: The immunobiology of eosinophils. *N Engl J Med* 1991;324: 1110.
12. Gabella G: Structure of muscles and nerves in the gastrointestinal tract. In: Johnson LE (ed). *Physiology of the Gastrointestinal Tract*, 2nd ed. New York: Raven Press, 1987, pp 335–342.
13. Faussone-Pellegrini MS: Histogenesis, structure, and relationships of interstitial cells of Cajal (ICC): from morphology to functional interpretation. *Eur J Morphol* 1992;30:137.
14. Granger DN, Kvietys PR, Korthuis RJ, et al: Microcirculation of the intestinal mucosa. In: Schultz SG, Wood JD, Rauner BB (eds). *Handbook of Physiology, Sect. 6: The Gastrointestinal System. Motility and Circulation.* Bethesda, MD: American Physiology Society, 1989, pp 1405–1420.
15. Vanner S, Surprenant A: Cholinergic noncholinergic submucosal neurons dilate arterioles in the guinea pig colon. *Am J Physiol* 1991;261: G136.
16. Vallance P, Collier J: Biology and clinical relevance of nitric oxide. *BMJ* 1994;309:453.
17. Vanhoutte PM, Boulanger CM, Mombouli JV: Endothelium-derived relaxing factors and converting enzyme inhibition. *Am J Cardiol* 1995;76:3E.
18. Mino-Kenudson M, Brugge WR, Puricelli WP, et al: Management of superficial Barrett's epithelium related neoplasms by endoscopic mucosal resection: clinicopathologic analysis of 27 cases. *Am J Surg Pathol* 2005;29:680.
19. Compton CC, Henson DE, Hutter RV, et al: Updated protocol for the examination of specimens removed from patients with colorectal carcinoma. A basis for checklists. *Arch Pathol Lab Med* 1997;121:1247.
20. Compton CC, Sobin LH: Protocol for the examination of specimens removed from patients with gastric carcinoma. A basis for checklists. *Arch Pathol Lab Med* 1998;123:9.
21. Compton CC: Protocol for the examination of specimens from patients with carcinoma of the ampulla of Vater. A basis for checklists. *Arch Pathol Lab Med* 1997;121:673.

The Nonneoplastic Esophagus

ESOPHAGEAL DEVELOPMENT

The esophagus develops from the cranial part of the primitive foregut, becoming recognizable at the 2.5-mm stage of development (approximately the third gestational week) as an annular constriction located between the stomach and pharynx (Fig. 2.1) (1). It elongates and grows in a cephalad direction becoming increasingly tubular. Early, the cephalad parts of both the esophagus and trachea lie within a single common tube. Lateral ridges of proliferating epithelium develop in the uppermost segment, dividing the lumen into anterior and posterior compartments. Primitive mesenchyme grows into the forming septum, eventually separating the esophagus and trachea. As soon as the esophagus and trachea divide, the esophagus lies dorsally, and the trachea and lung buds lie ventrally (Figs. 2.1 and 2.2).

The earliest identifiable esophagus consists of two to three layers of pseudostratified columnar cells (Fig. 2.3). The cell layers thicken and then vacuolate (Fig 2.4). Eventually the vacuoles disappear. Abnormalities in the vacuolation process account for the formation of some esophageal cysts. Mucin-secreting cells replace the ciliated cells (2). Glycogenated, nonkeratinized, stratified squamous cells then replace the mucinous epithelium. Squamous cells first appear in the midesophagus and extend both proximally and distally to line the remainder of the esophagus by the fifth gestational month. Submucosal glands appear following the development of the squamous epithelium; they fully mature after birth (2). The implication of these developmental changes is that residual nests of embryonic types of esophageal epithelium may persist in the adult esophagus giving rise to some congenital abnormalities.

GROSS ANATOMIC FEATURES

The esophagus begins in the pharynx at the cricopharyngeus muscle and ends at the gastroesophageal junction (GEJ) to the left of midline opposite the 10th or 11th thoracic vertebrae. The esophagus usually measures 25 to 35 cm in adults. For the endoscopist, the esophagus starts 15 cm from the incisor teeth; it ends with the appearance of gastric folds at the GEJ or Z line (Fig. 2.5). The esophagus follows the course of the vertebral column maintaining close proximity with the trachea, left mainstem bronchus, aortic arch, descending aorta, and left atrium (Fig. 2.6). It is customarily divided into thirds. The normal esophagus has constrictions (Fig. 2.7) at its cricoid origin, along its left side at the aortic arch, at the crossing of the left mainstem bronchus, at the fifth thoracic vertebra and left atrium, and where it passes through the diaphragm. These constrictions become clinically significant when food or pills lodge in them making them susceptible to ulceration. The esophagus enters the abdomen, passing through the esophageal hiatus formed by the diaphragmatic muscles. Its intra-abdominal portion measures 1.5 cm in length. The right side of the GEJ appears smooth, whereas the left side forms a sharp angle known as the *incisura* or *angle of His*.

Sphincters that maintain esophageal closure under resting conditions lie at the proximal and distal ends. The esophagus is mobile between the upper sphincter and its passage through the diaphragm, allowing it to be displaced by mediastinal or pulmonary diseases. Lower esophageal sphincter (LES) pressure involves a balance between neurogenic and tonic contraction of the musculature and various neural and possibly endocrine and paracrine influences that inhibit contraction resulting in relaxation. The LES keeps the esophageal lumen closed, preventing reflux during rest and regulating food passage into the stomach. The most distal portion of the LES defines the GEJ. The esophageal mucosa has a smooth, featureless, glistening, pink-tan appearance. The squamocolumnar junction appears as a serrated line known as the Z line (Fig. 2.5). Grossly, the Z line consists of small projections of red glandular epithelium measuring up to 5 mm in length and 3 mm in width extending through the pink-white squamous epithelium.

Four arterial groups regionally supply the esophagus: (a) the thyroidal arterial trunk and branches of the subclavian artery that supply the upper esophagus, (b) bronchial arteries and esophageal arch arteries from the upper descending aorta that supply the upper and midesophagus, (c) intercostal arteries and periesophageal arteries from the lower thoracic aorta that supply the distal esophagus, and (d) branches from the inferior phrenic, left gastric, and short gastric artery that supply the diaphragmatic part of the esophagus. The arteries run within the muscularis propria,

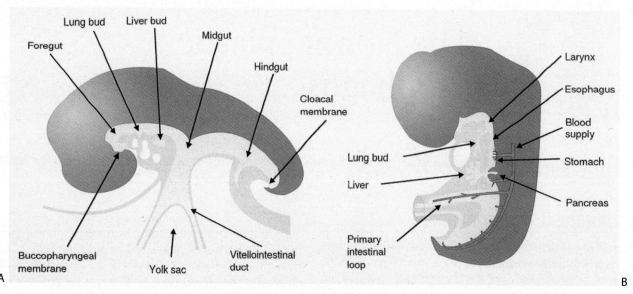

FIG. 2.1. Embryogenesis of the gut. **A:** Embryo at the end of first month shows a primitive gastrointestinal tract divided into the foregut, midgut, and hindgut. **B:** A 5-mm embryo. Note the development of primary intestinal loop.

giving rise to branches that course through the submucosal plexus (3). Extensive anastomoses among these arterial supplies account for the rarity of esophageal infarction.

Venous drainage also demonstrates a regional distribution. Esophageal veins form a well-developed submucosal plexus that drains into the thyroid, azygos, hemizygous, and left gastric veins, thereby providing links between the systemic and portal venous circulations. The lower esophagus drains into the systemic circulation through branches of the azygos and left inferior phrenic veins. The lower segment also drains into the portal system through the left gastric vein and into the splenic vein through the short gastric veins. The azygos veins ascend on either side of the thoracic segment and drain the midesophagus. The anterior and posterior hypopharyngeal plexus, the supe-

rior laryngeal and internal jugular veins, and the inferior thyroidal vein and intercostal veins drain the proximal esophagus. These eventually drain into the superior vena cava.

Seven lymph node groups drain the esophagus (Fig. 2.8). The nodes adjacent to the esophagus include paratracheal, parabronchial, paraesophageal, pericardial, and posterior mediastinal lymph nodes. The superior and inferior deep cervical lymph nodes lie further away from the esophagus. In general, the cervical esophagus drains into the internal jugular and upper tracheal lymph nodes. The thoracic esophagus drains into the superior, middle, and lower mediastinal lymph nodes. It also drains into the bronchial and posterior mediastinal paraesophageal lymph nodes and then to the thoracic duct. The distal esophagus drains

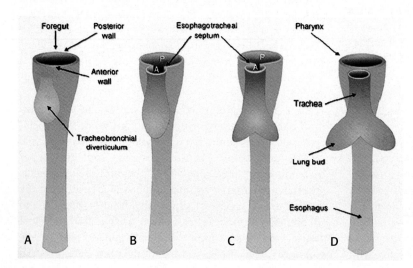

FIG. 2.2. Septation events. **A:** The embryonic foregut begins as a single tube from which the tracheobronchial diverticulum develops. **B:** The more proximal portion of the foregut divides into the posterior esophagus and the anterior tracheal tree. **C:** Septation results from ingrowth of epithelium and mesenchyme in the area of constriction. **D:** This ingrowth eventually forms a complete septum between the trachea and the esophagus.

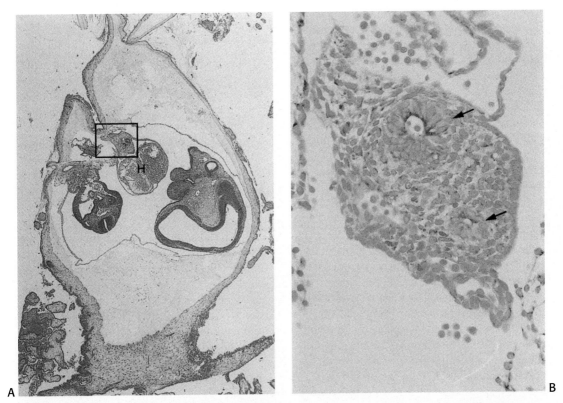

FIG. 2.3. Section through developing fetus at approximately 12 weeks of age by dates. **A:** Hematoxylin and eosin–stained section demonstrating fetus in the amniotic sac with the forming heart (*H*) and gastrointestinal tract. The section indicated in the box represents the separated trachea and esophagus. **B:** Higher magnification of the area outlined in the box in A. It is stained with an antibody to cytokeratin. Two distinct lumens representing the esophagus and the trachea are present (*arrows*). Immature mesenchyme surrounds the two lumina.

into the pericardial lymph nodes at the GEJ. The infradiaphragmatic portion drains to the left gastric and perigastric nodes (4). The two sets of intramural lymphatics lie in the submucosa and in the muscularis propria. The rich mucosal lymphatic plexus connects with a less extensive submucosal one and communicates with longitudinally oriented channels in the muscularis propria. Because of this arrangement, esophageal cancers tend to display early and extensive intramucosal and submucosal intralymphatic spread (see Chapter 3).

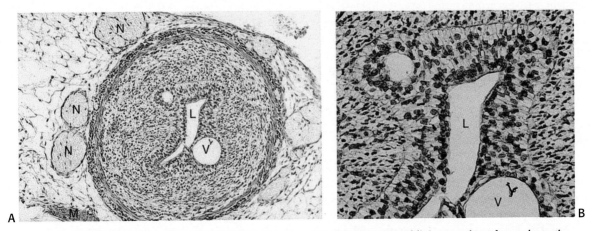

FIG. 2.4. Cross section of fetal esophagus at 60-mm stage. **A:** The mucosal lining consists of pseudostratified cells. *L* represents the central lumen; *N* represents developing neural tissue. Epithelial vacuoles (*V*) are beginning to form. **B:** Higher magnification of the pseudostratified epithelium. The epithelium appears clear due to intracytoplasmic glycogen accumulations. The underlying tissues consist of immature mesenchyme. Two intraepithelial vacuoles (*V*) are present.

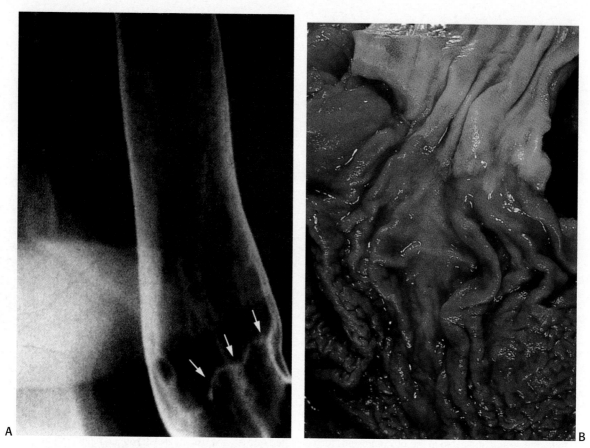

FIG. 2.5. Esophagogastric Z line. **A:** A double-contrast esophagogram demonstrates white zigzag line (*arrows*) representing the Z line. **B:** The Z line lies where the pinkish-gray squamous mucosa of the esophagus meets the velvety brown glandular gastric mucosa.

Parasympathetic and sympathetic nerves innervate the esophageal mucosa, glands, blood vessels, and musculature. Adrenergic, cholinergic, and peptidergic nerves richly supply the esophageal smooth muscle and serve several neurotransmitter functions, particularly in the LES (5–7). LES function is regulated in part by neural nitric oxide synthetase (8). Nitric oxide is a major mediator of LES relaxation. It also initiates the release of and enhances the effect of other transmitters. Intramuscular interstitial cells of Cajal also play an important role in nitric oxide–dependent neurotransmission in the LES (9).

MUCOSAL DEFENSES

Pre-epithelial, epithelial, and submucosal defenses protect the esophagus from injury. *Pre-epithelial defenses* include the coordinated actions of the LES and the esophageal muscles to minimize reflux of gastric contents and promote clearance of refluxed material. Microridges on squamous cells hold mucus on their surfaces, providing a protective coat (10). The esophageal epithelium is also protected by a luminal mucus–bicarbonate barrier and hydrophobic surfactants that derive from submucosal and salivary gland secretions. Other

salivary components, including mucin, nonmucin proteins, epidermal growth factor (EGF), prostaglandin E$_2$, and carbonic anhydrase also significantly enhance the *pre-epithelial barrier*.

Epithelial defenses include the glycocalyx, permeability properties of the cell plasma membrane, cells junctions, and ion transport processes that regulate intracellular pH (11). The multiple layers of squamous cells functionally resist damage from the passage of substances over the epithelial surface (Fig. 2.9). *Submucosal defenses* mainly involve regulation of blood supply via responses of nerves, mast cells, and the blood vessels themselves.

HISTOLOGIC FEATURES

The Squamous Mucosa

Most of the esophagus is lined by squamous epithelium, except at its distal end. The normal squamocolumnar junction (SCJ) lies at the level of the diaphragm. The squamous mucosa contains three components: Squamous epithelium, lamina propria, and a thick muscularis mucosae (Figs. 2.10 and 2.11). The squamous epithelium consists of nonkeratinizing stratified squamous epithelium (Figs. 2.10 to 2.12). The basal zone consists of several layers of cuboidal

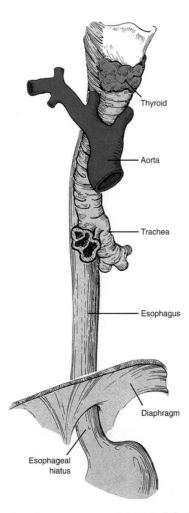

FIG. 2.6. The esophagus commences as an inferior extension of the pharynx. Superiorly it is related to the larynx and thyroid gland. Its middle region courses with the trachea, bronchi, and aortic arch, whereas the lower third descends with the aorta and passes through the esophageal diaphragmatic hiatus.

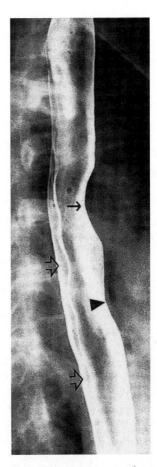

FIG. 2.7. Normal double-contrast esophagogram showing indentation from aorta (*arrow*), left mainstem bronchus (*arrowhead*) and indentation of spinal disc spaces (*open arrows*).

basophilic cells with dark nuclei arranged in an orderly fashion along the basement membrane. Its upper limit is defined as the level where the nuclei are separated by a distance equal to their diameter. It rarely contains mitoses unless some form of injury (esophagitis) is present. The basal layer gives rise to daughter cells that progressively differentiate as they move toward the surface and desquamate. Epithelial cell renewal takes an average of 7 days (12). The basal layer normally occupies the lower 10% to 15% of the epithelium, being one to four cells thick. However, most individuals without evidence of gastroesophageal reflux show basal cell hyperplasia >15% in the distal 3 cm of the esophagus (13). Above the basal cell layer the glycogenated cells progressively flatten as they approach the surface (Fig. 2.13). Periodic acid–Schiff (PAS) stains, which detect intracellular glycogen, facilitate their identification (Fig. 2.14). As one approaches the luminal surface, cell polarity changes from a vertical to a horizontal orientation. This change is accompanied by conversion of a round to an elliptical cell shape. The esophageal mucosa

may contain rare keratohyaline granules even though granular and keratinizing layers are usually absent; this finding suggests previous injury.

Endocrine cells lie scattered among the basal cells; they are not present in the mucous glands or ducts. Melanocytes are also present (Fig 2.15) (14). Occasional CD3+ intraepithelial lymphocytes populate the lower and middle squamous cell layers (15). As these lymphocytes interdigitate between the epithelial cells, their nuclei become convoluted, hence the term "squiggle cells." Antigen-presenting S100+ Langerhans cells lie in a suprabasal location (Fig. 2.16) (15).

Papillae, projections of lamina propria, extend into the squamous epithelium at regular intervals creating an irregular lower border of the squamous epithelium. These *papillae normally do not extend more than 50% to 60% through the epithelial height*. One measures the height of the papillae from the basal lamina of the surrounding squamous epithelium to the basal lamina at the top of the papilla. The papillae and lamina propria contain blood vessels, lymphatics, fibrovascular tissue, elastic tissue, and occasional inflammatory cells. The lamina propria rests on a two-layer, relatively thick muscularis mucosae. The mucosa is maintained in part by EGF, a mitogenic polypeptide that helps maintain tissue

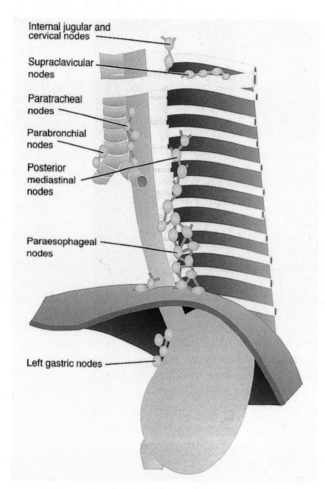

FIG. 2.8. Lymph nodes draining the esophagus. See text for further description.

Normal Histology at the Gastroesophageal Junction

The normal histology of the GEJ is a contentious topic. Traditional teaching suggests that the normal Z line is a junction between squamous epithelium and cardiac epithelium with the cardiac mucosa being the most proximal part of the stomach (17). The crux of the current controversy centers on whether the distal esophageal mucosa normally contains cardiac mucosa and whether cardiac mucosa can contain parietal cells. Some suggest that the presence of any parietal cells precludes a histologic diagnosis of cardiac epithelium (18). Others contend that cardiac glands can contain occasional parietal cells provided that other architectural features typical of cardiac mucosa are present (19). Some recommend terms such as *oxyntocardiac* or *cardio-oxyntic* or *transitional* mucosa to describe a cardiac mucosa with occasional parietal cells (18). The histologic controversies are complicated by the fact that there are no uniformly accepted criteria by which the GEJ can be recognized grossly. Thus, it is difficult to establish whether the Z line normally lies precisely at or slightly proximal to the GEJ (20). Furthermore, the upper gastrointestinal (GI) tract easily undergoes metaplastic changes as a result of injury.

Most current authors agree that the extent of the cardiac epithelium is shorter than had been previously suggested. If cardiac epithelium is present at all, it rarely extends more than a few millimeters below the Z line or a few millimeters into the esophagus. Some view the cardia as a normal structure that is present at birth (21,22), whereas others suggest that cardiac mucosa develops as a metaplastic response to gastroesophageal reflux disease (GERD) (23–25). Thus, it remains unclear whether there is a tiny band of cardiac mucosa that is a normal structure and whether it lines the esophagus, the proximal stomach, or both. When cardiac mucosa or cardio-oxyntic mucosa overlies submucosal esophageal glands or squamous epithelial-lined ducts, one can be certain that one is in the esophagus and not in the proximal stomach. In the absence

integrity and cell maturation. The epidermal growth factor receptor (EGFR) possesses tyrosine kinase activity (16) and binds EGF. This may make the esophageal mucosa vulnerable to the anti-EGFR therapies used to treat multiple types of cancer.

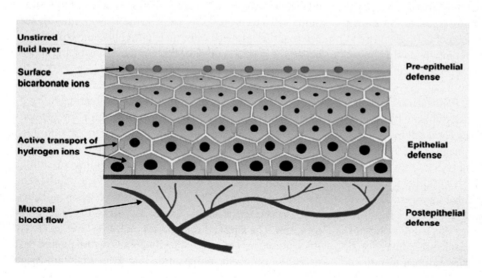

FIG. 2.9. Diagram of the normal protective mechanisms for the esophageal mucosa. See text for further description.

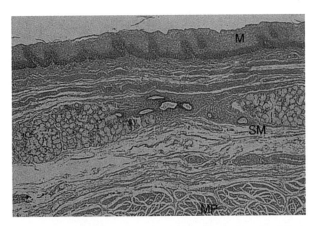

FIG. 2.10. Low-power view of the normal esophagus showing the mucosa (*M*), submucosa (*SM*), and muscularis propria (*MP*).

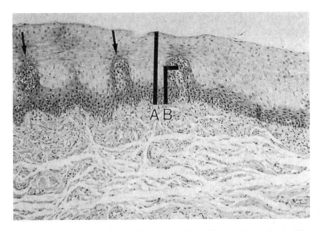

FIG. 2.12. Measurement of the height of esophageal papillae. The distance between the basal lamina of the adjacent flat squamous epithelium (*A*) and the basal lamina at the top of the papillae (*B*) is one-half the full measurement of the epithelium.

of this landmark, the location is less clear and it is perhaps best referred to as the area of the GEJ. Variability in the extent of the cardiac mucosa likely reflects the presence of underlying disorders such as GERD or *Helicobacter pylori* gastritis (25) and suggests that the area of the GEJ is a dynamic structure that may change over time.

In our view, cardiac mucosa consists of a surface mucus-secreting columnar epithelium similar to gastric foveolar epithelium. This epithelium dips down to form foveolae into which branched or compound tubular glands open. In the proximal end of the cardiac mucosa the glands branch freely and show a distinctly lobular architecture (Fig. 2.17). Distally

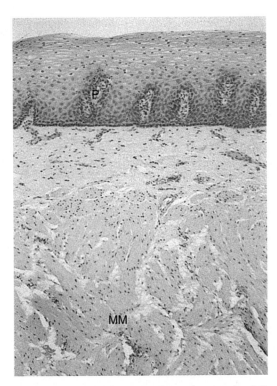

FIG. 2.11. Histology of the normal esophagus. The following layers of the esophageal stratified squamous epithelium can be identified: basal layer of oval cells, intermediate layers of cuboidal cells, and outer layers of squamous cells with flattened nuclei. The papillary lamina propria (*P*) invaginates halfway into the epithelium carrying small blood vessels and inflammatory cells. Smooth muscle fibers of the muscularis mucosae (*MM*) are seen at the bottom of the photograph.

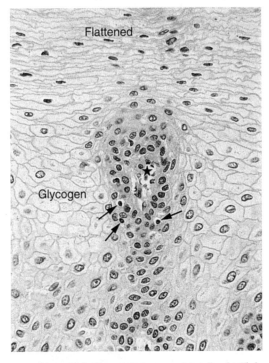

FIG. 2.13. Photograph of squamous mucosa stained with hematoxylin and eosin demonstrating the esophageal squamous lining. The *star* indicates the center of a papilla. It is surrounded by small basal cells with high nuclear-to-cytoplasmic ratios. The cells progressively enlarge, acquiring intracytoplasmic glycogen, and then eventually flatten out toward the surface. Normally, a small number of intraepithelial lymphocytes are present (*arrows*).

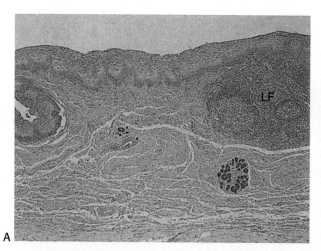

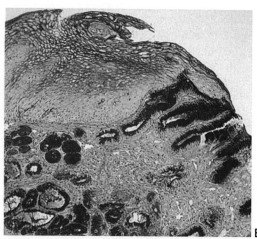

FIG. 2.14. **A:** The glycogenated superficial keratinocytes are demarcated from the basal epithelial layers by a periodic acid–Schiff (PAS) stain. The submucosal glands are also PAS positive. A lymphoid follicle (*LF*) is present. **B:** PAS-stained example of the gastroesophageal junction. Note the presence of the strongly PAS-positive glands both in the superficial portions as well as in the submucosa of the esophagus. The basal layer of the distal esophagus is thicker than elsewhere and is present in this photograph as a pale band underneath the pink-staining glycogenated epithelium superficial to it.

the glands are less branched and the lobular arrangement becomes less evident. The glands contain mucin-producing cells and may contain parietal cells or even rare chief cells. Abundant endocrine cells are also present. The cells may also blend with pancreatic exocrine cells, a change described in a later section.

Lamina Propria

The lamina propria constitutes the nonepithelial portion of the mucosa above the muscularis mucosae. It consists of loose areolar connective tissue containing blood vessels, nerves, inflammatory cells, and mucus-secreting glands. Lymphocytes (mostly immunoglobulin-producing B cells), plasma cells, and, occasionally, lymphoid follicles are present.

Muscularis Mucosae

The muscularis mucosae begins at the cricoid cartilage and becomes thicker distally. Proximally it consists of isolated or irregularly arranged muscle bundles rather than

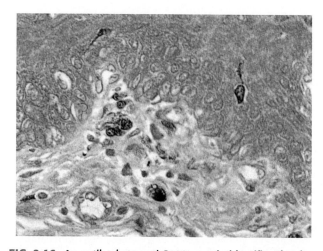

FIG. 2.16. An antibody to anti-S100 protein identifies the dendritic Langerhans cells scattered in the normal esophageal mucosa. Submucosal nerves and ganglia are also positive (diaminobenzidine–methylene blue).

FIG. 2.15. Melanocytes in the esophagus.

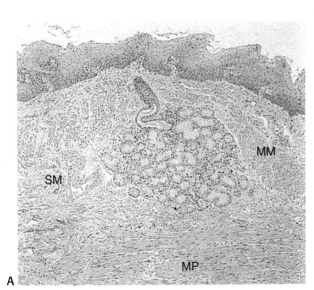
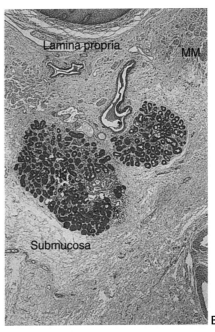

FIG. 2.17. Submucosal glands. **A:** Mucous glands empty their secretions into the esophageal lumen via ducts that penetrate the muscularis mucosae (*MM*). The submucosa is designated by the letters *SM*; the muscularis propria is designated by the letters *MP*. **B:** Periodic acid–Schiff (PAS)–stained esophagus. Note the PAS-positive acini in the submucosal glands.

being arranged in a continuous sheet. In the middle and lower esophagus, the muscularis mucosae forms a continuum of longitudinal and transverse fibers that may appear thicker than elsewhere in the GI tract (Fig. 2.11), especially at the GEJ. The muscularis mucosae may appear so thick as to be mistaken for the muscularis propria in biopsy specimens.

Submucosa

The submucosa is a wide zone that lies below the muscularis mucosae. It consists of loose connective tissue containing blood vessels, nerves, poorly formed submucosal ganglia, lymphatics, and submucosal glands (Fig. 2.17). The submucosa contains an extensive ramifying lymphatic plexus lying in a loose connective tissue network accounting for early and extensive submucosal spread of esophageal carcinomas. It also contains a rich vascular supply.

There are of two types of *submucosal glands*: Simple tubular mucous glands called superficial or mucosal mucous glands, and deep or submucosal glands. The former lie in the lamina propria, confined to narrow zones at the distal and proximal ends of the esophagus. They produce neutral mucins and because of their similarity to the glands of the gastric cardia, have also been termed cardiac glands. In contrast, deep or submucosal glands lie in the submucosa, along the length of the esophagus. These glands produce acidic mucins and drain their secretions via ducts lined by columnar epithelium surrounded by myoepithelial cells (26). Submucosal

glands contain acini and tubules. From two to four lobules drain into a common duct lined by stratified columnar epithelium that passes obliquely through the muscularis mucosae into the lumen. Loose connective tissue often surrounds these ducts. They vary in position and number from patient to patient and may be purely mucinous, purely serous, or mixed seromucinous in nature. Four types of cells line the submucosal glands: Mucous cells, serous cells, myoepithelial cells, and oncocytes. Mucous cells contain neutral sialated and sulfated mucins. The glands may be surrounded by lymphocytes.

Muscularis Propria

The muscularis propria consists of well-developed circular and longitudinal layers. In its upper part, the muscle fibers assume an oblique orientation and are striated in nature. The striated muscle gradually changes to smooth muscle in the middle third of the esophagus. The LES is not a clearly defined anatomic structure but consists of thickened smooth muscle fibers that extend approximately 2 cm above and 3 cm below the diaphragmatic esophageal hiatus.

Adventitia

The esophagus does not have a serosa as exists elsewhere in the GI tract. Rather, the external part is called the adventitia. It consists of loose connective tissue with longitudinally directed blood and lymph vessels and nerves; it gradually

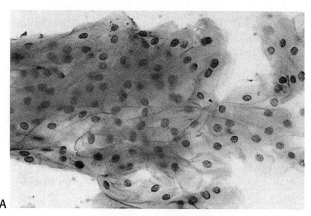

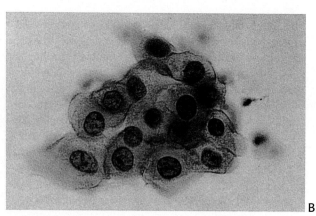

A   B

FIG. 2.18. Normal esophagus. **A:** Normal superficial squamous epithelial cells without keratinization. (Unless otherwise specified, all figures are taken from brushing material and stained with Papanicolaou.) **B:** Normal intermediate squamous epithelial cells.

merges into the loose connective tissue in the mediastinum. Numerous elastic fibers at the GEJ attach the esophagus to the diaphragm.

CYTOLOGY OF THE NORMAL ESOPHAGUS

Esophageal cells normally exfoliate from the esophageal mucosa. These include nonkeratinized superficial squamous cells, intermediate cells, and, rarely, parabasal cells (Fig. 2.18). Some squamous cells seen in esophageal cytology specimens derive from the oropharynx. Benign epithelial pearls may occasionally be found. The presence of large numbers of the latter suggests an inflammatory or erosive lesion. Metaplastic squamous cells may exfoliate from the subepithelial mucous glands and their ducts. Benign columnar gastric-type cells (Fig. 2.19) derive from the distal esophagus or from islands of gastric mucosa associated with inlet patches or Barrett esophagus (BE). Foreign material, particularly plant cells, may be present, especially if the esophageal lumen is obstructed. One may also find cells of respiratory origin, such as dust-containing

macrophages and ciliated bronchial cells. These usually represent cells that are swallowed, although esophagobronchial or esophagotracheal fistulae or the presence of congenital abnormalities containing bronchial mucosa may account for these cells as well.

HETEROTOPIAS
Cervical Inlet Patch

Inlet patches affect 1% to 21% of the population (27–29), with the highest incidence occurring during the first year of life. A subsequent decline in incidence suggests that some lesions regress with age. Two pathogenetic mechanisms have been advanced to explain inlet patches. As noted earlier, columnar epithelium lines the fetal esophagus and remnants of columnar or ciliated epithelium may persist leading to the formation of inlet patches. Others suggest that inlet patches represent metaplastic replacement of the squamous mucosa in adults with GERD (30). Those favoring an association with GERD cite similar mucin and cytokeratin patterns in both inlet patches and BE (30). Inlet patches lie in the subcricoid and upper sphincteric region, usually within 3 cm of the upper esophageal sphincter. Most lesions remain asymptomatic. Acid or pepsin secretion by the ectopic gastric mucosa may produce peptic symptoms, ulcers, granulation tissue, webs, strictures, esophagotracheal fistulae, or perforations (31). Adenocarcinomas may also develop, although this is rare (32).

Inlet patches are easily visible velvety, ovoid, pink-red mucosal areas with distinct borders that vary in diameter from a few millimeters to complete esophageal encirclement. Histologically, the lesions consist of cardiac, antral, and/or oxyntic glands covered by foveolar epithelium (Fig. 2.20). In patients with gastric *H. pylori* (*HP*) infections, the heterotopic epithelium may become colonized by *HP*. Intestinal or pancreatic metaplasia may develop (28,29). Large amounts of lymphoid tissue accompany

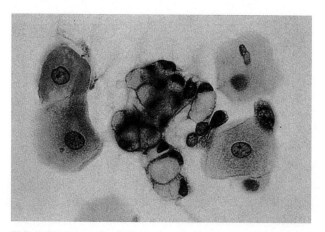

FIG. 2.19. Normal cells from the esophageal–gastric junction.

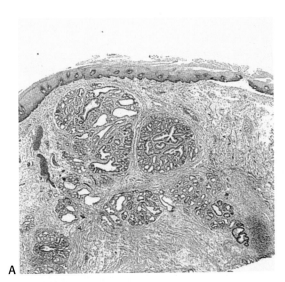
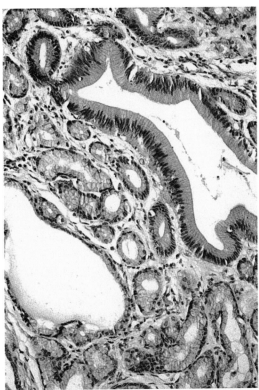

FIG. 2.20. Inlet patch. **A:** Low magnification of an upper esophageal "polyp" containing lobular nests of gastric epithelium. **B:** Higher magnification showing the gastric epithelium.

smaller lesions, as compared to larger ones, suggesting that the lymphocytes play a role in lesional regression. An intense inflammatory reaction may surround the lesion, especially following peptic ulceration.

Heterotopic Gastric Mucosa away from Inlet Patches

Ectopic gastric mucosa also occurs in the mid- or distal esophagus, usually in congenital malformations, including duplications or diverticula. It may also develop following atresia repair (33). Since it often contains oxyntic mucosa, it may present with peptic ulceration.

Heterotopic Pancreas

Heterotopic pancreas usually affects the distal esophagus. It may associate with trisomy 18, trisomy 13, esophageal atresia, and esophageal duplication. Complications include fat necrosis, bleeding, ulcers, diverticulum formation, cystic degeneration, inflammation, and, rarely, malignancy. Heterotopic pancreas usually presents as a submucosal mass and contains normal-appearing pancreatic acini and ducts (Figs. 2.21 and 2.22) without islets, although any pancreatic tissue component may be present. Injury due to heterotopic pancreas involves failure of the pancreatic ducts to empty into the esophageal lumen. Eventually the obstructed ducts dilate and rupture, releasing proteolytic enzymes into surrounding

tissues. Inflammation and necrosis follow. Heterotopic pancreas differs from pancreatic metaplasia, which is discussed in a later section. The latter is usually a focal change consisting only of pancreatic acini that blend into cardiac

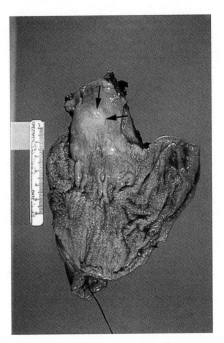

FIG. 2.21. Heterotopic pancreas at gastroesophageal junction presenting as a submucosal mass (*arrows*).

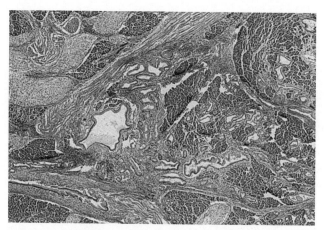

FIG. 2.22. Histologic appearance of the lesion illustrated in Figure 2.21 demonstrating the presence of pancreatic acini and ducts.

or oxyntic mucosa. Pancreatic ducts are never present in pancreatic metaplasia.

Other Heterotopic Tissues

Ectopic esophageal sebaceous glands present grossly as multiple small, yellowish, mucosal plaques, typically lying in the mid- or distal esophagus. Mature sebaceous glands underlie the squamous mucosa (Fig. 2.23). The lesion represents a developmental abnormality without any clinical significance (34). Patches of *ciliated columnar cells* may lie within the esophagus. These represent residual fetal remnants and are particularly common in premature infants. They are rarely seen in adults unless they are found in inlet patches, duplications, and/or bronchogenic cysts. *Heterotopic thyroid tissue* may be present in the esophagus either alone or in tracheobronchial hamartomas.

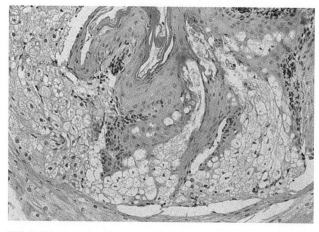

FIG. 2.23. Ectopic sebaceous glands underlying the esophageal squamous epithelium.

DEVELOPMENTAL CONGENITAL ANOMALIES

Congenital Esophageal Atresia, Fistula, and Stenosis (Tracheoesophageal Fistula)

Demography and Pathophysiology

Complete esophageal atresia affects 1 in 3,000 live births. Atresia with a common tracheoesophageal fistula occurs in 1 of every 800 to 1,500 live births. Esophageal stenosis affects only 1 in every 25,000 live births (35). Atresia is more common in males than in females. Premature babies and monozygotic twins have a higher risk of atresia than other infants. Occasionally esophageal atresia affects siblings (36). Risk factors include prenatal exposure to lead (37), drugs, and physical agents; maternal diabetes; and a maternal age <20 years (38). Genetic factors include Down syndrome, trisomy 18, and various other chromosomal alterations (39). Severe etiologic insults occur in the first trimester when major organogenesis occurs, often resulting in many associated abnormalities (40).

In esophageal agenesis the proximal primitive foregut develops primarily into a trachea rather than an esophagus (41). Esophageal atresia results from failure of the primitive foregut to recanalize; tracheoesophageal fistula results from failure of the lung bud to separate completely from the foregut. The fistulas that develop vary depending on the amount of epithelium left behind to maintain foregut epithelial continuity. The distal esophageal segment may contain respiratory elements representing a transition zone between the upper foregut, which differentiates into the trachea, and the lower part, which differentiates into the lower esophageal segment (41).

Studies in animal models and in patients with syndromic forms of esophageal atresia indicate the importance of altered genes in the sonic hedgehog signaling pathway. These genes include N-myc and SOX2, which encode transcription factors, and CHD7, which encodes a homeodomain helicase DNA-binding gene, important for chromatin structure and gene expression (42). There are also a number of other genes that are important for normal tracheoesophageal development (Table 2.1); abnormalities in these may also account for some cases of tracheoesophageal malformations.

TABLE 2.1 **Genes Necessary for Normal Tracheoesophageal Development**

Gene	Human Chromosomal Location
Foxf1	16q24
Gli2	2q14
Gli3	7p13
Hoxc4	12q13.3
RARα	17q21
RARβ	3p24
Shh	7q36
Tbx4	17q21-q22

Clinical Features

Esophageal atresia may be detected prenatally by finding a small or absent gastric bubble and maternal polyhydramnios or by the presence of a fluid-filled, blind-ending esophagus (Fig. 2.24). At birth, the presence of a single umbilical artery may alert clinicians to the possibility of esophageal atresia. Infants typically present in the first few hours or days of life with regurgitation, excessive drooling, choking, aspiration, cyanosis, and respiratory distress. Inability to pass a nasogastric tube into the stomach confirms the diagnosis. Air in the stomach and small bowel indicates the presence of a distal tracheoesophageal fistula. Most patients with esophageal stenosis present with dysphagia and regurgitation upon the introduction of solid food.

Approximately one third of infants with esophageal atresia have associated congenital anomalies involving the cardiovascular, gastrointestinal, neurologic, genitourinary, or orthopedic systems (43). Some of the more complex associations are described briefly. The *VATER syndrome* links **v**ertebral defects, **a**nal atresia, **t**racheo**e**sophageal fistula, and **r**enal dysplasia (44). The *VATER association* is defined by finding at least three of the VATER anomalies. A subset of infants with the VATER syndrome have other defects including diaphragmatic, genital, cardiovascular, and neural tube defects; oral clefts; bladder exstrophy; small intestinal atresias; and omphalocele. A variant syndrome, the *VACTERL anomaly,* combines the VATER syndrome with radial or other **l**imb defects (43). It affects approximately 1.6 of 10,000 live births (45). Defective development of the neural tube and preaxial mesoderm may result in the full spectrum of changes (45). Patients with VACTERL are most likely to be male, have a higher perinatal mortality rate, and have lower mean birth weights than control populations (46). Mothers of infants with VACTERL often exhibit a higher frequency of fetal loss in previous pregnancies than a control population. Patients with a familial form of X-linked VACTERL, X-linked VACTERL-H, develop hydrocephalus due to aqueductal stenosis.

Esophageal atresia also associates with the *CHARGE syndrome* (**c**oloboma, **h**eart disease, **a**tresia choanae, growth and developmental **r**etardation, **g**enital hyperplasia, and **e**ar anomalies) (47). The *oculodigitoesophageoduodenal syndrome,* also known as *Feingold syndrome,* is a dominantly inherited combination of hand and foot anomalies, microcephaly, esophageal/duodenal atresia, short palpebral fissures, and learning disabilities. The abnormality maps to chromosome 2p23-p24 (48). The *Bartsocas-Papas syndrome* consists of bilateral renal agenesis, esophageal atresia, hypoplastic diaphragm, unilateral renal agenesis, agenesis of the penile shaft, or anal atresia (49).

Pathologic Features

Six types of esophageal atresia and stenosis are recognized (Figs. 2.25 and 2.26). In esophageal atresia, hypertrophic esophageal and tracheal muscles intimately blend with one another and the muscle layer contains an extramyenteric plexus. This is a manifestation of incomplete tracheal–esophageal separation. Striated muscle is present in the upper esophagus but not in the lower. Accompanying congenital esophageal neural abnormalities contribute to esophageal dysmotility (50).

Several types of stenosis exist. The stenotic segment varies from 2 to 20 cm in length and is usually located in the mid- or distal esophagus. In the first type of stenosis, segmental narrowing and loss of esophageal mural elasticity produces a localized area of muscular hypertrophy. In rare cases, the muscular hypertrophy involves the entire esophagus. The muscular hypertrophy may result from inflammatory damage to the myenteric plexus, with loss of the muscle-relaxing nitric oxide–producing nerves (51), and may coexist with hypertrophic pyloric stenosis. In a *second form* of stenosis, cartilaginous tracheobronchial remnants and respiratory epithelium lie within the esophageal wall, as a result of sequestration of a tracheobronchial anlage during the period of cranial elongation before embryologic separation of the esophagus and trachea. In a *third form,* a membranous diaphragm or web arising from the esophageal wall, containing fibromuscular tissue with a small central perforation, obstructs the lumen. These anomalies are treated surgically but when the lesions are repaired, patients often suffer residual

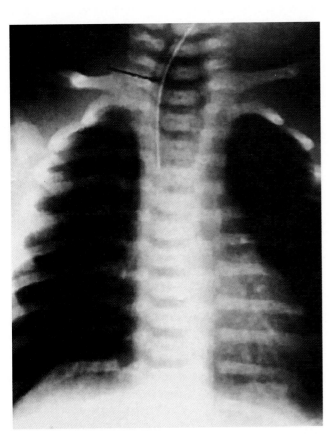

FIG. 2.24. Radiograph of esophageal atresia. The feeding tube (*arrow*) terminates in the air-distended proximal esophageal pouch.

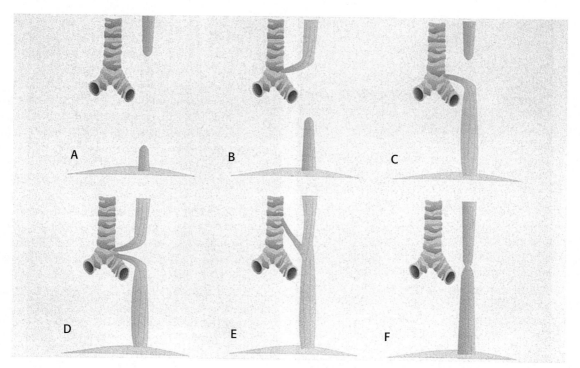

FIG. 2.25. Esophageal atresias and stenoses. **A:** In type I atresia, a segment of the esophagus is represented by only a thin, noncanalized cord with resultant formation of an upper blind pouch connecting with the pharynx and a lower pouch leading to the stomach. Most commonly, the atresia is located at or near the tracheal bifurcation. **B:** Rare type II atresia. The proximal and distal portions of the esophagus are completely separate. The upper part connects with the trachea. **C:** Type III is the most common anomaly. The lower pouch communicates with the trachea or mainstem bronchus. **D:** In type IV, both the upper and lower pouches connect to the trachea. **E:** Esophageal stenosis near tracheal bifurcation. Tracheoesophageal fistula is also illustrated. **F:** Simple esophageal stenosis.

esophageal dysmotility due to underlying neural abnormalities in the remaining esophagus. The abnormal motility often leads to GERD with all of its complications (52). Restenosis commonly occurs, leading to aspiration and respiratory infections.

Congenital Bronchoesophageal Fistulas

Bronchopulmonary malformations occur less commonly than tracheoesophageal abnormalities and result from imperfect separation of pulmonary and esophageal anlagen or from an accessory esophageal lung bud. If the communication between the pulmonary tissue and the esophagus is lost, the pulmonary tissue appears as a sequestration. Extralobar sequestrations remain anatomically separate from the lung and have their own pleura. They usually lie adjacent to the esophagus, with which they may communicate. Rarely, intralobar sequestrations communicate with the esophagus presenting as bronchoesophageal fistulas (53). Patients usually present in infancy with a mediastinal mass. *Tracheobronchial chondroepithelial hamartomas* represent an uncommon related lesion (54), which also results from the abnormal separation of the esophagus and trachea. They contain tracheobronchial lining epithelium, cartilage, and sometimes ectopic thyroid tissue or heterotopic pancreas. These lesions are extremely rare and usually lie in the distal esophagus (54).

Duplications

Esophageal duplications account for only 10% to 20% of all GI duplications. They affect approximately 1 of 8,000 persons (55). Duplications develop while columnar, ciliated columnar, or squamous epithelium lines the fetal esophagus and occur in three major forms: Cysts, diverticula (discussed in a later section), and tubular malformations. Cysts account for 80% of duplications. Duplications often present in infancy and childhood with dysphagia, nausea, vomiting, weight loss, pain, bleeding, anorexia, dyspnea, wheezing or recurrent coughing, and pneumonitis.

Duplication cysts are single, fluid-filled cysts (55) that lie posteriorly in a periesophageal location, develop within the esophageal wall (Fig. 2.27), or present as pedunculated intraluminal lesions (56). They average up to 5 cm in diameter. Duplication cysts typically demonstrate continuity of the esophageal muscularis propria with the muscle layer of the cyst wall. It may be difficult to distinguish between esophageal duplication cysts and other intrathoracic cysts

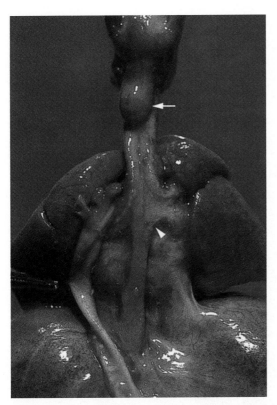

FIG. 2.26. Tracheoesophageal fistula. Thoracic and upper abdominal organs viewed from the posterior surface in a neonate born with esophageal atresia. The upper esophagus terminates blindly in a blunted esophageal pouch (*arrow*) and distal esophageal communication with the trachea at the carina (*arrowhead*).

lined by respiratory columnar (Fig. 2.28), cuboidal enteric, stratified squamous, or gastric epithelium. *Tubular duplications* usually lie within the esophageal wall paralleling the true esophageal lumen. Unlike duplication cysts, tubular duplications communicate with the true lumen at either or both ends of the tube. Duplications usually have a duplicated muscularis propria.

Bronchogenic Cysts

Bronchogenic cysts lie anteriorly, representing defective tracheoesophageal separation and aberrant bronchial budding from the foregut. They occur in the mediastinum, within the lung, or in the abdomen. Histologically, they contain cartilage, smooth muscle cells, and seromucinous minor salivary glands and are usually lined by ciliated, mucus-secreting, respiratory epithelium. Other bronchogenic cysts are lined by respiratory squamous epithelium but lack cartilage.

Esophageal Rings and Webs

The distal esophagus contains two rings that demarcate the proximal and distal borders of the esophageal vestibule (57). They occur alone or together. The *muscular ring* lies at its proximal border and corresponds to the upper end of the LES. It is a broad, 4- to 5-mm symmetric band of hypertrophic muscle covered by squamous epithelium that constricts the tubular esophageal lumen at its junction with the vestibule. The *mucosal ring* or *Schatzki ring* affects 6% to 14% of individuals and always associates with a hiatal hernia. Mucosal rings are thin, 2-mm transverse mucosal folds that protrude into the esophageal lumen. They usually lie at the SCJ with squamous epithelium covering the upper surface and columnar epithelium lining the lower. The core of the ring contains connective tissue, fibers of the muscularis mucosae, and blood vessels. The muscularis propria contributes little to its formation. Mucosal rings may progress to strictures due to coexisting inflammation (57). Mucosal webs and rings are compared in Table 2.2.

The incidence of *esophageal webs* ranges from 0.7% to 16%. Congenital esophageal webs are characterized by one or more thin horizontal membranes covered by stratified squamous epithelium arising in the upper and midesophagus. Unlike rings, webs rarely encircle the lumen, but instead protrude from the anterior wall, extending laterally. Webs rarely exceed 2 mm in thickness. Postinflammatory esophageal webs complicate many forms of esophagitis. As a result, they

TABLE 2.2	**Comparison of Rings and Webs**		
Type	Prevalence	Pathology	Pathogenesis
Postcricoid web	Association with iron deficiency anemia	Thin mucous membrane	• Autoimmune • Iron deficiency
Low esophageal mucosal ring	10% autopsies	Consists of center of loose areolar tissue covered on each side by thinned squamous epithelium	Associated with hiatus hernia • Congenital • Secondary to esophagitis
Low esophageal muscular ring	4% autopsies	Hypertrophy; muscle layer; mucosa thinned	Exaggeration of normal anatomy
Ringlike peptic stricture	Rare, complicates Barrett esophagus	Fibrous, inflamed tissue	Peptic esophagitis

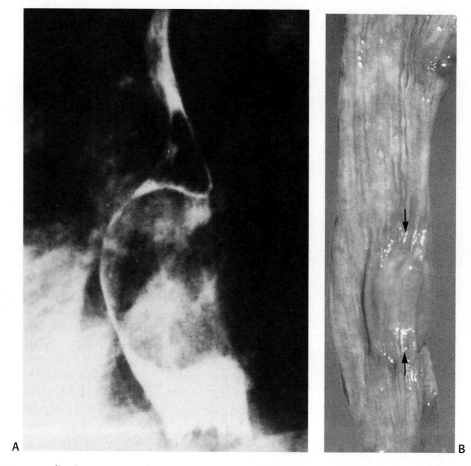

FIG. 2.27. Duplication cyst. **A:** Radiograph of a large intramural defect in proximal esophagus. **B:** Gross picture showing the presence of a bulging submucosal sausage-shaped mass from a different patient cyst (*arrows*).

tend to be multiple and distributed throughout the esophagus. Histologically, webs consist of a thin layer of variably inflamed connective tissue covered on both sides by stratified squamous epithelium. Gastric mucosa may line the undersurface of distal webs. The epithelium covering esophageal webs may undergo neoplastic transformation.

The association of cervical webs, dysphagia, and iron deficiency anemia is known as the *Plummer Vinson syndrome* or *Patterson Kelly syndrome* (58). It develops in middle-aged women with iron deficiency anemia, glossitis, splenomegaly, and oropharyngeal and esophageal inflammation. Not all patients with the syndrome have webs. Instead, they have nonpropulsive esophageal peristalsis (59) resulting from the iron deficiency, explaining symptom reversal following iron replacement therapy in patients without webs (59). The patients often have other abnormalities, some of which have autoimmune etiologies including autoimmune gastritis, ulcerative colitis, thyroid disease, Sjögren syndrome, and celiac disease (60). Shelflike mucosal webs arise from the anterior wall of the proximal esophagus, occasionally extending laterally or becoming circumferential. They are sometimes multiple. Most lie within 2 to 3 cm of the postcricoid area.

Diffuse Esophageal Intramural Pseudodiverticulosis

Diffuse esophageal intramural pseudodiverticulosis (DEIP) affects 15% to 17% of patients seen at autopsy. Patients range in age from 8 to 83 years (61); males are more commonly affected than females. The disease has several known associations but since many are common, the relationships may be fortuitous rather than etiologic. Possible predisposing factors include alcohol abuse, esophageal reflux, candidiasis, herpes esophagitis, motility disorders, and squamous cell carcinoma. The diverticula result from ductal obstruction caused by inflammation, mucin, or squamous debris. Strictures are present in approximately 75% of patients. Patients present with dysphagia and acute bolus obstruction. These symptoms probably result from coexisting esophagitis or strictures rather than the pseudodiverticula themselves (62).

Multiple cystically dilated submucosal glandular ducts produce innumerable 1- to 3-mm flask-shaped diverticula with pinpoint mouths lying evenly distributed in a linear fashion along the esophageal wall (Fig. 2.29). These are most numerous proximally. The intramural cysts extend 3 mm or

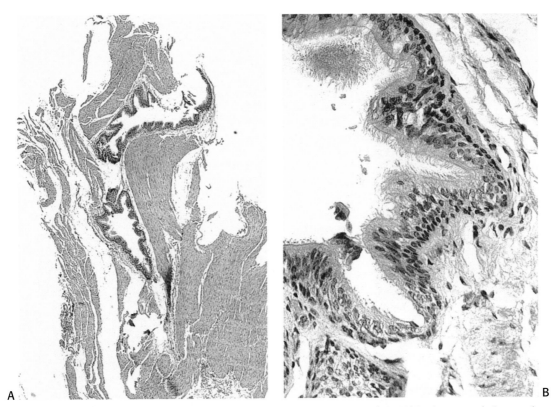

FIG. 2.28. Duplication cyst. **A:** An intramural cyst with epithelial lining lies within the muscularis propria. **B:** The lining is a ciliated respiratory epithelium.

less beyond the esophageal lumen. The dilated ducts are lined by stratified squamous epithelium, which may appear hyperplastic (Fig. 2.30). The lumen may contain desquamated squamous cells or inflammatory cells. Organisms, including bacteria, fungi, and parasites, can secondarily colonize the cysts. Nonspecific acute or chronic inflammation often surrounds the acini and the ducts. The inflammation may lead to subsequent submucosal fibrosis or stricture formation.

Diverticula

Esophageal diverticula are saccular outpouchings that contain all, or part, of the esophageal wall. One can classify them by their *location* (*pharyngoesophageal, thoracic,* or *epiphrenic*), their *pathogenesis* (*congenital, traction,* or *pulsion*), or their status as *true* or *false,* or *congenital* or *acquired* (Fig. 2.31). The most important feature distinguishing congenital versus acquired diverticula is the absence of an intact muscularis propria in acquired diverticula. *Zenker (hypopharyngeal) diverticulum* represents the most common (up to 70%) esophageal diverticulum. Twenty-one percent of diverticula originate in the midesophagus; 8.5% originate in the supradiaphragmatic region. Histologically, squamous epithelium lines all acquired esophageal diverticula unless they develop in an area of Barrett esophagus. Congenital diverticula contain all of the components of the esophageal wall, including the muscularis

propria, and may be lined by columnar, ciliated, or squamous epithelium.

Zenker Diverticulum (Pharyngoesophageal Diverticulum)

Patients with Zenker diverticula are generally in their 7th or 8th decades of life. There is a 2:1 male preponderance. The diverticulum originates in the proximal esophagus (Fig. 2.32) from mucosal outpouchings at points of weakness in the esophageal wall at its junction with the pharynx. Most develop posteriorly or posterolaterally between the inferior constrictor muscle and fibers of the cricopharyngeus muscle through a triangular zone of sparse musculature termed the Killian triangle. These pulsion diverticula result from uncoordinated muscular contractions during swallowing. As the diverticulum enlarges, it protrudes between the posterior wall of the esophagus and the vertebrae leading to anterior displacement of the proximal esophagus, sometimes causing esophageal compression.

Patients typically present with dysphagia, halitosis, and regurgitation of food consumed several days previously. Aspiration and secondary pneumonitis occur. Secondary bacterial colonization results in diverticulitis. Zenker diverticulum and cervical esophageal webs or hiatal hernias sometimes coexist. Perforation leads to mediastinitis. Squamous epithelium lines Zenker diverticula (Fig. 2.33).

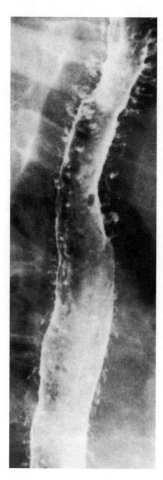

FIG. 2.29. Esophageal intramural pseudodiverticulosis. Double-contrast esophagram demonstrates numerous irregular thin outpouchings from the esophageal lumen, some of which have flask-shaped bases. These represent ectatic submucosal glands.

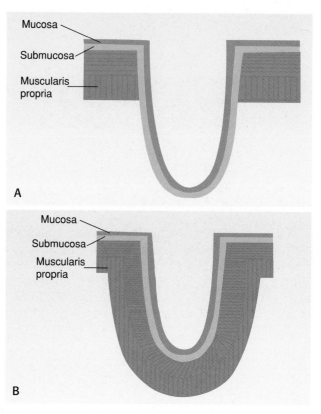

FIG. 2.31. Comparison of congenital versus acquired diverticula. **A:** False or acquired diverticula tend to demonstrate epithelial or mucosal outpouchings through the muscularis propria. In some instances, the submucosa follows the mucosa. **B:** In contrast, congenital or true diverticula represent herniations of the entire wall of the gastrointestinal tract, including the muscularis propria.

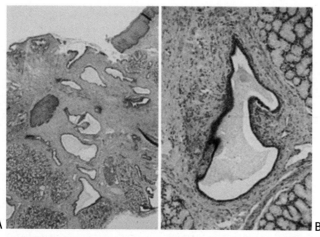

FIG. 2.30. Diffuse esophageal intramural pseudodiverticulosis. **A:** Low-power magnification demonstrating the presence of a cystically dilated duct, which passes between lobules of the submucosal glands. Some of the ducts have also undergone squamous metaplasia. **B:** Higher magnification of one of the ducts showing the presence of inspissated secretions and flattened cuboidal lining epithelium. A mild inflammatory infiltrate surrounds the duct.

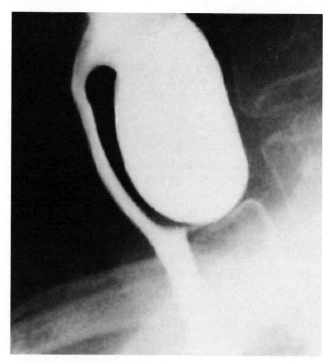

FIG. 2.32. Zenker diverticulum. Lateral view demonstrates the diverticulum as a large saclike structure containing barium.

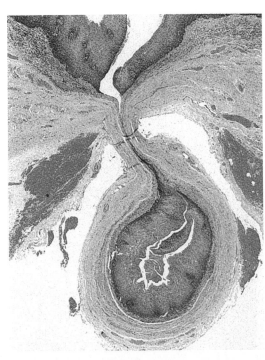

FIG. 2.33. Histologic appearance of Zenker diverticulum. Herniation of the mucosa, submucosa, and part of the muscularis propria into the paraesophageal tissues. The resulting diverticulum consists of muscular wall, submucosa, and a hyperplastic squamous epithelium.

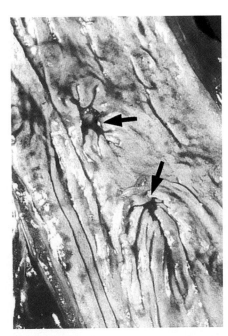

FIG. 2.34. Esophageal diverticulum. Mucosal view of two esophageal traction diverticula (*arrows*).

The muscle may appear attenuated and the wall is variably inflamed, sometimes with prominent lymphoid follicles. Ulcers may occur. There is a 0.31% to 0.7% incidence of squamous cell carcinoma secondary to longstanding inflammation (63).

Midesophageal Diverticula

Diverticula arising at the level of the tracheal bifurcation are less common than those in the cervical esophagus. Midesophageal diverticula almost always represent incidentally discovered lesions, unless there is coexisting diverticulitis. They are single or multiple (Fig. 2.34), and usually develop in association with mediastinal inflammation that causes traction on the esophageal wall, pulling it outward. Other diverticula result from motility disturbances, including achalasia or diffuse esophageal spasm. These wide-mouthed diverticula (Fig. 2.35) consist of a variably inflamed squamous mucosa and submucosa with an attenuated muscularis propria.

Epiphrenic Diverticula

Epiphrenic diverticula are rare, developing in middle age, supporting an acquired etiology. They are almost always of the pulsion type, resulting from increased intraesophageal pressure that pushes the mucosa outward in areas of muscular

weakness. They frequently coexist with other disorders including hiatal hernia, diaphragmatic eventration, and carcinoma and/or motility disturbances (64). The presence of hypertrophic muscle distal to the diverticula supports the concept that functional or anatomic obstructions are important in their pathogenesis. Patients present with substernal pain, dysphagia, and weight loss. Complications include aspiration pneumonia and lung abscesses, diverticulitis, esophageal obstruction, perforation, mediastinitis, or hemorrhage. Epiphrenic diverticula develop in the distal 10 cm of the esophagus. They appear globular and wide mouthed and, in contrast to midesophageal lesions, may become quite large. The diverticula contain a squamous mucosa and submucosa but no muscularis propria (Fig 2.36). Chronic inflammation is often present. Carcinomas may develop within epiphrenic diverticula for the same reason they do in other diverticula (i.e., stasis of luminal contents), leading to chronic inflammation.

PANCREATIC METAPLASIA

Pancreatic metaplasia develops in patients with BE (65), carditis, and inlet patches. Mean patient age is 52 years with a range of 18 to 89 years. It occurs in 24% to 60% of patients with biopsy specimens from the SCJ (65–67). These glands often lie in the deeper aspects of the mucosa and vary in size from 0.1 to 0.5 mm in greatest diameter (65). They form small clusters of compactly packed cells that either blend imperceptibly into the adjacent metaplastic gastric glands or form distinct nodules that can stand out prominently within

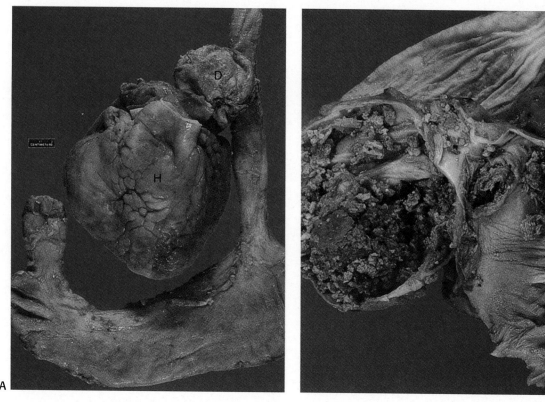

FIG. 2.35. Esophageal diverticulum. **A:** Unopened esophagus and stomach with the dissected-out heart (*H*). A large saccular dilation (*D*) extends from the midesophageal region and lies next to the heart on the photography table. **B:** Opened specimen demonstrating the presence of a large diverticulum containing necrotic debris. This diverticulum was attached to the pericardium.

the mucosa. The pyramidal pancreatic acinar cells have abundant apical and midcellular eosinophilic coarse granular cytoplasm and appear basophilic in the basal areas. The basally located nuclei are small, round, and uniform with occasional conspicuous but small nucleoli. The acinar cells are positive for pancreatic lipase and amylase. Mucous cells may intermingle with the pancreatic acinar cells within individual lobules. Endocrine cells may also be present. The foci of pancreatic metaplasia lack pancreatic ducts, periductal smooth muscle fibers, and islet cells.

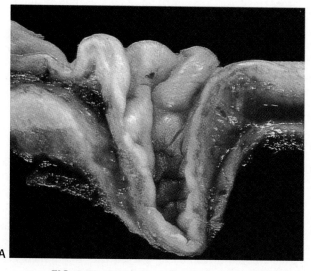

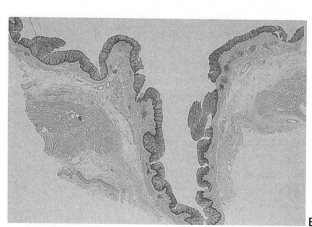

FIG. 2.36. Esophageal diverticulum. **A:** Midsagittal section of the diverticulum showing lining of tan squamous mucosa; the outer coat is thinned. **B:** Histologic section of A.

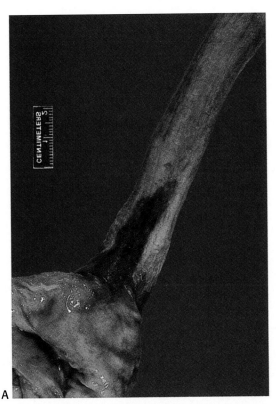
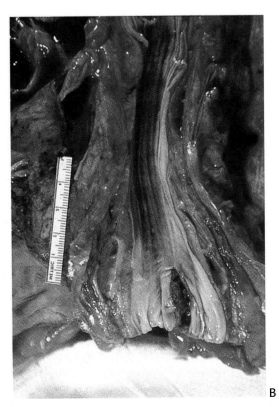

FIG. 2.37. Esophageal lacerations and perforations. **A:** Mallory-Weiss tear. This tear straddles the gastroesophageal junction. Deeper ulceration is present as well. This laceration occurred through an area of preexisting esophagitis. **B:** Boerhaave syndrome with spontaneous transmural rupture.

MUCOSAL LACERATIONS, ULCERATIONS, AND PERFORATIONS

Esophageal perforation complicates many settings (Fig. 2.37) (Table 2.3). A retrospective study of esophageal perforations in a large hospital found 26 instances in a 10-year time frame. Only six of these were spontaneous, while 19 were due

---

TABLE 2.3 **Causes of Esophageal Perforation**

Esophagitis regardless of cause
Penetrating wounds
Iatrogenic trauma
   Pneumatic dilation
   Intubation
      Intraoperative
      Endoscopic
Foreign bodies
Blast injury
Postemetic (Mallory-Weiss syndrome)
Blunt trauma (auto accidents, etc.)
Esophageal diverticula
Esophageal cancer
Corrosive injury
Sclerotherapy
Mucosal ablative therapies

---

to instrumentation with the largest number due to pneumatic dilation in cases of achalasia (68). Perforations due to foreign bodies occur in areas of physiologic narrowing. Spontaneous *transmural* perforations qualify for a diagnosis of *Boerhaave syndrome*. Spontaneous *intramural* tears qualify for a diagnosis of a *Mallory-Weiss tear*. When the esophagus perforates, free air enters the mediastinum and spreads to adjacent structures causing palpable cervical emphysema, mediastinal crackling sounds, and pneumothorax. Over time, secondary infections cause mediastinal abscesses, pyopneumothorax, and pleural-pulmonary suppurations.

Mallory-Weiss Syndrome

The term *Mallory-Weiss syndrome* refers to cases of painless GI bleeding resulting from esophageal or gastroesophageal mucosal lacerations (Fig. 2.37), usually following severe vomiting. Sometimes, vomiting precipitates tears of pre-existing ulcers. Less traumatic events, even snoring, can produce partial esophageal tears, usually above the cardia (69). Most patients are males with a history of alcohol and/or salicylate abuse or hiatal hernias. Rarely lacerations develop in children (70), even neonates. Risk factors for bleeding include portal hypertension or a coagulopathy. These tears account for 5% to 10% of cases of upper GI hemorrhage (71). Single or multiple lacerations lie along the long axis of the distal esophagus crossing the GEJ or lying in the gastric fundus. Over 75% of lacerations are limited to the stomach; they average 1.5 cm in length. The lacerations vary in depth, often only affecting the mucosa; they rarely extend into the muscularis propria. Submucosal hematomas may form and dissect for a distance beyond the tear. Histologic changes reflect the temporal relationship to the tear. If acute, there may be little in the way of acute inflammation. Over time, acute and then chronic inflammatory cells infiltrate the area around the tear. Previous lacerations may associate with scarring. Bleeding from Mallory-Weiss tears usually stops spontaneously; <5% of patients rebleed.

Boerhaave Syndrome

The typical patient with Boerhaave syndrome is a middle-aged male, and frequently an alcoholic individual. The disease may also affect children, even neonates (72). Severe vomiting followed by constant excruciating chest pain are the classic clinical signs. Hematemesis occurs at times. The clinical and radiologic findings point to an intrathoracic catastrophe. The nonspecific symptomatology often delays the correct diagnosis. The mortality rate is approximately 31%. The sudden development of a pressure gradient between an internal portion of a viscus and its external supporting tissues represents the common pathogenetic denominator in cases of gastrointestinal rupture (73). The antecedent background varies; the viscus may become overdistended by food, drink, gas, or any combination thereof. Other antecedent events include abdominal blows, straining at stool, parturition, seizures, asthma, prolonged hiccups, and neurologic diseases.

Characteristically, the rent is linear and longitudinal and occurs most commonly in a left lateral posterior location, 1 to 3 cm above the GEJ (Fig. 2.37). The tears measure 1 to 20 cm in length with an average length of 2 cm; the mucosal part of the tear is usually longer than the muscular part. Immediate surgical repair must occur if the patient is to survive. Persistent reflux often follows repair of the rupture (73).

ESOPHAGITIS
General Comments

Esophagitis has many causes (Table 2.4), the most common being gastroesophageal reflux, infections, and drugs. Esophageal biopsies are taken to determine the etiology of the esophagitis, to assess the consequences of the inflammation, to follow the course of the underlying disease, and to gauge therapeutic responses. Irrespective of its cause, most cases of esophagitis share common histologic features. Therefore, determining a specific etiology may be difficult unless one detects specific diagnostic features such as the presence of viral inclusions. Additionally, multiple etiologies may be present in any given patient.

Esophageal inflammation can be acute, chronic, or mixed. Mild esophageal injury results in reversible mucosal changes

TABLE 2.4   Causes of Esophagitis
Gastroesophageal reflux
Uremia
Ingested material
Drugs
Corrosive agents
Food
Graft vs. host disease
Infections
Radiation
Smoking
Systemic disorders
Behçet syndrome
Crohn disease
Epidermolysis bullosa
Pemphigus
Sarcoid
Scleroderma
Trauma
Intubation
Vascular disease
Motility disorders
Repaired tracheoesophageal fistula
Sclerotherapy

and transient inflammation. Changes associated with acute damage include the presence of balloon cells and inflammatory cells (particularly mononuclear cells) and eosinophils. Basal cell hyperplasia and papillary elongation develop and vascular lakes form. In severe esophagitis, ulcers, erosions, or neutrophils may be seen. Chronic damage leads to submucosal fibrosis or strictures. Patients with longstanding reflux esophagitis may develop Barrett esophagus.

Multinucleated epithelial giant cell changes develop in esophagitis of varying etiologies, representing a nonspecific reparative response. The mucosa contains multinucleated (mean three nuclei per cell, range two to nine) squamous epithelial cells. They are often confined to the basal zone, but sometimes they involve both the basal and superficial epithelium. The nuclei contain single or multiple eosinophilic nucleoli with a perinuclear halo but no inclusions, hyperchromicity, or atypical mitoses (74). Multinucleated cells can also be seen in viral infections, but the use of immunostains or genetic tests allows one to separate nonspecific giant cell changes from virally induced changes.

Cytologic material obtained from patients with esophagitis may show a nonspecific acute and chronic inflammatory infiltrate with mixtures of neutrophils, eosinophils, lymphocytes, plasma cells, histiocytes, and erythrocytes. Epithelial cells, when present, usually appear degenerative.

Reflux Esophagitis

The term *gastroesophageal reflux* (GER) refers to the retrograde flow of gastric and sometimes duodenal contents into the esophagus. The term *gastroesophageal reflux disease* is a symptomatic condition or histopathologic alteration resulting from episodes of GER. *Reflux esophagitis* describes a subset of GERD patients with histopathologic changes in the esophageal mucosa.

Demography/Epidemiology

GERD affects patients of all ages, even children and small infants. The prevalence of GERD ranges from 3% to 36%. GERD is equally present among men and women, but there is a male predominance of esophagitis and Barrett esophagus. GERD affects whites more frequently than members of other races. There is also geographic variability in the prevalence of GERD with very low rates in Africa and Asia and high rates in North America and Europe (75). However, GERD is increasing in frequency in Asians. Nonerosive reflux disease appears to be the commonest form of GERD among Asians. Ethnic and geographic demographic differences suggest that both genetic factors and environmental factors play a role in predisposition to GERD (76).

Conditions predisposing to GERD include smoking; increased intra-abdominal or intragastric pressure, including pregnancy, ascites, and obesity; and delayed gastric emptying. Motility disorders including diabetes, alcoholic neuropathies, achalasia, and scleroderma also predispose to GERD. Patients with hiatal hernias and strictures are especially prone to develop GERD. It also follows surgical procedures. Erosive esophagitis is particularly common in acid hypersecretors such as those with the Zollinger-Ellison syndrome (77). GER in infants and children complicates congenital esophageal or gastric abnormalities. GER also associates with cystic fibrosis (78).

Pathophysiology

GERD is a multifactorial disorder (Table 2.5). Most patients have a lower mean LES resting pressure than is seen in patients without GERD. This allows acid to reflux into the esophagus, leading to the development of esophagitis. The inflammation further impairs LES pressure, increasing acid exposure in the esophagus (79). Patients also have inadequate or slowed clearance of refluxed material and delayed gastric emptying and/or increased gastric volume. The nature and amount of refluxed material and the length of time it remains in contact with the esophageal mucosa as well as the number of reflux episodes determine whether GERD develops (80). GERD results from reflux of both acid and alkaline secretions (Fig. 2.38). Acid alone causes relatively few changes, but when combined with pepsin or bile acids, more severe damage results (81). Pepsin requires an acid pH to exert its full damaging effects (82). Patient age, nutritional status, and other less well-understood factors also influence the mucosal capacity to withstand injury and to repair itself following injury. Reflux esophagitis may also be enhanced by the genesis of free radicals during reflux. These free radicals damage cell membranes, thereby altering

TABLE 2.5	**Causes of, or Predisposition to, Gastric Reflux**

Loss of lower esophageal sphincter (LES) pressure gradient
Loss of esophageal closure pressure
Abnormal LES sphincter position
Hiatus hernia
Certain foods, drinks
Smoking
Pyloric stenosis
Smooth muscle medications
Atropine
β-Adrenergics
Aminophylline
Nitrates
Calcium channel antagonists
Smooth muscle relaxants
Iatrogenic destruction of the LES
Surgical resection
Myotomy
Balloon dilation
Gastroplasty
Gastrostomy feeding
Nasogastric intubation
Pregnancy
Esophageal dysmotility syndromes (inefficient mucosal clearing)
   Collagen vascular diseases
   Intestinal pseudo-obstruction syndromes
   Autoimmune neuropathies
   Diabetes
Zollinger-Ellison syndrome
Decreased esophageal mucosal resistance
Infections
Prior chemotherapy
Intubation (nasogastric)
Increased gastric pressure
Abnormally distended stomach
Refluxed duodenal contents
Esophageal and gastric structural abnormalities

the mucosal barrier. Lipid peroxidation increases with the increasing grade of esophagitis; it is highest in patients with BE (83).

Relationship of Reflux Esophagitis to Helicobacter pylori Infections

Studies addressing the relationship of *HP* infection to GERD often reach conflicting conclusions. This results from the fact that the interplay of *HP* infections and GERD is complex and complicated by the common use of proton pump inhibitor (PPI) therapy in these patients. At the heart of the debate is the link between gastric acid secretion, *HP* infection, and GERD. In patients with gastric ulcer and corpus gastritis, the impact of *HP* infection varies substantially producing wide variation in patterns of acid secretion. In many patients gastric acid is suppressed and is no longer produced in the

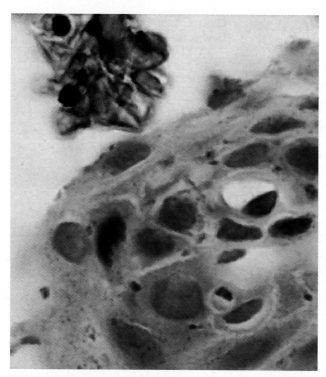

FIG. 2.38. Bile reflux esophagitis. Surface of the esophageal mucosa demonstrating the presence of bile crystals overlying the squamous epithelium.

amount necessary to induce GERD. Bacterial eradication in some of these individuals results in a substantial recovery of acid secretion with sufficient acid to increase the aggressiveness of refluxed gastric juice to the esophageal mucosa (84). In contrast, duodenal ulcer patients typically have antrum-predominant *HP* gastritis and a well-preserved acid-secreting mucosa. In these patients, *HP* infections may make the acid-secretory mechanism hyperresponsive to stimulation, increasing acid production. In this patient group, *HP* infections can increase the aggressiveness of the gastric juice to the esophageal mucosa.

Current epidemiologic trends indicate an inverse relationship in the Western world between the rising incidence of GERD and the decreasing incidence of *HP* infections (85). The lower prevalence of *HP* in GERD patients, the increase of GERD following *HP* eradication, and the association with certain gastritis patterns (atrophic corpus gastritis) have led to the widespread opinion that *HP* exerts a protective effect on the esophagus and may prevent the development of GERD and its complications (85). However, as noted, the data and their interpretations are conflicting, keeping this subject one of continuing interest.

Clinical Features

Transient mild reflux affects most individuals including children and adults. It is especially common in preterm infants (86). The degree of reflux must be severe for individuals to become symptomatic. Fifty percent of symptomatic patients have complications including esophagitis, strictures, or BE. Adults present with diverse symptoms including heartburn, regurgitation, bitter-tasting fluid in the mouth, dysphagia, odynophagia, nausea, vomiting, hiccups, anginalike chest, and hoarseness. The regurgitation can cause a spectrum of conditions, including asthma, chronic laryngitis or pharyngitis, subglottic stenosis, and dental disease. Some patients present with bleeding from esophageal ulcers. Complications peak between ages 50 and 70 years (87). The severest complication is carcinoma developing in the setting of BE.

The clinical course and prognosis of infants and children with GER differ depending on the age at onset. Some children present with symptoms of asthma. GERD may also cause obstructive apnea in infants. Severe dental caries are common. The most frequent complication of recurrent GER in children is failure to thrive as the result of caloric deprivation, vomiting, recurrent bronchitis, or pneumonia caused by repeated episodes of pulmonary aspiration. Some children require gastroesophageal fundoplication and/or pyloroplasty to alleviate the symptoms.

Gross and Endoscopic Features

The gross appearance of the esophagus varies with disease severity. Approximately one third of patients with chronic GERD symptoms are endoscopically normal (88). Low-grade esophagitis is only evident histopathologically. Areas of patchy erythema and red streaks are the first endoscopic abnormalities. Later erosions and ulcers develop; these predominate distally and taper off proximally. The esophagus appears friable, diffusely reddened, and hemorrhagic (Fig. 2.39); it bleeds easily. As the disease progresses, the ulcers become confluent, even circumferential. Strictures or BE characterize severe chronic disease. Prolonged reflux may result in esophageal shortening. Inflammatory polyps may be present. The distinction between the squamous and the columnar epithelium becomes less clear. Several endoscopic classifications have been developed to evaluate the esophageal mucosa. The two most common are the Savary-Miller MUSE system and "Los Angeles" classifications (89,90).

Histologic Features

Biopsies are performed to confirm the diagnosis of GERD; to document complications, including esophagitis, BE, or tumor development; and to rule out the presence of coexisting infections. Since esophagitis tends to be a patchy process, it is easy to miss diagnostic changes on a single biopsy. The current wisdom is that biopsies should be taken in the area just distal to the Z line to detect carditis (see below), just proximal to the Z line to detect esophagitis, and 3 cm proximal to the Z line to detect the hyperplastic changes that are more predictive of the presence of GERD than more distally derived biopsies.

Repetitive episodes of tissue injury and healing produce histologic features that reflect disease activity at the time of

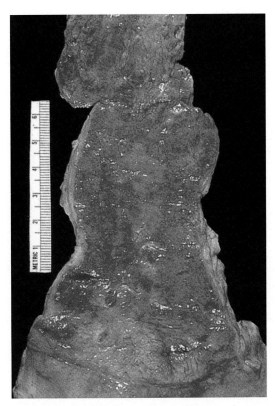

FIG. 2.39. Reflux esophagitis. Area of the Z line is destroyed. Acute hemorrhagic ulcerative reflux esophagitis demonstrating multiple areas of ulceration and erythema.

TABLE 2.6	Histologic Features of Acute Esophagitis

Basal zone hyperplasia (>15% to 20%)
Basal layer spongiosis (edema)
Nuclear enlargement
Mitoses in basal cell layer
Elongated papillae (>75%)
Venular dilation (vascular lakes)
Intraepithelial eosinophils
Polymorphonuclear leukocytes
Lymphocytes
Eosinophils
Acanthosis
Balloon cells
Erosions or ulcers

This change affects patients with an endoscopically normal mucosa as well as those with endoscopic evidence of esophagitis. Regenerative changes are characterized by nuclear enlargement, hyperchromasia, and mitoses that remain limited to the basal layer (Fig. 2.40). Prominent nucleoli may be present. EGFR expression is enhanced in the hyperplastic cells (92).

Accurate assessment of the basal and papillary height requires evaluating well-oriented specimens. *It is helpful to divide the epithelial thickness into thirds. Papillae should not extend into the upper third. When the lower third is divided in half, the basal cells should be confined to its lower half.* PAS stains may help distinguish the basal layer from the superficial layers enabling more accurate measurements of basal cell hyperplasia (Fig. 2.41). In less optimally oriented specimens, basal zone thickness can be evaluated if one sees at least three to four papillae arranged in parallel to one another and not cut tangentially. In tangentially cut sections, a helpful feature is an increase in the number of papillae, which can be evaluated in an en face section. In this setting one may see overlapping capillaries. Since the biopsies may be small or have minimal or no lamina propria or they may be inappropriately oriented and therefore difficult to evaluate for basal hyperplasia and papillary elongation, we recommend that the biopsies be examined at three levels to increase their diagnostic accuracy.

If marked squamous epithelial hyperplasia develops, the elongated epithelial pegs extend into the underlying lamina propria, in a process known as acanthosis (Fig. 2.42). Extensive acanthosis, also termed *pseudoepitheliomatous hyperplasia*, can suggest the presence of an invasive carcinoma. The epithelium may appear markedly regenerative with cytoplasmic basophilia, an increased nuclear-to-cytoplasmic ratio, glycogen depletion, and increased mitotic activity. However, the reactive cells more or less maintain their polarity and abnormal mitoses are absent. The individual cell keratinization seen in high-grade dysplasia is absent. The cell nuclei may have prominent nucleoli but the nuclei appear relatively uniform in size and one may see some evidence of

examination, superimposed on changes from previous injurious episodes. Esophagitis can heal completely or it may progress on to a number of the complications discussed later. Biopsies from patients with heartburn commonly show only basal cell hyperplasia without inflammation. The basal hyperplasia can progress to frank esophagitis. There are four stages of reflux esophagitis: (a) *acute* (necrosis, inflammation, and granulation tissue formation); (b) *repair* (basal cell hyperplasia and elongation of the papillae); (c) *chronic* (fibrosis and formation of Barrett esophagus); and (d) *complications* (dysplasia and adenocarcinoma).

Various histologic features should be assessed when examining the biopsy for GERD (Table 2.6). No single feature described below represents an absolute criterion for the presence of GERD, but each is helpful in suspecting the diagnosis. In the absence of a known drug history or the presence of specific microorganisms, biopsies, particularly distal biopsies showing esophagitis, are most likely to be due to GERD.

Epithelial Hyperplasia

The normal basal cell layer is only one to four cells high; it should not constitute more than 15% of the epithelial thickness. In the setting of GERD, the basal zone increases from 10% to more than 50%; papillary height can increase to more than 50% to 75% of the total epithelial thickness (91).

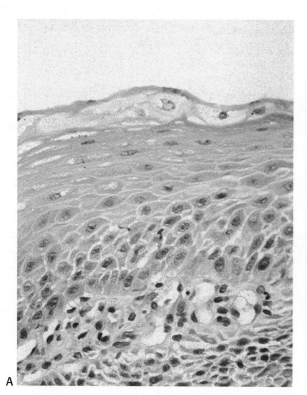
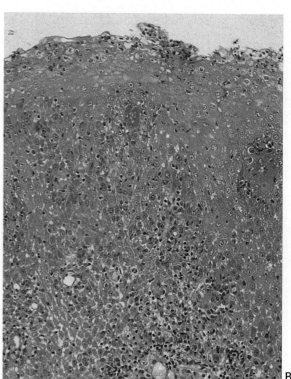

A

B

FIG. 2.40. Esophagitis. **A:** Esophagitis with basal cell hyperplasia and a bandlike inflammatory infiltrate in the lamina propria. **B:** The mucosal vessels are dilated and congested. This histology corresponds to the hyperemia seen endoscopically in esophagitis. Numerous intraepithelial inflammatory cells are present. The epithelium appears poorly glycogenated.

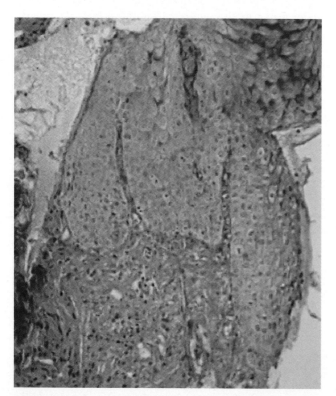

FIG. 2.41. Periodic acid–Schiff stain demonstrating the regularity of the underlying basement membrane and lack of glycogenation of the epithelium.

squamous cell maturation in the more superficial cell layers. The boundary between the epithelium and the underlying stroma appears smooth, unless extensive inflammation occurs.

The stroma underlying the epithelium may appear inflamed, but one should not see desmoplasia. Very small or poorly oriented biopsies, especially those with significant inflammation and associated inflammatory atypia, may be impossible to interpret. If one is completely unable to distinguish between reactive atypia and dysplasia, a diagnosis of indefinite for dysplasia can be made. In this situation, one may want to recommend repeat biopsies once the reflux has been treated, to rule out the presence of an ulcerated and inflamed carcinoma. The sensitivity of hyperplasia as a diagnostic feature is only 60% to 70% (93). Basal cell hyperplasia is a reversible change that disappears with treatment. Hyperplasia also complicates other forms of esophagitis so that it is not specific for GERD.

Balloon Cells

Balloon cells often develop in the midzone of the epithelium clustering around vascular papillae (94). These occur in approximately two thirds of cases of GERD (Fig. 2.43). The cytoplasm of the enlarged, globoid cells appears swollen; cells contain irregular pyknotic nuclei or demonstrate karyorrhexis.

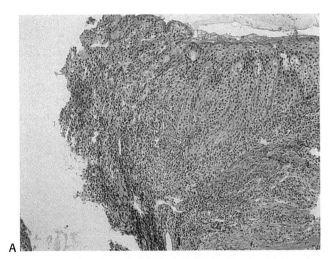
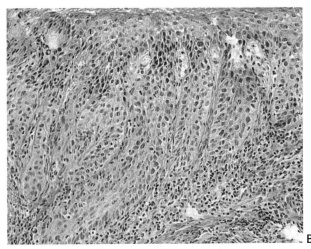

FIG. 2.42. Esophagitis. A: Acanthosis and immaturity of the squamous epithelium is present. Note the long prolongations of the epithelium into the underlying lamina propria. The lymphatics appear dilated and lymphocytes infiltrate the epithelium. **B:** Higher magnification of A demonstrating the elongated acanthotic, glycogen-depleted squamous epithelial prolongations. The flattened cells between the epithelial ridges represent compressed endothelium in the papillae. Chronic inflammation underlies the hyperplastic process.

Balloon cells can be accentuated by PAS stains since they lose the normal intensity of PAS staining characteristic of superficial epithelium. PAS stains also help distinguish balloon cells from the enlarged squamous cells seen in patients with glycogen acanthosis. The presence of balloon cells does not establish a diagnosis of GERD, since they develop in any damaged mucosa, irrespective of its cause. Nonetheless, in the absence of other more characteristic features, the presence of balloon cells may be the only clue to suggest that some form of injury has occurred.

Vascular Changes

Papillary capillary ectasia (sometimes called vascular lakes) (Fig. 2.44) and hemorrhage represent an early but nonspecific histologic sign of GERD. These lakes correspond to the red

streaks seen endoscopically. Capillary ectasia develops in up to 83% of patients with reflux, contrasting with its presence in only 10% of control patients (80). This change is often present in the absence of any inflammation. Dilated and congested venules are seen high up at the top of the lengthened papillae. This may be accompanied by mucosal red cell extravasation. This change develops in many other forms of esophagitis.

Inflammation

Lymphocytes. Small numbers of lymphocytes populate both the normal mucosa and the lamina propria so that their presence does *not* aid in making a diagnosis of esophagitis. However, they are very conspicuous in patients with GERD (95). Biopsies with esophagitis average greater than six lymphocytes per high-powered field (hpf) (96). Since the lymphocytes have irregular

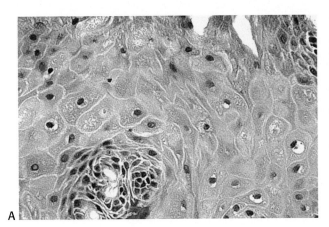
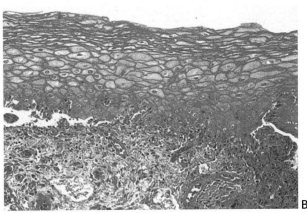

FIG. 2.43. Ballooning degeneration. A: Beginning hydropic degeneration of squamous epithelial cells is evidenced by vacuolization of the cytoplasm. **B:** The epithelium has become paler than usual. The underlying lamina propria appears hemorrhagic and the epithelium separates from the underlying lamina propria.

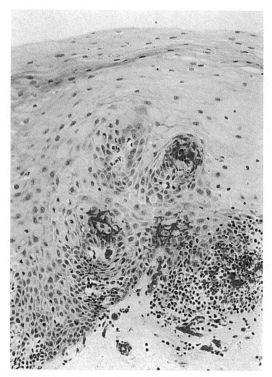

FIG. 2.44. Patients with esophagitis often develop vascular lakes and extravasated red cells. These begin at the area of the papillae and extend outward.

elongated nuclear contours, they are sometimes referred to as "squiggle cells" or as "cells with irregular nuclear contours." Squiggle cells contain scant to invisible cytoplasm. The nuclear shape often curves to fit between the squamous cells (Fig. 2.45). Squiggle cells exhibit a T-lymphocyte phenotype (96). They are part of the inflammatory response in GERD but are not an independent marker of reflux esophagitis (95). A small percentage of the lymphocytes are intraepithelial S100+ antigen-presenting cells. Occasionally, the mononuclear cell infiltration becomes severe enough to cause a focal lymphoid hyperplasia mimicking a lymphoma.

Neutrophils. The presence of isolated neutrophils, either in the squamous epithelium or in the lamina propria, serves as evidence for acute esophagitis of many etiologies. Neutrophils are present in the epithelium of 20% or less of patients with reflux esophagitis, making them a relatively insensitive marker. They tend not to appear until the inflammation becomes severe and the epithelium ulcerated. Large collections of neutrophils suggest that a biopsy comes from the area of an ulcer or erosion. Neutrophils decrease in number the further one goes away from the erosion or ulcer. Neutrophils are most commonly detected near the Z line.

Eosinophils. A modest number of eosinophils (at least six) in the epithelium or in the lamina propria strongly suggest

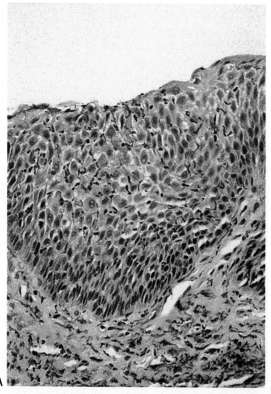

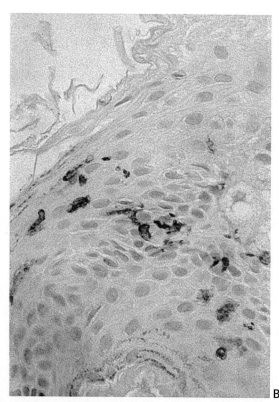

FIG. 2.45. Intraepithelial lymphocytes in reflux esophagitis. **A:** Increased numbers of lymphocytes insinuate themselves between the epithelium. **B:** Lymphocyte common antigen–immunostained sample demonstrating the presence of numerous intraepithelial lymphocytes (*brown*).

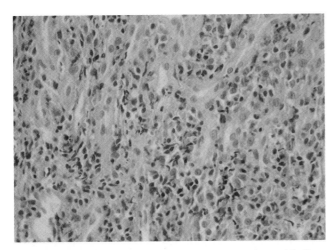

FIG. 2.46. Eosinophilia in reflux esophagitis. The epithelium appears immature and is glycogen poor. Numerous eosinophils infiltrate the epithelium.

the diagnosis of GERD (Fig. 2.46) (97). Infiltration by eosinophils in GERD is more common in children than in adults. It occurs early and may occur in the absence of basal cell hyperplasia. Other causes for mucosal eosinophilia include the entities listed in Table 2.7. One can easily appreciate eosinophils in small endoscopic biopsies, even when the biopsies are not well oriented. They affect up to 60% of adults with severe disease but the intraepithelial eosinophils may be focal in nature, necessitating a search for them on serial sections; their presence does not correlate with disease severity (95,97). Eosinophils are not a sensitive marker for GERD, since they are only found in 40% to 50% of individuals with GERD. Significant esophageal eosinophilia (>20 intraepithelial eosinophils per hpf) and eosinophilic microabscesses are not characteristic of GERD but are part of the entity known as eosinophilic esophagitis discussed in a later section.

Erosions, Ulcers, and Fistulas in Gastroesophageal Reflux Disease

The mucosal changes of reflux esophagitis range from the changes already described to acute esophagitis, erosions,

TABLE 2.7	Eosinophil-associated Esophageal Disorders

Primary eosinophilic disorders
  Eosinophilic esophagitis
Secondary eosinophilic disorders
  Eosinophilic gastroenteritis
  Hypereosinophilic syndrome
Secondary noneosinophilic disorders
  Infection
  Gastroesophageal reflux disorder
  Tumors
  Vasculitis
  Connective tissue disorders

superficial ulcers (Figs 2.47 to 2.49), and extension of the inflammatory process, leading to fistula formation. The depth of the process distinguishes an esophageal *erosion* from an ulcer. Erosions are superficial lesions that remain confined to the lamina propria and muscularis mucosae sparing all but the most superficial layers of the submucosa. The necrosis, hemorrhage, and inflammation associated with *ulcers* extend deeper into the underlying submucosa or muscularis propria. The epithelium close to erosions or ulcers often contains neutrophils, eosinophils, and many lymphocytes. The erosions or ulcers (Fig. 2.49) often contain granulation tissue, an inflammatory exudate, and fibrinoid necrosis in the ulcer base. Lymphoplasmacytic infiltrates, often forming lymphoid aggregates, tend to cluster around erosions and ulcers. Epithelium at the ulcer margin is usually attenuated. Marked basal cell hyperplasia may occupy the entire mucosal thickness and there may be marked acanthosis. These changes may be accompanied by occasional bizarre epithelial or stromal cells.

Erosions or ulcers may be isolated or confluent; they commonly coexist with one another. The damaged mucosa present in reflux esophagitis becomes prone to secondary infections. For this reason, both ulcers and adjacent tissues need to be carefully examined for the presence of coexisting fungal or viral infections. If appreciable ulceration has occurred, longitudinal ridges with crests develop (Fig. 2.48). The ridges consist of hyperplastic, hyperkeratotic, acanthotic, squamous epithelium and extensions of lamina propria; the troughs represent linear ulceration. The alternating ridges and ulcers end abruptly at the cardia; they usually taper away gradually into the surrounding squamous mucosa as one proceeds proximally. Pyogenic granulomas may develop.

Esophageal peptic ulcers also develop in the setting of reflux esophagitis; they resemble peptic ulcers occurring elsewhere. These may erode through the muscular layers, resulting in perforation. Peptic ulcers appear large, oval, and well circumscribed with elevated borders and deep necrotic centers. As these heal strictures develop. This occurs in about 10% of patients with severe reflux esophagitis. Fibrosis is usually present and may extend into the submucosa or beyond, sometimes extending into the periesophageal tissues. Although peptic strictures nearly always involve the distal esophagus, they occasionally develop more proximally. Proximal strictures average 2 to 4 cm in length. Extensive strictures complicate fulminant reflux esophagitis as well as nasogastric intubation in patients with reflux esophagitis or Zollinger-Ellison syndrome.

Differential Diagnosis

The differential diagnosis consists of the esophagitis itself as well as the distinction from neoplasia in very reactive-appearing lesions. The histologic features discussed in the preceding sections suggest the diagnosis of reflux esophagitis, but, as indicated, none is specific for this entity, since they

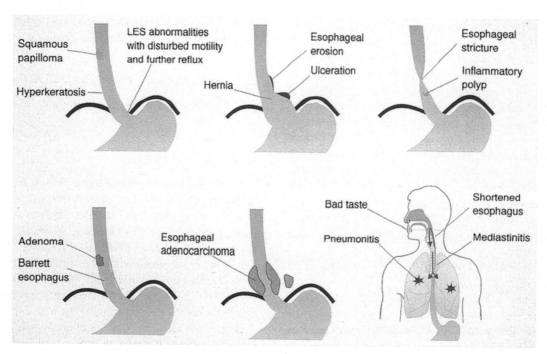

FIG. 2.47. Complications of reflux esophagitis. LES, lower esophageal sphincter.

represent a common pattern of response to diverse forms of injury. Entities to be considered in the differential diagnosis include those listed in Table 2.4.

Reactive changes in biopsies from patients with GERD may appear so atypical (Fig. 2.50) that the differential diagnosis includes both invasive and noninvasive neoplasia. When the basal cell hyperplasia occupies the full thickness of the mucosa and it is very reactive in appearance, it may mimic squamous cell dysplasia. The mucosa in reactive lesions remains architecturally uniform and orderly with relatively regular and uniform papillae. In contrast, dysplastic lesions tend to appear more disorderly (irregularly irregular) and lengthened papillae are generally not present, but if they are present, they are irregular in their configurations. Hyperplastic squamous epithelial cells may appear atypical, but they are uniformly atypical, resembling one another. The enlarged nuclei of hyperplastic cells have generally smooth nuclear membranes, prominent nucleoli, and open chromatin with little or no nuclear overlapping. The cells maintain their normal polarity and abnormal mitoses are absent.

Fragments or irregular nests of very regenerative-appearing squamous cells, areas of pseudoepitheliomatous hyperplasia, bizarre mesenchymal cells in ulcer bases, or enlarged reactive endothelial cells in the granulation tissue or ulcer bases can simulate an invasive carcinoma. Routine histologic examination and immunohistochemical stains using antibodies directed against endothelial cells and cytokeratin can distinguish between some reparative reactions and malignancy. The bizarre stromal cells are usually distributed singly or in groups of two to three cells, usually in obvious granulation tissue. The nuclei are normal or almost normal in size and are nonoverlapping. If the atypia remains confined to cells that mark with endothelial cell antibodies, one can be certain that the tissue is inflammatory in nature. The presence of isolated cytokeratin positive cells strongly suggests the presence of an invasive cancer, especially if the cytokeratin positive cells demonstrate significant nuclear atypia and lie within a desmoplastic stroma. However, care must be taken in interpreting the immunostains since some of the mesenchymal cells occasionally stain with antibodies to cytokeratin. Additionally, isolated benign epithelial cells can drop into a severely inflamed stroma. In some cases with significant atypia and severe inflammation a definitive diagnosis may need to be deferred until the inflammation subsides.

Pyogenic granulomas may mimic an esophageal carcinoma, especially if they are large and polypoid. These larger lesions may be removed by polypectomy. The use of cytokeratin stains and vascular markers allows one to make the correct diagnosis. Finally, marked lymphoid hyperplasia may simulate a lymphoma, but immunohistochemical stains serve to demonstrate the polyclonal nature of the inflammatory infiltrate.

Carditis

As noted earlier, there is debate about the cardia, where it is located, and whether it represents a normal structure or a metaplastic process. There is also debate as to whether cardiac mucosa contains parietal cells. We view the cardiac mucosa as one that contains lobular mucin-secreting glands, with or without parietal cells. Regardless of how one views the cardia, the diagnosis of carditis is usually straightforward. Carditis,

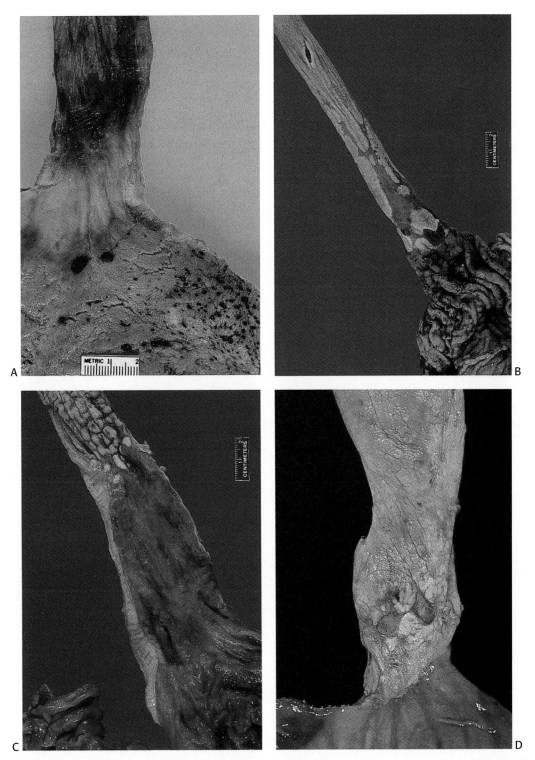

FIG. 2.48. Gross appearance of reflux esophagitis. **A:** This photograph demonstrates the presence of both stress gastritis and reflux esophagitis. The gastric folds extend over the brown discolored, more distal portions of the stomach and end in a hemorrhagic zone. The Z line has been destroyed. The overlying mucosa appears ulcerated, hemorrhagic, and eroded. **B:** Multiple linear continuous and noncontinuous erosions and ulcers are present. Histologically, the most distal lesion just above the Z line in the center of the esophageal mucosa demonstrated Barrett mucosa. The remaining erosive lesions appear more tan in the surrounding mucosa. The epithelium in the distal portion of the esophagus is also whiter than normal due to the presence of hyperkeratosis. **C:** Severe Barrett esophagus arising in the setting of reflux esophagitis. One can see the termination of the gastric folds and then the presence of more proximal red epithelium extending up into the esophagus. Just above the gastroesophageal junction are two linear ulcers lying in the longitudinal axis of the esophagus. Several more proximal erosions are seen. The more proximal portion of the mucosa demonstrates ridges and valleys. The tops of the ridges are associated with white epithelium consistent with areas of hyperkeratosis. **D:** Areas of hyperkeratosis and ulcerations. In this particular patient, the area of the Z line is maintained and there is no evidence of Barrett esophagus.

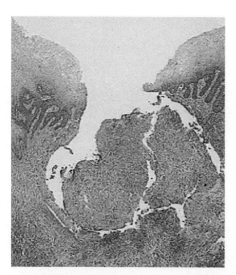

FIG. 2.49. Esophageal ulcer. The ulcer bed is filled with granulation tissue. Reactive hyperplasia is seen in the adjacent squamous mucosa.

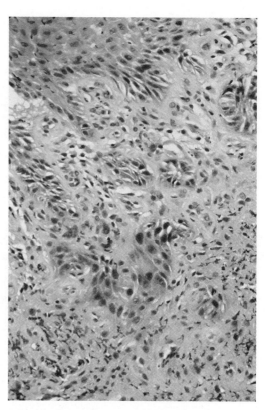

FIG. 2.50. In this example of severe reflux esophagitis, the epithelium is acanthotic and shows significant inflammatory atypia that mimics an invasive squamous cell carcinoma. However, the individual cells contain abundant cytoplasm, the nuclei are not overlapping, and there are no abnormal mitotic figures. There is also intercellular edema.

as the name implies, is an inflammation of cardiac-type epithelium, whether it be in the distal esophagus or proximal stomach. This inflammation is usually chronic in nature consisting of lymphocytes and plasma cells. In acute carditis, acute inflammatory cells are present.

The main question is whether the carditis is part of GERD, *HP* gastritis, or both. The answer is both since GERD and *HP* cause similar histologic features in cardiac epithelium and distinguishing the etiology requires evaluation of the carditis in the context of coexisting changes that may be present in either the esophagus or the stomach. Determining the etiology of the carditis is difficult if only a single biopsy is examined. In patients with multiple biopsies, one is often able to determine the etiology of the carditis by examining the histologic changes in the squamous epithelium and/or the gastric epithelium. If there are classic features of GERD in the esophageal squamous biopsies, then the carditis is most likely part of GERD. In this setting, the carditis occurs in the absence of similar changes in the stomach. Early studies suggest that chronic carditis may be a more sensitive marker for GERD than inflammation involving the squamous mucosa when compared with the results of pH monitoring studies (98). Carditis in this setting is characterized by the presence of lymphocytic, eosinophilic, or plasma cell infiltrates in the lamina propria (Fig. 2.51). Frequently there is foveolar hyperplasia. A villiform surface may be present. The inflammation tends to decrease with increasing distance from the SCJ. Pancreatic metaplasia is also common; this is not common in *HP* infections. The pancreatic acini imperceptibly merge with the cardiac glands.

Some suggest that if the SCJ appears normal endoscopically, then the carditis associates with *HP* infections, whereas an irregular SCJ with short columnar segments and tongues more commonly associates with carditis due to GERD (99).

Unfortunately, the appearance of the SCJ is frequently unknown to the pathologist interpreting the biopsy specimen. *HP* infections start in the distal stomach and move proximally. The presence of a chronic gastritis in gastric biopsies makes chronic carditis much more likely to reflect *HP* infections.

Infectious Esophagitis

General Comments

Infectious esophagitis is a major cause of morbidity, due to increased numbers of individuals with altered immune defenses as a result of organ transplantation, aggressive cancer treatments, an aging population, increased use of steroids and other immunosuppressive agents, and the AIDS epidemic. Various clinical settings predispose patients to infectious esophagitis. These include GERD, general debilitation, advanced age, immunodeficiency states, chronic alcoholism, diabetes, and motility disorders. Certain malignancies, especially hematologic malignancies, increase the risk of infections. GERD or an anatomic abnormality also predisposes patients to infectious esophagitis.

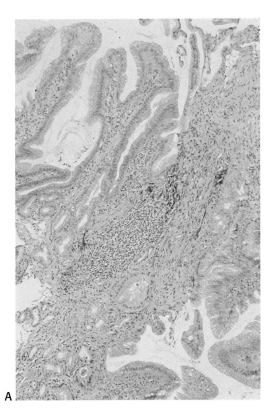
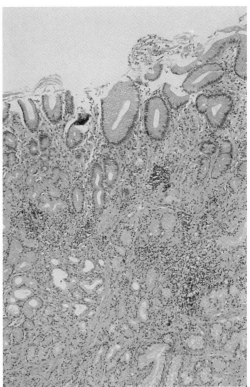

FIG. 2.51. Carditis. In both figures **(A, B)** cardiac mucosa is present that is heavily inflamed. The example in A has a villiform surface and the lobular appearance of the glands is less evident than in B. In B the surface is flatter and the glands are more obviously lobular.

The presence of bacteria within esophageal specimens does not always imply the presence of an infection. The bacterial biota of the normal esophagus resembles that of the oropharynx (100). Organisms are swallowed or carried into the esophagus by the endoscope. One commonly encounters round or small oval-shaped bacteria lying in pairs or tetrads in the esophageal lumen. Bacteria may be present in both the normal esophagus or in an esophagus affected by esophagitis due to other causes (Fig. 2.52). Bacteria lying free on mucosal surfaces or in the esophageal lumen are unlikely to be pathogenic. In contrast, bacteria invading the underlying tissues are usually pathogenic. Esophageal endoscopy with brushings and biopsies is the procedure of choice in the diagnostic workup of patients with suspected infections. Because different infections localize to different areas, ulcer bases as well as ulcer edges and intervening areas should be biopsied (Fig. 2.53). *Candida*, cytomegalovirus (CMV), and herpes infections are the commonest causes of infectious esophagitis in the Western world.

Bacterial Esophagitis

Bacterial esophagitis is defined as the presence of histopathologically demonstrable bacterial invasion of the esophageal mucosa or deeper layers without concomitant fungal, viral, or neoplastic disease. Esophageal bacterial infections are unusual and generally occur in profoundly granulocytopenic patients or they represent an extension of an infection from adjacent structures. Bacterial esophagitis often involves previous mucosal damage due to GERD, radiation, chemotherapy, or nasogastric intubation, processes that allow bacteria to invade the lamina propria, submucosa, or even the vasculature. The commonest causes of bacterial esophagitis include *Staphylococcus aureus, Staphylococcus epidermidis,* and streptococcus strains. Rare bacterial esophagitis results from *Klebsiella* or *Lactobacillus acidophilus* infections. Bacterial esophagitis may also complicate *diphtheria* (in which case, pseudomembranes form over the upper esophageal mucosa) anthrax (101), syphilis, brucellosis, or bacillary angiomatosis (102). Often, several bacterial species are present, supporting a polymicrobial nature of the infections.

Bacterial esophagitis presents with odynophagia, dysphagia, chest pain, or upper gastrointestinal bleeding. The most significant complications include perforation, fistulas, and sepsis; the risk of bacteremia correlates with the severity of the esophagitis. Bacteria are best seen by examining tissue sections stained with a Gram stain and examined under an oil immersion lens. Histologically, bacterial infections produce an intense neutrophilic exudate, cellular necrosis, and degeneration. However, ulcers and pseudomembranes without significant acute inflammation can be seen in severely granulocytopenic patients. Features of specific bacterial infections follow.

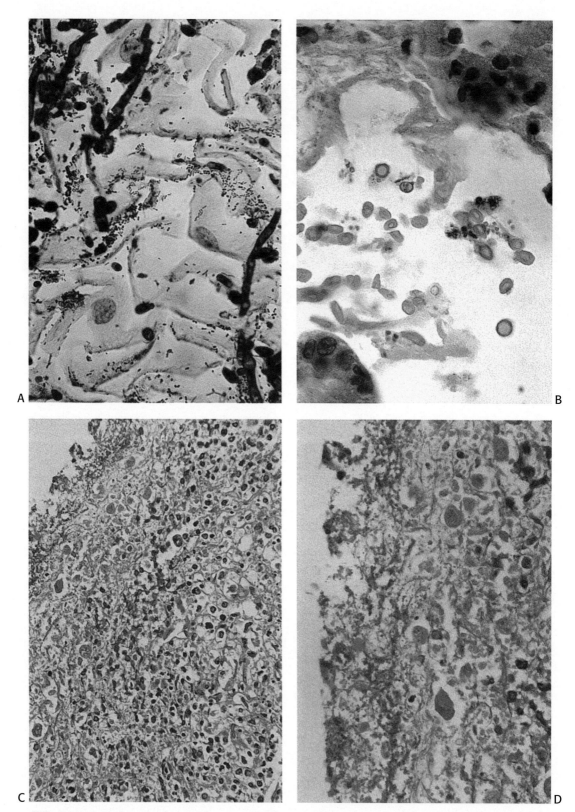

FIG. 2.52. Organisms in the esophagus. **A:** High magnification of desquamated epithelial cells, fungal hyphae, and spores, and numerous coccobacilli. **B:** Luminal contents demonstrating the presence of extravasated red cells and small clusters of Gram-negative diplococci belonging to the *Vionella* group. **C:** Necrotic debris overlying an area of an ulcer in the esophagus. The right-hand part of the picture demonstrates large amounts of necrotic debris with degenerating epithelial cells and pyknotic nuclei. **D:** Higher magnification of C at the edge of the lesion demonstrates a fringe of bacteria. None of the organisms illustrated in A–D are pathogenic and represent either the transmission of oral flora into the esophagus via swallowing or being carried on the endoscope, or in C and D represent nonspecific colonization of necrotic tissue.

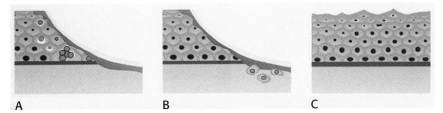

A　　　　　　　　　　B　　　　　　　　　　C

FIG. 2.53. Comparative features of viral infections of the esophagus. **A:** Herpes and varicella infections. Herpetic inclusions typically affect the epithelium in the area adjacent to the ulcer. The mesenchymal tissues at the ulcer base are negative. **B:** Cytomegalovirus (CMV). CMV inclusions typically occur in mesenchymal cells, especially macrophages, endothelial cells, and fibroblasts at the base of the ulcers. They are not found in the epithelium. **C:** In human papillomavirus infections, true viral inclusions are not seen in the same way they are seen in herpes or CMV infections. Instead, one sees koilocytotic atypia affecting the superficial portions of the epithelium. These differential localizations of the viral cytopathic effects dictate where biopsies should be taken, depending on the nature of the infection suspected.

Individuals at risk for developing *esophageal tuberculosis* include immigrants from underdeveloped countries and immunocompromised individuals. Patients present with dysphagia, weight loss, fever, chest pain, and cough. Rupture of mediastinal disease into the esophagus causes fistulae between the tracheobronchial tree and the esophagus (103). Mediastinal tuberculous lymphadenitis may present as an esophageal submucosal tumor. Typically, tuberculous esophagitis involves the midesophagus. Grossly, tuberculous lesions appear ulcerative, hyperplastic (pseudotumoral), or both (104). Since the esophagus is usually involved by direct extension of mediastinal or thoracic disease, the biopsy is often not deep enough to provide diagnostic material. When one is able to make the diagnosis in biopsy material, the histologic features resemble those seen elsewhere with caseating granulomas containing epithelioid histiocytes, giant cells, and acid-fast bacilli (Fig. 2.54). Cytologic smears of the esophagus may facilitate the detection of the infection. Polymerase chain reaction (PCR) evaluation may also yield a definitive diagnosis in cases without typical histologic features but in which the diagnosis is clinically suspected (105).

Actinomyces, anaerobic Gram-positive bacteria frequently present in the oral flora, may colonize a damaged mucosa. If tissue invasion occurs, sinuses, fistulous tracts, and abscesses may develop. The diagnosis depends on recognition of the characteristic sulfur granules. The filaments at the periphery of the colonies are club shaped with enlarged ends. Usually, an acute inflammatory exudate surrounds the colonies.

Viral Esophagitis

Viruses commonly infect the esophageal mucosa, especially in immunocompromised persons. These infections include herpes simplex virus (HSV), CMV, Epstein-Barr virus (EBV), varicella, and human papillomavirus (HPV). Multinucleated epithelial giant cells suggest the diagnosis of a viral infection. However, as noted earlier, giant cells can be seen in nonviral forms of esophagitis. Occasionally, some viral infections, particularly CMV and HSV, produce a vaguely granulomatouslike

lesion, which can be confused with other forms of granulomatous esophagitis.

Herpes Esophagitis

HSV-induced esophagitis affects 0.5% to 6% of patients, primarily those who are immunosuppressed due to AIDS, transplantation, or chemotherapy. However, immunocompetent individuals and neonates also acquire these infections. Primary infections are common in neonates with disseminated HSV (106); in adults the disease often represents reactivation of latent infection. The esophagus is the most commonly affected GI site. In immunocompetent individuals, HSV infections are self-limited; in immunocompromised

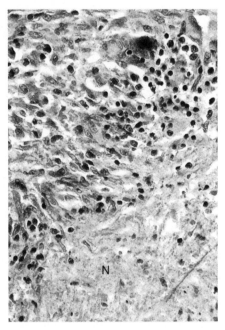

FIG. 2.54. Tuberculosis. Caseating granulomas with central necrosis (*N*) and peripheral multinucleated giant cells are the hallmark of mycobacterial infections.

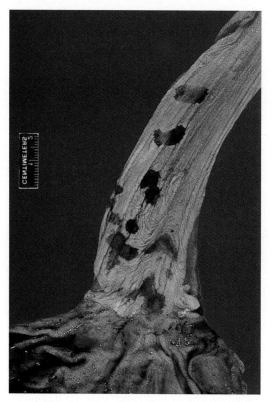

FIG. 2.55. Herpetic esophagitis with numerous punched-out ulcers.

individuals, the infections may be severe and prolonged. Patients present with acute-onset nausea and vomiting, odynophagia, fever, retrosternal pain, GI bleeding, or spontaneous esophageal perforation (107). Oral herpetic blisters may suggest the diagnosis. Up to 70% of patients have concurrent coinfections (108). Immunocompromised individuals develop serious complications, including mucosal necrosis, superinfections, hemorrhage, strictures, HSV pneumonia, tracheoesophageal fistulas, and disseminated infections (107).

The lesions begin as discrete vesicles with erythematous bases that break down to form erosions that progress to isolated or confluent targetoid or aphthous ulcers with discrete punched-out erythematous or yellow raised margins (Fig. 2.55). Typically, the ulcers are shallow and surrounded by normal-appearing mucosa. Large areas of denuded mucosa develop in severe disease. Pseudomembranes may be present. Herpetic ulcers usually stop at the GEJ. The changes of herpetic esophagitis occur alone or are superimposed on pre-existing damage resulting from nasogastric tubes, caustic injury, other infections, or GERD.

Since HSV preferentially infects squamous epithelium, the margins of esophageal ulcers and islands of residual squamous epithelium must be sampled to confirm the diagnosis. Herpetic changes may also be seen in submucosal gland ducts and acini. Biopsies from the base of herpetic ulcers reveal only nonspecific inflammation, necrotic debris, granulation tissue,

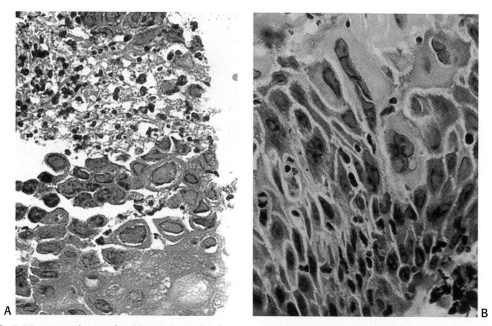

FIG. 2.56. Herpetic esophagitis. **A:** Superficial squamous epithelium demonstrating area of ulceration and discohesive squamous epithelial cells containing prominent ground-glass nuclei with margination of the nuclear chromatin. **B:** Epithelium demonstrating the typical multinucleated syncytial squamous cells with surrounding pyknotic nuclei, inflammation, and ground-glass nuclei. Cowdry type A inclusions are seen.

and desquamated epithelial cells. Characteristic lesions include the presence of nuclear molding, multinucleated giant cells, ballooning degeneration, and eosinophilic Cowdry type A intranuclear inclusions (Figs. 2.56 and 2.57). The latter have a clear zone with an outer dark margin of condensed chromatin. Cowdry A inclusions are less common than Cowdry type B inclusions, which show ballooning degeneration, enlarged nuclei, and a faintly basophilic, ground-glass appearance. Only a small number of viral inclusions are present in immunocompetent patients, contrasting with large numbers present in immunosuppressed patients (109). Acute and chronic inflammation may be present. Prominent collections of mononuclear cells consisting of aggregates of large mononuclear cells with convoluted nuclei near an ulcer may suggest the diagnosis (Fig. 2.58) (110). The histologic features are not specific for HSV, but also develop in patients with herpes zoster infections. Immunostains or genetic probes distinguish between the two. Herpetic ulcers may become secondarily infected by bacteria, fungi, or CMV infections, and in severely immunocompromised individuals, multiple infectious organisms may contribute to the esophagitis. It is important to distinguish herpetic esophagitis from other forms of infectious esophagitis because specific drugs exist to treat each infection.

Varicella Zoster Virus (Chickenpox)

Varicella zoster virus (VZV), a DNA virus morphologically identical to HSV, causes chickenpox and herpes zoster and severe esophagitis in profoundly immunocompromised adults. VZV infections in immunocompromised children are particularly severe and visceral dissemination has a mortality rate of 7% to 30% (111). Esophageal involvement may precede the development of skin lesions (112). The epithelium, endothelium, and stromal cells may contain numerous intranuclear eosinophilic inclusion bodies indistinguishable from those seen in HSV (Fig. 2.59). The cells swell with

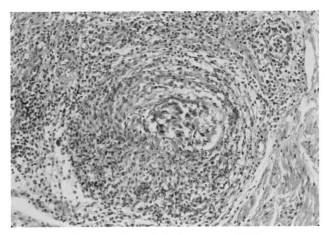

FIG. 2.58. Microgranulomalike lesion surrounded by numerous lymphocytes in herpes esophagitis.

rarefaction and vacuolization of the cytoplasm, and the basal layer separates from the lamina propria. Other characteristic morphologic features include edema and ballooning degeneration. Immunohistochemical staining using monoclonal antibodies to VZV antigens or molecular probes serves to differentiate HSV from VZV.

Cytomegalovirus

CMV infections commonly cause esophagitis, especially in debilitated, elderly, or immunocompromised individuals. However, they also affect immunocompetent individuals. Patients with disseminated CMV infections have circulating cytomegalic inclusion–containing endothelial cells in the peripheral blood. Nausea, vomiting, fever, epigastric pain, diarrhea, and weight loss constitute prominent symptoms, whereas odynophagia and retrosternal pain are less common than in HSV infections (113). CMV affects the entire GI tract; esophageal involvement may be the first manifestation of GI disease. Rarely, CMV infections cause massive esophageal bleeding.

CMV presents as multiple, discrete, well-circumscribed, superficial flat serpiginous or oval ulcers in the mid- or distal esophagus (Fig. 2.60). The ulcers may be quite extensive, extending for distances up to 10 to 15 cm. Giant ulcers may penetrate the esophagus causing fistulas. AIDS patients may develop pseudotumoral CMV esophagitis. Characteristic cytopathic effects include prominent eosinophilic, intranuclear inclusions, cellular enlargement, and occasional granular basophilic cytoplasmic inclusions. The histologic features differ from those seen in HSV infections (Table 2.8) in that CMV cytopathic effects typically develop in the glandular epithelium (Fig. 2.61), endothelial cells, macrophages, and fibroblasts in the granulation tissue of the ulcer bases rather than in the squamous cells. The cells in the stroma often appear enlarged (cytomegalic) with conspicuous intranuclear inclusions. For this reason, biopsies should be taken of

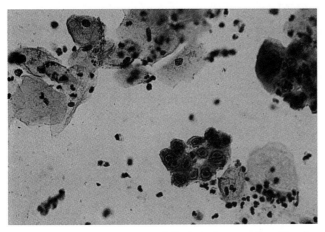

FIG. 2.57. Intranuclear eosinophilic inclusions and multinucleation are seen in this cytologic specimen of herpetic esophagitis.

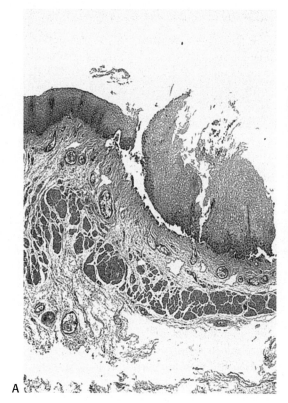
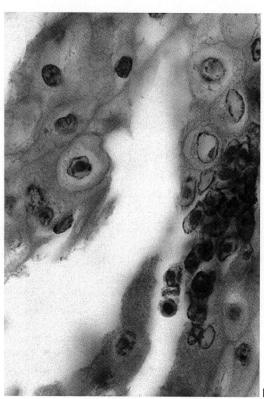

FIG. 2.59. Varicella zoster viral esophagitis from a young girl who died of disseminated chickenpox. Her varicella hepatitis was the immediate cause of death. However, this patient also demonstrated fulminant varicella esophagitis. **A:** One area of superficial ulceration demonstrating separation of the epithelium from the underlying tissues. **B:** Squamous epithelium in an area remote from active ulceration demonstrating multinucleated epithelial cells.

the ulcer base rather than of the epithelium. The virus can also be diagnosed on esophageal brushings (Fig. 2.62) by finding the characteristic viral inclusions. Perivascular macrophage aggregates may be present (110). As in HSV infections, the use of specific antibodies or genetic probes for the virus may establish the diagnosis (Fig. 2.63). In situ hybridization reactions usually disclose the presence of many probe-positive cells that would not have been predicted by examination of only the hematoxylin and eosin (H&E)-stained slides, especially in immunocompromised individuals.

Other Viral Infections

Papillomaviruses belong to a family of epitheliotropic DNA viruses primarily involving skin and mucous membranes. They produce hyperplastic lesions as well as the well-defined papillomas and condylomas. For this reason, they are discussed further in Chapter 3. *Epstein-Barr virus* is a double-stranded DNA virus of the herpesvirus family that causes infectious mononucleosis. Odynophagia and hematemesis may affect otherwise healthy patients with infectious mononucleosis. EBV infections are also found in AIDS patients (114). Patients develop 3- to 5-mm esophageal ulcers

with erythematous rims and gelatinous bases. In contrast to HSV, EBV ulcers are deep, linear, and located in the midesophagus. They resemble the lesions of oral hairy leukoplakia in AIDS patients (115). The virus is detectable by immunohistochemistry, ultrastructural examination, or in situ hybridization reactions.

Fungal Esophagitis

Like viral esophagitis, fungal esophagitis tends to affect debilitated or immunocompromised individuals. In cancer patients, radiation, chemotherapy, and neutropenia predispose to the infections. Motility disorders also predispose patients to fungal infections. Some patients acquire nosocomial fungal infections during hospitalization for serious illness. Fungal infections may be (and often are) superimposed on other infections, and one should diagnose all organisms that are present if the patient is to be optimally treated. Fungal esophagitis most commonly results from *Candida* species, although other organisms such as *Histoplasma, Paracoccidioides, Trichosporon, Aspergillus, Cryptococcus, Coccidioides, Fusarium, Blastomyces,* and *Mucor* can rarely cause esophagitis. The fungi may form large esophageal fungus balls.

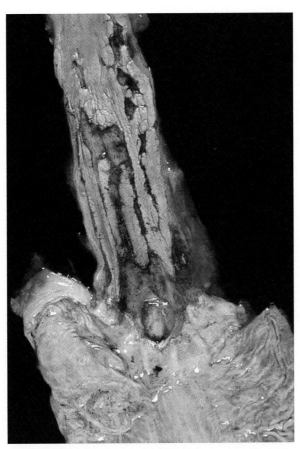

FIG. 2.60. Gross appearance of cytomegalovirus esophagitis. Linear ulcerations and discrete oval ulcers are present.

Candida Infections

Candida species are both commensal organisms (frequently found in the oral cavity) as well as pathogens. The yeasts grow as round to oval eukaryotic cells, reproducing asexually by budding. Other morphologic features include pseudohyphae (linear arrangements of buds or blastoconidia) and occasionally true septated hyphae. *Candida albicans* is the predominant cause of fungal esophagitis, but other *Candida* species including *Candida tropicalis, Candida glabrata, Candida parapsilosis, Candida stellatoidae,* and *Candida krusei* can be pathogenic. *C. tropicalis* tends to be more invasive than *C. albicans.*

Candida causes acute, subacute, and chronic disease. The most common form is *acute candidal esophagitis* with a sudden onset affecting immunocompromised individuals. Patients present with dysphagia, odynophagia, and chest pain. Rare complications include stricture or fistula formation, perforation, extensive necrosis that denudes the entire esophageal mucosa, and *Candida* sepsis. *Subacute candidal esophagitis* is uncommon and occurs as an indolent, often asymptomatic infection in immunocompetent patients. Patients present with symptoms relating to esophageal strictures or pseudodiverticulosis. *Chronic candidal esophagitis* is rare and generally affects patients with chronic mucocutaneous candidiasis. These patients have other gastrointestinal abnormalities including malabsorption and loss of parietal cell function (116). Candidal infections result in significant morbidity and death, especially in high-risk patients. Chronic mucocutaneous candidiasis associates with neoplasms, especially thymomas.

Fungal attachment, adhesion, morphogenesis (conversion of the spore to a filamentous growth phase), and aggregation constitute important events in fungal colonization and virulence. *C. albicans* encounters the host tissue, where it replicates (colonization) or moves deeper into the host tissues (invasion), a process facilitated by proteolysis (117). Patients with intact immune systems may show an inflammatory reaction around the infected site, which usually limits the *Candida* epithelial penetration. A number of complications follow *Candida* infections.

Typically, whitish, raised, longitudinally oriented, discrete or confluent plaques or membranes measuring <1 cm cover

TABLE 2.8	Histologic Features of Various Viral Infections		
Virus	**Gross Features**	**Location**	**Histology**
HSV VZV	Multiple discrete shallow ulcers	Esophagus (HSV) common site	Biopsy (BX) of base: Only granulation tissue; inflammation; necrosis; epithelial ballooning; inclusions in epithelium at ulcer edge
CMV	Resembles HSV	Tends to involve the stomach and intestines more frequently than esophagus	Cytopathic effects involve submucosal glands, endothelium, stromal fibroblasts; infection of squamous cells—rare
HIV	May resemble HSV and CMV	Esophageal involvement hard to document	No specific changes
HPV	Normal or papillomas	Esophagus occasionally involved	Koilocytosis, condyloma or normal appearing, and virus found by antigenic or molecular biologic tests
EBV	Deep, linear ulcers	Midesophagus	Resembles oral leukoplakia

CMV, cytomegalovirus; EBV, Ebstein-Barr virus; HSV, herpes simplex virus; HPV, human papilloma virus; VZV, varicella zoster virus; BX, biopsy.

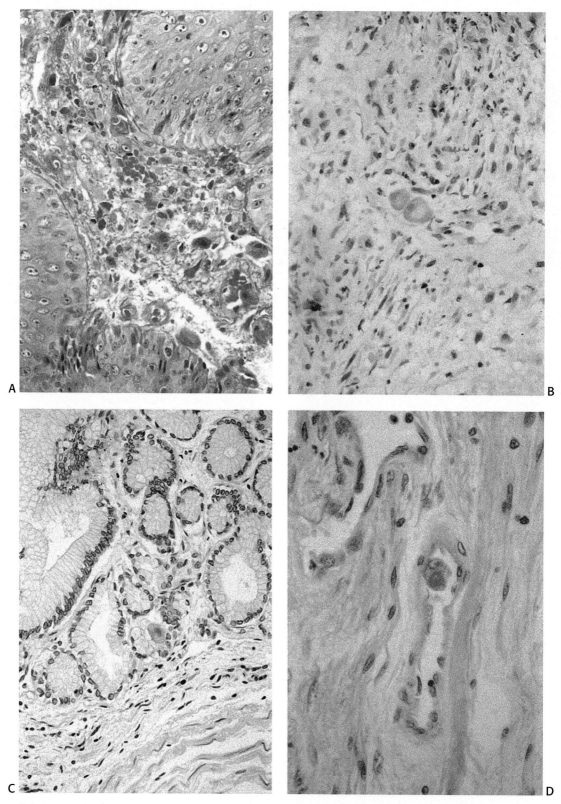

FIG. 2.61. Histologic features of cytomegalovirus (CMV). Severe esophagitis due to CMV infection. **A:** Numerous CMV intranuclear inclusions are present in the stroma. **B:** Higher magnification of stromal cell inclusions. **C:** Intranuclear inclusion in epithelium of submucosal glands. **D:** Intranuclear inclusion in endothelial cell.

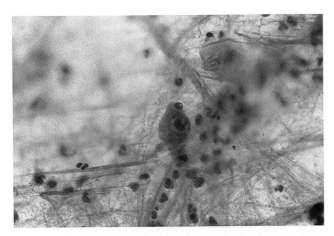

FIG. 2.62. Cytologic preparation of esophageal brushing demonstrating the presence of typical viral inclusions in the stromal cells from a patient with a cytomegalovirus infection.

a friable, erythematous, ulcerated mucosa, particularly in the mid- and distal esophagus (Fig. 2.64). Erosions, ulcers, and strictures may also develop. The fungi are densely adherent to the esophageal mucosa and are not easily removed. In advanced disease, the esophagus becomes narrow, with a shaggy or cobblestoned appearance easily confused grossly with pseudodiverticulosis, strictures, varices, or carcinoma. In chronic cases umbilicated wartlike lesions may be present. Rarely, fungal esophagitis assumes a polypoid multinodular shape resembling clusters of grapes. Mucosal bridges may also form. Severe esophageal candidiasis can cause necrosis of the entire esophageal mucosa (118).

In tissue, *Candida* species show a mixture of spores (4 μm in diameter) and pseudohyphae without true branching. They stain poorly with H&E, but PAS or methenamine silver stains may highlight their presence (Fig. 2.65). The nonbranching pseudohyphae may become quite large (up to 2 μm in diameter) and interdigitate, forming large clumps. Fungal plaques consist of pseudohyphae and budding spores embedded in a fibrinous exudate and necrotic debris. Pseudohyphal or true hyphal forms should be present to make the diagnosis of a true infection. Inflammatory exudates at the ulcer bases often contain budding yeast without pseudohyphae or evidence of tissue invasion. Surface colonization, particularly of devitalized tissue, does not imply clinically significant disease. Patients treated with antifungal agents may only have spores. Examination of cytologic brushings made directly from the plaques (Fig. 2.66) significantly increases fungal detection rate, but biopsies are required to determine whether the fungus is invasive. It is helpful to indicate in the pathology report the types of fungal forms that are present (i.e., whether it is a yeast or pseudohyphae and whether it is in the exudate or invades the tissue).

Candidal infections may resemble other fungal infections. The major distinguishing characteristics between *Candida* and *Aspergillus* are differences in hyphal width, the presence of true dichotomous branching in *Aspergillus*, and the presence of blastoconidia in *Candida* species. The major differential point between *Histoplasma* and *Candida* is the absence of pseudohyphae in the former. If there are only yeast forms and no pseudohyphae, *Candida* may be impossible to

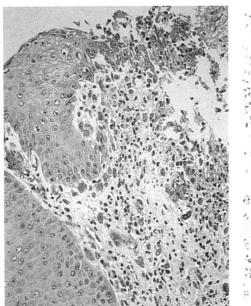

A   B

FIG. 2.63. Detection of cytomegalovirus. **A:** Hematoxylin and eosin (H&E) section demonstrating the presence of an esophageal ulcer. The epithelium, which remains intact, shows no evidence of viral inclusions. The stroma underlying the ulceration contains atypical cells. **B:** In situ hybridization detects many more cells that are positive for the virus than would be detected by H&E examination alone.

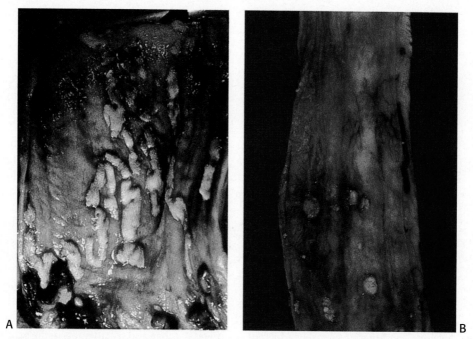

FIG. 2.64. Gross features of esophageal candidiasis. **A:** Characteristically, the esophageal mucosa is covered by densely adherent white plaques that are difficult to remove. One may also see erosions and ulcers. These may be confluent and produce linear streaks as seen in A. **B:** In some patients, the candidal lesions appear more discrete and complicate other disorders, in this case esophageal varices.

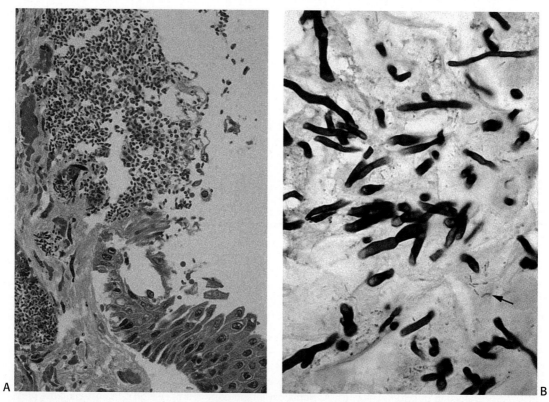

FIG. 2.65. *Candida.* **A:** Esophageal mucosa containing numerous *Candida* spores and rare hyphae. **B:** Silver stain demonstrating the presence of septated hyphae. The smaller rodlike structures represent bacilli derived from the mouth (*arrow*).

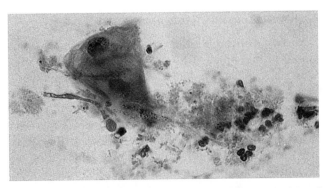

FIG. 2.66. Typical fungal hyphae are present in this esophageal brushing preparation from a patient with *Candida* esophagitis.

differentiate from *Histoplasma capsulatum* solely on a morphologic basis, since the morphologic features overlap.

Aspergillosis

Aspergillus species occur worldwide, being ubiquitous in the environment. They reproduce by spores termed conidia. Infections generally affect severely immunocompromised patients. Nosocomial *Aspergillus* infections affect hospitalized patients. Spore inhalation is the commonest route of infection. Several species of *Aspergillus* infect the esophagus, including *Aspergillus fumigatus*, *Aspergillus niger*, and *Aspergillus flavus*. Prerequisites for tissue invasion include expression of specific receptors that recognize host tissues and excretion of proteases that facilitate fungal invasion (119). Patients present with painful or difficult swallowing and weight loss. Concurrent mucosal candidiasis may be present. The lesions typically extend from the mucosa into the muscularis propria (Fig. 2.67). When vascular invasion occurs, thrombosis and infarction create secondary damage, including perforation. The fungi are characterized by the presence of 45-degree right-angle, dichotomously branching, slender, septate hyphae with smooth, parallel walls, ranging in size from 2 to 4 μm in diameter. Characteristic conidiophores, if present, aid in their identification. These contrast with phycomycetes, which are broad and nonseptate and branch at right or obtuse angles.

Other Fungal Infections

North American blastomycosis is caused by the fungus *Blastomycosis dermatitidis*. In the United States it is endemic to the Mississippi and Ohio River valleys. *Blastomycosis* predominantly infects the lungs, skin, bones, and genitourinary tract. GI involvement develops in patients with disseminated disease. Grossly, esophageal infections cause an edematous friable mucosa with linear ulcers or strictures (120). *Blastomyces* appear larger than *Histoplasma*. In well-fixed tissues, multiple nuclei can be seen. The lesion may occasionally stain weakly for mucin. Biopsies show exudates of polymorphonuclear leukocytes containing yeast forms and granuloma formation.

Histoplasmosis affects endemic areas in the central United States and in other areas of the world. The fungus grows in soil with a high nitrogen content enriched by bird and bat guano. Individuals living in endemic areas are probably repeatedly infected but generally remain asymptomatic. The fungi usually gain access to the body through inhalation. Extrapulmonary dissemination occurs frequently in immunosuppressed or debilitated patients. The disease also extends directly into the esophagus from the lungs or mediastinal lymph nodes. In patients with disseminated disease, the incidence of esophageal involvement may be as high as 13%.

Patients present with dysphagia secondary to esophageal compression by mediastinal lymphadenopathy or from sclerosing mediastinitis. Mediastinal granulomas may cause traction diverticula. Grossly, ulcers or nodular lesions may be present. The fungus infects humans in the mycelial phase but

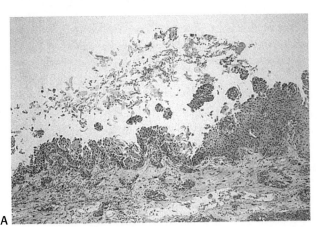

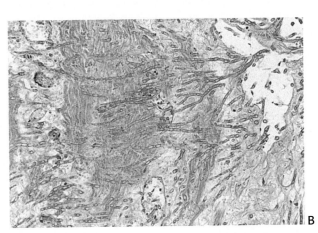

FIG. 2.67. Esophageal aspergillosis. **A:** Low-power magnification demonstrating the presence of an erosive esophagitis. **B:** Higher magnification demonstrating the presence of branching hyphae infiltrating the muscularis propria.

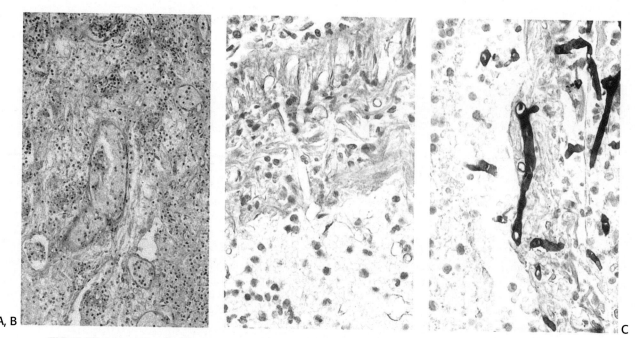

A, B   C

FIG. 2.68. Mucor esophagitis. A: Hematoxylin and eosin–stained section demonstrating the presence of inflamed, apparently necrotic esophageal tissues. The outlines of capillaries are identified. One can vaguely make out the irregularly shaped grayish structures in the infiltrate. **B:** Higher magnification demonstrating the presence of the edematous mucosa. Irregularly shaped fungi invade through the muscular wall of a vessel. The organisms are barely visible except as linear defects in the wall. **C:** Silver stains highlight the presence of the organisms, which in this case lie in the tissues. Branching hyphae are also present in a capillary.

converts to the yeast phase at body temperature. The yeast is ovoid, measuring 1.5 to 2.0 μm $\times$ 3.0 to 3.5 μm, and yeasts reproduce by budding within macrophages in the infected tissues. *Histoplasma* has a rigid cell wall. During fixation, the protoplasm retracts from the rigid wall leaving a clear space.

Infectious *Phycomycetes* include fungi from the genera *Absidia*, *Rhizopus*, and *Mucor*. *Mucor* usually causes more extensive necrosis and ulceration than other infections (Fig. 2.68). These infections are essentially limited to severely immunocompromised hosts. Esophageal infections result either from direct mucosal involvement from the lumen after swallowing inhaled organisms, from extension from contiguous structures, or following blood-borne dissemination. *Phycomycetes* are often difficult to see on H&E-stained sections but are easily delineated by mucin stains. They have irregular broad, nonseptated, haphazardly branched hyphae with obtuse to right-angle branches. Occasional hyphae may measure 3 to 4 μm in diameter but broad hyphae measuring 10 to 15 μm in diameter predominate. The irregular branching contrasts with the uniform acute angle branching of *Aspergillus*. Cross sections of large empty hyphae can be mistaken for empty spherules of *Coccidioides immitis*. The organism has a predilection for vascular invasion, leading to secondary ischemia.

Parasitic Infections

Esophageal parasitic infections are less common than other types of infections. They include Chagas disease (see Chapter

10), trichomoniasis, *Pneumocystis* (121), cryptosporidiosis (122), and leishmaniasis (123). Esophageal involvement also complicates amoebic liver abscesses and hepatic echinococcal cysts.

Esophageal Diseases in AIDS Patients

AIDS patients often first present with esophageal manifestations due either to the HIV infection itself or to the presence of another infection. Frequent clinical presentations include dysphagia and severe odynophagia. *Candida* esophagitis causes most esophageal disease followed by CMV and herpesvirus infections, idiopathic esophageal ulcers, and Kaposi sarcoma and lymphoma. Esophageal candidiasis is so common that esophageal *Candida* infection is a diagnostic criterion for AIDS (124). EBV and parasitic and bacterial infections (including *Mycobacterium avium*) must also be considered in the differential diagnosis of esophageal disease. The use of protease inhibitors in the treatment of HIV has had a major impact on improving the outcome of HIV-associated esophageal diseases (125).

Acute HIV infection produces multiple discrete esophageal aphthous ulcers (126). These develop in the first month or so following the HIV infection complicating a mononucleosislike febrile illness. Progressive weight loss results from the presence of multiple hypopharyngeal and esophageal ulcers. Dysphagia and odynophagia further compromise the patient's already compromised nutritional status. The esophagus

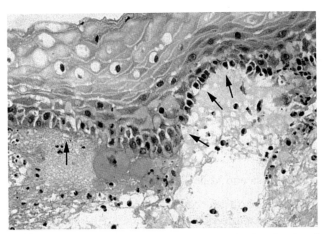

FIG. 2.69. Nonspecific esophageal changes. The basal stromal junction *(arrows)* shows prominent subepithelial edema. This area is also infiltrated with polymorphonuclear leukocytes.

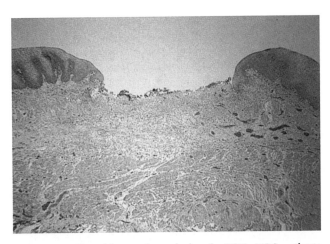

FIG. 2.71. Idiopathic esophageal ulcer in AIDS. AIDS patients often demonstrate well-demarcated, punched-out ulcers and erosions that do not contain obvious microorganisms.

exhibits variable inflammatory reactions, erosions, and esophageal ulcers (Figs. 2.69 to 2.71). The ulcers often become quite large and are sometimes termed *giant esophageal ulcers* (127). These ulcers affect both children and adults with HIV infections and may progress to a life-threatening size, eroding vessels and limiting oral nutrition. Alternatively, one may only see focal edema coexisting with rare apoptotic cells (Fig. 2.69). The submucosa becomes densely infiltrated with neutrophils and a few mononuclear cells extend to the level of the muscularis propria (128). Ultrastructurally, one finds retrovirallike virions measuring 120 to 160 nm in diameter that contain 60- to 100-nm bar-shaped nucleoids (128) within mononuclear cells. In situ hybridization also shows HIV sequences within the mononuclear cells and sometimes in the epithelium. Ulcers measuring up to 1.5 cm in diameter develop in patients taking zidovudine (AZT) and dideoxycytidine, antiviral agents capable of inhibiting HIV replication. GERD is uncom-

mon in HIV-infected patients, perhaps because many have hypochlorhydria in late-stage disease.

Eosinophilic Esophagitis

Eosinophilic esophagitis is well recognized in children, but it may also affect adults, in whom it is underdiagnosed (129). More than 75% of cases affect males. In adults, the peak incidence is in the 3rd and 4th decades of life. Most patients have personal family histories of allergic disorders, including asthma, food allergies, or atopic dermatitis. Its pathogenesis is poorly understood, although food and aeroallergens are suspected etiologic agents (130,131). Eosinophilic esophagitis often responds to dietary elimination, elemental diets, and corticosteroids. Some speculate that antigen sensitization occurs through the respiratory tract and that when sensitized individuals subsequently swallow or ingest aeroallergens, they develop a hypersensitivity response that leads to esophageal eosinophilic infiltrates. Alternatively, the esophageal eosinophilia may reflect a response to the lung inflammation by shared communicating T cells and eosinophils in both tissues. Eosinophilic infiltrates also occur in the lungs, but not in the stomach or intestine, suggesting that there is an intimate immunologic connection between pulmonary and esophageal abnormalities. There are also substantial increases in numbers of mast cells and CD3+ T cells. Eosinophilic esophagitis may be an interleukin (IL)-5–T$_H$2 cell– and mast cell–associated disease similar to asthma (132).

Adults present clinically with progressive dysphagia, refusal of food, vomiting, and abdominal pain. Children present with refusal to eat and failure to thrive (131). Some patients develop obstructive symptoms that may lead to food impaction. Peripheral eosinophilia is often present. Many patients with eosinophilic esophagitis are referred to gastroenterologists for refractory GERD symptoms that are unresponsive to acid blockade and/or prokinetic treatment.

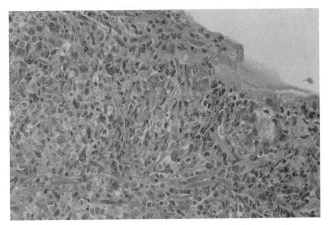

FIG. 2.70. Nonspecific ulceration with granulation tissue in an HIV-positive patient. Significant cytologic atypia is present in the stromal and endothelial cells.

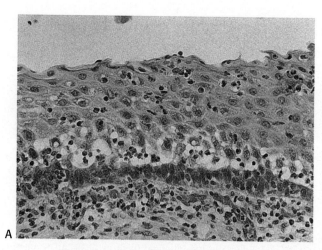
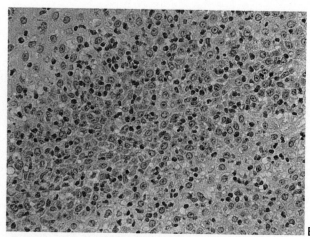

FIG. 2.72. Eosinophilic esophagitis. **A:** The mucosa is heavily infiltrated with eosinophils. They lie at all levels of the squamous epithelium and form small clusters and microabscesses. Prominent suprabasal edema is also present. **B:** Numerous eosinophils infiltrate the mucosa.

Endoscopically, the esophagus is abnormal in 91% of patients (133). Strictures are common and involve both focal as well as long-segment (small-caliber) esophagus. Corrugation, multiple esophageal rings, webs, vertical furrows, mucosal granularity, mucosal fragility white specks or exudates, and polypoid lesions (132) are other common findings. These represent inflammatory pseudomembranes containing numerous eosinophils breaking through the squamous mucosa (134). Some patients have white mucosal patches resembling *Candida* infections. The rings may also result from contraction of the fibers of the muscularis mucosae, perhaps in response to activation of acetylcholine by secretions from mast cells and eosinophils (135).

The key histologic feature is an intense eosinophilic infiltrate involving the proximal and distal esophageal squamous mucosa. Generally the eosinophil density is >20 eosinophils

per hpf (Fig. 2.72) (129). However, eosinophils can number up to 120/hpf (133). The eosinophils may show preferential clustering in both the superficial luminal portion of the mucosa as well as in the peripapillary area. Eosinophilic microabscesses frequently form and these correspond to the white specks seen at endoscopy. The eosinophilia is often accompanied by basal cell hyperplasia, edema, and papillary elongation (129).

The differential diagnosis of esophageal eosinophilic infiltrates centers around reflux esophagitis (Table 2.9), allergic esophagitis, parasitic infections, hypereosinophilic syndrome, idiopathic eosinophilic esophagitis, and eosinophilic gastroenteritis; there may be overlap among some of these entities. The histologic features help distinguish between GERD and eosinophilic esophagitis. The eosinophilia is greater in eosinophilic esophagitis than in GERD, with the eosinophil density usually exceeding 20 eosinophils per hpf. In contrast,

TABLE 2.9	Features Distinguishing Eosinophilic Esophagitis and Gastroesophageal Reflux Disease (GERD)	
Typical Features	**Eosinophilic Esophagitis**	**GERD**
Clinical		
Presence of atopy	Very common	Normal (possibly increased)
Sex preference	Male	Male
Abdominal pain, vomiting	Common	Common
Food impaction	Common	Uncommon
Endoscopic Findings		
Endoscopic furrowing	Very common	Occasionally
pH probe	Usually normal	Abnormal
Histologic Features		
Proximal involvement	Yes	No
Distal involvement	Yes	Yes
Epithelial hyperplasia	Yes	Yes
Number of eosinophils	>20–24/hpf	0–7/hpf

the eosinophil density in GERD is usually less than five eosinophils per hpf. Further, superficial layering of the eosinophils and/or superficial eosinophilic microabscesses (greater than four eosinophils in a cluster) is a hallmark of eosinophilic esophagitis and are unusual in GERD. Cases with deeper eosinophilic infiltrates may represent esophageal manifestations of a more generalized eosinophilic gastroenteritis, whereas those with only mucosal disease may represent pure eosinophilic esophagitis. Thus, in some patients, eosinophilic esophagitis may represent one end of the eosinophilic gastroenteritis spectrum with eosinophilia elsewhere in the gastrointestinal tract and peripheral eosinophilia.

Thermal Injury

Thermal injury follows consumption of boiling hot liquids or microwaved food due to the uneven heat distribution in the latter. Endoscopically, patients show bands of thin, white, densely adherent pseudomembranes alternating with bands of pink mucosa creating a candy-cane appearance that extends from the upper esophagus to the SCJ. Histologically, the mucosa is characterized by superficial mummified layers of gangrenous necrosis with anucleated, nonviable, squamous epithelium firmly adherent to the viable underlying squamous epithelial cells. The absence of inflammation suggests the diagnosis and differs from the inflammatory reactions seen in infectious or reflux esophagitis. The most important complications of thermal injury are seen in those who drink maté, a risk factor for the development of esophageal squamous cell carcinoma (see Chapter 3).

Radiation Esophagitis

Patients receiving radiation therapy for cancers of the lung, head and neck, esophagus, mediastinum, or vertebral column may develop radiation esophagitis. The extent of the injury is influenced by the type of radiotherapy; its dose; time course of administration; tissue sensitivity; use of other therapies, particularly radiosensitizing chemotherapy; and various patient-related factors (136,137). Injuries seldom occur at doses below 4,200 to 4,500 cGy. One hundred percent of patients with 6,000 rads to the esophagus develop esophagitis. Four periods of radiation-induced tissue damage include the *acute period* (first 6 months following treatment), the *subacute period* (second 6 months), the *chronic period* (2 to 5 years following radiation), and the *late period* (after 5 years).

The spectrum of injury ranges from acute self-limited esophagitis to life-threatening esophageal perforation. Patients with radiation esophagitis present with dysphagia, odynophagia, or dysmotility. Symptoms are common during initial radiation damage. The symptoms mimic those of peptic esophagitis, opportunistic infections, or drug-induced mucositis. *Esophageal strictures and webs* develop following large radiation doses (Fig. 2.73), typically between 13 and 21 months after the initiation of therapy. The length of the strictures depends on the size of the radiation field. It is important to distinguish radiation ulcers or strictures from cancer.

Acute radiation esophagitis involves any part of the esophagus. Patients present with multiple small discrete ulcers or they have a distinctive granular mucosa. Esophageal narrowing and thickening of esophageal folds also occurs. Severe

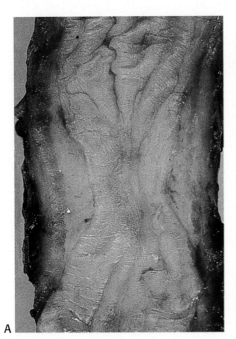
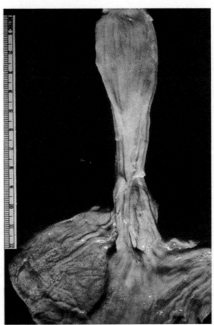

A   B

FIG. 2.73. Strictures following radiation therapy. **A:** Esophageal stricture that narrowed the mucosa. The radiotherapy was given for esophageal carcinoma. Note that the mucosa retracts into an hourglass shape over the underlying submucosal tissues. **B:** More advanced stricture following radiation for esophageal carcinoma. It almost completely blocks the lumen. The proximal esophagus has become dilated.

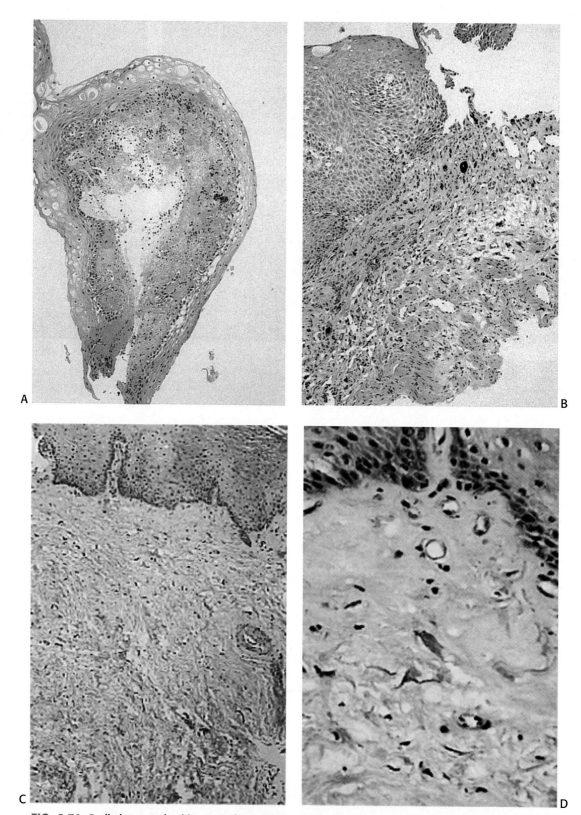

FIG. 2.74. Radiation esophagitis. **A:** Early esophageal damage demonstrating ballooning degeneration, edema, and acute and chronic inflammation. **B:** Higher magnification demonstrating the edge of an ulcer with prominent radiation fibroblasts. **C:** The lamina propria appears fibrotic and the vessels are hyalinized. **D:** Irregular stellate fibroblasts are present in the hyalinized tissue.

esophagitis, stricture formation, and rare fistulas develop in patients treated with both chemotherapy and radiation therapy. Motility abnormalities result from secondary neuronal damage. Late complications include primary esophageal cancer, which may develop many years after irradiation.

The different layers of the esophageal wall vary in their radiosensitivity. The squamous epithelium and the vasculature are the most radiosensitive. The muscularis propria and fibrous connective tissue are relatively radioresistant. Acute radiation esophagitis is characterized by basal cell necrosis, submucosal edema, capillary dilation, and endothelial swelling (Fig. 2.74). About 2 weeks after the initial dose, superficial erosions form. These may coalesce to form larger superficial ulcers. Prominent epithelial and endothelial cells lie in the edematous granulation tissue. Pseudomembranes may form. Occasional patients develop multinucleated epithelial giant cells that suggest a viral infection. Bizarre (radiation) fibroblasts suggest the diagnosis (Fig. 2.74). The regenerating epithelium may mimic dysplasia (138). Epithelial hyperplasia develops in an effort to re-epithelialize the mucosal surface. These changes resolve within 3 to 4 weeks following the last radiation dose (136). Deeper ulcers and esophageal fistulas develop during the subacute phase. The ulcers may become quite large, measuring up to 5 cm in diameter. They may also perforate into adjacent structures, possibly causing hemorrhage (139). Clues to the diagnosis at this stage include the presence of vascular changes and radiation fibroblasts. Mucosal bridges may develop. Histologically, they contain normal epithelium overlying the chronically inflamed lamina propria. These represent late sequelae of radiation esophagitis.

Most typically one sees radiation injury in its late stages. The epithelium shows nonspecific changes, including acanthosis, hyperkeratosis, and parakeratosis. The muscularis mucosae may appear normal or fibrotic. The submucosa commonly becomes fibrotic; frank areas of scarring or strictures may develop. The submucosal glands become atrophic and the acini disappear. Occasionally, the ducts contain inspissated secretions producing a lesion similar to intramural pseudodiverticulosis. Hyalinized blood vessels, submucosal fibrosis, and muscular degeneration are also present. Telangiectatic capillaries and thick-walled hyalinized arterioles sometimes showing foam cells are present in the submucosa (Fig. 2.75). The endothelial cells appear enlarged and bizarre. Chronic ulcers develop and may have granulation tissue at their base. Hemosiderin deposits follow previous hemorrhage from ischemia due to the arterial occlusion. Chronic arteriolitis may result in transmural ischemia, perforation, or fistula formation. Esophageal strictures demonstrate marked thickening of the esophageal wall and submucosal expansion.

Caustic Esophagitis

Caustic esophagitis results from ingestion of strong alkalis or acids usually following suicide attempts in adults or acciden-

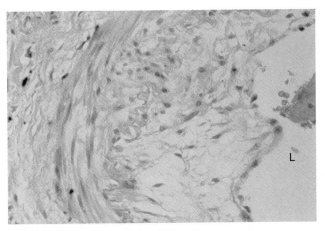

FIG. 2.75. The vessels develop foamy degeneration of the intima and media. *L*, vascular lumen.

tal ingestions in children. Commonly ingested agents include lye, sodium carbonate, ammonium hydroxide, and bleaches. Drain cleaners (NaOH), decalcifiers (formic acid), and detergents for automatic dishwashing machines (metasilicates) are also very caustic and responsible for the serious accidents in children. The extent of the injury depends on the type and amount of the ingested agent, its concentration, physical state, and exposure duration (140,141). The most severe injury occurs in areas of esophageal luminal narrowing. Severe, corrosive esophagitis leads to esophageal hemorrhage, perforation, and death. Liquids tend to produce extensive geographically continuous erosive esophagitis, whereas granular agents produce more localized lesions. Alkalis damage the esophagus more severely than acids because alkalis penetrate the tissue (142). A pH of 12.5 is the critical boundary for the ability to generate injury. Deep ulcers and strictures complicate injury caused by substances with a pH over 13. Alkalis produce liquefaction necrosis with intense inflammation and saponification of the mucosa, submucosa, and muscularis propria (142). Vascular thrombosis leads to ischemic necrosis followed by bacterial or fungal colonization. The superficial necrotic layers slough 2 to 4 days following the injury, sometimes creating deep ulcers with underlying granulation tissue (Fig. 2.76). Complete separation of the squamous mucosa results in the formation of a mucosal cast, which the patient vomits up in a situation referred to as "esophagitis desiccans superficialis" (143). Other changes include swelling and hemorrhage, inflammatory exudates, and ulcers. The overlying surface appears normal, inflamed, ulcerated, hypertrophic, or atrophic, depending on when one examines the tissues in relation to the acute event and whether recurrent damage has occurred. The cytologic features of the cells usually appear normal without much reactive atypia. Corrosive burns can be graded as shown in Table 2.10. If the patient survives, the mucosal re-epithelialization and fibrosis occur. Caustics cause coagulative necrosis (Fig. 2.77) that produces a firm protective eschar, which delays injury and limits acid penetration (144).

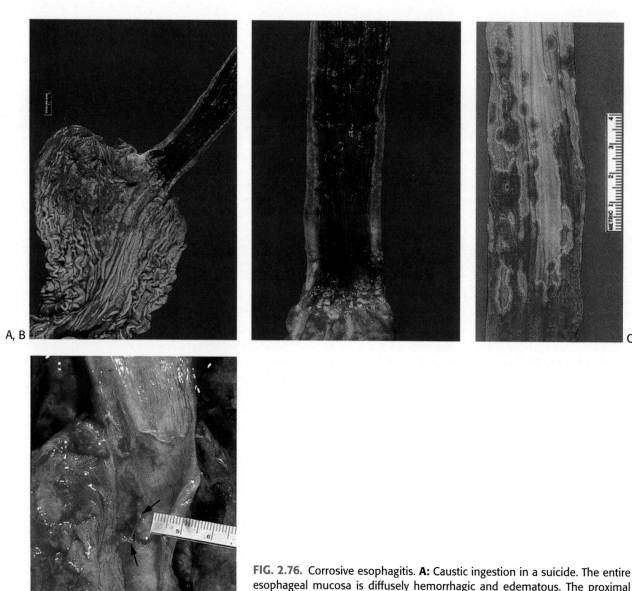

FIG. 2.76. Corrosive esophagitis. **A:** Caustic ingestion in a suicide. The entire esophageal mucosa is diffusely hemorrhagic and edematous. The proximal stomach also shows an erosive gastritis. **B:** Higher magnification demonstrating the hyperemia, congestion, and mucosal ulceration. The esophageal wall also appears thickened and edematous. **C:** Esophagus in young girl who had ingested arsenic-containing rat poison in a suicide. Multiple acute ulcers and erosions are present. **D:** Esophageal perforation following lye ingestion (*arrows*).

Strictures, especially focal ones, must be distinguished from carcinomas, since carcinomas may develop at these sites. Strictures demonstrate dense, uniform mucosal and submucosal fibrosis throughout the involved esophagus. One of the most effective ways of evaluating strictures is to perform endoscopic brushings of the surface of the stricture, since the densely fibrotic scar tissue may be exceedingly difficult to biopsy. Longstanding focal strictures cause dilation and hypertrophy of the proximal esophagus. Esophagobronchial fistula represents a late complication. Other long-term sequelae include motility disorders, GERD, BE, and carcinomas; the latter have a latent period of 12 to 40 years (145).

Drug-Related Esophagitis

The incidence of drug-induced esophagitis is unknown because many cases go unrecognized. It is estimated to affect 3.9 people per 100,000 population per year. Elderly patients are particularly at risk for developing drug injury for at least four reasons: They take more medications, they are more likely to have altered esophageal motility, saliva production decreases with age, and they spend more time in a recumbent position. Drugs commonly associated with esophageal injury are listed in Table 2.11. The remaining 10% result from a long list of other drugs, often described in single case

TABLE 2.10   Grading of Corrosive Esophageal and Gastric Burns

Grade	Pathologic Involvement
First degree	Superficial involvement of the mucosa
Second degree	Transmucosal involvement with or without involvement of the submucosa No extension into periesophageal or perigastric tissue
Third degree	Full-thickness injuries with extension into periesophageal or perigastric tissue Mediastinal or intraperitoneal organs may be involved

TABLE 2.11   Drugs Most Commonly Associated with Esophageal Injury

Antibiotics (Doxy-tetracycline, clindamycin, Bactrim)
Nonsteroidal anti-inflammatory drugs
Ferrous sulfate
Potassium chloride (slow release)
Ascorbic acid
Zidovudine (AZT)
Theophylline
Quinidine
Gluconate
Alendronate (Fosamax)
Empromium bromide (not available in the United States)

reports. The effects of the various drugs may be additive if combined. For example, bisphosphonates taken together with nonsteroidal anti-inflammatory drugs (NSAIDs) increase the risk of gastrointestinal injury.

Drug-induced injury results from three mechanisms: (a) a normal side effect of the pharmacologic action of the drug, (b) a complication of the therapeutic action of the drug, or (c) pill esophagitis (see below). Complications of therapeutic actions of drugs include viral or fungal esophagitis in patients treated with immunosuppressives, chemotherapeutic agents, or antibiotics, and immunologic reactions to certain drugs causing disorders such as Stevens-Johnson syndrome. Properties of drugs that cause esophageal injury include their chemical nature (acidity or alkalinity), their solubility, and their mucosal contact time. Many drugs cause damage because they are acidic in solution (iron salts, tetracycline, doxycycline, aspirin); others produce alkaline solutions (phenytoin). The effects of acidic drugs are made worse by acid reflux. Some drugs lower LES pressure, thereby predisposing to reflux esophagitis. Any condition that delays esophageal passage increases the risk of drug-induced damage. These include motility disorders, hiatal hernias, strictures, webs, and rings; taking pills while in a recumbent position; taking medication with small amounts of liquids; or extraneous structural abnormalities (cardiac enlargement, nodal disease, or enlarged thyroids). If drugs get stuck in the esophagus, there is prolonged mucosal contact with a high concentration of a toxic substance leading to local topical damage. These act as foreign bodies impacting in the esophageal lumen, especially if taken with minimal liquid. As the medication dissolves, localized esophageal damage, ranging from inflammation to severe hemorrhage and even perforation, develops (146).

The clinical features of drug injury reflect patient age, comorbidities, and the nature of the drug. The most common clinical symptoms are retrosternal pain and/or odynophagia. Severe complications include massive bleeding, perforation, and death. Strictures complicate ingestion of iron, NSAIDs, potassium salts, quinidine, and alprenolol (147). Chemotherapy-induced vomiting leads to Mallory-Weiss tears, intramural hematomas, and esophageal perforation.

The most common gross abnormalities are ulcers ranging in size from pinpoint aphthous ulcers to large (up to 10 cm) circumferential ulcers. These tend to involve the mid- to distal esophagus. Most ulcers remain superficial and heal readily, except for those associated with potassium chloride, which may be deep or even perforate. NSAIDs also induce large, shallow, discrete midesophageal ulcers with a normal surrounding mucosa. Patients taking bisphosphonates develop confluent erosions or multiple deep, large ulcers in the distal esophagus. Endoscopically, the ulcers sometimes contain pills within them. Charcoal deposits complicate administration of activated charcoal as a therapy for overdoses in patients who have attempted suicides. They appear as black linear lesions in the distal esophagus and stomach.

There are no characteristic pathologic findings for drug-induced esophagitis since different drugs damage the esophagus via different mechanisms. The histologic features of the ulcers are nonspecific and vary depending on the age of the lesion. If one is lucky, one may see pill residue in the form of crystals (bisphosphonates or iron) on the surface or admixed

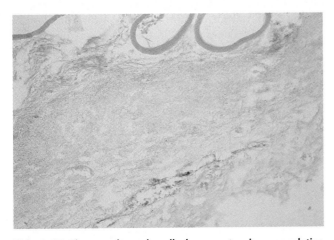

FIG. 2.77. The esophageal wall shows extensive coagulative necrosis without inflammation.

with an inflammatory exudate or a discolored mucosa (iron pills and Lugol). Apoptotic changes may be present as may mucosal eosinophilia. Enteric-coated potassium chloride tablets cause edema, ballooning degeneration, hemorrhagic erosions, and strictures. Tetracycline may cause marked spongiotic esophagitis (148). Allergic drug-induced esophagitis may associate with numerous degranulating eosinophils. Chemotherapeutic agents directly damage replicating cells, leading to mucositis (acute inflammation of the mucosa), ulcers, erosions, strictures, and fistulas. Early changes include increased numbers of apoptotic bodies in the basal mucosa. This is followed by a nonspecific esophagitis with or without ulcers. Basal cell hyperplasia, nuclear atypia, and numerous mitoses, some of which may appear atypical, characterize recovery from chemotherapeutic agents. The atypia affects both the epithelium and the mesenchymal cells, and the nuclear:cytoplasmic ratio is usually low, providing a clue to the fact that the lesion does not represent dysplasia or carcinoma. Taxol can be associated with striking mitotic arrest associated with necrosis and ulceration. The mitotic arrest associates with bundling of intermediate filaments secondary to the accumulation of polymerized microtubules causing ring-shaped mitoses. Vincristine causes myenteric plexus damage and pseudo-obstruction syndromes. Bisphosphonates cause an ulcerative and erosive esophagitis along with multinucleated giant epithelial cells simulating viral cytopathic effects. Excessive intake of vitamin E may lead to esophageal cornification and produce a histologic pattern similar to that seen in vitamin A–deficient individuals (149). Charcoal deposits appear as aggregates of coarse, black, foreign material in the underlying submucosal tissues where they can persist for decades. The esophagus may exhibit striking findings in colchicine toxicity where the basal layers show numerous mitotic figures and mitotic arrest (150).

Esophagitis in Otherwise Healthy Newborns

A very severe form of esophagitis characterized by the presence of circular esophageal ulcerations without evidence of accompanying gastroenteritis affects newborns. The lesions generally disappear within 48 to 72 hours after diagnosis with a very rapid clinical and histologic recovery. The etiology remains obscure, but the distribution of the lesions (more severe in the upper esophagus), their early onset (almost at birth), the very rapid healing, and the absence of gastric or intestinal lesions suggest a possible traumatic origin, perhaps from perinatal pharyngeal, esophageal, and/or gastric suction (151).

BARRETT ESOPHAGUS

Definitions

The old definition of BE included any columnar epithelium (gastric, cardiac, oxyntic, or intestinal) lining the distal esophagus. The current definition requires that both endo-scopic and histologic criteria be met. The endoscopic component requires the presence of columnar mucosa identified endoscopically by its salmon pink color, extending proximally from the GEJ into the tubular esophagus. The histologic component requires that biopsies taken from the endoscopically identified columnar pink mucosa contain metaplastic or intestinalized columnar epithelium with goblet cells (152). The reason for this approach is a practical one: Dysplasia and carcinoma virtually never develop in any columnar epithelium other than in an intestinal metaplastic one. BE is generally divided into long-segment BE (LSBE), in which the columnar mucosa extends 3 cm or more above the GEJ, and short-segment BE (SSBE), in which the specialized columnar epithelium is restricted to <2 to 3 cm above the GEJ (153).

Prevalence/Incidence

Like GERD, BE demonstrates geographic, temporal, and ethnic incidence differences. BE affects approximately 1.6% of the patient population (154). Its prevalence is approximately 9% in the elderly. However, BE was found in 25% of the asymptomatic male veterans over the age of 50 who underwent an upper endoscopy at the same time that they had a screening sigmoidoscopy (155). Most patients who seek medical help usually have underlying severe symptomatic GERD associated with esophageal ulcers, strictures, and hemorrhage. BE develops in up to 44% of patients with reflux esophagitis (153,156). It demonstrates a bimodal age distribution with one peak at 0 to 15 years and another at 40 to 80 years (153,157,158). BE preferentially affects white males; it is uncommon in blacks. The male:female ratio is 4:1 (153). Patients with complications of BE are usually older. Although BE is rare in Orientals, its incidence is increasing, perhaps due to westernization of the diet and rapid growth of an elderly and obese population (76). Familial cases also exist. These may result from either a familial genetic predisposition to BE or to common conditions associated with reflux. BE may also complicate chemotherapy (159) or lye ingestion (160). There is also an increased prevalence of BE in patients with celiac disease (161). The prevalence of BE in the asymptomatic population is probably much higher than might be expected from data based on endoscopic examinations of symptomatic patients. An autopsy study in Olmstead County, Minnesota, found BE in 7 of 733 (1%) cases. When adjusted for age and sex to correspond to the U.S. population, the true prevalence was 376 per 100,000 population, or 17 times that of the 27 cases per 100,000 diagnosed endoscopically during the study period (162).

Pathogenesis

BE is an acquired metaplastic change that results from long-standing GERD. It results from a combination of substances in the refluxate including acid, bile salts, lysophospholipids, and activated pancreatic enzymes. The interaction of these substances ultimately determines the degree of damage, repair, transformation, and eventual maturation of the clinical phenotype including esophagitis, BE, stricture, dysplasia, or carcinoma. In this abnormal milieu, multipotential immature stem cells differentiate into various epithelial types, including columnar epithelium, which is more resistant to acidic digestion and which is able to regenerate more rapidly than the native squamous epithelium (163,164). Once established, BE is a highly proliferative mucosa (165).

The development of BE is a multistep process with at least three distinct phases. During the *initiation phase,* genetically predisposed individuals (mostly white men) suffering from GERD develop reflux esophagitis. This leads to the formation of a metaplastic epithelium with features of intestinal columnar epithelium. The metaplastic columnar cells of BE could derive from three sources (166): (a) metaplasia of squamous epithelium, similar to that seen with vaginal mucinosis; (b) from the mixed squamous/columnar cell population at the transitional zone, as seen in cervical metaplasia; or (c) from the columnar cells of the esophageal glands, such as may be associated with ulcer repair. Circulating bone marrow–derived stem cells (BDSCs) have been proposed to be the source of metaplastic cells in the stomach in response to *HP* gastritis (167). Recruitment of BDSCs in response to reflux-induced inflammation might serve as another potential source of BE.

During the *formation stage,* the metaplastic epithelium, which continues to be exposed to the refluxate, establishes its presence and occupies a variable surface area of the distal esophagus. This results in the oral migration of the SCJ over time (168). A long and multifaceted *progression phase* follows, during which the metaplastic epithelium either remains dormant and clinically insignificant or progresses to dysplasia and eventually invasive adenocarcinoma. (The progression to dysplasia and invasive carcinoma is discussed in depth in Chapter 3.)

This multistep progression involves transient and permanent molecular alterations in the esophageal squamous cells or in the BE epithelium. These are under the influence of numerous factors and signal transduction cascades (169) that can be influenced by both host and environmental factors. It is not known why only a fraction of GERD patients develop BE or which host factors or combination factors in the refluxate lead to metaplasia. Prolonged acid exposure increases villin expression and correlates with the appearance of microvilli. Another factor important in intestinal differentiation is CDX2, a transcription factor that belongs to the caudal-related homeobox gene family (170). Its expression in the GI tract is intestine specific with a tightly regulated boundary in the duodenum (171).

Bile acids act as tumor promoters increasing cell proliferation. Activation of the CCK2 receptor may stimulate cell proliferation. It induces numerous humoral mediators, including EGF ligands (transforming growth factor-α [TGF-α], heparin-binding epidermal factorlike growth factor, and the trefoil peptide TFF1) (172–174) and growth of the BE, especially in patients treated with acid-suppressive therapies in whom gastrin levels may be increased (175). Gastrin also induces cyclooxygenase, which plays a role in the inhibition of apoptosis, promotion of cell proliferation, invasion of malignant cells, and promotion of angiogenesis (176). Another factor that plays a role in the proliferation of BE is activation of mitogen-activated protein kinase (MAPK) activities due to acid exposure (169). Activation of the MAPK pathways increases cell survival and decreases apoptosis (169). The molecular markers are discussed further in Chapter 3.

Gross and Endoscopic Features

BE appears beefy red and velvety, contrasting with the lighter pink-tan colored, smooth squamous mucosa. The SCJ often lies within 30 cm of the incisor teeth, and often coexists with a hiatal hernia, strictures, diffuse esophagitis, or esophageal ulcers. Grossly, there are several distinct patterns of BE: Circumferential, islands, and fingerlike projections or tongues (Fig. 2.78). The island type accompanies less severe epithelial injury than the circumferential type and probably represents an earlier stage, which then progresses to the circumferential lesion (177). Sometimes it is difficult to distinguish the distal border of the metaplastic epithelium from the adjacent gastric mucosa with which it may appear to merge. Locating the gastric folds helps delineate the beginning of the stomach. Patients with SSBE have short tongues or patches of red mucosa lying <2 cm above the GEJ.

Since it may be difficult to endoscopically distinguish areas of intestinal metaplasia from other columnar epithelium, various additional endoscopic approaches may be used to evaluate the mucosa. These include magnification endoscopy, endoscopic optical coherence tomography, chromoendoscopy, endoscopic confocal imaging, light-scattering spectroscopy, and in vivo fluorescence endomicroscopy. These advanced imaging methods may enable the endoscopist to detect intestinal metaplasia in a background of gastric epithelium; to detect foci of dysplasia and early neoplasia in a background of intestinal metaplasia; and to distinguish early invasive carcinoma from mucosal dysplasia (178,179).

Typically the endoscopist biopsies the following areas: The stomach just distal to the upper end of the gastric folds, particularly along the lesser curvature; 1 to 2 cm above the GEJ; tongues of mucosa or irregular areas above the SCJ; and the SCJ and squamous epithelium of the native esophagus. Biopsies at the upper end of the gastric folds may allow one to determine whether there is gastritis, particularly *HP*-induced gastritis and possibly intestinal metaplasia. This biopsy may be within a hiatal hernia. These biopsies can detect localized carditis, localized intestinal metaplasia, reactive changes, acute inflammation, and possibly eosinophils in the squamous mucosa.

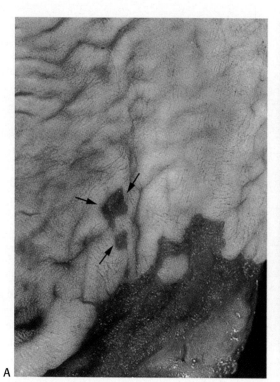 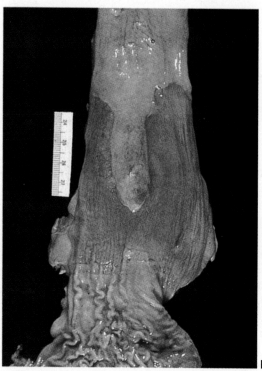

FIG. 2.78. Barrett esophagus. **A:** Islands of red-brown Barrett epithelium surrounded by white-gray squamous mucosa (*arrows*). **B:** Circumferential Barrett esophagus. In contrast to the island-type Barrett esophagus, the circumferential type completely surrounds the esophageal mucosa, although there may be tongues of squamous epithelium extending into it.

Histology of Barrett Esophagus

There are two major problems in the pathologic evaluation of patients with BE: Overdiagnosis of BE and overdiagnosis of dysplasia in the setting of BE. The diagnosis of BE is covered here. The diagnosis of dysplasia and its mimics is discussed in Chapter 3. The histology of the columnar-lined esophagus displays heterogeneous histologic features with respect to the types of glandular mucosa that are present and the surface architecture. As noted earlier, the definition of BE requires histologic confirmation of intestinal metaplasia in biopsies taken from the columnar regions of the esophagus (152). The metaplastic BE epithelium resembles either small intestinal absorptive cells (complete intestinal metaplasia) or incomplete intestinal metaplasia (resembling colonic epithelium). In the latter, the cells lack a distinct brush border and the associated enzymes that normally characterize small intestinal absorptive cells. There is debate over whether incomplete metaplasia poses a higher risk than the complete type, but since both types confer a neoplastic risk, subtyping is not indicated. If any goblet cells are seen, one can make the diagnosis of BE when the biopsy derives from the esophagus (Figs. 2.79 and 2.80).

Examination of multiple biopsies and multiple levels helps identify this patchy process. The epithelium covering the mucosal surface and pits commonly contains a mixture of gastric foveolar cells and intestinal cells (Fig. 2.79). The latter include goblet cells, intestinal columnar cells, endocrine cells

(containing serotonin, somatostatin, calcitonin, pancreatic polypeptide, and secretin) (180,181), and sometimes Paneth cells. The majority of the intestinal columnar cells are so-called intermediate, principal, or pseudoabsorptive cells that have characteristics of both absorptive and secretory cells. A villiform architecture may be present on the surface. *H. pylori* may be found in the esophagus of some patients with BE but only when it is also present in the stomach. It may contribute to the severity of the inflammation seen in BE.

Goblet cells are usually readily identifiable in H&E-stained sections by their round supranuclear mucin accumulation (Figs. 2.79 and 2.80). While goblet cells contain acidic mucin that stains intensely blue with Alcian blue staining at pH 2.5, routine Alcian blue staining is usually not necessary (181a). Alcian blue–positive cells are also found in normal esophageal submucosal glands and their ducts. These submucosal glands are readily distinguished from BE because of their rounded, grouped lobular configuration and their resemblance to minor salivary glands as well as by their diffuse positivity for Alcian blue at pH 2.5. The entire esophageal glandular lobules stain intensely contrasting with the individually scattered intensely positive goblet cells typical of BE.

Careful histologic attention should be paid to potential BE mimics, particularly pseudogoblet cells. These columnar cells are hyperdistended gastric foveolar cells. They contain a mucinous droplet that is larger than the typical foveolar cell

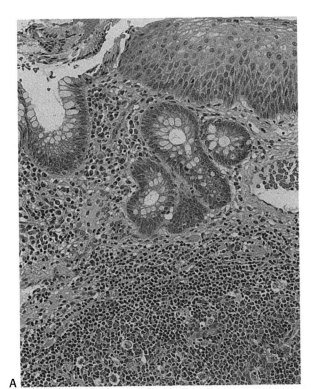
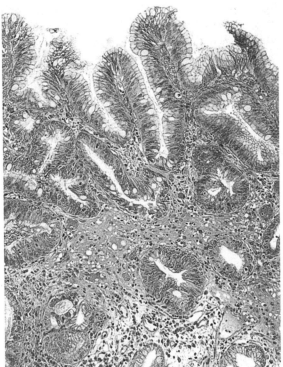

FIG. 2.79. Barrett esophagus. **A:** Specialized intestinal epithelium. Squamous epithelium at the surface merges with specialized epithelium as evidenced by the presence of goblet cells. A couple of intestinalized-type specialized epithelial glands are also present underlying the squamous epithelium. Prominent lymphoid aggregates containing both mature lymphocytes and histiocytes are present. **B:** Villous transformation in an area of specialized Barrett epithelium. Goblet cells intermingle with gastric foveolar cells.

but smaller than the usual goblet cell. They occur in the surface epithelium at the GEJ and distal esophagus. They may occur in the presence or absence of true goblet cells. The cells stain positively with Alcian blue at a pH 2.5; for this reason they are sometimes referred to as the "columnar blues" (Fig. 2.81). However, the pseudogoblet cells stain less intensely than true goblet cells. *If only Alcian blue–positive columnar cells are present in the absence of true goblet cells, the diagnosis of BE should not be made.* Because of the lack of specificity of Alcian blue staining for true goblet cells, there has been interest in finding a more specific marker of intestinal goblet cells. Markers of interest have included stains for sulphomucins and sialomucins. Sulphomucin expression is

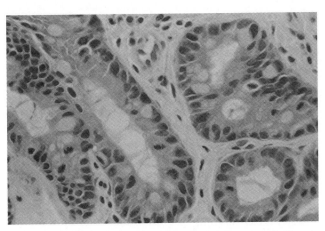

FIG. 2.80. Barrett esophagus. Only intestinal-type epithelium is present in this figure. There are several mitoses present.

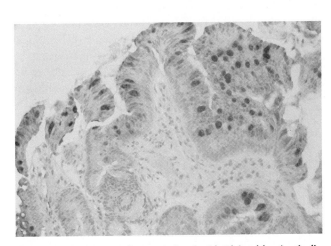

FIG. 2.81. Barrett esophagus stained with Alcian blue/periodic acid–Schiff at pH 2.5. Note that the goblet cells stain strongly blue and have a large distended mucous droplet. These cells contrast with the "columnar blues," which stain much less intensely and do not have the prominent mucinous droplet.

less sensitive (sensitivity 62%) but more specific (specificity 90%) for the presence of true goblet cells. However, sialomucins or sulphomucins can also be present in the surface epithelium of a small percentage of patients without goblet cells (182), contradicting the commonly held belief that gastric-type surface epithelial cells only contain neutral-type mucins. Another promising marker is MUC2, which may be specific for intestinal metaplasia in BE (183).

Of note, the muscularis mucosae is hyperplastic in the distal esophagus and in some areas collagen-rich fibrous tissue replaces the muscularis mucosae. An understanding of these features is important in two situations: The first is the correct interpretation of alterations that may affect the submucosal glands, and the second is in the correct staging of invasive malignancies (discussed in Chapter 3). The fibroblastic or muscular abnormalities may deform the ducts of the submucosal glands, causing the glands to dilate. The combination of irregular ductal compression in the presence of atypical epithelial cells lying in the fibrous tissue can cause difficulty in differentiating normal or dysplastic esophageal glands trapped in the collagen-rich fibrotic tissue from invasive cancer (184). Immunostaining the section may be helpful, especially if one can demonstrate the normal two-cell population of the submucosal glands.

Pathologic Features of Short-Segment Barrett Esophagus and Intestinal Metaplasia of the Cardia

Intestinal metaplasia at the GEJ is either SSBE, which has a cancer risk at most of 0.5% per year, or intestinal metaplasia of the proximal stomach, which appears to have a substantially smaller risk for malignancy (20). These two conditions cannot be distinguished reliably because the morphologic and histochemical features of gastric and esophageal intestinal metaplasia resemble one another and because the gross landmarks used to identify the GEJ do not have the precision necessary to localize a mucosa, whose extent may be measured only in millimeters. The significance of intestinal metaplasia in the cardia is currently unknown but it can be found in up to 25% of individuals without evidence of BE (153). Therefore, it is uncertain whether it reflects GERD or not. Recent immunohistochemical data show similar phenotypes in LSBE and SSBE and intestinal metaplasia at the GEJ, and a different phenotype from gastric antral intestinal metaplasia (185), suggesting that both LSBE and SSBE are related disorders and that they differ from the intestinal metaplasia resulting from *HP* infections. Intestinal metaplasia is relatively uncommon in North America as compared to other parts of the world so that the presence of intestinal metaplasia in the area of the cardia most likely represents GERD. This may be particularly true in white men, since this is the dominant demographic group that develops BE-associated carcinomas.

SSBE and endoscopically unsuspected intestinal metaplasia are far more common than LSBE; therefore, SSBE may represent the lesion in which most cancers develop (186). The risk of developing adenocarcinoma in these short intestinalized segments is unclear. Presumably, if intestinal metaplasia is found, the patient is at risk for neoplasia. The incidence of adenocarcinoma of both the esophagus and gastric cardia has increased at a rate far exceeding that of any other cancer, and short segments of intestinal metaplasia at the GEJ may underlie this phenomenon. Forty-two percent of all esophageal adenocarcinomas associate with SSBE because SSBE is more common than LSBE (187).

Rather than dealing with whether or not intestinal metaplasia at the GEJ represents BE or not, perhaps the more important questions are: Is the biopsy abnormal? Is it associated with GERD? Does it predispose to adenocarcinoma (153)? Intestinal metaplasia on either side of the GE junction is abnormal. Several approaches can be used practically. One approach utilizes three categories: (a) columnar-lined esophagus with specialized intestinal metaplasia, (b) columnar-lined esophagus without specialized intestinal metaplasia, and (c) specialized intestinal metaplasia at the GEJ (188). Using this classification, an association with adenocarcinoma is seen in columnar-lined esophagus with specialized epithelium and probably associated with specialized metaplasia at the GEJ. When using these three categories, it is unclear whether or not the specialized intestinal metaplasia at the GE junction represents an association with GERD (188). An alternative approach would be to consider any form of metaplasia detected in a biopsy regardless of where it comes from as a marker of a cell population at risk for transformation into a dysplastic cell population and therefore at least potentially able to become malignant. For patients found to have intestinal metaplasia at the GEJ, a conservative approach is to assume a worst-case scenario in which the condition is SSBE and to manage the patients according to guidelines established for Barrett esophagus (153). One could use the term *intestinal metaplasia of the GEJ* to describe the intestinal metaplasia found at the Z line (153). Once histologically confirmed, the presence of BE may serve as a marker for future cancer surveillance.

Immunohistochemical/Molecular Features of Barrett Esophagus

Cytokeratin staining (CK7/CK 20) has been proposed as a way to distinguish intestinal metaplasia of the cardia from SSBE (189,190). Specialized intestinal metaplasia of BE frequently exhibits strong immunoreactivity for CK7 in its superficial and deep glands and immunoreactivity for CK20 in the superficial glands and superficial epithelial cells (189,190). In contrast, intestinal metaplasia in the gastric body infrequently shows the so-called "Barrett CK7/20" pattern. However, BE and SSBE show marked variability in the cytokeratin staining patterns, resulting in a poor sensitivity and specificity (191,192).

Other markers that have been examined include reactivity with the antibody Das-1 (a monoclonal antibody raised

TABLE 2.12	MUC Gene Expression
MUC1	Intestinal goblet cells and enterocytes
MUC2	Intestinal goblet cells
MUC3	Intestinal enterocytes
MUC5AC	Gastric foveolar and mucous neck cells
MUC6	Gastric, antral, and fundic epithelium

against colonic epithelial cells) (185) and expression of colonic-type mucins such as MUC2 (193), CDX2 (194) villin, sucrase isomaltase (195), intestinal-type alkaline phosphatase (196), and dipeptidyl peptidase IV. At least 12 MUC genes, (MUC1 to 12), have been identified, each of which encodes a specific mucin core polypeptide (197) that is differentially expressed in different portions of the normal gut (Table 2.12). A recent study using gene expression arrays suggest that BE is an incompletely differentiated epithelium with similarities to both gastric and squamous epithelium. In addition, there are several uniquely expressed genes (198). However, a criticism of this study is that the epithelia were not microdissected and as noted earlier, Barrett mucosa contains heterogeneous cell populations. At present writing, it does not appear that specific biomarkers can distinguish SSBE from intestinal metaplasia of the gastric (199).

Squamous Metaplasia in the Distal Esophagus

Squamous metaplasia develops in the distal esophagus following treatment of BE. It appears as a normal-appearing neosquamous epithelium or as a multilayered immature squamous metaplasia. The neosquamous epithelium appears in areas previously occupied by BE, often appearing as squamous islands surrounding the Barrett epithelium. These squamous cells largely arise from a progenitor cell that differs from the cells responsible for self-renewal of the Barrett epithelium, although occasionally it arises from a stem cell that gives rise to either the squamous cells or the Barrett epithelium (199a).

Squamous metaplasia resembling that seen in the uterine cervix develops at the GEJ in patients with BE (200). It usually appears as a pseudostratified epithelium; cilia are often present on the luminal surface (201). The epithelium has morphologic and cytochemical characteristics of both squamous and columnar epithelium and may be a precursor of BE (200). It is possible that a multipotent stem cell is stimulated to differentiate toward a columnar phenotype after passing through an intermediate multiepithelial-layered phase.

Multilayered epithelium typically consists of four to eight cell layers (Fig. 2.82). The basal cells contain a small round to oval nucleus with a small centrally placed nucleolus and abundant eosinophilic cytoplasm, features similar to those of normal basal or suprabasal esophageal squamous cells. Nuclear pseudostratification is common. Intercellular bridges are absent. The suprabasal and superficial layers of the multilayered epithelium show increasing degrees of columnar

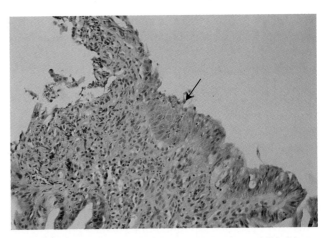

FIG. 2.82. Multilayered epithelium. The surface of this biopsy from the gastroesophageal junction shows columnar epithelium on the right side of the figure. The area underlying the *arrow* is an example of the multilayered epithelium.

differentiation characterized by cells with clear or slightly bubbly cytoplasm and a basally oriented nucleus having an appearance like that of basal cells. Most cases contain rare superficial columnar cells with distended cytoplasm similar in appearance to goblet cells. The epithelium expresses cytokeratin patterns characteristic of both stratified squamous and columnar epithelium (202). Ultrastructurally the surface cells show features of both squamous and columnar cells (200). This multilayered epithelium often lies contiguous to the mucosal gland duct epithelium. The multilayered epithelium shows a high proliferative capacity as demonstrated by Ki67 immunoreactivity and the strong expression of growth factors such as TGF-α and EGFR. This epithelium may also serve as a potential source of multipotential cells for the development of both the multilayered epithelium and BE. Others suggest that it is a metaplastic change and that the mature form of this change may be ciliated pseudostratified epithelium with an immunophenotype that resembles that of the bronchial mucosa (201).

Pathology of Treated Barrett Esophagus

The aim of therapeutic strategies for BE is to eliminate the abnormal epithelium, thereby removing the risk of progression to malignancy. Regression occurs following both surgical treatment and treatment with proton pump inhibitors and is more common in patients with SSBE than LSBE (203). Newer techniques for eradicating BE include photodynamic therapy, laser therapy, and endoscopic mucosal resection.

Biopsies are often taken after these therapies to evaluate their effectiveness. Restoration of squamous epithelium may occur if the established columnar tissue is ablated and the acid secretion is reduced while the esophageal epithelium heals. The histologic changes following treatment show partial squamous re-epithelialization of the previously metaplastic columnar epithelium. Squamous re-epithelialization results from the ingrowth of contiguous squamous epithelium, extension of epithelium from the submucosal glandular ducts, and growth of progenitor stem cells within the glandular mucosa. When regression occurs, one may see squamous epithelium overlying columnar epithelium, especially near the area of the squamocolumnar junction. The mucosa may also show evidence of scarring and mucosal hyperplasia with acanthosis. Many cases show intestinal-type epithelium underlying the squamous islands (Fig. 2.83). The Barrett epithelium under squamous islands shows a significantly lower KI67 proliferative index and a lower degree of cyclin D and p53 positivity compared to adjacent areas of BE, perhaps due to decreased exposure to the luminal contents (204). This raises the question as to the subsequent risk of neoplasia in the buried metaplastic epithelium. However, low-grade (Fig. 2.84) and high-grade dysplasia may be present in these buried regions (204). Patients with dysplasia in the Barrett epithelium under squamous islands often have coexisting dysplasia in other areas of the esophagus. In addition, adenocarcinomas arising in the esophageal wall and presenting as unresectable or metastatic cancers have been reported following argon plasma coagulation (205), photodynamic therapy (206), or laser treatment (207). All techniques using chemical or thermal measures to ablate the epithelium make it virtually impossible to detect occult carcinoma buried beneath the squamous epithelium during endoscopic surveillance. Residual glandular mucosa, both nonneoplastic and dysplastic, underlying the squamous epithelium may require histologic examination of deep biopsies in order to rule out the presence of the buried neoplastic glands (208). Because of the cancer risk, endoscopic mucosal resections are becoming more popular, particularly if the BE is associated with high-grade dysplasia or early invasive carcinoma.

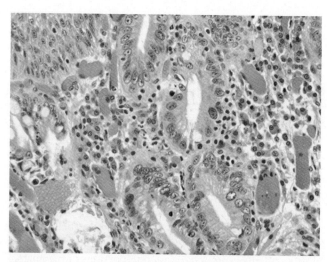

FIG. 2.84. Higher magnification of the area indicated by the *arrows* in Figure 2.83 shows glands with hyperchromatic, overlapping nuclei, some of which have irregular contours.

Tumor Development

Patients with BE develop hyperplastic polyps, squamous papillomas, dysplasia, and rarely adenomas. However, the major importance of BE lies in its propensity to develop into an adenocarcinoma (see Chapter 3). The management of patients with Barrett esophagus includes careful examination of endoscopic biopsies for evidence of dysplasia. Cytology may also have a role in assessing Barrett metaplasia in terms of monitoring it for the development of neoplasia. Cytology, however, should not be relied on without biopsy confirmation since one cannot assess either the exact location or the extent of the lesion using only cytology.

ESOPHAGEAL VARICES

Varices are portosystemic collaterals formed from pre-existing vascular channels that have become dilated by portal hypertension. The esophageal submucosal venous plexus, part of the portacaval collateral system, receives blood from the left coronary gastric vein; it drains chiefly through the azygous, although some vessels may drain through the inferior thyroidal veins into the superior vena cava. Typically, this plexus remains closed but it fills in response to increased portal venous pressure. The longer the duration is of the portal hypertension, the greater the risk is of developing large varices (209). In portal hypertension the number of lamina propria veins increases (210). The veins also enlarge with increasing flow resistance.

Portal hypertension also triggers overexpression of mucosal nitric oxide synthase, and this combined with the thinness of the muscularis mucosae and the epithelium may facilitate the development and rupture of esophageal varices (211). Venous stasis and subsequent anoxia also produce

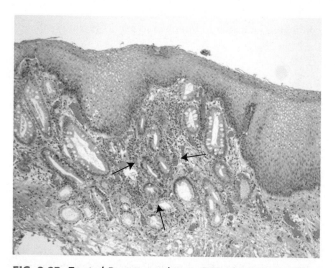

FIG. 2.83. Treated Barrett esophagus (BE). The Barrett epithelium lies under a parakeratotic squamous lining. The majority of the epithelium is nonneoplastic BE. However, there is a central area of low-grade dysplasia indicated by the *arrows*.

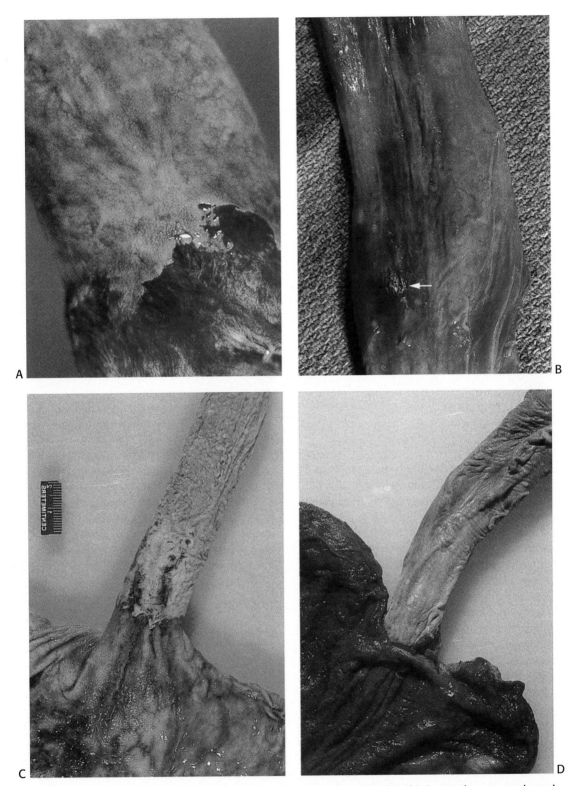

FIG. 2.85. Varices. **A:** Tortuous, dilated submucosal veins are visualized in this inverted gastroesophageal junction. **B:** Prominent small vessels are seen showing through the mucosa. On the left-hand portion of the esophagus, one also sees areas of hemorrhagic esophagitis. The area of the large bulge with the linear extension extending proximally (*arrow*) represents an area of hemorrhage around a varix producing a small submucosal hematoma. The proximal dilated vessel is also seen. **C:** Markedly dilated tortuous vessels are seen extending from the gastroesophageal junction where they involve both the proximal stomach and the distal esophagus. They taper proximally. Linear ulcers occur overlying the distended vessels. **D:** These varices appear even more distended and tortuous. The stomach shows an erosive gastritis.

epithelial necrosis and ulceration, thereby increasing the risk of a variceal bleed. An increase in intravariceal pressure leads to an expanding diameter so that the variceal wall thickness decreases. Bleeding occurs when the expanding force is no longer counterbalanced by the variceal wall tension. Varices almost always rupture on the unsupported luminal side of the varix (212).

Varices usually remain asymptomatic until they rupture, at which time they produce massive hematemesis. Variceal hemorrhage accounts for 10% to 30% of all upper GI bleeds (213).

Variceal hemorrhage occurs in 25% to 35% of patients with cirrhosis and accounts for 80% to 90% of bleeding episodes in these patients (214). Thirty-forty percent of initial bleeding episodes are fatal; as many as 70% of survivors have recurrent bleeding after the first hemorrhage (214). If patients survive the initial episode, their probability of remaining alive for 1 year remains about 30%. If bleeding from esophageal varices occurs, it usually stops spontaneously, at least temporarily, in up to two thirds of patients. However, 30% to 40% of these patients remain at risk for rebleeding within 2 to 3 days, and 60% rebleed within 1 week.

Variceal rupture may occur without an apparent triggering event. However, many patients have an antecedent history of vomiting. In some patients, the bleeding arises from concomitant gastritis, esophageal lacerations (Fig. 2.85), or peptic ulcer disease. Endoscopic predictors of bleeding include large varices and endoscopic red signs (215). Prolonged tube placement may weaken the esophageal wall, precipitating ulcer formation, and eventually leads to fistula development. Masses of varices may also produce esophageal pseudotumors (216).

Varices are endoscopically visible as areas of telangiectasia, cherry-red spots, red color signs, wale markings, minivarices, or varices. Red wale markings generally measure about 1 to 2 mm in diameter and, if present, lie on top of the large dilated subepithelial or submucosal vessels, which are usually >5 mm in size (215). Well-developed varices appear as bluish, sinuous, linear mucosal elevations that are most prominent below the aortic arch, especially as one approaches the distal esophagus. Occasionally, the vascular channels appear ruptured. Varices may be difficult to detect at the time of pathologic examination (autopsy or resection) because they collapse unless special efforts are made to keep them blood filled or to fill them with a plastic or gelatin-containing solution. In some cases, transillumination highlights their presence.

The dilated deep intrinsic veins displace the superficial venous plexus and assume a subepithelial position. Histologically, varices present as dilated intraepithelial or subepithelial blood-filled channels (Figs. 2.86 and 2.87). Vessels deeper in the esophageal wall may appear massively thickened and sclerotic. Thrombosis is rare but perivenous edema and necrosis of the adjacent epithelium are often present, as are hemorrhage and submucosal inflammation.

Evidence of old thrombosis, hemorrhage, hemosiderin deposition, inflammation, or fibrosis suggests previous rupture. Epithelial necrosis occurs over extremely dilated superficial submucosal varices. Patients who survive eventually develop fibrosis and re-epithelization of the ulcerated surface. Eventually, severe stenosis with stricture formation results.

Patients are often treated with sclerosing agents that are introduced perivariceally to incite inflammation, thrombosis, and fibrosis. Sclerotherapy results in severe necrosis initiated by venous thrombosis, particularly in the submucosa. This results in extensive superficial injury and less extensive deep tissue necrosis. Patients usually develop ulceration within the first week. The ulcers usually remain limited to the submucosa, but transmural ulcerations do occur. The organized thrombi can be difficult to identify by H&E stains, but their presence can be highlighted by the use of elastic tissue stains. Fibrosis occurs late and is often transmural. Destruction of neural plexuses may lead to subsequent esophageal dysmotility, and reduced LES tone predisposes the patient to GERD. Occasionally, one identifies the sclerosing agent within the tissues. Complications of sclerotherapy include esophagitis, necrosis, ulcer, tears (Fig. 2.88), perforations, and bacteremia.

Because of the high complication rate associated with sclerotherapy, endoscopic ligation offers an alternate therapy. In this therapy, varices are ligated and strangled with small elastic "O" rings. Changes following band ligation vary, depending on the proximity to the time of the ligation procedure. Shortly after ligation, the appearance is that of a polyp with its base compressed by a band. Thrombosis is present by day 2, resulting in mucosal and submucosal necrosis and superficial ulceration without involvement of the muscularis propria. Varying degrees of ischemic necrosis of the polyp are present on days 0 to 5. If there is premature loss of the bands, the polyp becomes necrotic and dilated variceal vessels develop. After complete healing, submucosal fibrosis occurs (217).

VASCULAR ABNORMALITIES

Esophageal vascular malformations, other than varices, are rare. They appear as an isolated, protruding, visible vessel in the middle or distal third of the esophagus covered by a normal-appearing surrounding mucosa (218). These are the esophageal counterpart of the Dieulafoy ulcer or caliber-persistent artery (see Chapter 4).

Ischemia

Esophageal ischemia (Fig. 2.89) is rare because the esophagus is well vascularized. However, ischemia may result from therapeutic agents used to treat varices, radiation, or manifestations of systemic diseases, such as atherosclerosis and anticardiolipin antibody syndrome. Esophageal small-vessel

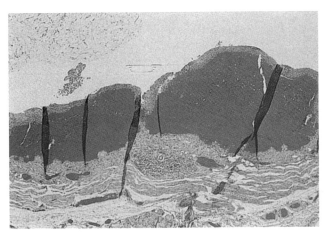

FIG. 2.86. Prominent subepithelial vascular lakes are present.

disease consists of submucosal arteriolar narrowing, a condition usually associated with advanced arteriolosclerosis (Fig. 2.90). The vascular lumen may be reduced by a hypertrophic smooth muscle wall or by intimal proliferation and fibrosis. Protein-rich edema fluid intermingles with fibrin in the adjacent connective tissue. Interstitial necrosis affects the epithelium from below, leading to local tissue necrosis and sloughing of the surface layers to expose the partially infarcted connective tissue stroma at the base of the shallow ulcers or erosions.

The entity known as *idiopathic acute esophageal necrosis* is thought to have an ischemic basis. Most patients have severe underlying diseases (hyperglycemia, significant cardiac problems, hypoxia, and shock) (219). The average age at diagnosis is 65.2, with a range of 26 to 83; men are much more likely to be affected than women (220). Grossly, the esophagus appears erythematous with a friable, denuded mucosa; whitish exudates; and superficial ulcers. The changes may progress to a black esophagus with blood clots on the surface. In severe cases, one sees full-thickness necrosis of the

esophageal wall, absence of stratified squamous epithelium, necrotic tissue, and deranged muscle fibers. The differential diagnosis includes severe reflux disease, exogenous dye ingestion, lye ingestion, malignant melanoma, melanosis, pseudomelanosis esophagi, and ischemia (219).

Vasculitis

A primary vasculitis, such as *periarteritis nodosa*, may produce esophageal vascular disease. The extent of the mucosal damage depends on the severity of the lesion. The pathologic features resemble those seen in the intestine (see Chapter 13). *Behçet syndrome* most commonly affects the terminal ileum or cecum. Exceptionally, it affects the esophagus; when it does it may cause a severe esophagitis with multiple small erosions, ulcers, and strictures involving the midesophagus (221). Esophageal ulcers can tunnel under the mucosa. Strictures and perforations may also develop (221). If biopsied, most cases show no distinctive features with only necrosis and inflammation. Vasculitis may be present (221). Granulomas are usually absent. The features of Behçet disease are discussed further in Chapter 6.

NUTRITIONAL AND METABOLIC DISORDERS

Amyloidosis and *diabetes* affect the esophagus, but since they largely alter esophageal motility they are discussed further in Chapter 10. Iron pigment becomes deposited in the submucosal glands of the esophagus in patients with advanced *hemochromatosis*. Dyskeratotic, degenerative epithelial alterations with nuclear enlargement and extreme vacuolar degeneration within, between, and beneath the epithelium develop in *uremia*. Necrobiosis leads to ulceration. Following this, the entire epithelial layer desquamates. A fibrinous exudate with neutrophils covers the ulcer. Granular eosinophilic

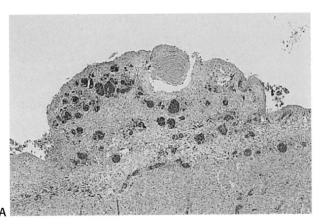
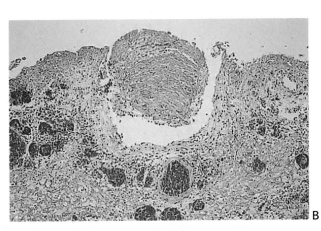

FIG. 2.87. Vascular ectasia in esophageal varices. **A:** Low-power magnification demonstrating the presence of a "polyp" of residual esophageal tissue. A central area of organizing fibrin is identified. **B:** Higher magnification demonstrating the organizing blood clot and vascular dilation.

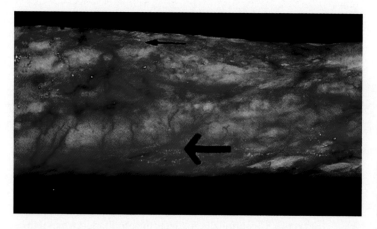

FIG. 2.88. The mucosa overlying the varices is eroded because of rupture of the dilated vessels. *Small arrow* shows a small tear, whereas a large tear is near the *larger arrow.*

degeneration suggests partial submucosal hydrolysis and necrosis. Hydropic degeneration and cytoplasmic zonation affecting the smooth muscle cells develop. Vascular ectasia with focal incomplete thrombosis of the capillaries and veins occurs. The damage results from circulating metabolites in the uremic patient.

INFLAMMATORY BOWEL DISEASE

Esophageal *Crohn disease* is rare and it is difficult to distinguish the esophageal lesions from other forms of esophagitis (Fig. 2.91), especially if one is unaware that the patient has Crohn disease. Rarely, Crohn disease manifests initially in the esophagus; intestinal disease becomes

apparent later. Grossly or endoscopically one or more erosions, aphthous ulcers, ulcers, inflammation, fistulas, or strictures are present. Histologically, one may see acute and chronic inflammation, ulcers, sinus tracts, and possibly granulomas (222). The granulomas should be compact sarcoidlike granulomas without necrosis. They may have inflammatory cells infiltrating them. If present, esophageal granulomas should prompt a differential diagnosis of possible etiologies so as not to miss specific, and perhaps rare, lesions. One must perform special stains for fungi and acid-fast bacilli to exclude the possibility that the granulomas result from an infectious process. Muscular hypertrophy and neural hyperplasia are also often present. In some cases only granulomas are seen. Many patients only show focal nonspecific inflammation

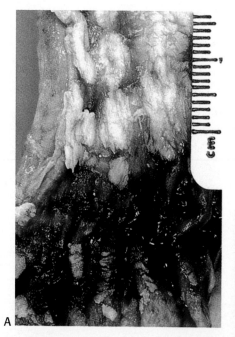

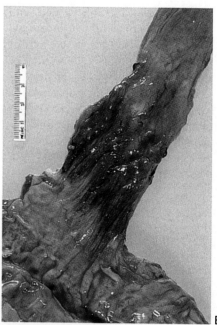

FIG. 2.89. Infarction of the gastroesophageal junction. **A:** A well-demarcated area of hemorrhagic mucosa contrasts with the intact squamous and glandular mucosa on either side. **B:** Appearance of an acute infarction in the fresh state as compared to the fixed state shown in A.

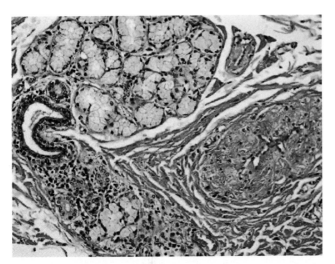

FIG. 2.90. Small muscular artery in the submucosa with thickened intima caused by arteriolosclerosis. A submucosal gland and duct are also present.

deep in the esophageal wall, and it may be impossible to make a definitive diagnosis. Irregular stenotic esophageal segments may mimic esophageal carcinoma.

Patients with ulcerative colitis may have esophagitis, but this is usually the result of coexisting GERD.

SARCOIDOSIS

Sarcoidosis may involve the esophagus and is in the differential diagnosis of granulomatous esophagitis. Intrinsic esophageal involvement shows characteristic noncaseating epithelioid granulomas usually in the lamina propria or submucosa. If sarcoid is suspected, the biopsy must be deep

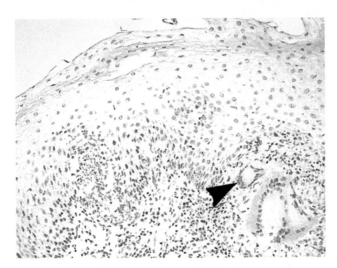

FIG. 2.91. Multinucleated giant cells (*arrowhead*) in the lamina propria are seen in this example of Crohn disease of the esophagus. (Courtesy of Dr. D. Schmutz-Moorman, Klinikun der Phillips Universität, Marburg, West Germany.)

enough to sample the submucosa. However, esophageal sarcoid is extremely rare and other causes of granulomas within the esophagus should be excluded first.

DERMATOLOGIC CONDITIONS INVOLVING THE ESOPHAGUS

A number of primarily dermatologic disorders affect the esophagus (Table 2.13), a fact not surprising since both the skin and mucous membranes are lined by squamous epithelium. These disorders include epidermolysis bullosa, drug-induced conditions such as Stevens-Johnson syndrome, and various forms of antibody-mediated pemphigoid and pemphigus. In some patients, esophageal disease develops in the absence of dermatologic evidence of the disease.

Pemphigus

Desmogleins (DSGs), glycoprotein components of the core regions of desmosomes in the squamous epithelium, represent the target antigens in the various forms of pemphigus (Fig. 2.92) (222). Antibodies against them interfere with their adhesive functions. The various forms of pemphigus can be distinguished by the autoantibody type as well as the clinical and histologic features. Antibodies in pemphigus foliaceous (PF) and pemphigus vulgaris (PV) are directed at the extracellular domains of DSG-1 and DSG-3, respectively (223). As stem cells migrate from their origin in the basal layer and move toward the surface, the epithelium forms, breaks, and reforms tight desmosomal connections with its neighbors while simultaneously undergoing a process of differentiation that culminates at the surface. This scaffolding of squamous cells is disrupted via impaired desmosomes due to the anti-DSG antibodies. Bullae develop from the fluid that accumulates in the mucosal gaps. Levels of circulating autoantibodies correlate with disease activity.

TABLE 2.13 Dermatologic Diseases Involving the Esophagus

Acanthosis nigricans
Behçet syndrome
Benign mucous membrane pemphigoid
Darier disease
Dermatitis herpetiformis
Epidermolysis bullosa
Erythema multiforme
Kaposi sarcoma
Lichen planus
Pemphigus
Scleroderma
Toxic epidermal necrolysis (Lyell disease)
Tylosis palmaris et plantaris

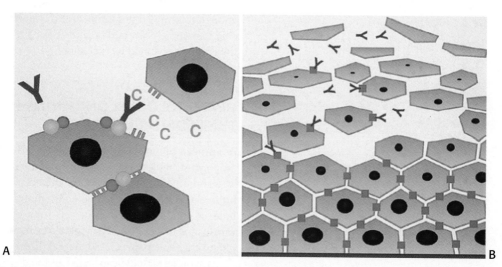

FIG. 2.92. Pathophysiology of pemphigus vulgaris. **A:** The targets of the autoimmunity as mediated by antibodies against cellular components are directed against two disulfide-linked proteins that function in cell-to-cell adhesion. Binding of autoantibodies to the cell surface antigen activates the complement cascade (*C*). **B:** As a result of the immunologic attack, acantholysis develops.

Pemphigus Vulgaris

PV, the most common type of pemphigus, predominates in middle-aged and elderly Jewish patients and is characterized by the formation of flaccid blisters and/or erosions. PV is an autoimmune disease as noted above, but it may also be induced by drugs, including D-penicillamine and angiotensin-converting enzyme inhibitors (224). All patients with PV initially have antibodies against DSG-3, but they may also develop antibodies against DSG-1 (225). Esophageal involvement is uncommon. Patients develop flaccid dermal and mucosal bullae. The latter involve various mucosae, including the esophagus (226). Typical esophageal lesions include exfoliative erosions, ulcers, and blisters. Esophageal bleeding, webs, strictures, and formation of epithelial casts may develop. The mucosa becomes acantholytic, causing the cells to separate from each other and resulting in a suprabasal cleft (Fig. 2.93). Eosinophilic spongiosis may also be present. Direct immunoelectron microscopic examination of esophageal biopsies discloses immunoglobulin (Ig) G and C3 localized to desmosomes on the free surfaces of acantholytic cells (227).

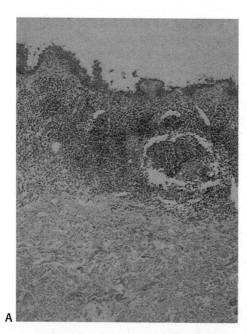
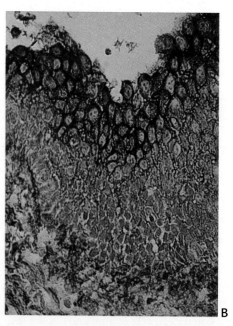

FIG. 2.93. Pemphigus vulgaris. **A:** Hematoxylin and eosin–stained section demonstrating the presence of mucous membrane that has lost the overlying layers due to the acantholysis and dissolution of the epithelium. **B:** Antibodies localize to the intracellular areas between the keratinocytes antibodies.

Pemphigus Foliaceous

PF, or superficial pemphigus, is also a disease of the middle-aged and elderly, but it does not preferentially affect Jewish persons. These patients develop antibodies to DSG-1 (225). Some cases result from exposure to sulfhydryl-containing drugs such as penicillamine (228). An endemic form known as fogo selvagem occurs in Brazil, Columbia, and Tunisia (229). The endemic and nonendemic forms of the disease are clinically, histologically, and immunologically similar (228). Features unique to the endemic form include the geographic, temporal, and familial clustering of cases; a higher frequency of cases among children and young adults; and an association with specific HLADR alleles (229). Antibodies to DSG-1 are high among normal subjects living in endemic areas, suggesting that antibody production is initiated by exposure to some environmental agent (229). The most characteristic lesions of PF are scaling and crested plaques. Intact blisters are uncommon. Mucosal involvement in PF is rare.

Pemphigus Vegetans

Pemphigus vegetans may affect the esophagus, presenting as severe odynophagia. Multiple white plaquelike lesions are present with erythematous bases in the esophageal mucosae. Biopsies from the mucosal esophageal layer show rounded epidermal cells with large nuclei and numerous inflammatory cells, including eosinophils.

Paraneoplastic Pemphigus

Paraneoplastic pemphigus (PNP) is an atypical form of pemphigus that shows features of PV and erythema multiforme but is clinically distinct from both. It associates with various malignancies and with Castleman disease (230). The autoantibodies are directed against desmoplakin 1, a protein common to the cytoplasmic plaque of desmosomes in all epithelia (230). Patients with PNP also develop antibodies to DSG-3 as well as several members of the plakin family of desmosomal plaque proteins. Features that characterize PNP include (a) painful mucosal erosions and a polymorphous skin eruption; (b) intraepidermal acantholysis, basal cell vacuolization, keratinocyte necrosis, and vacuolar interface reaction; (c) deposits of IgG and C3 along the epidermal basement membrane zone; (d) serum autoantibodies that bind to skin and mucous epithelium in a pattern characteristic of pemphigus and bind to simple columnar and transitional epithelia; and (e) immunoprecipitation of a complex of four proteins from keratinocytes by the autoantibodies (231).

Pemphigoid

Pemphigoid is a heterogeneous group of blistering disorders characterized by bullae and ulcers affecting mucous membranes and skin. Two types of pemphigoid are identified: Bullous pemphigoid and cicatricial (mucous membrane pemphigoid). Patients with bullous pemphigoid typically have skin lesions; approximately one third have mucosal lesions. All patients with cicatricial pemphigoid have mucosal lesions and one third have skin lesions. The disorder is rare and tends to affect the elderly. It affects men twice as frequently as women. Bullae form as the result of complement activation following IgG binding to basement membrane areas (232,233). The target protein is BP, a 180- to 230-kd protein associated with basilar membranes of basal keratinocytes (234). Eosinophils, neutrophils, and mast cells have all been implicated in the pathogenesis of bullous pemphigoid.

The mean age of onset of bullous pemphigoid is approximately 60 years, with most cases presenting between ages 41 and 80 (235). Esophageal lesions appear suddenly and may persist for days. They reappear at the same site, often following mild trauma induced by food ingestion. Gross findings include bullae, webs, and dense strictures, usually in the upper esophagus. Histologic findings are relatively nonspecific and include inflammation and multiple subepithelial bullae and basement membrane deposits of IgG and complement. In some cases, epithelial sloughing occurs. Patients with cicatricial pemphigoid have significant IgA in addition to IgG circulating anti–basement membrane antibodies.

Epidermolysis Bullosa

Epidermolysis bullosa (EB) is a heterogeneous group of heritable mechanobullous blistering diseases manifesting with fragility of the skin and mucous membranes. Gastrointestinal tract involvement is observed in different forms of EB, including esophageal involvement in dystrophic EB (DEB) or pyloric stenosis in junctional epidermolysis bullosa (JEB) (236). Even mild trauma splits off the mucosa from the underlying submucosa, resulting in severe scarring and chronic nonhealing wounds. EB associates with mutations in at least ten different genes, encoding proteins that form the basement membranes of skin and mucous membranes. These proteins include keratin intermediate filaments, laminin 5, collagen VII, and plectin (236,237).

Dystrophic epidermolysis bullosa is an inherited disorder caused by a structural abnormality in type VII collagen that prevents proper assembly of collagen and anchoring fibrils (238). Esophageal bullae develop at sites of trauma by food at the proximal and distal ends of the esophagus and at the level of the carina. The bullae develop in childhood. They lead to dysphagia, poor oral intake, and malnutrition. Both the skin and mucosal lesions heal by fibrosis, leading to mummification and recurrent esophageal strictures (239). Endoscopy is contraindicated because it can cause new bullae to form. Instead, the disease is diagnosed from skin manifestations and esophagograms. Dilation carries a high risk of perforation.

Junctional epidermolysis bullosa is a clinically and genetically heterogeneous autosomal disorder in which the phenotype depends on the specific gene/protein system affected as well as on the type and combination of genetic defects within these genes (237). Three major variants of JEB have been recognized (237): (a) the classic, lethal type of JEB associates with mutations in both alleles of one of the three genes LAMA3, LAMB3, or LAMC2 encoding the $\alpha3\beta$ and $\gamma2$ polypeptides of laminin 5; (b) a rare variant of JEB presenting with neonatal blistering together with congenital pyloric atresia (JEB-PA) (239) associated with genetic lesions in the plectin and $\alpha6$ and $\beta4$ integrin genes (237,238); and (c) generalized atrophic benign epidermolysis bullosa, a relatively rare nonlethal variant of JEB associated with widespread atrophic skin changes, alopecia, nail dystrophy, and dysplastic teeth in addition to skin fragility. The latter is inherited as an autosomal recessive disorder, and mutations in collagen type XVII, a transmembrane component of hemidesmosomes, is found in most patients. They may also show mutations in the LAMB3 gene (237).

Epidermolysis bullosa acquisita (EBA) is characterized by the presence of autoantibodies to type VII collagen. The disease primarily affects the skin. Esophageal disease results from bulla formation followed by ulceration and edema. This eventually predisposes to severe stricture or web formation (240). Perforation may also result (241).

Erythema Multiforme

Erythema multiforme is an acute, benign, self-limited mucocutaneous eruption associated with underlying infections, particularly HSV. It is preceded or accompanied by a low-grade fever, malaise, and symptoms suggesting upper respiratory tract infection. Erythema multiforme also results from drug reactions. Mucosal involvement is referred to as *Stevens-Johnson syndrome.* Diffuse erythema, friability, and whitish plaques that can be mistaken for candidiasis are seen endoscopically. The lesions may resemble peptic esophagitis. Esophageal disease ranges from mild to severe, with the severity of esophageal lesions corresponding to the severity of dermal disease. Keratinocytes become necrotic, containing a homogeneous pink cytoplasm and pyknotic nuclei. Biopsies reveal marked inflammation in the lamina propria, eosinophilia, and subepithelial bullae; severe ulceration; or inflamed granulation tissue.

Lichen Planus

Lichen planus is a common disease of unknown etiology that often affects the oral cavity. Esophageal disease is very rare. The lesion begins in adulthood; about two thirds of patients are women. Medications such as gold, thiazides, and antimalarials can induce the lesions (242). Patients develop dysphagia and odynophagia. The gross features include esophageal erythema, papules, ulcers, erosion, strictures, or webs. The lesions may appear as subtle papules involving the distal third of the esophagus; occasionally the entire esophagus is involved. A submucosal bandlike CD3+ T-cell–rich lymphocytic infiltrate develops with vacuolization,

degeneration of the basal epithelium, and superficial parakeratosis (243). The squamous epithelium is variably atrophic or acanthotic with elongation of the rete pegs. Fibroinflammatory exudates and granulation tissue indicate the presence of coexisting ulcers or erosions. Immunofluorescence examination shows dense fibrillar fibrinogen in the upper lamina propria (243).

Acanthosis Nigricans

Acanthosis nigricans is a distinctive dermatosis characterized by hyperpigmented velvety plaques. The lesions involve the skin and mucous membranes. Histologically the squamous epithelium displays hyperkeratosis, papillomatosis, and slight and irregular acanthosis in the valleys between the papillae. Esophageal lesions are usually not pigmented (244).

GRAFT VERSUS HOST DISEASE

Graft versus host disease (GVHD) typically affects the skin, liver, and GI tract. Severe acute GVHD occurs after mismatched allogenic transplants, after discontinuation of drugs such as cyclosporin and tacrolimus, or following allogeneic donor lymphocyte infusions. Chronic GVHD damages the esophagus, but the presentation of chronic GVHD is more subtle than that of acute GVHD. Esophageal symptoms include dysphagia, retrosternal pain, and aspiration. Acute GVHD may present as mucosal shedding ulcers or strictures. GVHD usually affects the upper third of the esophagus, producing focal or diffuse mucosal friability, vesicles, bullae, mucosal sloughs, ulcers, webs, and strictures (Fig. 2.94) (245). GVHD may also result in esophageal casts (246). The diagnosis is based on the history and presence of single cell necrosis (apoptosis) as well as the failure to identify specific infectious agents, although superinfection may be present. The mucosa becomes infiltrated with CD8+ T lymphocytes. Submucosal fibrosis may develop. Despite the fact that these findings are typical of the disorder, often all one sees is nonspecific inflammation and/or granulation tissue.

MELANOSIS

Melanocytes lie in the epithelial–stromal junction in 4% to 8% of normal esophageal specimens examined at the time of autopsy, 21% of consecutive upper endoscopies, and 29.9% of surgical cases with esophageal melanomas (247,248). They are more common in Asians than in Western populations and in patients with carcinomas. The latter may result from some factor induced or produced by tumors that stimulate melanocytic hyperplasia (Fig. 2.95) (248). Single or multiple, discrete, 1- to 3-mm, circular or oval, brown, or brown-black mucosal patches or linear streaks are present, usually in the midesophagus. The melanotic areas consist of

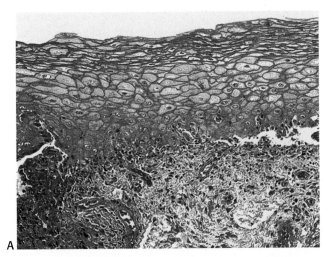
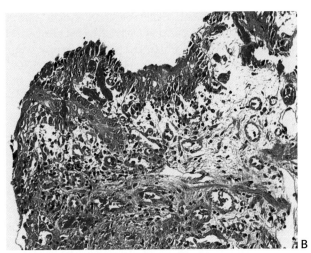

FIG. 2.94. Graft versus host disease (GVHD). **A:** Biopsy from a patient who underwent a bone marrow transplant. Single-cell necrosis is evident in the basal cell layer. **B:** The esophageal mucosa appears desquamated, inflamed, hyperemic, and edematous in this severe case of GVHD. (Case donated by Drs. Sale, Myerson, and Schulman, Fred Hutchinson Cancer Center, Seattle, WA.)

increased numbers of melanocytes in the basal mucosa as well as an increased number of melanosomes in individual melanocytes and increased melanin transfer to keratinocytes, stromal macrophages, and fibroblasts. The pigment is positive with melanin stains.

WHITE SPONGE NEVUS

White sponge nevus is a rare benign disorder of mucous membranes, with an autosomal dominant inheritance pattern (249). Most lesions exist at birth or have their onset in infancy,

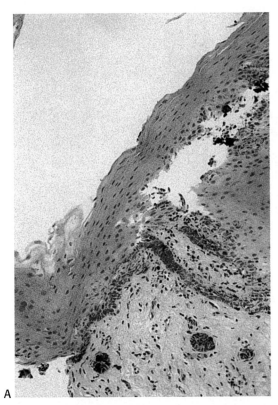
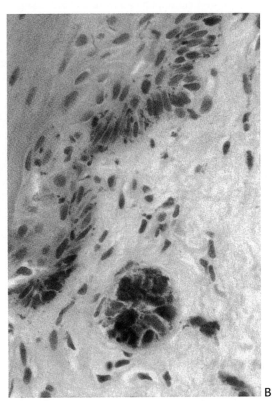

FIG. 2.95. Melanosis of the esophagus. **A:** Low-power magnification demonstrating the presence of prominent pigmentation at the basal layer. In the areas of acanthosis, the pigmentation is particularly prominent as it is in the cross sections through the acanthotic extensions. **B:** Higher magnification showing the presence of the melanin within the basal portion of the epithelium. Melanophages are also present in the underlying stroma.

childhood, or adolescence. The condition usually affects Caucasians of either sex. It is characterized by the presence of a thickened, deeply folded mucosa with a creamy white appearance. The mucosa is fragile and bleeds when touched. The lesions appear small and wartlike or large, moist, and white, resembling *Candida*. They increase in size and number after puberty and then stabilize. The lesions are characterized by irregular acanthosis with spongy hydropic squamous cells at all mucosal levels except for the uninvolved basal layer. Mitoses may be present but there is no nuclear atypia. The finding of parakeratotic plugs appears to be pathognomonic. Surface fragmentation leads the superficial squamous cells to appear shaggy (249). Inflammation is absent.

NEVI

Nevi are melanocytic lesions composed of dendritic melanocytes and subepithelial stromal tissue. They may develop in the esophagus (250), where they appear as linear patches of bluish pigmentation. Elongated, sometimes finely branched S100+ melanocytes are present in the lamina propria. They have long, dendritic processes and cytoplasmic brownish melanin granules. Chronic inflammation, fibrosis, and granulation tissue are also present. The overlying esophageal epithelium does not show melanin deposits. The differential diagnosis includes charcoal deposits following lye ingestion, pigmentation caused by hemosiderin, pseudomelanosis, heavy metal deposition, and melanosis.

WEGENER GRANULOMATOSIS

Wegener granulomatosis is characterized by granulomatous vasculitis, renal disease, and upper and lower respiratory tract disease. Esophageal involvement may present with severe odynophagia, secondary to severe necrotizing and erosive esophagitis due to the underlying vasculitis (251). Necrotizing granulomatous inflammation is present, as is necrotizing inflammation of the walls of small and medium-sized vessels. Variable numbers of multinucleated giant cells are present. Affected vessels may be occluded by organizing thrombi.

BENIGN POLYPS

Polypoid lesions of the esophagus and GEJ are uncommon and include giant fibrovascular polyps; squamous papillomas; polypoid mesenchymal tumors such as lipomas and smooth muscle tumors; fibroid polyps; pyogenic granulomas; and hyperplastic/inflammatory polyps. Mesenchymal lesions are discussed in Chapter 19.

Inflammatory Polyps

Inflammatory polyps are the most common esophageal polyps, often complicating reflux esophagitis. Most affect men, reflect-

ing their relationship to reflux esophagitis. Similar lesions occur at anastomotic sites, following irradiation or in any severe erosive or ulcerative esophagitis. They may be single or multiple and usually consist of granulation tissue. When they re-epithelialize, they resemble mucosal tags. These lesions bleed easily when eroded by the passage of food. They may be covered by squamous or glandular mucosa depending on the circumstances in which they arise. Some inflammatory polyps develop a pseudosarcomatous stroma. The presence of large, pleomorphic, atypical cells in the stroma can be quite alarming. However, they are strongly positive for vimentin and negative for cytokeratin, CD34, CMV, S100, and HMB45.

Inflammatory Fibroid Polyps

Inflammatory fibroid polyps (IFPs) complicate GERD (252) or HIV infections. These lesions are almost always single and the symptoms depend on lesional location. They present as solitary raised, often eroded or ulcerated lesions with a pedicle, often with a prominent submucosal component. The lesions may measure up to 5 cm in maximum diameter. Microscopically, the lesions appear variably cellular (Fig. 2.96), edematous, and highly vascular. IFPs contain fibrous tissue, proliferating blood vessels and inflammatory cells, fibroblasts, myofibroblasts, and histiocytes. They resemble their gastric counterparts, which are more common (see Chapter 4). These lesions must be differentiated from sarcomatoid carcinoma (see Chapter 3).

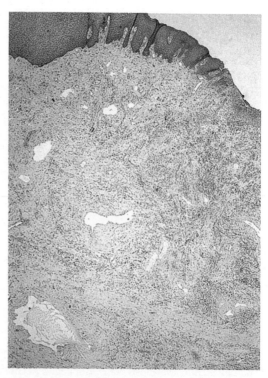

FIG. 2.96. Esophageal inflammatory polyp. The lesion is covered with squamous epithelium. The core consists of blood vessels, fibrous connective tissue, and inflammatory cells.

Giant Fibrovascular Polyps

Giant fibrovascular polyps account for 0.5% to 1% of all esophageal tumors. Seventy-five percent of patients are male, usually between the ages of 40 and 70. They are pedunculated, slow-growing, intraluminal tumorlike lesions usually arising in the upper esophagus (253), just below the upper esophageal sphincter. The clinical differential diagnosis includes carcinoma and intramural myoma. The lesions vary in size with an average length of 15 cm. Fibrovascular polyps consist of a core of mature fibrous tissue with an occasionally myxoid stroma that contains scattered, thin-walled vessels and variable amounts of fat covered by nonkeratinizing squamous epithelium. These are resected to avoid complications of obstruction of either the upper airway or the esophagus.

Hyperplastic Polyps

Hyperplastic polyps most typically complicate GERD and therefore usually arise in the distal esophagus and GEJ. They are usually associated with ulcers or erosive esophagitis. There is a moderate male predominance reflecting the fact that most lesions develop in patients with GERD. Other potential etiologies include medications, infection, anastomotic or polypectomy sites, vomiting, and photodynamic therapy. The lesions represent a regenerative response to surrounding mucosal injury (254). Average patient age is 53.9 years, although the lesion may occasionally be seen in children. Hyperplastic polyps may be single or multiple and they are typically <1 cm in size, but they may measure up to 3 cm. They are characterized by a proliferation of hyperplastic gastric-type foveolar epithelium, hyperplastic squamous epithelium, or admixture of these two mucosal types. Most contain variably inflamed predominantly cardiac mucosa; mixed types are the least common. These lesions frequently resemble their gastric counterparts. Intestinal metaplasia and low-grade dysplasia can be seen in a small number of cases.

GLYCOGEN ACANTHOSIS

Glycogen acanthosis appears as discrete raised, nodular, white plaquelike esophageal lesions usually measuring <1 cm in diameter (Fig. 2.97). They rarely measure more than 3 mm in diameter. When extensive, they coalesce into larger plaques. The presence of diffuse esophageal glycogen acanthosis represents an endoscopic marker of Cowden disease (see Chapter 12), and it is a characteristic component of the syndrome. Glycogen acanthosis may also be associated with celiac disease (255). The lesions appear as small, round, mucosal elevations, representing focal thickening of the squamous epithelium. The mucosa contains a collection of hyperplastic enlarged squamous cells containing increased amounts of intracellular glycogen (Fig. 2.98) distributed along the longitudinal ridges. The lesion can be accentuated by the use of PAS reactions since the cell cytoplasm contains abundant glycogen. There is no inflammation and no basal cell hyperplasia.

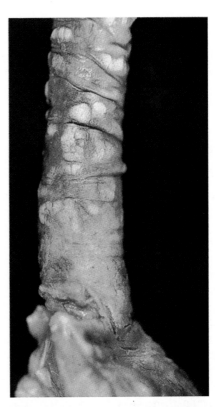

FIG. 2.97. Glycogen acanthosis. Everted esophagus showing characteristic pale-tan raised nodules of glycogen acanthosis. These lesions may be confused with the inflammatory pseudomembranes of candidiasis. They are unrelated to leukoplakia and have no malignant potential.

XANTHELASMA/XANTHOMA

Xanthelasmas, also known as *xanthomas* or *lipid islands*, are asymptomatic incidental lesions sometimes encountered during upper GI endoscopy. They most commonly develop in the stomach (see Chapter 4), but they can occur in the

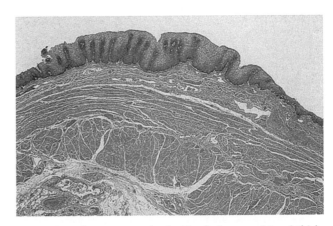

FIG. 2.98. Glycogen acanthosis. The lesion consists of thickened epithelium caused by both an increased number of squamous cells and an increased glycogen content of individual cells.

esophagus where they are quite rare (256). They appear as yellow-white well-demarcated single or multiple mucosal nodules or plaques. They consist of collections of large foamy histiocytes containing cholesterol and lipoproteins. They may be surrounded by chronic inflammatory cells. The cells have small central or slightly eccentric nuclei.

ABNORMALITIES ASSOCIATED WITH SURGICAL PROCEDURES

Esophageal replacement surgery is unavoidable in patients with long-gap esophageal atresia, esophageal resection, or severe *esophageal strictures* resulting from caustic or peptic injury. The small intestine and colon are favored organs for use for the interposition, although the stomach is also occasionally used. The transplants are placed in a subcutaneous or retrosternal location or in the left chest. Tissue-engineered esophagus created from esophagus organoid units, mesenchymal cores surrounded by epithelial cells, represents an attractive alternative for replacement of the native esophagus, since it can maintain normal histology (257).

Complications relate to luminal patency, conduit integrity, hemorrhage, ulceration, anastomotic leaks, fistula formation, strictures, and ischemia. The transplant may develop ischemic necrosis. The histology of the transplanted segment demonstrates the presence of normal, inflamed, or infarcted colonic or small intestinal histology. When the grafts are followed prospectively with mucosal biopsies, minimal histologic changes are found in uncomplicated patients. There may be congestion and neutrophilic infiltrates in the distal third. They may show a proliferation of fibrous tissue with reactive blood vessels and inflammatory cells that include histiocytes, lymphocytes, neutrophils, and eosinophils mixed with notable numbers of fibroblasts. The regional lymph nodes may show reactive hyperplasia.

REFERENCES

1. Langman J, ed: *Medical Embryology, Human Development—Normal and Abnormal,* 3rd ed. Baltimore: Williams and Wilkins, 1975.
2. Johns BAE: Developmental changes in the esophageal epithelium in man. *J Anat* 1952;86:431.
3. Potter SE, Holyoke EA: Observation of the intrinsic blood supply of the esophagus. *Arch Surg* 1950;61:944.
4. Akijama H, Tsurumaru M, Kawamura T, Ono Y: Principles of surgical treatment for carcinoma of the esophagus: analysis of lymph node involvement. *Ann Surg* 1981;194:438.
5. Aggestrup S, Uddma R, Jensen ST, et al: Regulatory peptides in the lower esophageal sphincter of pig and man. *Dig Dis Sci* 1986;31:1370.
6. Goyal RK, Rattan S: Neurohumoral, hormonal and drug receptors for the lower esophageal sphincter. *Gastroenterology* 1978;74:598.
7. Kravitz JJ, Snape WJ, Cohen S: The effect of histamine and histamine antagonists on human lower esophageal sphincter function. *Gastroenterology* 1978;74:435.
8. Ny L, Alm P, Ekstrom P, et al: Nitric oxide synthase-containing peptide-containing, and acetylcholinesterase-positive nerves in the cat lower oesophagus. *Histochem J* 1994;26:721.
9. Ward SM, Morris G, Reese L, et al: Interstitial cells of Cajal mediate enteric inhibitory neurotransmission in the lower esophageal and pyloric sphincters. *Gastroenterology* 1998;115:314.
10. Sperry DG, Wassersug RJ: A proposed function for microridges on epithelial cells. *Anat Rec* 1976;185:253.
11. Orlando RC: Esophageal epithelial resistance. *J Clin Gastroenterol* 1986;8:12.
12. Eastwood GL: Gastrointestinal epithelial renewal. *Gastroenterology* 1977;72:962.
13. Weinstein WM, Bogoch ER, Bowes KL: The normal human esophageal mucosa: a histological reappraisal. *Gastroenterology* 1975;68:40.
14. Ohashi K, Kato Y, Kanno J, Kasuga T: Melanocytes and melanosis of the oesophagus in Japanese subjects—analysis of factors effecting their increase. *Virchows Arch A Pathol Anat* 1990;417:137.
15. DeNardi FG, Riddell RH: The normal esophagus. *Am J Surg Pathol* 1991;15:296.
16. Sporn MB, Roberts AB: The epidermal growth factor family. In: Sporn MB, Roberts AB (eds). *Peptide Growth Factors and Their Receptors I.* Berlin: Springer-Verlag, 1990, pp 100–367.
17. Owen DA: Stomach. In: Sternberg SS (ed). *Histology for Pathologists.* New York: Raven Press, 1992, pp 533–545.
18. Chandrasoma P: Pathophysiology of Barrett's esophagus. *Semin Thorac Cardiovasc Surg* 1997;9:270.
19. Goldblum JR, Vicari JJ, Falk GW, et al: Inflammation and intestinal metaplasia of the gastric cardia: the role of gastroesophageal reflux and H. pylori infection. *Gastroenterology* 1998;114:633.
20. Spechler SJ: Intestinal metaplasia at the gastroesophageal junction. *Gastroenterology* 2004;126:567.
21. Glickman JN, Fox V, Antonioli DA, et al: Morphology of the cardia and significance of carditis in pediatric patients. *Am J Surg Pathol* 2002; 26:1032.
22. De Hertogh G, Van Eyken P, Ectors N, et al: On the origin of cardiac mucosa: a histological and immunohistochemical study of cytokeratin expression patterns in the developing esophagogastric junction region and stomach. *World J Gastroenterol* 2005;11:4490.
23. Chandrasoma P: Controversies of the cardiac mucosa and Barrett's oesophagus. *Histopathology* 2005;46:361.
24. Kilgore SP, Ormsby AH, Gramlich TL, et al: The gastric cardia: fact or fiction? *Am J Gastroenterol* 2000;95:921.
25. Oberg S, Peters JH, DeMeester TR, et al: Inflammation and specialized intestinal metaplasia of cardiac mucosa is a manifestation of gastroesophageal reflux disease. *Ann Surg* 1997;226:522.
26. Hopwood D, Logan KR, Milne G: Mucosubstances in the normal human oesophageal epithelium. *Histochemistry* 1977;54:67.
27. Borhan-Manesh F, Farnum JB: Incidence of heterotopic gastric mucosa in the upper oesophagus. *Gut* 1991;32:968.
28. Jacobs E, Dehou MF: Heterotopic gastric mucosa in the upper esophagus: a prospective study of 33 cases and review of literature. *Endoscopy* 1997;29:710.
29. Tang P, McKinley MJ, Sporrer M, Kahn E: Inlet patch: prevalence, histologic type, and association with esophagitis, Barrett esophagus, and antritis. *Arch Pathol Lab Med* 2004;128:444.
30. Lauwers GY, Mino M, Ban S, et al: Cytokeratins 7 and 20 and mucin core protein expression in esophageal cervical inlet patch. *Am J Surg Pathol* 2005;29:437.
31. Sanchez-Pernaute A, Hernando F, Diez-Valladares L, et al: Heterotopic gastric mucosa in the upper esophagus ("inlet patch"): a rare cause of esophageal perforation. *Am J Gastroenterol* 1999;94:3047.
32. von Rahden BH, Stein HJ, Becker K, et al: Heterotopic gastric mucosa of the esophagus: literature-review and proposal of a clinico-pathologic classification. *Am J Gastroenterol* 2004;99:543.
33. De La Hunt MN, Jackson CR, Wright C: Heterotopic gastric mucosa in the upper esophagus after repair of atresia. *J Pediatr Surg* 2002; 37:E14.
34. Hoshika K, Inoue S, Mizuno M, et al: Endoscopic detection of ectopic multiple minute sebaceous glands in the esophagus: report of a case and review of the literature. *Dig Dis Sci* 1995;40:287.
35. Katzka DA, Levine MS, Ginsberg GG, et al: Congenital esophageal stenosis in adults. *Am J Gastroenterol* 2000;95:32.
36. Hausmann PF, Close AS, Williams LP: Occurrence of tracheoesophageal fistula in three consecutive siblings. *Surgery* 1957;41:542.
37. Levine F, Muenke M: VACTERL association with high prenatal lead exposure: similarities to animal models of lead teratogenicity. *Pediatrics* 1991;87:390.

38. Depaepe A, Dolk M, Lechat MR: The epidemiology of tracheo-oesophageal fistula and oesophageal atresia in Europe. *Arch Dis Child* 1993;68:743.

39. Digilio MC, Marino B, Bagolan P, et al: Micro-deletion 22q11 and oesophageal atresia. *J Med Genet* 1999;36:137.

40. Kimble RM, Harding J, Kolbe A: Additional congenital anomalies in babies with gut atresia or stenosis: when to investigate, and which investigation. *Pediatr Surg Int* 1997;12:565.

41. Merei JM, Farmer P, Hasthorpe S, et al: Timing and embryology of esophageal atresia and tracheo-esophageal fistula. *Anat Rec* 1997;249:240.

42. Brunner HG, van Bokhoven H: Genetic players in esophageal atresia and tracheoesophageal fistula. *Curr Opin Genet Dev* 2005;15:341.

43. Jones KL: *Smith's Recognizable Patterns of Human Malformation,* 4th ed. Philadelphia: WB Saunders, 1988, pp 602–606.

44. Quan L, Smith DW: The VATER association: vertebral defects, anal atresia, tracheoesophageal fistulas with esophageal atresia, radial and renal dysplasia. A spectrum of associated defects. *J Pediatr* 1973;82:104.

45. Khoury MJ, Cordero JF, Greenberg F, et al: A population study of the VACTERL association: evidence for this etiologic heterogeneity. *Pediatrics* 1983;71:815.

46. Rittler M, Paz JE, Castilla EE: VATERL: an epidemiologic analysis of risk factors. *Am J Med Genet* 1997;73:162.

47. Valente A, Brereton RJ: Oesophageal atresia and the CHARGE association. *Pediatr Surg Int* 1987;2:93.

48. Celli J, van Beusekom E, Hennekam RCM, et al: Familial syndromic esophageal atresia maps to 2p23-p24. *Am J Hum Genet* 2000;66:436.

49. Hennekam RCM, Huber J, Variend D: Bartsocas-Papas syndrome with internal anomalies: evidence for a more generalized epithelial defect or new syndrome? *Am J Med Genet* 1994;53:102.

50. Cheng W, Bishop AE, Spitz L, et al: Abnormal enteric nerve morphology in atretic esophagus of fetal rats with adriamycin-induced esophageal atresia. *Pediatr Surg Int* 1999;15:8.

51. Singaram C, Sweet MA, Gaumnitz EA, et al: Peptidergic and nitrinergic denervation in congenital esophageal stenosis. *Gastroenterology* 1995;109:275.

52. Lindahl H, Rintala R, Sariola H: Chronic esophagitis and gastric metaplasia are frequent late complications of esophageal atresia. *J Pediatr Surg* 1993;28:1178.

53. Hruban RH, Shumway SJ, Orel SB, et al: Congenital bronchopulmonary foregut malformations. *Am J Clin Pathol* 1989;91:403.

54. Goldman RL, Ban JL: Chondroepithelial choristoma (tracheo-bronchial rest) of the esophagus associated with esophageal atresia: report of an unusual case. *J Thorac Cardiovasc Surg* 1972;63:318.

55. Arbona JL, Fazzi JG, Mayoral J: Congenital esophageal cysts: case report and review of literature. *Am J Gastroenterol* 1984;79:177.

56. Craig SR, Wallace WH, Scott DJ, et al: A pedunculated intraluminal foregut reduplication cyst of the proximal esophagus. *Ann Thorac Surg* 1998;65:1777.

57. Tobin RW: Esophageal rings, webs, and diverticula. *J Clin Gastroenterol* 1998;27:285.

58. Hoffman RM, Jaffe PE: Plummer-Vinson syndrome. A case report and literature review. *Arch Intern Med* 1995;155:2008.

59. Bredenkamp JK, Castro DJ, Mickel RA: Importance of iron repletion in the management of Plummer-Vinson syndrome. *Ann Otol Rhinol Laryngol* 1990;99:51.

60. Dickey W, McConnell B: Celiac disease presenting as the Paterson-Brown Kelly (Plummer-Vinson) syndrome. *Am J Gastroenterol* 1999;94:527.

61. Graham DY, Goyal RK, Sparkman J, et al: Diffuse intramural esophageal diverticulosis. *Gastroenterology* 1975;68:781.

62. Castillo S, Aburashed A, Kimmelman J, et al: Diffuse intramural esophageal pseudodiverticulosis. New cases and review. *Gastroenterology* 1977;72:541.

63. Huang B-S, Unni KK, Payne WS: Long-term survival following diverticulectomy for cancer in pharyngooesophageal (Zenker's) diverticulum. *Ann Thorac Surg* 1984;38:207.

64. Benacci JC, Deschamps C, Trastek VF, et al: Epiphrenic diverticulum—results of surgical treatment. *Ann Thor Surg* 1993;55:1109.

65. Krishnamurthy S, Dayal Y: Pancreatic metaplasia in Barrett's esophagus. An immunohistochemical study. *Am J Surg Pathol* 1995;19:1172.

66. Integlia MJ, Krishnamurthy S, Berhane R, et al: Pancreatic metaplasia of the gastric mucosa in pediatric patients. *Am J Gastroenterol* 1997;92:1553.

67. Doglioni C, Laurino L, Dei Tos AP, et al: Pancreatic (acinar) metaplasia of the gastric mucosa. Histology, ultrastructure, immunocyto-chemistry, and clinicopathologic correlations of 101 cases. *Am J Surg Pathol* 1993;17:1134.

68. Port JL, Kent MS, Korst RJ, et al: Thoracic esophageal perforations: a decade of experience. *Ann Thor Surg* 2003;75:1071.

69. Merrill JR: Snore-induced Mallory-Weiss syndrome. *J Clin Gastroenterol* 1987;9:88.

70. Powell TW, Herbst CA, Usher M: Mallory-Weiss syndrome in a 10-month-old infant requiring surgery. *J Pediatr Surg* 1984;19:596.

71. Wilcox CM, Clark WS: Causes and outcome of upper and lower gastrointestinal bleeding: the Grady Hospital experience. *South Med J* 1999;92:44.

72. Inculet R, Clark C, Girvan D: Boerhaave's syndrome and children: a rare and unexpected combination. *J Pediatr Surg* 1996;31:1300.

73. Salo JA: Spontaneous rupture and functional state of the esophagus. *Surgery* 1992;112:897.

74. Singh SP, Odze RD: Multinucleated epithelial giant cell changes in esophagitis: a clinicopathologic study of 14 cases. *Am J Surg Pathol* 1998;22:93.

75. Sonnenberg A, El-Serag HB: Clinical epidemiology and natural history of gastroesophageal reflux disease. *Yale J Biol Med* 1999;72:81.

76. Goh KL: Changing epidemiology of gastroesophageal reflux disease in the Asian-Pacific region: an overview. *J Gastroenterol Hepatol* 2004;19:S22.

77. Miller LS, Vinayek R, Frucht H, et al: Reflux esophagitis in patients with Zollinger-Ellison syndrome. *Gastroenterology* 1990;98:341.

78. Button BM, Roberts S, Kotsimbos TC, et al: Gastroesophageal reflux (symptomatic and silent): a potentially significant problem in patients with cystic fibrosis before and after lung transplantation. *J Heart Lung Transplant* 2005;24:1522.

79. Biancani P, Billett G, Hillemeier C, et al: Acute experimental esophagitis impairs signal transduction in cat lower esophageal sphincter circular muscle. *Gastroenterology* 1992;103:1199.

80. Jones MP, Sloan SS, Rabine JC, et al: Hiatal hernia size is the dominant determinant of esophagitis presence and severity in gastroesophageal reflux disease. *Am J Gastroenterol* 2001;96:1711.

81. Fiorucci S, Santucci L, Chiucchiu S, et al: Gastric acidity and gastroesophageal reflux patterns in patients with esophagitis. *Gastroenterology* 1992;103:855.

82. Kauer WK, Peters JH, DeMeester TR, et al: Mixed reflux of gastric and duodenal juices is more harmful to the esophagus than gastric juice alone. The need for surgical therapy re-emphasized. *Ann Surg* 1995;222:525.

83. Wetscher GJ, Hinder RA, Klingler P, et al: Reflux esophagitis in humans is a free radical event. *Dis Esophagus* 1997;10:29; discussion 33.

84. Dent J: Is Helicobacter pylori relevant in the management of reflux disease? *Aliment Pharmacol Ther* 2001;15:16.

85. Blaser MJ: Hypothesis: the changing relationships of Helicobacter pylori and humans: implications for health and disease. *J Infect Dis* 1999;179:1523.

86. Kaijser M, Akre O, Cnattingius S, Ekbom A: Preterm birth, low birth weight, and risk for adenocarcinoma. *Gastroenterology* 2005;128:607.

87. Nebel OT, Fornes MF, Castell DO: Symptomatic gastroesophageal reflux: incidence and precipitating factors. *Dig Dis Sci* 1976;21:953.

88. Biller JA, Winter HS, Grand RD, et al: Are endoscopic changes predictive of histologic esophagitis in children? *J Pediatr* 1983;103:215.

89. Armstrong D, Monnier P, Savary M, et al: Endoscopic assessment of esophagitis. *Gullet* 1991;1:63.

90. Kusano M, Ino K, Yamada T, et al: Interobserver and intraobserver variation in endoscopic assessment of GERD using the "Los Angeles" classification. *Gastrointest Endosc* 1999;49:700.

91. Ismail-Beigi F, Horton PF, Pope CE: Histological consequences of gastroesophageal reflux in man. *Gastroenterology* 1970;58:163.

92. Fujiwara Y, Higuchi K, Takashima T, et al: Increased expression of epidermal growth factor receptors in basal cell hyperplasia of the oesophagus after acid reflux oesophagitis in rats. *Aliment Pharmacol Ther* 2002;16:52.

93. Collins BJ, Elliott H, Sloan JM, et al: Oesophageal histology in reflux oesophagitis. *J Clin Pathol* 1985;38:1265.

94. Jessurun J, Yardley JH, Giardiello FM, et al: Intracytoplasmic plasma proteins in distended esophageal squamous cells (balloon cells). *Mod Pathol* 1988;1:175.

95. Wang HH, Mangano MM, Antonioli DA: Evaluation of T-lymphocytes in esophageal mucosal biopsies. *Mod Pathol* 1994;7:55.

96. Mangano MM, Antonioli DA, Schnitt SJ, et al: Nature and significance of cells with irregular nuclear contours in esophageal mucosal biopsies. *Mod Pathol* 1992;5:191.

97. Brown LF, Goldman H, Antonioli DA: Intraepithelial eosinophils in endoscopic biopsies of adults with reflux esophagitis. *Am J Surg Pathol* 1984;8:899.

98. Bowrey DJ, Williams GT, Carey PD, et al: Inflammation at the cardio-oesophageal junction: relationship to acid and bile exposure. *Eur J Gastroenterol Hepatol* 2003;15:49.

99. Wolf C, Seldenrijk CA, Timmer R, et al: Does carditis have two different etiologies? *Dig Dis Sci* 2001;46:2424.

100. Pei Z, Bini EJ, Yang L, et al: Bacterial biota in the human distal esophagus. *Proc Natl Acad Sci USA* 2004;101:4250.

101. Mansour-Ghanaei F, Zareh S, Salimi A: GI anthrax: report of one case confirmed with autopsy. *Med Sci Monit* 2002;8:CS73.

102. Chetty R, Sabaratnam RM: Upper gastrointestinal bacillary angiomatosis causing hematemesis: a case report. *Int J Surg Pathol* 2003;11:241.

103. Rubies-Prat J, Soler-Amigo J, Plans C: Pseudotumoral tuberculosis of the esophagus. *Thorax* 1979;34:824.

104. Damtew B, Frengley D, Wolinsky E, et al: Esophageal tuberculosis: mimicry of gastrointestinal malignancy. *Rev Infect Dis* 1987;9:140.

105. Fujiwara T, Yoshida Y, Yamada S, et al: A case of primary esophageal tuberculosis diagnosed by identification of Mycobacteria in paraffin-embedded esophageal biopsy specimens by polymerase chain reaction. *J Gastroenterol* 2003;38:74.

106. Whitley RJ: Neonatal herpes simplex virus infections. *J Med Virol* 1993;1:13.

107. Rattner HM, Cooper DJ, Zaman MB: Severe bleeding from herpes esophagitis. *Am J Gastroenterol* 1985;80:523.

108. McBane RD, Gross JB Jr: Herpes esophagitis: clinical syndrome, endoscopic appearance, and diagnosis in 23 patients. *Gastrointest Endosc* 1991;37:600.

109. Ashenburg C, Rothstein FC, Dahms BB: Herpes esophagitis in the immunocompetent child. *J Pediatr* 1986;108:584.

110. Greenson JK, Beschorner WE, Boitnott JK, et al: Prominent mononuclear cell infiltrate is characteristic of herpes esophagitis. *Hum Pathol* 1991;22:541.

111. Feldman S: Varicella zoster infections of the fetus, neonate and immunocompromised child. *Adv Pediatr Infect Dis* 1986;1:99.

112. Takatoku M, Muroi K, Kawano-Yamamoto C, et al: Involvement of the esophagus and stomach as a first manifestation of varicella zoster virus infection after allogeneic bone marrow transplantation. *Intern Med* 2004;43:861.

113. Weber JN, Thom W, Barrison I, et al: Cytomegalovirus colitis and oesophageal ulceration in the context of AIDS: clinical manifestations and preliminary report of treatment with foscarnet. *Gut* 1987;28:482.

114. Miller G: Epstein-Barr virus: biology, pathology and medical aspects. In: Fields BN, Knipe DM, (eds). *Virology*, 2nd ed. New York: Raven Press, 1990, pp 1921–1958.

115. Kitchen VS, Helbert M, Francis ND, et al: Epstein-Barr virus infections: biology, pathogenesis, and management. *Ann Intern Med* 1990;31:1223.

116. Kirkpatrick CH: Chronic mucocutaneous candidiasis. *J Am Acad Dermatol* 1994;31:S14.

117. Ogawa H, Nozawa Y, Rojanavanich V, et al: Fungal enzymes in the pathogenesis of fungal infections. *J Med Vet Mycol* 1992;30:189.

118. Abildgaard N, Haugaard L, Bendix K: Nonfatal total expulsion of the distal oesophagus due to invasive candida oesophagitis. *Scand J Infect Dis* 1993;25:153.

119. Tronchin G, Bouchara JP, Larcher G, et al: Interaction between aspergillus fumigatus and basement membrane laminin—binding and substrate degradation. *Biol Cell* 1993;77:201.

120. McKenzie R, Khakoo R: Blastomycosis of the esophagus presenting with gastrointestinal bleeding. *Gastroenterology* 1985;88:1271.

121. Grimes MM, LaPook JD, Bar MH, et al: Disseminated *Pneumocystis carinii* in a patient with acquired immunodeficiency syndrome. *Hum Pathol* 1987;18:307.

122. Kazlow PG, Shah K, Benkov KJ, et al: Esophageal cryptosporidiosis in a child with acquired immune deficiency syndrome. *Gastroenterology* 1986;91:1301.

123. Datry A, Similowski T, Jais P, et al: AIDS-associated leishmaniasis: an unusual gastro-duodenal presentation. *Trans R Soc Trop Med Hyg* 1990;84:239.

124. Centers for Disease Control: Revision of the case definition of acquired immunodeficiency syndrome for national reporting – United States. *Ann Intern Med* 1985;103:402.

125. Bini EJ, Micale PL, Weinshel EH: Natural history of HIV-associated esophageal disease in the era of protease inhibitor therapy. *Dig Dis Sci* 2000;45:1301.

126. Rabeneck L, Popovic M, Gartner S, et al: Acute HIV infection presenting with painful swallowing and esophageal ulcers. *JAMA* 1990;263:2318.

127. Blitman NM, Ali M: Idiopathic giant esophageal ulcer in an HIV-positive child. *Pediatr Radiol* 2002;32:907.

128. Bonacini M, Young T, Laine L: Histopathology of human immunodeficiency virus-associated esophageal disease. *Am J Gastroenterol* 1993;88:549.

129. Parfitt JR, Gregor JC, Suskin NG, et al: Eosinophilic esophagitis in adults: distinguishing features from gastroesophageal reflux disease: a study of 41 patients. *Mod Pathol* 2006;19:90.

130. Orenstein SR, Shalaby TM, Di Lorenzo C, et al: The spectrum of pediatric eosinophilic esophagitis beyond infancy: a clinical series of 30 children. *Am J Gastroenterol* 2000;95:1422.

131. Teitelbaum JE: Natural history of primary eosinophilic esophagitis: a follow up of 30 adult patients for up to 11.5 years. *J Pediatr Gastroenterol Nutr* 2004;38:358.

132. Khan S, Orenstein SR, Di Lorenzo C, et al: Eosinophilic esophagitis: strictures, impactions, dysphagia. *Dig Dis Sci* 2003;48:22.

133. Straumann A, Rossi L, Simon HU, et al: Fragility of the esophageal mucosa: a pathognomonic endoscopic sign of primary eosinophilic esophagitis? *Gastrointest Endosc* 2003;57:407.

134. Fox VL, Nurko S, Furuta GT: Eosinophilic esophagitis: it's not just kid's stuff. *Gastrointest Endosc* 2002;56:260.

135. Mann NS, Leung JW: Pathogenesis of esophageal rings in eosinophilic esophagitis. *Med Hypotheses* 2005;64:520.

136. Berthrong M, Fajardo LF: Radiation injury in surgical pathology. *Am J Surg Pathol* 1981;5:153.

137. Greco FA, Brereton HD, Kent H, et al: Adriamycin and enhanced radiation reaction in normal esophagus and skin. *Ann Intern Med* 1976;85:294.

138. Yang Z-Y, Hu Y-H, Gu X-Z: Non-cancerous ulcer in the esophagus after radiotherapy for esophageal carcinoma—a report of 27 patients. *Radiother Oncol* 1990;19:121.

139. Silvain C, Barrioz T, Besson I, et al: Treatment and long-term outcome of chronic radiation esophagitis after radiation therapy for head and neck tumors—a report of 13 cases. *Dig Dis Sci* 1993;38:927.

140. Cello JP, Fogel RP, Boland R: Liquid caustic ingestion spectrum of injury. *Arch Intern Med* 1980;140:501.

141. Zargar SA, Kochhar R, Nagi B, et al: Ingestion of corrosive acids. Spectrum of injury to upper gastrointestinal tract and natural history. *Gastroenterology* 1989;97:702.

142. Leape LL, Ashcraft KW, Scarpelli DH, et al: Hazard to health—liquid lye. *N Engl J Med* 1971;284:578.

143. Stevens AE, Dove GAW: Esophageal cast: esophagitis dessicans superficialis. *Lancet* 1960;ii:1279.

144. Ashcraft KW, Padula R: The effect of dilute corrosives on the esophagus. *Pediatrics* 1974;53:226.

145. Song HY, Han YM, Kim HN, et al: Corrosive esophageal stricture—safety and effectiveness of balloon dilation. *Radiology* 1992;184:373.

146. Schreiber JB, Covington JA: Aspirin-induced esophageal hemorrhage. *JAMA* 1988;259:1647.

147. McCord GS, Clouse RE: Pill-induced esophageal strictures: clinical features and risk factors for development. *Am J Med* 1990;88:512.

148. Banisaeed N, Truding RM, Chang C: Tetracycline-induced spongiotic esophagitis: a new endoscopic and histopathologic findings. *Gastrointest Endoscopy* 2003;58:292.

149. Wang CH: Cornification of esophagus induced by excessive vitamin E. *Nutrition* 1993;9:225.

150. Gilbert JD, Byard RW: Epithelial cell mitotic arrest—a useful postmortem histologic marker in cases of possible colchicine toxicity. *Forensic Sci Int* 2002;126:150.

151. Deneyer M, Goossens A, Pipeleersmrichal M, et al: Esophagitis of likely traumatic origin in newborns. *J Pediatr Gastroenterol Nutr* 1992;15:81.

152. Sampliner RE: Practice Parameters Committee of the American College of Gastroenterology. Updated guidelines for the diagnosis, surveillance, and therapy of Barrett's esophagus. *Am J Gastroenterol* 2002;97:1888.

153. Spechler SJ: Barrett's esophagus and esophageal adenocarcinoma: pathogenesis, diagnosis, and therapy. *Med Clin North Am* 2002;86:1423.

154. Ronkainen J, Aro P, Storskrubb T, et al: Prevalence of Barrett's esophagus in the general population: an endoscopic study. *Gastroenterology* 2005;129:1825.

155. Gerson LB, Shetler K, Triadafilopoulos G: Prevalence of Barrett's esophagus in asymptomatic individuals. *Gastroenterology* 2002;123:461.

156. Winters C Jr, Spurling TJ, Chobanian SJ, et al: Barrett's esophagus. A prevalent, occult complication of gastroesophageal reflux disease. *Gastroenterology* 1987;92:118.

157. Hassall E, Weinstein WM, Ament ME: Barrett's esophagus in children. *Gastroenterology* 1985;89:1331.

158. Qualman SJ, Murray RD, McClung HJ, et al: Intestinal metaplasia is age related in Barrett's esophagus. *Arch Pathol Lab Med* 1990;114:1236.

159. Peters FTM, Sleijfer DT, Vanimhoff GW, et al: Is chemotherapy associated with development of Barrett's esophagus. *Dig Dis Sci* 1993;38:923.

160. Spechler SJ, Schimmel EM, Dalton JW, et al: Barrett's epithelium complicating lye ingestion with sparing of the distal esophagus. *Gastroenterology* 1981;81:580.

161. Maieron R, Elli L, Marino M, et al: Celiac disease and intestinal metaplasia of the esophagus (Barrett's esophagus). *Dig Dis Sci* 2005;50:126.

162. Cameron AJ: Epidemiology of columnar-lined esophagus and adenocarcinoma. *Gastroenterol Clin N Am* 1997;26:487.

163. Skinner DB, Walther BC, Riddell RH, et al: Barrett's esophagus. Comparison of benign and malignant cases. *Ann Surg* 1983;198:554.

164. Hamilton SR, Smith RR: The relationship between columnar epithelial dysplasia and invasive adenocarcinoma arising in Barrett's esophagus. *Am J Clin Pathol* 1987;87:301.

165. Hong MK, Laskin WB, Herman BE, et al: Expansion of the Ki-67 proliferative compartment correlates with degree of dysplasia in Barrett's esophagus. *Cancer* 1995;75:423.

166. Jankowski J, Harrison RF, Perry I, et al: Barrett's metaplasia. *Lancet* 2000;356:2079.

167. Houghton J, Stoicov C, Nomura S, et al: Gastric cancer originating from bone marrow-derived cells. *Science* 2004;306:1568.

168. Hamilton SR, Yardley JH: Regeneration of cardiac type mucosa and acquisition of Barret's mucosa after esophagogastrostomy. *Gastroenterology* 1977;72:669.

169. Souza RF: Molecular and biologic basis of upper gastrointestinal malignancy—esophageal carcinoma. *Surg Oncol Clin N Am* 2002;11:257.

170. Suh E, Traber PG: An intestine-specific homeobox gene regulates proliferation and differentiation. *Mol Cell Biol* 1996;16:619.

171. Silberg DG, Swain GP, Suh ER, et al: Cdx1 and cdx2 expression during intestinal development. *Gastroenterology* 2000;119:961.

172. Miyazaki Y, Shinomura Y, Tsutsui S, et al: Gastrin induces heparin-binding epidermal growth factor-like growth factor in rat gastric epithelial cells transfected with gastrin receptor. *Gastroenterology* 1999;116:78.

173. Sun W, Tsuji S, Tsuji M: Gastrin upregulates HB-EGF and cyclooxygenase-2 in rate gastric mucosa. *Gastroenterology* 1999;116:1401.

174. Khan ZE, Wang TC, Varro A, et al: Transcriptional regulation of the TFF1 gene by gastrin. *Gastroenterology* 2001;120:A101.

175. Haigh CR, Attwood SE, Thompson DG, et al: Gastrin induces proliferation in Barrett's metaplasia through activation of the CCK2 receptor. *Gastroenterology* 2003;124:615.

176. Molina MA, Sitja-Arnau M, Lemoine MG, et al: Increased cyclooxygenase-2 expression in human pancreatic carcinomas and cell lines: growth inhibition by nonsteroidal anti-inflammatory drugs. *Cancer Res* 1999;59:4356.

177. Herlihy KJ, Orlando RC, Bryson JC, et al: Barrett's esophagus: clinical, endoscopic, histologic, manometric, and electrical potential difference characteristics. *Gastroenterology* 1984;86:436.

178. Chak A, Wallace MB, Poneros JM: Optical coherence tomography of Barrett's esophagus. *Endoscopy* 2005;37:587.

179. Georgakoudi I, Van Dam J: Characterization of dysplastic tissue morphology and biochemistry in Barrett's esophagus using diffuse reflectance and light scattering spectroscopy. *Gastrointest Endosc Clin N Am* 2003;13:297.

180. Layfield LJ, Ulich TR, Lewin KJ, et al: Serotonin and polypeptide hormone production in Barrett's esophagus. *Surg Path* 1988;1:131.

181. Buchan AMJ, Grant S, Freman HJ: Regulatory peptides in Barrett's oesophagus. *J Pathol* 1985;146:227.

181a. Wright CL, Kelly JK: The use of routine special stains for upper gastrointestinal biopsies. *Am J Surg Pathol* 2006;30:357.

182. Gottfried MR, McClave SA, Boyce HW: Incomplete intestinal metaplasia in the diagnosis of columnar lined esophagus (Barrett's esophagus). *Am J Clin Pathol* 1989;92:741.

183. Warson C, Van De Bovenkamp JH, Korteland-Van Male AM, et al: Barrett's esophagus is characterized by expression of gastric-type mucins (MUC5AC, MUC6) and TFF peptides (TFF1 and TFF2), but the risk of carcinoma development may be indicated by the intestinal-type mucin, MUC2. *Hum Pathol* 2002;33:660.

184. Rubio CA, Riddell R: Musculo-fibrous anomaly in Barrett's mucosa with dysplasia. *Am J Surg Pathol* 1988;12:885.

185. Glickman JN, Wang H, Das KM, et al: Phenotype of Barrett's esophagus and intestinal metaplasia of the distal esophagus and gastroesophageal junction: an immunohistochemical study of cytokeratins 7 and 20, Das-1 and 45 MI. *Am J Surg Pathol* 2001;25:87.

186. Riddell RH: The biopsy diagnosis of gastroesophageal reflux disease, "carditis," and Barrett's esophagus, and sequelae of therapy. *Am J Surg Pathol* 1996;20:S31.

187. Hirota WK, Loughney TM, Lazas DJ, et al: Specialized intestinal metaplasia, dysplasia, and cancer of the esophagus and esophagogastric junction: prevalence and clinical data. *Gastroenterology* 1999;116:277.

188. Spechler SJ, Goyal RK: The columnar-lined esophagus, intestinal metaplasia, and Norman Barrett. *Gastroenterology* 1996;110:614.

189. Ormsby AH, Vaezi MF, Richter JE, et al: Cytokeratin immunoreactivity patterns in the diagnosis of short-segment Barrett's esophagus. *Gastroenterology* 2000;119:683.

190. Ormsby AH, Goldblum JR, Rice TW, et al: Cytokeratin subsets can reliably distinguish Barrett's esophagus from intestinal metaplasia of the stomach. *Hum Pathol* 1999;30:288.

191. Mohammed IA, Streutker CJ, Riddell RH: Utilization of cytokeratins 7 and 20 does not differentiate between Barrett's esophagus and gastric cardiac intestinal metaplasia. *Mod Pathol* 2002;15:611.

192. Glickman JN, Ormsby AH, Gramlich TL, et al: Interinstitutional variability and effect of tissue fixative on the interpretation of a Barrett cytokeratin 7/20 immunoreactivity pattern in Barrett esophagus. *Hum Pathol* 2005;36:58.

193. Chinyama CN, Marshall RE, Owen WJ, et al: Expression of MUC1 and MUC2 mucin gene products in Barrett's metaplasia, dysplasia and adenocarcinoma: an immunopathological study with clinical correlation. *Histopathology* 1999;35:517.

194. Lord RV, Brabender J, Wickramasinghe K, et al: Increased CDX2 and decreased PITX1 homeobox gene expression in Barrett's esophagus and Barrett's-associated adenocarcinoma. *Surgery* 2005;138:924.

195. Wu GD, Beer DG, Moore JH, et al: Sucrase-isomaltase gene expression in Barrett's esophagus and adenocarcinoma. *Gastroenterology* 1993;105:837.

196. Matsukura N, Suzuki K, Kawachi T, et al: Distribution of marker enzymes and mucin in intestinal metaplasia in human stomach and relation to complete and incomplete types of intestinal metaplasia to minute gastric carcinomas. *J Natl Cancer Inst* 1980;65:231.

197. Corfield AP, Carroll D, Myerscough N, Probert CS: Mucins in the gastrointestinal tract in health and disease. *Front Biosci* 2001;6:D1321.

198. van Baal JW, Milano F, Rygiel AM, et al: A comparative analysis by SAGE of gene expression profiles of Barrett's esophagus, normal squamous esophagus, and gastric cardia. *Gastroenterology* 2005;129:1274.

199. Morales CP, Spechler SJ: Intestinal metaplasia at the gastroesophageal junction: Barrett's, bacteria, and biomarkers. *Am J Gastroenterol* 2003;98:759.

199a. Paulson TG, Xu L, Sanche C, et al: Neosquamous epithelium does not typically arise from Barrett's epithelium. *Clin Cancer Res* 2006;12:1701.

200. Shields HM, Zwas F, Antonioli DA, et al: Detection by scanning electron microscopy of a distinctive esophageal surface cell at the junction of squamous and Barrett's epithelium. *Dig Dis Sci* 1993;38:97.

201. Takubo K, Vieth M, Honma N, et al: Ciliated surface in the esophagogastric junction zone: a precursor of Barrett's mucosa or ciliated pseudostratified metaplasia? *Am J Surg Pathol* 2005;29:211.

202. Boch JA, Shields HM, Antonioli DA, et al: Distribution of cytokeratin markers in Barrett's specialized columnar epithelium. *Gastroenterology* 1997;112:760.

203. Gurski RR, Peters JH, Hagen JA, et al: Barrett's esophagus can and does regress after antireflux surgery: a study of prevalence and predictive features. *J Am Coll Surg* 2003;196:706.

204. Hornick JL, Blount PL, Sanchez CA, et al: Biologic properties of columnar epithelium underneath reepithelialized squamous mucosa in Barrett's esophagus. *Am J Surg Pathol* 2005;29:372.

205. May A, Gossner L, Gunter E, et al: Local treatment of early cancer in short Barrett's esophagus by means of argon plasma coagulation: initial experience. *Endoscopy* 1999;31:497.

206. Overholt BF, Panjehpour M, Haydek JM: Photodynamic therapy for Barrett's esophagus: follow-up in 100 patients. *Gastrointest Endosc* 1999;49:1.

207. Bonavina L, Ceriani C, Carazzone A, et al: Endoscopic laser ablation of nondysplastic Barrett's epithelium: is it worthwhile? *J Gastrointest Surg* 1999;3:194.

208. Biddlestone LR, Barham CP, Wilkinson SP, et al: The histopathology of treated Barrett's esophagus: squamous reepithelialization after acid suppression and laser and photodynamic therapy. *Am J Surg Pathol* 1998;22:239.

209. Cales P, Desmorat H, Vinel JP, et al: Incidence of large oesophageal varices in patients with cirrhosis: application to prophylaxis of first bleeding. *Gut* 1990;31:1298.

210. Arakawa M, Masuzaki T, Okuda K: Pathomorphology of esophageal and gastric varices. *Semin Liver Dis* 2002;22:73.

211. El-Newihi HM, Kanji VK, Mihas AA: Activity of gastric mucosal nitric oxide synthase in portal hypertensive gastropathy. *Am J Gastroenterol* 1996;91:535.

212. Terblanche J, Burroughs AK, Hobbs KEF: Controversies in the management of bleeding esophageal varices. *N Engl J Med* 1989;320:1393.

213. Laine L: Upper gastrointestinal tract hemorrhage. *West J Med* 1991;155:274.

214. North Italian Endoscopic Club for the Study and Treatment of Esophageal Varices: Prediction of the first variceal hemorrhage in patients with cirrhosis of the liver and esophageal varices. A prospective multicenter study. *N Engl J Med* 1988;319:983.

215. Paquet KJ: Causes and pathomechanisms of oesophageal varices development. *Med Sci Monit* 2000;6:915.

216. Jonsson K, Rian RL: Pseudotumoral esophageal varices associated with portal hypertension. *Radiology* 1970;97:593.

217. Polski JM, Brunt EM, Saeed ZA: Chronology of histological changes after band ligation of esophageal varices in humans. *Endoscopy* 2001;33:443.

218. Jaspersen D, Korner T, Schorr W, et al: Extragastric Dieulafoy's disease as unusual source of intestinal bleeding: esophageal visible vessel. *Dig Dis Sci* 1994;39:2558.

219. Haviv YS, Reinus C, Zimmerman J: "Black esophagus": a rare complication of shock. *Am J Gastroenterol* 1996;91:2432.

220. Benoit R, Grobost O: Black esophagus related to acute esophageal necrosis: a new case. *Presse Med* 1999;28:1509.

221. Yashiro K, Nagasako N, Hasegawa K, et al: Esophageal lesions in intestinal Behçet's disease. *Endoscopy* 1986;18:57.

222. Amagai M, Karpati S, Prussick R, et al: Autoantibodies against the amino-terminal cadherin-like binding domain of pemphigus vulgaris antigen are pathogenic. *J Clin Invest* 1992;90:919.

223. Anhalt GJ, Labib RS, Voorhees JJ, et al: Induction of pemphigus in neonatal mice by passive transfer of IgG from patients with the disease. *N Engl J Med* 1982;306:1189.

224. Kuechle MK, Hutton KP, Muller SA: Angiotensin-converting enzyme inhibitor-induced pemphigus: three case reports and literature review. *Mayo Clin Proc* 1994;69:1166.

225. Ishii K, Amagai M, Hall RP, et al: Characterization of autoantibodies in pemphigus using antigen-specific enzyme-linked immunosorbent assays with baculovirus-expressed recombinant desmogleins. *J Immunol* 1997;159:2010.

226. Rosenberg FR, Sanders S, Nelson CT: Pemphigus: a 20-year review of patients treated with corticosteroids. *Arch Dermatol* 1976;112:962.

227. Joly P, Thomine E, Dusade P, et al: Esophageal involvement in pemphigus vulgaris: a direct and indirect immunoelectron microscopic study. *Eur J Dermatol* 1994;4:320.

228. Stanley JR: Pemphigus. In: Freedberg IM, Eisen AZ, (eds). *Dermatology in General Medicine*. New York: McGraw-Hill, 1999, pp 690–702.

229. Warren SJ, Lin MS, Giudice GJ, et al: The prevalence of antibodies against desmoglein 1 in endemic pemphigus foliaceus in Brazil. *N Engl J Med* 2000;343:23.

230. Anhalt GJ: Paraneoplastic pemphigus. *Adv Dermatol* 1997;12:77.

231. Su WPD, Oursler JR, Muller SA: Paraneoplastic pemphigus: a case with high titer of circulating anti-basement membrane zone autoantibodies. *J Am Acad Dermatol* 1994;30:841.

232. Weigand DA, Clements MK: Direct immunofluorescence in bullous pemphigoid: effects of extent and location of lesions. *J Am Acad Dermatol* 1989;20:437.

233. Gammon WR, Merrit CC, Lewis DM, et al: Leukocyte chemotaxis to the dermal epidermal junction of human skin mediated by pemphigus antibody and complement: mechanism of cell attachment in the in vitro leukocyte attachment method. *J Invest Dermatol* 1981;76:514.

234. Venning VA, Frith PA, Bron AJ, et al: Mucosal involvement in bullous and cicatricial pemphigoid: a clinical and immunopathological study. *Br J Dermatol* 1988;118:7.

235. Ahmed AR, Newcomer VD: Bullous pemphigoid: clinical features. *Clin Dermatol* 1987;5:6.

236. Pfendner E, Rouan F, Uitto J: Progress in epidermolysis bullosa: the phenotypic spectrum of plectin mutations. *Exp Dermatol* 2005;14:241.

237. Pfendner EG, Nakano A, Pulkkinen L, et al: Prenatal diagnosis for epidermolysis bullosa: a study of 144 consecutive pregnancies at risk. *Prenat Diagn* 2003;23:447.

238. Lin MS, Mascaro JM Jr, Liu Z, et al: The desmosome and hemidesmosome in cutaneous autoimmunity. *Clin Exp Immunol* 1997;107:9.

239. Berger TG, Detlefs RL, Donatucci CF: Junctional epidermolysis bullosa, pyloric atresia, and genitourinary disease. *Pediatr Dermatol* 1986;3:130.

240. Stewart MI, Woodley DT, Briggaman RA: Epidermolysis bullosa acquisita and associated symptomatic esophageal webs. *Arch Dermatol* 1991;127:373.

241. Horan TA, Urschel JD, Maceachern NA, et al: Esophageal perforation in recessive dystrophic epidermolysis bullosa. *Ann Thorac Surg* 1994;57:1027.

242. Lefer LG: Lichen planus of the esophagus. *Am J Dermatopathol* 1982;4:267.

243. Abraham SC, Ravich WJ, Anhalt GJ, et al: Esophageal lichen planus: case report and review of the literature. *Am J Surg Pathol* 2000;24:1678.

244. Rogers DL: Acanthosis nigricans. *Semin Dermatol* 1991;10:160.

245. McDonald GB, Sullivan KM, Schuffler MD, et al: Esophageal abnormalities in chronic graft-vs-host disease in humans. *Gastroenterology* 1981;80:914.

246. Nakshabendi IM, Maldonado ME, Coppola D, et al: Esophageal cast: a manifestation of graft-versus-host disease. *Dig Dis* 2000;18:103.

247. Ohashi K, Kato Y, Kanno J, et al: Melanocytes and melanosis of the oesophagus in Japanese subjects—analysis of factors effecting their increase. *Virch Archiv A Pathol Anat* 1990;417:137.

248. Piccone VA, Klopstock R, Leveen HH, et al: Primary malignant melanoma of the esophagus associated with melanosis of the entire esophagus. *J Cardiovasc Surg* 1970;59:864.

249. Krajewska IA, Moore L, Howard-Brown J: White sponge nevus presenting in the esophagus—case report and literature review. *Pathology* 1992;24:112.

250. Lam KY, Law S, Chan GS: Esophageal blue nevus: an isolated endoscopic finding. *Head Neck* 2001;23:506.

251. Spiera RF, Filippa DA, Bains MS, et al: Esophageal involvement in Wegener's granulomatosis. *Arth Rheum* 1994;37:1404.

252. Staples DC, Knodell RG, Johnson LF: Inflammatory pseudotumor of the esophagus: a complication of gastroesophageal reflux. *Gastrointest Endosc* 1978;24:175.

253. Patel J, Kieffer RW, Martin M, et al: Giant fibrovascular polyp of the esophagus. *Gastroenterology* 1984;87:953.

254. Abraham SC, Singh VK, Yardley JH, et al: Hyperplastic polyps of the esophagus and esophagogastric junction: histologic and clinicopathologic findings. *Am J Surg Pathol* 2001;25:1180.

255. Suoglu OD, Emiroglu HH, Sokucu S, et al: Celiac disease and glycogenic acanthosis: a new association? *Acta Paediatr* 2004;93:568.

256. Gencosmanoglu R, Sen-Oran E, Kurtkaya-Yapicier O, et al: Xanthelasmas of the upper gastrointestinal tract. *J Gastroenterol* 2004;39:215.

257. Grikscheit T, Ochoa ER, Srinivasan A, et al: Tissue-engineered esophagus: experimental substitution by onlay patch or interposition. *J Thorac Cardiovasc Surg* 2003;126:537.

The Neoplastic Esophagus

sophageal tumors arise in any of the tissues comprising its four layers: The mucosa, submucosa, muscularis propria, and adventitia. Many types of carcinoma arise in the esophagus, but >70% to 95% are either squamous cell carcinomas (SCCs) and their variants or gastroesophageal junction (GEJ) adenocarcinomas arising in the setting of Barrett esophagus (BE). This chapter focuses on epithelial tumors. The World Health Organization (WHO) classification of epithelial tumors is shown in Table 3.1 (1). WHO staging for esophageal carcinomas is shown in Table 3.2. Mesenchymal tumors are discussed in Chapter 19. Hematologic tumors are discussed in Chapter 18. Neuroendocrine tumors are discussed in Chapter 17. Esophageal epithelial neoplasms are more likely to be malignant than benign. Esophageal squamous carcinomas are the eighth most common cancer worldwide and the sixth most common cause of cancer-related deaths (2). Adenocarcinomas at and proximal to the GEJ are less common, but are increasing in frequency in North America (3) and Europe (4).

BENIGN SQUAMOUS PAPILLOMAS

Squamous papillomas are benign exophytic esophageal tumors that fall into two major types: Those associated with human papillomavirus (HPV) infection, often referred to as condylomas, and those unassociated with HPV, usually referred to as squamous papillomas. Their prevalence ranges from 0.01% to 1% (5,6). Squamous papillomas may arise on a background of esophagitis due to reflux or other causes. Some result from the synergistic action of mucosal irritation (as from gastric acid reflux) and HPV infection (7). Evidence of HPV infection is most likely when the papillomas demonstrate a condylomatous histology (5,8,9). In this setting, HPV 16 is most commonly present followed by HPV types 18, 6b, and 11.

Esophageal squamous papillomas may be asymptomatic or present with dysphagia, heartburn, or hematemesis. Patients range in age from 2 to 86 years, with a male:female ratio of 24:9. Esophageal papillomatosis affects children with laryngeal papillomatosis, and is usually related to HPV infection (10). HPV-related esophageal papillomas are rare in adults. Acanthosis nigricans, a rare hereditary condition,

associates with multiple esophageal papillomas and late-onset hyperkeratosis (tylosis) of the palms and soles.

Squamous papillomas usually arise in the lower esophagus where they are generally single, exophytic, multilobulated, soft, semipedunculated, pinkish-white lesions with smooth or slightly rough surfaces. They measure from 0.2 to 1 cm in diameter with an average size of 0.4 to 0.5 cm (5,11). Some patients have multiple lesions, numbering from 2 to more than 20 (5). Benign, proliferating, hyperplastic (thickened and acanthotic) stratified squamous epithelium covers inconspicuous connective tissue cores containing stromal cells and thin-walled vessels (Fig. 3.1). The squamous cells demonstrate orderly cellular maturation from the basal layer toward the surface (Fig. 3.2). The basal cells may appear prominent but they lack significant cytologic atypia. The squamous epithelium of distal papillomas may exhibit the characteristic features of reflux esophagitis.

Esophageal papillomas demonstrate several distinct architectural patterns (5). *Exophytic lesions* have smooth, finger-like, papillary, and acuminate configurations with central fibrovascular cores extending to the surface of the papillae (Fig. 3.1). *Endophytic lesions* consist of benign squamous cell proliferations with an inward or papillomatous proliferation of the surface epithelium. The *spiked type* has a spiked surface configuration and invariably demonstrates a prominent granular cell layer and marked hyperkeratosis. These different histologic patterns exist alone or intermingle with one another (5).

Esophageal condylomas demonstrate the cytologic changes characteristic of HPV infection, including giant cells, multinucleated cells, superficial koilocytosis, and anisonucleosis (Fig. 3.3). Disturbances in squamous cell maturation and keratinization are present, including hyperkeratosis, acanthosis, papillomatosis, and dyskeratosis. Papillomas are benign lesions with little or no malignant potential.

PAPILLOMATOSIS

Papillomatosis consists of multiple minute esophageal squamous papillomas. It involves any part of the esophagus, most frequently affecting the distal esophagus. The lesion is rare,

TABLE 3.1 World Health Organization Classification of Esophageal Epithelial Tumors

Epithelial tumors
Squamous papillomas
Intraepithelial neoplasia
   Squamous
   Glandular
      Flat
      Adenoma
Carcinomas
   Squamous cell carcinoma
   Verrucous (squamous) carcinoma
   Basaloid squamous carcinoma
   Spindle cell (squamous) carcinoma
   Adenocarcinoma
   Mucoepidermoid carcinoma
   Adenoid cystic carcinoma
   Small cell carcinoma
   Undifferentiated carcinoma
   Others
Carcinoid tumor

TABLE 3.2 TNM Classification of Esophageal Carcinomas

T—Primary Tumor

TX	Primary tumor cannot be assessed
T0	No evidence of primary tumor
Tis	Carcinoma in situ
T1	Tumor invades lamina propria or submucosa
T2	Tumor invades muscularis propria
T3	Tumor invades adventitia
T4	Tumor invades adjacent structures

N—Regional Lymph Nodes

NX	Regional lymph nodes cannot be assessed
N0	No regional lymph node metastases
N1	Regional lymph node metastases present

M—Distant Metastases

MX	Distant metastases cannot be assessed
M0	No distant metastases
M1	Distant metastases present
	For tumors of the lower esophagus
	M1a Metastasis in celiac lymph nodes
	M1b Other distant metastases

Stage Groupings

Stage 0	Tis	N0	M0
Stage I	T1	N0	M0
Stage IIA	T2 or T3	N0	M0
Stage IIB	T1 or T2	N1	M0
Stage III	T3	N1	M0
	T4	Any N	M0
Stage IVa	Any T	Any N	M1a
Stage IVb	Any T	Any N	M1b

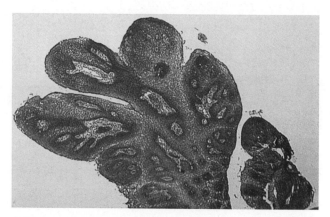

FIG. 3.1. Esophageal papilloma composed of vascular connective tissue cores covered by hyperplastic squamous epithelium with surface koilocytes. (Courtesy of Dr. Barbara Winkler, New York, NY.)

appearing in <1% of endoscopic examinations. The papillomas appear as multiple, small, irregular, wartlike mucosal projections. Their histology resembles that seen in isolated papillomas. Esophageal papillomatosis results from chronic inflammation from HPV infection, gastroesophageal reflux, prolonged nasogastric intubation, or the use of esophageal self-expanding metal stents. One unusual patient had multiple polyps showing synchronous HPV-16 and -33 infections. She also had a gastric carcinoma and once the gastric carcinoma was resected, the esophageal polyps completely regressed (12).

SQUAMOUS CELL CARCINOMA AND ITS PRECURSORS

Globally, esophageal SCC is the sixth most common cancer in males and the ninth most common in females (2). Esophageal SCCs show marked geographic (13) and ethnic

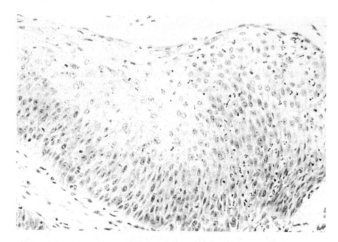

FIG. 3.2. Squamous papilloma in an adult with multiple lesions involving the upper respiratory tract due to human papilloma virus types 6 and 11. Cytopathic epithelial changes consist of koilocytosis and minimal nuclear atypia.

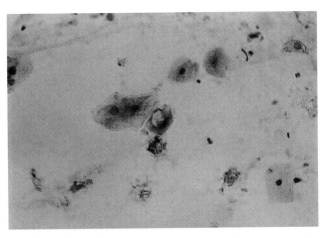

FIG. 3.3. Cytologic features of a squamous cell showing a koilocytic perinuclear halo.

(2,13) differences. Esophageal SCC is relatively uncommon in the United States (3) and Western Europe. Its annual incidence is 2.2 per 100,000 among white men in the United States compared to 13.2 among black men (3); 18.2 per 100,000 in Normandy, France (13); and 8.2 per 100,000 in Shanghai, China and 183.8 per 100,000 in Linxian, China (13). The most prominent cluster of elevated cancer rates occurs in north central China on the border of Henan, Hebei, and Shanxi provinces. Northeast China is the eastern pole of the Asian belt of SCC that begins in eastern Turkey and extends through the southern states of the former Soviet Union, Iran, and Iraq (14). Other high-risk areas include Chile, the Transkei region of South Africa, Japan, and Brazil (13). Because many risk factors interact with one another, their individual effects are difficult to weigh; however, antecedent esophagitis is common to all patients with esophageal carcinoma. Migrants from high-risk to low-risk countries retain their high risk through the first generation, but fall to the level of the host country in the second generation (15). This decline in rates may be attributed to diminished exposure to the environmental carcinogens peculiar to the country of origin. The persistence of risk in first-generation migrants, however, suggests that the anatomic changes induced by these carcinogens are not reversed in the new environment.

The male:female ratio varies from 1.5:1 in Linxian, China, to 17:1 in Normandy, France (13). In the United States, the age-adjusted incidence of esophageal cancer is highest among blacks (15 per 100,000) and Hawaiians (5,8) and is lowest among Filipinos (2.9) (16). The incidence of esophageal cancer increases with age and peaks in the 6th decade in high-risk areas (13). Patients 35 years or younger constitute approximately 7.4% of esophageal cancers in high-risk populations such as China. Time-trend studies show that incidence rates for SCC are stable or decreasing in most populations. For example, there has been a decrease in SCC incidence among U.S. blacks of 5.8% per year between 1992 and 2001 (17), while the rates of SCC in U.S. whites

have fallen below that of esophageal adenocarcinoma (3). A decrease in smoking in Western countries (18), combined with an increased consumption of fresh fruits and vegetables, may account for this decline (19).

The incidence of esophageal SCC closely correlates with a low socioeconomic status whatever the level of risk in any population (20); childhood economic status is a predictor of SCC risk in the adult (14). This suggests that increased tobacco consumption (21) and poor nutrition associated with poverty are common denominators in the genesis of this cancer. The increased incidence in U.S. black males has been attributed to increased tobacco and alcohol use, but the deleterious effects of these agents are amplified by the absence of the protective effects of fruits and vegetables (19).

Etiology

Both genetic and environmental factors play a role in the genesis of esophageal SCC. Environmental factors associated with esophageal SCC and adenocarcinomas are summarized in Table 3.3.

Alcohol and Tobacco

Heavy consumption of strong liquors, such as whiskey and calvados, shows a dose-dependent increased SCC risk (19,22). The combined use of alcohol and tobacco incurs a multiplicative increase in the risk of SCC. In Brittany, the relative risk is 49.6 for nonsmokers with the highest alcohol intake, 7.8 for nondrinkers with the highest tobacco use, and 155.6 for men at the maximum consumption level of both substances (23). Persons at high risk for SCC due to alcohol and tobacco consumption and poor nutrition may be vulnerable to field cancerization of

TABLE 3.3 Environmental Risk Factors for Esophageal Carcinoma

	Squamous Cell Cancer	Adenocarcinoma
Alcohol intake	Yes	Maybe
Tobacco use	Yes	Yes
HPV infection	Yes	No
Inadequate intake of fruits and vegetables	Yes	No
High intake of nitrate and nitroso compounds	Yes	No
Thermal injury	Yes	No
Caustic injury	Yes	No
Achalasia	Yes	No
Barrett esophagus	No	Yes
Obesity	No	Yes
Prior radiotherapy	Yes	Yes
Low birth weight	No	Yes

HPV, human papilloma virus.

the entire upper aerodigestive tract (UADT), including the esophagus (24). The frequency of developing a second UADT SCC in the 10 years following treatment of an index cancer is estimated to be from 5% to 40% (25). A prospective family study found the 10-year standardized incidence rates for esophageal cancer to be elevated after the diagnosis of an index cancer in the UADT (8.24) and lung (2.0) (26). Half of the multicentric cancers are synchronous. Most metachronous cancers develop within 3 years.

Dietary/Personal Factors

Patients with esophageal SCC can be divided into two overlapping risk groups: Those who smoke and consume large amounts of alcohol and those whose diets lack green, leafy vegetables, citrus fruits, micronutrients, and trace elements (27). The missing trace elements include molybdenum, manganese, zinc, iron, silicon, barium, titanium, and magnesium. Mineral deficiencies in the soil lead to increased fungal invasion and mycotoxin food contamination. Calcium, riboflavin, vitamin A, and vitamin C deficiencies may also play a role in esophageal carcinogenesis, since these vitamins play a role in maintaining mucosal integrity and normal epithelial differentiation. Deficiencies in these substances render the esophageal mucosa vulnerable to carcinogens in foods, such as mycotoxins in the Transkei (28) and N-nitroso compounds in China (29).

The influence of dietary supplements on SCC cancer risk has been studied among high-risk Chinese communities. These micronutrients have included β-carotene, vitamin E, selenium, zinc, molybdenum, retinol, riboflavin, and vitamin C. Overall, the evidence shows that these supplements cause a small, or borderline, reduction in the SCC risk (27). Since exposure to dietary carcinogens begins in childhood, it is not surprising that micronutrient supplements show only modest protection from this cancer in the adults in high-risk populations.

Thermal injury from hot drinks including hot tea in East Asia and maté consumption in South America has long been identified as a risk factor for SCC (27,30). It is difficult to separate the effects of thermal injury from the constituents of tea and maté, but the many studies strongly suggest that hot drinks do impose a risk of developing SCC (27).

The nitrosamine content of foods varies widely in high- and low-risk areas of China. Fermented, moldy, pickled food that contains high levels of nitroso compounds is a dietary staple in high-risk areas (27). The low molybdenum content of the soil in these high-risk areas yields crops with a high nitrate content that may be converted to potentially carcinogenic nitroso compounds. Nitrosamines are potent alkylating agents that can produce various alkyl DNA adducts, particularly involving O^6-methylguanine, which can preferentially mispair with thymine rather than cytosine, causing GC to AT mutations (31). O^6-methylguanine-DNA methyl transferase (MGMT) is a primary defense against alkylase-induced carcinogenesis. Some SCC patients have MGMT inactivation via aberrant promoter methylation (32). Vitamin C inhibits this conversion.

The dietary factors that increase or decrease the SCC risk vary from culture to culture. Thus, heavy chili consumption is an independent risk factor for SCC in India (33). Capsaicin, the active component of chili and its metabolites, may be a proximate carcinogen/mutagen. In contrast, a Mediterranean diet would appear to lower the risk of SCC, even when associated with moderate to high alcohol consumption (34).

Environmental and Genetic Interactions

Genetic polymorphisms in enzymes that metabolize alcohol render some individuals vulnerable to its deleterious effects. Acetaldehyde, the first metabolite of alcohol, is eliminated by aldehyde dehydrogenase-2 (ALDH2) (35). *ALDH2* polymorphisms influence blood acetaldehyde concentrations after drinking (36). An inactive mutant allele, *ALDH2*2*, is common in Orientals and is associated with increased circulating acetaldehyde levels, inducing painful facial flushing among occasional alcohol consumers (37). Alcoholics with this mutant allele develop tolerance to this reaction and the presence of this less active genotype in alcoholics enhances their SCC risk (38). The influence of alcohol on SCC risk may also be modified by an *XRCCI* polymorphism at codon 399. The XRCCI protein facilitates base excision repair or single-strand break repair. The odds ratio (OR) for SCC among alcoholics with the Arg/Arg *XRCCI* genotype compared to the Arg/Gln or Gln/Gln genotypes is 2.78 (1.15 to 6.67) (39). Recent data suggest that individuals with low selenium intake and *ALDH2* Lys/Lys and *XRCC1* 399 Gln/Gln genotypes associate with an increased risk of developing SCC, especially in the presence of exposure to tobacco and alcohol (40).

Aromatic hydrocarbons in tobacco smoke require metabolic activation by phase I enzymes (CYP450s), and are then subject to detoxification by phase II enzymes (GSTM1) (41). Patients with the Val/Val *CYP1A1* genotype are at increased risk of SCC (OR = 6.63, 95% confidence interval [CI], 1.86 to 23.7); this risk is enhanced when associated with *GSTM1*⁻ (OR = 12.7, CI 95%, 1.97 to 81.8) (47). The *cyclin D1* G870A polymorphism also influences the SCC risk in smokers (42). A study of North Chinese patients found that smokers with the G/G *cyclin D1* phenotype have a lower risk of SCC than those with the G/A or A/A phenotypes.

Low folate and impaired folate metabolism have also been implicated in the development of gastrointestinal cancers. Genetic polymorphisms in *5,10-methylenetetrahydrofolate reductase (MTHFR)* plays a central role in folate metabolism. This gene is polymorphic and the *MTHFR 677TT* genotype, which is associated with reduced enzymatic activity, significantly associates with increased esophageal SCC risk (43).

Occupational Factors

Certain occupations associate with an increased risk for SCC. These include warehouse workers and workers in miscellaneous food industries as well as those with occupational exposure to asbestos, metal dusts, vulcanization products, asphalt, petrochemicals, and combustion products (44). Persons engaged in the production and distribution of alcoholic beverages also have an increased SCC risk as seen in the Calvados region of France (45).

Radiation Exposure

Radiation therapy increases esophageal SCC in patients treated for various malignancies. As an example, the risk following treatment for breast cancer increases starting 5 years after exposure (46). Most radiation-induced cancers arise in the upper and midesophagus and the tumors may be multifocal in nature.

Infections

HPV DNA may be found in invasive SCC, areas of carcinoma in situ, the hyperplastic epithelium surrounding cancers, and histologically normal cells near these cancers (47). The areas with the highest incidence of HPV infections include China, Japan, and parts of South Africa. Although HPV types 6, 7, 9, 11, 13, 16, 18, 24, 30, 33, 51, 52, 57, and 73 have all been identified, HPV 16 is the most common (47). A *p53* codon 72 polymorphism significantly ($p = 0.001$) associates with HPV-related esophageal cancers in northern China (48). Fifty-three percent of patients with HPV positive were Arg/Arg carriers, compared to 26% of HPV-negative cancers and 23% of controls. The presence of HPV infection may be suspected in cytology preparations, as shown in Figure 3.3.

Fungi frequently contaminate the grains and foodstuffs consumed in high-risk geographic areas. The fungi belong to many genera, but *Fusarium* and *Aspergillus* are the two most common and their respective mycotoxins, fumonisin B1 and aflatoxin, act as carcinogens. They are found on maize (corn), millet, and other cultivated grains in Linxian and on pickled vegetables. The fungi reduce nitrates to nitrites and promote the formation of nitrosamines (22).

Chronic Chagas disease, resulting from infection by *Trypanosoma cruzi*, causes achalasia and associates with SCC development (49). Since the infection is frequently acquired in early childhood, the resulting carcinoma may appear as early as the 3rd decade of life.

Inherited Risk Factors

The autosomal dominant familial syndrome *palmoplantar keratoderma* (PPK) (tylosis) predisposes patients to the development of esophageal SCC. PPK results in defective mucosal keratinization (50) and altered mucosal integrity, increasing susceptibility to environmental mutagens. The mean age of onset for esophageal malignancies in these patients is 61 years. Members of PPK families have a 50% risk of developing esophageal cancer by age 50 and a 90% to 95% risk of developing esophageal cancer by age 65 (50).

These patients also have an increased risk of melanoma, breast and lung cancer, leukemia, hepatomas, malignant lymphomas, and colorectal adenomas (50,51). The presence of multiple carcinomas involving the oral cavity, tongue, oropharynx, and stomach suggests that exposure to a common environmental agent contributes to the genesis of all of the tumors. PPK patients who smoke are particularly likely to develop SCC (51). PPK results from a mutation in the *tylosis in esophageal cancer* (*TOC*) region of chromosome 17q25 (52). Loss of heterozygosity (LOH) of polymorphic microsatellite markers located near the *TOC* locus also occurs in sporadic esophageal cancers (52,53). PPK patients develop chronic esophagitis, followed by dysplasia, carcinoma in situ, and invasive carcinoma. Other histologic changes include abnormal keratinocyte maturation, the presence of basophilic inclusions, and surface keratinization (54). The neoplastic squamous cell lesions that develop resemble those arising in the absence of tylosis.

The recessive form of *dystrophic epidermolysis bullosa* due to a *type VII collagen* mutation is a less common source of inherited esophageal SCC (55). This condition is most common among people of Northern European origin.

Predisposing Diseases

Chronic esophagitis is the most common SCC precursor (56). The esophagitis has many causes, as discussed in Chapter 2. SCC arising in association with GERD originates in the mucosa bordering the upper limits of BE (57). The SCC associated with *caustic burns* emerges 30 to 45 years after the initial injury, usually in the midesophagus (58). *Motility disorders* that increase the risk of SCC include *achalasia* and *scleroderma*. Patients with achalasia develop esophagitis due to postprandial retention of solid foods (59). Food retention also increases the risk of SCC in *diverticula*, including Zenker (60) and the epiphrenic diverticula. The achlorhydria that accompanies *autoimmune atrophic gastritis* associates with an elevated SCC risk (61), as does the *multifocal gastritis* caused by CagA-positive *Helicobacter pylori*. This effect is strongest among patients with gastric atrophy, as measured by low pepsinogen group I levels (62). The association is supported by the parallel decline in the incidence of esophageal SCC and *H. pylori*–induced stomach cancer in migrants from Japan to the United States (63). The esophagitis that accompanies *Plummer-Vinson syndrome* also associates with an increased risk of SCC in the hypopharynx and cervical esophagus (64). There is also an association with *celiac disease* (64).

Dysplasia

Esophageal SCC passes through the sequence of chronic esophagitis, low-grade and high-grade dysplasia (also know as intraepithelial neoplasia), and invasive carcinoma. As a result, histologic or cytologic specimens may contain a constellation of histologic abnormalities, including normal, or

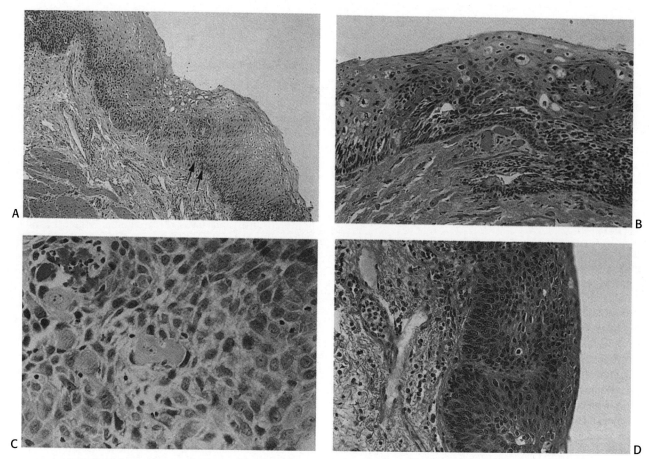

FIG. 3.4. Squamous dysplasia. **A:** Low-grade dysplasia. The changes are more severe on the right-hand side of the photograph. Note the beginning of irregular budding to the left of the *arrows* and the disorderly arrangement of the epithelium. **B:** Mild dysplasia. Disorderly atypical squamous epithelial cells localize to the basal epithelium. **C:** Moderate dysplasia. Dyskeratotic cells and cells with enlarged nuclear-to-cytoplasmic ratios and prominent nucleoli are present. **D:** Severe dysplasia. The atypical cells extend almost to the free surface.

near-normal esophageal mucosa, atrophy; esophagitis; parakeratosis; dyskeratosis; basal cell hyperplasia; simple hyperplasia; mixed basal spinous hyperplasia; variable degrees of dysplasia; and invasive cancer. In general, the epithelium increases in thickness and the papillae elongate as the process evolves (Figs. 3.4 and 3.5). *Dysplasia*, defined as

the presence of unequivocally neoplastic squamous cells that are confined to the mucosa above the basement membrane, is the immediate precursor lesion for SCC. Dysplasia was traditionally classified into mild, moderate, and severe degrees. However, since interobserver agreement in distinguishing the three grades is generally poor, most favor a two-tier

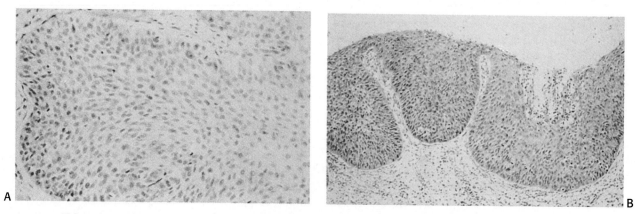

FIG. 3.5. Dysplasia of the esophageal epithelium. **A:** Moderate dysplasia. **B:** Severe dysplasia–carcinoma in situ.

system of low-grade and high-grade dysplasia. The latter classification scheme includes epithelial changes previously classified as carcinoma in situ. The higher the grade of dysplasia, the greater is the likelihood that the lesion will evolve into an invasive cancer.

The following facts support the concept that dysplasia is a step in SCC development. The frequency of dysplasia correlates with the level of risk. For example, endoscopically screened subjects in high-risk Linxian, China, show high-grade dysplasia in 7.9% of men and 9.8% of women. This contrasts with 2.4% and 2.5% in intermediate-risk Argentinean men and women, respectively, and 0% of screened subjects in low-risk areas of China (14). The age distribution of dysplasia and cancer supports a continuous progression from mild dysplasia to severe dysplasia to invasive carcinomas. Follow-up studies show that invasive cancers develop in areas of dysplasia. When assessed prospectively, 20% of 500 Chinese people with high-grade dysplasia progressed to carcinoma, compared with only 0.12% of 11,011 individuals with a normal mucosa (14). Areas of dysplasia share similar molecular abnormalities with the invasive cancers adjacent to them.

As in other tumors, there is a sequential acquisition of molecular abnormalities as the lesions progress from early precancerous lesions to invasive carcinoma (1). Those that are thought to be important are shown in Figure 3.6. A biopsy study from Chinese patients with dysplasia found genetic instability, including LOH and microsatellite instability (MSI) in the precursor lesions (65). LOH was identified at ten different markers on chromosomes 3p, 5q, 9p, 9q, 13q, 15q, and 17p. This study also found MSI in both low-grade and high-grade dysplasia, with its frequency increasing with the severity of the process. *p53* mutations can be found in dysplasia and in situ cancer (66). The same mutations are present in the adjacent invasive cancer, indicating that *p53* mutations are an early event in esophageal carcinogenesis. A Japanese study of field carcinogenesis found different p53 mutations in synchronous multicentric SCCs, but the identical *p53* mutations were found in the dysplastic epithelium adjacent to each invasive cancer (67,68). *p53* mutations may also be found in areas of transitions from esophagitis to dysplasia and are among the earliest changes seen in the development of esophageal SCC (1).

Areas of dysplasia generally remain symptomless, and it takes 3 to 5 years for carcinoma in situ to progress to more advanced stages of the disease. Up to 25% of patients with squamous dysplasia will develop cancer within 8 years. Because of the stepwise progression of SCC, cytologic esophageal screening has proven to be cost effective in asymptomatic patients in the high-risk areas. Cytology examination of 12,877 subjects in a high-risk Chinese population found high-grade dysplasia in 6% of cases and carcinoma in 3% (69). Population-based screening programs for esophageal cancer are not applicable to low-risk areas, such as North America or Europe. Selective cytologic screening of high-risk individuals, however, such as participants in alcohol abuse programs, may discover SCC at an earlier stage of progression than is usually the case in Western countries, as shown by Japanese studies that targeted alcoholics using endoscopy and iodine staining (70).

Dysplasia has several endoscopic appearances including a friable, irregular erosion and a raised polypoid lesion, with or without erosions or a hyperemic roughening that bleeds easily. Dysplasia usually involves the middle and lower esophagus and does not affect motility. Grossly visible areas of dysplasia vary in size from 0.5 to 5 cm in diameter. The dysplasia may be scanty in type with well-defined margins, extensive, or multifocal. Extensive lesions have ill-defined

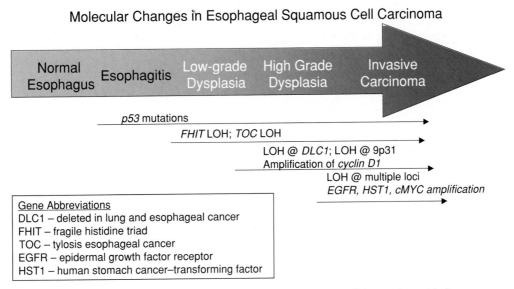

FIG. 3.6. Diagram of the progressive acquisition of molecular abnormalities as the epithelium progresses from normal to invasive cancer.

margins. The gross changes may be very subtle, showing only a slight mucosal depression, but mucosal staining with Lugol facilitates the detection of dysplasia since the normal mucosa is stained but the dysplastic mucosa is not (1). Dysplasia may merge with or be separate from an invasive cancer. Dysplasia is more likely to be identified in small or early cancers than in large or advanced neoplasms, since large cancers are more likely to overgrow their precursors.

Histologic examination is necessary to diagnose dysplasia. Dysplasia is characterized by both architectural and cytologic abnormalities. A disorderly proliferation of immature cells with hyperchromatic nuclei, abnormally clumped chromatin, and pleomorphic nuclei is present (Fig. 3.4). The cells typically have an increased nuclear:cytoplasmic ratio and demonstrate loss of polarity. The nuclei are frequently overlapping. Mitoses are frequent and are often abnormal. The dysplasia is considered to be *low grade* when the abnormal cells are limited to the middle third of the mucosa and *high grade* when they extend to the upper third of the epithelium or involve the full mucosal thickness and show more epithelial atypia than low-grade lesions. In *carcinoma in situ* (the high end of the spectrum of high-grade dysplasia), atypical cells extend through the full thickness of the epithelium without evidence of surface maturation. Dysplastic cells may also extend into the underlying submucosal glands and ducts. While ductal extension predisposes to deeper penetration (71), this finding by itself does not constitute invasion. Dysplastic squamous cells may also spread in a pagetoid manner into the adjacent normal esophageal mucosa. The pagetoid cells stain positively with low-molecular-weight keratin, do not stain for mucus, and have a high proliferative index.

Acanthotic epithelial buds containing atypical epithelial cells occur in both low-grade and high-grade dysplasia. They appear regular and the same size or vary in size, shape, length, and width (Fig. 3.5). Irregular buds are most common in areas of severe dysplasia adjacent to invasive cancer (72) and microinvasive cancer tends to develop from their tips. Dysplasia associated with HPV infection shows koilocytotic changes. Lymphocytic infiltrates in the surrounding lamina propria are common and correlate with the severity of the dysplasia.

Japanese and Western pathologists differ in their diagnostic criteria for esophageal squamous cell lesions. Invasion is the most important diagnostic criterion for a diagnosis of carcinoma for Western pathologists, whereas nuclear and structural features are more important for Japanese pathologists. In Japan, esophageal squamous cell carcinomas are diagnosed based on nuclear grade, and include cases judged to be noninvasive, low-grade dysplasia in the West. This difference may contribute to widely variant incidence rates and predictions of prognosis. In an effort to address these differences, the Vienna Classification was developed (Table 3.4) (73), although it has not been widely adopted. It corresponds to the treatment recommendation of local tumor ablation.

There are several diagnostic pitfalls with respect to early squamous neoplasias. Dysplasia must be distinguished from regenerative changes or areas of pseudoepitheliomatous hyperplasia. Herpes esophagitis, chemotherapy, or radiotherapy and areas of regeneration adjacent to ulcers may induce histologic changes that may be mistaken for early squamous neoplasia. The differences between regenerative and neoplastic changes are summarized in Table 3.5. Inflammation or ulceration, if extensive, may help identify the epithelium as regenerative in nature. However, caution must be exercised because dysplastic epithelium may become ulcerated or inflamed. If one is unable to distinguish between a truly dysplastic lesion and one that is regenerative in nature, one can use the term *indefinite for dysplasia* to diagnose the changes that are present. Subsequent biopsies, particularly those obtained once the inflammation has been treated, often help clarify the nature of the underlying process. Immunostaining for p53 may also help distinguish

TABLE 3.4	**Vienna Classification**

Category 1: Negative for dysplasia/neoplasia
Category 2: Indefinite for dysplasia/neoplasia
Category 3: Noninvasive neoplasia: Low grade (low-grade dysplasia)
     Low-grade dysplasia or adenoma includes mild and moderate dysplasia
Category 4: Noninvasive neoplasia: High grade (high-grade dysplasia)
     a. High-grade adenoma/dysplasia (severe dysplasia)
     b. Noninvasive carcinoma (carcinoma in situ)
     c. Suspicious for invasive malignancy
Category 5: Invasive neoplasia
     a. Intramucosal carcinoma: Invades the lamina propria
     b. Invasion into the submucosa or beyond

TABLE 3.5	**Features Useful in Distinguishing between Reactive and Neoplastic Squamous Epithelium**

Reactive Changes	Neoplastic Changes
Basal cell hyperplasia	Highly atypical cells
Glycogen depletion	Keratinizing epithelium
Vesicular hyperchromatic nucleoli	Bizarre cell shapes
Normal or increased N:C ratio	Increased N:C ratios
Prominent nucleoli	Prominent heterochromatin
Increased mitotic activity	Eosinophilic nucleoli
Basophilic cytoplasm	Irregular nuclear outlines
Presence of inflammation	
Presence of causative agent (i.e., HSV, etc.)	
Nonkeratinizing epithelium	
Epithelial edema	
Vascular congestion	

HSV, herpes simplex virus; N:C, nuclear:cytoplasmic.

dysplasia from reactive changes. While this test is by no means specific, the presence of large numbers of p53 immunoreactive cells (as opposed to only isolated positive cells) is much more likely to be present in areas of dysplasia than in reactive lesions.

Both radiation and/or chemotherapy, particularly in the setting of neoadjuvant therapy, may induce mucosal changes that mimic dysplasia. Individual cells may have irregular contours and contain hyperchromatic nuclei as well as abnormal mitotic figures. Often the latter have a ring shape, a feature not found in neoplastic cells, which helps avoid overdiagnosing dysplasia or carcinoma in this setting.

A final pitfall in the diagnosis is the examination of biopsies that are not representative of the mucosal changes. This generally results from superficial biopsies that do not contain lamina propria so that areas of invasive carcinoma cannot be excluded and very superficial biopsies that may miss pagetoid spread of a tumor along the basal part of the mucosa.

Early Esophageal Cancers

The term *early esophageal cancer* is used by the Japanese and Chinese to designate a neoplastic process that is confined to the mucosa or submucosa, regardless of the nodal status. For these pathologists, early esophageal cancers include both areas of dysplasia and superficially invasive cancer with and without nodal metastases. The small proportion of early cancers that become symptomatic and/or have abnormal radiographic features are most likely to be protruding lesions. The prognosis in early lesions is good and progression to advanced cancer is slow (74). It takes a little more than 1 year to progress from mucosal involvement to submucosal invasion, 6.6 ± 3.2 months to progress from submucosal invasion to advanced disease, and 21.1 ± 6.8 months to progress from mucosal to advanced disease (75).

Early cancers may be multicentric or consist of large fields of invasive or microinvasive cancer associated with varying degrees of epithelial dysplasia. Several macroscopic types of early carcinoma are recognized: Flat, coarse, verrucous, polypoid, and ulcerating infiltrating (76). Most appear as areas of redness, plaques, or maplike erosions. The frequency of multicentric esophageal SCC ranges from 7% to 28% (76,77). Flat, early lesions may be difficult to detect endoscopically or in resected specimens. Lugol staining of the specimen highlights the abnormal areas and allows one to assess the extent of the disease and to detect the presence of multiple lesions.

Several histologic patterns of early esophageal cancer exist: (a) conventional SCC, (b) SCC with basaloid features and expansile growth, and (c) SCC with spindle cell features (76,78). Tumor cells invading the submucosa appear larger than the dysplastic cells. Areas of dysplasia often surround the invasive foci. Basaloid tumors tend to show prominent peripheral nuclear palisading and the invasive cells tend to appear smaller than those of ordinary SCC. Basaloid tumors tend to be superficial and lack metastases, thus having a better prognosis than other histologic types (78). The earliest

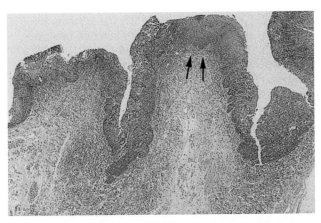

FIG. 3.7. Carcinoma in situ and early squamous cell carcinoma. The intraepithelial neoplasia sends short fingerlike extensions into the underlying lamina propria. A marked lymphocytic infiltrate accompanies the lesion. There is a small patch of nearly normal epithelium (*arrows*). (Case courtesy of Masaki Mori, Department of Surgical Oncology, Medical Institute of Bioregulation, Kyushu University, Beppu, Japan.)

invasive lesions appear to drop off the base of the mucosa. The overlying mucosa may or may not be involved by full-thickness replacement by intraepithelial neoplasia (Fig. 3.7). Progression from noninvasive to invasive disease associates with an increased lymphocytic reaction (Fig. 3.7).

Identifying superficially invasive cancers in resection specimens is usually not a diagnostic problem. However, the interpretation of small endoscopic biopsies may be challenging. The distinction of malignancy from pseudoepitheliomatous hyperplasia in regenerating squamous epithelium in the setting of esophagitis poses the greatest difficulty. Regenerating squamous cells generally do not show abnormal mitoses or loss of polarity.

When a cancer is superficial and not associated with nodal metastases, endoscopic mucosal resection (EMR) may be the treatment of choice since it incurs less morbidity and a smaller risk of mortality than esophagectomy. This procedure is now widely used in Japan. Single or multiple areas of the mucosa unstained by iodine identify resection targets. Recurrence after EMR varies from 2% to 4%, but may be treated by repeat EMR.

Patient survival with SCC correlates with the extent of the tumor, and there are several systems used to assess the stage of this disease. The different systems shown in Table 3.6 have been used to stage the SCCs and each has advantages in certain situations. The T (tumor) N (node) M (metastasis) system is used by the American Joint Committee for Cancer Staging and End Results (AJCC) (79) and the WHO classification (1). When preceded by a lowercase "p", the TNM values are based on pathology findings. When preceded by lowercase "yp", the TNM values represent pathology review of a tumor that has been previously treated (80). A simplified system used by the Surveillance, Epidemiology, and End Results (SEER) registries is frequently used in epidemiologic studies of incidence and

TABLE 3.6 Comparison of Staging Systems for Esophageal Squamous Cell Cancer

AJCC (6th ed.)	Modified Dukes[a]	SEER
Stage O TisN0M0	A	Localized
Stage I T1N0M0	A	Localized
Stage IIA T2N0M0	A	Localized
T3N0M0	B	Localized
Stage IIB T1N1M0	C1	Regional
T2N1M0	C1	Regional
Stage III T3N1M0	C1	Regional
T4 Any N M0	CII (>3+Nodes)	Regional
Stage IV Any T Any N M1	CII (>3+Nodes)	Distant

AJCC, American Joint Committee for Cancer; SEER, Surveillance, Epidemiology, and End Results.

[a] From Parenti AR, Rugge M, Frizzera E, et al: p53 overexpression in multistep process of esophageal carcinogenesis. *Am J Surg Pathol* 1995;19:1418.

mortality since it generates data comparable to those from the large, population-based international registries that are published by the International Agency for Cancer Research (13). Tachibana et al. (81) proposed a modified Dukes system to bypass international variations in the use of the TNM system. One variable not included in these systems is tumor size even though this is an independent predictor of 1- and 2-year survivals among patients with node-negative cancers (82). The number of involved lymph nodes also correlates with mortality (82).

In countries such as China and Japan, where a large proportion of SCCs are diagnosed at an early stage, a more discriminating assessment of prognosis of early cancers is achieved by dividing them into three levels of mucosal and submucosal penetration (Fig. 3.8) (83). The deeper the penetration, the greater the probability is of lymph node metastases, as shown by Araki et al. (84), who found nodal spread in 35.7% of *sm3* cancers, compared with 8.3% of *sm1* lesions. This staging system is commonly used to evaluate EMR specimens. Other Japanese studies have also found lymph node metastases in approximately 30% of tumors that penetrate to the submucosa (84).

Multivariate analysis indicates that factors that increase the relative risk of recurrence with submucosal cancer are intramural metastases, vascular invasion, and nodal metastases (85). The postresection 5-year survival rates of patients with submucosal SCC vary from 44% to 96%, with the most favorable prognosis occurring in patients without vascular invasion, intramural metastases, or nodal involvement. Patients with all three of these have the least favorable prognosis (85). If metastases are found in a patient with esophageal high-grade dysplasia, or if one detects vascular and/or lymphatic vessel invasion, an undetected invasive cancer is likely to be present. Resection specimens should be extensively sampled to find the invasive focus. If none is found the possibility remains that an invasive focus remains in the patient.

Superficial Spreading Carcinoma

Superficial spreading carcinoma is defined as a tumor >5 cm in length consisting mainly of intraepithelial carcinoma with or without limited submucosal invasion. The tumor can measure up to 14 cm in length and is frequently located in the midesophagus. Like other early squamous cell lesions, the lesions may be superficial and flat, slightly elevated, slightly depressed, or superficial and distinctly depressed (86). These tumors may show well-differentiated or moderately differentiated squamous cell histologies or may be basaloid in appearance. Superficial spreading carcinomas are likely to be multicentric. These lesions are important to recognize due to the difficulty in establishing clear resection margins at the time of esophagectomy (87). The mean age of patients with superficial spreading esophageal squamous carcinoma is 56 to 63 years, with the lesion being most common in females.

Advanced Squamous Cell Carcinoma

Clinical Features

Esophageal SCC usually grows slowly. The patients may remain asymptomatic with invasive disease because the esophagus is highly distensible and tumors can grow to a considerable size before the lumen becomes sufficiently narrowed to produce symptoms. Symptomatic esophageal SCC presents with dysphagia, odynophagia, weight loss, coughing, choking, pain, and dehydration (88). Frequently patients do not complain of dysphagia, but make subtle changes in their eating habits without realizing it. Other symptoms include fever, anemia, hematemesis, melena, hoarseness, or the sensation of food "becoming stuck in the throat." A persistent hiccup may indicate the presence of laryngeal nerve paralysis or aspiration, ominous signs of advanced disease. Local tumor extension beyond the esophagus often leads to

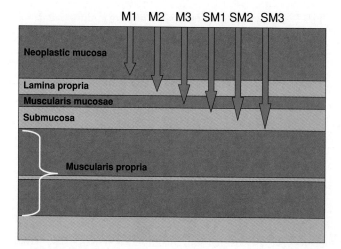

FIG. 3.8. Diagram of the system of staging mucosal and submucosal invasion.

substernal or high back pain. Aortic erosion results in rapid exsanguination. Aspiration of esophageal contents through a tracheoesophageal fistula is a common cause of death in patients with advanced SCC. Palpable lymph nodes in the cervical or supraclavicular regions may be noted.

Patients may also develop various paraneoplastic syndromes. Tumor-induced hypercalcemia is common (89). It results from the release of calcium from the bones due to tumor production of parathyroid hormone–related protein (PTHrP) (90). The presence of hypercalcemia is a poor prognostic sign (91). A hypertrophic osteoarthropathy affects some patients with esophageal SCC (92), but this may result from concomitant chronic obstructive lung disease, which shares an association with heavy tobacco consumption. An acute vasculitis developed in a patient with stage II SCC, a phenomenon attributed to circulating immune complexes or tumor-associated antigens (93). The vasculitis went into remission after tumor resection.

The AJCC divides the esophagus into three compartments (79). The cervical esophagus extends from the pharyngo-esophageal junction to the thoracic inlet, approximately 18 cm from the incisors. The middle esophagus extends from the thoracic inlet to a point 10 cm above the GEJ, approximately 31 cm from the incisors and at the level of the lower edge of the eighth thoracic vertebra. The lower esophagus extends from this point to the GEJ, or approximately 40 cm from the incisors. Carcinomas may develop in both the hypopharynx and cervical esophagus in men who are heavy consumers of alcohol and tobacco. SCCs complicating the Plummer-Vinson syndrome arise in the area of the cricopharyngeus muscle in women (male:femal ratio = 1:10) with a median age of 45 to 50 years. Cancers that appear after radiation therapy for breast cancer usually develop in the upper and mid-esophagus. Most SCCs in high-risk populations develop in the middle and lower thirds of the esophagus.

Pathologic Features

Esophageal SCCs appear as fungating, ulcerating, infiltrating, or stenotic lesions. Mixed gross growth patterns also occur. Advanced tumors may measure up to 10 cm in length. Fungating cancers present either as large, intraluminal, variably ulcerated masses with raised, everted margins or less commonly as polypoid, irregular, bulky tumor masses (Fig. 3.9).

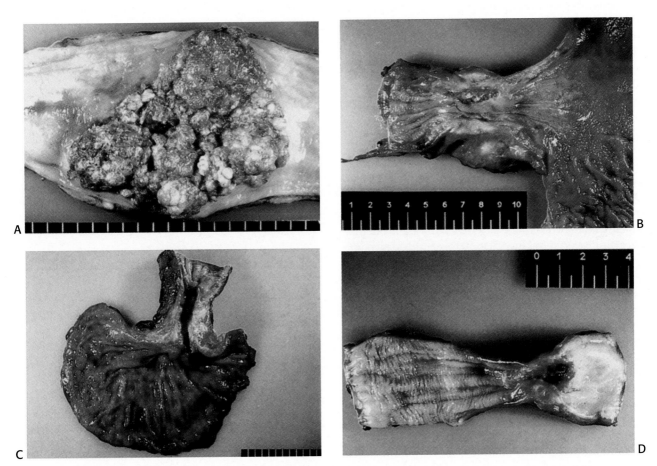

FIG. 3.9. Gross features of squamous cell carcinoma. **A:** Large fungating and polypoid excrescences of the midthoracic esophagus. **B:** Neoplastic oval ulcer of the lower thoracic esophagus. The wall of the esophagus is infiltrated and thickened. **C:** Ulcerating carcinoma of the lower thoracic esophagus with extension to the cardia. **D:** Stenosing ulcerated carcinoma with dilation proximal to the tumor.

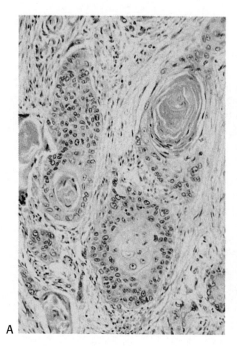
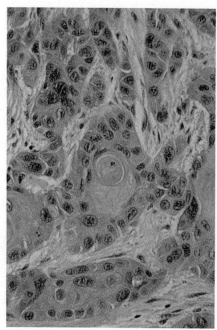

FIG. 3.10. Well-differentiated keratinizing squamous cell carcinoma. **A:** Note the infiltrating nests with prominent central keratinization. **B:** The high nuclear-to-cytoplasmic ratio is appreciated.

The lesions may have sharply defined borders; intramural sub-mucosal extension may be grossly inapparent. The extent of tumor infiltration at the tumor base varies and does not necessarily reflect the size of the protruding mass. Ulcerating cancers have irregular, noninverted, and sometimes serpiginous edges, and a shaggy, hemorrhagic central crater. The ulcers lie along the longitudinal esophageal axis and the tumors may extend into the surrounding viscera. Infiltrating carcinomas cause esophageal wall thickening. The esophagus appears rigid with slitlike areas of stenosis. The proximal esophagus dilates. Rarely, the pattern resembles the linitis plastica pattern seen in gastric carcinoma. Papillary or verrucous lesions usually develop in the proximal esophagus. Their differential diagnosis includes a papilloma, sarcomatoid carcinoma, and verrucous carcinoma.

Biopsies cannot determine the extent of invasion, but they yield a positive diagnosis in 81% to 100% of cases, depending on the number of biopsies obtained. Endoscopic ultrasonography (EUS) may identify tumor penetration to the submucosa or muscularis propria in up to 80% of early cases (94). EUS is most useful in identifying the superficial lesions that are best treated by surgery alone. Detection of nodal involvement is more accurate with EUS than with tomography (95). Fine needle aspirations enhance the ability of EUS to detect nodal disease, yielding an accuracy of more than 90% (96).

SCCs arise from areas of pre-existing dysplasia and invade through the basement membrane into the lamina propria or deeper tissues. Histologically, ordinary SCCs show varying grades of differentiation ranging from a well-differentiated keratinizing carcinoma containing well-formed squamous cell nests and keratin pearls to undifferentiated tumors without recognizable keratin or prickle cells. The tumors are classified into well-, moderately, and poorly differentiated lesions based on how closely they resemble mature nonneoplastic squamous

cells (Figs. 3.10 to 3.12). As the lesions become less mature, they show progressive degrees of pleomorphism and loss of keratinization and intercellular bridges. The degree of keratinization and the prominence of intercellular bridges inversely correlate with the degree of cytologic atypia and nuclear pleomorphism, although one occasionally sees marked keratinization of highly atypical cells. Most tumors are well- to moderately differentiated lesions. *Well-differentiated keratinizing* carcinomas have a high proportion of large differentiated squamous cells (Fig. 3.10) and a low proportion of small basal-type cells, which are typically located at the periphery of the tumor cell nests. The tumors contain squamous cell nests, dyskeratotic cells, and keratin pearls. Less well-differentiated tumors consist of cellular masses containing

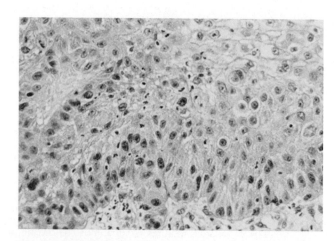

FIG. 3.11. Moderately differentiated invasive squamous cell carcinoma. Note the absence of marked atypia, keratinization, and pearl formation.

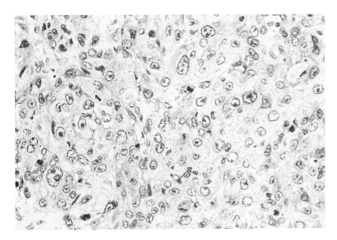

FIG. 3.12. Poorly differentiated invasive squamous cell carcinoma. Note the high degree of atypia and the brisk mitotic index.

polygonal, round, fusiform, or, rarely, small nonkeratinizing cells. *Poorly differentiated carcinomas* typically contain an abundance of basaloid cells and the degree of differentiation often varies throughout the tumor. Most poorly differentiated SCCs contain some foci of squamous differentiation such as dyskeratotic epithelial nests, keratin pearls, or intercellular bridges. They generally appear as invasive sheets of cells with prominent areas of central necrosis. Occasionally, areas of

individual cell necrosis in poorly differentiated tumors produce a pseudoacinar pattern, but mucicarmine stains are negative. Typically the degree of differentiation varies throughout the tumor. In *undifferentiated lesions*, one may not recognize keratin or prickle cells, and one has difficulty identifying the tumor as squamous in nature. Most tumors contain at least focal histologically identifiable squamous differentiation with evidence of epithelial nests, pearls, or intercellular bridges. Cytokeratin 14 immunostains may help identify a tumor as being squamous cell in origin (97).

As the tumor cells infiltrate the esophageal wall, they may form sheetlike nests with rounded margins or they may have an asteroid shape with spiculated margins. Tumors with an asteroid configuration are more likely to show deep penetration, lymphatic permeation, nodal metastases, and desmoplasia and have a worse prognosis than those with rounded borders (98). Tumors with downward penetration are more likely to show vascular and lymphatic invasion (Fig. 3.13).

Patients treated preoperatively with chemotherapy or chemoradiation may show complete tumor ablation, partial regression with a reduced tumor:stroma ratio, or residual unaltered tumor cells, sometimes resulting in a stricture (Figs. 3.14 and 3.15). Tissues examined within 3 to 6 days of preoperative treatment show pronounced apoptotic changes, with or without necrosis. Most tumor cells appear extensively degenerated. The tumor may completely disappear, creating a

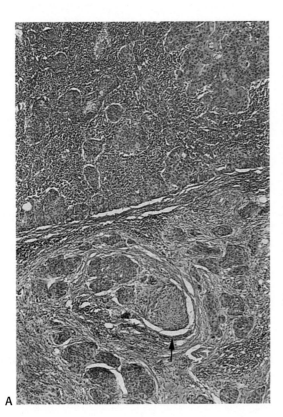
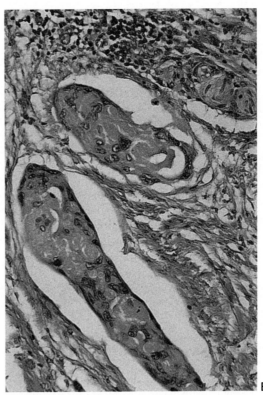

FIG. 3.13. Moderately differentiated squamous cell carcinoma involving the regional lymphatics and lymph node. **A:** The lymph node has become secondarily involved with a moderately to poorly differentiated tumor. The nerve outside of the lymph node is also surrounded by tumor (*arrow*). **B:** Tumor within lymphatic spaces.

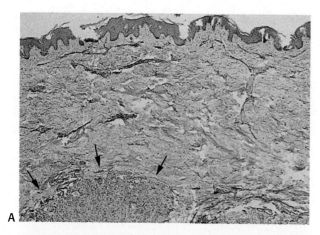

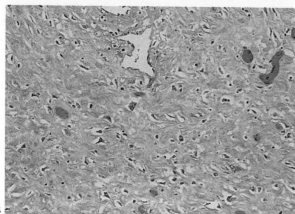

FIG. 3.14. Esophagus following radiotherapy. **A:** Low-power magnification showing the presence of a recurrent tumor (*arrows*) deep in the wall of the esophagus. The superficial tissues have become markedly sclerotic. The overlying epithelium is hyperplastic but nonneoplastic. **B:** Higher magnification shows the presence of the dense, sclerotic, submucosal tissues with atypical stellate-shaped radiation fibroblasts.

partially re-epithelialized ulcer containing granulation tissue heavily infiltrated by lymphocytes. Calcification may be present. Fibrosis in the muscularis propria causes shrinkage of the muscle bundles. Tumor regression can be graded (99), although this is not commonly done.

Cytologic Features

Cytologic evaluation of the esophagus is important as noted above. Exfoliated malignant cells from intraepithelial squamous cell carcinomas may be obtained by means of esophageal washings. These cells resemble those of carcinoma in situ of the cervix without evidence of keratinization. Abundant cell samples are usually obtained from SCCs. Paradoxically, large fungating growths frequently associate with inadequate material; false-positive results are rare in this setting. Well-differentiated carcinomas shed highly atypical and partly keratinized cells with bizarre

shapes, anisocytosis, and hyperchromatic nuclei (Fig. 3.16). Malignant pearl formations may be observed. Moderately and poorly differentiated squamous cell carcinomas exfoliate single or clustered immature atypical cells with increased nuclear:cytoplasmic ratios and either pale nucleoli or dark angulated nuclei containing large amounts of heterochromatin (Fig. 3.17).

Tumor Spread

SCC spreads within the esophageal wall, invading the muscularis propria and extending into the periesophageal tissues. Mediastinitis, pleural fistulas, and empyema may develop. Depending on tumor location, invasion into the trachea, bronchi, aorta, pleural cavity, lung, thyroid, lymph nodes, pericardium, major vessels, and/or nerves occur. Malignant tracheoesophageal fistulas develop in up to 28% of patients (100). Eventually the tumors become fixed to surrounding structures, including the diaphragm, mainstem bronchi, aortic arch, or the great veins of the neck. At this point, the lesion is unresectable.

Intramural intralymphatic vascular spread is common; lymphatic extension produces submucosal nodules distant from the main tumor in up to 16% of esophageal carcinomas (85). The esophageal lymphatics drain into the mediastinal lymphatics leading to regional spread early in the disease. In Western populations, up to 61% of patients show local extension and nodal involvement at the time of diagnosis (101). Cervical nodes become involved in 19% to 60% of cases, mediastinal nodes in 21% to 64%, and abdominal nodes in 47%. Tumors of the cervical region metastasize to infraclavicular, peritracheal, supraclavicular, paraesophageal, and posterior mediastinal lymph nodes. Tumors of the upper and midesophagus commonly involve the paraesophageal, posterior, and tracheobronchial nodes. Lower esophageal tumors disseminate to paraesophageal, celiac, and splenic and hepatic artery lymph nodes. However, the distribution of nodal metastases does not always reflect the site of the primary tumor, since 40% of cervical esophageal tumors metastasize to abdominal nodes; 38% of lower esophageal carcinomas metastasize to cervical nodes (101). Extrathoracic nodal metastases represent distant metastases. The number of positive nodes is higher in distal cancers than in upper or midesophageal cancers. Simultaneous metastases to lymph nodes in the neck, mediastinum, and abdomen occur far more commonly in lower esophageal cancers than in upper and midesophageal cancers. In some cases, the appearance of a supraclavicular, cervical, or abdominal metastasis may precede detection of the primary tumor.

Hematogenous metastases occur late in the disease, usually following nodal metastases. The most common metastatic sites include liver (35% to 72%), lungs (20% to 60%), adrenals (35%), kidneys (25% to 26%), bones (9% to 20%), adrenal gland (5%), peritoneum (2%), and, rarely, the central nervous system (2%) (101).

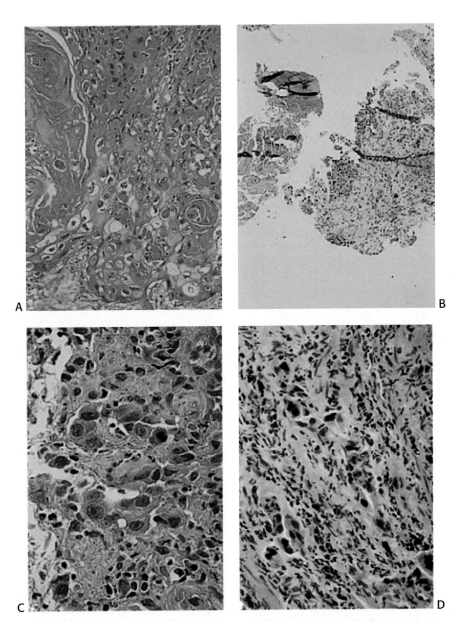

FIG. 3.15. Squamous cell carcinoma (SCC) following radiotherapy. **A:** Most of the tumor appears viable, although the cytoplasm is vacuolated and some nuclei appear pyknotic. **B:** Biopsy of a stenotic area in a patient several years after radiotherapy for SCC. The tissue fragments contain squamous epithelial cells and a highly cellular stroma. **C:** Higher magnification of the epithelial component of the tumor shows marked cytologic atypia and a disorderly architecture. **D:** The stroma contains infiltrating squamous cell nests as well as atypical stromal cells secondary to the radiation.

Molecular Alterations

SCC induction and progression result from genetic and epigenetic changes in genes controlling cell cycling, cell growth, DNA repair, and tumor dissemination (see Fig. 3.18). A brief summary of immunostains that may be useful in the diagnosis of dysplasia and in determining the prognosis of esophageal SCC follows. Abnormalities in p53 expression are common in esophageal SCCs occurring early in

tumor development (102). A significantly greater frequency of p53 expression occurs in high-grade dysplasia versus low-grade dysplasia and in low-grade versus normal esophageal mucosa (103). p53 expression had no influence on survival in one study (104), was a marker for radioresistance in another study (105), and in another had no predictive value in patients receiving either chemoradiation therapy or radiation alone (106). Cyclin D overproduction or production at the wrong time may stimulate

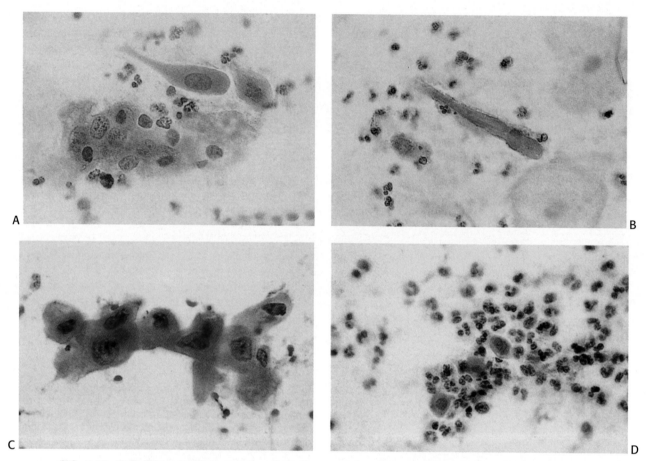

FIG. 3.16. Well-differentiated squamous cell carcinoma of the esophagus. **A–D:** Variably shaped cells are found singly and in small groups.

inappropriate cell division. Tumors showing *cyclin* amplification tend to invade deeply (107). Cyclin D overexpression increases in frequency from 22% in well-differentiated cancers to 54% in poorly differentiated tumors (107), but is not a useful prognostic marker. Cyclin B1 expression, however, associates with poor prognosis in both univariate and multivariate analyses (108).

Expression of epithelial growth factor receptor (EGFR), c-erbB2, Int-2, transforming growth factor-alpha (TGF-α), and human stomach cancer transforming factor (HST-1) has prognostic significance for SCC. EGFR overexpression occurs in 40.65% to 71% of esophageal SCC (109) (Fig. 3.18) and correlates with nodal metastases and depth of invasion. Immunoreactivity for TGF-α in esophageal SCC ranges from 35% to 78% (109,110) and associates with lower survival than seen in TGF-α–negative cancers ($p < 0.01$). Survival is poorest with cancers that overexpress both EGFR and TGF-α (111). Amplification of *HST-1* affects approximately 50% of SCCs, associating with hematogenous spread (112). Expression of vascular endothelial growth factor (VEGF), a selective mitogen for endothelial cells, correlates with microvessel density adjacent to the tumor. Shortened survival has been observed in VEGF-positive esophageal SCCs in most studies (113), but not all (114).

Degradation of extracellular matrix components by matrix serine proteinases (MSPs) is essential for tumor invasion. Esophageal SCC trypsin (an MSP) production correlates with the depth of invasion, TNM stage, and probability of recurrence (115). Matrix metalloproteinases (MMPs) also play a role in this process. Trypsin activates matrilysin, an MMP. Expression of both proteinases increases the probability of recurrence and mortality. Cytoplasmic overexpression of heparinase, an enzyme that cleaves the carbohydrate chains of heparin sulfate proteoglycans, associates with poor survival (116). Its expression is related to the depth of invasion, the TNM stage, and nodal metastases.

Prognostic Factors

The prognosis of esophageal SCC is influenced by patient age and gender (117); nutritional status (118); tumor location, size, and stage; proliferative rate (119); histologic differentiation; growth pattern; tumor resectability (120); and the presence of micrometastases, as determined by immunohistochemistry

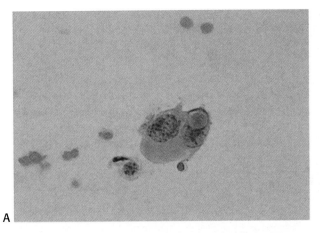

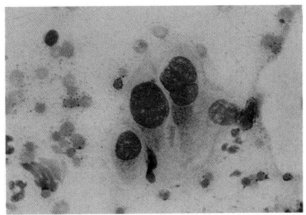

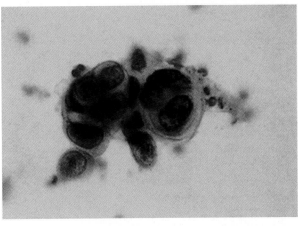

FIG. 3.17. Moderately to poorly differentiated squamous cell carcinoma of the esophagus. **A:** Two large hyperchromatic cells: one has ingested an erythrocyte. **B:** Cluster of hyperchromatic cells (May-Grunwald-Giemsa). **C:** Poorly differentiated squamous cell carcinoma.

(121). Esophageal SCCs in young adults are significantly larger and more likely to associate with nodal metastases when compared to older patients (122). Patients undergoing esophagectomy for SCC have a less favorable long-term prognosis than those with adenocarcinoma, experience higher postoperative mortality, and have more frequent lymph node metastases in early-stage tumors. In one study approximately 68% of esophageal cancers were resectable. Of these, 30.3% of SCCs were 5-year survivors, compared to 42.3% of adenocarcinomas (123).

Tumor stage is an important prognostic factor. Most esophageal SCCs in Western countries are detected at an advanced stage and have a very poor prognosis. The SEER registries note that only 23% of men and 29% of women with esophageal SCC have localized disease; only 7% of men and 10% of women are 5-year survivors (124). The 5-year survival rate exceeds 95% for stage 0 disease and is 50% to 80% for stage II, 30% to 40% for stage IIA, 10% to 30% for stage IIIB, and 10% to 15% for stage III disease (125). Patients with stage IV disease treated with palliative chemotherapy have a median survival of <1 year (126). Tumors that completely infiltrate the esophageal wall or extend beyond it have a very poor prognosis. Patients with a malignant tracheoesophageal fistula have a median survival

time of 1.4 months after the development of the fistula (127). Disease-specific survival also correlates with the presence and number of nodal metastases. The 5-year survival is 92.2% for node-negative patients compared to 58.4% for patients with one to four positive nodes and 21.3% for those with five or more positive nodes (128). In one study, 31.7% of esophageal SCCs originally classified as node-negative by routine histopathologic examination exhibited micrometastases when the nodes were examined immunohistochemically (129). Immunohistochemically detected micrometastases exhibit the same poor prognosis as those in which the metastases are detected by hematoxylin and eosin (H&E) stains. Gastric involvement affects 8% of patients and has an extremely poor prognosis.

Tumor growth patterns also affect patient prognosis. Papillary lesions are less aggressive and present at a lower stage than other squamous cell carcinomas. Their 5-year survival rate is 71% compared to 11% for other growth patterns. The frequency of *aneuploidy* ranges from 42% to 72% (130,131). Sixty-two percent of patients with diploid tumors are 5-year survivors, compared to 34% of those with aneuploidy tumors (130). Tumors with heterogeneous DNA patterns exhibit more frequent nodal metastases than those with homogenous DNA patterns (130). Ploidy also correlates

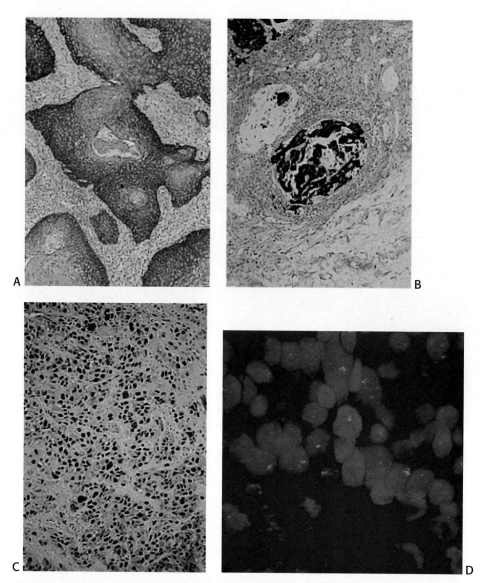

FIG. 3.18. Prognostic markers. **A:** Squamous cell carcinoma (SCC) stained for the epidermal growth factor receptor (EGFR). The tumor is strongly positive, especially at the tumor–stromal junctions. **B:** EGFR immunoreactivity of a poorly differentiated SCC present within vessels. **C:** p53 immunostain showing numerous immunoreactive cells. **D:** Fluorescence in situ hybridization for cyclin D showing the presence of multiple copies of the gene in the neoplastic cells. The nuclei are stained with propidium iodide and appear red. The cyclin D is labeled with a fluorescent probe and appears yellow. More than two copies (*yellow spots*) are seen in many cells.

with histologic grade (131), distant metastases (131), mitotic activity (131), and the presence of other genetic aberrations (132).

Treatment

The only therapy that can potentially cure esophageal SCC is complete surgical resection, including removal of the regional lymph nodes (133). Depth of tumor invasion and nodal status determine tumor resectability. Key findings that preclude esophagectomy are aortic and/or tracheobronchial invasion. Local invasion of the pericardium, diaphragm, or stomach does not preclude surgical resection in some medical centers (134). Advanced tumors with early infiltration of the tracheobronchial system may benefit from preoperative radiation to reduce tumor burden (135). Early postoperative mortality is about 10% (136) resulting from respiratory complications, pyothorax, surgical dehiscence, and hemorrhage.

In evaluating treatment data, it is important to recognize that esophagectomy with extended lymph node resection as performed in Japan differs significantly from that performed in other countries. This has implications both in terms of outcome and assignment of tumor stage. An extended lymph node dissection involving the neck, mediastinum, and abdomen (137) results in better detection of metastatic lesions. As a result, some recommend adding cervical lymph node status to the N category and combining stages IIA and IIB. The survival in the N stages can then be divided into N1 and N2 based on the number of involved lymph nodes (138).

The presence of systemic disease accounts for most treatment failures after esophagectomy. Supplemental adjuvant and neoadjuvant chemoradiation therapy may improve on the results of surgery alone. A review of 34 randomized controlled trials and six metaanalyses evaluating these approaches concluded that for patients with resectable esophageal cancer for whom surgery is appropriate, surgery alone (i.e., without neoadjuvant or adjuvant therapy) is appropriate (139). Preoperative cisplatinum-based chemotherapy trials show conflicting results (140,141). Chemotherapy may reduce SCC metastases (142). Shrinkage of the tumor by at least 50% may occur in 15% to 30% of patients treated preoperatively with fluorouracil, taxane (paclitaxel or docetaxel), or irinotecan (125). Similar results have been found in 35% to 55% of patients treated with cisplatin combined with these agents (143). While chemotherapy can palliate the symptoms in many patients, the response typically only lasts for a few months and survival is usually short.

Tumor recurrence is the most frequent cause of death in patients with resectable disease. The carcinoma may recur locally, in lymph nodes, or at distant sites or disseminate throughout the thorax and/or abdomen (144). Factors favoring recurrence include male sex, moderate to poor differentiation, presence of nodal metastasis, stage IIB or worse disease, and incomplete resection. A common reason for inadequate resection is the failure to recognize the extent of the submucosal spread. Submucosal extension to the resection margins associates with an increased risk of anastomosis dehiscence, a potentially fatal complication. Therefore, surgeons usually place the resection line well beyond the margins of visible carcinoma. Even with this approach, as many as 35% of patients have residual cancer in the tumor margins. For this reason, many surgeons monitor resection margins with frozen sections to detect unsuspected submucosal tumor extension.

Special Variants of Squamous Cell Carcinoma

There are several squamous cell carcinoma variants (Table 3.7).

Undifferentiated Carcinoma

Undifferentiated carcinomas lack definitive light microscopic features of differentiation, although some ultrastructural and immunohistochemical features of squamous differentiation may be present (1). The tumors constitute up to 20% of esophageal cancers (145) and belong in the group of

TABLE 3.7 Histologic Variants of Squamous Cell Carcinoma
Conventional squamous cell carcinoma
Sarcomatoid carcinoma
Verrucous carcinoma
Basaloid carcinoma
Carcinoma with lymphoid stroma
Carcinoma associated with Epstein-Barr virus
Adenoacanthoma
Adenosquamous carcinoma
Undifferentiated carcinoma

poorly differentiated SCCs (Fig. 3.19). Undifferentiated cancers tend to be large tumors that penetrate to the esophageal adventitia, spread to regional nodes, and associate with poor survival. The immunohistochemical profile of these cancers is consistent with their highly malignant properties and include reduced expression of cell–cell adhesion molecules (E-cadherin, thrombomodulin), high expression of Ki-67, and no expression of p21 (146). Poorly differentiated carcinomas may coexpress keratin and vimentin, desmin, or neurofilament proteins (147), especially after chemoradiation.

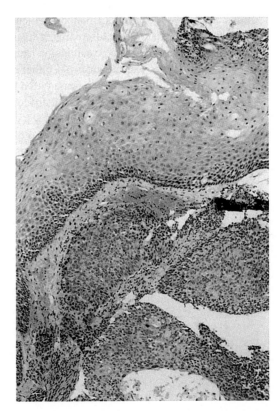

FIG. 3.19. Undifferentiated squamous cell carcinoma (SCC). An undifferentiated SCC dissects beneath the more or less normal squamous epithelium above it.

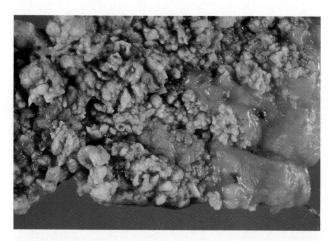

FIG. 3.20. Verrucous carcinoma. Note the multiple warty outgrowths of the tumor. Part of the lesion was a spike condyloma.

Verrucous Carcinoma

Verrucous squamous cell carcinoma is a distinct, well-differentiated SCC variant. This very rare tumor typically associates with chronic esophagitis, usually developing in the distal esophagus (148). Associated medical conditions include achalasia, gastroesophageal reflux disease, caustic injury, and esophageal diverticula. Because of its slow growth, symptom onset is insidious and there is usually a long delay between development of dysphagia and detection of the lesion. Grossly these tumors appear as exophytic warty, papillary, spiked, or cauliflowerlike masses (Fig. 3.20). The tumors consist of very well-differentiated keratinized squamous epithelium with cytologic atypia that may be so minimal that the pattern mimics benign squamous proliferations (Fig. 3.21). The tumors exhibit a pushing rather than an infiltrating margin. Superficial biopsies show only nonspecific acanthosis, parakeratosis, and hyperkeratosis, making it very difficult to make the correct diagnosis. Invasion of the wall of the esophagus is

its distinguishing feature and may be detected by ultrasonography. A fully resected specimen may be needed to confirm this. Morbidity and mortality result from local invasion. The tumors have a very low potential for metastases.

Squamous Cell Carcinoma with Lymphoid Stroma

SCC with lymphoid stroma is a rare variant of esophageal SCC and some tumors contain Epstein-Barr virus (EBV) DNA sequences (149). The tumors are poorly differentiated, penetrate into the muscularis propria, and may be focally necrotic (Fig. 3.22). Broad inflammatory cell infiltrates containing lymphocytes, plasma cells, neutrophils, macrophages, and eosinophils separate individual tumor cell nests. The infiltrating lymphocytes consist of a large number of T cells around tumor cell nests and a small number of B cells (149). Well-formed lymphoid follicles with and without germinal centers are present at the periphery. It may be difficult to distinguish the neoplastic epithelium from the lymphoid stroma without immunostains for epithelial and/or lymphocytic differentiation. These tumors resemble medullary carcinomas of the stomach.

Squamous Cell Carcinoma in Barrett Esophagus

SCCs may arise in the squamous mucosa just above Barrett esophagus (150), often in areas of high-grade squamous dysplasia. The invasive SCC and the squamous cell dysplasia are separated from the Barrett mucosa by normal squamous epithelium. These tumors resemble other SCCs.

Spindle Cell Carcinoma

Synonyms for spindle cell carcinoma include polypoid carcinoma with spindle cell features, pseudosarcoma, spindle cell carcinoma, carcinosarcoma, metaplastic carcinoma, carcinoma with mesenchymal stroma, and sarcomatoid carcinomas.

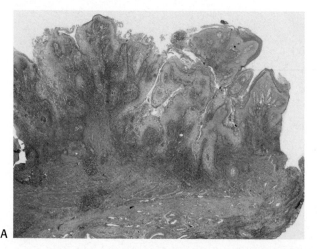

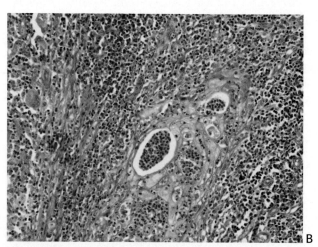

FIG. 3.21. Verrucous carcinoma. **A:** The lesion shows a well-differentiated squamous cell carcinoma (*left*) that arose in a condylomalike lesion (seen at the *right* of the picture). **B:** The metastases in regional lymph nodes are less well differentiated.

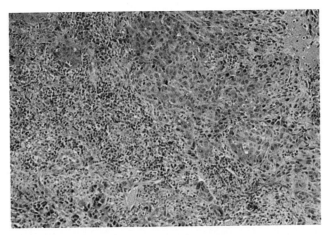

FIG. 3.22. Invasive carcinoma with lymphoid stroma. An invasive poorly differentiated squamous cell carcinoma is present. It is associated with large numbers of inflammatory cells.

Spindle cell carcinomas are biphasic tumors characterized by a typical SCC pattern or carcinoma in situ admixed with a spindle cell component. These carcinomas show varying degrees of "mesenchymal" differentiation (151–153). Most observers believe that the epithelial and mesenchymal components of the tumor arise by divergent differentiation from a common progenitor cell. Spindle cell carcinomas account

for 0.3% to 1.75% of esophageal malignancies (151). Some tumors arise on a background of BE. Most patients with spindle cell carcinomas present with slowly developing dysphagia and weight loss. Vomiting, regurgitation, and epigastric or retrosternal pain frequently occur. Because of their polypoid growth, they become symptomatic early and therefore present at a lower stage than typical SCCs. An unusual patient presented with leukocytosis and granulocytic hyperplasia due to high serum levels of granulocyte–colony-stimulating factor (G-CSF) produced by both the epithelial and sarcomatous components of the cancer. The peripheral white count and cerebrospinal fluid (G-CSF) levels reverted to normal after removal of the tumor (154).

Spindle cell carcinomas are typically polypoid, with 7% developing in the upper third and 82% to 93% arising in the middle and lower third of the esophagus. Most lesions are large lobulated masses with mucosal erosions (Fig. 3.23). They range in size from 1 to 15 cm (151,153). The tumors may have a broad base or, less frequently, are attached by a slender pedicle, measuring up to 2 cm in length. Occasionally, they may be flat with surface ulceration resembling a more typical esophageal SCC (153,155). Multiple satellite nodules may lie in the adjacent mucosa (155). On cut section, the tumors appear gray-white, soft, and fleshy. At the time of diagnosis, 80% are confined to the esophageal wall. Metastases of the regional lymph nodes, liver, and skin occur late in the disease (153).

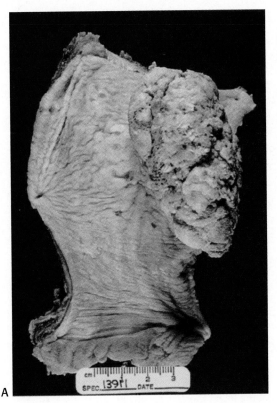
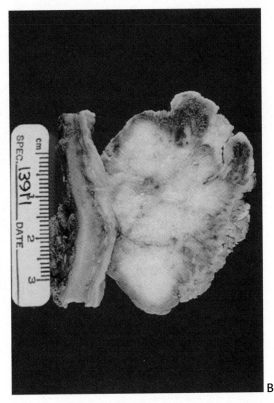

A   B

FIG. 3.23. Sarcomatoid carcinoma. **A:** A polypoid exophytic spindle cell carcinoma. **B:** Cross section shows the exophytic tumor to be confined to the area above the mucosa. It is attached to the mucosa by a small stalk.

Characteristically, spindle cell carcinomas have a clearly identifiable squamous cell component consisting of invasive SCC and/or squamous cell dysplasia in the adjacent mucosa. However, surface necrosis or tumor growth may erode any residual intraepithelial neoplasia. The invasive SCC may appear well- to poorly differentiated. Other types of carcinoma may be present, including those with basaloid, neuroendocrine, glandular, adenoid cystic, or undifferentiated growth patterns (151,155). The epithelial components of spindle cell carcinoma are best seen at its base and in the adjacent mucosa. Mitotic activity in different areas of the tumor can be quite brisk.

The spindle cell component typically forms the majority of the tumor mass (Figs. 3.24 to 3.26). It varies from a bland proliferation of spindle-shaped cells with little or no pleomorphism to areas showing marked pleomorphism with bizarre giant cells similar to those seen in malignant fibrous histiocytomas. Mitoses are frequent. Some tumors show cartilaginous,

osseous, or rhabdomyoblastic differentiation. Multinucleated cells resembling osteoclasts may also be present (153). The epithelial areas are often sharply demarcated from the more spindled areas. Transition zones between the two cell populations are frequently present. An edematous, myxoid, or collagenized stroma may be admixed with inflammatory cells and prominent blood vessels. There is a greater level of proliferation and a higher level of aneuploidy in the sarcomatous components than in the epithelial components, giving the sarcomatous phenotype a growth advantage, allowing it to become the predominant part of the tumor (156).

The squamous component typically expresses high-molecular-weight cytokeratin (Fig. 3.26), whereas the spindle cells variably express cytokeratin, vimentin (Fig. 3.26), desmin, and smooth muscle actin. Cytokeratin positivity is present in 50% to 65% of the spindle cell areas. Cytokeratin staining may be strong and diffusely positive, or may be scattered and faint. Vimentin antibodies strongly stain the sarcomatoid areas

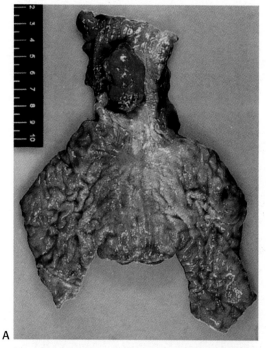

A

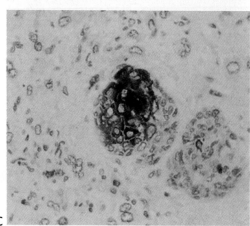

C

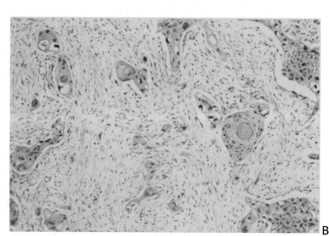

B

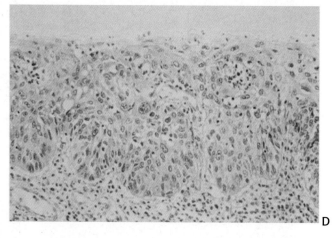

D

FIG. 3.24. Sarcomatoid carcinoma. **A:** Polypoid pedunculated lesion of the lower thoracic esophagus. **B:** Nests of squamous cell carcinoma (SCC) within a cellular moderately atypical stroma. **C:** Epithelial cell nest positive for keratin. Note the negativity of the stroma. **D:** Intraepithelial SCC adjacent to the tumor mass.

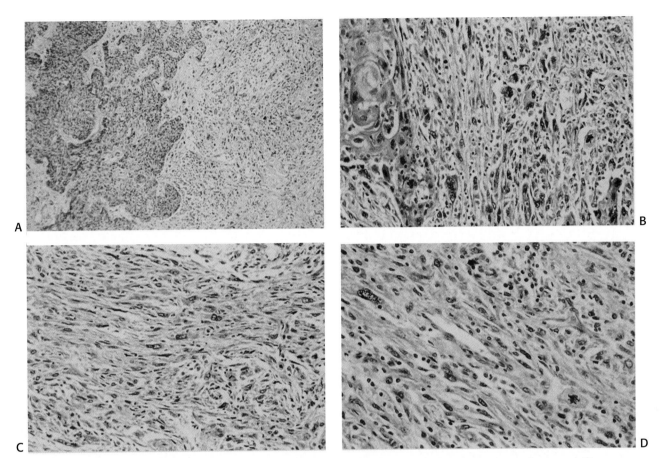

FIG. 3.25. Sarcomatoid carcinoma. **A:** The recognizable epithelial component shows varying degrees of differentiation. **B:** Areas of tumor cells show mesenchymal cell features with marked cytologic atypia. An epithelial component is on the *left*. **C:** In this area the sarcomatous component resembles a fibrosarcoma. **D:** Here the sarcomatous component resembles a malignant fibrous histiocytoma.

and sometimes stain the epithelial areas. E-cadherin is expressed in the epithelial cells and is absent from the spindle cells (159).

The differential diagnosis includes true sarcomas, malignant melanoma, and inflammatory pseudotumors. Diffuse strong staining for myogenous markers supports a diagnosis of leiomyosarcoma, although smooth muscle tumors can sometimes stain with antibodies to cytokeratin and some sarcomatoid carcinomas may express muscle antigens. Malignant melanoma markers include melan-A, HMB45, and S100. Inflammatory pseudotumors lack cytologic anaplasia and the abnormal mitotic figures that characterize sarcomatoid carcinomas.

The prognosis of patients with spindle cell carcinoma resembles that of patients with pure SCCs. The tumor metastasizes to regional lymph nodes and the lung, liver, brain, and adrenal glands. The metastases may consist of only sarcomatoid or epithelial elements or a mixture of the two (151).

Basaloid Carcinoma

Basaloid carcinoma is a rare SCC variant, being more common in the upper aerodigestive tract. This pattern occurs in approximately 0.3% to 4.5% of primary esophageal malignant

tumors (156,157) and is more common in men than in women (male:female ratio = 7:1). It often presents in the 6th decade, but does have a wide age range from 27 to 88 years with a mean of 62 years. Dysphagia is the most common presenting symptom. The gross and endoscopic features resemble those of typical SCC. The tumors arise throughout the esophagus (156). These tumors are frequently fungating, but they may also be ulcerative and infiltrative. The tumors range in size from 10 to 90 mm (156). Early lesions resemble submucosal tumors since they are frequently covered by normal epithelium, a feature that makes their diagnosis difficult by endoscopic biopsy.

These invasive tumors arise from totipotent stem cells in the basal layer of the squamous epithelium (158). The intermediate and superficial cells show normal maturation in noninvading areas, a feature that distinguishes basal cell intraepithelial neoplasia from squamous cell intraepithelial neoplasia. The palisading pattern that characterizes normal basal cells is retained in areas of invasion. The mitotic index is high (15 to 40 mitoses/10 high-powered field [hpf]). The lobular pattern is characterized by comedonecrosis and interlobular desmoplasia. The cribriform form is characterized by glandlike squamous hyalinosis and associates with

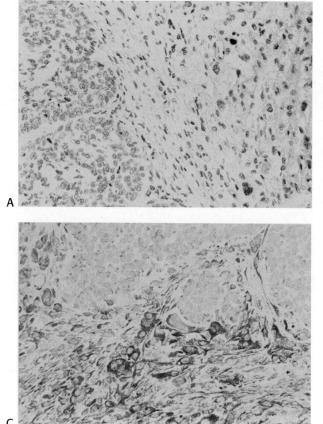

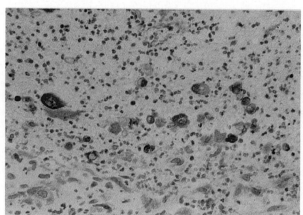

FIG. 3.26. Sarcomatoid carcinoma. **A:** Malignant epithelial (*left*) and stromal components (*right*). **B:** Antikeratin antibody stains single cells within stromal area. **C:** Antivimentin antibody localizes to more stromal cells and is also present in the epithelial cells.

the presence of basement membrane substance positive for collagen 4 and laminin (157). Comedonecrosis affects the intraepithelial component as well as its invasive nests. The lobules and nests have smooth rounded margins. Small nests tend to be solid, but large lobules frequently show central comedonecrosis. The nuclei demonstrate an open chromatin pattern and contain small nucleoli. Occasional serpentine or ribbonlike arrangements of the tumor cells remind one of neuroendocrine differentiation. The presence of squamous cell dysplasia, carcinoma in situ, or invasive cancer in the contiguous mucosa is common (158), but adenocarcinomatous or small cell carcinomatous components may also be present. Each component is usually clearly distinguishable from the others, and they metastasize separately.

Antibodies to a wide range of molecular-weight cytokeratins, such as AE1/AE3 and AE1, may show heterogeneous staining patterns with some areas being strongly positive and others being negative (78). CK14 stains 90% of the tumors (159). There is extensive to moderate neuron-specific enolase (NSE) reactivity when a small cell component is present (160), but chromogranin and other neuroendocrine markers are negative. The differential diagnosis of basaloid carcinoma includes small cell carcinoma. Both neoplasms may coexist with a squamous component and both are thought to arise from pluripotent stem cells or basal cells with multidirectional differentiating capabilities. The distinction between basal cell SCC and small cell undifferentiated carcinoma is important because of the therapeutic implications (157).

There is confusion between adenoid cystic carcinomas and the basaloid variant of SCC. These lesions may be separated from one another by the features shown in Table 3.8. Basaloid cancers are aggressive tumors with a prognosis

TABLE 3.8   Basaloid Carcinoma Versus Adenoid Cystic Carcinoma

Finding	Basaloid Carcinoma	Adenoid Cystic Carcinoma
Sex	Most common in males	Most common in females
Age	Tends to affect older individuals	Tends to affect younger persons
Clinical duration	Tends to be short	Tends to be prolonged
Myoepithelial cells	Very rare	Characteristically present
Cytologic features	Mild pleomorphism	Bland cytology
Mitoses	Numerous	Rare
Coexisting dysplasia	Present	Absent

similar to that of SCC (156). They form large tumors with lymph node metastases and commonly spread hematogenously to the lungs and liver (160). The poor prognosis of these tumors relates in part to their advanced clinical stage at the time of diagnosis. Their metastases may show only the basaloid component or may have basaloid and squamous components in different lymph nodes. The metastasis may consist only of the small cells if the small cell component is predominant in the main tumor (156).

ADENOCARCINOMA OF THE GASTROESOPHAGEAL JUNCTION

It may be impossible to determine whether a cancer straddling the GEJ arose from the gastric cardia or the distal esophagus. Cancers in both sites associate with gastroesophageal reflux disease (GERD) and BE. Cardia cancer shares the same secular trends, epidemiologic backgrounds, and molecular profiles as BE-associated adenocarcinoma (161–163) and differs in these respects from noncardiac gastric cancer (164). The following discussion bundles cardia cancer together with BE-associated esophageal adenocarcinoma as cancer at the GEJ.

Adenocarcinomas usually arise in the distal esophagus from BE. BE-associated cancers account for more than 90% of esophageal adenocarcinomas. The remainder arise from heterotopic rests or submucosal glands. The origin and morphology of BE are discussed in detail in Chapter 2. Not all GEJ cancers are of esophageal origin. Some arise from the gastric cardia or involve the esophagus by proximal extension from more distal gastric cancers. The presence of dysplasia in BE helps identify a cancer as originating in the esophagus, but this may be impossible to identify in advanced adenocarcinomas that replace the pre-existing BE.

Siewert et al separated GEJ cancer into three subgroups based on their relationship to the proximal end of the gastric folds: adenocarcinoma of an esophagogastric junction (AEG) I = cancers of the distal esophagus; AEG II = cancers of the true cardia; and AEG III = cancers of the subcardia (165). Types AEG II and III are categorized as gastric cancers in this treatment-based classification. However, as noted above, we believe that BE-associated cancers (AEG I) and cardia cancer (AEG II) are so similar with respect to patient characteristics (obese, middle-aged white men with reflux disease and no *H. pylori* gastritis), secular incidence trends, and molecular profiles that they are essentially the same cancer.

Epidemiology

The incidence of GEJ adenocarcinoma has increased by more than 350% in the United States since the mid-1970s (3). The increase has shown marked gender, geographic, and ethnic differences. The 3-year average incidence of this cancer among white males in the period 1996–1998 was 4.0 compared to 0.5 for women. A survey of 11 SEER registries found that white male rates in Seattle increased 800% from 1974–1975 to 1996–1998, compared to only 300% in Utah during the same timeframe (166). Black males had a small but significant increased incidence. The 3-year average incidence of this cancer among blacks is 0.8 compared to 4.0 among whites. A similar increased incidence occurred in Britain (167), and there was a 10-fold increased incidence in Finland since the 1970s. However, Finnish rates (1.1 per 100,000) are low compared to those in the United States or Britain (168). In contrast to Western countries, GEJ adenocarcinoma incidence rates have been stable over the past 40 years in Japan, where these tumors constitute only 0.67% of all esophageal cancers (169).

Predisposing Factors

The degree of *GERD* is more severe in BE patients with cancer than in those without it (170), and antireflux therapy does not decrease the cancer risk (171). The risk of cancer increases with the duration of GERD (172). This may explain an 11-fold increased risk of GEJ cancer among adults whose birth weights were <2,000 g (173), since GERD is very common in preterm infants. The presence and size of a *hiatal hernia* also directly correlates with the presence of both BE and adenocarcinoma (174). The presence of bile acids in the refluxate is thought to be critical to the generation of BE-associated adenocarcinomas (175,176).

Obesity consistently associates with esophageal adenocarcinoma (177), possibly due to the increased risk of GERD in this setting (178). Recent studies, however, found an independent positive association of obesity with GEJ cancer in patients without GERD (177,179). The association between the body mass index (BMI) and GEJ cancer is dose dependent in males (180), and in 17% of cases the BMI exceeds the value that defines the highest decile of the control population (181). *Smoking* and *alcohol* are consistently and directly related to GEJ cancer (247,248,251), but the risk is not as strong as that for SCC and in some studies does not reach statistical significance (172,177,181,182).

It has been proposed that interactions between salivary nitrite and gastric refluxate can activate mutagenic nitroso compounds within the Barrett mucosa (183). On entering the Barrett segment there is a substantial fall in nitrite levels, indicating a reduction of nitrite to nitric oxide (NO) at this site. High luminal NO concentrations exert nitrosative and oxidative stress, damaging DNA and inhibiting DNA repair. The decreased risk of GEJ carcinoma associated with a high intake of antioxidants (184) may result from suppression of this process (185).

H. pylori is a well-established risk factor for gastric cancer distal to the cardia (see Chapter 5). In contrast, *H. pylori* inversely correlates with GERD and GEJ cancer (186,187). As the frequency of distal gastric cancer decreased in Western countries, there was a reciprocal increase in GEJ cancers (3). The decreased gastric acidity resulting from *H. pylori*–induced gastritis prevents GERD development and its metaplastic and neoplastic consequences (188). Successful eradication of the *H. pylori* infection doubles the frequency of GERD when compared to untreated patients (189).

Medications that promote GERD through relaxation of the esophageal sphincter, such as anticholinergics, may increase the risk of esophageal adenocarcinoma (190), while medications that inhibit prostaglandin synthesis and block prostaglandin-induced immunosuppression may protect against BE-associated cancer (191).

Genetic Factors

It appears that there may be a genetic susceptibility to the development of carcinomas arising in the setting of BE. The fact that these cancers develop almost exclusively in white males suggests the involvement of an as yet unknown genetic factor in the development of the disease. In addition, there are familial forms of the disease that appear to have an auto-somal dominant mode of inheritance (192,193). Genetic polymorphisms may also play important roles in determining the risk of developing this tumor. An association has been shown for polymorphisms in *glutathione S-transferase P1* (*GSTP-1*) and BE-associated adenocarcinoma (194). *GSTP-1* is responsible for the detoxification of various carcinogens, and inherited differences in carcinogen detoxification may play an important role in the develop of BE and its associated carcinoma. There is also an association between the *MTHFR 677TT* variant and esophageal adenocarcinoma (43). A number of genetic alterations characterize the development of neoplasia in areas of BE. Among the most common and earliest are p53 and p16 alterations (195,196). Other alterations are listed in Table 3.9.

Dysplasia

Because dysplasia often lies adjacent to areas of invasive carcinoma, the presence of dysplasia represents both a marker of increased risk for the subsequent development of esophageal adenocarcinoma and a potential marker for the coexistence of an invasive carcinoma. The risk level correlates with the extent of high-grade dysplasia (197), but a recent study indicated that invasive cancer is as likely to accompany focal high-grade dysplasia as extensive diffuse dysplasia (198). Dysplasia is found in 5% to 10% of patients with BE (199), and increases in frequency as BE is followed over time. A cohort study of patients with BE followed for 20 years found the rate of cancer to be 1 in 274 patient-years in the presence of dysplasia, compared to 1 in 1,114 patient-years in patients without dysplasia (197). The diagnosis of dysplasia is a decisive factor in the management of patents with BE (199).

Problems in establishing a diagnosis of dysplasia include difficulties relating to sampling error, the distinction between reactive changes and dysplasia, differences in observer interpretation of the diagnosis of dysplasia, and difficulties in differentiating high-grade dysplasia from invasive carcinoma.

TABLE 3.9	**Genes and Genetic Products Involved in Barrett-associated Carcinogenesis**
Tumor Suppressor Genes	
p53	Commonly mutated in dysplasia and invasive carcinoma
p16	Hypermethylated in dysplasia
FHIT	Altered in dysplasia
APC	Mutations occur late in the dysplasia–carcinoma sequence
Rb	Loss in invasive carcinoma
Cell Cycle Regulatory Factors	
Cyclin D1	Frequently overexpressed in invasive adenocarcinomas
MDM2	Overexpression and/or amplification affect many invasive carcinomas
Growth Factor Receptors	
EGFR	Overexpressed in >75% of invasive carcinomas
TGF-A	Overexpressed in invasive carcinoma
c-erbB2	Amplified in invasive carcinomas; prognostic factor
Cell Adhesion Molecules	
E-cadherin	Loss of expression in dysplasia and invasive carcinoma
P-cadherin	Up-regulated in invasive carcinoma
α-Catenin	Loss of expression in invasive carcinoma
β-Catenin	Nuclear expression in invasive carcinoma
Proteases	
UPA	Prognostic factor in invasive carcinoma

Dysplasia has no specific gross or endoscopic features unless there is a mass lesion. Flat dysplasia is more common than a polypoid lesion. The dysplastic mucosa may be slightly raised, with or without areas of ulceration. Usually, the dysplastic foci cannot be distinguished grossly from the surrounding BE or from gastric-type mucosa. Therefore, multiple random biopsies are usually required for its detection. A protocol proposed by Levine et al (200) requires the endoscopist to obtain quadrant biopsies from three levels of the BE. However, this will sample only 3.5% of the affected mucosa, assuming that jumbo biopsy forceps are used and that a 2-cm segment of BE has a surface area of 14 cm^2 (201). It is therefore not surprising that reports of the prevalence of unsuspected invasive cancer found in resections for high-grade dysplasia esophagus vary from 0% to 75% (202).

The sampling problem is compounded by the lack of interobserver agreement on the histologic diagnosis of dysplasia, especially of low-grade dysplasia (see below). Since cytologic atypia is the defining characteristic of dysplasia, some endoscopists supplement biopsies with cytologic smears. Unfortunately, cytology may miss BE-associated adenocarcinomas that *drop off* the base of the mucosa in a manner analogous to that seen in ulcerative colitis. Because of the difficulty in recognizing dysplasia, newer imaging methodologies have been developed. These include high-resolution endoscopy, which enhances the ability to target small lesions for biopsy, and chromoendoscopy and optical coherence tomography (OCT), which are analogous to ultrasound but measure echo time delay of light rather than sound (203).

As noted, interpretation of dysplastic lesions can be quite difficult because the histologic and cytologic abnormalities form a continuous spectrum that extends from relatively mild atypia to overt dysplasia to invasive cancer. The boundaries separating negative and low-grade dysplasia, low-grade and high-grade dysplasia, and high-grade dysplasia and invasive cancer are therefore not always sharply definable. Histologically, dysplasia is defined as a benign neoplastic epithelial change that is confined within the basement membrane. The classification of dysplasia resembles that used for inflammatory bowel disease, with dysplasia being divided into high-grade, low-grade, and indefinite categories. The levels of inter- and intraobserver agreement are poor for the low-grade and indefinite categories. Although the level of agreement is better for high-grade dysplasia, substantial differences remain (204). Supplemental immunohistochemical (IHC) procedures may increase the ability to identify dysplastic mucosa (see below). However, IHC may not distinguish between low-grade and high-grade dysplasia, but may identify patients who require rebiopsy and/or careful follow-up.

A large cohort study found incidental cancer to be uncommon with BE, but the risk was significantly higher in men with low-grade dysplasia (205). Patients with low-grade dysplasia were free of cancer or high-grade dysplasia in 90% of cases at 6 years and in 80% of cases at 10 years. This suggests that there is no urgency in making a definitive diagnosis, and that careful follow-up may resolve doubts created by diverging interpretations. Inadequate sampling may result in

underdiagnosis of the degree of dysplasia. Approximately one third of resections for high-grade dysplasia have a previously unsuspected invasive cancer, even when the biopsy samples are taken according to recommended guidelines. The frequency of underdiagnosis with low-grade dysplasia cannot be determined because this diagnosis does not mandate resection. The diagnosis of low-grade dysplasia therefore establishes a need for long-term follow-up. A diagnosis of high-grade dysplasia is of critical importance. Overdiagnosis in an older, obese male (the usual BE patient) could generate substantial, but unnecessary, operative morbidity and mortality, while underdiagnosis could allow a cancer to progress from an early treatable stage to an inoperable one.

A diagnosis of dysplasia is based on both cytologic and architectural changes, including varying degrees and combinations of epithelial disarray, cytologic atypia, and architectural distortion. While both architectural and cytologic abnormalities characterize dysplastic areas, one or the other usually predominates (Figs. 3.27 and 3.28). The dysplastic epithelium may be tubular or villiform, and it may contain glands with papillary infoldings, irregular contours, or back-to-back configurations. Dysplastic crowded cells show decreased mucous secretion with nuclear irregularity, enlargement, hyperchromasia, and chromatin clumping. Increased nuclear:cytoplasmic ratios, abnormal mitotic figures, and nuclear stratification are also present. As low-grade lesions progress to high-grade dysplasia, architectural and cytologic abnormalities increase. A description of the specific lesions follows.

Negative for Dysplasia

Reactive metaplastic glands in BE may appear irregular in size and position with expanded proliferative zones containing cells with enlarged crowded nuclei and prominent centrally located nucleoli and numerous mitoses. Since a gradient of cellular differentiation extends from the base of the gland to the surface, the abnormalities remain confined to

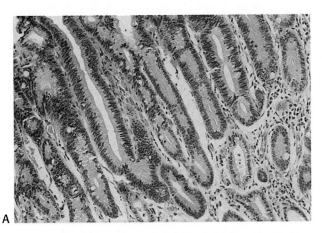
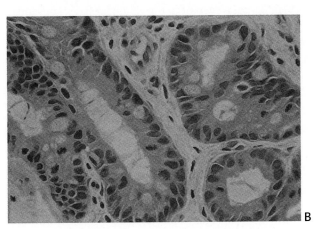

FIG. 3.27. Low-grade dysplasia in Barrett esophagus. **A:** Most of the glands are dysplastic. Some residual nondysplastic cells are seen in the lower right-hand corner. The dysplastic nuclei extend approximately halfway toward the lumen. **B:** Higher magnification of a different lesion showing loss of nuclear polarity and dysplastic goblet cells.

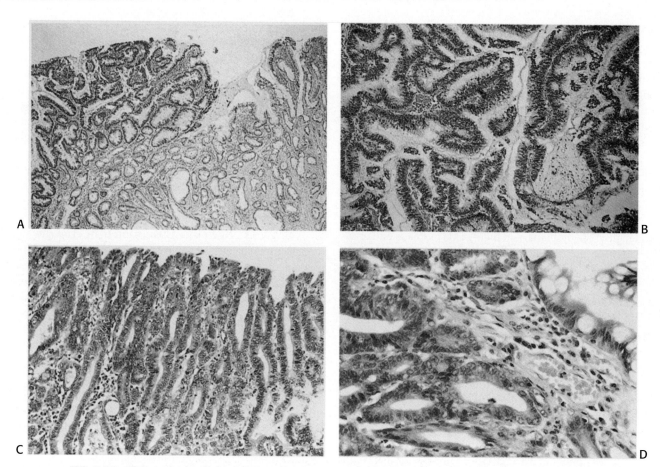

FIG. 3.28. High-grade dysplasia. **A:** Polypoid area of dysplasia resembling a colonic adenoma. It arises on a broad area of Barrett metaplasia. Note the villiform transformation on the right side of the figure. **B:** Higher magnification of the dysplastic part of lesion shown in A. Note the prominent nuclear stratification. **C:** Severe dysplasia affects the cells at the upper mucosa. The cells are beginning to lose their polarity and the glands are beginning to fuse with one another. **D:** Dysplastic glands on the left and Barrett esophagus on the upper right. Note the disorganized architecture.

the lower part of the glands while their upper portions show few abnormalities and the surface cells usually appear normal. However, it is important to note that when extreme cytologic atypia is present in the glandular bases and not at higher levels, a diagnosis of dysplasia is still warranted (see below). A diagnosis of dysplasia should not be made on the basis of villiform transformation or glandular branching since these changes may be present in either reactive or dysplastic lesions.

Indefinite for Dysplasia

Chronic reflux-induced inflammation generates overlapping inflammatory, regenerative, and dysplastic changes in BE. Therefore, it may be difficult to distinguish reactive changes from low-grade dysplasia in this setting, especially if ulceration has occurred, since both cytologic and architectural alterations may be present. The term *indefinite for dysplasia* describes the uncertainty engendered by these changes. Villiform hyperplasia with mild atypia may superficially resemble villous adenomas, creating diagnostic confusion,

especially when mucus-depleted foveolar cells resemble intestinal absorptive cells. There may also be an expansion of the proliferative zone. The glands usually show a differentiation gradient as the surface is approached in regenerative epithelium that contrasts with a shift of the proliferative zone to the surface in dysplastic lesions. However, in the face of proliferation that involves the full length of the crypt, it may be impossible to tell whether the proliferative cells are extending upward (as in regeneration) or downward (as in dysplasia). When doubt exists as to the true nature of the lesion, a diagnosis of indefinite for dysplasia is made and a repeat biopsy is performed following a course of antireflux therapy. Features that favor a reactive lesion over a dysplastic one are listed in Table 3.10.

Low-grade Dysplasia

Low-grade dysplasia is characterized by minimal or no architectural abnormalities, but the cells appear more atypical than in BE. The nuclei become elongated and stratified, but the nuclei do not reach the apical surfaces, remaining limited

TABLE 3.10	Reactive Versus Dysplastic Epithelial Features

Features shared by reactive and dysplastic epithelia
   Increased mitoses
   Nuclear enlargement
   Hyperchromasia
   Decreased intracellular mucin
   Expanded proliferative zone
Features that favor reactive changes
   Round to oval nuclei
   Smooth nuclear contours
   Evenly spaced and nonoverlapping nuclei
   Granular chromatin
   Uniform nucleolar appearance among the cells
   Nearby active inflammation
Features that favor dysplasia
   Cellular pleomorphism
   Irregular nuclear contours
   Variable hyperchromasia
   Nuclear stratification, overlapping, and crowding
   Loss of nuclear polarity
   Atypical mitoses
   Prominent apoptotic activity
   Glandular budding

to the lower three fourths of the cells. The enlarged nuclei are crowded and hyperchromatic. Goblet cell mucus is usually diminished and goblet cell dystrophy may be present (Fig. 3.27). (Goblet cell dystrophy does not, by itself, constitute a diagnosis of dysplasia.) Since the mucosa of the distal esophagus often resembles gastric mucosa, the lower portions of the glands normally exhibit a back-to-back configuration. When intestinal metaplasia involves these pre-existing glands, they will present a back-to-back appearance, which, when combined with reactive changes (increased mitoses and hyperchromatic nuclei), may prompt an erroneous diagnosis of high-grade dysplasia. This is less worrisome than a back-to-back configuration involving the upper mucosa where the mucous neck region and glandular crypts are normally separated by a loose stroma. The dysplasia often resembles early colonic tubular adenomas.

Since dysplasia usually affects the mucosal surface, mitotic figures and KI-67–labeled cells are characteristically present in this area (Fig. 3.29). p53 immunostaining may also be useful in identifying dysplasia if more than a few isolated cells are positive (Fig. 3.29).

High-grade Dysplasia

One may diagnose high-grade dysplasia by cytologic or architectural criteria, or both, since the cells have the features of malignancy. Nuclear stratification reaches the luminal surface and the nuclei lose their normal polarity. As a result, the long axis of the nucleus no longer remains perpendicular to the crypt basement membrane. Nuclear enlargement, hyperchromasia, variations in size and shape, nucleolar prominence, increased nuclear:cytoplasmic ratios, and increased numbers of abnormally shaped mitoses develop. Metaphases may exhibit horizontal rather than the usual vertical orientation relative to the cytoplasmic luminal surface. Goblet cells and mucous cells are usually absent. These abnormalities extend to the mucosal surface (Fig. 3.28). Architectural distortion may be quite marked, consisting of branching and lateral budding of the crypts, villiform configuration of the mucosal surface, or intraglandular epithelial bridging to form a cribriform back-to-back glandular pattern (Fig. 3.30). The architectural distortion of high-grade dysplasia may be so marked that it may be hard to distinguish from an invasive carcinoma. The pattern that usually prompts this diagnostic dilemma consists of back-to-back glands closely packed together or ill-defined glands present in the lamina propria. In this setting, one can make the diagnosis "high-grade dysplasia, cannot rule out an invasive carcinoma." Intramucosal carcinoma is recognized by the presence of single cells, small irregular cluster cells, or sheets of neoplastic cells infiltrating the lamina propria. Examination of multiple biopsies increases the chance of detecting invasive foci.

Crypt Dysplasia with Surface Maturation

We have seen a number of cases, especially among our consult material, in which the cells at the bases of the crypts display features consistent with those that are present in areas of dysplasia (Table 3.10) and yet the cells mature as they approach the mucosal surface. These areas occur in the absence of acute inflammation, ulcers, or erosions. The most common features

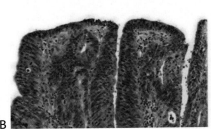
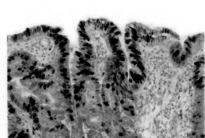
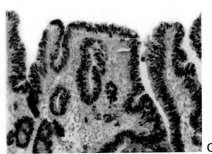

A, B   C

FIG. 3.29. Dysplasia in Barrett esophagus. **A:** Area of high-grade dysplasia. **B:** KI-67 stain shows the preferential staining of the epithelium at the surface. **C:** Many of the cells express p53.

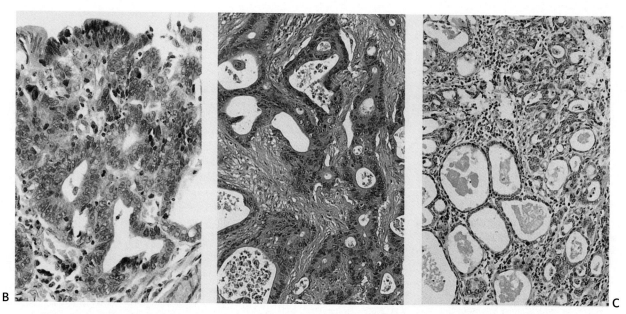

FIG. 3.30. Well-differentiated carcinoma. **A:** The lesion illustrated in this figure could represent either carcinoma in situ or severe dysplasia. Note the absence of desmoplasia surrounding the lesion. The glands are highly atypical and have lost their polarity. **B:** An infiltrating well-differentiated carcinoma surrounded by a desmoplastic stroma. The glands have acquired irregular shapes and back-to-back glandular formations. **C:** Microglandular pattern (*upper right corner*) of an invasive carcinoma.

of these basal cells include nucleomegaly, loss of nuclear polarity, marked variation in cell size and shape, overlapping of the nuclei, increased mitotic activity, and goblet cell dystrophy.

Similar lesions have been recently evaluated by Lomo et al, who termed the changes *basal crypt dysplasialike atypia* (BCDA). They found that this change had a prevalence of 7.3% and it was commonly associated with high-grade dysplasia, a high percentage of p53 immunoreactivity, a high proliferative rate, and aneuploidy (206). These authors concluded that BCDA is a possible variant of dysplasia that warrants further study. It is our practice to diagnose these lesions as at least low-grade dysplasia due to the nature of the cytologic changes, even though surface maturation does occur.

Adenomas (Polypoid Dysplasia)

Polypoid dysplasia is uncommon. Its precise frequency is unknown since most GEJ adenomas have been described as individual case reports. One retrospective study found only five adenomas among 250 cases of BE-associated dysplasia, corresponding to a prevalence of 2% in a highly selected population (207). Instances of multiple polyps have been reported (208). As in the colon, the polyps display a tubular, tubulovillous, or villous architecture; show varying degrees of dysplasia (Fig. 3.31); and may contain areas of invasive carcinoma.

Natural History of Dysplasia

The progression to malignancy in BE is a multistep process involving the transition from metaplasia to low-grade dysplasia to high-grade dysplasia to invasive carcinoma. The development of infiltrating carcinoma is rare in patients initially diagnosed as negative for dysplasia. This contrasts with the up to 60% of patients who have or will develop invasive carcinoma if their biopsies disclose the presence of development of high-grade dysplasia. Thus, high-grade dysplasia is the proximate precancerous lesion but it need not progress to full-blown invasive adenocarcinoma, and predicting which case will evolve into cancer is difficult. In some cases, high-grade dysplasia persists for years without progressing (209). The risk increases if high-grade dysplasia associates with a mass lesion (210). High-grade dysplasia found in biopsies associates with concurrent adenocarcinoma in approximately one third of cases; the presence of the associated invasive cancer may not be suspected until a resection specimen is examined (202,210). This is particularly true of well-differentiated tubular carcinomas. The glands forming these neoplasms may be so "benign" in appearance and rarely show tumor cell dissociation, even at the invasive front, that the only way to correctly diagnose the lesion is to see it invading into the lamina propria and beyond.

Early invasive adenocarcinoma may develop anywhere throughout the length of BE. The presence of high-grade dysplasia is an indication for surgical intervention, but there is no consensus as to how patients with high-grade dysplasia should be treated (211). Most agree that immediate rebiopsy should be performed to determine whether there is coexistent carcinoma. If a diagnosis of high-grade dysplasia with unassociated carcinoma is made, the diagnosis should be confirmed by a pathologist familiar with the changes in the setting of BE and with extensive experience in this area.

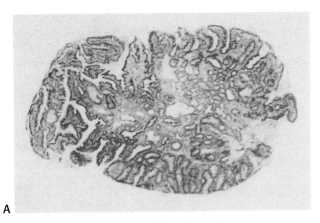

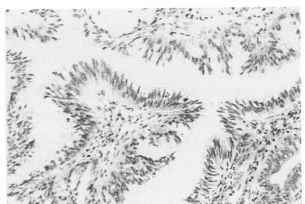

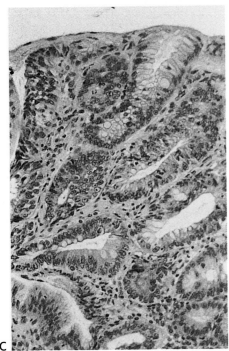

FIG. 3.31. Adenoma in Barrett esophagus. **A:** Round sessile adenoma without evidence of ulceration or much atypia. **B:** Low-grade tubular adenoma. **C:** Moderate dysplasia and numerous mitotic figures in adenoma.

Patients with high-grade dysplasia or early cancer arising in BE have the best chance of cure if handled in a careful multidisciplinary team approach involving the surgeon, gastroenterologist, and pathologist. The surgical procedure is determined by the length of the BE. Some individuals develop a second carcinoma following resection for the first one. The second tumor usually develops in the residual BE. These findings suggest that if the patient does undergo a resection, all of the BE should be resected to avoid the future development of another cancer.

Ancillary Techniques for Evaluating Dysplasia

Because of the difficulties in distinguishing regenerative changes from dysplasia and because not all individuals with dysplasia develop carcinomas, numerous adjunctive tests have been developed to predict which lesions are most likely to evolve into carcinomas. Some of the more promising are discussed below.

At least three *cell cycle abnormalities* develop in the dysplastic mucosa. These include mobilization of cells from the G0 into the G1 compartment of the cell cycle, loss of control of the G1/S-phase transition, and accumulation of cells in the G2 phase (212). Cell proliferation shifts from the lower parts of the glands into the upper mucosa and mucosal surface. Markers of cell proliferation, such as PCNA and Ki67, highlight this shift toward the superficial mucosa (Fig. 3.29).

Flow cytometric abnormalities correlate well with the presence of dysplasia and carcinoma (210). DNA aneuploidy increases as the severity of the neoplastic process increases (212). However, even specimens histologically negative or indefinite for dysplasia may contain aneuploid cells (213). Careful mapping studies demonstrate that early carcinomas arise within a single aneuploid population (212). An abnormal DNA pattern in a small biopsy may change a diagnosis from indefinite for dysplasia to frank dysplasia, or may prompt rebiopsy.

p53 immunoreactivity may help diagnose areas of dysplasia since its overexpression increases as dysplasia progresses toward invasive cancer. Patches of strongly positive cells occurs in 9% of low-grade dysplasia, 55% of high-grade dysplasia, and 87% of adenocarcinomas (214). The nonneoplastic mucosa may only show an isolated positive cell. p53 immunoreactivity may predict progression from low- to high-grade dysplasia (215).

Recently, it has been suggested that α-Methylacyl-CoA racemase (AMACR), which is overexpressed in a number of cancers, has a high sensitivity in its ability to detect areas of dysplasia, especially high-grade dysplasia (216). It is not yet clear how useful this marker will be in discriminating between reactive lesions and those that are truly dysplastic.

Distinguishing High-grade Dysplasia from Invasive Cancer

It can be difficult to distinguish an invasive cancer from dysplasia in small biopsies. The complex glandular arrangement that characterizes either low-grade or high-grade dysplasia may resemble that seen in invasive cancer. If BE becomes ulcerated, individual glands may drop into the ulcerated areas and mingle with the reduplicated muscularis mucosae, making it difficult to determine whether or not invasion has occurred. The presence of a mass in the esophagus is suggestive of an underlying carcinoma, even if none is demonstrated histologically.

Surveillance and Management of Patients with Barrett Esophagus

The object of surveillance programs is to identify adenocarcinomas at an early stage. BE-associated cancers of patients in surveillance programs are diagnosed at an earlier stage and have a better prognosis than cancers found because they are symptomatic. In one study the stage of surveillance cases versus symptomatic cases was as follows: stage 0 or I: 76% versus 15%; stage II: 17% versus 35%; stage II or IV: 6% versus 50% ($p < 0.001$). The 3-year survival of surveillance cases was 80% versus 31% of symptomatic cases ($p = 0.008$) (217), confirming similar findings in other studies (218). Therefore, it is now generally agreed that surveillance of BE patients helps detect adenocarcinomas at an early stage. The surveillance protocol recommended by the American Gastroenterological Association (AGA) (219) is as follows:

1. A program of regular endoscopic surveillance for dysplasia and early carcinoma is recommended for patients with BE unless contraindicated by a comorbidity.
2. Random biopsies should be taken from the involved segment of the esophagus with four sites sampled every 1 to 2 cm, with additional biopsies from endoscopically detectable lesions.
3. Patients without dysplasia or identifiable lesions on their initial evaluation should be re-examined again in 1 year to decrease the chance of sampling errors. If the second set of surveillance biopsies shows no evidence of dysplasia, the patient should be re-evaluated in 5 years.
4. If high-grade dysplasia is detected, treatment with either surgical resection or endoscopic mucosal resection is recommended.
5. Patients with multiple foci of high-grade dysplasia should undergo surgical resection of all of the esophagus that is lined by columnar epithelium. Surveillance may be offered to such patients if they are willing to undergo endoscopy every 3 months with at least eight random biopsies taken every 2 cm.
6. Surveillance should only be practiced if the patient is anticipated to have a reasonable life expectancy and can tolerate treatment for high-grade dysplasia or invasive cancer.

The recommendations of the American Society of Gastrointestinal Endoscopy (220) differ from these in the following respects:

1. For BE patients with no dysplasia in the first two examinations, follow-up examinations are recommended at 3-year, rather than 5-year, intervals.
2. Patients with low-grade dysplasia should be followed at 12-month intervals as long as dysplasia persists.
3. When the degree of dysplasia is indeterminate and there is evidence of acute inflammation, repeat biopsy should be performed after 8 weeks of acid-suppression therapy.

Various endoscopic ablative modalities are utilized to treat dysplasia in the setting of BE. These include photodynamic therapy, argon plasma coagulation, Nd-YAG laser, multipolar electrocoagulation, and EMR. In addition, other modalities such as cryotherapy and radiofrequency ablation are also currently in clinical trials (203). All of these methodologies, except for EMR, basically destroy the lesion without yielding a pathologic sample to evaluate the completeness of the ablative technique.

Invasive Adenocarcinoma at the Gastroesophageal Junction

The symptoms of patients with GEJ cancer typically relate to those caused by the underlying GERD. The dysphagia becomes progressive as tumors develop. Patients with advanced disease develop weight loss, bleeding, fatigue, chest pain, and vomiting. Most tumors arise distally and extend into the stomach at the GEJ. The cancer may arise anywhere within BE, although early Barrett carcinomas are often contiguous with both the specialized BE mucosa and the squamous epithelium (Fig. 3.32), suggesting that the mucosa at the squamocolumnar border is most vulnerable to cancer development. The majority of GEJ cancers are found at an advanced stage unless patients are in a surveillance program. Advanced lesions may be flat, ulcerated,

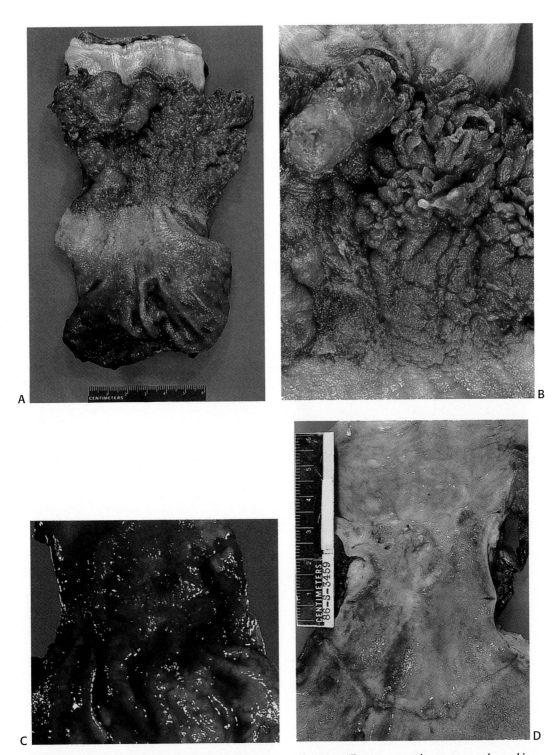

FIG. 3.32. Papillary esophageal adenocarcinoma. **A:** Exophytic papillary tumor at the gastroesophageal junction. The squamous mucosa is recognized by the pearly-white mucosal surface. **B:** Higher power shows numerous papillary fronds. **C:** A large fungating lesion occupies almost the entire circumference of the esophagus. The patient has a relatively short amount of Barrett esophagus, which appears beefy red and lies above the termination of the gastric folds. This lesion is difficult to see but is more easily appreciated by palpation of the specimen. **D:** Flat ulcerating lesion lies near the junction of the normal squamous epithelium with the Barrett epithelium. It is present on a large field of Barrett esophagus.

polypoid, or fungating. A diffusely infiltrative form resembling linitis plastica may also be present. Tumors vary in size, measuring up to 10 cm in greatest diameter.

Histologically, cancers arising in the setting of BE and those arising in the gastric cardia are virtually identical in terms of growth pattern (expansile or infiltrative), degree of differentiation, and extent of spread at the time of surgery. As in the stomach, the cancers may be either intestinal or diffuse in type. In the former, a tubular (Fig. 3.33), papillary (Fig. 3.34), or colloid microscopic pattern prevails. Well-differentiated intestinal-type carcinomas often mimic intraepithelial neoplasia on their surface and the diagnosis is determined by examining the base of the lesion. Poorly differentiated tumors often grow as solid sheets of cells without obvious glandular differentiation (Fig. 3.34). Diffuse cancers that produce a linitis plastica growth pattern infiltrate the esophageal wall and cause luminal stenosis (221). Signet ring cells predominate in diffuse cancers and associate with a desmoplastic stroma. Occasional tumors show a mixed intestinal and diffuse histology.

In contrast to carcinomas occurring in the gastric cardia, adenocarcinomas arising in BE may be multifocal and pleomorphic and may be accompanied by dysplasia in the contiguous BE (222). The surrounding epithelium may show a spectrum of premalignant epithelial changes ranging from hyperplasia, regeneration, and dysplasia of varying degrees, including adenocarcinoma in situ. Some tumors show extensive mucin production and occasional cases contain areas of squamous or endocrine differentiation. Squamous cell carcinomas may arise in BE, either alone or separate from the adenocarcinoma. These arise from residual squamous islands in the BE or from squamous epithelium immediately proximal to the squamocolumnar junction (223). Some tumors are so well differentiated that they are only recognized as carcinomas by their submucosal invasion. GEJ cancers may produce various hormones including gastrin, bombesin, substance P, somatostatin, and serotonin; somatostatin and serotonin are the most commonly detected (224).

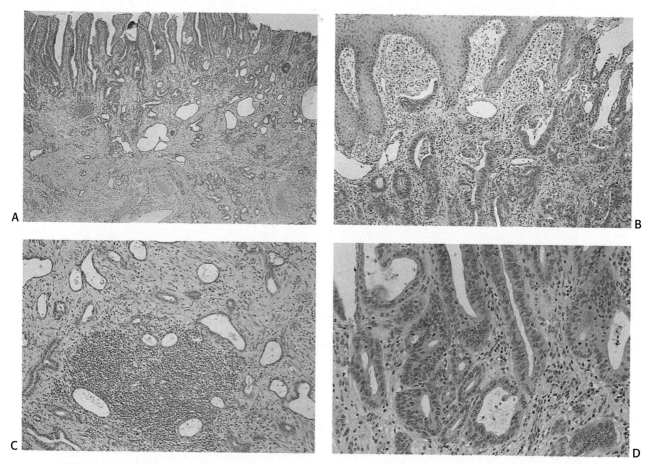

FIG. 3.33. Well-differentiated adenocarcinoma. **A:** The surface epithelium has become villous in architecture. A well-differentiated carcinoma drops off the bottom of the mucosa. Some glands are so well differentiated that making a cancer diagnosis would be difficult except for the obvious invasion into the esophageal wall. **B:** Extension of well-differentiated adenocarcinoma under the acanthotic hyperplastic squamous epithelium above it. **C:** Higher magnification of the well-differentiated areas shown in A. Note that desmoplasia surrounds individual glands. **D:** Higher magnification of another focus of the invasive carcinoma with more glandular crowding, cytologic atypia, and loss of polarity.

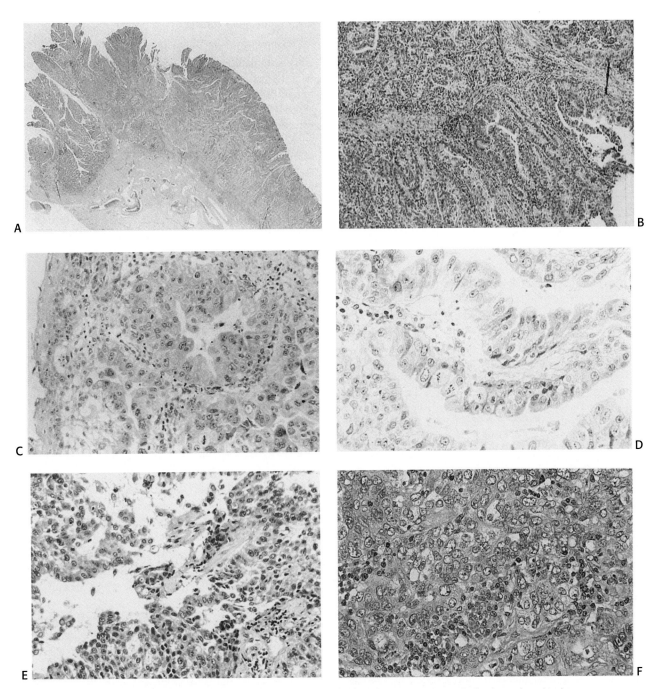

FIG. 3.34. Papillary adenocarcinoma. A: The overall architecture shows irregularly shaped projections or papillae. **B:** The fronds consist of mucus-secreting columnar epithelium supported by fibrovascular stalks. **C:** Areas of glandular differentiation. **D:** Areas of papillary differentiation. **E:** Moderately differentiated adenocarcinoma. **F:** Poorly differentiated adenocarcinoma consisting of sheets of cells and no obvious glandular spaces. This tumor produced mucin histochemically.

The tumors may arise underneath the squamous epithelium (Fig. 3.35) in patients who have been previously treated with various endoscopic ablative techniques. These tumors may not be grossly visible on the mucosal surface, since the squamous epithelium may be intact. They may be suspected by seeing or palpating a submucosal mass.

If ulceration occurs, exuberant granulation tissue containing prominent endothelial or mesenchymal cells may simulate an invasive cancer. Cytokeratin stains used to distinguish between invasive cells and mesenchymal cells can be misleading, since mesenchymal cells occasionally stain with these antibodies. Repeat esophageal biopsies after healing of the ulcer may show resolution of reactive atypia.

The histologic appearance of a GEJ cancer may be altered if the patient was treated prior to resection. Neoadjuvant chemoradiation may completely destroy a GEJ cancer leaving

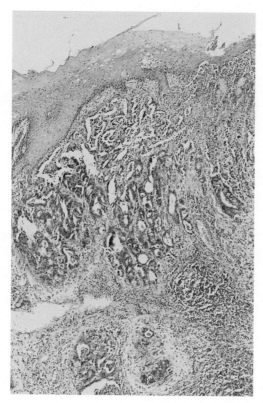

FIG. 3.35. Adenocarcinoma arising beneath the squamous epithelium.

only a dense acellular stroma, or it may have little impact on its histologic appearance. The presence of small islands of very bizarre tumor cells embedded in a dense stoma is a commonly encountered neoadjuvant effect (Fig. 3.36). Acellular mucous lakes in regional lymph nodes may mark the sites of no longer viable metastases from a mucoid carcinoma (Fig. 3.36). If the acellular lakes fail to contain viable cells, after examination at several levels the tumors are staged as ypN0.

Cytologic preparations may be useful in identifying the neoplastic changes associated with BE. Cells deriving from esophageal adenocarcinomas usually form groups and clusters (Fig. 3.37) and are recognizable if the primary tumor appears well differentiated and sheds papillary fragments. Less well-differentiated adenocarcinomas exfoliate cells that may be indistinguishable from poorly differentiated squamous cell carcinomas. Malignant cells from adenocarcinoma in situ of the esophagus do not differ morphologically from those of invasive adenocarcinoma. However, cytology has the advantage of obtaining diagnostic material safely from regions difficult to sample.

BE-associated adenocarcinomas may also contain areas of yolk sac and trophoblastic differentiation (225,226). These rare tumors appear as large, bulging, hemorrhagic, and necrotic masses (225). *Choriocarcinomas* usually contain both cytotrophoblasts and syncytiotrophoblasts. Areas of *yolk sac differentiation* exhibit glandular and papillary structures lined by columnar epithelium. Mucin is absent in these areas but diastase-resistant periodic acid–Schiff (PAS)-positive

cytoplasmic globules are present. Choriocarcinomatous areas produce both human placental lactogen and human chorionic gonadotropin (hCG). Areas of yolk sac differentiation produce α-fetoprotein. hCG production by carcinomas is not limited to choriocarcinomas. hCG production also occurs in squamous cell carcinomas, usually in the most infiltrative areas of the tumors where poorly differentiated and pleomorphic cells predominate.

Adenocarcinomas extensively infiltrate the esophageal wall and often show perineural invasion (Fig. 3.38), lymphatic (Fig. 3.39) and vascular invasion, and direct extension through the esophageal wall. Lymph node metastases are present in 51% to 74% of cases (227). The frequency of nodal metastasis correlates with the depth of tumor invasion. A study of 90 early cancers found no metastases among 36 mucosal tumors, 3 of 29 cancers that involved the muscularis mucosae or superficial submucosa (10%), and 9 of 25 cases that penetrated to the deep submucosa (36%; $p < 0.001$) (228). In another study, nodal metastases were present in 67% of intramural and 89% of transmural carcinomas (229). The paracardiac lymph nodes have the highest frequency of metastases (40%), followed by nodes along the lesser curvature of the stomach (29%), and splenic/pancreatic nodes in 11%. Intrathoracic nodes are involved in only 7% of cases (230). Metastases to distant sites, such as the celiac axis or upper mediastinum, almost exclusively affect patients with multiple positive regional nodes. Skipping of regional node occurs in <5% of cases (231).

Recurrences affect cervical (7.9%), mediastinal (21%), and abdominal lymph nodes (24%). Nodal recurrences develop at sites outside the resection margins in 60% of cases. The prognosis of patients with lymphatic metastases is enhanced if fewer than four nodes are involved (231). When a similar number of nodes show metastatic disease, patients with metastases limited to nodes within 3 cm of the primary cancer fare better than those with more distant nodal involvement (232).

The prognosis of BE-associated cancer correlates with tumor stage, the degree of differentiation, and the status of the lymphatics and other vascular structures. GEJ cancers are staged by the same systems used for esophageal SCC (Table 3.2). The deeper the penetration, the worse the prognosis is (229,233). The higher the tumor stage, the lower the survival rate is. The 3-year survival rates for stages 0, I, IIA, IIB, III, and IV tumors in one study were 100%, 85.7%, 53.6%, 45%, 25.2%, and 0%, respectively. The overall 5-year survival rate was 23.5% (171). Early cancers offer the best chance of cure. For example, the 5-year survival rates of patients with invasive tumors limited to the submucosa may be as high as 63% (234).

Patients under 55 years of age have a slightly poorer prognosis than the following 10-year cohort. After that, age shows an inverse relationship with survival (233). Other factors that unfavorably affect survival include the presence of vascular or perineural invasion and an infiltrative growth pattern. The chance of survival is enhanced if there is a Crohn-like lymphoid response and/or an intense peritumoral lymphoid

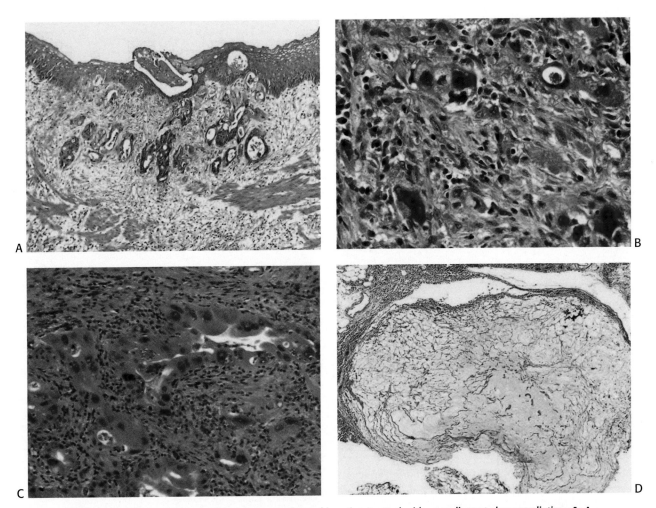

FIG. 3.36. Adenocarcinoma of the gastroesophageal junction treated with neoadjuvant chemoradiation. **A:** A small focus of invasive carcinoma remains. It and the overlying squamous epithelium show the effects of the chemoradiation. **B:** Higher magnification discloses the presence of isolated bizarre cells in a desmoplastic stroma. **C:** Higher magnification of the glandular areas. **D:** Acellular mucinous lake in a regional lymph node.

response (233). Lymphatic invasion relates to poor prognosis of GEJ cancers and shows statistically different subsite variations in frequency (235). Cancers limited to the esophagus are less likely to show lymphatic invasion than are cancers that also involve the cardia and proximal stomach.

There are now many immunohistochemical procedures that help pathologists identify the phenotype of a GEJ tumor and assess its prognosis. Many genes are altered in GEJ cancer (Table 3.9; Fig. 3.40). The literature on this subject is vast and expanding. A short, and necessarily incomplete, review of the subject follows.

A diagnosis of BE or BE-associated cancer requires identification of intestinal metaplasia in the affected tissue. Several markers fill this need, including two brush-border proteins: villin (236) and sucrase-isomaltase (SI) (237). Poorly differentiated cancers arising in BE are more likely to retain villin expression than SI (237). Cdx2, a homeobox gene regulating intestine-specific gene transcription, is uniformly expressed in the BE nuclei (238,239). As with villin and SI, progression to dysplasia and undifferentiated cancer is characterized by cases

that express this marker in the contiguous epithelium, suggesting that Cdx2 transcription is an early step in the generation of metaplasia. Cytokeratin 7/20 and mucin core protein (MUC) have been proposed as markers to distinguish between cancers arising in the distal esophagus from those arising in the proximal stomach, but they yield inconsistent results among different investigators (240,241). Invasive GEJ adenocarcinomas that express EGFR are more likely to be poorly differentiated and show more rapid progression than EGFR-negative cancers (242,243). Increasing cyclooxygenase (COX)-2 expression is a feature of BE progression to dysplasia and carcinoma (244,245). It significantly correlates with local recurrence ($p = 0.05$) and distant metastases ($p = 0.02$) (246).

The main treatment for advanced GEJ cancer is surgical resection in operable cases; however, as in SCC, patients with high-grade dysplasia and early cancers may have other options. Radical resection is the treatment of choice when the tumor penetrates into the submucosa. The levels of the resection are based on the length of the Barrett segment and the extent of gastric involvement. Careful intraoperative

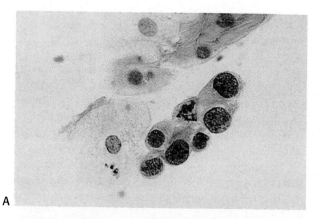

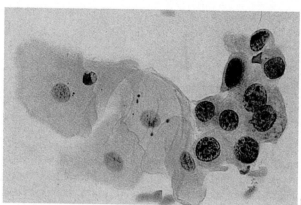

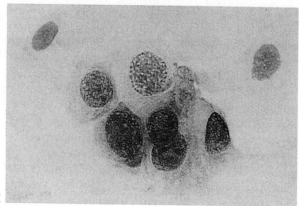

FIG. 3.37. Recurrence of esophageal adenocarcinoma at the esophagogastric anastomosis. **A:** Cancer cells with large nuclei and eccentrically placed granular cytoplasm. Mitoses are evident. **B:** Group of cancer cells with granular cytoplasm and uniform nuclei. **C:** Same case stained with May-Grünwald-Giemsa.

pathologic evaluation ensures that all of the Barrett mucosa is resected (247). EMR has been used to remove areas of high-grade dysplasia, mucosal cancers, and superficially invasive cancer (248). EMR has substantially less morbidity and negligible mortality than esophagectomy, but incompleteness of resection is a significant pitfall that dictates continued endoscopic surveillance. Patients with advanced disease may benefit from targeted EGFR therapy. The response is unrelated to the expression of the protein in the tumor and does not associate with EGFR mutations (249).

PROXIMAL ADENOCARCINOMA OF THE ESOPHAGUS

Developmental anomalies may be the sites of a small minority of adenocarcinomas in the proximal esophagus. The heterotopic gastric epithelium present in an inlet patch (see Chapter 2) may undergo metaplastic changes and may develop areas of dysplasia or invasive carcinoma (250,251). Adenocarcinoma can also arise in tracheobronchial rests in the upper esophagus (252).

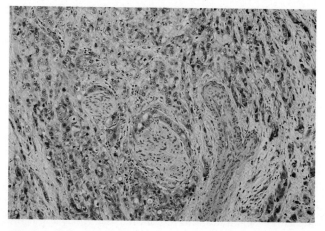

FIG. 3.38. Perineural invasion by a gastroesophageal junction adenocarcinoma.

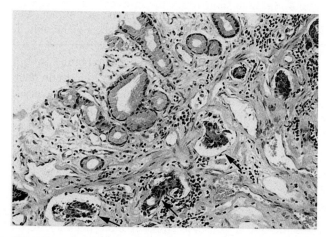

FIG. 3.39. Extension of carcinoma arising in a Barrett esophagus into the lymphatics (*arrows*).

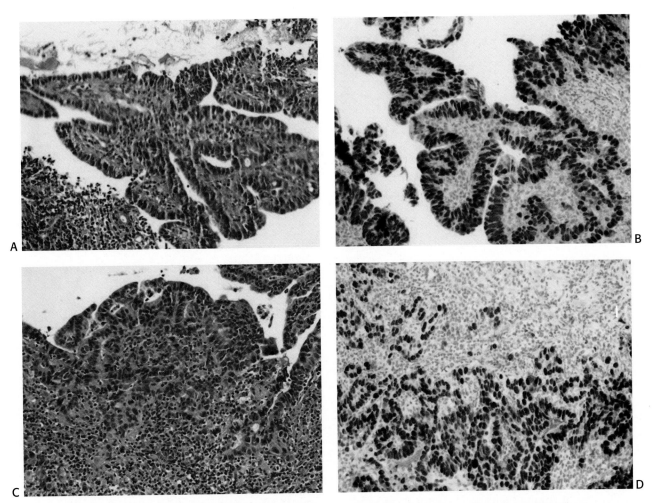

FIG. 3.40. Adenocarcinoma arising in an area of high-grade dysplasia. **A:** Hematoxylin and eosin (H&E) stain of the high-grade dysplasia. **B:** p53 immunostain of the same area. **C:** Area of invasive carcinoma stained with H&E. **D:** p53 immunostain. All the cells are positive.

TUMORS ARISING FROM SUBMUCOSAL GLANDS

Submucosal Adenomas

Submucosal adenomas arise from the ducts of submucosal glands independent of BE (253). They present as an esophageal polyp and are often covered by an intact squamous epithelial mucosa. The adenomas have a globoid shape and measure about 1 cm in diameter. Histologically, they retain the lobular architecture of submucosal glands but the acini appear hyperplastic and they may become cystic. Such lesions are sometimes termed serous cystadenomas because of their resemblance to pancreatic lesions. Histologically, they may show mild atypia (254).

Adenoid Cystic Carcinoma

Adenoid cystic carcinomas are rare esophageal neoplasms that resemble similar tumors that develop in salivary glands. However, they are more aggressive than their salivary counterparts. Less than 50 cases have been reported (255–258).

The tumors are more common in women than men. Progressive dysphagia and obstruction are common presenting symptoms and are typically present for 2 weeks to 6 months. The tumors have a high rate of distant metastases at the time of diagnosis, and the median survival is only 9 months following diagnosis. However, exceptions exist in which long-term survival has been reported. Such patients present early when the tumor is small and more localized. Additionally, such tumors tend to be better-differentiated lesions.

Most commonly, adenoid cystic carcinomas arise in the middle third of the esophagus (63%), less often in the lower third (30%), and rarely in the upper third (7%). They are typically fungating or polypoid lesions, although ulcerative and infiltrative growth patterns are sometimes seen. The histology of adenoid cystic carcinoma resembles that of analogous salivary tumors. They contain two cell types: Duct-lining epithelial cells and myoepithelial cells (257,258). The tumor has expansile or infiltrating margins. The tumors are subclassified based on their histologic pattern into tubular, cribriform, solid, or basaloid variants (Fig. 3.41). The tubular pattern is

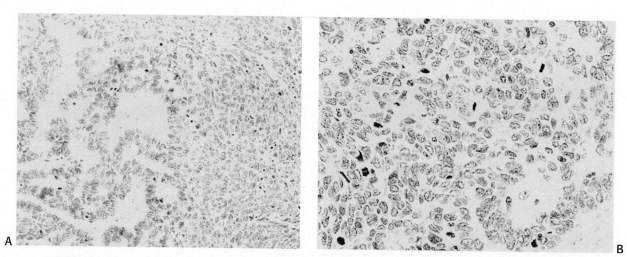

FIG. 3.41. Adenoid cystic carcinoma of the esophagus. **A:** Shows a basaloid and lacelike pattern. **B:** Note the high mitotic index.

characterized by ductlike structures or large cellular masses dispersed around microcystic spaces with a lacelike pattern. This pattern is more common than the cribriform pattern usually found in salivary gland lesions. The microcystic spaces are not true glandular lumina, but rather they consist of replicated, eosinophilic, PAS-positive, diastase-resistant basement membrane material. One may see coexisting squamous cell carcinoma in situ in the overlying epithelium. The esophageal tumors tend to show more cellular pleomorphism and a higher mitotic index than those arising in salivary glands.

Epithelial membrane antigen (EMA), carcinoembryonic antigen (CEA), and cytokeratin stains are focally positive, especially in cells around tubular and cribriform structures and also in some basaloid regions. S100 antibodies stain rare tubular structures and diffusely stain solid areas. The tumor cells are vimentin negative. Collagen IV and laminin are positive at the margins of the epithelial cells and luminal parts of cribriform and tubular structures.

Adenoid cystic carcinomas present certain challenges to the surgical pathologist, especially in biopsy specimens. Many of these lesions lie within the submucosa with an intact overlying squamous mucosa, and an endoscopic biopsy may miss the tumor. A second diagnostic difficulty results from the inability to classify the tumor correctly on the basis of a small unrepresentative biopsy. Because the esophageal tumor is so commonly solid or basaloid, a small biopsy may suggest the diagnosis of a small cell carcinoma or undifferentiated carcinoma unless the more cribriform or tubular areas are also present.

Mucoepidermoid Carcinoma

This uncommon esophageal cancer consists of a diffuse mixture of squamous and mucin-secreting cells (259) and most commonly arises in the middle and upper two thirds of the esophagus. Less than 100 cases of this type had been reported through 2000. These aggressive cancers uniformly express CEA. The infrequency of this cancer limits comparative studies

of its prognosis, but published reports suggest that its prognosis is similar to SCC with 1-, 2-, and 5-year survival rates of 46%, 39%, and 0%, respectively (260). Mucoepidermoid carcinomas are usually well-differentiated tumors and should not be confused with adenocarcinomas with squamous metaplasia (adenoacanthomas).

The tumors consist of solid nests of squamous cells, mucus-secreting cells (in glandular formations or as signet ring cells), and cells with histologic features that are intermediate between the two (Fig. 3.42). The approximately concentric structure of the epithelial cell nests is such that mucus-secreting cells lie in the center of the tumor cell nests and are surrounded by multiple layers of nonkeratinizing, or rarely keratinizing, squamous epithelium. Mucicarmine stains demonstrate mucin both in glandular lumina and in squamous cell nests. Tumor cells invade into the adventitia and patients die of widespread metastases (260).

ADENOSQUAMOUS CARCINOMA

Adenosquamous carcinomas are rare and the differential diagnosis includes mucoepidermoid carcinoma. Adenosquamous cancers may arise in esophageal submucosal glands or ducts, and in some cases, one can identify ductal epithelial origin. They may also arise as a result of multipotential cellular differentiation in BE. The tumor contains a mixture of adenocarcinoma and squamous cell carcinoma. Mucin stains show the histochemical profile of esophageal glands when they arise from these structures (261). These tumors are highly malignant, especially when poorly differentiated, and they can spread in a pagetoid fashion. They behave more aggressively than mucoepidermoid carcinomas, warranting a distinction between them (262). Several characteristics separate these two tumor types: (a) adenosquamous carcinoma tends to spread throughout the mucosal surface; (b) prominent separate foci of squamous cell carcinoma, often containing focal mucin production, occur in adenosquamous carcinomas (Fig. 3.43);

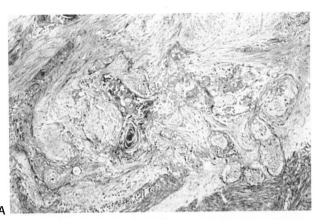

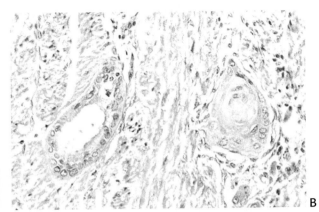

FIG. 3.42. Mucoepidermoid carcinoma. **A:** Nests of malignant cells with glandular and squamous differentiation. Pearl formations and intraluminal mucinous material are shown. Kreyberg stain. **B:** Intramural spread by two nests, one composed of squamous cells and the other having glandular features.

(c) keratinization, a characteristic feature of adenosquamous carcinoma, is rarely present in mucoepidermoid carcinomas; (d) invasive and metastasizing glandular formations with abundant mucin production occur in adenosquamous carcinoma, although mucin production is not a requirement for the diagnosis of adenosquamous carcinoma in the presence of well-formed glands; and (e) severe nuclear pleomorphism characterizes adenosquamous carcinomas.

PAGET DISEASE

Pagetoid spread accompanies squamous cell carcinoma, adenocarcinomas arising in Barrett esophagus (Fig. 3.44), adenosquamous carcinoma, or, more rarely, proximal spread of a gastric cancer. The pagetoid cell nests can extend away from the main tumor for considerable distances and may even involve the ducts of submucosal glands. Grossly, the lesions may appear as mucosal irregularities. Alternatively, Paget dis-

ease may arise as an intraepithelial neoplasm of the ducts of the submucosal glands. The cells grow singly or in clusters in the lower part of the epithelium and, unlike malignant melanoma, single cells usually do not appear in the upper mucosa. The tumor cells may contain mucin- or CEA-positive material if the primary tumor contains glandular or mucinous differentiation. The tumor cells may attach to neighboring keratinocytes by short, poorly formed desmosomes. Detection of Paget disease in a specimen indicates that an invasive carcinoma is likely to be present in the nearby mucosa.

MALIGNANT MELANOMA

Esophageal malignant melanomas represent 0.1% to 0.5% of primary malignant esophageal neoplasms (263,264), and approximately 0.5% of malignant melanomas originate in the esophagus (265). Cutaneous malignant melanomas metastatic to the esophagus are more common than primary esophageal malignant melanomas (266). Slightly more males are affected than females (267). Mean patient age is 60 years with a wide age range from 7 to over 80 years (268). The disease almost exclusively affects whites. Patients with esophageal melanoma usually complain of dysphagia and weight loss. Primary esophageal melanomas are most common in the lower and middle thoracic segments; mean tumor diameter is 7 cm (267). They usually appear as a polypoid intraluminal mass in a dilated esophageal segment. The tumors often appear gray or black in color. Satellite nodules are relatively uncommon.

Esophageal malignant melanomas resemble their cutaneous counterparts. The tumor cells vary in size and shape, both from neoplasm to neoplasm and within a given tumor. The tumor contains a mixture of variably pigmented epithelioid, spindle-shaped, and bizarre cells (Fig. 3.45) (267). Spindle cells arranged in fascicles may impart a sarcomalike pattern to the tumor. Occasional tumors show marked pleomorphism with numerous bizarre cellular forms. Small cell, signet ring cell, and balloon cell features

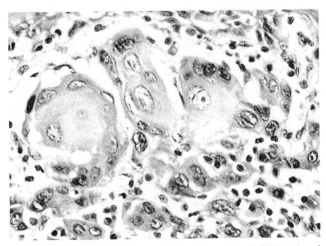

FIG. 3.43. Adenosquamous carcinoma. Foci of well-differentiated squamous metaplasia in an adenocarcinoma.

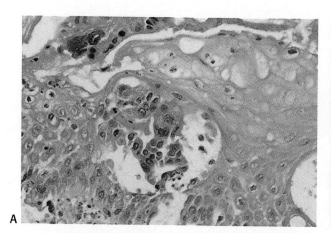
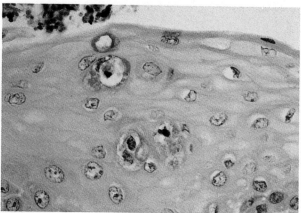

FIG. 3.44. Pagetoid spread. A: Intramucosal extension of an adenocarcinoma into the surrounding squamous epithelium. Tumor is also present in the underlying submucosa. **B:** Periodic acid–Schiff (PAS) stain of a biopsy showing the presence of atypical cells that are PAS positive within the upper layers of the squamous epithelium.

may also be present. The inflammatory host response is usually mild. A peripheral in situ lentiginous growth pattern often surrounds the main lesion. It is important to distinguish between primary and metastatic melanoma. Melanosis (Fig. 3.46), a nesting growth pattern and junctional change in the contiguous squamous mucosa, suggests the diagnosis, but absence of these changes does not exclude a primary esophageal malignant melanoma (269). If the tumor has overgrown these premalignant features, it may be extremely difficult to establish the fact that the tumor represents a primary esophageal neoplasm, even if a careful examination has been made of the skin, other mucosal membranes, and the eyes.

When contemplating the diagnosis of malignant melanoma, several antibodies are useful in confirming the diagnosis. These include melan-A, HMB45, and S100. Melan-A is specific for melanocytic lesions and is more sensitive than HMB45, but it has less value than S100 in detecting spindle cell and desmoplastic melanomas (270).

Prognosis is extremely poor and not much different from that of esophageal squamous cell carcinoma. The prognosis is worse than that seen in cutaneous melanoma perhaps due to the rich esophageal vascular and lymphatic supply. Esophageal melanomas are usually treated by esophagectomy and excision of any identifiable paraesophageal lymph nodes or regional metastases. Melanomas are radioresistant. Unfortunately, these distinctly uncommon neoplasms tend to present as advanced tumors with aggressive biologic behavior and a dismal prognosis. Survival after surgery averages about 8 months. The best survival rates appear to be those following radical surgical resection with 5-year survivals of 4.2%.

OTHER PRIMARY TUMORS

Primary malignant nonepithelial esophageal tumors constitute only 0.4% to 0.99% of esophageal tumors. These include

mesenchymal tumors as described in Chapter 19 and hematologic tumors as described in Chapter 18.

COLLISION TUMORS

Collision tumors occur when two tumors that have arisen independently lie adjacent to one another. One makes the diagnosis of a collision tumor when the component tumors are phenotypically different and there is clear separation of the two components. If both tumor types metastasize, the two types of growth also remain clearly separated in the metastasis. At the early stage of their evolution, the two components may appear as separate dual noncolliding carcinomas. With further growth, the tumors may become more intimately admixed with one another. Collisions occur between squamous cell carcinomas and/or adenocarcinomas, and with sarcomas, lymphomas, melanomas, or metastases (271,272). However, the simultaneous occurrence of mesenchymal and epithelial tumors in the esophagus is quite rare.

Spagnolo and Heenan proposed the following guidelines for diagnosing collision tumors: (a) two distinct topographically separate sites of origin for the two components must be present (e.g., squamous cell carcinoma arising from esophageal squamous epithelium and adenocarcinomas arising from the gastric mucosa), (b) there must be at least some separation of the two components so that despite intimate mixing at points of juxtaposition, the dual origin can be recognized, and (c) at the areas of the collision, in addition to intimate mixing of the two components, some transitional patterns may be seen such as a mucoepidermoid appearance as in the case of collisions between squamous carcinomas and adenocarcinomas (272).

Costa (273) proposed three possible explanations for collision tumors: A carcinogen could theoretically interact with two neighboring histologically distinct tissues causing tumors to arise in them both. This would be more likely to

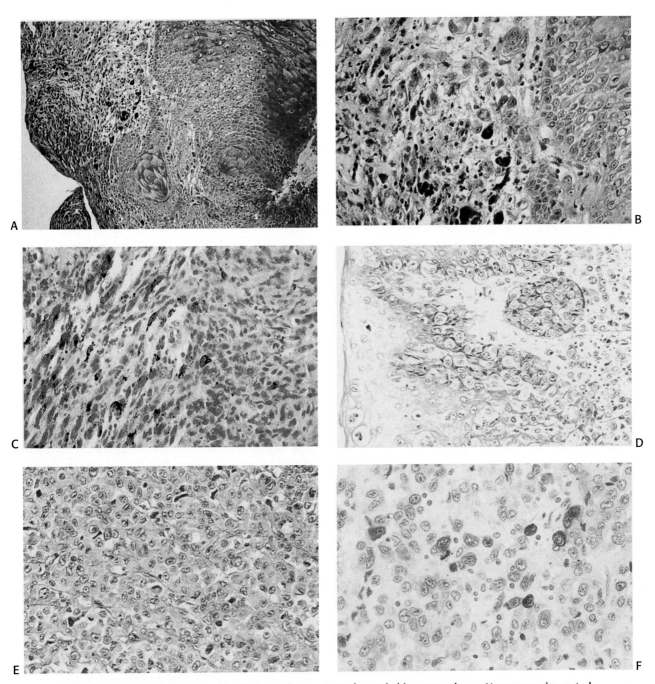

FIG. 3.45. Malignant melanoma of the esophagus. **A:** Endoscopic biopsy specimen. Numerous pigmented cells in the lamina propria suggest the diagnosis of melanoma. **B:** Bizarre tumor cells are variably pigmented. **C:** Spindle cell component stained with Fontana Masson. **D:** Pagetoid lentiginous radial growth at the periphery of a different esophageal melanoma. **E:** Epithelioid features of the melanoma cells. **F:** Immunoreactive S100 protein in scattered cells.

occur in patients suffering from inherited predispositions to tumors or from exposures to some agent that causes cancer in several tissue types. A second possibility would result from the phenomenon known as horizontal recruitment, which describes those tumors composed of host cells that are induced to become malignant adjacent to a pre-existing tumor. A third possibility is that the growth of one tumor creates circumstances that directly or indirectly favor the genesis of the second lesion. In addition, one lesion may represent a primary lesion and the second a metastasis.

SECONDARY MALIGNANT TUMORS

Secondary carcinomas involve the esophagus, either by direct extension or by metastasis. Carcinomas originating in

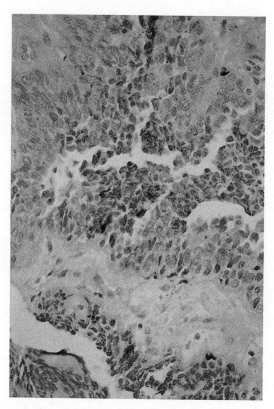

FIG. 3.46. Melanosis of the esophagus in an area adjacent to a malignant melanoma. The underlying submucosa also contains a malignant melanoma of the small cell type.

TABLE 3.11	Tumorlike Conditions of the Esophagus

Inflammatory fibroid polyps
Granuloma pyogenicum
Cysts/duplications
Pseudoepitheliomatous hyperplasia
Pancreatic metaplasia
Congenital rests producing masses
Heterotopic tissues (pancreatic, gastric, sebaceous, thyroid)

the lungs, pharynx, larynx, thyroid, or stomach may extend directly into the esophagus. Breast, kidney, testes, prostate, and pancreas tumors can all metastasize to the esophagus. Breast carcinoma, in particular, may be responsible for strictures (274) or concentric stenosis of the esophageal wall with an intact mucosa, due to the permeation of submucosal lymphatic vessels showing the typical picture of the so-called carcinomatous lymphangitis. Metastatic breast cancer can also present as achalasia. Melanoma metastasizes to the gastrointestinal tract in 43.5% of patients (248).

TUMORLIKE CONDITIONS

There are a number of esophageal conditions that create variably sized masses that may clinically or endoscopically mimic neoplasms (Table 3.11). These are discussed in Chapter 2.

HANDLING ESOPHAGEAL RESECTION SPECIMENS

Esophagectomy specimens should be opened longitudinally. The prosector should describe all lesions, including tumors, ulcers, or areas of Barrett esophagus or other discolorations.

The distance of a tumor from the proximal, distal, and radial margins should be measured. The depth of invasion should be estimated and extension beyond the esophagus should be documented, if present. A comment should be made as to whether or not the nodes appear to be grossly involved. It is a common practice to remove a fresh piece of tumor and normal mucosa for future research if this does not interfere with the pathology assessment. This should be in compliance with Health Insurance Portability and Accountability Act (HIPAA) regulations. If there is an interest in studying SCCs and their precursor lesions, the esophageal mucosa may be sprayed with a Lugol iodine solution or dipped in a Lugol solution so as to highlight areas of mucosal abnormality. This approach may allow one to detect small lesions that remain unstained by the Lugol iodine and that may represent areas of dysplasia or multicentric carcinomas. On completion of the gross examination the esophagus should be pinned out flat on a cork board and floated upside down in 10% formalin, and fixed overnight.

Once the resection specimen is handled for sectioning, attention should be given to documenting the size, appearance, and anatomic relationship of any lesions that are present. Blocks should be obtained to evaluate the nature and extent of those lesions. The gross evaluation should include measurements of tumor size, since this measurement helps determine prognosis. Specimen palpation helps delineate full tumor extent. The status of the resection margins, including the soft tissue (especially the submucosa) as well as proximal and distal margins must be established. Painting the margins with India ink can be useful in making these determinations. Lymph nodes should be carefully sought in the adipose tissue adjacent to the esophagus and cardia, and the distance of harvested nodes from the tumor should be identified. It is important that when sections are submitted, the origins of each section be noted in the gross description.

When dealing with squamous cell lesions, it is important to document the presence of multiple lesions, including areas of coassociated carcinoma in situ. The margins should be examined not only for the presence of invasive disease, but also for the presence of intramucosal disease or evidence of pagetoid spread.

With respect to adenocarcinomas, one should describe the extent of the tumor. If the Barrett epithelium is present in the resection margin, this should also be documented, since it is subject to the risk of subsequent development of carcinoma.

If the patient has been treated with preoperative radiation and/or chemotherapy, the presence of residual cancer may not be obvious and one may need to block an entire suspicious area in order to find remnants of tumor.

EMR specimens require special handling in order to determine whether the resection margins are microscopically complete. Intact specimens should be stretched and pinned to a block. Deep and lateral margins should be marked with India ink. The specimen should be sectioned longitudinally at 2-mm intervals after fixation for 24 hours in formaldehyde. Piecemeal resections should be handled in a similar way, although it is generally not possible to pin out the individual tissue pieces. A resection may be classified as being complete for neoplasia if the deep and lateral margins are negative, and complete for BE if the margins are composed of nonmetaplastic mucosa.

REFERENCES

1. Gabbert HE, Shimoda T, Hainaut P et al: Squamous cell carcinoma of the oesophagus in pathology and genetics. Tumours of the digestive system. In: Hamilton SR, Aaltonen LA (eds). *WHO Classification of Tumors.* Lyons, France: IARC Press, 2000, pp 10–19.
2. Parkin DM, Pisani P, Ferlay J: Estimates of the worldwide incidence of 25 major cancers in 1990. *Int J Cancer* 1999;80:827.
3. Devesa SS, Blot WJ, Fraumeni JF Jr: Changing patterns in the incidence of esophageal and gastric cancer in the United States. *Cancer* 1998;83:2049.
4. Newham A, Quinn MJ, Babb P, et al: Trends in the subsite and morphology of oesophageal and gastric cancer in England and Wales 1971-1998. *Alimen Pharmacol Ther* 2003;17:665.
5. Carr NJ, Monihan JN, Sobin LH: Squamous cell papilloma of the esophagus: a clinicopathologic and follow-up study of 25 cases. *Hum Pathol* 1994;25:536.
6. Orlowska J, Jarosz D, Gugulski A, et al: Squamous cell papillomas of the esophagus: report of 20 cases and literature review. *Am J Gastroenterol* 1994;89:434.
7. Odze R, Antonioli D, Shocket D, et al: Esophageal squamous papillomas: a clinicopathologic study of 38 lesions and analysis for human papillomavirus by the polymerase chain reaction. *Am J Surg Pathol* 1993;17:803.
8. Carr NJ, Monihan JM, Sobin LH: Squamous cell papilloma of the esophagus: a clinicopathologic and follow-up study of 25 cases. *Am J Gastroenterol* 1994;89:245.
9. Carr NJ, Bratthauer GL, Lichy JH, et al: Squamous cell papillomas of the esophagus: a study of 23 lesions for human papilloma virus by in situ hybridization and polymerase chain reaction. *Hum Pathol* 1994;25:536.
10. Sablich R, Benedetti G, Bignucolo S, et al: Squamous cell papilloma of the esophagus. Report of 35 endoscopic cases. *Endoscopy* 1988;20:5.
11. Mosca S, Manes G, Manaco R, et al: Squamous papilloma of the esophagus: long-term follow-up. *J Gastroenterol Hepatol* 2001;16:857.
12. Kato H, Orito E, Yoshinouchi T, et al: Regression of esophageal papillomatous polyposis caused by high risk type human papilloma virus. *J Gastroenterol* 2003;38:579.
13. Parkin DM, Whelan SL, Ferlay J, et al (eds). *Cancer Incidence in Five Continents,* Vol. VIII, IARC Publication No. 155. Lyon, France: IARC Press, 1998, pp 543–545.
14. Munoz N, Day NE: Esophageal cancer. In: Schottenfeld D, Fraumeni JE Jr (eds). *Cancer Epidemiology and Prevention.* New York: Oxford University Press, 1996, pp 681–706.
15. Thomas DB, Karagas MR: Cancer in first and second generation Americans. *Cancer Res* 1987;47:5771.
16. Miller BA, Kolonel LN, Bernstein L, et al: Racial/ethnic patterns of Cancer in the United States 1988-1992. SEER Monograph, National Cancer Institute. NIH Pub. 96-4104, Bethesda, MD, 1996.
17. Jemal A, Clegg LX, Ward E, et al: Annual report to the nation on the status of cancer. 1975-2001, with a special feature regarding survival. *Cancer* 2004;101:3.
18. Frank PI, Morris JA, Frank TL, et al: Trends in smoking habits. *Fam Pract* 2004;21:33.
19. Ziegler RG. Alcohol-nutrient interactions in cancer etiology. *Cancer* 1986;58:1942.
20. MacKillop WJ, Zhang-Salomans J, Boyd CJ, Groome PA: Associations between community income and cancer in Canada and the United States. *Cancer* 2000;89:901.
21. Jha P, Peto R, Zatonski W, et al: Social inequalities in male mortality from smoking: indirect estimation from national death rates in England and Wales, Poland and North America. *Lancet* 2006;368:367.
22. Valsecchi MG: Modeling the relative risk of esophageal cancer in a case-control study. *J Clin Pathol* 1992;45:347.
23. Tuyns AJ, Pequignot G, Jensen OM: Le cancer de l'oesophage en Ille-et-Vilaine en fonction des niveaux de consommation d'alcool et tabac. Des risques qui se multiplient. *Bull Cancer* 1977;64:45.
24. Pesko P, Rakic S, Milicevic M, et al: Prevalence and clinicopathologic features of multiple squamous cell carcinoma of the esophagus. *Cancer* 1994;73:2687.
25. Winn DM, Blot WJ: Second cancer following cancers of the buccal cavity and pharynx in Connecticut, 1935-1982. *Natl Cancer Inst Monogr* 1985;68:25.
26. Hemminki K, Jiang YW: Familial and second esophageal cancers: a nation-wide epidemiologic study in Sweden. *Int J Cancer* 2002;98:106.
27. Cheng KK, Day NE: Nutrition and esophageal cancer. *Cancer Causes Control* 1996;7:33.
28. Van Rensberg SJ, Benade AS, Rose EF, et al: Nutritional status of African populations predisposed to esophageal cancer. *Nutr Cancer* 1983;4:206.
29. Lu SH, Ohshima H, Fu HM, et al: Urinary excretion of N-nitrosamino acids and nitrate by inhabitants of high and low risk areas of esophageal cancer in northern China: endogenous formation of nitroso-orolin and its inhibition by vitamin C. *Cancer Res* 1986;46:1485.
30. Victora CG, Munoz N, Day NE, et al: Hot beverages and oesophageal cancer in southern Brazil: a case-control study. *Int J Cancer* 1987;39:710.
31. Toorchen D, Topal MD: Mechanisms of chemical mutagenesis and carcinogenesis: effects of DNA replication of methylation at the 06-guanine position of dGTP. *Carcinogenesis* 1983;4:1591.
32. Zhang L, Lu W, Miao X, et al: Inactivation of DNA repair gene 06-methylguanine-DNA methyltransferase by promoter hypermethylation and its relation to p53 mutations in esophageal squamous cell carcinoma. *Carcinogenesis* 2003;24:1039.
33. Gaur D, Arora S, Mathur M, et al: High prevalence of p53 gene alterations and protein overexpression in human esophageal cancer. *Clin Cancer Res* 1997;3:2129.
34. Bosetti C, Gallus S, Trichopoulou A, et al: Influence of Mediterranean diet on the risk of cancers of the upper aerodigestive tract. *Cancer Epid Biomarkers Prev* 2003;12:1091.
35. Bosron WF, Li TK: Genetic polymorphism of human liver alcohol and aldehyde dehydrogenases, and their relation to alcohol metabolism and alcoholism. *Hepatology* 1986;6:502.
36. Yokoyama A, Muramatsu T, Ohmori T, et al: Esophageal cancer and aldehyde dehydrogenase-2 genotypes in Japanese males. *Cancer Epidemiol Biomarkers Prev* 1996;5:99.
37. Yokoyama A, Muramatsu T, Ohmori T, et al: Reliability of a flushing questionnaire and the ethanol patch test in screening for aldehyde dehydrogenase-2 and alcohol-related cancer risk. *Cancer Epidemiol Biomarkers Prev* 1997;6:1105.
38. Yokoyama A, Muramatsu T, Ohmori T, et al: Alcohol and aldehyde dehydrogenase gene polymorphisms influence susceptibility to esophageal cancer in Japanese alcoholics. *Alcohol Clin Exper Res* 1999;23:1705.
39. Lee JM, Lee YC, Yang SY, et al: Genetic polymorphisms in XRCC1 and risk of esophageal cancer. *Int J Cancer* 2001;95:240.
40. Cai L, You N-C Y, Lu H, et al: Dietary selenium intake, aldehyde dehydrogenase-2 and x-ray repair cross-complementing 1 genetic polymorphisms and the risk of esophageal squamous carcinoma. *Cancer* 2006;106:2345.
41. Nimura Y, Yokoyama S, Fujimori M, et al: Genotyping of CYP1A1 and GSTM1 genes in esophageal cancer patients with special reference to smoking. *Cancer* 1997;80:852.

42. Zhang J, Li Y, Wang R, et al: Association of cyclin D1(G870A) polymorphism with susceptibility to esophageal and gastric cardia carcinoma in a northern Chinese population. *Int J Cancer* 2003;105:281.

43. Larsson SC, Giovannucci E, Wolk A: Folate intake, MTHFR polymorphisms and the risk of esophageal, gastric and pancreatic cancer: A meta-analysis. *Gastroenterology* 2006;131:1271.

44. Parent ME, Siemiatycki J, Fritschi L: Workplace exposures and esophageal cancer. *Occup Environ Med* 2000;57:325.

45. Pottier D, Launoy G, Cherie L, et al: Esophageal cancer at the department of Calvados. Geographic and social inequality factors. *Bull Cancer* 1989;76:1111.

46. Zablotska LB, Chak A, Das A, Neugat AI: Increased risk of squamous cell esophageal cancer after adjuvant radiation therapy for breast cancer. *Am J Epidemiol* 2005;161:330.

47. Syrjänen KJ: HPV infections and esophageal cancer. *J Clin Pathol* 2002;55:721.

48. Li T, Lu Z-M, Guo M, et al: p53 codon 72 polymorphism(C/G) and the risk of human papillomavirus-associate carcinomas in China. *Cancer* 2002;95:2571.

49. Lopes ER: Megaesophagus, megacolon and cancer. *Rev Soc Brasil Med Trop* 1988;21:91.

50. Marger RS, Marger D: Carcinoma of the esophagus and tylosis-a lethal genetic combination. *Cancer* 1993;72:17.

51. Stevens HP, Kelsell DP, Bryant SP, et al: Linkage of American pedigree with palmoplantar keratosis and malignancy (palmoplantar ectodermal dysplasia type III) to 17q24. Literature survey and proposed updated classification of keratodermas. *Arch Dermatol* 1996;132:640.

52. Risk JM, Mills HS, Garde J, et al: The tylosis esophageal cancer (TOC) locus: more than just a familial cancer gene. *Dis Esophagus* 1999; 12:173.

53. Langan JE, Cole C, Huckle E, et al: Novel microsatellite markers and single nucleotide polymorphisms refine the tylosis with oesophageal cancer (TOC) minimal region on 17q25 to 42.5kb: sequencing does not identify the causative gene. *Hum Genet* 2004;114:534.

54. Ashworth MT, Nash JRG, Ellis A, et al: Abnormalities of differentiation and maturation of the esophageal squamous epithelium of patients with tylosis: morphologic features. *Histopathology* 1991;189:303.

55. Horn HM, Tidman MJ: The clinical spectrum of dystrophic epidermolysis bullosa. *Br J Dermatol* 2002;146:267.

56. Crespi M, Munoz N, Grassi R, et al: Precursor lesions of oesophageal cancer in a low-risk population in China: comparison with high-risk populations. *Int J Cancer* 1984;34:559.

57. Ribet ME, Mensier EA: Reflux esophagitis and carcinoma. *Surg Gynecol Obstet* 1992;175:121.

58. Hopkins RA, Postlethwait RW: Caustic burns and carcinoma of the esophagus. *Ann Surg* 1981;194:146.

59. Brucher BLDM, Stein HJ, Bartels H, et al: Achalasia and esophageal cancer: incidence, prevalence and prognosis. *World J Surg* 2001;35:745.

60. Bradley PJ, Kochaar A, Quraishi MS: Pharyngeal pouch carcinoma: real or imaginary risks? *Ann Otol Laryngol* 1999;108:1027.

61. Ye W, Nyren O: Risk of cancers of the oesophagus and stomach in patients hospitalised for pernicious anemia. *Gut* 2003;52:938.

62. Ye W, Held M, Lagergren J, et al: Helicobacter pylori infection and gastric atrophy: risk of adenocarcinoma and squamous cell carcinoma of the esophagus and adenocarcinoma of the cardia. *J Natl Cancer Inst* 2004;96:388.

63. Goodman MT, Stemmermann GN: Cancer registration and incidence in Hawaii. *Eur J Cancer* 1991;27:1701.

64. Jessner W, Vogelsang H, Pűspők A, et al: Plummer-Vinson syndrome associated with celiac disease and complicated by postcricoid carcinoma and carcinoma of the tongue. *Am J Gastroenterol* 2003;98:1208.

65. Lu N, Hu N, Li W-J, et al: Microsatellite alterations in esophageal dysplasia and squamous cell carcinoma from laser capture microdissected endoscopic biopsies. *Cancer Lett* 2003;189:137.

66. Shi ST, Yang GY, Wang LD, et al: Role of p53 gene mutations in human esophageal carcinogenesis: results from immunohistochemical and mutation analyses of carcinomas and nearby cancerous lesions. *Carcinogenesis* 1999;20:591.

67. Ito S, Ohga T, Saeki H, et al: p53 mutation profiling of multiple esophageal carcinoma using laser capture microdissection to demonstrate field carcinogenesis. *Int J Cancer* 2005;113:22.

68. Yasuda M, Kuwano H, Watanabe M, et al: p53 expression in squamous dysplasia associated with carcinoma of the oesophagus: evidence for field carcinogenesis. *Br J Cancer* 2000;83:1033.

69. Shen O, Liu SF, Dawsey SM, et al: Cytologic screening for esophageal cancer: results from 12,877 subjects from a high-risk population in China. *Int J Cancer* 1993;54:185.

70. Yokoyama A, Ohmori T, Makuuchi H, et al: Successful screening for early esophageal cancer in alcoholics using endoscopy and mucosa iodine staining. *Cancer* 1995;76:926.

71. Takubo K, Takai A, Takayama S, et al: Intraductal spread of esophageal squamous cell carcinoma. *Cancer* 1987;59:1751.

72. Rubio CA, Liu F, Zhao H: Histologic classification of intraepithelial neoplasias and microinvasive squamous carcinoma of the esophagus. *Am J Surg Pathol* 1989;13:685.

73. Schlemper RJ, Riddell RH, Kato Y, et al: The Vienna classification of gastrointestinal neoplasia. *Gut* 2000;47:251.

74. Li J-Y, Ershow AG, Chen CJ, et al: A case-control study of cancer of the esophagus and gastric cardia in Linxian. *Int J Cancer* 1989;43:755.

75. Nabeya K: Markers of cancer in the esophagus and surveillance in high risk groups. In: Sherlock P, Morson BC, Barbara L, et al (eds). *Precancerous Lesions of the Gastrointestinal Tract*. New York: Raven Press, 1983, pp 71–86.

76. Bogomoletz, Molas G, Gayet B, Potet F: Superficial squamous cell carcinoma of the esophagus. A report of 76 cases and review of the literature. *Am J Surg Pathol* 1989;13:535.

77. Kanamoto A, Yamaguchi J, Nakanishi Y, et al: Clinicopathological study of multiple superficial oesophageal carcinoma. *Br J Surg* 2000;87:1712.

78. Tsang WY, Chan JKC, Lee KC, et al: Basaloid-squamous carcinoma of the upper aero-digestive tract and so-called adenoid cystic carcinoma of the oesophagus: the same tumour type? *Histopathology* 1991;19:35.

79. Greene FL, Balch CM, Page DL, et al (eds). *AJCC Cancer Staging Manual*. 6th ed. New York: Springer-Verlag, 2002, pp 91–95.

80. Brierley JD, Greene FL, Sobin LH, Wittekind C: The "y" symbol: an important classification tool for neoadjuvant cancer treatment. *Cancer* 2006;106:2526.

81. Tachibana M, Kinugasa S, Dhar DK, et al: Dukes' classification as a useful staging system in resectable squamous cell carcinoma of the esophagus. *Virchows Arch* 2001;438:350.

82. Eloubeidi MA, Desmond R, Arguedas MR, et al: Prognostic factors for the survival of patients with esophageal carcinoma in the US: the importance of tumor length and lymph node status. *Cancer* 2002; 95:1434.

83. Soetikno R, Kaltenbach T, Yeh R, et al: Endomucosal resection for early cancer of the upper gastrointestinal tract. *J Clin Oncol* 2005;23:4490.

84. Araki K, Ohno S, Egashira A, et al: Pathologic features of superficial squamous cell carcinoma with lymph node and distal metastases. *Cancer* 2002;94:570.

85. Tachibana M, Kinugasa S, Dhar DK, et al: Prognostic factors after extended esophagectomy for squamous cell carcinoma of the thoracic esophagus. *J Surg Oncol* 1999;72:88.

86. Yuasa N, Miyachi M, Yasui A, et al: Clinicopathological features of superficial spreading and nonspreading squamous cell carcinoma of the esophagus. *Am J Gastroenterol* 2001;96:232.

87. Soga A, Tanaka O, Sasaki K, et al: Superficial spreading carcinoma of the esophagus. *Cancer* 1982;50:1641.

88. Murray GF, Keagy B: Esophagus. In: Manning H, van Schaik M (eds). *Clinical Surgery*. St. Louis: Mosby, 1987, pp 1161–1169.

89. Geddes LG J, Dorn RA, Wadleigh RG: Hypercalcemia in patients with esophageal cancer. *J Exp Clin Cancer Res* 1999;18:61.

90. Broadus AE, Mangan M, Ikeda K, et al: Humoral hypercalcemia of cancer. Identification of novel parathyroid hormone-like peptide. *N Engl J Med* 1988;319:556.

91. Pinel N, Berthon C, Everad F, et al: Prognosis of hypercalcemia in aerodigestive tract cancers: a study of 136 cases. *Oral Oncol* 2005;41: 884.

92. Barber PV, Lechler R: Hypertrophic osteoarthropathy: two unusual causes. *Postgrad Med J* 1983;59:254.

93. Mita T, Nakanishi Y, Ochiai A, et al: Paraneoplastic vasculitis associated with esophageal carcinoma. *Pathol Int* 1999;49:643.

94. Dittler HJ, Siewert JR: Role of endoscopic ultrasonography in esophageal carcinoma. *Endoscopy* 1993;25:561.

95. Van Dam J. Endosonographic evaluation of the patient with esophageal cancer. *Chest* 1997;112:184S.

96. Vasquez-Sequeiros E, Norton ID, Clain JE, et al: Impact of EUS-guided fine-needle aspiration on lymph node staging in patients with esophageal carcinoma. *Gastrointest Endosc* 2001;53:751.

97. Chu PG, Lyda MH, Wess LM: Cytokeratin 14 expression in epithelial neoplasms: a survey of 435 cases with emphasis on its value in differentiating squamous cell carcinomas from other epithelial tumours. *Histopathology* 2001;39:9.

98. Nakanishi Y, Ochiai A, Kato H, et al: Clincopathologic significance of tumor nest configuration in patients with esophageal squamous cell carcinoma. *Cancer* 2001;91:1114.

99. Mandard AM, Dailbard F, Mandard JC, et al: Pathologic assessment of tumor regression after preoperative chemoradiotherapy of esophageal carcinoma. *Cancer* 1994;73:2680.

100. Altorki NK, Migliore M, Skinner DB: Esophageal carcinoma with airway obstruction: evolution and choices of therapy. *Chest* 1994;106:742.

101. Sons HU, Borchard F: Esophageal cancer: autopsy findings. *Arch Pathol Lab Med* 1984;108:983.

102. Fagundes RB, Mello CR, Tollens P, et al: p53 protein esophageal mucosa of individuals at high risk of squamous cell carcinoma of the esophagus. *Dis Esophagus* 2001;14:185.

103. Parenti AR, Rugge M, Frizzera E, et al: p53 overexpression in multistep process of esophageal carcinogenesis. *Am J Surg Pathol* 1995;19:1418.

104. Takeno S, Nogichi T, Kikuchi R, et al: Prognostic value of cyclin B1 in patients with esophageal squamous cell carcinoma. *Cancer* 2002;94:2974.

105. Miyata H, Doki Y, Shiozaki H, et al: CDC25B and p53 are independently implicated in radiation sensitivity for human esophageal cancers. *Clin Cancer Res* 2000;6:4839.

106. Kajiyama Y, Hattori K, Amano T, et al: Histopathologic effects of neoadjuvant therapies for advanced squamous cell carcinoma of the esophagus: multivariate analysis of predictive factors and p53 overexpression. *Dis Esophagus* 2002;15;61.

107. Jiang W, Kahn SM, Tomita N, et al: Amplification and expression of human cyclin D gene in esophageal cancer. *Cancer Res* 1992;51:2980.

108. Nozoe T, Korenaga D, Kabashima A, et al: Significance of cyclin B1 expression as an independent prognostic indicator of patients with squamous cell carcinoma of the esophagus. *J Cancer Res Clin Oncol* 2002;129:691.

109. Yoshida K, Kuniyasu H, Yasui W, et al: Expression of growth factors and their receptors in human esophageal carcinoma: regulation of expression by epidermal growth factor and transforming growth factor alpha. *J Cancer Res Clin Oncol* 1993;119:401.

110. Yoshida K, Kyo E, Tsuda T, et al: EGF and TGF-α, the ligands of hyperproduced EGFR in human esophageal carcinoma cells, act as autocrine growth factors. *Int J Cancer* 1990;45:131.

111. Ozawa S, Ueda M, Ando N, et al: High incidence of EGF receptor hyperproduction in esophageal squamous cell carcinoma. *Int J Cancer* 1987;39:333.

112. Chikuba K, Saito T, Uchino S, et al: High amplification of hst-1 gene correlates with haematogenous recurrence after curative resection of oesophageal carcinoma. *Br J Surg* 1995;82:364.

113. Kitadai Y, Haruma K, Tokutomi T, et al: Significance of vessel count and vascular endothelial growth factor in human esophageal carcinoma. *Clin Cancer Res* 1998;4:2195.

114. Rosa AR, Schirmer CC, Gurski RR, et al: Prognostic value of p53 protein expression and vasular endothelial growth factor expression in resected squamous cell carcinoma of the esophagus. *Dis Esophagus* 2003;16:112.

115. Yamamoto H, Iku S, Itoh F, et al: Association of trypsin expression with recurrence and poor prognosis in human esophageal squamous cell carcinoma. *Cancer* 2001;91:1324.

116. Ohkawa T, Naomoto Y, Takaoka M, et al: Localization of heparanase in esophageal cancer cells: respective roles in prognosis and differentiation. *Lab Invest* 2004;84:1289.

117. Lu JP, Xian MS, Hayashi K, et al: Morphologic features in esophageal carcinoma in young adults in North China. *Cancer* 1994;74:573.

118. Vanoverhagen H, Berger MY, Meijers H, et al: Influence of radiologically and cytologically assessed distant metastases on the survival of patients with esophageal and gastroesophageal junction carcinoma. *Cancer* 1993;72:25.

119. Kawamura T, Goseki N, Koike M, et al: Acceleration of proliferative activity of esophageal squamous cell carcinoma with invasion beyond the mucosa. Immunohistochemical analysis of Ki-67 and p53 antigen in relation to histopathologic findings. *Cancer* 1996;77:843.

120. Chan KW, Chan YET, Chan CW: Carcinoma of the esophagus. An autopsy study. *Pathology* 1986;18:400.

121. Izbiki JR, Hosch SB, Pichlmeier U, et al: Prognostic value of histochemically identifiable tumor cells in lymph nodes of patients with completely resected esophageal cancer. *N Eng J Med* 1997;337:1188.

122. Nozoe T, Saeki H, Ohga T, Sugimachi K: Clinicopathologic characteristics of esophageal carcinoma in younger patients. *Ann Thorac Surg* 2001;72:1914.

123. Siewert JR, Stein HJ, Feith M, et al: Histologic tumor type is an independent prognostic parameter in esophageal cancer: resections from a single center in the western world. *Ann Surg* 2001;234:360.

124. Miller RA, Ries LAG, Hankey BF, et al: Cancer Statistics Review 1973-1989, National Cancer Institute. NIH Pub. No. 92-2789. Washington, DC: National Institutes of Health, 1992, pp VIII.3-9.

125. Enzinger PC, Mayer RJ: Esophageal cancer. *N Eng J Med* 2003;349:2241.

126. Enzinger PC, Ilson DH, Kelson DP: Chemotherapy in esophageal cancer. *Semin Oncol* 1999;26:12.

127. Gschossmann JM, Bonner JA, Foote RL, et al: Malignant tracheoesophageal fistula in patients with esophageal cancer. *Cancer* 1993;72:1513.

128. Tachibana M, Kinugasa S, Yoshimura H, et al: Clinical outcomes of extended esophagectomy with three-fold lymph node dissection for esophageal squamous cell carcinoma. *Am J Surg* 2005;189:98.

129. Natsugoe S, Mueller J, Stein HJ, et al: Micrometastasis and tumor cell microinvolvement of lymph nodes from esophageal squamous cell carcinoma: frequency, associated tumor characteristics, and impact on prognosis. *Cancer* 1998;83:858.

130. Böttger T, Störkel S, Stöckle M, et al: DNA image cytometry, a prognostic tool in squamous cell carcinoma of the esophagus? *Cancer* 1991;67:2290.

131. Kaketani K, Saito T, Kobayashi M: Flow cytometric analysis of nuclear DNA content in esophageal cancer. Aneuploidy as an index of highly malignant potential. *Cancer* 1989;64:887.

132. Watanabe M, Kuwano H, Tanaka S, et al: Flow cytometric DNA analysis is useful in detecting multiple alterations in squamous cell carcinoma of the esophagus. *Cancer* 1999;2322.

133. Natsugoe S, Shimazu H, Baba M, et al: Recurrence of thoracic esophageal cancer after lymph node dissection in three areas with special reference to the relationship between recurrence and the number of metastatic lymph nodes. *Jpn J Gastroenterol Surg* 1991;24:2888.

134. Takashima S, Takeuchi N, Shiozaki H, et al: Carcinoma of the esophagus: CT vs. MR imaging in determining resectability. *AJR Am J Roentgenol* 1991;156:297.

135. Siewert JR, Holscher AH, Dittler HJ: Preoperative staging and risk analysis in esophageal carcinoma. *Hepatogastroenterology* 1990;37:382.

136. Isono K, Onoda S, Ishikawa T, et al: Studies on the causes of death from esophageal carcinoma. *Cancer* 1982;49:2173.

137. Isono K, Sato H, Nakayama K: Results of nation-wide study of the three field lymph-node dissection of esophageal cancer. *Oncology* 1991;48:411.

138. Kato H, Tachimori Y, Watanabe H, Toshifumi T: Evaluation of the new (1987) TNM classification for thoracic esophageal tumors. *Int J Cancer* 1993;53:220.

139. Malthaner RA, Wong RKS, Rumble RB, et al: Neoadjuvant and adjuvant therapy for resectable esophageal cancer: a systematic review and meta-analysis. *BMC Med* 2004;2:35.

140. Kelsen DP, Ginsberg R, Pajak TF, et al: Chemotherapy followed by surgery compared with surgery alone for localized esophageal cancer. *N Eng J Med* 1998;339:1979.

141. Medical Research Council Oesophageal Cancer Working Party: Surgical resection with or without chemotherapy in oesophageal cancer: a randomized control trial. *Lancet* 2002;359:1727.

142. Ilson DH, Sirott M, Saltz L, et al: A phase II trial of interferon alpha-2, 5-fluorouricil, and cisplatin in patients with advanced esophageal cancer. *Cancer* 1995;75:2197.

143. Ilson DH, Forastiere A, Arquette M, et al: A phase II trial of paclitaxel and cisplatin in patients with advanced carcinoma of the esophagus. *Cancer* 2000;6:316.

144. Carlisle JG, Quint LE, Francis IR, et al: Recurrent esophageal carcinoma-CT evaluation after esophagectomy. *Radiology* 1993;189:271.

145. Dawsey SM, Lewin KJ, Liu FS, et al: Esophageal morphology from Linxian, China—squamous histologic findings in 754 patients. *Cancer* 1994;73:2027.

146. Matsumoto M, Natsugoe S, Nakashima S, et al: Biological evaluation of undifferentiated carcinoma of the esophagus. *J Surg Oncol* 2000;7:204.

147. Fischer HP, Wallner F, Maier H, et al: Coexpression of intermediate filaments of squamous cell carcinoma of upper aerodigestive tract before and after radiation and chemotherapy. *Lab Invest* 1989;61:433.

148. Osborn NK, Keate RF, Trastek VF, Nguyen CC: Verrucous carcinoma of the esophagus. Clinicophysiologic features and treatment of a rare entity. *Dig Dis Sci* 2003;48:463.

149. Mori M, Watanabe M, Tanaka S, et al: Epstein-Barr virus carcinoma of the esophagus and stomach. *Arch Path Lab Med* 1994;118:998.

150. Rosengard AM, Hamilton SR: Squamous cell carcinoma of the esophagus in patients with Barrett esophagus. *Mod Pathol* 1989;2:2.

151. Iezzoni JC, Mills SE: Sarcomatoid carcinomas (carcinosarcomas) of the gastrointestinal tract. *Semin Diag Pathol* 1993;10:176.

152. Gal AA, Martin SE, Kernan JA, et al: Esophageal carcinoma with prominent spindle cells. *Cancer* 1987;60:2244.

153. Handra-Luca A, Terris B, Couvelard A, et al: Spindle-cell squamous carcinoma of the oesophagus: an analysis of 17 cases, with new immunohistochemical evidence of clonal origin. *Histopathology* 2001;39:125.

154. Ota S, Kato A, Kobayashi H, et al: Monoclonal origin of an esophageal carcinosarcoma producing granulocyte-colony stimulating factor. *Cancer* 1998;82:2102.

155. Robertson NJ, Rahmin J, Smith ME: Carcinosarcoma of the oesophagus showing neuroendocrine, squamous and glandular differentiation. *Histopathology* 1997;31:236.

156. Lauwers, Grant LD, Scott GV, et al: Spindle cell squamous carcinoma of the esophagus: analysis of the ploidy and proliferative activity in a series of 13 cases. *Hum Pathol* 1998;29:863.

157. Takubo K, Mafune K, Tanaka Y, et al: Basaloid-squamous carcinoma of the esophagus with marked deposition of basement membrane substance. *Acta Pathol Jap* 1991;41:59.

158. Guarino M, Micoli G: Basaloid-squamous carcinoma of the upper aerodigestive tract. *Histopathology* 1992;20:462.

159. Ohashi K, Horiguchi S, Moriyama S, et al: Superficial basaloid squamous carcinoma of the esophagus. A clinicopathological and immunohistochemical study of 12 cases. *Path Res Pract* 2003;199:713.

160. Cabrera E, Fernandes F, Gomez-Roman J, Val-Bernal JF: Basaloid squamous carcinoma of the esophagus: immunohistochemistry and flow cytometric DNA analysis in two cases. *Int J Surg Pathol* 1996;3:267.

161. Dolan K, Morris AI, Gosney JR, et al: Three different subsite classifications for carcinomas in the proximity of the GEJ, but is it all one disease? *J Gasatroenterol Hepatol* 2004;19:24.

162. Flucke IJ, Steinborn E, Dreis V, et al: Immunoreactivity of cytokines (CK7, CK29) and mucin peptide care antigens (MUC1, MUC2, MUC5AC) in adenocarcinomas, normal, and metaplastic tissues of the distal oesophagus, oesophago-gastric junction and proximal stomach. *Histopathology* 2003;43:127.

163. Ectors N, Driessen A, De Hertog G, et al: Is adenocarcinoma of the esophagogastric junction or cardia different from Barrett adenocarcinoma? *Arch Path Lab Med* 2005;128:183.

164. Stemmermann GN, Nomura AMY, Kolonel LN, et al: Gastric carcinoma in a multiethnic population. *Cancer* 2002;95:744.

165. Siewert JR, Holscher AH, Becker K, et al: Cardia cancer: attempt at a therapeutically relevant classification. *Chirurg* 1987;58:25.

166. Kubo A, Corley DA: Marked regional variation in adenocarcinomas of the esophagus and gastric cardia in the United States. *Cancer* 2002;95:2096.

167. Newnham A, Quinn MJ, Babb P, et al: Trends in subsite and morphology of oesophageal and gastric cancer in England and Wales. *Aliment Pharmacol Ther* 2003;17:665.

168. Voutilainen ME, Juhola MT: The changing epidemiology of esophageal cancer in Finland and the impact of the surveillance of Barrett's esophagus in detecting esophageal adenocarcinoma. *Dis Esophagus* 2005;18:221.

169. Hongo M: Barrett's esophagus and carcinoma in Japan. *Aliment Pharmacol Ther* 2004;20:50.

170. Blot W: Esophageal cancer trends and risk factors. *Semin Oncol* 1994;21:403.

171. Streitz JM, Ellis FH, Gibb P: Adenocarcinoma in Barrett's esophagus: a clinicopathologic study of 65 cases. *Ann Surg* 1991;213:122.

172. Pera M, Pera M: Recent changes in the epidemiology of esophageal cancer. *Surg Oncol* 2001;10:81.

173. Kaijser M, Akre O, Cnattingius S, Ekbom A: Preterm birth, low birth weight and risk of esophageal adenocarcinoma. *Gastroenterology* 2005;128:607.

174. Avidan B, Sonnenberg A, Scnell TG, et al: Hiatal hernia size, Barrett's length, and severity of acid reflux are all risk factors for esophageal adenocarcinoma. *Am J Gastroenterol* 2002;97:1930.

175. Pera M, Trastek VF, Carpenter HA, et al: Influence of pancreatic and biliary reflux on the development of esophageal carcinoma. *Ann Thorac Surg* 1993;55:1386.

176. Miwa K, Hattori T, Miyazaki I: Duodenogastric reflux and foregut carcinogenesis. *Cancer* 1995;75:1426.

177. Lindblad M, Rodriguez LAG, Lagergren J: Body mass, tobacco and alcohol risk of esophageal, gastric cardia and gastric non cardia adenocarcinoma among men and women in a nested case-control study. *Cancer Causes Control* 2005;16:285.

178. La Vecchia C, Negri E, Lagiou P, Trichopolous D: Oesophageal adenocarcinoma: a paradigm of mechanical carcinogenesis? *Int J Cancer* 2002;102:269.

179. Chow WH, Blot WJ, Vaughn TL, et al: Body mass index and risk of adenocarcinoma of the esophagus and gastric cardia. *J Natl Cancer Inst* 1998;90:150.

180. Ryan A, Rowley S, Fitzgerald A, et al: Adenocarcinomas of the oesophagus and gastric cardia: male preponderance in association with obesity. *Eur J Cancer* 2006;42:1151.

181. Vaughn TL, Davis S, Kristal A, Thomas DB: Obesity, alcohol and tobacco as risk factors for cancers of the esophagus and gastric cardia: adenocarcinoma versus squamous cell carcinoma. *Cancer Epidemiol Biomarkers Prev* 1995;4:85.

182. Kim R, Weissfeld JL, Reynolds JC, Kuller LH: Etiology of Barrett's metaplasia and esophageal adenocarcinoma. *Cancer Epidemiol Biomarkers Prev* 1997;6:369.

183. Suzuki H, Iijima K, Scobie G, et al: Nitrate and nitrosative chemistry within Barrett's esophagus during acid reflux. *Gastroenterology* 2001;120:387.

184. Terry P, Jagergren J, Weimin YE, et al: Inverse association between intake of cereal fiber and risk of gastric cardia cancer. *Gastroenterology* 2001;120:387.

185. Sihvo EIT, Salminen JT, Rantanen TK, et al: Oxidative stress has a role in malignant transformation in Barrett's oesophagus. *Int J Cancer* 2002;102:551.

186. Chow WH, Blaser MJ, Blot WJ, et al: An inverse relation between cagA(+) strains of Helicobacter pylori infection and risk of esophageal and gastric cardia adenocarcinoma. *Cancer Res* 1998;58:588.

187. Yamaji Y, Mitsushima T, Ikuma H, et al: Inverse background for Helicobacter pylori antibody and pepsinogen in reflux oesophagitis compared with gastric cancer: analysis of 5732 Japanese subjects. *Gut* 2001;49:335.

188. El-Serag HB, Sonnenberg A: Opposing time trends of peptic ulcer and reflux disease. *Gut* 1998;43:327.

189. Labens J, Blum AL, Bayerdorfter E, et al: Curing Helicobacter pylori infection in patients with duodenal ulcer may provoke reflux esophagitis. *Gastroenterology* 1997;112:1412.

190. Lagergren L, Bergstrom R, Adami HO, Nyren O: Association between medications that relax the lower esophageal sphincter and risk of esophageal adenocarcinoma. *Ann Int Med* 2000;133:165.

191. Vaughn TL, Dong LM, Blount P, et al: Nonsteroidal anti-inflammatory drugs and risk of neoplastic progression in Barrett's oesophagus: a prospective study. *Lancet Oncol* 2005;6:945.

192. Eng C, Spechler SJ, Ruben R, Li FP: Familial Barrett esophagus and adenocarcinoma of the gastroesophageal junction. *Cancer Epidemiol Biomarkers Prev* 1993;2:397.

193. Jochem VJ, Fuerst PA, Fromkes JJ: Familial Barrett's esophagus associated with adenocarcinoma. *Gastroenterology* 1992;102:1400.

194. van Lieshout EM, Roelofs HM, Dekker S, et al: Polymorphic expression of the glutathione-S-transferase P1 gene and its susceptibility to Barrett's esophagus and esophageal carcinoma. *Cancer Res* 1999;59:586.

195. Barrett MT, Sanchez CA, Prevo LJ, et al: Evolution of neoplastic cell lineages in Barrett oesophagus. *Nat Genet* 1999;22:106.

196. Neshat K, Sanchez CA, Galipeau PC, et al: p53 mutations in Barrett's adenocarcinoma and high grade dysplasia. *Gastroenterology* 1994;106:1589.

197. Buttar NS, Wang K, Sebo TJ, et al: Extent of high grade dysplasia in Barrett's esophagus correlates with risk of adenocarcinoma. *Gastroenterology* 2000;120:1630.

198. Dar MS, Goldblum JR, Rice TW, Falk GW: Can extent of high grade dysplasia in Barrett's oesophagus predict the presence of adenocarcinoma at esophagectomy? *Gut* 2003;52:486.

199. Spechler SJ. Barrett's esophagus. *Semin Oncol* 1994;21:431.
200. Levine D, Haggit R, Blount P, et al: An endoscopic biopsy protocol can differentiate high-grade dysplasia from early adenocarcinoma in Barrett's esophagus. *Gastroenterology* 1993;105:40.
201. Boyce HW. Barrett esophagus-endoscopic findings and what to biopsy. *J Clin Gastroenterol* 2003;36:S6.
202. Tschanz ER: Do 40% of patients resected for Barrett esophagus with high-grade dysplasia have unsuspected adenocarcinoma? *Arch Pathol Lab Med* 2005;129:177.
203. Canto MI: Diagnosis of Barrett's esophagus and esophageal neoplasia: East meets West. *Dig Endosc* 2006;18:S36.
204. Montgomery E: Is there a way for pathologists to decrease interobserver variability in the diagnosis of dysplasia? *Arch Pathol Lab Med* 2005;129:174.
205. Dalai GS, Shakelle PG, Jensen DM, et al: Dysplasia and risk of further neoplastic progression in a regional Veterans Administration Barrett's cohort. *Am J Gastroenterol* 2005;100:775.
206. Lomo LC, Blount PL, Sanchez CA, et al: Crypt dysplasia with surface-maturation. A clinical, pathologic and molecular study of a Barrett's esophagus cohort. *Am J Surg Pathol* 2006;30:42.
207. Thurberg BL, Duray PH, Odze RD: Polypoid dysplasia in Barrett's esophagus: a clinicopathologic, immunohistochemical, and molecular study of five cases. *Hum Pathol* 1999;30:745.
208. Wong RS, Temes RT, Follis FM, et al: Multiple polyposis and adenocarcinoma arising in Barrett's esophagus. *Ann Thorac Surg* 1996;61:216.
209. Haggitt RC: Barrett's esophagus, dysplasia and adenocarcinoma. *Hum Pathol* 1994;25:982.
210. Rice TW, Falk GW, Achcar E, Petras RE: Surgical management of high grade dysplasia in Barrett's esophagus. *Am J Gastroenterol* 1993;88:536.
211. Spechler SJ: Dysplasia in Barrett's esophagus: limitations of current management strategies. *Am J Gastroenterol* 2005;100:927.
212. Reid BJ, Sanchez CA, Blount PL, et al: Barrett's esophagus: cell cycle abnormalities in advancing stages of neoplastic progression. *Gastroenterology* 1993;105:119.
213. Fennery MB, Sampliner RE, Way D, et al: Discordance between flow cytometric abnormalities and dysplasia in Barrett's esophagus. *Gastroenterology* 1989;97;815.
214. Younes M, Lebovitz RN, Lechago LV, et al: p53 protein accumulation in Barrett's metaplasia, dysplasia and carcinoma: a follow-up study. *Gastroenterology* 1993;105:1637.
215. Keswani RN, Noffsinger A, Waxman I, Bissonnette M: Clinical use of p53 in Barrett's esophagus. *Cancer Epidemiol Biomarkers Prev* 2006;15:1243.
216. Dorer R, Odze RD: AMACR immunostaining is useful in detecting dysplastic epithelium in Barrett's esophagus, ulcerative colitis and Crohn's disease. *Am J Surg Pathol* 2006;30:871.
217. Fountoulakis A, Zafirellis KD, Dolan K, et al: Effect of surveillance of Barrett's oesophagus on the clinical outcome of oesophageal cancer. *Br J Surg* 2004;91:997.
218. Corley DA, Levin TR, Habel LA, et al: Surveillance and survival in Barrett's adenocarcinoma: a population-based study. *Gastroenterology* 2002;122:633.
219. Wang KK, Wongkeesong M, Buttar NS: American Gastroenterological Association medical position statement: role of the gastroenterologist in the management of esophageal carcinoma. *Gastroenterology* 2005;128:1468.
220. ASGE guideline: the role of endoscopy in the surveillance of premalignant conditions of the upper GI tract. *Gastrointest Endosc* 2006;63:570.
221. Chejfec G, Jablokow VR, Gould VE: Linitis plastica carcinoma of the esophagus. *Cancer* 1983;51:2139.
222. Kalish RJ, Clancy PE, Orringer MB, et al: Clinical, epidemiologic and morphologic comparison between adenocarcinomas arising in Barrett's esophageal mucosa and in the gastric cardia. *Gastroenterology* 1984;86:451.
223. Paraf F, Flejou JF, Potet F, et al: Esophageal squamous carcinoma in five patients with Barrett's esophagus. *Am J Gastroenterol* 1992;87:746.
224. Banner BF, Memoli VA, Warren WH, et al: Carcinoma with multi-directional differentiation arising in Barrett's esophagus. *Ultrastruct Pathol* 1983;4:205.
225. Kikuchi Y, Tsuneta Y, Kawai T, et al: Choriocarcinoma of the esophagus producing chorionic gonadotropin. *Acta Pathol Jpn* 1988;38:489.
226. Wasan HS, Schofield JB, Krausz T, et al: Combined choriocarcinoma and yolk sac carcinoma arising in Barrett's esophagus. *Cancer* 1994;73:514.
227. Paraf F, Flejou J, Pignon J, et al: Surgical pathology of adenocarcinoma arising in Barrett's esophagus. Analysis of 67 cases. *Am J Surg Pathol* 1995;18:183.
228. Liu L, Hofstetter WL, Rashid A, et al: Significance if the depth of tumor invasion and lymph node metastasis in superficially invasive (T1) esophageal adenocarcinoma. *Am J Surg Pathol* 2005;29:1079.
229. Clark GWB, Peters JH, Ireland AP, et al: Nodal metastasis and sites of recurrence after en-bloc esophagectomy for adenocarcinoma. *Ann Thorac Surg* 1994;58:646.
230. Aikou T, Shimazu H, Takao T, et al: Significance of lymph nodal metastases in the treatment of esophagogastric adenocarcinoma. *Lymphology* 1992;25:31.
231. Feith M, Stein HJ, Siewert JR: Pattern of lymphatic spread of Barrett's cancer. *World J Surg* 2003;27:1052.
232. de Manzoni G, Pedrazzani C, Verlato G, et al: Comparison of old and new TNM systems for nodal staging in adenocarcinoma of the gastro-oesophageal junction. *Br J Surg* 2004;91:296.
233. Torres C, Turner JR, Wang HH, et al: Pathologic prognostic factors in Barrett's-associated adenocarcinoma. *Cancer* 1999;85:52.
234. Menke-Pluymers MB, Schoute NW, Mulder AH, et al: Outcome of surgical treatment of adenocarcinoma of Barrett's oesophagus. *Gut* 1992;33:1454.
235. von Rahden BHA, Stein HJ, Feith M, et al: Lymphatic vessel invasion as a prognostic factor in patients with primary resected adenocarcinomas of the esophagogastric junction. *J Clin Oncol* 2005;23:874.
236. Regalado SP, Nambu Y, Iannettoni MD, et al: Abundant expression of the intestinal protein villin in Barrett's metaplasia and esophageal adenocarcinoma. *Mol Carcinog* 1998;22:182.
237. Wu GD, Beere DG, Moore JH, et al: Sucrase-isomaltase expression in Barrett's esophagus and adenocarcinoma. *Gastroenterology* 1993;105:837.
238. Phillips RW, Frierson HF, Moshaluk CA: CDx2 as a marker of epithelial intestinal differentiation in the esophagus. *Am J Surg Pathol* 2003;27:1442.
239. Moons LMG, Bax DA, Kuipers EJ, et al: The homeodomain protein CDX2 is an early marker of Barrett's oesophagus. *J Clin Pathol* 2003;57:1063.
240. Taniere P, Borghi-Scoazec G, Saurin JC, et al: Cytokeratin expression in adenocarcinoma of the esophagogastric junction—a comparative study of adenocarcinomas of the distal esophagus and of the proximal stomach. *Am J Surg Pathol* 2002;26:1213.
241. van Lier MGF, Bomhof FJ, Leenderste, et al: Cytokeratin phenotyping does not help in distinguishing oesophageal adenocarcinoma from cancer of the gastric cardia. *J Clin Pathol* 2005;58:722.
242. Gramlich TL, Fritsch C, Cohen C, et al: Oncogene expression and amplification in Barrett adenocarcinoma. *Int J Surg Pathol* 1997;4:203.
243. Wilkinson NW, Black J, Roukhadze E, et al: Epidermal growth factor receptor expression correlates with histologic grade in resected esophageal adenocarcinoma. *J Gastrointest Surg* 2004;8:448.
244. Lagorce C, Paraf F, Vidaud D, et al: Cyclooxygenase-2 is expressed frequently and early in Barrett's oesophagus and associated adenocarcinoma. *Histopathology* 2003;42:457.
245. Shimizu D, Vallböhmer D, Kuamochi H, et al: Increasing cyclooxygenase-(cox-2) gene expression in the progression of Barrett's esophagus to adenocarcinomas correlates with that of Bcl-2. *Int J Cancer* 2006;119:765.
246. Buskens CJ, van Rees BP, Sivula A, et al: Prognostic significance of elevated cuclooxygenase-2 expression in patients with adenocarcinoma of the esophagus. *Gastroenterology* 2002;122:1800.
247. Rusch VW, Levine DS, Haggit R, Ried BJ: The management of high-grade dysplasia and early cancer in Barrett's esophagus: a multidiscipline problem. *Cancer* 1994;74:1225.
248. Mino-Kenudson M, Brugge W, Puricelli W, et al: Management of superficial Barrett's epithelium-related neoplasms by endoscopic mucosal resection: clinicopathologic analysis of 27 cases. *Am J Surg Pathol* 2005;29:680.
249. Dragovich T, McCoy S, Urba S, et al: Phase II trial of erlotinib in gastroesophageal (GEJ) and gastric carcinoma: SWOG 0127. *J Clin Oncol* 2006;24:4922.
250. Lauwers GY, Scott GV, Vauthey JN: Adenocarcinoma of the upper esophagus developing in cervical ectopic gastric mucosa: rare evidence of malignant potential of so-called inlet patch. *Dig Dis Sci* 1998;43:901.
251. Sperling RM, Grendell JH: Adenocarcinoma arising in an inlet patch of the esophagus. *Am J Gastroentrol* 1995;90:150.
252. Bergmann M, Charnas RM: Tracheobronchial rests in the esophagus: their relation to some benign strictures and certain types of cancer in the esophagus. *J Thorac Surg* 1958;35:97.

253. Takubo K, Esaki Y, Watanabe A, et al: Adenoma associated by superficial squamous cell carcinoma of the esophagus. *Cancer* 1993;71:2435.

254. Tsutsumi M, Mizumoto K, Tsujiuchi, et al: Serous cystadenoma of the esophagus. *Acta Pathol Jpn* 1990;40:153.

255. Akamatsu T, Honda T, Nakayama J, et al: Primary adenoid cystic carcinoma of the esophagus. Report of a case and its histochemical characterization. *Acta Pathol Jpn* 1986;36:1707.

256. Epstein JI, Sears DL, Tucker RS, et al: Carcinoma of the esophagus with adenoid cystic differentiation. *Cancer* 1984;53:1131.

257. Bell-Thompson J, Haggit RC, Ellis FH Jr: Mucoepidermoid and adenocystic carcinomas of the esophagus. *J Thorac Cardiovasc Surg* 1980;79:438.

258. Sweeney EC, Cooney T: Adenoid cystic carcinoma of the esophagus: a light and electron microscopic study. *Cancer* 1980;45:1516.

259. Hagiwara N, Tajiri T, Miyashita M, et al: Biological behaviour of mucoepidermoid carcinoma of the esophagus. *J Nippon Med Sch* 2003;70:401.

260. Sasajima K, Watanabe M, Takubo K, et al: Mucoepidermoid carcinoma of the esophagus. Report of two cases and review of the literature. *Endoscopy* 1990;22:140.

261. Azzopardi JG, Menzies T: Primary oesophageal adenocarcinoma; confirmation of its existence by the finding of mucus gland tumors. *Br J Surg* 1962;49:497.

262. Ming S-C: *Tumors of the Esophagus and Stomach. An Atlas of Tumor Pathology.* 2nd Series, Fasc. 7, Washington, DC: AFIP, 1973.

263. Caldwell CB, Bains MS, Burt M: Unusual malignant neoplasms of the esophagus: oat cell carcinoma, melanoma and sarcoma. *J Thorac Cardiovasc Surg* 1991;1-1:100.

264. Guzman RP, Wightman R, Ravinsky E, et al: Primary malignant melanoma of the esophagus with diffuse melanocytic atypia and melanoma in-situ. *Am J Clin Pathol* 1989;92;802.

265. Scotto J, Fraumeni JF, Lee JAH: Melanomas of the eye and other noncutaneous sites: epidemiological aspects. *J Natl Canc Inst* 1976;56:489.

266. Patel JK, Didolkar MS, Pickren JW, et al: Metastatic pattern of malignant melanoma. A study of 216 autopsy cases. *Am J Surg* 1978;135:807.

267. Mills SE, Cooper PH: Malignant melanoma of the digestive system. In: *Pathology Annual*, Part 2, Vol. 18. Norwalk, CT: Appleton-Century-Crofts, 1983, pp 1–26.

268. Basque GJ, Boline JE, Holyoke JB: Malignant melanoma of the esophagus: first report in a child. *Am J Clin Pathol* 1970;53:609.

269. Chello M, Marchese AR, Panza A, et al: Primary malignant melanoma of the oesophagus with left atrial metastasis. *Thorax* 1993;48:185.

270. Blessing K, Sanders DS, Grant JJ: Comparison of immunohistochemical staining of the novel antibody melan-A with S-100 and HMB-45 in malignant melanoma and melanoma variants. *Histopathology* 1998;323:139.

271. Manier JW, Reyes CN: Collision tumour of the stomach. Report of two cases. *Gastroenterology* 1974;67:1011.

272. Spagnola DV, Heenan PJ: Collision carcinoma at the esophagogastric junction: report of two cases. *Cancer* 1980:46:2702.

273. Costa J: Critical commentary to: Collision tumors of squamous cell carcinoma and leiomyoma of the esophagus. *Pathol Res Pract* 1993;189:475.

274. Polk HC Jr, Camp FA, Walker AW: Dysphagia and esophageal stenosis. Manifestation of metastatic mammary cancer. *Cancer* 1967;20;2002.

The Nonneoplastic Stomach

EMBRYOLOGY

The stomach develops from a fusiform foregut swelling at approximately 4 weeks' gestation. It originates in the neck and descends into the abdomen during the next 8 weeks. The enlarging thoracic contents push the stomach caudally. The gastric curvature develops during the 6th to 7th fetal week. Simultaneously, the dorsal stomach rotates to the left. In the ninth week, a diverticulum appears in the upper stomach, which subsequently merges with and lengthens the greater curvature. The stomach rotates 90 degrees so that the greater curvature lies on the left, and the distal end becomes anchored by a short ventral mesentery, the bile duct, and the vitelline artery (1).

Gastric development is more complex than other parts of the gut due to the different epithelial types that populate different areas of the stomach. These areas constitute a complex epithelial system organized in a highly structured, continually renewing architecture. Embryonal differentiation is regulated via several signaling cascades, an important one of which starts with the transcription factor Sonic hedgehog (Shh), which binds to its receptor Patched (Ptc). The Shh signaling system helps maintain normal gastric glandular architecture (2). Shh is expressed in parietal cells and its receptor Ptc is present in chief cells (3).

The stomach is initially lined by stratified or pseudostratified epithelium; later, cuboidal cells replace it. As secretions accumulate, droplets and vacuoles coalesce to form the gastric lumen. The first differentiated cell type to appear is the mucous neck cell, which acts as a progenitor for the other cell types. Gastric pits are well developed by 5 to 7 weeks. Gastric glands begin to develop at 11 to 14 weeks (1); they grow by progressively branching, a process that continues until birth. Parietal cells appear by 9 to 11 weeks (Fig. 4.1). Endocrine cells begin to appear at the second week of fetal life; a full spectrum of endocrine cells is present by week 11. Mesoderm surrounding the stomach differentiates into the gastric connective tissue and the muscularis propria by the end of the second fetal month. The muscularis mucosae forms by the 20th week.

GASTRIC PHYSIOLOGY

The stomach exhibits major motor, secretory, digestive, hormonal, and mucosal barrier functions, some of which will be briefly summarized here.

Mucosal Barrier

One of the incredible facets of gastric physiology is that the acid-containing stomach is able to withstand the detrimental effects of its intraluminal contents. In order to do this, a complex mucosal cytoprotection system has evolved that protects the stomach without inhibiting gastric acid secretion. Mucosal defenses include pre-epithelial, epithelial, and postepithelial mechanisms (Fig. 4.2). Adherent mucus provides a stable unstirred layer that supports surface neutralization of acid by mucosal bicarbonate and acts as a permeability barrier to luminal pepsin (4). (Surface mucus is hydrophobic and water repellent.) Surface-active phospholipids are produced by mucous neck cells and parietal cells. Parietal cells pump one HCO_3^- ion across the basal membranes for every H^+ they secrete into the canaliculi (5). HCO_3^- is picked up by mucosal capillaries and carried to the basal part of surface foveolar cells. The bicarbonate ions are then secreted into the overlying mucous layer, where they are trapped by glycoproteins in the mucus, increasing the pH in the unstirred layer from approximately pH 2.0 in the gastric lumen to approximately 7.0 at the mucosal surface. This creates a pH gradient that traps and neutralizes most hydrogen ions as they enter the unstirred mucous layer (6). Maintenance of the pH gradient depends on both the secretion rate of bicarbonate and the thickness of the mucous gel layer (6). Mucus also lubricates the stomach facilitating food movement along the gastric lining, without causing mucosal abrasions. Its glycoproteins play a major role in resistance to injury by maintaining the viscoelastic and permeability properties of the mucous gel. Foveolar cells secrete lipid into the mucus that coats the epithelium lining the gastric lumen with a nonwettable surface, protecting the mucosa against the action of water-soluble H^+ and pepsin (7). (Pepsin can destroy the polymeric structure of this glycoprotein layer, solubilizing the surface mucous gel and liberating degraded glycoprotein subunits into the gastric lumen.)

An adequate mucosal blood flow is critical to maintaining the mucosal barrier since it brings oxygen and nutrients to the luminal surface and removes hydrogen ions from the same region (8). The autonomic nervous system, peptidergic nerves (8), nitric oxide (9), prostaglandins (10), epidermal growth factor (EGF), and transforming growth factor-alpha

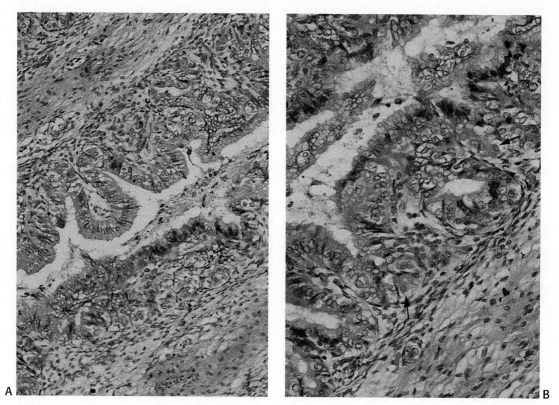

FIG. 4.1. Gastric mucosa of a 10-week-old fetus. **A:** Medium power showing the presence of a well-defined lumen lined by columnar epithelial cells with primitive glands. The muscularis mucosae is just beginning to form. **B:** Higher magnification showing the presence of parietal cells (*arrows*).

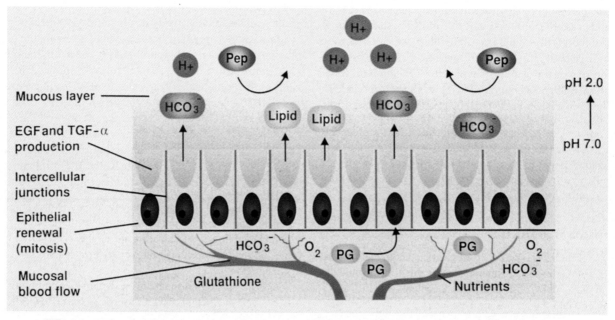

FIG. 4.2. Mucosal defenses. A mucous layer that contains a pH gradient overlies the surface epithelium. Bicarbonate ions are pumped into this layer along with lipids secreted by the lining epithelium. The epithelium is bound together by intercellular tight junctions. The epithelial cells lie on intact basement membrane and produce the epidermal growth factor (EGF) and transforming growth factor-α (TGF-α). The underlying blood supply in the lamina propria brings bicarbonate to the surface-lining cells from the parietal cells where it was produced. The mucosal blood flow also brings oxygen and nutrients. Prostaglandins (PGs) are made within the stroma. The stroma contains antioxidants such as glutathione. Pep, pepsin.

(TGF-α) all regulate mucosal blood flow. Interruption of the mucosal blood flow (as occurs in stress gastritis) results in decreased intramucosal pH and ulceration. Junctional complexes, basolateral membranes, and the basal lamina are also major structural components of the gastric mucosal barrier (11). Cytoprotectants (prostaglandins, immunoglobulins, sulfhydryl donors such as glutathione, and neuropeptides) are also naturally present in the gastric mucosa (10,12). Prostaglandins aid in mucosal protection (10) by mediating mucus and bicarbonate secretion, inhibiting acid secretion, regulating mucosal blood flow, maintaining surface-active phospholipids, and mediating the protective actions of EGF and TGF-α (13). Prostaglandins also modulate the inflam-

matory response by inhibiting release of tumor necrosis factor (TNF) from macrophages (14) and TNF plus other inflammatory mediators from mast cells (15).

Another aspect that protects the gastric mucosa is its ability to proliferate and rapidly replace damaged surface epithelial cells. The gastric epithelium maintains a dynamic equilibrium between cell production and cell loss (Figs. 4.3 and 4.4) (16). The surface epithelium is renewed every 4 to 8 days. Gastrointestinal and nongastrointestinal hormones, growth factors, neural mediators, secretions, luminal food, and absorbed nutrients all modulate gastric mucosal growth (17). EGF, TGF-α, and insulinlike growth factor directly stimulate gastric mucosal growth (17,18). EGF is ideally suited to participate in gastric repair because it is acid stable and stimulates epithelial migration, DNA synthesis, and gastric mucus production. TGF-α shares 35% homology with EGF and mimics its mitogenic effects (19). EGF and TGF-α also modulate parietal cell function and inhibit gastric hydrochloric secretion (20).

Cell progenitors reside in the mucous neck region giving rise to multiple cell types. One type migrates toward the luminal surface and differentiates into foveolar cells. Other cell lineages migrate downward from the mucous neck region slowly differentiating into parietal, chief, mucous, and endocrine cells (Fig. 4.3). Mature parietal cells and chief cells do not divide. Parietal, chief, and endocrine cells turn over more slowly than surface cells, renewing themselves every 1 to 3 years.

Acid and Pepsin Secretion

Three separate pathways stimulate acid secretion: (a) a neural pathway, which delivers transmitters such as acetylcholine

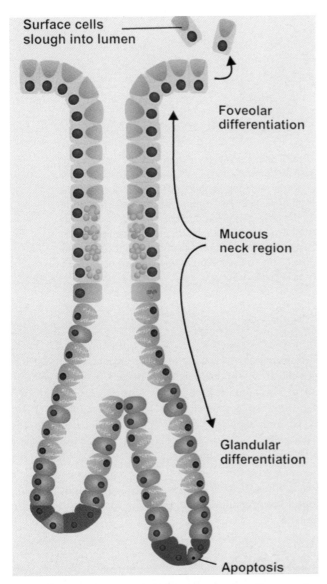

FIG. 4.3. Mucosal renewal. The mucous neck region contains stem cells and is the generative zone. From here, foveolar cells begin to differentiate and migrate toward the surface to be exfoliated. Other cells developing in this area migrate downward to form the epithelium of the oxyntic, cardiac, and antropyloric glands. These glandular cells die by apoptosis.

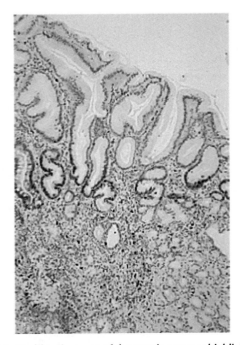

FIG. 4.4. Proliferative zone of the gastric mucosa highlighted by Ki-67 immunostain.

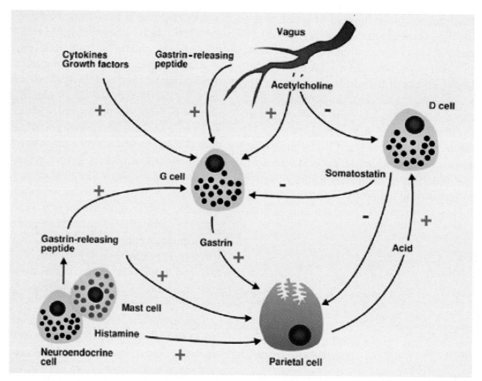

FIG. 4.5. G cells are central to parietal cell secretion. The G cell is positively influenced by acetylcholine release and gastrin-releasing peptide from the vagus as well as from cytokines and growth factors in the gastric mucosa. Mucosal neuroendocrine cells also produce gastrin-releasing peptide, positively influencing the G cell. Vagal stimulation releases acetylcholine, negatively influencing D cells, suppressing somatostatin function. Somatostatin negatively regulates G-cell activity, suppressing gastrin production. G cells, once stimulated, act directly on parietal cells through release of gastrin or indirectly through enterochromaffinlike cells that produce histamine. Histamine released from mast cells or neuroendocrine cells positively influence parietal cells to secrete acid. Somatostatin has a negative influence on acid secretion and forms part of the feedback loop in which acid secretion by parietal cells enhances D-cell function.

(ACH) released from postganglionic nerves in the stomach wall; (b) an endocrine pathway, which delivers hormones such as gastrin; and (c) a paracrine pathway, which delivers tissue factors such as histamine (Fig. 4.5) (21). Potentiating interactions between two or three gastric secretagogues amplify oxyntic secretory responses. Histamine released from lamina propria mast cells and from enterochromaffinlike (ECL) cells binds to H_2 receptors on oxyntic cells, resulting in up-regulation of cholinergic and gastrin receptors, making them more sensitive to subsequent stimulation by their respective secretagogues. ACH binds to muscarinic cholinergic receptors on oxyntic cells, stimulating acid secretion. ACH in the antral mucosa inhibits somatostatin production, a peptide that inhibits gastrin release (22).

Antral G cells release gastrin when the antrum becomes alkalinized, stimulating acid secretion via gastrin receptors on parietal cells and histamine release from ECL cells (23). Vagal stimuli also liberate gastrin-releasing peptide, prompting G cells to produce gastrin and stimulating ECL cells to release histamine. Pepsinogens synthesized by gastric chief cells (24)

have no digestive capacity until they are broken down into pepsin, a reaction that maximally occurs in an acid environment. The stomach produces two immunologically distinct pepsinogens: Pepsinogen 1 (PG1) and pepsinogen 2 (PG2). PG1 is only present in fundic chief and mucous neck cells, whereas PG2 is produced by chief cells, fundic mucous neck cells, cardiac and pyloric glands, and Brunner glands (25). Serum levels of PG1 and PG2 reflect the volume of the cells that produce them. PG1 levels below 20 mg/dL indicate a profound loss of fundic gland volume, as occurs in autoimmune gastritis.

Gastric Motor Functions

In addition to its secretory, digestive, hormonal, and mucosal barrier functions, the stomach has three specific motor functions: (a) storage and volume adaptation, (b) mixing of gastric contents, and (c) forward propulsion of its contents, or gastric emptying. When empty, the stomach is at its smallest possible size. Filling the stomach with fluid or food increases the gastric luminal volume without increasing gastric pressure. Gastric motility is regulated by the extrinsic nerves and by the intrinsic myenteric plexus, which contains cholinergic nerves, adrenergic nerves, and nonadrenergic, noncholinergic nerves.

ANATOMY

The stomach lies intraperitoneally, extending from the lower end of the esophagus at the Z line at the level of the 11th thoracic vertebrae, crossing to the right of the midline, and ending in the duodenum. The opening that connects the esophagus to the stomach is known as the *cardiac orifice*; the opening from the stomach to the intestine is known as the *pyloric orifice*. The stomach has two curvatures: The greater curvature, the inferior border of the stomach, is convex in shape, extending from the gastroesophageal junction to the duodenum. It is more freely movable than the lesser curvature. The concave lesser curvature is the upper margin of the stomach. The size and shape of the usually J-shaped stomach (Fig. 4.6) depends on body position and the degree of filling. Its anterior surface abuts the abdominal wall and the inferior surface of the left lobe of the liver. Posteriorly, it abuts the pancreas, splenic vessels, left kidney, and adrenal gland. The lesser curvature is suspended from the inferior aspect of the liver by the hepatogastric ligament and the lesser omentum. The greater omentum extends caudally from the greater curvature. The gastric fundus touches the dome of the left diaphragm and the upper left margin of the greater omentum rests against the spleen to which it is attached by the gastrosplenic ligament.

The stomach has four layers: Mucosa, submucosa, muscularis propria, and serosa (Fig. 4.7). The gastric wall is slightly firm but pliable and, with the exception of the pylorus, usually does not measure more than 0.5 cm in thickness. The stomach is often divided into four anatomic regions: Cardia,

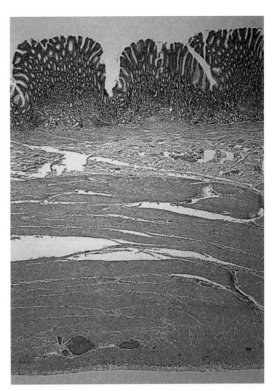

FIG. 4.7. Full-thickness section of the normal stomach. The four layers are easily discerned.

fundus, body, and antropyloric region (Fig. 4.8). The cardia, a narrow, ill-defined region, is not grossly distinctive and is identified histologically by the presence of cardiac glands. Its anatomy is discussed in Chapter 2. The fundus is that portion of the gastric body that protrudes over a horizontal line drawn from the esophagogastric junction (Fig. 4.8). It blends into the gastric body, which constitutes most of the stomach. The body is demarcated from the distal portion, called the pyloric antrum, by a notch in the lesser curvature, the incisura angularis. Numerous longitudinal, grayish pink mucosal folds (called rugae) lie parallel to the lesser curvature (Fig. 4.9) and characterize the mucosa of the gastric body.

The triangularly shaped antrum occupies the distal third of the stomach proximal to the pyloric sphincter extending further along the lesser curvature (5 to 8 cm) than along the greater curvature (6 cm), often almost reaching the cardia (26). The antrum is more firmly anchored to the underlying submucosa than the remainder of the stomach. A greatly thickened distal muscular wall forms the pyloric sphincter. A narrow lumen passes through the pyloric sphincter. The *pyloric canal*, or *pyloric channel*, measures 2.5 cm in length. The various gastric zones are not fixed anatomic entities; their extent varies between individuals, with age, and with disease processes.

The gastric muscularis propria differs from that of the rest of the gastrointestinal (GI) tract in that it consists of

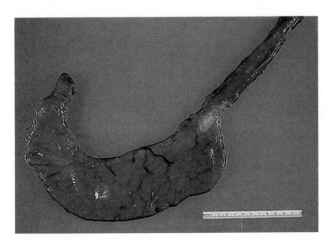

FIG. 4.6. Unopened stomach demonstrating its classic J shape. Esophagus and duodenum is also present.

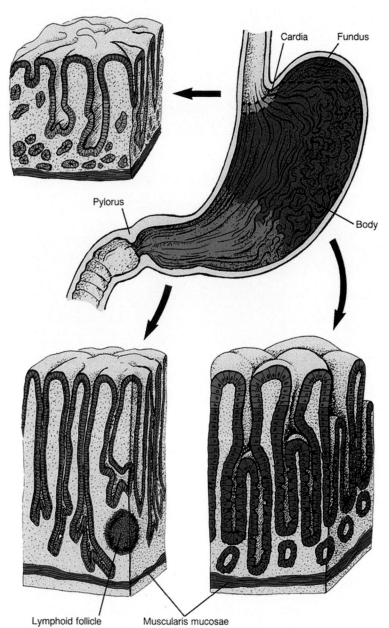

FIG. 4.8. Diagram of the four anatomic and three histologic regions of the stomach. The depths of the gastric pits (*red*) and the glandular composition are different in the various areas of the stomach. The color of the glands corresponds to the color of the anatomic regions. The histology of the glands differs in the pink, green, and blue areas. The gastric pits are similar (*red*) throughout the entire stomach.

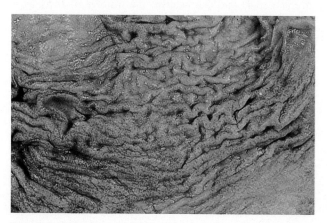

FIG. 4.9. Gastric rugae. When the normal stomach is opened the rugae appear as coarse folds of the mucosa.

muscle fibers oriented in three different directions: The outer longitudinal, the middle circular, and the inner oblique layer. Only the middle circular layer is complete. It is the strongest of the three muscle layers and it becomes hypertrophic proximally and distally at the sphincters. The pyloric musculature consists of two layers: A thick inner circular layer and a thin outer longitudinal layer. The muscularis mucosae consists of two or three muscle layers.

The stomach has a rich blood supply that derives from the celiac, hepatic, and splenic arteries. Mucosal capillaries lie beneath the epithelium. The capillary networks drain into subepithelial venules, which converge into submucosal veins. Venous drainage is through the portal system to the liver. Right and left gastric veins drain the lesser curvature. The left gastric vein arises on the anterior and posterior gastric surfaces. Esophageal veins enter before it reaches the portal vein. Venous drainage from the anterior and posterior surfaces of the antropyloric region forms the right gastric vein, which empties directly into the portal vein. The abundant blood supply explains why gastric ischemia is unusual and why gastric hemorrhages are so life threatening.

Gastric lymphatic distribution resembles that of the colon. Lymphatics are absent from the superficial mucosa but are present in the deep interglandular region (27). They converge into thicker channels piercing the muscularis mucosae and enter the larger submucosal plexus. From there, they drain into the lymphatic plexus between the inner and outer layers of the muscularis propria (27). The lymphatic distribution generally follows that of the main arteries and veins. Gastric lymphatics drain into numerous lymph nodes situated in chains along the greater and lesser curvatures, the cardia, and the splenic hilum. There are four drainage areas. The largest drainage area comes from the lower esophagus and most of the lesser curvature (Fig. 4.10). It follows the left gastric artery and drains into the left gastric lymph nodes. The pylorus drains to the right gastric and hepatic lymph nodes (Fig. 4.10). Lymphatics from the cardia drain into pericardial lymph nodes surrounding the gastroesophageal junction, and efferent channels from the left gastric lymph nodes drain into the celiac lymph nodes. The proximal greater curvature drains into the pancreaticosplenic lymph nodes in the splenic hilum. The distal greater curvature drains into right gastroepiploic lymph nodes in the greater omentum and to the pyloric lymph nodes at the pancreatic head. The pyloric portion of the lesser curvature drains into the right gastric lymph nodes, which then drain into hepatic nodes located along the course of the common hepatic artery. Efferents from all four lymph node groups ultimately pass to the celiac nodes around the main celiac axis.

The stomach is innervated by sympathetic and parasympathetic components of the autonomic nervous system as well as by the peptidergic neural system. The parasympathetic nerve supply derives from the vagus and its branches. Numerous neuropeptides produced and released from nerve fibers in the stomach wall regulate gastric function (28).

A thin translucent serosa (the visceral peritoneum) invests the outer portion of the stomach. The serosa normally appears pink-tan, smooth, and glistening.

NORMAL GASTRIC HISTOLOGY

Histologically, the stomach contains three major epithelial compartments: The gastric pits and surface lining, the mucous neck region, and the glands. The nature and relative thickness of the glands and pits (Fig. 4.8) defines each gastric zone. Foveolar (or surface) epithelium lines the entire gastric surface and short, straight, narrow gastric pits (foveolae) that lie parallel to one another. Gastric glands empty into the bottom of the pits. The stomach is divided into the cardiac, oxyntic, and pyloric areas based on its glandular components. The oxyntic mucosa, which secretes acid and pepsinogen, occupies the proximal 80% of the stomach, including the mucosa of the body and fundus. It is thicker than the cardiac and pyloric mucosa due to the presence of specialized acid-secreting glands. Fundic gastric pits are shorter than elsewhere, occupying only 25% of the mucosal thickness (Fig. 4.8). The antropyloric mucosa constitutes the distal 20% of the stomach and contains mucus-secreting glands and endocrine cells. Cardiac mucosa extends distally from the lower esophagus. Transitional zones between the different areas are gradual and junctional mucosa showing mixed histologic features commonly measures up to 1 cm in width. Each of the gastric epithelial cell types produces a specific cell product (Table 4.1).

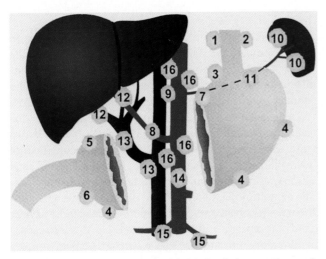

FIG. 4.10. Regional gastric lymph node drainage. The node groups are perigastric nodes (*1–6*), left gastric (*7*), along the splenic artery (*10,11*), along the hepatoduodenal ligament (*12*), para-aortic (*9,16*), and intra-abdominal nodes (*8,13–15*).

TABLE 4.1	Gastric Epithelial Cells and Their Products
Cell Type	**Product**
Surface cells	Mucin, carbonic anhydrase, TGF-α, EGFR
Mucous neck cells	Mucin, pepsinogens, weak lipase, TGF-α
Parietal cells	HCl, intrinsic factor, carbonic anhydrase, TGF-α, cathepsins
Chief cells	Pepsinogen, carbonic anhydrase, lipase
Endocrine cells	Numerous hormones (see Chapter 17)
Cardiac and antral cells	Mucin, proteinases, cathepsins, lysozymes

EGFR, epithelial growth factor receptor; TGF-α, transforming growth factor-α.

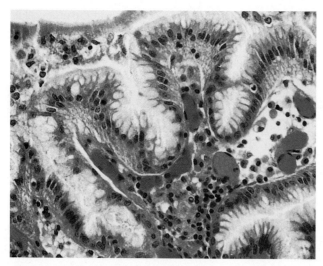

FIG. 4.11. Mucus-secreting foveolar cells cover the gastric surface and line the upper gastric pits.

Surface Epithelium (Foveolar Epithelium)

Tall, columnar, foveolar epithelium covers the entire gastric mucosa. It consists of a single layer of mucus- and bicarbonate-secreting cells with irregular, basally situated nuclei and a single inconspicuous nucleolus (Figs. 4.11 and 4.12). Ovoid, spherical, mucin-containing, membrane-bound granules

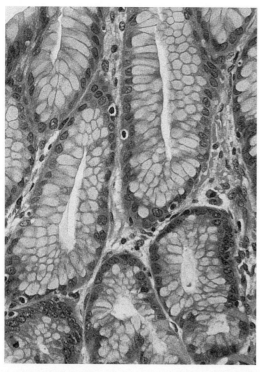

FIG. 4.12. Lining of the gastric pits. Variably mature foveolar cells populate the pits. The mucinous contents increase in size as the cells progress toward the surface. Foveolar epithelia characteristically have basal nuclei with supranuclear mucin collections.

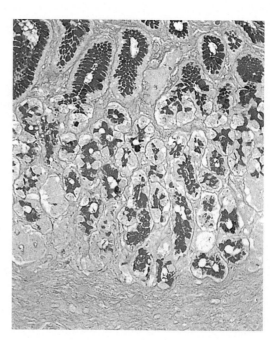

FIG. 4.13. Alcian blue–periodic acid–Schiff stain of cardia.

pack the supranuclear cytoplasm. The mucin stains strongly with the periodic acid–Schiff (PAS) stain (Fig. 4.13); it is negative or only weakly positive with mucicarmine stains. Numerous spot desmosomes and gap junctions maintain intercellular communication between the surface mucous cells, regulate cell differentiation (29), and help maintain mucosal barrier integrity. The surface mucous cells are produced in the mucous neck region, migrate upward, and extrude from the surface.

Gastric Glands

The three types of gastric glands are fundic, cardiac, and pyloric glands. Cardiac and antral glands contain mucin and are compared in Table 4.2. The cardiac mucosa is discussed in detail in Chapter 2. Both cardiac and pyloric glandular cells have ill-defined borders and a bubbly vesicular cytoplasm containing neutral mucin (Figs. 4.14 and 4.15). Unlike foveolar cells, the mucin fills the basal cytoplasm displacing and flattening the nuclei. Pyloric glands contain two major cell types: Tall columnar cells, which secrete neutral mucin, and scattered endocrine cells. Rare parietal and chief cells may also be present. The oxyntic mucosa characteristically contains long, tightly packed oxyntic glands and short foveolae. In contrast to cardiac and pyloric glands, oxyntic glands are straight rather than coiled. Up to three gastric glands empty into the base of a gastric pit. Oxyntic mucosa contains six different cell types: Surface foveolar cells, isthmus mucous cells, parietal cells, mucous neck cells, chief cells, and endocrine cells (Figs. 4.16 and 4.17). The gland neck contains undifferentiated, mucous neck, and parietal

TABLE 4.2 Comparison of Antral and Cardiac Glands

	Cardiac	Antral
Contents	Neutral mucin	Neutral mucin
Structure	Coiled, occasionally branched, loosely packed	Coiled, extensively branched, more compact than cardiac glands
Lamina propria	Abundant	Less abundant than cardiac glands
Cell types	Tall columnar mucinous cells, some endocrine cells	Tall columnar mucinous G cells, enterochromaffin cells
Cystic dilation	May be present	Usually absent
Gastric pits	Length variable up to 50% of mucosa	One third of the mucosal height

cells; the glandular bases contain parietal, chief, and endocrine cells.

Mucous Neck Cells

Mucous neck cells reside in the neck and isthmic region of the gastric glands (Fig. 4.18). They are continuous with, and resemble, foveolar epithelium, but they contain fewer cytoplasmic mucous granules. They derive from mitotically active stem cells in the neck region. These tall, irregularly shaped cells with basal nuclei produce acid glycoproteins, which differ from the neutral mucins secreted by foveolar epithelium. Mucous neck cells may be difficult to recognize in routine sections but they can be highlighted using a PAS stain. The major function of mucous neck cells is mucosal proliferation and regeneration. However, mitoses are rare unless regeneration is occurring.

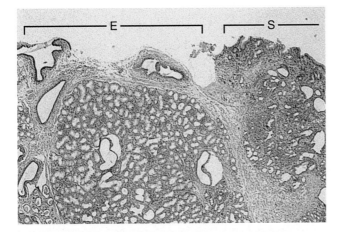

FIG. 4.14. Low magnification showing the junction of the esophagus bracketed by the band labeled *E* and cardiac glands bracketed by the band labeled *S*. Submucosal glands lie both underneath the esophageal-lining epithelium and the gastric-lining epithelium. The esophageal lining has been denuded, although major ducts remain. Note that the glandular configuration underlying the S resembles those underlying the E.

Parietal Cells

Parietal cells constitute approximately one third of the cells in oxyntic glands. They arise from progenitor cells in the lower isthmus and slowly migrate down into the deeper parts of the gland. Intermediate forms exist between immature and mature parietal cells. Parietal cells are easily identifiable by their large size, pyramidal shape, central nuclei, and intensely eosinophilic or clear cytoplasm. Their tapered apical ends tend to bulge into the glandular lumen, whereas their broader basal surfaces rest against the basement membrane (Fig. 4.19). Parietal cells produce hydrochloric acid, intrinsic factor, TGF-α, and cathepsins B and H. In the nonsecretory state, an extensive closed system of smooth membranes, the tubulovesicular system, occupies the cytoplasm adjacent to intracellular canaliculi. Stimulation of acid secretion causes the tubulovesicles to fuse with the canaliculi and the apical secretory membrane, resulting in up to a 40-fold expansion of the apical membrane area. The microvilli become more prominent (30). The canaliculi derive from the smooth endoplasmic reticulum and contain the hydrogen ion pump, a unique H^+,K^+-ATPase that exchanges H^+ for K^+ across the apical membrane (31). When acid secretion is inhibited, the situation reverses. The canaliculi collapse, the microvilli recede, and cytoplasmic tubulovesicular structures become prominent again as the cell returns to its resting state.

The basolateral membranes of parietal cells carry receptors for histamine, gastrin, and acetylcholine (Fig. 4.20). Ligand binding to these receptors stimulates hydrogen ion secretion into the lumen and bicarbonate ions into the interstitium. There is a simultaneous appearance of pathways for K^+ and Cl^- movement coordinated with exchange of H^+ for K^+ powered by the proton pump located in the membranes. Basolateral uptake of chloride by parietal cells is mediated by an HCO_3^- Cl^- anion exchange mechanism (31).

Chief Cells

Chief (zymogenic) cells arise from isthmic stem cells. These triangular low columnar cells contain a coarsely granular, pale gray-blue, basophilic cytoplasm with one or more small nucleoli. Chief cells constitute 20% to 26% of oxyntic glands lying

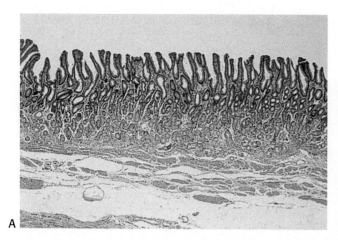

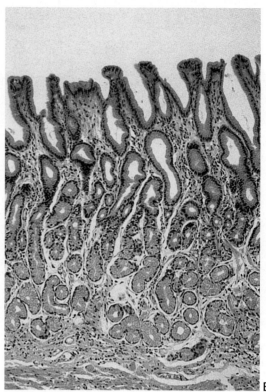

FIG. 4.15. Normal antral glands. **A:** Low magnification of a normal antrum. **B:** Higher magnification showing the mucous glands.

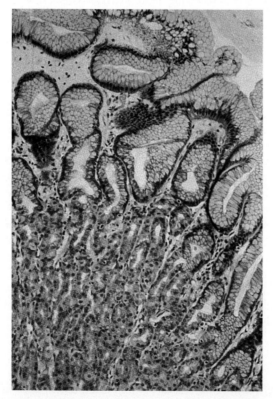

FIG. 4.16. Normal oxyntic mucosa. The bottom portion of the photograph contains densely packed oxyntic glands containing chief cells, parietal cells, and endocrine cells.

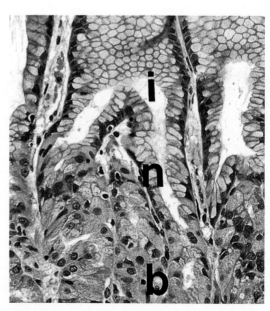

FIG. 4.17. Oxyntic gland showing its base (*b*), neck (*n*), and isthmus (*i*).

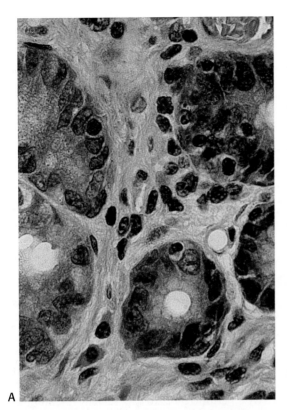
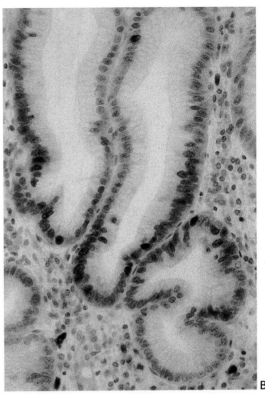

FIG. 4.18. Mucous neck cells. **A:** High magnification of the mucous neck region showing the presence of tall cells lacking the differentiated features of either foveolar epithelium or underlying glandular epithelium. Mitoses are absent. **B:** Ki-67 immunostaining showing the proliferative nature of this region.

deep within them (Fig. 4.19). The basal cytoplasm contains an extensive rough endoplasmic reticulum, which appears as a striated basophilic region. Chief cells produce lipase and pepsinogen, the pepsin precursor. Pepsinogen secretion is stimulated by the same agents that stimulate acid secretion.

Secretory granules form in the Golgi complex and are released by exocytosis. Zymogenic cells degenerate via necrosis or apoptosis. Apoptotic cells are phagocytosed by neighboring zymogenic cells or by lamina propria macrophages that break through the basement membrane of oxyntic glands.

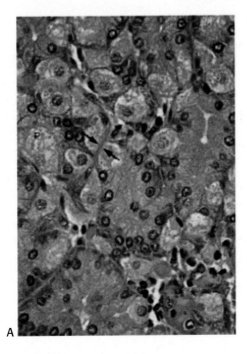
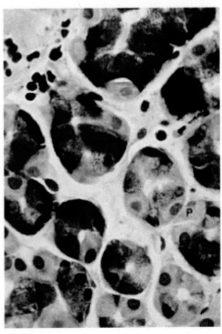

FIG. 4.19. Normal oxyntic glands. **A:** The plump eosinophilic cells are parietal cells, and the chief cells are basophilic. Note the prominent capillaries lying beneath the parietal cells (*arrow*). **B:** Oxyntic mucosa stained with Giemsa. The parietal cells (*P*) are particularly prominent.

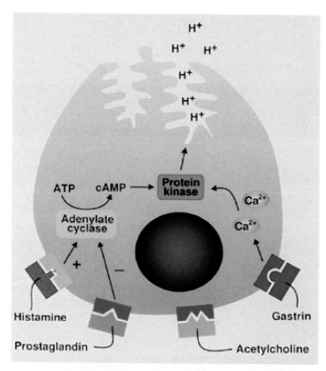

FIG. 4.20. Parietal cells have various receptors along their basolateral membranes. These include those for histamine, prostaglandin, acetylcholine, and gastrin. Ligands bind their respective receptors and activate protein kinase through cyclic adenosine monophosphate (cAMP). The process involves calcium ions. These events result in cellular secretion of H$^+$ ions. ATP, adenosine triphosphate.

Antral and Pyloric Glands

In the antral and pyloric region, the pits occupy approximately 40% of the mucosa. These branch and may not always lie perpendicular to the surface. The deep mucosa contains coiled tubular glands that are lined by faintly granular mucin-secreting cells, often resembling mucous neck cells.

Endocrine Cells

The stomach contains a prominent and diverse endocrine cell population that is discussed further in Chapter 17.

Gastric Transitional Zones

Gastric transitional zones are the junctional zones between the different types of mucosae: Antral/body, body/cardia, and antrum/duodenum. They are dynamic areas that involve a gradual merging of mucosal types so that it may be difficult to determine the exact location of each of the transitional zones. The antral/body transitional zone is usually located approximately two fifths of the way along the lesser curvature; on the greater curvature it is closer to the pylorus (26). The most useful criteria to determine when one crosses from

body into antrum are the absence of chief cells and the change from single tubular glands in the body to branched glands in the antrum (32). It may be difficult to determine the site of origin of the gastric mucosa, particularly when it is altered by inflammation, atrophy, and/or metaplasia. In particular, it may be difficult to differentiate between a nonatrophic antral gastritis and an atrophic body gastritis with pyloric metaplasia.

Lamina Propria and Mononuclear Cells

The surface, pits, and glands are supported by a well-developed lamina propria that contains a fine reticulin meshwork with occasional collagen and elastic fibers condensed beneath epithelial basement membranes and blood vessels. The lamina propria is more abundant in the superficial mucosa between the pits than in the lower mucosa. It contains numerous cell types including fibroblasts, macrophages, plasma cells, and lymphocytes. The lymphocytes are predominantly immunoglobulin (Ig) A–producing B cells. IgG- and IgM-secreting cells are also present. Intraepithelial T lymphocytes are present but they are much less frequent than in the small bowel. These may have a perinuclear halo superficially resembling endocrine cells. There are also a small number of lamina propria T cells, neutrophils, and mast cells. Lymphoid follicles suggest the diagnosis of chronic gastritis. The lamina propria also contains capillaries, arterioles, and nonmyelinated nerve fibers.

Lymphatics appear in the deep lamina propria adjacent to and within the muscularis mucosae. The upper and mid–lamina propria lacks lymphatics. In contrast, the entire mucosa contains a rich supply of capillaries, many of which lie adjacent to the basal lamina of the gastric glands and surface epithelium.

Neuromuscular Relationships

The muscularis mucosae varies from 30 to 200 μm in thickness. It becomes hyperplastic and extends into the overlying mucosa in certain conditions as discussed later. The muscularis propria consists of smooth muscle cells and contains nerve fibers and a myenteric plexus. There are also interstitial cells of Cajal (ICC), which have contacts with each other and with the smooth muscle cells and nerve endings in the muscularis propria (33). They lie in the myenteric plexus and in the circular muscle (33). They serve as gastric pacemakers.

Serosa

The serosa, the outermost gastric layer, consists of connective tissue and a mesothelial lining continuous with the peritoneum.

STRUCTURAL ABNORMALITIES

Duplications

Gastric duplications constitute only 3.8% to 10% of all gastrointestinal duplications (34). They affect females more commonly than males. Sixty-five percent of patients present during the first year of life, often with respiratory distress or as an intrathoracic or extragastric mass (34). Occasionally, the lesions present in adults (35). Thirty-five percent of patients have associated developmental anomalies (Table 4.3) (36). Complications include ulceration, bleeding, rupture, fistula formation, and, rarely, carcinoma (37). Distal duplications cause gastric outlet obstruction, pain, vomiting, fever, weight loss, or hemorrhage (34).

Gastric duplications appear as intramural cylindrical or cystic masses ranging in size from 1.3 to 12 cm. They share a common blood supply with the rest of the stomach; a common musculature invests them. Most duplications occur on the greater curvature (34); one third affect the distal stomach. They may be complete or incomplete, communicating or noncommunicating. Alimentary mucosa lines gastric duplications. This lining resembles and/or differs from that of the normal stomach. Gastric and small intestinal epithelium may coexist within a single duplication. Pancreatic tissue may also be present, as may respiratory mucosa, cartilage, or submucosal glands.

Dextrogastria

In patients with situs inversus, the stomach lies to the right of the midline, a condition known as dextrogastria. The esophageal diaphragmatic hiatus also lies on the right side; the first part of the duodenum lies on the left side. Dextrogastria affects approximately 1 of every 6,000 to 8,000 births (38). Situs inversus affecting only the stomach and duodenum (with the remainder of the thoracic and abdominal viscera lying in their normal positions) is extremely rare (38). The stomach either lies completely behind the liver or above it. Although abnormally positioned, gastric structure and function are normal.

Gastroschisis

The incidence of gastroschisis increased from 0.006 per 1,000 in 1968 to 0.089 per 1,000 in 1977. Young, socially dis-advantaged women have the highest risk of giving birth to a child with gastroschisis (39). Gastroschisis presumably results from vascular injury to the abdominal wall causing defective somatopleural mesenchymal differentiation during the 5th to 11th fetal weeks (40). Gastroschisis may complicate premature atrophy or abnormal persistence of the right umbilical vein (40). Portions of the stomach, small intestine, and colon herniate through an abdominal wall defect lateral to the umbilicus. Since no peritoneal sac or sac remnant covers the eviscerated abdominal contents, the herniated organs are exposed to amniotic fluid leading to gastric wall thickening, serosal edema, and fibrinous exudates.

Congenital Hiatal Hernia

A congenital periesophageal gap or congenital elongated esophageal hiatus can result in a congenital hiatal hernia with invagination of abdominal contents into the thorax (Fig. 4.21). The defect results from failure of the pleuroperitoneal folds to develop or from failure of the pleuroperitoneal canal to close. Urinary tract abnormalities are common in patients with congenital posterolateral diaphragmatic defects including renal agenesis, dysplasia, hypoplasia, or hydronephrosis.

Acquired Hiatal Hernia

The freely movable stomach can prolapse through natural and surgically created diaphragmatic defects, coming to lie in the thoracic cavity. Clues that a biopsy may come from the area of a hiatal hernia include the presence of variably inflamed cardiac or oxyntic mucosa with edema, lymphatic

TABLE 4.3	Lesions Coexisting with Gastric Duplications
Esophageal duplications	Accessory spleen
Heterotopic pancreas	Abnormally shaped spleen
Gastrointestinal malrotations	Urinary tract anomalies
Meckel diverticulum	Turner syndrome
Thoracic vertebral anomalies	Patent ductus arteriosus
Pulmonary sequestration	Ventricular septal defect

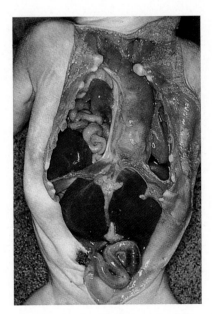

FIG. 4.21. Congenital right diaphragmatic defect. The small intestine has herniated into the right thoracic cavity with partial collapse of the right lung and deviation of the trachea to the left. A large thymus overlies the trachea.

dilation, and pronounced muscle hyperplasia, splaying, or stranding. Squamous metaplasia may be present.

Diverticula

Congenital Diverticula

Gastric diverticula are rare, ranging in incidence from 0.02% to 0.18% (41). Most arise on the posterior wall, in a juxtacardiac position (41). Congenital diverticula appear as solitary, sharply defined, round, oval, or pear-shaped pouches communicating with the gastric lumen via a narrow or broad-based mouth (Fig. 4.22).

Acquired Diverticula

Acquired diverticula almost always originate in the distal stomach as a complication of antral inflammation. Fibrosis following acute inflammation causes traction on the tissues and mucosa herniates through the gastric wall. Therefore, antral diverticula should be carefully evaluated to exclude the presence of an underlying pathologic process such as gastritis, peptic ulcer disease, or neoplasia.

Atresia, Webs, and Diaphragms

Congenital gastric outlet obstruction due to a membranous antral web is extremely rare with an incidence of 0.0001% to 0.0003% of live births (42). A high incidence of associated extraintestinal anomalies and a strong familial history for

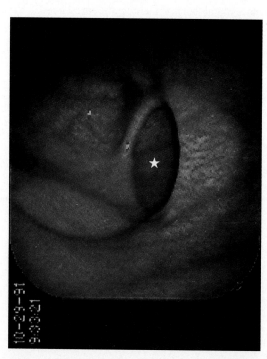

FIG. 4.22. Gastric diverticulum. Endoscopic appearance. The orifice of the diverticulum is indicated by a *star*. Note the similarity of the mucosal lining in both the native stomach as well as in the diverticulum.

pyloric atresia support the theory that atresias and webs result from underlying genetic alterations. Polyhydramnios affects more than 50% of cases. Gastric atresia may associate with trisomy 21, epidermolysis bullosa, or esophageal and anal atresia (43,44). Hereditary multiple gastrointestinal atresias affect the GI tract from the pylorus to the rectum and are inherited in an autosomal recessive fashion. They may associate with immunodeficiency syndromes (44,45).

Most patients with gastric atresia present in the first few days of life with bile-free vomiting and abdominal distention. Type 1 gastric atresia (the most common type) consists of an internal web or diaphragm that completely separates the stomach from the duodenum. Type 2 atresia (the rarest type) consists of a thin, fibrous cord that connects a blind gastric pouch to a distal blind small intestinal segment. Type 3 atresia consists of a blind gastric pouch and a blind distal intestinal pouch without intervening tissue (44,45).

A variably inflamed distal antral mucosal fold with a central aperture measuring from 1 to 10 mm in diameter lies perpendicular to the long axis of the antrum. The serosa may appear indented at the level of the diaphragm. Antral mucosa lines both sides of the diaphragm covering a submucosal core. Heterotopic pancreatic tissue sometimes lies within webs and diaphragms (44,45). In adults, diaphragms and webs complicate inflammatory conditions (35).

Pyloric Stenosis

Pyloric stenosis affects both children and adults and assumes several forms.

Infantile Hypertrophic Pyloric Stenosis (Congenital Pyloric Stenosis)

This disorder is discussed in Chapter 10 since it is primarily a motility-related disorder.

Acquired Pyloric Stenosis

Adult forms of hypertrophic pyloric stenosis result from inflammation associated with antral gastritis and/or peptic ulcer disease, or from inherent neuromuscular abnormalities. Partial gastric obstruction leads to an increased stomach size and weight due to localized or diffuse gastric muscular hypertrophy and hyperplasia, increased mucosal thickness, and G-cell hyperplasia. The pyloric deformity leads to bile reflux and secondary alkaline reflux gastritis.

Torus Hyperplasia

The very rare condition known as focal pyloric hypertrophy (torus hyperplasia) appears as a localized area of circular muscle hypertrophy affecting the lesser curvature near the pyloric torus. The lesion may represent a form of acquired pyloric stenosis or it may represent persistence of congenital pyloric stenosis into adulthood. Some speculate

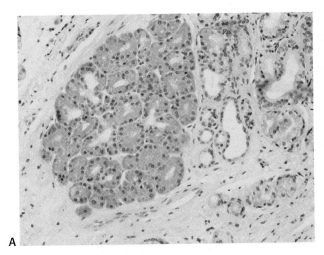

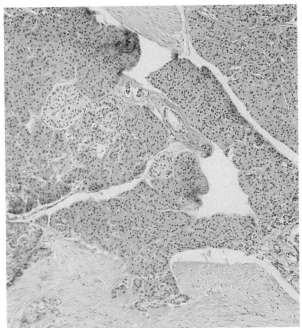

FIG. 4.23. Pancreatic metaplasia versus heterotopic pancreas. **A:** Pancreatic metaplasia consists of pancreatic acini that merge with the surrounding gastric mucosa. **B:** Heterotopic pancreas usually involves the submucosa and may contain pancreatic lobules, islets, and ductules (not shown).

that the lesion results from chronic gastritis or from repeated spastic pyloric contractions (46).

Heterotopias

Normal tissues lie in abnormal locations due to a congenital heterotopia or secondary to a metaplasia. Congenital heterotopias differ from metaplastic (acquired) lesions in that they usually retain a normal organizational structure, whereas metaplastic processes tend to consist of a single cell type lacking normal tissue patterns (Fig. 4.23). Congenital heterotopias result from cellular entrapment during embryonic morphogenetic movements. The congenitally displaced tissues then differentiate along the lines of normal organs in response to the local environment.

Heterotopic Pancreas

Heterotopic pancreas is the most common gastric heterotopia. It accounts for 25% to 30% of all pancreatic heterotopias (47). It is usually an incidental finding, commonly found in the antrum, and followed by the pylorus, greater curvature, and esophagogastric junction. If a tumor or pancreatitis develops, the heterotopic tissue may become symptomatic. Heterotopic pancreas usually appears as a solitary submucosal, hemispheric, umbilicated mass measuring 0.4 to 4.0 cm in diameter. The entry of single or multiple ducts into the gastric lumen produces a symmetric cone or short, cylindric, nipplelike projection (Fig. 4.24). Heterotopic pancreas may also present as large submucosal mucinous cysts. Multiple or pedunculated

pancreatic heterotopias are uncommon. Approximately 75% of pancreatic heterotopias lie in the submucosa (Fig. 4.25), with the remainder involving the muscularis propria. Cross section of larger lesions reveals the typical tan, lobulated tissue characteristic of eutopic pancreas. The deeper the lesion, the more disorderly it tends to appear. The pancreatic lobules contain variable mixtures of pancreatic acini, ducts, islets, glands resembling Brunner glands, and hypertrophic smooth muscle fibers. The islets contain variable numbers of pancreatic polypeptide and insulin-producing cells (48). If only pancreatic acini are present, the lesion may represent foci of pancreatic metaplasia (see below), especially if the cells lie within the mucosa. Sometimes one sees both heterotopic pancreatic and gastric tissue lying side by side in the submucosa (Fig. 4.26).

Heterotopic pancreatic tissue does not pose a diagnostic problem when both pancreatic acini and ducts are present. However, lesions containing only smooth muscle and/or pancreatic ducts have been misinterpreted as adenomyomas. A clue that the lesion represents heterotopic pancreatic tissue, rather than an adenomyoma, is the finding of hypertrophic circular and longitudinal smooth muscle cells arranged circumferentially around the ducts in a more or less normal fashion (Fig. 4.25). Secondary changes such as pancreatitis, cyst formation, or neoplasia (islet cell tumors, ductal dysplasia [Fig. 4.27], and adenocarcinoma) may also cause confusion, particularly when they distort the underlying tissue (49). Dilated ducts forming submucosal mucin pools containing epithelial clusters and variable degrees of inflammation, without obvious pancreatic tissue adjacent to the mucin, may suggest a diagnosis of colloid carcinoma. One should not

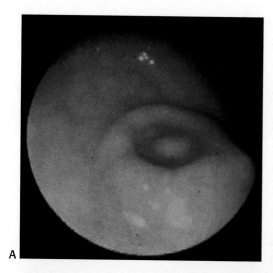

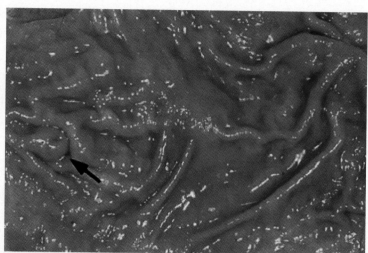

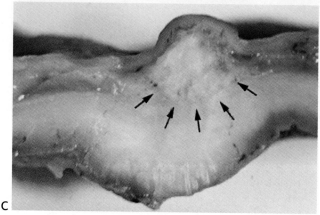

FIG. 4.24. Heterotopic pancreas. The heterotopic pancreas produces a well-defined submucosal mass that is visible endoscopically **(A)** as well as grossly **(B)**. The submucosal mass distorts the gastric folds (*arrow*) and appears as a hemispheric lesion with a central umbilication. **C:** Cross section of the gastric wall demonstrating the presence of a whitish, firm mass lying within the submucosa as indicated by the *arrows*.

make a diagnosis of invasive cancer in the absence of significant cytologic atypia and stromal desmoplasia.

Heterotopic Gastric Glands

Diffuse or localized submucosal gastric heterotopias occur in up to 14% of stomachs (50). These are either congenital in origin or represent areas of gastritis cystica profunda (discussed below). Congenital gastric heterotopia usually contains oxyntic mucosa with foveolar epithelium arranged in a normal architectural pattern.

Heterotopic Brunner Glands

Heterotopic Brunner glands can accompany heterotopic pancreas, or the heterotopia may contain only Brunner glands and smooth muscle. The heterotopic glands lie in the pylorus and gastric antrum and histologically resemble duodenal Brunner gland hyperplasia (see Chapter 6).

Double Pylorus

Double pylorus is an acquired condition in patients with peptic ulcer disease. Prepyloric ulcers penetrate the pyloric wall, perforate into the duodenum, and create a new mucus-

lined channel. Rare examples of congenital double pylorus also exist (51).

Pyloric Mucosal Prolapse

Antral mucosa may prolapse into the duodenum, sometimes forming a mushroom-shaped duodenal or gastric pseudopolyp (Fig. 4.28). It occurs sporadically or complicates gastritis or previous gastric surgery. Submucosal edema (as the result of an underlying inflammation) predisposes to mucosal prolapse. As the edema increases, the tissues fail to return to their normal position; progressive gastric outlet obstruction develops. Patients with mucosal prolapse usually develop crampy abdominal pain, delayed gastric emptying, or vomiting due to the gastric outlet obstruction. The prolapsed mucosa appears variably inflamed, edematous, and necrotic, depending on the duration and severity of the obstruction and the degree of vascular compromise. Pit hyperplasia, pit distortion with cystic serrated branched villiform surfaces, a hyperplastic muscularis mucosae with a muscular lamina propria, erosions, ulcers, glandular atrophy, and variable inflammation may all develop.

Volvulus

Gastric volvulus, also known as gastric torsion, affects both children and adults, usually in the presence of a left

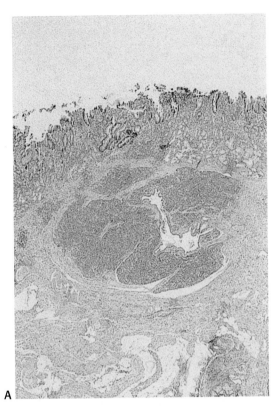
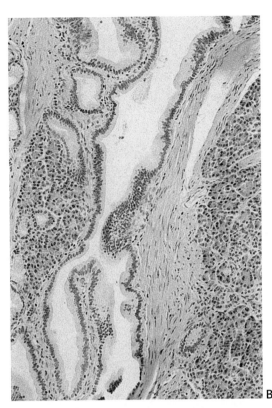

FIG. 4.25. Heterotopic pancreas. **A:** A lobulated submucosal glandular structure with a central duct. Delicate strands of fibrovascular tissue separate individual lobules. **B:** Higher magnification of the duct and pancreatic acini on either side of the duct. Prominent smooth muscle fibers also surround the duct.

diaphragmatic abnormality (52,53). It presents acutely or chronically. Acute presentations include hemorrhage, ischemia, and infarction (52,53). Most patients are elderly with a chronic form of the disease. They have recurrent epigastric pain, vomiting, and occasional hematemesis.

Gastric volvulus occurs in several forms. The most common type, *organoaxial volvulus*, accounts for approximately 60% of cases. The stomach twists around the longitudinal axis of its lesser curvature, causing the stomach to turn upside down (Fig. 4.29), producing both proximal and distal

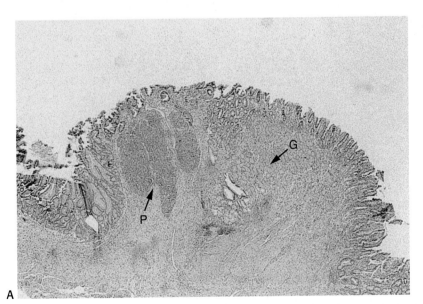
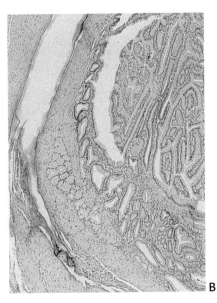

FIG. 4.26. Heterotopic pancreas combined with heterotopic gastric tissue. **A:** Low-power magnification demonstrating the side-by-side arrangement of heterotopic pancreatic tissue (*P*) (*arrow*) and gastric foveolar epithelium (*G*) (*arrow*). **B:** Higher magnification demonstrating the histologic features of the gastric epithelium.

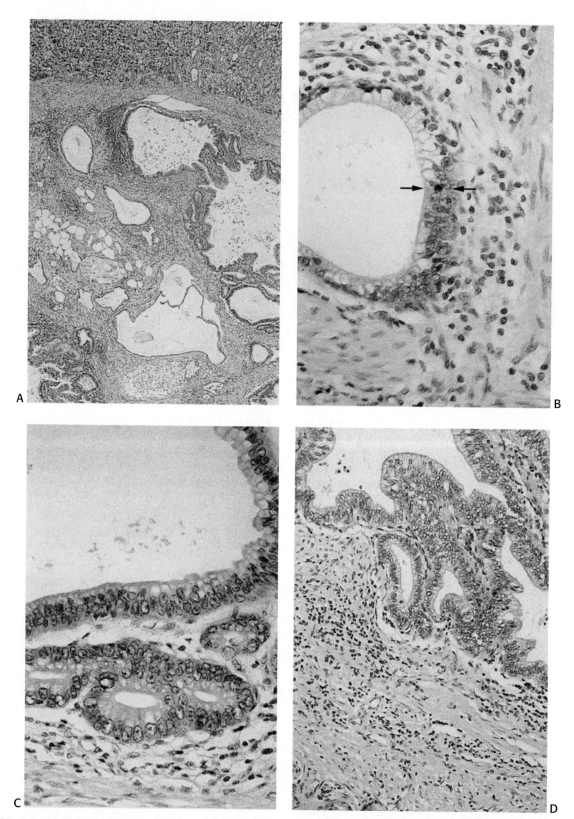

FIG. 4.27. Heterotopic pancreas with dysplastic epithelium. **A:** Numerous cystic structures lie within the gastric wall. Some are lined by flattened epithelium and contain prominent mucinous collections. Others are lined by benign neoplastic epithelial cells. **B:** Higher magnification of one of the glands showing the junction of more or less normal epithelium with basal nuclei above the *arrows* with the benign neoplastic hyperchromatic epithelium with an increased nuclear:cytoplasmic ratio and prominent nucleoli beneath the arrows. **C:** Higher magnification of the neoplastic epithelium showing cytologic atypia, nuclear stratification, and prominent nucleoli. **D:** Another area with a more complicated glandular architecture. Note the absence of invasion into the surrounding tissues and the absence of a desmoplastic response. The glands are still surrounded by intact smooth muscle fibers.

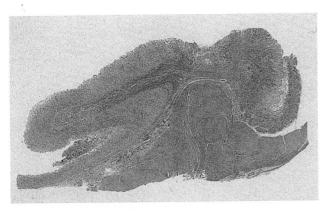

FIG. 4.28. Mucosal prolapse. The prolapsed mucosa assumes a mushroom-shaped configuration overlying the area of the pylorus.

obstructions. Anterior rotation is more common than posterior rotation. *Mesenteroaxial volvulus* represents 30% of cases. It occurs around a line that runs from the center of the greater curvature to the porta hepatis. Mesenteroaxial and organoaxial volvulus can coexist. The stomach can also twist about the vertical axis of the gastrohepatic omentum producing torsion rather than a true volvulus. As a volvulus develops, the stomach progressively distends, due to accumulated secretions that cannot pass forward or be regurgitated because the volvulus produces both distal and proximal obstruction. Death results from the sequence of obstruction, strangulation, and ischemic necrosis, the latter resulting from compression of the gastric vasculature.

Microgastria

Microgastria, a rare congenital anomaly, often coexists with other anomalies such as midgut malrotations, cardiac abnor-

malities, and asplenia (54). The underdeveloped lower esophageal sphincter becomes incompetent and gastroesophageal reflux develops. Symptoms appear in infancy and include failure to thrive, vomiting, and recurrent aspiration pneumonia. Barium swallows demonstrate a small tubular stomach. Histologically, the gastric wall appears hypoplastic (55). The stomach is small, often nonrotated without a clear definition of the various zones. The disorder may result from failed development of the mesogastrium.

MUCOSAL BIOPSY

Endoscopic examination with mucosal biopsy and/or cytologic sampling is regularly employed for the initial identification and monitoring of patients with various gastric conditions including gastritis, gastric atrophy, peptic ulcer disease, and neoplastic proliferations. Gastric biopsies are also commonly used to evaluate the stomach for the presence or absence of *Helicobacter pylori (HP)*. Routine gastric biopsies may also show special forms of gastritis (eosinophilic, lymphocytic, and granulomatous), giant fold disease, or polyps. Gastric biopsies can provide information about the grade, extent, and topography of gastritis-related and atrophy-related lesions, information that provides the opportunity to assess the patient's risk for developing gastric carcinoma. As noted previously, gastric histology varies from area to area and since many gastric diseases are patchy in their distribution, an adequate evaluation often requires examining biopsies from the body, antrum, and any endoscopically visible lesions. The Sydney system requires that biopsies be obtained from five locations in the stomach (the greater and lesser curvature in the antrum, the greater and lesser curvature in the corpus, and the incisura) (56), although this seldom happens in routine clinical practice.

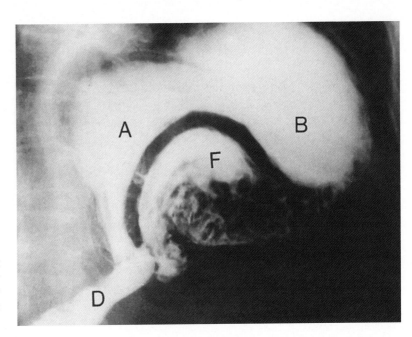

FIG. 4.29. Barium examination showing a gastric organoaxial volvulus. Large thick radiolucent curvilinear defect represents the superiorly located lesser curvature wall and the inferiorly located greater curvature wall. F, fundus; B, body; A, antrum; D, duodenum.

Typically gastroenterologists take a couple biopsies from the antrum and a couple from the corpus. Ideally these should be submitted in separate containers, although this does not always happen either.

It is important to note that endoscopic procedures may cause variable degrees of edema, vascular dilation, focal lamina propria hemorrhage, and surface cell flattening. These changes are usually easily distinguishable from mucosal disease because of the absence of both epithelial degeneration and acute inflammation. A systematic examination of gastric biopsies facilitates the diagnosis of various gastric diseases and provides the discipline of establishing a differential diagnosis so that specific diagnostic entities are considered and important entities are not overlooked. One should determine where the biopsy comes from by looking at various mucosal components. However, it may be difficult to determine the precise location of a biopsy because of the presence of atrophy and/or metaplasia. Gastric epithelium may appear in the duodenum in peptic duodenitis; intestinal metaplasia occurs in the setting of gastritis and Barrett esophagus, and pyloric glands develop in the proximal stomach in certain forms of gastritis.

One can broadly divide gastric inflammatory diseases into gastritis and gastropathy. The major distinction between the two is the presence of inflammation in gastritis and its absence in gastropathies. Gastritis typically results from infections, autoimmune or hypersensitivity reactions, or drugs. Determining whether gastritis is a pangastritis or affects only the antral or corpus, whether it is focal or diffuse, and whether it is superficial or occupies the entire mucosal thickness helps distinguish among these etiologies. Other changes that may be assessed include a determination of whether any of the following are present: Surface epithelial damage, superficial stromal hemorrhage, metaplasia (intestinal, pancreatic, or antral), endocrine cell hyperplasia,

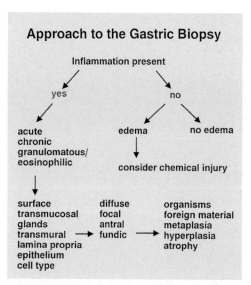

FIG. 4.30. Diagnostic algorithm. One can use this approach once one has determined the subsite localization for the changes that are present. One makes an assessment as to whether or not inflammation is present and, if so, what type and where it is. If inflammation is absent, then one might consider a chemical injury.

intraepithelial lymphocytosis, granulomas, apoptosis, or microorganisms. Gastropathies result from hypovolemia, stress, ischemia, drug or alcohol ingestion, chronic congestion, or alkaline reflux from the duodenum. Diagnostic approaches we find useful are shown in Figures 4.30 and 4.31. We do not believe that it is necessary to routinely order special stains to determine whether *HP* infections or intestinal metaplasia are present, a view shared by others (57). A more detailed evaluation can be used by applying the Sydney system as discussed further in a later section.

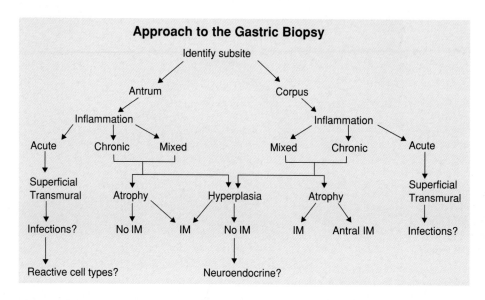

FIG. 4.31. Diagnostic approach to interpreting gastric biopsies. In this approach, one starts by identifying the portion of the stomach that is primarily affected because different entities preferentially affect the antrum and corpus. One then goes through a decision tree based on the character of the inflammation and whether the mucosa appears normal, atrophic, or hyperplastic and contains other cell types. IM, intestinal metaplasia.

TABLE 4.4 Causes of Acute Gastritis			
Drugs	Radiation	Acute alcoholism	Multiorgan failure
Uremia	Certain foods	Severe burns	Portal hypertension
Ischemia	Sepsis	Alkaline reflux[a]	Congestive heart failure
Shock	Trauma	Bile reflux[a]	Respiratory failure
Corrosive agents	Certain infections	Major surgery	Increased intracranial pressure

[a] Acute inflammation uncommon.

ACUTE GASTRITIS

Acute gastritis (accompanied by acute mucosal injury) results from many disorders with multifactorial etiologies and diverse histologic patterns (Table 4.4). The clinical symptoms, endoscopic findings, and histologic features rarely correlate with one another due to the nonspecificity of the symptoms, the diverse etiologies, and the diffuseness (or focality) of the process. Acute gastritis appears hemorrhagic, nonhemorrhagic, erosive, or nonerosive.

Acute Hemorrhagic, Erosive Gastritis (Stress Gastritis)

Acute erosive gastritis complicates major physiologic disturbances including sepsis, extensive burn injury, head injury, severe trauma, and multiorgan failure. It also develops following ingestion of nonsteroidal anti-inflammatory drugs (NSAIDs), aspirin, or alcohol. Acute gastritis often presents as abdominal discomfort, pain, heartburn, nausea, vomiting, and hematemesis. Bleeding begins 3 to 7 days following a stressful event. It ranges from occult blood loss to massive hemorrhage that originates from innumerable foci of mucosal damage to smaller, more discrete ulcers (Fig. 4.32). Curling ulcers develop in severe burn patients within 24 to 72 hours, predominantly in the proximal stomach.

Pathophysiology

Major factors implicated in the development of stress ulcers include hyperchlorhydria and decreased mucosal protection.

The latter results from decreased mucus secretion, mucosal blood flow, and DNA and prostaglandin synthesis, and mucosal barrier breakdown. Indeed, mucosal ischemia is the common denominator of stress-associated injury. Cardiac dysfunction, hemorrhage, shock, and sepsis redistribute blood flow away from the subepithelial capillaries, causing mucosal hypoxia. The hypoxia may persist after recovery from the initial injury, especially as mucosal arterioles contract, further reducing tissue oxygenation (58). An adequate microcirculation that provides nutrients and removes waste products, particularly oxygen-free radicals, is required to maintain the mucosal barrier. A damaged mucosal barrier allows back-diffusion of acid, resulting in tissue acidosis, vascular compromise, mucosal congestion, and necrosis. The mucosal injury increases significantly during the reperfusion that follows ischemia due to the production of toxic oxygen-free radicals (59) by infiltrating neutrophils (60). In addition, activated leukocytes release mediators that reduce mucosal blood flow and increase vascular permeability (61,62). The oxygen-free radical-induced injury is further enhanced by mucosal depletion of the endogenous antioxidant reduced glutathione (GSH) (63). The GSH oxidation/reduction cycle, catalyzed by glutathione peroxidase, reduces H_2O_2 and breaks the chain reaction that generates highly reactive hydroxyl radicals. GSH acts as a natural scavenger whose superoxide anion protects proteins against oxidation. GSH also plays a major role in restoring other free radical scavengers and antioxidants such as vitamins E and C to their reduced state (64). Prostaglandins limit the initial injury (65). Oxidative stress leads to epithelial growth factor receptor (EGFR) phosphorylation and increased production

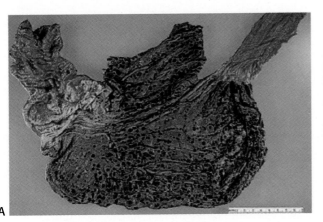
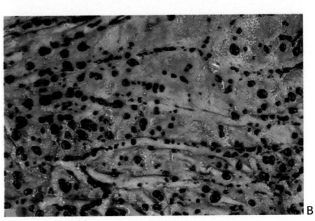

FIG. 4.32. Stress ulcers. **A:** Multiple small punctate hemorrhagic ulcers in a patient who died of severe head trauma. Scattered small petechiae are also visible. **B:** Higher power magnification of individual lesions.

of its ligands, EGF and amphiregulin (66). A mucoid cap promotes mucosal restitution by protecting the lamina propria from luminal acid, limiting the extent of the injury (65).

Various factors contribute to the repair of acute gastric mucosal injury. Re-epithelialization requires epithelial migration across an intact basal lamina. This occurs within minutes to hours of the injury to ensure quick restoration of surface epithelial continuity and inhibiting acid back-diffusion (65). In addition, cells in the mucous neck region migrate out of the proliferative zone and progressively differentiate into mature foveolar cells. Gastric mucosal blood flow increases (65). If this is inhibited, mucosal cytoprotective events fail and the mucosal injury progresses with deeper ulceration than would otherwise result from the initial injury.

Pathologic Features

Erosive gastritis and stress ulcers typically appear as multiple lesions located anywhere in the stomach, although they tend to predominate in the oxyntic mucosa (Fig. 4.32). When severe, they extend to the antrum. Stress ulcers tend to be superficial and usually measure <15 mm in diameter. The ulcer bases appear grayish yellow and hemorrhagic with slightly raised, congested, regenerative margins. The intervening gastric mucosa appears diffusely congested and contains numerous small petechial hemorrhages. Alternatively, the mucosa is diffusely hemorrhagic without discrete areas of damage. Early lesions center around intensely congested blood vessels, which leak blood into the surrounding tissues (Fig. 4.33). Extensive hemorrhagic mucosal erosions or ulcers develop in more severe cases. Rare cases present with deep linear ulcers coexisting with more discrete, round, superficial lesions. Curling and Cushing ulcers tend to be deep and single.

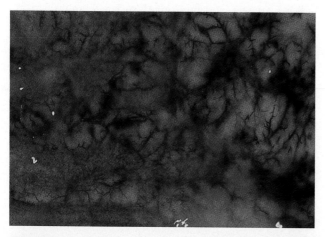

FIG. 4.33. Close-up gross photograph of the gastric mucosa in a patient who died of multiorgan failure. Note the intensely congested vessels as well as the areas of neovascularization. Pinpoint hemorrhages extend from vessels of all sizes contributing to the diffuse leakage of blood from the gastric surface.

TABLE 4.5	Pathology of Acute Erosive Gastritis

Acute phase
  Vascular engorgement
  Lamina propria hemorrhage
  Superficial necrosis
  Polymorphonuclear leukocytes in pits and glands
  Ulcers and erosions
  Superficial fibrin deposits
Healing phase
  Epithelial regeneration with nuclear enlargement
  Pit elongation
  Mucus depletion
  Numerous mitoses

The histologic features depend on the severity and duration of the underlying insult; they are often not as dramatic as the gross features. Features associated with acute gastritis are listed in Table 4.5. Mucosal changes range from hyperemia, surface erosions, and acute inflammation to massive mucosal necrosis (Fig. 4.34), sloughing, and eventual scarring. Lesions seen in biopsies are typically early. More severe changes are usually seen at the time of autopsy. Mild stress gastritis may be difficult to distinguish from biopsy trauma. More severe disease shows extreme vascular congestion with dilation and hemorrhage into the superficial lamina propria (Fig. 4.34) often associated with acute inflammation (Fig. 4.34).

Erosions appear as discrete, superficial oval or circular areas of mucosal necrosis and tissue loss that do not extend deeper than the muscularis mucosae and have sharply defined, often raised edges; edema; and superficial epithelial necrosis (Fig. 4.34). Numerous neutrophils infiltrate the gastric pits and glandular lumina (Fig. 4.35). The inflammation usually spares the deepest glands. True granulation tissue is absent. Rather, the eroded cavity contains an exudate of proteinaceous fluid, debris, neutrophils, and red cells. The mucosa contains superficial fibrin deposits (Fig. 4.34). Chronic inflammation is absent in the acute phase. Only a minimal reparative fibroblastic response occurs when the injury is minor. Healing occurs in days to weeks following removal of the causative factor(s).

The healing phase (Table 4.5) is characterized by proliferation of pluripotential stem cells in the mucous neck region, pit elongation, a pseudostratified or syncytial appearance of the superficial epithelium, and vascular congestion (Fig. 4.35). The stem cells differentiate into foveolar cells above and specialized glandular epithelial cells below, reconstituting a normal mucosal architecture within a few days. Proliferating mucous neck cells contain abundant basophilic cytoplasm, increased mitoses, and an increased nuclear:cytoplasmic ratio, and appear mucin depleted. Despite their potentially alarming cytologic features (Fig. 4.35), the nuclei of the regenerating epithelium retain a basal orientation and contain vesicular chromatin and a prominent solitary eosinophilic nucleolus. The nuclear

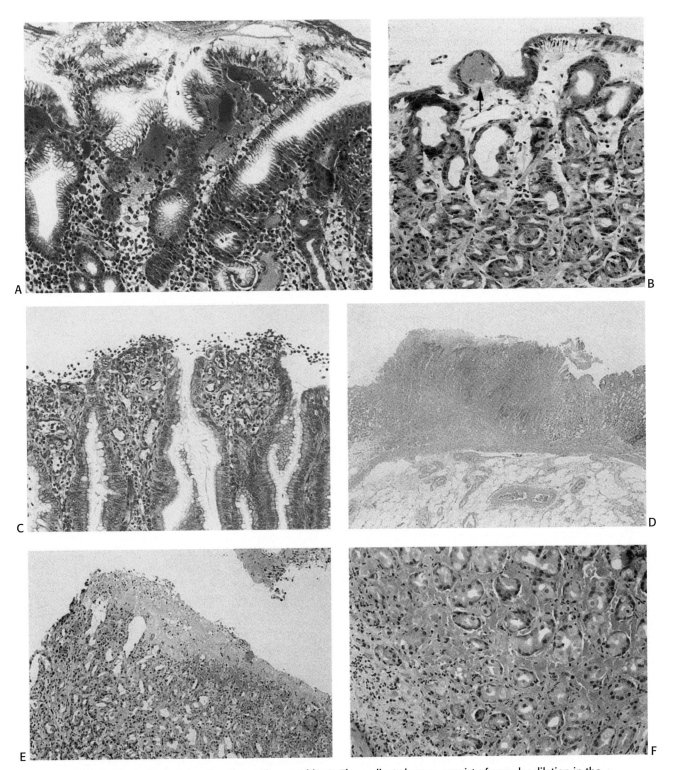

FIG. 4.34. Early changes of acute erosive gastritis. **A:** The earliest changes consist of vascular dilation in the superficial lamina propria. The overlying epithelium remains intact. **B:** Small thrombi develop (*arrow*) and the superficial lamina propria becomes increasingly edematous. **C:** With further disease progression, the tops of the gastric surface become eroded with loss of the surface epithelium. **D:** In larger lesions, extensive areas of transmucosal necrosis are present. **E:** Portions of the superficial epithelium degenerate, forming amorphous pinkish fibrinous debris on the surfaces of the mucosa. The glands become widely dilated and the surrounding lamina propria is infiltrated with extravasated red cells. **F:** Higher magnification of the extravasated red cells.

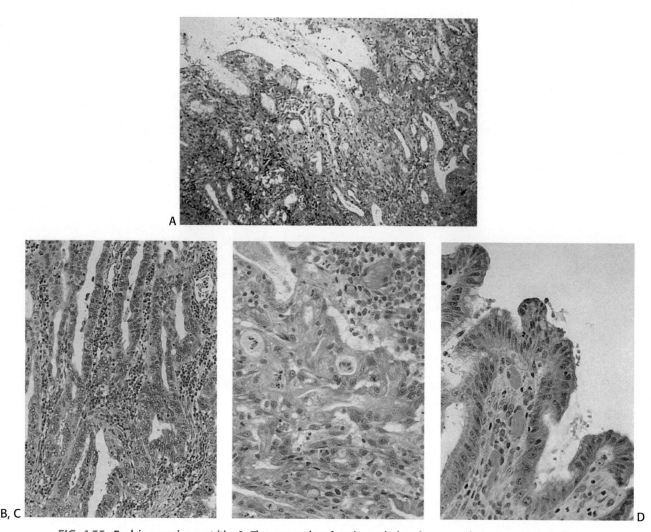

FIG. 4.35. Evolving erosive gastritis. **A:** The mucosal surface is eroded and as a result mucous neck regions become hyperchromatic and appear regenerative. **B:** With further disease progression, one sees a marked expansion of the mucous neck region with the regenerative cells showing significant reparative atypia. **C:** The surface cells acquire a syncytial appearance. **D:** Eventually, the entire surface becomes re-epithelialized, although the epithelium appears immature and has a large nuclear:cytoplasmic ratio. Some residual syncytial knots remain.

pleomorphism and atypical mitoses characteristic of neoplasia are usually absent. Residual clusters of neutrophils may reside within the pits and the surrounding lamina propria may be inflamed. One must be careful not to mistake regenerative changes for carcinoma. Atypical regenerative epithelium still retains a normal glandular architecture. If one can line the glands up parallel with one another in a regular fashion, perpendicular to the mucosal surface, if there is acute inflammation and if lamina propria separates the glands, one should be extremely cautious before making a diagnosis of malignancy, even in the face of extreme epithelial atypia.

Superficial erosions usually heal completely, without evidence of scarring, providing the inciting agent disappears. In patients with deeper lesions, complete regeneration of the gastric glands rarely occurs. Rather, mild mucosal scarring results (Fig. 4.36).

Ethanol-Induced Gastritis

The extent of alcohol-induced injury results from the quantity of alcohol ingested as well as its mucosal contact time (67). Injury usually requires gastric alcohol concentrations >10%. The presence of a concurrent *HP* infection may augment the alcohol-induced injury. Alcohol contacting the superficial gastric mucosa impairs mucus synthesis and secretion and damages epithelial cells, causing them to become necrotic and slough, leaving the underlying mucosa exposed to the alcohol and to gastric luminal acid (68). Acid back-diffusion increases mucosal blood flow, capillary permeability, and acid secretion. Increased capillary permeability leads to interstitial edema. Vasoactive mediator release from mast cells, endothelial cells, and neutrophils triggers venoconstriction and plasma transudation. The neutrophils generate superoxide anion and hyperchlorous acid in a manner similar

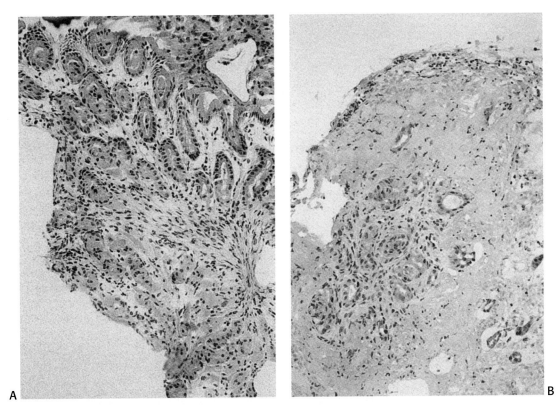

FIG. 4.36. Healed erosion. **A:** A focal area of fibrosis of the lamina propria distorts the glands. **B:** This figure shows more extensive lamina propria fibrosis and collagenization with only a few atrophic glands remaining. The surface has not re-epithelialized in this particular specimen, indicating the presence of both acute and more chronic recurrent damage.

to that seen in stress gastritis (69). Arterial and arteriolar dilation rapidly follow, leading to marked congestion, edema, hemorrhage, cellular translocation, ischemia, and cell membrane damage sufficient to cause local edema, hypoxia, hemorrhage, and cellular necrosis (Fig. 4.37). Alcohol penetration

into the congested tissues causes hemolysis, vascular congestion, protein precipitation, vascular stasis, thrombus formation, and capillary leakage (70). Neuropeptides stimulated by the alcohol affect blood vessels, leukocytes, and epithelium, and aid in activating inflammatory mediators (71).

FIG. 4.37. Alcohol-induced gastric injury. **A:** Low magnification demonstrates the presence of superficial damage in the oxyntic mucosa. **B:** Higher magnification shows the presence of superficial loss of the epithelium, edema, vascular congestion, and almost no inflammation.

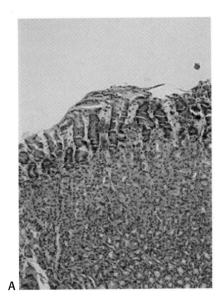

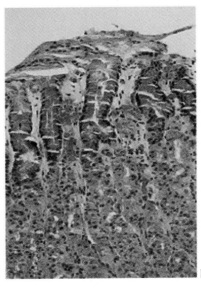

Actively drinking alcoholics predominantly show multiple areas of subepithelial hemorrhage, prominent mucosal edema in the adjacent nonhemorrhagic mucosa, and only mild inflammation. The edema may be severe enough to extend into the submucosa (72). The foveolar epithelium overlying the lamina propria hemorrhage may appear mucus depleted and show focal loss of nuclear polarity. Tiny erosions may be present in some patients, especially those consuming large quantities of alcohol in a short period of time. These resemble the lesions seen in stress gastritis and predominantly involve the proximal stomach. In these patients there may be focal necrosis of the foveolar epithelium along with focal neutrophilic infiltrates in the gastric pits. Chronic ethanol ingestion increases mucosal expression of EGF and other growth factors (68) leading to increased cell proliferation. Differentiation of cells in the proliferating mucous neck region replaces the damaged cells.

DRUG-INDUCED GASTRITIS AND GASTROPATHY

Many drugs produce gastric erosions, hemorrhage, and necrosis, the most common of which are NSAIDs and aspirin. The pathogenesis of the injury varies. Some drug-induced and stress-induced ulcers share common pathogenetic events, but the factors that lead to the initial cellular damage may differ. The fact that many drugs produce similar changes whether administered intravenously or orally suggests that mucosal contact need not occur to produce the damage.

Aspirin/Nonsteroidal Anti-Inflammatory Drugs

The nature of aspirin-related injury depends on whether the drug ingestion is acute or chronic. One-time aspirin ingestion causes subepithelial hemorrhages within an hour, and regular intake over a 24-hour period leads to gastric erosions in many individuals. Chronic ingestion often results in less severe damage than acute ingestion because mucosal adaptation occurs, making the mucosa resistant to injury. The adaptive response involves decreased neutrophilic infiltration and extensive epithelial proliferation (73). Aspirin-induced damage results from its toxic effects as well as by decreasing mucosal defenses (74). The physicochemical property of aspirin aids in its rapid absorption, mucosal accumulation, and mucosal barrier breaking effects. Salicylates in aspirin become trapped inside gastric epithelia interfering with ATPase-dependent processes and leading to increased membrane permeability. Eventually osmotic swelling and cell death develop. Additionally, small aspirin fragments may become embedded in the mucosa. These produce circular erosions or ulcers surrounded by hemorrhagic zones. Adjacent erosions become linked by linear mucosal cracks. The aspirin particles then fall into the cracks and become walled off in mucus until they dissolve.

Nonsteroidal Anti-Inflammatory Drugs

NSAIDs are a common cause of grossly visible gastric injury and are responsible for some of the most severe drug injury seen in the United States (75). Gastric injury typically complicates the use of NSAIDs prescribed by physicians. However, consumption of high-dose over-the-counter NSAIDs also causes significant gastrointestinal injury (76). Gastroduodenal lesions develop in 31% to 68% of patients on chronic therapy; up to 25% have gastric ulcers (77). The vast majority of individuals utilizing NSAIDs are 60 years of age or older. These patients are particularly susceptible to develop GI hemorrhage and gastric ulcers, in part due to the fact that mucosal prostaglandin levels decrease in the elderly (78).

NSAIDs cause direct local mucosal toxicity and inhibit hydrogen sulfide generation (79) and cyclooxygenase enzymes. The latter leads to reduced prostaglandin synthesis. As noted earlier, prostaglandins are critical to maintaining the integrity of the mucosal barrier. Most NSAIDs are weak organic acids and in the highly acidic stomach, are un-ionized so that they are lipid soluble and diffuse freely into the epithelium elevating intracellular pH. The damaged mucosa becomes leaky allowing acid back-diffusion, peptic injury, erosions, hemorrhage, and other damage to occur. Coexisting *HP* infections increase mucosal susceptibility to NSAID-mediated damage and increase the risk of ulceration and bleeding (80).

NSAIDs produce acute mucosal lesions within 7 days of administration by the mechanisms shown in Figure 4.38. Altered blood flow and increased leukocyte–endothelial interactions in the gastric microcirculation occlude microvessels, further reducing mucosal blood flow. The inflammatory cells also release various procoagulants, inflammatory mediators, proteases, and oxygen-free radicals that further damage the endothelium and the underlying connective tissue (81). NSAID effects are summarized in Table 4.6 (74).

NSAIDs cause several types of injury: Acute hemorrhagic gastritis, erosions, chemical gastropathy (discussed in a later section), ulcers, and perforation. Because of the direct local toxicity caused by NSAIDs, the damage is patchy and is increased in areas of mucosal contact. Thus, injury is more common in dependent parts of the stomach (antrum and body along the greater curvature). Gastric ulcers are of greater clinical significance than erosions because of their chronicity and their potential for perforation and significant bleeding.

The acute hemorrhagic gastritis is characterized by a damaged surface epithelium with edema, hemorrhage into the superficial lamina propria, and variable inflammation, resembling stress gastritis. The degree of inflammation tends to be minimal. However, neutrophilic infiltrates are present if erosions or ulcers develop. The hemorrhagic erosions usually heal within a few days. Prominent eosinophilia may also be present, as may increased epithelial apoptosis. Biopsies

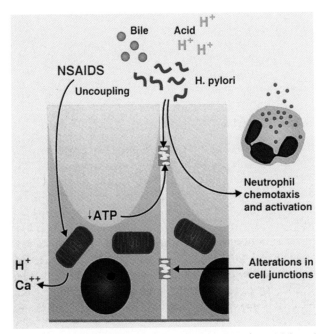

FIG. 4.38. Diagram of the mechanism of nonsteroidal anti-inflammatory drug (NSAID) damage. Following NSAID absorption, there is uncoupling of mitochondrial oxidative phosphorylation leading to reduced adenosine triphosphate (ATP) levels, which in turn result in the loss of intercellular junctional integrity and increased mucosal permeability. Also as a result of the mitochondrial oxidative phosphorylation uncoupling, an efflux of calcium and hydrogen ions from mitochondria occurs, further depleting ATP stores and promoting oxygen radical damage. The damaged cell releases arachidonic acid, but the conversion of arachidonic acid to prostaglandins is prevented by the NSAID inhibition of cyclooxygenase. As a result, the damage of the gastric mucosa is more prolonged than would ordinarily be the case. As a result of the damage, the mucosa becomes vulnerable to luminal aggressive factors, which include acid, pepsin, bile, and *Helicobacter pylori.*

taken of antral lesions thought to be erosions by endoscopists are frequently areas of chemical gastropathy with moderate to marked capillary dilation. The epithelium may appear very atypical (Figs. 4.39 and 4.40). The diagnosis of NSAID-induced gastritis can be problematic in the absence of a history of NSAID ingestion, but the presence of changes resembling stress gastritis, or a chemical gastropathy, especially if increased eosinophils are present, may suggest the diagnosis.

Proton Pump Inhibitors

Proton pump inhibitor (PPI) therapy may induce changes in G cells, ECL cells, and parietal cells. Mild G-cell and ECL-cell hyperplasias (but not carcinoid tumors) occur and may be diffuse, linear, or micronodular (82). The micronodular hyperplasia is more likely to occur in patients with *HP* infections. Parietal cell changes include increases in cell size and

TABLE 4.6	Nonsteroidal Anti-inflammatory Drug Effects

Break gastric mucosal barrier
Alter cell membrane permeability, allowing H^+ back-diffusion
Increase acid secretions
Concentrate in epithelial cells due to ion trapping
Alter transmural electrical potential differences
Cause surface cell damage and loss
Alter cell junctions
Inhibit gastric mucosal secretions
Increase pepsin-mediated proteolysis of mucin
Increase permeability of mucus to H^+
Inhibit active bicarbonate secretion
Alter surface phospholipids
Alter mucosal blood flow
Inhibit prostaglandin synthesis
Reduce surface hydrophobicity

number, leading to swelling (Fig. 4.41) and convex bulging of the apical cell membranes into the glandular lumens, which imparts a serrated appearance to the normally round or tubular glandular lumens (83). This change affects over 90% of patients treated for 1 year with daily doses of 20 to 40 mg of omeprazole. The parietal cell protrusions appear to be related to the hypergastrinemia (83,84). For this reason, parietal cell protrusions are not specific for PPI therapy. They can also be seen in patients with *HP* gastritis, gastric ulcers, morbid obesity, Zollinger-Ellison syndrome, or gastric cancer (83).

Patients on long-term treatment may develop tiny fundic gland polyp (FGP)-like lesions. They contain glandular cysts measuring between 0.25 and 7 mm in diameter (Fig. 4.41). These are lined by flattened parietal and chief cells; they may also contain foveolar cells. The lesions may disappear after PPI therapy is withdrawn and reappear after the reintroduction of the therapy (85). While there appears to be a relationship between FGPs and PPIs, the data are inconsistent and not all patients develop the polyps. Additionally, some PPI-associated fundic gland cysts lack superficial foveolar dilation, a hallmark of FGPs. PPIs also slightly increase the number of apoptotic bodies in the antral mucosa (86).

Steroids

The association between peptic ulcer disease and corticosteroids has been debated for years. There appears to be a small increased risk of gastric ulceration and bleeding in steroid users; the concomitant use of steroids and NSAIDs associates with an up to 10-fold increased risk of an upper GI bleed. Steroids stimulate G-cell hyperplasia (87), indirectly increasing acid production by parietal cells. They also decrease epithelial turnover and mucin secretion, thereby impairing mucosal barrier protection. There may be acute inflammatory cells in the lamina propria and apoptotic debris in the glandular lumens (Fig. 4.42).

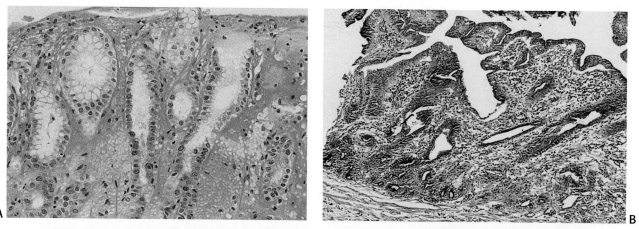

FIG. 4.39. Nonsteroidal anti-inflammatory drug (NSAID) damage. **A:** A gastric biopsy from the body region of a patient on NSAIDs. The patient showed endoscopic evidence of multiple petechial hemorrhages. The biopsy shows that the changes mainly affect the superficial mucosa with edema, telangiectasia, and little or no inflammatory infiltrate. **B:** The mucosa appears regenerative with loss of glands and irregularity of the remaining pits.

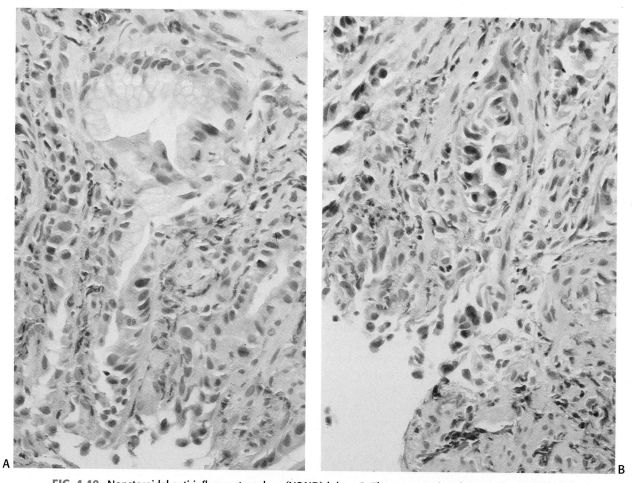

FIG. 4.40. Nonsteroidal anti-inflammatory drug (NSAID) injury. **A:** The regenerative changes that develop following NSAID-induced injury can be cytologically alarming. The atypia primarily affects the cells in the mucous neck region. A clue to their regenerative, nonneoplastic nature is evidence of maturation in the foveolar cells. **B:** When the biopsy is fragmented without the ability to see the foveolar cell maturation, the diagnosis is more difficult.

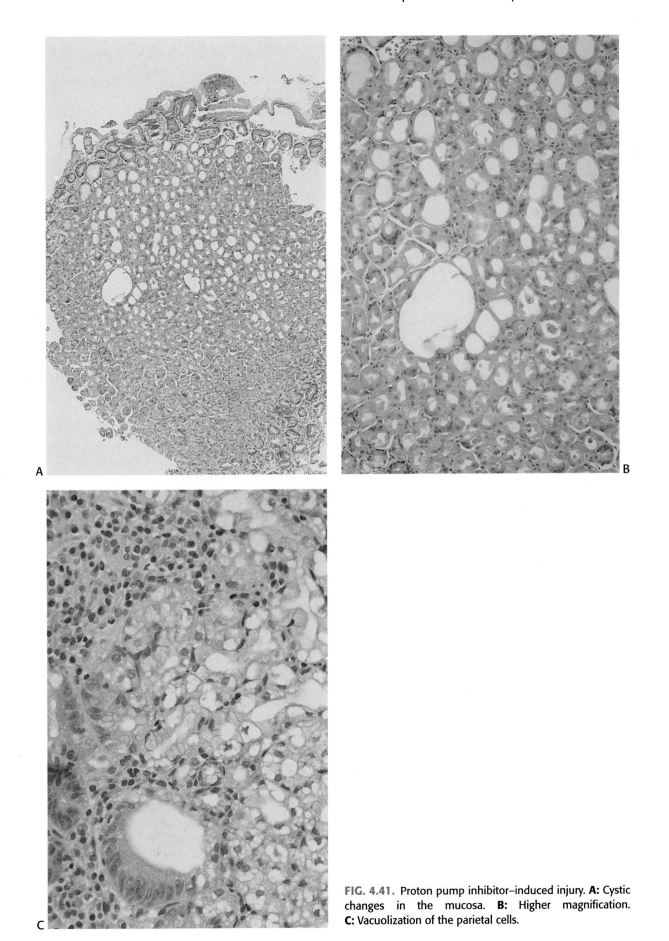

FIG. 4.41. Proton pump inhibitor–induced injury. **A:** Cystic changes in the mucosa. **B:** Higher magnification. **C:** Vacuolization of the parietal cells.

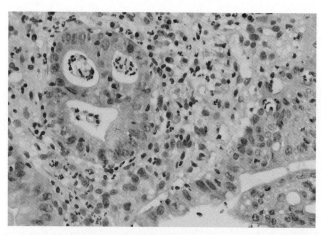

FIG. 4.42. Patient with aplastic anemia treated with steroids. There is acute inflammation in the lamina propria and the gland, and the glands contain apoptotic debris.

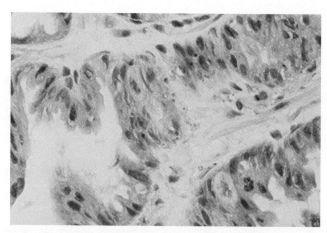

FIG. 4.43. Chemotherapy-associated gastric changes showing increased mitotic activity and enlarged atypical cells. The nuclear:cytoplasmic ratio is not increased.

Chemotherapy

Patients undergoing chemotherapy develop many complications due to direct mucosal injury, vomiting (leading to potential esophagogastric tears), drug-induced immunosuppression, and thrombocytopenia. Cisplatin, doxorubicin, nitrosoureas, and vincristine are notorious for inducing nausea and vomiting. Chemotherapy-induced immunosuppression can lead to multiple gastric infections. Hepatic arterial infusion chemotherapy (HAIC) can produce gastric ulcers and alarming epithelial regenerative atypias easily confused with carcinoma (88,89) because of the presence of binucleated or multinucleated cells containing massive nuclei (Fig. 4.43). Features of the atypia of HAIC and neoplasia are compared in Table 4.7. The presence of ring mitoses, which are not characteristic of neoplasias, suggests drug injury. Floxuridine causes epithelial necrosis with the inflammation and epithelial regeneration (90). The epithelial cytoplasm becomes vacuolated and foamy. Other drugs causing severe epithelial atypia include combinations of 5-fluorouracil (5-FU) with either leucovorin or mitomycin. These drug-induced atypias become most difficult to accurately diagnose

in superficial gastric mucosal brushing specimens. Vinorelbine predisposes to bezoar formation (91), probably due to toxic myenteric plexus damage.

Iron Pill Gastritis

Acute gastritis develops in individuals consuming large amounts of oral iron. Iron supplements may cause erosions, ulcers, an almost infarctlike gastric mucosal necrosis, and strictures as the ulcers heal. Grossly, grayish or bluish mucosal patches may be present. Superficial edema, inflammation, and necrosis characterize the histologic changes. A layer of brownish pigment that stains positively with iron stains (Fig. 4.44) may cover the epithelial surface and extend into the superficial gastric pits. Some of the pigment may appear crystalline. The majority of the iron that is present is in an extracellular location. Iron pigment may lie in granulation tissue, on the top of damaged epithelium, in the glands or lamina propria, or in the submucosa (Fig. 4.45) (92). Focal epithelial or stromal cell deposition is less common than deposits in the lamina propria and surface unless the

TABLE 4.7	Comparison of Hepatic Arterial Infusion Chemotherapy (HAIC) and Neoplasia	
Feature	HAIC	Neoplasia
Cytologic features	Bizarre enlarged cells	Uniform anaplasia
Nuclear:cytoplasmic ratio	Low	High
Mitoses	Few or none	Many
Location of the atypia	Glands	Mucous neck region and foveolae
Atypia in granulation tissue	Yes	No
Atypia in stromal cells	Yes	No
Glandular architecture	Preserved	Distorted
Cytoplasmic vacuolization	Present	Absent

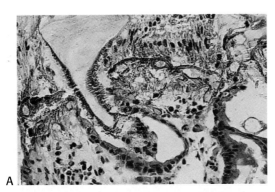
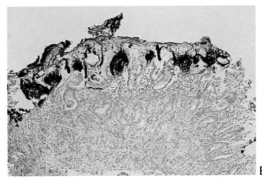

FIG. 4.44. Changes associated with high-dose iron ingestion. **A:** Note the superficial damage and edema of the lamina propria. A layer of iron is deposited on the surface of the gastric mucosa as well as extending into the upper portions of the gastric pits. **B:** Prussian blue stain of the same biopsy at a lower magnification showing the prominent coating of the gastric mucosa with iron and extension into the pits.

patient has also had transfusions or has alcoholic liver disease. Features of chemical gastropathy may also be present (93). The changes differ from those seen in hemosiderosis in that patients with hemosiderosis or hemochromatosis lack significant inflammation (unless there is a coexisting gastritis) and the iron predominantly localizes within cells, especially the epithelium of deeper glands. Erosions are not present.

Prostaglandin Therapy

Prostaglandin E infusions, used to treat congenital heart disease and other neonatal and adult disorders, induce gastric outlet obstruction secondary to foveolar hyperplasia and elongation of the gastric pits that results in marked antral hyperplasia (94).

Cocaine Use

Cocaine abuse can cause gastric injury with the newer forms being more toxic than cocaine hydrochloride (95). Affected

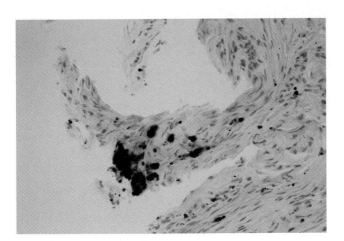

FIG. 4.45. Iron-pill gastritis. Note the prominent iron deposits in the submucosa.

patients tend to be young males. Cocaine causes intense vasoconstriction, focal ischemia, and perforation (95,96). Granulomas may be present, presumably due to cutting the drugs with foreign materials (Fig. 4.46).

Gastric Mucosal Calcinosis

Rare patients have crystalline deposits in the superficial gastric mucosa that consist of aluminum, phosphorus, calcium, and chlorine. They occur in transplant patients on long-term aluminum-containing antacid therapy or sucralfate therapy (97). The deposits lie just below the foveolar epithelium, sometimes rimmed by macrophages. They show variable degrees of calcification and often appear refractile (Fig. 4.47). There may be coexisting gastritis.

Other Drugs

Kayexalate resin crystals can be present in the stomach in patients treated for hyperkalemia. Sodium cations are released from the resin and exchanged for hydrogen ions in the gastric acid milieu. As the resin passes through the intestines, hydrogen is exchanged for potassium, which is then eliminated in the feces along with the remainder of the altered resin, thereby lowering serum potassium levels. The crystals have a characteristic refractile crystalline mosaic pattern that resembles fish scales that distinguishes Kayexalate crystals from cholestyramine crystals, which they resemble (98,99). This pattern is faintly seen in hematoxylin and eosin-stained sections and is better demonstrated with acid fast, Alcian blue, or Diff-Quik stains. The crystals do not polarize. The crystals are always located in a luminal location, either adherent to intact surface epithelium or admixed with inflammatory exudates in patients with ulcers or erosions (98,99). In some cases, Kayexalate crystals aggregate with mucous secretions and clotted blood to form gastric bezoars.

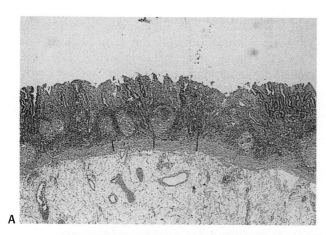
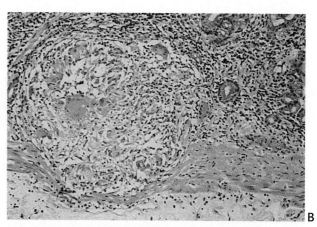

FIG. 4.46. Granulomatous gastritis in a cocaine addict. **A:** Numerous granulomas lie in the basal portion of the mucosa just above the muscularis mucosae. They are surrounded by a prominent mononuclear cell infiltrate. **B:** Higher magnification of one of these granulomas shows the basal location and the presence of a granulomatous response containing giant cells.

Some patients on *colchicine* develop gastritis or antral erosions. The most discriminating feature indicating colchicine damage is the presence of abundant epithelial mitotic figures in metaphase arrest (100), particularly in the proliferative zone in the mucous neck region. Metaphase mitoses appear as enlarged epithelial cells with condensed chromatin in a ring formation in the center of the cell (ring mitoses). These changes are accompanied by marked foveolar cell hyperplasia resulting in crowded, enlarged, distorted epithelial cells; epithelial pseudostratification; and loss of cellular polarity. However, in contrast to the large size of the cells, the nuclei are small, hyperchromatic, and compressed to the cellular periphery. The changes are more prevalent in the gastric antrum than in the gastric body (100).

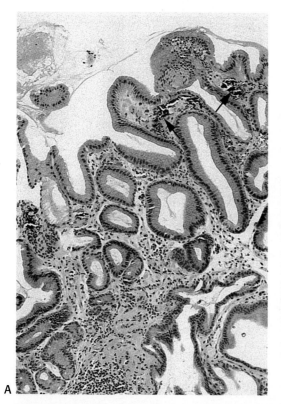
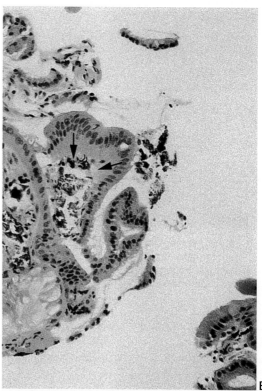

FIG. 4.47. Mucosal calcinosis. **A:** Low-magnification photograph of the gastric mucosa showing the presence of superficial aggregates of deeply pigmented crystalline material (*arrows*) that were positive with Von Kossa stains. **B:** Higher magnification showing the details of these mucosal deposits (*arrows*).

Ticlopidine sometimes causes lymphocytic gastritis, and *methyldopa* treatment sometimes leads to the development of autoimmune gastritis (101). Both *interleukin-4* (IL-4) and *tumor necrosis factor* (TNF), agents used to treat patients with advanced cancer, cause acute gastric mucosal injury and hemorrhagic necrosis (102). Some drugs alter gastric motility, including anticholinergics, adrenergic agents, dopaminergic agents, narcotics, and erythromycin.

ACUTE CORROSIVE GASTRITIS

Extensive acute gastritis results from ingestion of corrosive agents (Fig. 4.48), be it accidental or suicidal. The types of agents that cause injury resemble those damaging the esophagus (see Chapter 2). Ingestion causes rapid and widespread gastric mucosal necrosis. The mucosal surface may appear black due to digested blood and mucosal necrosis. The damage often localizes to the prepyloric region, due to the stasis that occurs there allowing longer mucosal contact times with injurious agents than would otherwise exist. However, if only small quantities of the corrosive agent are consumed, then the injury may be more proximal in location. Initially there is mucosal hemorrhage and edema. The injury may extend deep into the gastric wall and patients with myonecrosis may perforate. Severe acute changes consist of coagulative necrosis (Fig. 4.49). The damage is patchy, with the most severe damage occurring in the areas of mucosal contact. Alkalis usually injure the esophagus more severely than the stomach; the reverse occurs with acids.

If the patient survives the acute event, fibrosis causes progressive stricturing. If the process progresses, complete obstruction may result. Perforation, peritonitis, or massive hemorrhage complicates corrosive gastritis. One classifies corrosive gastritis into three grades, in a manner similar to that used for corrosive esophageal burns (Table 2.10).

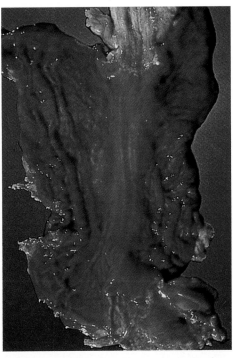

FIG. 4.48. Corrosive gastritis from a suicidal ingestion of acid.

ISCHEMIC GASTRITIS

While focal ischemia mediates many of the changes seen in acute (stress) gastritis, gastric infarction is rare because of the rich gastric vasculature. Severe, diffuse arterial sclerosis coupled with smoking and systemic hypertension (103) can lead to severe gastric damage and even gastric infarction (Fig. 4.50). Less severe ischemia develops secondary to vasculitis, bacterial gastritis, previous gastric surgery, disseminated intravascular coagulation (DIC), or volvulus (103). The features of ischemic gastritis include a coagulative

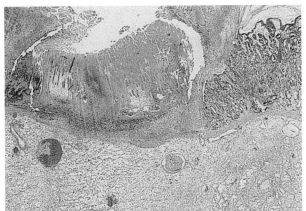
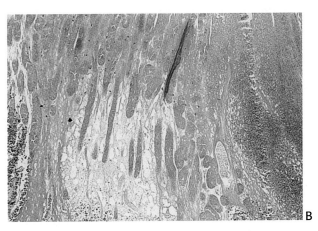

FIG. 4.49. Lye ingestion in suicide attempt. **A:** Much of the stomach had become completely necrotic. The lesions were focally distributed throughout the gastric mucosa as seen in A. **B:** Higher magnification demonstrating the coagulative necrosis and edema of the gastric mucosa.

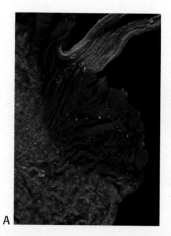
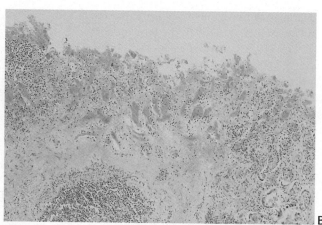

FIG. 4.50. Ischemic necrosis of the cardia and upper part of the fundus. **A:** This patient died of severe cardiovascular collapse. The patient was a known smoker, was hypertensive, and had previously undergone a surgical procedure. The death occurred during the postoperative period. **B:** Coagulative necrosis is seen affecting the gastric glands.

necrosis (Fig. 4.50), the extent of which reflects the degree and duration of the ischemia. Transmural infarction is a rare and usually terminal event. The histologic features resemble those seen in the intestines and are discussed more extensively in Chapter 6.

RADIATION GASTRITIS

Patients receiving radiation in doses in excess of 4,000 rads demonstrate both acute and chronic gastritis with areas of epithelial necrosis and shallow ulcers (104). Gastric radiation injury assumes one of three forms:

1. *Acute radiation gastritis* develops a few days to a few months following the radiation exposure. Inflammation is present early but it eventually diminishes. Extensive mucosal necrosis and superficial ulcers may be present. The endothelium swells, reducing vascular luminal caliber. Submucosal capillary ectasia is present. As the mucosa heals, it regenerates, but variable degrees of atrophy, fibrosis, edema, and endarteritis persist. The cytologic features may resemble those induced by many chemotherapeutic agents. Indeed, many cancer patients show the effects of combined chemoradiation.
2. One to two months following radiation exposure, some patients develop a deep *acute ulcer*, which usually walls off before perforation occurs. The ulcer represents the long-term effects of vascular damage and ischemia. Stigmata of radiation damage are histologically evident as evidenced by the vascular alterations and the presence of radiation fibroblasts in the surrounding fibrotic stroma (104).
3. A month to several years following radiation exposure, a *chronic ulcer*, indistinguishable from a peptic ulcer, may develop. The only clues to its etiology are the clinical history, an unusually prominent antral fibrosis with oblit-

erative endarteritis or foamy macrophages involving the submucosal blood vessels, and the presence of atypical hyperchromatic fibroblasts ("radiation fibroblasts"). The submucosa develops capillary telangiectasia and arterial wall hyalinization with intimal fibrosis. Patients may also develop severe atrophic gastritis. Even though mucosal regeneration occurs, gastric acid output remains reduced; many patients develop hypochlorhydria.

INFECTIOUS GASTRITIS

The stomach normally contains $<10^3$ organisms/mL, with most coming from the oral cavity. Gastric pH determines the gastric bacterial content; pH levels below 4.0 kill most bacteria. If the pH is not at or below this level, the stomach does not sterilize itself and an abnormal flora may become established. Normal gastric motility and emptying also protect against bacterial infections. When dysmotility or pyloric obstruction develops, anaerobic organisms may accumulate. Not uncommonly one finds oral bacteria lying in the gastric lumen. They have a typical diplococcal or tetrad morphology and reach the stomach when swallowed with other oral contents or when they are carried there via the endoscope. These organisms have no clinical significance.

Helicobacter Pylori

Transmission

HP infections occur worldwide, although there are marked geographic variations in their incidence. The prevalence of *HP* infections in adults ranges from $<15\%$ in some populations to virtually 100% in less well-developed areas. There are also substantial variations among different ethnic groups in the same geographic locale (105). In developing countries, people become infected much earlier in life than in developed countries. The prevalence of *HP* infections correlates with lower socioeconomic status (106). The human stomach is the primary reservoir for the organism and it is transmitted via an oral–oral route and possibly via a gastric–oral and fecal–oral route (107). The infection is easily passed from one family member to another, particularly in areas of dense housing. Children under the age of 5 are most susceptible to *HP* infections. *HP* infections are present in gastric biopsies of 16.8% to 55% of children with abdominal pain, upper gastrointestinal symptoms, and histologic evidence of acute and/or chronic gastritis (106). The infection prevalence in developing countries can be as high as 75% by age 25. There has been a recent decline in the incidence of *HP* infections in the developed world, largely due to improved living conditions and a decrease in living density and family size. Even though the prevalence of *HP* infections is currently decreasing, at least 50% of the world population is infected with the organism (108).

Recurrent infections are usually a persistent infection rather than the acquisition of new infections. Infection with more than one *HP* strain can also occur (109). When AIDS patients become infected, the disease may exhibit particularly virulent characteristics and large numbers of organisms may be present.

Pathogenesis

HP is highly adapted to occupy a special ecologic gastric niche with unique features that allow it to enter the mucus of the mucosal barrier, attach to the epithelium, evade immune responses, proliferate, and colonize the gastric mucosa. The eventual outcome of *HP* infections reflects strain-specific, environmental, and host-related factors. After they are ingested, *HP* organisms must evade the bactericidal activity of the gastric lumen and enter the mucous layer. Corkscrewlike bacterial movement and enzyme production (particularly urease and lipase) are important early in the infection (110,111). Bacterial proteases digest gastric mucin (194–197) facilitating bacterial movement and urease protects the *HP* from the luminal acid by creating an alkaline microenvironment around the bacterium (110,111).

HP bacteria normally reside in the unstirred layer of gastric mucus. They wind down to the epithelial surface, moving easily through the viscous environment above it, to attach themselves to the apical membranes of foveolar cells (Fig. 4.51). Bacterial adhesins recognize cell surface–specific proteins facilitating epithelial colonization. The best characterized adhesin, BabA, is a 78-kD outer bacterial membrane protein that binds to the fucosylated Lewis B blood group antigen (112). The Lewis blood group terminal carbohydrate structures are present on the ends of MUC1 carbohydrate side chains as well as on secreted mucins. MUC1 is highly polymorphic and evidence suggests that functional allelic differences affect infection susceptibility (113). *HP* bacteria also bind to MUC5AC, a major mucin produced by foveolar

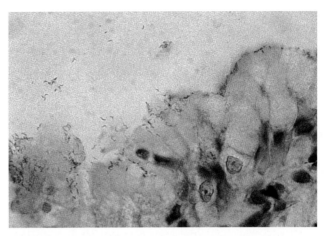

FIG. 4.51. *Helicobacter pylori* gastritis. Diff-Quik–stained section demonstrating spirally shaped bacteria intimately adherent to the surfaces of the epithelium as well as lying in the intercellular spaces. Both coccoid and spiral forms are present at the free surface.

cells (114). The specificity of the binding, together with the limited distribution of the receptors, results in a restricted range of *HP*-colonized tissues. Bacteria unable to adhere to the epithelium are rapidly cleared from the mucosa. *HP* bacteria preferentially attach at or near intercellular junctions, penetrating the junctional complexes moving down along the lateral cell membranes. This disrupts intercellular tight junctions between viable cells, allowing luminal contents, including acid, to flow between the cells.

Most *HP* strains secrete the vacuolating cytotoxin VacA (115). The toxin inserts itself into the epithelial cell membrane and forms a hexameric anion-selective, voltage-dependent channel through which bicarbonate and organic anions can be released, possibly providing *HP* bacteria with their nutrients (116). VacA (117) also inhibits T-lymphocyte activation (118). Certain *vacA* gene variants produce more severe disease than others (119).

Most *HP* bacteria possess the *cag* pathogenicity island (*cag* PAI) that contains 29 distinct genes (120). Some of these genes facilitate translocation of the CagA protein into foveolar cells (121). Once in the cells, CagA is phosphorylated and binds to the SHP-2 tyrosine phosphatase (122), leading to host growth factor–like cellular responses, cytokine production, and cell proliferation (123). These cytokines mobilize leukocytes to areas of immune challenge. An EPIYA-repeat polymorphism influences the magnitude and duration of phosphorylation-dependent CagA activity (124). CagA also plays a major role in disruption of the apical junctional complexes (125). *cagA*-positive strains associate with increased epithelial cell apoptosis (126).

The *oipA* (outer inflammatory protein) gene encodes one of the outer membrane proteins and is an inflammation-related gene near, but not in, the *CagA* PAI. *oipA* functional status correlates with clinical presentation, *HP* density, and gastric inflammation. *Cag* PAI, *babA2*, and *vacA* status may be a surrogate marker for a functional *oipA* gene (127). OipA and the *cag* PAI are both necessary for full activation of the IL-8 promoter (128). Nitric oxidase synthase and cyclooxygenase-2 are induced by *HP* infections; these enzymes modulate the inflammatory responses.

Host Responses to Helicobacter pylori

HP infections cause gastric inflammation (gastritis) in almost all infected persons, although the severity of the changes varies among individuals. The injury results from both the infection and its associated inflammation. Bile reflux and dietary irritants may further enhance the deleterious bacterial effects. Additionally, anti-*HP* antibodies that cross-react with the gastric mucosa induce further damage (129). Some *HP*-infected patients develop an autoantibody response directed at the H^+-K^+-ATPase pump in parietal cells leading to atrophy of the corpus (129).

Initially neutrophils are recruited to the infected site, followed by the recruitment of T and B lymphocytes, plasma cells, and macrophages. The neutrophilic infiltrate and mononuclear phagocytic activation may be facilitated by bacterial urease production and induction of nitric oxide synthase and cyclooxygenase (130). *HP* infections generate significant cellular and humoral responses via antigenic stimulation of mucosal monocytes and T cells. The inflammatory cells produce numerous cytokines (TNF-α, interferon-γ, and interleukins 1, 6, and 8), prostaglandins, proteases, and reactive oxygen metabolites that cause epithelial necrosis and mucosal injury. IL-8, a potent neutrophil-activating chemokine expressed by gastric epithelium, plays a central role in the inflammatory response (127,128). *HP* bacteria containing the *cag* PAI induce a stronger IL-8 response than *cag*-negative strains (131). Some cytokines promote leukocyte adhesion to endothelial cells and others recruit additional leukocytes to the infected site. Mediators of local humoral responses, such as mucosal IgA, attract eosinophils, which then degranulate. Stimulated B cells differentiate into IgM, IgA, and IgG antibody–producing cells (132). IgA promotes complement-dependent phagocytosis and *HP* killing by polymorphonuclear neutrophils (PMNs). Secretory IgA synergizes with IgG to promote antibody-dependent cell-mediated cytotoxicity induced by PMNs, monocytes, and lymphocytes. High anti-*HP* IgG antibody levels correlate with severe antral gastritis and dense *HP* antral colonization (132).

HP infections result in hyposecretion, hypersecretion, or normal acid secretion, depending on disease stage. Hypochlorhydria develops when the gastritis extends proximally to involve (and destroy) the oxyntic mucosa. Acid secretion increases via several mechanisms (133). Patients with an increased parietal cell mass and hyperchlorhydria exhibit antral restriction of the gastritis because the high acid levels protect the corpus from bacterial adhesion and inflammation.

Helicobacter pylori Identification

HP, a Gram-negative, nonsporulated microaerophilic motile bacterium, measures 1 to 3 μm in length and 0.3 to 0.6 μm in width and has distinctive sheathed flagella that terminate in a bulbous disc structure. *HP* bacteria assume a curved, sinuous, or gently spiraled shape (Fig. 4.51). They lie freely in the mucous layer, are attached to surface foveolar cells, or lie between epithelial cells (Fig. 4.51). The faintly eosinophilic organisms closely resemble and may be obscured by mucus, contaminating oral flora or epithelial cell membranes. During treatment, *HP* bacteria may lose their typical spiral shape and assume new forms, including U shaped, circular, irregular rod shaped, or coccoid (134). Histologically, coccoid forms appear as solid, round, basophilic, dotlike structures ranging from 0.4 to 1.2 μm in diameter. They resemble nonpathogenic bacteria, fungal spores, and cryptosporidia (134), but can be correctly diagnosed using immunohistochemical stains.

Diagnostic tests for *HP* include microbial cultures, histologic or cytologic examination, rapid urease-based tests, and serologic studies. Histologic examination equals or even surpasses culture, especially when positive. However, the patchy nature of the infection requires examination of a minimum of two biopsies: One from the gastric antrum and one from the fundus. The greater the number of biopsies examined, the greater the diagnostic yield, especially in individuals with light infections. Mucosal biopsies have the advantage of allowing one to examine the mucosa for the presence of gastritis or other lesions. Careful examination of four specimens, two from the antrum and two from the corpus, has a high probability of establishing the correct diagnosis of the infection (135). *HP* bacteria are generally readily apparent on H&E-stained sections but the infection may be focal and patchy or there may be only sparse organisms, especially if intestinal metaplasia is present (136).

A number of special stains aid in *HP* detection including Dieterle silver, Warthin-Starry, Gram, toluidine blue, Giemsa, Wright-Giemsa, Brown-Hopps, acridine orange, or Diff-Quik stains. In addition, there are good immunohistochemical reagents that detect the organism. These are particularly useful in detecting the coccoid forms of the bacteria. Each laboratory has its favorite stain for detecting *HP*. While some laboratories routinely use special stains on most gastric biopsies to highlight the organism, we routinely only examine H&E-stained sections since the organism is generally readily appreciated, especially in heavy infections. Special stains only increase the diagnostic yield by 1% (137). If we use a special stain, we favor an immunohistochemical stain to detect the organism. We will use this if there is a chronic active gastritis and no organisms are seen in the H&E-stained section or if we are asked by the clinicians to specifically rule out an *HP* infection and *HP* bacteria are not seen in the H&E-stained preparation.

One can also identify *HP* in routinely prepared cytology specimens. Gastric mucosal brushings sample larger surface

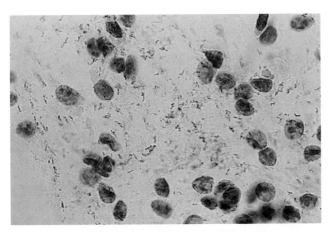

FIG. 4.52. Numerous *Helicobacter pylori* bacteria amidst naked nuclei in a gastric smear.

TABLE 4.8	*Helicobacter pylori*–related Diseases
Acute gastritis	
Chronic gastritis	
Chronic active gastritis	
Follicular gastritis	
Atrophic gastritis	
Lymphocytic gastritis[a]	
Granulomatous gastritis[a]	
Gastric and duodenal ulcers	
Some forms of autoimmune gastritis	
Hyperplastic polyps[a]	
Intestinal metaplasia	
G-cell hyperplasia	
Giant fold gastritis	
Gastric adenocarcinoma	
Gastric MALToma	
Menetrier disease[a]	

[a]Uncommon.
MALT, mucosa-associated lymphoid tissue.

areas than a biopsy, thus serving as a useful adjunctive diagnostic test. *HP* bacteria are easily detected microscopically in smears stained with H&E, (modified) Giemsa, Papanicolaou (Fig. 4.52), and silver-based stains (Warthin-Starry and Steiner). The availability of an anti-*HP* polyclonal antibody allows immunohistochemical identification.

Since culture, cytologic and histologic examination, and rapid urease-based examinations all require endoscopy, less expensive and noninvasive diagnostic tests have been developed; the most popular is the urea breath test. The *HP* bacteria produce urease following orally administered carbon-labeled urea. The urease activity releases carbon, which is absorbed into the blood and converted to bicarbonate and expired as radiolabeled CO_2. Such tests are rapid and reasonably easy to perform. They are indicated for the initial diagnosis of the infection and to follow patients for infection eradication.

HP bacteria elicit antibody responses, allowing serologic testing. Serum enzyme-linked immunosorbent assays (ELISA) tests detect *HP* antibodies and indicate current or past infection. The test has a sensitivity of 80% to 100% and a specificity of 75% to 100% (138). There may be variations in the sensitivity based on strain differences. Serologic testing is not useful for detecting infection elimination. Stool antigen tests can be used to follow patients to determine if the infection has been eradicated if used after 8 weeks following treatment. They are particularly useful in children (139).

Relationship of Helicobacter pylori to Gastric Diseases

HP infection plays a significant role in the genesis of several gastric diseases (Table 4.8). The risk for developing gastric ulcers is highest in the nonatrophic forms of gastritis, whereas cancer associates with severe atrophic gastritis. Patient outcomes reflect differences in host susceptibility, organism virulence, or both. The development of gastritis, ulcer, and gastric cancer all involve an interplay between environmental, host, genetic, and microbial factors.

Gastritis

HP bacteria preferentially colonize the antrum, but they may infect any part of the stomach where they cause gastritis. When treated, the bacteria migrate from the antrum to the corpus with decreasing activity of the antral gastritis. Corpus gastritis is significantly more pronounced in patients with gastric cancer or a family history of gastric cancer (140). Infections with *vacA*-positive *HP* strains result in *acute gastritis* with cytoplasmic swelling and vacuolization, micropapillary changes, mucin loss, erosion of the juxtaluminal cytoplasm, and desquamation of surface foveolar cells. Regenerating cells form a multicellular layer with indistinct intercellular borders, creating syncytial polypoid excrescences (Fig. 4.53). Marked neutrophilic infiltrates

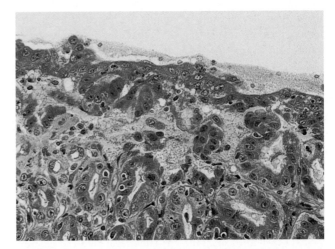

FIG. 4.53. Regenerating epithelium at the surface of an active chronic gastritis. This epithelium resembles that seen in an acute gastritis and occurs when chronic gastritis becomes active and loses the superficial epithelium.

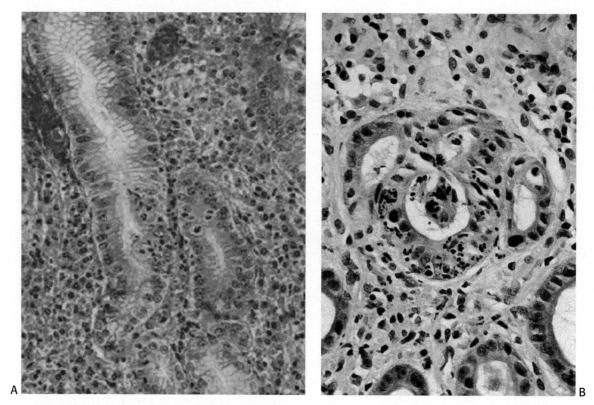

FIG. 4.54. Active *Helicobacter pylori* gastritis. Large numbers of neutrophils infiltrate the mucous neck region causing pit abscesses and cytotoxic damage to the cells. **A:** Pits seen in longitudinal section. **B:** Pits seen in cross section.

appear in the mucous neck region (Fig. 4.54) and lamina propria in early acute gastritis; when severe, they aggregate in the pit lumens to form pit abscesses. The mucosa appears normal in thickness or even slightly expanded due to the lymphoplasmacytic cell infiltrate in the superficial lamina propria. At this point the lesion can be termed *chronic active gastritis* or *active chronic gastritis*. Eosinophils may also be present. The regenerative pit bases are characterized by mucin loss, cytoplasmic basophilia, increased mitoses, and hyperchromatic nuclei (Fig. 4.55) that are sometimes severe enough to mimic dysplasia. If the pits and glands appear parallel to one another with intervening lamina propria, one should be extremely hesitant before making a diagnosis of carcinoma, even in the presence of severe glandular or cellular atypia.

Both the neutrophils and the *HP* destroy the epithelium, causing the mucous neck cells to proliferate in an effort to replace the dying cells. Other changes in severe infections include epithelial cell dropout, microerosions, larger erosions, and ulcers. Erosions forming in the setting of *HP* infections typically lack the homogeneous eosinophilic necrosis seen in patients with stress ulcers or aspirin- or NSAID-related ulcers. One virtually never sees *HP* in individuals with a histologically normal gastric mucosa. However, it is not unusual to find significant quantitative differences in the amount of inflammation present relative to the number of *HP* bacteria that are present.

The acute foveolitis may associate with an epithelial alteration known as the "malgun" (clear) cell change. Malgun cells have enlarged euchromatic nuclei, abundant cytoplasm, and increased expression of proliferating cell nuclear antigen (PCNA) and cytokeratin 8, indicating that they are mitotically and metabolically active. Malgun cells

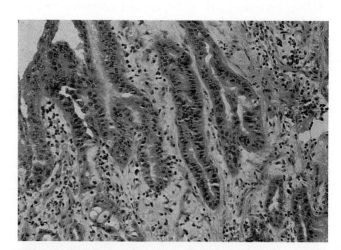

FIG. 4.55. Regeneration in active chronic gastritis. The mucous neck region of the oxyntic mucosa demonstrates marked regeneration. The superficial surface has become completely eroded. An intense bandlike infiltrate of lymphocytes and plasma cells occupies the superficial mucosa.

may be morphologic indicators of genomic damage and repair (141).

HP eradication causes rapid neutrophil disappearance. Eosinophils disappear more slowly. The surface changes reverse rapidly, and the epithelial cells acquire their normal shape and spatial organization within a few days of *HP* eradication. However, any atrophy that had developed remains, as do the lymphoid aggregates. These features become a permanent component of the once-infected gastric mucosa.

In *quiescent superficial gastritis*, the acute inflammation, edema, and vascular congestion disappear, and the epithelium returns to normal. However, the lamina propria contains increased numbers of mononuclear cells. Chronic superficial gastritis progresses to the next stage, chronic atrophic gastritis, over a period of 15 to 20 years (142). Since chronic gastritis develops as a patchy process, all stages in the evolution of chronic gastritis often coexist in a single stomach leading to the term *multifocal atrophic gastritis*, an entity discussed below with other forms of chronic gastritis. Lymphoid aggregates appear and sometimes lymphoid follicles develop. These are located deep in the mucosa, near the muscularis mucosae. When lymphoid follicles develop, with or without follicular centers (Fig. 4.56), the lesion is termed *follicular gastritis* (143). Antral lymphoid follicles can become quite prominent, sometimes causing mucosal nodularity, especially in children (144). The lymphoid aggregates represent an immune response to the bacteria. Their pres-

ence provides a useful marker for *HP* infections. Their number may decrease when the *HP* infections are treated. The features of *HP*-related mucosa-associated lymphoid tissue (MALT) lesions and the lymphomas that develop from them are discussed further in Chapter 18.

Granulomatous gastritis develops in approximately 1% of *HP*-infected patients, usually in patients with small numbers of organisms. The small sarcoid-type granulomas lie in the gastric lamina propria and *HP* bacteria can sometimes be found within them (145). The granulomas develop late in the disease, after the host has become sensitized to the organism. Antibody-coated bacteria ingested by macrophages may stimulate a histiocytic response (145).

Diffuse antral gastritis (DAG) is often considered to represent part of the peptic ulcer disease spectrum with antral and duodenal ulcers since it associates with increased gastrin, acid, and pepsin secretion (146). The hyperacidity creates a hostile environment for *HP* bacteria, restricting them to the antrum. The gastritis is characterized by an intense antral mononuclear infiltrate consisting of mature lymphocytes and plasma cells. Follicular gastritis is common. The epithelium may appear mucin depleted and there may be pit elongation.

Occasionally *HP* infections lead to the development of enlarged gastric folds in the gastric body, creating an endoscopic pattern suggestive of a hypertrophic gastritis/gastropathy (147). The *HP*-induced mucosal fold thickening is termed *giant fold gastritis*. This differs from Menetrier disease (discussed in a later section) in that the mucosa is thinner in giant fold gastritis and there is less foveolar hyperplasia (148). Additionally, there are ultrastructural parietal cell alterations (148).

Gastric Ulcer

About 95% of patients with duodenal ulcer and 70% to 93% of patients with gastric ulcer have an *HP* infection (149). The mucosa, weakened by *HP* infection, becomes susceptible to peptic injury, especially in the face of increased gastric acid production, explaining the relationship between *HP* infection and peptic ulcer disease (149) as discussed further below.

Gastric Cancer

There is a well-established relationship between *HP* infection and gastric carcinoma, as discussed in detail in Chapter 5, and MALT lymphomas, as discussed in Chapter 18.

Gastroesophageal Reflux Disease

Some have suggested that *HP* infections may actually be beneficial to some humans. This assumption is based on the increased incidence of gastroesophageal reflux disease, Barrett esophagus, and adenocarcinoma of the esophagus following the eradication of *HP* in some countries. This aspect is discussed further in Chapter 2.

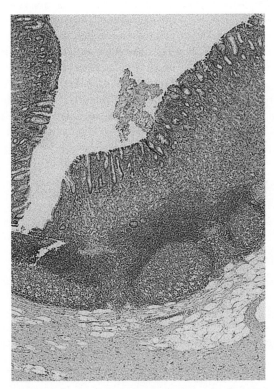

FIG. 4.56. Follicular gastritis. The gastric mucosa is infiltrated by mononuclear cells. The basal portion of the mucosa is expanded by a marked lymphocytic proliferation with the presence of prominent germinal centers.

TABLE 4.9	Comparison of *Helicobacter heilmannii* and *Helicobacter pylori* Infection	
	H. heilmannii	*H. pylori*
Organism differences	3.5–7.5 μm in length	3 μm in length/0.5 μm width
	0.5 μm width	Curved or spiral
	Up to 12 bipolar sheathed flagella	Four to six unipolar sheathed flagella
	Tightly coiled, regular helical structure	Less tightly coiled
	Urease producing	Urease producing
	No in vitro culture available	Cultured under microaerophilic conditions
Location of the gastritis	Antrum/fundus	Antrum/fundus
	No adherence to gastric epithelial cells	In gastric mucus/adherent to epithelium
Pathologic features	Mild chronic active gastritis	Chronic active gastritis
	Seen with same stains as *H. pylori*	Seen with silver staining, H&E, Diff-Quik, Giemsa, immunostains
Host species	Dogs, cats, pigs, primates	Humans, ferrets, cats, dogs, pigs, rabbits

H&E, hematoxylin and eosin.

Treatment

The goal of *HP* treatment is complete elimination of the organism. Triple therapy combines two or more antimicrobials with an antisecretory agent. The chief antimicrobials are amoxicillin, clarithromycin, metronidazole, tetracycline, and bismuth. However, some patients develop resistance to the antimicrobial drugs, with the frequency of this resistance differing depending on the drug that is used. Organism eradication is more difficult when a first treatment attempt has failed, usually due to the development of antibiotic resistance. Second-line therapy using quadruple therapies combines a proton pump inhibitor or H$_2$-receptor antagonist with a bismuth-based triple regimen therapy and high-dose metronidazole (150).

Other *Helicobacter* Infections

Helicobacter heilmannii, previously known as *Gastrospirillum hominis*, belongs to the *Helicobacter* family (151) and is found in up to 1.1% of gastric biopsies (152). The infection may be acquired from pets (153). It is a Gram-negative, urease-producing bacterium that is twice as long as and more tightly coiled than *HP* (154). The organisms tend to have five to eight prominent spiral turns making the organisms distinguishable from *HP*. The features listed in Table 4.9 differentiate it from *HP*. *H. heilmannii* infections affect both children and adults, with a frequency of 0.3% to 0.7% (154,155). However, unlike *HP* bacteria, which closely adhere to the gastric epithelium, *H. heilmannii* bacteria usually lie freely in the lumen or deep in the gastric pits and necks of the pyloric glands with little or no epithelial attachment (Fig. 4.57). The organisms tend to be

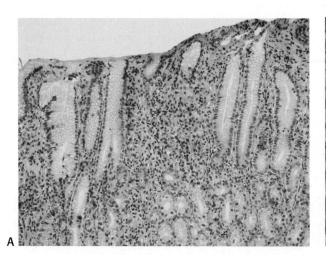
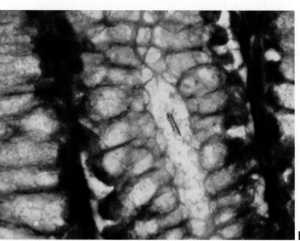

FIG. 4.57. *Helicobacter heilmannii* gastritis. **A:** Hematoxylin and eosin–stained section showing the presence of a chronic active gastritis. **B:** Diff-Quik stain highlighting the tight coils of the bacterium.

less numerous than in *HP* infections and therefore, they can be easily missed. In one study, examination of touch cytology specimens had a higher rate of diagnosis than the examination of biopsy specimens (156). The organism produces a chronic active gastritis but it is usually milder than that produced by *HP*. Prominent lymphoid aggregates may be present (157) and ulcers may develop. Gastric colonization is focal and restricted to the antrum. The organism is detectable with the same stains used to detect *HP*. Other changes that may be present include foveolar hyperplasia, vascular congestion, and edema, changes mimicking a chemical gastropathy (156). The infection rarely results in gastric carcinoma or MALT lymphomas.

Suppurative Gastritis

Most cases of suppurative (phlegmonous) gastritis antedate the antibiotic era. The disease typically affects severely debilitated individuals. Patients present with dramatic episodes of nausea, vomiting, and severe, acute, noncolicky, epigastric pain. Commonly, peritonitis or pleural effusions develop. The clinical course resembles that of patients with a perforated viscus. The mortality rate approaches 100% unless the affected part of the stomach is resected. Some patients develop abscesses. The most common offending organisms belong to *Streptococcus* species.

The stomach appears dilated and the wall is thickened, rigid, and purplish. Marked submucosal brawny edema leads to flattening of the rugal folds and hyperemia; fibrinous serous adhesions are also present. In some cases the mucosa contains focal necrosis; in others, a mucopurulent exudate completely replaces the mucosa. Acute inflammation with or without microabscesses and hemorrhage affects the submucosa. Widespread intravascular thrombosis involving the mural vessels results in secondary ischemic gangrenous necrosis with transmural inflammation. The muscularis propria appears variably inflamed and necrotic. A Gram stain demonstrates bacteria in the tissues.

Emphysematous Gastritis

Emphysematous gastritis, a form of suppurative gastritis, results from infections by gas-forming organisms, most commonly *Clostridium*, *Escherichia coli*, *Streptococcus*, *Enterobacter*, and *Pseudomonas aeruginosa* (158). Predisposing conditions include previous surgery, alcohol abuse, corrosive ingestion, pancreatitis, and cancer (158). Clinical features include an acute abdomen, systemic toxicity, and radiographic evidence of air bubbles in the gastric wall. Approximately two thirds of patients die of their disease; long-term complications include gastric fibrosis with stricture formation.

The gastric wall feels crepitant due to the presence of numerous, variably sized, air-filled, intramural spaces. In advanced cases, the gastric wall appears thickened, gangrenous, and necrotic.

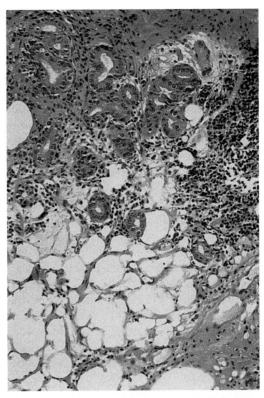

FIG. 4.58. Emphysematous gastritis. Photograph of the gastric mucosa showing the presence of an inflamed, partially necrotic, gastric mucosa. Deep in the mucosa one sees large, dilated, air-filled spaces.

The most prominent histologic findings consist of submucosal thickening, edema with transmural neutrophilic collections, a purulent serosal surface, patchy mucosal necrosis, and pneumatosis (Fig. 4.58). The infection rarely spreads to adjacent organs.

Syphilis

Syphilis affects the stomach in both its secondary and tertiary stages, but <1% of patients with syphilis develop gastric disease (159). Patients develop erosive gastritis or gastric ulcers with heaped, nodular edges. Erosions first develop in the pylorus, causing patients to present with gastric outlet obstruction. An infiltrative disease pattern causes thickened, edematous, rugal folds. Usually, the histologic features of H&E-stained slides are suggestive, but not diagnostic, of syphilis. One sees a diffuse gastritis containing a dense plasmocytic infiltrate, sometimes with prominent perivascular cuffing. Variable numbers of neutrophils and lymphocytes accompany the plasma cells. The lymphocytes may create lymphoepithelial lesions mimicking a MALToma. Neutrophils invade the gastric pits (Fig. 4.59). Variable degrees of glandular destruction and reactive atypia result. The inflammation extends into the submucosa with concomitant edema and fibrosis. A vasculitis is often present (160). However, the marked proliferative endarteritis or

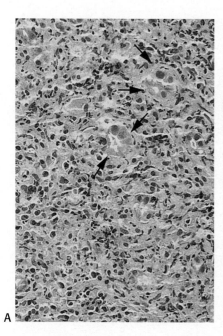
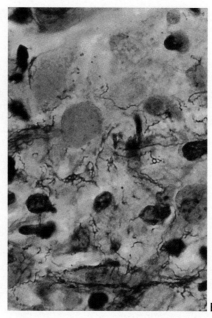

FIG. 4.59. Syphilitic gastritis. **A:** The tissue appears to consist almost exclusively of inflammatory cells. There are rare residual glands (*arrows*). The inflammatory infiltrate consists of plasma cells and lymphocytes. **B:** Silver stain on this biopsy demonstrating numerous silver-stained spirochetes within the lamina propria. (Case courtesy of Dr. D. Schwartz, Department of Pathology, Emory University, Atlanta, GA.)

proliferative endophlebitis typical of syphilitic lesions elsewhere is often absent. This may reflect the superficial nature of most gastric biopsies, which do not include the submucosa where these vessels are located. An ill-defined granulomatous process may be present. Silver stains (Fig. 4.59), dark-field examination, immunohistochemical stains, and polymerase chain reactions (PCRs) all demonstrate the spirochetes (161). The silver stains are not specific for the spirochetes since they also stain *Helicobacter*, but the morphology of the organisms is sufficiently different that they should not be easily confused.

The lesions of tertiary syphilis appear infiltrative, ulcerative, or gummatous. In later-stage disease, the muscularis propria and submucosa become more severely involved and the stomach acquires a fibrotic, hourglass, or leather bottle (linitis plastica) appearance. Squamous metaplasia with the subsequent development of squamous cell carcinoma may complicate syphilitic gastritis (162).

Tuberculosis

Tuberculous gastritis occurs much less commonly in North America and Western Europe than it did decades ago. Less than 1% of individuals with pulmonary or disseminated disease (Fig. 4.60) develop gastric involvement. Primary gastric tuberculosis is even rarer (163). The relative rarity of gastric tuberculosis results from three factors: The scarcity of lymphoid follicles in the stomach, the high gastric acidity, and the rapid passage of organisms through the stomach.

Gastric tuberculosis produces multiple shallow ulcers and confluent caseating granulomas that cause local tissue destruction with little reactive fibrosis. The gastric wall becomes thickened and ulcerated, and fistulas develop. Tuberculosis usually affects the antrum and duodenum in a distribution similar to that seen in syphilis and Crohn

disease. Rarely, extensive confluent granulomas thicken the pylorus, causing gastric outlet obstruction. The granulomas involve the mucosa, submucosa, or serosa. Perigastric lymph nodes frequently contain granulomas. The diagnosis rests on finding acid-fast organisms in the granulomas, although they may be very sparse. PCRs identify the bacterial DNA in cases that are negative on special stains.

Viral Infections

One can diagnose gastric viral infections histologically, cytologically, or by culture. Immunohistochemical reagents and genetic probes aid in their detection and specific diagnosis.

Patients previously exposed to *cytomegalovirus* (CMV) often maintain latent virus in many organs without evidence

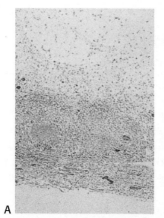
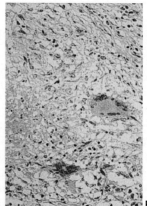

FIG. 4.60. Tuberculosis involving the serosal aspect of the stomach. **A:** Note the presence of caseating granulomas. **B:** Higher magnification showing the area of caseous necrosis and giant cells. Acid-fast stains (not shown) demonstrated the presence of rare organisms.

of tissue damage. The latent infections reactivate when patients age, develop serious disease, or become immunosuppressed. The infections are most common in transplant and AIDS patients. Infections affect children as young as 22 months (164). Patients present with epigastric pain, nausea, and vomiting. Complications include bleeding, ulcers, gastric outlet obstruction, and perforation. Unusual presentations include gastrocolic fistula (165) and pediatric forms of Menetrier disease (164). The stomach may appear normal or there may be an erosive gastritis. When severe, the gastric folds appear thickened and edematous with reduced antral distensibility simulating antral malignancy (166).

Gastric CMV infections display one of two major histologic patterns: Either a subtle infection or an obvious CMV gastritis. In more subtle forms of the disease, the mucosa appears almost normal with rare cells containing viral inclusions. CMV inclusions affect mucous neck cells and mesenchymal cells, including endothelial cells, macrophages, fibroblasts, and smooth muscle cells (Fig. 4.61). Usually one must examine multiple serial sections to find the viral inclusions. One can also routinely perform immunohistochemical stain in patients with a strong likelihood of having the infection. Patients with severe CMV infections demonstrate an obvious gastritis with inflammation and ulcers, and numerous prominent nuclear and cytoplasmic viral inclusions. Deep biopsies or resection specimens may disclose the presence of CMV-containing smooth muscle or ganglion cells; these patients may develop disordered gastric motility.

Herpes simplex virus rarely infects the gastric mucosa, contrasting with frequent esophageal involvement. Herpetic gastritis presents as yellowish plaques or edematous mucosal nodules separated by criss-crossed ulcers. Biopsies from vesicle and ulcer bases disclose epithelial cells containing typical eosinophilic intranuclear inclusions and ballooning cytoplasm (Fig. 4.62). The infection remains restricted to epithelium; it does not affect mesenchymal cells. Herpes zoster may also infect the stomach.

Fungal Infections

Fungal infections often present as an acute gastritis, although some fungal organisms cause a granulomatous gastritis. Table 4.10 lists entities in the differential diagnosis of granulomatous gastritis. Death results from disseminated infection or from hemorrhage following fungal invasion of gastric blood vessels, especially in patients with peptic ulcer disease.

Candida *Infections*

Candida infections account for most cases of fungal gastritis. Infections develop in debilitated, immunosuppressed, alcoholic, or achlorhydric individuals (167). The infection grossly appears localized, sometimes presenting as discrete, gray-yellow, creamy, mucosal plaques, or it is seen in peptic ulcers (Fig. 4.63) where it represents either a *Candida* infection or secondary colonization of a peptic ulcer. Most often, fungi colonize superficial parts of ulcer beds, a finding with

TABLE 4.10	Gastric Granulomatous Disorders
Foreign body granulomas	Food granulomas
	Suture granulomas
	Barium granulomas
	Kaolin granulomas
	Talc granulomas
	Beryllium granulomas
	Material used to cut drugs by drug addicts
Infectious granulomas	Tuberculosis
	Syphilis
	Mycobacterium intracellulare
	Whipple disease
	Histoplasmosis
	Mucor
	South American blastomycosis
	Anisakiasis
	Helicobacter pylori
Idiopathic	Crohn disease
	Sarcoidosis
	Isolated granulomatous gastritis
Neoplastic	Associated with gastric carcinoma
	Associated with gastric lymphoma
	Langerhans cell histiocytosis
Miscellaneous	Chronic granulomatous disease of childhood
	Eosinophilic granuloma
	Allergic granulomatosis and vasculitis
	Plasma cell granulomas
	Tumoral amyloidosis
	Rheumatoid nodules

little clinical significance since the organism does not infect adjacent viable tissues. In healthy persons, the *Candida* disappears when the ulcer heals. Alternatively, the fungus aggravates the peptic ulcer by invading arterial walls in the ulcer base, causing arterial rupture and massive hemorrhage. In this situation, the fungus plays a significant role in patient morbidity and mortality.

Histologic examination discloses the presence of fungal spores and/or pseudohyphae on the surface of peptic ulcers. The pseudohyphae invade the underlying tissues in invasive disease (Fig. 4.64). Grossly visible nodules result from microabscesses in which pseudohyphae invade and thrombose adjacent vessels and then coalesce to produce linear ulcerations presumably secondary to ischemia. Rarely, *fungal bezoars* develop. When diagnosing gastric *Candida*, a comment should be made as to whether the fungi invade the tissues or merely colonize the mucosal or ulcer surface and whether the organisms are spores, pseudohyphae, or both.

Other Fungal Infections

Other gastric fungal infections include *Aspergillus, Mucor, Coccidioides, Histoplasma* (168), *Cryptococcus neoformans*

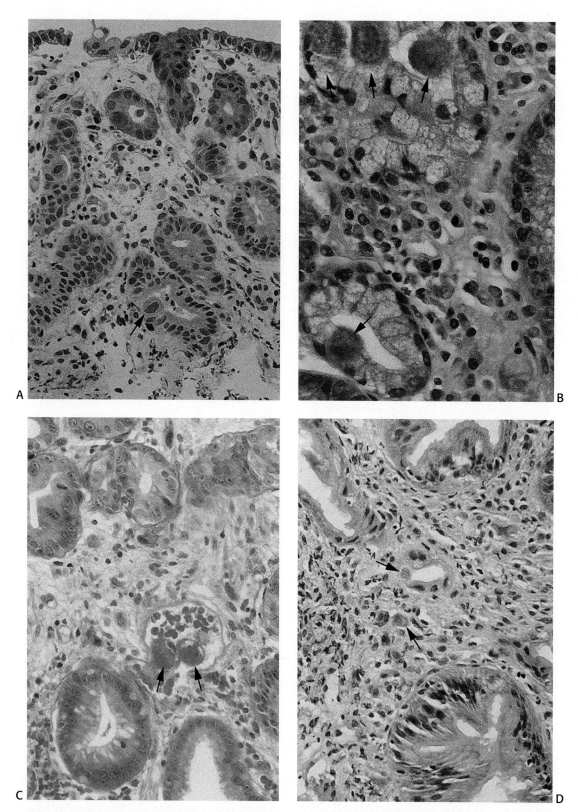

FIG. 4.61. Cytomegalovirus (CMV) gastritis. **A:** Renal transplant patient with subtle CMV infection. A small intranuclear inclusion is noted in the mucous neck cells (*arrow*). **B:** Gastric biopsy in a patient who had undergone a liver transplant. Numerous CMV inclusions are present (*arrows*). These are both cytoplasmic as well as intranuclear. **C:** Gastric biopsy in a renal transplant patient demonstrating the presence of intranuclear inclusions within the endothelial cells (*arrows*). **D:** Subtle infection demonstrating the presence of a diffuse gastritis. Rare intranuclear inclusions are evident both in the epithelium as well as in the stromal cells (*arrows*).

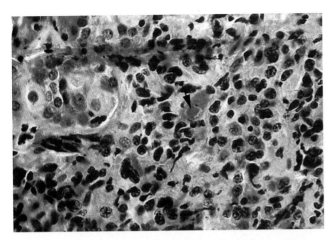

FIG. 4.62. Herpes simplex viral inclusion (*arrow*) in a degenerating epithelial cell associated with chronic gastritis in a patient with AIDS.

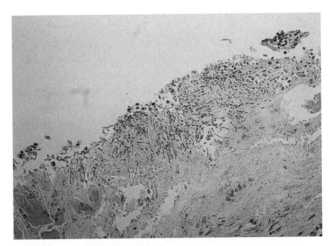

FIG. 4.64. Gastric candidiasis. Hyphae at the base of a necrotic gastric ulcer.

(169), *Pneumocystis carinii* (170), and *Torulopsis glabrata* (169). These organisms, like *Candida*, sometimes produce fungal bezoars. Zygomycotic gastric infections, formerly known as phycomycoses or mucormycoses, complicate chronic malnutrition. Gastric histoplasmosis complicates disseminated disease, producing a picture that mimics gastric carcinoma, gastric ulcer, polyps, or hypertrophic gastropathy. Vascular invasion causes hemorrhage and death. Both tumorlike nodules and perforated ulcers develop. The histologic features of these infections resemble those seen elsewhere.

Parasitic Infections

Patients with parasitic gastric infections may exhibit mucosal eosinophilia or only a nonspecific gastritis. The diagnosis rests on demonstrating the specific organism.

Anisakiasis

Gastric anisakiasis develops in individuals consuming raw or poorly cooked fish (171) or pickled herring (172). The infected fish spend part of their time in freshwater and part in salt water, such as salmon, herring, cod, pollack, and mackerel. When people eat infected fish, the larvae penetrate the gastric, small intestinal, or colonic mucosa, causing acute focal inflammation. Patients present with intolerable abdominal pain, usually within 12 hours of larval ingestion. Unlike other worms, anisakiasis preferentially affects the

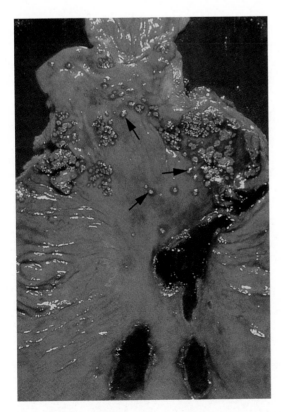

FIG. 4.63. Gastric candidiasis. Three ulcers are present, each of which was colonized by the fungi. In addition, numerous whitish plaques were densely adherent to the mucosa. The *arrows* point to three of these. Note that prominent atrophy is present.

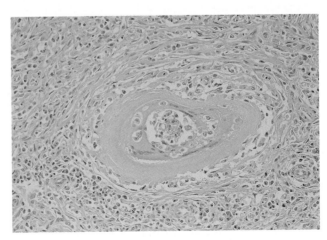

FIG. 4.65. Gastric anisakiasis.

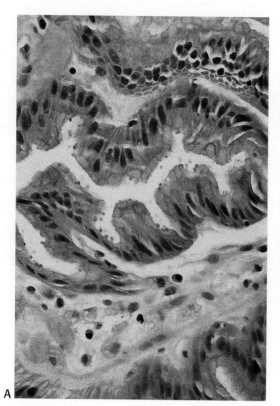
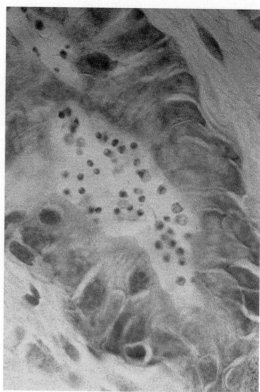

A   B

FIG. 4.66. Gastric cryptosporidia. **A:** Hematoxylin and eosin–stained section. **B:** Giemsa-stained section.

stomach rather than the intestines. Gastric perforation may cause omental granulomas. Endoscopy allows removal of the larvae (173). Severe, acute infections appear phlegmonous and the gastric wall becomes infiltrated with numerous eosinophils, neutrophils, plasma cells, lymphocytes, histiocytes, and sometimes giant cells.

Other Parasitic Infections

Gastric *cryptosporidiosis* (Fig. 4.66) represents a legacy of the AIDS epidemic and the pathologic features resemble those seen in the intestines. *Ascaris lumbricoides* infects sites adjacent to the small bowel, including the stomach. Patients may present with gastric outlet obstruction due to an antral roundworm mass (174). *Giardia* can be found in the gastric antrum in approximately 9% of patients with duodenal infections (175). Patients with gastric *Diphyllobothrium latum* infections present with megaloblastic anemia. The gastric mucosa shows variable degrees of chronic gastritis and atrophy. Other rare gastric parasitic infections include *Strongyloides* (Fig. 4.67), toxoplasmosis, schistosomiasis, and filaria.

Rickettsial Infections

Rickettsial infections affect the stomach in patients with generalized disease. The histologic changes are subtle and easily overlooked if one is unaware of the patient's condition. The

mucosa develops petechial hemorrhages. A mild nonspecific chronic inflammatory response affects small vessels. The organism can be demonstrated within the endothelium ultrastructurally or by immunohistochemistry (176,177).

Gastric Changes Present in AIDS Patients

AIDS patients develop several gastric abnormalities, the most common of which is CMV gastritis. Patients with *HP* infections often have severe disease with a large number of

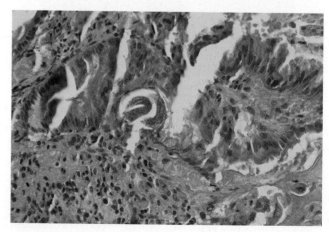

FIG. 4.67. Gastric *Strongyloides* in a patient with a widely disseminated infection.

organisms present. *HP* bacteria colonize cell surfaces and also the lamina propria, producing a prominent inflammatory response. The infection may also cause marked enlargement of the gastric folds. The inflammation resolves with treatment. Phlegmonous gastritis sometimes causes a fatal fulminant gastritis. Cryptosporidial or syphilitic infections of the antral mucosa cause isolated antral narrowing. Other rare infections of the stomach include those due to *Pneumocystis* and *Toxoplasma*.

Some patients develop *AIDS gastropathy*, a disorder characterized by a reduction in parietal cell mass, gastric acid, and pepsinogen secretion and an increase in mucus secretion. The disease is mediated by the presence of antiparietal cell antibodies. Hypochlorhydria predisposes the patient to gastrointestinal bacterial infection.

CHEMICAL GASTROPATHIES (REACTIVE GASTROPATHIES)

Chemical gastropathy is the second most common diagnosis made on gastric biopsies (178). Chemical gastropathies result from surface-damaging agents in the gastric lumen. NSAIDs and alkaline reflux are its commonest causes. Endoscopically, gastritis is present, but there is little histologic evidence of inflammation. All chemical gastropathies resemble one another, making it impossible to determine the exact etiology in the absence of identifiable bile or a pertinent clinical history. Clues that suggest the presence of a chemical gastropathy are listed in Table 4.11. The most diagnostic features include gastric pit elongation and tortuosity, often with reactive changes and foveolar mucin depletion. There is only minimal chronic inflammation and no acute inflammation, unless that the patient has coexisting *HP* gastritis, NSAID-induced ulcers, or stress gastritis.

Uremic Gastropathy

Uremic patients may develop gastric mucosal abnormalities since urea and other metabolites disrupt the mucosal barrier

---

TABLE 4.11 Clues That Suggest the Presence of a Chemical Injury

Pit expansion
Mucus depletion
Superficial edema
No organisms present[a]
No metaplasia
No polyps
No enlarged folds
Muscle fibers extending into the mucosa from the muscularis mucosae
Villiform transformation

---

[a] *Helicobacter pylori* infection may be superimposed on a chemical gastropathy confounding the histologic features.

(179). Uremia preferentially stimulates differentiation of mucous neck region stem cells into parietal cells and ECL cells, leading to an increased parietal cell mass, decreased production of foveolar cells, a thinned mucous gel layer, and increased acid secretion. Abnormalities in bile salt formation and hypergastrinemia enhance the acid injury. The stomach contains intramucosal hemorrhages varying in size from petechiae to large ecchymoses. Uncommonly, gastric mucosal necrosis with superimposed active ulceration develops. The histologic features overlap with those seen in stress gastritis. Superficial gastritis, erosions, and ulcers may be present. Uremic patients may also have the Kayexalate crystals described earlier in the mucosa.

Alkaline Reflux (Bile Reflux) Gastritis

Alkaline reflux gastritis develops in patients with abnormal pyloric sphincter function, often resulting from previous surgical interventions, chronic alcohol ingestion, or aging. Both alkaline duodenal secretions and bile damage the gastric mucosa. Bile salts increase mucosal permeability to hydrogen ions (180), resulting in H^+ back-diffusion. The most severe injury occurs in the antrum. The amount of reflux often correlates with symptom severity, but the endoscopic and histologic features rarely correlate with one another.

The histologic features of alkaline reflux gastritis are quite subtle and often overlooked. They include glandular elongation, tortuosity, and hypercellularity of the gastric pits; foveolar hyperplasia; and mucosal villiform transformation (Fig. 4.68).

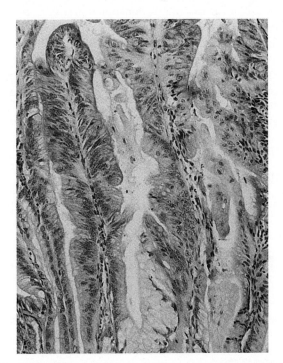

FIG. 4.68. Alkaline reflux gastritis. Some patients develop prominent villiform transformation of the surface with foveolar hyperplasia that can be quite pronounced, as in this photograph. The hyperplastic epithelium almost appears adenomatous.

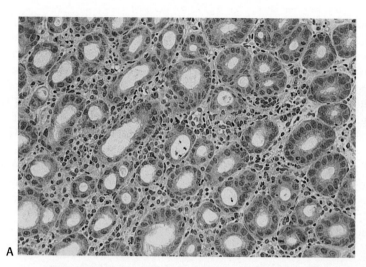
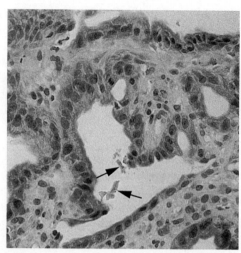

FIG. 4.69. Alkaline reflux gastritis. **A:** At first glance, the mucosa does not appear to be abnormal, although there might be a slight increase in the number of chronic inflammatory cells within the mucosa. **B:** Higher magnification of a different area of the same biopsy demonstrating the presence of an irregular gland containing bile crystals (*arrows*). The glandular epithelium appears regenerative both within the mucous neck region and at the free surface. The lamina propria contains a very mild increase in the number of mononuclear cells.

The regenerative glands may appear more angular than usual. The foveolar cells show mild mucin depletion and vacuolization. Other changes include capillary congestion and vasodilation in the superficial lamina propria, edema, and increased numbers of smooth muscle fibers that sometimes extend quite high in the lamina propria. The number of chronic inflammatory cells and neutrophils is generally sparse (181). The lack of inflammation is in striking contrast to the degree of epithelial hyperplasia. Bile may be present on the luminal surface or within glands (Fig. 4.69). Glandular atrophy develops in patients who have had an antrectomy, due to loss of the gastrin-producing G cells in the antral mucosa. The output of gastric acid, however, remains unchanged (181). Intestinal metaplasia and/or atrophy may develop in longstanding disease.

CHRONIC GASTRITIS

Nonspecific chronic gastritis has many etiologies (Table 4.12) that produce similar or overlapping histologic features.

TABLE 4.12 Etiology of Chronic Gastritis

Chronic alcoholism
Increased age
Smoking
Reflux of bile and alkaline secretions
Autoimmune injury
Hypersecretion
Gastric resection
Environmental factors including diet
Helicobacter pylori infection

For this reason, the correlation between clinical symptoms, endoscopic features, and histologic evidence of chronic gastritis is poor. However, three distinct forms of chronic gastritis can be delineated: Diffuse antral, fundic, and multifocal (Fig. 4.70). Diffuse antral and multifocal gastritis are sometimes referred to as type B gastritis, and both share *HP* as an etiologic factor. The major difference between the two is that diffuse antral gastritis is nonatrophic, whereas multifocal gastritis progresses to atrophic gastritis. These forms of gastritis show specific histologic, clinical, epidemiologic, and etiologic parameters (Table 4.13) (182,183). Chronic gastritis can be further classified as active or quiescent depending on its histologic features. Multifocal atrophic gastritis usually

TABLE 4.13 Fundic Versus Antral Gastritis

Fundic	Type B Antral
Fundal, antral sparing	Antral, then spreads proximally
Immunologic factors	Dietary, intraluminal factors
Pernicious anemia	Pernicious anemia rare
Hypo- or achlorhydria	Hyperchlorhydria
Parietal cell antibodies	No parietal cell antibodies
Intrinsic factor antibodies	No intrinsic factor antibodies
Hypergastrinemia (due to antral sparing)	Gastrin levels low or normal
No familial tendency	Familial tendency
Parietal and chief cell destruction	No parietal and chief cell destruction
Tends to persist and progress	Progression less rapid
Gastric atrophy common	Peptic ulcers common
Helicobacter pylori does not play a role	*H. pylori* plays a role

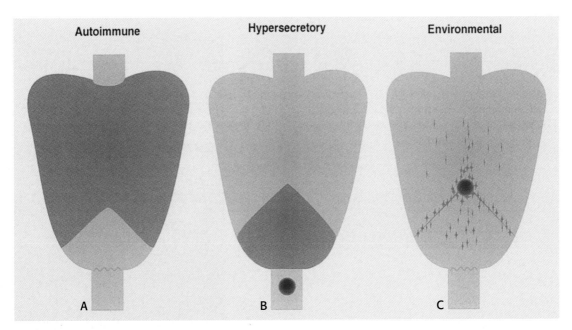

FIG. 4.70. The different forms of chronic gastritis show different gastric localizations. **A:** Autoimmune gastritis predominantly affects the fundus and body and spares the antrum. **B:** Hypersecretory gastritis predominantly affects the antrum and is associated with duodenal ulcers. **C:** Multifocal atrophic gastritis starts at the corpus–antral junction spreading proximally and distally. This form associates with gastric ulcers along the lesser curvature.

complicates longstanding *HP* infections, it although rarely complicates other conditions.

Helicobacter pylori–Associated Chronic Gastritis

Following *HP* infection the mucosa may become inflamed producing acute gastritis and then chronic active gastritis (Fig. 4.71). Early, the chronic inflammation remains confined to the superficial mucosa (Fig. 4.72). Superficial lamina propria lymphoplasmacytosis then extends for variable

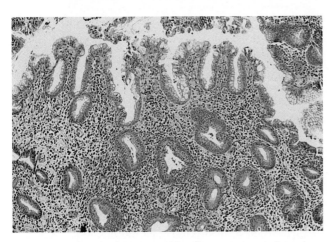

FIG. 4.71. Chronic active gastritis. The mucous neck regions appear hyperchromatic and are infiltrated with acute inflammatory cells.

distances into the glandular compartment. With time, the inflammation becomes confluent until it occupies the full thickness of the mucosa. T cells increase in number in both the epithelium and the lamina propria. Neutrophils, eosinophils, basophils, B cells, macrophages, monocytes, plasma cells, and mast cells infiltrate the mucosa resulting in mucosal damage. When the infection is treated, the mucosa regenerates and returns to normal; if the destroyed glands fail to regenerate, the space that they previously occupied in the lamina propria may be replaced by fibroblasts and extracellular matrix leading to an irreversible loss of functional mucosa and a change diagnosable as *atrophy* (Figs. 4.73 and 4.74). As atrophy develops, areas of intestinal metaplasia replace the native gastric mucosa. This may represent an adaptive response because *HP* bacteria cannot colonize the metaplastic cells since they lack the necessary bacterial adhesion factors discussed earlier. However, attachment of *HP* to areas of what appears to be incomplete intestinal metaplasia has been documented (184). These cells in fact represent a hybrid epithelium whose cells share characteristics of both gastric surface mucous cells and intestinal metaplastic cells (185). The intestinal metaplasia decreases the sites hospitable to the growth of the *HP*. However, the inflammation and its associated reparative processes continue in sites of persisting infection. As a result, the stomach acquires a mixed pattern of architecturally normal but inflamed areas (gastritis) alternating with expanding patches of atrophy and metaplasia producing multifocal atrophic gastritis (MAG) (186).

MAG is the most common form of chronic atrophic gastritis among populations at high risk for developing gastric

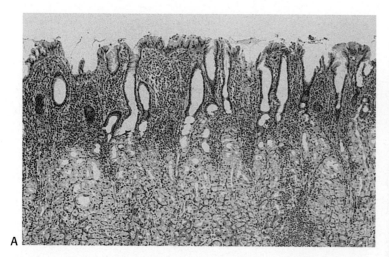

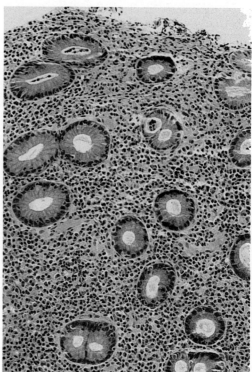

FIG. 4.72. Superficial gastritis. A: The superficial portion of the gastric mucosa is populated with a bandlike infiltrate of mononuclear cells. **B:** Higher magnification showing the presence of large numbers of lymphocytes and plasma cells.

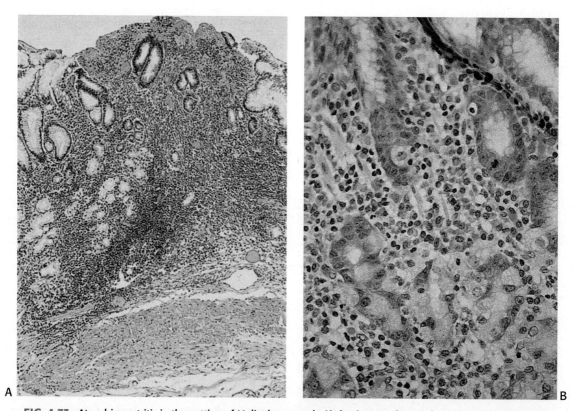

FIG. 4.73. Atrophic gastritis in the setting of *Helicobacter pylori* infection. **A:** There is loss of pit, mucous neck, and glandular areas of the mucosa associated with a mononuclear and neutrophilic cell infiltrate. There is also a lymphocytic aggregate at the base of the mucosa. **B:** Higher magnification of the area of glandular destruction showing epithelial dropout.

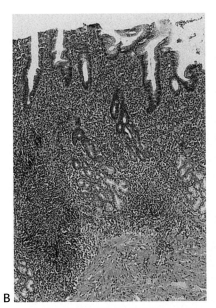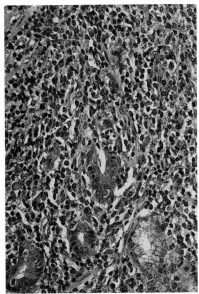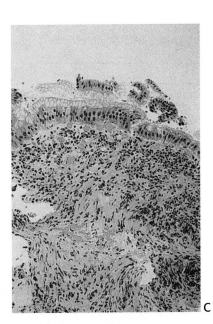

A, B
C

FIG. 4.74. Atrophic gastritis. These three figures show varying degrees of atrophic gastritis. **A:** Active chronic gastritis with glandular dropout. The mucosa contains prominent lymphocytic collections. **B:** Higher magnification of the lesion shown in A demonstrating the intense infiltration of the lamina propria by mononuclear cells and active destruction of the mucous neck region by polymorphonuclear leukocytes. **C:** This biopsy comes from a stomach that has become so atrophic that gastric pits and glands have both disappeared and all that remains is a simple mucosal lining covered by foveolar epithelium.

cancer, and it strongly associates with the presence of *HP* infections (187). A high intake of salt and nitrate and smoking contribute to its development (188,189). The development of atrophy determines the two main divergent outcomes of *HP*-related gastritis. Individuals who do not develop atrophy have an increased risk of duodenal ulcers but not of gastric cancer (187). Those who develop atrophy are at risk of gastric ulcers, mainly located on the lesser curvature around the incisura angularis, and they may develop intestinal metaplasia, dysplasia, and intestinal-type gastric adenocarcinoma (187). The progression of the gastritis to carcinoma involves a series of well-defined stages as discussed in detail in Chapter 5.

MAG first appears on the lesser curvature at the incisura (187). Later, atrophic foci appear along the lesser curvature and on both sides of the antral–corpus junction in the shape of an inverted V. In untreated patients the atrophy may spread to the corpus. Histologically, MAG consists of superficial gastritis, regenerative epithelial changes, glandular loss, intestinal metaplasia, and atrophy.

Atrophic Gastritis

Gastric atrophy, a preneoplastic condition (56), especially in populations where gastric carcinoma is prevalent, develops following gastric injury induced by various factors. There are substantial geographic and ethnic variations in the prevalence and severity of atrophic gastritis and its distribution within the stomach. Its features differ, primarily determined by the clinical setting in which it arises, the lesion location,

and etiologic, environmental, and host factors. One may also grade chronic atrophic gastritis as active or quiescent based on the presence or absence of acute inflammation.

Because extensive atrophy and metaplasia appear to increase the risk of gastric cancer, it is important to determine the severity of these lesions in biopsies (187). However, the definition of gastric atrophy is controversial and there is poor agreement in grading its severity, especially when it is only mild or moderate in nature (190). It is more difficult to appreciate minor degrees of atrophy in the antrum than in the corpus. This is due to the fact that in the antrum the gastric pits tend to be long and the antral glands normally lie in a loose connective tissue stroma. The interpretation is made more difficult due to the presence of an intense antral inflammatory infiltrate that typically complicates *HP* gastritis and expands the lamina propria. In contrast, the glands of the oxyntic mucosa are normally tightly packed and lined by a population of parietal and chief cells that occupy well-established positions from the neck zone to the deepest portion of the gland. In advanced atrophic gastritis, the glands disappear, the inflammation recedes, and the cellularity of the lamina propria returns to normal. Pre-existing reticulin fibers collapse on one another between the pits.

There is a large section of literature devoted to defining and quantifying gastric atrophy (56,186,191), particularly since atrophy is an early step in the carcinogenic process (187). It has been recommended that the term *atrophic gastritis* be restricted to those cases in which there is glandular loss that is replaced by extracellular matrix and fibroblasts, and/or when intestinal metaplasia is present (186). We agree with this approach.

TABLE 4.14 Definitions and Grading Guidelines for Each of the Histologic Features to Be Graded in the Sydney System

Feature	Definition	Grading Guidelines
Chronic inflammation	Increased lymphocytes and plasma cells in the lamina propria	Mild, moderate, or severe increase in density
Activity	Neutrophilic infiltrates of the lamina propria, pits, or surface epithelium	Less than one third of pits and surface infiltrated = mild; one third to two thirds = moderate; more than two thirds = severe
Atrophy	Loss of specialized glands from either antrum or corpus	Mild, moderate, or severe loss
Intestinal metaplasia	Intestinal metaplasia of the epithelium	Less than one third of mucosa involved = mild; one third to two thirds = moderate; more than two thirds = severe.
Helicobacter pylori	*H. pylori* density	Scattered organisms covering less than one third of the surface = mild colonization; large clusters or a continuous layer over two thirds of surface = severe; intermediate numbers = moderate colonization

The revised Sydney classification for gastritis provides guidelines for grading different histopathologic changes in gastric biopsies (56). It aims to produce a standardized, consistent histologic interpretation of gastritis based on topography, morphology, and etiology and includes a morphologic component by which five histologic variables (chronic inflammation, neutrophil activity, glandular atrophy, intestinal metaplasia, and *HP* density) are graded (Table 4.14) (56). If one chooses to use this system, the pathology report should note the presence or absence of each variable and when present, each of these variables can be graded on a mild, moderate, or marked scale using the published visual guidelines (56). The *HP* density should be evaluated in nonmetaplastic areas.

The degree of atrophy can be graded as mild, moderate, or severe by estimating the thickness of the glands in relationship to the entire mucosal thickness. This is facilitated by examining properly oriented biopsies containing the muscularis mucosae. Increasing degrees of atrophy associate with glandular cystic dilation, epithelial atypia, and intestinal metaplasia. Loss of all the glands qualifies for the diagnosis of *severe atrophic gastritis* (Fig. 4.75). Intestinal and pyloric metaplasia commonly develop. A confident diagnosis of atrophy can be made when epithelial metaplasia and/or gastric gland loss affects at least 50% of the total area of gastric biopsy material (192), assuming that there has been adequate mucosal sampling as recommended by the updated Sydney classification (56). Three features, the ratio of the glandular

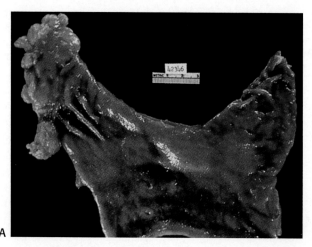

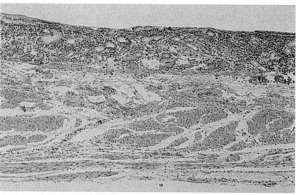

FIG. 4.75. Severe atrophic gastritis. **A:** The stomach has an almost complete loss of rugal folds. **B:** There is significant glandular loss and thinning of the mucosa. A few residual glands remain.

length to total mucosal thickness, the proportion of the secretory compartment area occupied by glands, and the number of glandular cross sections per 40× microscopic fields, consistently discriminate atrophic from nonatrophic lesions, particularly if one avoids areas of intestinal metaplasia and lymphoid follicles (191). Most patients with intestinal metaplasia have enough nonmetaplastic areas that the degree of atrophy can be evaluated. In patients in whom the entire stomach has been replaced by intestinal metaplasia, the patients are given the highest atrophy score (191). One factor that may call attention to the presence of atrophy is the presence of intestinal metaplasia, since the two lesions are commonly found together, but in its absence, mild or focal atrophy is easily missed.

Both antral and autoimmune gastritis show a marked inflammatory infiltrate consisting of plasma cells, lymphocytes, and variable numbers of eosinophils in all levels of the lamina propria. Initially, chronic inflammation fills the spaces left by glandular destruction and loss, thereby maintaining normal mucosal thickness. Plasma cells tend to lie superficially in the lamina propria, whereas lymphocytes lie deeper in the mucosa. Chronic progressive atrophy of the specialized epithelium results in an almost total loss of acid- and pepsinogen-secreting cells in the body of the stomach in autoimmune (type A) gastritis and of the antral glands in type B gastritis. As the mucosa thins and glands disappear, the bases of the pits come to rest on the muscularis mucosae. One must be careful not to mistake isolated residual cells seen in the setting of a gland-poor, stromal-rich mucosa, especially on a biopsy, as evidence of an early diffuse carcinoma.

Autoimmune Gastritis

The minority (approximately 20%) of cases of chronic gastritis fall into type A or autoimmune gastritis. Autoimmune gastritis results from immune-mediated destruction of parietal cells and is therefore restricted to the body and fundus. It shows a characteristic hypochlorhydria and an associated neuroendocrine cell hyperplasia discussed in Chapter 17. The classic form of the disease tends to affect individuals of Scandinavian or northern European descent. It is rare among other ethnic groups. The predilection for autoimmune gastritis to affect blue-eyed individuals with blood group A suggests a genetic predisposition to the disease.

Patients with autoimmune gastritis often have pernicious anemia and intrinsic factor autoantibodies and autoantibodies directed against other organs (Table 4.15) (193–196). Patients receiving methyldopa treatment may develop Parietal Cell Antibodies (PCAs) (101) and chronic autoimmune gastritis. The changes disappear upon cessation of the drug. Recently *HP* infections have been recognized as a cause of autoimmune gastritis. The majority of patients with *HP* infections have autoantibodies directed against the canalicular membranes of parietal cells or the luminal membrane of

TABLE 4.15	Autoimmune Diseases Associated with Autoimmune Gastritis
Graves disease	Idiopathic hypoadrenalism
Hashimoto thyroiditis	Idiopathic hypoparathyroidism
Thyrotoxicosis	Insulin-dependent diabetes
Dermatitis herpetiformis	Juvenile autoimmune thyroid disease
Celiac disease	

foveolar epithelium (129,197). The canalicular antibody targets the H^+,K^+-ATPase proton pump (197).

Patients with autoimmune gastritis have PCAs, autoantibodies to intrinsic factor, and the gastrin receptor (198,199). The PCAs target the catalytic subunit of the H^+,K^+-ATPase proton pump. The antibodies against intrinsic factor are of two types. The most common inhibits the attachment of vitamin B_{12} to intrinsic factor and the other binds the intrinsic factor–vitamin B_{12} complex, interfering with its small intestinal absorption (200). Therefore, many patients with autoimmune gastritis develop pernicious anemia secondary to a vitamin B_{12} deficiency.

Pathologic Features

Destruction of the oxyntic mucosa occurs over a period of years, ultimately leading to mucosal atrophy with hypo- or achlorhydria and decreased serum PG1 levels. PG1 levels below 20 mg/dL characterize the disease (201). Patients with severe disease often have mucosal flattening that stops abruptly at the antrum. Mucosal mononuclear cell infiltrates containing lymphocytes (both T and B lymphocytes), plasma cells, and eosinophils center around the oxyntic glands, eventually leading to their destruction (Fig. 4.76). Neutrophils are not a prominent component of the inflammation. The degree of parietal and chief cell loss and atrophy varies with disease stage. In the preatrophic phase of the lesion biopsies reveal cellular lamina propria infiltrates rich in plasma cells. T cells infiltrate the oxyntic glands resulting in lymphoepithelial lesions (202). The changes progress from a superficial gastritis to atrophic gastritis and eventually gastric atrophy. The patchy loss of parietal cells and chief cells is accompanied by an increased space between the glands that is readily appreciated when the atrophy is moderate or severe. As the oxyntic glands are lost, the lymphoepithelial lesions disappear and the lamina propria inflammation tends to be mild in nature. Eventually, the fundic mucosa becomes replaced by pyloric and/or intestinal glands (Figs. 4.77 and 4.78), foveolae may become hyperplastic (Fig. 4.77), and pancreatic metaplasia may develop. If the patient has coexisting untreated pernicious anemia, the epithelial cells may appear megaloblastic. Retention cysts may be present in the mucosa and superficial submucosa. In severe disease the entire gastric wall becomes atrophic, including even the musculature. Patients

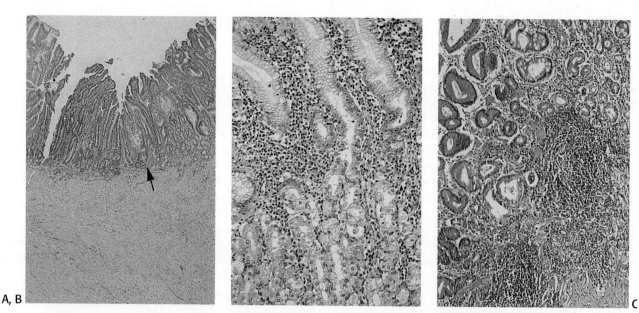

FIG. 4.76. Autoimmune gastritis. **A:** Low-magnification photograph showing the presence of a gastric mucosa that exhibits lengthened pits and glandular loss. Focal intestinal metaplasia (*arrow*) is also noted. **B:** Higher magnification of the oxyntic mucosa demonstrating the loss of parietal cells. **C:** The mucosa also contains evidence of *Helicobacter pylori*–associated gastritis with the presence of dense lymphocytic aggregates arranged in a follicular pattern.

with coexisting *HP* infections exhibit histologic features of both diseases.

Gastric adenocarcinoma affects 1% to 3% of patients with autoimmune gastritis via intervening steps of intestinal metaplasia and dysplasia (Figs. 4.77 and 4.79) (203). Autoimmune gastritis also leads to G-cell hyperplasia, multifocal gastric ECL hyperplasia, ECL micronests, and multifocal carcinoid tumors as discussed in Chapter 17 (Fig. 17.12).

Juvenile Forms of Pernicious Anemia

Juvenile pernicious anemia is rare and has three distinct forms. One occurs in late childhood and adolescence and appears to resemble the adult form of the disease in all respects except the age of patient presentation. So-called "true" juvenile pernicious anemia results from the failure of the parietal cells to produce intrinsic factor. The stomach is histologically normal and acid is produced by the parietal

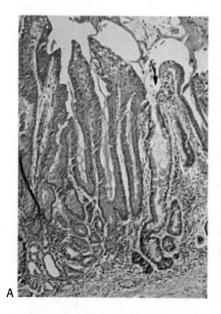

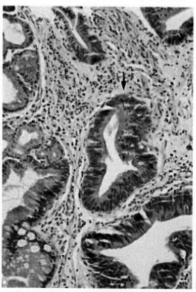

FIG. 4.77. Autoimmune gastritis. **A:** Patients often develop foveolar hyperplasia presumably in response to the gastrin secretion. A metaplastic gland lies to the right of the hyperplastic foveolae (*arrow*). **B:** Dysplasia (*arrows*) sometimes develops in the areas of intestinal metaplasia. A metaplastic gland is seen at the lower left-hand corner of the photograph.

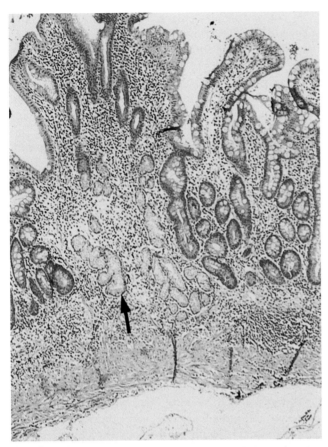

FIG. 4.78. Gastric body mucosa with focus of pyloric metaplasia (*arrow*). Villiform intestinal metaplasia makes up the remainder of the mucosa. Unless the location of this section is known, it would be difficult to identify it as body mucosa.

cells. The cause of the failure to produce intrinsic factor is not understood. The third type results from failed absorption of the vitamin B_{12}–intrinsic factor complex (204).

Atrophic Autoimmune Pangastritis

Atrophic autoimmune pangastritis is a distinctive form of antral and fundic gastritis associated with systemic autoimmune disease. This gastritis is characterized by intense mucosal inflammation that persists even into the phase of severe glandular atrophy. This differs from the other two major forms of chronic atrophic gastritis in which the inflammation tends to diminish as the mucosa becomes atrophic. The stomach shows a pangastritis with diffuse involvement of the body and antrum that is unassociated with either *HP* infections or the neuroendocrine cell hyperplasia associated with autoimmune gastritis. Patients range in age from 1 to 75 years and show a slight female predominance. All patients have systemic autoimmune diseases that include autoimmune enterocolitis, systemic lupus erythematosus, refractory sprue, autoimmune hemolytic anemia, and disabling fibromyalgia (205). The mucosal inflammation involves the mucosal thickness with a slight tendency to preferentially affect the deep glands, frequently accompanied by apoptotic bodies in a pattern resembling graft versus host disease (205). Glandular atrophy, lymphoplasmacytic infiltrates, and neutrophilic infiltrates diffusely involve the stomach. Microabscesses may be present in the gastric glands. There may also be areas of overt ulceration. These patients are not hypergastrinemic and do not develop neuroendocrine cell lesions.

FIG. 4.79. Autoimmune gastritis with diffuse gastric dysplasia. **A:** Low magnification demonstrating the presence of extensive replacement of the glands by dysplastic epithelium. **B:** Higher magnification demonstrating the presence of dysplastic glands showing abnormally shaped nuclei with prominent nucleoli and numerous mitoses, some of which are atypical.

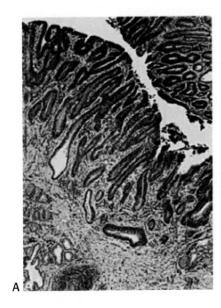

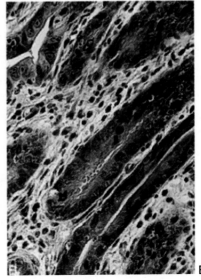

Corpus Atrophy

Corpus atrophy also follows antrectomy. The loss of antral G cells results in a selective loss of parietal cells, atrophy, and pyloric and/or intestinal metaplasia.

Metaplasias in Gastritis

Morphologic, histochemical, and enzymatic patterns enable one to recognize five major types of metaplasia occurring in the stomach: Intestinal, pyloric, pancreatic, ciliated, and squamous. The first three types are the most common.

Pyloric Metaplasia

Pyloric metaplasia (also sometimes referred to as pseudopyloric metaplasia) most commonly occurs in the setting of autoimmune gastritis. It begins with loss of specialized cells in the oxyntic mucosa (Fig. 4.78). As the cells are lost, they are replaced by a simpler glandular epithelium. Ultimately, the metaplastic glands become indistinguishable from antral glands. Pyloric metaplasia first affects glands closest to the antral junction, producing antral expansion at the expense of the oxyntic mucosa. There is some debate whether the metaplastic cells are indeed metaplastic or are a novel cell lineage that develops in the stomach and other gastrointestinal sites following ulceration. The cells appear adjacent to the ulcers and are thus termed *ulcer-associated cell lineage* (UACL). The UACL produces EGF and trefoil peptides that promote mucosal proliferation and healing (206,207).

Intestinal Metaplasia

Gastric intestinal metaplasia (IM) is quite common. It is believed to represent a response to chronic injury, often caused by *HP* infections. The risk factors for developing IM resemble those of gastric cancer in high-risk populations. Thus, IM is more frequent in smokers and in Asians than in other nationalities. Diets deficient in fresh fruits and vegetables combined with a high salt and nitrite content are common to both conditions (208). Thirteen percent of consecutive American Caucasians undergoing upper endoscopy and 50% of Hispanics and Blacks had evidence of gastric IM when routine protocol-mapping biopsies of the normal appearing mucosa were performed (209).

One of the more contentious issues is the significance of IM at the cardia. IM has been implicated in the development of both gastric and esophageal carcinoma. However, while gastric IM increases the risk of gastric cancer, with the increased risk being proportional to the extent of the metaplasia (208), the risk is much lower than Barrett esophagus (BE) progressing to cancer (210), at least in the United States. Thus, it is important to try to distinguish the IM of BE from the gastric type of IM. IM at the gastroesophageal junction is discussed in detail in Chapter 2.

As noted earlier, IM often complicates MAG. Over time, widened areas of gastric atrophy, often accompanied by gastric IM, replace the chronic active gastritis associated with *HP* infections. IM begins at the antral–corpus junction in a patchy (Fig. 4.80), multifocal fashion, and then spreads both distally and proximally to involve the antrum and fundus. The areas of IM increase with patient age and often become confluent, replacing large areas of the gastric mucosa. This process can be highlighted by staining gastric resection specimens for alkaline phosphatase activity since only intestinal-type epithelium expresses the enzyme (Fig. 4.80). IM more frequently coexists with gastric cancer than with gastric ulcer, but it shows the same distribution when associated with either condition.

IM may result from mutations caused by nitrosative deamination of DNA by nitric oxide generated by inflammatory cells in stem cells in the replicating compartment of gastric glands in response to *HP* infection (208). IM may also represent a change that raises gastric pH by replacing the oxyntic mucosa with an epithelium that favors the growth of bacteria capable of generating endogenous mutagens. Down-regulation of Sox2 and ectopic expression of Cdx2, an intestine-specific transcription factor belonging to the *caudal*-related homeobox gene family (211), are important in the development of IM (212). Cdx2 expression may lead to activation of intestine-specific gene transcripts, thereby directing intestinal epithelial development and differentiation in the metaplastic areas.

In IM the cells that normally line the gastric mucosa (surface epithelium, foveolar epithelium, and glands) are replaced by an epithelium resembling that of the small or large intestine. The earliest metaplastic changes consist of the appearance of mucin-negative absorptive enterocytes with a brush border alternating with Alcian blue–positive goblet cells (Figs. 4.81 and 4.82). In young individuals with less extensive IM, the metaplastic glands resemble normal small intestinal epithelium. Initially, only the epithelial type changes, but later the mucosal architecture acquires a small intestinal villiform architecture, often containing Paneth cells at the base of the pits (Fig. 4.83). Paneth cells in areas of IM do not have the same uniform distribution seen in the intestine. In some cases, they are limited to the antral corpus border and are lacking in IM in the distal stomach. They may lie in the superficial portions of the metaplastic gland; ultrastructurally some Paneth cells contain both Paneth cell granules and mucinous vacuoles (208).

Goblet cells are easily seen on H&E-stained sections. However, an Alcian blue/PAS stain is commonly used to identify the goblet cells since it stains all acidic mucins blue-purple and neutral mucins magenta and is easy to perform and interpret. Some metaplastic cells exclusively secrete sialomucins and contain a "complete" set of normal small intestinal digestive enzymes (sucrase, trehalase, and alkaline phosphatase). This type of metaplasia is characterized by weak expression of (intestinal) MUC2 and absence of gastric

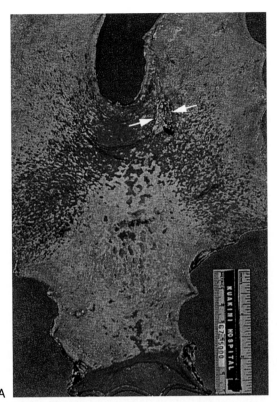

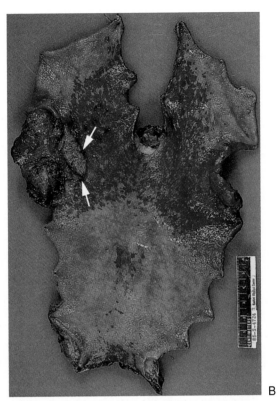

A

B

FIG. 4.80. Intestinal metaplasia. Both gastric specimens have been opened along the greater curvature and were stained with alkaline phosphatase to highlight areas of intestinal metaplasia. **A:** Note the inverted V-shaped configuration of the metaplastic process at the corpus–antral junction with areas of punctate staining as one moves away from this border. The duodenum also stains intensely with the enzyme. There is a benign gastric ulcer (*arrows*) at the junction zone of the metaplastic epithelium with the native oxyntic mucosa. **B:** A similar preparation in which the gastritis has extended far more proximally. Patchy metaplastic lesions are also seen in the antral region along the greater curvature. With the extensive replacement of the oxyntic mucosa, it is easy to see how hypo- or achlorhydria can develop. A polypoid carcinoma is present in the metaplastic area (*arrows*).

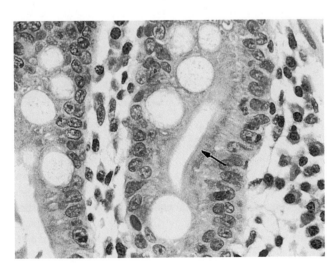

FIG. 4.81. Type I intestinal metaplasia. The brush border (*arrow*) of the absorptive cells is present, as are numerous goblet cells.

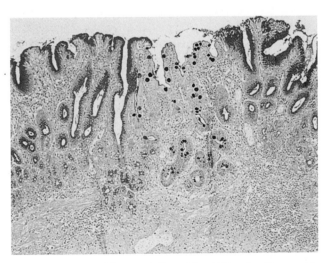

FIG. 4.82. Alcian blue–periodic acid–Schiff stain. The gastric mucosa stains red, indicating that neutral mucins are present. The acidic mucins of intestinal metaplasia are blue.

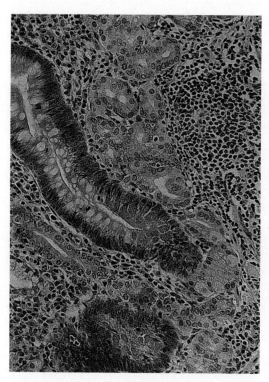

FIG. 4.83. Chronic gastritis with intestinal metaplasia. This metaplastic gland demonstrates the presence of goblet cells, absorptive cells, and prominent Paneth cells.

(MUC1, MUC5AC, and MUC6) mucins and cytokeratin (CK) immunoreactivity (213). These cells have a complete switch in their differentiation program from a gastric to an intestinal phenotype, and they have been termed small intestinal, complete, or type I IM.

Later, as the disease becomes more extensive, the enterocytes disappear and are replaced by columnar cells containing abundant mucous droplets in their cytoplasm. These metaplastic cells lack a well-developed brush border and secrete both sialomucins and sulfomucins (214). They lack the complete set of digestive enzymes. This type of metaplasia has been termed enterocolonic, colonic, type II, or incomplete metaplasia. Incomplete metaplasia strongly expresses MUC1, MUC5AC, MUC6, MUC2, Das-1 (a large intestinal antigen), and CK 7. Incomplete IM shows a mixed gastric and intestinal phenotype reflecting aberrant differentiation programs that do not reproduce any phenotype occurring in normal adult gastrointestinal epithelia (213). Several types of metaplastic epithelium may develop within the same stomach. IM occurs concurrently with atrophic gastritis or independently. Incomplete IM frequently associates with areas of dysplasia and carcinoma.

The endocrine cell population in the different types of metaplasia changes with the phenotype of the nonendocrine cells. In patients with antral gastritis, the proportion of gastrin and somatostatin neuroendocrine cells decreases as the glands pass from a mixed gastric–intestinal phenotype to a pure intestinal phenotype. There is a corresponding increase in intestinal-type endocrine cells that produce glicentin, gastric inhibitory polypeptide, and glucagonlike peptide 1 (215). Gastrin-positive cells emerge in the areas of pyloric metaplasia.

A distinct cellular subset consisting of groups of undifferentiated columnar cells lies on the interfoveolar crests of the gastric mucosa (216). These cells differ from both normal foveolar cells and metaplastic cells, and they show a close association with atrophic gastritis, particularly in the presence of sulfomucin-secreting IM. This lesion, termed *gastric tip lesion*, may provide a link between this type of metaplasia and the intestinal variant of gastric adenocarcinoma that develops in intestinalized areas (216). Histologically the large, columnar, pseudostratified cells have central nuclei and lack the prominent cup-shaped mucus collection typical of foveolar cells. The cells cluster in groups of up to 25 cells and they show an abrupt transition with the adjacent normal foveolar epithelium.

There is no consensus on the role of the various IM subtypes and subsequent risk of developing carcinoma, and the question then arises as to what to do with a patient with a diagnosis of gastric IM. The answer to this depends on whether the patient has a family history of gastric cancer, has migrated from a high-risk geographic location, lives in a high-risk location, or is a member of an ethnic population with a high risk of developing carcinoma, and whether there is evidence of dysplasia on the biopsy. It can be assumed that any person with an increased cancer risk as defined by the factors noted in the previous sentence or those with extensive metaplasia is at high risk for gastric cancer and should be subject to periodic screening. The extent of the IM is probably more important than the metaplastic subtype (208). The prudent thing to do if IM is detected in a biopsy is to describe the type of metaplasia that is present, to make some estimate as to whether the process is focal or diffuse in nature, and to note whether or not dysplasia is also present. The guidelines of the Sydney System (56) can be used to grade the intestinal metaplasia. The relationship of IM to gastric cancer is discussed in greater detail in Chapter 5.

Ciliated Cell Metaplasia

Ciliated cells may develop deep to areas of intestinal metaplasia; in the mucosa of patients with gastric ulcers, dysplasia, or adenocarcinomas; and at sites away from the main lesion (Fig. 4.84) (217). The ciliated cells show some evidence of an antral phenotype, as demonstrated by their pepsinogen group II activity (208). The cilia in the cells often are structurally abnormal. The ciliated cells line cystically dilated glands, where they may represent an adaptive mechanism aimed at expelling semifluid viscous material and inflammatory cells from the cysts. As cysts enlarge, the intrinsic pressure of the retained mucus results in cellular atrophy and ciliary disappearance (217).

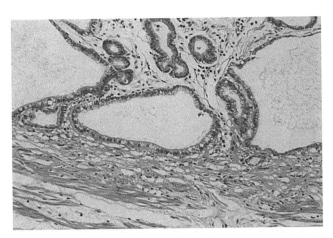

FIG. 4.84. Ciliated metaplasia. Ciliated metaplastic cyst located near the muscularis mucosae. The cilia are difficult to see on hematoxylin and eosin stain.

Pancreatic (Acinar) Metaplasia

Pancreatic metaplasia is present in 12% of patients with autoimmune gastritis, usually developing in the cardia and often coexisting with other types of metaplasia (218). Pancreatic acinar cells can also develop in the gastric antral mucosa in areas of IM or atrophy. The metaplastic foci contain single or multiple pancreatic nests and lobules measuring up to 1.7 mm in diameter (Fig. 4.85). The metaplastic tissue imperceptibly merges with the gastric glands. Less commonly, acinar cells lie scattered individually or in small cellular foci among the gastric glands. Larger lobules contain tubules or small cystic spaces reminiscent of dilated ductules. The layers of smooth muscle cells that circumferentially surround the ducts in heterotopic pancreas are absent. The acinar cells have a truncated pyramidal shape with a rim of deeply basophilic basal cytoplasm and numerous small, acidophilic, weakly PAS-positive, refractile granules in the mid- and apical cytoplasm. These granules contain trypsin, amylase, and lipase. The

nuclei appear round, relatively small, and centrally or basally located, with a prominent nucleolus. Endocrine cells positive for somatostatin, gastrin, or serotonin intermingle with the acinar cells. Amphicrine cells containing both zymogen and neurosecretory granules are also present.

The metaplastic cells probably result from aberrant stem cell differentiation (219). PDX-1, a homeodomain transcription factor, plays a key role in both endocrine and exocrine pancreatic differentiation and differentiation of endocrine cells in the gastric antrum. Therefore, it is of interest that both the pancreatic metaplasia and endocrine cell hyperplasia associated with atrophic corpus gastritis express PDX-1 (220).

GRANULOMATOUS GASTRITIS

Since gastric granulomas complicate many conditions (Table 4.10) (221), the diagnosis depends on the clinical presentation, the histologic appearance, and sometimes the use of special stains or other ancillary diagnostic techniques to determine whether the patient has a primary gastric granulomatous disease or some other entity. The granulomas contain epithelioid macrophages and lymphocytes with occasional giant cells, eosinophils, and neutrophils with or without necrosis. There are generally two types of granulomas in the stomach: Those that are a reaction to inert foreign material (like food) and those that form as part of a T-cell immune response to microorganisms. The products of activated T lymphocytes transform macrophages into epithelioid cells and multinucleated giant cells.

Idiopathic Granulomatous Gastritis

The diagnosis of idiopathic granulomatous gastritis is made when other entities associated with granuloma formation have been excluded. Symptomatic patients usually present over the age of 40 with epigastric pain, bleeding, weight loss, and vomiting secondary to pyloric obstruction. The histologic changes

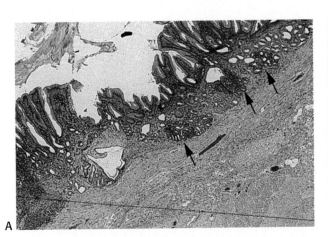
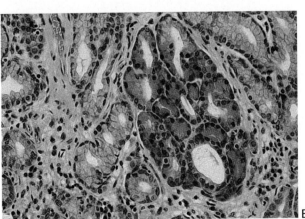

FIG. 4.85. Pancreatic metaplasia in autoimmune gastritis. **A:** This stomach shows the presence of prominent pancreatic metaplasia as well as cystic change. Numerous pancreatic lobules lie at the basal portion of the mucosa (*arrows*). **B:** Higher magnification of one of the metaplastic areas showing pancreatic acini-surrounded antropyloric glands.

parallel those seen in sarcoid disease, so that a definitive morphologic diagnosis may be impossible. The predominant findings consist of antral narrowing and rigidity caused by transmural, noncaseating granulomas. The inflammation and fibrosis rarely extend beyond the mucosa. Ulcers similar to peptic ulcers may develop, but the slit-shaped ulcers and fissures typical of Crohn disease are absent. In a third of cases,

regional lymph nodes become involved. Controversy exists as to whether idiopathic granulomatous gastritis represents a distinctive entity or whether it represents an isolated or limited form of gastric sarcoid or Crohn disease. In the United States, most patients with gastric granulomas will eventually be shown to have inflammatory bowel disease (IBD) or sarcoid disease. The latter diagnoses may become evident over time.

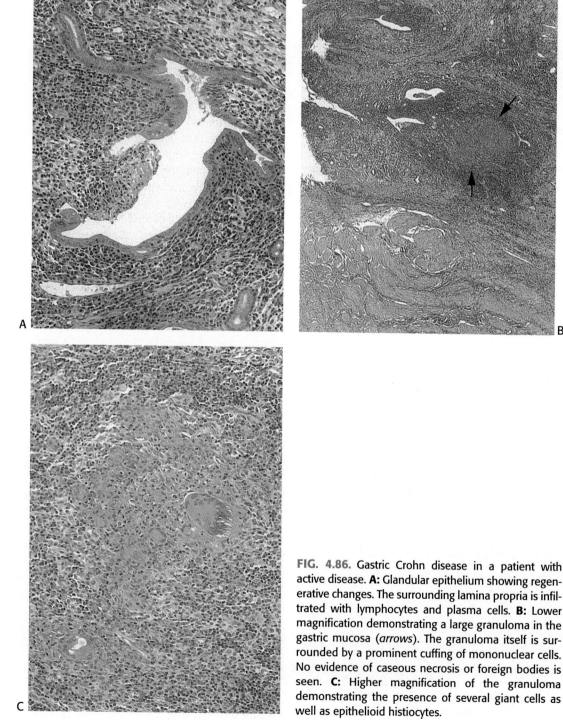

FIG. 4.86. Gastric Crohn disease in a patient with active disease. **A:** Glandular epithelium showing regenerative changes. The surrounding lamina propria is infiltrated with lymphocytes and plasma cells. **B:** Lower magnification demonstrating a large granuloma in the gastric mucosa (*arrows*). The granuloma itself is surrounded by a prominent cuffing of mononuclear cells. No evidence of caseous necrosis or foreign bodies is seen. **C:** Higher magnification of the granuloma demonstrating the presence of several giant cells as well as epithelioid histiocytes.

Crohn Disease

Crohn's patients with gastric involvement often also have duodenal disease. Endoscopic abnormalities, including mucosal nodularity with cobblestoning, aphthous ulcers, linear or serpiginous ulcers, thickened antral folds, antral narrowing, hypoperistalsis, and duodenal strictures, are present in patients with severe gastric Crohn disease (222). The diagnosis of gastric Crohn disease is easy in the presence of florid disease and in the setting of disease elsewhere in the gut. However, the diagnosis is more difficult if gastric involvement is the first disease manifestation. Well-developed gastric Crohn disease shows patchy, focal inflammation associated with acute inflammation in the pits (pit abscesses) or glands. Neural hyperplasia and lymphoid aggregates may be present (Fig. 4.86). A prominent lymphoplasmacytic infiltrate often surrounds the granulomas, contrasting with both sarcoid and isolated granulomatous gastritis, which tend to lack the associated nonspecific inflammation. Gastric Crohn disease is discussed further in Chapter 11.

Sarcoidosis

Gastric sarcoidosis is unusual and can only be diagnosed with confidence when gastric granulomas occur in the setting of documented sarcoid in other organs, such as in the liver, lungs, or hilar lymph nodes, and in the absence of microorganisms in the granulomas. Asymptomatic gastric involvement affects approximately 10% of sarcoid patients. Symptomatic patients present with gastric ulcers, hemorrhage, pyloric stricture, and gastric outlet obstruction. Endoscopic changes range from a distal gastritis with or without nodularity to ulceration and pyloric stenosis (223). The histologic features of the granulomas resemble those seen elsewhere in the body. They tend to associate with fewer lymphocytes and plasma cells than one sees in patients with Crohn disease, unless the patient has coexisting chronic gastritis (Fig. 4.87).

Food Granulomas

The presence of a gastric granuloma should always prompt the search for a foreign body. *Foreign body granulomas* form when mucosal defects allow small food particles or other substances access to the submucosa. These foreign body granulomas are usually easily distinguished from the granulomas seen in the disorders discussed above. They frequently have palisades of histiocytes and foreign body giant cells. Acid leads to necrosis, increasing the size of the mucosal defect, thereby allowing more food to enter. These food particles (particularly insoluble cereals) lying deep in the gastric wall elicit the granulomas (Figs. 4.88 and 4.89). They appear

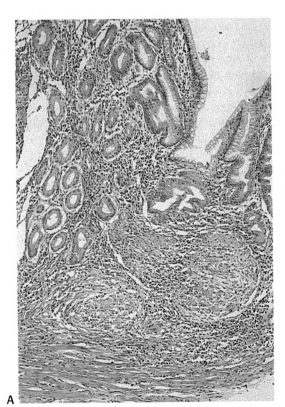

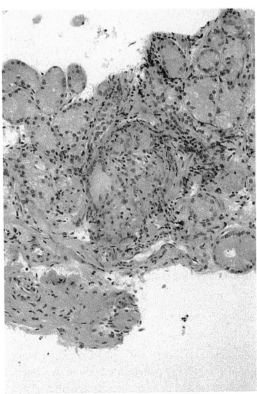

A   B

FIG. 4.87. Gastric sarcoid. A: Low magnification demonstrating the presence of several noncaseating granulomas within the gastric mucosa. Note that the mucosa lacks the intense infiltrate that surrounded the granulomas illustrated in Crohn disease in Figure 4.86. **B:** Another granuloma from a different patient in which almost no associated inflammation is present.

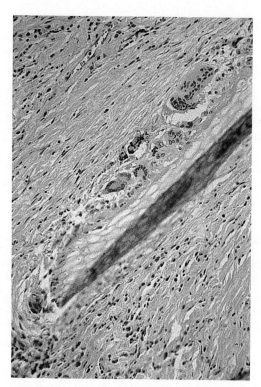

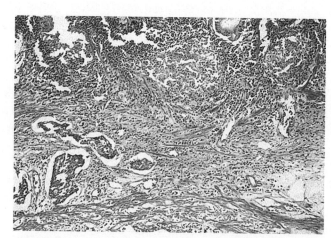

FIG. 4.90. Granulomatous gastritis complicating gastric carcinoma.

FIG. 4.88. Food granuloma in the muscularis propria. Note the presence of the bricklike architecture of the vegetable fiber in the center of the photograph surrounded by prominent multinucleated giant cells.

as amorphous eosinophilic masses, sometimes containing vegetable cells recognizable by their thick, bricklike cell walls. Palisading epithelioid histiocytes and foreign body giant cells surround the food particles. The granulomas may become fibrotic or calcified.

Other Granulomas

Barium granulomas also develop in the stomach. Collections of macrophages containing refractile, greenish gray, foamy cytoplasm develop. Granulomas may also form around parasites.

A marked granulomatous gastritis may also complicate gastric malignancies (carcinomas or lymphomas) (Fig. 4.90). The granulomas resemble sarcoid granulomas and may affect all levels of the gastric wall or the draining regional lymph nodes. The granulomas likely result from an immune response to the tumor.

EOSINOPHILIC GASTROENTERITIS

Eosinophilic gastroenteritis, an uncommon condition, affects one or more gastrointestinal segments, commonly involving the stomach and small bowel (224). It usually presents between the 2nd and 5th decades of life. Seventy-five percent of patients present under age 50; some patients have an underlying connective tissue disorder (225) or an infection with *Eustoma rotundatum*, a parasite of North Sea herring (224). Many patients have a history of allergy, peripheral eosinophilia, asthma, eczema, or food sensitivity (226).

The eosinophilic infiltrates tend to affect specific layers of the bowel wall. They may involve only the mucosa, the submucosa (the most common location), the muscularis propria, or the serosa. Symptoms differ depending on the site and extent of involvement. Patients with predominantly mucosal disease experience postprandial nausea, vomiting, abdominal pain, and food intolerance. Disease predominantly affecting the muscular layer results in thickening and rigidity of the muscularis propria and gastric outlet obstruction. The least common disease pattern predominantly involves the serosa. Usually, one of these patterns

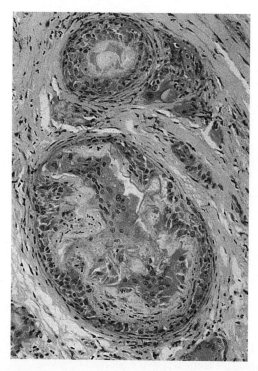

FIG. 4.89. Food granuloma. Granulomas demonstrating the presence of palisading epithelioid histiocytes and a thin eosinophilic line in the center of the lesion. This represents a dissolved material, which deposits in the granulomatous wall.

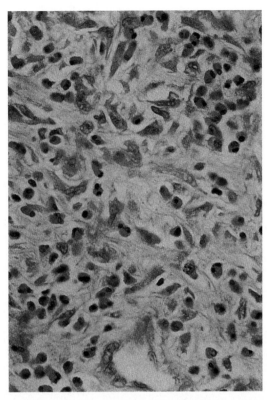

FIG. 4.91. Eosinophilic gastroenteritis. Note the prominent number of eosinophils distributed throughout the lamina propria.

predominates; some patients have a mixed disease pattern. Patients often have a prompt response to steroid treatment.

Mucosal edema, capillary lymphatic dilation, and an intense but patchy eosinophilic infiltrate displace and destroy gastric pits and glands (Fig. 4.91). The infiltrate typically contains 10 to 50 eosinophils per high-powered field (hpf) (227). One often sees a concomitant increase in IgE-secreting plasma cells. Epithelial necrosis and degeneration develop, but ulcers are rare. Mucosal eosinophilic gastritis can be diagnosed in gastric biopsies, but due to its patchy distribution, multiple biopsies should be evaluated, including deeper biopsies that sample the submucosa, since each biopsy may show striking variations in the intensity of the eosinophilic, lymphocytic, and histiocytic infiltrates. The muscularis propria may show pronounced hyperplasia with the muscle fibers separated by dense eosinophilic aggregates. Charcot-Leyden crystals are present in areas of eosinophilic infiltrates. Some patients develop loose

TABLE 4.16   Gastric Eosinophilia

Allergic reactions	Peptic ulcers
Drug reactions	Crohn disease
Parasite reactions	Foreign bodies
Allergic granulomatosis	Adenomas
Chronic granulomatous disease	Carcinomas
	Langerhans cell histiocytosis
Varioliform gastritis	T-cell lymphoma
Inflammatory fibroid polyp	Eosinophilic gastroenteritis

granulomas and acute vasculitis affecting small arteries, features characteristic of allergic granulomatosis (227). Postinflammatory strictures complicate muscularis propria involvement. Table 4.16 lists the differential diagnosis of gastric eosinophilia.

Allergic Gastritis

The stomach is commonly involved in food-induced hypersensitivity reactions, especially in children (228). It is usually a manifestation of a more extensive allergic gastroenteritis. Patients present with anorexia, nausea, vomiting, diarrhea, weight loss, peripheral eosinophilia, elevated serum IgE, a personal or family allergic history, and epigastric pain. Direct mucosal challenge with a specific antigen in allergic individuals produces gastric mucosal edema, erythema, and petechial hemorrhages (228). Mast cell degranulation recruits neutrophils followed by mononuclear cells (229). A diffuse eosinophilic infiltrate involving the lamina propria and the superficial and pit epithelium causes epithelial damage with focal denudation and erosions, mucin depletion, and concurrent regeneration. The mucosa surrounding the erosions shows foveolar hyperplasia (Fig. 4.92). Excessive histamine release can lead to gastric gland hyperplasia.

LYMPHOCYTIC AND VARIOLIFORM GASTRITIS

A recently described form of gastritis consists of an intense T-cell infiltrate in the gastric pits and surface epithelium. The stomach may appear grossly normal, but in its most severe form *varioliform gastritis* is seen endoscopically (230). Lymphocytic gastritis affects 0.83% to 4.5% of individuals, mainly middle-aged and elderly men (230). The disorder complicates various diseases, including celiac disease, *HP* infections, Crohn disease, HIV infections, Menetrier disease, lymphocytic enterocolitis, inflammatory polyps, hypersensitivity reactions, autologous hematopoietic cell transplantation, ticlopidine use, lymphoma, and esophageal carcinoma (230–235). However, the change is most common in celiac disease and in patients with *HP* infections (235). In approximately 20% of cases, the etiology is unknown. Some patients develop ulcers or hypoproteinemia (236).

The stomach appears normal or it may present with thickened gastric folds, often with multiple discrete mucosal nodules, ulcers, erosions, or elevations measuring 3 to 10 mm in diameter. These are covered with mucus and have central umbilications surrounded by hyperemia, leading to the name varioliform gastritis (230,231). The mucosal elevations persist after the erosions heal, resembling sessile hyperplastic polyps. The disorder affects the entire stomach. Some patients develop hypertrophic lymphocytic gastritis.

Lymphocytic gastritis is characterized by an intraepithelial lymphocytosis with at least 25 lymphocytes/100 epithelial cells and mild foveolar hyperplasia (230,231). Usually the intraepithelial lymphocytosis is obvious so that counting the number of lymphocytes present is seldom required. The intraepithelial

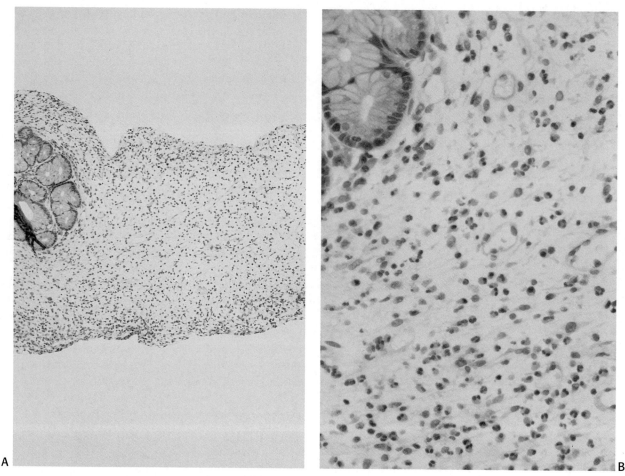

FIG. 4.92. Allergic gastritis in a child. **A:** Low-power view of the focal destruction that has occurred as the result of the inflammation. **B:** Higher magnification showing the intense mucosal eosinophilia.

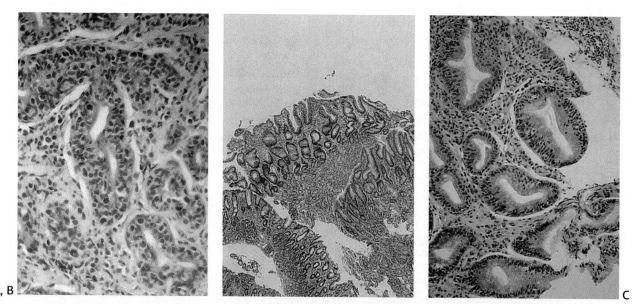

FIG. 4.93. Lymphocytic gastritis. **A:** Low-power magnification of this biopsy shows an intensely cellular mucosa. Increased numbers of cells are found both within the lamina propria and within the epithelium. **B:** Low-power magnification of another biopsy showing similar changes although less intensely inflamed. **C:** Higher magnification of B showing the details of the intraepithelial lymphocytic populations.

TABLE 4.17 Lymphocytic Gastritis Versus Mucosa-associated Lymphoid Tissue (MALT) Lymphomas

Feature	Lymphocytic Gastritis	MALT Lymphomas
Lymphocyte number	Significantly increased	Significantly increased
Lymphocyte distribution	Single cells or linear arrangement in the epithelium	Clusters of three or more lymphocytes in the epithelium
Lymphocyte type	Mature T cells	Malignant B cells
Perilymphocytic halo	Common	Uncommon
Significant epithelial destruction	No	Yes
Cytologic atypia of the lymphocytes	No	Yes
Diffuse lamina propria infiltration and destruction by atypical lymphocytes	No	Yes

lymphocytes are small and round, sometimes surrounded by a clear halo. They infiltrate the basal part of the surface epithelium and the gastric pits (Fig. 4.93). The process spares the deeper glands. The lymphocytosis may be patchy so that different biopsies may vary in the intensity of the intraepithelial lymphocytosis. The intraepithelial lymphocytosis may be greater in the antrum in celiac disease, whereas it is greater in the corpus in *HP* infections (235). In patients with celiac disease, the number of gastric intraepithelial lymphocytes correlates with the histologic severity of small intestinal disease and gluten restriction results in a marked reduction in intraepithelial lymphocytes. An intense lamina propria lymphoplasmacytic infiltrate may accompany the intraepithelial lymphocytosis. The pits acquire a corrugated and dilated appearance and their lumina may contain abundant mucus admixed with neutrophils forming pit abscesses. Neutrophils are usually not present unless there are ulcers or erosions. Foveolar hyperplasia may create giant gastric folds. The intraepithelial lymphocytes cause the epithelium to appear vacuolated and acquire a clear cell appearance, particularly in the subnuclear region. Other entities that mimic this pattern include endocrine cell hyperplasia, dystrophic goblet cells, and fixation artifact. Immunohistochemical stains distinguish among these possibilities. Additionally, one must distinguish the lesions present in lymphocytic gastritis (particularly if lymphoepithelial lesions are present) and MALT lymphomas (see Chapter 18) (Table 4.17). The lack of cytologic atypia in lymphocytic gastritis and the fact that the cells are T cells readily differentiates lymphocytic gastritis from the B-cell lesion of MALT lymphoma.

GRAFT VERSUS HOST DISEASE

Graft versus host disease (GVHD) follows allogeneic bone marrow transplant or transfusions, especially in immunocompromised patients (237). Upper gastrointestinal GVHD pre-

cedes lower gastrointestinal GVHD (238). Patients with isolated gastric GVHD present with nausea, vomiting, and upper abdominal pain without diarrhea. Early, the stomach appears endoscopically normal; 30% to 80% of patients have histologic evidence of GVHD after a normal endoscopy (237,238). In more severe disease, the stomach appears variably congested and atrophic. Histologically, the mucosa contains apoptotic cells (Fig. 4.94) predominantly in the mucous neck region; gland abscesses may also develop. The apoptotic bodies are present in both the antral and oxyntic mucosa and are small and less conspicuous than those seen in the colon (see Chapter 13). Sparse inflammation is present and granular eosinophilic material may be present in the glands. Even though apoptotic bodies may be present in small numbers, their presence is diagnostic of GVHD in the appropriate setting (237,239).

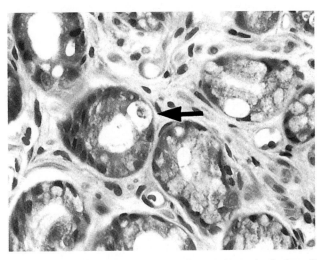

FIG. 4.94. Gastric graft versus host disease (GVHD). Single-cell necrosis (*arrow*) is the sine qua non of GVHD. (Case courtesy of Drs. Sale, Schulman, and Myerson, Fred Hutchinson Cancer Research Center, Seattle, WA.)

TABLE 4.18	Conditions Associated with Increased Apoptoses in the Gastric Mucosa

Graft versus host disease
Cytomegalovirus infections
Severe T-cell immunodeficiency
HIV infections
Conditioning chemotherapy
Cancer chemotherapy
Radiation
Crohn disease
Proton pump inhibitors
Nonsteroidal anti-inflammatory drugs

An interpretative problem complicating the diagnosis of GVHD results from the changes induced by the transplant cytoreduction regimen that can produce histologic features identical to those seen in GVHD. However, the changes due to the cytoreductive regimen are more diffuse than those typically seen in GVHD (237). Because of this confounding feature, it is prudent to avoid the diagnosis of GVHD early in the immediate posttransplant period. Another confounding feature is the use of PPI therapy, which can increase the number of apoptotic bodies seen in the antrum but not in the fundus (240). Table 4.18 lists entities associated with increased apoptotic bodies in gastric biopsies. GVHD may coexist with concurrent gastritis resulting from an *HP* or other infection and/or a chemical gastropathy.

COLLAGENOUS GASTRITIS

Collagenous gastritis is rare, affecting men and women, children and adults (241–244). The disease occurs as an isolated disorder or it may coexist with collagenous colitis (245) and/or collagenous duodenitis, lymphocytic colitis (241), Sjögren syndrome (243), and ulcerative colitis (244). Patients range in age from 11 to 77 with a mean age of 40 (242). It appears that there are two subsets of patients with collagenous gastritis: (a) collagenous gastritis occurring in children and young adults who present with severe anemia, a nodular endoscopic pattern, and disease limited to the gastric mucosa; and (b) collagenous gastritis associated with collagenous colitis in adults with chronic watery diarrhea (242). Some patients present with vomiting or upper GI bleeding, whereas others are asymptomatic or have nonspecific symptoms. Rare patients improve on gluten-free diets (241). Other patients have slowly progressive disease (246). We have seen a patient with severe collagenous gastritis, duodenitis, and colitis who required total parenteral nutrition to maintain his nutritional requirements. The cause of collagenous gastritis is unknown, but it may result from immune-mediated processes. In the stomach, signs of local immune activation include epithelial overexpression of HLA-DR and increased numbers of CD3+ intraepithelial lymphocytes and CD25+ cells in the lamina propria (247).

Endoscopic abnormalities include erythema, mucosal hemorrhage, and mucosal nodularity involving the corpus and body and sparing the antrum. The stomach shows histologic changes resembling those present in collagenous sprue (in the small bowel) or collagenous colitis. The diagnostic criteria consist of a subepithelial collagen layer >10 μm in thickness, lamina propria lymphoplasmacytosis, intraepithelial lymphocytes, and epithelial damage (246). The distribution and thickness of the subepithelial collagen bands varies within and between biopsy specimens and can be highlighted by trichrome stains. Its thickness ranges from 13 to 96 μm, averaging close to 40 μm. It is discontinuous and irregular and contains entrapped dilated capillaries and mononuclear cells. Intraepithelial CD3+ T lymphocytes range from 14 to >30 per 100 surface epithelial cells with a mean of 20. A patchy chronic active gastritis may be present.

The lamina propria contains variable numbers of neutrophils, eosinophils, and mast cells. Patchy epithelial damage with surface cell flattening, reactive epithelial changes, and focal sloughing are present. Rare abscesses form. The regenerative surface epithelial changes may be severe enough to warrant a diagnosis of indeterminate for dysplasia (246). The stomach may also show patchy glandular atrophy with shortening of the oxyntic glands. However, parietal and chief cells are still present. There may also be linear or micronodular endocrine cell hyperplasia in the corpus (246), a change that may result from treatment with proton pump inhibitors. In addition, intestinal metaplasia may develop in longstanding disease. Smooth muscle hyperplasia deep in the lamina propria increases over time with extension to the surface.

PEPTIC ULCER

A "peptic ulcer" refers to any deep mucosal break resulting from exposure to gastric acid or pepsin. These ulcers develop adjacent to sites containing oxyntic mucosa. Rarely, they arise in the acid-secreting mucosa itself. Peptic ulcers fall into several major etiologic groups: Those resulting from acid hypersecretion, as in Zollinger-Ellison syndrome; those due to NSAIDs; and those associated with *HP* infection. Previously, most peptic ulcers resulted from *HP* infections. Urease and other factors produced by the *HP* break the mucosal barrier, allowing ulcers to develop. Not all *HP* infections lead to ulcer development. *VacA-* and *CagA*-positive *HP* are more likely to produce peptic ulcers than *VacA-* and *CagA*-negative HP (159,248). Specifically, colonization with *vacA2m2/cag A*-positive *HP* strains correlates with peptic ulcer disease (PUD) risk (249). Smoking also increases ulcer incidence. In Western countries the importance of *HP* in gastric PUD has declined and has been replaced by NSAID use.

Multiple environmental and genetic factors associate with peptic ulcer risk. The incidence of gastric ulcers varies depending on geographic locale, age, and sex. Evidence supporting a genetic contribution to gastric and duodenal peptic ulcers include increased family aggregation (more for blood relatives than spouses), twin studies (250), blood group studies, and elevated pepsinogen levels among relatives (251). A marked decline in peptic ulcers has resulted from decreased smoking (252), a decreased incidence of *HP* infections, and the widespread use of aggressive acid suppressive therapies. Today in Western countries, peptic ulcers tend to affect the elderly using NSAIDs. The probability of developing a peptic ulcer is highest in middle-aged men (age 41 to 60) with chronic antral gastritis or chronic pangastritis (253). Peptic ulcers also develop as sporadic lesions, in patients with gastrinomas or systemic mastocytosis (due to increased histamine secretion), and in rare genetic syndromes including multiple endocrine neoplasia type 1 (MEN-1). A specific pepsinogen C gene polymorphism may predict gastric ulcer risk (254). Peptic injury may also complicate any disorder in which the mucosal barrier is compromised and mucosal ulcers form including infectious or drug injury.

Prepyloric and duodenal ulcers arise in the setting of increased acid secretion and antral gastritis, whereas gastric ulcers associate with decreased gastric acid secretion and diminished mucosal defenses (Fig. 4.95). There is a close association between the ulcer site and the severity of the gastritis. Antral ulcers most commonly develop along the lesser curve; with increasing severity of corpus gastritis, the ulcer location moves proximally. The further a gastric ulcer is from the pylorus, the more likely one is to find atrophic gastritis involving the body. This contrasts with duodenal and prepy-

loric ulcers, which associate with an antral-predominant gastritis without progressive body gastritis (255,256).

Episodic epigastric pain that is aggravated by meals or alcohol, often occurring at night, is the most prominent clinical feature of PUD. Bleeding develops in about 20% of patients and is massive in 5%. Bleeding is particularly likely in older individuals on NSAIDs (257). Endoscopic visualization of a bleeding vessel or other signs of recent hemorrhage predict further bleeding and increased mortality. Juxtapyloric ulcers cause obstruction due to coexisting edema and pyloric stenosis as the ulcer heals and fibrosis develops. Ulcer depth varies; it may perforate through the wall, extending into adjacent structures. The risk of perforation is increased in those who smoke and the risk correlates with the number of cigarettes smoked (258).

Gastric ulcers are usually solitary, although about 30% of patients have associated duodenal ulcers and 6% to 13% have multiple gastric ulcers (259). Gastric peptic ulcers arise anywhere in the stomach, but they typically develop on its lesser curvature, usually at the antral–corpus junction. The consequences of peptic ulceration include hemorrhage secondary to vascular erosion, perforation, ulcer penetration into contiguous structures, and pyloric outlet obstruction due to inflammation or scarring. Perforations typically appear as a round hole in the ulcer base. The serosal surface appears congested and fibrinous adhesions may be present. Occasionally, a large gastric ulcer high on the lesser curvature

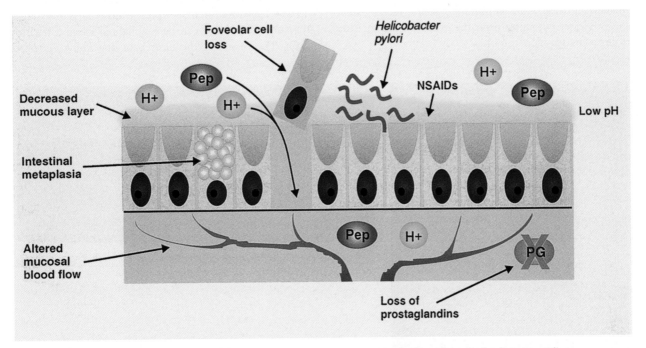

FIG. 4.95. Aggressive factors and etiology of peptic ulcer disease. A number of aggressive factors predispose the gastric mucosa to peptic damage. Two major causes involve infections with *Helicobacter pylori* or the use of nonsteroidal anti-inflammatory drugs (NSAIDs), both of which damage the mucosa by mechanisms discussed elsewhere. This leads to weakening of the intercellular junctions and foveolar damage that then allows pepsin and acid to diffuse into the underlying lamina propria. Prostaglandins (PGs) that play a major role in maintaining mucosal integrity are inhibited by the NSAIDs and therefore further predispose the mucosa to damage and failure to repair itself. Pep, pepsin.

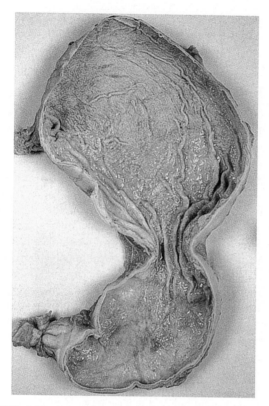

FIG. 4.96. Gross photograph of an hourglass stomach.

heals to produce a scarred, constricted, hourglass-shaped stomach (Fig. 4.96). Less commonly, gastric ulcers extend along the lesser curvature from the cardia to the incisura, forming a "trench ulcer" (260).

Acute peptic ulcers are often deep, measure >0.5 cm in diameter, penetrate the muscularis mucosae, and have little fibrous tissue at their base. Those that measure >3 cm in diameter are sometimes referred to as *giant gastric ulcers*. These are more likely to penetrate than smaller gastric ulcers (261). Additionally, the risk of microscopic malignancy is significantly greater in giant ulcers than in the smaller ones (261). Chronic ulcers evolve from the acute ulcers. However, the acute stage is rarely seen unless a major blood vessel becomes eroded early in the disease, resulting in significant hemorrhage. Chronic ulcers that undergo repeated ulceration exhibit both acute and chronic features.

Benign ulcers are typically round to oval, sharply punched-out lesions with perpendicular walls (Fig. 4.97). The surrounding congested, edematous mucosa overhangs the ulcer margin, sometimes forming a lip and giving the ulcer a flask-shaped appearance. This lip should not appear rolled or heaped up. The mucosa away from the ulcer also often appears atrophic with flattened mucosal folds (Fig. 4.98). Ulcer bases appear smooth, cream colored or pearly gray, and clean, and are surrounded by thick fibrous tissue (Fig. 4.99) unless hemorrhage has occurred. Scarring at the ulcer base causes puckering of the surrounding mucosal folds, causing them to radiate away from the ulcer in a spokelike fashion (Fig. 4.98).

Four zones characterize chronic ulcers: (a) polymorphonuclear leukocytes, (b) coagulation necrosis, (c) granulation tissue, and (d) fibrosis of the ulcer base (Figs. 4.100 and 4.101). The latter often disrupts the muscularis mucosae and the submucosa, and can be highlighted using a trichrome stain. The vessels at the ulcer base may show endarteritis

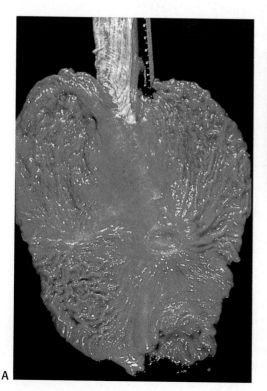

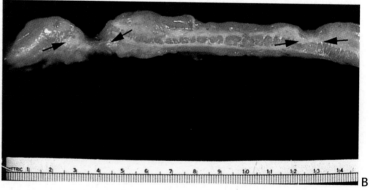

FIG. 4.97. Gastric ulcers. **A:** Two peptic ulcers in body of stomach. **B:** Cross section of the stomach shows penetration of the muscularis propria by the larger ulcer on the left (*arrows*). The smaller ulcer on the right (*arrows*) penetrates the submucosa.

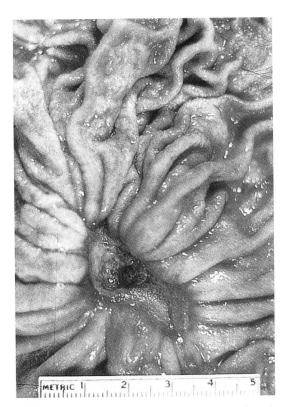

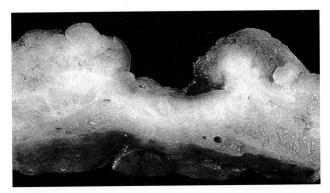

FIG. 4.99. Cross section of ulcer surrounded by white fibrous tissue.

FIG. 4.98. Prominent gastric folds radiate from this chronic benign ulcer.

obliterans; the extent of this change governs the magnitude of hemorrhage should the vessels become eroded (Fig. 4.102). The muscularis propria may be interrupted by the acute inflammation and tissue loss or by scar tissue. *Candida* may colonize the ulcer base. If the organism does not invade the underlying tissues, it has no clinical significance.

Acute peptic ulcers do not contain the four zones described above. A polymorphonuclear exudate replaces the epithelium and moderate amounts of granulation tissue fill the ulcer center. The remaining mucosa appears regenerative with immature cells and occasional mitotic figures. Scarring is absent. These are seldom examined histologically unless an acute bleed has resulted in death or surgical resection. Histologic examination of bleeding gastric ulcers usually

reveals a small eroded artery in the ulcer crater. The mean diameter measures 0.7 mm with a range of 0.8 to 3.4 mm. The larger the size of the eroded artery, the more likely that death will result (458). The vessels may show aneurysmal dilation, intense arteritis, and/or endarteritis obliterans.

Peptic ulcers begin to heal by epithelial migration from the ulcer margin over the vascular granulation tissue of the ulcer base with mucosal replacement by the inward migration of a single epithelial layer at the ulcer edge (Fig. 4.103). The proliferating mucosa grows downward and extends over the ulcer surface. This single cell layer can extend to cover the entire surface of smaller ulcers (<2 cm). Epithelial migration is stimulated by multiple factors, including spasmolytic polypeptide, EGF, and TGF-β and by inhibition of E-cadherin expression (262). Simple mucous glands and areas of pyloric metaplasia develop. As noted earlier, the pyloric metaplasia may not be a metaplastic process at all, but rather the development of a novel cell lineage from stem cells called ulcer associated cell lineage, the cells of which produce a number of products that promote mucosal healing and repair (207). The cells grow in proliferating cell buds until they reach the mucosal surface (207). A number of genes are up-regulated following ulcer development, leading to the production of an integrated cascade of gene products that promote vasculogenesis, mucosal restitution, and healing (263). Later, other growth factors produced by the stromal cells stimulate epithelial proliferation and differentiation.

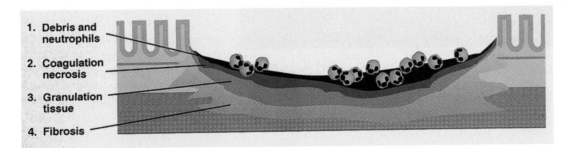

FIG. 4.100. Four zones characterize the histology of chronic gastric peptic ulcers. The first layer consists of debris and neutrophils. Underlying this is an area of coagulation necrosis followed by granulation tissue and then fibrosis.

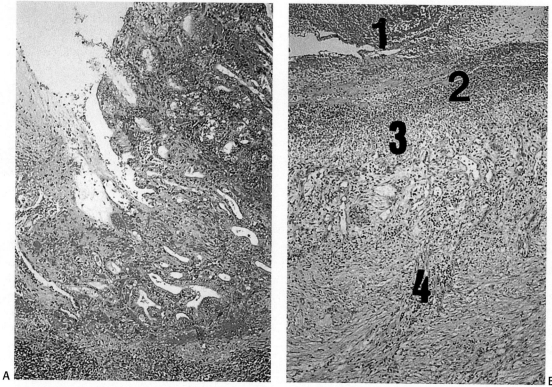

FIG. 4.101. Histologic section of gastric ulcer. **A:** Edge of the ulcer demonstrating gastritis and regenerative epithelium. **B:** Base of ulcer demonstrating the typical four zones seen in most peptic ulcers: (*1*) fibrinopuru-lent debris, (*2*) inflammatory layer, (*3*) granulation tissue, and (*4*) fibrosis.

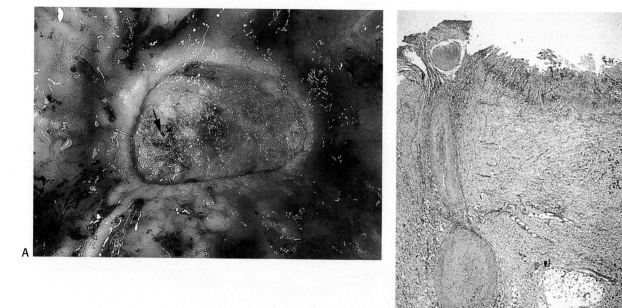

FIG. 4.102. Large artery penetrating an ulcer base. **A:** Large gastric ulcer eroding into gastric artery (*arrow*) causing massive gastrointestinal bleeding. **B:** Endarteritis obliterans is present, and there is fibrin clot at the surface.

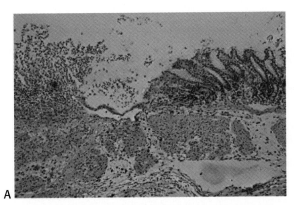

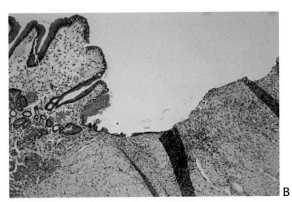

A   B

FIG. 4.103. Healing gastric ulcer. **A:** Ulcers heal by the migration and ingrowth of epithelium from the ulcer edges. In this photograph, one can see the single layer of epithelial cells extending from the mucosa on the right-hand portion of the picture overlying the muscle and extending toward the inflammatory debris. **B:** Further progression of the healing process demonstrates an almost completely intact lining at the base of the ulcer. The acute inflammation has disappeared but the surrounding mucosa appears edematous and congested.

The cell cycle is suppressed in the migrating cells until they meet cells from the opposite side of the ulcer, at which time there is a proliferative spurt coinciding with a downward penetration of new glands. Mucosal islands may become entrapped in areas of submucosal fibrous or granulation tissue, and may be mistaken for an invasive carcinoma. Away from the ulcer, the mucosa appears normal or exhibits chronic gastritis (Fig. 4.104). There may also be prominent collections of chronic inflammatory cells (a Crohn-like reaction) associated with neural hyperplasia (Fig. 4.105) in a pattern that could suggest a diagnosis of Crohn disease, if one were unaware of the presence of an old ulcer.

The serosa underlying a peptic ulcer often appears fibrotic, demonstrates fat necrosis, or shows mesothelial

hyperplasia. The fibrosis and fat necrosis thicken the gastric wall. Adhesions develop and one may see extensive areas of mesothelial hyperplasia trapped within the inflammatory process. These can mimic a carcinoma, but the lack of cytologic atypia and positive immunostains for calretinin

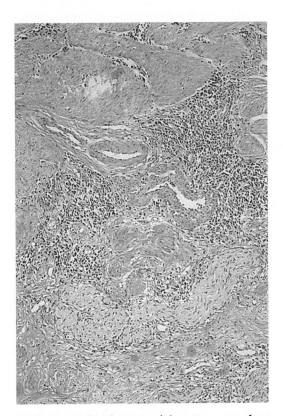

FIG. 4.105. The wall of the stomach in areas remote from peptic ulcers often demonstrate secondary changes, including collections of chronic inflammatory cells, fibrosis, and neuromuscular hyperplasia. The neuromuscular changes may lead to motility abnormalities.

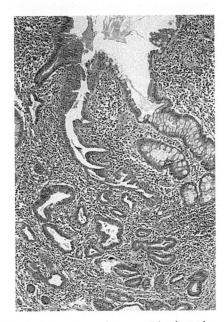

FIG. 4.104. Gastritis surrounding a gastric ulcer. The ulcer is not shown.

TABLE 4.19 Benign Versus Malignant Gastric Ulcers

Feature	Benign	Malignant
Age	Younger	Older
Length of history	Long, may be short	Short, may be long
Ulcerlike symptoms	Usually present	May be present
Location	Antrum or lesser curvature 100% benign	Cardiac and body 50% malignant
Radiologic appearance	Ulcer base outside gastric wall	Ulcer base inside gastric wall
Gastric pH	Tends to be low	Variable
Gross appearance	Punched out with overhanging edges	Bowl shaped with sloping edges
Rugal folds	Terminate in ulcer	Do not terminate in ulcer

provide the correct diagnosis. Regional lymph nodes become enlarged and reactive in appearance.

Histologic Distinction of Gastric Ulcers from Gastric Cancer

Ulcerated carcinomas tend to be shallow, irregular, bowl-shaped lesions with rolled or heaped-up sloping borders and a necrotic base that often flattens out and distorts the rugal folds in such a way that they do not converge toward the ulcer or, if they do, they terminate short of it. Table 4.19 compares the gross features of benign and malignant gastric ulcers.

One of the most difficult tasks facing the pathologist is to distinguish malignant cells from the regenerative atypia invariably present in areas of gastritis adjacent to ulcers. Marked desmoplasia at the base or sides of a chronic ulcer crater can distort regenerating glands suggesting invasion from a carcinoma. In these circumstances it is imperative that one recognize classic cytologic hallmarks of malignancy before one makes a diagnosis of cancer.

When one cannot unequivocally distinguish regenerative epithelium from a carcinoma in a biopsy specimen, a rebiopsy, once the inflammation subsides, may be warranted if a strong clinical suspicion for cancer exists. However, if the clinical features suggest that the lesion is benign and reactive, the patient can be treated medically for 4 to 6 weeks, then re-evaluated and additional biopsies taken at that time. A useful rule of thumb is that any chronic ulcer that has been histologically diagnosed as benign should be followed by the gastroenterologist until ulcer healing is complete.

The use of cytokeratin immunostains may help to determine whether or not individual cells have invaded into the lamina propria. However, one must be careful in interpreting these because isolated nonneoplastic cells can remain entrapped from necrotic glands in the granulation or fibrous tissue at the base of gastric ulcers. Alternatively, residual epithelial remnants from the associated gastritis may be present. Additionally, cytokeratin positivity is occasionally found in nonepithelial cells, especially near the peritoneal surface, due to the presence of subserosal mesothelial cells. These cytokeratin-positive spindled submesothelial cells do not communicate with the gastric mucosa and usually fail to show other epithelial features, such as epithelial membrane antigen (EMA) immunoreactivity. The mesothelial cells are also vimentin and calretinin immunoreactive.

The distinction between chronic ulcers and ulcerating cancers can be further facilitated by examination of the muscularis propria. Deep ulcers and their scars result in fibrous replacement of the muscle layer, whereas the muscularis propria deep to a cancer usually remains intact and nonfibrotic, and may even become accentuated.

HYPERTROPHIC HYPERPLASTIC GASTROPATHIES

The gastric mucosa contains two epithelial compartments: The superficial foveolar epithelium and gastric pits and a deeper glandular compartment that contains the specialized epithelium unique to each gastric region. If the mucosa measures >1.5 mm in thickness, it is considered to be hypertrophic or hyperplastic. Diffuse mucosal expansions result in giant rugal folds (hypertrophic gastropathies) producing dramatic gross (Fig. 4.106) abnormalities. In contrast, localized expansions produce discrete polypoid lesions. Hyperplasia may affect either or both mucosal compartments. When a single component becomes hyperplastic, the remaining compartment may appear normal, hyperplastic, or atrophic. Thus, the surface can appear hyperplastic with concomitant glandular hyperplasia, atrophy, or normal numbers of glands (Fig. 4.107). Similarly, the glands may appear hyperplastic beneath normal, hyperplastic, or atrophic pits (Table 4.20). Gastric mucosal expansions are classified by the compartments that are expanded and by whether the expansion appears diffuse or localized.

Four well-defined hypertrophic gastropathies exist: Classic Menetrier disease with protein loss and hypochlorhydria, hypertrophic hypersecretory protein-losing gastropathy, hypertrophic hypersecretory gastropathy, and hypersecretory

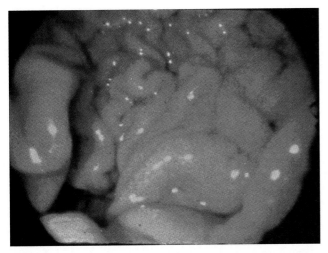

FIG. 4.106. Endoscopic view of hypertrophic gastric mucosa. The gastric folds appear increased in size and number.

hypergastrinemia with protein loss (Zollinger-Ellison syndrome). Distinct clinical features often define the underlying process, but individual patients may exhibit incomplete manifestations of a particular syndrome. Other patients have classical clinical or laboratory findings but discordant histologic features. Additionally, some patients with hypertrophic gastric folds are not easily classified.

The surgical pathologist plays a limited role in the diagnosis of gastric giant fold diseases because most patients present with a classic clinical syndrome as detected by laboratory (264), radiographic, and endoscopic examinations. Mucosal biopsies document the presence or absence of classic forms of one of the diseases and rule out the presence of tumors that may expand the gastric wall. However, gastric biopsies are inadequate for complete diagnosis because all giant fold disorders share an expanded mucosae and it is difficult to obtain a full-thickness mucosal biopsy unless giant forceps are used. Usually in Menetrier disease either a biopsy contains pure foveolae, suggesting focal foveolar hyperplasia or the top of a hyperplastic polyp, or the mucosa appears normal. In Zollinger-Ellison syndrome or hypertrophic/hypersecretory gastropathy, the biopsy may

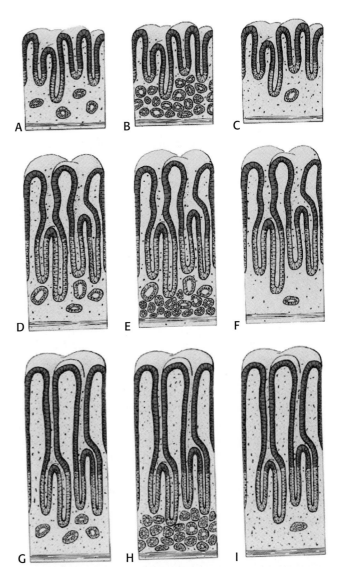

FIG. 4.107. Diagram illustrating the options for atrophy and hyperplasia in the stomach. **A:** Pit atrophy, normal gland. **B:** Pit atrophy, hyperplastic gland. **C:** Pit atrophy, gland atrophy. **D:** Normal pit, normal glands. **E:** Normal pit, gland hyperplasia. **F:** Normal pit, gland atrophy. **G:** Pit hyperplasia, normal gland. **H:** Pit hyperplasia, gland hyperplasia. **I:** Pit hyperplasia, gland atrophy. (Pits are *red*, glands are *yellow*.)

TABLE 4.20 **Morphologic Clinical Manifestation of Giant Gastric Folds**

Condition	Surface Mucous Cells	Body Glandular Component	Gastrin	Ulcers	Protein Loss
Normal variants	Normal	Normal	−	−	−
Zollinger-Ellison syndrome	Normal	Hyperplastic	+	+	−
Hypertrophic hypersecretory gastropathy	Hyperplastic	Hyperplastic	−	+	−
Menetrier disease	Hyperplastic	Atrophy	−	−	+
Hypertrophic hypersecretory protein-losing gastropathy	Hyperplastic	Hyperplastic	−	−	+

appear normal because the pits are likely to be normal and the expanded glandular component is not easily appreciated. The only hint of Zollinger-Ellison syndrome is the finding of hyperplastic parietal cells high in the mucosa even near the surface, a phenomenon not usually observed in other conditions.

Normal Variants of the Gastric Mucosa

Hypertrophic, but otherwise well-formed, rugae may occur in some individuals. When these are examined histologically, one finds that the gastric folds consist of prominent submucosal cores covered by a normal mucosa without evidence of hyperplasia or inflammation.

Menetrier Disease

Menetrier disease usually affects men in the 4th through 6th decades of life (265). Some cases are familial in nature (266). Exceptionally, the lesion coexists with colonic and gastric juvenile polyposis. Menetrier disease begins insidiously and gradually becomes increasingly symptomatic. Symptoms including epigastric pain, bloating, anorexia, vomiting, weight loss, anemia, and peripheral edema wax and wane. Diffusely enlarged gastric folds and marked mucus hypersecretion are present. Severe hypoproteinemia; hypoalbuminemia; hypochlorhydria, even to the point of achlorhydria; and a tendency to develop peripheral edema may all be present. Not all manifestations are present at the same time. Eosinophilia affects up to 61% of adults. In adults, Menetrier disease may resemble lymphocytic gastritis (265), especially since about one third of patients with lymphocytic gastritis present with weight loss, anorexia, protein loss, and peripheral edema. Extraintestinal phenomena include severe or recurrent pulmonary infections and pulmonary edema. Some patients have premature thrombotic cardiovascular disease, predisposing them to myocardial infarcts, pulmonary emboli, small bowel infarcts, and venous throm-

boses. Other associations include coexisting esophageal or gastric cancer.

Menetrier disease may affect children and young infants, although it is rare in infants (267). The pediatric form associates with CMV infection, allergies, and autoimmune reactions (268). Proteins, such as cow's milk, sometimes precipitate the disease. Children with CMV infections develop atypical lymphocytosis and transient hepatosplenomegaly, and have CMV demonstrable in the blood, urine, and gastric tissues (269). In young children, the disease is usually self-limited with spontaneous reversal of the protein loss, contrasting with the adult form of the disease, which is generally so prolonged and severe that it may require gastrectomy. Marked periorbital or facial edema affects 88% of children with the disease. Vomiting (78% of cases), abdominal pain (45% of cases), and anorexia are other common symptoms. Frank upper GI bleeding develops in only 12% of children, contrasting with an incidence of 20% to 40% in adults. Eosinophilia may also develop, presumably due to mucosal allergen penetration following viral damage.

A bulky, thickened gastric wall characterized by marked enlargement of the mucosal folds is present in all cases. The enlarged folds vary from 1 to 3 cm in height and resemble cerebral convolutions with an occasional nodular or polypoid appearance (Fig. 4.108). The disease mostly affects the body and greater curvature, generally sparing the antrum, except in children where the reverse is true. The enlarged gastric folds can occur in both a localized and a diffuse form.

The most striking histologic feature of Menetrier disease is foveolar hyperplasia and glandular atrophy. Foveolar cells line elongated, tortuous, and dilated hyperplastic gastric pits. Excessive mucus spills onto the luminal surface. Mucus-secreting cells replace the glands and the elongated pits extend to the base of the mucosa, where they become cystic (Fig. 4.109). They may also extend into the superficial submucosa creating *gastritis cystica profunda*. The cysts further increase the mucosal thickness. The expanded mucosa covers lengthened submucosal cores. There is also superficial edema

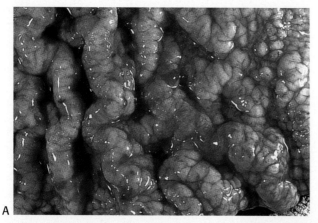
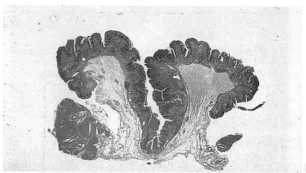

FIG. 4.108. Menetrier disease. **A:** Prominent cerebriform folds characterize the gastric mucosa of this patient. **B:** Low-power magnification of a section of the gastric wall corresponding to two of the cerebriform folds. The mucosa is markedly expanded and covers edematous exaggerated submucosal cores.

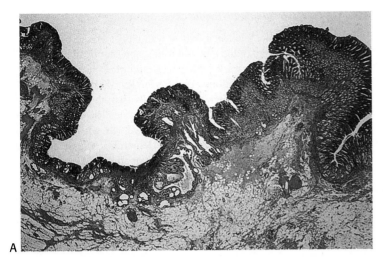

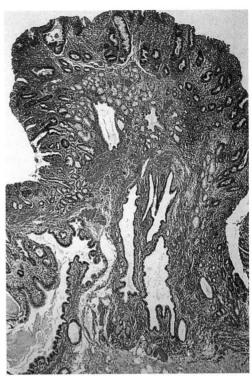

FIG. 4.109. Resection from a patient who clinically had Menetrier disease. **A:** Elongated foveolae characterize the tissue. Cysts are present in the glandular portions of the stomach. **B:** The cysts extend into the submucosa.

and variable lamina propria inflammation. The inflammatory infiltrate consists of neutrophils, eosinophils, lymphocytes, and occasional plasma cells. The muscularis mucosae becomes hypertrophic and hyperplastic, sending smooth muscle extensions into the lamina propria. Protein loss correlates with the pit hyperplasia, edema, and superficial inflammation. As the disease runs its course, mucosal atrophy develops with loss of the superficial inflammation and edema. Progressive hypochlorhydria results from gradual replacement of the glandular compartment by expanding pit compartments, thereby compromising the parietal cell mass and resulting in decreased acid secretion. Intestinal metaplasia occurs uncommonly and dysplasia is rare. Gastric adenocarcinoma complicates Menetrier disease, but the frequency of this event is hard to estimate.

Mucosal biopsies confirm the foveolar hyperplasia and exclude other causes of enlarged rugae. Biopsies from the tips of the expanded folds show pit hyperplasia and pit distortion, as well as superficial inflammation. However, the presence of the hyperplastic mucosal cells is not sufficient to establish the diagnosis of Menetrier disease since foveolar cell hyperplasia occurs in other settings (Table 4.21). For this reason, it is important to correlate the histologic and clinical findings.

TGF-α overexpression in Menetrier disease leads to upregulation of the antral transcription factor Pdx-1 in the gastric fundus. Pdx-1 is expressed in the cells of the affected glands and scattered gastrin cells appear, suggesting a repro-gramming of the oxyntic mucosa to a more antral pattern (220). A disorder resembling Menetrier disease is seen in TGF-α transgenic mice and TGF-α overexpression induces Pdx-1 expression (270). These findings are of interest because of the report of a patient treated by EGFR blockade who went into disease remission with re-emergence of parietal cells (271).

Zollinger-Ellison Syndrome

Gastric mucosal hypertrophy and acid hypersecretion secondary to hypergastrinemia characterize Zollinger-Ellison syndrome (ZES), the prototypic hypersecretory gastropathy. The hypergastrinemia often results from a gastrin-secreting tumor (gastrinoma) located either in the pancreas or in the bowel wall (272). Five percent of patients with ZES have gastric G-cell hyperplasia rather than a true hyperplasia (272). For a further description of gastrinomas

TABLE 4.21	Causes of Foveolar Hyperplasia
Chemical gastropathy	
Hyperplastic polyps	
Menetrier disease	
Juvenile polyposis	
Cronkite-Canada syndrome	
Regeneration adjacent to ulcers and stomas	

and G-cell hyperplasia, see Chapter 17. The increased gastrin levels stimulate acid secretion as well as the growth of parietal cells, peptic cells, ECL cells, and foveolar epithelium.

ZES affects 0.1% of all patients with duodenal ulcer disease and has an incidence of between 0.2 and 0.4 case per million population per year. The disease affects patients ranging in age from 7 to 90 (272), with most patients being diagnosed between the 3rd and 5th decades of life. There is no major gender predominance. The most common presenting symptom is abdominal pain. Diarrhea develops in 33% to 75% of patients. Some patients lack all features of ZES. Peptic ulcers may be absent, and diarrhea with steatorrhea may be the only clinical manifestation. The acid hypersecretion may be mild and indistinguishable from that seen in ordinary duodenal ulcer.

ZES causes profound alterations in the oxyntic mucosa, including mucosal hyperplasia with formation of prominent rugal folds, and an increased number and total mass of parietal and proliferation of ECL cells, potentially leading to the development of carcinoid tumors, especially in patients with MEN-1 (see Chapter 17). Giant rugal folds cover the body and fundus and spare the antrum. The surfaces of the folds appear uniformly exaggerated, coarsely granular, or finely cobblestoned. Ulcers, particularly multiple ulcers, may be present. Histologic examination of the hypertrophic gastric folds reveals substantial glandular lengthening due to the parietal cell hyperplasia. The increased parietal cell mass comprises a progressively larger share of the glands, filling their entire length down to their bases. Parietal cells also extend into the neck regions or higher, coming closer to the surface than usual. In some cases, parietal cells completely populate the mucosal glands. Large numbers of parietal cells can also be present in the antrum, an area that usually lacks them. The foveolae appear normal in length or shortened (Fig. 4.110).

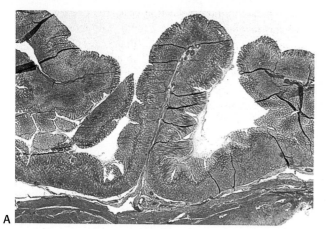

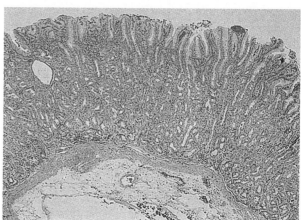

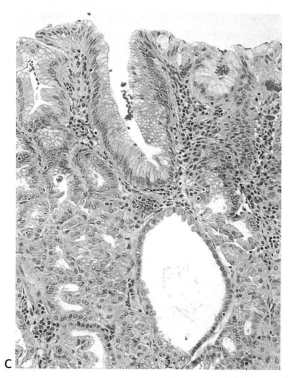

FIG. 4.110. Zollinger-Ellison syndrome. **A:** A thick nodular mucosa with expanded glands covers the enlarged folds. **B:** The mucosa contains a hyperplastic glandular compartment and shortened pits. **C:** The parietal cells are hypertrophic, hyperplastic, and located higher than normal in the gastric necks.

Fundic gland polyps also may be present, probably not as the result of the disease itself but due to long-term administration of proton pump inhibitors. Intramucosal cysts of the oxyntic mucosa are found in over 70% of patients with ZES, even in the absence of endoscopically recognizable polyps or nodules (272). These mucosal cysts range in size from 0.3 to 1.1 mm in diameter. The severity of the cystic change correlates with the serum gastrin levels (272a), and the cysts are more common than fundic gland polyps, which likely arise from them. They are typically lined by parietal cells, tall foveolar cells, and/or cuboidal or flattened cells of unrecognizable lineage. The upper parts of the cysts lie near the foveolar epithelium of the gastric pits, but occasionally they have an inverted deep localization.

Hypertrophic, Hypersecretory Gastropathy

Hypertrophic, hypersecretory gastropathy combines corpus glandular hyperplasia, normal surface components, and peptic ulcer disease without hypergastrinemia. The stomach appears as diffusely nodular mucosa with prominent rugal folds, resembling ZES. However, the extensive parietal cell hypertrophy and hyperplasia that characterize ZES is absent.

Hypertrophic, Hypersecretory Gastropathy with Protein Loss

Hypertrophic, hypersecretory gastropathy with protein loss, the rarest giant fold disease, exhibits giant gastric folds, hypersecretion, protein loss, and a clinical presentation that resembles a cross between Menetrier disease and ZES. Most patients complain of epigastric pain, asthenia, anorexia, weight loss, edema, and vomiting. By definition, hypoalbuminemia and enteric protein loss exist in most cases. Occasionally, a concomitant gastric ulcer is present. Histologically, foveolar hyperplasia is present with deep cysts, mild glandular atrophy, and increased numbers of lymphocytes and plasma cells. It is not clear if this disorder differs from Menetrier disease or if it represents a stage in the evolution of the disease in which protein loss and edema become excessive and clinically important before the glandular compartment is compromised by loss of parietal cells and hypochlorhydria occurs.

Helicobacter pylori–Associated Hypertrophic Gastropathy

Hypertrophic gastropathies with features of Menetrier disease may complicate *HP* infections, leading to the speculation that the hypertrophic gastropathy is a special form of *HP* gastritis. Patients exhibit hypertrophic gastric folds and protein-losing enteropathy (273). Antibiotic treatment restores the normal architecture (274). Biopsies demonstrate the presence of a chronic or chronic active gastritis with or without ulceration. The pit-to-gland ratio is normal and the

TABLE 4.22	Differential Diagnosis of Enlarged Gastric Folds
Menetrier disease	Systemic mastocytosis
Zollinger-Ellison syndrome	Prostaglandin therapy
Varioliform gastritis	Infections (tuberculosis, syphilis)
Carcinoma (linitis plastica)	
Lymphoma	Sarcoid
Granulomatous disease	Crohn disease
Allergic gastritis	Eosinophilic gastritis

increased mucosal thickness results from the edema and inflammation. The differential diagnosis of enlarged gastric folds is listed in Table 4.22.

Localized Hypertrophic Disorders

A number of entities cause localized mucosal hyperplasia. Localized polypoid reparative mucosal proliferations occur sporadically, at sites of healed gastric ulcers, or near surgically created stomas.

Focal foveolar hyperplasia is a nonneoplastic regenerative process that compensates for increased epithelial cell turnover and surface cellular exfoliation in situations of mucosal injury, most commonly *HP infections* or chemical gastropathy. The process creates antral lesions measuring up to 5 mm in diameter (Fig. 4.111) that are frequently multiple (275). Foveolar cells line elongated, but architecturally normal, gastric pits. The cells contain hyperchromatic nuclei and there is an expanded proliferative zone with increased mitotic activity. Foveolar cellular immaturity is present as evidenced by mucin depletion, a cuboidal shape, and a high nuclear:cytoplasmic ratio. There may be up to more than four cross sections of the same pit in a well-oriented gastric biopsy specimen. The major entity in the differential diagnosis is a hyperplastic polyp (see below).

GASTRIC POLYPS

Gastric polyps are usually incidental findings. They may be neoplastic or nonneoplastic, with most (80% to 90%) being nonneoplastic. They may be multiple or solitary, and some complicate polyposis syndromes (see Chapter 12). The two main types of nonneoplastic polyps are hyperplastic polyps and fundic gland polyps. Neoplastic polyps are described in Chapter 5.

Fundic Gland Polyp

In our experience, FGPs are the most common benign polyps encountered in a surgical pathology practice. They occur sporadically, develop in the setting of familial adenomatous polyposis (FAP), or complicate the use of proton pump inhibitors (see the dug injury section). Sporadic and

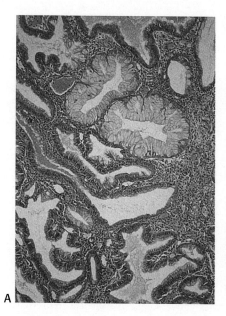
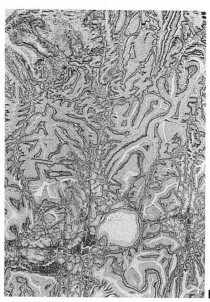

FIG. 4.111. Localized foveolar hyperplasia. **A:** A microscopic area of foveolar hyperplasia in a patient with gastritis. **B** comes from a patient with a wider area of foveolar hyperplasia that has branching, very irregularly shaped glands.

FAP-associated polyps result from separate and distinct *wnt* signaling pathway alterations. Sporadic polyps contain activating *β-catenin* mutations, whereas FAP-associated polyps have biallelic *APC* mutations (276,277).

FGPs are sessile polyps arising in the oxyntic mucosa that can be single or multiple. FGPs developing in the setting of FAP may result in a carpet of several hundred polyps usually measuring <5 mm in diameter with a sessile base and a smooth-domed surface. Some of these polyps may be adenomas and others are FGPs. Unlike adenomas, FGPs are the same color as the surrounding mucosa (278). FGPs can develop and disappear within weeks. Torsion or mechanical traction resulting in autoamputation may cause some polyps to disappear (278).

FGPs are localized hyperplastic expansions of the deep glandular compartment of the oxyntic mucosa (Fig. 4.112). The overlying pits appear shortened or absent. They contain cystically dilated, irregularly deformed oxyntic glands with or without glandular proliferations, increased smooth muscle in the lamina propria, and a lack of hyperplastic foveolar cells. The glands are lined by normal oxyntic cells, including a mixture of parietal, chief, and mucous neck cells. The glands appear almost to be tacked onto the surface of a normal or slightly atrophic mucosa. FGPs probably develop from the progressive dilation and infolding of glandular buds to produce irregular tortuous glands and microcysts. These lesions are generally benign. However, in the setting of FAP, they may contain areas of dysplasia.

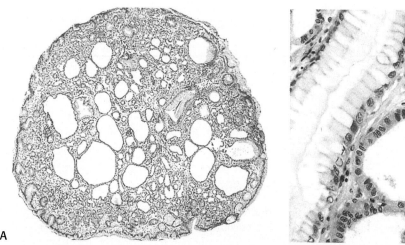
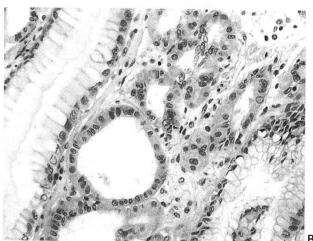

FIG. 4.112. Fundic gland polyp. **A:** The fundic glands are dilated and form numerous small microcysts. **B:** Higher power view of microcysts lined by both parietal and chief cells.

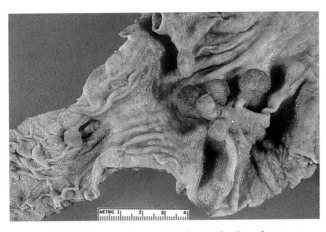

FIG. 4.113. Multiple gastric hyperplastic polyps.

Hyperplastic Polyps

Hyperplastic polyps develop in response to gastric injury such as from *HP* infections or autoimmune gastritis or around gastric remnants, ulcers, or surgically created stomas. They may also develop in the proximal stomach in patients with chronic gastroesophageal reflux. Most hyperplastic polyps develop in the gastric body (Fig. 4.113) and antrum. Hyperplastic polyps are typically small, smooth, sessile lesions, measuring <2.0 cm in diameter. Rare polyps are large (up to 13 cm) and simulate carcinoma (279). Larger polyps may appear lobulated and/or pedunculated, often with superficial erosions. These may twist on their stalks, leading to superficial ulceration, hemorrhage, pyloric prolapse, or intermittent obstruction.

Most hyperplastic polyps arise on a background of chronic gastritis. Intestinal metaplasia (as part of the surrounding atrophic gastritis) may be present. It is believed that they represent an exuberant regenerative response of gastric foveolar cells. The glands do not normally participate in the formation of the polyps. Two major features categorize hyperplastic polyps. The first is marked elongation, infolding, and branching of the gastric pits leading to a corkscrew or serrated appearance. Tall mucin-secreting foveolar cells line exaggerated, elongated, and distorted pits that extend from the surface deep into the stroma. Hypertrophic foveolar cells resembling goblet cells can be present. The pits also dilate to form variably sized and shaped cysts (Fig. 4.114), which can be quite prominent. Glandular epithelium may be found in the deeper parts of the polyps. The glands are often antral in type, even when the polyps arise in the body or fundus. Occasionally one sees oxyntic glandular mucosa.

The second major change is an excess of an edematous stroma that is infiltrated by plasma cells, lymphocytes, eosinophils, mast cells, macrophages, and variable numbers of neutrophils (Fig. 4.115). Smooth muscle fibers arborize in the lamina propria. These lesions are highly vascularized. Vascular proliferations resembling granulation tissue develop superficially near areas of erosion. The glands may acquire an apparent back-to-back configuration near areas of ulceration, but epithelial atypia is either absent or minimal and often regenerative in nature, especially in areas of surface erosion (Fig. 4.115). Neutrophils are prominent in ulcerated areas. Reparative changes can superficially resemble low-grade dysplasias or adenomas.

The polyps may contain areas of epithelial dysplasia, which may be high grade or low grade (Fig. 4.116). The prevalence of dysplasia ranges from 1% to 20% and is most frequently found in larger polyps (280). Dysplastic changes are generally more extensive than the atypias seen in focally eroded polyps. These areas of dysplasia may give rise to invasive carcinomas. The polyps may contain clonal *ras* mutations, in the neoplastic as well as the nonneoplastic regions (281). The overall malignant potential is probably <2%. If dysplasia is found in a hyperplastic polyp at the time of biopsy, it is important to determine whether the dysplasia is confined to the hyperplastic polyp or is part of a more diffuse neoplastic process. If the lesion is confined to the polyp and the polyp has been removed by a polypectomy, then the lesion is likely cured.

The differential diagnosis of hyperplastic polyps includes Menetrier disease, juvenile polyposis, and Cronkite-Canada

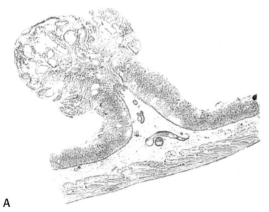

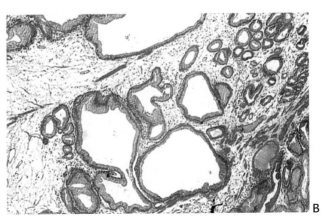

A   B

FIG. 4.114. Hyperplastic polyp. **A:** Note that the multiple cysts are present in an edematous stroma. **B:** Higher power magnification illustrates cystic glands lined by gastric mucous cells.

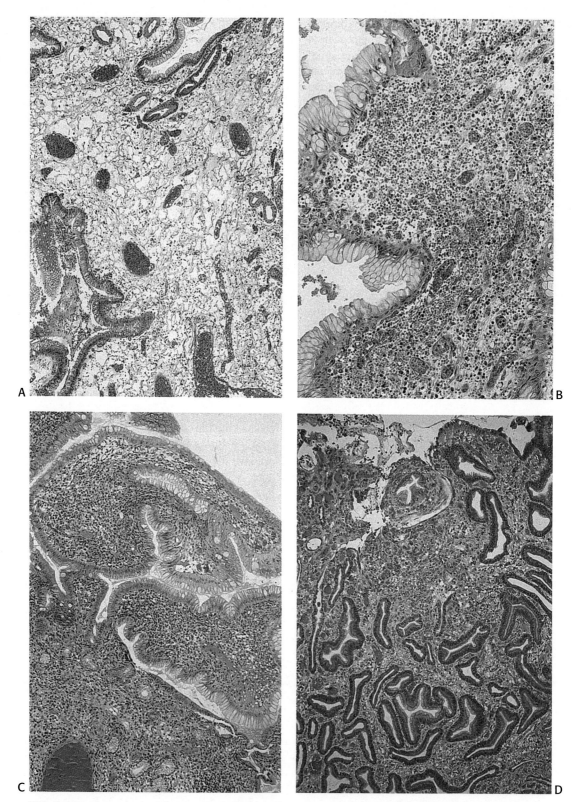

FIG. 4.115. Hyperplastic polyp. A: Hyperplastic polyps often contain an edematous stroma widely separating the hyperplastic and irregular glands that are frequently lined by foveolar epithelium. The vessels appear congested. **B:** In some instances, hyperplasia of the foveolar epithelium causes papillary infoldings. Additionally, severely congested lesions may associate with extravasated red cells in the lamina propria. **C:** Other lesions have a more cellular lamina propria due to the absence of the edema and an infiltrate of inflammatory cells. **D:** Hyperplastic polyps become eroded and may contain prominent areas of granulation tissue and acute inflammation.

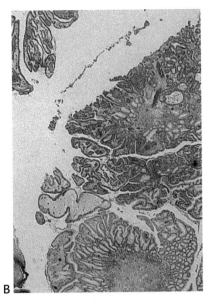
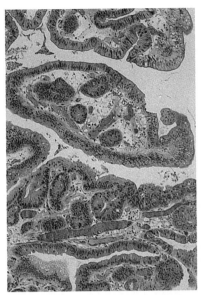
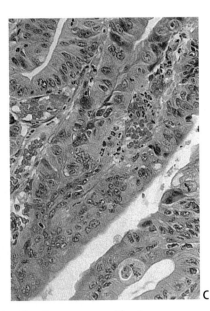

A, B   C

FIG. 4.116. Hyperplastic polyp containing dysplasia. **A:** Low magnification showing the presence of benign polypoid fragments (*lower*). Other parts of the polyp exhibit a more complex architectural pattern. **B:** Higher magnification of one of the more cellular areas demonstrates the presence of what appears to be adenomatous epithelium. **C:** In other areas, frank cytologic malignancy is evident and diagnosable as high-grade dysplasia.

syndrome. Menetrier disease is usually a more extensive process and has characteristic clinical features. The distinction from juvenile polyposis usually relies on the presence of colonic polyps and the clinical features. The distinction from Cronkite-Canada syndrome may be very difficult, although it is a very rare disorder and does have characteristic ectodermal features (see Chapter 12).

Isolated Hamartomatous Polyps

Isolated hamartomatous polyps consist of a prominent submucosal mass of haphazardly arranged oxyntic glands in a framework of smooth muscle tissue and occasional focal accumulations of mature lymphoid tissue. The entire lesion is supported by normal lamina propria. The glands may appear normal or be cystically dilated. One also sees mucous cells resembling foveolar epithelium as well as rare antral or cardiac-type glands containing endocrine cells indigenous to the mucosal site. The lesions differ from those seen in Peutz-Jeghers syndrome, which are usually not submucosal lesions but more mucosally based with possible submucosal extensions (see Chapter 12). Additionally, the arborizing muscle bundles seen in Peutz-Jeghers polyps are typically absent in isolated gastric hamartomas.

Inflammatory Fibroid Polyps

Inflammatory fibroid polyps (IFPs) affect all areas of the GI tract (282). Most lesions develop in adults, although some occur in children (282). The average patient is 63 years old. IFPs may remain asymptomatic or cause abdominal pain

due to gastric outlet obstruction (283). The lesions are reactive in nature. Associated lesions include *HP* gastritis (284), gastric ulcer, adenoma (285), or carcinoma (286). Grossly, IFPs present as sessile, firm, gray-tan polypoid or semipedunculated lesions that can be solitary or multiple. Most lesions arise in the antrum, ranging in size from <1 to 12 cm. IFPs originate in the submucosa, are usually covered by normal mucosa (Fig. 4.117), and grossly mimic leiomyomas or GI stromal tumors. The mucosa overlying the polyp is eroded in approximately a quarter of the cases. The lesions extend into the muscularis propria and may reach the serosa.

Histologically, IFPs consist of loosely structured stromal tissue. The predominant cell type consists of spindled fibroblastlike cells intermingled with inflammatory cells and proliferating vessels, arranged in an edematous stroma. Whorls of fibroblasts or myofibroblasts surround thin-walled vessels in a concentric or onion skin–like fashion. Vascularity and cellularity vary (Fig. 4.118) and may be striking. Proliferating cells appear uniform and contain abundant cytoplasm and pale spindle-shaped nuclei. Varying numbers of eosinophils and lymphocytes infiltrate the tissues. The numerous vessels vary in their appearance and some appear thickened with hyalinized walls. Multinucleated giant cells can be present. IFPs gradually merge into the surrounding tissues.

The lesions evolve through several stages. The nodular stage (average size 0.4 cm) contains nodules of immature fibroblasts in a loose myxoid stroma. The fibrovascular stage (average size 1.5 cm) demonstrates concentric aggregations of mature fibroblasts with endothelial proliferation and eosinophilic infiltrates. In larger polyps (average

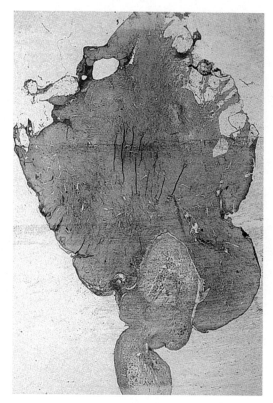

FIG. 4.117. Inflammatory fibroid polyp. This pedunculated lesion consists almost exclusively of mesenchymal tissues; no glands are identified. The cellularity varies from area to area, depending on the degree of edema and inflammatory infiltrate.

size 4.8 cm), the histologic pattern evolves into the sclerotic or edematous stage by either collagenization or vascular compromise.

The differential diagnosis of this lesion includes eosinophilic gastroenteritis, which typically affects younger patients and is characterized by diffuse eosinophilic infiltrate

that may involve long bowel segments as opposed to being relatively restricted lesions. Additionally, there is peripheral eosinophilia, and the lesions of eosinophilic gastroenteritis do not show the marked fibroblastic or vascular proliferation seen in IFPs. Other entities in the differential diagnosis include GI stromal tumors (GISTS) and other mesenchymal lesions. The spindle cells in IFPs are diffusely immunoreactive for vimentin and CD34. They may be focally positive for histiocytic makers. They may show focal immunoreactivity for α smooth muscle actin. Cytokeratin, desmin, S100, factor VIII, and Ki67 are negative in the spindle cells.

GASTRITIS CYSTICA PROFUNDA

This rare condition primarily affects elderly men and is often encountered in a previously operated on stomach. Cysts develop in the submucosa or muscularis mucosae of the gastric body and antrum (Fig. 4.119). They arise from displaced mucin-producing gastric glands. Sometimes chief and parietal cells lie scattered among the mucin-secreting epithelium. Foveolar cells may also be present. The abnormality results from previous ulceration or gastric surgery that allows the mucosa to gain access to the submucosa (287). A normal-appearing lamina propria usually surrounds the displaced glands providing a clue to the diagnosis. Coexisting hemosiderin deposits and fibrosis support episodes of previous injury. *Heterotopic pyloric glands with an inverted downgrowth pattern*, a lesion consisting of foveolar epithelium and tubular glands with abundant gastrin immunoreactive cells (60), represent a variant of this process.

VASCULAR ABNORMALITIES

Gastric vascular lesions include both neoplastic and nonneoplastic entities (Table 4.23). All typically present with upper

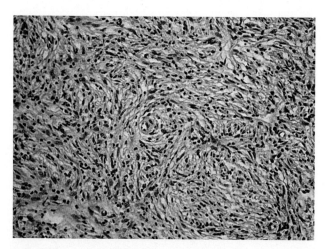

FIG. 4.118. Inflammatory fibroid polyp. Proliferation of loose fibrovascular tissue and chronic inflammatory cells. Eosinophils are admixed with the chronic inflammatory cells.

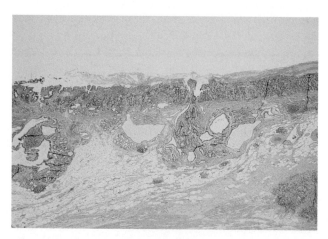

FIG. 4.119. Gastritis cystica profunda in a patient with gastric cancer. Lobules of gastric mucosa lie in the upper submucosa. Part of the surface appears dysplastic.

TABLE 4.23	Gastric Vascular Lesions
Nonneoplastic	Neoplastic
Varices	Kaposi sarcoma
Portal hypertensive gastropathy	Angiomas
Gastric antral vascular ectasia	Angiosarcomas
Angiodysplasia	Glomus tumor
Persistent caliber artery	Hemangiopericytoma
Telangiectasias	

GI bleeding. Only the nonneoplastic conditions are discussed here. Vascular neoplasms are discussed in Chapter 19.

Gastric Varices

Gastric varices are less common than esophageal varices and affect approximately 20% of patients with portal hypertension (288), usually accompanying esophageal varices. Gastric varices typically surround the cardioesophageal junction and they commonly bleed. Their histologic features resemble esophageal varices, which are discussed in detail in Chapter 2.

Portal Hypertensive Gastropathy (Congestive Gastropathy)

Portal hypertensive gastropathy (PHG) is a vasculopathy involving the gastric microvasculature in both adults and

children with portal hypertension (289). Mild PHG is highly prevalent in cirrhotics, while severe changes are only seen in 10% to 25% of these patients (289). The disorder presents with bleeding in severe cases. A hallmark of the condition is mucosal and submucosal capillary and venous ectasia that in severe PHG imparts a typical mosaic appearance. The mucosa appears "beefy" red with multiple petechial hemorrhages, red spots, ulcers, and erosions. Patients exhibit increased mucosal blood flow. Vascular congestion, rather than erosions, damages the mucosa.

Histologically, mucosal capillary (Figs. 4.120 and 4.121) and venous ectasia and submucosal venous dilation are present. The submucosal vessels may appear thickened and abnormal. These changes occur in the absence of erosions or inflammation. Propranolol and various jugular intrahepatic portosystemic shunts are used to treat PHG (289). The differential diagnosis includes gastric vascular ectasia, another condition that is common in cirrhotic patients.

Gastric Antral Vascular Ectasia (Watermelon Stomach)

Gastric antral vascular ectasia (GAVE) differs from PHG in its clinical features, gross appearance, and histologic features. However, both conditions are common to patients with cirrhosis. GAVE presents clinically with bleeding and typically affects elderly females with an average age of 66.5 years (290). GAVE associates with various conditions, including

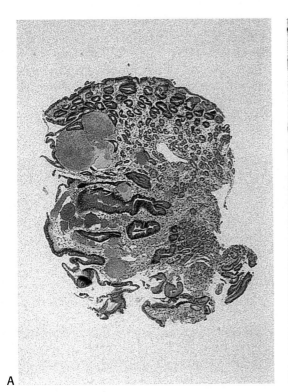
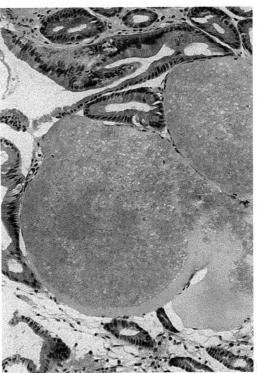

FIG. 4.120. Portal gastropathy. **A:** Low-power magnification demonstrating the presence of markedly dilated and congested mucosal capillaries. **B:** Higher magnification of the lesion shown in A demonstrating the presence of markedly dilated spaces lined by endothelial cells and filled with unclotted blood.

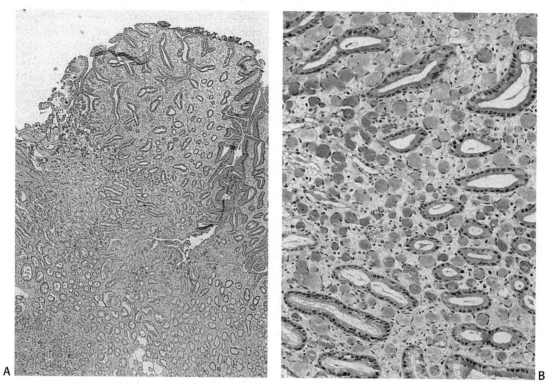

FIG. 4.121. Portal gastropathy. **A:** In some patients, portal gastropathy takes the form of multiple dilated mucosal capillaries that diffusely affect the gastric mucosa. **B:** Higher magnification.

cirrhosis, chronic heart disease, bulimia, bone marrow transplantation, and autoimmune connective tissue disorders. In contrast to the hemodynamic disturbances seen in PHG, motility disturbances may play a role in the pathogenesis of GAVE. It is conceivable that antral mucosal prolapse into the duodenum causes some of the changes that are present.

GAVE is characterized by aggregates of mucosal red spots in the distal stomach. The ectatic red spots may be more diffuse and occasionally involve the proximal stomach. If the red spots are present on a background mosaic pattern, the disorder is more likely to be PHG than GAVE, in which the background mucosa appears normal without the mosaic appearance. Its most distinctive appearance consists of nearly parallel, intensely red, longitudinal stripes situated at the crests of hyperplastic mucosal folds traversing the gastric antrum creating the pattern of a "watermelon stomach" (291). These stripes correspond to markedly dilated, tortuous mucosal capillaries (Figs. 4.122 and 4.123). The ectatic mucosal capillaries often contain fibrin thrombi, and they are surrounded by fibrohyalinosis with fibromuscular

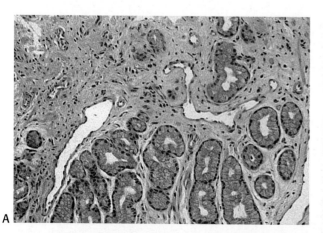

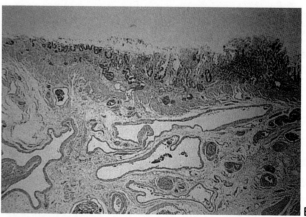

FIG. 4.122. Gastric antral vascular ectasia. **A:** A gastric biopsy demonstrating a wider than normal separation of the glands in part of the biopsy. This separation results from sclerosis around the mucosal capillaries and also affects the lamina propria. **B:** Similar lesions may be encountered in the submucosa. One sees irregular thickening and hyalinosis of the vasculature. Mucosal congestion may also be present.

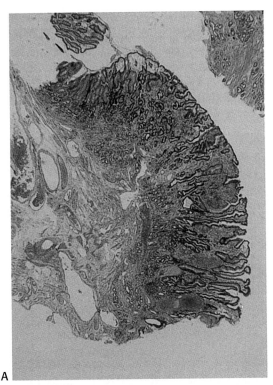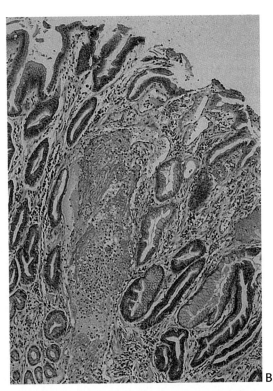

A   B

FIG. 4.123. Gastric antral vascular ectasia (GAVE). **A:** Gastric biopsy showing prominent vascular congestion with thrombosis of the vasculature. The surrounding glands appear regenerative. The vessels in the submucosa are dilated and sclerotic. **B:** Higher magnification of one of the thrombosed vessels.

hyperplasia of the lamina propria. The fibrohyalinosis appears as a homogeneous light pink substance surrounding ectatic capillaries in the lamina propria and submucosa. The presence of the hyalinosis and the fibrin thrombi are important in differentiating GAVE from severe PHG (Table 4.24) (291). Epithelial damage from gastric acid, intraluminal food, or other factors can disrupt the mucosal barrier in mucosal areas overlying engorged vessels and may explain the presence of the fibrin thrombi. The lesions usually show patchy mild chronic inflammation in the superficial lamina propria. One may also see coexisting atrophic gastritis with

intestinal metaplasia. The muscularis mucosae often appears thickened and hyperplastic, perhaps reflective of mucosal prolapse. Submucosal vessels appear dilated and congested, but no vascular malformations are evident.

Angiodysplasia

Patients with angiodysplasia present with overt gastrointestinal bleeding or anemia. Bleeding from the lesions can be massive and recurrent. If the lesions are visible endoscopically, they appear bright red, flat, and well circumscribed, or

TABLE 4.24	A Comparison of Portal Gastropathy and Gastric Antral Portal Ectasia (GAVE)	
Feature	**Portal Gastropathy**	**GAVE**
Location	Fundus and corpus	Antrum
Degree of ectasia	Mild–moderate ectasia	Marked ectasia
Presence of cirrhosis	Always	30% of patients
Presence of fibrohyalinosis	No	Yes
Presence of thrombosis	No	Yes
Vascular spindle cell proliferation	No	Yes
Anemia and hemorrhage	Low incidence	High incidence
Endoscopic lesions	Diffuse erythema	Appear as microvessels
Sex	More commonly affects men	Predominantly affects women

fernlike. Selective arteriography is the preferred way to establish the diagnosis. Controversy surrounds the etiology of angiodysplasia. Arguments favoring an acquired origin include its association with aortic stenosis, underlying inflammatory gastrointestinal conditions, and von Willebrand disease. Mechanical factors such as vascular destruction may play a role in some cases, with vigorous peristalsis or increased intraluminal pressure causing shunting of blood into the submucosal arteriovenous system. The lesions may also result from progressive dilation of normal vascular structures secondary to vascular degenerative changes present in the elderly.

Most angiodysplasias are mucosal and submucosal lesions that are not always grossly visible. A helpful way to identify the vascular abnormality in resection specimens is to inject an India ink–radiopaque dye combination into the specimen and then to radiograph the specimen and then section it. Angiodysplasia consists of abnormal numbers of dilated, distorted arteries and veins lined by endothelium and rarely by a small amount of smooth muscle between the pre-existing ectatic arteries, veins, venules, and capillaries (Fig. 4.124). The vessels have an abnormal distribution and aberrant morphology and probably represent true arteriovenous malformations.

The earliest abnormality consists of dilated submucosal veins, which may be present in the absence of mucosal disease. As the disease progresses, the mucosal abnormalities become more pronounced with increased numbers of dilated and deformed mucosal and submucosal vessels, eventually leading to distortion of the mucosal architecture and erosions. The vascular channels may be separated from the gastric lumen by a single layer of endothelial cells. The walls of the vessels in the submucosa appear irregularly thickened. The presence of distorted and dysplastic vessels distinguishes this lesion from a hemangioma or telangiectasia.

Caliber-Persistent Artery (Dieulafoy Lesion)

The entity variously termed caliber-persistent artery, cirsoid aneurysm, or Dieulafoy lesion tends to affect middle-aged

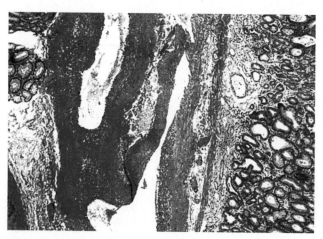

FIG. 4.124. Angiodysplasia affecting the gastric mucosa. Abnormal arteriovenous connections occur.

and elderly men. Median patient age is 52 to 54 years, with patients ranging in age from 16 to 91 (292). The disorder presents as recurrent, massive, and sometimes fatal hematemesis. Massive hemorrhage and rupture occur when a large submucosal artery impinges on the mucosa while pursuing its tortuous course through the submucosa. The lesion is thought to represent a congenital anomaly related to defective arterial involution or elongation and even curling of a deep elongated submucosal vessel (293).

Because the lesions are flat, they are hard to detect. However, the angiographic appearance is characteristic. The lesion is often not visible endoscopically, although one may see an area of bleeding. When endoscopically identifiable, the lesion presents as a volcanic crater with a central whitish discoloration projecting from an otherwise normal gastric mucosa. An abnormally large submucosal vessel protrudes through a minute mucosal defect (Fig. 4.125). Ulceration is usually not present in the region surrounding the place where the vessel breaks through the mucosa. In most cases, the bleeding site lies within the first 6 cm of the gastroesophageal junction, usually on the lesser curvature (293).

Histologically, an abnormally large oversized tortuous muscular artery measuring about 1.5 mm in diameter runs through the submucosa and approaches the mucosa (Fig. 4.126), often with superficial erosion (Fig. 4.127). Veins often accompany the lesion. The arterial wall may show medial hypertrophy and adventitial fibrosis, but the lesion typically lacks inflammation, aneurysm formation, atherosclerosis, or dystrophic calcification. An elastic tissue stain demonstrates the normal architecture of an arterial wall with only slight intimal hyperplasia and reduplication of the internal elastic lamina. If the wall of the artery is eroded at the base of a mucosal ulcer, hemorrhage ensues. The ulcer is often minute even though the hemorrhage is massive. The overlying ulcer usually lacks the intense inflammation typical of peptic ulcer disease and is superficial with no involvement of the muscularis propria or associated mural fibrosis. The part of the artery at the base of the ulcer usually shows focal necrosis and rupture. A thrombus may be attached to a protruding open artery. The artery forces the mucosa upward and a wide submucosal area characteristically exists between these arteries and the true muscularis propria.

Hemodialysis-Associated Telangiectasias

Telangiectasia generally refers to the dilation of pre-existing vessels, whereas angiomatosis refers to new vessel growth. Gastric telangiectasias develop in some patients on long-term hemodialysis (294). The telangiectatic areas appear small, flattened, and reddish with fernlike margins. Several factors may predispose to its development. Chronic sodium and water overload may result in venous hypertension, causing submucosal venous dilation. Additionally, dialysis patients receive aluminum hydroxide on a long-term basis to control hyperphosphatemia. Aluminum compounds are

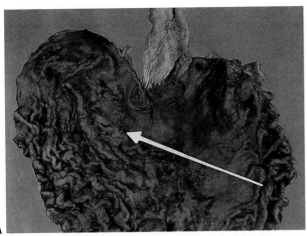
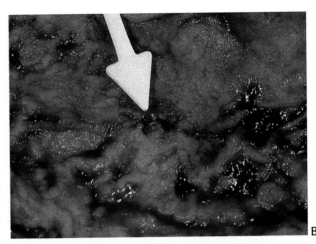

FIG. 4.125. Caliber-persistent artery. **A:** Opened specimen seen from the mucosal side is not very dramatic. The stomach was completely filled with blood and the *arrow* points to the lesion. **B:** Higher magnification demonstrates the eroded surface of the prominent vessel. Such lesions must be carefully sought. They characteristically lie in the proximal stomach and are usually very difficult to see.

known to cause skin telangiectasias (295). Patients on hemodialysis also develop accelerated atherosclerosis (296), which may predispose the gastrointestinal vasculature to develop abnormalities.

with eating disorders due the repeated episodes of induced vomiting. The cause of gastric rupture in infants is not always clear, although endotoxins and muscular defects are postulated etiologic factors. Intramural gastric hematomas may develop in patients with coagulopathies, prior surgery, bleeding benign gastric ulcer, or trauma.

GASTRIC TEARS, PERFORATIONS, FISTULAE, RUPTURES, AND HEMATOMAS

The upper portion of the stomach is subject to the same types of tears, perforations, and linear erosions and fistulae as seen in the lower esophagus (see Chapter 2) (Fig. 4.128). They complicate surgical treatment, foreign bodies, trauma, peptic ulcer disease, severe or persistent vomiting, infections, neoplasms, chemical injury, and lung infections. They can affect adults as well as newborns. They are seen in young women

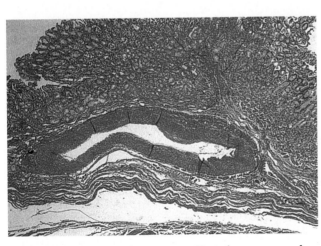

FIG. 4.126. Caliber-persistent artery. Note the presence of an unusually large vessel underlying the gastric mucosa. In this case, the overlying mucosa remains intact.

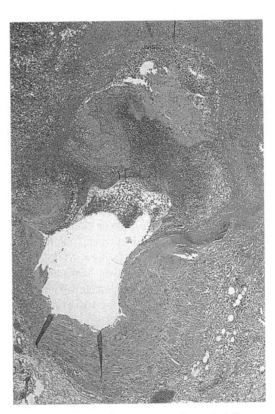

FIG. 4.127. Histologic section through the vessel illustrated in Figure 4.125. Note the unusually large size. Fresh blood and organizing thrombus are present.

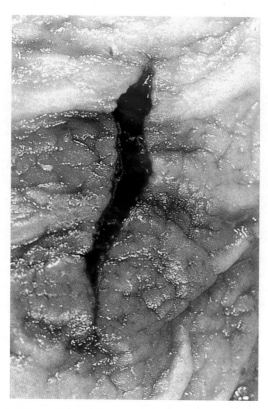

FIG. 4.128. Mallory-Weiss tear of the stomach in a patient who had a previous Nissen fundoplication.

GASTRIC SIDEROSIS

Approximately 4% of gastric biopsies will demonstrate evidence of gastric siderosis (93). Three patterns of gastric siderosis have been identified: (a) a nonspecific gastric siderosis with predominant iron deposits in the stromal cells including macrophages and focally in the epithelium, (b) an iron pill gastritis (discussed previously in the drug-induced gastritis section of this chapter), and (c) a predominant deposition in antral and fundic glandular epithelium. The first two types of siderosis are focal and patchy and associate with variable inflammation; the third is strong and diffuse and is characteristic of the iron deposition that is seen in hemochromatosis (93).

Hemochromatosis is an iron overload disorder that causes prominent damage to the liver and pancreas. It is diagnosed on the basis of the clinical triad of a micronodular pigmented cirrhosis, diabetes mellitus, and skin pigmentation. The most severe iron overload occurs in a genetic disorder, whereas secondary hemochromatosis results from excessive iron overload. Patients with hemochromatosis have a susceptibility gene located on chromosome 6 closely linked with the HLA locus. The excessive iron accumulates preferentially in the cytoplasm of parenchymal cells (Fig. 4.129). This contrasts with iron deposition in the mononuclear cells in patients with systemic hemosiderosis.

GASTRIC INVOLVEMENT IN SYSTEMIC DISEASES

Inflammatory Bowel Disease

The stomach may be abnormal in patients with IBD. The changes associated with Crohn disease were discussed in the section on granulomatous gastritis. Ulcerative colitis patients may also develop gastritis (297). The changes include multiple tiny ulcers, glandular abscesses, and intraepithelial lymphocytosis. The intensity of the changes reflects the activity of the colonic disease.

Amyloid

Gastric amyloid deposits occur in approximately 1% of patients with systemic amyloidosis. Some patients have coexisting small bowel amyloidosis (298). GI involvement may lead to vascular compromise, tumoral deposits, intramural thickening, prolonged nausea and vomiting, weight loss, gastroparesis, and gastric outlet obstruction (298). Other patients remain completely asymptomatic only to have the amyloid demonstrable on gastric biopsies performed for other reasons. In its earliest stages, amyloid tends to accumulate in the intima and media of small submucosal and serosal blood vessels (Fig. 4.130). The lamina propria and muscularis propria are variably involved, and the epithelium appears normal. Amyloid deposition is more massive in primary than in secondary types of amyloidosis. Parenchymal deposits primarily affect the muscularis mucosae and muscularis propria (298), causing thickened gastric folds. Amyloid also surrounds gastric glands. In tumoral amyloidosis, the entire gastric wall becomes replaced by large acellular eosinophilic masses that completely destroy the underlying histology (Fig. 4.131). The amyloid aggregates may be surrounded by macrophages.

Diabetes

By far the most common gastric complication of diabetes is diabetic gastroparesis, a condition that results from a peripheral autonomic neuropathy. It is discussed further in Chapter 10.

Mastocytosis

Accumulations of mast cells in the skin and parenchymal organs characterize systemic mastocytosis (299). Gastrointestinal symptoms include nausea, vomiting, abdominal pain, and diarrhea. Parietal cell mass increases due to increased histamine levels from the mast cells and results in hyperchlorhydria and peptic ulceration (299). Endoscopic features include the presence of erosions and gastroduodenal ulcers with a bleeding tendency, thickening of the gastric folds, mucosal edema, urticarialike

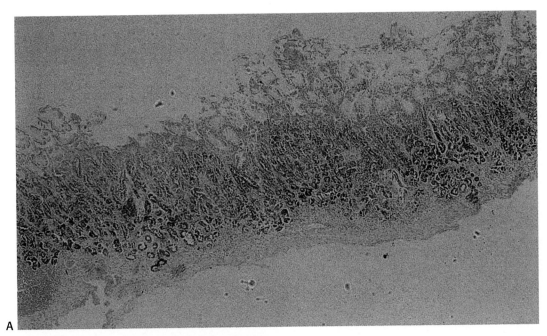

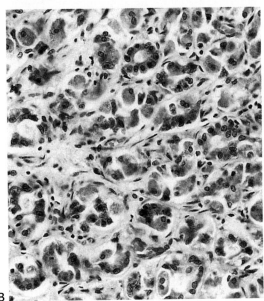

FIG. 4.129. Hemochromatosis. **A:** Patients with hemochromatosis often exhibit marked iron deposition within the epithelium of the gastrointestinal tract. In the stomach, iron deposits in the glandular component of the mucosa, as is demonstrated by this Prussian blue stain. **B:** Hematoxylin and eosin section showing the presence of pigmented glandular epithelium.

lesions, and, occasionally, varices due to portal hypertension. Because the gastric folds appear hypertrophic, mastocytosis is included in the differential diagnosis of giant fold diseases. Histologically the gastric wall is infiltrated by increased numbers of mast cells. These can be highlighted using an immunohistochemical reaction for tryptase.

Sjögren Syndrome

Gastric involvement in primary Sjögren syndrome is present in approximately 50% of patients (300). Some individuals show moderate chronic atrophic gastritis, whereas most show superficial gastritis. Antibodies to gastric parietal cells are detectable in approximately 10% of cases.

Hypercalcemia

Patients with hypercalcemia often demonstrate dystrophic calcification in various sites. In the stomach, this takes the form of deposits within the mucosa often surrounding individual gastric glands or occasionally lying free in the lamina propria. Slender areas of calcification are visible histologically (Fig. 4.132). Their true nature can be confirmed with the use of a Von Kossa stain .

TUMORLIKE LESIONS (PSEUDOTUMORS)

A number of lesions may present as pseudotumors. Some of the more common ones are discussed below.

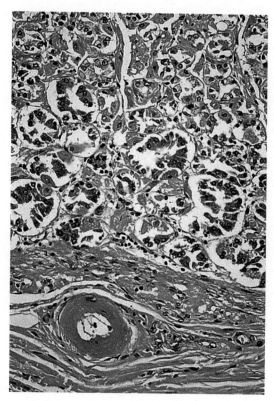

FIG. 4.130. Amyloidosis involving the submucosal blood vessels, lamina propria, and muscularis mucosae.

Gastric Xanthelasma (Xanthoma)

Xanthelasmas appear to the endoscopist as single or multiple, well-demarcated, circular-oval, whitish yellow lesions measuring 1 to 2 mm and rarely exceeding 5 mm. They may develop in the setting of cholestasis and hypercholes-

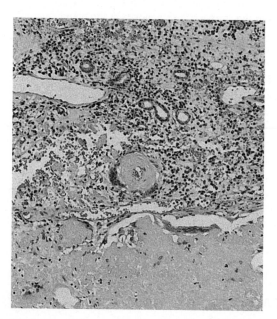

FIG. 4.131. Tumoral amyloidosis of the stomach. Eosinophilic acellular material concentrically surrounds blood vessels.

terolemia. Histologically, the lesions consist of collections of lipid-containing macrophages (xanthoma cells) arranged in pavementlike patterns in the upper lamina propria immediately beneath the surface epithelium (Figs. 4.133 and 4.134). Lymphocytes, plasma cells, and macrophages associate with the foam cells. The macrophages contain a foamy, finely vacuolated cytoplasm and the cells are PAS negative. The etiology of the lipid islands is unknown, but they never occur in a normal stomach. Patients often have evidence of duodenal reflux, varying degrees of gastritis, gastric surgery, or even associated cancer. These lipid islands stain with the macrophage marker KP1 and the foam cells contain low-density lipoproteins (LDLs) and oxidized LDLs.

Regenerative Lesions with Pseudosarcomatous Stroma

Regenerative lesions, whether they appear polypoid or surround an area of ulceration, may contain a stroma that appears pseudosarcomatous due to prominent reactive endothelial cells and/or myofibroblasts. In the stomach, the lesions usually affect middle-aged or elderly individuals. The reactive cells contain large nuclei and prominent nucleoli. Often, inflammatory cells associate with the reactive cells. The reactive cells are cytokeratin negative, allowing one to distinguish the lesion from an undifferentiated carcinoma. The overall reactive appearance of the lesion distinguishes it from a mesenchymal tumor in that the cells are typically large and lack mitoses. Vimentin immunostains are usually strongly positive.

BEZOARS AND FOREIGN BODIES

Multiple factors predispose to bezoar development. Motility disturbances or obstructions predispose to their formation. As a result, bezoars complicate diabetes mellitus, myotonic muscular dystrophy, sclerotherapy, and medications that impair GI motility, such as opioids or neuromuscular blockers. Most foreign objects are swallowed accidentally by children, intentionally by psychiatric patients, or as contraband by smugglers. Patients with bezoars complain of anorexia, epigastric fullness, nausea, or vomiting. Ulceration, bleeding, and peritonitis complicate ingestion of pointed objects such as needles or toothpicks. Bezoars consist of accumulated ingested material that forms a gastric intraluminal mass. Most result from consumption of indigestible organic substances such as hair (trichobezoars), vegetables (phytobezoars), drugs, or a combination thereof (trichophytobezoars). Trichobezoars typically develop in emotionally disturbed young girls chewing and swallowing long hair with the ultimate formation of a hair ball that leads to pyloric outlet obstruction.

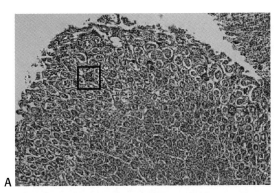
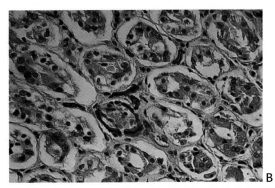

FIG. 4.132. Mucosal calcification in hypercalcemia. **A:** Low magnification shows several glands that appear to stand out due to prominent basophilic staining. One such gland is outlined in the box. This area is shown at higher magnification in **B:** Dystrophic calcification lies in the lamina propria as well as in a periglandular distribution. The patient had hypercalcemia from parathyroid hyperplasia.

CONSEQUENCES OF GASTROINTESTINAL SURGERY

A number of histologic changes complicate the postsurgical stomach. *Marginal, anastomotic, stomal,* and *surgical ulcer* are terms that refer to the ulcers developing at surgically created gastric outlets. They usually follow duodenal ulcer operations. Today stomal ulcers are uncommon and have largely disappeared with the abandonment of simple gastroenterostomy as the primary ulcer operation.

Chronic gastritis is common, particularly if the stomach is connected to the jejunum in a Billroth II operation. The gastritis is often severe with atrophy, pyloric and intestinal metaplasia, and sometimes dysplasia. Proximal to the anastomosis, there is pit hyperplasia, superficial edema, a muscular lamina propria, minimal inflammation, and glandular atrophy secondary to gastrin loss from the antrectomy. Numerous factors contribute to the genesis of these lesions, including chronic bile reflux, stomal ischemia secondary to mucosal prolapse, or mucosal deformities that occur when the anastomosis is constructed. Increased G-cell proliferation after the procedure perhaps explains the increased risk of cancer development in the gastric remnant. These lesions

may start as foveolar hyperplasia in response to pancreatic or duodenal secretions.

Repetitive injury may lead to release of proinflammatory agents, which may stimulate smooth muscle and later fibroblastic proliferations. The first macroscopically visible lesion is polypoid foveolar hyperplasia, which then evolves into

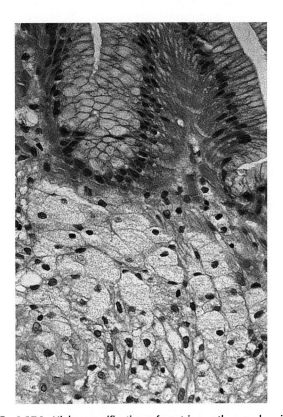

FIG. 4.134. High magnification of gastric xanthoma showing the collection of foam cells in the lamina propria. These cells are distinguishable from signet ring cell carcinomas by virtue of the small nucleus and large amount of cytoplasm. Additionally, the nuclei are often centrally placed. In cases of doubt, they can be stained with the antibody KP1 to confirm their true nature.

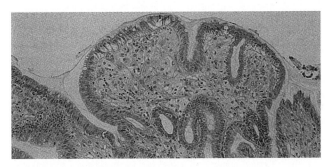

FIG. 4.133. Gastric xanthelasma. A prominent lamina propria collection of xanthoma cells distorts the architecture of the mucosa, filling it up and widening the interglandular regions.

TABLE 4.25   Gastric Remnant Changes

Chronic alkaline reflux gastritis
Cystic glandular dilatation (similar to fundic gland polyps)
Surface (foveolar) hyperplasia
Atrophic gastritis
Intestinal metaplasia
Hyperplastic polyps
Gastric cystica profunda
Gastric xanthelasma
Dysplasia
Carcinoma
Stomal ulcers

larger masses of hyperplastic polyps found at the gastrectomy site. Grossly, the lesions present as a solitary sessile polyp or as a linear arrangement of polyps encircling the gastric side of the stoma. The gastric pits have an increased depth or diameter with saccular dilations, and the increased stroma appears edematous and/or inflamed, widely separating the gastric glands. The base of the lesion contains fibrous connective tissue replacing or extending through the muscularis mucosae. Histologically, these proliferative lesions resemble hyperplastic polyps in that they contain proliferating nondysplastic foveolar cells. The hypertrophic muscularis mucosae appears irregularly frayed, with penetration of cystic glands into the submucosa, producing gastritis cystica profunda. The lesion microscopically represents a localized rugal hypertrophy, often resembling Menetrier disease. The natural history of these lesions is controversial, and it remains unclear as to whether they represent an intermediate stage between chronic stromal gastritis and stomal cancer.

REFERENCES

1. Arey LB: *Developmental Anatomy*. Philadelphia: WB Saunders, 1974, p 245.
2. Van den Brinck GR, Hardwick JCH, Nielsen C, et al: Sonic hedgehog expression correlates with fundic gland differentiation in the adult gastrointestinal tract. *Gut* 2002;51:628.
3. Dimmler A, Brabletz T, Hlubek F, et al: Transcription of sonic hedgehog, a potential factor for gastric morphogenesis and gastric mucosa maintenance is upregulated in acidic conditions. *Lab Invest* 2003; 83:1829.
4. Allen A, Flemstrom G, Garner A, Kivilaakso E: Gastroduodenal mucosal protection. *Physiol Rev* 1993;73:823.
5. Engel E, Peskoff A, Kauffman GL Jr, Grossman MI: Analysis of hydrogen ion concentration in the gastric gel mucus layer. *Am J Physiol* 1984;247:G321.
6. Wallace JL, Whittle BJR: The role of extracellular mucus as a protective cap over gastric mucosal damage. *Scand J Gastroenterol* 1986;21:79.
7. Allen A, Cunliffe WJ, Pearson JP, Venables CW: The adherent gastric mucus gel barrier in man and changes in peptic ulceration. *J Intern Med* 1990;732:83.
8. Holzer P, Livingston EH, Guth PH: Sensory neurons signal of an increase in rat gastric mucosal blood flow in the face of pending acid injury. *Gastroenterology* 1991;101:416.
9. Jacobson E: Circulatory mechanisms of gastric mucosal damage and protection. *Gastroenterology* 1992;102:1788.
10. Robert A: Role of endogenous and exogenous prostaglandins in mucosal protection. In: Allen A, Flemstrom G, Garner A, et al (eds). *Mechanisms of Mucosal Protection in the Upper Gastrointestinal Tract.* New York: Raven Press, 1984, pp 377–393.
11. Pabst MA, Wachter C, Holzer P: Morphologic basis of the functional gastric acid barrier. *Lab Invest* 1996;74:78.
12. Konturek PK, Brzozowski T, Konturek SJ, Dembinski A: Role of epidermal growth factor, prostaglandin, and sulfhydryls in stress-induced gastric lesions. *Gastroenterology* 1990;99:1607.
13. Ishikawa T, Sarfeh IJ, Tarnawski A, et al: Epidermal growth factor protects portal hypertensive gastric mucosa in ischemia/reperfusion: the role of capillary endothelia and prostaglandins. *Surgery* 1992;112:341.
14. Kunkel SL, Wiggins RC, Chensue SW, Larrick J: Regulation of macrophage tumor necrosis factor production by prostaglandin E2. *Biochem Biophys Res, Commun* 1986;137:404.
15. Hogaboam CM, Bissonnette KY, Chin, BC, et al: Prostaglandins inhibit inflammatory mediator release from rat mast cells. *Gastroenterology* 1993;104:122.
16. Silen W, Ito S: Mechanisms for rapid re-epithelilization of the gastric mucosal surface. *Ann Rev Physiol* 1985;47:217.
17. Chen MC, Lee AT, Soll AH: Mitogenic response of canine fundic epithelial cells in short-term culture to TGFα and IGF-1. *J Clin Invest* 1991;87:1716.
18. Beauchamp RD, Barnard GA, MacCutchen CN, et al: Localization of TGFα and its receptor in gastric mucosal cells. Implications for regulatory role in acid secretion and mucosal renewal. *J Clin Invest* 1989;84:1017.
19. Sporn MB, Roberts AB: Autocrine growth factors and cancer. *Nature* 1985;313:745.
20. Marti U, Burwen SJ, Jones AL: Biological effects of epidermal growth factor, with emphasis on the gastrointestinal tract and liver: an update. *Hepatology* 1989;9:126.
21. Hirschowitz BL: Neural and hormonal control of gastric secretion. In: Schultz SG, Forte JG (eds). *Handbook of Physiology*, Vol. III. Washington, DC: American Physiology Society, 1989, p 128–146.
22. Uvnas-Wallensten K, Efendic S, Johansson C, et al: Effect of intraluminal pH on the release of somatostatin and gastrin into antral, bulbar and ileal pouches of conscious dogs. *Acta Physiol Scand* 1980;110:391.
23. Modlin IM, Tang LH: The gastric enterochromaffin-like cells: an enigmatic cellular link. *Gastroenterology* 1996;111:783.
24. Samloff IM: Pepsinogens I and II: purification from gastric mucosa and radioimmunoassay in serum. *Gastroenterology* 1982;82:26.
25. Sano J, Miki K, Ichnose M, et al: In situ localization of pepsinogens I and II mRNA in human gastric mucosa. *Acta Pathol Jpn* 1989;39:765.
26. Stave R, Bandtzaeg P, Nygaard K, Fausa O: The transitional body-antrum zone in resected stomachs. Anatomical outline and parietal-cell and gastrin-cell characteristics in peptic ulcer disease. *Scand J Gastroenterol* 1978;13:685.
27. Listrom MB, Fenoglio-Preiser CM: The lymphatic distribution of the stomach in normal, inflammatory, hyperplastic and neoplastic tissues. *Gastroenterology* 1987;93:506.
28. Neutra MR, Padykula HA: The gastrointestinal tract. In: Weiss L (ed). *Modern Concepts of Gastrointestinal Histology.* New York: Elsevier, 1984, pp 1–30.
29. Kyoi T, Ueda F, Kimura K, et al: Development of gap junctions between gastric surface mucous cells during cell maturation in rats. *Gastroenterology* 1992;102:1930.
30. Helander HF: The cells of the gastric mucosa. *Int Rev Cytol* 1981;70:217.
31. Jons T, Warrings B, Jons A, Drenckhahn D: Basolateral localization of anion exchanger 2 (AE2) and actin in acid-secreting (parietal) cells of the human stomach. *Histochemistry* 1994;102:255.
32. Grossman MI: The pyloric gland area of the stomach. *Gastroenterology* 1960;38:1.
33. Faussone-Pellegrini MS, Pantalone D, Cortesini C: An ultrastructural study of the smooth muscle cells and nerve endings of the human stomach. *J Submicrosc Cytol Pathol* 1989;21:421.
34. Bartels RJ: Duplication of the stomach: case report and review of the literature. *Am Surgeon* 1967;33:747.
35. Luks FI, Shah MN, Bulauitan MC, et al: Adult foregut duplication. *Surgery* 1990;108:101.
36. Ildstad ST, Tollerud DJ, Weiss RG, et al: Duplication of the alimentary tract. Clinical characteristics, preferred treatment and associated malformations. *Ann Surg* 1988;208:184.
37. Kay S, Mills S: The stomach. In: Sternberg S (ed). *Diagnostic Surgical Pathology.* New York: Raven Press, 1994, pp 1071–1085.

38. Hewlett PM: Isolated dextrogastria. *Br J Radiol* 1982;55:678.

39. Torfs CP, Velie EM, Oechsli FW, et al: A population-based study of gastroschisis: demographic, pregnancy, and lifestyle risk factors. *Teratology* 1994;50:44.

40. de Vries PA: The pathogenesis of gastroschisis and omphalocele. *J Pediatr Surg* 1980;15:245.

41. Kurgan A, Hoffman J: Aetiology of gastric diverticula—an hypothesis. *Med Hypoth* 1981;7:1471.

42. Moore CC: Congenital gastric outlet obstruction. *J Pediatr Surg* 1989;24:1241.

43. Achiron R, Hamiel-Pinchas O, Engelberg O, et al: Aplasia cutis congenita associated with epidermolysis bullosa and pyloric atresia: the diagnostic role of prenatal ultrasonography. *Prenat Diagn* 1992;12:765.

44. Bell MJ: Infantile pyloric stenosis. Experience with 305 cases at Louisville Children's Hospital. *Surgery* 1968;64:983.

45. Bell JM, Ternberg JL, Keating JP, et al: Prepyloric gastric antral web: a puzzling epidemic. *J Pediatr Surg* 1978;13:307.

46. Aaron JM, Newman A, Heaton JW: Torus hyperplasia of the pyloric antrum presenting as a gastric pseudotumor. *Gastroenterology* 1973;64:634.

47. Dolan RV, Remine WH, Dockerty MB: The fate of heterotopic pancreatic tissue: a study of 212 cases. *Arch Surg* 1974;109:762.

48. Tomita T, Kanabe S: Islet tissue in the heterotopic pancreas. *Arch Pathol Lab Med* 1983;107:469.

49. Barbosa J, Dockerty MB, Waugh JM: Pancreatic heterotopia: review of the literature and report of 41 authenticated surgical cases of which 25 were clinically significant. *Surg Gynecol Obstet* 1946;82:527.

50. Yamagiwa H, Matsuzaki O, Ishihara A, Yoshimura H: Heterotopic gastric glands in the submucosa of the stomach. *Acta Pathol Jpn* 1979;29:347.

51. Sufian S, Ominsky S, Matsumoto T: Congenital double pylorus. *Gastroenterology* 1977;73:1154.

52. Miller D, Pasquale M, Seneca R, Hodin E: Gastric volvulus in the pediatric population. *Arch Surg* 1991;126:1146.

53. Patel NM: Chronic gastric volvulus: report of a case and review of the literature. *Am J Gastroenterol* 1985;80:170.

54. Shackelford GD, McAlister WH, Brodeur AE, et al: Congenital microgastria. *Am J Roentgenol Radium Ther Nucl Med* 1973;118:72.

55. Neifeld JP, Berman WF, Lawrence W Jr, et al: Management of congenital microgastria with a jejunal reservoir pouch. *J Pediatr Surg* 1980;15:882.

56. Dixon MF, Genta RM, Yardley JH, et al, and the Participants of the International Workshop on the Histopathology of Gastritis, Houston 1994: Classification and grading of gastritis: the updated Sydney system. *Am J Surg Pathol* 1996;20:1161.

57. Wright CL, Kelly JK: The use of routine special stains for upper gastrointestinal biopsies. *Am J Surg Pathol* 2006;30:357.

58. Stark ME, Szurszewski JH: Role of nitric oxide in gastrointestinal and hepatic function and disease. *Gastroenterology* 1992;103:1928.

59. McCord JM: Oxygen-derived free radicals in postischemic tissue injury. *N Engl J Med* 1985;312:159.

60. Hernandez LA, Grisham MB, Twohig B, et al: Role of neutrophils in ischemia-reperfusion-induced microvascular injury. *Am J Physiol* 1987;253:H699.

61. Kozol R, Kopatsis A, Fligiel SEG, et al: Neutrophil-mediated injury to gastric mucosal surface cells. *Dig Dis Sci* 1994;39:138.

62. Andrews FJ, Malcontenti C, O'Brien PE: Sequence of gastric mucosal injury following ischemia and reperfusion: role of reactive oxygen metabolites. *Dig Dis Sci* 1992;37:1356.

63. Stein HJ, Hinder RA, Oosthuizen MJ: Gastric mucosal injury caused by hemorrhagic shock and reperfusion: protective role of the antioxidant glutathione. *Surgery* 1990;108:467.

64. Ross D: Glutathione, free radicals and chemotherapeutic agents: mechanism of free radical induced toxicity and glutathione-dependent protection. *Pharmacol Ther* 1988;37:231.

65. Silen W, Ito S: Mechanisms for rapid re-epithelialization of the gastric mucosal surface. *Annu Rev Physiol* 1985;47:217.

66. Miyazaki Y, Hiraoka S, Tsutsui S, et al: Epidermal growth factor receptor mediates stress-induced expression of its ligands in rat gastric epithelial cells. *Gastroenterology* 2001;120:108.

67. Kvietys PR, Twohig B, Danzell J, Specian RD: Ethanol-induced injury to the rat gastric mucosa. *Gastroenterology* 1990;98:909.

68. Trier JS, Szabo S, Allan CH: Ethanol-induced damage to mucosal capillaries of rat stomach. *Gastroenterology* 1987;92:13.

69. Masuda E, Kawano S, Nagano K, et al: Endogenous nitric oxide modulates ethanol-induced gastric mucosal injury in rats. *Gastroenterology* 1995;108:58.

70. Pihan G, Rogers C, Szabo S: Vascular injury in acute gastric mucosal damage: mediatory role of leukotrienes. *Dig Dis Sci* 1988;33:625.

71. Holzer P, Livingston EH, Guth PH: Sensory neurons signal an increase in rat gastric mucosal blood flow in the face of pending acid injury. *Gastroenterology* 1991;101:416.

72. Laine L, Weinstein WM: Histology of alcoholic hemorrhagic "gastritis": a prospective evaluation. *Gastroenterology* 1988;94:1254.

73. Romano M, Lesch CA, Meise KS, et al: Increased gastroduodenal concentrations of transforming growth factor a in adaptation to aspirin in monkeys and rats. *Gastroenterology* 1996;110:1448.

74. Schoen RT, Vender RJ: Mechanisms of nonsteroidal anti-inflammatory drug-induced gastric damage. *Am J Med* 1989;86:449.

75. Levy M, Miller DR, Kaufman DW, et al: Major upper gastrointestinal tract bleeding: relation to the use of aspirin and other nonnarcotic analgesics. *Arch Intern Med* 1988;148:281.

76. Lewis JD, Kimmel SE, Localio AR, et al: Risk of serious upper gastrointestinal toxicity with over-the-counter nonaspirin nonsteroidal anti-inflammatory drugs. *Gastroenterology* 2005;129:1865.

77. Langman MJS: Epidemiologic evidence on the association between peptic ulceration and antiinflammatory drug use. *Gastroenterology* 1989;96:640.

78. Lee M, Feldman M: Age-related reductions in gastric mucosal prostaglandin levels increase susceptibility to aspirin-induced injury in rats. *Gastroenterology* 1994;107:1746.

79. Fiorucci S, Antonelli E, Distrutti E, et al: Inhibition of hydrogen sulfide generation contributes to gastric injury caused by anti-inflammatory nonsteroidal drugs. *Gastroenterology* 2005;129:1210.

80. Aalykke C, Lauritsen JM, Hallas J, et al: Helicobacter pylori and risk of ulcer bleeding among users of nonsteroidal anti-inflammatory drugs: a case control study. *Gastroenterology* 1999;116:1305.

81. Wallace JL, McKnight W, Miyasaka M, et al: Role of endothelial adhesion molecules in NSAID-induced gastric mucosal injury. *Am J Physiol* 1993;265:G993.

82. Klinkenberg-Knol EC, Nelis F, Dent J, et al: Long term omeprazole treatment in resistant gastroesophageal reflux disease. Efficacy, safety and influence on gastric mucosa. *Gastroenterology* 2000;118:661.

83. Krishnamurthy S, Dayal Y: Parietal cell protrusions in gastric ulcer disease. *Hum Pathol* 1997;28:1126.

84. Aprile MR, Azzoni C, Gibril F, et al: Intramucosal cysts in the gastric body of patients with Zollinger-Ellison syndrome. *Hum Pathol* 2000;31:140.

85. Choudhry U, Boyce HW Jr, Coppola D: Proton pump inhibitor-associated gastric polyps: a retrospective analysis of their frequency and endoscopic, histologic and ultrastructural characteristics. *Am J Clin Pathol* 1998;110:615.

86. Welch DC, Wirth PS, Goldenring JR, et al: Gastric graft-versus-host disease revisited. Does proton pump inhibitor therapy affect endoscopic gastric biopsy interpretation? *Am J Surg Pathol* 2006;30:444.

87. Delaney JP, Michel HM, Bonsack ME, et al: Adrenal corticosteroids cause gastrin cell hyperplasia. *Gastroenterology* 1979;76:913.

88. Petras RE, Hart WR, Bukowski RM: Gastric epithelial atypia associated with hepatic arterial infusion chemotherapy. Its distinction from early gastric carcinoma. *Cancer* 1985;56:745.

89. Weidner N, Smith JG, LaVanway JM: Peptic ulceration with marked epithelial atypia following hepatic arterial infusion chemotherapy. A lesion initially misinterpreted as carcinoma. *Am J Surg Pathol* 1983;7:261.

90. Doria MI, Doria LK, Faintuch J, Levin B: Gastric mucosal injury after hepatic arterial infusion chemotherapy with floxuridine-a clinical and pathologic study. *Cancer* 1994;73:2042.

91. Ferrero JM, Francois E, Frenay M, Namer M: Occurrence of a gastric phytobezoar after chemotherapy with vinorelbine. *Presse Med* 1993;22:638.

92. Haig A, Driman DK: Iron-induced mucosal injury to the upper gastrointestinal tract. *Histopathology* 2006;48:808.

93. Marginean EC, Bennick M, Cyczk J, et al: Gastric siderosis. Patterns and significance. *Am J Surg Pathol* 2006;30:514.

94. Peled N, Dagan O, Babyn P, et al: Gastric-outlet obstruction induced by prostaglandin therapy in neonates. *N Engl J Med* 1992;327:505.

95. Lee HS, LaMaute HR, Pizzi WF, et al: Acute gastroduodenal perforations associated with use of crack. *Ann Surg* 1990;211:15.

96. Escobedo LG, Ruttenber J, Agocs MM, et al: Emerging patterns of cocaine use and the epidemic of cocaine overdose deaths in Dade County, Florida. *Arch Pathol Lab Med* 1991;115:900.

97. Greenson JK, Trinidad SB, Pfeil SA, et al: Gastric mucosal calcinosis. Calcified aluminum phosphate deposits secondary to aluminum-containing antacids or sucralfate therapy in organ transplant patients. *Am J Surg Pathol* 1993;17:45.

98. Abraham SC, Bhagavan BS, Lee LA, et al: Upper gastrointestinal tract injury in patients receiving Kayexalate (sodium-polysterene sulfonate) in sorbitol: clinical endoscopic and histopathologic findings. *Am J Surg Pathol* 2001;25:637.

99. Rashid A, Hamilton SR: Necrosis of the gastrointestinal tract in uremic patients as a result of sodium-polysterene sulfonate (Kayexalate) in sorbitol: an underrecognized condition. *Am J Surg Pathol* 1997;21:60.

100. Iacobuzio-Donahue CA, Lee EL, Abraham SC, et al: Colchicine toxicity: distinct morphologic findings in gastrointestinal biopsies. *Am J Surg Pathol* 2001;25:1067.

101. Feltkamp TE, Mees EJD, Niewenhuis MG: Autoantibodies related to treatment with chlorthalidone and methyldopa. *Acta Med Scand* 1970;187:219.

102. Krigel RL, Padavic-Shaller KA, Rudolph AA, et al: Hemorrhagic gastritis as a new dose-limiting toxicity of recombinant tumor necrosis factor. *J Natl Cancer Inst* 1991;83:129.

103. Casey KM, Quigley TM, Kozarek RA, Raker EJ: Lethal nature of ischemic gastropathy. *Am J Surg* 1993;165:646.

104. Goldgrabber MB, Rubin CE, Palmer WL, et al: The early gastric response to irradiation. A serial biopsy study. *Gastroenterology* 1954;27:1.

105. Malaty HM, Evans DG, Evans DJ, Graham DY: Helicobacter pylori in Hispanics: comparison with blacks and whites of similar age and socioeconomic class. *Gastroenterology* 1992;103:813.

106. Kilbridge PM, Dahms BB, Czinn SJ: Campylobacter pylori-associated gastritis and peptic ulcer disease in children. *Am J Dis Child* 1988;142:1149.

107. Parsonnet J, Shmuely H, Haggerty T: Fecal and oral shedding of Helicobacter pylori from healthy infected adults. *JAMA* 1999;282:2240.

108. Smith VC, Genta RM: Role of *Helicobacter pylori* gastritis in gastric atrophy, intestinal metaplasia and gastric neoplasia. *Microsc Res Tech* 2000;48:313.

109. Hirschl AM, Richter M, Makristathis A, et al: Single and multiple strain colonization in patients with Helicobacter pylori associated gastritis: detection by microrestriction DNA analysis. *J Infect Dis* 1994;170:473.

110. Slomiany BL, Bilski J, Sarosiek J, et al: Campylobacter pyloridis degrades mucin and undermines gastric mucosal integrity. *Biochem Biophys Res Commun* 1987;144:307.

111. Smoot DT, Mobley HLT, Chippendale GR, et al: Helicobacter pylori urease activity is toxic to human gastric epithelial cells. *Infect Immun* 1990;58:1992.

112. Ilver D, Arnqvist A, Ogren J, et al: Helicobacter pylori adhesin binding fucosylated histo-blood group antigens revealed by retagging. *Science* 1998;279:373.

113. Vinall LE, King M, Novelli M, et al: Altered expression and allelic association of the hypervariable membrane mucin MUC1 in *Helicobacter pylori* gastritis. *Gastroenterology* 2001;123:41.

114. Linden S, Nordman H, Hedenbro J, et al: Strain and blood group-dependent binding of *Helicobacter pylori* to human gastric MUC5AC glycoforms. *Gastroenterology* 2002;123:1923.

115. Montecucco C, Papini E, de Bernard M, et al: *Helicobacter pylori* VacA vacuolating cytotoxin and HP-Nap neutrophil activating protein. In: Achtman M, Suerbaum S (eds). *Helicobacter Pylori: Molecular and Cellular Biology.* Wymondham, United Kingdom: Horizon Scientific Press, 2001, pp 245–263.

116. Szabo I, Brutsche S, Tombola F, et al: Formation of anion-selective channels in the cell plasma membrane by the toxin VacC of Helicobacter pylori is required or its biological activity. *EMBO J* 1999;18:5517.

117. Galmiche A, Rassow J, Doye A, et al: The n terminal 34 kDa fragment of *Helicobacter pylori* vacuolating cytotoxin targets mitochondria and induces Cytochrome c release. *EMBO J* 2000;19:361.

118. Gebert B, Fischer W, Weiss E, et al: *Helicobacter pylori* vacuolating cytotoxin inhibits T lymphocyte activation. *Science* 2003;301:1099.

119. Atherton JC, Peek RM Jr, Tham KT, et al: Clinical and pathological importance of heterogeneity in vacA, the vacuolating cytotoxin gene of *Helicobacter pylori. Gastroenterology* 1997;112:92.

120. Censini S, Lange C, Xiang Z, et al: *cag,* a pathogenicity island of *Helicobacter pylori* encodes type-I specific and disease-associated virulence factors. *Proc Natl Acad Sci USA* 1996;3:14648.

121. Segal ED, Cha J, Lo J, et al: Altered states: involvement of phosphorylated CagA in the induction of host cellular growth changes by *Helicobacter pylori. Proc Natl Acad Sci USA* 1999;96:14555.

122. Higashi H, Tsutsumi R, Muto S, et al: SHp-2 tyrosine phosphatase as an intracellular target of *Helicobacter pylori* CagA protein. *Science* 2002;295:683.

123. Mimuro H, Suzuki T, Tanaka J, et al: Grb2 is a key mediator of Helicobacter pylori CagA protein activities. *Mol Cell* 2002;278:745.

124. Naito M, Yamazaki T, Tsutsumi R, et al: Influence of EPIYA-repeat polymorphism on the phosphorylation-dependent biological activity of Helicobacter pylori CagA. *Gastroenterology* 2006;130:1181.

125. Amieva MR, Vogelmann R, Covacci A, et al: Disruption of the epithelial apical junctional complex by Helicobacter CagA. *Science* 2003;1430.

126. Moss SF, Sordillo EM, Abdalla AM, et al: Increased gastric epithelial apoptosis associated with colonization with CagA+ *Helicobacter pylori* strains. *Cancer Res* 2001;61:1406.

127. Yamaoka Y, Kikuchi S, El-Zimaity HMT, et al: Importance of *Helicobacter pylori* oipA in clinical presentation, gastric inflammation and mucosal interleukin 8 production. *Gastroenterology* 2002;123:414.

128. Yamaoka Y, Kwon DH, Graham DY: A M_r34,000 proinflammatory outer membrane protein (oipA) of Helicobacter pylori. *Proc Natl Acad Sci USA* 2000;97:7533.

129. Negrini R, Savio A, Appelmelk BJ: Autoantibodies to gastric mucosa in *Helicobacter pylori* infection. *Helicobacter* 1997;Suppl 1:S13.

130. Fu S, Ramanujam KS, Wong A, et al: Increased expression and cellular localization of inducible nitric oxide synthase and cyclooxygenase 2 in *Helicobacter pylori* gastritis. *Gastroenterology* 1999;116:1319.

131. Naumann M, Wessler S, Bartsch C, et al: Activation of activator protein I and stress response kinases in epithelial cells colonized by *Helicobacter pylori* encoding the *cag* pathogenicity island. *J Bol Chem* 1999;274:31655.

132. Kreuning J, Lindeman J, Biemond I, Lamers CBHW: Relation between IgG and IgA antibody titres against Helicobacter pylori in serum and severity of gastritis in asymptomatic subjects. *J Clin Pathol* 1994;47:227.

133. Hunt RH: Hp and pH: implications for the eradication of Helicobacter pylori. *Scand J Gastroenterol* 1993;196:12.

134. Chan WY, Hui PK, Leung KM, et al: Coccoid forms of Helicobacter pylori in the human stomach. *Am J Clin Pathol* 1994;102:503.

135. Bayerdorffer E, Oertel H, Lehn N, et al: Topographic association between active gastritis and Campylobacter pylori colonization. *J Clin Pathol* 1989;42:834.

136. Warren JR: Gastric pathology associated with Helicobacter pylori. *Gastroenterol Clin North Am* 2000;29:705.

137. Appelman HD: Gastritis: terminology, etiology and clinicopathological correlations. *Hum Pathol* 1994;25:1006.

138. Taha AS, Boothman P, Nakshabendi I, et al: Diagnostic tests for Helicobacter pylori: comparison and influence of non-steroidal anti-inflammatory drugs. *J Clin Pathol* 1992;45:8.

139. Suerbaum S, Michetti P: *Helicobacter pylori* infection. *New Engl J Med* 2002;347:1175.

140. Stolte M, Meining A: Helicobacter pylori gastritis of the gastric carcinoma phenotype: is histology capable of identifying high risk gastritis? *J Gastroenterol* 2000;35:98.

141. Jang J, Lee S, Jung Y, et al: Malgun (clear) cell change in *Helicobacter pylori* gastritis reflects epithelial genomic damage and repair. *Am J Pathol* 2003;162:1203.

142. Sobala GM, Axon ATR, Dixon MF: Morphology of chronic antral gastritis: relationship to age, Helicobacter pylori status and peptic ulceration. *Eur J Gastroenterol Hepatol* 1992;4:825.

143. Genta RM, Hamner HW: The significance of lymphoid follicles in the interpretation of gastric biopsy specimens. *Arch Pathol Lab Med* 1994;118:740.

144. Hassall E, Dimmick JE: Unique features of *Helicobacter pylori* disease in children. *Dig Dis Sci* 1991;36:417.

145. Dhillon AP, Sawyer A: Granulomatous gastritis associated with Campylobacter pylori. *APMIS* 1987;97:723.

146. Faraji EI, Frank BB: Multifocal atrophic gastritis and gastric carcinoma. *Gastroenterol Clin North Am* 2002;499.

147. Niemala S, Karttunen T, Kerola T: *Helicobacter pylori*-associated gastritis. Evolution of histologic changes over 10 years. *Scand J Gastroenterol* 1995;30:542.

148. Murayama Y, Mayagawa J, Shinomura Y, et al: Morphological and functional restoration of parietal cells in *Helicobacter*-associated enlarged fold gastritis after eradication. *Gut* 1999;45:653.

149. Nomura A, Stemmermann GN, Chyou P-H, et al: Helicobacter pylori infection and the risk for duodenal and gastric ulceration. *Ann Intern Med* 1994;120:977.

150. Hojo M, Miwa H, Nagahara A, Sat N: Pooled analysis on the efficacy of the second line treatment regimens for Helicobacter pylori infections. *Scand J Gastroenterol* 2001;36:690.

151. O'Rourke J, Grehan M, Lee A: Non-pylori *Helicobacter* species in humans. *Gut* 2001;49:601.

152. Hilzenrat N, Lamoureux E, Weintraub I, et al: *Helicobacter heilmannii*-like spiral bacteria in gastric mucosal biopsies. Prevalence and clinical significance. *Arch Pathol Lab Med* 1995;119:1149.

153. Meining A, Kroher G, Stolte M: Animal reservoirs in the transmission of Helicobacter heilmannii. *Scand J Gastroenterol* 1998;33:795.

154. McNulty CAM, Dent JC, Curry A, et al: New spiral bacterium in gastric mucosa. *J Clin Pathol* 1989;45:585.

155. Oliva MM, Lazenby AJ, Perman JA: Gastritis associated with Gastrospirillum hominis in children: comparison with Helicobacter pylori and review of the literature. *Mod Pathol* 1993;6:513.

156. Debongnie JC, Domnnay M, Manesse J: Gastrospirillum hominis (Helicobacter heilmanii). A cause of gastritis, is sometimes transient, better diagnoses by touch cytology? *Am J Gastroenterol* 1995;90:411.

157. Singhal AV, Sepulvada AR: *Helicobacter helmannii* gastritis. A case study with review of the literature. *Am J Surg Pathol* 2005;29:1537.

158. Moosvi AR, Saravolata LD, Wong DH, Simms SM: Emphysematous gastritis: case report and review. *Rev Infect Dis* 1990;12:848.

159. Sachar DB, Klein RS, Swerdlow F, et al: Erosive syphilitic gastritis: dark-field and immunofluorescent diagnosis from biopsy specimen. *Ann Intern Med* 1974;80:512.

160. Fyfe B, Poppiti RJ, Lubin J, Robinson MJ: Gastric syphilis—primary diagnosis by gastric biopsy: report of four cases. *Arch Pathol Lab Med* 1993;117:820.

161. Chen CY, Chi KH, George RW, et al: Diagnosis of gastric syphilis by direct immunofluorescence staining and real-time PCR testing. *J Clin Microbiol* 2006;44:3452.

162. Sexton RL, Dunkley RE, Kreglow AF: Gastroscopic study of 100 cases of early syphilis. *Trans Am Ther Soc* 1937;87:73.

163. Bhansali AK: Abdominal tuberculosis: experiences with 300 cases. *Am J Gastroenterol* 1977;67:324.

164. Khoshoo V, Alonzo E, Correa H, et al: Menetrier's disease with cytomegalovirus gastritis. *Arch Pediatr Adol Med* 1994;148:611.

165. Aqel NM, Tanner P, Drury A, et al: Cytomegalovirus gastritis with perforation and gastrocolic fistula formation. *Histopathology* 1991;18:165.

166. Garcia F, Garau J, Sierra M, Marco V: Cytomegalovirus mononucleosis-associated antral gastritis simulating malignancy. *Arch Intern Med* 1987;147:787.

167. Gotlieb-Jensen K, Andersen J: Occurrence of Candida in gastric ulcers. Significance for the healing process. *Gastroenterology* 1983;85:535.

168. Schulz DM: Histoplasmosis: a statistical morphologic study. *Am J Clin Pathol* 1954;24:11.

169. Washington K, Gottfried MR, Wilson MI: Gastrointestinal cryptococcosis. *Mod Pathol* 1992;4:707.

170. Dieterich DT, Lew EA, Bacon DJ, et al: Gastrointestinal pneumocystosis in HIV-related patients on aerosolized pentamidine: report of five cases and literature review. *Am J Gastroenterol* 1992;87:1763.

171. Yokogawa M, Yoshimura H: Clinicopathologic study on larval anisakiasis in Japan. *Am J Trop Med Hyg* 1967;16:723.

172. Verhamme MA, Ramboer CHR: Anisakiasis caused by herring in vinegar: a little known medical problem. *Gut* 1988;29:843.

173. Rosset JS, McClatchey KD, Knisely AS: Anisakis larval type I in fresh salmon. *Am J Clin Pathol* 1982;78:54.

174. Siurala M: Gastric lesion in some megaloblastic anemias with special reference to the mucosal lesion in pernicious tapeworm anemia. *Acta Med Scand* 1954;151:1.

175. Oberhuber G, Kastner N, Stolte M: Giardiasis: a histological analysis of 57 cases. *Scand J Gastroenterol* 1997;32:48.

176. Weber DJ, Walker DH: Rocky Mountain spotted fever. *Infect Dis Clin North Am* 1991;5:19.

177. Ruiz-Beltran R, Herrero-Herrero JI, Walker DH, Cunado-Rodriguez A: Mechanisms of upper gastrointestinal hemorrhage in Mediterranean spotted fever. *Trop Geogr Med* 1990;42:78.

178. Carpenter HA, Talley NJ: Gastroscopy is incomplete without biopsy: clinical relevance of distinguishing gastropathy from gastritis. *Gastroenterology* 1995;108:917.

179. Quintero E, Kaunitz J, Nishizaki Y, et al: Uremia increases gastric mucosal permeability and acid back diffusion injury in the rat. *Gastroenterology* 1992;103:176.

180. Bushnell L, Bjorkman D, McGreevy J: Ultrastructural changes in gastric epithelium caused by bile salt. *J Surg Res* 1990;49:280.

181. Dixon MF, O'Connor HJ, Axon ATR, et al: Reflux gastritis: distinct histopathological entity? *J Clin Pathol* 1986;39:524.

182. Sipponen P, Kekki M, Siurala M: Age-related trends of gastritis and intestinal metaplasia in gastric carcinoma patients and in controls representing the population at large. *Br J Cancer* 1984;49:521.

183. Villako K, Siurala M: The behaviour of gastritis and related conditions in different population samples. *Ann Clin Res* 1981;13:114.

184. Genta RM, Gürer IE, Graham DY, et al: Adherence of *Helicobacter pylori* to areas of incomplete intestinal metaplasia in the gastric antrum. *Gastroenterology* 1996;111:1206.

185. Ota H, Katsuyama T, Nakajima S, et al: Intestinal metaplasia with adherent Helicobacter pylori: a hybrid epithelium with both gastric and intestinal features. *Hum Pathol* 1998;29:846.

186. Genta RM: Helicobacter pylori, inflammation, mucosal damage and apoptosis: pathogenesis and definition of gastric atrophy. *Gastroenterology* 1997;113:S51.

187. Correa P: Human gastric carcinogenesis; a multistep and multifactorial process – first American Cancer Society award lecture on cancer epidemiology and prevention. *Cancer Res* 1992;52:6735.

188. Nomura A, Yamakawa H, Ishidate, et al: Intestinal metaplasia in Japan: association with diet. *J Natl Cancer Inst* 1982;68:401.

189. Tredaniel J, Boffeta P, Buiatti A, et al: Tobacco smoking and gastric cancer: a review and metaanalysis. *Int J Cancer* 1997;72:565.

190. Offerhaus GJA, Price AB, Haot J, et al: Observer agreement on the grading of gastric atrophy. *Histopathology* 1999;34:320.

191. Ruiz B, Garay J, Johnson W, et al: Morphometric assessment of gastric antral atrophy: comparison with visual evaluation. *Histopathology* 2001;39:235.

192. Genta RM: Atrophy and atrophic gastritis: one step beyond the Sydney system. *Ital J Gastroenterol Hepatol* 1998;20:S273.

193. Irvine WJ: The association of atrophic gastritis with autoimmune thyroid disease. *Clin Endocrinol Metab* 1975;4:351.

194. Valnes K, Brandtzaeg P, Elgjo K, et al: Local immunoglobulin production is different in gastritis associated with dermatitis herpetiformis and simple gastritis. *Gut* 1987;28:1589.

195. Sengi M, Brrelli O, Pucarelli I, et al: Early manifestations of gastric autoimmunity in patients with juvenile autoimmune thyroid diseases. *J Clin Endocrinol Metab* 2004;89:4944.

196. De Block CE, De Leeuw IH, Bogers JJ, et al: Autoimmune gastropathy in type I diabetic patients with parietal cell antibodies: histological and clinical findings. *Diabetes Care* 2003;26:82.

197. Claeys D, Faller G, Appelmelk BJ, et al: The gastric H^+K^+ ATPase is a major autoantigen in *Helicobacter pylori* gastritis with body mucosal atrophy. *Gastroenterology* 1998;115:340.

198. Carmel R: Reassessment of the relative prevalences of antibodies to gastric parietal cell and to intrinsic factor in patients with pernicious anemia—Influence of patient age and race. *Clin Exper Immunol* 1992;89:74.

199. DeAizpurua HJ, Ungar B, Toh B-H: Autoantibody to the gastrin receptor in pernicious anemia. *N Engl J Med* 1985;313:479.

200. Ardeman S, Chanarin I: Intrinsic factor antibodies and intrinsic factor mediated vitamin B12 absorption in pernicious anemia. *Gut* 1966;6:436.

201. Samloff IM, Varis K, Ihamaki T, et al: Relationships among serum pepsinogen I, serum pepsinogen II and gastric mucosal histology. A study in relatives of patients with pernicious anemia. *Gastroenterology* 1982;83:204.

202. Torbenson M, Abraham SC, Boitnott J, et al: Autoimmune gastritis: distinct histological and immunohistochemical findings before complete loss of oxyntic glands. *Mod Pathol* 2002;15:102.

203. Elsborg L, Mosbech J: Pernicious anaemia as a risk factor in gastric cancer. *Acta Med Scand* 1979;206:315.

204. Imerslund O, Bjorrstad P: Familial vitamin B12 malabsorption. *Acta Haematol* 1963;30:1.

205. Jevremovic D, Torbenson M, Murray JA, et al: Atrophic autoimmune pangastritis: a distinctive form of antral and fundic gastritis associated with systemic autoimmune disease. *Am J Surg Pathol* 2006;30:1412.

206. Plaut AG: Trefoil peptides in the defense of the gastrointestinal tract. *N Engl J Med* 1997;336:506.

207. Wright NA, Pike C, Elia G: Induction of a novel epidermal growth factor secreting cell lineage by mucosal ulceration in human gastrointestinal stem cells. *Nature* 1990;343:82.

208. Stemmermann GN: Intestinal metaplasia of the stomach. *Cancer* 1994;74:556.

209. Fennerty MB, Emerson JC, Sampliner RE, et al: Gastric intestinal metaplasia in ethnic groups in the southwestern United States. *Cancer Epidemiol Biomarkers Prev* 1992;1:293.

210. Fennerty MB: Gastric intestinal metaplasia on routine endoscopic biopsy. *Gastroenterology* 2003;125:586.

211. James R, Erler T, Kazenwadel J: Structure of the murine homeobox gene cdx-e. Expression in embryonic and adult intestinal epithelium. *J Biol Chem* 1994;269:15229.

212. Tsukamoto T, Inada K, Tanaka H, et al: Down-regulation of agastric transcription factor, Sox2 and ectopic expression of intestinal homeobox genes, Cdz1 and Cdx2: inverse correlation during progression from gastric/intestinal-mixed to complete intestinal metaplasia. *J Cancer Res Clin Oncol* 2004;130:135.

213. Piazuelo MB, Hague S, Delgado A, et al: Phenotypic differences between esophageal and gastric intestinal metaplasia. *Mod Pathol* 2004;17:62.

214. Siurula M, Lehtola J, Ihamaki T: Atrophic gastritis and its sequelae. Results of 19-23 years' follow-up examinations. *Scand J Gastroenterol* 1974;9:441.

215. Otsuka T, Tsukamto T, Mizoshita T, et al: Coexistence of gastric- and intestinal-type endocrine cells in gastric and intestinal mixed intestinal metaplasia of the human stomach. *Pathol Int* 2005;55:170.

216. Newbold KM, MacDonald F, Allum WH: Undifferential columnar cells on the gastric interfoveolar crest: a previously undescribed observation. *J Pathol* 1988;155:311.

217. Rubio C, Hayashi T, Stemmermann G: Ciliated gastric cells: a study of their phenotypic characteristics. *Mod Pathol* 1990;3:720.

218. Doglioni C, Laurino L, Dei Tos AP, et al: Pancreatic (acinar) metaplasia of the gastric mucosa. Histology, ultrastructure, immunocytochemistry, and clinicopathologic correlations of 101 cases. *Am J Surg Pathol* 1993;17:1134.

219. Krishnamurthy S, Integlia MJ, Grand RJ, Dayal Y: Pancreatic acinar cell clusters in pediatric gastric mucosa. *Am J Surg Pathol* 1998;22;100.

220. Leys CM, Nomura S, Rudzinski E, et al: Expression of PDX-1 in human gastric metaplasia and gastric adenocarcinoma. *Hum Pathol* 2006;37:1162.

221. Fenoglio-Preiser C: Creating a framework for diagnosing the benign gastric biopsy. *Curr Diag Pathol* 1998;5:2.

222. Danzi JT, Farmer RG, Sullivan BH, et al: Endoscopic features of gastroduodenal Crohn's disease. *Gastroenterology* 1976;70:9.

223. Gould SR, Handley AJ, Barnardo BE: Rectal and gastric involvement in a case of sarcoidosis. *Gut* 1973;14:971.

224. Johnstone JM, Morson BC: Eosinophilic gastroenteritis. *Histopathology* 1978;2:335.

225. Caldwell JH, Mekhjian HS, Hurtubise PE, et al: Eosinophilic gastroenteritis with obstruction: immunological studies of seven patients. *Gastroenterology* 1978;74:825.

226. Cello JP: Eosinophilic gastroenteritis: a complex disease entity. *Am J Med* 1979;67:1097.

227. Talley NJ, Shorter RG, Phillips SF, Zinsmeister AR: Eosinophilic gastroenteritis: a clinicopathological study of patients with the disease of the mucosa, muscle layer, and subserosal tissues. *Gut* 1990;31:54.

228. Goldman H, Proujansky R: Allergic proctitis and gastroenteritis in children. Clinical and mucosal biopsy features in 53 cases. *Am J Surg Pathol* 1986;10:75.

229. Wershil BK, Furuta GT, Wang ZS, Galli SJ: Mast cell-dependent neutrophil and mononuclear cell recruitment in immunoglobulin E-induced gastric reactions in mice. *Gastroenterology* 1996;110:1482.

230. Haot J, Jouret A, Willette M, et al: Lymphocytic gastritis-prospective study of its relationship with varioliform gastritis. *Gut* 1990;31:282.

231. Wolber R, Owen D, DelBuono L, et al: Lymphocytic gastritis in patients with celiac sprue or sprue-like intestinal disease. *Gastroenterology* 1990;98:310.

232. Dixon MF, Wyatt JI, Burke DA, Rathbone DI: Lymphocytic gastritis—relationship to Campylobacter pylori infection. *J Pathol* 1988;154:125.

233. Haot J, Bogomoletz QV, Jouret A, Mainguet P: Menetrier's disease with lymphocytic gastritis. *Hum Pathol* 1991;22:379.

234. Wolber RA, Owen DA, Anderson FH, Freeman HJ: Lymphocytic gastritis and giant gastric folds associated with gastrointestinal protein loss. *Mod Pathol* 1991;4:13.

235. Wu T-T, Hamilton SR: Lymphocytic gastritis: association with etiology and topology. *Am J Surg Pathol* 1999;23:153.

236. Farahat K, Hainaut P, Jamar F, et al: Lymphocytic gastritis: an unusual cause of hypoproteinaemia. *J Int Med* 1993;234:95.

237. Snover DC, Weisdorf SA, Vercellotti GM, et al: A histopathologic study of gastric and small intestinal graft-versus-host disease following allogeneic bone marrow transplantation. *Hum Pathol* 1985;16:387.

238. Weisdorf DJ, Snover DC, Haake R, et al: Acute upper gastrointestinal graft-versus-host disease: clinical significance and response to immunosuppressive therapy. *Blood* 1990;76:624.

239. Washington K, Bentley RC, Green AM, et al: Gastric graft-versus-host disease: a blinded histologic study. *Am J Surg Pathol* 1997;21:1037.

240. Welch DC, Wirth PS, Goldenting JR, et al: Gastric graft-versus-host disease revisited. Does proton pump inhibitor therapy affect endoscopic gastric biopsy interpretation? *Am J Surg Pathol* 2001;30:444.

241. Stancu M, Petris G, Palumbo TP, Lev R: Collagenous gastritis associated with lymphocytic colitis and celiac disease. *Arch Pathol Lab Med* 2001;125:1579.

242. Lagorce-Pages C, Fabiani B, Bouvier R, et al: Collagenous gastritis: a report of six cases. *Am J Surg Pathol* 2001;25:1174.

243. Freeman HJ: Topographic mapping of collagenous gastritis. *Can J Gastroenterol* 2001;475.

244. Vesoulis Z, Lozanski G, Ravichandran P, Esber E: Collagenous gastritis: a case report, morphologic evaluation and review. *Mod Pathol* 2000;13:591.

245. Castellano VM, Munoz MT, Colina F, et al: Collagenous gastrobulbitis and collagenous colitis. Case report and review of the literature. *Scand J Gastroenterol* 1999;34:632.

246. Winslow JL, Trainer TD, Colleti RB: Collagenous gastritis: a long term follow-up study with the development of endocrine cell hyperplasia, intestinal metaplasia and epithelial changes indeterminate for dysplasia. *Am J Clin Pathol* 2001;116:753.

247. Cote JF, Hankard GF, Faugre C, et al: Collagenous gastritis revealed by severe anemia in a child. *Hum Pathol* 1998;29:883.

248. Peek R, Miller G, Tham T, et al: Heightened inflammatory response and cytokine expression in vivo to cagA- Helicobacter pylori strains. *Lab Invest* 1995;73:76.

249. Tham KT, Peek RM, Atherton JC, et al: *Helicobacter pylori* genotypes, host factors and gastric mucosal histopathology in peptic ulcer disease. *Hum Pathol* 2001;32:264.

250. Fiocca R, Villani L, Luinetti O, et al: Helicobacter colonization and histopathological profile of chronic gastritis in patients with or without dyspepsia, mucosal erosion and peptic ulcer-a morphological approach to the study of ulcerogenesis in man. *Virch Arch A Pathol Anat Histopathol* 1992;420:489.

251. Rotter JI, Peterson G, Samloff IM, et al: Genetic heterogeneity of hyperpepsinogenic I and normopepsinogenic in duodenal ulcer disease. *Ann Intern Med* 1979;91:372.

252. Stemmermann GN, Marcus EB, Buist AS, MacLean CJ: Relative impact of smoking and reduced pulmonary function on peptic ulcer risk. A prospective study of Japanese men in Hawaii. *Gastroenterology* 1989;96:1419.

253. Sipponen P, Seppala K, Aarynen M, et al: Chronic gastritis and gastroduodenal ulcer: a case control study on risk on coexisting duodenal or gastric ulcer in patients with gastritis. *Gut* 1989;30:922.

254. Azuma T, Teramae N, Hayakuma T, et al: Pepsinogen C gene polymorphisms associated with gastric body ulcer. *Gut* 1993;34:450.

255. Hopkins R, Girardi L, Turney E: Relationship between Helicobacter pylori eradication and reduced duodenal and gastric ulcer recurrence: a review. *Gastroenterology* 1996;110:1244.

256. Stadelmann K, Elster K, Stolte M, et al: The peptic gastric ulcer – histophotographic and functional investigations. *Scand J Gastroenterol* 1971;6:613.

257. Hawkey CJ: Review article: aspirin and gastrointestinal bleeding. *Aliment Pharmacol Ther* 1994;8:141.

258. Svanes C, Sereide JA, Skarstein A, et al: Smoking and ulcer perforation. *Gut* 1997;41:177.

259. Oi M, Oshida K, Sugimora S: The location of gastric ulcer. *Gastroenterology* 1959;36:45.
260. Kamada T, Fusamoto H, Majuzawa M, et al: "Trench ulcer" of the stomach. *Am J Gastroenterol* 1975;63:486.
261. Chua C, Jeyaraj P, Low C: Relative risks of complications in giant and nongiant gastric ulcers. *Am J Surg* 1992;164:94.
262. Playford RJ: Peptides and gastrointestinal mucosal integrity. *Gut* 1995;37:595.
263. Wong WM, Playford RJ, Wright NA: Peptide gene expression in gastrointestinal mucosal ulceration: ordered sequence or redundancy? *Gut* 2000;46:286.
264. Meuwissen SM, Ridwan BU, Hasper HJ, Innemee G: Hypertrophic protein-losing gastropathy. *Scand J Gastroenterol* 1992;27:1.
265. Wolfsen HC, Carpenter HA, Talley NJ: Menetrier's disease: a form of hypertrophic gastropathy or gastritis? *Gastroenterology* 1993;104:1310.
266. Cantanzaro C: Chronic hypertrophic gastritis: report of two cases in siblings. *Am J Gastroenterol* 1962;37:525.
267. Knight J, Matlak M, Condon V: Menetrier's disease in children: report of a case and review of the pediatric literature. *Pediatr Pathol* 1983;1:179.
268. Fishbein M, Kirschner BS, Gonzales-Vallina R, et al: Menetrier's disease associated with formula protein allergy and small intestinal injury in an infant. *Gastroenterology* 1992;103:1664.
269. Eisenstat D, Griffiths A, Cutz E, et al: Acute cytomegalovirus infection in a child with Menetrier's disease. *Gastroenterology* 1995;109:592.
270. Goldenring JR, Ray GS, Soroka CJ, et al: Overexpression of transforming growth factor-alpha alters differentiation of gastric cell lineages. *Dig Dis Sci* 1996;41:773.
271. Burdick JS, Chung E, Tanner G, et al: Treatment of Menetrier's disease with a monoclonal antibody against the epidermal growth factor receptor. *N Engl J Med* 2000;343:1697.
272. Isenberg JI, Walsh JH, Grossman MI: Zollinger-Ellison syndrome. *Gastroenterology* 1973;65:140.
272a. Aprile MR, Azzoni C, Gibril F, et al: Intramucosal cysts in the gastric body of patients with Zollinger-Ellison syndrome. *Hum Pathol* 2000;31:140.
273. Chaloupka JC, Gay BB, Caplan D: Campylobacter gastritis simulating Menetrier's disease by upper gastrointestinal radiography. *Pediatr Radiol* 1990;20:200.
274. Bayerdorffer E, Ritter MM, Brooks W, et al: Healing of protein losing hypertrophic gastropathy by eradication of Helicobacter pylori: is Helicobacter pylori a pathogenic factor in Menetrier's disease? *Gut* 1994;35:701.
275. Koch HK, Lesch R, Cremer M, Oehlert W: Polyps and polypoid foveolar hyperplasia in gastric biopsy specimens and their precancerous prevalence. *Front Gastrointest Res* 1979;4:183.
276. Abraham SC, Park SJ, Mugartegui L, et al: Sporadic fundic gland polyps with epithelial dysplasia: evidence for preferential targeting for mutations in the adenomatous polyposis coli gene. *Am J Pathol* 2002;161:1735.
277. Torbenson M, Lee JH, Cruz-Correa M, et al: Sporadic fundic gland polyposis: a clinical histological, and molecular analysis. *Mod Pathol* 2002;15:718.
278. Hizawa K, Iida M, Matsumoto T, et al: Natural history of fundic gland polyposis without familial adenomatosis coli: follow-up observations in 31 patients. *Radiology* 1993;189:429.
279. Mukada T, Kashiwagura J, Itasaka K, et al: Giant hyperplasiogenous polyp of the stomach simulating malignant polyp. *Tohoku J Exp Med* 1984;142:125.
280. Ginsberg GG, Al-Kawas FH, Fleischer DE, et al: Gastric polyps: relationship of size and histology to cancer risk. *Am J Gastroenterol* 1996;91:714.
281. Dijkhuisen SMM, Entius MM, Clement MJ, et al: Multiple hyperplastic polyps in the stomach: evidence for clonality and neoplastic potential. *Gastroenterology* 1997;112:561.
282. Johnston JM, Morson RC: Inflammatory fibroid polyp of the gastrointestinal tract. *Histopathology* 1978;2:349.
283. Stolte M, Finkenzeller G: Inflammatory fibroid polyp of the stomach. *Endoscopy* 1990;22:203.
284. Nishiyama Y, Koyama S, Andoh A, et al: Gastric inflammatory fibroid polyp treated with Helicobacter pylori eradication therapy. *Int Med* 2003;42:263.
285. Kim YI, Kim WH: Inflammatory fibroid polyps of gastrointestinal tract: evolution of histologic patterns. *Am J Clin Pathol* 1988;89:721.
286. Mori M, Tamura S, Enjoji M, Sugimachi K: Concomitant presence of inflammatory fibroid polyp and carcinoma or adenoma in the stomach. *Arch Pathol Lab Med* 1988;112:829.
287. Fonde EC, Rodning CB: Gastritis cystica profunda. *Am J Gastroenterol* 1986;81:459.
288. Furuse A, Koseni K, Takeshita M, et al: Retrograde gastric varices in a patient with total cavopulmonary. *Ann Thorac Surg* 1993;55:1574.
289. Pique JM: Portal hypertensive gastropathy. *Bail Clin Gastroenterol* 1997;11:257.
290. Ma CK, Rosenberg BF, Wong D, et al: Gastric antral vascular ectasia: the watermelon stomach. *Surg Pathol* 1988;1:231.
291. Jabbari M, Cherry R, Lough JI, Daly DS, et al: Gastric antral vascular ectasia: the watermelon stomach. *Gastroenterology* 1984;87:1165.
292. Miko TL, Thomazy VA: The caliber persistent artery of the stomach: a unifying approach to gastric aneurysms, Dieulafoy's lesion and submucosal arterial malformation. *Hum Pathol* 1988;19:914.
293. Eidus LB, Rasuli P, Manion D, Heringer R: Caliber-persistent artery of the stomach (Dieulafoy's vascular malformation). *Gastroenterology* 1990;99:1507.
294. Dave PB, Romeu J, Antonelli A, Eiser AR: Gastrointestinal telangiectasias. A source of bleeding in patients receiving hemodialysis. *Arch Intern Med* 1984;144:1781.
295. Theriault G, Cordier S, Harvey R: Skin telangiectases in workers at an aluminum plant. *N Engl J Med* 1980;303:1278.
296. Lindner A, Charra B, Sherrard DJ, et al: Accelerated atherosclerosis in prolonged maintenance hemodialysis. *N Engl J Med* 1974;290:697.
297. Tobin JM, Siha B, Ramani P, et al: Upper gastrointestinal mucosal disease in pediatric Crohn's disease and ulcerative colitis. A blinded control study. *J Pediatr Gastroenterol Nutr* 2001;32:443.
298. Menke D, Kyle RA, Fleming CR, et al: Symptomatic gastric amyloidosis in patients with primary systemic amyloidosis. *Mayo Clin Proc* 1993;68:763.
299. Cherner JA, Jensen RT, Dubois A, et al: Gastrointestinal dysfunction in systemic mastocytosis. *Gastroenterology* 1988;95:657.
300. Ostuni PA, Germana B, Dimario F, et al: Gastric involvement in primary Sjogren's syndrome. *Clin Exp Rheumatol* 1993;11:21.

The Neoplastic Stomach

Gastric neoplasms constitute a heterogeneous group of tumors; most are adenocarcinomas. Less common gastric cancers, such as lymphomas, neuroendocrine tumors, and stromal tumors, are discussed in Chapters 17 to 19.

ADENOCARCINOMA DISTAL TO THE CARDIA AND ITS ANATOMIC PRECURSORS

The stomach is divided into three subsites: The cardia, the corpus, and the pyloric antrum. Cancers of the cardia and Barrett-associated adenocarcinomas of the esophagus share similar backgrounds, temporal trends, molecular profiles, and behavioral patterns. These two cancers constitute gastroesophageal junction (GEJ) cancer and are discussed in Chapter 3. The epidemiologic backgrounds and temporal trends of cancers arising distal to the cardia are distinctly different from those arising in the cardia. Noncardia stomach cancer was once the most common human cancer worldwide, but it has shown a steep decline in frequency in the United States and Western Europe, where it is now less common than cancer of the GEJ in white males (1). Distal stomach cancer is still very common in developing countries and among migrants from them.

Epidemiology

Gastric carcinoma shows striking temporal and geographic variations in frequency (2), with a more than 10-fold difference in incidence between countries with high and low rates (Table 5.1). England and Wales offer a good example of the temporal decline in noncardia gastric cancer incidence, with male rates falling from 8.5 to 4.1 between 1971 and 1998, and female rates falling from 3.8 to 1.7 over the same time period (3). First-generation migrants from high-risk countries to low-risk countries continue to experience the high rates of their motherland, whereas their children and grandchildren show rates that approach those of the host country (4). This supports the concept that environmental exposures in early life generate cancer precursors that persist into adulthood and are not reversed by a more favorable environment.

The age-specific gastric cancer incidence rates rise steeply after 50 years of age in all populations, peaking at 673 per 100,000 at age 80 in Miyagi, Japan, compared to 103 per 100,000 for 80-year-old white males in low-risk Los Angeles (2). The wide incidence differences in high- and low-risk populations is already apparent at age 25 when the Miyagi and Korean male rates stand at 2.1 and 4.1, respectively, compared to the Los Angeles white male rate of 0.3 per 100,000. This supports the concept that exposure to environmental hazards begins early in life among people in high-risk populations. Gastric cancer incidence rates for men are approximately twice those of women in all populations for persons over 50 years of age, but the male:female incidence ratio is 1 or less at younger ages. The age-related variation in the male:female incidence ratio suggests that host factors may influence the level of risk of acquiring this cancer.

The rapid decline in the frequency of gastric cancer in the United States since World War II is best appreciated by following the age-adjusted mortality rates for this tumor in white males: 16.34 per 100,000 for the years 1950–1969 and 7.33 per 100,000 for the years 1970–1994 (5). A decrease in gastric cancer incidence since 1973 has occurred in both high- and low-risk countries as is shown in Table 5.2 (2). The earlier decrease in stomach cancer in Western countries was unplanned, resulting from modern refrigeration of foods, year-round access to fresh fruits and vegetables, and, more recently, the treatment of *Helicobacter pylori* infections.

Gastric cancer arising distal to the cardia does not behave as a single disease, but as several diseases that affect different parts of the stomach and vary in their histologic presentations. Lauren (6) first recognized that distal stomach cancers occur in two forms that differ in their structure and behavior: An intestinal type that consists of intestinal-type glands and a diffuse type that consists of discohesive cells supported by a desmoplastic stroma. The intestinal type is more likely to show vascular spread and hepatic metastases. The diffuse form has a less favorable prognosis, is less likely to have hepatic metastases, and is prone to transperitoneal spread. Both types have decreased in frequency in developed countries and share similar environmental exposures. Age, sex, and blood type, as well as inherited predispositions, determine whether a patient will develop an intestinal or diffuse cancer. The distinction between intestinal and diffuse types of gastric cancer has proven to be valuable in epidemiologic studies and in assessing tumor prognosis. Mixed forms of

233

TABLE 5.1 Geographic Variation, Male, Age-standardized Gastric Cancer Incidence Rates per 100,000

High incidence:	China, Changle	145.0
	Japan, Yamagata	91.6
	Korea, Busan	72.5
Intermediate incidence:	Costa Rica	40.1
	Belarus	40.5
	Italy, Romagna	32.3
	Portugal	38.3
	Colombia, Cali	30.5
Low incidence:	United States, Utah	4.6
	United States, New Mexico	4.4
	Switzerland, Geneva	7.8

these cancers occur, as well as distinctive subtypes of these tumors, but the practical advantages of this simple classification have held up over time.

Both types of gastric cancer occur in high-risk populations, but the proportion of diffuse tumors is increased in low-risk groups. A retrospective analysis of gastric cancer in the SEER (Surveillance, Epidemiology, and End Results) registries of the United States found that diffuse cancers have increased in frequency between the years 1973 and 2000, while intestinal-type cancers have decreased over the same time period (7). A similar trend may account for a recent decrease in antral carcinomas relative to those in the middle third of the stomach in Japan (8), since the proportion of diffuse cancers is higher in the more proximal stomach. The typical differences in intestinal and diffuse gastric cancers are summarized in Table 5.3.

Predisposing Factors and Conditions

The persons at highest risk of acquiring gastric cancer are concentrated in the lower economic strata of developing countries. The initial steps in cancer induction occur in childhood with infection by *H. pylori* (9). The youngest children of large families living in crowded, unsanitary conditions are at highest risk (10). Familial clusters of stomach cancer result from a shared exposure to environmental hazards (11) and to inherited factors (12).

Genetic Factors

There are a number of types of genetic and epigenetic changes that play a role in the predisposition to or the development of gastric carcinoma (Table 5.4). These include activation of oncogenes, growth factors and growth factor receptors, inactivation of tumor suppressor genes, DNA repair genes, and cell adhesion molecules, as well as alterations in cell cycle regulatory genes. Inherited factors interact with environmental hazards to increase gastric cancer risk in two ways: (a) germline mutations account for well-defined, but infrequent, familial cancer syndromes; and (b) polymorphisms in genes that govern cell cycling or enzymes that catalyze carcinogen detoxification may also influence gastric cancer risk. Other types of changes occur in sporadic tumors.

Inherited gastric cancer predisposition syndromes account for approximately 10% of gastric cancers. The genetic events are known for some but not all of the predispositions. The *hereditary nonpolyposis colon cancer syndrome* (HNPCC) is an example of the interaction of environmental hazards with germline mutations. Persons with this autosomal dominant condition are at increased risk of developing

TABLE 5.2 Temporal Trends in Gastric Cancer Incidence Rates, Selected National Registries

	Male		Female	
	1973–1977[a]	1993–1997[b]	1973–1977	1993–1997
Brazil (Sao Paulo)	45.7	21.2	19.0	10.3
Colombia (Cali)	46.3	30.5	27.3	18.8
United States (Iowa)	7.5	6.0	3.1	2.1
Japan (Miyagi)	88.0	69.0	42.0	27.1
Finland	29.7	12.6	15.5	7.0
Poland (Warsaw)	31.4	22.9	12.9	8.4
Italy (Varese)	38.5	23.6	19.1	11.2
Spain (Navarre)	34.8	12.7	18.2	6.4
United Kingdom (Oxford)	20.0	10.7	10.7	4.0

[a]From Kolonel LN, Hanken J, Nomura AMY, et al: Multiethnic studies of diet, nutrition and cancer in Hawaii. In: Hayashi Y, Nagao M, Sugimura T (eds). *Diet, Nutrition and Cancer.* Tokyo, Japan: Scientific Societies Press, 1986, pp 29–40.
[b]From Henson DE, Dittus C, Younes M, et al: Differential trends in the intestinal and diffuse types of gastric carcinoma in the United States, 1973–2000. *Arch Pathol Lab Med* 2004;128:765.

TABLE 5.3   **Intestinal Versus Diffuse Gastric Cancers**

	Intestinal	Diffuse
Epidemiologic type	"Epidemic" Type seen in high-risk populations	"Endemic" Incidence similar in most countries
Characteristic subsite	Antrum	Corpus
Gross appearance	Polypoid, fungating	Linitis plastica
Histology	Cohesive, gland-forming cells	Discohesive, signet ring cells
Distant disease	Discrete hepatic metastases	Diffuse, transperitoneal spread
Precursor lesions	Multifocal atrophic gastritis	Superficial gastritis
Age, gender	Males >60 years of age	Females, younger men
Prognosis	Better survival	Poor

cancer at sites other than the colon, including the stomach. HNPCC is due to a germline mutation in mismatch repair genes. The risk of gastric cancer in Korean patients who carry these mutations is 3.2-fold greater than the general population of Korea, where gastric cancer accounts for 25% of all male cancers (12). In occidental countries HNPCC-associated gastric cancer has decreased in frequency in parallel with the decline in sporadic cancer (13), as might be expected if a DNA repair defect is not challenged by genotoxic hazards. The Finnish HNPCC registry has identified 45 patients with gastric cancer in 51 HNPCC families (14), and gastric cancer was the only cancer found in 22 of these. The mean age of gastric cancer development was 6 years older than colon cancer in these HNPCC families. Like sporadic stomach cancer, but unlike most Finnish familial stomach cancers, the HNPCC cancers were intestinal in type and arose in the distal stomach.

Familial adenomatous polyposis (FAP) may involve the stomach as well as the large bowel. As in the colon, gastric cancers are preceded by the development of dysplasia. The dysplasia may be flat or in polypoid lesions including adenomas, hyperplastic polyps, and fundic gland polyps. An environmental influence is suggested by the observation that Japanese patients with FAP have more frequent gastric adenomas and cancers than westerners with FAP (15,16). This may reflect the higher Japanese exposure to gastric cancer risk factors.

Germline mutations in the E-cadherin/CDH1 gene were first recognized as a source of familial stomach cancer in a

TABLE 5.4   **Types of Genetic Alterations in Gastric Carcinogenesis**

Mutations
Chromosomal losses
Amplification and/or overexpression
CpG island methylation
Microsatellite instability
Genetic polymorphisms
Telomerase activation

New Zealand Maori family (17), and have since been shown to have a worldwide distribution (18,19). This form of familial cancer is now termed *hereditary diffuse gastric cancer* (HDGC). E-cadherin is a cell adhesion protein. The loss of its function (and loss of its normal expression on the cell membrane; Fig. 5.1) due to gene mutations results in the discohesive cells that characterize sporadic diffuse gastric cancers and lobular breast cancers. It is not surprising, therefore, that familial gastric cancers associated with germline mutations in this gene are diffuse in type and that HDGC kindreds also show an increased frequency of lobular breast cancer (20). Asymptomatic patients who carry the HDGC mutation are treated with prophylactic gastrectomy since the early lesions are undetectable at the time of endoscopy (21). Multiple superficial mucosal cancers may be found at the time of gastrectomy (Fig. 5.1). The chance discovery of similar lesions in an endoscopic biopsy should alert the pathologist to a possible HDGC mutation (22). Lynch et al (13) suggest that these superficial neoplastic foci represent a widespread field effect due to promoter hypermethylation and that dysregulation of genes required for invasion and metastases are much less common.

Carriers of *BRCA1/2 mutations* have a substantial increase in the lifetime risk of breast and ovarian cancer. These mutations have been related to a variety of other sites as well, including the stomach. The Swedish Family Cancer Database assessed the cancer incidence in classified family members (n = 944,723) and compared their cancer experience with that of the general population of Sweden and found a twofold increase in the risk of acquiring stomach cancer before age 70 among male members of families with breast and ovarian cancer (23).

Germline *p53 mutations* are inherited among families diagnosed with the Li-Fraumeni syndrome. Cancers arise at diverse sites in these families (24). Interaction with environmental factors is suggested by the more common prevalence of stomach cancer in Japanese families with this syndrome than among affected American families (25). Patients with the Peutz-Jeghers syndrome are at very high relative and absolute risk for gastrointestinal and other cancers. The relative risk of stomach cancer risk with this syndrome is 213

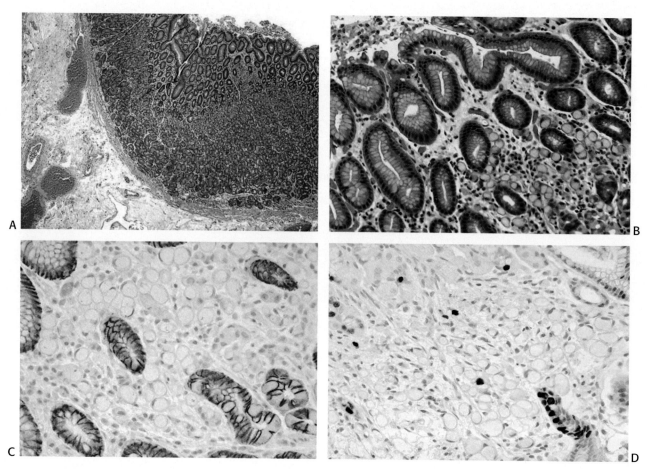

FIG. 5.1. Hereditary diffuse gastric cancer in a young male with a strong family history of diffuse gastric cancer. **A:** At a low-power cursory glance the mucosa appears to be more or less normal. **B:** Higher magnification discloses multiple foci of intramucosal diffuse (signet ring cell) gastric carcinoma. **C:** E-cadherin immunostain showing staining of the nonneoplastic gastric glands and absence of staining in the tumor cells in the lamina propria and a few isolated tumor cells in the glands (*lower right*). **D:** Ki-6 immunostain showing the low proliferative index of the tumor cells. A portion of a nonneoplastic gland shows some proliferation (*lower right*).

(95% confidence interval [CI] = 96 to 368) (26). A mucoid gastric adenocarcinoma associated with germline mutation in the STK11 gene has been identified in a Japanese Peutz-Jeghers family (27).

Interaction between the Environment and Inherited Polymorphisms

By 1966 a large number of studies had found a consistent relationship between the diffuse type of stomach cancer and blood type A (28). It seems unlikely that blood type A has a direct role in the carcinogenic process, but it may serve as a marker for an as yet unidentified mutation, or a genetic polymorphism that increases the cancer risk by modulating the host reaction to environmental hazards. For example, the *interleukin-1 (IL-1) B* gene that encodes a proinflammatory cytokine is highly polymorphic (29). Gastric cancer patients are more likely to have the IL-1B-31T/IL-1RN* phenotype. Such persons mount an especially strong inflammatory

response to *H. pylori* infection through IL-1 overexpression. The level of gastric cancer risk varies greatly depending on the association of specific genotypes of the infecting organism with different IL-B phenotypes, with an odds ratio (OR) of 87 (CI = 11 to 697) when the vacAs1 strain associates with IL-B-511*T (30). In contrast, when *H. pylori* strain vacAm1 associates with this phenotype, the OR is substantial but falls to 7.4 (CI = 3.2 to 17). Tumor necrosis factor-α (TNF-α), another proinflammatory protein, is increased in the gastric mucosa of persons infected with *H. pylori*. The TNF-α-308* allele increases TNF-α production. The risk of acquiring multifocal atrophic gastritis and gastric cancer increases in persons with the high-risk IL-1B and TNF-α genotypes (31).

Variations in glutathione-S-transferase (GST-1), an enzyme that catalyzes the conjugation of numerous carcinogens, may modify the stomach cancer risk from smoking or ingested carcinogens. The null variant of the μ form of GST-1 constitutes 40% of the Japanese population and associates with a modest increased risk of gastric carcinoma (32). A similar association has been identified between gastric cancer and a variation in the *N-acetyl transferase* gene (*NAT-1*) (33). Aromatic and heterocyclic amine carcinogens are acetylated by NAT-1, but persons with a variant form of this enzyme lack this function. Cytochrome 450 2E1 (CYP2E1) is involved in the metabolism of environmental carcinogens. Two reports suggest that polymorphisms in this gene interact with smoking to increase the risk of gastric cancer (34). Finally, the lining of the stomach is protected from environmental insults by mucin. The *MUC1* gene is polymorphic and individuals with small *MUC1* genotypes have an increased risk of gastric cancer (35).

A recent Korean study has shown that polymorphisms in the DNA repair gene *XRCC1* may either enhance or reduce the risk of gastric cancer in this high-risk population (36). Carriers of one haplotype (194/Trp, 280/Arg, 399Arg) are at decreased risk of gastric cancer, while those with another haplotype (194/Arg, 280/Arg, 399Arg) are at increased risk of antral cancer. The polymorphism in *XRCC1* interacts with a polymorphism in *adenosine diphosphate ribosyl transferase* (*ADPRT*) in such a way that *ADPRT* and *XRCC1* polymorphisms confer host susceptibility to gastric carcinoma possibly from reduced *ADPRT–XRCC1* interactions and attenuated base excision repair, particularly in smokers (36a).

Other Genetic Factors

In addition to the genetic factors listed above, there are a number of somatic alterations that play a role in gastric cancer development. These include sporadic alterations in oncogenes, tumor suppressor genes, and mismatch repair genes. These genetic alterations include many that are altered in other cancers. Genetic instability, CpG island methylation, telomerase activation, and p53 mutations tend to occur early in the development of gastric cancer. Some of the more common alterations are listed in Table 5.5.

Epigenetic alterations, the most common of which is CpG island methylation of the promoter regions of cancer-related genes, are also common in gastric carcinoma. There is global DNA methylation and subsequent gene silencing in gastric cancers and its precursors and tumors showing these changes fall into the CpG island methylator (CIMP) phenotype. When the CIMP phenotype occurs, there is frequently an absence of mutation in genes that are commonly mutated in gastric cancer, such as *p53* (36b). Genes that are frequently hypermethylated in the setting of Ebstein-Barr virus (EBV) include *p16* and *hMLH1* (36c). Promoter methylation of *E-cadherin* is common in the setting of *H. pylori* infection (36d). *Sonic hedgehog*, a gene important in foregut development, is also frequently hypermethylated (36e).

Environmental Factors

Environmental factors may affect gastric cancer risk directly or inversely. Several environmental hazards combine to induce distal stomach cancer; other environmental factors

TABLE 5.5 Selected Genetic Alterations in Sporadic Gastric Carcinoma

Tumor Suppressor Genes

p53	Commonly mutated in dysplasia and invasive carcinoma
p16	Loss or hypermethylated in dysplasia and carcinomas
FHIT	Altered in dysplasia and invasive carcinoma
APC	Mutations occur early in the dysplasia-carcinoma sequence
Rb	Loss in invasive carcinoma
DCC	Loss in invasive carcinomas

Mismatch Repair Genes (Altered by Mutation or Hypermethylation)

hMLH1	Results in MSI phenotype
hMLH2	Results in MSI phenotype
hMSH2	Results in MSI phenotype
hMSH3	Results in MSI phenotype
hMSH6	Results in MSI phenotype

Oncogenes

Cyclin D1	Frequently overexpressed in invasive adenocarcinomas; amplification prognostic

Growth Factors and Their Receptors

EGFR	Overexpressed in >75% of invasive carcinomas
TGF-α	Overexpressed in invasive carcinoma
c-erbB2	Amplified in a small percentage of invasive carcinomas; prognostic factor
c-met	Frequently amplified and overexpressed in invasive cancer
K-sam	Often abnormal in diffuse cancers

Cell Adhesion Molecules

E-cadherin	Loss of expression in dysplasia and invasive carcinoma, especially diffuse cancers
α-catenin	Loss of expression in invasive carcinoma
β-catenin	Nuclear expression occurs in some invasive carcinomas reflecting abnormal Wnt signaling

protect the stomach from exposure to these hazards. The risk of acquiring stomach cancer ultimately depends on which prevails.

Helicobacter pylori *Infection*

H. pylori infection is usually the step leading to the development of gastric cancer. The infection is acquired in childhood (37). Infected children carry the infection and its anatomic consequences into middle and old age (9). *H. pylori* gastritis may affect 75% of persons in high-risk populations, but no more than 5% of infected individuals develop stomach

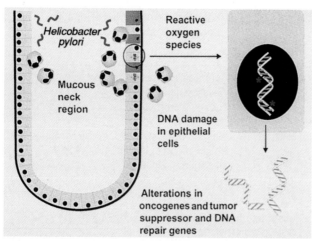

FIG. 5.2. Mechanisms by which *Helicobacter pylori* increases gastric cancer risk.

cancer (38), indicating that infection does not act alone. Prospective studies have shown a consistent association between the presence of distal gastric cancer and high antibody levels against *H. pylori* (39). Asymptomatic persons with the highest *H. pylori* antibody levels are the most likely to develop gastric cancer in these studies. When compared to other *H. pylori* strains, the *cagA* strain is associated with heightened antibody levels, a more robust inflammatory response, and a higher risk of gastric cancer (39). One mechanism by which *H. pylori* infection may increase stomach cancer risk is through exposure of replicating cells to reactive oxygen species derived from the inflammatory cells that are part of *H. pylori* gastritis (Fig. 5.2).

The initial manifestation of *H. pylori* infection is severe superficial gastritis, followed by the development of multifocal atrophic gastritis and intestinal metaplasia (see Chapter 4). The process begins at the antral–corpus junction and along the lesser curvature of the antrum. Over time the atrophic foci expand and fuse so that in old age much of the oxyntic mucosa is replaced by intestinalized tissue. Cancer risk is highest in *H. pylori*–infected persons at the nadir of acid production (40). The achlorhydria favors a bacterial flora that may generate carcinogens through the nitrosation of dietary amines (41).

Diet

The pattern of food consumption may increase or reduce the risk of acquiring stomach cancer. The addition of nitroso compounds to the diet of experimental animals produces gastric cancer and its precursor, intestinal metaplasia (42). Epidemiologic studies show a direct association between the development of intestinal metaplasia and nitrate/nitrite consumption in humans (43). Salt intake also directly relates to stomach cancer risk in humans (44). The consumption of dried, salted fish in Japan and the consumption of salted, nitrosated foods through the winter months in northern

countries are examples of dietary practices that increase the stomach cancer risk. In contrast, fresh fruits and vegetables provide antinitrosating effects that protect the stomach from both exogenous and endogenous mutagenic nitroso compounds. Fresh fruits and vegetables function as antioxidants and contain substantial amounts of folate, ascorbic acid, carotene, and tocopherol. Epidemiologic studies of Japanese and European populations suggest that raw green and yellow vegetables protect against the development of gastric cancer (45), and a Japanese cohort study showed that increased fresh produce consumption and reduced consumption of pickled food reduced the gastric cancer risk, even in the presence of atrophic gastritis (46). The year-round availability of fresh produce eliminates the need to use salt to preserve vegetables. Smoking and salting of meat is no longer a necessity with the advent of universal household refrigeration. These two factors have contributed to the dramatic decrease in stomach cancer rates in Western countries after World War II.

Smoking

A meta-analysis of 37 case control studies on the relationship of smoking to gastric cancer yielded inconsistent results (47). This inconsistency is surprising and contrasts with the strong association of smoking with gastric ulcer (48), a disease that is closely related to intestinal metaplasia, *H. pylori* gastritis, and gastric cancer. The same analysis, however, found that each of ten prospective cohort studies showed a significantly increased risk of gastric cancer in the order of 1.5 to 2.5, four of the studies showing a dose response. Thus, the magnitude of smoking-related risk is low, but may account for 11% of stomach cancers worldwide (47).

Radiation

A dose-dependent increase in gastric cancer frequency has occurred among Japanese atomic bomb survivors, suggesting that ionizing radiation may play a role in gastric carcinogenesis (49). Additionally, radiotherapy in young patients increases their risk of gastric cancer when lymph nodes of the upper abdomen are included in the radiation field, as may occur in the treatment of lymphoma and testicular cancer (50).

Previous Gastric Surgery

The creation of a gastroenterostomy after subtotal gastrectomy for peptic ulcer is a well-established risk factor for the development of cancer in the gastric stump (Fig. 5.3) (51). The cancer may not be apparent until 17 to 20 years after the creation of the anastomosis. It is preceded by the appearance of gastritis and hyperplastic polyps at the anastomotic line (52). The cause of the increased risk is attributed to the reflux of bile and pancreatic juice into the gastric remnant, a hypothesis that is supported by rodent experiments that show the sequential development of gastritis, hyperplasia, metaplasia, and adenocarcinoma after duodenal contents

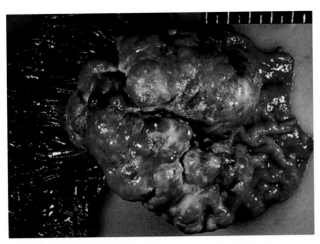

FIG. 5.3. Large polyploid gastric cancer originating in the gastric stump. The small bowel mucosa is seen on the left.

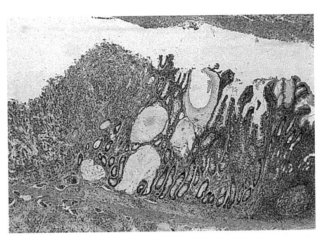

FIG. 5.4. Neoplastic progression in the stomach. A prominent area of follicular gastritis is present on the right side of the photograph. There is a transition to intestinal metaplasia as one moves toward the center of the figure. Dysplasia develops in the areas of intestinal metaplasia, until finally an invasive carcinoma of the intestinal type develops as seen on the far left side of the photograph. Note the tumor within the lymphatics under the muscularis mucosae.

were diverted into the stomach (53). Since subtotal gastrectomy is no longer commonly employed to treat peptic ulcer, this risk factor will disappear in the near future. Its place may be taken by subtotal gastrectomy for early antral cancer, a procedure that has become quite common in Asian high-risk countries with active screening programs of asymptomatic subjects (54). The interval between surgery for early cancer and the development of stump cancer may be shorter than after peptic ulcer surgery. Another potential source of postenterostomy stomach cancer is the Roux-en-Y gastrojejunostomy used to treat morbid obesity. Gastric cancer has been reported in four women at 5, 5, 13, and 22 years after surgery (55). Since bariatric surgery has become a very common procedure, we may expect increasing numbers of such cancers. The defunctionalized gastric segment is subject to the reflux of bile and alkaline secretions and the subsequent development of gastritis (56).

Predisposing Gastric Lesions

Gastric cancer does not arise de novo from a normal mucosa. Gastritis is usually the first step in cancer induction, whatever the underlying cause. In persons with polymorphisms that render them especially vulnerable to exogenous or endogenous carcinogens, an intense superficial gastritis may be the only anatomic precursor to cancer induction.

Multifocal Atrophic Gastritis and Intestinal Metaplasia

The intestinal-type cancer so characteristic of high-risk populations is preceded by a sequence of changes that begins with inflammation and passes through atrophy and intestinal metaplasia (IM) to dysplasia and ultimately to invasive cancer (57) (Figs. 5.4 and 5.5). These changes are initiated in childhood by *H. pylori* infection. The dense leukocytic response that affects the superficial lamina propria and the epithelium of the mucous neck region of the gastric glands, as discussed

in Chapter 4, is followed by the appearance of foci of atrophic, intestinalized mucosa at the antral–corpus junction. These changes become apparent in adolescents and young adults. The metaplastic glands and the mucosa adjacent to them show increased cell proliferation. The foci of multifocal atrophic gastritis (MAG) enlarge, fuse, and expand proximally and distally so that, by the 6th or 7th decade of life, all but a small portion of the proximal greater curvature of the corpus may be lined by intestinalized mucosa. Two forms of IM are recognized: The "complete" form faithfully reproduces small intestinal-type cells. There are subsite-dependent variations that diverge from this pattern. Some intestinalized glands lack Paneth cells, lose the ability to make some glycocalyceal enzymes, or may produce mucins similar to those of the colon, the so-called "incomplete" form of IM (58). There is a widely held view that incomplete IM carries a higher risk of carcinoma than the complete form, but the most common site for early cancer is the antral–corpus junction, where the complete form predominates. The incomplete form is best seen on the distal greater curvature of the antrum, an area that is involved in the later stages of intestinalization. Cancer risk increases with the extent of the IM; the presence of incomplete IM is synonymous with extensive IM.

The mechanisms that underlie the development of IM in MAG are complex. The development and maintenance of specific organ structures and functions in the gastrointestinal tract are regulated by *CDX*, a homolog of the *Drosophila* caudal gene, during intestinal development (59). *CDX1* and *CDX2* are not expressed in the normal stomach, but their mRNAs are expressed in metaplastic glands. *CDX2* precedes *CDX1* expression and appears to trigger IM. Transgenic mice that express *CDX2* in gastric parietal cells have complete replacement of gastric mucosal glands by the full array of intestinal cells,

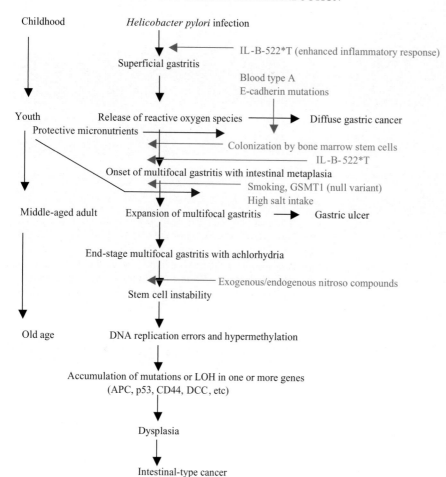

PATHWAYS OF GASTRIC CANCER INDUCTION

FIG. 5.5. Diagram of the pathways of gastric cancer induction. LOH, loss of heterozygosity.

including goblet cells and absorptive cells (60). A mechanism for the activation of this gene has been suggested by Houghton and Wang (61). They found that, in the presence of *H. pylori*–generated gastritis, circulating bone marrow stem cells are recruited and engrafted into the replicating zone of the gastric mucosa. The presence of these stem cells in the gastric mucosa in patients with *H. pylori* gastritis may account for the extreme heterogeneity of gastric cancer and the presence of cells with a hybrid intestinal/gastric phenotype (62,63).

Serum pepsinogen levels reflect the extent of gastric mucosal intestinalization. Pepsinogen is a proenzyme activated by gastric acid to produce pepsin. It is produced in two forms: Pepsinogen group I (PGI) is only produced in the oxyntic mucosa, while pepsinogen group II (PGII) is made throughout the stomach and in Brunner glands. Replacement of oxyntic mucosa by IM results in decreasing PGI serum levels (64). A PGI level $<$30 ηg/mL or a PGI:PGII ratio $<$2 are established cut-points used in screening programs to identify patients with extensive IM and who are at especially high risk of gastric cancer (65). The predictive value of the PGI level is improved when it is combined with the *H. pylori* serum antibody levels, as shown in Table 5.6, adapted from a case control study (66). Similar trends are observed with the PGI:PGII ratio.

Autoimmune Gastritis

Autoimmune gastritis, as discussed in Chapter 4, is a well-recognized, but less common, gastric cancer precursor than MAG. Autoimmune gastritis and *H. pylori* gastritis may coexist in most patients with pernicious anemia and the titers of both antibodies inversely relate to disease duration (67). It may be distinguished from late-stage MAG by the absence of antral inflammation and atrophy. The cancers associated with this form of gastritis arise in the antrum or the atrophic corpus, with a relative risk ranging from 2.2 to 5.6 (68). The increased risk stems from several factors: (a) Loss of gastric acidity favors the growth of bacteria that may generate endogenous nitroso compounds from dietary amines. (b) Gastrin production is greatly increased in response to prolonged achlorhydria. The trophic effects of hypergastrinemia result in accelerated cell turnover in a replicating compartment already expanded due to the loss of parietal and chief cells. (c) These replicating cells are exposed to reactive oxygen species from inflammatory cells.

Gastric Ulcer

A stage is reached in the early phases of the expansion of MAG when the proximal antral intestinalized mucosa is

TABLE 5.6 Age-, Sex-, and Ethnicity-adjusted Odds Ratios for Serum Pepsinogen Group I (PGI) Levels and *Helicobacter pylori* (*HP*) Antibody Status, According to Histologic Types of Gastric Cancer

All Cancers	Intestinal	Diffuse	Distal to Cardia
HP/CagA negative, PGI normal	1.0	1.0	1.0
HP/CagA negative, PGI low	5.4 (2.61–11.2)	5.06 (2.43–10.97)	8.92 (1.48–53.6)
HP/CagA positive, PGI normal	4.86 (2.9–8.13)	3.64 (2.05–6.45)	14.84 (9.51–54.4)
HP/CagA positive, PGI low	9.21 (4.95–17.13)	6.91 (3.53–13.53)	40.74 (9.51–174.6)

exposed to the acid produced by the still intact oxyntic mucosa. The intestinalized mucosa lacks the protective mucous barrier of the normal antrum, so that it is vulnerable to peptic ulceration. Patients with gastric ulcer are at greatly increased risk of gastric cancer. This is not surprising since gastric ulcer and gastric cancer share the same risk factors: *H. pylori* gastritis, a diet rich in salt, smoking (48), and a declining frequency in Western countries (69). As may be expected among patients who have retained the ability to make acid, the mean age of gastric ulcer patients is 10 years younger than the mean age of patients with cancer. Re-epithelialization

of the ulcer associates with expansion of the replication zone of the glands bordering the ulcer, exposing a larger number of vulnerable proliferating cells to genotoxic hazards. In contrast, the regenerating epithelial cells that migrate over the ulcer base are arrested in the postmitotic phase of the cell cycle, accounting for the observation that the gastric mucosa bordering the ulcer, rather than the ulcer base, is a common site of early cancer.

The term *ulcer cancer* defines a gastric carcinoma that arises in a pre-existing peptic ulcer (Figs. 5.6 and 5.7). Tumors arising in this setting account for <1% of all gastric

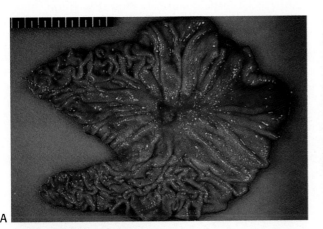

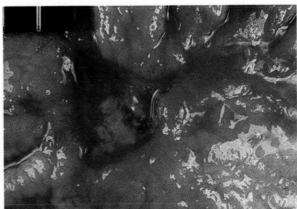

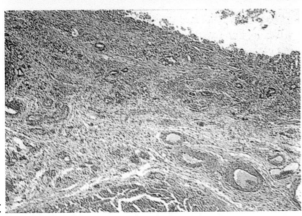

FIG. 5.6. Ulcer cancer. **A:** Large, centrally located gastric ulcer. **B:** Closer view. **C:** Ulcer base. Malignant glands are within and below the muscularis mucosae.

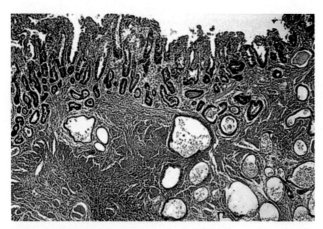

FIG. 5.7. Invasive carcinoma in healed gastric peptic ulcer. Well-differentiated adenocarcinoma infiltrates the muscularis propria, which is fused with the muscularis mucosae.

carcinomas. In order to be accepted as an ulcer cancer, the case must show definite evidence of pre-existing chronic peptic ulcer and evidence of coexisting malignancy. About 5% of endoscopically benign ulcers eventually prove to be malignant, but some lesions may require more than one biopsy to detect the underlying malignancy (70). Under-estimation of the depth of invasion may occur when the tumor develops from the epithelium of a healed ulcer in which the submucosa and muscularis propria are no longer recognizable because of scarring.

Hyperplastic Polyps

Hyperplastic polyps used to constitute from 75% to 90% of all gastric polyps (71). They arise from the foveolar hyperplasia that frequently accompanies atrophic gastritis, whether of the multifocal or autoimmune type. They may

also appear on the gastric side of gastroenterostomy stomas. Patients with hyperplastic polyps are at increased risk of gastric cancer, but the cancers very rarely arise in them. Rather, they are byproducts of the chronic gastritis that is the underlying cause of cancer induction. In the unusual event that a cancer does arise in a hyperplastic polyp, it is preceded by the development of dysplasia (Fig. 5.8).

Dysplasia

Dysplasia is the first microscopically detectable anatomic change in the neoplastic process. The dysplastic changes may represent cytologic alterations or disorganized architecture. Gastric dysplasia shows two major growth patterns: A flat, grossly inconspicuous dysplasia or polypoid lesions recognizable as adenomas. The dysplastic cells may be gastric or intestinal in type, or they may be hybrid forms from each lineage.

Nonpolypoid Dysplasia

Areas of mucosal dysplasia are characterized by histologic and cytologic abnormalities that must be distinguished from regenerative (reactive) atypia. Atypical regenerative changes are usually accompanied by active inflammation without significant architectural or differentiation abnormalities (Fig. 5.9). In contrast, dysplastic cells show one or more nuclear abnormalities (increased size, hyperchromasia, irregular shape, abnormal mitoses) and form abnormal glands with branching and occasional back-to-back configuration (Figs. 5.10 and 5.11) (71). The identification of dysplasia is critical to the management of patients in high-risk populations, but the assignment of grades is subjective, with wide inter- and intravariations in grade selection. A workshop convened to resolve international differences in the

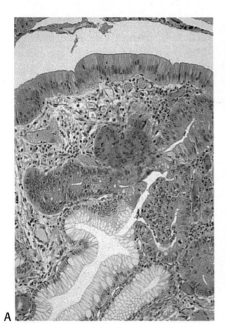

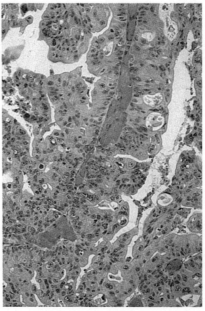

FIG. 5.8. Dysplasia arising in a hyperplastic polyp. **A:** Low-grade dysplasia spreads from the surface to the deeper portions of gland, replacing the normal foveolar epithelium. **B:** Higher power view of another area of high-grade dysplasia. The cells are hyperchromatic, pleomorphic, and disorganized. The glands are beginning to develop a back-to-back arrangement suggestive of intramucosal carcinoma.

A   B

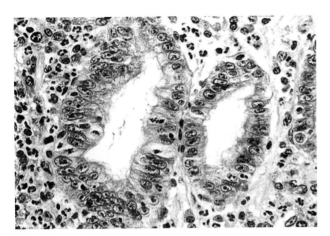

FIG. 5.9. Regenerative hyperplasia. An increased nuclear-to-cytoplasmic ratio and mitotic rate, along with large nucleoli and stromal inflammatory cells, are all present.

TABLE 5.7	The Padova Classification of Gastric Dysplasia and Related Lesions

Negative for dysplasia
   Reactive foveolar hyperplasia
Intestinal metaplasia (IM)
   IM, complete type
   IM, incomplete type
Indefinite for dysplasia
   Foveolar hyperproliferation
   Hyperproliferative IM
Noninvasive neoplasia (flat or elevated [synonym, adenoma])
   Low grade
   High grade
      Including suspicious for carcinoma without invasion (intraglandular)
      Including carcinoma without invasion (intraglandular)
      Suspicious for invasive carcinoma
Invasive carcinoma

definitions of different grades of gastric epithelial dysplasia resulted in the Padova classification (72), as summarized in Table 5.7.

Pathologists achieve fairly high levels of agreement in the diagnosis of high-grade dysplasia, but the agreement is only "fair" for low-grade dysplasia and "poor" for indefinite for dysplasia (73). We believe that it is sufficient to identify dysplasia and to classify it as high or low grade. In low-grade dysplasia, the gastric mucosal architecture is generally preserved, although abnormalities sometimes occur, including pseudovilli, irregular branching papillary infoldings, crypt lengthening with serration, and cystic changes (Fig. 5.10). Dystrophic goblet cells may also be seen. The pyloric glands branch at the crypt base and range from normal in appearance to frankly dysplastic. We have also seen cases in which dysplasia occurred in gastric foveolar cells (Fig. 5.12). The term high-grade dysplasia replaces "carcinoma in situ." Severe gastric dysplasia shows nuclear stratification, increased abnormal mitoses, dis-

ordered polarity, and glandular crowding. Problems associated with diagnosing gastric epithelial dysplasia are threefold: (a) one must be able to separate dysplasia from atypical regenerative changes, (b) one should be able to characterize high-grade from low-grade dysplasia, and (c) the dysplasia should be separable from invasive carcinoma. Immunohistochemical detection of p53 overexpression and Ki-67 (Fig. 5.13) stains to detect expansion of cell proliferation to the mucosal surface and abnormal tumor suppressor gene function may help to distinguish dysplastic from atypical regenerative changes.

Gastric Adenomas

Gastric adenomas are less common than hyperplastic polyps and, unlike colonic adenomas, they are uncommon in the

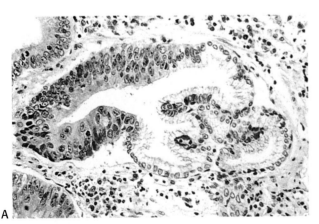
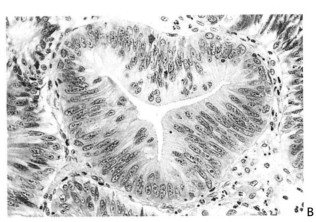

FIG. 5.10. Gastric dysplasia. **A:** The gastric gland is partially replaced by neoplastic epithelium. **B:** Mild dysplasia as illustrated here is characterized by cellular crowding and elongation, generally basally located nuclei, few mitoses, little cellular stratification, and nuclear pleomorphism.

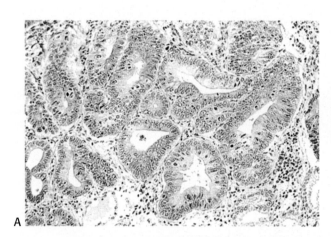
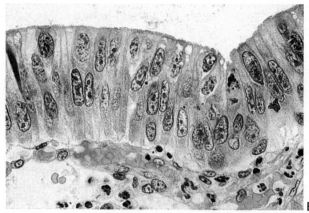

FIG. 5.11. Severe dysplasia. **A:** Gastric dysplasia with distorted architecture and severely dysplastic epithelium. There are numerous mitoses. **B:** The cells are so stratified that the nuclei reach the luminal surface.

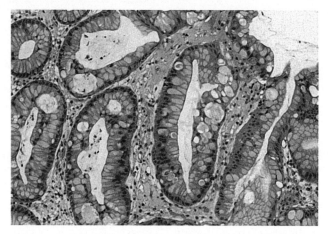

FIG. 5.12. Foveolar dysplasia. The foveolar epithelium is disorganized with some loss of polarity and the nuclei are pseudostratified. No inflammation is present.

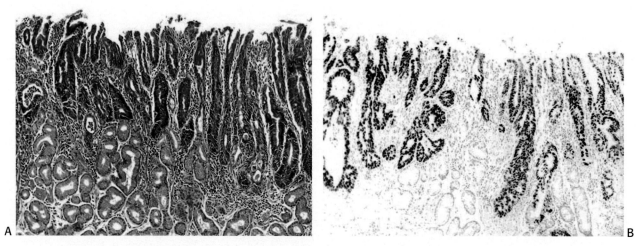

FIG. 5.13. High-grade dysplasia replacing the gastric pits. **A:** Hematoxylin and eosin–stained section. **B:** p53 immunostain shows nuclear labeling in virtually all of the neoplastic cells.

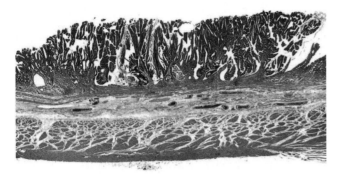

FIG. 5.14. Flat villous adenoma.

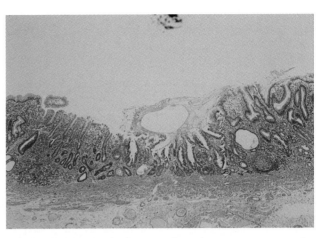

FIG. 5.16. Depressed adenoma. The adenoma appears as the central mucosal depression.

absence of FAP. They may be flat (Fig. 5.14) or pedunculated (Fig. 5.15). An endoscopic study in high-risk Korean patients found that 74.5% of these lesions arose in the distal third of the stomach. Focal areas of malignancy were found in 6.7% of adenomas, all but one arising in the distal stomach (74).

Gastric and colon polyps share some features. Grossly they have a lobulated or mamillated surface and are often covered by a reddened, velvety mucosa (Fig. 5.15). Abnormal epithelium occupies the surface and the luminal portions of the pit. With increasing degrees of dysplasia there is cellular stratification, progressive loss of nuclear polarity, and increased cellular crowding. The nuclei appear close to the lumina of the tubules and eventually secondary lumina form. A villous configuration may predominate in larger lesions (Fig. 5.14). When traumatized, adenomas may acquire surface changes resembling those seen in hyperplastic polyps. Gastric adenomas contain many dysplastic cell types, including enterocytes, goblet cells, endocrine cells, and Paneth cells. The World Health Organization (WHO) classification subdivides gastric adenomas into three subtypes: Tubular, papillary, and papillary–tubular. In contrast, Japanese authors recognize two types of adenoma: Protruding and depressed (75). Depressed adenomas (Fig. 5.16) are significantly larger than protruding

adenomas and are more likely to contain high-grade dysplasia than protruded adenomas. We have also seen serrated adenomas arising in the stomach (Fig. 5.17). These lesions are far too rare to know whether this morphology reflects the underlying genetic alterations as it does in the colon (see Chapter 14).

Histogenesis of Gastric Cancer

Areas of dysplasia may remain stable, regress (76), or take several years to progress to invasive intestinal-type cancer (77). In contrast, invasive diffuse cancers in young persons may arise in a mucosa that does not appear overtly dysplastic (Fig. 5.1), although in situ carcinoma may be present as discussed below. The factors that determine the cancer phenotype and the speed of its progression from normal gastric epithelium are complex. An invasive cancer might arise directly from the replicating compartment in the neck region of gastric glands, from the crypts of intestinalized glands, or from replicating surface cells in areas of dysplasia. The cells

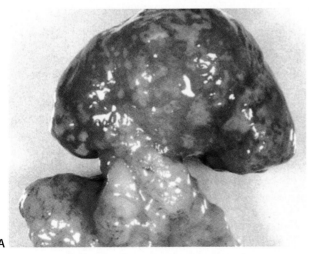

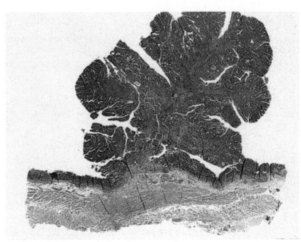

A   B

FIG. 5.15. Gastric adenoma. **A:** The pedunculated adenoma is covered by a reddened mucosa. **B:** Whole mount section of the adenoma depicted in A showing the proliferation of the neoplastic cells.

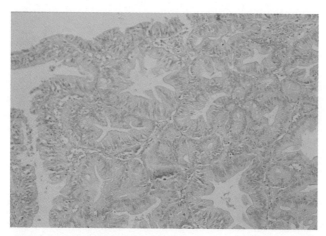

FIG. 5.17. Serrated adenoma that arose on a background of intestinal metaplasia.

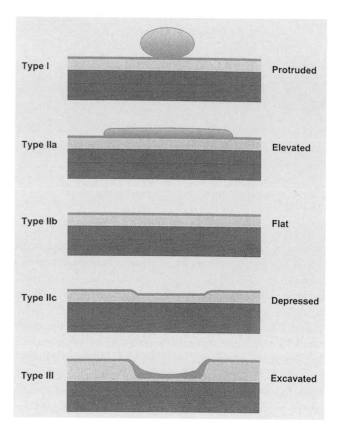

FIG. 5.19. Macroscopic classification of early gastric cancer.

of origin may determine the phenotype of an early cancer, but postinduction mutations may introduce so much heterogeneity that the mother cells of advanced cancers cannot be determined. The types and numbers of genetic and epigenetic changes in the cancer influence the speed of its progression from an early superficial lesion to a widely disseminated one.

Early Gastric Cancer

Early gastric cancer is defined as a cancer that is limited to the mucosa or submucosa, regardless of the presence of lymph node metastases (Fig. 5.18). This concept evolved in Japan, where community screening programs discovered many early cancers in asymptomatic patients. In recent years early cancers have come to constitute the majority of gastric cancers among Japanese (78). In the period 1965–1970, early cancers constituted <20% of gastric cancers, but by 1988 the proportion reached 57%. Between 1962 and 1991 there was a marked decrease in the size of early cancers in these screening programs (78).

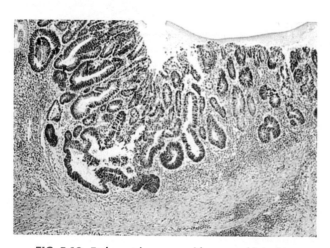

FIG. 5.18. Early gastric cancer with mucosal invasion.

There is a considerable variation in the configuration of early cancers. The macroscopic classification of the different forms of early cancer, as proposed by the Japanese Endoscopic Society (79), is now accepted worldwide. This classification divides early cancers into three main types, one having three subtypes, as shown in Figure 5.19. The gross appearance of two such tumors is shown in Figure 5.20. Superficial-spreading cancer is a subtype of early cancer and is defined as a tumor >4 cm in diameter that is confined to the mucosa or with minimal invasion of the submucosa (80).

Endoscopic biopsies often permit a straightforward diagnosis of early gastric cancer, but occasional problems arise. The most common of these include the following: (a) a small number of signet ring cells in the lamina propria may be easily missed (Fig. 5.21), and (b) the distinction of high-grade dysplasia from intestinal-type carcinoma and from atypical glandular regeneration may be difficult. Multiple biopsies, particularly from the edges of the lesion and cytologic brush sampling, are usually adequate for diagnosis, even of minute (<5 mm in diameter) carcinomas. Truly malignant cells are most reliably recognized by their pleomorphic and hyperchromatic nuclei, combined with a large hypertrophic nucleolus. Mitoses are uncommon. Histiocytes containing phagocytosed mucin or lipid (Fig. 5.22) may mimic intramucosal malignant signet ring cells. Granulation tissue may simulate malignancy in gastric biopsies when large, bizarre

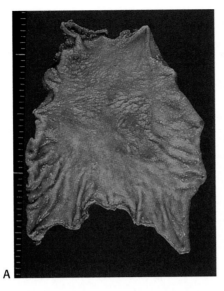
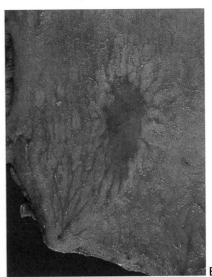

FIG. 5.20. Early gastric cancer. **A:** Type IIa cancer. The neoplasm is a slightly elevated, plaquelike lesion in the center of the specimen. **B:** Type IIc cancer. The lesion is slightly depressed below the level of the surrounding mucosa. (Photographs courtesy of Dr. Onja Kim, ANSA Medical Center, Seoul, Korea.)

endothelial cells are present. Special stains for intracytoplasmic mucin or cytokeratin immunostains sometimes help resolve these problems.

One must identify penetration of the muscularis mucosae, with invasion of the submucosa, to make a diagnosis of invasive cancer. The depth of invasion cannot be ascertained with endoscopic biopsies. Lesions detected as early

cancers may be tumors with an indolent behavior or may be aggressive lesions that happen to be detected at an early stage. In one series of 56 patients with early cancer, 16 showed no progression during a mean follow-up of 29 months, indicating an unexpectedly slow evolution (81). This is supported by the observation of two men who had gastrectomies 6 and 8 years after the diagnosis of mucosal

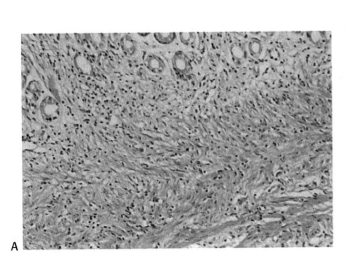
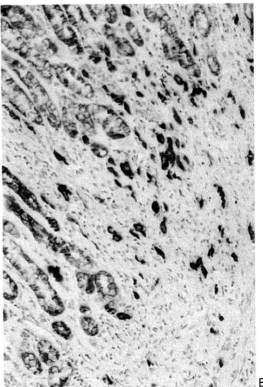

FIG. 5.21. Diffuse carcinoma. **A:** Scattered minimally atypical cells lie deep in the lamina propria. These cells could easily be mistaken for chronic inflammatory cells. **B:** Cytokeratin stain confirms the presence of an infiltrating carcinoma.

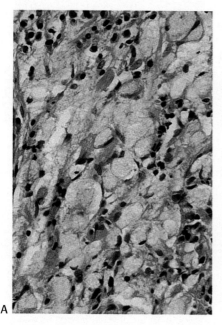
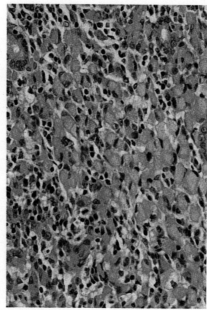

A   B

FIG. 5.22. Comparison of lamina propria macrophages and diffuse cancer. **A:** The lamina propria macrophages contain abundant foamy cytoplasm and small peripherally located nuclei. **B:** Diffuse carcinoma. Infiltrating signet ring cells are present in the lamina propria. These cells have foamy eosinophilic cytoplasm and peripherally placed nuclei. There is more nuclear atypia in these cells than in those shown in A. In cases where there is doubt, immunohistochemistry using histiocytic markers and cytokeratin allows characterization of the cell type present.

cancer without deeper penetration occurring in the interval (82).

Nodal metastases may accompany early gastric cancers (78), and, as may be expected, their frequency correlates with the depth of tumor penetration into the submucosa (83). Nodal metastases also directly relate to tumor size and the presence of ulceration (79). The frequency of nodal metastases varies from 15% to 30% in Japan (79), but may be from two to three times higher than this if immunohistochemical stains for cytokeratin are used to detect occult micrometastases (84). Although the biologic significance of occult metastases is unclear at the present time, the presence of overt metastases is unfavorable in all studies. Other factors that increase the risk of recurrence of early gastric cancer include vascular invasion (85) and poor differentiation (86). In Japan, the 10-year postoperative survival of patients with early cancer is 99% for patients with mucosal cancer and 91% for those with submucosal cancer (78). The 7-year survival rates for a French study of early gastric cancer were 93% for mucosal cancers and 83% for submucosal cancers, indicating that the value of early diagnosis is not an exclusively Asian phenomenon (87).

The ability to diagnose early gastric cancer allows clinicians to devise function-preserving treatment methods that give the patient a better quality of life than would be seen following gastric resection and eliminates the risk of cancer developing in the proximal stomach after a subtotal gastrectomy. These treatment options include endoscopic mucosal resection (EMR) (88) and wedge resection, with or without lymphadenectomy (89). Selection of either approach depends on the probability that the tumor will recur. The currently acceptable indications for EMR include well-differentiated carcinoma without ulceration, measuring <2 cm if elevated (type IIa) or <1 cm if flat (types IIb and IIc). In examining an EMR specimen, the pathologist must ascertain the tumor-free status of the lateral and deep margins. Patients treated with EMR require periodic surveillance for recurrences of residual tumor or for the development of metachrononous cancer, since it must be assumed that the anatomic precursors of the original tumor will be present in the residual stomach.

Following EMR, follow-up biopsies are performed to ensure that there is no residual neoplasia. Mitsuhashi et al performed a retrospective analysis of post-EMR biopsies. The histologic changes included inflammation, stromal edema, foveolar hyperplasia, vascular ectasia, epithelial atypia, increased mitotic activity, clear cell changes, and signet ring–like changes. Many of the alterations were secondary to ischemia following the EMR. Among the most worrisome were areas of clear cell–like changes and signet ring–like changes, since these were the most difficult to distinguish from neoplasia. However, these reactive features were often embedded in a nondesmoplastic stroma (89a).

Advanced Gastric Cancer

Gross Features

The first classification of gastric cancer, the Borrmann classification, is based on the gross appearance of the tumor (90). Four growth patterns are recognized: Polypoid, fungating, ulcerated, and infiltrating (Figs. 5.23 to 5.26). Any of the four types may coexist. Polypoid cancers protrude into the lumen without major areas of ulceration. Fungating tumors are irregularly shaped exophytic growths showing areas of ulceration. Ulcerated tumors are irregular in outline and have raised edges. The ulcer margins appear hard and stiff, the ulcer base necrotic. Infiltrating tumors are flat, plaquelike lesions with or without shallow areas of ulceration. Transmural infiltration associates with a characteristic desmoplastic reaction,

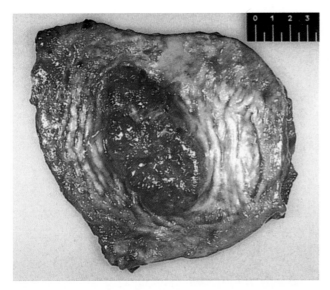

FIG. 5.23. Borrmann type I. Polypoid carcinoma of the stomach. A large vegetating mass without much hemorrhage or necrosis is present.

giving the stomach wall a marked rigidity. In one large gastric cancer series the percentage for each subtype was as follows: Polypoid, 7%; ulcerated, 25%; fungating, 36%; and infiltrating, 26% (91).

Ulcerated gastric cancers can be differentiated from benign peptic ulcers in several ways: They have irregular margins with raised edges. The surrounding tissues are firm, thick, and uneven. The ulcer base is necrotic, shaggy, and often nodular. The mucosal folds surrounding the ulcer have a more irregular shape and distribution than is seen adjacent to benign ulcers (see Chapter 4). Additionally, benign ulcers usually penetrate through and replace the muscularis propria, whereas cancers infiltrate between the muscle bundles, so that the muscularis propria is thickened. Malignant ulcers are usually larger than their benign counterparts. Unfortunately, some malignant ulcers are indistinguishable

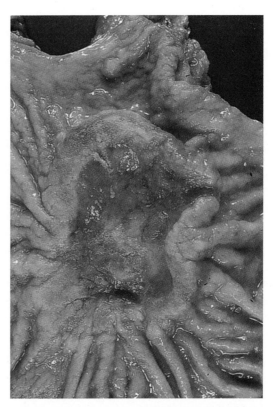

FIG. 5.25. Borrmann type III. Ulcerated gastric carcinoma with heaped-up margins, but without significant intraluminal growth.

from benign ulcers based solely on their gross appearance, and it is important that all endoscopically detected ulcers be systematically biopsied, even if they are healing.

Diffuse (infiltrating) tumors spread superficially in the mucosa and submucosa, tending to flatten the mucosal folds. As they extend into the stomach wall they associate with a dense connective tissue reaction that fixes the mucosa to the muscularis propria. Frequently the infiltrating cells involve the entire stomach, producing the picture of linitis plastica, or "leather bottle" stomach. Linitis plastica often involves the pylorus (Fig. 5.26). The gastric rigidity induced by neoplastic infiltration combined with marked desmoplasia accounts for the early satiety that commonly occurs with this tumor.

An analysis of the subsite location of resected gastric cancers among 171,721 Japanese patients between 1975 and 1985 found the distal third to be the most frequent site of cancer development, followed by the middle third, the upper third, and the entire stomach (92). Women are more likely to have tumors involving the entire stomach, as might be expected since the diffuse cancer that produces this growth pattern is most common in women. The subsite distribution is what may be expected in any high-risk population, but there was an increase in the proportion of middle and upper third cancers at the expense of the distal third in later years. The basis of this temporal trend is unclear. It could result from finding more proximal lesions at an operable stage as a result of screening programs, or technical improvements

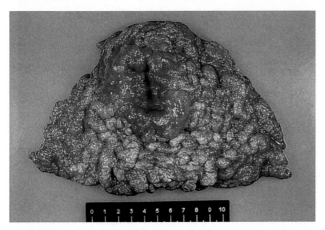

FIG. 5.24. Borrmann type II. Fungating carcinoma with extensive surface ulceration and hemorrhage.

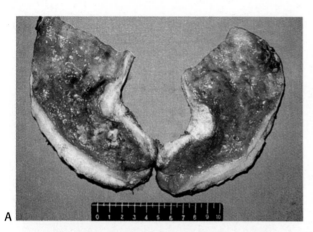 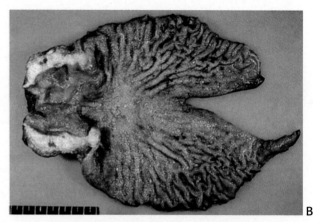

FIG. 5.26. Borrmann type IV. **A:** The gastric wall is thickened with irregularly ulcerated mucosa. **B:** Cancer involving the antrum showing a uniform thickening of the gastric wall.

that allowed more aggressive selection of advanced proximal cancer for surgery. The increase in the number of operated cases in each 5-year period is compatible with either explanation.

The extensive surface area of the stomach affected by late-stage multifocal gastritis lends itself to the development of multiple primary cancers. This is a special concern in patients selected for EMR treatment. Multicentric tumors affect from 3.5% to 15% of gastric cancer patients. Two, three, and four or more early cancers may be found in the same stomach (78). Multiple gastric cancers are most frequently seen in men over 65 years of age in high-risk populations. Chromoendoscopy may help identify unsuspected synchronous multicentric tumors; continuing posttreatment surveillance is necessary to discover metachronous cancers.

Clinical Features

Gastric cancers that elicit symptoms are usually late-stage tumors and are more likely to precede the diagnosis of cancer in Western, unscreened populations than in Asia or other high-risk areas. The early cancers that may accompany chronic gastric ulcers are exceptions to this rule. A review of 18,265 stomach cancers by the American College of Surgeons (93) found the following frequently overlapping symptoms to be the most common: Weight loss (61.6%), abdominal pain (51.6%), nausea (34.3%), dysphagia (26.1%), and melena (20.2%). Weight loss is an ominous presenting symptom and associates with poor survival. Early satiety may result from either pyloric obstruction or the ability of the stomach to expand. Blood loss from an ulcerated tumor may induce anemia and fatigue. Infection of necrotic, fungating tumors may cause fever. Spread of gastric cancer to a distant site is the presenting symptom in some cases. This may take the form of an enlarged supraclavicular lymph node. Ascites or vaginal bleeding due to endometrial metastases may be the presenting symptom in premenopausal women with diffuse cancer (94).

Endoscopy, Biopsy, and Cytology

Upper gastrointestinal endoscopy provides the initial method of evaluating a gastric cancer. Winawer et al studied 63 patients with gastric adenocarcinoma (95) and found that the correct diagnosis was made endoscopically in 90% of patients. Combined brush cytology and biopsy studies were histologically accurate in 92% of exophytic cancers, contrasting with only 50% accuracy in infiltrating lesions. The cardia and the antrum distal to the incisura are more difficult to sample than other parts of the stomach. The diagnostic yield from endoscopy in a population at moderate risk of gastric cancer was assessed in an Asian population, and 10 gastric cancers among 905 (1.1%) symptomatic patients were found (96). The biopsy diagnostic accuracy increases with the number of samples taken. When there is uncertainty as to the distinction between benign or malignant ulcer, quadrant biopsies of the ulcer margin are indicated. Once a diagnosis of gastric carcinoma has been made, endoscopic ultrasonography (EUS) may be employed to estimate tumor stage prior to definitive therapy. This procedure yields 82% accuracy as to the depth of tumor invasion (97), but is less accurate in detecting lymph node metastases (98).

Brushing cytology plays a key role in the diagnosis of gastric malignancy. The cytologic sampling is often supplemented by multiple biopsies in order to increase the diagnostic sensitivity. However, the role of cytology has been questioned because of the possible occasional false-positive results and the very high sensitivity of biopsies (99). Overt gastric adenocarcinoma, regardless of its subtype, has distinctive cytopathologic features (Fig. 5.27). Malignant epithelial cells usually appear larger than normal cells and reveal anisocytosis, anisokaryosis, pronounced nuclear atypia including marked irregular indentations of the nuclear outline, hyperchromasia, irregularly distributed heterochromatin, multinucleation, nucleolar hypertrophy, occasionally abnormal mitotic figures, signet ring features (Fig. 5.27), and microvacuolized cytoplasm. The chromatin often appears very coarse or sharply granular (100) in contrast to abnormal benign cells in gastritis. Nuclear molding also represents

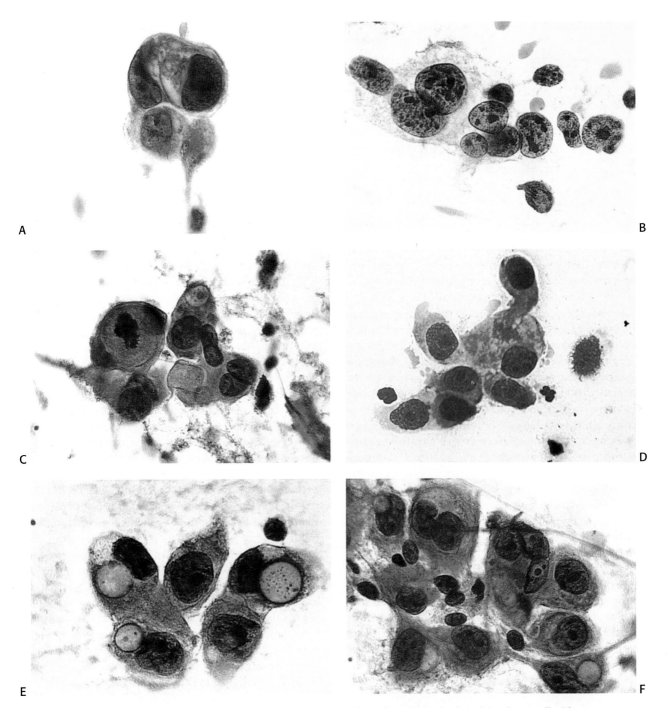

FIG. 5.27. Gastric adenocarcinoma. **A:** Group of cancer cells with variably sized nuclei. A large cell with vacuolated cytoplasm and smaller cells with granular cytoplasm is visible. **B:** Extreme variation in nuclear size is seen in these single cancer cells. Note the large nucleoli. **C:** Intracytoplasmic secretory vacuoles are present as well as overlapping nuclear borders. **D:** May-Grünwald-Giemsa stain of intestinal-type gastric cancer. The cells are retaining their columnar appearance. The nucleoli are large and basophilic. **E:** Signet ring cancer cells with prominent nucleoli. **F:** Scattered signet ring cells are visualized.

a valuable malignant feature that may be appreciated in cell groups. The cell-in-cell (cannibalism) phenomenon might be prominent as might the finding of naked nuclei. Occasionally, features of squamous metaplasia are displayed (Fig. 5.28).

The background is often studded with debris and damaged red blood cells. The tumor cells may be predominantly single when derived from poorly differentiated carcinomas or may be present in sheets of more cohesive cells when derived from papillary or well-differentiated adenocarcinomas.

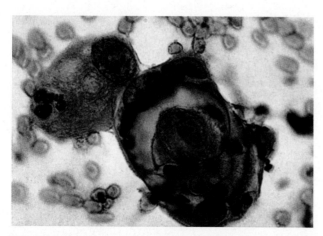

FIG. 5.28. Gastric adenoacanthoma. A keratinizing cell-in-cell arrangement is seen as well as single glandular cells with foamy cytoplasm.

Cytologic subtyping of gastric cancer is not essential (101). If one equates papillary, tubular, and some mucinous carcinomas with Lauren's intestinal-type and signet ring cell carcinoma with the diffuse type, then a specificity rate for cytologic typing of >90% for the former and of 85% for the latter may be obtained (102,103). However, vacuolized cells should be evaluated with special care because signet ring cells are easily simulated by goblet cells. The size of the nucleolus and the nuclear outline are helpful differential diagnostic features. Unless fine needle aspiration is combined with the endoscopic examination, early gastric carcinoma cannot be identified cytologically because no features exist that allow one to distinguish between early and advanced gastric cancer (104). Advanced carcinomas with extensive necrosis and stenosis may not yield sufficient diagnostic material.

Fine needle aspiration during endoscopy providing a somewhat higher sensitivity than that of brush cytology of gastric and esophageal cancer is reported for biopsy touch smear cytology (105,106). With this method, gastric endoscopic biopsies are gently pressed several times on clean glass slides and the imprints processed routinely. Cell features are different from those of brush preparations, so that cytopathologists should be familiar with the difference in the two approaches. In addition to cytologic abnormalities, the percentage of single cells is taken into consideration because malignant tumors yield more than 20% single cells in touch smears (107). The same imprint technique can be used to stage gastric cancer during resections since bisected lymph nodes may be evaluated in this way for the presence of malignant cells.

Microscopic Features

Gastric cancers exhibit considerable heterogeneity from tumor to tumor, and also within a given tumor. This heterogeneity results from the complex cellular composition of the gastric and intestinalized glands from which the cancers arise (108,109). Additionally, postinduction mutations in gastric cancers produce diverging clones of cell types that increase

in number as tumors evolve from early (86) to advanced stages. Intestinal characteristics may be evident if goblet cells or Paneth cells are identified in hematoxylin and eosin (H&E)-stained sections or neuroendocrine cells specific to the intestine are found. An intestinal origin may also become apparent when the tumor cells are examined for their secretion products, biologic markers, or ultrastructural features. In some cases the tumor cells are gastric in type (Fig. 5.29), or may revert to a gastric phenotype from intestinalized precursors (110). Thus, although many histologic classifications have been proposed, none satisfactorily accounts for the cellular variability that may be encountered in an individual tumor. They are most useful for making rough estimates of the expected behavior of broad classes of tumor types.

Gastric Cancer Classifications

The Lauren classification divides gastric cancers into two major histologic types: Intestinal (Fig. 5.30) and diffuse (Fig. 5.31) (6). From 85% to 90% of gastric cancers fit into these categories. The remainder consist of carcinomas with mixed intestinal–diffuse features and uncommon subtypes (e.g., germ cell carcinomas, squamous cell carcinomas). Cohesive tumor cells that form recognizable glands, regardless of their degree of cytologic differentiation or cell of origin, fall into the intestinal category. They constitute approximately 60% of gastric cancers in high-risk populations, are most common in the antrum, and usually arise in an intestinalized mucosa. They associate with discrete distant metastases since they are likely to show lymphatic channel and/or vascular invasion.

Diffuse carcinomas consist of discohesive cells that penetrate through the stomach wall as individual cells embedded in a desmoplastic stroma. They appear as layered signet ring cells in the superficial portions of the mucosa, but signet ring cells are less numerous in the deeper portions of the wall, where more pleomorphic cells predominate. Cell cycle markers may fail to label superficial signet ring cells, in contrast to the discohesive cells that infiltrate deeper into the gastric wall. A few inconspicuous, abortive glands may be present (Fig. 5.32). The desmoplastic reaction that accompanies diffuse cancer may be more conspicuous than the cancer cells that elicit it. The infiltrating cells may show so little differentiation that they resemble histiocytes and can only be identified with certainty by immunostains for cytokeratin (Fig. 5.33). These stains should be used when it is uncertain whether dense connective tissue in the stomach wall is a scar from a healed ulcer or a desmoplastic reaction has been elicited by a diffuse cancer. Diffuse cancers seldom form discrete metastases and show a tendency for transperitoneal spread. When they spread into the mesentery and peritoneum, the cells can be very inconspicuous and difficult to detect unless the sections are stained with cytokeratin antibodies (Fig. 5.34). They account for most of cases that present with ascites or Krukenberg ovarian metastases.

Diffuse gastric cancers arise in the setting of germline mutations in the E-cadherin gene, as noted earlier. This

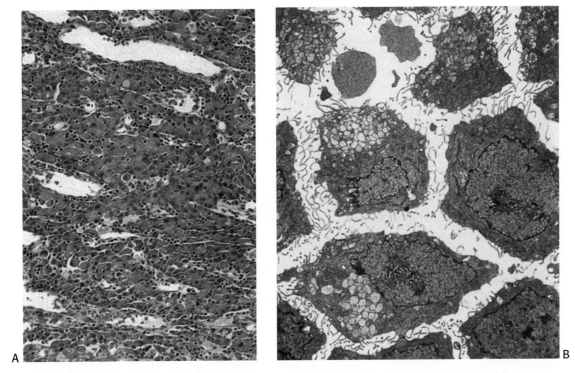

FIG. 5.29. Foveolar differentiation in gastric cancer. **A:** The cytoplasm of the neoplastic cells appears eosinophilic. The nuclei are peripherally placed. **B:** Ultrastructurally the cells resemble foveolar cells with prominent apical mucin globules and lateral cytoplasmic extensions.

genetic syndrome may be suspected when the specimen is examined if the tumor arises in a very young individual and shows multiple foci of intramucosal diffuse (signet ring cell) carcinoma. In addition, tumors associated with this form of the disease may show in situ changes that are characterized by signet ring cells with hyperchromatic nuclei and a lack of polarity with respect to the basement membrane lining the foveolae and glands. In addition, the glands and foveolae

may demonstrate pagetoid spread that is characterized by the presence of a two-layer structure, an inner layer consisting of benign mucous cells under which is a continuous or discontinuous layer of signet ring cells (Fig. 5.35). Furthermore, the tumors arising in this setting lose their membrane staining of E-cadherin (Fig. 5.1), unlike many diffuse carcinomas that are not hereditary in nature and retain their E-cadherin immunoreactivity (Fig. 5.36).

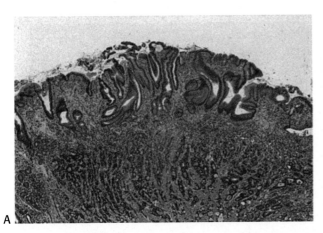
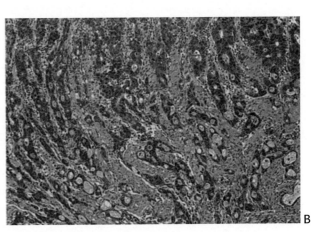

FIG. 5.30. Intestinal-type adenocarcinoma. **A:** Intestinal carcinoma invading the submucosa and infiltrating the muscularis propria. Note that the tumor is composed of well-formed glands similar to carcinomas arising in the small or large intestine. **B:** Higher power view showing well-formed glands and cohesive clusters of neoplastic cells.

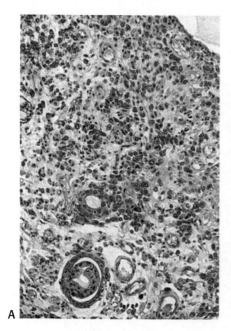
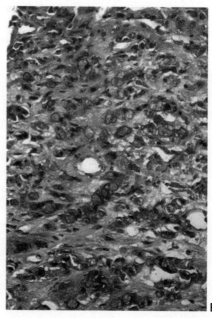

FIG. 5.31. Diffuse-type adenocarcinoma. **A:** The lamina propria contains individual infiltrating, discohesive cells. A few regenerating residual gastric glands are present in the bottom of the photograph. **B:** A digested periodic acid–Schiff (PAS) stain demonstrates diastase-resistant PAS staining in the cytoplasm of the neoplastic cells.

The simplicity of the Lauren classification that makes it useful for large epidemiologic studies makes it less useful for predicting the outcomes of histologic subsets of gastric cancers. The *WHO International Reference Histologic Classification of Gastric Cancer* (110), as listed in Table 5.8, has evolved to meet this need. In this classification adenocarcinomas are graded as well, moderately well, and poorly differentiated. *Well-differentiated carcinomas* produce recognizable, well-formed glands. *Poorly differentiated* tumors have poorly formed glands composed of very pleomorphic cells arranged in small clusters or solid sheets. *Moderately well-differentiated* tumors are intermediate between these extremes. WHO subtyping takes into account traditional histopathologic features, with most tumors falling into four types: Papillary, tubular, mucinous, and signet ring forms.

Tubular carcinomas (Fig. 5.37) contain dilated or branching tubules. Acinar structures may be present. Individual tumor cells may be columnar, cuboidal, or flattened by intraluminal mucin. Clear cells may be present. The degree of cytologic atypia varies from low grade (111) to high grade (112). A poorly differentiated variant is sometimes called solid carcinoma.

Papillary carcinomas (Fig. 5.38) are well-differentiated exophytic tumors with fingerlike processes, lined by cylindric or cuboidal cells supported by slender vascular cores. The cells tend to maintain their polarity. The degree of cellular atypia varies and may be severe. The invading tumor margin is usually sharply defined from the surrounding structures. The tumor may be infiltrated with acute and chronic inflammatory cells.

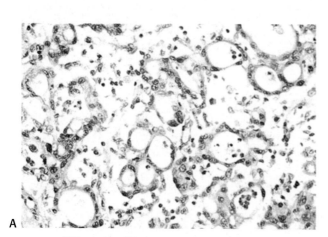
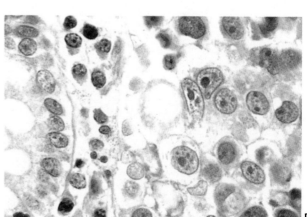

FIG. 5.32. Diffuse-type carcinoma. **A:** Microglandular structures of a diffuse-type carcinoma. **B:** Huge nucleoli in diffuse-type carcinoma.

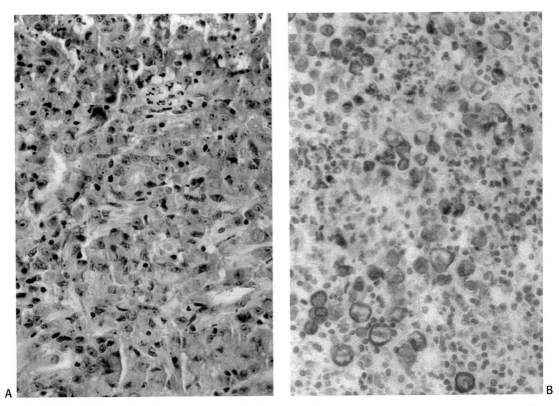

FIG. 5.33. Signet ring cell carcinoma. **A:** The neoplastic cells are highlighted with a mucicarmine stain. **B:** Immunohistochemical staining for cytokeratin demonstrates numerous infiltrating signet ring cells.

Mucinous carcinomas (Fig. 5.39) are sometimes referred to as colloid carcinomas. By definition, >50% of the tumor contains extracellular pools of mucin. They may present in one of two forms: (a) glands lined by mucus-secreting epithelium surrounding collections of extracellular mucin, and (b) irregular clusters of cells floating freely in mucinous lakes. Signet ring cells, if present, do not dominate the histologic pattern. Sometimes the tumors consist of large acellular pools of mucin (Fig. 5.40).

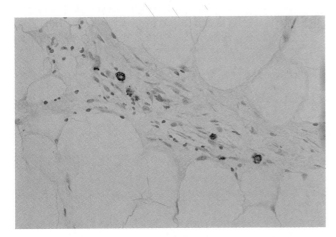

FIG. 3.34. Single cancer cells infiltrating the mesentery stained with an antibody to cytokeratin.

Signet ring carcinomas are tumors in which >50% of the mass consists of cells containing mucin that compresses the nucleus to the periphery of the cell walls. The classic signet ring cells are most numerous in the superficial portions of the tumor where they are stacked in a layered fashion. Signet ring cancers usually exhibit the infiltrating growth pattern and desmoplasia that is called diffuse cancer in the Lauren classification. Infiltrating Borrmann type IV carcinomas are usually signet ring tumors. The tumor cells in the deeper portions of the stomach wall have less cytoplasmic mucin and more centralized nuclei. They may be so widely dispersed through the stroma that they may be difficult to detect in routine H&E-stained preparations. Some form of mucin stain (periodic acid–Schiff [PAS], Alcian blue, mucicarmine) or immunohistochemical staining with cytokeratin antibodies may be used to detect these cells. We prefer the latter method since it detects a greater percentage of the neoplastic cells.

Less Common Types of Stomach Cancer

Medullary Carcinoma. Medullary carcinomas of the stomach with lymphocytic infiltration associate with two conditions: EBV infection (113) and microsatellite instability (MSI) (114). It is now well recognized that from 5% to 15% of gastric cancers contain EBV DNA and that these cancers have distinct clinicopathologic features (Fig. 5.41). They are most frequent

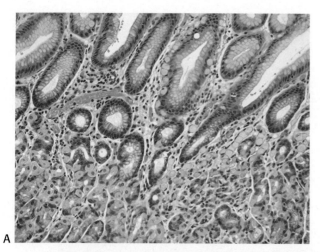
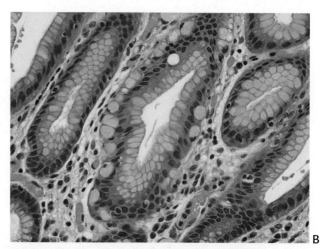

FIG. 5.35. Hereditary diffuse gastric carcinoma. **A:** This photograph shows the presence of an early infiltrating diffuse gastric cancer along with areas of pagetoid spread in the gastric glands. **B:** Higher magnification of the pagetoid spread. Signet ring cells are seen infiltrating beneath the nuclei of the intact gastric glands.

in men, arising in the corpus, but may occur in any part of the stomach. Grossly, many of these cancers present as ulcerated plaquelike lesions, although papillary forms also occur. An EBV association with gastric cancer may be suspected in H&E-stained sections if one of two growth patterns are present, but the diagnosis must be confirmed by in situ hybridization, which demonstrates the virus in the nuclei of the cancer cells (Fig. 5.42). A conspicuous lymphocytic infiltration is present in both types, and in approximately half of the cases this infiltrate may be so dense that the neoplastic epithelial cells are best recognized by cytokeratin stains (Fig. 5.41). EBV-associated tumors of this type probably account for 90% of medullary cancers. The other growth pattern seen with these cancers consists of slender, interlacing glands supported by a delicate stroma, the so-called lacelike pattern (115). If both patterns are present in the same cancer, the lacelike pattern is best seen in the superficial portions of the tumor, a distribution that could

be explained by the lacelike pattern being a feature of the early stages of this cancer (116). Patients have been observed with synchronous, multicentric cancers in which EBV DNA sequences were found in only one cancer (113), suggesting that the association is limited to a specific cancer phenotype. The survival of patients with EBV-associated cancers is similar to that of other stomach cancers when assessed on a stage-by-stage basis. EBV-containing gastric cancers, however, are diagnosed at a lower stage than other cancers because they show fewer lymph node metastases than EBV-negative tumors ($p = 0.0018$) (117). It is not unusual for EBV-associated cancers to exceed 10 cm in diameter without acquiring nodal metastases (Fig. 5.41).

Abundant T-cell lymphocytic infiltration is a feature of sporadic, poorly differentiated gastric cancers that display MSI (118). These tumors are most common in the antrum among elderly patients and carry a relatively good prognosis.

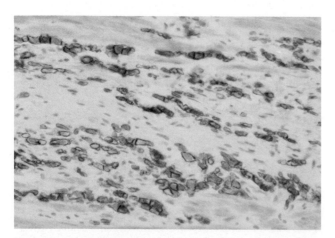

FIG. 5.36. Diffuse gastric cancer stained for E-cadherin. Note that the tumor cells are positive, contrasting with the tumor shown in Figure 5.1.

TABLE 5.8	**World Health Organization Histologic Classification of Gastric Epithelial Tumors**

Intraepithelial neoplasia-adenoma
Carcinoma
   Adenocarcinoma
      Intestinal type
      Diffuse type
   Papillary adenocarcinoma
   Tubular adenocarcinoma
   Mucinous adenocarcinoma
   Signet ring adenocarcinoma
   Adenosquamous carcinoma
   Squamous cell carcinoma
   Undifferentiated carcinoma
   Others
Carcinoid (well-differentiated endocrine neoplasm)

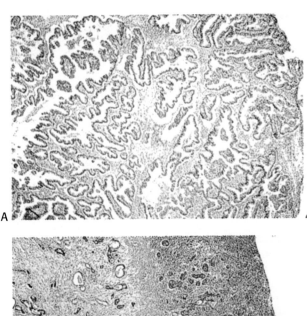

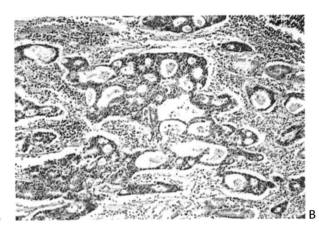

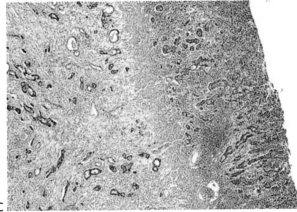

FIG. 5.37. Adenocarcinoma, tubular subtype. **A:** Well differentiated. **B:** Moderately differentiated. **C:** Marked desmoplasia.

The survival advantage of patients with this type of cancer has been attributed to an enhanced immune response generated by abnormal tumor-specific peptides that recruit lymphocytes to the tumor (114).

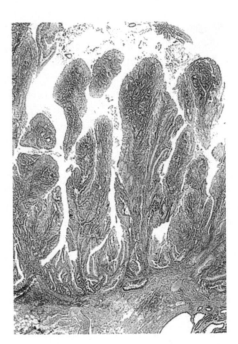

FIG. 5.38. Adenocarcinoma, papillary subtype. Long papillary fronds are the primary feature.

Paneth Cell Carcinoma. Paneth cell carcinomas arise from areas of complete intestinal metaplasia (119) and associate with a conspicuous desmoplastic reaction. The tumor cells contain bright red cytoplasmic granules that are highlighted by antilysozyme antibodies (Fig. 5.43). These cancers are too uncommon to assess their impact on survival. The patient with the illustrated cancer showed no nodal metastases, but died with peritoneal metastases 7 years after a subtotal gastrectomy.

Pylorocardiac Carcinoma. The pylorocardiac gland–type carcinoma may represent a distinct microscopic variant. This type of carcinoma is typically well demarcated and fungating, ulcerated, or fibrotic, and tends to arise either in the antrum or at the cardia. Microscopically, the cells appear predominantly clear (Fig. 5.44) because of the presence of cytoplasmic vacuoles containing PAS-positive diastase-resistant neutral mucin. Papillary infoldings of the glandular lining cells may be a prominent feature.

Gastric Parietal Cell and Parietal Cell-like Carcinoma (Oncocytic Adenocarcinomas). Gastric cancers that contain cells resembling parietal cells are very uncommon. The tumors tend to be large with lymph node metastases. Histologically, the tumor has a solid, or medullary, appearance with occasional tubular differentiation. The tumor cells contain abundant granular cytoplasm that lacks mucin and neuroendocrine granules (Fig. 5.45). The cell stains with antibodies directed toward the H^+,K^+-ATPase pump and human milk fat

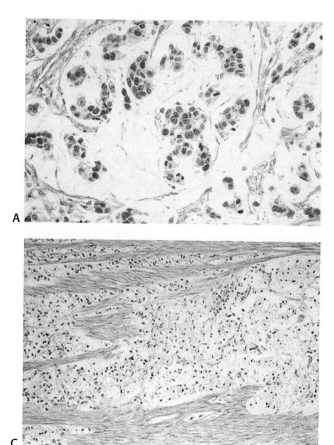

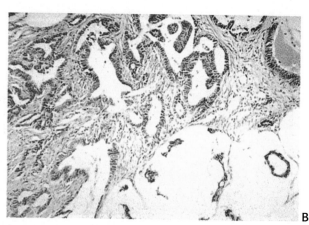

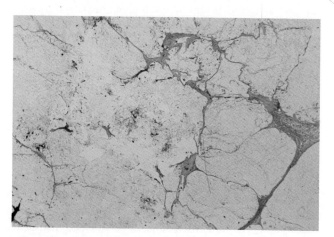

FIG. 5.39. Mucinous carcinoma. **A:** Lakes of mucus-containing clusters and strands of tumor cells. **B:** Mucinous carcinoma combined with tubular carcinoma. **C:** Poorly differentiated carcinoma with a signet ring cell component and infiltration of the muscle coat.

globulin-2. The tumor cells also contain prominent intracytoplasmic canaliculi that can be identified ultrastructurally (120). As with Paneth cell cancers, clinical observations of these cancers are too few to assess their expected behavior. A favorable prognosis has been observed in some reports (121), but aggressive dissemination occurs in others (120). Well-differentiated adenocarcinomas that are rich in mitochondria have been termed *oncocytic adenocarcinoma* and are distinguished from parietal cell cancers by the absence of antiparietal cell antibodies (122).

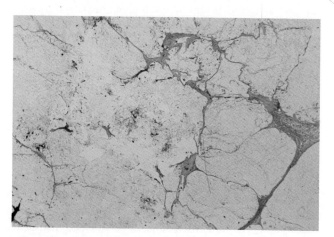

FIG. 5.40. Colloid carcinoma. This tumor contains large paucicellular mucin pools infiltrating the gastric wall.

Adenosquamous and Squamous Cell Carcinoma. Adenosquamous carcinoma is a rare tumor in which adenocarcinomatous and squamous components coexist (Fig. 5.46). Transitions exist between the two components. Adenosquamous carcinomas differ from tumors that contain discrete foci of benign-appearing squamous metaplasia. The latter are referred to as adenoacanthomas with squamous metaplasia. The prognosis of adenosquamous carcinoma is less favorable than adenocarcinoma, probably because these cancers are usually diagnosed at an advanced stage and show evidence of vascular invasion (123). A pure squamous cell carcinoma at the gastric cardia is likely to represent extension of an esophageal primary lesion into the stomach. The remaining squamous cell carcinomas are either tumors that arise in areas of squamous metaplasia in the gastric mucosa or adenosquamous carcinomas in which the squamous component has become the predominate histologic feature. Pure squamous cell cancers develop in association with tertiary syphilis, after cyclophosphamide therapy (124), and in stump cancers (125). All forms of gastric cancer that express a squamous phenotype probably amount to <0.5% of gastric carcinomas.

Gastric Adenocarcinomas with Features of Germ Cell Tumors. Most tumors with features of choriocarcinoma are combinations of variably differentiated adenocarcinoma and choriocarcinoma (Fig. 5.47). Slightly <30% of these tumors are pure choriocarcinomas, otherwise indistinguishable

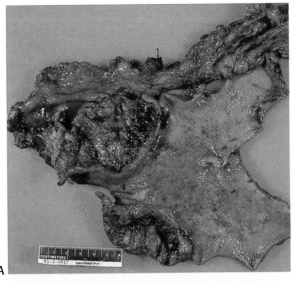

FIG. 5.41. Medullary carcinoma. A: Gastrectomy specimen containing a large, fungating mass with surface ulceration and hemorrhage. B: An intense lymphocytic infiltrate surrounds cords of neoplastic cells. C: The neoplastic cells are easily seen in cytokeratin-stained sections.

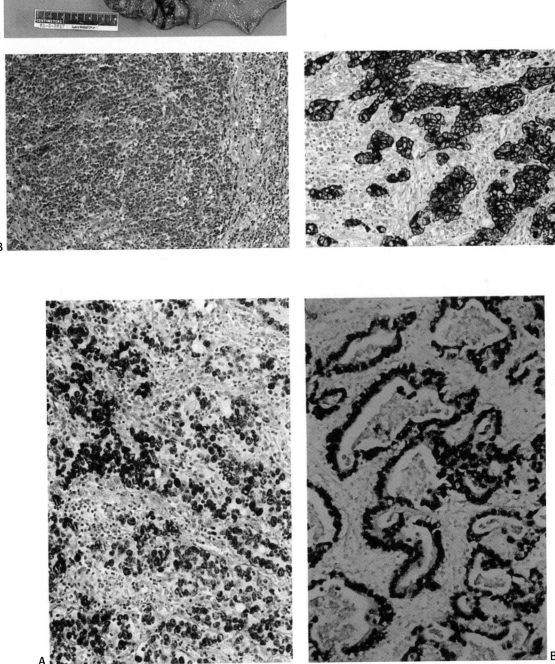

FIG. 5.42. Epstein-Barr virus (EBV) in gastric carcinoma. A: In situ hybridization for EBV in a medullary carcinoma. B: EBV DNA is present in a small proportion of gastric cancers without lymphoid stroma.

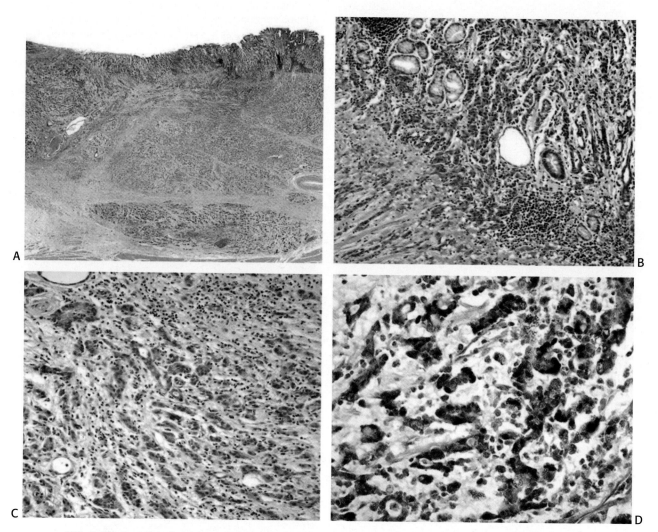

FIG. 5.43. Paneth cell carcinoma. **A:** Low magnification showing an infiltrating carcinoma. **B:** The mucosa shows adjacent areas of intestinal metaplasia. **C:** Higher magnification showing the eosinophilic granules of the Paneth cells. **D:** The tumor cells stain with an antibody to lysozyme.

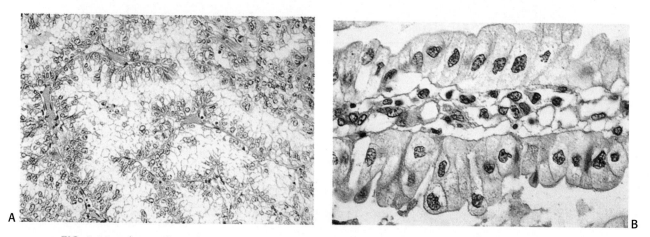

FIG. 5.44. Pylorocardiac subtype. **A:** The glands are lined by large cells with clear cytoplasm. **B:** The cytoplasm is diffusely vacuolated.

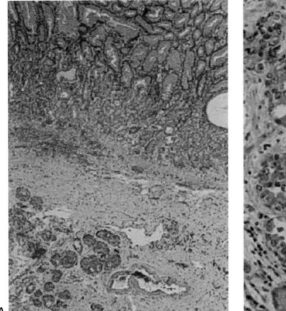
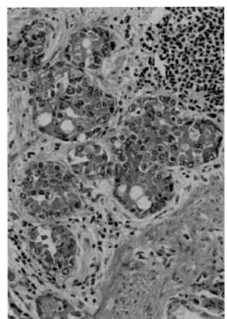

FIG. 5.45. Parietal cell differentiation in gastric cancer. **A:** An infiltrating carcinoma is seen extending into the submucosa. **B:** These glands are lined by cells with brightly eosinophilic, granular cytoplasm resembling that of the nonneoplastic parietal cells in the overlying mucosa.

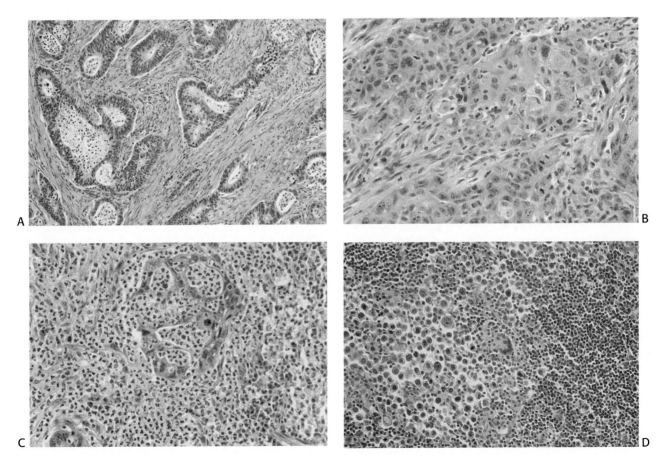

FIG. 5.46. Adenosquamous cell carcinoma. **A:** Area of adenocarcinoma. **B:** Area of squamous differentiation. **C:** Another area showing both glandular and squamous carcinoma. **D:** The nodal metastases were poorly differentiated, simulating a mantle zone lymphoma.

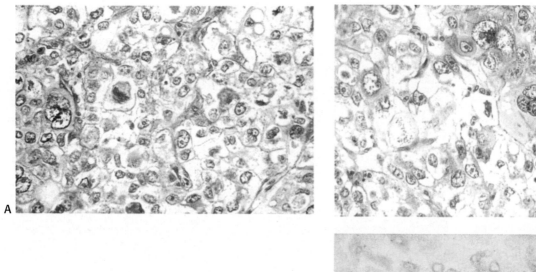

FIG. 5.47. Carcinoma with choriocarcinoma. **A:** Poorly differentiated adenocarcinoma admixed with choriocarcinoma. **B:** A large trophoblasticlike cell is seen on the right. **C:** These cells are human chorionic gonadotropin positive.

from gestational and gonadal cancers. Rarely, the glandular component may be an early carcinoma. Histologically, transitions occur from the trophoblastic areas to the more classic glandular phenotype. The tumors arise in both sexes (male-to-female ratio = 2.1), affecting individuals between the ages of 25 to older than 80 years, with a mean age of 55 to 58 years (126). High circulating human chorionic gonadotropin (hCG) levels may cause gynecomastia and Leydig cell hyperplasia in men or secretory mammary changes and abnormal uterine bleeding in women. The nonneoplastic antral mucosa contains hCG-producing cells (127), and cells that contain hCG may be seen in as many as 8.2% of advanced cancers and 6% of early cancers (128). The adenocarcinomatous component of this tumor is usually negative for hCG (Fig. 5.47), but positive for cytokeratin, carcinoembryonic antigen (CEA), and α-fetoprotein (AFP). It is known that many human malignancies can produce hCG or its subunits, so that the presence of hCG immunoreactivity is insufficient to diagnose a choriocarcinoma. Gastric carcinomas that express hCG have a poor prognosis (128).

Rare gastric cancers contain components resembling endodermal sinus tumors (129) and embryonal carcinoma. They may occur in males or females. Like choriocarcinomas, they may be associated with adenocarcinoma. Transitions occur between the germ cell and epithelial components of the cancer. The presence of Schiller-Duval bodies and hyaline droplets allows the recognition of the endodermal sinus component.

Hepatoid Carcinoma and α-Fetoprotein-producing Gastric Cancer. Hepatoid carcinomas have the histologic and immunohistochemical features of hepatocellular carcinomas. They arise from various organs, including the stomach (130,131). Since the fetal liver is a principal source of AFP, and because hepatocellular carcinomas are characteristically associated with AFP production, this protein has been widely accepted as a marker for hepatic differentiation at other sites (131). Albumin (ALB) mRNA also indicates hepatocellular differentiation (132). Not all primary gastric hepatoid carcinomas produce AFP (133), however, and not all AFP-producing gastric cancers show hepatoid differentiation (133). Most hepatoid carcinomas contain distinctive areas of tubular carcinoma that produce intestinal-type mucins (131). The tubular and hepatoid components of these cancers share common p53 mutations and common patterns of chromosome X inactivation (131). Similarly, hepatoid carcinomas that produce ALB mRNA may or may not produce AFP (132), indicating that the diagnosis of hepatoid adenocarcinoma should be made on the basis of its morphology, irrespective of its AFP production. When compared to AFP-negative cancers, AFP-producing cancers show higher Ki-67 labeling indices and lower apoptosis indices, reflecting the aggressive behavior and poor prognosis of these tumors (133).

Carcinosarcoma and Osseous Stromal Metaplasia. Carcinosarcomas are very uncommon and are usually encountered among elderly men (134). As in the esophagus, they usually present as large polypoid or fungating masses containing areas of carcinoma and sarcoma. The sarcomatous component usually has spindle cell morphology and, when differentiated, most often shows smooth muscle features. Chondrosarcoma and rhabdomyosarcomas have been reported on several occasions. Recent reports of gastric carcinosarcomas that show neuroendocrine differentiation highlight the heterogeneity of these tumors (135). The sarcomatous components sometimes stain with epithelial markers. The presence of osteoid and mature bone in the desmoplastic stroma of a gastric cancer must be distinguished from carcinosarcoma (136). Stromal ossification occurs in gastrointestinal cancers from the stomach to the rectum and appears to result from tumor production of bone morphogenic protein (137).

Gastric Carcinomas with Unusual Host Reactions. Gastric cancers, like those at other primary sites, may associate with intense eosinophilia. *Tumor-associated tissue eosinophilia* has been observed frequently in cancer tissues, but its cause is unknown (138). A study of 25 early gastric cancers found that eosinophils were more numerous in the stroma of these tumors than in the adjacent normal-appearing mucosa (139). The intensity of the infiltrate does not relate to the size of the tumor, its histologic type, or the presence of necrosis in the tumor. Tumor cells in intimate contact with activated eosinophils exhibited cytopathic changes. This might explain

the observation that stage-adjusted gastric cancers with numerous stromal eosinophils carry a lower risk of death than those with none (140).

Sarcoidlike granulomas have been observed in the stroma adjacent to many cancers and in the regional nodes that drain them, including gastric carcinoma (141,142). A recent study found four gastric adenocarcinomas among 14 cancers (28.5%) that associated with this sarcoidlike reaction (142). The carcinoma-associated granulomas resemble those seen in sarcoidosis with respect to their morphology and angiotensin I–converting enzyme expression, but show some differences. CD4+ helper T lymphocytes generally outnumber CD8+ T lymphocytes in sarcoidosis, while the sarcoid reaction to tumors associates with a greater proportion of CD8+ T cells, to the extent that they may even outnumber CD4+ cells. Although the sarcoid reaction may represent a T cell–mediated immune response to the tumors, too few gastric cancers have been observed with this reaction to assess its impact on survival.

Spread of Gastric Cancer

Most patients in unscreened populations, and a significant minority of patients in screened populations, are diagnosed when their cancer is already advanced. There may be direct extension to adjacent organs, including the pancreas, transverse colon, hilum of the liver, abdominal wall, or esophagus (143). Intramural spread beneath the intact mucosa is common (Fig. 5.48), as is lymphatic invasion (Fig. 5.48).

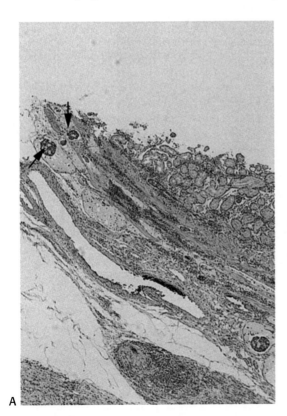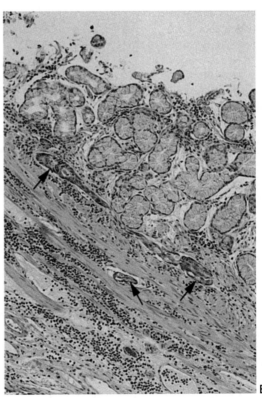

FIG. 5.48. Intramural spread of gastric cancer. **A, B:** Intact overlying epithelium is seen in both of the illustrated cases. The presence of gastric cancer within lymphatics (*arrows*) at these resection margins was not appreciated grossly.

Lymphatic spread occurs early, and as noted above, may even be observed with small submucosal cancers. Lymphatic and vascular invasion carries a poor prognosis (144) and is frequently seen in advanced cases (145). Surgical resection margins should be monitored by frozen section because gross assessment is inaccurate and margin involvement occurs in 15% of cases.

The failure rate of adjuvant postoperative treatment of gastric cancer has prompted investigators to better define the surgical potential of influencing patient prognosis. Intense interest centers on assessment of the extent of mural invasion, because this correlates with the presence of tumor at the resection margins. Infiltration of the proximal margin of the resection is significantly more frequent when the tumor penetrates the serosa than when the lesion is confined to the mucosa, submucosa, or muscularis propria. Proximal or distal infiltration >3 cm does not occur with lesions confined to mucosa, submucosa, or muscularis propria. The pathologist should take pains to identify the proximity of the cancer to the radial margin, which is defined as the surgically dissected surface adjacent to the deepest point of tumor invasion. A deeply penetrating cancer that centers on the lesser or greater curvature may have a radial margin that lies in the connective tissue of the lesser or greater omentum, rather than the serosal surface. Microscopic involvement of a resection margin is almost synonymous with early recurrence or death.

The extent of lymphadenectomy is another area of interest. Lymphatic spread occurs early. The purpose of nodal dissection is to detect and remove metastases, so as to improve the chances of survival and to accurately stage the disease. The Japanese Research Society for Gastric Cancer divides the regional nodes of the stomach into four groups (143), as shown in Table 5.9. Some of the decline in gastric cancer mortality in Japan has been attributed to the widespread practice of extended lymph node resections to include all N1 and N2 node groups (R-2 resections). These node groupings roughly overlap with those defined in the current American Joint Committee on Cancer (AJCC) staging manual (146),

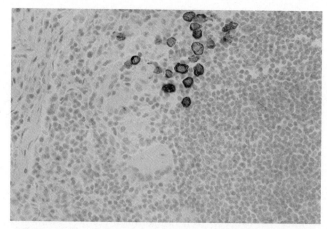

FIG. 5.49. Micrometastases of a diffuse gastric carcinoma in a regional lymph node highlighted by a cytokeratin immunostain.

although the number of involved nodes, rather than the node subsite, is the basis for assigning an N level in the AJCC system. It is therefore important that the pathologist search for as many nodes as possible within a resection specimen and that the location of these nodes be accurately documented. Sentinel node technology has the potential of predicting the extent of lymph node involvement (147). One sentinel node mapping study, using both radioisotope and dye labeling, found the sentinel node to be positive in 40 of 41 (98%) of cases with regional node involvement (148). These promising results need to be confirmed by much larger studies.

Micrometastases, unsuspected by standard H&E stains, can be identified with immunochemical (Fig. 5.49) (148) and molecular markers (149), but their clinical significance is uncertain. One study suggests that identification of micrometastases in lymph nodes may predict prognosis (148). In another study immunohistochemical stains discovered micrometastases to the bone marrow in 44 of 50 (88%) patients undergoing resection for GEJ cancer (150). This is far more frequent than the clinical frequency of bone metastases from this site. Large, prospective studies will be required to determine the prognostic value of detecting nodal and bone marrow micrometastases.

Age, gender, and histologic type strongly influence the patterns of spread to distant sites. The intestinal-type cancers that typically arise in the distal third of the stomach in older men frequently metastasize to the liver, where they form discrete masses (151). The diffuse cancers that predominate in premenopausal women show a predilection for transperitoneal spread. Ovarian metastases from gastric cancer (Krukenberg tumors) are acquired by this route (Fig. 5.50). While Krukenberg tumors classically result from the spread of diffuse gastric carcinomas, ovarian metastases of intestinal-type tumors also occur, usually in older women with widespread disease (151a). Transperitoneal spread also accounts for metastases to the endometrium and uterine cervix in the same age group (152). Peritoneal involvement,

TABLE 5.9	Regional Lymph Groups, Cancers at All Gastric Subsites

Group 1 (N1): Right and left cardinal nodes
  Nodes along lesser curvature
  Nodes along greater curvature
  Suprapyloric nodes
  Infrapyloric nodes
Group 2 (N2): Nodes along left gastric artery
  Nodes along common hepatic artery
  Nodes around celiac artery
  Nodes at splenic hilum
Group 3 (N3): Nodes in hepatoduodenal ligament
  Nodes behind pancreas head
  Nodes at root of mesentery
Group 4 (N4): Nodes along middle colic artery
  Para-aortic nodes

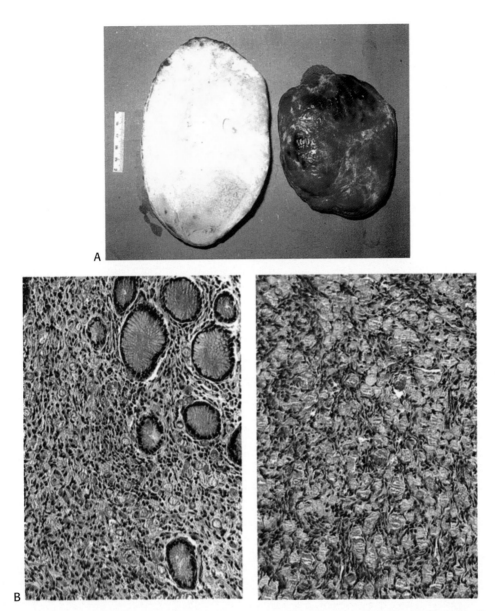

FIG. 5.50. Krukenberg tumor. **A:** Enlarged ovaries in a 46-year-old woman with diffuse signet ring cell carcinoma of the stomach. **B:** Microscopic appearance of the primary tumor (*left*) and metastasis (*right*).

combined with lymphatic obstruction, may result in the development of ascites, a presenting symptom in some cases. Blood-borne metastases occur even in the absence of lymphatic involvement with seeding to the liver, lungs, bone, and skin. Direct extension to the pancreas, the colon, and other neighboring organs is common. When the cancer penetrates the serosal surface, peritoneal implants may flourish in the greater omentum and pelvic cul-de-sac.

The prognosis of gastric carcinoma is best estimated by assessing its stage at the time of diagnosis. The TNM system (T, extent of primary tumor; N, extent of lymph node metastases; M, presence of distant metastases), as published by the WHO (110), is now the standard stage classification worldwide and is summarized in Table 5.10. The age-adjusted 5-year survival of patients with stage I cancer approximates

95% (78), but only 7% of patients with stage IV cancers are 5-year survivors (153). The presence and number of nodal metastases are important determinants of survival (154), and the correct assignment of an N stage clearly depends on the number of nodes removed by the surgeon (155). More extensive lymph node dissection probably accounts for much of the difference in the 5-year survival of patients with stage I cancer in Japan (95%) versus in the United States (78%) (153).

The standard of care in the treatment of gastric cancer in the United States is reflected by an analysis of 50,169 patients treated by gastrectomy during the years 1985–1996. Less than half of these patients could be staged by the WHO system (153). This study found that only 33,806 (67%) cases had sufficient node data for TNM staging, and of those with

TABLE 5.10   World Health Organization TNM Classification of Gastric Tumors

T—Primary Tumor	Stage	Grouping
TX—Primary tumor cannot be assessed	Stage 0	TisN0M0
T0—No evidence of primary tumor	Stage IA	T1N0M0
Tis—Carcinoma in situ	Stage IB	T2N0M0
Intraepithelial tumor without invasion of lamina propria		T1N1M0
T1—Tumor invades lamina propria or submucosa	Stage II	T1N2M0
T2—Tumor invades muscularis propria or subserosa		T2N1M0
T3—Tumor penetrates serosa (visceral peritoneum)		T3N0M0
T4—Tumor invades adjacent structure*	Stage IIIA	T2N2M0
*Spleen, transverse colon, liver, diaphragm, pancreas, abdominal wall, adrenal gland, kidney, small intestine, retroperitoneum		T3N1M0
		T4N0M0
	Stage IIIB	T3N2M0
	Stage IV	Any T Any N M1
		T4N1–3M0
		T1–3N3M0

N—Regional Lymph Nodes

NX—Regional nodes cannot be assessed
N0—No lymph node metastases
N1—Metastases in one to six lymph nodes
N2—Metastases to 7 to 15 lymph nodes
N3—Metastases to more than 15 lymph nodes

M—Distant Metastases

MX—Distant metastases cannot be assessed
M0—No distant metastases
M1—Distant metastases

counted nodes, 25% had less than seven nodes examined. None of these patients could be assigned to stage IIIB, since this stage is defined by having metastases in seven or more nodes. The conclusion of the report was that undertreatment of patients with gastric cancer is a problem in the United States. It should be emphasized, however, that perfunctory pathology reporting may have made significant contributions to staging errors as well. Lymph node harvesting is noticeably better in American hospitals that specialize in cancer treatment than in the country as a whole, but a direct comparison between one of them and two Japanese institutions found that more accurate staging contributed to the more favorable outcome of gastric cancer patients in Japan (155). The depth of invasion is the most important TNM variable for gastric cancer staging (144), and this is fortunately less subject to error than nodal appraisal.

Pathology variables not included in the TNM system also influence survival with stomach cancer, including tumor size, location, and histologic type. A Japanese retrospective, multivariate analysis of survival after curative resection found that, in addition to the depth of invasion, the size of the cancer and location in the proximal third of the stomach were independent predictors of the time interval between treatment and recurrence (156).

Immunohistochemical Markers

It is now common practice to use immunohistochemical stains to assess the phenotypic heterogeneity of gastric cancers, to identify tumor characteristics that might influence prognosis, and to determine whether these characteristics might make them more, or less, responsive to chemotherapeutic agents.

Phenotypic Markers

Markers are available that identify the different gastric and intestinal cells from which cancers may arise, but loss of specific traits through dedifferentiation and the accumulation of other traits through postinduction alterations complicate attempts to identify the progenitor cells of specific cancers. Analysis of large numbers of cancers, however, provides levels of probability that a cancer in the proximal stomach derives from the cardia, the distal esophagus, or the corpus, or that a distal gastric cancer derives from metaplastic intestinal cells or residual antral glands. Cytokeratin 20 (CK20) is a marker for antral epithelium, while CK7 generally labels the columnar cells of the cardia (157). Adenocarcinomas of the gastroesophageal junction are more likely to express CK7,

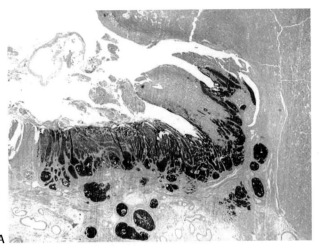
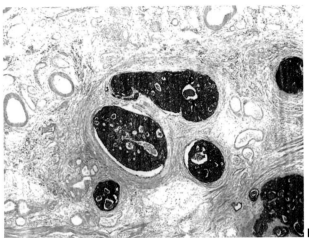

FIG. 5.51. Epithelial growth factor receptor (EGFR) positivity of a gastric adenocarcinoma. **A:** Note that not all the tumor cells are positive. There is an area in the middle of the tumor which is completely EGFR negative. **B:** The EGFR-positive clones have a propensity for vascular invasion.

and those in the antrum are more likely to express CK20 (158). The mucin core peptide cores (MUC) vary from site to site in the gastrointestinal tract. Two of these, MUC1 and MUC5AC, are more frequent in carcinomas distal to the cardia than in cardia cancers (159).

Sucrase, a disaccharidase normal to the glycocalyx of small bowel epithelium, is present in the intestinalized gastric mucosa. Its expression in gastric cancer is less consistent. Its expression is most frequent in well-differentiated intestinal-type cancers, suggesting that these cancers derive from metaplastic intestinal cells. Sucrase expression increases in frequency with the depth of invasion for both well- and poorly differentiated tumors, but this phenomenon is unexpectedly stronger for the less differentiated tumors (160). This suggests that some late-stage tumors that arise from gastric stem cells may undergo postinduction metaplasia.

PGII is produced in all gastric glands. Approximately 40% of gastric cancers express this product (161,162), suggesting a gastric, rather than metaplastic, origin of these cancers. This may be misleading, since PGII expression is most frequent in poorly differentiated, high-stage cancers arising in a totally intestinalized gastric mucosa. This suggests that, as in the case of sucrase, postinduction alterations may change a cancer phenotype, in this case by reversion from an intestinal to a gastric phenotype.

Prognostic and Therapeutic Markers

Amplification of growth factors, such as epithelial growth factor (EGF) and its receptor (EGFR), associate with higher proliferative indices, an effect that is enhanced when coexpressed with other growth factors, such as TGF-α and p185[c-erb-2] (163). EGFR overexpression associates with more frequent metastases and less favorable prognosis (164). The influence of growth factors on tumor progression is augmented by abnormalities in cell cycling. Thus, adenocarcinomas dependent on the TGF-α–EGFR autocrine loop exhibit increased aggressiveness in the presence of aberrant p53 expression (165). Clonal heterogeneity of EGFR and other tumor markers in advanced cancer is especially ominous, with the amplified components showing a selective advantage in vascular invasion (Fig. 5.51).

The *met* oncogene is a tyrosine kinase that encodes the hepatocyte growth factor receptor and stimulates mitogenesis, motogenesis, vasculogenesis, and morphogenesis in a wide range of cellular targets. Abnormalities in this gene are implicated in gastric carcinoma (165a). Importantly, like other tyrosine kinases that become abnormal in cancer, it represents an attractive therapeutic target (165a).

The Wnt signaling pathway is also commonly abnormal in gastric cancer. TC1, a novel regulator of the Wnt signaling pathway, is up-regulated in gastric cancers. It plays a role in poor differentiation and aggressive biologic behavior in gastric cancer (165b). Cyclin D1, a Wnt signaling target, regulates cell cycle progression from the G1 to S phase (166). It is not expressed in normal gastric mucosa, but is expressed in 40% of gastric cancers (167). Patients whose tumors show cyclin D amplification, but not overexpression, have a less favorable 5-year survival than those who do not, although there is no correlation between cyclin D1 amplification and either nodal metastases or histologic grade (unpublished observations).

One would predict that loss of tumor suppressor factors also spurs abnormal cell growth, but the results of numerous studies on p53 are conflicting in this regard (168). p53 expression does not exactly correlate with mutational status since it does not detect deletions or nonsense mutations in this gene. Observed differences respecting the influence of p53 immunohistochemical expression on prognosis (168) are less consistent than growth or cell cycle factors. A higher cancer stage is more likely, however, when p53 expression accompanies an amplified growth factor than with the growth factor alone.

As may be expected, factors that mark the transition from preinvasive to invasive cancer are also associated with less favorable prognosis. Immunohistochemical expression of MMP7 associates with lymphatic invasion and poor survival (169,170). Expression of two motility factors, fascin (171,172) and autocrine motility factor (AMFr) (173), also associates with poor survival. A cancer enhances its chances of dissemination by stimulating angiogenesis with vascular endothelial growth factor (VEGF). Expression of two members of the VEGF family, VEGF-C and VEGF-D, in gastric cancer correlates with lymphatic invasion and increased mortality (174,175).

Several other biomarkers have been associated with aggressive growth and poor prognosis with gastric cancer, including thioredoxin, a putative oncogene (176); microsatellite stability; and the non-CIMP phenotype (36b). As noted above, *met* abnormalities independently associate with gastric cancer progression, especially when coexpressed with AMFr and urokinase-type plasminogen activator receptor. Androgen receptor (AR) activation enhances VEGF gene transcription and may have antiapoptotic activity as well. Approximately 17% of gastric cancers express AR, with no gender difference in frequency. AR-expressing gastric cancers are more likely to have nodal metastases and less favorable prognosis than those that do not (177). Overexpression of cyclooxygenase-2 (COX-2) associates with deep invasion and nodal metastases (178). COX-2 frequently associates with HER-2 or tumors with reduced expression of Smad4 (an intracellular transducer), suggesting that signal transduction through the HER-2 and SMAD system may regulate COX-2 expression. There are polymorphisms in this gene, some of which associate with reduced gene expression. There is a greater than twofold higher risk for progressing to gastric cancer among patients with chronic gastritis who have the homozygous variant 1195AA *COX2* genotype than heterozygotes and those who are homozygous wild type (178a).

Treatment

The almost limitless heterogeneity of most advanced gastric cancers creates a barrier to the development of customized chemotherapeutic approaches. Surgery remains the mainstay of treatment of advanced gastric cancers. Palliation, rather than cure, is the primary goal of adjuvant therapy (177). Most patients who have had a resection for gastric cancer with extensive lymph node metastases will have a disease relapse. No randomized trial has shown a benefit for this subset of patients and no single agent has proved effective for postoperative chemotherapy (179). This is not unexpected since successful response to treatment with drugs that target specific oncogenes allows subsets of other cells to survive and serve as the seedbeds for recurrent tumors.

METASTASES TO THE STOMACH

The stomach may be the recipient of cancers from other sites, the most common primary sources being melanoma, lung

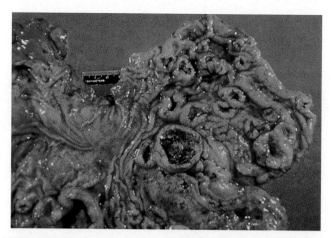

FIG. 5.52. Metastatic melanoma in the stomach. The mucosal surface contains numerous ulcerated and hemorrhagic tumor nodules.

cancer, and breast cancer. If the tumor produces multiple, discrete, ulcerated nodules such as may occur with disseminated melanoma (Fig. 5.52), the diagnosis is fairly obvious. In contrast, metastases from breast cancer may mimic linitis plastica, both clinically and anatomically (180), and a gastric metastasis may be the presenting symptom of a primary breast cancer (180,181). In one recent study of 51 breast cancers metastatic to the stomach, this was the metastatic site in 14 cases (180). Lobular cancer is a frequent type of breast cancer that metastasizes to the stomach (Fig. 5.53). Endoscopic biopsies may be negative in up to a quarter of these cases, because the metastases may be localized to the deep layers. The desmoplasia associated with lobular carcinoma and its discohesive growth pattern may so closely resemble diffuse gastric cancer that distinction between the two tumors may be difficult. The fact that gastric cancers, irrespective of gender, may be estrogen receptor (ER) positive (182) and that diffuse gastric cancer may metastasize to the breast (183) does not make the problem any easier. A study that compared primary gastric cancers with positive gastric biopsies from

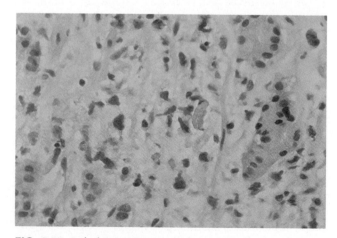

FIG. 5.53. Lobular carcinoma of the breast metastatic to the gastric mucosa. It simulates a primary diffuse gastric cancer.

patients with a history of breast cancer found that the tumors in 14 of 28 (50%) patients with breast cancer were ER positive, compared to only 1 of 46 (2%) gastric cancers (184). Stains for E-cadherin expression are more likely to be negative with breast than gastric cancer, even when the comparison is limited to diffuse gastric cancer and lobular breast cancer ($p = 0.01$). These findings indicate that a gastric biopsy that yields an ER-positive, E-cadherin–negative cancer is diagnostic of a metastatic breast cancer rather than a primary stomach cancer.

HANDLING OF GASTRIC RESECTION SPECIMENS

The gastrectomy specimen should be sent to the pathology department as soon as possible after its removal from the patient. The stomach should be opened along the greater curvature and pinned to a cork board or paraffin plate and floated upside down in 10% neutral buffered formalin for at least 12 hours. The gross limits of the tumor are more easily assessed if the specimen is well fixed, and small, unsuspected multicentric tumors may be more easily identified. However, if alkaline phosphatase staining is performed, the specimen should be fixed in formalin prechilled to 4°C because this enzyme is thermolabile. This procedure is usually reserved for investigational purposes and need not be performed in routine cases.

The gross description of the fixed specimen should include the type of resection (proximal subtotal, distal subtotal, or total), the lengths of the greater and lesser curvatures, the length of attached esophagus and/or duodenum, the axial and transverse diameters of the tumor, and the location of the tumor within the stomach. The gross configuration of the tumor should also be noted (i.e., fungating, ulcerated, diffuse, etc.). All lesions should be described and sampled, including areas of ulceration and polypoid or elevated lesions. The location of such lesions should be accurately described in relation to the main tumor mass. In many cases, an explanatory diagram or photograph is useful for documenting the distance of the tumor from resection margins and its relationship to other lesions present in the stomach.

The cut edges of the specimen should be marked with India ink before sectioning. Circumferential blocks are obtained from the margins of resection to rule out grossly inapparent intramural spread to the surgical margin. Two to four sections should be taken from the tumor, depending on its size. At least one of these sections should include the full thickness of the gastric wall so that the maximum depth of penetration can be determined. A generous sample of the intact nonneoplastic mucosa on the proximal and distal sides of the tumor should be included with the neoplasm in order to identify precursor lesions, including intestinal metaplasia, atrophic gastritis, and areas of dysplasia. The pathologist should harvest as many nodes as possible from the lesser curvature and the distal and proximal greater curvature, separately identifying those <3 cm or >3 cm from the tumor.

Histologic examination should include the following: (a) the TNM status of the tumor; (b) the histologic type of the cancer using the Lauren or WHO classification, and its degree of differentiation; (c) the presence and extent of vascular and perineural invasion; (d) the histologic findings in the nonneoplastic gastric mucosa; and (e) the presence or absence of lymph node metastasis. Each report should contain, as a minimum, the information needed to assign an accurate TNM stage, the gastric subsite location of the tumor, a histologic classification of the tumor, and an estimate of its degree of differentiation. EMR specimens should be handled as discussed in Chapter 3.

REFERENCES

1. Devesa SS, Blot WJ, Fraumeni JF Jr: Changing patterns in the incidence of esophageal and gastric carcinoma in the United States. *Cancer* 1998;83:2049.
2. Parkin DM, Whelan SL, Ferlay, et al: *Cancer Incidence in Five Continents*, Vol. VIII, No. 155. Lyon, France: IARC Scientific Publications, 2002, pp 546–548.
3. Newnham A, Quinn MJ, Babb P, et al: Trends in the subsite and morphology of oesophageal cancer in England and Wales 1971–1998. *Aliment Pharmacol Ther* 2003;17:665.
4. Kolonel LN, Hanken J, Nomura AMY, et al: Multiethnic studies of diet, nutrition and cancer in Hawaii. In: Hayashi Y, Nagao M, Sugimura T (eds). *Diet, Nutrition and Cancer*. Tokyo, Japan: Scientific Societies Press, 1986, pp 29–40.
5. Devesa SS, Grauman DJ, Blot WJ, et al: *Atlas of Cancer Mortality in the United States 1950–94*. NIH Publication No. 99-4564. Washington, DC: National Institutes of Health, 1999, pp 36–37.
6. Lauren T: The two histologic main types of gastric carcinoma: diffuse and so-called intestinal type. *Acta Pathol Microbiol* 1965;64:31.
7. Henson DE, Dittus C, Younes M, et al: Differential trends in the intestinal and diffuse types of gastric carcinoma in the United States, 1973–2000. *Arch Pathol Lab Med* 2004;128:765.
8. Liu Y, Kaneko S, Sabue T: Trends in reported incidences of gastric cancer by tumor location, from 1975–1989 in Japan. *Int J Epidemiol* 2004;33:808.
9. Stemmermann GN, Fenoglio-Preiser CM: Gastric carcinoma distal to the cardia: a review of the epidemiological pathology of the precursors to a preventable disease. *Pathology* 2002;34:494.
10. Mendall MA, Goggin PM, Molineaux N, et al: Childhood living conditions and Helicobacter pylori seropositivity in adult life. *Lancet* 1992;39:896.
11. El-Omar EM, Oien K, Murray LS, et al: Increased prevalence of precancerous changes in relatives of gastric cancer patients: critical role of H. pylori. *Gastroenterology* 2000;118:22.
12. Park YJ, Shin K-H, Park J-G: Risk of gastric cancer in hereditary nonpolyposis colorectal cancer in Korea. *Clinical Cancer Res* 2000;6:2994.
13. Lynch HT, Grady W, Suriano G, Huntsman D: Gastric cancer: new genetic developments. *J Surg Oncol* 2005;90:114.
14. Aarnio M, Salovaaro R, Aaltonen LA, et al: Features in gastric cancer in hereditary non-polyposis colorectal cancer syndrome. *Int J Cancer* 1997;89:1021.
15. Utsonomiya Y, Maki T, Iwanuma T, et al: Gastric lesions in familial polyposis coli. *Cancer* 1974;34:745.
16. Iida M, Yao T, Ito H, et al: Natural history of fundic gland polyposis in patients with familial polyposis coli/Gardener's syndrome. *Gastroenterology* 1985;89:1021.
17. Guilford P, Hopkins J, Harraway J, et al: E-cadherin germline mutations in familial gastric cancer. *Nature* 1998;392:402.
18. Gayther SA, Gorringe KL, Ramus SJ, et al: Identification or germ-line E-cadherin mutations in gastric cancer family of European origin. *Cancer Res* 1998;58:1086.
19. Keller G, Vogelsang H, Becker I, et al: Germline mutations of E-cadherin (CDH1) and TP53 genes rather than RUNX and HPP1, contribute to genetic predisposition of German gastric cancer patients. *J Med Genet* 2004;41:401.

20. Brooks-Wilson AR, Kaurah P, Suriano G, et al: Germline E-cadherin mutations in hereditary diffuse gastric cancer: assessment of 42 families and review of genetic screening data. *J Med Genet* 2004;41:508.

21. Newman EK, Mulholland MW: Prophylactic gastrectomy for hereditary diffuse gastric cancer syndrome. *J Am Coll Surg* 2006;202:612.

22. Oliveira C, Moreira H, Seruca R, et al: Role of pathology in the identification of hereditary diffuse cancer: report of a Portuguese family. *Virchows Archiv* 2005;446:181.

23. Bermejo JL, Hemminki K: Risk of cancer at sites other than breast in Swedish families eligible for BRCA1 or BRCA2 mutation testing. *Ann Oncol* 2004;15:1834.

24. Varley JM, McGown G, Thorncroft M, et al: An extended Li-Fraumeni kindred with gastric-carcinoma and a codon 175 mutation on TP53. *J Med Genet* 1995;32:942.

25. Horio Y, Suzuki H, Ueda R, et al: Predominantly tumor-limited expression of a mutant allele in a Japanese family carrying a germline p53 mutation. *Oncogene* 1994;9:1231.

26. Giardiello FM, Brensinger JD, Tersmette AC, et al: Very high risk of cancer in familial Peutz-Jeghers syndrome. *Gastroenterology* 2000;119:1447.

27. Shinmura K, Goto M, Tao H, et al: A novel STK11 germline mutation in two siblings with Peutz-Jeghers syndrome complicated by primary gastric cancer. *Clin Gen* 2005;67:81.

28. Correa P, Sasano N, Stemmermann GN, Haenszel W: Pathology of gastric carcinoma in Japanese populations: comparison between Miyagi Prefecture, Japan and Hawaii. *J Natl Cancer Inst* 1973;51;1449.

29. El-Omar E, Carrington M, Chow WH, et al: Interleukin-1 polymorphism associated with increased risk of gastric cancer. *Nature* 2000; 404:398.

30. Figueiredo C, Machado JC, Carlos J, et al: Helicobacter pylori and interleukin 1 genotyping: an opportunity to identify individuals at high risk for gastric carcinoma. *J Natl Cancer Inst* 2002;94:1662.

31. Machado JC, Figueiredo C, Canado P, et al: A proinflammatory genetic profile increases the risk of chronic atrophic gastritis and gastric cancer. *Gastroenterology* 2003;125:364.

32. Katoh T, Nagata N, Kuroda, et al: Glutathione S-transferase M1(GSTM1) and T1(GSTT1) genetic polymorphism and susceptibility of gastric and colorectal cancer. *Carcinogenesis* 1996;17;1855.

33. Boissey RJ, Watson MA, Umbach DM, et al: A pilot study investigating the role of NAT-1 and NAT-2 polymorphisms in gastric adenocarcinoma. *Int J Cancer* 2000;87:507.

34. Park GT, Lee OY, Kwon SJ, et al: Analysis of CYP1E1 polymorphism for the determination of genetic susceptibility to gastric cancer in Koreans. *J Gastroenterol Hepatol* 2003;18:1257.

35. Carvalho F, Seruca R, David I, et al: MUC1 polymorphism and gastric cancer-an epidemiological study. *Glycoconj J* 1997;14:107.

36. Lee SG, Kim B, Choi J, et al: Genetic polymorphisms of XRCC1 and risk of gastric cancer. *Cancer Lett* 2002;187:53.

36a. Miao X, Zhang X, Zhang L, et al: Adenosine diphosphate ribosyl transferase and x-ray repair cross-complementing 1 polymorphisms in gastric cardia cancer. *Gastroenterology* 2006;131:420.

36b. Kusano M, Toyota M, Suzuki H, et al: Genetic, epigenetic and clinicopathologic features of gastric carcinomas and the CpG island methylator phenotype and an association with Epstein-Barr virus. *Cancer* 2006;106:1467.

36c. Chang M-S, Uozaki H, Chong J-M, et al: CpG island methylation status in gastric carcinoma with and without infection of Epstein-Barr virus. *Clin Cancer Res* 2006;12:2995.

36d. Leung WK, Man EPS, Yu J, et al: Effects of Helicobacter pylori eradication on methylation status of e-cadherin gene in noncancerous stomach. *Clin Cancer Res* 2006;3216.

36e. Wang L-H, Choi Y-L, Hua X-Y, et al: Increased expression of sonic hedgehog and alteration methylation of its promoter region in gastric cancer and its related lesions. *Mod Pathol* 2006;19:675.

37. Goodman KJ, Correa P: The transmission of Helicobacter pylori: a critical review of the evidence. *Int J Epidemiol* 1995;24:875.

38. Nomura AMY, Stemmermann GN, Chyou H, et al: Helicobacter pylori infection and gastric cancer among Japanese Americans in Hawaii. *N Engl J Med* 1991;325:1132.

39. Forman D: Gastric cancer and Helicobacter pylori: a combined analysis of 12 case-control studies nested in prospective cohorts. *Gut* 2001;49:347.

40. Nomura AMY, Kolonel L, Miki K, et al: Helicobacter pylori, pepsinogen and gastric adenocarcinoma in Hawaii. *J Infect Dis* 2005;191:2075.

41. Mirvish SS: Etiology of gastric cancer. Intragastric nitrosamide formation and other theories. *J Natl Cancer Inst* 1983;71:629.

42. Sugimura T, Fujimura S: Tumor production in the glandular stomach of rat by N-methyl-N′-nitro-N-nitrosoguanadine. *Nature* 1967;216:943.

43. Stemmermann GN, Nomura AMY, Chyou PH, et al: Impact of diet and smoking on the risk of developing intestinal metaplasia of the stomach. *Dig Dis Sci* 1990;35:433.

44. Nomura AMY: Stomach cancer. In: Schoenfeld D, Fraumani J (eds). *Cancer, Epidemiology and Prevention*, 2nd ed. Oxford University Press, 1996, pp 707–724.

45. Butiatti E, Palli D, De Carli A, et al: A case-control study of gastric cancer in Italy: association with nutrients. *Int J Cancer* 1990;45:896.

46. Inoue M, Tajima K, Kobayashi S, et al: Protective factor against progression of atrophic gastritis to gastric cancer—data from a cohort study in Japan. *Int J Cancer* 1996;66:309.

47. Tridaniel J, Boffeta P, Butiatti E, et al: Tobacco smoking and gastric cancer: a review and meta-analysis. *Int J Cancer* 1997;72:565.

48. Stemmermann GN, Marcus EB, Buist AS, et al: Relative impact of smoking and reduced pulmonary function on peptic ulcer risk. *Gastroenterology* 1989;96:1413.

49. Kato H, Schull WJ: Studies of mortality of A-bomb survivors. *Radiat Res* 1982;90:395.

50. Brumback RA, Gerber JE, Hicks DJ, et al: Adenocarcinoma of the stomach following radiation and chemotherapy in young patients. *Cancer* 1984;54:994.

51. Stael von Holstein CCS, Anderson H, Eriksson SBS, Huldt B: Mortality after remote surgery for benign gastroduodenal disease. *Gut* 1995;37:612.

52. Stemmermann GN, Hayashi T: Hyperplastic polyps of the gastric mucosa adjacent to gastroenterostomy stomas. *Am J Clin Pathol* 1979;71:341.

53. Mukaisho KI, Miwa K, Kumagai H, et al: Gastric carcinogenesis by duodenal reflux through gut regenerative cell lineage. *Dig Dis Sci* 2003;48:2153.

54. Kamanishi M: How is it possible to prevent gastric mucosal injury and remnant cancer after distal gastrectomy? *J Gastroenterol* 2005;40:661.

55. Toledano MT, del Olmo JCM, Castano JG, et al: Gastric pouch carcinoma after gastric bypass for morbid obesity. *Obes Surg* 2005;15:1215.

56. Flickinger EG, Sinar DR, Pories WJ, et al: The by-passed stomach. *Am J Surg* 1985;149:151.

57. Correa P, Haenszel W, Cuello C, et al: A model for gastric cancer epidemiology. *Lancet* 1975;2:58.

58. Matsukura N, Suzuki K, Kawachi T, et al: Distribution of marker enzymes and mucin in intestinal metaplasia of the stomach and relation of complete and incomplete types of metaplasia to gastric cancer. *J Natl Cancer Inst* 1980;65:231.

59. Chiba T: Key molecules in metaplastic gastritis: sequential analysis of CDX1/2 homeobox gene expression. *J Gastroenterol* 2002;38:2975.

60. Mutoh H, Hakamoto Y, Sato K, et al: Conversion of gastric mucosa to intestinal metaplasia in CDX2-exoressing transgenic mice. *Biochem Biophys Res Commun* 2002;294:470.

61. Houghton J, Wang TG: Helicobacter pylori and gastric cancer: a new paradigm for inflammation-associated epithelial cancers. *Gastroenterology* 2005;128:1567.

62. Ota H, Katsuyama T, Nakajima S, et al: Intestinal metaplasia and adherent Helicobacter pylori: a hybrid epithelium with gastric and intestinal features. *Hum Pathol* 1998;29:846.

63. Otsuka T, Tsukamoto T, Mizoshita T, et al: Coexistence of gastric and intestinal-type endocrine cells in gastric and mixed intestinal metaplasia of the stomach. *Pathol Int* 2005;55:170.

64. Stemmermann GN, Samloff IM, Nomura AMY, Walsh JH: Serum pepsinogen and gastrin in relation to extent and location of intestinal metaplasia in patients with atrophic gastritis. *Dig Dis Sci* 1980;25:680.

65. Urita Y, Hike K, Torii N, et al: Serum pepsinogens as a predictor of the topography of intestinal metaplasia in patients with atrophic gastritis. *Dig Dis Sci* 2004;49:795.

66. Nomura AMY, Kolonel L, Miki K, et al: Helicobacter pylori, pepsinogen and gastric carcinoma in Hawaii. *J Infect Dis* 2005;191:2075.

67. Ma JY, Bork K, Sjostrand E, et al: Positive correlation between H,K adenosine triphosphatase auto-antibodies and Helicobacter pylori antibodies in patients with pernicious anemia. *Scand J Gastroenterol* 1994;29:961.

68. Brinton LA, Gridley G, Hrubec R, et al: Cancer risk following pernicious anemia. *Br J Cancer* 1989;59:810.

69. Sonnenberg A: Changes in physicians visits for gastric and duodenal ulcer in the United States during 1958–84. *Dig Dis Sci* 1987;32:1.

70. Graham DY, Schwartz JT, Cain D, et al: Prospective evaluation of biopsy number in the diagnosis of esophageal and gastric cancer. *Gastroenterology* 1982;82:228.

71. Jarvis LR, Whitehead R: Morphometric analysis of gastric dysplasia. *J Pathol* 1985;147:143.

72. Rugge M, Correa P, Dixon MF, et al: Gastric dysplasia. The Padova classification. *Am J Surg Pathol* 2000;24:167.

73. Montgomery E: Is there a way for pathologists to decrease the interobserver variation in the diagnosis of dysplasia? *Arch Pathol Lab Med* 2005;129:174.

74. Park DI, Rhee Pl, Kim JG, et al: Risk factors suggesting malignant transformation of gastric adenoma: univariate and multivariate analysis. *Endoscopy* 2001;33:501.

75. Tamei N, Kaise M, Nakayoshi T, et al: Clinical and endoscopic characterization of depressed gastric adenoma. *Endoscopy* 2006;38:391.

76. Saraga E-P, Gardiol D, Costa J: Gastric dysplasia. A histologic follow-up study. *Ann Surg Pathol* 1987;11:788.

77. Coma del Corral MJ, Pardo-Mindan FJ, Razquin S, et al: Risk of cancer in patients with gastric dysplasia. *Cancer* 1990;65:2078.

78. Hirota T, Ming SC, Itabashi M: Pathology of early gastric cancer. In: Nishi M, Ichikawa H, Nakajima Y, et al (eds). *Gastric Cancer*. Tokyo: Springer-Verlag, 1993, pp 66–85.

79. Murakami T: Pathomorphologic diagnosis. Definition and gross classification of early gastric cancer. In: *Early Gastric Cancer*. Gann Monograph on Cancer Research, No. 11. Tokyo: University Press, 1972, pp 53–55.

80. Kodama Y, Inokuchi K, Soejima K, et al: Growth patterns and prognosis in early gastric cancer. *Cancer* 1983;51:320.

81. Tskuma H, Mishima T, Oshima A: Prospective study of "early gastric cancer." *Int J Cancer* 1983;31:421.

82. Adachi Y, Mori M, Sugimachi K: Persistence of mucosal gastric carcinomas for 8 and 6 years in two patients. *Arch Pathol Lab Med* 1990;114:1046.

83. Son HJ, Song SY, Kim S, et al: Characteristics of submucosal gastric carcinoma with lymph node metastases. *Histopathology* 2005;46:158.

84. Arigami T, Natsugoe S, Uenosono Y, et al: Lymphatic invasion using D2-40 monoclonal antibody and its relation to lymph node micrometastasis in pN0 gastric cancer. *Brit J Cancer* 2005;92:688.

85. Maehara Y, Kakeji Y, Oda S, et al: Tumor growth patterns and biological characteristics of early gastric cancer. *Oncology* 2001;102.

86. Nakamura T, Yao T, Kabashima A, et al: Loss of phenotypic expression is related to tumor progression in early gastric differentiated adenocarcinoma. *Histopathology* 2005;47:357.

87. Borie F, Rigau V, Fingerhut A, et al: Prognostic factors for early gastric cancer in France: Cox regression analysis of 332 cases. *World J Surg* 2004;28:686.

88. Otsuka K, Murakami M, Aoki T, et al: Minimally invasive treatment of stomach cancer. *Cancer J* 2005;11:63.

89. Shimomiya S, Seo Y, Yasuda H, et al: Concepts, rationale and current outcomes of less invasive strategies for early gastric cancer: data from a quarter-century of experience. *World J Surg* 2005;29:58.

89a. Mitsuhashi T, Lauwers GY, Ban S, et al: Post-gastric endoscopic mucosal resection surveillance biopsies: evaluation of mucosal changes and recognition of potential mimics of residual adenocarcinoma. *Am J Surg Pathol* 2006;30:650.

90. Bormann R: Makroskopischen formen des vorschritteten Magenkrebses. In: Henke-Lubarsch O (ed). *Handbuch der speziellen pathologischen Anatomie und Histologie*, Vol 4/1. Berlin, 1926.

91. Ming SC: Classification of gastric carcinoma. In: Filipe MI, Jass J (eds). *Gastric Carcinoma*. Edinburgh: Charleston-Livingston, 1986, pp 197–199.

92. Liu Y, Kaneko S, Sabue T: Trends in reported incidences of gastric cancer by tumour location, from 1975 to 1989. *Int J Epidemiol* 2004;33:808.

93. Wanebo HJ, Kennedy BJ, Chmiel J, et al: Cancer of the stomach: a patient case study by the American College of Surgeons. *Ann Surg* 1993;218:583.

94. Stemmermann GN: Extrapelvic carcinoma metastatic to the uterus. *Am J Obstet Gyn* 1961;82:1261.

95. Winawer SJ, Sherlock P, Hajdu SI: The role of gastrointestinal endoscopy in patients with cancer. *Cancer* 1976;37:440.

96. Chan Y-M, Goh K-L: Appropriateness and diagnostic yield of EGD: a prospective study in a large Asian hospital. *Gastrointest Endosc* 2004;59:517.

97. Willis S, Truong S, Gribnitz S, et al: Endoscopic ultrasonography in the preoperative staging of gastric cancer: accuracy and impact on surgical therapy. *Surg Endosc* 2000;14:951.

98. Karpeh M, Brennan M: Gastric carcinoma. *Ann Surg Oncol* 1998;3:650.

99. Cook IJ, de Carle DJ, Haneman B, et al: The role of brushing cytology in the diagnosis of gastric malignancy. *Acta Cytol* 1988;32:4.

100. Drake M: Gastric cytology: normal and abnormal. In: *Gastroesophageal Cytology*. Basel: Karger, 1985, p 125.

101. Moreno-Otero R, Marron C, Cantero J, et al: Endoscopic biopsy and cytology in the diagnosis of malignant gastric ulcers. *Diag Cytopathol* 1989;5:366.

102. Thompson H: Gastric cytology. In: Filipe MI, Jass JR (eds). *Gastric Carcinoma*. Edinburgh: Churchill Livingstone, 1986, pp 217–220.

103. Rilke F: Malignant lesions of the stomach: cytohistologic correlations. *Acta Cytol* 1979;23:517.

104. Drake M: Early cancer and precancer of esophagus and stomach. In: *Gastroesophageal Cytology*. Basel: Karger, 1985, pp 211–215.

105. Young JA, Hughes HA: Three year trial of endoscopic cytology of the stomach and duodenum. *Gut* 1980;21:241.

106. Yoshii Y, Takahashi J, Tamaoka Y, et al: Significance of imprint smears in cytologic diagnosis of malignant tumours of the stomach. *Acta Cytol* 1970;14:249.

107. Young JA, Hughes HE, Dole DJ: Morphological characteristics and distribution patterns of epithelial cells in the cytological diagnosis of gastric cancer. *J Clin Pathol* 1982;35:585.

108. Stemmermann GN: A comparative study of the histochemical patterns of non-neoplastic and neoplastic gastric epithelium. *J Natl Cancer Inst* 1967;39:375.

109. Sasano N, Nakamura K, Arai M, et al: Ultrastructural cell patterns in human gastric carcinoma compared with normal gastric mucosa. Histogenic analysis of mucin histochemistry. *J Natl Cancer Inst* 1969;43:783.

110. Fenoglio-Preiser CM, Carneiro F, Correa P, et al: Gastric cancer. In: Hamilton SR, Aaltonen LA (eds). *World Health Organization Classification of Tumours. Pathology and Genetics. Tumours of the Digestive System*. Lyon, France: IARC Press, 2000, pp 38–52.

111. Endoh Y, Tamura G, Motoyama T, et al: Well-differentiated adenocarcinoma mimicking complete type metaplasia in the stomach. *Hum Pathol* 1999;30:826.

112. Nishikura Y, Watanabe H: Gastric microcarcinoma: its histopathological characteristics. In: Siewert JH, Roder JD (eds). *Progress in Cancer Research*. Bologna, Italy: Monduzzi Editore, 1997.

113. Shibata D, Tokunaga M, Uemura Y, et al: Association of Epstein-Barr virus with undifferentiated gastric carcinomas with intense lymphoid infiltration. *Am J Pathol* 1991;139:10.

114. Chiaravalli AM, Feltri M, Bertolini V, et al: Intratumor T cells, their activation status and survival in gastric carcinomas characterized for microsatellite instability and Epstein-Barr virus infection. *Virch Arch* 2006;488:344.

115. Uemura Y, Tokunaga M, Arikawa J, et al: A unique morphology of Epstein-Barr virus-related early gastric carcinoma. *Cancer Epidemiol Biomarkers Prev* 1994;3:607.

116. Moritani S, Kushima R, Sugihara H, Hattori T: Phenotypic characteristics of Epstein-Barr-virus-associated gastric carcinoma. *J Cancer Res Clin Oncol* 1996;122:750.

117. Tokunaga M, Land CE: Epstein-Barr virus involvement in gastric cancer: biomarker for lymph node metastases. *Cancer Epidemiol Biomarkers Prev* 1998;7:449.

118. Serruca R, Santos NR, David L, et al: Sporadic gastric carcinomas with microsatellite instability display a particular clinicopathological profile. *Int J Cancer* 1995;64:32.

119. Lev R, De Nucci TD: Neoplastic Paneth cells in the stomach. *Arch Pathol Lab Med* 1989;113:129.

120. Yang GY, Liao J, Casai ND, et al: Parietal cell carcinoma of the gastric cardia: immunophenotype and ultrastructure. *Ultrastruct Pathol* 2003;27:87.

121. Byrne D, Holley MP, Cuschieri A: Parietal cell carcinoma of the stomach: association with long-term survival after curative resection. *Br J Cancer* 1998;58:85.

122. Takubo K, Honma N, Sawabe M, et al: Oncocytic adenocarcinoma of the stomach. *Am J Surg Pathol* 2002;26:458.

123. Mori M, Iwashima A, Enjoji M: Adenosquamous carcinoma of the stomach. *Cancer* 1986;57:333.

124. McClaughlin GA, Cave-Bigely DFJ, Tagore V, et al: Cyclophosphamide and pure squamous carcinoma of the stomach. *Br Med J* 1080;1:524.

125. Ruck P, Wehrmann M, Campbell M, et al: Squamous cell carcinoma of the gastric stump: case report and review of the literature. *Am J Surg Pathol* 1989;13:317.

126. Jindrak K, Bochetto JF, Alpert LI: Primary gastric choriocarcinoma. Case report with a review of the world literature. *Hum Pathol* 1976;7:595.

127. Manabe T, Adachi M, Hirao K: Human chorionic gonadotropin in normal, inflammatory and carcinomatous tissue. *Gastroenterology* 1985;89:1319.

128. Ito H, Tahara E: Human chorionic gonadotropin in human gastric cancer. *Acta Pathol Jap* 1983;33:287.

129. Motoyama T, Saito K, Iwafuchi M, et al: Endodermal sinus tumor of the stomach. *Acta Pathol Jap* 1985;35:497.

130. Kodama, Kameya T, Hirota T, et al: Production of alpha-fetoprotein, normal serum proteins and human chorionic gonadotropin in stomach cancer: histologic and immunohistochemical analyses of 35 cases. *Cancer* 1981;48:1647.

131. Akiyama S, Tamura G, Endoh Y, et al: Histogenesis of hepatoid adenocarcinoma of the stomach: molecular evidence of identical origin with coexistent tubular carcinoma. *Int J Cancer* 2003;103:510.

132. Supriatna Y, Kishimoto T, Uno T, et al: Evidence for hepatocellular differentiation in alpha fetoprotein negative gastric adenocarcinoma with hepatoid morphology: a study with *in situ* hybridisation for albumin mRNA. *Pathology* 2005;37:211.

133. Koide N, Nishio A, Igarashi J, et al: α-Fetoprotein-producing gastric cancer: histochemical analysis of cell proliferation, apoptosis and angiogenesis. *Am J Gastroenterol* 1999;94:1658.

134. Cho KJ, Myong MH, Choi DW, et al: Carcinosarcoma of the stomach: a case report with light microscopic, immunohistochemical and electron microscope study. *APMIS* 1990;98:991.

135. Kuroda N, Oonishi K, Iwamura S, et al: Gastric carcinosarcoma with neuroendocrine differentiation as the carcinoma component and leiomyomatous and myofibroblastic differentiation as the sarcomatous component. *APMIS* 2005;114:234.

136. Yasuma T, Hashimoto K, Miyazawa R, Hiyama Y: Bone formation and calcification in gastric cancer. Case report and review of the literature. *Acta Pathol Jap* 1973;23:155.

137. Kypson AP, Morphew E, Jones R, et al: Heterotopic ossification in rectal cancer: rare finding with a novel proposed mechanism. *J Surg Oncol* 2003;82:132.

138. Ercan I, Cakir B, Basak T, et al: Prognostic significance of stromal eosinophilic infiltration in cancer of the larynx. *Otolaryngol Head Neck Surg* 2005;132:869.

139. Caruso RA, Giuffre G, Inferrera C: Minute and small early gastric carcinoma with special reference to eosinophilic infiltration. *Histol Histopathol* 1993;8:155.

140. Cuschieri A, Talbot IC, Weeden S: Influence of pathological tumour variables on long-term survival with resectable gastric cancer. *Br J Cancer* 2002;86:674.

141. Bigotti G, Coli A, Magistrelli P, et al: Gastric adenocarcinoma associated with granulomatous gastritis. Case report and review of the literature. *Tumori* 2002;88:163.

142. Kurata A, Terado Y, Schulz A, et al: Inflammatory cells in the formation of tumor-related sarcoid reactions. *Hum Pathol* 2005;36:546.

143. Japanese Research Society for Gastric Cancer: The general rules for gastric study in surgery and pathology. *Jpn J Surg* 1981;11:127.

144. Okada M, Kojima S, Murakami M, et al: Human gastric carcinoma: prognosis in relation to macroscopic and microscopic features of the primary tumor. *J Natl Cancer Inst* 1983;71:275.

145. Noguchi Y: Blood vessel invasion in gastric carcinoma. *Surgery* 1990;107:140.

146. Greene FL, Page DL, Fleming ID, et al (eds): *American Joint Committee on Cancer Staging Manual,* 6th ed. New York: Springer Verlag, 2002, pp 99–102.

147. Gipponi M, Solari N, Di Somma FC, et al: New fields of application of the sentinel node biopsy in pathologic staging of solid neoplasms: a review of the literature and surgical prospectives. *J Surg Oncol* 2004; 85:171.

148. Karube T, Ochiai T, Shimada H, et al: Detection of sentinel lymph node micrometastases in gastric cancer based on immunohistochemical analysis. *J Surg Oncol* 2004;87:32.

149. Pelise M, Castells A, Gines A, et al: Detection of lymph node micrometastases by gene promoter hypermethylation in samples obtained by endosonography-guided fine-needle aspiration biopsy. *Clin Cancer Res* 2004;10:4444.

150. O'Sullivan GC, Sheehan D, Clarke A, et al: Micrometastases in esophagogastric cancer: high detection rate in resected rib segments. *Gastroenterology* 1999;116;543.

151. Esaki Y, Hirayama R, Hirokawa K, et al: A comparison of patterns of metastasis in gastric cancer by histologic type and age. *Cancer* 1990;65:2086.

151a. Lerwill MF, Young RH: Ovarian metastases of intestinal-type gastric carcinoma. A clinicopathologic study of 4 cases with contrasting features to those of the Kruckenberg tumor. *Am J Surg Pathol* 2006;30:1382.

152. Imachi M, Tsukamoto N, Amagase H, et al: Metastatic adenocarcinoma of the uterine cervix from gastric cancer. *Cancer* 1993;71:3472.

153. Hundahl SA, Phillips JL, Menck HR: The National Cancer Data base report on poor survival of US gastric carcinoma patients treated with gastrectomy. *Cancer* 2000;88:921.

154. Siewert JR, Bottcher K, Stein HJ, et al: Relevant prognostic factors of gastric cancer: ten-year results of the German Cancer Study. *Ann Surg* 1998;228:449.

155. Noguchi Y, Yoshikawa T, Tsuburaya A, et al: Is gastric carcinoma different between Japan and the United States? A comparison of patient survival in three institutions. *Cancer* 2000;89:2237.

156. Otsuji E, Toshiaki K, Ichikawa D, et al: Time of death and pattern of death in the recurrence following curative resection of gastric carcinoma: analysis based on depth of invasion. *World J Surg* 2004;28:866.

157. Ectors N, Driessen A, De Hertog G, et al: Is adenocarcinoma of the esophagogastric junction or cardia different from Barrett adenocarcinoma? *Arch Pathol Lab Med* 2005;128:183.

158. Taniere P, Borghi-Scoazec G, Saurin J-C, et al: Cytokeratin expression in adenocarcinomas of the esophagogastric junction. A comparative study of adenocarcinomas of the distal esophagus and proximal stomach. *Am J Surg Pathol* 2002;103:1439.

159. Kim MA, Lee SH, Yang H-K, Kim WH: Clinicopathologic and protein expression differences between cardia carcinoma and noncardia carcinoma of the stomach. *Cancer* 2005;103:1439.

160. Nakamura W, Inada K, Hirano K, et al: Increased expression of sucrase and intestinal type phosphatase in human gastric carcinoma with progression. *Jpn J Cancer Res* 1998;89:186.

161. Stemmermann GN, Samloff IM, Hayashi T: Pepsinogens I and II in carcinoma of the stomach: an immunohistochemical study. *Appl Path* 1985;3:375.

162. Fiocca R, Cornsaggia M, Villani L, et al: Expression of pepsinogen II in gastric cancer, its relation to local invasion and lymph node metastases. *Cancer* 1988;61:956.

163. Suzuki T, Tsuda T, Haruma K, et al: Growth of gastric carcinomas and expression of epidermal growth factor. Transforming growth factor-a, epidermal growth factor receptor and p185[c-erb-2]. *Oncology* 1995;52:3856.

164. Tokunaga A, Onda M, Okuda T, et al: Clinical significance of epidermal growth factor (EGF), EGF receptor and c-erB-2 in human gastric cancer. *Cancer* 1995;75:1418.

165. Espinoza J, Tone LG, Beto JB, et al: Enhanced TGFα-EGFR expression and p53 alterations contributes to gastric tumor aggressiveness. *Cancer Lett* 2004;212:33.

165a. Peruzzi B, Bottaro DP: Targeting the c-met signaling pathway in cancer. *Clin Cancer Res* 2006;12:3657.

165b. Kim B, Koo H, Yaang S, et al: TC1 (C8orf4) correlates with Wnt/β-catenin target genes and aggressive biological behavior in gastric cancer. *Clin Cancer Res* 2006;12:3541.

166. Tam SW, Theodorus AM, Shay JW, et al: Differential expression and regulation of cyclin D1 in normal and human gastric tumor cells: association with Cdk4 is required for cyclin D function in G! progression. *Oncogene* 1994;9:2663.

167. Gao P, Zhou GY, Liu Y, et al: Alteration in cyclin D1 in gastric carcinoma and its clinicopathologic significance. *World J Gastroenterol* 2004;10:2933.

168. Fenoglio-Preiser CM, Wang CM, Stemmermann GN, Noffsinger A: Tp53 and gastric cancer: a review. *Hum Mutat* 2003;3:258.

169. Kitoh T, Yanai H, Saitoh T, et al: Increased expression of matrix metalloproteinase-7 in invasive early cancer. *J Gastroenterol* 2004;39:434.

170. Liu XP, Kawachi S, Oga A, et al: Prognostic significance of matrix metallopreinase-7(MMP-7) expression at the invasive front in gastric cancer. *Cancer Res* 2002;93;291.

171. Hashimoto Y, Skcel M, Adams JC: Roles of fascin in human carcinomas motility and signaling: prospects for a novel biomarker. *Int J Biochem Cell Biol* 2005;37:1787.

172. Hashimoto K, Shimada Y, Kawamura J, et al: The prognostic relevance of fascin expression in human gastric carcinoma. *Oncology* 2004;67: 262.

173. Taniguchi K, Yonemura Y, Nojima, et al: The relation between the growth patterns of gastric carcinoma and the expression of hepatocyte growth factor (c-met), autocrine motility factor and urokinase-type plasminogen activator factor. *Cancer* 1997;82:2112.

174. Jüttner S, Weissmann C, Jones T, et al: Vascular endothelial growth factor-D and its receptor VEGFR-3: two novel independent prognostic markers in gastric adenocarcinoma. *J Clin Oncol* 2006:24:228.

175. Kitadai Y, Kodama M, Cho S, et al: Quantitative analysis of lymphangiogenic markers for predicting human gastric cancer in lymph nodes. *Int J Cancer* 2005;115:388.

176. Grogan TM, Fenoglio-Preiser CM, Zeheb R, et al: Thioredoxin, a putative oncogene product, is expressed in gastric cancer and associated with increased cell proliferation and increased cell survival. *Hum Pathol* 2000;31:475.

177. Kominea A, Konstantinopoulos N, Kapranos N, et al: Androgen receptor (AR) expression is an independent unfavorable prognostic factor in gastric cancer. *J Cancer Res Clin Oncol* 2004;130:253.

178. Okano H, Shinohara H, Miyamoto A, et al: Concomitant overexpression of cycloexygenase-2 in Her-2-positive and Smad-reduced human gastric carcinoma is associated with poor outcome. *Clin Cancer Res* 2004;10:6938.

178a. Liu F, Pan K, Zhang X, et al: Genetic variants in cyclooxygenase expression and risk of gastric cancer and its precursors in a Chinese population. *Gastroenterology* 2006;130:1975.

179. Catalano V, La Bianca R, Beretta GD, et al: Gastric cancer. *Oncol Hematol* 2005;54:209.

180. Taal BG, Peterse H, Boot H: Clinical presentation, endoscopic features and treatment of gastric metastases from breast cancer. *Cancer* 2000;89:2214.

181. Clavien PA, Laffer U, Torhorst J, Harder F: Gastrointestinal metastases as the first manifestation of disseminated breast cancer. *Eur J Surg Oncol* 1990;16:121.

182. Matsuyama S, Ohkura Y, Eguchi H, et al: Estrogen receptor beta is expressed in human stomach adenocarcinoma. *J Cancer Res Clin Oncol* 2002;128:319.

183. Quereshi SS, Shrikhande SV, Tanuja S, Shukla PJ: Breast metastases of gastric signet ring cell carcinoma. *J Post Grad Med* 2005;51:125.

184. VanVelhuysen M-LF, Taal BJ, van der Hoeven JJM, Peters JL: Expression of estrogen receptor and loss of E-cadherin are diagnostic of metastases of breast cancer. *Histopathology* 2005;46:153.

The Nonneoplastic Small Intestine

EMBRYOLOGY AND DEVELOPMENT

Gastrulation occurs 2 weeks after fertilization, inducing a massive rearrangement of the embryo. It transforms a relatively uniform cell ball into a multilayered organism with recognizable body plans. Some cells divide faster than others, resulting in a change in embryonic shape. Cells converge on the embryonic midline. As they crowd together, they push each other toward the future head and tail, and the embryo lengthens.

There are two major steps in gastrointestinal (GI) development: The formation of the gut tube and the formation of individual organs each with their own specialized cell types (1). These events are regulated by homeobox or Hox genes (2), particularly *Cdx1* and *Cdx2*, which are only expressed in the intestine. These two genes are important in the anterior to posterior patterning of the intestines and in defining patterns of proliferation and differentiation along the crypt–villus axis (3). Their importance in intestinal differentiation is important not only in normal intestinal development, but also in the development of intestinal metaplasia in the stomach and in Barrett esophagus as discussed in Chapters 2 to 4. Other signaling cascades also play a major role in gut development. These include the Hedgehog, Hh, Bmp, FGF, and Wnt signaling pathways (4–8). They are used at multiple steps of the developmental process. Congenital abnormalities, including malrotations, associate with germline mutations/deletions of genes encoding hedgehog signaling components as reviewed in reference 8.

The endoderm is the precursor to the gastrointestinal epithelial lining, and endodermal development requires the expression of the homeotic genes *MIXER, SOX17α* and *SOX17β* (9). Multiple interactions occur between the endoderm, mesoderm, and ectoderm during development. The endoderm induces the mesoderm, conferring on it a dorsal–ventral pattern. Endoderm and ectoderm contact one another in the 2- to 4-week embryo, with the endoderm forming the yolk sac roof. This contact results in up-regulation of growth factors, including transforming growth factor (TGF)-α, TGF-β, epidermal growth factor (EGF), and hepatocyte growth factor (HGF), all of which stimulate cell proliferation. A primitive gut forms in the third to eighth weeks secondary to cephalocaudal and lateral foldings that incorporates the dorsal endodermally lined yolk sac cavity. The amnion and yolk sac communicate through the neuroenteric canal (Fig. 6.1). The neuroenteric canal closes and the notochord grows forward, becoming intercalated within the endoderm. The neural tube then separates from the ectoderm. Mesoderm surrounds the notochord, separating the ectoderm and endoderm (10). (Gastrointestinal duplications associate with a defective spinal cord and/or vertebra if mesodermal ingrowth does not occur and neural and gastrointestinal elements fail to separate.) Splanchnic mesoderm surrounding the primitive gut forms the muscular and connective tissue layers. The former yolk sac elongates under the developing nervous system to form the primitive foregut anteriorly and the primitive hindgut posteriorly. The central portion develops into the midgut, which has a free communication with the yolk sac (the vitellointestinal duct). The anterior abdominal wall develops by simultaneous cranial, caudal, and lateral infoldings, which attenuate the yolk sac, causing it to become intracoelomic in location (Fig. 6.1). The foregut is short at first, lying closely apposed to the developing vertebrae, and it becomes suspended by a short mesentery. The foregut gives rise to the esophagus, stomach, duodenum as far as the ampulla of Vater, liver, pancreas, and respiratory system, and it has its own arterial blood supply deriving from the celiac axis (11).

The duodenum distal to the bile duct, and the jejunum, ileum, cecum, ascending colon, and proximal one half to two thirds of the transverse colon derive from the midgut and are supplied by the superior mesenteric artery. At about the 5- to 12-mm stage, the midgut lengthens, becoming tubular and growing away from the vertebral axis. It then coils, inducing dorsal mesenteric development. During the fifth fetal week the midgut is U-shaped and suspended by a dorsal mesentery distributed around the superior mesenteric artery. The apex of the intestinal loop communicates with the vitelline duct, which rapidly decreases in size. During the fifth to sixth fetal weeks, increases in intestinal length, along with the disproportionate amount of abdominal space occupied by the fetal liver, cause the intestines to herniate into a mesothelial-lined sac within the umbilical cord (11). The cecum develops on the caudal limb and the vitellointestinal duct lies at the apex. A small portion of the caudal limb, between the attachment of the vitellointestinal duct and cecum, forms the

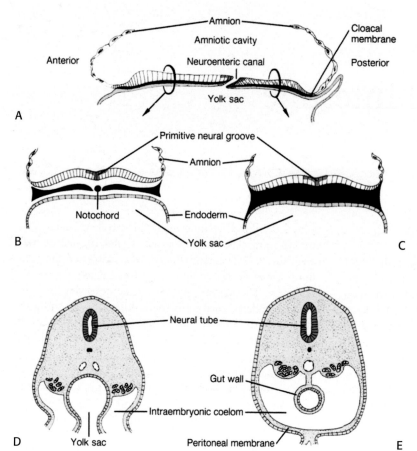

FIG. 6.1. Diagram of early embryogenesis. **A–E** show the progressive formation of the gut.

terminal ileum. The midgut starts sliding back into the abdomen between the 10th and 12th fetal weeks, a process accomplished in three phases (Fig. 6.2). The first is a 90-degree counterclockwise rotation around the superior mesenteric artery. The second occurs at about the 10th week, when there is enough room for the bowel to return to the abdominal cavity. The cranial loop of the small bowel re-enters the abdomen, first passing to the right of the superior mesenteric artery and rotating a further 180 degrees, thereby making the total rotation 270 degrees. Small intestinal loops fill the central abdomen.

Although an anatomically distinguishable intestinal tract develops early in embryonic life, functional absorptive cells do not appear until later in gestation. Intestinal differentiation occurs along a proximal-to-distal gradient. The epithelium develops from simple endodermal tubules early in embryogenesis (12) appearing as a multilayered sheet of undifferentiated endodermal cells with short microvilli. Deeper cells do not demonstrate any polarity; mitoses occur throughout the epithelium. Villous formation with mesenchymal infiltration into the villous core begins at the ninth gestational week. Between 9 and 10 weeks, the stratified epithelium converts to a simple columnar epithelium (13). The progenitor cell region, which gives rise to the crypts, localizes to the intervillous area (14). Villi are long and tapering by 20 weeks and the muscle coats are obvious at this time.

Enterocyte proliferation occurs along the entire villous length until several days before birth.

The diverse small intestinal functions require multiple cell types arranged in specific locations. Enterocyte differentiation depends on the cell's location along both a vertical and a horizontal axis. It parallels the pattern of cellular migration from the base of the crypts to the tips of the villi. The horizontal axis refers to a cell's position in the intestine as one progresses from the duodenum distally to the ileum (Fig. 6.3). Functional differences along both the vertical and the horizontal axes (15) reflect both different patterns of gene expression and different epithelial cell types. Fully differentiated cells of a given lineage may express a different spectrum of gene products depending on their location along the gut (15). The pattern of brush border enzyme gene expression in the distal small intestine resembles that in the proximal gut, but it is delayed by several days. This establishes a proximal-to-distal gradient of gene expression (9). The basis for regional differences in gene expression results from differences in the transcription factors that interact with the promoter and enhancer region of these genes. Homeobox genes participate in establishing differentiation gradients during development and then maintaining these patterns in adult tissues. The epithelium finishes its morphologic differentiation into enterocytes, goblet cells, endocrine cells, and Paneth cells in the 4 to 5 days prior to birth (16).

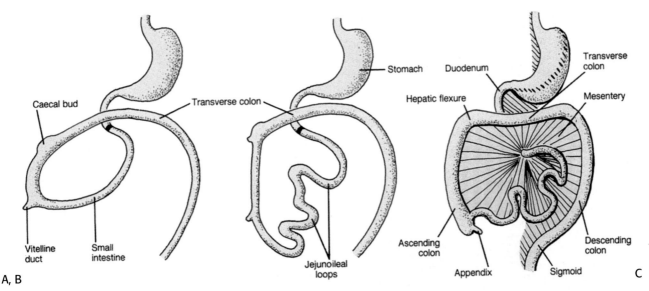

FIG. 6.2. A: Intestinal rotations. Schematic drawing of the primitive intestinal loop after a 180-degree counterclockwise rotation. The transverse colon passes in front of the duodenum. **B:** Intestinal loop after a 270-degree counterclockwise rotation. Note the coiling of the intestinal loops. **C:** Intestinal loops in final position and their associated mesenteries.

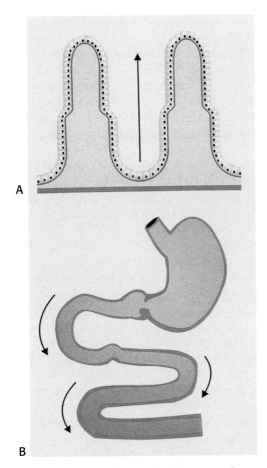

FIG. 6.3. Comparison of the vertical and horizontal axes of differentiation. **A:** Vertical axis of differentiation from the base of the crypts to the tip of the villus. **B:** Horizontal axis of differentiation from the proximal duodenum to the ileocecal valve.

This differentiation process appears to rely on *Math1* and *Cdx2* expression (17,18).

Primordial intestinal lymphoid structures appear approximately halfway through gestation. At the time of birth, Peyer patches have the greatest density of any proliferating lymphoid tissue in the body. T- and B-cell aggregates form early Peyer patches by 16 weeks' gestation, and by 19 weeks organized Peyer patches are present. T cells populate the lamina propria and epithelium from 11 weeks' gestation and increase in number thereafter. Following birth, there is a marked increase in the number of Peyer patches, reflecting the initial response of the host immune system to environmental antigens passing through the intestinal tract.

SMALL INTESTINAL MUCOSAL BARRIER

The mucosal surfaces are regions where individuals and the environment meet. The gut mucosa is in continuous contact with food antigens, the enteric commensal bacteria that constitute the normal gut flora, and potential pathogens that enter the host through the intestine. The upper intestinal bacterial count is normally low and it increases as one progresses distally. Bacterial numbers are kept low by intestinal motility, mucus, and the antibacterial effects of pancreatic and biliary juice and gastric acid (Fig. 6.4). This resident microflora maintains a stable environment and eliminates pathogenic organisms by producing antimicrobial substances and short-chain fatty acids. It also stimulates mucosal epithelial growth (19).

The small intestinal mucosa forms a barrier to the unimpeded movement of antigens, pathogens, and other noxious

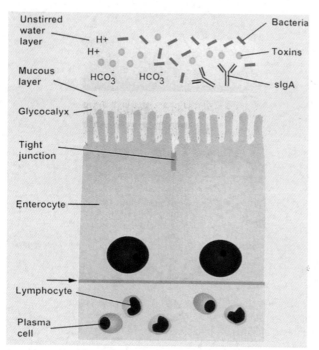

FIG. 6.4. Mucosal barrier. The mucosal barrier consists of several nonspecific defenses, including the epithelium, which forms an intact single cell layer. It lies above an intact basement membrane (*arrow*) and tight junctions seal the upper intercellular spaces. The microvilli are covered by a glycocalyx. Overlying this is a mucous layer followed by the unstirred water layer. The epithelium pumps bicarbonate, water, hydrogen ions, and mucus, as well as secretory immunoglobulin into the unstirred layer above it. These substances interact with bacteria, toxins, or antigens in the lumen. Underlying the epithelium is the lamina propria, which contains abundant immune cells.

substances from the exterior world to the internal environment. A single layer of columnar epithelium, held together by tight junctions, lies on an intact basement membrane. Intercellular tight junctions, which are impermeable to large molecules and bacteria, help maintain epithelial integrity and prevent the entry of foreign material. The tight junctions are specialized membrane domains at the apical pole of the cells that not only create a primary barrier to prevent paracellular transport of solutes (barrier function), but also restrict the lateral diffusion of membrane lipids and proteins to maintain cellular polarity (gate function) (20). The tight junction complexes form a complete ring around the apical pole of the cells. Tight junction permeability is plastic and can be altered by extracellular stimuli including bugs and drugs (21). An unstirred layer, which measures 400 to 500 μm in thickness, covers the epithelium. Molecules diffuse into this layer (22).

The proximal duodenum transports bicarbonate into an adherent mucus layer in a manner similar to that seen in the stomach, providing a protective barrier from damage caused by pepsin and acid. The alkaline pH environment beneath the mucin layer acts as a buffer and a lubricant. The mucus protects against microbial adherence to the epithelium and

resists digestion by intraluminal enzymes. Mucus secretion is stimulated by immune complexes, chemical agents, soluble mediators, histamine, lymphokines, and neurotransmitters (23). Nitric oxide plays an important role in modulating epithelial fluid secretion (24). The secreted mucus contains albumin; immunoglobulin, particularly secretory IgA; α_1-antitrypsin; lysozyme; lactoferrin; and EGF. Secretory IgA in the intestinal lumen acts in concert with nonspecific host defenses, including mucin, bacteriocidins, defensins, and lytic cells (25), to protect the host by neutralizing or excluding antigens, toxins, and organisms (26). Granulocytes, macrophages, and Paneth cells act as intramucosal phagocytes.

Intestinal epithelium is vulnerable to enteric pathogens that express specific adhesion molecules, enzymes, and other specialized mechanisms for colonizing epithelial surfaces as described in a later section. As a result, the intestines have evolved protective mechanisms in which the lamina propria reacts to microbes and other foreign material by mounting an immunologic barrier. This immunologic barrier includes the gut-associated lymphoid tissues and the systemic immune system. The mucosa is at the leading edge of the immunologic barrier. The intestinal mucosa contains more lymphoid cells and produces more antibodies than any other site in the body. These immunologic responses lead to a cascade of events aimed at inactivating and removing offending antigens or microbes.

Specific immunologic responses include IgA production and lymphocyte sensitization in Peyer patches or in the epithelium (27). Enterocytes can present antigen, express secretory component, and transport immunoglobulin into the intestinal lumen. Enterocytes also can produce and secrete interleukinlike substances that activate T cells in response to luminal antigens (28). Secretory IgA coats microbes and toxins, inhibiting mucosal attachment or interaction, and facilitates their rapid expulsion. IgA also mediates antibody-dependent, cell-mediated cytotoxicity resulting in pathogen killing and also activates complement, mainly via the alternate pathway (29).

Intestinal mucosal function is immature in the newborn. Immaturity of the microvillous membrane, low outputs of gastric acid, decreased proteolytic activity, and altered mucin production all contribute to an impaired intestinal barrier that facilitates macromolecular uptake and sepsis. Intestinal immune mechanisms at this stage are also underdeveloped (Fig. 6.5). IgA concentrations in saliva, stool, and serum are low compared to those seen in adults (30). As a result, neonates are particularly prone to develop enteric infections. After 1 month of age, IgA assumes its role as the main immunoglobulin in the lamina propria. The importance of GI immune defenses is dramatically illustrated in immunocompromised patients, especially those with AIDS, who become overwhelmed by GI infections.

Because of the importance of small intestinal barrier functions and transport, small intestinal injury must be repaired as rapidly as possible. The GI mucosa heals by both restitution and proliferation (31). The extracellular matrix,

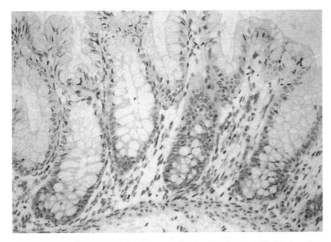

FIG. 6.5. Lamina propria of a newborn. The hypocellular lamina propria contains few lymphocytes and plasma cells.

pericryptal myofibroblasts, and growth factors regulate these processes. Initial phases of mucosal restitution involve rapid migration of linked sheets of enterocytes from the epithelium shouldering the wound over the denuded basement membrane across mucosal defects. Once the migrating cells are free of the shoulder of the wound, they begin to proliferate (Fig. 6.6). Matrix–cytoskeletal links participate in this cellular migration. Surviving epithelial cells phagocytose adjacent dead cells. If the progenitor cells are damaged, as in radiation injury, atrophy results. Conversely, if the surface cells are damaged, cell proliferation increases and the cells migrate out of the crypt at a faster rate, leading to a population of immature cells lining the crypts.

GROSS FEATURES

The human small intestine, which extends from the gastric pylorus to the ileocecal valve, measures about 7 m in length.

The C-shaped duodenum encloses the head of the pancreas in its concavity. It measures approximately 20 to 25 cm in length and, except for its first part, lies in the retroperitoneum. The first part of the duodenum measures approximately 5 cm in length, and it ascends posteriorly from the pylorus to the right. It lies above and anterior to the head of the pancreas, below the gallbladder, and anterior to the common bile duct, gastroduodenal artery, and portal vein. The second portion measures approximately 7 cm in length and is covered by the peritoneum of the infracolic compartment of the peritoneal cavity, which separates it from coils of the small bowel. The transverse colon and its mesentery cross it. The hilum of the right kidney and right renal vessels lie behind it, and the bodies of the lumbar vertebrae and inferior vena cava lie medially.

The common bile duct and pancreatic duct enter the second part of the duodenum posteromedially at the ampulla of Vater approximately 9 to 10 cm from the pyloric ring (Fig. 6.7). In most patients, the common bile duct and pancreatic duct join before draining into the ampulla (Fig. 6.8), but in about 10% of cases, the bile duct and pancreatic duct open separately into the intestinal lumen. In about 30% of patients, an accessory, more proximal pancreatic duct drains into the duodenal lumen. Both the bile duct and the pancreatic duct have their own muscular coats. A cross section through this area of the duodenum contains numerous ramifying ducts in all layers of the duodenal wall (Fig. 6.9). The sphincter of Oddi at the ampulla of Vater measures approximately 9.5 mm in length (32).

The third part of the duodenum arches transversely across the vena cava and aorta at the level of the body of the third lumbar vertebra. It is 7 to 9 cm in length. The root of the mesentery obliquely crosses its terminal portion. It is also crossed by the superior mesenteric artery and vein. Superiorly, it relates to the pancreatic uncinate process. The fourth part of the duodenum varies in length and is difficult

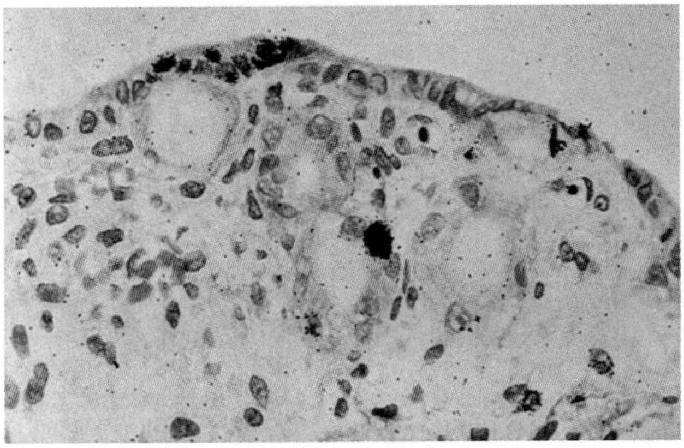

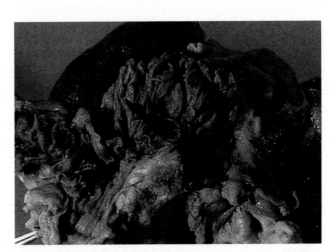

FIG. 6.6. Radioautograph from a damaged region of the small intestine. The normal villous architecture is lost, and the surface epithelial cells now covering the mucosal defect appear immature and cuboidal. Goblet cells are absent. Proliferating cells are present as indicated by the radioactive grains covering them.

FIG. 6.7. Normal ampulla of Vater. Opened duodenum with gallbladder posteriorly. The common bile duct is shown by adjacent green and blue probes at ampulla of Vater. The solitary blue probe is an accessory duct of Wirsung.

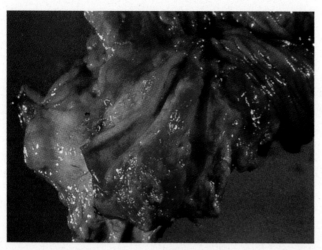

FIG. 6.8. Ampulla of Vater. The pancreatic and bile ducts enter separately and have been opened, showing their entrance into the duodenum.

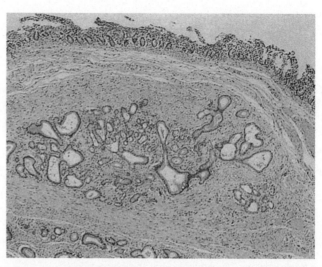

FIG. 6.9. Ramifying ducts in the submucosa are surrounded by a muscular coat. The architecture in this area can normally be very complex.

to distinguish from the third part. It curves up to the left to the duodenojejunal flexure, where it is attached by a suspensory duodenal ligament, the ligament of Treitz.

Although the duodenum has a fairly constant length, the length of the rest of the small intestine is not as clearly established. Measurements taken at autopsy suggest adult lengths between 300 and 900 cm with a mean of approximately 600 cm. Other measurements taken during life give a much shorter length of 280 cm. The mesentery supporting the small intestine fans out from an origin only 15 to 20 cm long. The mesentery runs along an oblique line crossing the posterior abdominal wall from the left to right, from the duodenojejunal flexure to the right iliac fossa.

There is no recognizable line of division between the three parts of the small intestine: Duodenum, jejunum, and ileum. Traditionally, the jejunum represents the proximal 40 cm after the ligament of Treitz and the ileum the distal 60 cm

of the small intestine. The lumen of the jejunum is wider than that of the ileum, and its wall is thicker due to prominent circular mucosal folds, known as folds of Kerckring (Fig. 6.10). These folds run parallel to the longitudinal axis of the bowel, are most prominent between the midduodenum and jejunum, and are absent in the distal ileum. They contain both the mucosa and the underlying submucosa.

BLOOD SUPPLY

The duodenum is supplied by the celiac and superior mesenteric arteries (Fig. 6.11). The celiac trunk branches into the gastroduodenal artery. The superior mesenteric artery supplies the jejunum, cecum, and appendix, traveling through the mesentery in several major branches (Fig. 6.12). Ten to fifteen jejunoileal arteries arise from the left side of the

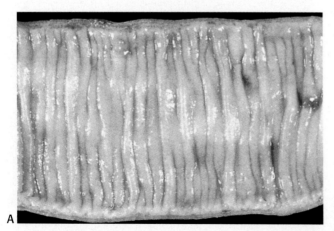

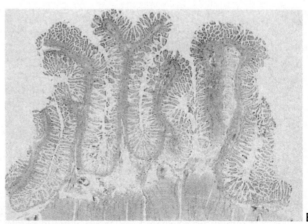

FIG. 6.10. Normal small intestine. **A:** The surface of the small intestine is covered by numerous regular folds (plicae circulares) with a submucosal core. **B:** Convolutions of mucosa and submucosa are the histologic equivalent of the folds of Kerckring.

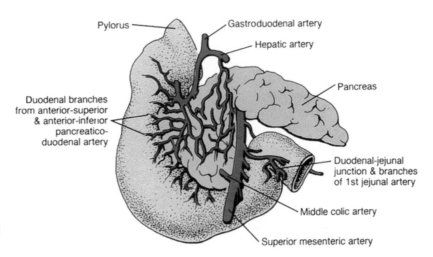

FIG. 6.11. Diagram of duodenal arterial supply.

superior mesenteric artery, which originates 1 to 2 cm below the celiac artery. Each divides into two branches, which join adjacent branches to form a series of arcades. These in turn branch and form a second series of arcades before the vasa recta penetrate the intestinal wall (33). The ileocolic artery, which arises from the lower superior mesenteric artery, supplies the terminal ileum, cecum, appendix, and proximal ascending colon. It anastomoses with the right colic artery. This and subsequent branches form complex arcades.

Intramural arteries enter the intestinal serosa and pierce the muscularis propria to form an extensive submucosal vascular plexus (Fig. 6.13). The submucosal arterial plexus gives rise to arterioles, which supply the mucosa, submucosa, and muscular layers. However, the mucosal capillary bed is isolated from that of the muscularis propria. The capillary bed in the muscularis mucosae has two layers (34). These two

groups of arteries make their way into the mucosa. Some ramify on the luminal side of the muscularis mucosae and give rise to a capillary network that surrounds the crypts. Others continue into the villus, entering it at its base before arborizing into a dense capillary network. A rich network of blood capillaries ramifies through the lamina propria and is closely apposed to the epithelial basement membranes (Figs. 6.14 and 6.15). Villi are more highly vascularized than are the crypts (35). The mucosa receives approximately 75% of the blood flow. The bowel can autoregulate its blood flow, which means that it maintains a constant blood flow in the face of fluctuating arterial pressures. Following eating, small intestinal blood flow increases by over 100%, with the majority of the blood flow being diverted to the mucosa.

Villous capillaries drain into a single venule that starts high in the villus. One or two veins form in each villus. These

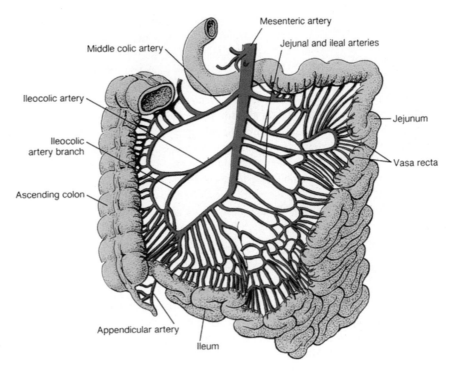

FIG. 6.12. Distribution of superior mesenteric artery.

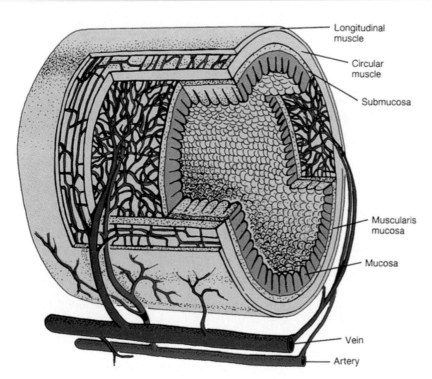

FIG. 6.13. Diagram of the submucosal vascular plexus.

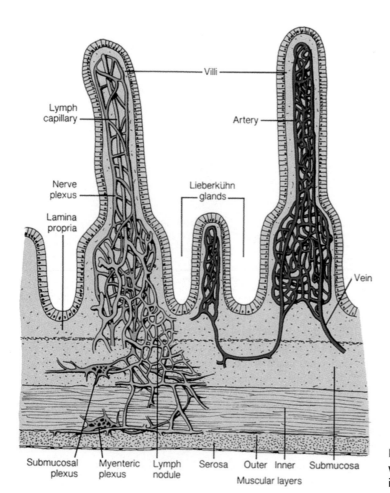

FIG. 6.14. Diagram of distribution of arteries (*red*), veins (*blue*), lymphatics (*yellow*), and nerves (*green*) in the small intestine.

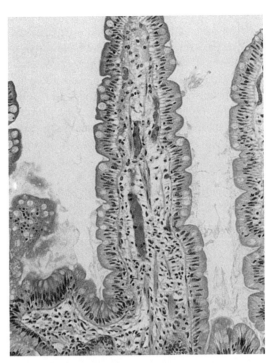

FIG. 6.15. Dilated capillaries in a small intestinal villus showing the prominent capillary structure.

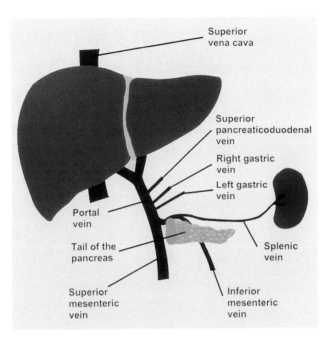

FIG. 6.16. Diagram of the portal system.

course downward, eventually joining veins at the crypt bases and merging with veins draining into the submucosal plexus. These vessels continue on through the muscularis propria and serosa, merging with other veins draining into the portal vein via the superior mesenteric vein. The superior mesenteric vein receives its drainage from the distal duodenum, jejunum, ileum, appendix, and cecum, as well as the ascending and transverse colon. Venous drainage of the duodenum parallels its arterial supply. Inferior pancreaticoduodenal veins drain to the right gastroepiploic vein. The major veins draining the GI tract form the portal system (Fig. 6.16). The portal vein forms by the junction of the splenic vein and the superior mesenteric vein. The portal vein receives direct input from the right and left gastric veins, superior pancreaticoduodenal vein, accessory pancreatic vein, and pyloric vein. Blood in the portal vein is carried to the liver, where nutrients are absorbed and processed.

LYMPHATICS AND LYMPHOID FOLLICLES

Lymphatic drainage starts with the central lacteal, which drains into the submucosal lymphatic plexus (Figs. 6.14 and 6.17). CD 38, a type II transmembrane glycoprotein involved in signaling and adhesion, is a novel marker of small intestinal lacteals (36). The broad proximal villi contain from two to five lacteals, whereas more distal thin villi contain only one. Lacteals measure 5 to 15 μm in diameter and run parallel to one another in the longitudinal direction of the villus. The endothelial lining contains gaps and has overlapping areas

with adjacent endothelial cells. Chylomicrons and fatty droplets can pass through the gaps (Fig. 6.18) (37). The wall of the lacteal consists of endothelium and a reticulin fiber sheath to which smooth muscle fibers attach (Figs. 6.17 and 6.19) (38). Villi intermittently contract and shorten due to the activity of the smooth muscle cells. These contractions force lymph from the central lacteal into the basal lymphatics. The

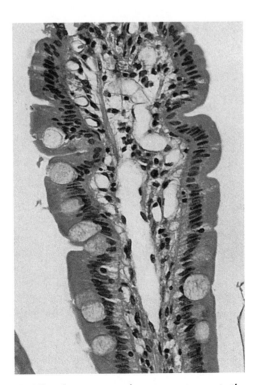

FIG. 6.17. Dilated empty vascular space represents the central lacteal of this villus.

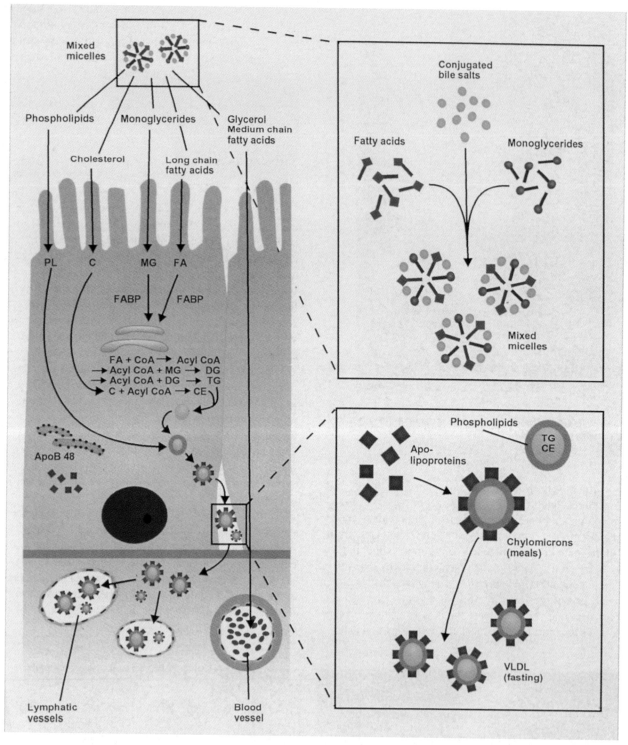

FIG. 6.18. The lipolytic products—fatty acids (*FAs*) and monoglycerides (*MGs*)—form small molecular aggregates with bile salts, called micelles. The micelles provide an ideal shuttle between the bulk water phase and the water–microvillus interface separated by the unstirred water layer. Phospholipids (*PLs*) and cholesterol (*C*) are also transported into the cell after hydrolysis in the lumen. Within the enterocytes, FAs and cholesterol are transported to the endoplasmic reticulum by fatty acid–binding proteins and a sterol carrier protein (*SP*). The assembled prechylomicron, composed of triglycerides and cholesterol esters, moves to the Golgi stacks, where a final glycosylation occurs. The triglyceride and cholesterol ester core is coated with a thin layer of protein to form the chylomicron. The chylomicrons then migrate to the lateral membrane, cross it by a process of membrane fusion, and enter the extracellular space. The chylomicrons pass through the basement membrane and interstitium of the lamina propria to enter the lacteals. The endothelial cells of the lacteals separate during feeding, facilitating chylomicron translocation. VLDL, very-low-density lipoprotein.

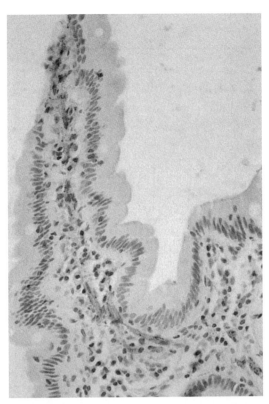

FIG. 6.19. Muscle fibers in the lamina propria. They are stained with an antibody to smooth muscle actin and counterstained with hematoxylin.

central lacteal is also completely surrounded by the subepithelial blood capillary network (Fig. 6.17). Lacteals anastomose with each other, which forms an expanded sinus. In the fasted state, lacteals are difficult to see.

There are many blind-ending lymphatics in the upper part of the interfollicular area. These gradually fuse and form perifollicular lymphatic sinuses surrounding the lateral surfaces and bottoms of Peyer patch follicles. Between the perifollicular lymphatic networks and the interfollicular area are many high endothelial venules (HEVs) that connect to capillaries in the dome and follicle. The close association of HEVs with perifollicular lymphatics facilitates prompt drainage of fluid and keeps macromolecules from leaking out of HEVs during lymphocyte migration into the lymphatics. At the villous base, lymphatics empty into thicker lymphatics that then connect to form a flat, wide sinus (the intravillous lymphatic sinus). From the base of each sinus, several lymphatics descend perpendicularly to drain into submucosal lymphatics that run transversely beneath the muscularis mucosae to form a two-layer meshwork. The submucosal lymphatic plexus drains into large subserosal lymphatics (39) that drain into large conducting mesenteric lymphatics eventually flowing into the cisterna chyli.

Draining lymph nodes consist of the pancreaticolienal group lying along the splenic artery, the pyloric group lying along the gastroduodenal artery, and the superior mesenteric nodes. Small pancreaticoduodenal nodes lie scattered along

the artery of the same name. The lymphatics also drain into the small pyloric nodes superiorly and preaortic lumbar nodes inferiorly. Pyloric nodes drain to the hepatic nodes along the common hepatic artery. Others drain to the root of the superior mesenteric lymph nodes, following the distribution of the superior mesenteric artery and draining the areas supplied by it. Small mesenteric lymph nodes lie along the vasa recta of the mesentery, adjacent to the bowel wall, and larger ones lie along the primary arcades and the intestinal arteries. There are about 200 mesenteric lymph nodes. Two major groups of ileocolic lymph nodes drain the terminal ileum and cecum: One near the bowel wall and another at the origin of the ileocolic artery.

INNERVATION

The innervation of the small bowel resembles that of the large intestine described in Chapter 13. The intrinsic innervation is discussed in Chapter 10.

HISTOLOGIC FEATURES

General Structure

Small intestinal epithelium is organized into two morphologic and functionally distinct compartments: The crypts of Lieberkühn and the villi. Villi that are unique to the adult small intestine are fingerlike or leaflike mucosal evaginations lined by epithelium overlying a connective tissue core that contains a highly cellular lamina propria, a capillary network, lacteals, and nerves. Simple tubular invaginations (crypts of Lieberkühn) at the base of the villi extend down toward the muscularis mucosae but do not penetrate it (Figs. 6.20 and 6.21). Several crypts open into the intervillous basin.

Villi vary in height and form in different regions of the small bowel. The duodenum has the greatest villous variability. Villi in the proximal duodenum are shorter and broader than elsewhere, not infrequently showing increased numbers of stunted and leaf-shaped or branched forms when compared to the jejunum. Jejunal villi vary little in their width from their base to their apex. In the ileum, the villi become broader and shorter than in the jejunum (Fig. 6.21). Villous morphology also varies among different ethnic groups and geographic locales. Villi in persons from Thailand, Africa, India, South Vietnam, and Haiti are shorter and thicker and have an increased portion of leaf-shaped forms with a more intensely cellular lamina propria when compared to biopsies from the English or Northern Americans (40). It is unclear whether this variation represents true racial differences or results from exposure to the infections endemic to the former areas.

The ratio of villous height to crypt length, a feature best appreciated in well-oriented sections, allows one to assess

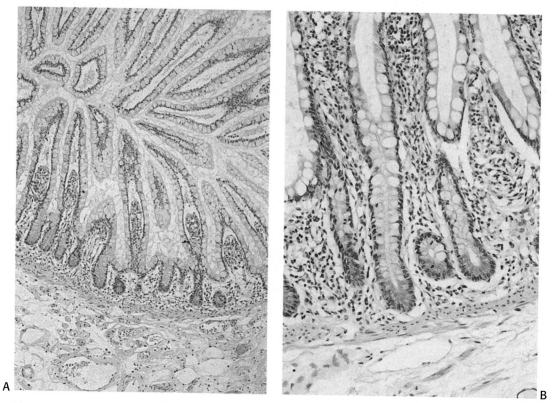

FIG. 6.20. Ileal mucosa. **A:** Crypts and villi. The crypts contain numerous goblet cells, allowing one to identify this area as ileal. **B:** Higher magnification of the crypts shows prominent Paneth cell differentiation.

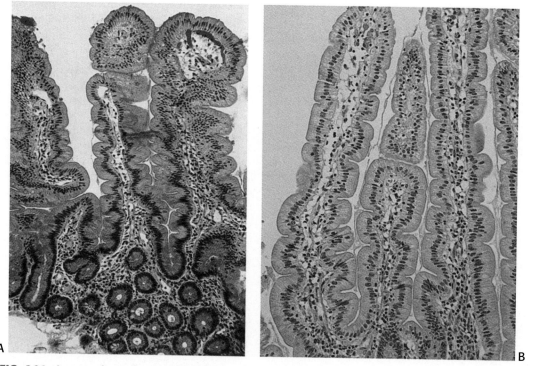

FIG. 6.21. A comparison of proximal ileal **(A)** versus jejunal **(B)** villi. The more distal villi are more irregular in shape than those of the proximal region.

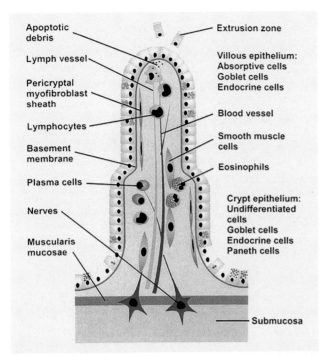

FIG. 6.22. Diagrammatic summary of the structures found in the villus.

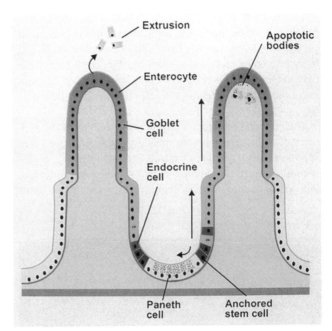

FIG. 6.23. Mucosal renewal. The mucosa continuously generates new epithelial cells from a population of anchored stem cells. These give rise to all of the epithelial cell types lining the crypts and villi. Most of the cells migrate upward, undergoing progressive differentiation into enterocytes, goblet cells, and endocrine cells, as well as a minor population of other cells. At the surface, the mature and effete cells either undergo extrusion into the lumen via shedding from the basement membrane or undergo apoptosis and apoptotic bodies are passed into the underlying lamina propria, where macrophages ingest them. In contrast to the upward migration, some cells migrate downward, differentiating into Paneth cells and endocrine cells.

small intestinal absorptive function. In adults, villous height is approximately three or more times the length of the crypts, whereas in children this ratio is lower, more typically being 2:1. Villous height is also lower in the elderly (41). The duodenal crypt:villus ratio is 3:1 to 7:1, whereas the ileal crypt:villus ratio is 4:1. Villi overlying lymphoid areas are often stubby or absent. Each villus contains an arteriole with capillary network veins and a central lymphatic as well as numerous nerve fibers (Fig. 6.22).

Each crypt consists of a single clone of cells; several crypts contribute cells to each villus. The epithelial lining harbors a heterogeneous cell population, including Paneth cells, undifferentiated crypt cells, endocrine cells, cup cells, tuft cells, goblet cells, absorptive cells (enterocytes), and M cells. Each cell type possesses distinctive structural features and functions (see below). The epithelium maintains a close association with the underlying stroma.

Cell Proliferation and Differentiation

Maintaining the integrity of the gut epithelium as well as ensuring its continuous turnover is essential for mucosal defense. As a result, the gut has one of the most rapid proliferative rates in the body (42). Regular cellular renewal maintains an equilibrium between cell birth and cell death. When the mucosa is damaged, replacement of the injured cells guarantees mucosal integrity. New epithelial cells arise from a fixed proliferating stem cell population located in the lower part of the crypt (Figs. 6.23 and 6.24) (43–45). These pluripotential stem cells give rise to descendants that

undergo three or four divisions while migrating up the villus or to the top of the lymphoid dome (44).

The duration of cellular proliferation and migration is approximately 5 to 6 days in most of the human small intestine and 3 days in the ileum. Differentiated enterocytes live for little more than 2 days (46). Cells at the villous tip undergo Fas-mediated apoptosis (47) and slough off and are extruded into the lumen; sloughing cells can also be seen on the edges of the villi (48). Apoptotic cell death occurs without any apparent disruption of the mucosal barrier integrity (49).

Mitotic figures are present in the deep crypt, but they are never normally present on the villi. Stem cells give rise to four major epithelial cell types: Absorptive cells (enterocytes), goblet cells, endocrine cells, and Paneth cells (44). The production and maturation of these cells is under the control of homeobox genes including *MATH1*, *Cdx1*, and *Cdx2* (3,17,18) and the Wnt signaling pathway (45). The MYC-MAD-MAX network is another key regulator of intestinal cell maturation (45).

Newly produced cells migrate out of the crypt, differentiate, and assume the functional characteristics of mature surface cells. Precursors of absorptive enterocytes comprise 90%

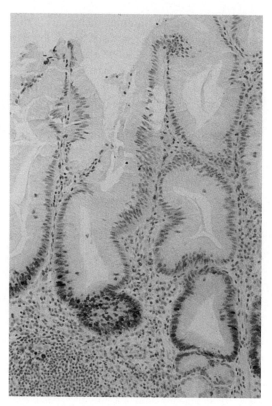

FIG. 6.24. Mucosal proliferation. The epithelium at the base of the duodenal crypts shows a population of brown-stained nuclei corresponding to the proliferating cells. Additionally, proliferating cells are seen in the lamina propria.

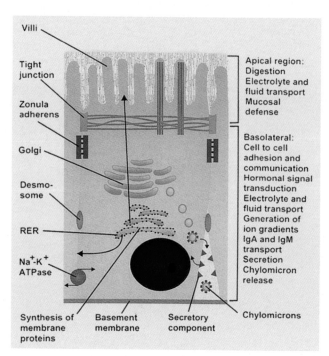

FIG. 6.25. Enterocytes are highly polarized cells with distinct apical, lateral, basolateral, and basal portions, each of which serves special roles.

of the cells in the crypt and mature absorptive cells comprise 95% of the cells located on proximal intestinal villi (43,44). The other three primary epithelial phenotypes constitute a small but important percentage of the total cell number. Cell migration occurs in a linear fashion, with cells moving directly vertically upward or downward from their site of genesis in the crypt bases. The process of proliferation and cellular differentiation are topologically well organized and maintained within this progressively differentiating epithelium. As the cells mature, enterocytes gain digestive enzymes. Gene expression profiling studies show that different genes are differentially expressed in the crypt and on the villi. Genes that are up-regulated in the crypt and down-regulated at the villous tip include those related to the cell cycle, RNA processing, and protein translation. In contrast, genes related to cytoskeletal assembly, lipid uptake, and enzyme biosynthesis show the opposite pattern (50).

There are also specific specializations of intestinal cells, such as the M cell, which derive from the multipotential stem cell. M cells play a major role in antigen sampling from the GI mucosa and are described in a later section.

Enterocytes (Absorptive Cells)

Enterocytes are highly polarized cells with two structurally and functionally distinct plasma membrane domains: The apical microvillous membrane and the basolateral membrane. The apical domain includes the brush border and extends to the tight junction that forms a band around the membrane, creating a relatively impermeable joint between adjacent epithelial cells. The remainder of the cell membrane constitutes the basolateral domain. The basolateral membranes contain abundant Na$^+$, K$^+$-ATPase and adenylate cyclase and are the site of the receptor for dimeric IgA attachment before its transport to the apical membrane. It is also the transfer site for chylomicrons and other foodstuffs from the enterocyte into the intercellular space and the lamina propria (Fig. 6.25). This activity is restricted from the apical surface by tight junctions that maintain these differences and prevent lateral movement of membrane components (51).

Enterocytes continuously synthesize new components of the cell membrane and surface coat and transport them to the microvillous surface. Microvilli exhibit bidirectional cell trafficking with various metabolites being absorbed and transported inward while the hydrolytic enzymes are synthesized in the endoplasmic reticulum, glycosylated in the Golgi, and transported to the brush border for insertion into the brush border membranes (Fig. 6.25). Some intestinal diseases result from impaired membrane protein trafficking including microvillous inclusion disease, congenital sucrase-isomaltase deficiency, and adult lactase deficiency disease.

The mature brush border, which covers the cell apex, consists of closely packed microvilli and the terminal web (Fig. 6.26). Microvilli vary in length, increasing in height as the cells migrate up the crypt–villus axis. Mature microvilli

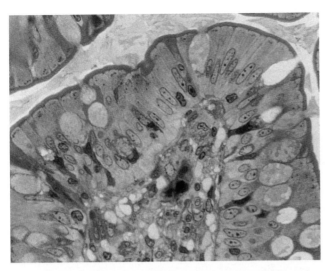

FIG. 6.26. Enterocytes. This photograph is from a thick section showing mature enterocytes and goblet cells at the free surface. The enterocytes are covered by a prominent purple fringe, which corresponds to the brush border.

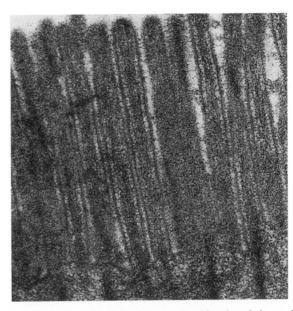

FIG. 6.28. Normal small intestine. Striated border of absorptive cells is made of large numbers of closely packed parallel microvilli.

measure approximately 1.5 to 2 μm in length and 100 nm in diameter. These structures are periodic acid–Schiff (PAS) positive (Fig. 6.27). Each microvillus contains a core bundle of approximately 20 vertically oriented, polarized actin filaments extending from the tip of the microvillus to the base of the terminal web (Fig. 6.28). These are cross-linked by the actin-bundling proteins fimbrin and villin. The other major actin-binding protein of the microvillous core is

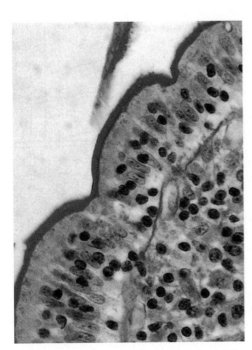

FIG. 6.27. Normal jejunum. The brush border is highlighted by a periodic acid–Schiff stain.

myosin 1 (52). Myosin 1, coupled with calmodulin, forms a double spiral of bridges cross-linking the actin bundles to the plasma membrane (53). The microvilli house a wide array of brush border enzymes that play critical roles in the digestion and absorption of proteins, fats, and carbohydrates. A complex anastomosing meshwork of filaments called the *terminal web* surrounds the microvillous rootlets. It consists of a network of actin filaments cross-linked with myosin 2, nonerythroid spectrins, α-actinin, and tropomyosin (52). The filamentous network links with the junctional complex at the edge of the cell.

The intercellular space is a dynamic area. When the cell is in a resting state, it remains collapsed and represents a potential space. In contrast, the intercellular space dilates in actively transporting cells, particularly at its most basal part (54). The junctional complex, a series of intercellular junctions, is present at the apical end of the intercellular space. The most basal member of this complex is usually the desmosome, a macular structure resembling a spot weld or adhesion point between adjacent epithelial cells (55). The zonula adherens (ZA), or intermediate junction, is a more apically located circumferential adhesive structure. Filaments from the ZA extend into the terminal web to form part of the cytoskeleton. The tight junction or zonula occludens lies at the most apical aspect of the lateral cell surface and it surrounds each epithelial cell, forming a gasketlike seal that restricts the movement of substances through the paracellular pathway by forming semipermeable barriers (56). Signaling via interactions of the cytoskeleton with the tight junctions may regulate paracellular permeability of solutes and water. Diverse microfilament-associated proteins contribute to the cellular morphology, motility, and other cellular specialized functions.

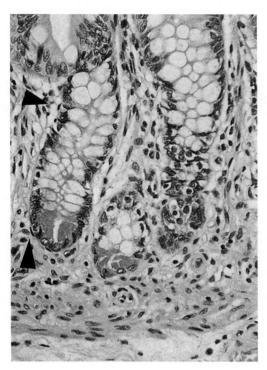

FIG. 6.29. Pericryptal fibroblasts are flattened fusiform cells closely apposed to the crypt basement membrane (*arrows*). Notice the Paneth cells in the crypt base identified by their eosinophilic apical granules.

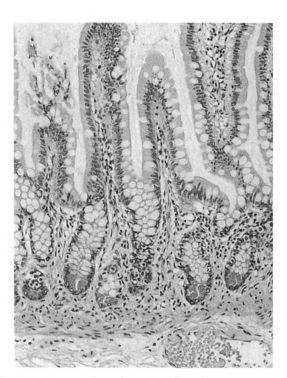

FIG. 6.30. Decreased numbers of goblet cells are present at the luminal surface.

Goblet Cells

Goblet cells play an important role in mucosal protection. They secrete mucus, ions, and water into the overlying mucous gel that protects epithelial cell surfaces. Goblet cells also produce trefoil peptides (57), which are important in preventing intestinal injury and promoting wound healing (58). They occur in both the crypts (Fig. 6.29) and among the surface absorptive cells, but they progressively decrease in number as one progresses toward the villous tip (Fig. 6.30). At the tip of the villus the ratio of enterocytes to goblet cells is about 8:1. Goblet cells increase in frequency along the length of the small intestine, being most numerous in the lower ileum. Goblet cells are primarily columnar in shape and mucus droplets accumulate in the supranuclear cytoplasm. This area also contains the Golgi apparatus at its center and rough endoplasmic reticulum at its periphery. As the mucus droplets accumulate, the supranuclear cytoplasm bulges so this part of the cell appears like a barrel or a wine goblet. When the vacuole opens into the intestinal lumen, mucus pours out (Fig. 6.31). The microvilli resemble those on enterocytes, although they are fewer in number. The terminal web of goblet cells is poorly developed, facilitating mucus release from the apical cytoplasm. The nucleus lies in a basal location and its superficial part is flattened by cytoplasmic mucin droplets (Fig. 6.31).

Follicle-Associated Epithelium

Follicle-associated epithelium (FAE), a one-cell-thick layer, forms the interface between intestinal lymphoid aggregates and the intestinal luminal environment (Figs. 6.32 and 6.33). This area has fewer goblet cells, no endocrine cells, and abundant intraepithelial lymphocytes (IELs) when compared with the epithelium of the crypts and the villi (59–61). FAE has a different differentiation program than cells along the crypt–villus axis. The FAE and villous enterocytes are also functionally different since absorptive and digestive

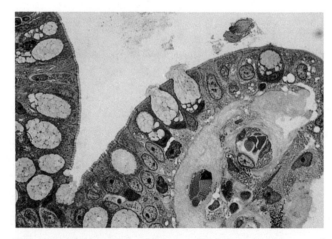

FIG. 6.31. Thick section of the superficial mucosa with several prominent goblet cells, two of which are extruding mucus into the overlying lumen.

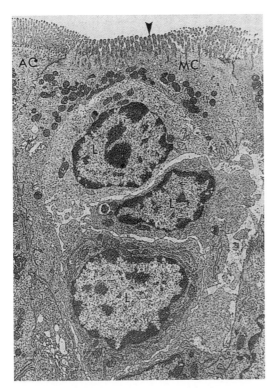

FIG. 6.32. Electron micrograph of an M cell (*MC*) flanked on the left by an absorptive cell (*AC*). M cells characteristically have microvilli that are shorter and wider (*arrowhead*) than those of neighboring absorptive cells. Lymphoid cells (*L*) are often found within the central hollow of M cells. (Courtesy of Dr. James L. Madara, University of Chicago, Chicago, IL. Reprinted with permission from the author.)

functions are down-regulated in the FAE (62). The epithelium of the FAE originates from crypts and differentiates into FAE enterocytes and M cells as they move toward the apex of the dome of the lymphoid follicle. The FAE lacks the subepithelial myofibroblasts seen in the crypts and villi, and

the basal lamina underlying the FAE differs from that of the rest of the mucosa (63).

M (membranous) cells are a unique epithelial subtype that only exists in the FAE, where they are seen at the periphery of the dome at sites where the epithelial cells exit the crypts (64). Intestinal M cells derive their name from the luminal microfolds or membranous projections formed by lymphocytes invaginating their basolateral surfaces (Fig. 6.32). Their key structural features include the following: Fewer, shorter, and more irregular microvilli, less glycocalyx, and fewer lysosomes than found on adjacent absorptive cells; a close spatial association with immunocompetent cells that reside in pocketlike extensions of the intercellular space between M cells and adjacent epithelium; a thin apical cytoplasmic rim created by intrusive lymphocytes and macrophages (there are no junctions between the M cells and their enclosed lymphocytes and plasma cells; this thin cytoplasmic rim is the only epithelial barrier between the intestinal lumen and the immunocompetent cells); and numerous endocytic vesicles that are especially abundant in the apical cytoplasmic rim. These features allow the approach of microorganisms and other intestinal luminal particles that are normally kept at bay by the closely packed microvilli and thick glycocalyx of enterocytes. Additionally, M-cell apical membranes contain abundant glycoconjugates that serve as binding sites for cationic molecules and possibly for lectinlike microbial surface interactions. As a result, certain pathogenic microorganisms selectively adhere to M cells, such as rotaviruses.

Recent data suggest that the M-cell phenotype is transiently expressed by cells as they migrate to the dome surface (63). M cells increase in number in chronic ileitis or when individuals are exposed to pathogens or antigens (65). Vimentin and cytokeratin 18 expression identifies M cells in tissue sections (Fig. 6.33) (66) since adjacent enterocytes are vimentin negative.

M cells facilitate uptake and transport a wide variety of macromolecules and microorganisms (67). The endocytosed

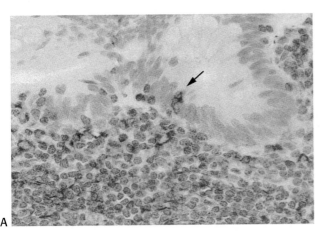

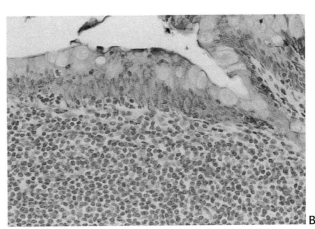

FIG. 6.33. M cells. **A:** M cells (*arrow*) are present in the epithelium overlying Peyer patches. They are highlighted with a vimentin immunostain. **B:** Cytokeratin staining is positive in absorptive cells, but not M cells in the dome epithelium.

material is delivered into apical endosomal tubules and vesicles (68), which then deliver the particles to lymphoid cells nestled in invaginations in their basolateral membranes (69). Antigens transported by the M cells first interact with antigen-presenting cells and lymphocytes in the intraepithelial pocket (70). This transepithelial transport delivers immunogens directly to organized mucosal lymphoid tissues, the inductive sites for mucosal immune responses (71). Thus, M cells form a crucial component of the afferent limb of the intestinal immune system, but they also provide a site through which potential pathogens and other noxious substances can breach the epithelial barrier. M cells may also rupture, releasing lymphocytes into the GI lumen. The bursting of the M cells at the top of the lymphoid follicles interrupts epithelial lining and allows access of the luminal contents to the lymphoid tissues. This mechanism may be responsible for the genesis of aphthous ulcers (72). Also, enterocyte attachment overlying lymphoid follicles is more labile than that of other cells, and this too may be physiologically important during the development of pathologic processes such as the development of aphthous ulcers (73).

Paneth Cells

Paneth cells populate the crypt bases and their number differs along a cranial–caudal gradient, with a greater number of Paneth cells seen caudally. Paneth cells constitute approximately 1% of small intestinal cells (74) and they arise from a common stem cell in the crypt base (74). Intermediate cell types can be encountered during their development. Paneth cells are renewed every 30 days, a rate much slower than that of other crypt cells. These strongly eosinophilic, pyramidal cells have the cytologic characteristics of zymogenic or secretory cells (Fig. 6.34). Irregular microvilli cover their apical ends. The supranuclear Golgi complex contains large, apical, membrane-bound, eosinophilic, refractile granules. The red staining quality of Paneth cells depends on the fixative used. If an acidic fixative such as Bouins is used, the cells may appear less eosinophilic. Paneth cells release granules into the crypt lumen where they participate in mucosal immunity. The granules contain various proteins involved in host defenses including lysozyme, secretory phospholipase A_2, and α-defensins, also known as cryptdins (75).

Endocrine Cells

At least 16 different subpopulations of endocrine cells are present in the small intestines. This cell population is discussed in Chapter 17, along with the proliferative lesions that arise from them.

Undifferentiated Crypt Cells

Undifferentiated crypt cells are the most abundant cells in the lower crypt. They are columnar cells with basally located nuclei and short microvilli that are less numerous than those

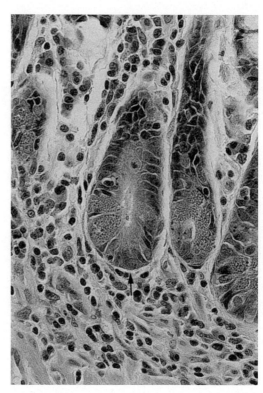

FIG. 6.34. Paneth cells. Cross sections of several crypts demonstrating the presence of Paneth cells with their prominent supranuclear granules.

seen on absorptive cells. The terminal web and glycocalyx are not well developed. Secretory granules may be present in the apical cytoplasm.

Pericryptal Myofibroblasts

Intestinal subepithelial myofibroblasts are present immediately subjacent to the basement membrane and close to the basal surface of the epithelium (Fig. 6.29). These cell underlie the epithelium of the crypts and the villi but they are absent from the FAE (63). The subepithelial myofibroblasts replicate and migrate in synchrony with the replicating and migrating epithelium, thereby enhancing mucosal structural integrity and functional efficiency (76). Myofibroblasts play a crucial role in the differentiation of villous epithelium by elaborating the basal lamina (77). They also play a role in the maintenance of the intestinal mucosa via the secretion of proinflammatory cytokines and arachidonic acid metabolites. Their paracrine effects on other mucosal cells are also important in mucosal immunophysiology and the regulation of a number of epithelial functions including epithelial restitution and barrier function (78–80).

Lymphoid Tissues

The gut-associated lymphoid tissues are thought to function as secondary lymphoid organs (81), although recent evidence suggests that the small intestinal epithelium is a site of primary extrathymic T-cell differentiation (82). The organized gut-associated lymphoid tissue in the small intestines primarily consists of Peyer patches (PPs) and the mesenteric lymph nodes (81). Other forms of lymphoid aggregations include *isolated lymphoid follicles* (ILFs), which lie within the mucosa, and *submucosal lymphoid aggregations* (SLAs), which lie within the muscularis mucosae. Both ILFs and SLAs are thought to represent normal components of the small intestinal mucosa and they are assumed to represent solitary PPs. The numbers of all of these lymphoid structures increases in the distal small intestine. SLAs are submucosal extensions from an overlying ILF (83). The typical ILF resembles the follicular units that comprise PPs. There are variants of ILFs that are either completely confined to the mucosa or extend into the superficial fibers of the muscularis mucosa. In most cases, these mucosal variants do not contain a germinal center, suggesting that they are inactive under normal circumstances. These structures may represent a reserve of mucosal lymphoid tissue that can be activated under conditions of mucosal antigenic stimulation. These lymphoid aggregates and Peyer patches differ from lymph nodes because they lack a capsule, do not have a medulla, and do not have afferent lymphatics or a capsule. The most recently described lymphoid structures are the lymphocyte-filled villi described below.

Peyer Patches and Lymphoid Aggregates

PPs are lymphoid aggregates that are randomly distributed around the circumference of the small intestinal wall (84). They split the muscularis mucosae, being partially mucosal and partially submucosal, often with a central germinal center (Fig. 6.35). The number and size of PPs increases for the first 10 years of life and reaches a maximum at puberty (84). They increase in number as one proceeds distally in the small intestine, becoming confluent in the ileum. The duodenum may also contain well-formed lymphoid nodules that extend from the surface to the base of the mucosa. The most obvious parts of the PPs are their germinal centers and a surrounding corona of B cells. Germinal centers (Figs. 6.36 and 6.37) are much more common in children than in adults.

Peyer patches contain three major domains: The follicular B-cell area, the parafollicular T-cell area, and the FAE described above (Fig. 6.38). The epithelial basement membranes overlying lymphoid follicles within Peyer patches are very porous. This porosity may facilitate bidirectional passage of lymphocytes during immune responses (85). Lymphocytes and other mononuclear cells are constantly migrating into and out of the spaces in the dome epithelium. The subepithelial tissue immediately beneath the FAE contains IgM+ B cells, CD4+ T cells, Ia+ dendritic cells, and macrophages, allowing for efficient antigen processing and antibody production (86).

PPs are important sites of lymphocyte recirculation (81). Peyer patch–derived lymphocytes give rise to lamina propria plasma cells. There are also circulating small lymphocytes within the Peyer patches. The localization of B cells and T cells to Peyer patches is mediated by interactions between these cells and endothelial cells lining postcapillary HEVs (87).

PPs contain at least three different populations of non-lymphoid cells: Scavenger macrophages in the dome areas,

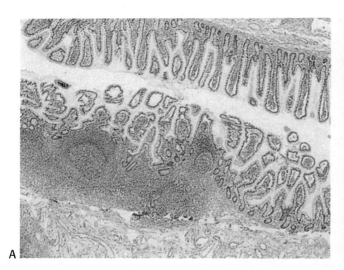

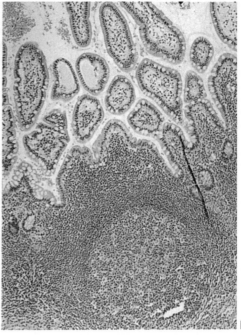

FIG. 6.35. Normal ileum. **A:** The ileum contains aggregated lymphoid nodules of Peyer patches. **B:** Higher power illustrates a germinal center with a prominent cuff of small lymphocytes.

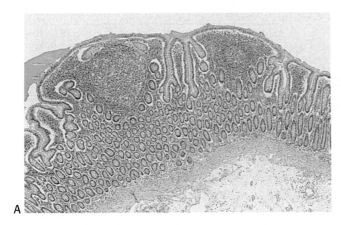

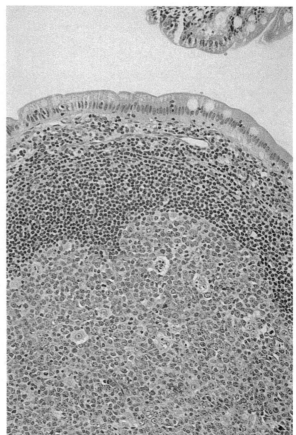

FIG. 6.36. Lymphoid follicles. **A:** Slightly tangentially cut mucosa with several lymphoid follicles. **B:** The prominent germinal centers containing tingible body macrophages and a prominent lymphocytic rim.

dendritic cells just beneath the epithelium in the dome in the T-cell area, and tingible body macrophages in the germinal centers of the B-cell follicles. Macrophages, particularly those near the dome of the lymphoid tissue, may contain bacteria. A mixed cell zone that contains follicular center B cells, numerous helper T cells, and human leukocyte antigen (HLA)-DR+ macrophages lies between the M

cells and the small lymphocytes that form the mantle of the follicle. The overlying epithelium contains intraepithelial B cells and suppressor T lymphocytes. The distribution of lymphocytes in the PP epithelium differs from IELs in the villi in that the dome epithelium lymphocytes cluster in groups and frequently occur above the level of the enterocyte nuclei.

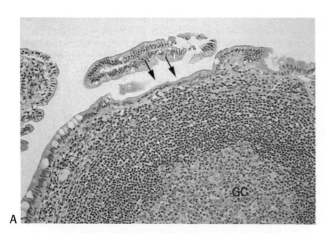

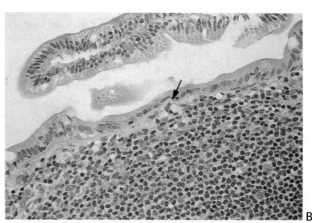

FIG. 6.37. Peyer patch. **A:** A flattened epithelium lies over the surface of the Peyer patch (*arrows*). A prominent lymphocyte mantle is present and the germinal center (*GC*) is seen at the lower portion of the photograph. **B:** Higher magnification shows the intraepithelial lymphocytes (*arrow*).

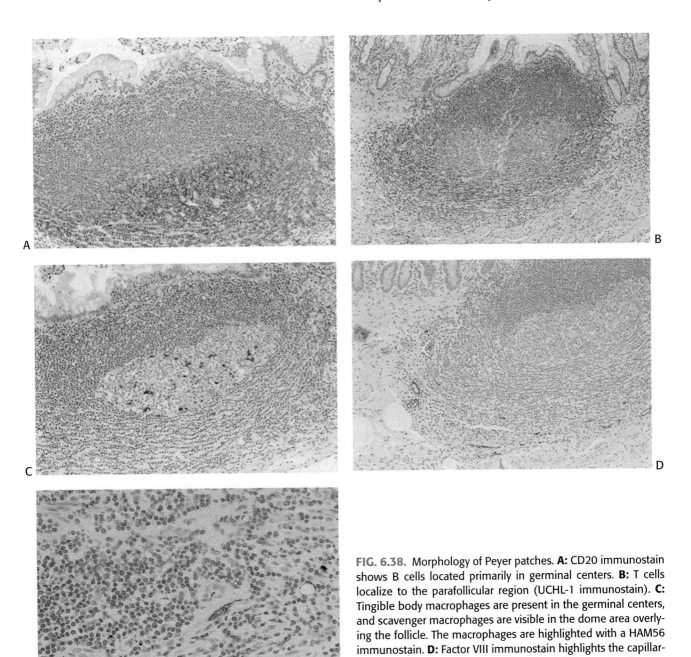

FIG. 6.38. Morphology of Peyer patches. **A:** CD20 immunostain shows B cells located primarily in germinal centers. **B:** T cells localize to the parafollicular region (UCHL-1 immunostain). **C:** Tingible body macrophages are present in the germinal centers, and scavenger macrophages are visible in the dome area overlying the follicle. The macrophages are highlighted with a HAM56 immunostain. **D:** Factor VIII immunostain highlights the capillaries and small vessels surrounding the follicle. **E:** Small nerve twigs populate the lamina propria surrounding the lymphoid follicles (synaptophysin immunostain).

The sides of the follicles are populated by a diffuse population of small lymphocytes, macrophages, and plasma cells. Variable numbers of eosinophils are also present. Underlying the follicles, there is a T-cell–rich population with a T-helper:T-suppressor ratio of 8:1. The lamina propria and Peyer patch immune cells participate in immunoglobulin synthesis and T-cell functions.

CD4+ and CD8+ cells are both present in the dome of Peyer patches, the site where B cells are preferentially found. The B cells may cluster in aggregates. B cells migrate more rapidly to the center of the Peyer patch follicles than do T cells. In contrast, CD4+ T cells accumulate in the interfollic-

ular zones. The distribution of cells in the dome epithelium differs from non–Peyer patch areas of the mucosa where T cytotoxic/suppressor cells predominate and B cells are few. Lymphocytes are usually absent from the crypts outside Peyer patches.

If migrating lymphocytes do not engage in an immune response, they continue their migration through the PPs and exit via the efferent lymphatics (88). The lymphocytes then move toward the submucosal lymphatics under the Peyer patches. Peyer patches have the potential capacity to store lymphocytes and modulate lymphocyte migration (89). Lymphocytes from PPs follow a migratory pattern from mesenteric lymphatics to the mesenteric lymph nodes, the superior mesenteric duct, and the thoracic duct before draining into the peripheral circulation. This dynamic lymphocyte recirculation facilitates effective surveillance for foreign invaders and alterations within the body's own immune system (89).

Lymphocyte-filled Villi

Lymphocyte-filled villi (LFV) are recently described structures that resemble Peyer patches. Morphologic features that distinguish LFV from classical villi are the presence of tightly packed lymphocytes that fill most of the lamina propria and a high concentration of IELs in the overlying epithelium. These IELs are enriched for CD4+ T cells that are often found in clusters, but the majority of the cells do not express surface immunoglobulin, CD3, or the T-cell receptor. Many of the cells are CD25+. They also contain major histocompatibility complex (MHC) class II–positive dendritic cells and a variable B-cell component. The epithelium overlying these structures resembles that of the FAE and includes the presence of M cells. These features suggest that the epithelium of LFV resembles the FAE. However, LFV lack HEVs and obvious lymphoid follicles. These structures are confined to the jejunum (83).

Intraepithelial Lymphocytes

IELs constitute a distinct and heterogeneous lymphocyte population nestled among the epithelium (90). They express the T-cell receptor (TCR)-$\alpha\beta$ and -$\gamma\delta$ with functional and phenotypic features that differ from cells in peripheral lymphoid tissues. There is also an intraepithelial population of functional killer lymphocytes (91). Cellular and molecular cross-talk between epithelial cells and IELs appears to play a key role in the reciprocal growth and activation of these cells and in the maintenance of intestinal homeostasis. IELs contribute to cytokine secretion, expression of MHC and adhesion molecules, and the integrity of mucosal defenses (92,93). They also possess cytotoxic activity, which is important in protecting against the invasion of luminal pathogens and the destruction of transformed epithelium (94,95).

IELs typically lie in the basal portion of the epithelium. They range from 3 to 11 μm in diameter and possess small dense nuclei, contrasting with the paler, more vesicular enterocyte nuclei (Figs. 6.39 and 6.40). IELs have a small nuclear:cytoplasmic ratio. They lack any junctional attachments to the surrounding epithelium, so that they can easily migrate in and out of the epithelium (96). The small intestine contains a large number of IELs, estimated to be approximately one IEL per six to ten epithelial cells (97). Fewer numbers are present in the ileum. In contrast to the IELs in the villi, IELs overlying lymphoid follicles are predominantly of B-cell derivation. There appear to be differences in the IEL populations of the crypt and the villus that facilitate different types of interactions of the IELs with the enterocytes.

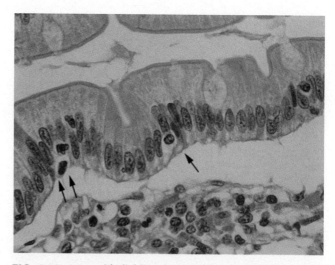

FIG. 6.39. Intraepithelial lymphocytes. The photograph has an artifact in which the epithelium has become separated from the underlying lamina propria. A single intraepithelial lymphocyte is present, as indicated by the *arrow,* and several lymphocytes are indicated by the *double arrows.*

Specifically, there is an increased frequency of $\gamma\delta$ TCR-carrying T cells in the villus as compared to the crypts (98).

Lamina Propria

The lamina propria provides the scaffolding on which the intestinal epithelium rests. It contains the blood vessels that nourish the epithelium and supplies a support structure for the immune cells. The majority of the cells are in the crypt region rather than in the villous region. These cells consist of immunocytes, particularly plasma cells and lymphocytes (Fig. 6.40). The majority are IgA-containing plasma cells, although IgM-, IgD-, IgG-, and IgE-containing cells are also present. IgM-containing cells are the second most numerous (99). The ratio of IgA to IgM cells in the intestinal mucosa is 15 to 20:1.

Plasma cells never normally infiltrate the epithelium. The increased number of plasma cells seen in the lamina propria following antigenic challenge results from recruitment of circulating lymphocyte pools and proliferation of newly recruited cells in the lamina propria. The majority of the lamina propria T lymphocytes exhibit a helper-inducer phenotype, whereas only 30% to 40% are suppressor cytotoxic T cells.

Numerous macrophages aggregate in the lamina propria at the tips of the villi. They extend pseudopods into the epithelial lining and internalize components of apoptotic aging enterocytes. The basal lamina propria, especially in the small bowel, contains large numbers of dendritic cells. These present antigens to mucosal CD4+ T cells. Polymorphonuclear leukocytes (PMNs) are uncommon.

It is estimated that there are between 100 and 200 eosinophils per millimeter of lamina propria in the jejunum (Fig. 6.41) (100). However, this figure varies significantly

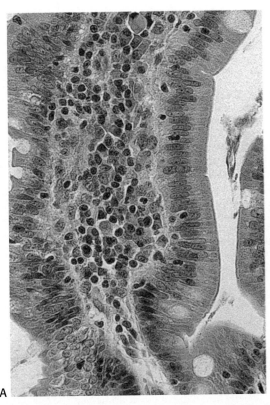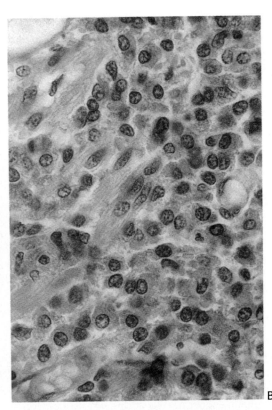

FIG. 6.40. Lamina propria immunocytes. **A:** The lamina propria contains a large number of lymphocytes and plasma cells, as well as eosinophils and mast cells. Additionally, intraepithelial lymphocytes are present. **B:** Higher magnification of the area of the lamina propria showing plasma cells and lymphocytes.

depending on the geographic locale in which one lives. In those parts of the world associated with a high incidence of environmental allergies, such as to pollens, eosinophils may increase in number, particularly during the height of the allergy seasons. Basophils are not very prominent.

In the normal adult jejunum, there are up to 300 mast cells/mm^2 of mucosa (101) compared with 750 mast cells/mm^2 of the ileal lamina propria in children (102).

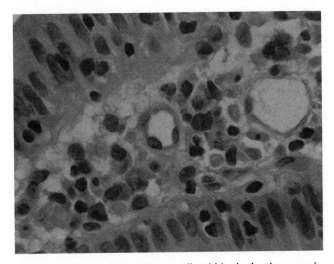

FIG. 6.41. Eosinophils and mast cells within the lamina propria.

Abundant mast cells lie in the superficial aspect of the mucosa. Mast cells may be highlighted by CD25, CD117, or tryptase immunostains. The cells are evenly distributed throughout the bowel wall and some maintain a relationship with neural structures.

Brunner Glands

Brunner glands form a continuous series of branched or coiled tubular glands in the submucosa and basal mucosa of the first part of the duodenum. In the first part of the duodenum, where Brunner glands are relatively large, bands of smooth muscle from the muscularis mucosae occasionally lie between the acinar lobules. Ducts of individual glands open either directly into the duodenal lumen or into the crypts of Lieberkühn. Occasionally, small groups of glands occur within the superficial epithelium, particularly in patients with peptic duodenitis. Their size and number gradually decrease from the proximal to the distal duodenum (Fig. 6.42). In the second portion, at the level of the ampulla of Vater they are scattered. In the third portion, only a few small glands are present (103).

Three morphologically distinctive cell types are present in Brunner glands: Cells with a central nucleus and uniform glassy eosinophilic basal cytoplasm, similar cells with a clear basal cytoplasm, and cells with basal nuclei and small clear perinuclear vacuoles. The glands produce neutral glycoproteins

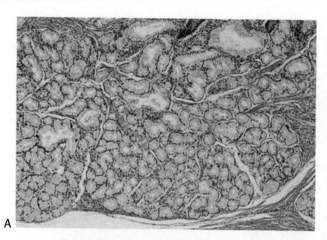
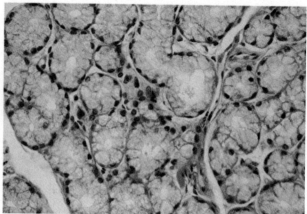

FIG. 6.42. Brunner glands. A: The submucosa of the duodenum is almost completely filled with highly branched tubular duodenal glands (Brunner glands). The muscularis mucosae may be disrupted as these glands penetrate into the deep lamina propria of the mucosa. **B:** Higher magnification showing the clear cytoplasm of the Brunner glands.

that do not stain with mucicarmine but are PAS positive. Brunner glands produce MUC6, bicarbonate, epidermal growth factor, trefoil peptides, bactericidal factors, proteinase inhibitors, and surface active lipids (104). Brunner glands also contain endocrine cells storing somatostatin, gastrin, cholecystokinin (CCK), and peptide YY.

Neural Structure

A complex neuronal circuitry regulates GI function. The overall mucosal and submucosal neural organization is described in Chapter 10.

Ampulla of Vater

The ampulla of Vater lies in the second part of the duodenum. The common bile duct and major pancreatic duct pass through this structure. The mucosa overlying this area appears highly variable. A complex collection of glands lies in the submucosa and passes through the muscularis mucosae into the overlying mucosa. They are surrounded by smooth muscle cells and a loose stroma (Fig. 6.43). This area is the weakest part of the duodenum and hence the most common site for diverticula to develop.

CONGENITAL ABNORMALITIES
Intestinal Malpositions

Intestinal malpositions include disorders of malrotation, malfixation, reversed rotation, incomplete rotations, fixation abnormalities, and situs inversus. Intestinal malrotations or nonrotations (Fig. 6.44) result from disordered or interrupted embryonic intestinal counterclockwise rotations around the superior mesenteric artery. The normal

rotations and fixations are either incomplete or occur out of order. Nonrotations result from an interruption early in the rotation, so that the duodenal–jejunal loop remains on the right side of the abdomen. The cecal position varies, but it usually lies in the upper abdomen on the left side (Fig. 6.44). Incomplete rotations reflect interruptions occurring after the duodenal–jejunal loop has partially rotated around the superior mesenteric artery. Variants of classic rotation also occur. These include reversed duodenal and colonic rotation and reversed duodenal rotation and normal colonic rotation. In reversed rotation, the dorsal and ventral loops rotate to the left rather than to the right. The cecum lies in the right iliac fossa but the small bowel lies superficial to the transverse colon (Fig. 6.44), often herniating into the right colonic mesentery (104). The small bowel may also fail to rotate fully. As the intestine returns to the abdominal cavity, the small intestine rotates 180 degrees but fails to continue rotating to the normal point of fixation at the ligament of Treitz. Considerable variations exist in the degree of rotation beyond 180 degrees. A short small intestinal and mesenteric segment often becomes fixed to the retroperitoneum along a line generally confined to the right upper quadrant. This line of fixation, rather than anchoring the small bowel securely, becomes a new point of rotation, substituting for the superior mesenteric artery as a rotation point. Fibrous bands or adhesions form between the bowel and other abdominal structures in an attempt to secure the mobile bowel (Fig. 6.45). These commonly cross and compress the duodenum, obstructing it. Rotational abnormalities also complicate developmental defects when the intestine occupies an extra-abdominal position, as occurs in congenital diaphragmatic hernias or in abdominal wall defects (105).

Intestinal malrotations affect approximately 1 in 6,000 live births (106). Three percent of patients have associated abnormalities (Table 6.1). Patients present with signs and symptoms

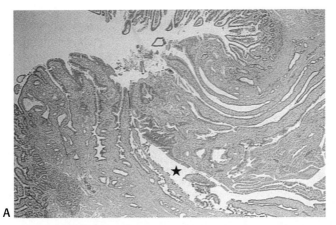

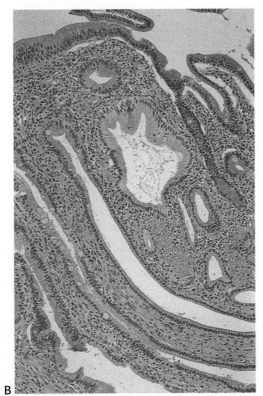

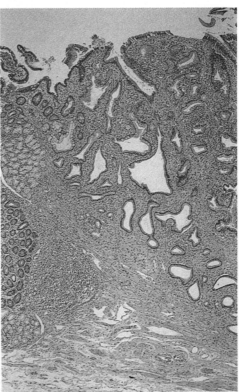

FIG. 6.43. Ampulla of Vater. **A:** Low magnification demonstrating the presence of numerous branching glands that enter at the area of the ampulla. A cross section of a larger duct is indicated by the *star*. **B:** Derives from the area to the right of the star in A. **C:** Higher magnification from the area to the left of the star.

of duodenal obstruction, intermittent volvulus, or acute life-threatening midgut volvulus characterized by bilious vomiting, abdominal distention, rectal bleeding, or intussusception. Infants may also develop malabsorption with steatorrhea and protein-losing enteropathy resulting from mesenteric lymphatic obstruction. Adults with malrotations often have a lifetime history of nonspecific abdominal complaints, including acute symptoms when they were children (107).

Malrotations exhibit obvious intestinal misplacement within the abdominal cavity. The intestines often lie to one side, appearing as a large mass of nonrotated bowel (Fig. 6.44). The entire bowel, from the duodenum to splenic flexure, remains unanchored and supported by a single mesen-

tery with a very narrow base, predisposing the intestines to torsion and volvulus.

Situs Inversus

In *situs inversus*, the organs lie in mirror image locations of their normal positions. When *complete*, it affects both thoracic and abdominal organs. When *incomplete*, it affects only the abdominal organs. *Limited situs inversus* affects only the stomach and duodenum. Situs inversus affects 1 in 1,400 live births and it forms part of Kartagener syndrome.

Many children with situs inversus and a neural tube defect have mothers with insulin-dependent diabetes mellitus. Partial

TABLE 6.1 **Abnormalities Associated with Small Intestinal Malrotation**

Biliary atresia or stenosis
Duodenal atresia or stenosis
Prune belly syndrome
Diaphragmatic hernia
Annular pancreas
Internal hernias
Paraduodenal hernia
Midgut volvulus and facial anomalies
Omphalocele and gastroschisis
Intestinal atresia
Craniofacial anomalies (especially in infants with intrauterine opiate or heroin exposure)
Trisomy 13, 18, and 21
Situs inversus

situs inversus usually associates with other malformations, including asplenia, duodenal stenosis, and cardiac defects. Major associated gastrointestinal anomalies include annular pancreas, midgut volvulus, duodenal atresia, and mucosal duodenal diaphragms. Situs inversus does not change organ function or histology. One group of patients that may have a somewhat worse prognosis than others are those with *Kartagener syndrome*. These patients have abnormal cilia and as

a result they produce thick, tenacious bronchial and sinus secretions that lead to chronic sinusitis and bronchiectasis.

Omphaloceles

Omphaloceles consist of an external mass of abdominal contents covered by a variably translucent peritoneal and/or amniotic membrane. They result from the failure of the anterior abdominal wall to form completely during fetal development combined with the failure of the abdominal viscera to return to the abdomen at the end of the 10th fetal week. Omphaloceles affect 2.52 per 60,000 to 2 per 3,000 live births. Significant heterogeneity exists in the prevalence rates among different geographic regions, with especially high prevalence rates occurring throughout the British Isles. In the United Kingdom and Ireland, there is a tendency for omphaloceles to associate with anencephaly and spina bifida. The male-to-female incidence is 3:1; however, a significant female excess exists among the cases of omphalocele associated with neural tube defects. Up to 54% of infants with omphaloceles have associated anomalies (Table 6.2) compared with only 5% of those with gastroschisis (108,109). Many fetuses with an omphalocele have an abnormal karyotype. Chromosomal anomalies are particularly common in omphaloceles that do not contain the liver (110).

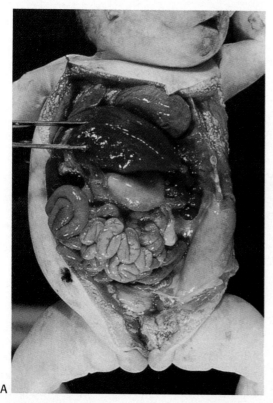
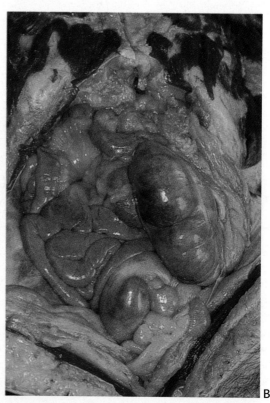

A   B

FIG. 6.44. Malrotation. **A:** The small intestines lie matted together in the lower abdomen, pushing the colon to the right side. **B:** A mass of unrotated small intestine lies on the right side of the abdominal cavity. The cecum lies on the left side.

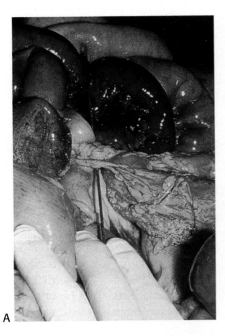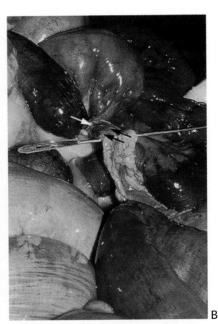

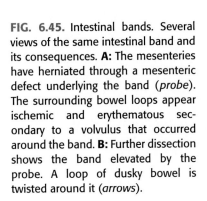

FIG. 6.45. Intestinal bands. Several views of the same intestinal band and its consequences. **A:** The mesenteries have herniated through a mesenteric defect underlying the band (*probe*). The surrounding bowel loops appear ischemic and erythematous secondary to a volvulus that occurred around the band. **B:** Further dissection shows the band elevated by the probe. A loop of dusky bowel is twisted around it (*arrows*).

The rare *OEIS* (*omphalocele, cloacal exstrophy, imperforate anus, spinal defects*) complex affects 1 per 200,000 to 400,000 pregnancies. OEIS occurs sporadically or it affects twins or siblings from separate pregnancies, suggesting that some cases have a genetic basis. Some patients with omphalocele and the Miller-Dieker syndrome have a deletion at 17p13.3, suggesting that a gene in this region plays a major role in lateral fold closure or the return of the midgut from the body stalk to the abdomen. Trisomy 18 affects some patients. OEIS

associates with a history of maternal diabetes mellitus or hydantoin or diazepam administration (111,112).

The OEIS complex arises from a single localized mesodermal defect early in development that contributes to infraumbilical mesenchymal, cloacal septum, and caudal vertebral abnormalities. Four somatic folds (a cephalic fold, two lateral folds, and a caudal fold) define the anterior thoracic and abdominal walls during the third fetal week. These folds migrate centrally to fuse at the umbilical ring, usually by the 18th gestational week. Arrested fold migration or development results in anterior wall defects and a widening of the umbilical ring.

The average birth weight and gestational age of infants with omphalocele is low. The amniotic membrane and peritoneum protect the developing intestinal loops from the damaging effects of exposure to amniotic fluid seen in gastroschisis. Omphaloceles range in size from only a few centimeters to lesions involving almost the entire anterior abdominal wall (Fig. 6.46). Abdominal viscera are present within a sac that initially is moist and transparent but with time becomes dry, fibrotic, opaque, friable, and prone to rupture with secondary evisceration. One often can see its contents through the glistening membrane. Abdominal skin may cover the sac base and the umbilical cord is usually attached to its apex or slightly to the side. Large omphaloceles, measuring 5 cm or more in greatest dimension, may contain the stomach, liver, spleen, pancreas, and intestines. They may also contain segments of duplicated bowel. Smaller omphaloceles usually only contain intestines.

The function and histology of the displaced organs tends to be normal unless there is a coexisting congenital abnormality. The lining of the sac that covers the eviscerated organs consists of peritoneum internally and amnion externally.

TABLE 6.2 **Defects Associated with Omphaloceles**

Heart anomalies
Intestinal atresia
Chromosomal defects
Genitourinary anomalies (cloacal or bladder exstrophy)
Craniofacial defects
Diaphragmatic abnormalities
Liver and bile duct abnormalities
Beckwith-Wiedemann syndrome
   Macroglossia
   Gigantism
   Hypoglycemia
   Umbilical abnormalities
Cantrell pentalogy
   Ectopia cordis
   Sternal cleft
   Diaphragmatic defect
   Cardiac disease
   Omphalocele
OEIS complex
   Omphalocele
   Cloacal exstrophy
   Imperforate anus
   Spinal defects

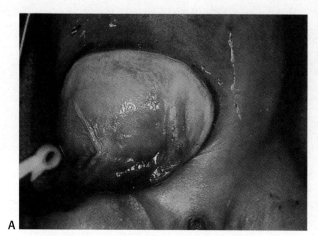
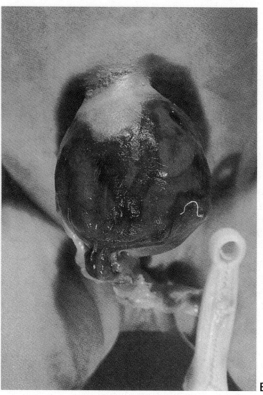

FIG. 6.46. Omphalocele. **A:** A large abdominal defect is covered by a thick white membrane extending into the base of the umbilical cord (dark red structure with clamp across it). The organs inside the omphalocele cannot be seen. **B:** The abdominal wall defect is smaller than that seen in A, and a clear sac covers the herniated intestines. A whitish membrane is forming near the abdominal wall attachment. At the periphery of this whitish lesion and within the clear membranous sac is an erythematous zone. The lesion continues into the umbilical cord, which has an umbilical clamp on it.

Gastroschisis

Gastroschisis is the persistent herniation of abdominal viscera through an abdominal wall defect at the base of the umbilicus. The abdominal organs remain outside the abdominal cavity. No peritoneal sac or amniotic remnant covers the eviscerated abdominal contents. The incidence of gastroschisis has risen, increasing from 0.48 per 10,000 births in 1980 to 3.16 per 10,000 in 1993 (113,114). Young, socially disadvantaged women have the highest risk of having a child with gastroschisis (115). An increased risk of gastroschisis also associates with intrapartum use of recreational drugs or smoking (113), exposure to salicylates, and radiation (116). Gastroschisis predominates among male infants. It is often an isolated lesion (109). Sixteen to twenty percent of infants have associated congenital malformations, including total intestinal atresia (113,117,118).

Gastroschisis probably results from vascular injury and ischemia of the abdominal wall during the 5th to 11th fetal weeks, leading to defective somatopleural mesenchymal differentiation (118). The ischemia results from intrauterine disruption of the right omphalomesenteric artery. Exposure of the bowel to inflamed amniotic fluid (119) leads to perivisceritis and premature birth. The damaged bowel frequently

develops secondary motility problems and malabsorption, which may present even following surgical repair. Other complications include obstruction due to coexisting malrotation, diverticulitis, ischemia, and perforation. Patients with ectopic gastric mucosa in the eviscerated bowel may develop a GI hemorrhage.

Gastroschisis may involve only the intestines or it may affect many other organs. Parts of the stomach, small intestine, and colon herniate through an abdominal wall defect, usually to the right of the umbilical cord (Fig. 6.47). All infants with gastroschisis have coexisting nonrotation and abnormal intestinal fixations. The small intestines typically appear thickened and shortened.

Omphalocele and gastroschisis are both associated with increased maternal serum and amniotic fluid α-fetoprotein (AFP) levels. Acetyl cholinesterase is also nearly always detectable in the amniotic fluid, albeit at much lower concentrations than in open neural tube defects (120). Antenatal ultrasound often allows an accurate diagnosis of gastroschisis.

The histology of the various organs may be normal (rarely) or changes may be present reflecting the presence of associated congenital abnormalities, heterotopias, atresia, meconium peritonitis, or perivisceritis. The last two entities lead to gastrointestinal wall thickening, serosal edema, and

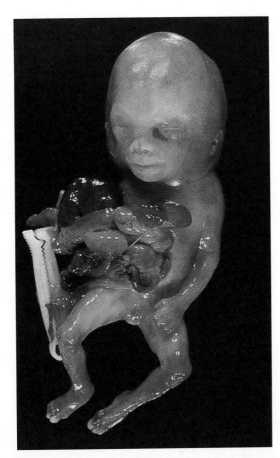

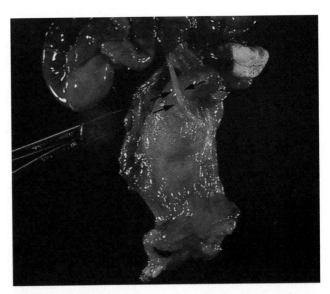

FIG. 6.48. Amniotic band syndrome. The fetus shows numerous abnormalities, including loss of limbs, an abdominal wall defect, gastroschisis, and an amniotic band (*arrows*).

FIG. 6.47. Gastroschisis. This infant shows external herniation of most of the abdominal contents, including the liver, spleen, and intestinal tract.

fibrinous exudates and fibrosis. The intestinal muscularis propria may also become hypertrophic. Acute inflammation consisting predominantly of neutrophils and mononuclear cells may be present in gastroschisis and may lead to postnatal bowel dysfunction. Functionally, there is often malabsorption and hypomotility as the result of the inflammation.

Long-term outcome in the absence of major chromosomal and structural abnormalities is excellent (121). Patient prognosis depends in part on whether the gastroschisis is an isolated lesion or whether there are associated abnormalities. The goal of the surgeon in both gastroschisis and omphalocele is to accomplish abdominal wall closure in a single stage. An alternate approach is to perform a staged closure using prosthetic materials while maintaining adequate nutritional support.

Bands

Peritoneal bands, known as Ladd bands, extend from the cecum, ascending colon, or posterior wall transduodenally to the subhepatic region, compressing the duodenum and causing partial obstruction, vascular compression, and intestinal ischemia. The bands represent incomplete absorption of the cecal and ascending colonic mesentery. Limb–body wall

malformations, also known as amniotic band syndrome (Fig. 6.48), cause body wall, limb, and intestinal malformations.

Atresia and Stenosis

Intestinal atresia and stenosis cause intestinal obstruction. Atresia occurs more often than stenosis. Their incidence varies from 1 per 2,000 to 6,000 live births (122). Atresia results from an occluding mucosal diaphragm, whereas stenosis represents either a narrowed intestinal segment or a luminal diaphragm with a small central opening. Duodenal atresia is the most common small intestinal atresia, followed by jejunal and ileal lesions. Duodenal atresia is less common than duodenal stenosis. Jejunoileal atresias affect 1 per 500 to 2,000 live births. Some patients have multiple atresias (123).

Intestinal atresia occurs on both a sporadic and a familial basis. Most intestinal atresias follow some form of ischemic injury (124) or intrapartum asphyxia (125) occurring after the intestine has developed and produce segmental intestinal necrosis with subsequent fibrosis or tissue loss (125). The presence of meconium, bile, squames, and lanugo hair in the atretic areas (Fig. 6.49) supports an intrauterine injury. Small intestinal atresia may complicate midtrimester amniocentesis (126), intrauterine intussusception due to Meckel diverticulum, or fetal infections (varicella and syphilis). Fetal exposure to cocaine in the mother may predispose to intestinal atresia due to vascular disruptions (127). Twins have a higher rate of small intestinal atresia than single-birth infants, possibly due to vascular disruption in monozygotic twins. Associated congenital abnormalities affect fewer than 10% of patients with jejunoileal atresia, contrasting with a 35% incidence of associated congenital anomalies in patients with small intestinal atresia (Table 6.3) (128,129). Familial

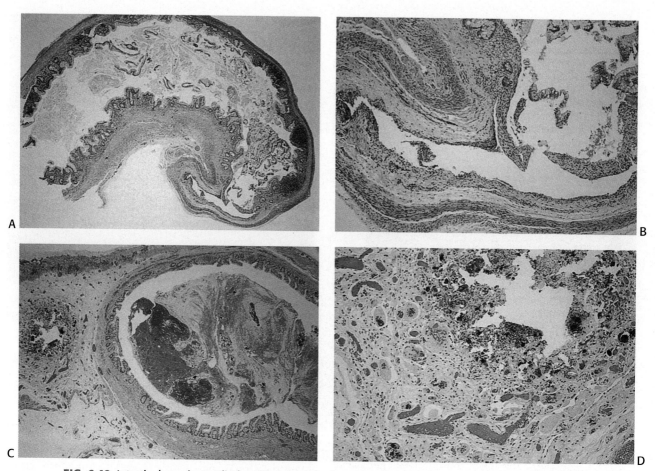

FIG. 6.49. Intestinal atresia. **A:** Blind-ending atresia is shown on the right. **B:** Fibrosis in atretic wall. **C:** Blind area of atresia on the right with stenotic area on the left. The atretic area is filled with meconium. **D:** Granulomatous reaction surrounding stenotic area.

jejunal atresia may associate with renal dysplasia. Apple-peel atresia probably results from a narrow mesenteric attachment, volvulus, and occlusion of the superior mesenteric artery distal to its proximal branches (130). Of all types of jejunoileal atresias, the apple-peel variety has the highest rate of associated anomalies (130). There is an increased frequency of cystic fibrosis among infants with small intestinal atresia (131). Ileal atresia may coexist with colonic aganglionosis (132).

Most duodenal atresias lie in a postampullary location or at the ampulla of Vater. Duodenal atresia can be diagnosed ultrasonographically at 15 weeks' gestation by finding polyhydramnios, a lack of amniotic fluid, intestinal dilation proximal to the atretic intestine, meconium peritonitis, and ascites. Elevated maternal serum AFP levels and polyhydramnios occur in the second trimester of pregnancy in 50% of cases (133). Signs of distress or ischemia are frequent. Approximately 50% of infants with intestinal atresia are premature.

Small intestinal atresias present in the neonatal period. Bilious vomiting (unless a coexisting esophageal atresia is also present) usually occurs during the first few hours of birth. Partial obstruction causes intermittent symptoms. The

vomitus lacks bile staining when the obstruction lies proximal to the ampulla of Vater. Duodenal atresia is also suggested radiographically by the presence of a double bubble on a plain abdominal x-ray, particularly when gas is present in a distended stomach and proximal duodenum.

In contrast, because stenoses allow passage of some enteric contents, they present later in life. Some patients with *duodenal stenosis* remain asymptomatic, whereas others present with an intermittent or delayed history of duodenal ulcer, symptoms associated with hiatal hernia, gastritis, duodenogastric reflux, a motility disturbance, duodenal diverticula, and bezoars (134).

Atresia results from a complete occlusion, whereas *stenosis* represents either a narrowed intestinal segment or a luminal diaphragm with a small central aperture. In atresia, a bowel segment is entirely missing, leaving a proximal segment with a blind end separated some distance from the distal segment. Alternately, the proximal and distal segments are united by a solid fibrous cord, or there is an occluding mucosal diaphragm. Some patients have multiple atresias (135). Intestinal atresia falls into four major types (Figs. 6.50 and 6.51). Two main types of stenosis exist. In type 1, a septum identical to that seen in type 1 atresia is present, but

TABLE 6.3 Lesions Associated with Small Intestinal Atresia and Stenosis

Malrotation of the gut
Meckel diverticulum
Volvulus
Esophageal atresia
VACTERL associations
Other small intestinal atresias
Imperforate anus
Biliary atresia
Annular pancreas
Perforation
Pancreatic lipomatosis
Ocular abnormalities
Microcephaly
Spina bifida
Gastrourinary abnormalities
Immunodeficiency states
Hirschsprung disease
Congenital heart disease
Cytogenetic changes
   Internal deletion on chromosome 13
   Ring chromosome 4
   Trisomy 21 (Down syndrome)
Maternal lesions
   Polyhydramnios
   Intrapartum hemorrhage

instead of being complete it has a central hole within it. In type 2 lesions, the GI lumen appears uniformly narrowed over a variable length of intestine (Fig. 6.52). All bowel layers form normally.

Normal small intestinal mucosa lines both sides of the atretic or stenotic intestinal segment. The height of the circular folds declines and the muscularis mucosa thickens as one approaches the blind segment. In complex atresia, the proximal bowel appears dilated and gangrenous. The circular folds widen due to stromal edema. The villi may appear shortened or only simple tubular glands may be present. The villi and crypts also often appear necrotic or ulcerated, with only a few residual intestinal glands. As a result, the mucosa contains granulation tissue, granulomas, foreign body giant cells, fibroblasts, and hemosiderin-laden macrophages. Dystrophic calcification and inflammation at or near the atretic site suggest previous injury. The blind segment may contain dense fibrosis, meconium, keratinizing squamous cells, lanugo hair, bile pigment, and mucin. The intervening mucosa between atretic areas is histologically normal. The muscularis propria eventually becomes markedly hypertrophic and the myenteric plexus may show inflammatory or degenerative changes.

Annular Pancreas

Annular pancreas, a congenital disorder of failed duodenal development, consists of a ring of pancreatic tissue sur-

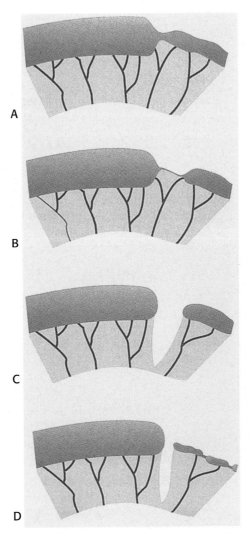

FIG. 6.50. Different types of atresia. **A:** In type 1, an imperforate septum, covered on each side by mucosa, stretches across an otherwise continuous bowel. **B:** In type 2, a thin fibromuscular cord with or without an associated mesenteric defect replaces the bowel. **C:** In type 3, a complete gap and a corresponding mesenteric defect separate the two blind intestinal ends. **D:** Type 4 atresia is characterized by the presence of atretic areas. The different forms of atresia may coexist and may be single or multiple.

rounding the second part of the duodenum (Fig. 6.53) that presents in the neonatal period or in the 4th and 5th decades of life (136). The incidence of annular pancreas is 1 in 20,000 persons. Annular pancreas may be part of a more generalized embryogenic disorder associated with trisomy 21, tracheoesophageal fistulae, or cardiorenal abnormalities (136), or it occurs alone. Eighty percent of infants with annular pancreas have associated anomalies, in contrast to 20% of adults. Neonates present with duodenal obstruction. Adults present with duodenal stenosis, peptic ulcers, upper abdominal pain, and chronic pancreatitis, or the lesion is found incidentally. Peptic symptoms result from gastric stasis and antral overdistention due to partial duodenal obstruction and

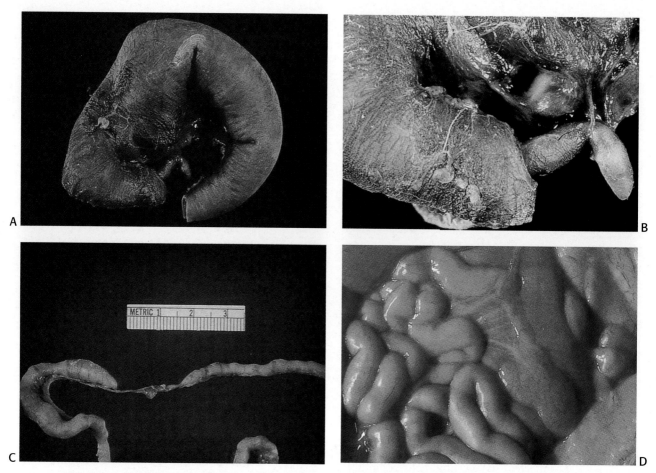

FIG. 6.51. Intestinal atresia. **A:** Resected portion of small intestine showing intestinal dilation proximal to the atretic area. **B:** Close-up of atretic portion of small bowel showing a marked narrowing of a segment partially encircled by a fibrous band. **C:** Type 2 atresia with thin fibromuscular core. **D:** Type 2 atresia in situ. No mesenteric defect is present.

secondary hypergastrinemia, hyperchlorhydria, and peptic ulceration. Although the pancreatic location is abnormal, the pancreatic histology is completely normal. Secondary inflammatory changes occur if the patient develops duodenal stenosis or peptic ulceration.

Enterogenous Cysts, Congenital Diverticula, and Duplications

Congenital diverticula, duplications, and enterogenous cysts are related lesions that contain all three bowel layers (Fig. 6.54). A *duplication* is a complete or partial doubling of a variable length of bowel. *Duplication cysts* are localized duplications that become incorporated into the bowel wall or embedded within its serosa. They often coexist with rotational disorders or vertebral body defects. These congenital malformations involve the mesenteric side of the intestine and they share a common blood supply with the native bowel. They may possess their own mesentery, but more commonly they are included in the mesentery of the normal bowel. The major distinction that separates this group of lesions is their gross appearance (Figs. 6.54 and 6.55). Duplications tend to be longer in their axial length than cysts or diverticula and they appear as tubular intestinal reduplications that may or may not communicate with the native intestinal lumen. They have thick walls and are filled with mucus. Initial manifestations include obstruction, intussusception, and volvulus. Duplication cysts may be single or multiple and vary widely in size. Spherical duplications do not communicate with the intestine and are usually filled with clear secretions. Fistulae may result from the inflammation and necrosis.

Duplications

Thirty-nine percent of duplications involve the foregut; 61% originate in the midgut or hindgut. Approximately 50% of cases affect the ileocecal valve. Small bowel duplications are occasionally multiple. Most patients are boys. Duplications may communicate with the intestinal lumen by opening proximally, distally, or both (Figs. 6.54 and 6.56). In other cases, the duplicated segment fails to communicate with the

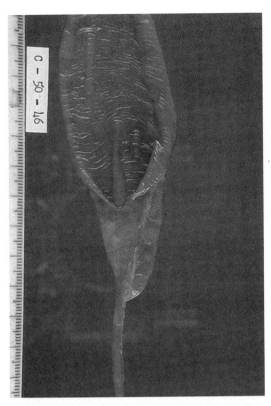

FIG. 6.52. Type 2 intestinal atresia that has been opened.

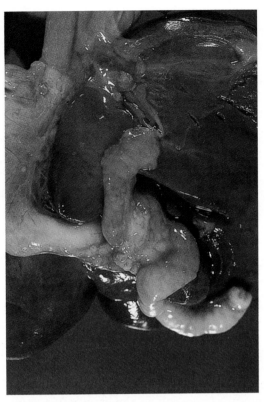

FIG. 6.53. Annular pancreas. The annular pancreas wraps around the first portion of the duodenum. Note the lobulated appearance of the pancreatic tissue.

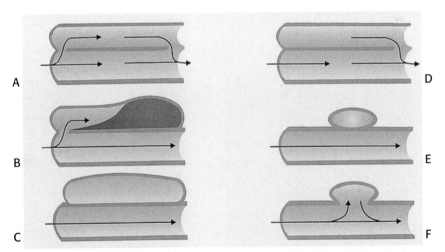

FIG. 6.54. Comparison of duplications, enterogenous cysts, and congenital diverticula. Panels A through D represent true duplications in which a significant portion of the intestinal length is duplicated. The *arrows* indicate the flow of intestinal contents. **A:** Both the proximal and distal ends of the duplicated segment communicate with the native intestinal lumen. This results in a free flow of intestinal contents through both lumens. **B:** The proximal portion of the duplication communicates with the native intestine. The distal portion of the duplication ends blindly. As a result, the intestinal contents pass into the duplication but then accumulate, causing dilation and inflammation. **C:** The duplicated segment fails to communicate with the native intestine, and as a result no intestinal contents flow into the duplicated lumen. If the lining of the duplicated segment produces significant secretions, these may accumulate and form a cystic dilation. **D:** Intestinal duplication in which the proximal end fails to communicate with the native intestinal lumen but the distal portion of the duplication does communicate with it. Intestinal contents do not enter the duplication and secretions produced by the duplicated segment are free to exit the duplicated segment and enter the main lumen. **E:** Enterogenous cyst. In this setting, the duplicated bowel represents a localized segment of duplicated bowel embedded within the intestinal wall. It fails to communicate with the native intestine. The enterogenous cyst may enlarge as the result of accumulated secretions. **F:** Congenital diverticulum. The duplication in this situation is relatively localized but it communicates freely with the intestinal lumen. The wall of the diverticulum contains all of the usual layers of the intestinal wall, distinguishing it from an acquired diverticulum.

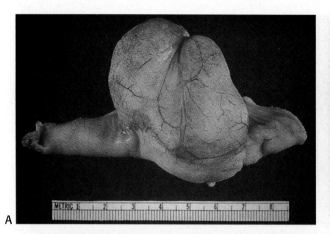
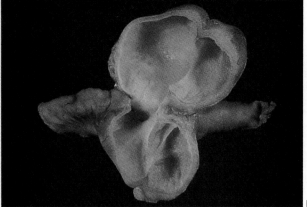

FIG. 6.55. Enterogenous cyst. **A:** A large, cystically dilated mass extends from the mesenteric portion of the bowel. It fails to communicate with the intestinal lumen. It was filled with mucinous secretions. **B:** Same specimen opened to show its internal structure.

intestinal lumen (Fig. 6.56). The clinical manifestations depend on the form the duplication takes. Patients present with an abdominal mass, bouts of abdominal pain, vomiting, distention, chronic rectal bleeding, intussusception, perforation, and obstruction. Bleeding is especially likely if the anomaly contains ectopic gastric epithelium. Ileocecal duplications act as lead points for chronic or recurrent intussusception. Grossly, two intestinal lumens are present. Triplications also occur.

Hypotheses to explain duplications include persistence of embryonic diverticula, fusion of embryologic longitudinal folds (the most popular theory) (137), abortive twinning (138), intrauterine intestinal ischemia (139), endodermal––neurodermal adhesions, and sequestration of embryonic tissues during embryonic movements. Small diverticula and epithelial islands in the mesentery of the developing small intestine may explain the presence of isolated intestinal duplications. Extensive intestinal duplications associated with multiple anomalies including the urinary bladder presumably result from teratogenic insults affecting several developing organs.

Duplications can be complete or incomplete, long or short segment, communicating or noncommunicating. Communicating duplications open proximally, distally, or at

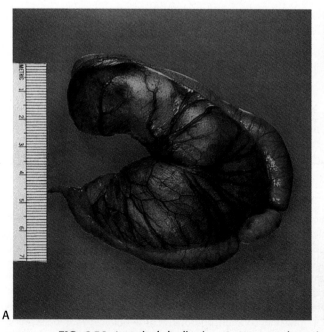
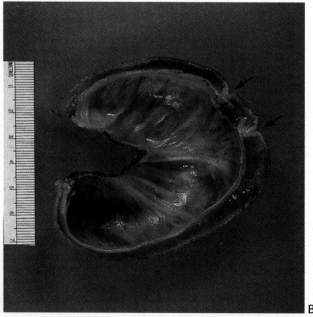

FIG. 6.56. Intestinal duplication. **A:** Unopened specimen. The native intestinal lumen that communicates with the rest of the gastrointestinal (GI) tract lies to the left of the smaller lumen. **B:** Both structures are opened, showing the wide dilated native GI lumen and a smaller lumen at the periphery and edge of the C-shaped structure. Several atretic areas are present in the duplicated bowel (*arrows*).

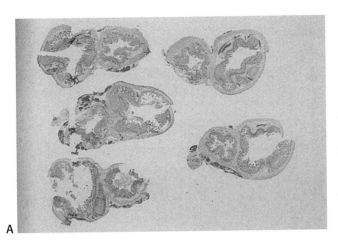

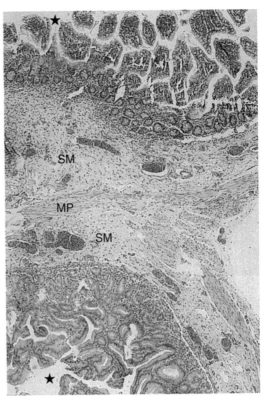

FIG. 6.57. Intestinal duplication. **A:** Cross section through duplicated segments shows two complete intestinal walls lying side by side. They share a common muscularis propria. **B:** Higher magnification showing strands of muscularis propria extending into the septum between the duplicated segments. The lumen of each segment is illustrated by the *star* and the attenuated muscularis propria (*MP*) separates the two submucosae (*SM*).

both ends. Grossly, duplications appear as hollow, cylindric, oval, or spheric cystic masses ranging in size from a few millimeters to up to 15 cm (140).

The three criteria for the diagnosis of a duplication are the presence of an intimate attachment to the GI tract, a smooth muscle coat, and an alimentary mucosal lining. Of these criteria, only the presence of a smooth muscle coat is absolutely necessary to define the lesion. Pressure within a cyst may lead to atrophy of the muscle component, causing it to appear incomplete. Generally, intestinal epithelium lines a duplicated segment (Fig. 6.57), but it may also contain heterotopic tissues, including thyroid stroma, pancreas, gastric mucosa (Fig. 6.58), lymphoid aggregates resembling Peyer patches, ciliated bronchial epithelium, lung tissue, and cartilage. A normal submucosa and inner circular muscle layer and myenteric plexus are present.

Congenital Diverticula

Duplication cysts that widely communicate with the lumen are termed *congenital diverticula*. Of the three related lesions, duplications, enterogenous cysts, and congenital diverticula, the latter are the rarest, affecting 1% to 2% of all individuals. Patients with congenital diverticula present with one of the following: Abdominal pain, distension, pressure, pain, and possibly perforation due to diverticulitis; ulceration and bleeding, usually from the presence of acid-secreting heterotopic gastric mucosa; or intussusception leading to sudden pain and bleeding. Duodenal diverticula may become large,

causing obstructive jaundice, pancreatitis, duodenal obstruction, fistulas, hemorrhage, and perforation (141). Congenital diverticula may also remain asymptomatic, only to be discovered incidentally in adults.

Congenital diverticula present as localized outpouchings (Fig. 6.59), sometimes being multiple. Some congenital duodenal diverticula pass upward behind the stomach through a separate opening in the diaphragm to enter the right thoracic cavity, where they attach to defective thoracic vertebrae.

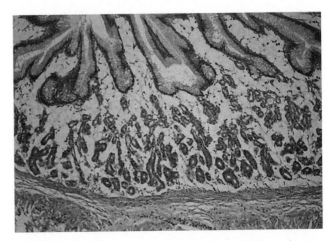

FIG. 6.58. Small intestinal duplication. Aberrantly formed crypts are present. The glands superficially resemble those seen in the gastric foveolae. Histochemical stains showed that the mucin was small intestinal mucin. Gastric glands are present.

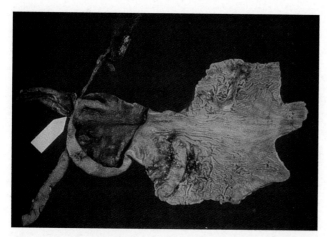

FIG. 6.59. Congenital duodenal diverticulum proximal to an intestinal band (*arrow*).

Congenital diverticula consist of all three bowel layers (Fig. 6.60). The lining epithelium is usually that of the site of origin. Some diverticula contain heterotopic tissues, similar to those found in duplications and enterogenous cysts. Diverticula containing oxyntic mucosa may develop peptic ulcers within them. If the diverticular orifice becomes blocked, diverticulitis develops.

Meckel Diverticulum

Meckel diverticulum, which represents a persistent omphalomesenteric or vitellointestinal duct, affects 1% to 4% of the population. Complete failure of the duct to atrophy produces a patent vitellointestinal duct with free communication between the ileal lumen and the umbilicus.

Meckel diverticulum affects males and females equally, but males are more likely to become symptomatic. Overall, only 5% of Meckel diverticula produce symptoms. A Meckel diverticulum has no clinical consequences unless complications develop (Figs. 6.61 and 6.62). Hemorrhage occurs if the diverticulum contains acid-secreting epithelium causing peptic ulceration. Diverticulitis develops secondary to peptic ulcerations or obstruction of the diverticular orifice. Intestinal obstruction, without diverticulitis, affects 25% of symptomatic patients. The obstruction results from intussusception, volvulus, adhesions, compression by a mesodiverticular band, or the presence of a tumor or heterotopic tissue, enteroliths, or bezoars.

Meckel diverticulum always lies on the antimesenteric ileal border (Fig. 6.63). In the infant, it usually lies about 30 cm proximal to the ileocecal valve; in the adult, it usually lies within 100 cm of the ileocecal valve. An apical fibrous band may connect the diverticulum to the umbilicus or to other abdominal structures. Meckel diverticulum may also be connected to other intestinal loops or mesenteries by a congenital band or by adhesions resulting from previous episodes of diverticulitis.

Meckel diverticulum varies in length from 2 to 15 cm (Fig. 6.63), but it usually measures <2 cm in width and has a narrow lumen. Variations in size, location, and shape are common. Meckel diverticulum may coexist with a duplication. Sometimes, a giant Meckel diverticulum develops. These appear as rounded, fusiform dilations resembling duplications rather than as saclike diverticula, and they are sometimes referred to as omphalomesenteric cysts.

Normal small intestinal epithelium lines the diverticulum, and heterotopic pancreatic tissue is common (Fig. 6.64). The latter usually appears as a nodular mass close to

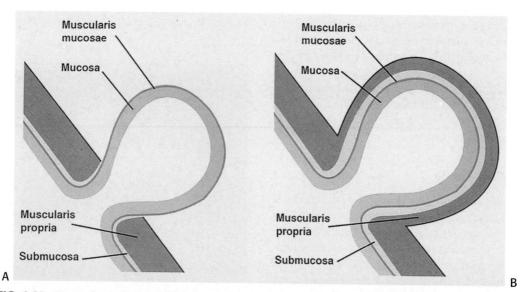

FIG. 6.60. Comparison of an acquired diverticulum versus a congenital diverticulum. **A:** An acquired diverticulum in which the mucosa and submucosa, and variable amounts of the muscularis propria and serosa (*not shown*), herniate through the bowel wall at areas of weakness. **B:** Congenital diverticulum. It is lined by all three layers of the bowel wall.

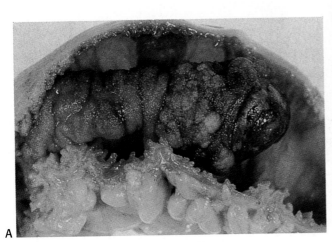
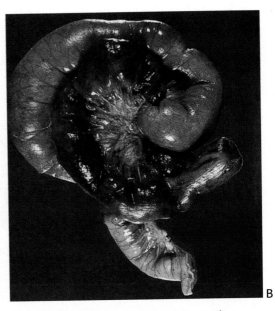

FIG. 6.61. Complications of Meckel diverticulum. **A:** Inverted Meckel diverticulum causing intussusception. **B:** External appearance of an intussusception in which a Meckel diverticulum acted as the lead point.

the diverticular tip. The pancreatic tissue sometimes acts as the lead point of an intussusception or it may cause obstruction. Heterotopic gastric mucosa (Fig. 6.65) leads to peptic ulceration, bleeding, or perforation, especially if oxyntic mucosa is present. Other heterotopic tissues include duodenal, jejunal, colonic, or biliary epithelium. Tumors may also form in the diverticulum.

Umbilical Fistula

Umbilical fistula represents a persistent vitelline duct. The fistula tract communicates from the umbilicus to the small bowel. It represents 2% of vitelline duct anomalies. The umbilical cord represents the fusion of the yolk sac containing the vitelline duct and the body stalk with its paired umbilical arteries, the umbilical vein, and the allantois. It contains primitive mesenchymal tissue (Wharton jelly) and is covered by an outer layer of amnion. Normally, the vitelline duct obliterates between the fifth and ninth weeks of intrauterine life. When it fails to obliterate, an umbilical fistula results. Umbilical fistula presents with persistent umbilical drainage. The diagnosis is confirmed when the dye is visualized in the lumen of the small bowel.

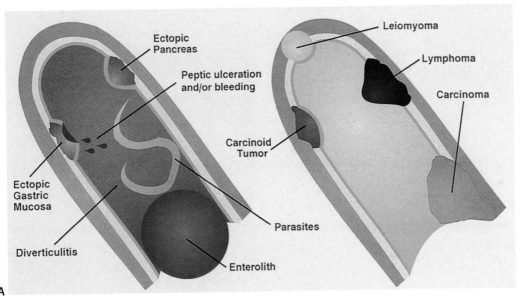

FIG. 6.62. Complications of Meckel diverticulum. **A:** Complications that lead to obstructions and diverticulitis and/or bleeding. **B:** Some of the tumors that may develop in the diverticula.

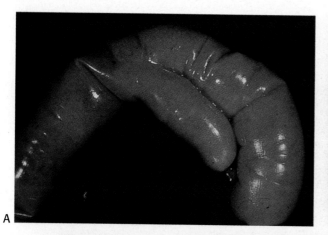

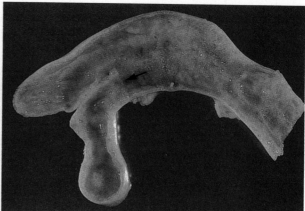

FIG. 6.63. Meckel diverticulum. **A:** Typical Meckel diverticulum arising from antimesenteric border of distal ileum. **B:** Cross section through an opened Meckel diverticulum. The diverticulum lies in a plane perpendicular to the long axis of the intestine. The mouth of the diverticulum is illustrated by the *arrow*. The lining of the diverticulum resembles that of the native intestine.

Congenital Heterotopic Gastric Mucosa

Heterotopic gastric epithelium occurs in the small intestine as the result of a congenital abnormality or a metaplasia. Acquired gastric mucosa (foveolar or pyloric metaplasia) usually associates with peptic duodenitis or chronic inflammatory disorders. Congenital heterotopic gastric mucosa exists alone (Fig. 6.66) or it complicates other congenital anomalies such as Meckel diverticulum (Fig. 6.65), duplications, and heterotopic pancreas.

Congenital heterotopic gastric epithelium often remains asymptomatic only to be discovered incidentally. Most cases of heterotopic gastric mucosa present as duodenal polyps at the time of upper endoscopy. However, an exceptional example of extensive gastric heterotopia that presented as multiple, carpetlike, nonpolypoid lesions that involved a large part of the small intestine in a child was recently reported (142).

Typically, the duodenal bulb appears nodular, often with small sessile polyps measuring <1.5 cm in maximum diameter. They are usually surrounded by normal-appearing mucosa. Symptomatic lesions present with intestinal obstruction, peptic ulceration, or intussusception. The ectopic tissue may appear solid or cystic. Larger lesions with central depressions may mimic a superficial ulcerating duodenal cancer (143).

Duodenal biopsies typically demonstrate intact duodenal villi and Brunner glands interrupted by discrete masses of gastric glands covered by foveolar epithelium. Congenital gastric mucosa usually consists of oxyntic mucosa. It appears well organized, consisting of superficial foveolar epithelium and glands. The latter contains chief and parietal cells. Antral glands may also be present. The glandular elements display their normal topographic relationships (Fig. 6.66). Rarely, the ectopic tissue develops

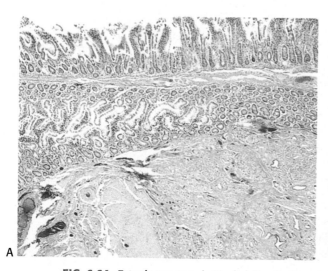

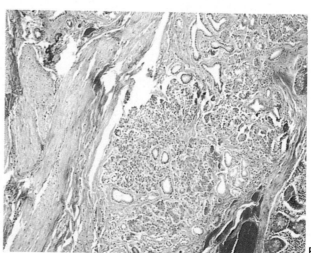

FIG. 6.64. Ectopic pancreas in Meckel diverticulum. **A:** Ectopic pancreatic tissue subjacent to mucosal lining. **B:** Pancreatic acini and ducts in ectopic pancreatic tissue.

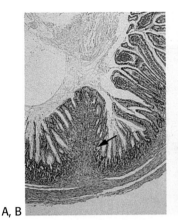
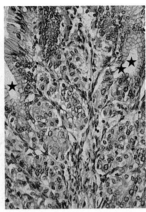
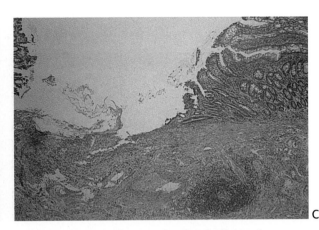

A, B

C

FIG. 6.65. Ectopic gastric mucosa within a Meckel diverticulum. **A:** Low magnification showing the lining of the Meckel diverticulum. The majority consisted of small intestinal epithelium. The *arrow* indicates the junction of the intestinal epithelium with gastric epithelium. **B:** Higher magnification of the gastric epithelium showing the foveolar epithelium lining the surface (*star*), a well-developed mucous neck region (*double star*), and well-formed glands containing parietal cells and chief cells. **C:** Portion of another Meckel diverticulum with a peptic ulcer in the mucosa adjacent to an area with oxyntic gastric epithelium.

diseases resembling those of the native stomach. These include areas of foveolar hyperplasia, hyperplastic polyps (Fig. 6.67), and oxyntic glandular mucosal cysts. Figure 6.68 compares the appearance of heterotopic gastric mucosa and gastric metaplasia.

Heterotopic Pancreas

Heterotopic pancreatic tissue affects 0.55% to 13.7% of duodenal or jejunal strictures, duplications, and Meckel diverticulum. It is particularly common in autosomal trisomy, especially involving chromosomes 13 and 18. Most

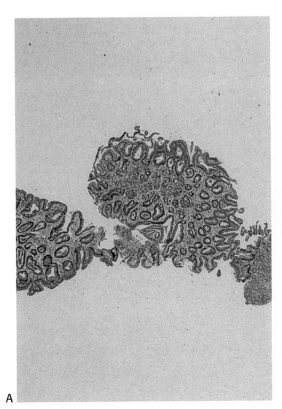
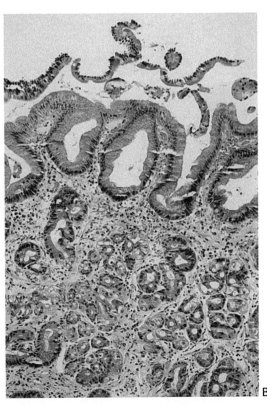

A

B

FIG. 6.66. Congenital heterotopic gastric epithelium. **A:** Biopsy of a duodenal "polyp." The tissue consists of typical oxyntic mucosa. **B:** Higher magnification showing the surface lined by foveolar epithelium and the presence of oxyntic glands with parietal cells and chief cells.

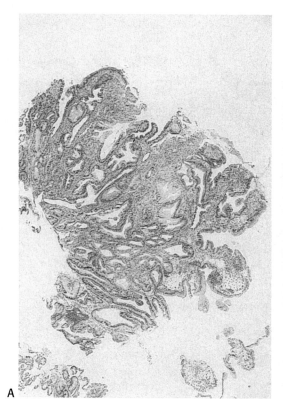
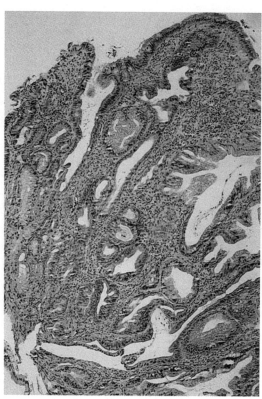

FIG. 6.67. Hyperplastic polyp arising in ectopic gastric mucosa. **A:** Low-power picture of the polypectomy specimen. **B:** Higher magnification showing irregular gastric glands.

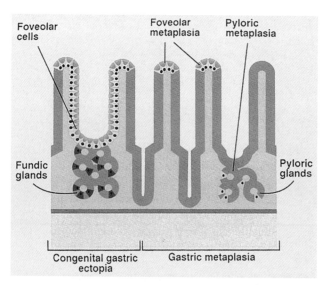

FIG. 6.68. Comparison of congenital gastric ectopia versus gastric metaplasia. Congenital gastric epithelium usually shows an orderly arrangement of the foveolar epithelium usually covering oxyntic glands. In contrast, gastric metaplasia lacks the three components of surface epithelium, gastric pits, and glands. It comes in two forms: The foveolar metaplasia commonly associated with peptic duodenitis and pyloric metaplasia commonly complicating chronic inflammatory diseases such as Crohn disease. In foveolar metaplasia, a mucous neck region and glands are completely absent. In pyloric metaplasia, foveolar cells and the mucous neck region are absent.

cases remain asymptomatic. Grossly and endoscopically, the lesion usually appears well demarcated. Heterotopic pancreas presents as a mass lesion that, on cut surface, has a solid, tan or cystic, lobular appearance, depending on whether or not the pancreatic ducts are dilated. The presence of a central mucosal dimple usually corresponds to the entrance of pancreatic ducts into the intestinal lumen. The lesion lies in the mucosa, in the submucosa, transmurally, or on the serosa (Figs. 6.69 and 6.70), and may coexist with heterotopic Brunner glands and/or gastric tissue (144).

Pancreatic acini, ducts, or islets occur alone or in combination with one another. When the lesion contains only ducts surrounded by the circular and longitudinal muscle of pancreatic ducts (Fig. 6.70), they are sometimes erroneously referred to as adenomyomas. However, the orderly arrangement of the two muscle layers around the ducts distinguishes the two lesions. Heterotopic pancreas can become inflamed or develop malignancies, often leading to variably sized and shaped duodenal wall cysts. In the setting of chronic pancreatitis, the cysts are surrounded by smooth muscle and myofibroblastic proliferations and may result in duodenal stenosis (145).

Brunner Gland Hamartomas

Brunner gland hamartomas are very unusual polypoid or nodular lesions that occur in the 4th to 6th decades of life. It

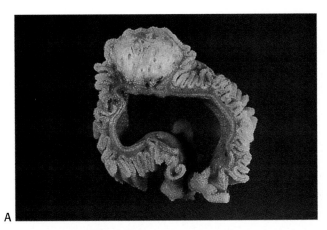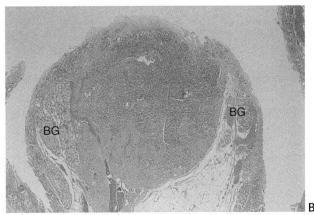

A   B

FIG. 6.69. Heterotopic pancreas. **A:** Cross section of a duodenal "polyp" produced by heterotopic pancreatic tissue in the submucosa. Prominent pancreatic ducts can be seen within the lesion. **B:** Histologic features. *BG* indicates surrounding Brunner glands.

is difficult to ascertain their true incidence because the lesions are confused with Brunner gland hyperplasia. They contain an admixture of muscular, glandular, and fatty elements including heterotopic pancreatic acini and ducts. Rarely, they cause massive upper GI bleeding. These lesions usually lie entirely beneath the muscularis mucosae. Dilation of the glandular acini or ducts gives them a cystic appearance.

Peritoneal Encapsulation

Peritoneal encapsulation is intestinal encasement by a peritoneal membrane. It probably results from the formation of an accessory peritoneal membrane from the mesocolon during the return of the intestinal loop to the abdomen following its herniation into the umbilical cord at the 10th fetal week. The dorsal mesentery covers most of the small intestine. It eventrates and moves counterclockwise, fusing with

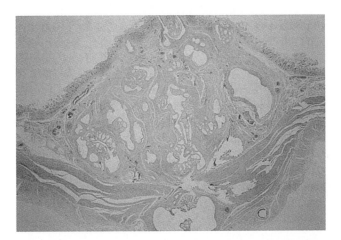

FIG. 6.70. Heterotopic pancreas. This lesion, originally diagnosed as an adenomyoma, represents heterotopic pancreas. It consists of pancreatic ducts surrounded by smaller ductules and a prominent proliferation of muscle fibers. No acini or islets are present.

the posterior abdominal wall. Alternatively, the accessory membrane forms from part of the yolk sac peritoneum as it is drawn back into the abdominal cavity with the intestine (146).

The lesion usually remains asymptomatic and is detected incidentally. However, patients may present with cramps, obstruction, abdominal pain, vomiting, and constipation alternating with diarrhea (146). Peritoneal encapsulation may mimic a left mesocolic hernia. Peritoneal encapsulations can measure up to 20 cm. A thin, peritoneumlike sac encases the entire small bowel. The sac lies freely and does not adhere to the mesentery, the parietal peritoneum, or other abdominal organs. The encased intestinal loops often have their own mesenteries. The histology of the encapsulated organs is normal. The histology of the membrane is that of a fibrous band.

The differential diagnosis includes *sclerosing encapsulated peritonitis,* usually a complication of peritoneal dialysis or other abdominal interventions. Sclerosing encapsulating peritonitis is characterized by a thick, grayish white fibrous membrane covering the small intestinal wall. It must also be differentiated from the *abdominal cocoon,* in which the small bowel is found totally or partially curled up in a concertinalike fashion encased in a dense white membrane.

ACQUIRED ANATOMIC VARIATIONS
Duodenal Diverticula

Duodenal diverticula are found in 1% to 6% of radiologic examinations and in an average of 8.6% of autopsies (147). They complicate peptic ulcer disease, choledocholithiasis (148), duodenal obstruction, and genetic or systemic disorders such as Marfan syndrome. Most duodenal diverticula develop as a result of chronic peptic ulcer disease (149). The ulcerating process causes fibrosis of the muscularis propria and abnormal contractility. Their frequency increases with

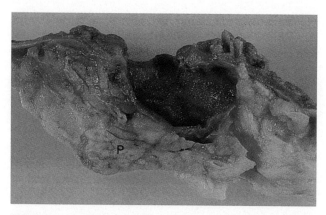

FIG. 6.71. Congenital duodenal diverticulum. A large duodenal diverticulum extends into the underlying pancreas (*P*). The overlying duodenal mucosa appears ulcerated and flattened at the edges of the ulcer.

age; they rarely develop before age 40. The diverticula usually involve the second portion of the duodenum in a juxtapapillary location and are usually solitary and medial in location. Diverticula arise in weakened areas of the bowel wall that gradually balloon out, causing the diverticula to enlarge over time. The diverticular wall consists of variably inflamed mucosa and submucosa with only scattered muscle cells.

Jejunal and Ileal Diverticulosis

Jejunal diverticulosis is a heterogeneous disorder affecting 1.3% to 4.6% of the population (150). It consists of single or multiple diverticula predominantly involving the jejunum (Fig. 6.72). However, both the duodenum and the ileum may be involved (150). Jejunal diverticula develop seven times more commonly than ileal diverticula (151); men are affected twice as frequently as women. Most affected individuals are over age 40 (150); 82% of patients remain asymptomatic. The diverticula become evident as an incidental find-

ing at the time of surgery, autopsy, or radiographic examination. Neuromuscular disorders typically coexist with jejunal diverticulosis, including Fabry disease, visceral myopathies or neuropathies, scleroderma, and neuronal inclusion disease (150). As a result, patients often suffer from pseudo-obstruction or malabsorption secondary to bacterial overgrowth. Diverticular resection cures the malabsorption. Small intestinal diverticula perforate, bleed, become inflamed, and undergo other complications. These complications lead to morbidity and mortality rates as high as 40%.

Small intestinal diverticula begin as a pair of small outpouchings along the mesenteric border. The mucosa herniates through the muscle layer along the path of the penetrating vessels. Alternatively, localized areas of muscular fibrosis and atrophy may weaken the bowel wall, creating localized mural sacculations. Uncoordinated muscular contractions from an underlying motility disorder lead to focal areas of increased intraluminal pressure and mucosal herniation through the weakened areas. The pair of outpouchings then enlarges until the outpouchings meet and they may fuse in the line of the mesentery, thereby forming a single thin-walled diverticulum. The diverticula usually measure <1 cm in size, although they may be larger. Jejunal diverticula tend to be larger in the proximal jejunum and become smaller and fewer as one progresses distally in the GI tract. As many as 400 diverticula ranging in size from 1 to 22 cm in diameter can exist in a single patient (150).

Histologically, diverticula are lined by mucosa, muscularis mucosae, and submucosa, but they usually lack a muscularis propria. The mucosa usually shows some degree of crypt hyperplasia, villous atrophy, and chronic inflammation, probably resulting from intestinal stasis and bacterial overgrowth. Lipid-containing histiocytes often lie in the mucosa, in the submucosa, and along lymphatics close to the collar of muscularis propria surrounding the diverticular neck (152). The histology of the bowel wall sometimes shows an underlying myopathy or neuropathy (see Chapter 10) or only fibrosis of the muscularis propria (150).

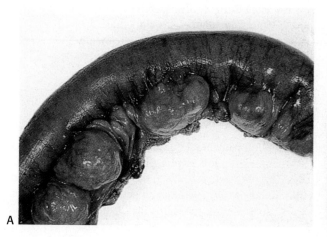
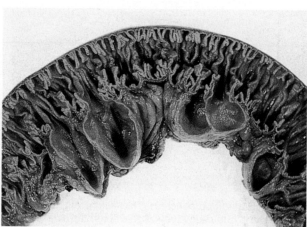

FIG. 6.72. Jejunal diverticulosis. **A:** Multiple outpouchings along mesenteric border of jejunum characteristic of jejunal diverticulosis. **B:** Cut section demonstrating thin-walled diverticular outpouchings.

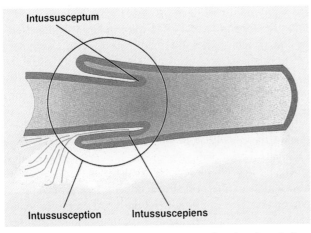

FIG. 6.73. Diagram of an intussusception showing the relationship of the intussusceptum with the intussuscipiens and the overall intussusception.

Intussusception

An intussusception results from invagination of an intestinal segment (the *intussusceptum*) into the next part of the intestine that forms a sheath around it (the *intussuscipiens*) (Figs. 6.73 to 6.76). Intussusceptions are classified as primary (without an identifiable cause) or secondary (due to a preexisting lesion). They are one of the most common abdominal emergencies in early childhood. Two thirds of cases occur in infancy, with a peak incidence between 3 and 5 months of age (153,154). Intussusception is the most common cause of intestinal obstruction in children (155,156), affecting 1.5 to 3.8 cases per 1,000 live births a year. The incidence varies considerably in different parts of the world (157). Some patients have strong family histories of intussusception (158). Paradoxically, there appears to be a high incidence of intussusception in doctors' families (159). In the United States, there is a male predominance of 2:1 and a seasonal prevalence with two peaks, one in the winter and one in the

summer (160). Patients are typically well nourished, without a history of gastrointestinal disease.

Lead points are common in children 6 years of age or older. Predisposing factors include masses, bezoars, Meckel diverticula, motility disorders, inflammatory fibroid polyps, or localized lymphoid hyperplasia secondary to adenovirus or other infections (Figs. 6.76 and 6.77). It also develops in some patients following rotavirus vaccination (161) and AIDS infections (162).

The intussusception constricts the mesentery between the inner intussusceptum and the ensheathing intussuscipiens blocking both venous outflow and the arterial supply, leading to secondary ischemia. As a result, the intussusception continues to swell, causing bowel obstruction and possibly gangrene and perforation. Some intussusceptions reduce spontaneously. The intussuscepted bowel may show the features of the intussusception, the pathology of the predisposing cause, and secondary ischemia.

The histology differs depending on whether the intussusception is acute, chronic, or acute superimposed on chronic intussusception. In patients with chronic or recurrent intussusceptions, the muscularis mucosa sometimes buckles upward, indicating the lead point of the intussusception, and the subserosal or even intramural vessels may show evidence of a "pulling artifact" with tethering in the same direction as the muscularis mucosae. One can imagine similar traction forces acting on the mucosa, muscularis propria, and subserosal vessels. Recurrent intussusceptions can produce florid submucosal vascular proliferations that may be so pronounced as to raise the possibility of a primary vascular neoplasm (163). Characteristically, there is also prominent muscular hypertrophy and neural hyperplasia. Most intussusceptions show variable degrees of ischemia. The histologic features of the ischemia resemble gastrointestinal ischemia due to other causes. They reflect the length of time that the injury lasted and the degree of vascular compromise that occurred. In children with adenovirus infections, the lymphoid tissue appears markedly hyperplastic and the

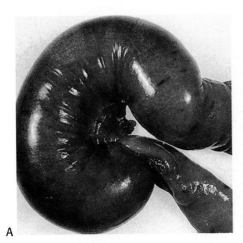
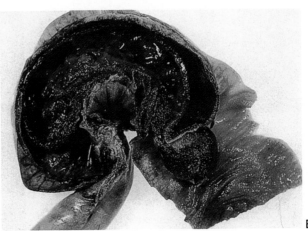

FIG. 6.74. Intussusception. **A:** External appearance of small bowel intussusception with secondary gangrenous necrosis. **B:** Opened specimen.

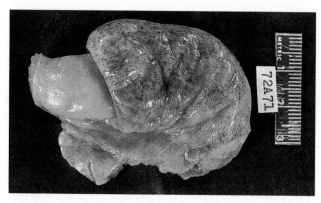

FIG. 6.75. Intussusception. The intussuscipiens exhibits early ischemic changes as demonstrated by the presence of the mottled speckling on the serosal surface and the dusky color in comparison to the paler intussusceptum.

epithelium overlying the lymphoid hyperplasia at the lead point appears damaged or even necrotic. Intranuclear viral inclusions appear as reddish globules surrounded by halos or as poorly demarcated purple nuclear smudges.

Volvulus

Volvulus accounts for 5% to 10% of all cases of intestinal obstruction. It develops when any portion of the intestine

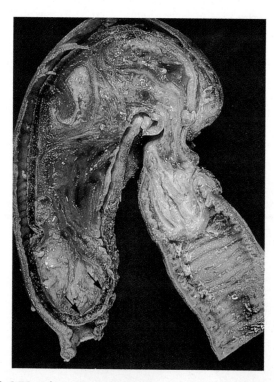

FIG. 6.76. Adenovirus-induced intussusception in an 8-year-old child. The lead point of the intussusception (*arrows*) is an area of lymphoid hyperplasia secondary to an infection. One loop of bowel completely telescopes into another.

loops around itself (Fig. 6.78). Intestinal volvulus is divided into primary and secondary forms. Primary volvulus develops in patients lacking a predisposing cause. Secondary volvulus affects patients with an acquired or congenital structural abnormality that predisposes the bowel to rotate on itself (Fig. 6.79). Underlying abnormalities include a congenitally long mesentery with a narrow base, the presence of congenital bands, an elongated small intestine, Meckel diverticulum, or inflammatory diseases.

Small bowel volvulus is a rare but life-threatening surgical emergency. Volvulus occurs acutely, causing complete obstruction, or intermittently, producing partial or complete obstruction with compromise of the blood supply, ischemia, gangrene, perforation, and peritonitis. The intestinal obstruction presents with severe abdominal pain, nausea, bilious vomiting, abdominal distension, and rectal bleeding. Often the patient collapses due to occlusion of the venous return by the mesenteric twist while arterial perfusion continues. As much as 50% of the blood volume may accumulate within the volvulus. Obstipation, tachycardia, and fever occur less commonly (164). A history of recurrent minor attacks of similar problems is present in approximately 50% of patients (165). Approximately 37% of patients present with a frankly gangrenous small bowel at the time of resection. Histologically, the tissues manifest variable degrees of ischemia.

Fistulae

Fistulae develop between the small intestine and adjacent organs or skin as a result of underlying diseases or previous surgery. *Enteroenteric fistulae* represent communications between two portions of the GI tract. *Bouveret syndrome* consists of a cholecystoduodenal or choledochoduodenal fistula due to the passage of a gallstone into the duodenal bulb and subsequent gastric outlet obstruction. Most patients spontaneously pass the eroding gallstone(s) without any complications. However, if the stone measures >2.5 cm in greatest diameter, it may lodge in the bowel, producing symptoms of obstruction, perforation, or "gallstone ileus." Peptic ulcers or duodenal carcinomas may also erode into the gallbladder or bile duct, forming a fistula.

Primary fistulae between the abdominal aorta and the gut are rare and fatal. *Aortoenteric fistulae* usually result from disorders involving either the aorta (usually atherosclerosis or following the insertion of an aortic bypass graft) or the GI tract (cancer, peptic disease, infections, or trauma). Fistulae may also develop in an ulcerating disease, regardless of the etiology.

Perforations

Intestinal perforations occur spontaneously or following trauma. The basis of the perforations differs from country to country. In countries with poor hygiene, underlying infectious diseases, including typhoid ulcers, intestinal tuberculosis, and

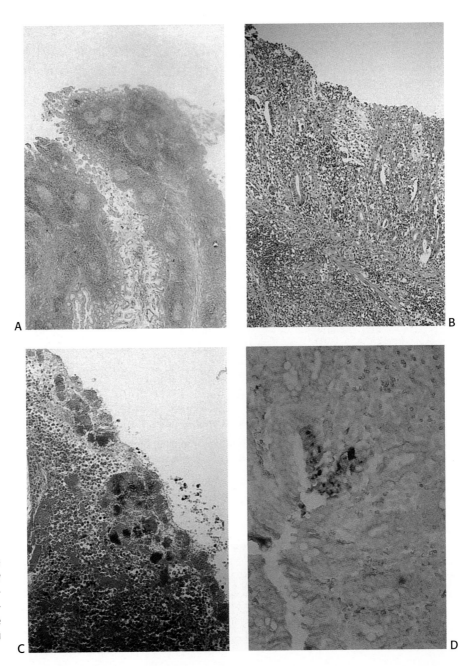

FIG. 6.77. Histologic features of the lesion shown in Figure 6.76. **A:** Low magnification showing marked lymphoid hyperplasia. **B:** Ischemic necrosis of the epithelium. **C:** The presence of bacterial overgrowth. **D:** The in situ hybridization (*red*) for adenovirus.

parasitic diseases, result in perforation. In Western countries, foreign bodies, ischemia, Crohn disease, tumors, diverticula, trauma, and radiation therapy represent the most common causes of perforation.

Adhesions

Any time the peritoneal or serosal surfaces of the bowel become inflamed, fibrous or fibrinous bands can form causing loops of bowel to become adherent to one another (Fig. 6.80) or to become adherent to any peritoneal surface. Adhesions commonly complicate previous transmural small intestinal inflammation as seen in ischemia, perforation, Crohn disease, previous surgery, or radiation therapy. Intestinal obstruction, volvulus, and ischemia all complicate

adhesions. The adhesions appear as strands of variably fibrotic or inflamed tissue on the serosal aspect of the bowel wall. These changes may associate with variable degrees of mesothelial hyperplasia.

Stenosis of the Ampulla of Vater (Papillary Stenosis)

Papillary stenosis complicates impacted gallstones, biliary tract infections, inflammation of the ampulla, previous endoscopic retrograde cholangiopancreatography, endoscopic sphincterotomy, and heterotopic pancreas. Traumatizing the papillae by repeated attempts at cannulation leads to edema and sphincter spasm and temporarily occludes the outflow of pancreatic juice, thereby increasing

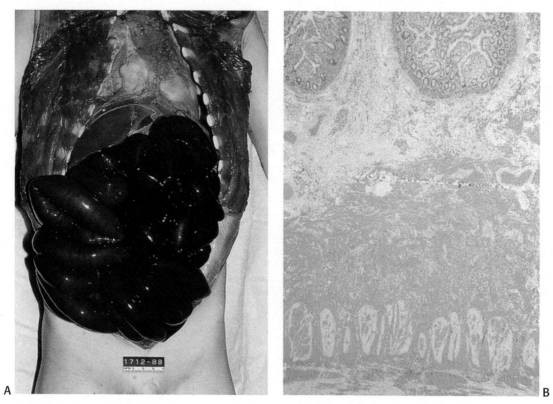

FIG. 6.78. Volvulus. **A:** The intestines rotated around an intestinal band, causing infarction of both the large and small intestine. **B:** Acute coagulative necrosis. The tissues lack an inflammatory response.

the intrapancreatic pressure and the risk of complications. Most patients are middle-aged women.

The histologic features of papillary stenosis include edema with acute and/or chronic inflammation, glandular hyperplasia, granulation tissue, granulomatous inflammation, and submucosal fibrosis (Fig. 6.81). One often sees a hyperplastic, regenerative mucosa with marked atypia. One must be careful to avoid making a diagnosis of malignancy in

this setting unless all of the histologic features of unequivocal malignancy are present. The presence of a desmoplastic response suggests that cancer is present. However, as a note of caution, healed diverticulitis may associate with a fibrotic response. One should be especially wary of establishing a diagnosis of malignancy if one sees evidence of acute and chronic inflammation, marked hyperplasia, and/or stromal edema (Fig. 6.81).

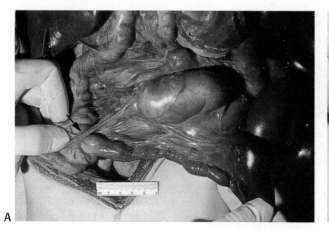

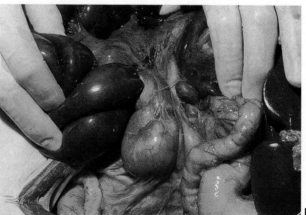

FIG. 6.79. Volvulus around intestinal band. **A:** This adult died from gangrenous necrosis of the small bowel. The cause of the necrosis was a torsion and volvulus around a congenital band demonstrated by the linear structure lying next to the thumb (*arrow*). **B:** The tissues are spread apart to show the bands and adhesions between various intra-abdominal structures.

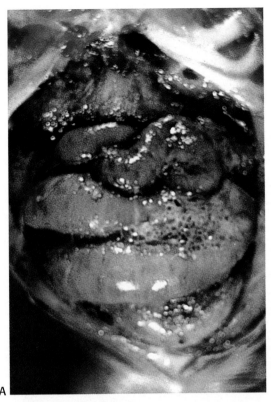
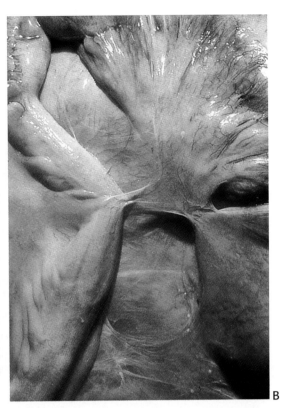

FIG. 6.80. Adhesions. **A:** Opened abdomen in a child with necrotizing enterocolitis. The bowel is dusky and appears hemorrhagic and infarcted. Additionally, fibrinous adhesions attach the bowel loops to one another. The bubbly areas are patches of pneumatosis intestinalis. **B:** Well-formed fibrous adhesions in a patient with previous surgeries.

Other Stenoses

Small intestinal stenosis complicates a number of conditions, including heterotopic pancreas; ischemia; peptic injury; radiation; drug injury, especially nonsteroidal anti-inflammatory drugs (NSAIDs); Crohn disease; infections; and trauma.

EROSIVE DUODENITIS

Erosive duodenitis may develop in patients subjected to severe stress or in those consuming large quantities of alcohol. The first part of the duodenum is most susceptible to a stress-induced injury that resembles stress gastritis (see Chapter 4). The duodenum appears diffusely hemorrhagic and reddened, usually in conjunction with similar changes in the stomach (Fig. 6.82). Bleeding may be present. Erosive duodenitis begins as areas of localized interstitial edema (Fig. 6.83). These evolve with red cell extravasation and the development of erosions and full-blown ulcers. Ulcers are particularly prone to develop in situations of marked stress. Early enterocyte damage consists of cytoplasmic vacuolization with eventual epithelial loss. Enterocytes contain enlarged, hyperchromatic nuclei with prominent nucleoli, syncytial changes, and cytoplasmic tufting. The villi degener-

ate and the epithelium becomes mucin depleted and cuboidal in shape. The villi shorten and the crypts become hyperplastic to accommodate for the cell loss. The crypt:villus ratio approaches 1:1. Neutrophils, lymphocytes, plasma cells, and sometimes eosinophils infiltrate the mucosa and the lamina propria (Fig. 6.84). Eventually, the inflammation progresses to crypt abscesses (Fig. 6.85). The stroma may exhibit prominent telangiectasia. One may also see prominent lymphoid follicles. Often, it is very difficult to distinguish the nonspecific effects of stress duodenitis from those of peptic duodenitis.

CHRONIC DUODENITIS ASSOCIATED WITH *HELICOBACTER PYLORI* INFECTION

Gastric *Helicobacter pylori* infections associate with various changes in the duodenal bulb. These include intraepithelial lymphocytosis (166), chronic duodenitis, chronic active duodenitis, gastric metaplasia-associated duodenitis (167), and duodenal ulcer (discussed in a later section). Endoscopically, the duodenum may appear normal or there may be mucosal edema, erythema, petechial hemorrhages, or erosions. These changes may be especially prominent in areas adjacent to peptic ulcers.

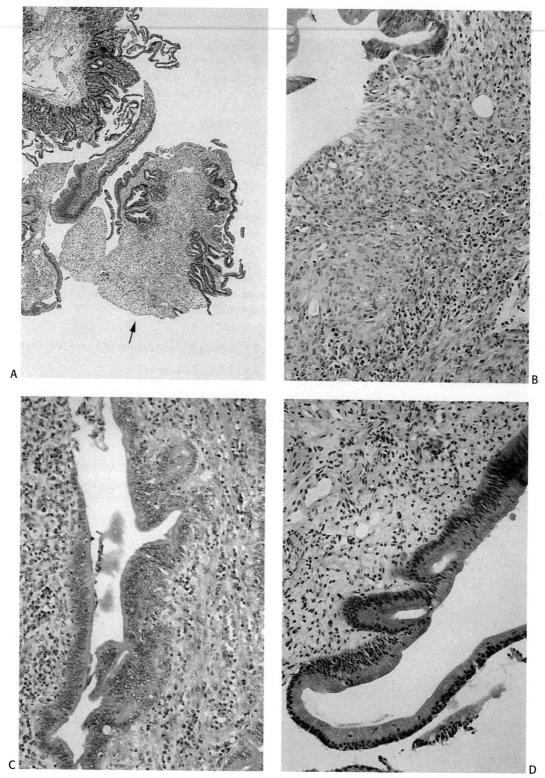

FIG. 6.81. Sclerosing papillitis. **A:** Low magnification of tissue removed endoscopically as a polyp. It came from the area around the ampulla of Vater. In the upper portion of the photograph, one sees more or less normal duodenal mucosa. The three lower fragments are abnormal. The largest piece (*arrow*) consists of edematous tissue covered by small intestinal epithelium. In some places, glandular crowding is evident. **B:** Higher magnification of the edematous, inflamed tissue. **C, D:** Higher magnifications of the epithelium from these tissue pieces that, if examined in isolation, might be interpreted as representing an area of dysplasia. One might be worried about severe dysplasia in C due to the tangential cutting of the specimen. Features that suggest dysplasia are the glandular crowding, the nuclear palisading, and the high nuclear:cytoplasmic ratio. The intensity of the associated inflammatory changes and the gradual transition to more mature epithelium indicate that this is a reactive process, not a neoplastic one. **D:** Glands superficially resembling adenomatous epithelium lining the upper portion of the gland gradually merge with more normal-appearing epithelium.

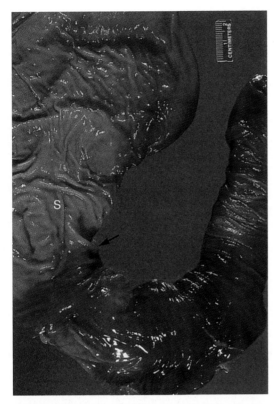

FIG. 6.82. Erosive duodenitis. The stomach (*S*) lies in the upper left-hand portion of the photograph; the *arrow* indicates the gastroduodenal junction. The first portion of the duodenum appears markedly erythematous and there are several punctate erosions.

The diagnosis of chronic duodenitis is fairly subjective since the criteria for the diagnosis are not well established and the architecture of duodenal villi is normally quite variable. However, one has the sense that the overall cellularity of the lamina propria is increased. The diagnosis is more cer-

tain if acute inflammation is present, if there is an intraepithelial lymphocytosis, or if there is foveolar metaplasia. Since the acute inflammation is usually patchy in nature, one may need to examine multiple sections or levels to detect its presence. The surface epithelium may appear degenerated and the crypts regenerative secondary to the inflammation. The number of duodenal IELs ranges from 3 to 42 per 100 enterocytes with a mean of 18.5. This contrasts with a mean of 6.6 in a control population (166). The IELs are T cells and their increase is patchy in nature. This level of intraepithelial lymphocytosis resembles that seen in celiac disease but the villous architecture is normal. The increased duodenal IELs occur even when the *H. pylori* is restricted to the stomach (166). Treatment of the gastric infection leads to a decrease in IELs (168).

DUODENAL PEPTIC DISEASES

Peptic Duodenitis

Peptic duodenitis and peptic duodenal ulcers represent different phases in the response to increased acid secretion often as the result of antral predominant *H. pylori* gastritis. The incidence of duodenal ulcers also increases in cigarette smokers, patients with chronic renal disease, and alcoholics. Disturbed motility also predisposes to active duodenal ulceration due to prolonged mucosal contact with the acid. Factors associated with refractory ulcers are listed in Table 6.4. Severe peptic duodenitis also occurs in patients with Zollinger-Ellison syndrome.

Peptic duodenitis is typically confined to the duodenal bulb. Endoscopic appearances vary from simple erythema to mucosal friability and nodularity. The erythema results from shunting of blood to the villous tips, a change induced by the hydrochloric acid (169). Severe cases exhibit erosions and

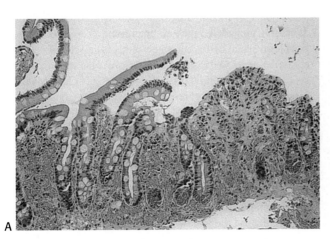

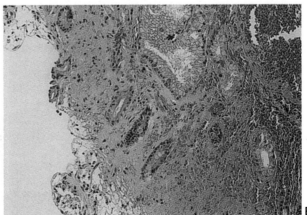

FIG. 6.83. Erosive duodenitis due to alcohol. **A:** A congested duodenal mucosa shows artifactual denudation of the superficial epithelium. Red cells have extravasated into the lamina propria. There is also focal glandular dropout. **B:** A more severe form of the disease in which amorphous eosinophilic material fills the area of the lamina propria, and the tissues are diffusely congested and infiltrated with red cells. The superficial epithelium is destroyed.

TABLE 6.4   **Factors Associated with Refractory Ulcers**

Zollinger-Ellison syndrome
Intestinal wall penetration by the ulcer
Smoking
Use of nonsteroidal anti-inflammatory drugs
Gastric outlet obstruction or duodenal stenosis
Postsurgical bypassed antrum without vagotomy

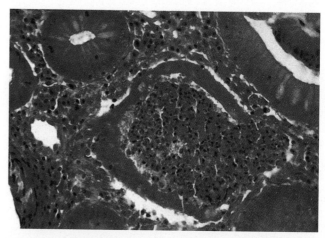

FIG. 6.85. Crypt abscess in a patient with active duodenitis and associated active regeneration.

ulcers. Alternatively, mucosal atrophy, thickening, or irregularity is present.

The principal findings of peptic duodenitis include any or all of the following: (a) inflammatory cells in the epithelium or lamina propria; (b) altered enterocyte morphology due to degeneration, regeneration, or the presence of foveolar metaplasia; (c) mucosal hemorrhage and edema; and (d) Brunner gland hyperplasia (Fig. 6.86) and foveolar metaplasia. The foveolar metaplasia may be extensive or patchy in its distribution. The inflammation may include neutrophils, lymphocytes, plasma cells, and eosinophils. Patients may also develop lymphoid hyperplasia (Fig. 6.87). Whitehead et al proposed dividing duodenitis into three grades based on the severity of the inflammation and the villous architecture (170). In the severest form of duodenitis, the villi appear flat (Fig. 6.87). The superficial epithelium and the brush border become progressively less distinct, with nuclear pseudostratification, mucosal erosions, and foveolar metaplasia. Neutrophils extend into the crypts and Brunner gland ducts.

Lymphoid aggregates and hyperplasia, vascular dilation, and edema may all be present.

The presence of *foveolar cell metaplasia* (gastric surface epithelial metaplasia) provides a helpful clue to the diagnosis of peptic duodenitis (Fig. 6.87). Foveolar metaplasia probably represents an adaptive response to either duodenal hyperacidity or *H. pylori* infection (171) and may protect against ulceration because this epithelium has the ability to transport hydrogen ions out of the mucosa back into the GI lumen (see Chapter 4). If *H. pylori* bacteria are *present* in the stomach, some may colonize areas of foveolar cell metaplasia in the duodenum via the same specific adherence mechanisms used in the stomach (see Chapter 4). The metaplastic cells are histologically identical to foveolar cells in the stomach, and not surprisingly, they express a gastric mucinous phenotype rather than an intestinal one (171). *H. pylori* attached to the foveolar cells then contribute to an acute or chronic active duodenitis and the development of duodenal peptic ulcer disease (172). A high density of cagA-positive strains of the bacteria in the patients with severe duodenitis is an important determinant of duodenal ulcer disease (173). The most persuasive argument supporting the dominant role of *H. pylori* in duodenal ulcer disease is the dramatic decrease in relapse rates after successful cure of the infection, with subsequent healing of the mucosa (174).

Brunner gland hyperplasia is common in patients with *H. pylori* infections and peptic duodenitis. It is characterized by a nodular proliferation of normal-appearing Brunner glands that have a lobular architecture accompanied by ducts and stromal elements. Voluminous Brunner glands may extend high into the overlying mucosa. Histologically, the glands appear identical to normal Brunner glands except that they are increased in number and size. They retain their lobular architecture, but the lobules vary in size and fibromuscular strands course through the lesion. Larger polypoid lesions may become superficially eroded or they may bleed or cause obstruction, requiring endoscopic or surgical removal (175). Exceptionally, areas of dysplasia may develop in the

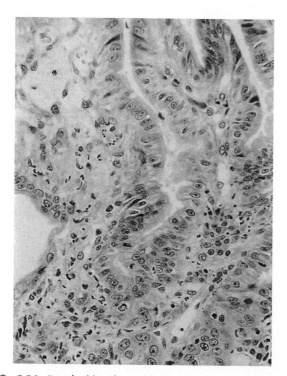

FIG. 6.84. Duodenitis. The epithelium appears very reactive and inflamed. There is syncytial formation.

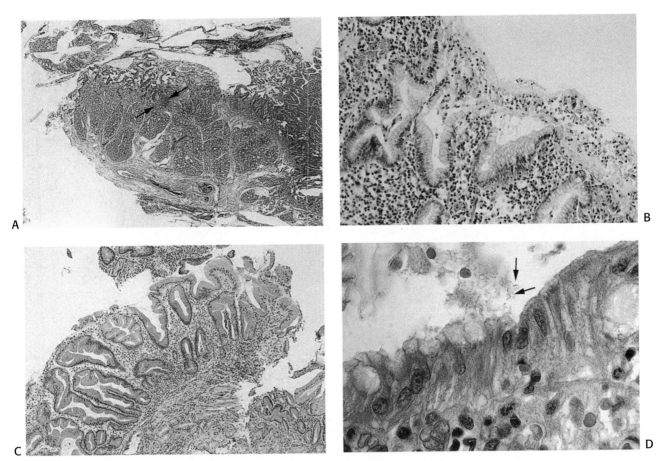

FIG. 6.86. Peptic duodenitis. **A:** Low magnification showing Brunner gland hyperplasia, erosion and distortion of the overlying epithelium, and a lymphoid aggregate (*arrows*). **B:** Higher magnification of the lining epithelium demonstrates eroded foveolar metaplasia. No goblet cells or enterocytes are identified. **C:** Almost complete replacement of the duodenal villi by gastric surface (foveolar) epithelium. **D:** Higher magnification of the foveolar epithelium showing various degrees of metaplastic change. *Helicobacter pylori* is present in the overlying exudate (*arrow*).

hyperplastic Brunner glands (176). When the latter occurs in patients with areas of foveolar metaplasia and Brunner gland hyperplasia, both the metaplastic and hyperplastic glands may show cytologic atypia, leading some to suggest that these lesions may be precursors of Brunner gland carcinoma (176).

It should be noted that many of the histologic features of peptic duodenitis are nonspecific, except for the foveolar metaplasia. Similar findings occur in patients with Crohn disease, stress-induced duodenitis, celiac disease, NSAID-induced injury, and certain infections.

Peptic Ulcer Disease

A major insight in the last decade or so is that gastric peptic ulcers primarily result from altered mucosal defenses, whereas duodenal ulcers (DUs) result from hyperchlorhydria. *H. pylori* plays a vital role in peptic ulcer development in both sites. A complicated relationship exists between host defense mechanisms and the presence of elevated acid,

pepsin levels, and *H. pylori* (Fig. 6.88). Indeed, *H. pylori* is found significantly more often in patients with peptic ulcer disease and duodenitis than in patients with normal endoscopic findings. *dupA* is a novel *H. pylori*–encoded gene that associates with an increased risk for the development of duodenal ulcer disease (177). The decline in duodenal ulcer disease in recent decades is likely the result of two factors, the decline in the incidence of *H. pylori* infections as discussed in Chapter 4 and the widespread use of acid-suppressive therapies.

Peptic duodenitis progresses from erosive peptic duodenitis with superficial mucosal loss to frank peptic DUs. The sequence of events leading to DU formation includes mucosal inflammation, weakening of the mucous bicarbonate barrier, superficial epithelial cell damage, increased serum gastrin levels with defective feedback control, a possible increase in parietal cell mass, and the development of gastric metaplasia in the duodenal cap. Colonization by *H. pylori* further weakens mucosal defenses and plays a major role in the genesis of the peptic ulcer disease (178).

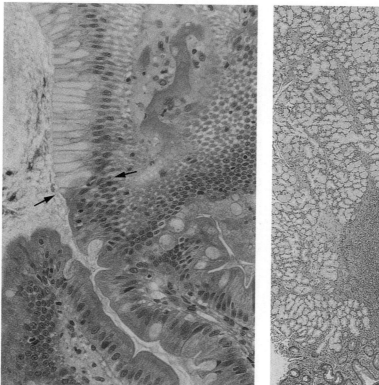
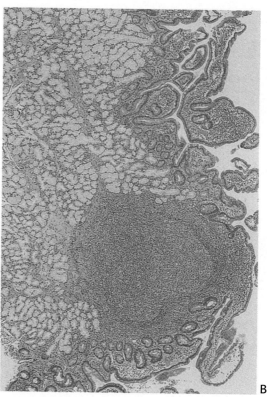

FIG. 6.87. Peptic duodenitis. **A:** Fully developed metaplastic epithelium above the *arrows* merges with well-developed small intestinal lining cells containing enterocytes and goblet cells. **B:** Prominent lymphoid follicle presenting as a polyp.

Patients with DUs experience dyspepsia and intermittent abdominal pain. DUs are more prone to perforate (Fig. 6.89), hemorrhage, or cause obstruction than are gastric ulcers. Bleeding causes massive upper GI hemorrhage in a significant number of cases. Rebleeding, sometimes massive, affects 13.6% to 32% of patients, tends to affect older patients (especially those on NSAIDs), and occurs more commonly in patients with a visible vessel (Fig. 6.89) (179). DUs in children may present in atypical ways. Only about 50% of children experience dyspepsia, approximately 61% have nocturnal pain, abdominal pain occurs in 70%, and bleeding affects about 33% of patients. Children with cystic fibrosis are particularly prone to develop DUs due to decreased duodenal bicarbonate secretion. Most duodenal ulcers develop in the first part of the duodenum, usually immediately distal to the pylorus.

Multiple DUs have different clinical features and pathophysiologies, and represent a more aggressive side of the ulcer spectrum (180). Peptic ulcers in the second and third portions of the duodenum or jejunum, repeated penetrating or perforating ulcers in the third portion of the duodenum or first portion of the jejunum, or the presence of multiple ulcers (Fig. 6.89) should arouse suspicion of Zollinger-Ellison syndrome.

Refractory ulcers heal slowly, recur rapidly after initial healing, or follow a prolonged course of exacerbation and short or absent remissions. Scarring leads to deformation of

the duodenal bulb and stricture formation. Larger ulcers take longer to heal and recur more often once they have healed.

Grossly, DUs appear circular or oval, usually measuring <3.0 cm in maximum diameter (Fig. 6.90). Ulcers located posteriorly in the bulb are more likely to bleed than those situated elsewhere (181) because two sizable arteries (i.e., the pancreaticoduodenal and the gastroduodenal) lie in the vicinity. Penetration of the duodenal wall by an ulcer results in erosion of one or both vessels (Fig. 6.91), producing massive hemorrhage. Perforation gives rise to generalized peritonitis. Ulcer scarring may lead to the formation of a prestenotic diverticulum. The histologic features of DUs resemble those of gastric ulcers (see Chapter 4). The surrounding mucosa usually shows evidence of peptic duodenitis. Antral gastritis is also usually present, as is *H. pylori*. These may be restricted to the stomach but they may also colonize areas of foveolar metaplasia.

ISCHEMIC ENTERITIS

When the blood supply to a tissue is interrupted, a sequence of chemical events leads to cellular dysfunction, edema, and ultimately cell death. Tissue anoxia results in anaerobic metabolism and lactic acidosis. Fewer high-energy bonds are created, and the cell is deprived of the

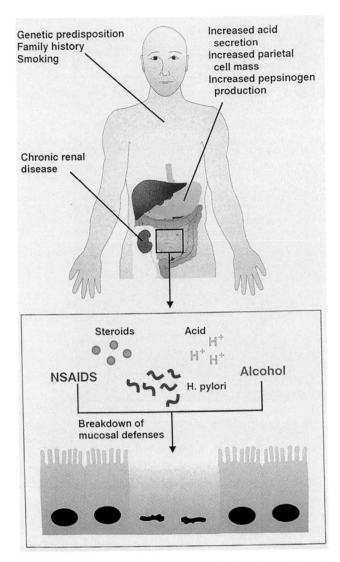

FIG. 6.88. The pathogenesis of duodenal ulcer disease is multifactorial and involves host factors as well as environmental factors. Most patients exhibit increased acid secretion, increased parietal cell mass, and increased pepsinogen production. Environmental agents such as steroids, nonsteroidal anti-inflammatory drugs (NSAIDs), alcohol, or *Helicobacter pylori* further contribute to the injury by breaking down mucosal defenses.

energy needed to maintain homeostasis (182) (Fig. 6.92). Ischemic injury forms a continuum of changes that range from increased mucosal permeability to frank necrosis. The clinical severity of ischemic enteritis varies widely from massive and sometimes fatal hemorrhagic infarctions to silent transient minimal ischemic episodes. Vascular occlusion and periods of hypotension or vasoconstriction account for most cases of intestinal ischemia. The ischemia may therefore be caused by diseases intrinsic or extrinsic to the bowel. Small intestinal ischemic necrosis predominantly affects elderly individuals with underlying cardiovascular disease. However, intestinal ischemia may affect individuals of any age, including infants. Intestinal ischemia complicates

peripheral vascular disease, various vasculopathies, some infections, intussusception and torsion, and certain drug therapies.

All forms of ischemic damage (see Table 6.5) share the underlying feature that the blood supply fails to meet the local tissue demands required to fulfill normal functions and/or maintain normal structure. Prolonged cessation of blood flow inevitably results in cell death because of the diminished delivery of oxygen and metabolic substrates and the accumulation of potentially cytotoxic end products of anaerobic metabolism. Small intestinal blood supply has to be reduced by >50% to induce detectable tissue injury (183). The extent and duration of the ischemia depends on several factors, including the nature of the intestinal vasculature, luminal bacterial virulence, and the duration of the ischemic episode. The first detectable sign of ischemic injury is increased capillary permeability. With continuing ischemia, detectable epithelial cell injury occurs. Mucosal cells are shed at an increased rate, and damage to the plasma membrane of unshed cells results in leakage of cytoplasmic digestive enzymes and tryptic digestion of the mucosa. Arteriolar spasm and decreased perfusion pressure accentuate the extent of the ischemic damage. Necrosis and subsequent bacterial invasion develop when the mucosal barrier becomes defective. The basic pathologic response to ischemia is mucosal coagulative necrosis. If reflow is reestablished, acute inflammation develops.

No single process represents the critical event in ischemic injury. Depletion of cellular energy stores and accumulation of toxic metabolites both contribute to cell death. Re-establishing the blood flow (reperfusion) is required to reverse the injury because it allows cellular regeneration and washout of toxic metabolites. However, reperfusion of ischemic tissues also paradoxically injures the tissues (Fig. 6.93) (184). In fact, most of the injury that occurs in intestinal ischemia occurs during the reperfusion period due to the production of reactive oxygen metabolites by activated neutrophils and other inflammatory cells. The severity of reperfusion injury depends on the duration of the preceding hypoxia, with it being more severe following partial rather than total intestinal ischemia (185). The sudden reintroduction of oxygen into the anoxic tissues unleashes oxygen-free radical cascades that overwhelm endogenous defenses. Many derive from the hypoxanthine-xanthine oxidase system (186). Superoxide and hydrogen peroxide increase mucosal and vascular permeability, recruit and activate neutrophils, and act as the precursors of more damaging hydroxyl radicals via the Fenton and myeloperoxidase reactions (Fig. 6.93) (186). Aggressive luminal factors (such as pancreatic proteases, especially trypsin) contribute to the mucosal damage and potentiate bacterial translocation and sepsis.

Neutrophil–endothelial cell interactions are a prerequisite for ischemic microvascular injury (187). The hypoxia induces endothelial cells to produce various adhesion molecules, including integrins, members of the immunoglobulin superfamily, and selectins. These powerful chemoattractants

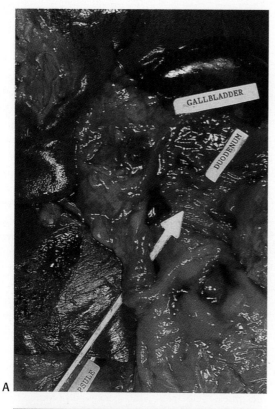

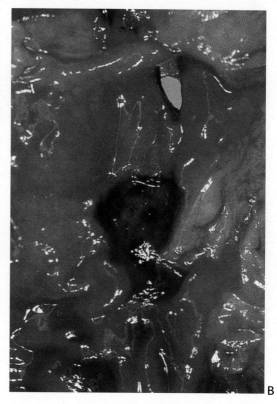

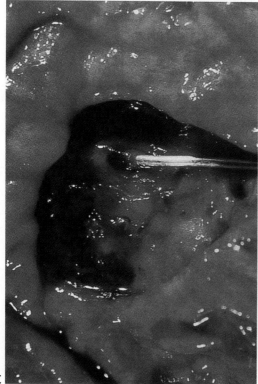

FIG. 6.89. Gross appearance of peptic duodenal ulcers. **A** and **B** derive from the same specimen dissected at the time of autopsy. The patient had numerous ulcerations involving the stomach, esophagus, and duodenum. The plastic *arrow* is inserted through a perforating duodenal ulcer. **B:** Higher magnification of a different ulcer showing the presence of a granular base. The specimen illustrated in A and B is from a patient with Zollinger-Ellison syndrome. **C:** Image from a different patient showing the presence of a large visible vessel containing a probe.

and chemoactivators attract leukocytes and platelets to reperfused sites and promote their adherence, transendothelial migration, and activation. As a result, one sees a massive mucosal influx of neutrophils. The infiltrating neutrophils are also a major source of reactive oxygen metabolites

(ROMs), including O_2^-, H_2O_2, OH·, HOCl, and certain *n*-chloramines.

Acute mesenteric infarctions result from mesenteric arterial occlusion (Fig. 6.94), nonocclusive low-flow states, mesenteric vein thrombosis (Fig. 6.95), or vasculitis.

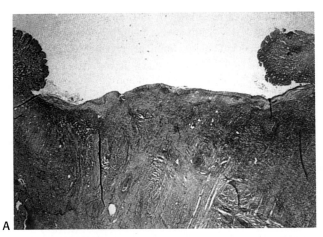
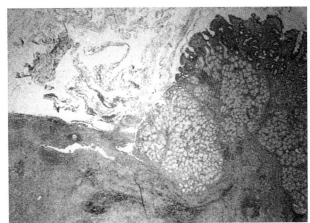

FIG. 6.90. Duodenal ulcer. **A:** An ulcer with typical overhanging margins is seen. It has the same zones as gastric peptic ulcers (see Chapter 4). **B:** Ulceration extends deep into the duodenal wall. Brunner gland hyperplasia is seen.

Mesenteric artery thrombosis and embolization (Figs. 6.96 and 6.97) occur with about equal frequency. Thrombi almost invariably overlie atheromatous plaques occupying the proximal few centimeters of the vessel. In contrast, emboli lodge at bifurcation points or in a distal branch. Ischemia also complicates numerous other conditions that ultimately obliterate the intestinal vascular supply (Table 6.5).

TABLE 6.5 Causes of Intestinal Ischemia

Acute vascular occlusion
  Arterial or venous thrombosis
  Embolus
Low-flow states (low cardiac output, hypotension/
  shock)
Atherosclerosis
Mechanical
  Intussusception
  Volvulus
  Hernias
Necrotizing enterocolitis
Vasculitides and vasculopathies
Hypercoagulable states
Drugs
  Oral contraceptives
  Cocaine
  Digitalis and vasopressors
  Potassium chloride
Vascular compression
  Volvulus
  Intussusception
  Celiac axis compression
Amyloidosis
Collagen vascular diseases
Radiation damage
Diabetes mellitus

Ischemia in Low Flow States (Nonocclusive Ischemia)

Low flow states usually result from decreased cardiac output following primary cardiac disease (infarction or arrhythmia), hypovolemia, shock, vascular shunting, or a combination of low mesenteric flow and mesenteric arterial vasoconstriction. Patients who develop low-flow states are typically elderly and they often have concomitant atherosclerotic vascular disease. Even though the blood supply to the superficial mucosa is fairly well maintained during shock, hypoxic injury still develops within 1 to 2 hours. Several pathogenic mechanisms account for the ischemic necrosis including vasoconstriction with increased resistance to blood flow, redistribution of the blood flow away from the mucosa, increased capillary filtration via relaxation of the precapillary sphincter smooth muscle fibers, and intestinal countercurrent mechanisms in the villi that shunt oxygen away from the villous tips (Fig. 6.98) (188). This explains why the villous tips become anoxic first and explains why early and minimal injury always occurs first at the villous tip (Fig. 6.99).

Arterial Occlusive Disease

Arterial occlusive disease occurs secondary to narrowing, thrombosis, embolism, or hemorrhage under an atheromatous plaque. Occlusions also result from aortic aneurysms, aortic dissections, obstruction by mural thrombi, and tumors that externally compress the vessels. The occlusion may involve one or all of the intestinal arterial trees. Atheromatous occlusion progresses slowly enough for collateral circulation to develop, and as a result patients often have severe disease involving all the mesenteric arteries before they become symptomatic. Intestinal infarction secondary to atheromatous occlusion of a single vessel is rare (189). (About 50% of patients over the age of 50 have atheromatous

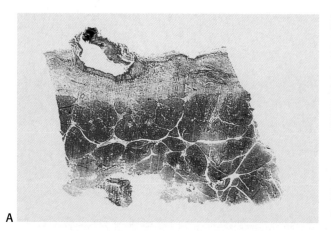
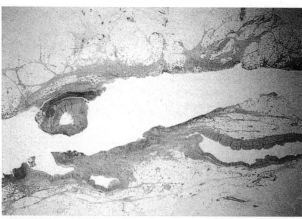

FIG. 6.91. Penetrating duodenal ulcer. **A:** The bottom of an ulcer bed has eroded a large extraintestinal vessel. The structure at the base is the pancreas, the periphery of which has become fibrotic due to the inflammatory response. **B:** Erosion into the serosal fat, exposing several branches of a major vessel.

narrowing or occlusion of the celiac axis.) The disease is most likely to be most severe in patients with diabetes. The superior mesenteric artery is affected more commonly than the inferior mesenteric artery. The most severe atherosclerotic lesions affect the proximal 2 cm of the superior and

inferior mesenteric arteries. Embolic occlusion accounts for one third of cases of mesenteric vascular occlusion (190). Massive, acute, and often fatal embolism usually results from migration of an intracardiac mural thrombus complicating heart disease. Cholesterol emboli migrate from aortic

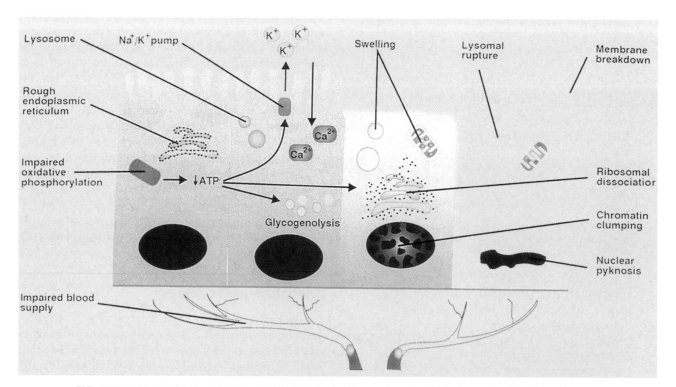

FIG. 6.92. Intestinal ischemia. Intestinal ischemia develops when insufficient arterial blood reaches the intestinal mucosa through the presence of a thrombus, an embolus, an atheromatous plaque, a vascular spasm, low-flow states, or obstruction of venous outflow. As a result, oxidative metabolism becomes impaired, leading to decreased adenosine triphosphate (ATP), increased glycolysis, acidosis, and changes in nuclear chromatin, as well as in other cellular organelles. The decreased ATP also leads to decreased functioning of the sodium-potassium pump with an influx of calcium ions and water and an efflux of potassium. As a result, the cells swell, as do intracellular organelles. As the organelles become damaged, ribosomes decrease and protein synthesis decreases, interfering with reparative processes.

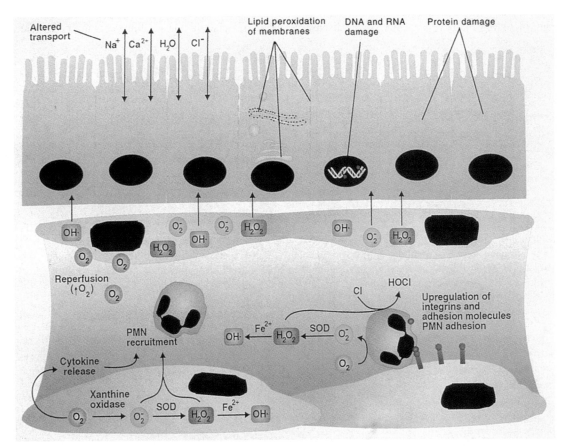

FIG. 6.93. During ischemia, cellular adenosine triphosphate (ATP) is converted to adenosine monophosphate and further catabolized to hypoxanthine, which serves as an oxidizable substrate for xanthine oxidase. The enzyme xanthine oxidase (XO) is the rate-limiting enzyme in nucleic acid degradation. XO generates H_2O_2 and O^{2-} during the oxidation of hypoxanthine or xanthine. Free radicals are also generated via the Fenton reaction, especially during cell reperfusion. The free radicals recruit polymorphonuclear leukocytes (PMNs) to the reperfused area. The neutrophils adhere to the endothelial cells secondary to increased transcription of integrins and adhesion molecules on both neutrophils and endothelial cells. Free radicals also diffuse into the local tissues, causing abnormalities in the enterocytes with lipid peroxidation of membranes and damage to DNA, RNA, and proteins, and alterations in cellular transport mechanisms.

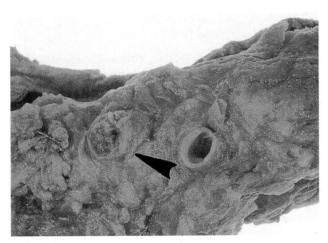

FIG. 6.94. Thrombosed superior mesenteric artery. The *arrowhead* points to the orifice of the superior mesenteric artery as it exits the aorta.

plaques, especially following catheterization, resulting in localized or widespread intra-abdominal ischemia. Valvular endocarditis may shed small mycotic emboli. Intestinal damage develops within minutes of total circulatory arrest.

Sudden occlusion of the superior mesenteric artery produces hemorrhagic infarction in the area supplied by the occluded vessel (as modified by the presence of a collateral blood supply). The infarcted area may extend from the proximal jejunum to the transverse colon, producing a pattern of ischemic enterocolitis (36). However, usually a small area is involved, and there is a sharp dividing line between the normal and ischemic parts of the bowel (Fig. 6.100).

Generally, one has little difficulty in diagnosing patients with acute, diffuse, transmural ischemic necrosis. These patients abruptly become symptomatic. The most common manifestation is poorly localized colicky abdominal pain that becomes constant and unremitting as the disease progresses. The pain results from spasm of the muscularis

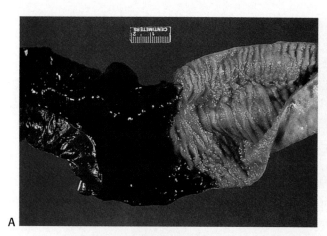
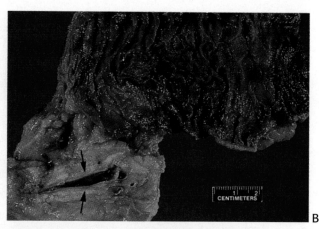

FIG. 6.95. Intestinal infarction secondary to portal vein thrombosis. **A:** Gross photograph of the junction of the infarcted intestinal segment with normal mucosa. There is a sharp line of demarcation between the infarcted tissue (black tissue on the left) and the viable, noninfarcted tissue on the right. **B:** Dissection through the peri-intestinal fat showing a branch of the portal venous system, which has been opened and contains a long thrombus (*arrows*).

propria. Diarrhea develops and stools become overtly bloody. As the ischemic muscle loses its contractile functions, much of the spasm ceases. The patient then experiences abdominal tenderness, positive rebound signs, and evidence of peripheral circulatory collapse. At this point, the bowel is usually beyond recovery and requires surgical resection. With further disease progression, the abdomen distends and bowel signs disappear. As the ischemia persists and infarction develops, the patients often develop an elevated white blood count, fever, and signs of peritonitis.

Mesenteric Venous Thrombosis

Mesenteric venous thrombosis is a relatively rare disease primarily affecting the elderly in their 6th and 7th decades of life (191). The prevalence of mesenteric vein thrombosis ranges from 0.003% in the general hospital population to 0.05% of autopsied populations (192). Venous thrombosis accounts for 5% to 15% of all cases of mesenteric ischemia and infarction (Fig. 6.101) (193). Multiple etiologic factors may exist in any one patient. For example, a patient requiring splenectomy may have a pre-existing abnormality involving the coagulation system, experience intraoperative trauma to regional veins, and develop a transient thrombocytosis caused by the splenectomy. Its presence in younger persons suggests that the patient has a hypercoagulable state. Twenty-five to fifty percent of cases have no predisposing cause; these are classified as *primary venous thrombosis*. Regardless of the cause of the thrombosis, egress of blood from the intestine becomes impaired, causing the mesenteric arterial pressure to rise and arterial blood flow to slow, leading to the development of ischemia. Increased intraluminal pressure further interferes with mucosal viability.

Approximately 95% of all mesenteric thromboses involve the superior mesenteric vein and lead to ischemia or infarction of the small bowel or proximal colon (191). In a small number of cases, the thrombosis develops over an extended period, permitting the development of collateral venous drainage from the involved intestinal segments. Depending on the cause, mesenteric venous thrombosis may begin in the portal vein and extend back into the mesenteric vein and its branches, or it may begin in smaller peripheral mesenteric venous branches and proceed up into the portal vein.

FIG. 6.96. Histologic section through the portal vein showing the presence of an organized thrombus.

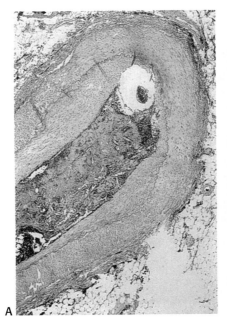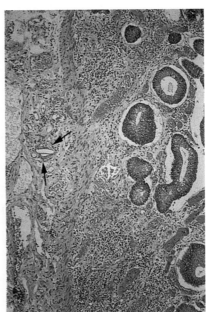

FIG. 6.97. Atheromatous emboli. **A:** Cross section through the superior mesenteric artery demonstrating the presence of a large atheromatous embolus. **B:** Emboli extend into the smaller vessels just beneath the muscularis mucosae (*arrows*).

Propagating portal vein thrombosis causes portal hypertension. Thrombi often arise in the distal arcades and propagate proximally.

Patients present with a constellation of nonspecific findings. The clinical presentation is characterized by gradually increasing colicky abdominal pain. With increased blockage of the collaterals by new thromboses, the patient develops nausea and vomiting, an acute abdomen, and rectal bleeding. At this time, surgical intervention is required. Involvement of the splenic or portal vein with a propagating thrombus may

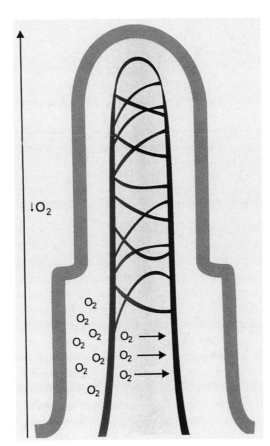

FIG. 6.98. Diagram of countercurrent mechanism demonstrating shunting that occurs at the villous base. It diverts oxygen from the villous tips to the base of the crypts during anoxic periods.

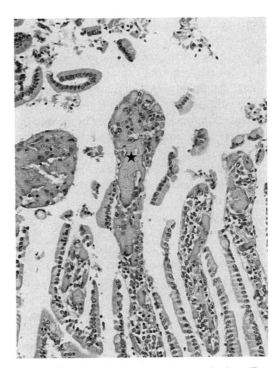

FIG. 6.99. Early ischemia demonstrating marked capillary congestion and loss of epithelium from the villous tips. One of these denuded villus tips is indicated by the *star*. Taken in isolation, the changes may resemble those seen in autolysis. No reperfusion has occurred and therefore acute inflammatory cells are absent.

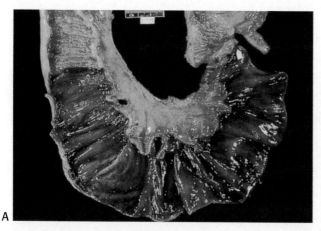

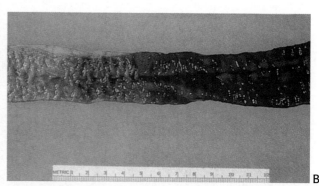

FIG. 6.100. Small bowel ischemia. **A:** Hyperemic infarcted areas with adjacent friable pink-tan mucosa. **B:** Area of infarction with gradual hyperemia of adjacent lesser involved mucosa.

result in portal hypertension (191). Patients with venous occlusion tend to have a subacute course producing days or weeks of abdominal pain. Bloody ascites is common.

The diagnosis of mesenteric venous thrombosis is usually made during laparotomy for an acute abdomen. At the time of surgery, the serosal and mucosal surfaces appear mottled, hemorrhagic, and discolored with fibrinous exudates deposited on them. The bowel appears thinned in areas of transmural hemorrhagic infarction. Adjacent areas show patchy ischemia. The mesentery usually appears thickened, hemorrhagic, and edematous, and it contains numerous cordlike thrombosed veins. The arteries usually appear normal. Numerous recent, organizing, and partially recanalized thrombi are observable in the mesenteric venous vasculature, and the bowel wall shows intramural hemorrhage and variable degrees of edema and ischemic necrosis with ulceration and acute inflammation. The thrombosis occurs in the absence of phlebitis. The arteries remain uninvolved. Patients may develop Budd-Chiari syndrome.

Mechanical Obstruction of Venous Return

Venous return becomes impeded when the bowel undergoes torsion, volvulus, or intussusception, or when it becomes strangulated and herniates. External compression of the vasculature causes obstruction of the relatively thin-walled and low-pressure venous system before the arterial supply is affected. As a result, the bowel becomes congested with blood, hemorrhagic, and edematous. Ischemic necrosis then develops rapidly. The histologic features resemble those of mesenteric venous thrombosis, except that thrombi are absent.

Gross Features of Ischemic Injury

The pathologic features of intestinal ischemia are similar, no matter what the underlying cause. Ischemia characteristically appears segmental in nature. Early on, the ischemic

bowel is edematous and pale with submucosal congestion, hemorrhage, and focal mucosal sloughing (Fig. 6.102). As the disease progresses, the serosa becomes dusky and purple or dark red due to the presence of large amounts of intraluminal blood. The serosa loses its normal glistening appearance and appears dull. The mucosa appears necrotic, nodular, and ulcerated. Extensive submucosal hemorrhage may be present. In early lesions, only the mucosa and sometimes the submucosa are affected; the muscularis propria usually remains normal. As the necrosis progresses, all of the bowel wall layers become damaged and the serosa becomes purplish green. With increasing damage, the intestinal wall thins and becomes friable and membranous exudates form. If the ischemia results from mesenteric venous thrombosis, one sees old and new thrombi extruding from the veins. Ulcers may be present that may be superficial or deep. Perforation may develop. Patients with chronic damage may have mural fibrosis and strictures.

Histologic Features of Ischemic Injury

The histologic features of ischemia depend on whether the changes are acute and minimal or whether they result from transmural infarction. They also depend on whether there is a total vascular occlusion without reperfusion or whether the blood flow is merely reduced below the local needs and reflow has occurred. Therefore, ischemic lesions vary from patchy congestion and ulceration to extensive infarction, gangrene, and perforation.

Most pathologists encounter small intestinal ischemia when they examine large resected segments of necrotic bowel. In this situation, it is easy to diagnose the ischemia. Diagnostic difficulties only occur when one encounters early lesions or when complications develop. Biopsies to establish a diagnosis of ischemia or to rule out other etiologies of enterocolitis are much less common than colonic biopsies for the same purposes. Therefore, the biopsy features of intestinal ischemia are extensively discussed in Chapter 13.

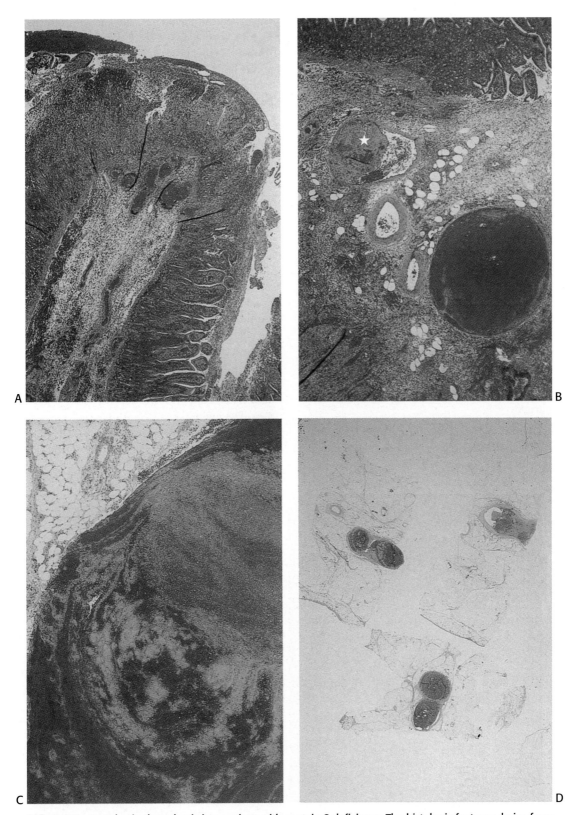

FIG. 6.101. Portal vein thrombosis in a patient with protein S deficiency. The histologic features derive from the specimen illustrated in Figure 6.95. **A:** The patient developed ischemia with reperfusion injury. There is glandular dropout, loss of villous epithelium, villous congestion, and inflammation. **B:** Higher magnification of the submucosa showing the presence of a congested and a thrombosed (*star*) submucosal vein. **C:** Higher magnification of one of the vessels showing the lines of Zahn in the thrombus. **D:** The mesenteric fat contains numerous thrombosed branches of the portal vascular system.

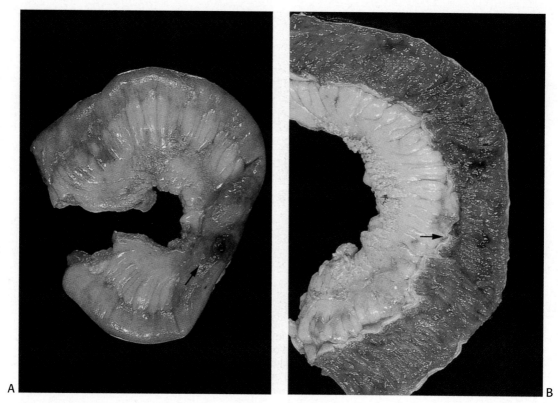

FIG. 6.102. Gross features of intestinal ischemia. **A:** Unopened specimen with a perforation (*arrow*). **B:** Opened specimen showing a localized area of ischemia (*arrow*).

Because the mucosa is the most vulnerable part of the intestinal wall, it is damaged first (Fig. 6.103). Early epithelial damage results from loss of energy-dependent processes, causing intercellular edema, and epithelial detachment. Membrane-enclosed cytoplasmic blebs develop on the basal side of the enterocytes where they attach to the basement membrane. This begins the epithelial detachment process. This process starts before the enterocytes display signs of

irreversible damage. The process advances from the villous tips to the crypt bases. With more severe or more prolonged ischemia, or both, the epithelium lining the sides of the villi lifts off the basement membrane until the epithelial cells are lost completely (Fig. 6.104). Within 1 hour of total vascular occlusion the upper two thirds of the villi becomes denuded. Then, the villous core disintegrates. The crypt cells often remain intact with little histologic evidence of damage. In

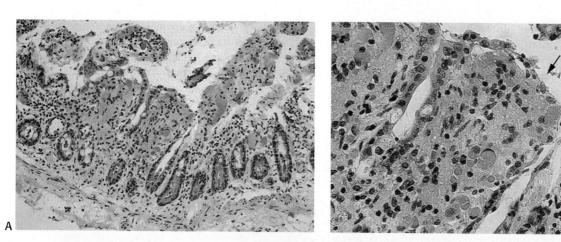

FIG. 6.103. Ischemic enteritis. **A:** Medium magnification showing loss of superficial epithelial lining from the villi. Large numbers of the crypts are identifiable only by residual cells at the base of the glands. **B:** Higher magnification of the superficial area showing edema, vascular congestion, and degeneration and sloughing of the epithelium from the tips (*arrow*).

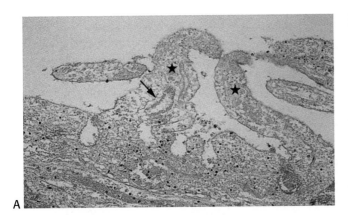

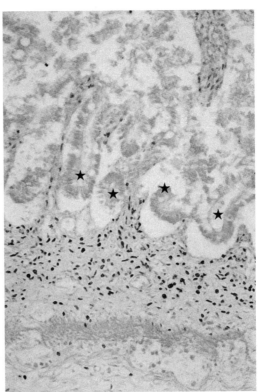

FIG. 6.104. Intestinal infarction. **A:** The small intestine is completely necrotic with transmural coagulative necrosis. The ghosts of the preexisting villous cores are present (*stars*). Ghosts of dead enterocytes are indicated by the *arrow*. There is no inflammation because reperfusion did not occur. **B:** Coagulative necrosis associated with anoxia. Sections of several crypts are indicated by the *stars*. The epithelium is sloughing and the nuclei lack their typical basophilia. This photograph shows the increased sensitivity of the epithelium to anoxic effects. The underlying stroma still contains intact nuclei in the stromal cells.

other cases, one sees crypt hypoplasia–villous atrophy interfering with normal cellular turnover. Occasionally, crypt dilation becomes prominent. Later, the epithelial cells become markedly attenuated and the crypts appear compressed and atrophic as the lamina propria swells and hemorrhages. After 5 hours of total acute occlusion, almost the entire intestinal wall appears necrotic.

In cases of total occlusion, the capillaries appear congested with red cell extravasation and coagulation necrosis unaccompanied by acute inflammation. The pathologic findings are definitive but mimic autolysis because of the absence of neutrophilic infiltrates. Longer periods of ischemia eventually destroy the crypt bases and the underlying musculature. Overt perforation occurs when the ischemic process involves the entire thickness of the bowel wall. The presence of fibrin thrombi in mucosal capillaries serves as a useful diagnostic feature of ischemia (Fig. 6.105), but it only becomes evident once epithelial breakdown occurs. In severe injury the crypts drop out completely, and if the damage heals the area becomes fibrotic. The degree of fibrosis that develops depends on the extent of the ischemic damage.

If partial blood flow is maintained, then the effects of the reperfusion are superimposed on the ischemic damage. Early stromal changes consist of edema of the lamina propria, often associated with hemorrhage and emigration of neutrophils through the epithelial surface, especially at the villous tips. There is often prominent telangiectasia. A pseudomembrane composed of necrotic epithelium, fibrin, and inflammatory cells develops (Fig. 6.106). In cases of severe injury, the

ischemic process extends into the submucosa and muscularis propria and serosa (Fig. 6.106). If the ischemia only affects a small segment, collateral circulation may allow healing to begin even as the infarction is proceeding at a smaller focus,

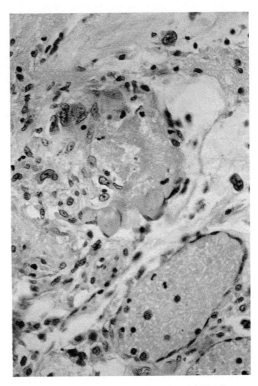

FIG. 6.105. Ischemia with focal fibrin thrombi in the vasculature.

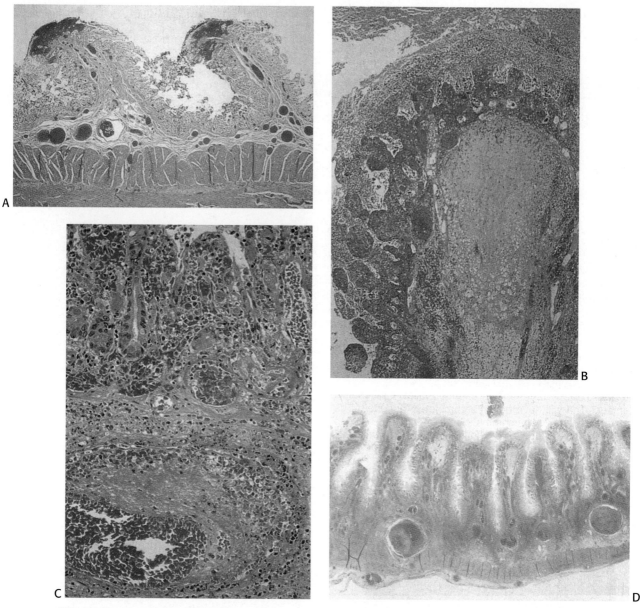

FIG. 6.106. Acute ischemia. **A:** Early hemorrhagic necrosis of the tips of the folds is seen. The epithelium is extensively denuded. **B:** Extensive hemorrhagic infarction of the tip of the folds. The entire mucosal structure is completely infarcted. A pseudomembrane covers the surface of the bowel. The submucosal structures are edematous and hemorrhagic. **C:** Marked necrosis is seen in the small bowel. The mucosa appears hemorrhagic and telangiectatic. An organizing thrombus is seen in the underlying blood vessel. **D:** Severe extensive transmural infarction of the small bowel.

resulting in regenerative changes superimposed on degenerative ones.

It is unusual for the etiology of the ischemic damage to be evident from an intestinal resection or biopsy specimen, unless one finds a vasculitis or thrombi. It is important to make a distinction between the damaged vessels that result from ischemia and ulceration and primary vascular disease. In trying to make this distinction, one must examine those parts of the intestine that are not ulcerated or show only minimal signs of ischemic damage to establish whether underlying vascular disease or another change is present.

Isolated intramucosal goblet cells may be present in patients with subacute ischemic enteritis and these may mimic signet ring cell carcinoma, particularly since gastrointestinal signet ring cell tumors may have a deceptively benign appearance (194). These are typically found in areas of extensive necrosis with mucosal sloughing. They typically lie within the crypt lumens along with inflammatory debris, near dying cells of the crypt. There is often continuity between the dying cells and the sloughed signet ring–like cells at the crypt bases. The signet ring–like cells represent degenerating goblet cells and are usually accompanied by other dying cells with the features of enterocytes, endocrine cells, and Paneth cells. These cells are confined to the ischemic areas in the partially viable mucosa.

Recovery from Ischemic Damage

Even when the villi are extremely damaged, healing begins quite rapidly if the tissues become adequately reoxygenated (195). Recovery takes place in several phases. In the first phase, a new epithelial layer regenerates from the crypts and the lower third of the villi (Fig. 6.107). The cells proliferate and migrate upward to cover whatever residual villous core remains. If the villous cores are completely destroyed, the mucosa will become simplified, resembling colonic tissue, or even appear as an area completely lacking crypts. After 12 hours, a flat epithelium is present, but by 24 hours the epithelium and cells appear cuboidal or columnar and incipient development of small intestinal villi is apparent. After 8 days, the regenerated small intestinal mucosa shows a variably normal morphology (196), depending on the extent of the original injury and architectural loss.

Complications

Reparative changes following ischemia can lead to stricture formation as early as 2 to 8 weeks after the initial injury.

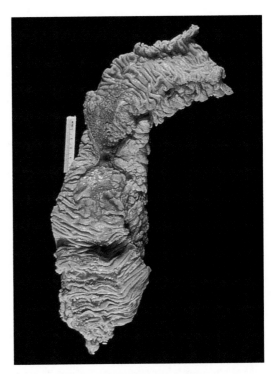

FIG. 6.108. Ischemic stricture.

Transmural infarction with serosal ischemia induces adhesions between adjacent structures. Extensive intestinal infarction leads to systemic acidosis and hypotension, with secondary cardiac, renal, or pulmonary failure; sepsis; strictures; and death (Fig. 6.108).

Ischemic strictures may be single or multiple and can measure many centimeters in length. They are usually sharply delimited concentric lesions. The bowel wall appears thickened, fibrotic, and whitish in color. There is usually mucosal necrosis. The submucosa may contain granulation tissue and abundant new vessels. The mucosa may be ulcerated, contain inflammatory polyps, or appear healed with distortion of the mucosal folds. There may also be fissures. The wall shows scattered inflammation and lymphoid aggregates may present throughout the bowel wall. All of these features mimic the strictures present in patients with Crohn disease. Hemosiderin deposits may be present in areas of previous hemorrhage and may serve to distinguish ischemia from Crohn disease. Other features that help distinguish between the two entities are listed in Table 6.6.

Necrotizing Enterocolitis

Necrotizing enterocolitis (NEC) affects all age groups, ranging from premature neonates to the very elderly. Ischemia is the underlying cause of the pathologic process, but the mechanisms are poorly defined and vascular occlusion is not usually demonstrable. Often there is a coexisting bacterial infection. Frequently this is due to *Clostridium* species. Disseminated intravascular coagulation may occur secondary to the presence of bacterial toxins.

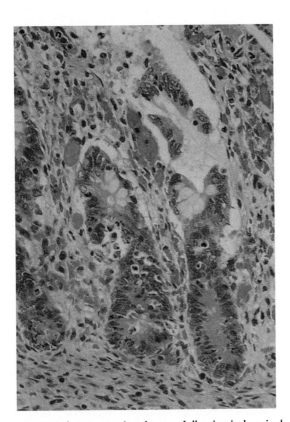

FIG. 6.107. Early regenerative changes following ischemic damage. The villi have become completely denuded. The crypts are lined by hyperchromatic cells that are beginning to proliferate and replace the previously destroyed epithelium.

TABLE 6.6 Ischemic Strictures Versus Crohn Disease

Feature	Ischemia	Crohn Disease
Stricture location	Usually distal ileal	Located away from the distal ileum
Sharp delineation from normal bowel	Present	Absent
Aphthous ulcers away from stricture	Absent	Often present
Transmural inflammation	Can be present	Characteristically present
Submucosal lymphoid aggregates	Can be present	Characteristically present
Hemosiderin deposits	May be present	Absent
Vasculitis	May be present	May be present
Fissures	May be present	May be present

Neonatal Necrotizing Enterocolitis

Neonatal NEC is a devastating neonatal disease with a rapid onset that affects 6% of all premature infants (197). Twenty to forty percent of cases are fatal. Surviving babies suffer from short bowel syndrome and/or malabsorption later in life. Stricture formation occurs as early as 5 weeks after the acute episode in infants who survive. Four major factors play critical roles in the pathogenesis of neonatal NEC, including prematurity, establishment of enteral feeding, intestinal mucosal ischemia, and the presence of luminal bacteria (Fig. 6.109). Some patients have a Paneth cell deficiency (198). Contributing factors include intestinal dysfunction and endotoxemia. In most cases the intestinal ischemia results from decreased cardiac output due to fetal asphyxia.

The neonatal intestine has a limited capacity to maintain oxygen uptake during periods of reduced perfusion pressure and arterial hypoxia, especially during feeding (199). Additionally, the enzymatic composition of the immature neonatal intestine does not allow complete digestion of fats, carbohydrates, and casein, leaving a large amount of protein in the intestinal lumen in the form of curd. This favors intestinal bacterial growth, particularly those that produce potent toxins. Mucosal injury permits proteins and bacterial toxins to pass into the portal circulation and then into the liver, injuring hepatocytes and Kupffer cells. If liver function becomes sufficiently impaired, endotoxin enters the systemic circulation, causing shock. Gram-negative bacterial colonization also occurs, further intensifying the circulatory insufficiency and the shock (197). The terminal ileum and right colon are preferentially affected.

The gross findings of neonatal NEC may be dramatic, with the affected bowel segments appearing dilated, necrotic, hemorrhagic, friable, and gangrenous (Fig. 6.110). The external surface shows shaggy serosal exudates and adhesions between adjacent loops of bowel. Because the injury is ischemic in nature, the changes are either diffuse or focal. Pneumatosis intestinalis may be present (Figs. 6.110 and 6.111).

Tropical Necrotizing Enterocolitis

Tropical necrotizing enterocolitis affects patients of all ages in tropical and subtropical areas. Dietary factors and infec-tions contribute to its pathogenesis. Ischemia is always the initial insult. Pig bel, seen in Papua, New Guinea (Fig. 6.111), represents an example of this group of lesions. This entity is described further in a later section.

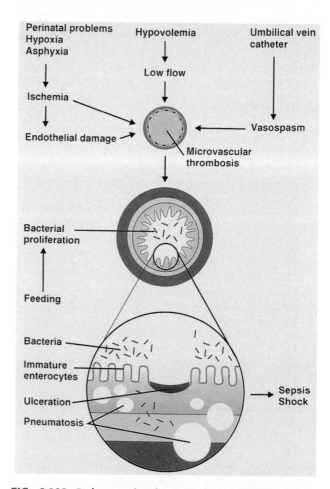

FIG. 6.109. Pathogenesis of neonatal enterocolitis. Multiple factors play a role in the etiology of this pediatric disorder. Common to most cases is a period of hypoxia leading to ischemia. Coexisting hypovolemia leads to low-flow states and complicates the underlying anoxia. Umbilical vein catheterization may cause localized vasospasm and further compromise luminal flow. At the same time as anoxic injury is progressing, the small intestinal epithelium loses its normal barrier function and bacteria that are present gain access to the underlying tissues, leading to sepsis and shock.

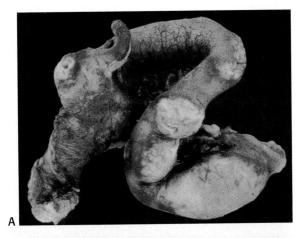

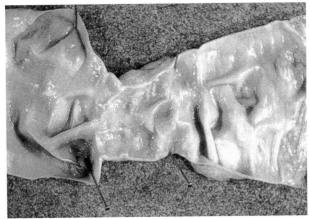

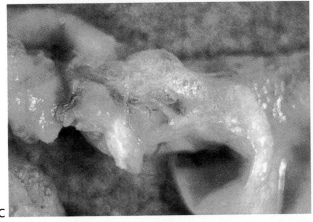

FIG. 6.110. Necrotizing enterocolitis. **A:** Resection specimen from a child with severe necrotizing enterocolitis. The bowel is dusky in many areas, representing areas of hemorrhagic infarction. In addition, multiple areas of transmural gangrene with pseudomembrane formation are represented by the multifocal whitish areas. **B:** Pneumatosis intestinalis is present in area of stricture. **C:** Higher power magnification demonstrates the bubbly quality of the mucosal surface representing entrapped air within the bowel wall.

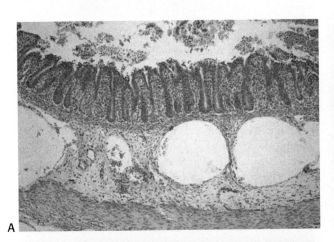

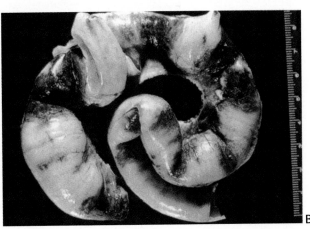

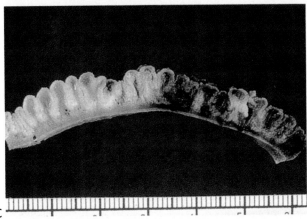

FIG. 6.111. Necrotizing enterocolitis. **A:** The mucosa has regenerated. The villi are markedly shortened. The crypts are hyperplastic with a regenerative appearance. Some residual pseudomembranes are seen dissolving in the bowel lumen. Gas-filled cysts are present in the submucosa and correspond to pneumatosis intestinalis. **B:** Pig bel showing the patchy segmental involvement as seen from the serosal surface. **C:** Pig bel. Cross section of the bowel wall demonstrating submucosal edema. Brownish green spots coalesce to form larger area of necrosis. (B and C courtesy of Robin Cooke, M.D., Department of Pathology, Royal Brisbane Hospital, Brisbane, Australia.)

Acute Segmental Obstructing Enteritis

Acute segmental obstructing enteritis is characterized by fever, leukocytosis, copious bilious vomiting, severe abdominal pain, and signs of intestinal obstruction. Many patients eventually recover from the disorder following antibiotic treatment. The disease may be self-limited. Some patients undergo surgical exploration with the demonstration of segmental ischemia. This pediatric disorder may account for some subsequent cases of shortened bowel syndrome with segmental transmural fibrosis (200).

Celiac Axis Compression Syndrome

Celiac axis compression syndrome (mesenteric vessel compression) results in abdominal pain, vascular narrowing, and ischemia. It results from mesenteric vessel compression (Table 6.7). The intestines develop typical ischemic injury. If the compression results from a neoplasm compressing the vasculature, the tumors may also extend into the bowel wall.

Intestinal Ischemia Following Atheromatous Embolization

Cholesterol emboli arising from complicated atheromatous plaques produce a wide range of clinical syndromes

TABLE 6.7	Mesenteric Vessel Compression
Retroperitoneal hematoma
Retroperitoneal fibrosis
Retroperitoneal tumors
Enlarged mesenteric lymph nodes
Metastatic carcinoma
Lymphoma
Infectious processes

depending on the organs and size of the vessels involved. Emboli usually arise from the aorta and patients present with abdominal pain and melena secondary to intestinal ischemia. Abdominal aortic catheterization in such patients sometimes results in a showering of atheromatous emboli throughout the abdominal arterial circulation. Such an unfortunate event may produce dramatic changes not only in the GI tract, but also in the spleen, kidneys, and adrenals. Because the emboli lodge in small vessels, it is rare for full-thickness infarction to develop due to the presence of collateral circulation. Patients with healed disease develop strictures. The vessels in the affected areas undergo various changes. Initially, they are plugged by atheromatous emboli, cholesterol crystals, or amorphous debris. This elicits a foreign body giant cell reaction followed by concentric intimal fibrosis, luminal reduction, and variable degrees of recanalization (Fig. 6.112) (201).

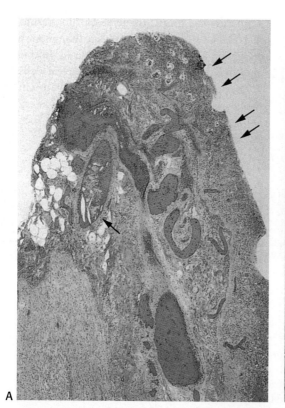
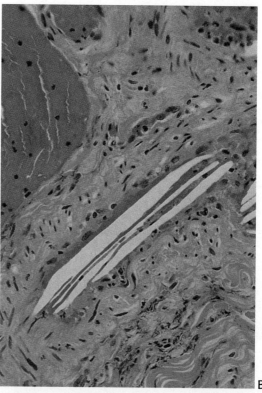

FIG. 6.112. Ischemia due to atheromatous emboli. **A:** A portion of ischemic small intestine with focal complete loss of the epithelium (*arrows*). The vessels are extremely dilated. One vessel contains an embolus with slitlike spaces corresponding to cholesterol emboli (*arrow*). **B:** Higher magnification of the cholesterol clefts in the emboli in a medium-sized vessel.

Bowel Infarctions in Dialysis Patients

Patients with end-stage renal disease who undergo dialysis are at increased risk for nonocclusive intestinal infarction due to the presence of hypertension, severe underlying heart disease, and the frequent removal of large volumes of fluid during ultrafiltration dialysis. Patients develop a hypotensive episode; an anion gap and metabolic acidosis are frequently present. Multiple infarctions may develop.

Gastrointestinal Ischemia in Vasculitis

Vascular inflammation complicates many disorders leading to ischemic enteritis, perforation, hemorrhage, infarcts, ulcers, and strictures. Both the small and large intestine may be involved. Larger vessel disease is exemplified by polyarteritis nodosa. The intestines are also affected by other forms of vasculitis, including Henoch-Schönlein disease, Wegener granulomatosis, and Churg-Strauss disorder. Venous disease leading to ischemia not caused by primary thrombotic processes may occur in systemic lupus erythematosus (202), Behçet disease (203), necrotizing giant cell granulomatous phlebitis (204), enterocolic lymphocytic phlebitis (205), and idiopathic myointimal hyperplasia of mesenteric veins (206). Vasculitides are often classified based on the size of the vessels that are involved as shown in Table 6.8.

Polyarteritis Nodosa

Twenty-five to seventy-nine percent of patients with polyarteritis nodosa (PAN) present with abdominal pain, diarrhea, positive fecal occult blood, nausea, vomiting, and hematemesis (207). Steatorrhea, perforation, strictures, ulcerative enteritis, ischemia, and intussusceptions may all occur (208). Thirty-six percent of patients with PAN exhibit only GI manifestations. Males are afflicted four times more often than women, most commonly between the ages of 20 and 40. Patients often have other autoimmune diseases, with rheumatoid arthritis and systemic lupus erythematosus being the most common. Deposition of immune complexes in the blood vessels leads to fibrinoid necrosis and thrombotic, occlusive, ischemic, and hemorrhagic events in the affected tissues. Microaneurysms and vascular stenoses develop in the medium-sized mesenteric arteries. The mesenteric vessels are involved in 25% to 30% of cases. Nodular swellings along the course of the mesenteric arteries represent a characteristic but uncommon finding.

A resection specimen often shows patchy necrosis, well-demarcated mucosal ulcers along the antimesenteric border, strictures, and possibly perforation. The major histologic findings usually remain confined to the smaller mesenteric arteries as well as small and medium-sized submucosal arteries. Vascular edema occurs first, followed by acute inflammation of all layers of the vessel walls (Fig. 6.113). Fibrinoid necrosis of the media and elastic intima occurs later, causing stretching and fragmentation. This predisposes the abnormal vessel to undergo thrombosis and luminal narrowing. Elastic tissue destruction results in aneurysmal dilation or rupture. The whole circumference of the artery may be involved, but more often the involvement is eccentric or segmental in nature. Elastic tissue stains demonstrate disruption and dissolution of the elastic fibers. Lymphocytes, histiocytes, polymorphonuclear cells, and eosinophils infiltrate the intestinal wall in response to the vasculitis. Giant cells are absent.

Henoch-Schönlein Purpura

Henoch-Schönlein purpura (HSP) is a multisystemic disorder characterized by a symmetric, nontraumatic, nonthrombotic, painless purpuric rash largely involving the skin of the legs and buttocks with arthritis, nephritis, hematuria, and GI injury (209). The disorder is primarily a pediatric disease characterized by IgA immune complex deposits beneath the

TABLE 6.8 Gastrointestinal Vasculitis

Affecting large vessels
  Takayasu arteritis[a]
  Giant cell arteritis[a]
  Polyarteritis rheumatica[a]
Predominantly affecting large and medium-sized vessels
  Crohn disease
Predominantly affecting small and medium-sized blood vessels
  Radiation damage
  Polyarteritis nodosa
  Kawasaki disease[a]
  Arterial fibromuscular dysplasia of childhood
  Buerger disease
  Fungal vasculitis
  Danlos-Ehlers syndrome
Predominantly affecting small-sized vessels, ANCA-associated
  Wegener granulomatosis
  Churg-Strauss syndrome
  Microscopic polyangiitis
Predominantly affecting small vessels
  Henoch-Schönlein syndrome
  Behçet syndrome
  Hypersensitivity vasculitis
  Thromboangiitis obliterans[a]
  Leukocytoclastic vasculitis
  Systemic lupus erythematosus
  Rheumatoid arthritis
  Hypocomplementemic vasculitis
  Cytomegalovirus vasculitis
  Rickettsial vasculitis
  Cryoglobulinemia
Predominantly affecting veins and venules
  Mesenteric inflammatory venoocclusive disease
  Diffuse hemorrhagic gastroenteropathy

ANCA, anticytoplasmic neutrophil antibody.
[a] Very rarely affects the gastrointestinal tract.

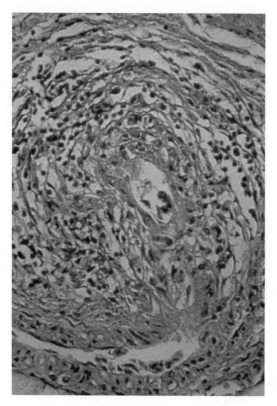

FIG. 6.113. Polyarteritis nodosa. The vessels are inflamed.

may be involved but the jejunum and ileum are most frequently affected. Patients present with acute abdominal symptoms, including pain and GI bleeding (210).

Grossly, the bowel exhibits small, superficial infarcts with diffuse edema, mottling, congestion, and hemorrhage. A white purulent exudate covers an erythematous mucosa (211). Erosions and ulcers may be present. Several ischemic areas of varying ages may be present. Transmural infarctions and perforations are rare. The mesentery may appear focally congested.

Histologically, there is vascular congestion, hemorrhage, necrosis, and inflammation (Fig. 6.114). The necrotizing small vessel vasculitis predominantly affects capillary venules in the mucosa and upper submucosa, sparing larger mesenteric vessels. The venules of involved portions of the bowel demonstrate an acute leukocytoclastic vasculitis, fibrinoid necrosis of the vascular walls, and polymorphonuclear leukocytic infiltrates in surrounding tissues (211). Fibrinoid necrosis can be seen within the lumens of involved venules subjacent to the areas of ischemic mucosal necrosis (Fig. 6.115) (211). The demonstration of IgA deposits in the vascular walls by immunofluorescence is diagnostic.

Hypersensitivity Vasculitis

Hypersensitivity vasculitis involves inflammation of the small blood vessels (arterioles, capillaries, and venules) and represents an allergic response to a precipitating antigen such as a drug, vaccine, microorganism, or foreign protein. Immune complexes deposit in the walls of small vessels, activating the complement cascade. Neutrophils infiltrate the vessel walls, releasing lysosomal enzymes, which results in

vascular basement membranes. Antigenic stimulation may result from respiratory tract infections, stings, immunizations, and drugs. The gut is involved in up to 85% of patients. Patients may initially manifest isolated GI disease but subsequently other organs become involved. Any bowel segment

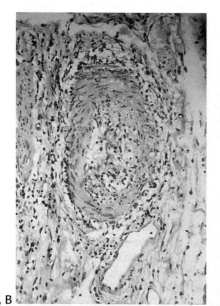
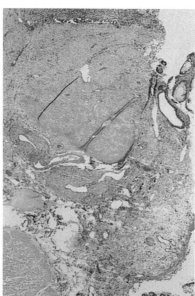
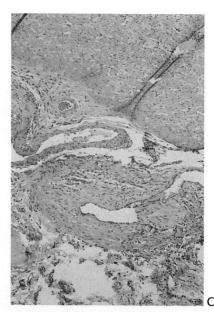

A, B   C

FIG. 6.114. Henoch-Schönlein purpura. **A:** A leukocytoclastic vasculitis is seen in a submucosal vessel. **B:** Low-power photograph demonstrating the presence of mucosa on the right side of the photograph and distorted, penetrating vessels with fibrosis and inflammation. **C:** Higher magnification of the penetrating vessel.

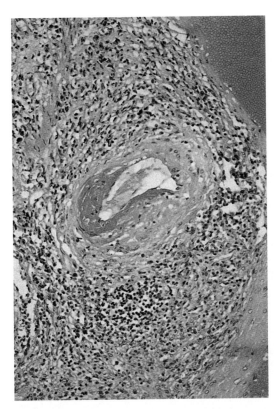

FIG. 6.115. Henoch-Schönlein purpura. Vessel demonstrating fibrinoid necrosis.

fibrin deposition and necrosis (212). Biopsies usually show ischemia, fragmentation of white cells (leukocytoclastic), and fibrinoid necrosis of the walls of the small blood vessels. Specific involvement of small vessels in contrast to medium-sized muscular arteries distinguishes hypersensitivity vasculitis from polyarteritis nodosa, the two kinds of vasculitis that most frequently involve the GI tract.

Wegener Granulomatosis

Persistent inflammatory sinonasal disease coexisting with systemic fevers, malaise, and migratory arthritis typifies the clinical presentation of Wegener granulomatosis. The disease, which affects males and females equally, classically involves the upper and lower respiratory tracts and the kidney, but it may affect any organ system. Wegener granulomatosis is characterized by a granulomatous vasculitis involving small or medium-sized arteries and veins. The granulomatous inflammation consists of palisading epithelioid histiocytes arranged around necrotic foci (213). Multinucleated giant cells constitute a prominent feature of the vascular inflammatory infiltrate. Antineutrophilic cytoplasmic antibodies (c-ANCAs) are diagnostic, especially in patients with concomitant renal disease.

Sjögren Syndrome

Sjögren syndrome associates with hypersensitivity vasculitis. The major histologic findings fit into four major vasculitic

categories: Acute necrotizing vasculitis, leukocytoclastic vasculitis, lymphocytic vasculitis, and endarteritis obliterans. The acute necrotizing vasculitis affects small and medium-sized arteries. The entire vascular wall becomes infiltrated with acute and, to a lesser extent, chronic inflammatory cells. Fibrinoid necrosis of the walls is characteristically present. The lesions simulate those seen in PAN during the acute phase, but they lack the aneurysmal formation seen in PAN. Patients with leukocytoclastic vasculitis demonstrate a polymorphonuclear infiltration in capillaries and venules and fibrinoid necrosis of the vessel wall with extravasated red blood cells. Patients with lymphocytic vasculitis exhibit a lymphoplasmacytic infiltrate in capillaries and venules. Vascular wall necrosis is absent. The noninflammatory obliterative vasculitis affects medium-sized vessels.

Rheumatoid Arthritis and Other Collagen Vascular Diseases

Approximately 10% of patients with *rheumatoid arthritis* (RA) have GI involvement. Patients with vasculitis usually have severe arthritis, rheumatoid nodules, and high titers of rheumatoid factor. They usually display signs of cutaneous vasculitis. Patients also develop complications from their NSAID or gold therapy. Intestinal infarction in RA patients usually results from the presence of a systemic vasculitis that also involves the vessels of the intestinal wall or mesenteries (Fig. 6.116). Occasionally, RA patients also have proliferative endarteritis characterized by intimal proliferation without vascular wall necrosis or inflammation. RA may also manifest as polyneuropathy, or skin infarction with ulceration, and digital gangrene. In severe cases, the vasculitis affects virtually any organ (214). GI tract involvement is rare but catastrophic when it occurs. GI bleeding, intraperitoneal bleeding, ischemic mucosal ulceration, small and large bowel infarction, bowel perforation, and pancolitis have all been reported. Patients with *scleroderma*, especially the form associated with Raynaud disease, may develop ischemic enterocolitis on the basis of an underlying vasculitis.

Arteritis and venulitis in *systemic lupus erythematosus* may result in massive lower intestinal hemorrhage. Histologic examination shows mucosal ulceration with necrotizing vasculitis (215). Rare complications include infarction and sepsis. Fibrinoid necrosis may be present. Hemorrhagic blebs result from intramucosal hemorrhage oozing from ruptured mucosal capillaries.

Ehlers-Danlos Syndrome

Ehlers-Danlos syndrome is an autosomal dominant disorder with abnormalities affecting the cardiovascular, gastrointestinal, and respiratory systems. Vessels become very fragile in the type IV form of the disease. The disorder results from a deficiency in type III collagen. GI vascular involvement presents with intramural hemorrhage, massive bleeding, ischemic necrosis, and perforation (216). The cardinal

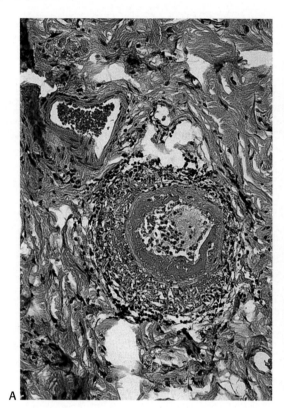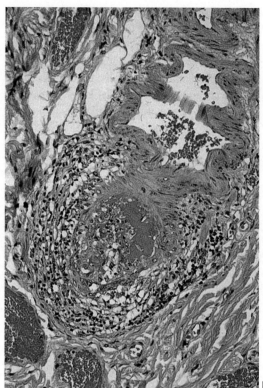

FIG. 6.116. Vasculitis in rheumatoid arthritis. A and B come from the same resection specimen that was removed for ischemic enterocolitis. **A:** Cross section through a small arteriole demonstrating the presence of prominent, predominantly concentric perivascular inflammation with a necrotizing vasculitis. Prominent fibrin deposition is present within the lumen. Desquamating cells are seen. **B:** Another vessel with an endoluminal proliferation and occlusion by proliferating reactive cells. Inflammatory cells surround the bottom portion of the photograph.

histologic features include arterial dilation with aneurysm formation and aneurysmal rupture, usually limited to medium-sized and smaller arteries (the muscular arteries), although multiple aneurysmal dilations may also affect major muscular arteries, including those in the mesentery. Collagen fibers appear disorderly and loose, disrupting the media of the muscular arteries. Medial hemorrhages occur at the site of the structural damage. Increased acid mucopolysaccharides deposit around the abnormal collagen defects in the arterial walls, suggesting the presence of interactions between the two. Muscular and collagen fiber abnormalities also lead to disintegration of the muscularis mucosae, which becomes practically unrecognizable, especially in the small intestine, and diverticula may develop.

Kawasaki Disease

Kawasaki disease is an acute systemic vasculitis of early childhood characterized by fever, rash, mucosal inflammation, and coronary artery damage (217). Most patients are under age 3. The acute phase of the illness is marked by a profound immunoregulatory change that includes a reduction in CD8+ cells, an increase in activated (DR+) circulating CD4+ cells, and marked polyclonal B-cell activation in the peripheral blood. GI tract involvement, manifesting as diarrhea and/or protein-losing enteropathy, is often the initial symptom.

Diffuse Hemorrhagic Gastroenteropathy

Diffuse hemorrhagic gastroenteropathy presents as a small vessel vasculopathy that involves the gastric and small intestinal mucosa, which appear diffusely hemorrhagic (218). Biopsies demonstrate luminal narrowing of capillaries and postcapillary venules in the lamina propria due to swelling and proliferation of endothelial cells, neutrophilic margination, and emigration and partial vascular occlusion by fibrin thrombi. These changes remain restricted to the mucosa and are not found in the submucosa, muscularis propria, or serosa. The endothelial cells are histologically abnormal in that they show redundant basal lamina and abnormal endothelial cells with myoid features (218).

Segmental Mediolytic Arteritis

GI segmental mediolytic arteritis (SMA) affects the abdominal muscular arteries and arterioles in the serosa and bowel wall of elderly patients. The lesion results from an inappropriate vasospastic response to shock or severe hypoxemia (219). Histologically, SMA is characterized by transformation of the arterial smooth muscle cytoplasmic contents into a maze of dilated vacuoles containing edema fluid. The vacuoles rupture, disrupting the smooth muscle cells. Fibrin deposits and hemorrhage occur at the adventitial–medial junction within the media. Inflammation is inconstant and limited to the periadventitial tissues. Transmural medial lysis leads to the formation of arterial wall gaps that become bridged by a serofibrinous layer (219).

Mesenteric Inflammatory Veno-occlusive Disease (Lymphocytic Phlebitis)

Nonthrombotic mesenteric occlusion is a rare cause of intestinal infarction. Patients are typically hypertensive, elderly individuals with a recent onset of abdominal symptoms. The patients often lack evidence of systemic diseases. It complicates rutoside therapy, a drug used to treat varicose veins in Europe. Histologically, there are prominent, dense, perivascular sheets of lymphocytes in both the grossly abnormal ischemic areas as well as in grossly normal areas. The disorder selectively affects veins and venules in the submucosa, subserosa, and peri-intestinal tissues (220). Arteries and arterioles remain completely unaffected. The phlebitis exhibits various stages of progression. Some veins have lymphocytic infiltrates in their walls without luminal compromise; others have intense transmural lymphocytic infiltrates accompanied by subintimal, focally occlusive fibroproliferative lesions and intraluminal thrombi (Fig. 6.117). Some veins recanalize. Sparse neutrophilic or eosinophilic infiltrates may accompany the lymphocytes (220,221). Focally necrotic areas and isolated giant cells may be present in the fibroproliferative process. The differential diagnosis of enterocolitic lymphocytic phlebitis includes a drug-induced hypersensitivity reaction, vasculitis affecting small veins as seen in systemic lupus erythematosus and Behçet disease, secondary effects of enterocolic inflammation, a benign lymphoproliferative disorder, myointimal hyperplasia of mesenteric veins, and necrotizing granulomatous phlebitis.

Idiopathic myointimal hyperplasia of mesenteric veins may represent an end stage of lymphocytic phlebitis. Idiopathic myointimal hyperplasia of mesenteric veins is characterized by the presence of bizarre, thick-walled, hypertrophic veins in the submucosa and mesentery. It develops in patients with venous hypertension. Veins become arterialized. Patients often recover following surgery, suggesting that the process is self-limited or indolent in nature (220,221). It is often very difficult to be certain whether the inflammatory venous changes are the cause or the result of the ischemia.

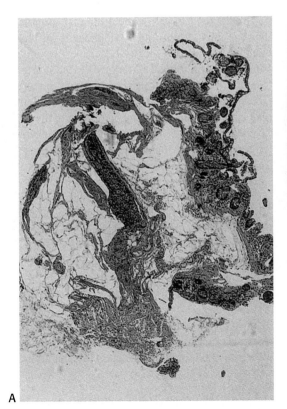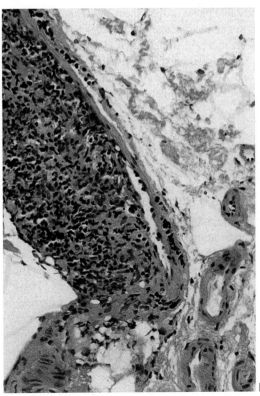

FIG. 6.117. Lymphocytic venulitis. **A:** Low magnification showing the mucosa to the right and a prominent submucosal vessel with intense basophilia due to mononuclear cell infiltration. **B:** Higher magnification showing complete obliteration of the vascular wall by a mixed mononuclear cell infiltrate.

Cryptogenic Multifocal Ulcerating and Stenosing Enteritis

The lesions of cryptogenic multifocal ulcerous stenosis enteritis (CMUSE) are isolated to the intestines. Its pathophysiology is unknown, although there is an association with a complement 2 deficiency and a possible relationship with polyarteritis nodosa (222,223). One hundred percent of patients have intestinal symptoms; 70% exhibit extraintestinal symptoms. Twenty percent of patients experience weight loss and 10% experience fever, altered well-being, polyarteritis, and mesenteric artery aneurysms (222,223). Asthma and sicca syndrome may coexist with the disease. Characteristic digestive lesions include 1- to 25-cm jejunal or proximal ileal areas of stenosis. The remainder of the small intestine appears normal. In all cases, the ulcers are superficial, affecting only the mucosa and submucosa. The stenoses associate with nonspecific inflammatory infiltrates containing eosinophils. Fifty-five percent of cases exhibit vascular wall degeneration with fibrous endarteritis. Patients who undergo surgical resection may experience a complete recovery. However, many patients require steroid therapy. CMUSE differs from chronic ulcerative nongranulomatous jejunitis because of the absence of villous atrophy and malabsorption.

Thromboangiitis Obliterans

Most patients with thromboangiitis obliterans (Buerger disease) are heavy-smoking men who present with progressive peripheral arteriolar disease and migratory thrombophlebitis. Buerger disease has a worldwide distribution but it is more prevalent in the Middle East and Far East than in North America or Western Europe (224). The disease typically affects small and medium-sized arteries and veins of the upper and lower extremities and patients have a history of recurrent episodes of thrombophlebitis involving both the upper and lower extremities. GI vascular lesions affect the smaller submucosal and serosal vessels. Larger mesenteric vascular involvement, although rare (225), causes low-grade intestinal ischemia with crampy abdominal pain or an acute abdominal emergency secondary to ischemic necrosis, skip ulcers, and intestinal perforation (225). The lesion occasionally affects the small bowel.

The histologic features reflect disease stage. During the acute stage, the thrombosis is accompanied by angiitis and microabscesses within the thrombus. There is a highly cellular and inflammatory thrombus with relative sparing of the vessel wall. GI lesions demonstrate endothelial cell proliferation, concentric vascular intimal thickening, mild fibrosis, marked transmural inflammation or degeneration (Fig. 6.118), and organizing thrombi. There is usually interruption of the internal elastic lamina. Subacute lesions appear less distinctive than the acute ones, and end-stage lesions may be difficult to distinguish from old organized thrombi. There may be mild perivascular inflammation. The internal elastic lamina is intact (distinguishing the lesion from other forms of vasculitis) and it and the media lack atheromas or calcification. Patients may have superimposed areas of acute and/or chronic ischemia. The absence of medial necrosis and

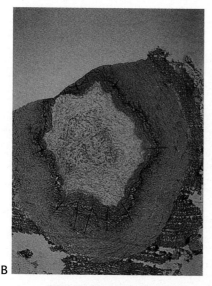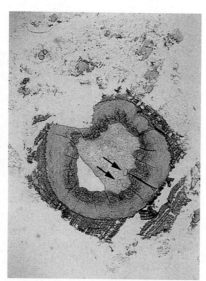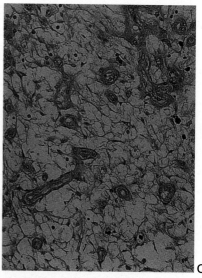

A, B   C

FIG. 6.118. Buerger disease. A through C show portions of a medium-sized vessel from a small intestinal resection in a patient with Buerger disease. **A:** Complete obliteration of the lumen by loose, edematous tissue. **B:** Cross section through another vessel demonstrating almost complete occlusion (van Gieson stain). It shows reduplication of the internal elastic membrane. The material within the vascular lumen represents an area of recanalizing thrombus. Several dilated vascular structures are seen (*arrows*). **C:** Higher magnification of the material within the central portion of the vessel shown in A demonstrating the presence of a loose reparative tissue containing numerous proliferating capillaries.

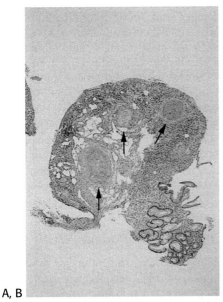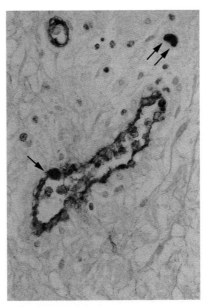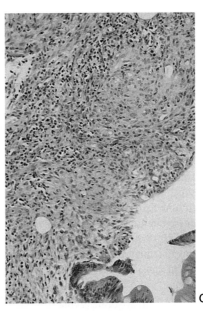

A, B   C

FIG. 6.119. Cytomegalovirus (CMV) vasculitis. **A:** A biopsy from the terminal ileum showing large abnormal vascular structures within the submucosa (*arrows*). The superficial portion of the mucosa is completely denuded and ulcerated. **B:** Immunostain of one of the smaller vessels from the specimen utilizing a dual stain for vessels (factor VIII–related antigen) and CMV. The CMV-infected cell is an endothelial cell (*arrow*). A second infected cell is seen at the top right-hand portion of the photograph (*double arrows*). This cell represents a mononuclear cell. **C:** CMV enterocolitis. The specimen demonstrates a loose, vaguely granulomatous appearance due to the collections of histiocytes that are obliterating underlying vascular structures. CMV immunostains disclosed the presence of immunoreactive cells in the surrounding tissues.

the involvement of medium-sized vessels distinguish these lesions from those seen in polyarteritis nodosa.

Vascular Diseases Caused by Infections

Several infections involve the GI vasculature, damaging the vessel walls and inducing secondary ischemia. Fungi and cytomegalovirus (CMV) are the most frequent offenders. Debilitated patients with *Aspergillosis* and *Candidiasis* may develop fungal vascular invasion and mycotic aneurysms. The fungi completely occlude the vascular lumens, becoming coated with platelets and fibrin, and eventually the vessels thrombose. The intravascular fungi induce an inflammatory response that leads to secondary damage of the vascular wall and extravasation of red blood cells and vasculitis.

CMV is notorious for its ability to invade endothelial cells, causing endothelialitis and predisposing the vessels to thrombosis. A granulomatouslike lesion characterized by histiocytic collections without giant cells may surround the vascular wall (Fig. 6.119). Viral inclusions are not always identifiable within the endothelium of the affected vessels, probably due to sampling problems. However, they are present elsewhere in the nearby vicinity. Viral inclusions may be highlighted by immunostains.

Diabetic Microangiopathy

The most consistent morphologic feature of diabetic microangiopathy is the presence of arteriolosclerosis (Fig. 6.120) and

hyalinized PAS-positive thickened vessel walls and variable degrees of luminal narrowing in smaller caliber submucosal vessels (226). The vascular thickening is secondary to the deposition of basement membrane material. The small bowel may be extensively involved, resulting in diarrhea and malabsorption. The vessels are uninflamed and Congo red stains are negative. There is no endothelial proliferation.

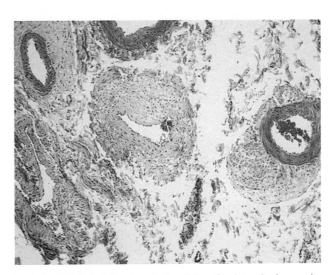

FIG. 6.120. Arteriolosclerosis involving the intestinal vasculature. These markedly thickened and fibrotic vessels were present in the submucosa of the small intestine.

Behçet Disease

A syndrome of orogenital and ocular inflammation (or ulceration) was first reported in 1937 by Behçet (227). The disease affects both genders of all ages from infants to the elderly. It has high prevalence rates in the area along the ancient Silk Road from Far East Asia to Turkey. The site of organ involvement is somewhat geography dependent, with ileocecal disease being relatively more common in the Japanese (228). Some cases are familial in nature (229), although no predisposing genetic abnormality has been identified. Possible etiologic associations include CMV (230) or Epstein-Barr (231) infections. Others suggest that the presence of high levels of truncated actin in the neutrophils of these patients may be specific for the disease (232,233). Gastrointestinal involvement occurs in about 5% of patients and about 1% to 2% have small intestinal disease (234).

Common wisdom is that the disease results from a vasculitis affecting both small and large vessels. However, more recent data suggest that the disorder is primarily a neutrophilic vasculitis that targets the vasa vasorum (235). Intestinal involvement most commonly affects men in their 4th and 5th decades of life. Patients preferentially develop ulcers in the terminal ileum and cecum. Enlarging ulcers or newly formed ulcers coexist with healed ulcers. The ulcers are localized or diffuse, often penetrating the serosa, leading to intestinal perforation. They have a tendency to irregularly undermine surrounding tissues. Edemalike swelling with crater formation around the ulcer margins produces a characteristic "collar-stud" appearance. Perforation and severe hemorrhage are the most severe complications of the disease.

Pathologically, the disease is characterized by a vasculitis that is usually lymphocytic in nature and affects small veins and venules to a greater extent than arteries. Mononuclear infiltrates surround capillaries and venules, and some vessels demonstrate intimal thickening. Occasionally, there may be more severe necrotizing inflammation with leukocytoclasis. Often the vasculitis is difficult to demonstrate, making the diagnosis challenging. Small intestinal involvement typically affects the terminal ileum, particularly in the area of lymphoid aggregates and Peyer patches (236). Behçet ulcers contain nonspecific chronic inflammation, and the submucosal connective tissue appears disrupted (Fig. 6.121). Granulomas are absent. The mucosa around the ulcers is usually normal in appearance. Patients treated surgically have a high rate of recurrent disease (236). The histologic features of recurrent disease resemble the primary disease. The preferred treatments are combined drug therapy with any or all of the following: Steroids, NSAIDs, and immunosuppressive and cytotoxic agents. Thalidomide, tacrolimus interferon, and antitumor necrosis factor monoclonal antibody have all attracted recent attention (237,238).

The presence of focal ulcers, fistulae, and strictures and the ileocecal location may mimic Crohn disease, and since the histologic features are nonspecific, one must rely on the clinician to suggest the diagnosis based on the presence of characteristic oral, genital, and eye lesions. The diagnosis of Behçet disease requires the presence of recurrent oral ulceration. Other helpful clinical features include ocular involvement, arthritis, erythema nodosum, and recurrent genital ulceration. Unfortunately, some of these may also be present in Crohn disease as discussed in Chapter 11.

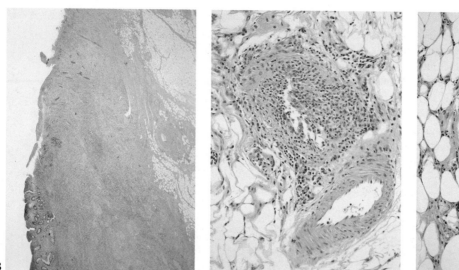

FIG. 6.121. Behçet disease. **A:** The ileum shows an area of ulceration and the adjacent mucosa shows ischemic changes. **B:** Acute vasculitis. **C:** Healing vasculitis.

Other Vasculitides

Other disorders affecting mesenteric arteries include *Takayasu arteritis* (pulseless disease), *Crohn disease* (see Chapter 11), and *cryoglobulinemia*. These disorders affect children and adolescents, and are usually heralded by severe abdominal pain. Takayasu disease may associate with inflammatory bowel disease.

Patients with *Churg-Strauss syndrome* sometimes develop GI involvement. These patients often have allergic rhinitis, nasal polyposis, and asthma as well as eosinophilic pulmonary infiltrates. Peripheral neuropathy is also common (239,240). This small-vessel ANCA-positive vasculitis resembles that seen in several other diseases, but the presence of eosinophils as part of the vasculitic infiltrate or an extravascular infiltrate into the surrounding tissues strongly favors the diagnosis. Extravascular granulomas may be present in this disorder and in Wegener granulomatosis (241). A number of drugs also cause vasculitis and ischemic complications. *Köhlmeier-Degos syndrome* affects the skin and gastrointestinal tract. The intima of small and medium-sized arteries undergoes progressive occlusive sclerosis leading to small intestinal infarction (242). Necrotizing angiitis may complicate AA amyloid (243).

Gastrointestinal Ischemia Secondary to Thrombotic Events

Hemolytic uremia syndrome (HUS) affects young adults who present with anemia, thrombocytopenia, and renal failure. Patients who develop intestinal involvement present with enterocolitis resulting from intravascular microthrombi. The GI effects of HUS and *thrombotic thrombocytopenic purpura* (TTP) are similar. HUS is discussed in greater detail in Chapter 13. TTP is an idiopathic disorder consisting of thrombocytopenia, microangiopathic hemolytic anemia (without significant consumption of clotting factors), fever, renal insufficiency, and profound neurologic dysfunction. The condition causes thrombosis of intestinal vessels with secondary ischemic injury (Figs. 6.122 and 6.123).

Homocystinuria, a recessively inherited inborn error of metabolism, may simulate Marfan syndrome. Vascular abnormalities develop, characterized by episodic thrombosis followed by fibroelastic reorganization of medium-sized arteries. This results in a fibroblastic intimal proliferation and luminal narrowing in the absence of inflammation or fibrinoid necrosis. Homocysteine in the urine is diagnostic of the disease.

Köhlmeier-Degos disease (malignant atrophic papulosis) primarily affects the skin, but small intestinal disease occurs in about 50% of cases (244). The disease usually presents in young adults, although it has been diagnosed in infancy and after age 55. Young men are primarily affected. Patients may develop severe abdominal pain, sometimes with vomiting, suggesting peritonitis, intestinal obstruction, or pancreatitis. Intestinal perforation is the most common cause of death.

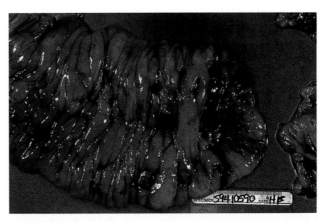

FIG. 6.122. Thrombotic thrombocytopenic purpura. Resection specimen removed due to uncontrollable intestinal bleeding. The bowel shows ischemic enteritis. Numerous ulcers are present throughout the small intestine.

Malabsorption due to widespread intestinal involvement also develops (242). The characteristic GI lesions consist of conical infarcts associated with thrombi. The arteries and veins appear thrombosed. Other vessels may show evidence of fibrinoid necrosis and perivascular hemorrhage. The intima of small and medium-sized blood vessels undergoes progressive occlusive sclerosis, leading to localized areas of infarction (242). Larger arteries develop proliferative changes resembling those seen in a thrombotic end arteriopathy.

Patients with *hypercoagulable states* often have anticardiolipin antibodies (245), lupus anticoagulants (246), protein C or S deficiencies (247), a dysfunction of antithrombin III or heparin cofactor II, (248), Leiden factor V mutations, and fibrinolytic dysfunction (249). These patients can present as a primary abdominal emergency due to the presence of ischemic necrosis. Typically, the patients present with diffuse intravascular venous thrombosis. Exceptionally, a *multiple myeloma* patient presented with an intestinal infarction due to crystallized immunoglobulins in the vasculature (250).

Patients with various bacterial infections may develop septicemia and widespread *disseminated intravascular coagulation* manifested by the presence of a petechial rash and mucosal hemorrhages. In severe cases, an entire segment of GI tract may become ischemic. This then predisposes the patient to additional septic events, with seeding of the blood by intestinal bacteria due to the disruption of the mucosal barrier. Toxigenic bacteria, such as enterohemorrhagic *Escherichia coli* and clostridia, damage capillary endothelial cells, causing severe mural edema, red cell extravasation, and hemorrhage. Ischemic necrosis then develops.

Handling Resection Specimens for Ischemia

Intestines are resected in ischemia either due to the presence of a perforation or due to life-threatening complications of intestinal ischemic necrosis. When the bowel infarcts or

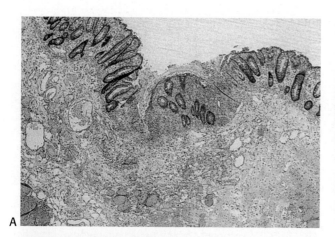

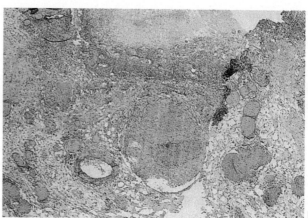

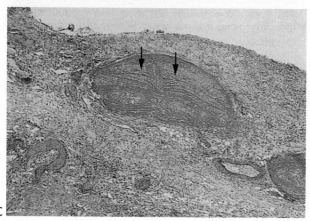

FIG. 6.123. Thrombotic thrombocytopenic purpura. **A:** Small bowel with ischemia and marked atrophy. Villi are completely obliterated. Focal glandular dropout is present. **B:** A portion of the submucosa immediately underlying an ulcer. The vessels are markedly dilated and contain laked blood. **C:** A portion of the submucosa underlying an ulcer. The oval-shaped vessel contains prominent lines of Zahn (*arrows*).

perforates, the clinician is already aware of the presence of ischemia. However, there are certain pieces of information that the resection specimen provides that the clinician may or may not know and may be extremely useful to future patient management. Sections should always be taken from the resection margins of the specimen whether or not they have been designated as to which is proximal and distal by the surgeons since the presence of nonviable tissue in either resection margin may lead to future surgical complications. Sections should also be taken through the most severely affected portion of the bowel to determine the extent of the ischemic damage and the depth of its involvement in the bowel wall. Perforation sites should be sampled. Sections should always be taken through the mesenteric vessels to determine whether the following are present: (a) atherosclerotic changes involving the vasculature, (b) other major vessel pathologies, (c) thrombi, and (d) emboli. If a thrombus or embolus is present, an effort should be made to determine its age.

When one examines the histologic sections from the bowel wall, an effort should be made to determine the cause of the ischemia. Therefore, the submucosal vessels should be examined carefully for the presence of vasculitis, thrombi, or emboli. The mucosa and submucosa should also be examined for the presence of viral inclusions. Special efforts should be made to assess the etiology in individuals who

would otherwise not be expected to have intestinal ischemia, particularly in younger patients. An intestinal resection often provides the first clue as to the presence of underlying disease. Perhaps the most difficult disorder to recognize is CMV-induced ischemia in an individual without the traditional risk factors for this infection. Viral inclusions should be sought in mononuclear cells and endothelium. If vaguely granulomatouslike lesions are seen around vessels, one may wish to perform immunostains for the presence of the virus. Subtle viral inclusions are often seen near perforations and/or deep ulcers, and in an individual without an obvious cause for the ischemia, one might want to stain such areas as well. The report should specifically state the viability of the resection margins, the depth of the involvement, and the presence of thrombi, emboli, vasculitides, or CMV.

CHRONIC ULCERATIVE JEJUNITIS

Numerous diseases cause small intestinal ulcers (Table 6.9). The rare disorder, chronic ulcerative jejunitis, also known as nongranulomatous chronic idiopathic enterocolitis and chronic ulcerative nongranulomatous jejunoileitis (251), is usually rapidly fatal and has a controversial etiology. Patients are typically middle-aged individuals who present with abdominal pain, anorexia, weight loss, fever, diarrhea,

TABLE 6.9 Causes of Small Intestinal Ulcers

Infections: Bacterial, fungal, viral parasitic
Crohn disease
Acute jejunoileitis
Celiac disease
Tumors: Carcinomas, lymphomas, sarcomas, metastases
Ischemia
Uremia
Hyperacidity syndromes
Drugs
   Arsenic
   Gold
   Mercury
   Nonsteroidal anti-inflammatory drugs
   Potassium chloride
   Corticosteroids
Radiation
Behçet syndrome
Peptic ulcer
Idiopathic mucosal enteropathy
Graft vs. host disease

malabsorption, steatorrhea, hypoalbuminemia, protein-losing enteropathy, celiac disease, lymphoma, hypogammaglobulinemia, pulmonary fibrosis, and polymyositis. Features shared with celiac disease include generalized severe malabsorption, profuse diarrhea, villous atrophy, and an intense mucosal mononuclear infiltrate, but dietary gluten exclusion does not ensure clinical improvement because the changes typically occur in refractory sprue. The clinical features mimic those of Crohn disease due to the presence of granulomas in some biopsies and a clinical response to anti-inflammatory drugs in some patients.

The patients develop well-demarcated but nonspecific ulcers in the duodenum and proximal jejunum (Fig. 6.124). They resemble those seen in ischemia or other ulcerating

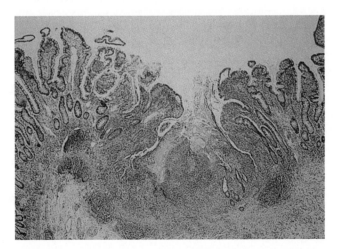

FIG. 6.124. Ulcerative jejunitis. A well-demarcated superficial ulcer extending into the upper portion of the submucosa is identified.

diseases. Polymorphonuclear and chronic inflammatory cells infiltrate the lamina propria, and the mucosa demonstrates varying degrees of villous atrophy (Fig. 6.124). Enterocytes lack significant cellular abnormalities. Gastric metaplasia may develop (252). Rarely, patients exhibit colonic lesions resembling those seen in the small bowel. These patients have a T-cell lymphoma as discussed further in Chapter 18.

DRUG EFFECTS

Drugs affect small intestinal structure and function in many ways. They may act as direct mucosal toxins, inhibit mucosal enzymes, interfere with micelle formation, alter the physicochemical state of dietary ions or other drugs, cause ischemia, alter bowel motility by interfering with neural transmission or blocking receptor sites, and produce structural alterations. Drug injuries result from the drugs themselves or from byproducts of food–drug interactions.

Drugs that Inhibit Intestinal Transport or Cause Malabsorption

Drugs associated with malabsorption include arsenic, biguanides, methotrexate, methyldopa, azathioprine, and neomycin (253,254). Neomycin induces villous clubbing, brush border fragmentation, microvillous loss, lamina propria inflammation, and ballooning degeneration. Micelle disruption and decreased pancreatic lipase leads to malabsorption. Some progestational agents cause crypt atrophy of the hypoplastic type, resulting in an immaturity of the intestinal epithelium and giving rise to secondary malabsorption. Alcohol causes both mucosal and microvascular injury (255). It directly damages the crypts and villi, leading to malabsorption. Cyclamates cause reversible malabsorption. Histologically, the bowel is inflamed and shows crypt hypoplasia and slight villous atrophy and goblet cell depletion. Erythromycin produces diarrhea, increases GI motor activity, and inhibits intestinal absorption. Colchicine given regularly causes steatorrhea, megaloblastic anemia, and abnormal xylose absorption (256). Chemotherapeutic agents may induce lactose intolerance (257).

The eosinophilia-myalgia syndrome (EMS) usually follows ingestion of L-tryptophan. Patients present with profound eosinophilia, an abnormal hepatic profile, and myalgia. Some patients develop a connective tissue disease that resembles scleroderma (258) with dysmotility and diarrhea. GI involvement leads to significant malabsorption with steatorrhea, hypoalbuminemia, and weight loss. Diffuse eosinophilic infiltrates occur in the small bowel, stomach, and colon (259). The differential diagnosis of the GI eosinophilia usually includes parasitic infection, lymphomas, polyarteritis nodosa, allergic gastroenteritis, eosinophilic gastroenteritis, systemic mastocytosis, and Crohn disease.

Drugs Causing Vasculitis or Inhibiting Intestinal Blood Flow

Cyclosporine therapy following renal transplantation causes generalized microvascular small intestinal disease (260). High concentrations of potassium salts and hydrochlorothiazide cause venous smooth muscle spasm, producing ischemic ulcers, fibrosis, and strictures. Ingestion of oral contraceptives predisposes to superior mesenteric vein thrombosis. Ergotamine-induced vasoconstriction leads to small intestinal ulceration. Cocaine abuse results in bowel ischemia by blocking the reuptake of released norepinephrine and causing vasoconstriction and decreased blood flow. Patients experience sudden crampy abdominal pain and bloody diarrhea. Severe and prolonged ischemic episodes eventually result in bowel necrosis, perforation, peritonitis, or abscess formation. A different form of cocaine damage occurs in the so-called cocaine body packer syndrome. Body packers, or "mules," ingest multiple small drug packets, which may rupture and cause death. Cocaine can also leak out from semipermeable wrappings to be absorbed through the mucosa (261).

Antineoplastic Agents and Antiproliferative Agents

Antineoplastic drugs often induce anorexia, diarrhea, and small intestinal morphologic changes secondary to massive cell death in the proliferative compartment. Cell death becomes apparent as apoptoses within an hour; the number of dead cells peaks within the first 8 hours (262). The dead cells or dead cell fragments are phagocytosed by neighboring healthy enterocytes and mucosal macrophages (263). Antineoplastic drugs also decrease crypt mitotic rate, villous height, and villous width. The morphologic changes superficially resemble those present in celiac disease. The epithelium becomes mucin depleted. Surface epithelial cells become foamy, brush borders are lost, and the enlarged pleomorphic nuclei contain prominent nucleoli. After a few days, lymphocytes and eosinophils infiltrate the lamina propria. In cases of severe damage, all crypts are affected and frank erosions or ulcers develop. Regeneration, recognizable by a burst in mitotic activity and marked variation in nuclear size, follows therapy cessation. Mitoses are present at all levels of the mucosa, even on the villous surface. These changes usually occur within 2 weeks, but inflammation and telangiectasia persist for up to a month. Megaloblastic nuclei develop in patients with vitamin B_{12} or folate deficiency, particularly in patients on extended chemotherapeutic protocols (Fig. 6.125). Patients treated with adjuvant CTLA-4 monoclonal antibodies develop an autoimmune panarteritis that is characterized by aphthous ulcers, larger ulcers, intraepithelial lymphocytosis in the crypt bases, increased apoptoses, and a mononuclear cell infiltrate in the lamina propria (264).

Duodenal lesions may complicate the hepatic artery infusion therapy typically used to treat primary or metastatic

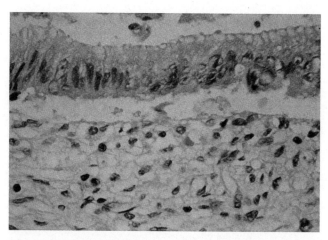

FIG. 6.125. Megaloblastic changes in a patient with cancer who received long-term chemotherapy.

liver tumors. The lesions consist of large solitary ulcers or polypoid inflammatory areas that cause a characteristic striking structural distortion and cellular pleomorphism. The changes affect the epithelium, stroma, and endothelial cells.

Nonsteroidal Anti-Inflammatory Drugs

NSAIDs cause various small intestinal lesions (Table 6.10) (265). Sixty to seventy percent of patients develop an enteropathy associated with bleeding and protein loss. Patients most at risk for the development of intestinal disease are the elderly and those who have had prior GI abnormalities while on NSAIDs (266). Even in control populations, endoscopic abnormalities develop within 2 weeks of the start of NSAID therapy (267). The development of NSAID enteropathy is a multistep process involving biochemical and subcellular organelle damage, followed by a relatively nonspecific tissue reaction. There is increased intestinal permeability in most patients. It also likely involves decreased mucosal blood flow and prostaglandin levels and diminished neutrophil function (265), all of which can interfere with mucosal barrier integrity. NSAIDs also induce dose-dependent drug–enterocyte adducts (268). These

TABLE 6.10 NSAID-induced Small Intestinal Lesions

Aggravates duodenal peptic ulcer disease
Diaphragm (strictures)
Ulcers
Perforation
Bleeding
NSAID enteropathy
  Protein-losing enteropathy
  Bile acid malabsorption
Enhanced intestinal permeability
NSAID, nonsteroidal anti-inflammatory drug

relationships are modified in each patient by specific host responses, drug dose, route of administration, choice of drug, and concomitant consumption of aspirin, alcohol, and other drugs. The nonselective cyclooxygenase (COX) inhibitors such as indomethacin or naproxen are more likely to cause intestinal damage than the more recently introduced selective COX-2 inhibitors (269).

In the duodenum, the drugs cause erosions, ulcers, and nonspecific inflammation. If *H. pylori* is present, the effects may be additive. Distal erosions, ulcers, and strictures may be seen at the time of endoscopy (270). Multiple mucosal diaphragmatic strictures, also known as *mucosal diaphragm disease,* are now thought to be pathognomonic for NSAID injury. Circumferential linear ulcers may be the precursors to the diaphragms. Smaller ulcers often surround larger ones. Three patterns of diaphragmlike strictures exist: (a) extreme exaggeration of the normal plica circularis in which delicate, elongated folds composed of minimally eroded mucosa, muscularis mucosae, and submucosa containing dense collagen bundles obstruct the lumen; (b) broad-based rigid strictures consisting of dome-shaped accumulations of hyalinized collagen occupying the submucosa and interdigitating with the muscularis mucosae; and (c) conventional flat strictures. The mucosa may show nonspecific inflammation, mucosal eosinophilia, increased numbers of intraepithelial lymphocytes, and increased numbers of apoptoses in the crypt bases. In patients who have had ulcers, there may be areas of pyloric metaplasia underlying a distorted and chronically damaged mucosa.

Immunosuppressive Agents

Patients on immunosuppressive therapies experience various GI complications, some of which have an ischemic basis. Ulceration and hemorrhage, with superimposed infection and perforation, also occur. *Indomethacin* inhibits mucosal bicarbonate production and causes localized ulcers, intestinal perforations, and tissue eosinophilia. Villous necrosis, hemorrhage, and neutrophilic infiltration also develop. This predisposes the duodenal mucosa to peptic ulceration and to enhanced bacterial translocation. *Corticosteroids* deplete lymphoid tissues, including gut-associated lymphoid tissues. Lymphoid follicles and domes decrease in size. The dome epithelium develops focal small erosions with M-cell necrosis (271). The follicular regions of Peyer patches become severely B-cell depleted. These histologic effects have a profound impact on the mucosal immune response and host resistance to microbial infections because of the important role played by M cells in mucosal defense.

Heavy Metals

Clinical features of heavy metal toxicity include nausea, vomiting, abdominal cramps, and severe, watery, bloody diarrhea. *Iron* damages the intestinal tract after prolonged contact and may cause intestinal perforation. Other heavy metals, including cadmium, mercury, and zirconium, cause degenerative changes. *Gold* produces enterocolitis, deep ulcers, and tissue eosinophilia (see Chapter 13). *Lead* causes small bowel toxicity by modifying the biochemical properties of the enterocyte surface coat, which then leads to microvillous damage (272). *Aluminum* toxicity occurs at low levels of ingestion. Patients develop enteropathy, encephalopathy, bone disease, and anemia (273). *Cadmium* toxicity results in a decrease in the number of Paneth cells; those that remain appear vacuolated (274).

Other Drug- and Chemical-Induced Injuries

Enterocolitis may complicate the use of *levetiracetam* in patients with refractory epilepsy (275). The use of *povidone iodine* for peritoneal lavage may result in sclerosing encapsulating peritonitis (276). Intestinal hematomas may complicate the use of anticoagulants (277). *Clofazimine* used to treat leprosy may cause a crystal-storing histiocytosis that may mimic hematologic malignancies. The crystals appear red on frozen sections and they show a bright red birefringence (278).

FOOD-ASSOCIATED ILLNESSES

Patients with food-related complaints pose a diagnostic challenge to their physicians because it is often difficult to document the underlying nature of the offending agent(s). Patients tend to report vague symptoms that are often chronic and delayed in onset. The patients generally fall into several distinct clinical groups: (a) patients with IgE-dependent mediated hypersensitivity allergic reactions, (b) patients who consume infected foods, (c) patients who consume food containing metals or toxins, and (d) infants on certain formulas.

Infants who receive hydrolysate formulas may develop necrotizing enterocolitis. This formula activates intestinal mast cells, thereby stimulating local immune mechanisms and inflammatory cells and increasing epithelial permeability (279). The mucosa becomes infiltrated with chronic inflammatory cells. Certain food additives induce GI disease via allergic reactions. Yellow dye No. 6, an artificial coloring found in candy, foods, and many drugs, serves as a GI allergen and results in allergic gastroenteritis with mucosal infiltration by large numbers of eosinophils (280,281).

Heavy metal intoxication may occur when foods are stored or cooked in tin, antimony, or copper containers. Patients develop GI symptoms, including diarrhea. Patients who consume poisonous mushrooms develop GI symptoms 1 to 8 hours following their consumption. Rapid-acting toxins usually affect a patient within 1 hour, and patients develop diarrhea and abdominal pain. Patients often remember consuming food with a metallic taste.

Seafood Neurotoxins

There are three similar syndromes produced by neurotoxins ingested in seafood: *Paralytic shellfish disease, ciguatera,* and *puffer-fish intoxication*. The neurotoxins are produced by dinoflagellates, the marine algae responsible for red tides (282). The toxins block voltage-gated sodium channels in myelinated and nonmyelinated nerves. These disorders are often misdiagnosed and attributed to fish allergies, gastroenteritis, or nonspecific neurologic disorders. *Paralytic shellfish poisoning* results from ingestion of bivalve mollusks (mussels, clams, oysters, and scallops) that contain toxins produced by the *Gonyaulax* species of dinoflagellates. GI symptoms include nausea, vomiting, abdominal pain, and diarrhea. *Ciguatera* is the most common fish-borne illness worldwide and is the most common type of nonbacterial food poisoning reported in the United States. Ciguatera follows consumption of fish, oysters, or clams. GI symptoms occur within the first 3 to 6 hours and include nausea, watery diarrhea, vomiting, and abdominal pain. It results from toxin or toxins produced by the dinoflagellate *Gambierdiscus toxicus*. *Puffer-fish intoxication* occurs within 4 to 10 hours of ingesting toxin-contaminated seafood. The toxins in these related disorders cause severe congestion of the villous and submucosal vessels with red cell extravasation into the lamina propria. Degeneration of microvilli also develops followed by localized desquamation of cells from the villous tips.

Scombroid Poisoning

The highest morbidity worldwide from fish poisoning results from ingestion of spoiled scombroid fish such as tuna, mackerel, and jacks. The syndrome is produced by Gram-negative enteric bacteria usually of the *Proteus* or *Klebsiella* species with decarboxylate histidine-producing saurine, a histaminelike substance (283). The scombroid toxins represent metabolic byproducts of bacterial degradation of fish flesh (284). GI symptoms include nausea, diarrhea, and, less commonly, vomiting. The diagnosis is made clinically, and there are no specific laboratory tests to diagnose the disorder. Affected patients invariably report a metallic, sharp, or peppery taste of the consumed fish.

Bacterial Food-Borne Diseases

Many food-related disorders result from the consumption of infected foods as discussed in a later section.

THERMAL INJURY

Erosive duodenitis and duodenal ulcers develop in severely burned patients (Fig. 6.126). The inflammatory lesions have an ischemic basis and their pathophysiology resembles that seen in stress ulcers. Gastroduodenal erosions occur within 5 hours of injury (285). Within the first 24 hours the mucosal

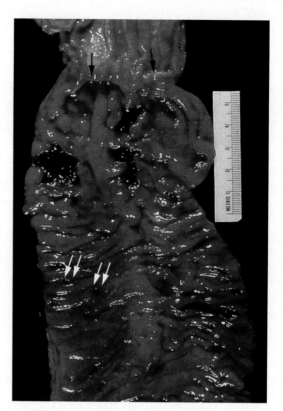

FIG. 6.126. Curling ulcers in a patient who was caught in a house fire. The *arrows* mark the gastroduodenal junction. Several large geographic ulcers are present within the duodenum, as evidenced by the dark, irregular, geographic areas. Additionally, smaller punctate ulcers (*double arrows*) are present. The duodenal mucosa also demonstrates marked hyperemia.

barrier breaks down, mediated in part by transient intestinal hypoperfusion and increased intestinal permeability. Early ischemia results in enterocyte membrane disruption. Bacterial and luminal endotoxins gain access to the systemic circulation. Another form of thermal injury occurs in GI gunshot wounds. Coagulation necrosis develops along the bullet path, due to the heat.

RADIATION INJURY

The small intestine is more sensitive to radiation injury than is the large intestine. The degree of radiation damage reflects many factors (Table 6.11) (286). Patients who receive radiation often have acute but temporary diarrhea, nausea, vomiting, and abdominal cramps. These symptoms usually subside within weeks, due to rapid mucosal regeneration. A small percentage of patients experience a chronic deteriorating disease course, referred to as *severe late radiation enteropathy*. It is characterized by diarrhea, pain, malabsorption, small bowel obstruction, acute or chronic GI bleeding, intestinal perforation, and pseudo-obstruction. The intestinal pseudo-obstruction develops secondary to neuromuscular damage, vascular obliteration, and intestinal wall fibrosis (286).

TABLE 6.11	Factors that Enhance Radiation Injury

Radiation doses given ≥45,000 rads
The way radiation is given (accelerated fractionation increases the incidence of late radiation enteropathy)
Presence of other disease
    Diabetes
    Hypertension
    Severe atherosclerosis
    Previous intestinal injury
    Cardiovascular disease
Prior surgery
Prior radiation
Adriamycin and other chemotherapeutic affects
An empty intestinal lumen during radiation therapy

The severity of the acute radiation enteritis determines the severity of subsequent chronic disease. The outcome is mediated by mucosal and vascular damage as well as by host defenses to intraluminal antigens and pathogens. The damage is usually most severe in those parts of the small intestine that are fixed because this part of the gut receives a constant maximal radiation dose. Therefore, the duodenum, proximal jejunum, and terminal ileum are most likely to show maximum damage.

Patients with acute ischemic damage have an intestinal mucosa that appears reddened and inflamed, with edema and fibrinous peritonitis. The serosa acquires a matte-white appearance as serosal adhesions develop. Eventually the bowel appears markedly thickened, fibrotic, and indurated with stricture formation (Fig. 6.127). The bowel proximal to the strictures distends. The abnormal bowel merges imperceptibly with the noninjured bowel, making it difficult to identify the exact junction of the injured and uninjured bowel.

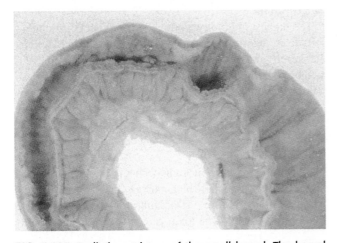

FIG. 6.127. Radiation stricture of the small bowel. The bowel superficially resembles Crohn disease (CD), except for the fact that the bowel wall is not as thickened as commonly seen in patients with CD and the specimen lacks creeping fat.

Acute radiation effects are predominantly mucosal in nature and range from mild epithelial degeneration to massive intestinal necrosis and ulceration. Endothelial apoptosis is the primary lesion initiating the bowel damage. Vascular damage ranges from isolated endothelial cell injury to complete capillary and venule obliteration. Capillary endothelium swells and the vessels become telangiectatic. Increases in vascular permeability immediately following radiation lead to edema and fibrin deposition in the interstitial spaces and blood vessel walls. The vascular damage leads to epithelial stem cell dysfunction (287).

The acute epithelial changes vary in severity. In some cases, one sees little damage, whereas in others, frank ulceration develops. Morphologic changes include loss of the columnar shape and nuclear polarity of enterocytes, epithelial degeneration, mucosal epithelial denudation, nuclear pyknosis and karyorrhexis, crypt disintegration, mucosal edema (Fig. 6.128), enlarged bizarre nuclei, absent mitoses, mucin depletion, prominent apoptoses in the crypt bases, and crypt abscesses with prominent eosinophilic infiltrates. The decreased mitotic activity occurs early and persists for at least 72 hours following the radiation event. Because of the decreased mitotic activity, there is no cellular migration from the crypt bases to replace cells lost from the mucosal surface. This results in surface erosions, ulcerations, and mucosal atrophy. Paneth cells are often unusually prominent. There is also a relative increase in the number of endocrine cells. Whether this represents a true hyperplasia or an apparent increase in endocrine cells due to endocrine cell sparing from the radiation remains unclear. The lamina propria becomes depleted of lymphocytes and is infiltrated by neutrophils. Later other chronic inflammatory cells appear. Because the mechanisms of radiation injury resemble those seen in ischemia and reperfusion injury, it is not surprising that the histologic features of both ischemia and acute radiation injury overlap. After 7 to 10 days of therapy the epithelial surface may be reduced by up to 40%.

Following the radiation injury there is an increase in the proliferative activity in the crypts, a process regulated in part by increased expression of EGF and TGF-α and -β (288). Areas of villous hypertrophy may surround localized ulcers. Complete structural recovery usually occurs within 2 to 3 weeks of cessation of the therapy but villous atrophy and abnormal crypts may persist, resulting in subclinical malabsorption. Distorted villi and ulcerations are characteristic of advanced injury.

TGF-β is produced by the epithelium, inflammatory cells, fibroblasts, endothelium, and smooth muscle cells and contributes to the generation of chronic radiation enteropathy (289). Chronic radiation enteropathy is a progressive disease resulting from the underlying vascular damage that develops months to years following the radiation event. Characteristic changes include fibrosis and hyalinization of the submucosal and serosal connective tissues, the presence of telangiectasia, and hyalinized blood vessels with subendothelial foam cells and mucosal damage (Fig. 6.129). Numerous enlarged,

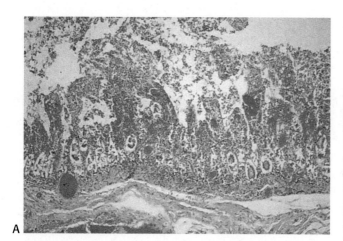

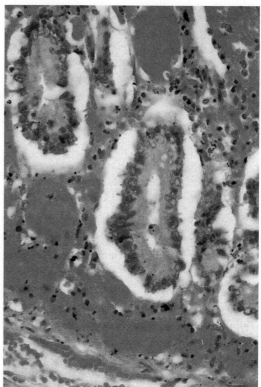

FIG. 6.128. Acute radiation damage. **A:** The mucosa appears hemorrhagic, necrotic, and telangiectatic. The villi are being sloughed. **B:** High-power magnification demonstrates the severe hemorrhagic necrosis involving the lamina propria. If one did not have the history of radiation, the features could be interpreted as being ischemic in nature. They share a common pathophysiology (see text).

atypical mesenchymal cells with bizarre hyperchromatic nuclei lie scattered throughout the fibrotic submucosa and serosa. These "swallow-tailed" or "radiation fibroblasts" contain abnormal nuclei, sometimes simulating nuclear inclusions. Muscular arteries develop marked intimal thickening with fibrosis and luminal narrowing that leads to endarteritis obliterans. Smaller vessels exhibit marked hyaline sclerosis and obliterative vasculitis. Progressive vascular damage, with increasing intimal fibrosis, leads to ischemia. Complications of the ischemia include ulcers, strictures, perforation, fistulae, malabsorption, and pseudo-obstruction.

Other changes include atrophy of the muscularis propria with interstitial fibrosis. Fibrosis and parenchymal atrophy subsequently replace the tissues and are characteristic of late phases of the disease. Epithelial displacement into the submucosa produces *enteritis cystica profunda*. Lymphangiectasia results from lymphatic obstruction, presumably due to the submucosal fibrosis. Neuronal proliferation, altered ganglia, and muscular changes are prominent in patients who present with pseudo-obstruction (290). The abnormal motility may facilitate bacterial colonization of the bowel (291). In addition, strictures predispose to intestinal

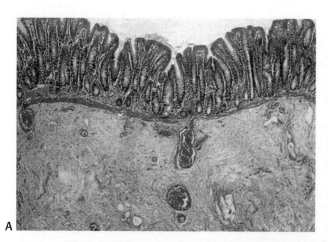

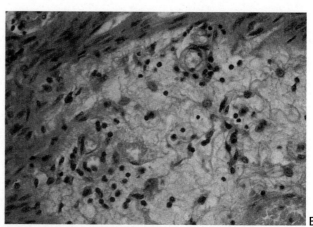

FIG. 6.129. Chronic radiation damage. **A:** The mucosal surface appears mildly distorted. The submucosa is markedly thickened and fibrotic. **B:** High-power magnification demonstrates the presence of small vessels, a fibrotic submucosa, and atypical fibroblasts.

stasis and the blind loop syndrome. These effects may be augmented in patients with hypochlorhydria secondary to the effects of gastric radiation injury and in those who are partially immunosuppressed by concomitant chemotherapy.

Because of the important role played by TGF-β overexpression in the induction of the chronic damage, the chronic changes may be preventable by the use of interferon treatment (292). Prophylactic use of EGF may also reduce ischemic injury (293). Additionally, the endothelial cell damage can be prevented by treatment with basic fibroblast growth factor (287).

INFECTIOUS DISEASES

Mechanisms of Bacterial Injury

Numerous factors predispose to microbial intestinal colonization and contribute to diarrhea, malnutrition, sepsis, and extraintestinal infections. Vigorous peristaltic forward propulsion of intestinal contents into the colon discourages bacterial colonization. This peristaltic defense is enhanced by

TABLE 6.12	Mechanisms of Bacterial Pathogenicity in Small Intestinal Injury

Ingestion of preformed bacterial enzyme or toxin (i.e., *Staphylococcus*)
Elaboration of an enterotoxin following gastrointestinal colonization (i.e., *Cholera, Shigella, Salmonella, Yersinia*)
Elaboration of a tissue-damaging cytotoxin (i.e., *Shigella*)
Mucosal invasion (i.e., *Shigella, Salmonella*)

the continuously secreted mucous layer that bathes the mucosal surface and mechanically prevents organisms from contacting enterocyte surfaces and adhering to them. Pancreatic enzymes in the intestinal lumen degrade bacterial toxins. Bacterial enteropathogens possess several distinct virulence properties (Table 6.12). The specific bacterial virulence pattern determines the way it interacts with the intestinal mucosa and influences the clinical syndromes that result.

Since *bacterial adherence* to epithelial cells is an important prerequisite for intestinal colonization and virulence (Fig. 6.130), bacteria have developed several mechanisms to attach

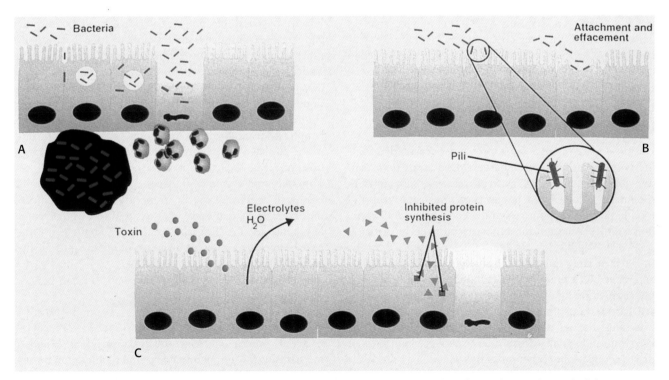

FIG. 6.130. Bacterial interactions with intestinal mucosa. **A:** Bacteria may directly invade into the epithelial cells or the intercellular junctions to become enclosed within phagocytic vesicles, where they multiply. Eventually, when a critical number of organisms are present, the cell lyses, reinitiating the process. Some bacteria pass directly into the underlying lymphoid follicle, where they are sequestered and multiply. The lysis of the cells attracts an inflammatory infiltrate, usually consisting of neutrophils. **B:** Bacteria may also attach directly to the epithelium without invading the enterocytes. They do this either by attaching via pili that recognize specific receptors on the enterocyte membranes or they produce attaching and effacing lesions. **C:** Bacteria also produce some of their effects by producing toxins. The two major groups of toxins either cause increased electrolyte and water secretion (represented by the *circles*) as exemplified by cholera toxin or inhibit protein synthesis leading to cellular death, as indicated by the *triangles*.

to enterocytes (294). Enterocyte adherence results from specific interactions between a ligand expressed on the bacterial surface (sometimes called an adhesin) and a receptor on the epithelial cell surface (295). Various bacteria produce plasmid-encoded adhesive pili that radiate from the bacterial surface and recognize specific glycoconjugates on mucosal cells (296). Other bacteria attach to epithelial cells in such a way that the outer membrane of the enterocyte appears to wrap around it. This gives the impression that the bacterium is perched on an enterocyte pedestal. *Bacterial toxins* interact with receptors on the enterocytes surfaces and activate cellular signal transduction mechanisms, causing fluid and electrolyte secretion and toxigenic diarrhea.

Bacterial translocation implies the passage of viable bacteria from the gastrointestinal lumen through the mucosa to distant sites, such as mesenteric lymph nodes, spleen, liver, kidney, and blood (296). Mechanisms inducing bacterial translocation include disruption of the normal ecologic microbial balance with overgrowth of Gram-negative enteric bacilli, impaired host defenses, and physical disruption of the mucosal barrier. Some invasive bacteria cross the intestinal barrier via M cells (296). Others enter cells and remain trapped inside phagocytic vacuoles, where they utilize antiphagocytic strategies to continue to multiply and resist cellular defense mechanisms (297). Still others, such as *Shigella,* escape from phagocytic vacuoles to invade the cytoplasmic compartment. The pathogens then pass from cell to cell.

Epidemiologic Settings in which Infections Occur

Diarrheal diseases are a global problem, particularly affecting populations living in underdeveloped areas. Both children and immunologically naive travelers are susceptible to the enteric pathogens that heavily contaminate the water and food in places with poor sanitation. Food-borne and water-borne illnesses account for significant numbers of diarrheal outbreaks worldwide. The pathogenic bacteria must be ingested in large numbers to cause clinical disease. Food- and water-borne illnesses develop not only in countries with poor sanitation, but also on cruise ships, at picnics, and at fast-food restaurants. Diarrheal illnesses also lead the list of infectious diseases that affect the military. Travelers of all ages from industrialized countries experience high rates of diarrheal illness and other infections when they visit developing tropical areas (298). Regional differences in the consumption of unpasteurized milk or raw or undercooked fish, shellfish, or meat increase the risk of certain bacterial, parasitic, and viral infections. Mass production of eggs also plays a role in bacterial enterocolitis. Globalization of the food supply also increases the opportunity for widespread food contamination. Table 13.11 lists factors that should trigger suspicion of widespread food contamination. Diarrheal illnesses are also increasing in daycare centers, hospitals, and extended-care facilities. Nosocomial diarrhea is particularly prevalent in intensive care units and pediatric wards, and is an increasingly difficult problem for bedridden patients and their caregivers.

The synthesis of large numbers of antibiotics over the past several decades has resulted in increased bacterial antibiotic resistance (299). The emergence of drug-resistant bacterial strains has contributed significantly to the increase in nosocomial infections (300). Increased international travel offers new opportunities for outbreaks and plagues to develop, and offers opportunities for the genesis of new bacterial genetic variations (301). Finally, the increased frequency of immune deficiencies, whether from AIDS, immunosuppressive therapy, aging, or other alterations, places patients at risk for life-threatening infections.

Patterns of Gastrointestinal Infection

Most diarrheal illnesses are noninflammatory, usually arising in the upper small bowel from the action of an enterotoxin or other process that specifically alters the absorptive function of the villous tip. Patients with toxigenic bacterial infections present with dysenteric syndromes characterized by fever, abdominal pain, and numerous small-volume stools containing blood, mucus, and neutrophils. In contrast, patients with invasive bacterial infections usually have a colonic infection and diarrhea dominates the clinical picture. Neutrophilic mucosal infiltrates are the hallmark of acute invasive disease. Toxigenic organisms tend to produce less severe morphologic damage than invasive bacteria. Another type of enteric infection results in enteric fever, often with constipation early in its course. The organisms enter Peyer patches and regional lymph nodes and then become systemic infections, returning to the gut later. In order to establish the diagnosis of infectious diarrhea, the organism must be found in, or cultured from, the stool or intestinal tissues. Alternatively, one should be able to demonstrate a rise in specific serum antibodies to the organism. With the advent of recombinant DNA technology, genes for the heat-labile and heat-stable enterotoxins have been cloned, allowing diagnosis of the toxin-producing bacterial strains.

Bacterial Overgrowth Syndromes (Blind Loop Syndromes)

Bacterial overgrowth leads to malabsorption. Proposed mechanisms for the abnormal bacterial proliferation include (a) failure to clear bacteria from the upper GI tract, usually due to achlorhydria; (b) continuous seeding of the small bowel with colonic contents as a result of jejunal-colic fistulae or reflux following abnormalities of the ileocecal valve; and (c) motility disturbances. The diagnosis of bacterial overgrowth relies on three criteria: (a) presence of an increased intestinal volume, (b) demonstration of increased bacterial concentrations, and (c) a positive response to antibiotic therapy. Multiple conditions predispose to bacterial overgrowth (Table 6.13).

TABLE 6.13	Conditions Predisposing to Bacterial Infection and Overgrowths	
Strictures (congenital, radiation, tuberculosis, Crohn disease, vascular)	Immunodeficiency states	
Small intestinal stagnation	Entities that destroy mucosal barrier function	
Afferent loop of Billroth II partial gastrectomy	Drugs	
Duodenal diverticula	Alcohol	
Small intestinal diverticulosis	Radiation	
Surgical blind loops (end-to-side anastomoses)	Infections	
Surgical recirculating loops (end-to-end anastomoses)	Ischemia	
Multiple laparotomies resulting in adhesions	Toxemia	
Obstructions	Thermal injury	
Intestinal pseudo-obstruction	Hypothyroidism	
Inflammatory lesions	Pancreatic insufficiency	
Tumors	Ileal valve resection	
Ganglionic blockers	Connective tissue disorders	
Amyloidosis	Nodular lymphoid hyperplasia	
Pancreatic insufficiency	Fistulae between bowel loops	

Most mucosal biopsies appear normal, but careful studies eventually demonstrate patchy mild histologic abnormalities that are easily missed by a single random biopsy or are so mildly abnormal as to be easily overlooked. In severe cases, one sees a spectrum of changes ranging from patchy, villous broadening and flattening to complete villous atrophy with crypt hyperplasia or hypoplasia. Numerous microorganisms, including bacteria and protozoa, adhere to the mucosa and are embedded in the unstirred mucous layer overlying the epithelium (Fig. 6.131). There is often an increase in the number of lamina propria mononuclear cells.

The recognition of specific pathogens may result from their localization in specific tissue sites, as in the colon (Table 13.12).

Specific Bacterial Infections

Escherichia coli Infections

E. coli bacteria are Gram-negative organisms that constitute part of the normal GI flora. They spread to contiguous structures when the mucosal barrier is damaged. The organisms tend to settle in necrotic tissues. Patients often have decreased host defenses as a result of underlying diseases. Several types of *E. coli* infections exist (Table 6.14) (302). However, they cannot be differentiated from one another on Gram stain or routine culture. The characterization of a strain of *E. coli* as an enteropathogen requires serotyping, tissue culture, immunochemical methods, or DNA hybridization studies, techniques that are not always routinely available.

Enteropathogenic E. coli (EPEC) account for outbreaks of severe fatal diarrhea in newborns (303), are a major bacterial cause of dehydrating infant diarrhea in developing areas, and cause traveler's diarrhea. The organism is acquired by ingesting contaminated food or water. Risk factors for death include a young patient age and the virulence of the bacterial

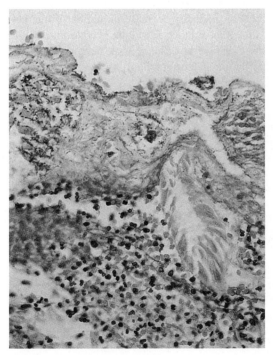

FIG. 6.131. Bacterial overgrowth. Note the presence of prominent collections of bacteria in the pyogenic membrane that was overlying an area of devitalized tissue.

TABLE 6.14	Types of Pathogenic *Escherichia coli*
Enteropathogenic	Attaches to epithelium; mechanism of injury unknown
Enterotoxigenic	Produces toxins that activate adenylate cyclase and guanylate cyclase
Enteroinvasive	Invades colonic epithelium
Enteroadherent	Adheres to brush borders and destroys microvilli; no invasion; rare villous atrophy
Enterohemorrhagic	Mechanism of action unknown

strain. Almost all deaths occur before age 2. The organisms are not invasive; nor do they produce toxins. They colonize the proximal small intestine via specific attachment mechanisms, producing characteristic attachment–effacement lesions on the enterocyte plasma membrane. Because EPEC colonizes the duodenum, it can be detected by culturing duodenal aspirates (304).

Enterohemorrhagic E. coli (EHEC) cause hemorrhagic colitis, hemolytic uremia syndrome, and thrombotic thrombocytic purpura; they are discussed in Chapter 13.

Enteroadherent E. coli are nontoxigenic and does not invade the mucosa (302). They avidly adhere to the epithelial brush border via specific receptors (Fig. 6.132). Often the histology of the small intestine in infected individuals is normal. Children with this infection develop chronic prolonged diarrhea (305). Rarely, villous atrophy results. The lesions may resemble celiac disease.

Enterotoxigenic E. coli (ETEC) elaborate an enterotoxin similar to cholera toxin (306). They represent a major cause of traveler's diarrhea and infant diarrhea in underdeveloped countries. The disease is initiated by consumption of contaminated food or water or by contact with infected persons. Once the bacteria are ingested, they pass to the small bowel, where they colonize the surface epithelium. ETEC adhere to

enterocyte brush borders without damaging them. The adhesion is specific, and pili and fimbrial colonization factor antigens determine host specificity. Once in the small intestine, the bacteria produce two toxins: A heat-labile toxin resembling cholera toxin and a heat-stable toxin that activates guanylate cyclase and stimulates active fluid secretion without injuring the enterocytes (307). The disease often begins with upper intestinal distress followed by watery diarrhea. The clinical course may be extremely mild or very severe, mimicking cholera and producing severe dehydration and rice water stools. Symptoms consist of the sudden onset of abdominal cramps, nausea, borborygmi, and malaise. Acute watery diarrhea then develops, followed by dehydration with low-grade fever and chills.

The presenting symptoms of *enteroinvasive E. coli* (EIEC) infection include diarrhea, tenesmus, fever, and cramps. The organism penetrates and multiplies within epithelial cells. Clinically, most patients manifest watery, nonbloody diarrhea. This organism is unusual in the United States, although it is relatively common in Thailand (308).

Enteroaggregative E. coli (EAEC) have been implicated as an important agents of persistent diarrhea among infants in the developing world and as a cause of traveler's diarrhea. A plasmid encodes the gene for the aggregative adherence

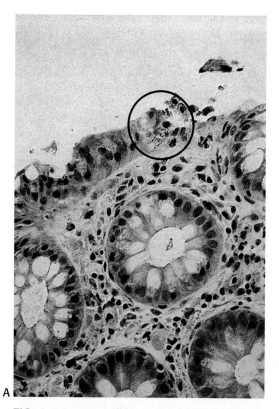 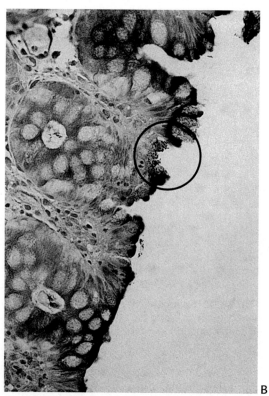

FIG. 6.132. Enteroadherent *Escherichia coli*. **A:** Hematoxylin and eosin–stained section showing bacteria adhering to the surface epithelium in an area of mucosal denudation. The area of epithelial loss with adherent organisms is contained within the *circle*. The underlying lamina propria and crypts appear normal. **B:** Giemsa-stained section showing the presence of attached bacteria in the denuded area. The area of epithelial loss with adherent organisms is contained within the *circle*. (This particular picture is from the colon, but similar lesions occur in the terminal ileum.)

properties of EAEC. Ultrastructurally, one can show that the EAEC strains have four morphologically distinct kinds of fimbriae that mediate cellular adhesion and induce mucosal damage (309). The typical illness presents with a watery mucoid secretory diarrhea with low-grade fever and little or no vomiting. The diarrhea may last for several weeks. The disease is diagnosed by isolating the organism from the stool and the demonstration of an aggregative adherent pattern on HEp-2 assay.

Salmonella *Infections*

Salmonella organisms are Gram-negative bacilli that produce five clinical syndromes: (a) gastroenteritis (70% of infections); (b) bacteremia with or without GI involvement (10%); (c) typhoid or enteric fever; (d) localized infections in joints, bones, and meninges (5%); and (e) an asymptomatic carrier state. Most *Salmonella* species can produce any of these syndromes, but certain serotypes more commonly associate with specific clinical presentations (310). Usually, *Salmonella* causes a mild self-limited illness, but very young, elderly, and immunocompromised patients develop serious complications, sepsis, and death. The disease pattern reflects the inherent bacterial virulence, the number of organisms ingested, their ability to survive and/or replicate, the presence of a normal flora in the upper intestinal tract, and host status. *Salmonella* species are generally divided into typhoid and nontyphoid species.

Infection with *Salmonella typhi* is almost always transmitted person to person (311). Infections with most other *Salmonella* species, except for *Salmonella paratyphi,* derive from environmental sources, principally poultry and livestock. The current rarity of typhoid fever in the United States reflects good hygiene, lack of crowding, and high public standards for home and industrial sewage.

Typhoid fever is spread by contaminated food or water. Humans are the only known reservoir for *S. typhi,* which is transmitted via a fecal–oral route. Its annual incidence in the United States is 0.2 cases per 100,000 population. Higher incidence rates occur in areas with contaminated water supplies and inadequate waste disposal. The usual victims are children and young adults. However, recently a nosocomial outbreak of fluoroquinolone-resistant *Salmonella enterica* was described among elderly individuals in a nursing home (312). Typhoid fever may also be sexually transmitted among men having sex with men (312a).

Patients usually remain relatively asymptomatic during an incubation period of a week followed by a 2- to 3-week period of illness. Then the patients present with fever, abdominal pain, and headache. Abdominal rash, delirium, hepatosplenomegaly, and leucopenia are common. Diarrhea begins in the second and third weeks of the infection. It is watery at first but may become bloody, and perforation may occur. Typhoid fever is a chronic systemic illness with a mortality rate of 15% in untreated individuals and 1% in treated individuals. A prolonged convalescent stage of 3 months is

usual. GI complications include perforation, massive intestinal hemorrhage (4% to 7%), peritonitis, and paralytic ileus (313). Perforation causes death in 25% to 33% of patients who die of the disease (314). If the patient recovers, intestinal lesions heal with minimal fibrosis so that stricture formation is unusual.

Nontyphoid species (*Salmonella enteritidis, Salmonella typhimurium, Salmonella muenchen, Salmonella anatum, S. paratyphi,* and *S. give*) result in a milder, more self-limited gastroenteritis with nausea, vomiting, fever, and watery diarrhea.

Salmonella organisms are facultative intracellular parasites capable of penetrating, invading, surviving, and multiplying in many cells. Plasmids encode the virulence factors involved in adherence to, invasion of, and growth within the epithelium (315). *Salmonella* organisms adhere to M-cell and enterocyte surfaces, where they induce almost complete destruction (316) as described in Chapter 13. When two or more cells are destroyed, the resulting mucosal defect predisposes to deeper infection (317). If bacteria pass between enterocytes, the tight junctions separate and then reseal following bacterial passage. Internalization of *Salmonella* is receptor mediated, possibly involving the epidermal growth factor receptor. Once inside the cells, the bacteria become enclosed by membrane-bound cytoplasmic vacuoles and they then multiply. Following their release from the vacuoles, they disseminate to the regional lymph nodes, spleen, and liver, sites where the bacteria multiply further (316).

Salmonella may infect any part of the gastrointestinal tract, but the ileum, appendix, and right colon are preferentially affected. The bowel wall appears thickened. Swollen, raised, ulcerated Peyer patches produce the typical gross appearance of small, longitudinally oriented (oval) terminal ileal ulcers (Fig. 6.133). Other ulcers appear aphthous, linear, discoid, or full thickness in nature. Ulcers are less prominent in the proximal small bowel. With progressive bowel wall involvement, it becomes paper thin and susceptible to perforation. In some cases, the bowel may appear grossly normal or only mildly erythematous in nature.

Shortened edematous villi contain neutrophilic infiltrates coexisting with crypt hyperplasia. There is marked vascular

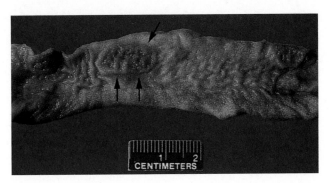

FIG. 6.133. *Salmonella* enteritis. Note the presence of the prominent longitudinal ulcer overlying the Peyer patches (*arrows*).

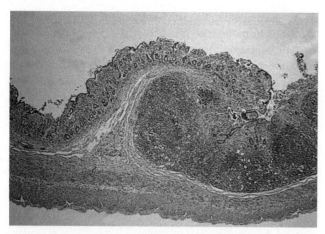

FIG. 6.134. Histologic lesion of the specimen shown in Figure 6.133 showing prominent lymphoid hyperplasia in the Peyer patches surrounded by atrophic small intestine and demonstrating superficial ulceration with surrounding regeneration.

congestion and lymphoplasmacytic infiltrates along with histiocytes with abundant eosinophilic cytoplasm containing nuclear debris and red blood cells. Peyer patches become hyperplastic (Fig. 6.134) followed by acute inflammation of the follicle-associated epithelium. Edema, fibrinous exudates, and vascular thromboses herald the onset of tissue necrosis and ulceration, causing the lymphoid follicles to appear elevated over the mucosal surface (Fig. 6.135). As the follicle-associated epithelium ulcerates, the lymphoid tissue extends from the submucosa to the mucosal surface, discharging large numbers of bacilli into the intestinal lumen. Eventually the lymphoid follicles become infiltrated and obliterated by macrophages. Architectural distortion severe enough to mimic irritable bowel disease (IBD) may be present.

The proliferation of monocytic elements is arranged in both a diffuse and nodular pattern. The nodular areas lie at the periphery of the lesions and the diffuse proliferations are in the center. The nodules are of two types. One contains a germinal center and consists of a mixture of centrocytes, centroblasts, and macrophages surrounded by a ragged compressed mantle zone. The second and predominant type of nodule consists of uniform sheets of monocytes/macrophages, many containing numerous apoptotic bodies and cellular debris rimmed by small lymphocytes. Some of these areas may contain foci of amorphous eosinophilic debris and cells with peripherally displaced nuclei. The interfollicular and diffuse areas are dominated by phagocytic macrophages with a round to irregular (occasionally crescenteric) shape and also contain intermingled small, mature-appearing lymphocytes. Occasional plasma cells and immunoblasts are also present. Neutrophils are surprisingly rare, even in the areas of ulceration. This inflammatory reaction extends into the muscularis propria and may even reach the serosa. Small mucosal erosions in areas of nonthickened bowel wall also consist of lymphoid infiltrates with germinal center formation and clusters of monocytes/macrophages, likely representing the early lesions (318).

The regional lymph nodes may show a necrotizing lymphadenitis and a marked sinusoidal and paracortical expansion due to a proliferation of monocytes/macrophages identical to those present in the involved bowel segments. Subcapsular sinuses are distended by monocytes in many areas and compressed or obliterated centrally. Actively phagocytic macrophages are present, many of which contain apoptotic fragments. The necrotic areas are rounded rather than stellate in shape and are rimmed by foamy macrophages that blend smoothly with the cellularity in the remainder of the lymph node (318).

The closest mimic of these changes are induced by *Yersinia* infections. Both diseases center around the ileocecal region and both the mucosa and the regional lymph nodes are distorted by lymphoid and histiocytic hyperplasia.

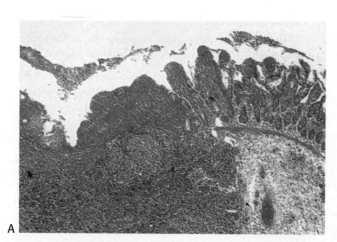

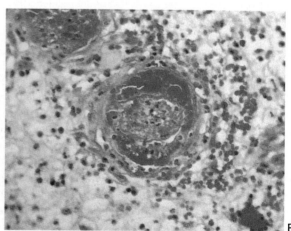

FIG. 6.135. *Salmonella* enteritis. **A:** The area overlying the Peyer patches is intensely inflamed, congested, and ulcerated. Part of the damage results from ischemia due to the presence of small thrombi in the specimen, such as that illustrated in B. Intense inflammation with ulceration of the mucosa. **B:** Thrombosed blood vessel in submucosal bowel.

However, penetrating ulcers and epithelioid granulomas only occur in *Yersinia* and the areas of necrosis in *Yersinia* are usually stellate in shape rather than being rounded.

Staphylococcal Infections

Staphylococcal food poisoning is an explosive but self-limited gastroenteritis associated with food poisoning. Staphylococci cause acute diarrheal disease by their ability to produce exotoxins that act as potent enterotoxins. In severe cases, patients have nonspecific enterocolitis with intense mucosal congestion, necrosis, and ulceration (319). Viable bacteria are absent.

Campylobacter *Infections*

Campylobacter species are spiral and highly motile Gram-negative rods. Numerous species exist within the genus *Campylobacter,* although classically only three are pathogenic for humans: *Campylobacter jejuni, Campylobacter coli,* and *Campylobacter fetus.* The frequency of the different *Campylobacter* infections differs from one country to another. *Campylobacter* is one of the most frequently isolated enteric stool pathogens. In one study it was found in 134 cases per 100,000 persons with diarrhea (320). The incidence in the United States is highest in children under 1 year of age and in persons 10 to 29 years of age (321). Because the disorder affects young adults, the initial clinical picture is easily confused with ulcerative colitis or Crohn disease. Water-borne outbreaks of *Campylobacter* enteritis associate with municipal water systems and with surface water. *C. jejuni* is a common cause of traveler's diarrhea and of diarrheal illnesses suffered by hikers who drink untreated water in mountainous areas. Currently, Rocky Mountain *Campylobacter* enteritis occurs three times more frequently than does giardiasis (322). The disease incidence is highest in the summer. Outbreaks also associate with consumption of contaminated milk, meat, poultry, and vegetables (323); person-to-person transmission; and transmission from pets. Infected chickens currently account for 70% of disease risk (323).

Campylobacter produces several disease patterns: (a) asymptomatic infections, (b) acute enteritis, and (c) acute colitis; the disease pattern reflects the type of organism infecting the patient. For example, *C. jejuni* is more likely to cause an acute self-limited gastroenteritis, whereas *C. fetus* causes systemic illnesses that are often fatal. Acute enteritis is the most common presentation. The incubation period between organism ingestion and symptom onset ranges from 1 to 7 days. A typical episode begins with fever and malaise followed within 24 hours by nausea, vomiting, abdominal pain, and diarrhea. Enlarged mesenteric lymph nodes become symptomatic in some patients (324). Grossly bloody stools are common, and many patients have at least 1 day with eight or more bowel movements. Headache and myalgia, which tend to be more severe than in other forms of infective enterocolitis, develop in some patients. Severe com-

plications, including sepsis, meningitis, toxic megacolon, pseudomembranous colitis, massive GI hemorrhage, arthritis, endocarditis, and genital and urinary infections, affect debilitated individuals. However, the illness is usually self-limited. Twenty percent of patients experience a relapse. The organism also causes death (325), especially in immunocompromised persons. A complication of *Campylobacter* infection is the Guillain-Barré syndrome. It results from cross-reactivity between neural and *C. jejuni* antigens (326). Most patients recover fully from their infections, either spontaneously or after antibiotic therapy.

Campylobacter enterocyte adhesion is critical to the development of the enteritis. When the organisms invade the cell surface, the epithelium becomes damaged and bacteria invade the cells. The organism also produces toxins that bind to specific receptors on cell membranes, damaging the cells (327).

Endoscopic features of *Campylobacter* infections include patchy mucosal inflammation, hyperemia, bloody exudates, segmental mucosal edema, loss of a normal vascular pattern, and ulceration. The changes mimic inflammatory bowel disease. Grossly, one sees a diffuse, bloody, edematous enterocolitis with multiple, superficial ileal ulcers measuring up to 1 cm in diameter just proximal to the ileocecal valve and involving the valve itself. The ulcers sometimes coincide with the region of Peyer patches.

Biopsies of both the enteritis and the colitis show nonspecific acute and chronic changes resembling other infections. Small intestinal lesions include inflammation and edema of the lamina propria, neutrophilic infiltrates, goblet cell depletion with crypt abscesses, and hemorrhagic necrosis. Other histologic features include hemorrhagic ulcers, erythema, cryptitis, broadening and flattening of the villi, mucosal atrophy, and features similar to those seen in chronic ulcerative colitis, nonspecific colitis, or infective colitis. The ulcer bases have acute inflammation, granulation tissue, and prominent vascularity, but they lack fibrosis (328). Rectal lesions are also often present. Unlike chronic ulcerative colitis, the changes tend to be segmental in nature. Poorly formed mucin granulomas can be seen. Suppurative foci in the granulomas distinguish the lesion from Crohn disease. If tissue is examined during the necrotizing phase, the epithelium will appear regenerative in nature. Because biopsies are usually nonspecific, bacterial culture or other diagnostic techniques are usually necessary to establish the diagnosis.

Vibrio *Infections*

Eleven *Vibrio* species cause human infections (329–334), but most infections result from *Vibrio parahaemolyticus, Vibrio cholerae, Vibrio vulnificus,* and *Vibrio cholerae. Vibrio* organisms are motile, Gram-negative, curved, rod-shaped bacteria, living in marine or brackish water. The seasonality of cholera relates in part to the presence of viable, noncultivatable forms of the organism in marine life and algae. In this environment, *V. cholerae* assume sporelike forms; when they are re-exposed to a more favorable environment, they revert to an infectious state. The sporelike form of *Vibrio* is consumed by fish, mollusks, and crustaceans. Infections with *V. vulnificus* commonly occur among persons who work in the shellfish industry, especially among individuals who sustain a puncture wound while handling fresh seafood. *V. parahaemolyticus* infections are a major cause of food poisoning, transmitted by sashimi or infected oysters. Rising ocean temperature waters appear to be contributing to continuing disease outbreaks (335).

V. cholerae infections may be mild or may be an extremely deadly disease. Disease virulence relates to the genes that encode the toxin responsible for cholera's life-threatening diarrhea. Cholera enterotoxin is the prototype for secretory enteritis and toxigenic diarrhea. The cholera toxin induces elevated mucosal levels of cyclic adenosine monophosphate (AMP). This has a direct secretory effect on crypt cells and an antiabsorptive effect on villous cells, producing the most overwhelming feature of the disorder: extreme fluid loss.

The clinical spectrum of cholera varies from asymptomatic carriers to patients with extremely severe diarrhea. In the acute phase, water secretion from the small intestine is greater than the capacity of the colon to absorb the water loss, resulting in large fluid, sodium, potassium, and bicarbonate losses. Cholera is a leading cause of death in some parts of the world because the large volume depletion leads to acidosis and renal failure. Death can occur within 3 to 4 hours of onset, with fecal output exceeding 1 L/hr at the height of the disease. Daily outputs of 15 to 20 liters have been observed when adequate fluid replacement is given. Incubation periods range from 6 to 48 hours and recovery occurs in 2 to 7 days. Untreated, the mortality ranges between 50% and 75% (336).

Although cholera is widespread, the histopathologist plays less of a role in its diagnosis than the microbiologist. Grossly, the bowel appears slightly edematous and only mildly abnormal. The intestinal mucosa appears intact with mucus-depleted dilated crypts. If goblet cells are present, they appear empty, and the lamina propria exhibits mild edema and vascular dilation. Occasional inflammatory cells are present but significant inflammation is absent. Widening of intercellular spaces is most prominent in the villous epithelium, whereas blebbing of microvillous border and mitochondrial changes usually occur in the crypts (337).

Three major clinical syndromes result from the *V. vulnificus* infections: Primary septicemia, wound infections, and GI illness without septicemia or wound infection (338). The disease is characterized by a 24-hour incubation period followed by the sudden onset of septicemia, fever, chills, hypotension, nausea, vomiting, bloody diarrhea, and a rash. Infection symptoms and duration are not as severe as in cholera. Skin lesions are distinctive. Large hemorrhagic bullae progress to necrotic ulcers.

Aeromonas *Infections*

Aeromonas organisms are facultative anaerobic Gram-negative bacteria ubiquitous in fresh and brackish water and soil.

The infection may also be acquired through consumption of untreated water or trauma, usually involving soil exposure in individuals with lacerations on the extremities. The organism has been isolated from children with acute diarrhea in daycare centers and from adults with traveler's diarrhea. The disease also affects neonates. *Aeromonas hydrophila, Aeromonas sobria,* and *Aeromonas caviae* cause a spectrum of GI diseases, ranging from a self-limited diarrhea to acute persistent dysentery (339). Typical symptoms include low-grade fever, watery stools often with occult blood, and abdominal cramps. Children present with severe diarrhea, whereas the adult disease tends to be chronic in nature with patients presenting with vomiting and abdominal cramps. *Aeromonas* produces enterotoxins, cytotoxins, and hemolysins. Histologic changes range from changes that resemble celiac disease, to edema of the lamina propria, to a full-blown enterocolitis (Fig. 6.136). The diagnosis is made by stool culture.

Plesiomonas *Infections*

Plesiomonas shigelloides, a facultative anaerobic Gram-negative rod-shaped bacterium, is recoverable from the stool in up to 17% of individuals with diarrhea (339). It associates with eating uncooked fish and with foreign travel, usually to Mexico. Most infected individuals experience a self-limited diarrhea with blood and mucus in the stool. Rarely, severe enterocolitis, pseudoappendicitis, osteomyelitis, and bacteremia develop.

Clostridial Infections

Various clostridial strains normally inhabit the large bowel and occasionally the ileum. Because clostridial infections more commonly involve the colon than the small bowel, the infections are discussed in Chapter 13. However, there are several unique forms of small intestinal clostridial diseases that will be covered in this chapter.

Enteritis Necroticans

Enteritis necroticans is a life-threatening infectious disease caused by *Clostridium perfringens* type C, a β-toxin–producing strain of clostridia causing necrosis and sepsis (340). The disease is characterized by segmental necrosis of the proximal jejunum and is associated with a high mortality rate if not diagnosed and treated early. It was first reported in Northern Germany after World War II among previously starved children and adults who ate large meals of meats and vegetables. The disease rarely occurs in developed countries; when it does it typically affects diabetics (341).

This disorder is also known as *Darmbrand enteritis* (342), *necrosis jejunitis,* or *jejunitis acta.* The lesion starts abruptly in the proximal jejunum and usually extends distally into the ileum. It presents as abdominal pain, vomiting, diarrhea, and progressive dehydration. The affected bowel becomes dilated,

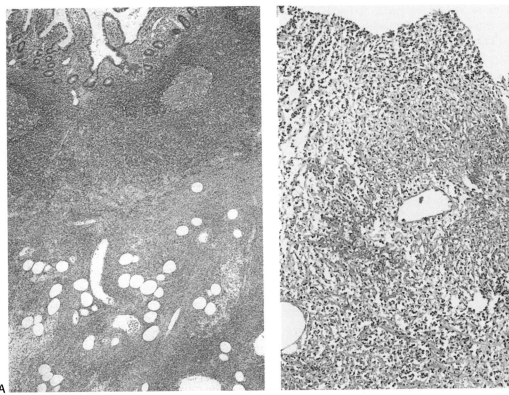

FIG. 6.136. *Aeromonas* enteritis. **A:** This case shows the presence of prominent lymphoid hyperplasia and a marked inflammatory infiltrate containing large numbers of acute inflammatory cells. These are seen at higher magnification in **B.**

edematous, thickened, rigid, and markedly congested. Valvulae conniventes become very prominent, imparting a washboard appearance to the mucosal surface. When the necrotic mucosa sloughs, extensively ulcerated areas remain. More severe cases have transmural inflammation.

Histologically, one sees severe mucosal necrosis with hemorrhage, mural thickening due to marked submucosal edema, and fibrinous or fibrous serosal exudate. Pseudomembranes and fibrin thrombi may be present in the inflamed areas. The mucosa between the thickened valvulae may appear normal, whereas the surfaces of the valvulae are more damaged. This pattern suggests a clostridial infection. There is little in the way of a neutrophilic response (342).

Pig Bel

A similar disease, pig bel, is endemic in Papua, New Guinea. It results from *Clostridium welchii* and *C. perfringens* infections (343), and it is the most common cause of death in children. Individuals become ill from eating infected pigs during ceremonial occasions. Patients present with symptoms lasting for a few days. These consist of severe, progressive abdominal pain, vomiting, blood-stained feces, and constipation. The small intestine shows segmental necrosis starting at the villous tips and progressing toward the base. The disease affects the duodenum to cecum. Alternatively, multiple segments of small intestine are involved, separated by normal-appearing unaffected segments. Kinking and adhesions between adjacent loops of bowel affect 50% of cases. At the time of surgery, the small intestine appears dilated and the distended bowel has a thickened wall and a red serosal surface. In about 25% of cases one or more yellow patches exist on the serosal surfaces. These represent areas of full-thickness infarction (Fig. 6.111).

Histologically, one sees ischemic changes with necrotic villi. Numerous bacteria are present. A clearly defined junctional zone exists between the necrotic mucosa and the submucosa. The vessels at this junction are thrombosed. Neutrophils accumulate at the edges of infarction. The mucosa becomes infiltrated with neutrophils, mononuclear cells, and eosinophils. Arterial walls appear edematous and infiltrated by inflammatory cells, and they demonstrate a homogeneous or granular eosinophilic appearance classically linked with fibrinoid necrosis.

Yersinia *Infections*

Yersinia enterocolitica (YE) and *Yersinia pseudotuberculosis (YP)* are facultative, anaerobic, non–lactose-fermenting, Gram-negative coccoid bacilli. The incidence of infection is highest in the cold months and in cold climates. *YE* and *YP* are a common cause of bacterial enteritis in Western and Northern Europe, but increasing numbers of cases have been reported in North America and Australia. Transmission usually follows ingestion of contaminated meats, vegetables, water, and milk (344). Swine constitute an important reservoir for human infections. However, the organism has also been isolated from numerous other animals. Transmission also occurs from dogs and cats and from person-to-person transmission via blood transfusion. Belgium is the country with the highest reported increase of the disease, strongly correlating with the consumption of raw pork. Most infections are self-limited. However, immunocompromised and debilitated patients as well as patients with iron overload are at a risk of serious disease.

The pathogenicity of *Yersinia* species is determined by a number of virulence factors encoded by the bacterial chromosomes or by the virulence plasmid pYV (345,346). Chromosomally encoded proteins facilitate bacterial intestinal attachment, mucosal penetration, survival, and proliferation. Virulence factors include various adhesins, invasin, and attachment-invasion locus. In addition, the pYV proteins make up a type III secretion system similar to that seen in pathogenic *E. coli* and *Salmonella*. A "high pathogenicity island" (HPI) is present in only highly pathogenic strains of *Yersinia*. The *Yersinia* HPI carries a cluster of genes involved in the biosynthesis, transport, and regulation of the siderophore yersiniabactin. The major function of the island is to acquire the iron molecules essential for bacterial growth and dissemination (347). Luminal bacteria adhere to M cells or absorptive cells in areas of the follicle-associated epithelium. Once inside the cell, the bacteria become enclosed by membranous vesicles (348). *YE* penetrate into the lamina propria by passing through the enterocyte cytoplasm in a manner similar to that exhibited by *Salmonella*. Only potentially pathogenic strains invade the lamina propria. *YE* organisms multiply within lymphoid follicles in Peyer patches, then drain into the mesenteric lymph nodes, eventually giving rise to systemic infections.

Yersinia preferentially involves the ileocecal and appendiceal regions and causes a wide spectrum of clinical and pathologic changes, ranging from self-limited enterocolitis to potentially fatal systemic infections. Diffuse enterocolitis, the most common clinical manifestation, usually affects children younger than 5 years of age (349). Patients present with gastroenteritis, diarrhea, low-grade fever, abdominal pain, ileitis, colitis, diffuse mesenteric lymphadenitis, pseudoappendicitis, sepsis (350,351), intestinal perforation, and the hemolytic uremia syndrome. Older children and adults develop mesenteric adenitis mimicking acute appendicitis. Immunosuppressed hosts often develop severe, fatal, *Yersinia* bacteremia. Patients who are in iron-overloaded states such as those with hemochromatosis or transfusional siderosis develop particularly virulent infections (352). Postinfection manifestations result from bacteremia and include erythema nodosum, bullous skin lesions, and reactive arthritis.

Grossly, *Yersinia* infections mimic Crohn disease. The bowel wall appears thickened, inflamed, congested, ulcerated, and edematous. Patients develop diffuse, focal, or aphthous mucosal ulcers. Even though numerous ulcers may be present, they are usually not very deep. The intestinal serosa

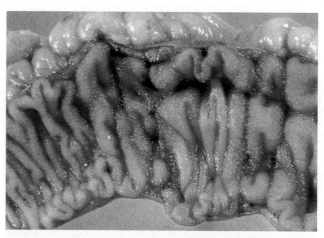

FIG. 6.137. *Yersinia.* Gross appearance in a patient with culture-proven *Yersinia* infection. The mucosal folds are unduly prominent due to the presence of the granulomas.

appears dull and hyperemic (Fig. 6.137). The muscularis propria thickens. Massively enlarged lymph nodes may become matted, and they may contain yellowish microabscesses. The enlarged mesenteric lymph nodes may become matted and contain yellowish microabscesses. Both the small and large intestines are involved, with the most severe changes centering on the ileocecal region and appendix.

There is considerable overlap in the histologic features of *YE* and *YP*. Both infections can produce mucosal ulceration, cryptitis, granulomatous inflammation with prominent lymphoid cuffing, lymphoid hyperplasia, transmural lymphoid aggregates, and nodal involvement. The affected bowel appears congested, edematous, and ulcerated with massively enlarged lymphoid follicles. Sharply demarcated areas of lymphoid hyperplasia contain prominent germinal centers. The follicular ileitis may persist for months. The mucosa overlying the follicles develops small punctate aphthoid ulcers measuring 1 to 2 mm in diameter (351) resembling similar lesions in Crohn disease. These ulcers are covered by fibrinopurulent exudates and large numbers of Gram-positive coccobacilli. Sharply demarcated lymphoid hyperplasia is present with prominent germinal centers and small aphthoid ulcers overlying the hyperplastic lymphoid follicles. Epithelial granulomas with central necrosis may be seen in the bowel wall and in the lymph nodes. The bowel and lymph nodes contain epithelioid granulomas with central necrosis (Fig. 6.138). Granulomas are located in the mucosa and submucosa, but they can also occur on the serosa. The muscularis propria and serosa become infiltrated by pleomorphic cellular infiltrates including eosinophils. Acute vasculitis or intussusception may cause ischemia (Fig. 6.139). Crypt hyperplasia occurs throughout the small intestine with villous atrophy (351). Strictures are rare. The changes superficially resemble those found in cat-scratch fever.

The most important entity in the differential diagnosis is Crohn disease, which may be very difficult to distinguish from *Yersinia* infections histologically. Culture, serologic

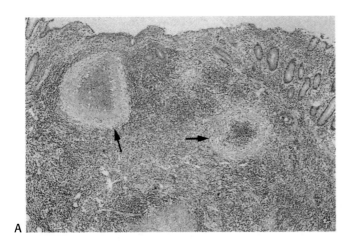

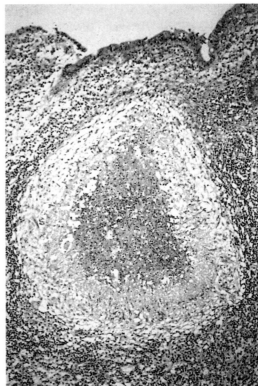

FIG. 6.138. *Yersinia* enterocolitis. A and B show the prominent necrotizing granulomas that characterize *Yersinia* infections. **A:** Contains two granulomas (*arrows*). The overlying epithelium appears atrophic and ulcerated. **B:** Higher magnification showing palisading histiocytes without foreign body giant cells. The entire granuloma is surrounded by a prominent cuff of lymphocytes.

studies, and polymerase chain reaction (PCR) assays may confirm *Yersinia* as the cause of the disease. Features that favor a diagnosis of Crohn disease include prominent neural hyperplasia and evidence of chronic changes including crypt distortion and hyperplasia of the muscularis mucosae.

Tuberculosis

In the 1980s, after decades of steadily declining rates of tuberculosis, ambitious plans were made to eliminate the disease in the United States. However, despite these plans, the

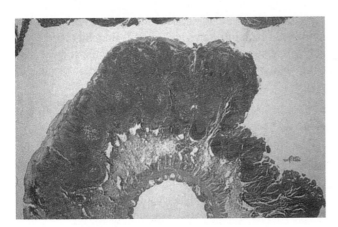

FIG. 6.139. *Yersinia* enteritis. *Yersinia* granulomatous enterocolitis causing intussusception and secondary ischemic necrosis.

control of tuberculosis was neglected, resulting in a resurgence of the disease (353). Between the mid-1980s and the early 1990s, the synergistic combination of a deteriorating public health infrastructure, inadequate institutional control of infection, urban crowding, the HIV epidemic, and immigration resulted in a resurgence of tuberculosis including infections with multidrug-resistant strains.

Tuberculosis is currently uncommon in North America but it remains endemic in Asia, where it constitutes a major health problem. In 2000, 16,377 cases (5.8 cases per 100,000 population) were reported to the Centers for Disease Control and Prevention (CDC), representing a 45% decrease in the incidence rate and the lowest rate in U.S. history (354). In the United States, 50% of all cases of tuberculosis occur in foreign-born individuals (355), who represent only 10% of the total population (356). Tuberculosis in the immigrant population is largely attributed to the importation of latent infection with subsequent reactivation of the disease (357). The rate of tuberculosis among immigrants who have lived in the United States for 5 years or less is three times as high as that among immigrants who have lived here for more than 5 years (358). Recognizing that existing public health practices are inadequate, both the CDC and the Institute of Medicine have called for stronger measures to detect and treat latent infection in immigrants to the United States (359). In addition to immigrants, HIV-infected persons, minorities, the homeless, incarcerated, alcoholics, and the poor have increased infection rates. Others at risk for the infection may include hospital workers and the military. Blacks are more likely to contract tuberculosis than persons of other races (360). Recent developments in bacterial genotyping are providing a better understanding of the pathogenesis, transmission, drug resistance, and reinfection of tubercular infections (361).

The severity of GI involvement relates to the severity of pulmonary infections and is most common in individuals with cavitary lung lesions and a positive sputum. Swallowed organisms pass through the small bowel mucosa without causing a local lesion, only to arrest in the regional lymph nodes. Ulcerative small intestinal lesions develop as the result of retrograde spread.

Complications of intestinal tuberculosis include severe enterocolitis, hemorrhage, perforation, obstruction, fistula formation, strictures, malabsorption, and severe secretory diarrhea. The latter results from bacterial overgrowth in dilated intestinal loops lying proximal to points of obstruc-

tion. It may also result from obstruction of the mesenteric lymphatics by granulomas in the regional lymph nodes. Chronic nonspecific abdominal pain is the most common complaint. Other findings include fever, weight loss, and malaise. The clinical differential diagnosis includes carcinoma, tuberculosis, Crohn disease, and *Yersinia* infections.

AIDS patients may develop generalized tuberculosis, and up to 50% of patients who die are undiagnosed premortem (362). This is due to the fact that generalized tuberculosis in the setting of AIDS often lacks the typical features of the disease. Inflammatory foci show areas of necrosis with numerous neutrophils, numerous acid-fast bacilli, few or no epithelioid histiocytes, and no Langhans giant cells (362).

The ileocecal region is affected in 90% of patients (Figs. 6.140 and 6.141); other affected locations in decreasing order of frequency include the ascending colon, appendix, jejunum, duodenum, stomach, sigmoid, and rectum. This distribution follows the distribution of the lymphoid tissues.

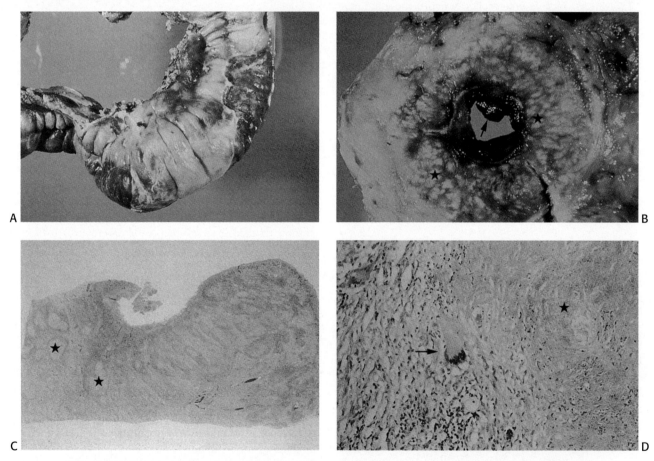

FIG. 6.140. Ileocecal tuberculosis. **A:** Gross photograph of the resection specimen showing transmural inflammation. It is difficult to delineate the ileocecal valve. The serosal tissues are markedly congested and edematous, and show fibrinous adhesions. **B:** Cross section through the specimen showing transmural necrosis and replacement of the intestinal wall by numerous granulomas, several of which are indicated by the *stars*. The intestinal lumen is severely compromised and narrowed. A hypertrophic lesion protrudes into the lumen (*arrow*). **C:** Low-magnification photograph of the wall showing confluent granulomas, some of which are indicated by *stars*. Granulomas appear centrally pale and surrounded by a bluer rim. **D:** Higher magnification showing the presence of a portion of a granuloma with central caseous necrosis (*star*) and a surrounding giant cell (*arrow*).

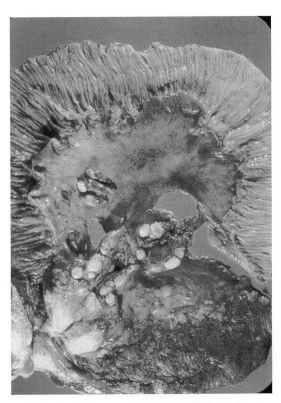

FIG. 6.141. Tuberculous ileocolitis exhibits extensive lymph node involvement.

The area of the ileocecal valve is frequently obscured by a mass that consists of mesenteric fat, fibrotic tissue, lymph nodes, and other inflammatory changes. The appendix and distal terminal ileum are usually thickened and strictured, with mucosal ulceration and surface fibrin deposits. The wall of the colon may be so extensively destroyed by the inflam-

matory process that one cannot tell which side of the ileocecal valve one is on.

Classically, intestinal tuberculosis assumes one of three forms: (a) the *ulcerative* form (60% of cases), which exhibits multiple superficial ulcers and has a virulent course with a high mortality; (b) the *hypertrophic* form (10% of cases), which grossly mimics Crohn disease because of the scarring, fibrosis, and heaped-up mass lesions; and (c) the *ulcerohypertrophic* form (30% of cases), in which the intestinal wall becomes thickened and ulcerated by an inflammatory mass centering around the ileocecal valve (363). The cut surface of the bowel appears friable, and necrotizing granulomas are easily seen.

Tubercles always begin in Peyer patches or lymphoid follicles and may give the mucosa a cobblestoned appearance. As the disease progresses, tubercles encircle the entire bowel wall (Fig. 6.140). Multiple tubercles may also stud the serosa and mesentery (Fig. 6.142). The ulcerative form of the disease begins as ragged, undermining ulcers. The ulcers may be single or multiple, large or small (Fig. 6.143). In contrast to Crohn disease, tuberculous ulcers tend to be circumferential with their long axis perpendicular to the lumen without fissuring. The ulcers may contain acid-fast bacilli (AFB), even in the absence of granulomas. The nonulcerated mucosa usually appears markedly edematous and focally hemorrhagic. Hyperplastic lesions cause pronounced intramural thickening with ulceration and obstruction (Fig. 6.140). Fibrosis, strictures, and stenosis result when the ulcers heal. Areas of irregular stenosis may measure several centimeters in length. This leads to the hypertrophic form of the disease. Giant cell granulomas with obvious caseation occur more frequently in ulcerative than hyperplastic lesions. They are distributed throughout the entire thickness of the intestinal wall (Fig. 6.140). Although tuberculosis classically associates with granulomas, it is only one of several causes of ileocecal

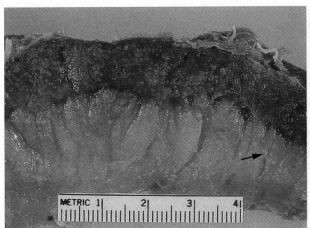

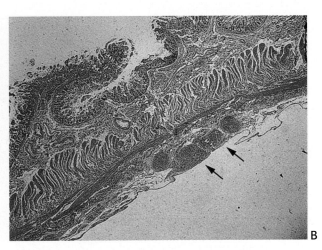

FIG. 6.142. Miliary tuberculosis. Gross and microscopic features of miliary tuberculosis. **A:** Gross resection specimen with numerous whitish mucosal nodules representing tubercles within the Peyer patches. The fat in the surrounding bowel also shows large numbers of 1- to 2-mm whitish nodules, one of which is indicated by an *arrow.* Fine adhesions are also present. **B:** Histologic section through several of the serosal tubercles (*arrows*). Mucosal and submucosal tubercles are not seen in this photograph.

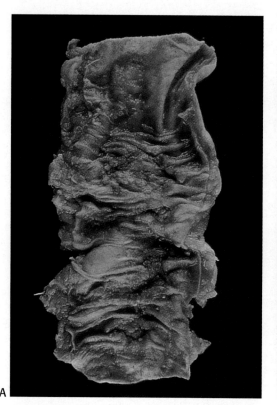
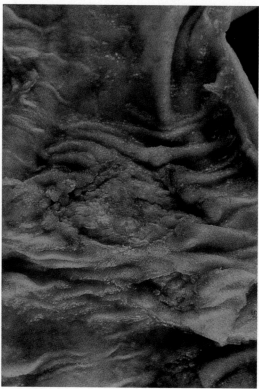

FIG. 6.143. Tuberculous enteritis. **A:** Resection specimen demonstrating the presence of the ulcerative form of tuberculosis. **B:** The ulceration at higher magnification.

granulomas (Table 6.15). Regional mesenteric lymph nodes become enlarged, containing areas of caseous necrosis (Fig. 6.144). Isolated organisms can be visualized in the tubercles and lymph nodes with the use of special stains, or they are recoverable from tissue culture.

TABLE 6.15   **Intestinal Granulomas**
Sarcoid
Crohn disease
Infections
Tuberculosis
Actinomyces
Histoplasmosis
Yersinia
Schistosomiasis
Hyperinfective strongyloidiasis
Mycobacterium avium-intracellulare
Mycobacterium tuberculosis
Mycobacterium bovis
Salmonella
Campylobacter
Brucella
Foreign material (talc, sutures, barium)
Feces due to perforation or fistulae
Pneumatosis intestinalis
Histiocytosis
Malakoplakia
Cell injury with mucin release

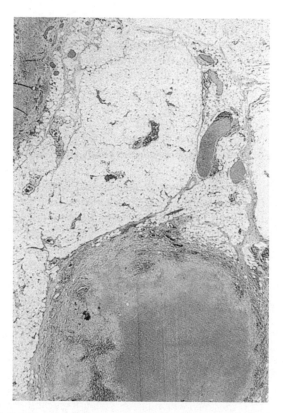

FIG. 6.144. Histologic section of the lymph node removed from the resection specimen shown in Figure 6.143. The lymph node is almost completely replaced by a caseating granuloma.

Sometimes it is difficult to detect the bacteria in suspected cases of tuberculosis, even in AFB-stained sections, due to the scarcity of the organisms. In this setting the detection of mycobacterial DNA in formalin-fixed paraffin-embedded tissue by duplex PCR reactions may prove valuable in the management of patients with granulomatous enterocolitis (364).

Mycobacterium avium-intracellulare *Infections*

Mycobacterium avium-intracellulare (MAI), a highly prevalent (ubiquitous) AIDS-associated pathogen, affects 15% to 40% of AIDS patients. Persons acquire the organisms through environmental exposure to aerosols, water, food, and soil. Unlike tuberculosis, which appears to result from reactivation of a previously contracted infection, disseminated *MAI* usually results from a primary infection. A period of asymptomatic colonization of the respiratory or GI tract often precedes disseminated disease, suggesting that the organism is acquired from the environment via the gut and then disseminates. The GI tract is involved twice as frequently as the lungs. Disseminated disease usually follows the primary infection within months.

Healthy people who become colonized by *MAI* do not normally develop active disease. The major risk factor for the infection is the level of immune dysfunction, as reflected by the CD4+ cell count. Between 76% and 90% of *MAI* infections develop late in the course of AIDS when other AIDS-defining diagnoses have already been established and CD4 counts measure <60/mm^3. *MAI* may be excreted in the stool of AIDS patients without GI symptoms.

Virulence factors for *MAI* are not well established. The organisms penetrate the gastrointestinal mucosa by unknown mechanisms and are phagocytosed by macrophages in the lamina propria. The macrophages cannot kill the bacteria and they become stuffed with mycobacteria as they multiply within the cells. With continued bacterial replication the host cell ruptures. The process leads to the presence of sheets of macrophages laden with AFB. The bacteria spread through the submucosal tissues, where the lymphatic drainage carries them to the regional lymph nodes. In the lymph nodes, the same process is again repeated. The mycobacteria replicate in macrophages, eventually breaking loose and again forming sheets of infected cells that eventually replace the normal histology of the lymph node. Tissue destruction is rare and most signs and symptoms of *MAI* result from the elaboration of cytokines (365).

Symptomatic *MAI* infections typically present indolently with nausea, chronic diarrhea, abdominal pain, malabsorption resembling Whipple disease, fever, sweats, chills, weight loss, lymphadenopathy, hepatosplenomegaly, and pancytopenia. Obstructive jaundice develops secondary to massive involvement of the peripancreatic and porta hepatis lymph nodes. Intestinal obstruction may result from intussusception secondary to hyperplasia of Peyer patches and lymph node involvement (366). Death may result from malnutri-

tion or superinfections. *MAI* also produces clinical and radiologic pictures resembling Crohn disease, especially in patients with terminal ileitis. At the time of autopsy, up to 60% of patients with *MAI* infection have GI involvement, even though the organism is rarely recognized antemortem (366). Numerous bacilli are seen in acid-fast–stained sections, both within macrophages and extracellularly.

MAI infections occur throughout the GI tract but they are most common in the duodenum (365). The mucosa appears edematous, erythematous, and friable, sometimes with multiple yellowish linear and oval erosions and/or 2- to 3-mm white or erythematous maculopapular nodules and prominent mucosal folds (Fig. 6.145). Fine white mucosal nodules may also be present. Regional lymph nodes become enlarged (Fig. 6.145). Hematoxylin and eosin (H&E)-stained sections reveal an atrophic mucosa with villous blunting, distortion, and widening due to a diffuse lamina propria infiltrate composed of large numbers of plump PAS-positive macrophages with granular or foamy cytoplasm. The glandular architecture usually remains intact, although the crypts become widely separated by a diffuse interstitial infiltrate of large cells with pale cytoplasm. Lymphocytes, plasma cells, and neutrophils are sparse, if present at all. Regional lymph nodes contain similar infiltrates. Occasionally, one sees poorly circumscribed epithelioid granulomas that contain lymphocytes and rare multinucleated giant cells. Small areas of necrosis may be present in up to 30% of cases (367).

When the changes are marked, the infiltrates are easily recognized on H&E stains using low-power microscopy (Fig. 6.146). The organism may also be detectable in duodenal brushings. Detection of focal involvement may require the use of special stains. *MAI* histologically resembles Whipple disease (see below), and the mucosa in both diseases contains macrophages with PAS-positive cytoplasmic granules. However, mycobacteria are several times larger than the Whipple bacillus and differ from Whipple bacillus in that they are acid fast. In contrast to traditional tuberculous infections, the macrophages in MAI teem with acid-fast microorganisms. The organisms form tight clusters in the cytoplasm. Giant cells and areas of caseous necrosis are usually absent in *MAI*.

Actinomycosis

Actinomyces israelii is a filamentous bacterium that is part of the normal oral flora. Abdominal infections result when swallowed organisms escape destruction in the stomach. *A. israelii* can cause serious small intestinal infections, particularly at the ileocecal valve. Changes in bowel habits, low-grade fever, malaise, weight loss, abdominal pain, and a palpable abdominal mass may lead to a misdiagnosis of carcinoma. The affected bowel appears thickened with multiple suppurative foci and scar tissue. Infections usually involve the full thickness of the bowel wall with extension into surrounding tissues. Ulceration may be minimal, but

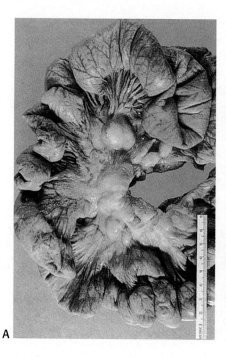

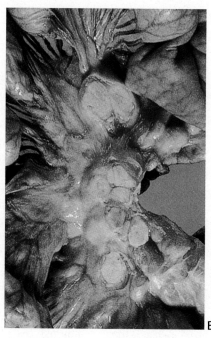

FIG. 6.145. *Mycobacterium avium-intracellulare.* **A:** Gross specimen showing marked atrophy of the mesenteric fat and prominence of the regional lymph nodes, which appear enlarged and matted. **B:** Higher magnification showing confluent matted mesenteric lymph nodes that have been sliced open.

fistulae often develop. Histologically, there is extensive fibrosis and granulation tissue containing foamy histiocytes, abscesses, and fistulous tracts. The typical bacterial colonies stain darkly with hematoxylin, often exhibiting a classic sulfur granule arrangement.

Brucellosis

Brucellosis, a fairly common disease in some parts of the world, is transmitted to humans via consumption of contaminated raw milk, through contact with the afterbirth products

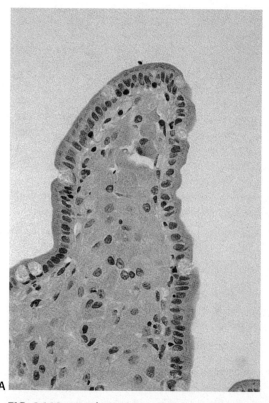

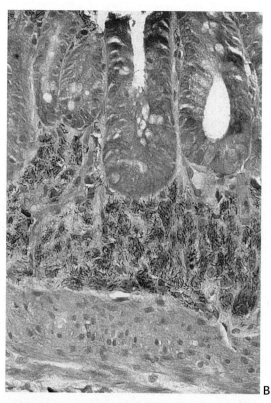

FIG. 6.146. *Mycobacterium avium-intracellulare.* **A:** The lamina propria of the small intestine contains massive collections of mononuclear cells with the histologic features of macrophages. These completely distend and replace the normal lamina propria. **B:** Acid-fast stain showing prominent collections of mononuclear cells containing organisms lying between the bases of the intestinal glands and the muscularis mucosae.

of infected animals, via transplacental transmission (368), or possibly via breast milk (369). In the United States, the disease usually presents in Hispanics, possibly related to the illegal importation of unpasteurized dairy products from Mexico, where the disease is endemic. Brucellosis is caused by *Brucella melitensis, Brucella abortus, Brucella suis,* and *Brucella canis* (370). Bacteria colonize the inoculation site or secondary sites causing chronic granulomatous infections.

The organism differs from other bacteria in that it does not exhibit the classic virulence factors such as exotoxin or endotoxin production (370). Rather, it has a tendency to invade and persist in the human host through inhibition of apoptosis (371). The bacteria invade the mucosa after which phagocytes ingest the organism. After ingestion, most bacteria are eliminated by phagolysozyme fusion. Surviving bacteria gradually evolve in bacteria-containing compartments in which rapid acidification occurs. Replication takes place in the endoplasmic reticulum, following which the bacteria are released with the help of a hemolysin and induced cell necrosis. Following their release they are transferred to the regional lymph nodes and then seeded throughout the body (370).

The disease has protean manifestations, with fevers, malodorous perspiration, and osteoarticular disease being the most common presentations. The reproductive system is also commonly affected (370). It rarely affects the small intestine (372). The changes consist of a chronic nonspecific inflammation and vasculitis. The diagnosis of the disease requires isolation of the bacterium from blood or tissue (370).

Listeriosis

Listeria monocytogenes is a Gram-positive bacterium that can be a serious food-borne pathogen. It primarily affects pregnant women, neonates, immunodeficient persons, and the elderly (373). The organism can be isolated from the intestinal tracts of humans, but it is more commonly found in the GI tract of ruminants. The disease follows consumption of contaminated salads, Mexican-style cheese, raw milk, ice cream, raw meat, sausages, and seafood (374,375). Once ingested, the bacteria breach the intestinal barrier, sometimes causing gastroenteritis in their human hosts. The organisms then travel throughout the body causing septicemia, meningitis, intrauterine infections, and, occasionally, diarrhea (375). *Listeria* enters the gut epithelium through the binding of its surface protein internalin to the transmembrane protein E-cadherin expressed on epithelial basolateral surfaces (376). *Listeria* bacteria are obligate intracellular pathogens that inhabit the cytoplasm. The secreted pore-forming protein listeriolysin O of the organism is an essential virulence determinant that allows the bacterium to escape the host vacuole and reach the host cytosol.

Whipple Disease

Whipple disease is an uncommon multisystem disease (Fig. 6.147) that results from a systemic infection with the recently

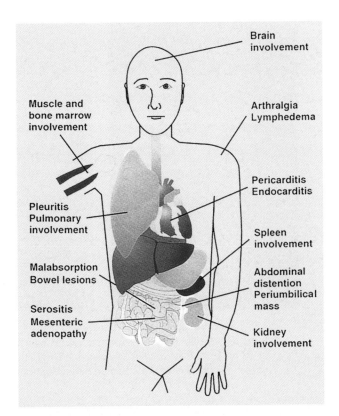

FIG. 6.147. Diagram showing the various manifestations of Whipple disease.

identified bacterium that was originally named *Tropheryma whippelii* (377). Subsequently, the name was changed slightly to *Tropheryma whippeli*. In autopsy studies its frequency is <0.1%. Whipple disease occurs in people of all ages throughout the world, but the typical patient is a middle-aged white male (378). Whipple disease may occur in regional clusters or in sibling pairs, but the spread of Whipple disease and the role of genetic susceptibility remain obscure. Sequencing studies suggest that immune evasion and host interaction play an important role in the lifestyle of this persistent bacterial pathogen. Persistent monocytic or macrophage dysfunction may predispose to the infection since the macrophages appear to be unable to degrade the bacteria once they are phagocytosed (379). This inability to degrade bacterial antigens may relate to decreased production of interleukin (IL)-12, which may lead to decreased interferon-γ production by T cells and defective macrophage activation. A decrease in IL-12 might prevent the development of an effective type 1 helper T-cell immune response (378). Additionally, the bacterium has a unique cell wall and it localizes in the lamina propria, where it elicits a cellular response that consists almost entirely of macrophages with the accumulation of bacterial wall remnants in these cells. Replication of the organism in the macrophages associates with apoptosis of the host cell with expression and release of IL-16. Elevated serum IL-16 levels and markers of apoptosis correlate with the activity of Whipple disease, decreasing to normal levels after successful therapy (378).

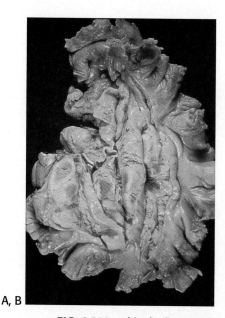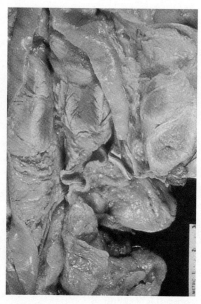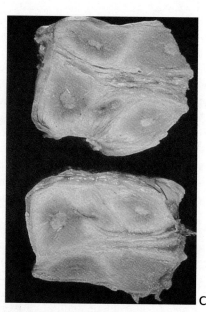

A, B   C

FIG. 6.148. Whipple disease. This disorder also used to be termed *intestinal lipodystrophy* due to gross presentations similar to those illustrated in this figure. **A:** Resection specimen with matted lymph nodes and loops of bowel that are markedly distended. **B:** Higher magnification of the specimen showing the induration of the intestinal fat. **C:** Cross section through lymph nodes replaced by fatty infiltrates.

Whipple disease is characterized by two stages: A prodromal stage and a much longer steady-state stage. The prodromal stage is characterized by the presence of migrating polyarthralgia and arthritis. The steady state is typified by diarrhea, abdominal pain, weight loss, malabsorption, low-grade fever, dermal hyperpigmentation, pericarditis, aortic valve vegetations, peripheral lymphadenopathy, anemia, and edema. The diarrhea is usually watery, malodorous, and often associated with steatorrhea (380,381). Lymphadenopathy affects approximately 50% of patients. Central nervous system disease affects approximately 10% of patients. The average time between the prodromal and steady-state stage is 6 years (378). However, if a patient had received previous immunosuppressive therapy, a more rapid clinical progression can occur. Macrophage infiltrations of the endocardium lead to valvular stenosis or insufficiency. The abdomen may be distended or slightly tender, and a periumbilical mass representing the enlarged mesenteric lymph nodes is sometimes palpable. Hepatosplenomegaly affects some patients. Approximately 15% of patients do not have the classic signs and symptoms of the disease. The disease is fatal if left untreated (378).

Whipple disease frequently involves the jejunum and ileum, but it usually spares the duodenum (381). The edematous mucosa acquires a coarse, granular appearance and it may contain yellow-white plaques. The intestinal wall thickens and subepithelial yellowish lipid deposits are seen. One may also see rare mucosal ulcers and petechial hemorrhages (Figs. 6.148 and 6.149) (381). Mesenteric and retroperitoneal nodes become grossly enlarged and pale, sometimes measuring as much as 3 to 4 cm in diameter (Fig. 6.150). Yellowish peritoneal plaques and massive infil-

tration of the mesenteric fat are characteristic of late-stage disease.

The diagnosis depends on the demonstration of multiple rounded, rod, or sickle-shaped PAS-positive diastase-resistant inclusions stuffing lamina propria macrophages. Some bacilli are seen within and between epithelial cells (379). PAS-positive material is also seen in smooth muscle, endothelium, and fibroblasts. The villi appear blunted and distorted by macrophage collections (Fig. 6.151). In severe cases, there may be subtotal or total villous atrophy. Most commonly, the macrophages lie just beneath the luminal epithelial basement membrane and decrease in number as one progresses toward the submucosa. This pattern of involvement supports the concept that the bacteria invade the tissues from the intestinal lumen. Lymphocytes, neutrophils, eosinophils, and macrophages may infiltrate among the macrophages. Rarely, one sees necrosis and fibrosis. Widespread fatty deposits and granulomas are present in the mucosa and intra-abdominal lymph nodes. The lymph nodes lose their normal architecture and become fibrotic. Three types of granulomas are seen (i.e., foreign body, lipogranulomas, and epithelioid granulomas). Granulomas may also be present in other tissues such as spleen, muscles, bronchial mucosa, lung parenchyma, kidney, GI mucosa, and bone marrow. Lymphatic obstruction causes dilation of the lacteals. Although the macrophages may resemble one another in several diseases (Table 6.16), fatty deposits are usually only present in Whipple disease. *MAI* infections are compared with Whipple disease in Table 6.17. In one study, the histology was characteristic with these features in only 90% of patients (382). The diagnosis may be confirmed using antibodies to the bacillus or by PCR reactions (377).

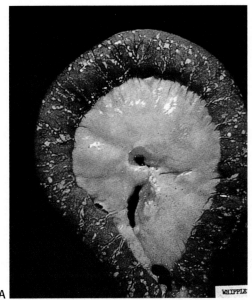

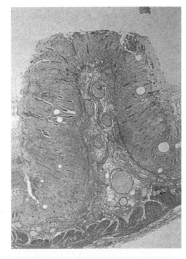

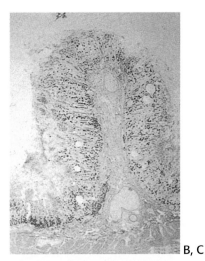

B, C

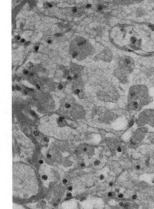

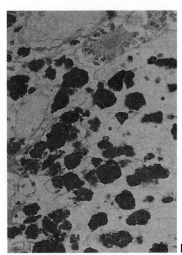

D, E

FIG. 6.149. Whipple disease. **A:** Hyperemic bowel, indurated mesentery, and prominent serosal lymphatic channels. **B:** Small bowel involvement demonstrating marked obliteration of the normal architecture with thickening of the mucosa and loss of normal crypts and villi. **C:** Same area stained with a periodic acid–Schiff (PAS) stain demonstrating the collections of dark fuchsinophilic macrophages within the mucosa. **D:** High magnification of the mucosal infiltrate showing histiocytic cells. **E:** Higher magnification of the infiltrate stained with PAS stain.

Treatment may affect the histology of the disease, with the principal changes consisting of a decrease in the number of PAS-positive macrophages and the pattern of mucosal inflammation changing from diffuse to patchy. In addition, the cytologic aspects of the PAS-positive macrophages change (382).

Tropical Sprue

Tropical sprue results from one or more of the following: (a) a nutritional deficiency, (b) a transmissible organism, and/or (c) a toxin elaborated by a microorganism or contained in the diet. Most believe the disease to be infectious in nature

TABLE 6.16   **Macrophage Collections in the Lamina Propria**

	PAS	Silver Stains	Acid-fast Stains	Architecture	Material in Macrophages
MAI infections	+	+	+	Normal	Bacteria
Whipple disease	+	−	−	Atrophy	Bacteria
Histoplasmosis	+	+	−	Variable	Fungi
Chronic granulomatous disease	+	−	−	Normal	Ceroid
T-cell defects	+	−	−	Partial villous atrophy	?
Transplant patients	+	−	−	Usually normal	?
Xanthomas	+	−	−	Normal	Lipid
Storage disease	+	−	−	Normal	Fat or glycoprotein depending on the disease
Combined immune deficiency	+	−	−	Villous atrophy	Cellular debris

MAI, *Mycobacterium avium-intracellulare;* PAS, periodic acid–Schiff.

TABLE 6.17 *Mycobacterium Avium-Intracellulare (MAI) Infections Versus Whipple Disease*

	MAI	Whipple Disease
Villi	Widened	Widened
Lacteals	Not dilated	Dilated
PAS	+	+
AFB	+	−
Appearance	Yellow–white granular appearance of small bowel	Erythema macular
Lipid deposits	−	+
Response to tetracycline	None	Good
Malabsorption, fever, cachexia	+	+
Migrating arthritis	−	+

PAS, periodic acid–Schiff; AFB, acid-fast bacillus.

(Table 6.18). Several microorganisms are the suspected pathogen, but none is common to all patients. Characteristic clinical features include the presence of nutritional deficiencies, anorexia, abdominal distention, and persistent diarrhea. Patients develop pallor, weakness, oral edema, and night blindness. Many patients develop milk intolerance because of a lactase deficiency; other patients develop alcohol intolerance (383). When severe, chronic diarrhea, steatorrhea, macrocytic anemia, glossitis, and emaciation occur, all due to fat, carbohydrate, vitamin B_{12}, and folic acid malabsorption.

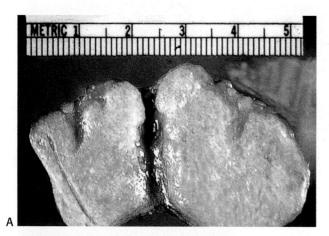

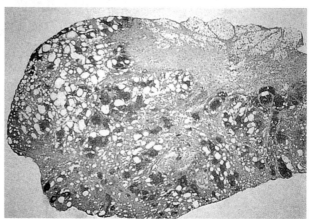

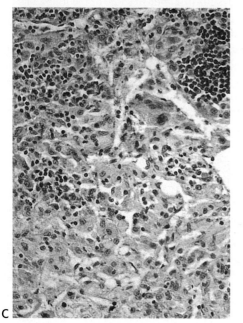

FIG. 6.150. Whipple disease in the mesenteric lymph nodes. **A:** Gross appearance with yellowish discoloration. **B:** Histiocytic collections and fatty replacement of lymph nodes. The normal underlying lymph node architecture has been destroyed. **C:** Histiocytic cells filled with foamy cytoplasm.

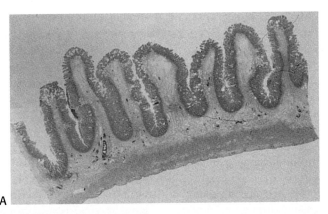

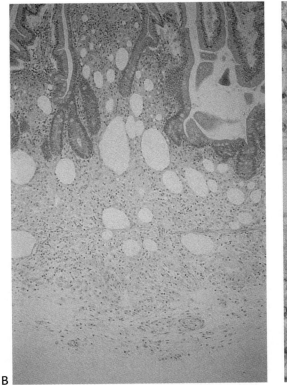

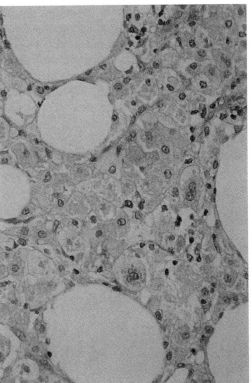

FIG. 6.151. Whipple disease. **A:** Whole mount section showing Whipple disease occupying the mucosa and the submucosa. **B:** Higher magnification of the base of the mucosa with the histiocytic infiltrates and prominent lipid collections. The histiocytic cells resemble those seen in patients with *Mycobacterium avium-intracellulare (MAI)* infections. However, the presence of the open spaces resulting from the organic chemical extraction of fats only occurs in Whipple disease and is virtually never seen in *MAI* infection. **C:** Higher magnification of the lipid-filled histiocytes.

TABLE 6.18	Factors Favoring an Infectious Origin of Tropical Sprue

Pattern with relapses and remission
Epidemic nature
Association in particular households; in spectrum of
  traveler's disease
Carriage to temperate zone by people from endemic areas
Large reservoir in indigenous populations
Seasonal epidemics
Disorder of expatriates

Tropical sprue has a striking geographic distribution affecting four groups of individuals: (a) indigenous populations of the world where the disease is endemic and epidemic, (b) travelers and tourists from temperate climates returning from visits to endemic areas, (c) Caucasian ex-residents of endemic areas returning to live in temperate zones, and (d) inhabitants of endemic areas who migrate to temperate climates. Most expatriates can pinpoint the disease onset, which usually consists of acute, watery, nonbloody diarrhea; malaise; fever; and weakness (383). Diagnostic evaluation of tropical sprue requires its differentiation from parasitic diarrheal diseases. In contrast to bacterial or viral infections, which are short lived, tropical sprue usually fails to improve after returning to a temperate climate. Jejunal biopsies are necessary to establish the presence of the characteristic morphologic abnormalities and to exclude other disorders such as celiac disease, Whipple disease, or lymphoma. The lesion first appears in the jejunum, spreading distally to involve the ileum. Early on, the jejunal mucosa appears normal or only slightly abnormal with increased numbers of intraepithelial lymphocytes. Chronic tropical sprue occurs if the acute phase does not completely remit.

Histologic features of tropical sprue consist of villous atrophy, crypt hyperplasia, and epithelial infiltration by chronic inflammatory cells, particularly plasma cells, lymphocytes, eosinophils, and histiocytes. The villi appear thickened, shortened, and broadened to form leaflike structures. Less than 10% of patients develop a completely flattened mucosa (Fig. 6.152). Enterocytes acquire abnormal shapes and orientations. A marked mononuclear infiltration develops in the lamina propria and epithelium. Lymphocytic infiltrates are distributed focally in the upper crypt and crypt villus in zones. Nuclei of crypt enterocytes appear megaloblastic. The basement membrane usually thickens and creates an increased collagen table.

Other Bacterial Infections

Extranodal cat-scratch disease, which is caused by *Bartonella henselae* infection, rarely involves the bowel but it may

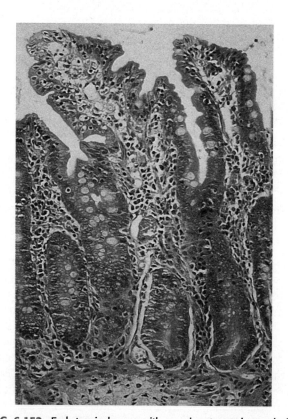

FIG. 6.152. Early tropical sprue with prominent crypt hyperplasia.

produce changes histologically identical to those seen in typhoid enteritis. The presence of a neutrophil-rich, macrophage-poor quality to the necrotic areas provides a clue to the diagnosis, as does the identification of microorganisms on a Warthin-Starry or other silver stain. Life-threatening chronic enteritis may complicate Gram-negative *Stenotrophomonas maltophilia* infections (384). To date, it only causes diarrheal disease in immunocompromised hosts or those with malignancies. The infection is characterized by small intestinal erosions.

Bacillus cereus is a spore-forming Gram-positive rod that causes both gastrointestinal and nongastrointestinal infections. *B. cereus* is responsible for an increasing number of food-borne diseases in industrialized countries (385). The incidence of *B. cereus* differs geographically and causes from 0.8% to 17.8% of bacterial food poisonings; in the United States it has only been reported in 1.3% of food poisonings (386). Many diverse types of foods can become contaminated as summarized in reference 385. Patients develop abdominal pain, cramps, and watery diarrhea after an 8- to 16-hour incubation period. Symptoms last for 12 to 24 hours. Vegetative cells of the bacterium in the small intestine produce an enterotoxin and the emetic toxin can be isolated directly from the food products (387).

Fungal Diseases

Candida *Infections*

Small intestinal candidal infections affect as many as 20% of autopsied patients with disseminated *Candida* infections (388). However, it is extremely rare to find an infection limited to the small bowel (388). Historically, candidemia affects patients on antibiotics, hemodialysis, or chemotherapeutic agents; immunocompromised individuals; immunocompetent patients with serious postoperative complications, cancer, and penetrating abdominal trauma; and patients with indwelling vascular access devices. More recently, increasing numbers of cases result from nosocomial infections (389). Symptoms are more common in hospitalized patients, particularly in children. Rarely, *Candida* species associate with neonatal necrotizing enterocolitis (390).

Autoimmune polyendocrinopathy-candidiasis-ectodermal dystrophy is an autosomal recessive disease characterized by (a) variable endocrine failure involving parathyroid glands, the adrenal cortex, gonads, pancreatic β cells, gastric parietal cells, and the thyroid gland; (b) chronic mucocutaneous candidiasis; and (c) dystrophy of dental enamel and nails, alopecia, vitiligo, keratopathy, and hepatitis. Eighteen percent of patients experience malabsorption (391). Patients develop candidiasis sometime during the course of their disease. Probably all species of *Candida* infect the immunocompromised host, although there is a higher frequency of disseminated *Candida tropicalis* than *Candida albicans*. The greater virulence of *C. tropicalis* causes their increased invasiveness (392). These two infections are compared in Table 6.19.

TABLE 6.19 Comparison of *Candida tropicalis* and *Candida albicans*

Characteristic	C. tropicalis	C. albicans
Simultaneous involvement of stomach, small intestine, colon	Common	Less common
Submucosal involvement	Common	Less common
Vascular involvement	Common	Less common
Necrotic band at invasive border in bowel wall	Present	Absent
Neutropenia	Less common	Common

Candida has difficulty colonizing nonsquamous cell sites such as the small intestine. In the small bowel, the rapid passage of feces due to peristalsis and the prevention of *Candida* mucosal interactions by bacterial antagonism reduce the likelihood of fungal colonization (393). Symptoms due to gastrointestinal *Candida* infections primarily relate to tissue invasion, although hypersensitivity mechanisms and possibly byproducts of fungal growth may induce functional abnormalities.

Fungal involvement falls into two broad categories: Noninvasive (Fig. 6.153) and invasive disease (Fig. 6.154). In noninvasive infection, the fungus grows in devitalized tissues. *Candida* commonly colonizes blind loops, sites of bacterial stasis, and necrotic areas. The fungus does not cause damage; the fungal spores and hyphae just lie in the fibrinopurulent exudate overlying the necrotic or devitalized tissues without invading intact tissues. Patients present with nausea, acute and chronic diarrhea, abdominal pain, and a host of allergic reactions. Invasive infections affect immunocompromised or chronically debilitated patients or patients in whom the mucosal integrity is destroyed. Such patients develop systemic fungal infections. The organism often invades the vasculature (Fig. 6.155), leading to ischemia and candidal sepsis. If the patient had pre-existing ischemia, the disease may worsen. Monilial enteritis may involve multiple intestinal sites, and multiple candidal ulcers or perforations can be seen. Histologically, *Candida* organisms appear as

4-to 6-μm budding yeastlike forms admixed with nonseptate pseudohyphae that stain positively with PAS and silver stains (Fig. 6.154).

Histoplasmosis

Histoplasma capsulatum is a dimorphic fungus with a worldwide distribution. It is the most common systemic endemic mycosis in the United States, occurring in the central regions of the country from the Gulf Coast to the Great Lakes. The fungus grows in soil that contains a high nitrogen content, particularly in soil enriched by bird and bat guano. Macrophages ingest the yeast after opsonization with antibody and/or complement or following direct binding of the organism to integrins on the surface of phagocytes (394) via the fungal adhesin HSP60s (395). The organism is internalized via a phagosome that subsequently fuses with lysosomes within the macrophage cytoplasm. Once inside the lysosome, *Histoplasma* employs several mechanisms to escape destruction. The major *Histoplasma*-secreted antigen, the M antigen, is thought to be a hydrogen peroxide–degrading catalase (396) that may neutralize the harmful effect of host cell–generated hydrogen peroxide. Survival of intact viable fungus in the hostile environment of phagolysosomes within the macrophages requires *Histoplasma* protein synthesis, indicating an active role of the organism in promoting its own survival. It may accomplish this by moderating the microenvironmental pH, reducing its acidity. This function may occur through a fungal protein pump (397). Additionally, the mode of entry of the *Histoplasma* into macrophages via alternative nonopsonophagocytic mechanisms may help the organism avoid or suppress host defenses against it.

Heavy inhalation of spores results in systemic illnesses, even in immunocompetent individuals. Immunosuppressed patients develop particularly severe infections. Gastrointestinal involvement is frequent in disseminated disease and may affect any site, including the esophagus, stomach, and small and large bowel. Patients present with crampy abdominal pain, nausea, vomiting, diarrhea, dysphagia, anorexia, vomiting, hematemesis, melena, and constipation. Intestinal ulceration develops in disseminated disease, often leading to perforation and peritonitis. Pulmonary symptoms are uncommon in patients with GI disease (398).

Terminal ileal involvement predominates in one third of the cases. In severe disease, perforation and peritonitis may

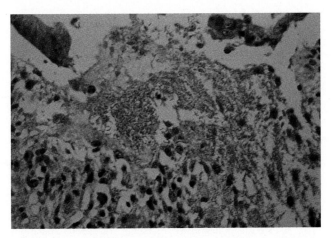

FIG. 6.153. Candidal colonization of necrotic intestinal tissues. Numerous candidal spores and young hyphae are present.

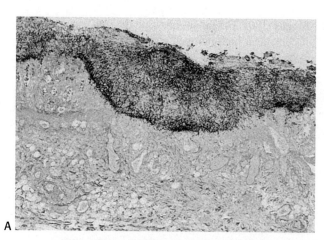

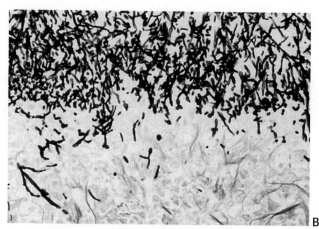

FIG. 6.154. Superficially invasive candidiasis. **A:** Low magnification showing a prominent monilial membrane overlying the ulcerated surface. The branching hyphae are beginning to invade the tissues. **B:** Higher magnification. A and B are stained with Grocott stain.

occur. Gastrointestinal masses or ulcers may mimic inflammatory bowel disease or carcinoma. Systemic manifestations often accompany these symptoms including gradual weight loss, fatigue, and weakness. AIDS patients with disseminated histoplasmosis often develop acute severe symptoms associated with shock, respiratory failure, and disseminated intravascular coagulation (399).

Grossly, ulcers, localized and diffuse granulomas, pseudopolyps (Fig. 6.156), and areas resembling xanthomas are present. The lesions usually assume the form of discrete, yellowish, raised plaques that undergo secondary ulceration and produce widespread tissue destruction and even perforation. The histologic response ranges from little response (in immunocompromised patients or those treated with cytotoxic drugs) to severe mononuclear cell infiltrates with fibrosis. The organism lies within well-formed granulomas (Fig. 6.157) or in scattered lamina propria macrophages, producing a pattern resembling Whipple disease. However, the organisms are large, round, and easily distinguishable from Whipple bacilli. In severe disease, fungi fill the macrophages. The capsule of *H. capsulatum* is PAS positive and diastase resistant.

Other Fungal Infections

Aspergillus species are ubiquitous environmental pathogens occurring worldwide. They pose particular problems in hospitalized populations when patients are exposed to organisms present in the ventilation or near construction sites. The infection generally affects severely debilitated or immunocompromised hosts, particularly those with severe neutropenia. The fungi tend to invade vessels, causing vasculitis, thrombosis, ischemia, and infarction (Figs. 6.158 and 6.159). When the tissues become ischemic, perforation and peritonitis develop. Identification of the characteristic hyphae leads to the diagnosis.

Mucor is widely distributed in nature and belongs to the phycomycetes with nonseptate hyphae. *Mucor* infections

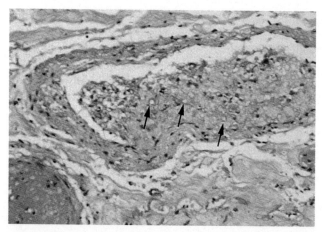

FIG. 6.155. Invasive *Candida* in a vessel. The vascular wall is partially destroyed in its lower margin. Numerous clear spaces (*arrows*) correspond to the cross section of hyphae.

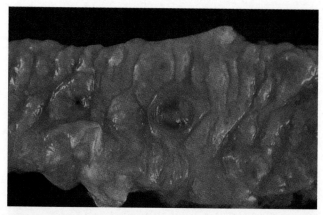

FIG. 6.156. Histoplasmosis. Intestinal resection specimen showing nodular ulcerated lesions diffusely throughout the bowel wall obliterating the normal mucosal fold pattern.

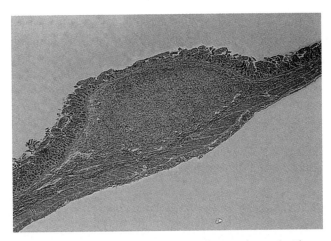

FIG. 6.157. Histologic section of the lesion shown in Figure 6.156 indicating the presence of a submucosal granuloma.

preferentially affect chronically debilitated individuals, diabetics, and severely malnourished children (400). Histologically, the pleomorphic, irregularly right-angled branched hyphae of *Mucor* appear broad and aseptate, measuring 10 to 20 μm in diameter. They are usually well seen in H&E-stained sections. The fungus tends to invade blood vessels, causing thrombosis and ischemia. *Mucor* produces discrete mucosal erosions and deep ulcers, causing hemorrhage, necrosis, and perforation as the infection spreads into the bowel wall. Histologically, the ulcer bases contain necrotic tissue with a surrounding rim of neutrophils and occasional giant cells, unless patients are on chemotherapy, in which case the inflammation may be negligible.

Paracoccidioidomycosis infects both the large and small intestines (401). The ulcerative lesions of paracoccidioidomycosis have a characteristic rolled border with a white exudative base and small hemorrhagic dots. These are due to

the formation of multiple granulomas. The draining lymph nodes are often involved. The fungi are easily seen in H&E-stained sections due to their large size, but they can be highlighted by fungal stains. The fungi are often surrounded by a granulomatous reaction combined with pyogenic inflammation. The distinctive feature of the fungus in tissue is an occasional large cell that, when hemisected, reveals peripheral buds protruding from a thin-walled, round mother cell that sometimes resemble a ship's wheel.

Penicillium marneffei is a thermally dimorphic fungus that can cause disseminated infections in individuals residing in, or traveling to, areas where the organism is endemic including Southeast Asia, Southern China, and Hong Kong (402). The disease infects both immunocompetent and immunocompromised hosts, but most cases occur in AIDS patients. It is the third most common opportunistic infection in HIV-infected patients in Thailand (403). The most common manifestations are fever, anemia, weight loss, and skin lesions, but GI symptoms are also common (403). The organisms infect the gut from the esophagus to the colon. Endoscopy demonstrates the presence of mucosal ulcers or bleeding tumorlike masses (404). Biopsies from the margins of the ulcers show lymphocytes and macrophages distended with yeasts in a pattern mimicking that of histoplasmosis. However, *P. marneffei* shows much more morphologic variation than *Histoplasma*. The demonstration of characteristic central septation and elongated sausage-shaped forms by silver stains and the absence of buds attached by a narrow neck distinguish *P. marneffei* from *H. capsulatum* (402).

Viral Infections

Numerous viral classes cause gastroenteritis (Table 6.20); some are compared in Table 6.21. Diagnostic methods used to identify GI viral infections include viral culture, electron microscopy, immunoelectron microscopy, enzyme-linked immunosorbent assay (ELISA) of stool specimens, genetic probes, and, rarely, biopsies.

Rotavirus Infections

Rotaviruses are a prominent cause of severe diarrhea in children under the age of 2 years. Most infected patients are between 5 months and 4 years in age (405). Annually, they

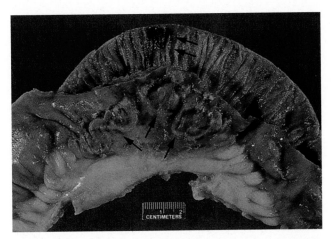

FIG. 6.158. Aspergillosis infection in a patient with acute myelogenous leukemia. The irregular, necrotic areas outlined by the *arrows* represent areas of ischemic necrosis due to invasive aspergillosis. The mucosal lesion is highlighted by the *double arrows*.

TABLE 6.20	**Etiologies of Viral Enteritis**
Rotavirus family of viruses	Coronavirus
Norwalk family of viruses	Dengue fever
Reovirus	Measles
Echoviruses	Human immunodeficiency
Adenoviruses	virus
Cytomegalovirus	Parvoviruses
Herpes simplex virus	Toroviruses
Calicivirus	Reoviruses
Astrovirus	Pestiviruses

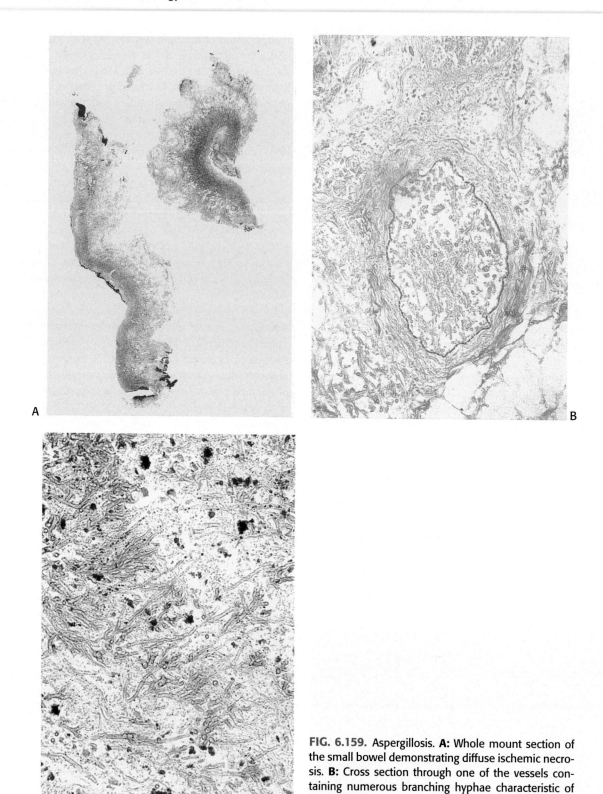

FIG. 6.159. Aspergillosis. **A:** Whole mount section of the small bowel demonstrating diffuse ischemic necrosis. **B:** Cross section through one of the vessels containing numerous branching hyphae characteristic of *Aspergillus*. **C:** Higher magnification of the *Aspergillus* hyphae in the lumen.

account for an estimated 140 million cases and 1 million deaths in young children. Child daycare increases the risk of diarrhea due to rotavirus infections (406). Rotavirus infections also affect immunosuppressed adults and transplant and geriatric patients. The infection is highly contagious so

that it only takes a small inoculum to infect a child. The viruses survive well on environmental surfaces and are difficult to inactivate. Rotaviruses are cosmopolitan in their distribution. Patients develop fever, severe vomiting, and watery diarrhea, often leading to dehydration and acidosis. Fatal

TABLE 6.21 Virologic Characteristics of Human Gastroenteritis Viruses

Virus	Virion Diameter (nm)	Virologic Features	Genomic Nucleic Acid	Medical Importance Demonstrated	Epidemiologic Characteristics	Clinical Characteristics	Laboratory diagnostic Tests
Rotavirus, group A	70–75	Double-shelled, wheel-like capsid; segmented; four common serotypes	RNA	Yes	Major cause of endemic severe diarrhea in infants and young children worldwide (in winter in temperate zone)	Dehydrating diarrhea for 5–8 days; vomiting and fever very common	Immunoassay, electron microscopy, PAGE
Enteric adenovirus	70–80	Morphologically like other adenoviruses; types 40 and 41 cause gastroenteritis	DNA	Yes	Endemic diarrhea of infants and young children	Prolonged diarrhea lasting 5–12 days; vomiting and fever	Immunoassay, electron microscopy, PAGE
Norwalk virus	27–32	Round with ragged surface outline; single structural protein similar to caliciviruses	RNA	Yes	Epidemics of vomiting and diarrhea in older children and adults; occurs in families, communities, and nursing homes; often associated with shellfish, other food, or water	Acute vomiting, diarrhea, fever, myalgia, and headache lasting 1–2 days	Immunoassay, immune electron microscopy
Norwalk-like viruses (small, round, structured viruses)	27–35	Examples are Snow Mountain, Hawaii, Taunton, and Otofuke	RNA	Yes	Similar to characteristics of Norwalk virus	Acute vomiting, diarrhea, fever, myalgia, and headache lasting 1–2 days	Immunoassay, electron microscopy
Calicivirus	27–38	Round, classically structured, cup-shaped indentations on surface	RNA	Partially	Usually pediatric diarrhea; associated with shellfish and other food in adults	Rotaviruslike illness in children; Norwalk-like in adults	Immunoassay, electron microscopy
Astrovirus	27–32	Round, classically structured, unbroken surface with pointed star	RNA	Partially	Diarrhea in children and nursing homes	Watery diarrhea, often lasting 2–3 days, occasionally longer	Immunoassay, electron microscopy

PAGE, polyacrylamide gel electrophoresis.

385

cases exhibit severe cardiac and central nervous system involvement (407).

The infection usually spreads from the proximal small bowel to the ileum over a period of 1 to 2 days. Rotaviruses infect mature enterocytes on the villous tips and differentiated enterocytes in the dome epithelium overlying Peyer patches, particularly M cells (408). The viruses mature in enterocytes, multiplying within the endoplasmic reticulum. As the viral particles accumulate, they lyse the cells, causing epithelial shedding, crypt hyperplasia, and round cell infiltration in the lamina propria (408). The crypt depth:villous height ratio increases. Severe infection causes gross destruction of villous architecture, leading to malabsorption. The changes persist for 3 to 8 weeks.

The diagnosis is usually made by examining the stool. Negative contrast electron microscopy demonstrates the presence of 70-nm wheel-like particles (Fig. 6.160). Immunoelectron microscopy increases the sensitivity of conventional ultrastructural examination. Other diagnostic tests include immunoelectrophoresis, complement fixation, viral RNA electrophoresis, radioimmunoassay, and rapid latex agglutination technique. PCR amplification provides a way of identifying the organism in stool specimens. There is also an antibody directed against the virus that can detect it in tissues.

In 1998, a tetravalent rotavirus vaccine was licensed in the United States for vaccination of infants, following the demonstration of its efficacy in a trial in South America (409). Following that, the American Academy of Pediatrics and the American Academy of Family Medicine recommended routine vaccination of healthy infants. To date, the only complication has been rare cases of intussusception (410). Since then additional highly effective vaccines have been developed that do not seem to be associated with an increased rate of intussusception (411).

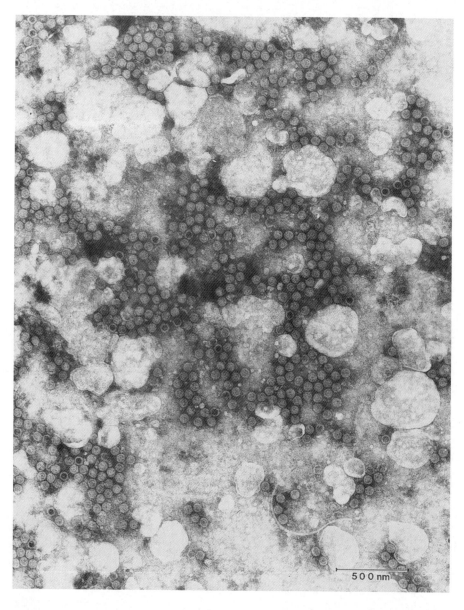

500 nm

FIG. 6.160. Electron microscopy (EM) photograph of rotavirus particles from a stool preparation.

Infections with Norwalk and Related Viruses

Caliciviruses cause more than 90% of outbreaks of acute gastrointestinal illness in the United States (412). Norwalk virus is the prototype of the human caliciviruses and is found in human feces by immunoelectron microscopy (413). The virus has a cosmopolitan distribution, infecting adults and school-age children, but not infants and young children. Norwalk virus and related viruses cause approximately 40% of gastroenteritis outbreaks in recreational camps and the military; on cruise ships; in communities or families; at elementary schools, colleges, and nursing homes; in hospital wards; in cafeterias; and among members of sports teams. The disease mainly spreads by person-to-person contact and by ingestion of contaminated drinking or swimming water, poorly cooked or raw shellfish, and contaminated food (414). Air-borne transmission also occurs. The virus has an incubation period of 12 to 48 hours, and the disease runs its course in 1 to 2 days. Symptoms of Norwalk virus infection include low-grade fever and combinations of diarrhea, anorexia, malabsorption, nausea, vomiting, abdominal cramps, malaise, myalgia, and headache. Unlike rotavirus infections, the gastroenteritis induced by Norwalk viruses is more epidemic in nature, usually resulting in shorter and milder illness, and the infections occur throughout the year.

Norwalk viruses invade the upper intestinal mucosa by binding to specific histo-blood group antigens present on the epithelium (415). Damage is limited to the small intestine in the area of the duodenal–jejunal junction. Volunteers who received the Norwalk agent developed histologic abnormalities within 12 to 48 hours following viral inoculation. These included mucosal inflammation, enterocyte changes, villous shortening, crypt hyperplasia, and increased epithelial mitoses. The lamina propria cellularity increased, containing both mononuclear cells and neutrophils. The changes persisted for at least 4 days and cleared by 6 to 8 weeks after the acute illness (416). Diagnostic tests include immunoelectron microscopy, radioimmunoassay for the virus and its antibodies, and PCR for the detection of Norwalk virus DNA.

Enteric Adenovirus Infections

Enteric adenovirus types 40 and 41 are readily transmitted from child to child and are the second most common cause of viral diarrhea in infants and young children requiring hospitalization. The virus has a worldwide distribution. Adenoviral illnesses usually affect children younger than 2 years old, particularly in the first year of life (417), and they may originate in daycare centers. Severe infections affect immunodeficient individuals and bone marrow transplant recipients, sometimes causing death. The infection also affects children following small bowel transplantation (418). The infections do not demonstrate seasonality. Adenovirus infections typically last from 5 to 12 days, producing protracted, watery diarrhea. Vomiting and fever are less prominent than with rotavirus infections (417). Rare infections associate with fatal disease and intussusception. The diagnosis is usually established by ultrastructural examination of the stool, viral cultures, radioimmunoassay, or the use of DNA probes. Ultrastructurally, the epithelial cells contain irregular hexagonal virions averaging 73 to 80 mm in diameter, often forming paracrystalline arrays.

Adenovirus infections tend to localize to the ileum because of the viral proclivity to infect lymphoid tissues (Fig. 6.77). Pathologists are unlikely to receive a specimen from a patient infected with an adenovirus unless the patient develops an intussusception, in which case the associated lymphoid hyperplasia acts as the lead point. Histologic changes are relatively nonspecific and include villous atrophy and inflammation. Neutrophils and mononuclear cells infiltrate the epithelium and lamina propria. Most of the changes remain confined to the villi, but rare glands also become necrotic and inflamed. Many villous epithelial cells contain intranuclear eosinophilic inclusions surrounded by a clear halo. In situ hybridization (Fig. 6.77) or PCR confirms the viral presence. Patients with intussusceptions may have ischemic changes superimposed on the viral changes.

Astrovirus Infections

Astroviruses occur worldwide and may be associated with both epidemic gastroenteritis and endemic childhood diarrhea (419). Astroviruses cause diarrheal outbreaks in newborn nurseries and pediatric wards, in community settings, and in nursing homes. Outbreaks sometimes affect daycare workers. Diarrhea due to astrovirus infections is more common in young children up to age 7 than in adults. Infants who are younger than 1 year of age are particularly vulnerable. Diarrhea usually develops in the winter months (420). Clinically, the infections resemble rotaviral illness, although the disease is less severe.

The virus infects the enterocytes along the upper parts of the villi and subepithelial macrophages. The viral particles are then released when the desquamated cells are released into the intestinal lumen and disintegrate. The epithelium restores itself within 5 days (421). Ultrastructurally, astroviruses measure 27 to 30 nm in diameter and exhibit a very characteristic five- or six-pointed star-shaped surface structure without a central hollow. Astroviral antibodies are detectable using indirect fluorescence. Most children acquire antiviral antibodies by age 5 years.

Cytomegalovirus Infections

CMV, a ubiquitous herpes virus, causes diverse clinical symptoms in many organs. Populations at highest risk for disseminated GI infection include neonates, allograft recipients, HIV-infected individuals, immunosuppressed patients, pregnant women, the very young or very old, or those with malnutrition or malignancy. Patients who undergo intestinal transplantation for short bowel syndrome are particularly vulnerable to CMV infections (422). In these patients, PCR analysis of intestinal biopsies may be useful for preemptive therapy in the selected patients (423).

The presentation of CMV enteritis in patients with isolated GI involvement ranges from mild anorexia to frank hemorrhage and perforation. The usual clinical manifestations are nonspecific and include fever, abdominal pain, diarrhea, vomiting, anorexia, weight loss, diarrhea, GI bleeding, and, occasionally, perforation. Mortality in CMV enteritis is adversely associated with age older than 65 and increased time to the institution of therapy but is not affected by the anatomic site of the infection (424). The entire small bowel may be involved, although some patients have limited ileocecal involvement. Histologically, the changes range from isolated inclusions with no accompanying tissue reaction to frank ulceration, toxic megacolon, and perforation. The pathologic features of CMV are discussed further in Chapter 13.

HIV Infections

More than 30 million people are infected with HIV-1 worldwide. Epidemiologically, the major risk groups for developing AIDS vary depending on geographic locale. In Africa and Asia, the major risk group is sexually active heterosexuals; women are more often infected than men (425). In contrast, in the United States, over 70% of cases affect homosexual or bisexual men. Another 15% develop in intravenous drug users. Other high-risk groups include prostitutes, hemophiliacs, children born to HIV-positive mothers, patients transfused with infected blood or blood products, and heterosexual contacts of any of the above groups (426). HIV-infected mothers pass the virus transplacentally, at the time of delivery through the birth canal, or through breast milk. AIDS especially affects Hispanics and African Americans (427). The AIDS patient population in the United States is disproportionately male, black, and poor. Women represented 18% of all cases in the United States in 1994. Sexual transmission is now the dominant route by which women become infected (428).

Substantial declines have occurred in AIDS incidence and death in recent years, probably due to an increased awareness in at-risk populations and the introduction of highly active antiretroviral treatment (HAART). Gastrointestinal complications were universally recognized during the course of HIV infection; however, in the era of HAART, these complications have dramatically decreased. There is a substantial reduction in the number of opportunistic infections associated with HIV infection in patients on HAART (429). Although substantially effective in suppressing opportunistic infections, the antiretroviral medications associate with GI side effects in up to 10% of cases. Currently, drug-induced side effects and nonopportunistic diseases are among the most common causes of GI symptoms in HIV-positive patients (430).

Multiple enteric pathogenic bacteria also cause diarrhea in AIDS patients. Patients may have one or more infections,

including *C. jejuni* or *C. fetus*, *C. difficile*, *Enterobacter aerogenes*, *Salmonella*, *S. flexneri*, *Klebsiella*, other Gram-negative bacilli, and *M. avium*. The most common virus to be detected is CMV. Patients may also have fungal or parasitic infections. The degree of inflammation seen in AIDS enteropathy correlates with mucosal levels of p24 antigen and clinical symptoms, supporting an etiologic role for HIV.

Disruption of the villous architecture with a reduction in villous height and crypt hyperplasia commonly occurs in patients with HIV enteropathy. This change alters the crypt:villus ratio and results in a decreased surface area in the small bowel. In addition, the epithelium converts from a columnar to a cuboidal morphology, consistent with epithelial cell injury. These epithelial changes associate with lamina propria inflammation, intraepithelial lymphocytosis, epithelial vacuolization, and increased apoptoses (Fig. 6.161) (431).

Some of the epithelial changes result from concomitant infections, and others are thought to be immune mediated. HIV can be found within the intestinal mucosa and the virus itself may be important in the enteropathy. In addition, nutritional factors may cause the enteropathy secondary to deficiencies of key nutrients (431). Other aspects of intestinal HIV infections are discussed in Chapter 13.

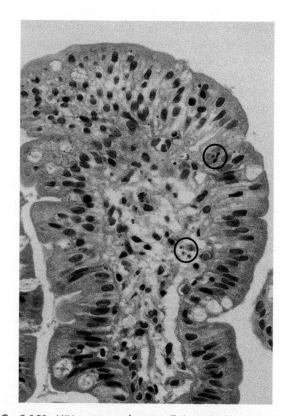

FIG. 6.161. HIV enteropathy. Small intestinal mucosa with increased number of intraepithelial lymphocytes and apoptosis within the epithelium as well as in the lamina propria mononuclear cells. The apoptotic areas are outlined by *circles*.

Parasitic Infections

Protozoans and helminths are responsible for considerable human morbidity and mortality (Table 6.22). Intestinal parasites infect more than 25% of the world's population. The infections are most frequent in developing countries due to overcrowding, poor nutrition, and inadequate sanitation. In a 1987 survey of 216,275 stool specimens examined by state diagnostic laboratories in the United States, parasites were found in 20.1%. Percentages were highest for protozoans (*Giardia lamblia*) (7.2%), *Entamoeba coli*, and *Endolimax nana* (4.2% each), *Blastocystis hominis* (2.6%), *Entamoeba histolytica* (0.9%), and *Cryptosporidium* spp. (0.2%). The most commonly identified helminths were nematodes: Hookworm (1.5%), *Trichuris trichiura* (1.2%), and *Ascaris lumbricoides* (0.8%). Other less commonly identified helminths included *Clonorcus* and *Opisthorchis* spp. (0.6%), *Strongyloides stercoralis* (0.4%), *Hymenolepis nana* (0.4%), *Enterobius vermicularis* (0.4%), and *Tinea* spp. (0.1%) (432,433).

Parasites have complex life cycles, with each stage exhibiting unique biochemical, antigenic, and morphologic features. Humans acquire protozoan and helminthic infections via multiple routes, including ingestion, direct penetration of the intact skin, or insect bites. The parasites then inhabit specific locations within their hosts. They reside intracellularly, intravascularly, in tissues, or in the GI lumen. Humans serve as both intermediate and definitive hosts for many parasites. Passage through intermediate hosts plays a significant role in the life cycle of many parasites.

Protozoal Infections

Giardia

G. lamblia has a worldwide distribution and is the most commonly reported parasitic disease in the United States and Canada (434). It is a leading cause of water-borne diarrheal outbreaks. *Giardia* infections increase in the summer and fall. In the United States, giardiasis commonly occurs in residents of, and travelers to, the Rocky Mountains. The surface waters become contaminated by the fecal material from wild animals. Most community-acquired infections occur where surface water (streams, rivers, and lakes) serves as the principal water source and chlorination is the principal disinfection method. Cysts remain viable in cold or tepid water for 1 to 3 months and can survive the chlorine concentrations present in municipal water systems. *Giardia* oocysts can also be found in the soil in up to 40% of parks, places where children commonly play (435). Infections occur by fecal–oral transmission, ingestion of contaminated food or drink, and person-to-person transmission in daycare centers and among homosexuals (436). *Giardia* also spreads among participants in swimming classes (437). Domestic pets, especially dogs, carry the organism (438). Patients with hypogammaglobulinemia, immunodeficiency syndromes, hypochlorhydria, or achlorhydria have an increased risk of acquiring the infection.

The infections may remain self-limited and asymptomatic or may last for years, causing severe diarrhea, cramps, malabsorption, and failure to thrive in children. The most common presentation is the onset of 5 to 7 days of acute diarrhea following an incubation period of 1 to 3 weeks. The acute illness varies in severity. Some patients experience an abrupt, explosive onset of frequent watery, foul-smelling stools, whereas others have only a few loose bowel movements. Other patients present with abdominal cramps, abdominal pain or distention, passage of flatus, lassitude, progressive weight loss, and malabsorption (439). Less often, fever and vomiting develop. Patients with chronic giardiasis have intermittent diarrhea that is less severe than that seen in the acute illness. Occasionally, allergic and other inflammatory phenomena develop.

TABLE 6.22	Small Intestinal Parasite Infections

Protozoa

Giardia lamblia
Cryptosporidium parvum
Isospora belli
Sarcocystis species
Coccidianlike bodies
Microsporidia
Trypanosoma cruzi
Visceral leishmaniasis

Helminths

Nematodes (round worms)
Ascaris lumbricoides
Trichuris trichiura
Capillaria philippinensis
Enterobius vermicularis
Trichostrongylus species
Trichinella species
Toxocara infections
Ancylostoma duodenale
Strongyloides stercoralis
Eustrongylus
Angiostrongylus costaricensis
Anisakis species

Cestodes (tapeworms)

Taenia saginata
Taenia solium
Diphyllobothrium latum
Hymenolepis nana

Trematodes

Schistosomal species
Intestinal flukes
Fasciolopsis buski
Echinostoma caprovi
Heterophyes heterophyes
Metagonimus yokogawai

Giardia exists in two morphologic forms: The motile trophozoite or feeding stage and the infective cyst (Fig. 6.162). Following ingestion, the cysts excyst in the duodenum, forming two daughter trophozoites. The oval, thick-walled cysts of *G. lamblia* initially contain two nuclei. These divide, forming four nuclei as the cysts pass through the intestinal tract. Mature cysts are shed in the stool. The cytoplasm often retracts from the cyst wall, imparting a double-walled appearance.

Giardia can be diagnosed by examining stool, duodenal aspirates, or duodenal biopsies. The diagnosis is most commonly made by finding characteristic cysts in the stool. However, stool examinations are only diagnostic in some patients with known infections. In contrast, most duodenal aspirates are positive. The number of trophozoites in these aspirates tends to be high during the acute phase of the infection and declines with the clearance phase (440). The sensitivity of *Giardia* detection increases if both stool specimens and duodenal aspirates are examined. Immunologic tests specific for the organism can supplement stool examination since most individuals develop antibodies to the parasite.

Giardia organisms are pear shaped, about the size of an epithelial cell nucleus, with two nuclei. One nucleus is visible when seen in profile. The parasites are often numerous. In H&E sections, *Giardia* appears gray or faintly basophilic

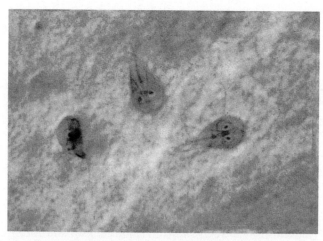

FIG. 6.163. Giardiasis. The *Giardia lamblia* trophozoites seen here in a trichrome-stained smear are distinguished by their pear shape and paired nuclei resembling eyeglasses.

(Figs. 6.163 and 6.164). The organism attaches itself to the microvilli of absorptive cells with its ventral suction disc and feeds through its dorsal surface. *Giardia* covers the enterocyte surface (Fig. 6.164), interfering with the microvillous layer and preventing interaction of digestive enzymes with luminal substrates. Rarely, trophozoites are found in the mucosa and lamina propria.

Small intestinal biopsies from immunocompetent patients show one of three patterns: (a) no alterations even though organisms are present; (b) a normal villous architecture, but increased numbers of intraepithelial lymphocytes and immunoglobulin containing cells in the lamina propria with a relative increase in the number of IgA- and IgG-containing cells; and (c) complete villous atrophy with brush border enzyme deficiencies, crypt hyperplasia, variable inflammation, large numbers of intraepithelial lymphocytes, and IgA- and IgM-containing cells in the lamina propria. Focally, neutrophils infiltrate the mucosa. The cellular infiltrate of the lamina propria tends to be highest in individuals with high trophozoite counts (440). A flat mucosa similar to that seen in celiac disease may occur, but it is rare. The incidence of partial villous atrophy ranges from 23% to 50% depending on a number of factors, including geography and the phase of the infection. When trophozoite numbers decline, the crypts lengthen to repair the villous atrophy. Patients may develop nodular lymphoid hyperplasia. Patients whose biopsies lack lamina propria plasma cells usually have coexisting hypogammaglobulinemia. Rarely, the organisms may be seen in the stomach or colon (439).

Cryptosporidial Infections

Cryptosporidium, a coccidial organism, infects the gastrointestinal epithelium, causing a diarrhea that is self-limited in immunocompetent persons but is potentially life threatening in those with AIDS (441). It accounts for 6% of all diarrheal diseases in immunocompetent persons and is found in

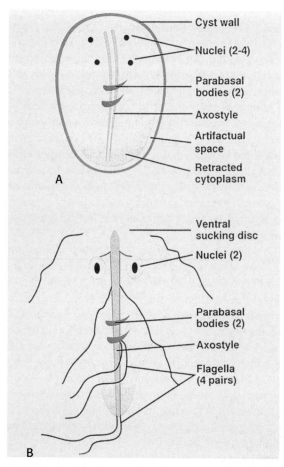

FIG. 6.162. *Giardia.* **A:** Cyst. **B:** Trophozoite.

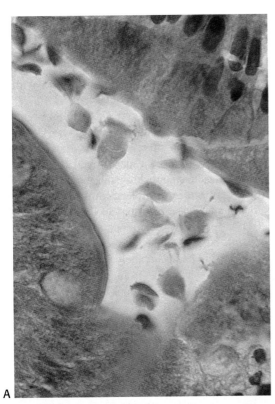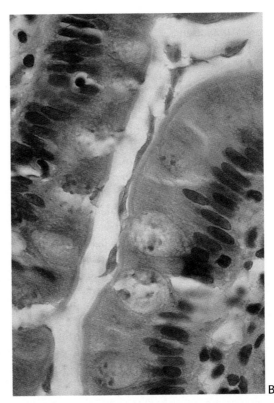

FIG. 6.164. Duodenal biopsy in a patient with giardiasis. **A:** Shows many trophozoites demonstrating their typical flattened appearance. **B:** Shows numerous trophozoites seen on their sides adherent to the glycocalyx of the enterocytes.

up to 24% of persons with AIDS and diarrhea worldwide (442). HIV-positive patients with self-limited infections have significantly higher CD4 counts than patients with persistent infections. The latter frequently have CD4 counts measuring <100 cells/mm³; they usually measure <50 cells/mm³. Although *Cryptosporidium parvum* is the most common species in humans, *Cryptosporidium felis, Cryptosporidium muris,* and *Cryptosporidium meleagridis* have also been identified in immunocompromised persons (443,444). *C. parvum* causes self-limited diarrhea in children, animal handlers, residents of developing countries, and travelers to tropical countries (445). Cryptosporidia have been added to the growing list of organisms causing diarrhea in daycare centers. Food, water, and other sources play a role in oocyst transmission (446). The organism is transmitted by fecal–oral or hand–mouth contamination, person to person, via pets, via contaminated food, and by water-borne outbreaks. Many community infections originate from public water sources, even when they are chlorinated since the cryptosporidia are resistant to chlorine treatment.

Humans are infected once they ingest the oocysts, which preferentially migrate to the GI tract where they begin their life cycle releasing infective sporozoites. Cryptosporidia can complete all stages of their development (sexual and asexual) within a single host cell (441). The sporozoite attaches to the apical membrane of enterocytes in a process mediated by specific ligands on the host cell (447). This attachment

induces reorganization of the host cell actin cytoskeleton and protrusion of the host cell membrane around the sporozoite to form a vacuole in which the organisms remain intracellular but extracytoplasmic (447). At the base of each vacuole an electron-dense band of host cell cytoskeletal elements facilitates the uptake of nutrients by the parasite from the host cell. The internalized sporozoite then matures and undergoes asexual reproduction to produce merozoites. After release into the intestinal lumen, the merozoites can either infect other epithelial cells or mature into gametocytes, the sexual form of the parasite. The life cycle is repeated after fertilization occurs in the intestinal tract, yielding thin-walled oocysts that sporulate to release sporozoites again. This cycle leads to autoinfection and heavy persistent infections with massive shedding of oocysts in the feces of an infected patient (441).

In immunocompetent individuals, the disease usually presents as an acute, mild to moderate, self-limited illness lasting 3 to 4 days (446), although it may persist for up to 4 weeks. Patients have nonspecific clinical manifestations including passage of watery, nonbloody stools; vomiting; anorexia; abdominal cramps and pain; and possibly malabsorption and weight loss. AIDS patients, unlike immunocompetent patients, cannot clear the organism, so that the infection often persists for the remainder of the patient's life. Patients with proximal small intestinal infections typically begin with a mild diarrhea that progresses to voluminous, debilitating, watery diarrhea associated with dehydration, malabsorption, and profound weight loss. Secondary malabsorption often occurs and is related to a decreased absorptive surface area in heavily infested individuals. Gastroduodenal involvement may produce partial gastric outlet obstruction. AIDS patients often have coexisting gastrointestinal infections; the intensity of the symptoms and histologic findings reflect the nature and intensity of all of the organisms that are present.

The clinical diagnosis primarily relies on detection of 5-μm acid-fast oocysts in fresh stools (Fig. 6.165). Immunofluorescence methods provide enhanced sensitivity and specificity over conventional staining methods. Enzyme immunoassay kits are simple, rapid, and less subjective ways to detect cryptosporidia in fecal samples (448).

Cryptosporidia can involve the esophagus, stomach, bile ducts, and intestines. The diagnosis of cryptosporidial infection requires close scrutiny of all epithelial surfaces, including those in the lumina of intestinal glands for the presence of the characteristic organisms (Fig. 6.165). The organisms can be recognized as clusters of spherical or ovoid basophilic (bluish) or golden brown bodies measuring 2 to 4 μm in diameter attached to the epithelial surfaces. The sensitivity of endoscopy with mucosal biopsy in detecting the organism varies by anatomic location as follows: Stomach (11%), duodenum (53%), terminal ileum (91%), and colon (60%) (449). Low-density infections may associate with normal duodenal histology, whereas severe inflammation and villous atrophy complicate high-density infections. The mucosa may contain acute inflammation and an intraepithelial lymphocytosis. The infected cells show a range in cell injury from only minimal injury and fragments of organisms in the cells to focal necrosis that results in variable villous and crypt atrophy.

In tissue sections, cryptosporidia are best seen with a modified Kinyoun stain. The organism stains deep blue with Giemsa and Gram stains, positively with PAS stains, and negatively with the Gomori methenamine silver (GMS) stain. A combined acid fast–trichrome stain may be useful in detecting the organism (450). A fluorescein-labeled IgG monoclonal antibody to the wall of cryptosporidial oocysts is very sensitive and can detect small numbers of organisms in tissue sections or GI brushings.

Cryptosporidia can be easily overlooked or mistaken for mucous droplets. Conversely, cellular debris and mucus clinging to the epithelium can be mistaken for cryptosporidia. However, unlike the apical mucin droplets that they resemble, cryptosporidia are mucicarmine negative. There is currently no effective treatment for the disease (441).

Microsporidial Infections

Microsporidia constitute a separate phylum of ubiquitous, spore-forming, obligate intracellular protozoans that cause a wide range of diseases, including enteritis and encephalitis. Distinctive features of the phylum *Microspora* include (a) a lack of mitochondria; (b) a merogonic and sporogonic life cycle, which gives rise to generations of sporoblasts that become mature spores; and (c) spores with a coiled polar filament; the number of coils is unique to each species (451). Microsporidiosis has an extensive host range, including most invertebrates and all classes of vertebrates. Microsporidia are pathogens in birds, arthropods, fish, and a few mammals. Most animals acquire the infection through ingestion. Microsporidia are primarily water borne, but food-borne disease also occurs. These infections predominantly, but not exclusively, affect severely immunocompromised persons with AIDS. The prevalence of microsporidial infection in AIDS patients varies from 15% to 39% (452,453). Patients with microsporidial infections are usually homosexual with a history of foreign travel or

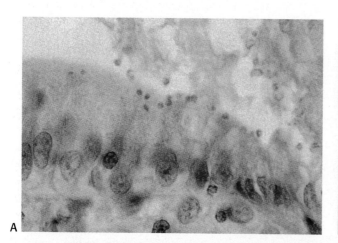
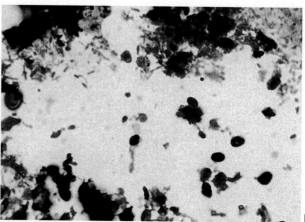

FIG. 6.165. *Cryptosporidium.* **A:** The cryptosporidial organisms appear as small (2 to 3 μm) round hematoxylinophilic bodies adjacent to or attached to the mucosal surface. **B:** In cryptosporidial diarrhea, the diagnosis can be made by demonstrating characteristic oocysts in the stools on modified acid-fast stains of the smear preparation. The oocysts typically measure 3 to 6 μm in diameter and stain bright pink-red and have a discernible outer wall.

residence in tropical regions. Microsporidia contribute significantly to the overall morbidity in HIV-infected patients. Human infections result from the following organisms: *Enterocytozoon bieneusi, Enterocephalitozoon cuniculi, Nosema, Pleistophora,* and *Encephalitozoon.* There are three currently recognized *Encephalitozoon* species: *Encephalitozoon hellem, Encephalitozoon cuniculi,* and *Encephalitozoon intestinalis.* Enterocytozoons and Encephalitozoons account for most microsporidial infections.

The clinical manifestations of microsporidiosis are diverse and include intestinal, biliary, pulmonary, ocular, muscular, and renal disease (453). The organisms also cause asymptomatic disease. Endoscopically, patients with microsporidial infections do not usually demonstrate discrete ulcerations or mass lesions, but the villi often appear abnormal under the dissecting microscope. *E. hellem* and *E. intestinalis* behave more like classic mammalian microsporidia. *E. cuniculi, E. hellem,* and *E. intestinalis* not only spread contiguously, but also infect macrophages and disseminate from their points of entry to the respiratory tract and other organs (454).

Enterocytozoon bieneusi *Infection*

The cardinal features of *E. bieneusi* infections are persistent diarrhea with increased fecal volumes measuring up to several liters per 24 hours. The chronic diarrhea (lasting up to 30 months) causes severe wasting (451) and fluid and electrolyte imbalance. Its prevalence ranges from 10% to 34% in AIDS patients with diarrhea. Patients with microsporidial infections are usually men having sex with men with a history of foreign travel or residence in tropical regions. CD4 counts typically measure <50 cells/mm^3. Although *E. bieneusi* infects the entire length of the small intestine, it preferentially involves the proximal small intestine. The lesion may go undetected if the infection does not produce enteritis, ulceration, or other histologic abnormalities. The infection is usually focal and spores may be very sparse. Mucosal biopsies may show an increase in mucosal macrophages or plasma cells.

Two phases of the life cycle of *E. bieneusi* are identified ultrastructurally: (a) a proliferative phase (merogony) and (b) a spore-forming phase (sporogony). During the proliferative phase, the organisms appear as small, electron-lucent round objects containing one to six nuclei. The spore-forming phase begins with the presence of stacks of electron-dense discs that later aggregate end to end to form the curved profiles of polar tubes. The nuclei continue to divide, resulting in larger organisms with up to 12 nuclei surrounded by several coils of the polar tube. These large multinucleated forms break up into sporoblasts (immature spores) that then develop into mature spores. The mature spores are very electron dense with a single nucleus and possess an exceptional tubular extrusion apparatus for injecting spore contents, termed *sporoplasm,* into host cells. It consists of several coils of polar tube, an anchoring tube, and a polarplast. Each

spore also contains a posterior polar vacuole and a polar filament with five to seven overlapping coils of the polar tubules that appear in cross section as a series of doublets. Spores are infective when released in the feces. Intracellularly, spores differentiate into trophozoites that undergo asexual multiplication to form merozoites. The merozoites invade new host cells and certain types develop into male and female microgametes. Fertilization produces oocysts that are either excreted or produce sporozoites in situ to repeat the cycle.

Microsporidia can be diagnosed by identifying the spores in the stools, small bowel biopsies, intestinal aspirates, or mucosal brushings with touch preparations. Stool examination for spores using the modified chromophobe stain is the simplest method and perhaps the most sensitive for diagnosing the intestinal infection (455).

Typically, the parasite has a focal distribution in the duodenal mucosa, although massive infestations may occur (Fig. 6.166). The degree of cellular injury parallels the intensity of the infection. Some patients develop villous atrophy, crypt hyperplasia, intraepithelial lymphocytosis, and loss of brush border enzyme activity. Involved villi may appear blunted or have a bulbous shape. The enterocytes may contain irregular hyperchromatic nuclei and a vacuolated cytoplasm. In heavy infections, disorganized aggregates of crowded, irregularly shaped, degenerating necrotic cells often containing merozoites and spores populate the villous tips. The tips of the villi and strips of infected mucosa eventually slough into the lumen. A variable lymphocytic infiltrate accompanies the epithelial changes, but neutrophils are usually absent. The organisms lie clustered in the supranuclear cytoplasm and may indent the enterocyte nucleus, making them easier to identify when screening at low power. The clustered, dark, refractile, oval spores measure approximately 0.7 to 1.0 μm in width and 1 to 1.6 μm in length and are less frequent than the parasite. They are surrounded by an inner unit membrane, an electron-lucent endospore, and a thin electron-dense exospore. Spores are often seen in degenerating enterocytes.

A helpful diagnostic feature is the presence of a PAS-positive polar cap at one end of the spore. The spores are also positive with acid-fast stains. Gram stains also are useful for detecting the organism. They are readily identified because of the contrasting dark blue or reddish staining against a brown-yellow background. Some use Warthin-Starry, modified trichrome, or Giemsa stains to identify the parasite. A combined acid-fast–trichrome stain may be useful in detecting the organism (450). The use of semithin sections (Fig. 6.167) gives better histologic definition and is helpful in identifying the organism in individuals with sparse infections and in identifying the earlier stages of the parasitic development because of the visualization of the characteristic clefts. The diagnosis is based on the ultrastructural features of the spores in the proliferative forms, the method of division, and the nature of the host cell–parasite interface. Ultrastructural examination is particularly useful in

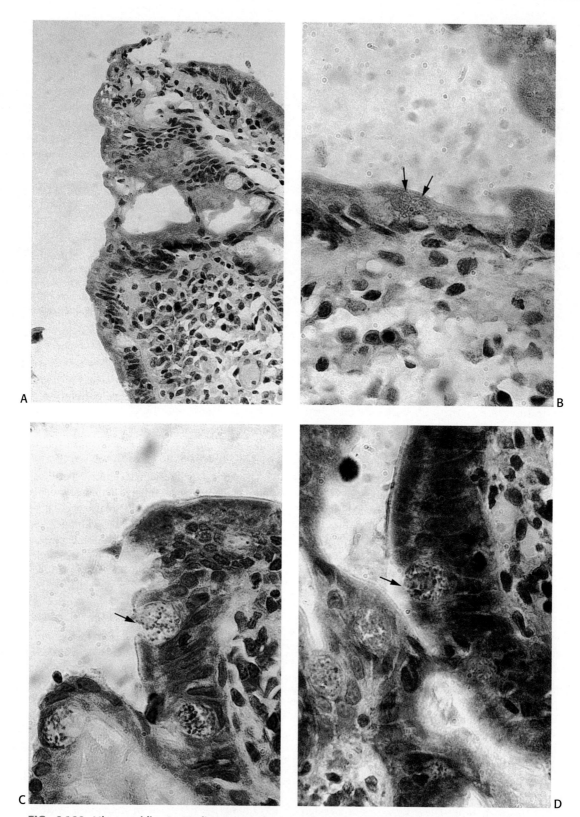

FIG. 6.166. Microsporidia. A: Medium-power hematoxylin and eosin–stained section showing a small intestinal mucosa with atrophy and a minimal increase in chronic inflammatory cells. **B:** Higher magnification shows a flattened epithelium with mild increased basophilia (*arrows*). **C:** Gram stain showing parasitophorous vesicles (*arrow*) containing a large number of organisms. **D:** Giemsa-stained specimen showing the azure blue organisms within the epithelium (*arrow*).

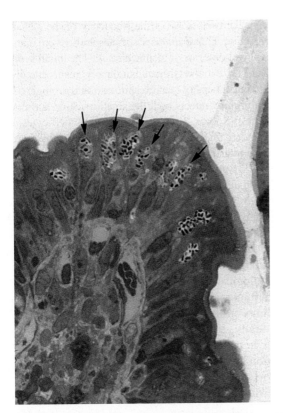

FIG. 6.167. Microsporidia. Thick Epon-embedded section stained with toluidine blue demonstrating numerous parasitophorous vesicles (*arrows*) in a supranuclear location.

differentiating between intestinal microsporidiosis due to *E. bieneusi* and *E. intestinalis* as described in reference 455. The organism may also be detected by the use of antibodies or PCR amplification of small-subunit RNA.

Microsporidia are often missed, even on careful examination, because of their small size, intracellular location, and poor staining with usual tissue stains. The stains discussed above may produce distinctive contrasts between the very small microsporidial spores and other cellular contents and background debris.

Because of the propensity of some microsporidia to disseminate and because of their differences in drug sensitivities, there is an increasing demand for pathologists and microbiologists to classify the microsporidia. The infection can be treated with fumagillin (456).

Enterocytozoon intestinalis *Infection*

Enterocytozoon intestinalis is the second most prevalent microsporidian infection reported in AIDS patients. *E. intestinalis* produced severe diarrhea, a wasting syndrome, and systemic disease. The initial symptoms usually localize to the GI tract, but the organisms can disseminate and infect hepatobiliary, respiratory, and urologic tissues leading to renal failure and rhinosinusitis (457).

E. intestinalis has a life cycle with four stages: Meront, sporont, sporoblast, and spore. Like *E. bieneusi*, the spores

contain a polar tube that injects membrane-bound sporoplasm into uninfected host cells. The earliest stage, the meront, is an ovoid, uninucleate organism measuring 2.7 × 1.5 μm that replicates by binary fission. The nuclear division sometimes outstrips cytoplasmic division, leading to binucleate and tetranucleate forms. As a result, a cluster of organisms aggregates within a vacuole in the host cell cytoplasm. The second stage, the sporont, divides by binary fission, each producing two or four sporoblasts (455). Sporoblasts are uninucleate organisms that develop a polar tube and as these mature, these organelles become more conspicuous. Transformation to the final or fourth stage of the spore is marked by the development of a thick coat. The spores measure approximately 2.0 × 1.2 μm in size and contain a single nucleus and a polar tube, as well as some other organelles. They infect target cells by sticking to the cell membrane by means of the anterior attachment organ and injecting sporoblasts into the host cell via the polar tube. This is followed by merogony.

E. bieneusi and *E. intestinalis* may be differentiated by their location in the intestine. *E. bieneusi* only infects the epithelial cells, usually at the villous tips. In contrast, *E. intestinalis* also infects the epithelium at the tips of the villi and deeper in the crypts and also infects fibroblasts, macrophages, and endothelial cells in the lamina propria.

Histologically, one sees the typical features of a microsporidia. The degree of villous blunting and inflammation varies considerably, and may be present or absent. Ultrastructurally, parasites in various stages of development cluster in parasitophorous vacuoles that appear to undergo septation by a fibrillar matrix so that each spore appears to lie in its own compartment. The spores contain a polar filament with five to seven coils.

Isospora belli *Infection*

Most *Isospora belli* infections affect patients in tropical and subtropical countries, particularly in Africa and South America. *I. belli* accounts for diarrhea in 15% of Haitian and 0.2% of U.S. patients with AIDS. The organism spreads by ingestion of contaminated food or water or via homosexual transmission. In the immunocompetent host, the disease manifests itself as a self-limited malabsorption lasting 3 to 5 weeks (458). Fever, malaise, colicky abdominal pain, nausea, weight loss, and watery diarrhea usually occur in immunocompromised patients. The diarrhea in AIDS patients may last for months and is more severe than that which affects the immunocompetent host, and these patients may become wasted (459). About 50% of patients develop peripheral eosinophilia. Malabsorption appears later in the disease course. Symptoms resemble those seen in cryptosporidial infections, but the distinction between the two infections is important because *Isospora* infections are easily treated by appropriate antibiotic therapy.

Like cryptosporidiosis, *I. belli* infections follow ingestion of infective forms (sporulated oocysts). Excystation occurs in the proximal small bowel, resulting in the release of eight sporozoites from each cyst. The latter invade epithelial cells and mature into trophozoites. During the schizogonous (asexual) phase, each trophozoite divides into numerous merozoites, which, when released from parasitized cells, invade other epithelial cells. Each merozoite may then pass through one or more repetitive cycles of asexual division or proceed to the sexual phase by maturing into macro- (female) and micro- (male) gametes. Zygotes, resulting from fertilization of the gametes, mature into oocysts that are then released into the bowel lumen. These then pass into the stools (Fig. 6.168), or during their transit in the bowel, undergo sporulation, and release trophozoites that parasitize enterocytes downstream to start the cycle over again. All stages of both asexual (trophozoite, schizont, and merozoite) and sexual (macrogametocyte) phases of the life cycle of the parasite are found in the epithelial cytoplasm, always enclosed within a parasitophorous vacuole. The nonsporulated (immature) oocytes excreted in stool mature into infective mature oocysts within 48 to 72 hours but can also remain dormant for long periods.

Because patients with isosporiasis intermittently shed oocysts, multiple stool specimens should be examined to increase the likelihood of detecting the organism. The oocysts are concentrated from fresh stool samples by sucrose flotation and highlighted by the Kinyoun acid-fast stain. *Isospora* oocysts are larger (25 to 30 μm in length) than *Cryptosporidium* (4 to 5 μm), with a thin wall enveloping two large sporoblasts or a single large zygote (an immature oocyst) when shed in the feces. Fecal specimens are best examined after 1 to 2 days at room temperature, allowing oocysts to mature. Although the organism preferentially infects the small bowel, it can spread to the stomach, esophagus, biliary tree, and large intestine, but it only rarely disseminates to extraintestinal lymph nodes, liver, or spleen.

This pathogen can be seen within enterocytes of the small intestine or, less commonly, in the colonic mucosa. *I. belli*

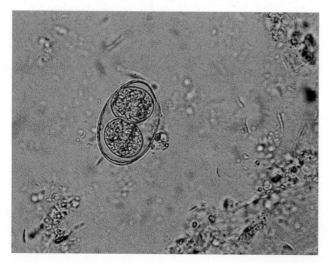

FIG. 6.168. *Isospora.* The relatively large (15 to 20 μm) oocyst of *Isospora* is thin walled and contains sporocysts after sporulation.

causes moderate mucosal villous atrophy, crypt hyperplasia, and lamina propria infiltration by lymphocytes, plasma cells, neutrophils, and eosinophils. Eosinophils may be so plentiful as to suggest a diagnosis of eosinophilic enteritis. The flattened mucosa may show clubbed villous tips, marked dilation of the vascular spaces, and excessive collagen deposits in the lamina propria. The epithelium generally appears well preserved except for foci of vacuolization. Closer examination usually discloses the presence of organisms in different stages of sexual and asexual life cycles. The parasitized cells are destroyed and adjacent cells are left intact, appearing normal. Occasional extracellular merozoites may be seen in the intestinal lumen and in the lamina propria near or within lymphatic vessels (460). Rarely, schizonts are present in the lamina propria and the submucosa. Mesenteric lymph nodes may also become involved.

The organisms are difficult to see on routine H&E sections, but Giemsa staining highlights them. Often one sees large numbers of unsuspected coccidial organisms within the epithelium. The organisms stain faintly with H&E, and dark blue with Giemsa or H&E plus Alcian blue. They are also strongly PAS positive but are difficult to differentiate from host goblet cells. The large schizont stage is best seen in overstained Giemsa preparations. The merozoite has a banana shape and occurs at all levels in the enterocyte cytoplasm. The central nucleus, large nucleolus, perinuclear halo, and location within a thick parasitophorous (PAS-negative) vacuole give it a characteristic appearance. Free merozoites and gametocytes are more difficult to detect than intracellular organisms.

Eimeria *Infections*

Eimeria infections resemble other coccidial infections. The clinical features and histologic features are essentially similar. The terminal web of microfilaments in the epithelial cells infected by the merozoites of *Eimeria tenella* becomes disrupted and cell extensions are present on the enterocyte surface. Marked morphologic alterations result in microvillous loss and extensive cytoplasmic bulging into the crypt lumen. Invasion of enterocytes and invasion of goblet cells also occurs. Large numbers of mast cells infiltrate the mucosa. Merozoites are also found within mast cells and lymphocytes in the lumen (461). Ultrastructurally, the organism lacks the crystalloid body found in Isospora.

Cyclospora *Infection*

Cyclospora infections affect up to 11% of Haitian AIDS patients (462), and they also commonly affect North American travelers returning from Haiti and Mexico. The organisms have been implicated in large diarrheal outbreaks and community infections originate from public water sources since the organism can withstand the chlorination process. The illness develops in both normal and immunocompromised individuals, and is characterized by severe

TABLE 6.23	Comparison of Helminths		
Characteristic	Nematodes	Cestodes	Flukes
Shape	Round, without segments	Tapelike, segmented	Leaflike, without segments
Body cavity	+	−	−
Sexes	Separate	Hermaphroditic	Hermaphroditic
Hooklets	−	+	−
Suckers	−	+	+

intermittent watery diarrhea, nausea, and anorexia and fatigue, which wax and wane for weeks to months before spontaneous recovery (463). Resolution occurs abruptly after 2 to 12 weeks of illness and the organism disappears from stool specimens. The symptoms resemble those seen in patients with *Isospora* or cryptosporidial infections.

The cysts measure 10 μm in diameter and in freshly passed stool are readily identified by their blue autofluorescence under ultraviolet light (463). This identification method may be more sensitive and reliable than the modified acid-fast stain or iodine stains. The organisms stain with modified acid-fast stain but not with hematoxylin, methenamine silver, or PAS stain.

The organism is not usually found in intestinal biopsies, although it is found in duodenal aspirates (463). Patients with these infections exhibit mild to moderate acute and chronic inflammation, surface epithelial disarray, variable villous atrophy and crypt hyperplasia, increased plasma cells in the lamina propria, and focal neutrophilic infiltrates. Surface enterocytes, especially their villous tips, appear focally vacuolated and lose their brush border. The enterocytes become columnar in shape and crypts become hyperplastic.

Helminthic Infections

Table 6.23 compares nematodes (round worms), trematodes (flukes), and cestodes (tapeworms).

Ascaris Infections

Ascaris infections are the most prevalent intestinal helminth, infecting approximately 25% of the human population (464). The worms have a worldwide distribution, although they are most common in tropical and subtropical regions of Asia, Africa, and America. Ascariasis is acquired by ingesting mature eggs from contaminated soil when children play on the ground or when ova are ingested in fecally contaminated food and water (Fig. 6.169). The number of worms harbored determines morbidity and transmission dynamics. The balance between exposure rates and rate of loss of the infection due to host immune defenses determines the intensity of infection. Environmental factors also play a role in disease transmission. *Ascaris* eggs remain dormant under dry conditions.

Ascaris lumbricoides is the largest of the round worms, measuring up to 40 cm in length. These worms have a lifespan of 1 year or less and females generally live longer than males. The worm has a constricted area known as a vulvar waist (genital girdle) located at the junction of the anterior and middle thirds of the body. A coiled tail forms copulatory spicules. Each female releases about 200,000 ova. Fertile eggs are ovoid, measure 6 to 40 μm in length, have a golden brown color due to bile staining, and consist of an albuminous

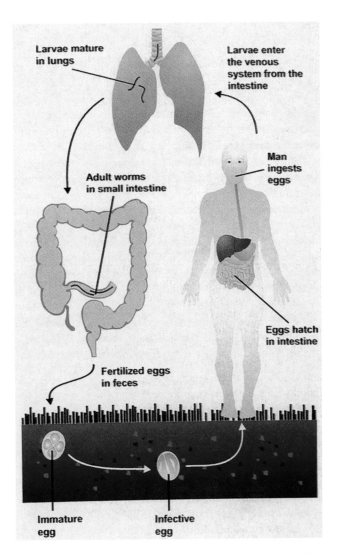

FIG. 6.169. Life cycle of the *Ascaris lumbricoides* (see text).

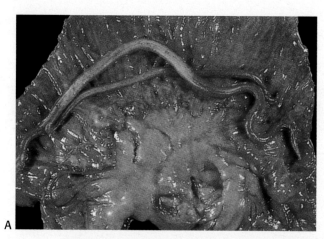
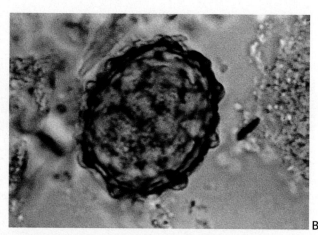

FIG. 6.170. *Ascaris lumbricoides.* **A:** This organism measures up to 35 cm in length, much larger than other intestinal roundworms, and resembles an earthworm. **B:** Diagnosis of *Ascaris* infection is usually made by demonstration in the stool of the characteristic egg with its corrugated outer surface. (B courtesy of Dr. Dickson Despommier, Department of Parasitology, Columbia University, NY.)

outer coat, a thick inner shell, and one or more yolk cells. Infertile eggs are longer, measuring 40 to 90 μm with irregular albuminous coats and no yolk cells. The organisms mature inside their egg shells before becoming infective. Eggs become infective in soil 3 to 4 weeks after excretion. It takes 2 to 3 weeks following ingestion for infective larvae to develop in the intestine and to penetrate the mucosa, reaching the portal venous system. Following migration, the adult worms (one to several hundred) develop in the small intestine (usually midjejunum), where they anchor themselves to mucosal surfaces (Fig. 6.170).

Clinical features include epigastric pain resembling peptic ulcer disease, duodenitis, and malnutrition. When present in large numbers, clumps of *Ascaris* obstruct the small intestinal lumen, causing an acute abdomen. Masses of worms also obstruct the common bile and pancreatic ducts, which leads to perforation and volvulus. When these long worms migrate into the common bile duct and pancreatic duct, they produce cholangitis and pancreatitis. In severe cases, the liver may be involved. Ascariasis has particularly adverse effects in malnourished populations. The worms may be evident within the intestinal lumen. Once the infection clears, one may only see residual traces of their presence. These may present as small polypoid structures lying within the submucosa and surrounded by fibrotic reactive tissue (Fig. 6.171).

Hookworm Infections

Hookworm infections rank second to ascariasis in incidence of intestinal helminthic infections. The parasites infect approximately 900 million individuals worldwide (465). The most significant nematodes in the hookworm group include *Ancylostoma duodenale* and *Necator americanus.* Hookworms cause chronic blood loss, intestinal malabsorption, abdominal pain, and bloody diarrhea. Patients with chronic infections present with iron deficiency anemia (which may be severe when the worm burden is high and

iron intake is limited), hypoalbuminemia, blood loss, and vague abdominal discomfort or pain. Patients often have peripheral eosinophilia as well as eosinophilic enteritis. The eosinophilia results from an allergic response to larval secretions.

Ancylostoma caninum (dog hookworm) causes disease in patients who own dogs. Infectious filariform larvae invade the skin through bare feet or other exposed skin surfaces (Fig. 6.172). A purpuric, papular, or vesicular eruption develops at the entry site. After passing through a series of developmental stages, the hookworm migrates through the lungs, occasionally causing pulmonary symptoms, infiltrates, and eosinophilia. Adult worms, measuring 8 to 10 mm in length, emerge in the proximal small intestine and anchor themselves to the mucosa (Fig. 6.173). *A. caninum* is often diagnosed by identifying the 1-cm long worm in GI biopsies or duodenal aspirates, especially in patients with heavy parasitic infections. The mucosa may appear hemorrhagic, eroded, congested, and edematous. The diagnosis is also made by stool examination and identification of characteristic ova (Fig. 6.173). Histologically, besides the presence of the worm, the most significant pathologic findings are a focal or diffuse eosinophilia and mural edema. Increased numbers of lamina propria eosinophils are particularly prominent near areas of parasitic attachment. Ulcers result from the hookworm bite sites. Some patients develop focal crypt hyperplasia, villous atrophy, and inflammation. Patients may exhibit regional lymphadenopathy due to the presence of granulomas with central eosinophilic degranulation and degradation products. The worms are often found within the short stenotic ileal segments.

Strongyloidiasis

Infections by *Strongyloides stercoralis* are widely prevalent throughout the world. Five million people harbor the nematode (466). Infections are most likely to occur in areas where

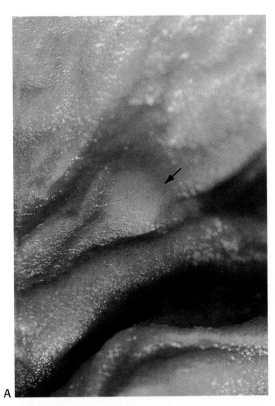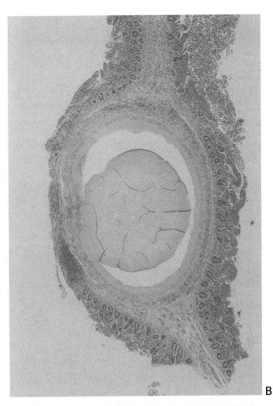

A   B

FIG. 6.171. Chronic parasitic infection in a patient who died of a myocardial infarction. **A:** Translucent elevated lesion is present (*arrow*). **B:** Histologic features demonstrating a submucosal cyst lined by centric rings of fibrous tissue and inflammatory cells. The center contains eosinophilic material.

waste is used as fertilizer. Principally found in tropical and subtropical areas, *S. stercoralis* is also endemic elsewhere. In the United States, the highest prevalence of strongyloidiasis occurs in Kentucky and eastern Tennessee (467). Endemic areas are also present in central and southern Europe (468). *Strongyloides,* the most common intestinal parasite in Southeast Asia, causes chronic debilitating illnesses. Individuals or military personnel returning from this area may experience symptoms for a long time (469). Prisoners of war are particularly prone to develop these infections. In the United States, parasitic infections emerged in World War II and Vietnam veterans years after exposure. Disseminated strongyloidiasis becomes manifest as the veteran population ages or undergoes immunosuppressive and/or cytotoxic therapy for other disorders. Disseminated hyperinfection affects subjects with immunocompromised T-cell immunity associated with steroid use, neoplasms, malnutrition, aging, or AIDS.

The rhabditiform larvae are found in soil contaminated by human feces where they go through four stages to become male (0.7 mm in length) and female (1 to 2 mm in length) adults. If the climatic conditions are unfavorable, the rhabditoid larvae change directly into filariform or strongyloid larvae, measuring approximately 400 μm in length. These are incapable of surviving for more than a couple of weeks in the external environment but they can continue development in humans (Fig. 6.174). The filariform larvae enter humans by penetrating the skin. The larvae reach the lungs through vessels. In the lung, they pass through the alveoli, reaching the bronchi, trachea, and larynx. They then enter the esophagus and migrate to the duodenum and jejunum, their preferred sites, where they transform into adults. After fertilizing the females, males are rapidly expelled with the feces, whereas the females penetrate the intestinal mucosa. Here they deposit up to 30 eggs a day. These develop into rhabditoid larvae. Only when they hatch do they leave the mucous membrane to reach the intestinal lumen from which they are excreted with the feces. It is for this reason that eggs are very rarely found in the stools. The rhabditoid larvae can transform into filariform larvae within 24 hours and then may reinvade the host either through the intestinal mucosa (internal autoinfection) or through the perianal skin (external autoinfection).

Adult females inhabit the duodenal and jejunal mucosa. However, adults can be found throughout both the small and large intestine in heavy infections. The worm perpetuates itself in the host for decades by autoinfection. Chronic infection results from the inability of the host to eliminate the adult worms from the small bowel, the inability to prevent colonic reinfection by filariform larvae, or the inability to destroy larvae that are in transit back to the intestine. Most filariform larvae lie within the intestinal lymphatics, and they concentrate in the mesenteric and retroperitoneal lymph nodes. Larvae may be found in many tissues.

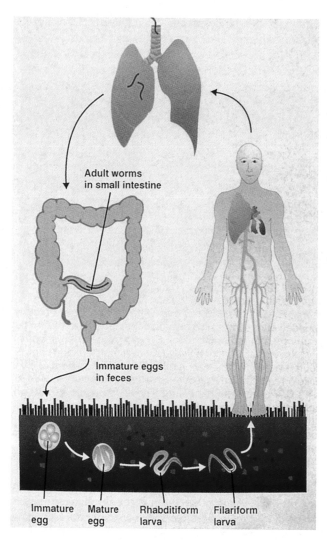

FIG. 6.172. Hookworm life cycle (see text).

Strongyloides infections range from asymptomatic cases to the presence of severe disease, especially in patients with heavy infections. Symptoms include diarrhea, malabsorption, weight loss, eosinophilia, abdominal pain, nausea, vomiting, constipation, gastrointestinal bleeding, and pruritus ani (469). A rash (creeping eruptions) results from dermal penetration. Patients with disseminated strongyloidiasis show the heaviest parasite burden in the proximal small intestine and lungs. Some patients die secondary to extensive small and large intestinal ulceration. Hyperinfection syndrome is diagnosed by finding parasites on stool examination, duodenal aspiration, sputum, bronchoalveolar lavages, cerebrospinal fluid, ascites fluid, or urine, or in biopsies. Serologic tests also detect the disease.

The intestines acquire hemorrhagic and ragged mucosal surfaces covered by a friable, greenish tan pseudomembrane. Larvae, adult worms, and eggs may be seen within the crypts. At the time of laparotomy or autopsy, one may find a mass in or attached to the bowel wall, often wrapped around the greater omentum. The lesions frequently center around the ileocecal valve. Occasionally, the changes mimic Crohn disease.

Biopsies show cross section of the worms. The posterior regions of the adult females exhibit a characteristic single intestine and double reproductive tubes (Fig. 6.175). The mucosa may show superficial segmental ulceration and the lamina propria may appear congested and edematous, containing numerous neutrophils and eosinophils early in the infection. Later, mononuclear cells, including lymphocytes and plasma cells, infiltrate the mucosa. If the inflammation becomes transmural, peritonitis develops. Most acute lesions affect the small intestine but similar changes occur both in the stomach and colon. Crypt hyperplasia with varying degrees of villous atrophy associates with inflammation of the lamina propria. In patients with severe malabsorption, the intestinal villi become atrophic, swollen, or fused, and one may see granulomas and fibrosis. Crypt distortion and erosions relate to the presence of adult worms, rhabditiform larvae, and ova. Some patients develop inflammatory pseudotumors or "helminthomas," usually in the ileocecal area. Smaller granulomas with necrotic centers are characterized by a cuff of eosinophils (Fig. 6.176). The presence of Charcot-Leyden crystals in the necrotic center should alert the examiner to the possibility of chronic hyperinfective strongyloidiasis. Worm tracks can be found within the masses as the worms try to migrate further into the bowel wall.

Angiostrongyloidiasis

Abdominal angiostrongyloidiasis results from infections with the nematode *Angiostrongylus costaricensis,* an organism prevalent in Central and South America. Its life cycle involves a definitive host (wild rodents) and an intermediate host (the slug). Human infections occur when persons ingest vegetables contaminated with third-stage larvae from the slugs. Larvae penetrate the GI wall and mature in lymphatics and lymph nodes to migrate through the vasculature of the ileocecal region. *A. costaricensis* causes an intense eosinophilic necrotizing arteritis associated with thrombosis and ischemic necrosis due to an arteritis and arterial thrombosis and the presence of numerous eosinophilic granulomas (470).

Capillaria philippinensis *Infections*

Capillaria philippinensis is a tiny nematode that causes severe diarrhea in humans. Persons infected with this parasite often live in the Philippines and Thailand, where it is common to eat raw freshwater fish. A fish–bird cycle plays a role in the infection. The worms inhabit both the large and small intestines. Male worms measure 1.5 to 3 mm in length and females measure 2.5 to 5 mm in length. Capillarids are closely related to *Trichuris* and *Trichinella* species (471). The organism is diagnosed by the presence of characteristic ova. The barrel-shaped eggs have flattened bipolar plugs (Fig. 6.177)

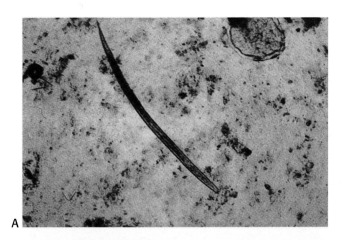

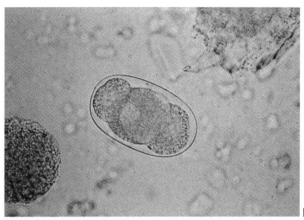

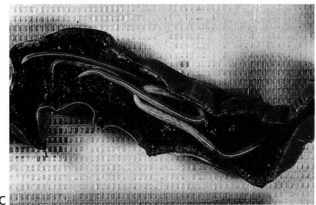

FIG. 6.173. Hookworm. A: The first-stage rhabditiform hookworm larva develops from the egg and is usually found in the stool. **B:** The hookworm egg with its thin shell, bluntly rounded ends, and multilobulated contents is typical of hookworm eggs found in the stool. Eggs of *Necator americanus* and *Ancylostoma duodenale* are indistinguishable. **C:** Patient with pig bel and incidental *Ascaris* infection and hookworm. The hookworm lies at the tip of the curved tail of the *Ascaris.* (A and B courtesy of Dickson Despommier, Ph.D., Department of Parasitology, Columbia Presbyterian Medical Center, New York, NY. C courtesy of Robin Cooke, M.D., Department of Pathology, Royal Brisbane Hospital, Brisbane, Australia.)

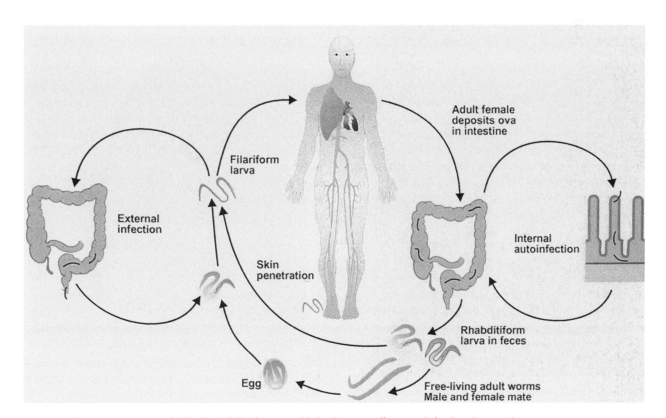

FIG. 6.174. Strongyloidiasis with both external infection as well as autoinfection (see text).

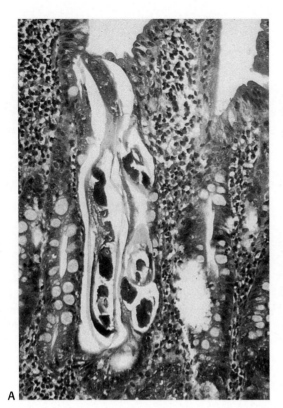

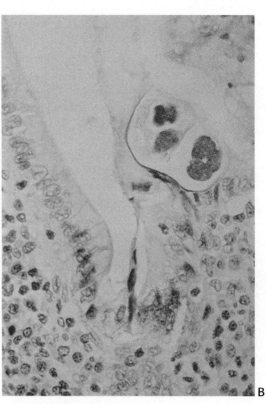

FIG. 6.175. *Strongyloides* infection of the small intestine. **A:** Longitudinal cross section of several worms lying within a crypt. **B:** Transverse cross section showing the paired intestinal tracts (see text).

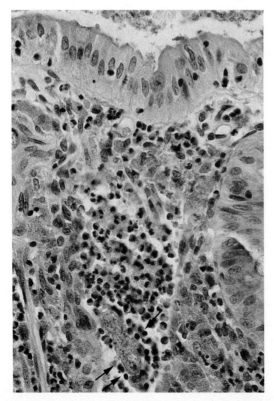

FIG. 6.176. Prominent eosinophilia in a patient with disseminated strongyloidiasis. Portions of a worm are present (*arrows*). Note the intense lamina propria eosinophilia.

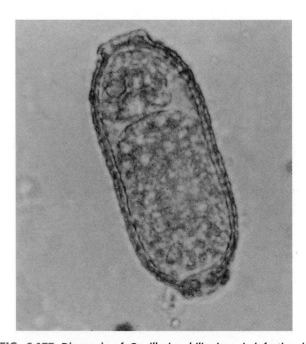

FIG. 6.177. Diagnosis of *Capillaria philippinensis* infection is made by demonstration of the characteristic egg with subtle flattened polar prominences in the stool. (Courtesy of Dickson Despommier, Ph.D., Department of Parasitology, Columbia Presbyterian Medical Center, New York, NY.)

and the presence of fully developed larvae. The eggs of *C. philippinensis* average 36 × 19 to 45 × 21 μm and they resemble those of *T. trichiuria*, which average 50 × 20 μm. Some patients have both infections.

Disease onset is acute with severe malabsorption and it has a 35% mortality. Patients develop diarrhea, malaise, anorexia, nausea, and vomiting, and they may die of extreme malnutrition, dehydration, or secondary bacterial infections. The period between symptom onset and death is usually 2 to 3 months.

Grossly, the small intestine appears thickened, indurated, and hyperemic and contains large amounts of fluid (472). Thousands of adult worms, larvae, and ova are seen within the jejunum and the upper portion of the ileum. Occasionally, they are also present in the duodenum. Infrequently, parasites are found in the stomach, esophagus, and colon. Patients with severe infections have many worms embedded in the small bowel mucosa. Histologically, one sees the parasites in the intestinal lumen, within the crypts of Lieberkühn, and in the lamina propria. The intestinal villi develop secondary changes, including villous atrophy, obliteration, and epithelial sloughing. Approximately 50% of biopsies disclose the presence of worms.

Tapeworm Infections

Tapeworms are ribbon-shaped, segmented, hermaphroditic worms that inhabit the intestinal tract of many species. Species that commonly infect humans in the West include the beef tapeworm, *Taenia saginata,* and the pork tapeworm, *Taenia solium.* Mucosal attachment occurs via suction cups or grooves located on the head or scolex. One can distinguish the various species of tapeworms by counting the number of teeth or cutting plates on the buccal cavity. *T. saginata* has a small unarmed scolex with four prominent suckers and 1,000 to 2,000 proglottid segments.

The proglottids (Fig. 6.178) develop to form the chainlike strobila of the worm. As each proglottid becomes gravid, eggs are released. Adult worms produce up to 20,000 eggs per

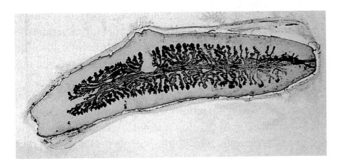

FIG. 6.178. The proglottid of *Taenia saginata* can be distinguished from that of *Taenia solium* by the number of primary lateral uterine branches. This proglottid injected with India ink shows the >15 branches characteristic of *T. saginata.* (Courtesy of Dickson Despommier, Ph.D., Department of Parasitology, Columbia Presbyterian Medical Center, New York, NY.)

day, which disseminate into the environment via stool. Once stuck to the mucosa, the worms suck blood from it. The amount of blood lost varies with the parasite species. Because the worms lack a GI tract, adults absorb predigested food across the tegumental surface of each segment (473).

Adult *T. saginata, T. solium,* and *Diphyllobothrium latum* are among the largest parasites to infect humans; they can reach lengths of 10 to 15 m. These three worms are acquired via ingestion of larvae. Pea-sized larvae (cysticerci) of the beef and pork tapeworms infect various tissues, including the musculature of cattle and pigs, respectively. Cysts are released into the small intestine of humans when raw or undercooked infected meat is consumed. Ingestion of tissues containing cysts with viable scolices allows larvae to develop into mature worms. It takes approximately 3 months for *T. solium, T. saginata,* and *D. latum* to become gravid. Humans are the only definitive host for the adult stage of *T. saginata,* which inhabits the upper jejunum for as long as 25 years. The intermediate hosts (cattle and pigs) acquire their infection by ingesting human feces contaminated with tapeworm ova.

Mild epigastric discomfort, nausea, and hunger sensations are the most common symptoms. Weight loss, diarrhea, irritability, and increased appetite also occur. Impacted proglottid segments cause obstruction, jaundice, or pancreatitis, depending on their location.

T. solium, the pork tapeworm, inhabits the human intestinal lumen, its only definitive host. When larvae invade humans, the condition is referred to as cysticercosis. *T. solium* infections occur most commonly in Mexico, Africa, Southeast Asia, South America, and Eastern Europe. It has recently been found in swine in New Mexico and Colorado. When the eggs of *T. solium* are ingested either by pigs or humans, the larvae hatch in the small intestine (upper jejunum), penetrate the gut wall, and enter the circulation. They are then carried by the blood to any organ in the body. Once in the capillaries, they encyst. No further development occurs while the worm is encysted, and it can remain in this stage for the life of the pig or for up to 10 years in humans. The adult worm measures about 3 m in length. The globular scolex contains a rostellum with two rows of hooklets; there are usually <1,000 proglottids.

Diphyllobothriasis is common in many countries, especially in those that dispose of raw sewage into freshwater lakes. The life cycle begins with the contamination of the freshwater by human feces containing the eggs of the parasites (Fig. 6.179). *D. latum* has various intermediate hosts, the last of which is many freshwater fish. The disease is acquired by eating raw or poorly cooked fish. The adult worm attaches to the ileal and jejunal mucosa by a pair of sucking grooves located on the scolex. It can live for decades and attain a length of 10 m with 3,000 to 4,000 proglottids attached to the neck.

Dwarf Tapeworm Infections

Hymenolepis nana, the dwarf tapeworm, is the most common autochthonously acquired tapeworm disease in the

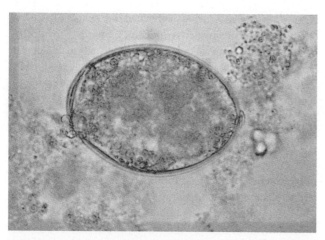

FIG. 6.179. The *Diphyllobothrium* egg passed in the stool is ovoid with a barely discernible operculum. It resembles the egg of *Paragonimus westermani,* which is larger. (Courtesy of Dickson Despommier, Ph.D., Department of Parasitology, Columbia Presbyterian Medical Center, New York, NY.)

United States. Most infections affect children and institutionalized individuals. The infection spreads by an oral–fecal route. Feces of infected children and rats are the most common reservoirs. In some countries, 25% of the rural population has an *H. nana* infection, presumably due to consumption of contaminated water (474). Most infections remain asymptomatic or associate with only mild infections. Proglottids and eggs (Fig. 6.180) are shed into the stool. Some patients develop severe crampy abdominal pain, diarrhea, constipation, vomiting, weakness, or weight loss. A

small percentage of patients develop anemia. About 40% of patients with the infection have low vitamin B_{12} levels because the tapeworm successfully competes with the host for the vitamin.

Fasciolopsiasis

Fasciolopsiasis results from infections by the large fluke *Fasciolopsis buski.* Fasciolopsis infections usually affect the biliary tree but occasionally they present in other organs (475). The diagnosis is made by finding ova in the stool (Fig. 6.181) (475). The disorder remains mainly confined to Southeast Asia, but with the travel patterns of many individuals, it is seen in other countries. Several flukes, including *F. buski,* are acquired when people ingest contaminated water plants such as the water chestnuts (Fig. 6.182).

F. buski inhabits the upper intestine. The hermaphroditic, 20-mm-diameter, flat flukes produce unembryonated ova that hatch 3 to 7 weeks later in water having a temperature of 80°C to 90°C. After infective forms of the organism are ingested, the parasites enter the peritoneal cavity through the intestinal wall, reach the liver where the young flukes enter the parenchyma through the capsule, and find a bile duct where they grow to adulthood. Aberrant localization of *Fasciolopsis* and other flukes occur while the parasite is migrating within the host tissues to its normal location

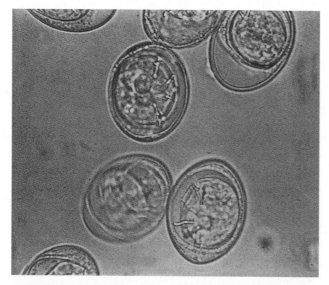

FIG. 6.180. *Hymenolepis nana* egg passed in the stool is distinguished by the presence of six hooklets on the embryo and the polar filaments that encircle the embryo. (Courtesy of Dickson Despommier, Ph.D., Department of Parasitology, Columbia Presbyterian Medical Center, New York, NY.)

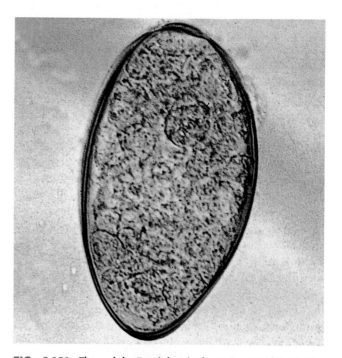

FIG. 6.181. The adult *Fasciolopsis hepatica* resides in the hepatic bile ducts and passes eggs, which may be found in the stool. The egg seen here is large (130 to 150 μm), is ovoid, and has a barely discernible operculum. (Courtesy of Dickson Despommier, Ph.D., Department of Parasitology, Columbia University, New York, NY.)

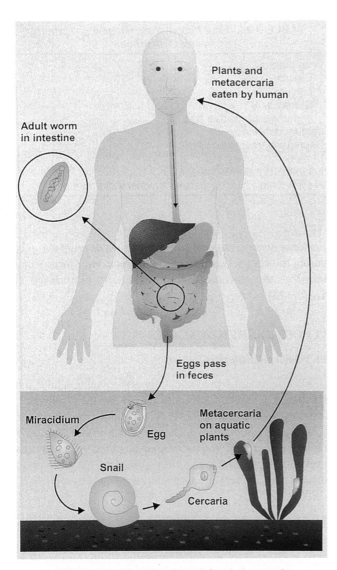

FIG. 6.182. Life cycle of *Fasciolopsis* (see text).

(476). The life cycle is shown in Figure 6.182. Pigs and humans act as the reservoirs for the infections.

The infection usually remains asymptomatic. However, patients with hundreds or thousands of flukes may develop intestinal obstruction, allergic responses to parasitic metabolites, or mucosal injury. Symptoms include nausea, diarrhea, epigastric pain, and GI hemorrhage. Histologically, the most severe lesions affect the duodenum and jejunum. Exceptionally, the ileum, stomach, and colon become involved. Large adults attach themselves to the intestinal mucosa, eliciting an intense inflammatory reaction with abscess formation. One may see cystic masses containing necrotic material, inflammatory debris, and hemosiderin-tinged exudates without grossly recognizable parasites. Eosinophils may surround dead worms. Other presentations include the presence of masses in the anterior abdominal wall, periumbilical area or iliac fossa, or intestinal intussusception. Peripheral eosinophilia is frequently present.

Schistosomiasis

Schistosomal infections occur within both the small and large intestine. Pathologists are much more likely to encounter the organism in colonic specimens than small intestinal ones; therefore, this infection is discussed in Chapter 13.

Helminthomas (Helminthic Pseudotumors)

Helminthoma is the term used to describe tumorlike inflammatory intestinal swellings caused by penetration of the intestinal wall by nematodes, usually in the area of the ileocecal valve (477). The worms usually belong to the genus *Oesophagostomum* and other closely related species in the *Strongyloides* family. Hookworms *Sparganum* and *Oxyuris* also occasionally bury themselves into the mucosa and submucosa causing circumscribed hemorrhages, but they do not usually penetrate the tissues any further (478).

Multiple nodules are present in the terminal ileum, cecum, and ascending colon (Fig. 6.183). Adhesions develop to surrounding structures and the greater omentum is frequently attached to the inflammatory mass. Sometimes the mass resides completely outside the bowel wall. Masses vary in size but usually they measure 4 to 6 cm in diameter. On sectioning, an abscess or fistulous tract is usually present. Often, a worm still resides inside the mass. Occasionally, the tract presents as a sausage-shaped lump resembling a double

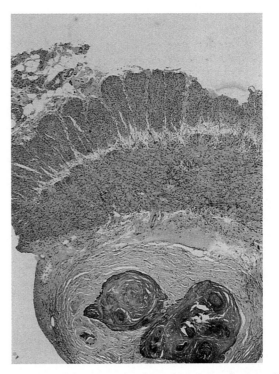

FIG. 6.183. Cross section through a small intestinal helminthoma. All that remains are nodular concentric fibrous regions containing areas of calcification. The patient had disseminated schistosomiasis and chronic *Ascaris* infections. The structures of the offending parasites are no longer visible.

appendix. Fat necrosis may occur. Patients present with symptoms resembling appendicitis, ileocecal tuberculosis, or Crohn disease or carcinoma. The histologic features of an inflammatory pseudotumor are present, often containing numerous eosinophils.

Traveler's Diarrhea

Between 20% and 70% of people who travel from the industrialized world to the developing world each year report some illness related to their travel (479,480). Diarrhea is the most common health problem of travelers to developing countries. Its incidence varies depending on the travel destination and the number of dietary indiscretions made by the traveler (481). High-risk destinations include most of the developing countries of Latin America, the Middle East, and Asia. Intermediate destinations include southern European countries and a few Caribbean islands. Low-risk destinations include Canada, northern Europe, Australia, New Zealand, the United States, and a number of Caribbean islands. Various infections are implicated (Table 6.24); these produce

a diverse clinical spectrum. The causative agents are identified in 50% to 75% of travelers with diarrhea that lasts <2 weeks. However, as the duration of the diarrhea increases, the likelihood of identifying the causative agent decreases (482). Seasonal variations exist in the etiology of traveler's diarrhea. Acquisition of multiple pathogens is much less common among individuals who travel in the winter than in the fall. *Campylobacter* strains are the leading cause of traveler's diarrhea in the winter, contrasting with enterotoxigenic *E. coli* and *Salmonella* in the fall (483). Because of Mexico's popularity and proximity to the United States, its version of traveler's diarrhea, popularly called "Montezuma's revenge," is the most extensively studied form of traveler's diarrhea in the United States (484).

Traveler's diarrhea occurs slightly more commonly in young people, perhaps due to their more adventurous travel styles or to different eating habits. Traveler's diarrhea is acquired through ingestion of fecally contaminated food and/or water. Both cooked and uncooked foods may be implicated. Particularly risky foods include raw vegetables, salads, raw meat and seafood, and foods left at room temperature and served buffet style. Other high-risk foods include tap water, ice, unpeeled fruits, unpasteurized milk, and dairy products. Episodes of generally self-limited diarrhea develop abruptly during travel or soon after returning home. Host factors that influence the outcome of traveler's diarrhea are listed in Table 6.25.

MALABSORPTION SYNDROMES

Malabsorption results from premucosal, mucosal, and postmucosal diseases (Table 6.26). In premucosal diseases, defective digestion and absorption results from pancreatic or other systemic diseases and reduced bile salt concentrations. Mucosal defects result from anatomic or biochemical epithelial alterations, the presence of microorganisms, and inflammatory or infiltrative processes. Postmucosal diseases include malabsorption due to lymphatic obstruction, vascular disease, or congestive heart failure. Mucosal diseases are the most common disorders that a surgical pathologist is likely to encounter. Malabsorption syndromes affect patients

TABLE 6.24	Causes of Travelers' Diarrhea
Bacterial	
Enterotoxigenic *Escherichia coli*	
Salmonella	
Shigella	
Campylobacter jejuni	
Vibrio parahaemolyticus	
Aeromonas hydrophilia	
Yersinia enterocolitica	
Plesiomonas shigelloides	
Vibrio cholerae	
Vibrio fluvialis	
Parasitic	
Giardia lamblia	
Entamoeba histolytica	
Cryptosporidium	
Dientamoeba fragilis	
Isospora belli	
Balantidium coli	
Strongyloides stercoralis	
Viral	
Rotavirus	
Norwalk-like virus	
Adenoviruses	
Astroviruses	
Caliciviruses	
Coronaviruses	
Enteroviruses	
Fungal	
Blastomyces hominis	

TABLE 6.25	Host Factors that Influence Outcome of Travelers' Diarrhea
Drugs	
Digitalis	
Lithium	
Diuretics	
Immunosuppressive agents	
Immunodeficiency	
Decreased gastric acidity	
Stroke	
Inflammatory bowel disease	
Previous high susceptibility to travelers' diarrhea	

TABLE 6.26	**Causes of Malabsorption**

Inadequate digestion
    Postgastrectomy steatorrhea
    Deficient activation of pancreatic lipase
    Chronic pancreatitis
    Pancreatic carcinoma
    Cystic fibrosis
    Pancreatic resection
Reduced intestinal bile salt concentration (with impaired micelle formation)
    Parenchymal liver disease
    Cholestasis (intrahepatic or extrahepatic)
    Blind loop syndrome
    Interrupted enterohepatic circulation of bile salts
    Ileal resection or inflammation
    Drugs that sequester or precipitate bile salts
Inadequate absorptive surface secondary to surgical procedures
Lymphatic obstruction
    Intestinal lymphangiectasia
    Whipple disease
    Lymphoma
Primary mucosal absorptive defects
Inflammatory or infiltrative disorders
    Regional enteritis
    Amyloidosis
    Scleroderma
    Lymphoma
    Radiation enteritis
    Eosinophilic enteritis
    Tropical sprue
    Infectious enteritis
    Collagenous sprue
    Nonspecific ulcerative jejunitis
    Mastocytosis
    Dermatologic disorders (e.g., dermatitis herpetiformis)
Biochemical or genetic abnormalities
    Celiac disease
    Disaccharidase deficiency
    Hypogammaglobulinemia
    Abetalipoproteinemia
    Monosaccharide malabsorption
Failed cell division
    Radiation
    Colchicine
Endocrine and metabolic disorders
    Diabetes mellitus
    Hypoparathyroidism
    Adrenal insufficiency
    Hyperthyroidism
    Zollinger-Ellison syndrome
    Pancreatic insufficiency (Zollinger-Ellison syndrome, gastrinoma)
    Carcinoid syndrome
Cardiovascular disorders
    Constrictive pericarditis
    Congestive heart failure
    Mesenteric vascular insufficiency
    Vasculitis

of all ages and the age incidence depends on the etiology. Celiac disease, the most common cause of malabsorption in developed countries, is detected at almost any age. Infectious disease, lactase deficiency, and nutrient deficiencies are the most common causes of malabsorption in the developing world. In an ideal world, the pathologist should be supplied with relevant clinical information, including results of laboratory or serologic tests, before attempting to arrive at a specific diagnosis. Information that allows the pathologist to make the most useful interpretation of the biopsy specimens is listed in Table 6.27.

Small intestinal biopsies can be obtained by either a suction capsule or by forceps after endoscopic visualization. The suction capsule method requires radiographic guidance and is more expensive than the more commonly used forceps biopsy. Focal or patchy lesions can be visualized and biopsied by the endoscopic method. This technique also permits visualization of the gastrointestinal tract and avoids the radiation exposure associated with suction biopsy. However, capsule biopsies are still preferred over endoscopic biopsies by some gastroenterologists, particularly in children younger than 2 years of age.

Either the duodenum or the jejunum is an appropriate site for biopsy, but the biopsy should be procured no more proximal than the second part of the duodenum to avoid artifacts due to prominent Brunner glands or the nonspecific or peptic duodenitis commonly seen in the bulb and proximal duodenum. Unfortunately, more often than not the biopsies derive from the proximal duodenum, a site that is not ideal for the interpretation of villous architecture. It is important to note that the presence of a normal small intestinal biopsy does not exclude many malabsorptive conditions. Conditions with malabsorption and a normal small bowel villous architecture are listed in Tables 6.28 and 6.29.

Certain factors optimize the diagnostic accuracy of the biopsy interpretation, including (a) careful biopsy handling and orientation, (b) provision of accurate clinical information

TABLE 6.27	**Information To Be Provided to Pathologists Interpreting Small Bowel Biopsies for Malabsorption**

Patient age
Patient sex
Ethnicity
Country of domicile
Travel history
Reason for the biopsy
Drug use
History of associated diseases
    AIDS
    Neoplasias
    Infections
    Metabolic diseases
    Immune deficiencies
    Prior surgery

TABLE 6.28   **Malabsorption with Normal-appearing Proximal Jejunal Biopsy**

Dermatosis other than dermatitis herpetiformis
Pancreatitis
Alcoholism
Cirrhosis
Hepatitis
Iron deficiency anemia
Ulcerative colitis
Postgastrectomy without bacterial overgrowth
Malignancy outside the gastrointestinal tract
Cholera
Biliary obstruction

to the pathologist, (c) an understanding by the pathologist of the spectrum of normal intestinal histology, and (d) familiarity with the spectrum of small intestinal diseases that may present as malabsorption.

Handling of Small Intestinal Biopsies

It is the clinician who decides when an intestinal biopsy needs to be obtained, but the pathologist and the clinician should work together to decide the best way to utilize and/or fix a given tissue specimen. Once it is decided that histologic interpretation will provide the optimal information, the optimal fixation can be decided, including a decision as to whether it is necessary to perform biochemical, microbiologic, electron microscopic, or immunophenotypic studies.

A nonfragmented, well-oriented biopsy specimen aids in establishing an accurate diagnosis. Immediate orientation by the gastroenterologist is ideal, but impractical in regular clinical practice. The optimal method of orienting the specimen is to put the base of the mucosa on filter paper and float it upside down in a bottle of fixative, allowing the specimen to float freely with the villi to hang down in a dependent way, thereby minimizing artifactual distortion. This facilitates a more accurate evaluation of the height of the villi and length

of the crypts to determine the ratio of these two measurements. Appropriate orientation can also be achieved by scanning under a dissecting microscope. An initial impression of the villous architecture can also be obtained by this method. However, its applicability in clinical practice is limited. In most institutions, adequate orientation is achieved by asking an experienced histotechnologist to embed the biopsies on edge.

Although Bouin, Hollande, or B5 fixatives yield little shrinkage artifact and optimal nuclear detail, most pathology departments use neutral buffered formalin as the fixative. Adequate fixation for histology and superior preservation of DNA for ancillary studies is possible with formalin fixation. Formalin is also inexpensive and easy to discard. There is a lack of consensus among pathologists regarding the number of slides and levels that should be prepared and examined histologically. Examination of multiple sections and levels increases the likelihood of finding patchy changes and well-oriented villi.

Evaluating the Small Intestinal Biopsy

When assessing a biopsy, it is usually best to follow a standardized format so as not to miss disease that may cause the underlying clinical syndrome (Fig. 6.184). This includes an examination of (a) villous height, crypt length, and overall architecture; (b) the lumen; (c) the surface epithelium; (d) crypts; (e) lamina propria constituents; (f) the presence of abnormal deposits; and (g) changes in other layers of the bowel wall. The histologic findings may allow the diagnosis of specific diseases (Table 6.30).

Villus Assessment

Villus assessment involves evaluating the ratio between crypt length and villous height. Since villi bend in various directions and their structure varies from slender fingerlike to leaflike, one should follow the rule that if a row of four fingerlike villi is present in any section, then the biopsy should be considered to be

TABLE 6.29   Malabsorption with Normal Villi but with Diagnostic Features

Disease	Specific Histologic Features
Abetalipoproteinemia	Vacuolated enterocytes containing lipids involving upper two thirds of the villi; acanthocytes
Crohn disease	Noncaseating granulomas
X-linked immunodeficiency	Absent lamina propria plasma cells
Lipid storage disease	Vacuolated ganglion cells, capillaries, and macrophages
Amyloidosis	Congo red–positive material in muscularis and blood vessels
Chronic granulomatous disease	Pigmented vacuolated macrophages in lamina propria
Melanosis	Brown pigmented macrophages in lamina propria
Systemic mastocytosis	Mast cell infiltrates in lamina propria
Hemochromatosis	Iron deposits in epithelium and macrophages
Mycobacterium avium-intracellulare	PAS-positive diastase-resistant macrophages containing acid-fast organisms

PAS, periodic acid–Schiff.

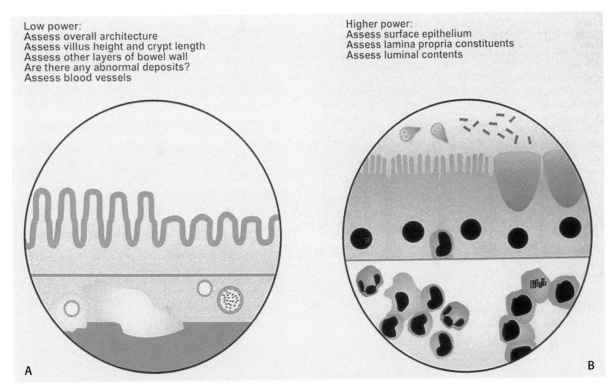

FIG. 6.184. Diagram of the approach to interpreting a mucosal biopsy. **A:** Low-power assessment. During this assessment, one determines the overall architecture and whether the villi appear normal or demonstrate one of the mucosal patterns of injury such as the villous atrophy shown on the right. One also examines the biopsy for the presence of abnormal infiltrates, such as the amyloid shown in the submucosa and surrounding the blood vessel. Other assessments are noted in the diagram. **B:** At higher magnification, one examines the lumen for the presence of bacteria or parasites, as shown by the trophozoites and *Helicobacter pylori*. One looks at the epithelium for evidence of metaplasia such as the two foveolar epithelial cells illustrated on the right. One examines the epithelium for the presence of intraepithelial lymphocytes and the lamina propria for neoplasms or inflammatory infiltrates.

TABLE 6.30	Specific Histologic Findings in Small Bowel Biopsies
Disease	**Diagnostic Histology**
Whipple disease	PAS positive (non–acid-fast); characteristic macrophages in lamina propria
Eosinophilic gastroenteritis	Eosinophilic infiltrates (50–70/hpf)
Intestinal lymphoma	Malignant lymphoid cells in lamina propria
Parasitic diseases	Identification of the parasite
Fungal diseases	Identification of the fungus
Viral diseases	Identification of the virus
Macroglobulinemia	Hyaline masses in lamina propria
Common variable hypogammaglobulinemia	Absent plasma cells in lamina propria, lymphoid hyperplasia
Severe B_{12} or folate deficiency	Epithelial macrocytosis
Intestinal lymphangiectasia	Dilated lymphatics
Acute radiation enteritis	Macrocytosis, increased apoptosis
Graft vs. host disease	Large numbers of apoptotic figures
Hemochromatosis	Iron deposits in epithelium and stroma
Transfusional siderosis	Iron deposits in macrophages
Crohn disease	Cryptitis, crypt abscesses, granulomas
Peptic duodenitis	Foveolar metaplasia
Mastocytosis	Increased numbers of mast cells
Amyloidosis	Amyloid deposits in intestinal wall
Collagenous sprue	Variably thick subepithelial collagen bands

PAS, periodic acid–Schiff.

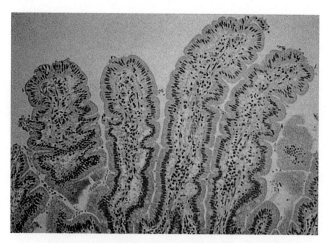

FIG. 6.185. Jejunal biopsy with four normal villi.

TABLE 6.31 Villous Atrophy
Hypoplastic type
Malnutrition
Untreated pernicious anemia
Paneth cell deficiency
Hypopituitarism
Gluten-sensitive enteropathy
Tropical sprue
Radiation
Chemotherapy
Patients with tumors
Hyperplastic type
Celiac disease
Chronic trauma
Urinary ileal conduits
Areas adjacent to ulcers
Patients with glucagonomas
Following extensive small bowel resections

normal (Fig. 6.185) (485). In adults, villous height is approximately three or more times the length of the crypts, whereas in children this ratio is lower, more typically being 2:1. Villous height is also lower in the elderly. The duodenal crypt:villus ratio is 3:1 to 7:1, whereas the ileal crypt:villus ratio is 4:1. Villi overlying lymphoid aggregates are often stubby or absent, and should not be evaluated in these areas. Tangentially sectioned villi are a common source of misinterpretation since they appear broadened and shortened. Tangential sectioning is recognized by the presence of multilayered nuclei in the crypts or villi or fused villi (Fig. 6.186). Villous changes occur in three different patterns as outlined below.

Villous Atrophy and Crypt Hyperplasia. This is the most common type of injury pattern seen by surgical pathologists since it is typical of celiac disease, as well as many other disorders (Table 6.31). The villous enterocytes are the target of the injury and are shed more rapidly from the villi than are normal enterocytes, leading to a reduction in the number of enterocytes per unit area of intestinal mucosa. The enterocyte loss is accompanied by increased apoptosis. The epithe-

lial cell loss results in a compensatory crypt hyperplasia with increased mitoses in the crypt bases. When epithelial replacement fails to keep up with the cellular loss, villous atrophy develops and the villus:crypt ratio decreases (Fig. 6.187). As villous height diminishes, the villi become morphologically abnormal. Shortened leaves and ridges replace the normal fingerlike villi, and in severe cases, mucosal mounds surrounding individual crypt openings are all that remain of the villi. Crypt length may increase to such an extent that the total mucosal height may remain normal despite marked villous atrophy. However, it is much more common to see a reduction in total mucosal thickness. (485). A system for grading the degree of villous atrophy is shown in Table 6.32. It is also useful to apply the Marsh classification in celiac disease (see below).

TABLE 6.32 Grades of Villous Atrophy
Mild
• Most villi appear branched, broadened, or fused; some remain normal
• Surface epithelium appears abnormal; loss of polarity; increased intraepithelial lymphocytes
• Increased mitoses outside the normal proliferative compartment
• Increased acute and chronic inflammatory cells in lamina propria
Moderate (partial villous atrophy)
• Villi broadened and shortened
• Cuboidal surface epithelium
• Large numbers of intraepithelial lymphocytes
• Increased mononuclear cells in the lamina propria
Severe (subtotal villous atrophy)
• Villi almost completely absent
• Marked mononuclear cell infiltrates

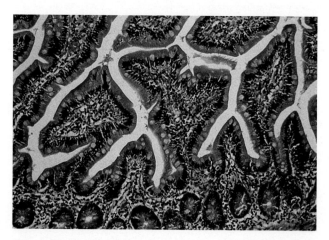

FIG. 6.186. Tangentially cut villi. As a result of the tangential cutting, the villi appear fused.

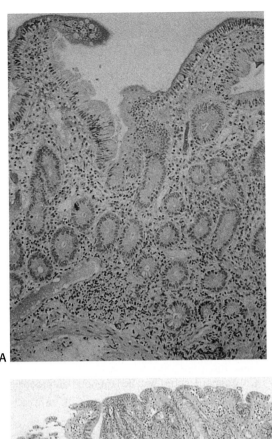

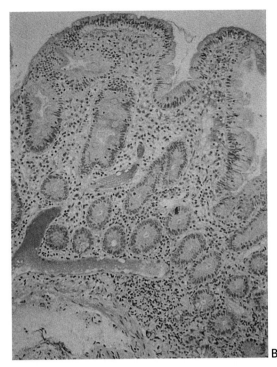

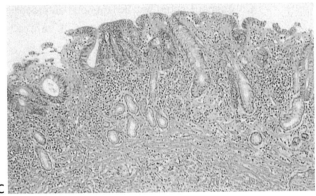

FIG. 6.187. Villous atrophy. **A:** Mild. **B:** Moderate. **C:** Severe.

Villous Atrophy with Crypt Hypoplasia. In this pattern of injury, the crypt is the primary site of damage. Crypt destruction leads to reduced numbers of cells that can mature and populate the villi. As a result, both villous and crypt atrophy occur. An abnormally low villous height and reduced crypt length give the impression of overall mucosal atrophy. However, the crypt:villus ratio may remain normal because the measurements of both portions of the crypt:villus axis are abnormal and reduced. This pattern is seen in advanced celiac disease, radiation damage, cytotoxic drug-induced injury, and vitamin B_{12} and folic acid deficiency (Table 6.31).

Villous Hyperplasia. This unusual pattern is seen following intestinal resection, in patients with glucagonomas, or in areas adjacent to ulcers or stenoses. It has also been recently described in hypertrophic eosinophilic gastroenteropathy (486). As in villous atrophy/crypt hypoplasia, the crypt length:villus height ratio tends to remain normal but, unlike villous atrophy/crypt hypoplasia, the overall height of the mucosa increases. The villi may appear thickened and the lamina propria may contain increased mononuclear cells.

Enterocyte Changes

Enterocyte changes include variations in cell shape and size as well as brush border alterations. Enterocytes may appear cuboidal or flattened due to a reduction in their height. They may also show nuclear irregularity, loss of polarity, basophilia, vacuolization, and syncytial formation. Regenerating superficial cells may become tufted. Neutrophils infiltrating the epithelium suggest inflammatory disorders such as Crohn disease, NSAID-induced injury, or peptic inflammation. Increased intraepithelial lymphocytes suggest a primary villous abnormality mediated by T lymphocytes or infection. Stainable iron is seen in transfusional siderosis, hemochromatosis, rare abnormalities in iron transport, and AIDS. In abetalipoproteinemia, the enterocytes develop characteristic vacuoles. Foveolar metaplasia occurs in peptic duodenitis. The apical borders of the enterocytes or the intestinal lumen may contain parasites. Enterocytes may also contain viral inclusions. The collagen table immediately underlying the epithelium may appear thickened.

Severe vitamin B_{12} and folic acid deficiency, acute radiation injuries, and chemotherapy all inhibit DNA synthesis and result in impaired epithelial replacement and macrocytosis (Fig. 6.125). Crypt mitotic activity is reduced, epithelial cells become enlarged, and villous abnormalities varying from mild to complete villous loss ensue. The macrocytosis may be irregularly distributed, varying from crypt to crypt or villus to villus. The mucosa reverts to normal following folic acid or vitamin B_{12} therapy or cessation of drug therapy. Radiation changes may also revert to normal, depending on the radiation dose and the degree of underlying vascular damage.

Crypt Changes

Crypts elongate and exhibit increased mitoses in the hyperplastic pattern of mucosal atrophy (Fig. 6.188), contrasting with shortened crypts and macrocytosis in the hypoplastic

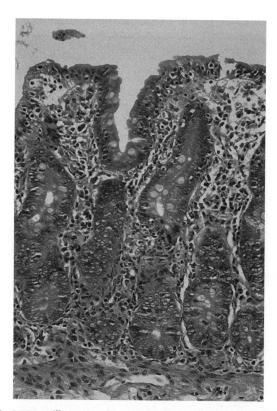

FIG. 6.188. Villous atrophy crypt hyperplasia. Note that the villi are hardly recognizable as such. They are broadened and flat. The epithelial lining at the surface contains large numbers of intraepithelial lymphocytes. The crypts are lengthened and contain mitotic figures. This biopsy is from a patient with celiac disease.

pattern of mucosal atrophy. Crypt abscesses may signify the presence of peptic disease, drug injury, infection, or Crohn disease. Increased apoptosis characterizes chemotherapy-induced disease, graft versus host disease (GVHD), AIDS enteropathy, and T-cell–mediated cell injury. Other crypt changes include variations in the number of Paneth cells and endocrine cells. Morphologic abnormalities of Paneth cells occur in acrodermatitis enteropathica (487).

Lamina Propria Changes

The lamina propria should be assessed for alterations in the normal cell populations, for changes in the lymphatics and vessels, and for the presence of abnormal deposits. The character of any lamina propria inflammatory infiltrate may help to determine the etiology of the patient's malabsorption. It is important to note that a mild degree of lymphoplasmacytosis is normally seen in duodenal biopsies. A marked increase in chronic inflammatory cells occurs in many conditions including celiac disease, peptic duodenitis, drug injury, infection, and nonspecific chronic duodenitis. Acute inflammation suggests peptic duodenitis, drug-induced injury, and Crohn disease. Crypt abscesses indicate acute enteritis or Crohn disease. Eosinophils (Table 6.33) complicate Crohn disease as well as many other disorders. (There is a recently developed web site creating a database for gastrointestinal eosinophilic disorders at www.cincinnatichildrens.org/eosinophils.) Viruses or parasites may be present. Mast cells increase in mastocytosis, allergic reactions, and Crohn disease. Plasma cells are altered in many small intestinal disor-

TABLE 6.33	Intestinal Lesions Characterized by Prominent Eosinophilia

Inflammatory fibroid polyps
Parasitic infections
Lymphomas
Hodgkin disease
Crohn disease
Eosinophilic gastroenteritis
Allergic enteritis
Gluten-sensitive enteropathy
Magnesium deficiency
Vitamin E deficiency
Selenium deficiency
Peptic duodenitis
Inflammatory pseudotumors
Toxic oil syndrome
L-Tryptophan–associated myalgia syndrome
Hypereosinophilic syndrome and eosinophilic leukemia
Allografts with rejection
Cow's milk intolerance and related entities
Granulomas
Peritoneal dialysis
Brown bowel syndrome
Hyperimmunoglobulinemia E

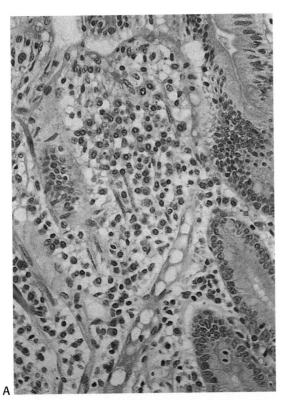 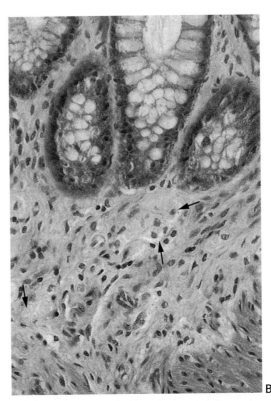

FIG. 6.189. Lamina propria infiltrates. **A:** Celiac disease with increased lamina propria plasma cells. **B:** Foamy histiocytes expanding the lamina propria and compressing the glands and crypts (*arrows*) in a patient with *Mycobacterium avium-intracellulare.*

ders, but they become the predominant cell type in patients with celiac disease (Fig. 6.189). When they increase significantly enough to cause villous abnormalities, the diagnosis of a lymphoproliferative disorder should be considered. Increases in lymphocyte populations also complicate many disorders, including celiac disease, Crohn disease, autoimmune diseases, and some infections. When lymphocytes appear atypical, a lymphoma may be present. Lymphoid follicles may be encountered and, when associated with reduced numbers of plasma cells, suggest the presence of an immunodeficiency syndrome. The number of macrophages may be increased in nonspecific inflammatory reactions. If they form, granulomas, Crohn disease, *Yersinia* infection, Whipple disease, histoplasmosis, or a mycobacterial infection should be considered (Table 6.15). Increased mucosal macrophages also complicate storage diseases. Dilated lymphatics characterize lymphangiectasia and intestinal obstruction. Blood vessels become abnormal with radiation, amyloid, certain infections, and thrombotic or embolic disorders.

It is also important to determine which cells types are not present in the biopsy. For example, an absence of plasma cells is a strong indicator of immunodeficiency disease, particularly common variable immunodeficiency. A decreased number of chronic inflammatory cells is seen in patients who are on steroids or who have other types of immunodeficiency.

Abnormal Acellular Infiltrates

Abnormal acellular infiltrates may lie in the lamina propria (Table 6.34). In collagenous sprue, collagenous duodenitis, or collagenous enteritis, a dense collagen band underlies the surface epithelium (Fig. 6.190). In Waldenstrom macroglobulinemia, amorphous eosinophilic masses lie within the lamina propria. Amyloidosis causes characteristic eosinophilic deposits.

TABLE 6.34   **Intestinal Mucosal Deposits**

Amyloid light chains
Macroglobulins
Collagenous sprue and collagenous enterocolitis
Infantile systemic hyalinosis
Lipid proteinosis
Melanosis
Pseudomelanosis
Xanthomas
Storage diseases
   Tangier disease
   Fabry disease
   Tay-Sachs and other gangliosidoses
   Niemann-Pick disease
   Wolman disease
   Cystinosis
   Mucopolysaccharidoses

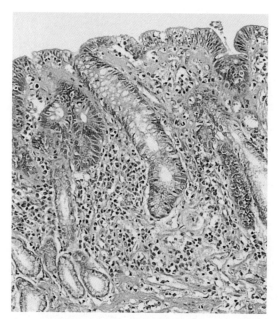

FIG. 6.190. Collagenous sprue demonstrating the presence of a thickened basement membrane underlying luminal surface.

Submucosal Changes

The submucosa is not always present in intestinal biopsies, but if it is present it should be evaluated. Changes affecting the submucosa include fibrosis, changes in number or thickness of blood vessels, the presence of thrombi or emboli, alterations in lymphatics and nerves, and the presence of abscesses, granulomas, parasites, amyloid deposits, or neoplastic infiltrates. Of note, it is not uncommon to encounter ganglion cells in the muscularis mucosae or the lower mucosa in the proximal small intestine. Their presence should not be interpreted as representing neuronal dysplasia.

Metaplasias

Patients with small intestinal diseases may develop several types of metaplasia. Intestinal crypts may be replaced by gastric mucous cells of the pyloric type. This process almost always occurs just above the muscularis mucosae and is referred to as *pyloric metaplasia*. Its presence indicates that chronic damage has occurred. The cells of pyloric metaplasia are sometimes referred to as *ulcer-associated cell lineage cells*, or UACL cells (488). Three-dimensional reconstruction studies suggest that these cells form by extrusion from crypt bases with the formation of a coiled acinar component and an elongated ductular component that extends to the surface. Ulceration appears to be cue for the development of UACL cells, suggesting that the lineage has a reparative function. This is supported by the presence of epidermal growth factor/urogastrone and heat-shock protein in the acini (488). The metaplastic cells also produce trefoil factors that help restore mucosal integrity. Pyloric metaplasia can occur throughout the small intestine. In contrast to pyloric meta-

plasia, the superficial duodenal epithelium undergoes foveolar metaplasia as discussed earlier in this chapter.

CELIAC DISEASE

Celiac disease (CD), also known as gluten-sensitive enteropathy and celiac sprue, is a malabsorptive disease in which the intestinal mucosa is injured as a result of ingestion of gluten-containing foods in genetically predisposed individuals. Withdrawal of dietary gluten causes prompt improvement of nutrient absorption and improvement of the characteristic mucosal lesions unless refractory sprue has developed.

Epidemiology

Celiac disease is the most common cause of malabsorption in Western populations. The prevalence of CD in Europe and North America is 0.5% to 1% (489–491). Celiac disease is rare in Japanese, Chinese, and African patients. The disorder is more common in women than men. It is now recognized that there is a substantial number of undiagnosed cases in the general population possibly ten times as many as actually have been diagnosed (492).

Celiac disease appears to have a strong genetic component, demonstrating a higher incidence in siblings than in the general population (493). There is 70% concordance for CD in identical twins (494). About 10% of first-degree relatives of celiac patients also have the disease (495), although a significant proportion (about 50%) remain asymptomatic and are said to have latent CD. The incidence of CD increases 10- to 30-fold in patients with other autoimmune disorders when compared with the normal population (496).

Pathogenesis

Celiac disease has a complex etiology that results from the interaction of environmental agents, genetic predispositions, and immunologic factors (497).

Gluten and Other Prolamines

Celiac disease is an autoimmune enteropathy triggered by ingestion of wheat gluten (gliadins), barley (hordeins), rye (secalins), and possibly oats (avenins). Gluten is found in grains such as wheat and buckwheat. Gluten is also found in many processed foods such as gravies, sausage, beer, ale, bread, and bread products. It can be separated electrophoretically into four major fractions: α-, β-, γ-, and ω-gliadins. Gliadins are prolamines with a high proline and glutamic acid content. All four types appear to be toxic, although α-gliadin is the most pathogenic (498). Toxic gliadins contain pro-ser-gln-gln and gln-gln-gln-pro sequences. These sequences are absent from nontoxic peptides (499). A 33-mer peptide generated by digestion of α-gliadin by intestinal enzymes is highly stimulatory for CD4+ T cells (500). This peptide is resistant to further digestion by intestinal brush border enzymes and is a highly specific substrate for deamidation by tissue transglutaminase. This 33-mer peptide is not present in cereal proteins that do not cause CD.

CD may be triggered in genetically susceptible individuals by activation of the immune system by a virus, usually an adenovirus. Later the mucosal system mistakenly reacts against gliadins bound to the intestine. α-Gliadin contains an amino acid region that is homologous to the 54-kDa E1b protein coat of adenoviruses. In addition, CD patients have a significantly higher prevalence of past adenovirus 12 infections than control subjects (501).

CD has the strongest association of any illness with a specific class II HLA molecule. The disorder is triggered by an environmental insult (gluten consumption), and the HLA haplotype acts as a classic immune response gene that operates at either the T-cell or antigen-presenting cell level to favor gliadin-specific responses. The primary HLA association in most CD patients is with DQ2. Fewer patients are of haplotype DQ8. An increased risk for CD also exists among individuals who are DR3-DQ2 homozygous and DR3-DQ2/DR7-DQ2 heterozygous (497).

In addition to the HLA linkage, CD has also been linked to several other chromosomal regions. Linkage to 2q33, an area of regulation for T-lymphocyte activation, has been seen in a Finnish family (502). Linkage to other regions on other chromosomes has also been reported, but linkage to 5p31-33 is the most consistently identified (503).

Gluten-reactive T cells can be isolated from small intestinal biopsies of celiac patients but not from nonceliac controls. These T cells are CD4+ and express the α/β TCR. A number of distinct T-cell epitopes within gluten exist. Lamina propria antigen-presenting cells that express HLA-DQ2 or -DQ8 present gliadin peptides bound to their α/β heterodimer antigen, presenting grooves to sensitized T lymphocytes that express the α/β TCR. These lymphocytes then activate B lymphocytes to produce immunoglobulins and stimulate other T cells to produce cytokines including interferon (IFN)-γ, IL-4, IL-5, IL-6, IL-10, IL-15, tumor necrosis factor (TNF)-α and TGF-β.

Tissue Transglutaminase and Other Autoantigens

Tissue transglutaminase (tTG) is expressed in many different tissues and is found both extra- and intracellularly. tTG is expressed just beneath the epithelium in the gut wall. Calcium-dependent tTG catalyzes selective cross-linking or deamidation of protein-bound glutamine residues. Deamidation of the glutamine residues of gliadin by tTG prepares the gliadin molecule to bind with HLA-DQ molecules (504). In addition, tTG can also cross-link glutamine residues of peptides to lysine residues in other proteins, including tTG itself. This may result in the formation of gluten–tTG complexes. These complexes may permit gluten-reactive T cells to stimulate tTG-specific B cells, thereby explaining the occurrence of gluten-dependent tTG autoantibodies that are a characteristic feature of active CD. Furthermore, tTG-catalyzed cross-linking and consequent haptenization of gluten with extracellular matrix proteins allows for storage and extended availability of gluten in the mucosa. tTG is necessary for activation of TGF-β, which is involved in differentiation of intestinal epithelium, regulates IgA expression, and modulates immune responses (505). Antibodies to tTG in CD patients interfere with fibroblast-induced differentiation of epithelial cells, possibly by inhibiting the cross-linking activity of tTG.

Cell-mediated and Antibody-mediated Immune Responses

Gluten ingestion in untreated CD induces nonproliferative activation of CD4+ TCR-α/β–positive cells in the lamina propria accompanied by proliferative activation of intraepithelial lymphocytes (α/β- and γ/β-positive T cells) in the epithelial compartment. CD patients harbor a population of DQ2+ (or DQ8+) antigen-presenting dendritic cells that efficiently capture and present deamidated gluten peptides leading to the activation of gluten-reactive T cells (506). Activated CD4+ T cells activate B lymphocytes and plasma cells that produce autoantibodies and T lymphocytes to secrete cytokines. These cytokines not only damage the enterocytes, but also induce expression of aberrant HLA class II cell surface antigens on the luminal surface of enterocytes, facilitating additional direct antigen presentation by these cells to the sensitized lymphocytes. Cytokines produced by DQ2- restricted T cells are of the Th1 type and are dominated by the secretion of IFN-γ. Cytokines produced by DQ8-restricted T cells have a Th0 profile. Increased γ/δ- cells in the epithelium and lamina propria of the small intestine have also been observed in CD patients, and these cells persist even after gluten withdrawal. These cells may play a protective role through activation of a nonspecific immune response that helps to lessen the antigen-specific immune response (497).

Celiac disease characteristically results in accumulation of IgA-, IgM-, and IgG-producing plasma cells within the mucosa. The antibodies produced by them are directed against gliadin, transglutaminase, endomysium, reticulin, and enterocyte actin. The exact physiologic role of these antibodies is still unclear.

Recent evidence also suggests that gliadin or its metabolites may directly injure the intestinal mucosa. Up-regulation of mucosal HLA-DR and intercellular adhesion molecule within 2 hours of in vitro exposure to gliadin suggests an early effect that may not be immune mediated (507). This early effect is followed by activation of CD4+ CD25+ T cells, producing the immunologic injury.

There may also be a role for intraepithelial lymphocytes in the pathogenesis of CD (508). In fact, these cells may play a key role in the development of refractory sprue and the development of enteropathy-associated T-cell lymphomas (509).

Clinical Features

Celiac disease is well known to be associated with gastrointestinal manifestations and malabsorption. However, over the years there has been increasing awareness of nongastrointestinal manifestations of the disease such as osteoporosis, cancer, and infertility. The clinical spectrum of CD is diverse and includes the following forms:

- *Typical CD:* This is fully expressed gluten-sensitive enteropathy associated with classic features of malabsorption. The full expression includes positive serology for endomysial and tTG antibodies and a diagnostic biopsy. This form of the disease usually affects younger patients.
- *Atypical CD:* This is fully expressed gluten-sensitive enteropathy found in association with atypical manifestations including short stature, anemia, infertility, etc.
- *Latent CD:* Patients have normal small bowel villous architecture on biopsy, but villous atrophy develops later on. Two variants have been described. The first includes patients in whom CD was diagnosed in childhood and who recovered completely with a gluten-free diet. The disease then remains latent in these individuals even after a normal diet is adopted. In the second variant, a normal mucosa is present in early biopsies while the patient is consuming gluten, but more typical features of CD develop later. The conversion of the latent state to active disease is often precipitated by nutritional deficiencies, by the effects or complications of a tumor, or by other environmental triggers, especially intracurrent infections, changes in the environment, or physiologically imposed stresses such as surgery, trauma, or pregnancy. Such patients exhibit abnormal jejunal permeability and high levels of antiendomysial antibodies. Such patients may have increased numbers of IELs in their biopsies (510) in the absence of villous changes.
- *Potential CD:* This includes patients who never had biopsy changes but have characteristic serologic abnormalities. HLA-DQ2 is more frequent in these patients and they frequently have a first-degree relative affected by CD.
- *Silent CD:* This includes asymptomatic patients with positive serologic autoantibodies and diagnostic biopsy.
- *Refractory CD:* These patients have severe, symptomatic, intestinal atrophy not responding to at least 6 months of a strict gluten-free diet.

The clinical presentation of any given patient with CD depends on the severity of the damage and patient age at presentation. The classic presentation of CD is that of steatorrhea with abdominal cramps and vomiting. In infants, the symptoms begin after weaning, when cereals are first introduced into the diet. Signs of nutritional deficiency, such as anemia, are the next most common presenting findings affecting children. Other manifestations include growth retardation, failure to thrive, short stature, muscle wasting, hypotonia, abdominal distension, and watery diarrhea. Celiac disease should be suspected in children with mild GI symptoms who have signs of nutritional deficiencies or a first-degree relative with celiac disease. It should also be suspected in children with IgA deficiency, dental enamel hypoplasia, or dermatitis herpetiformis or in children who have other diseases known to be associated with celiac disease (Table 6.35).

Celiac disease in adults is most often diagnosed in the 3rd and 4th decades of life, but it may develop at any age.

TABLE 6.35   Diseases Commonly Associated with Gluten-sensitive Enteropathy

Dermatitis herpetiformis
Ulcerative colitis
Sarcoid
Primary biliary cirrhosis
Pericarditis
Autoimmune chronic active hepatitis
Vasculitis
Dental enamel defects
Pseudohypoaldosteronemia
Selective Ig deficiency
Cystic fibrosis
Arthritis
IgA nephropathy
Splenic atrophy
Posterior cerebral calcifications
Epilepsy
Floating harbor syndrome
  Speech impediment
  Developmental delay
  Short stature
  Facial anomalies
Polyglandular autoimmune syndrome III
  Autoimmune thyroid disease
  Insulin-dependent diabetes
  Hypoparathyroidism
  Sarcoid
Autoimmune eye lesions
  Choroiditis
  Papillitis
Lung lesions
  Cavitary lung lesions
  Bronchiolitis
  Interstitial pulmonary fibrosis
Alopecia areata
α_1-Antitrypsin deficiency
Cavitary lymph nodes
Tumors
Enteropathy-associated T-cell lymphoma
Small intestinal carcinoma
  Oropharyngeal
  Breast
  Esophagus (squamous cell carcinoma)

Approximately 20% of cases are diagnosed in individuals over the age of 60 (511). Women are more frequently affected than men and are generally diagnosed at a younger age. Many adults with CD present with diarrhea, but as many as 50% do not (512). The classic presentation includes prolonged diarrhea, flatulence, weight loss, and fatigue. The degree of weight loss reflects the severity of the steatorrhea and an individual's ability to compensate for the nutritional deficit by increasing caloric intake. Patients with celiac disease may only have subtle signs of chronic malnutrition or nonspecific GI complaints. Patients may also present with anemia, short stature, nutritional deficiencies, or motility disturbances in the absence of diarrhea. Since the introduction of highly sensitive autoantibody tests, the number of patients presenting with classic features of CD has decreased. In fact, iron deficiency anemia, formerly regarded as an atypical presenting sign, is now the most common presentation of adult patients with CD (512). Iron deficiency is primarily due to iron malabsorption. Changes attributable to malabsorption and mineral, vitamin, and other essential nutrient deficiencies are listed in Table 6.36. The clinical presentation often reflects the degree of malabsorption present.

Atypical presentations include neurologic manifestations, osteopenia, and dermatitis herpetiformis without gastrointestinal manifestations. The most common neurologic finding is ataxia followed by epilepsy, cerebral calcification, cerebral white matter lesions on magnetic resonance imaging (MRI), myelopathy, peripheral neuropathy, seizures, and myopathy. CD also associates with an adverse fetal outcome in women with undiagnosed CD (513). Gastrointestinal bleeding occurs occasionally, and may represent an indicator of complications such as ulcerative jejunoileitis or malignancy.

Other extraintestinal features of the disease include vague abdominal pain, bone disease, abnormal peripheral blood smear findings, infertility (both male and female), amenorrhea, recurrent abortion or low-birth-weight babies, and hypoglycemia (494). Up to 8% of patients are detected due to mucosal changes on duodenal endoscopy performed for other conditions (494). From 7% to 15% of patients are detected through serum antibody tests performed because of a family history of CD.

Symptoms and histologic features improve while the patient follows a gluten-free diet. Gluten rechallenge causes symptom recurrence in many patients with uncertain diagnoses, especially those patients who lack typical GI symptoms.

Associated Diseases

Table 6.35 shows the wide variety of systemic diseases that are associated with celiac disease. Dermatitis herpetiformis and CD both associate with IgA-mediated epithelial injury. Initially, dermatitis herpetiformis was considered a skin disease occurring often concomitantly with CD, but currently it is believed that dermatitis herpetiformis is a cutaneous manifestation of celiac disease, affecting approximately 25% of patients. tTG also represents the autoantigen in dermatitis herpetiformis (514,515). Dietary restriction is essential in the treatment of both conditions.

Another IgA-mediated autoimmune disease associated with CD is IgA nephropathy. Patients with IgA nephropathy carry a risk of contracting CD. However, there is no increase in CD-type HLA-DQ in IgA nephropathy patients. It has been hypothesized that the increased intestinal permeability in IgA nephropathy may predispose genetically susceptible patients to celiac disease.

A wide spectrum of hepatobiliary diseases occurs in association with CD, including asymptomatic elevations of liver enzymes, nonspecific hepatitis, nonalcoholic fatty liver disease, and autoimmune and cholestatic liver disease (516). Increased alanine aminotransferase, aspartate aminotransferase, and/or alkaline phosphatase are seen in up to 47% of celiacs (516). Two main mechanisms underlying the development of the liver damage have been proposed. First, CD may result in increased intestinal permeability to toxins and antigens injurious to the liver. Second, chronic intestinal mucosal inflammation may represent a primary trigger. Prompt diagnosis and dietary treatment may prevent the progression to hepatic failure in patients with severe liver disease (517).

Associated autoimmune disorders include insulin-dependent diabetes, autoimmune thyroid disease, Addison disease, Sjögren syndrome, alopecia areata, and rheumatoid arthritis. Approximately 5% of insulin-dependent diabetics have associated CD, and one third of insulin-dependent diabetics with DQ2 have CD (518). The prevalence of the autoimmune disorders is related to the duration of the exposure to gluten (519). It is possible that chronic autoimmune stimulation of lymphocytes in the intestine predisposes to increased formation of other autoantibodies. Another important association is with trisomy 21 (Down syndrome). The prevalence of CD is 20 times that of the general population in patients with Down syndrome.

Some patients with CD develop lymphocytic colitis and/or lymphocytic gastritis (see Chapters 4 and 13). Patients with

TABLE 6.36	Extraintestinal Symptoms in Celiac Disease
Deficiency	**Symptoms**
Iron	Hemorrhage, hemolysis
Vitamin B_{12}	Anemia
Calcium	Osteomalacia, bone pain, compression fractures
Vitamin E	Night blindness
Vitamin A	Follicular hyperkeratosis of the skin
Vitamin B	Neuropathies
Pituitary, adrenal, parathyroid	Endocrine gland hypofunction

CD and microscopic colitis share certain predisposing HLA-DQ genes. However, these are not exactly related conditions. The intraepithelial lymphocytes in lymphocytic colitis are predominantly CD8+, unlike the IELs of CD. In addition, epithelial abnormalities and increased mononuclear inflammation are more prevalent in lymphocytic colitis than in CD patients. Furthermore, the watery diarrhea that is characteristic of lymphocytic colitis often does not respond to a gluten-free diet.

Patients with CD have an increased risk of cancer including lymphomas, oropharyngeal carcinomas, esophageal carcinoma, and small intestinal adenocarcinoma (520). There is also a small increased risk of colorectal carcinoma and liver cancer (520). Indeed, the primary cause of mortality in CD is malignancy (521). Abnormal lymphoid proliferations and lymphomas represent the most common malignant complication of celiac disease, affecting 5% to 10% of patients (522). An average of 8 years of celiac disease precedes the discovery of the malignant lymphoma, but both diseases may be discovered simultaneously or a diagnosis of celiac disease may follow the lymphoma diagnosis (522). Most celiac disease–associated lymphomas derive from mucosal T cells (521) and celiac disease is the most common setting in which enteropathy-associated T-cell lymphoma (EATL) is likely to occur. There is good evidence that uncontrolled IL-15 overexpression promotes the emergence of clonal T-cell proliferations (523). A strict gluten-free diet may lead to decreased cancer incidence and increased survival (521). An example of a duodenal somatostatinomas has also been reported in the setting of CD (524).

Diagnosis of Celiac Disease

The single most important step in diagnosing CD is to consider the disorder by recognizing its myriad clinical features. There is no one test that can definitively diagnose or exclude celiac disease in every individual. Just as there is a clinical spectrum of CD, there is also a continuum of laboratory and histopathologic results. IgA endomysial antibody and IgA tissue transglutaminase antibody are based on the target antigen tTG. *Antireticulin* and *antismooth muscle actin antibodies* are additional autoantibodies that may be seen in celiacs, but are not generally evaluated in routine clinical practice. All tests must be performed while the patient is on a gluten-containing diet. With concordant serologic tests and a positive biopsy, a diagnosis of CD can be made.

Endomysial antibodies bind to connective tissue surrounding smooth muscle cells (525). In the laboratory, IgA endomysial antibody (EMA) is most often detected by indirect immunofluorescence examination of sections of human umbilical cord. The test is reported as either positive or negative. The IgA endomysial antibody test has a sensitivity of 85% to 90% and a specificity of 97% to 100% (525). Antibody levels decrease when the patient is placed on a gluten-free diet, and may become undetectable in

treated patients (526). The sensitivity of this test is lower in children younger than 2 years of age than it is in older patients.

IgA tTG antibodies are detected by an automated enzyme-linked immunosorbent test. This test is less expensive and easier to perform than the test used to detect IgA endomysial antibodies. IgA tTG has a sensitivity of 95% to 98% and a specificity of 94% to 95% (512). Like endomysial antibody tests, sensitivity is lower in children younger than 2 to 3 years of age.

The *IgA antigliadin* assay has a sensitivity of 75% to 90% and a specificity of 82% to 95%. The *IgG antigliadin* assay has a sensitivity of 69% to 85% and a specificity of 73% to 90% (512). Most reports suggest that tests for antigliadin antibodies are more sensitive than EMA studies in infants and children younger than 2 to 3 years of age. High antigliadin antibody levels, however, have been reported in some normal individuals (527).

IgA endomysial antibodies and IgA tTG are used interchangeably as first-line tests for the diagnosis of celiac disease. In patients with IgA deficiency, IgG tTG testing is recommended as the first-line serologic test. Antibody levels decrease during treatment with a gluten-free diet and are useful in assessing dietary compliance. An IgA antigliadin antibody test is the most commonly used marker to monitor response to a gluten-free diet. A normal baseline value is reached within 3 to 6 months of dietary restriction. Currently, experience with IgA tTG in assessing dietary response is limited.

In a patient with suggestive symptoms and a negative serology test, three scenarios are possible: (a) the patient does not have CD, (b) the patient may have a selective IgA deficiency, and (c) the test is a "false negative" and should be repeated.

Other Laboratory Tests

Biochemical tests to be performed in the evaluation of CD patients include serum iron, folate, albumin, calcium, and potassium. Liver function studies should also be performed since serum transaminases are elevated in up to 40% of patients with untreated CD (516). Peripheral blood smears show features of iron deficiency anemia in the form of hypochromic microcytic anemia with low mean corpuscular volume (MCV), mean corpuscular hemoglobin (MCH), and mean corpuscular hemoglobin concentration (MCHC). Many target cells, siderocytes, Heinz bodies, and Howell-Jolly bodies are seen in patients with splenic atrophy. Patients with folic acid or vitamin B_{12} (unusual) deficiency will show macrocytosis and ovalocytosis with hypersegmented neutrophils on peripheral blood smears.

Microscopic stool examination to detect steatorrhea as a screening test for malabsorption is useful in the early stages of patient evaluation. Quantitative estimation of stool fat content is necessary to document steatorrhea. However, this and the D-xylose absorption test do not provide a specific

TABLE 6.37	Modified Marsh Classification of Celiac Disease		
Marsh Type	IEL/100 Surface Epithelial Cells	Crypts	Villi
Type 0 (normal)	<30–40	Normal	Normal
Type I (infiltrative)	>40	Normal	Normal
Type II (hyperplastic)	>40	Hyperplastic	Normal
Type IIIA (partial villous atrophy)	>40	Hyperplastic	Mild atrophy
Type IIIB (subtotal villous atrophy)	>40	Hyperplastic	Marked atrophy
Type IIIC (total villous atrophy)	>40	Hyperplastic	Absent
Type IV (hypoplastic)		Hypoplastic	Absent

IEL, intraepithelial lymphocyte.

diagnosis and are not routinely performed in the workup of celiac patients.

Endoscopic Findings

Endoscopic examination with biopsy is considered the "gold standard" for the diagnosis of celiac disease. Celiac disease can be patchy in its early stages and targeted biopsy of affected areas is necessary. Endoscopic findings include loss of villi, a mosaic mucosal pattern, scalloping of the duodenal folds, micronodularity, and visible vascularity. The endoscopic findings are not specific for CD, as similar changes may be seen in patients with eosinophilic gastroenteritis, giardiasis, tropical sprue, and other diseases (528). A biopsy is necessary to define the presence and extent of injury.

Histologic Features while on a Gluten-containing Diet

Small intestinal biopsies are used to diagnose or exclude celiac disease, to assess the severity of the damage, and to identify life-threatening complications of the disease. The presence of an abnormal biopsy while the patient is on his or her usual diet and improvement in the histologic features while he or she is on a gluten-free diet are diagnostic. Subsequent gluten challenge damages the mucosa. Since the histologic changes of CD are often patchy in their distribution, multiple biopsies from endoscopically normal and abnormal areas should be examined in order to establish the diagnosis. The histologic changes are most pronounced in the second and third parts of the duodenum. The microscopic features become less severe and patchier in the distal small bowel, particularly in the ileum.

Major histologic features of celiac disease include villous flattening, blunting, or absence; crypt hyperplasia; enterocyte degeneration; an intraepithelial lymphocytosis; and increased mononuclear cells and eosinophils in the lamina propria. However, the changes of celiac disease are not specific because similar lesions occur in patients with infections, allergies, and other immunologic conditions. Therefore, the pathology report should specify the degree of crypt hyperplasia and villous atrophy as well as assess the number of

intraepithelial lymphocytes. Standardization using the modified Marsh criteria (Table 6.37) facilitates communication with clinicians.

The histologic features vary depending on the presence or absence of gluten in the diet (Table 6.38). Two extremes of lesions occur in celiacs: A flat lesion with marked mucosal atrophy (Figs. 6.190 and Fig 6.191) and a relatively normal architecture with an intraepithelial lymphocytosis in the surface epithelium, with or without crypt hyperplasia and villous atrophy (Figs. 6.192 and 6.193). The histologic changes are highly characteristic, and when full-blown always suggest the diagnosis of celiac disease to the pathologist. However,

TABLE 6.38	Histopathologic Features in Relation to Diet

On a normal diet

- Malabsorption syndrome
- Flat jejunal biopsy (absent or severely blunted villi) with:
  Damaged surface epithelium
  Numerous intraepithelial lymphocytes
  Chronic inflammation in lamina propria
  Increased crypt mitoses
  Crypts elongated (hyperplastic pattern)

Short-term gluten-free diet

- Early onset of clinical improvement
- Within days, evidence of diminished surface epithelial damage
- Reduced number of intraepithelial lymphocytes
- Reduced chronic inflammation
- Mild to moderate villous atrophy

Gluten-free diet >3 months

- Villi gradually become normal
- No crypt hyperplasia
- Decreased mitoses
- Chronic inflammation diminished

Gluten challenge

- Early increase in intraepithelial lymphocytes and epithelium
- Eventual return of all lesions
- Malabsorption returns

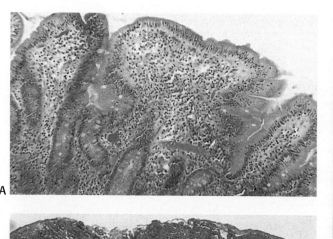

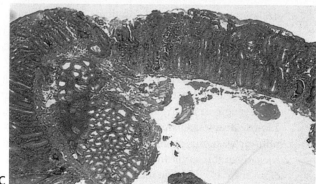

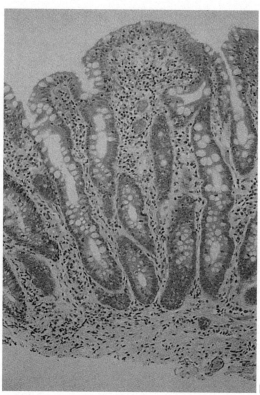

FIG. 6.191. Celiac disease **A:** Mild disease with blunted shortened villi and increased inflammatory cells. **B:** Blunted villi in celiac disease demonstrating more severe villous change than seen in A. Crypt hyperplasia is evident. **C:** Severe villous atrophy. A small portion of duodenum is seen.

this diagnosis should not be made purely on histologic findings because other diseases mimic CD (Table 6.39).

The severity of the histologic changes does not correlate well with the clinical signs and symptoms. However, the extent of the small intestinal disease does correlate with the clinical severity of the disease. Celiac patients with severe villous atrophy can be asymptomatic provided that the length of small bowel involvement is short. On the other hand, minimal histologic changes involving a longer segment of intestine can be associated with clinical symptoms.

A hallmark of CD is intraepithelial lymphocytosis (Fig. 6.192) and may be seen in celiacs in the absence of villous atrophy. It is a sensitive marker of CD, particularly when the IELs lie evenly within the villi (529), but it has relatively low specificity, thereby limiting its usefulness. Disorders associated with elevated IEL counts are listed in Table 6.40. IEL counts should be performed on 3 to 4 micron, well-oriented sections. Normal small bowel epithelium contains up to 20 lymphocytes per 100 enterocytes on H&E-stained sections (530). Slightly greater numbers of lymphocytes may be

TABLE 6.39   **Conditions Associated with a Flat Mucosa That Mimic Celiac Disease**

Infectious gastroenteritis	Giardiasis
Cow's milk intolerance	Radiation enteropathy
Soy or soy protein sensitivity	AIDS enteropathy
Malnutrition	Crohn disease
Tropical sprue	Eosinophilic gastroenteritis
Kwashiorkor	Zollinger-Ellison syndrome
Microvillous inclusion disease	Dermatitis herpetiformis
Familial enteropathy	Viral enteritis
Collagenous sprue	Lymphoma
Bacterial overgrowth syndromes	Ischemic enteritis
Graft vs. host disease	Drug effects
Common variable hypogammaglobulinemia	Autoimmune enteritis
	Cow's milk and soy protein enteropathy

TABLE 6.40   **Disorders Associated with Increased Intraepithelial Lymphocytes**

Celiac disease	*Helicobacter pylori* infection
Giardiasis	Collagen vascular diseases
HIV enteropathy	Autoimmune enteropathy
IgA deficiency	Lymphocytic enteritis
Blind loop syndrome	Nonsteroidal anti-inflammatory drugs
Tropical sprue	Viral infections
Cow's milk protein intolerance	Luminal stasis
Hypogammaglobulinemia	

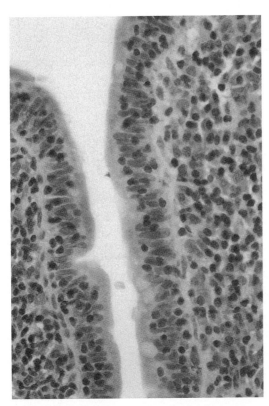

FIG. 6.192. Celiac disease. The biopsy is hypercellular due to epithelial crowding and infiltration of the epithelium by T lymphocytes. The lamina propria contains a dense infiltrate of mononuclear cells and plasma cells.

observed in immunostained sections. Higher numbers of lymphocytes are also seen overlying lymphoid follicles and lymphoid aggregates. As a result, counts of intraepithelial lymphocytes should not be performed in these areas. According to the modified Marsh classification for the diagnosis of celiac disease (Table 6.37), a significant increase in intraepithelial lymphocytes is defined as more than 40 lymphocytes per 100 surface or upper crypt enterocytes. Some authors suggest that clustering of lymphocytes (>12) in the epithelium at the tips of the villi also strongly indicates the disease (529). Others have observed a significant increase in villous tip lymphocytes in early celiac disease compared to controls, but did not find any difference in distribution of intraepithelial lymphocytes between controls and patients with early celiac disease (531).

Small bowel IELs consist of a heterogeneous population of T lymphocytes. In normal individuals, most IELs are CD3+ CD8+ T-cells, mostly TCR-$\alpha\beta$+, while CD4+ IELs are only a small component. In contrast, patients with untreated CD have an increase in CD3+ CD8− cells expressing TCR$\gamma\delta$. Since an intraepithelial lymphocytosis is not specifically diagnostic for CD, there may be a role for immunophenotyping of the IELs to show a preponderance of CD3+ CD8− cells (532).

Enterocytes show nonspecific changes in CD including attenuation of the brush border, a cuboidal appearance,

supranuclear cytoplasmic vacuolation, cytoplasmic basophilia, loss of polarity, and loss of basal nuclear orientation. They may also become pseudostratified as the cells become more crowded together (Figs. 6.194 and 6.195). Surface erosion is uncommon, but can be seen in severe cases of CD. Goblet cells are normal or occasionally increased in number. The subepithelial basement membrane may appear normal or thickened. Early histologic changes include a slight shortening of the villous height with an apparent increase in the villous width. Enterocyte destruction, associated with a marked increase in enterocyte proliferation and turnover, causes the villous changes. A mucosal hyperkinetic state with increased crypt mitoses (sometimes abnormal ones) compensates for the surface damage, maintaining the total mucosal thickness early in the disease. The proliferative zone of the crypt is expanded and there is an increase in enterocyte mitotic activity. The enterocytes at the bases of the crypts appear regenerative and goblet cells are decreased in number. The accepted normal ratio of villous length:crypt depth is 1:3 or greater, usually being even 1:4 or 1:5. Ratios less than this are considered to represent villous atrophy. Endocrine cells and Paneth cells are often increased in number and irregularly distributed within the crypt (Fig. 6.196). These changes progress with increased mucosal flattening and expansion of the crypt cells. It has been postulated that the increase in endocrine cells is a selective process to meet the demands of a small intestinal mucosa with a decreased absorptive area. The endocrine cell hyperplasia may contribute to the diarrhea present in celiacs. Pyloric metaplasia may develop. Gastric metaplasia as evidenced by the presence of gastric markers in the goblet cells may occur in untreated pediatric celiacs (533).

Edema, vascular congestion, and variable degrees of lamina propria inflammation are present (Fig. 6.187). The inflammatory infiltrate consists predominantly of lymphocytes and plasma cells, although eosinophils, mast cells, basophils, and, sometimes, neutrophils may also be seen. The presence of cryptitis and crypt abscesses are unusual in CD, and may point to another etiology such as infection or Crohn disease. IgA-, IgG-, and IgM-producing cells are increased two- to sixfold, with IgA-producing cells predominating. Patients with IgA deficiency and CD show a lower intensity of chronic inflammatory infiltration in the lamina propria. Lamina propria nerves may increase.

Histologic Features on a Gluten-free Diet

Morphologic recovery of the small intestine following consumption of a gluten-free diet and subsequent relapse upon gluten challenge represents the ultimate diagnostic criterion adopted by many. Repeat biopsies following gluten withdrawal usually demonstrate features of healing enteritis without evidence of active disease. If biopsies fail to return to normal, two alternatives should be considered: The patient is noncompliant with the dietary restriction or some other disease is present. Adults usually experience a prompt clinical improvement

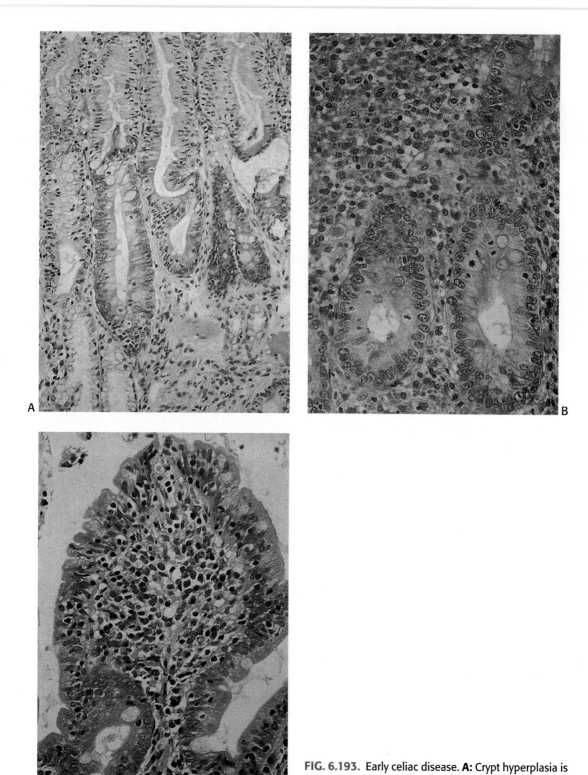

FIG. 6.193. Early celiac disease. **A:** Crypt hyperplasia is prominent. **B:** Numerous mitoses are present. **C:** Increased lamina propria and intraepithelial lymphocytes.

in their symptoms with gluten withdrawal and therefore fail to have a repeat biopsy following dietary modification. In contrast, children often have a more confusing diagnostic picture, and therefore biopsies are more regularly employed to evaluate the response to gluten withdrawal from the diet.

The most immediate effect of dietary gluten restriction is a change in the enterocytes lining the villi. As the mucosa heals, the inflammatory infiltrate decreases and the epithelial cells reassume their columnar shape and surface microvilli reappear. The cells become taller and one sees a progressive reduc-

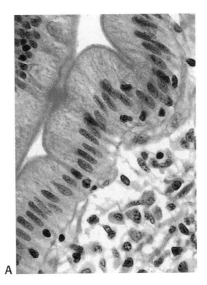
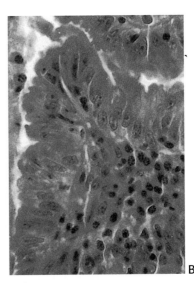

FIG. 6.194. Comparison of the normal mucosa **(A)** with celiac disease **(B)**. The hypercellularity of both the lamina propria and the lining epithelium is evident. The cells in celiac disease are palisaded, and there is an increase in lymphocytes.

tion in the number of intraepithelial lymphocytes. Patients clinically improve during this period of time. It takes villi several months to recover. If biopsies are obtained during the recovery period, the enterocytes may lack some of the classic features, including the intraepithelial lymphocytosis and subtle epithelial damage, but the crypts may appear somewhat hyperplastic and the villi somewhat atrophic. Several years may be required for lesions located at the duodenal–jejunal junction to return to normal on strict gluten-free diets.

Table 6.38 shows the chronology of the clinical and histologic responses to a gluten-free diet.

Treatment and Prognosis

Removal of gluten from the diet is essential for treatment of patients with CD, and generally is required lifelong. Symptomatic response to the institution of a gluten-free diet is often rapid, with many patients responding within 48 hours (534). In others, weeks or even months may be required before clinical remission is achieved. In addition to a gluten-free diet, patients with severe celiac disease may require supplemental therapy to correct nutritional deficiencies related to malabsorption.

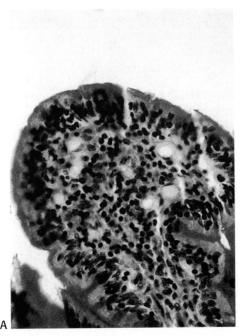
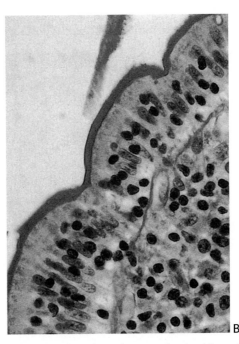

FIG. 6.195. Celiac disease **(A)** versus normal **(B)**. Both specimens have been stained with periodic acid–Schiff stain to accentuate the brush border, the site of the digestive enzymes. Note the absence of prominent brush border in the celiac specimen.

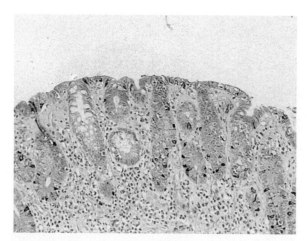

FIG. 6.196. Endocrine cell hyperplasia demonstrated by chromogranin stain.

The prognosis is excellent for patients who are diagnosed early and adhere strictly to the gluten-free diet. Late diagnosis or noncompliance with dietary restrictions may result in malnutrition and debilitation. In general, both treated adult and pediatric patients have life expectancies similar to those of the general population (535).

Refractory Sprue

Refractory sprue is defined as symptomatic severe villous atrophy that does not respond to a strict gluten-free diet for at least 6 months. Refractory sprue strongly associates with partial trisomy at 1q22-q44 (536). Since refractory sprue is a diagnosis of exclusion, the possibilities of inadvertent gluten ingestion and other causes of villous atrophy including disaccharidase deficiency, protein enteropathy, autoimmune enteropathy, and bacterial overgrowth should be ruled out. Refractory sprue in some patients suggests that the patient has developed ulcerative ileojejunitis or a neoplasm. Recent evidence suggests that refractory sprue may represent a manifestation of an aberrant clonal IEL-mediated neoplastic process. Cellier et al demonstrated that intraepithelial lymphocytes in patients with refractory

sprue are a monoclonal population that lacks CD8, a marker found in normal intraepithelial lymphocytes (506). These histologically undetected monoclonal T cells may be designated *cryptic intestinal T-cell lymphoma*. Others suggest that CD30 expression by the IELs in refractory sprue may indicate a poor prognosis including the occurrence of overt lymphoma (537). The lymphocyte-induced injury leads to intestinal ulceration and lymph node cavitation in some patients. In some but not all cases, the condition progresses to full-blown lymphoma.

At present, patients with suspected refractory sprue are given a trial of glucocorticoids. In steroid-unresponsive cases, a search for clonal TCR gene rearrangements and immunostains for CD8 are advised.

Collagenous Sprue

Collagenous sprue is diagnosed histologically and is characterized by the development of a subepithelial collagen band thicker than 10 microns. Collagenous sprue typically affects patients with a long history of CD, but has been regarded by some as a distinct entity. The disorder most commonly affects adults with a long history of celiac disease and may be barely perceptible or be quite prominent. The typical clinical history is of a patient with celiac disease who initially responded to a gluten-free diet but subsequently becomes refractory to treatment. The small bowel biopsy shows variable villous atrophy and other features typical of celiac disease. In addition, a prominent subepithelial collagen band is present, a change highlighted by trichrome stains (Fig. 6.197). When marked, the mucosa shows variable crypt hypoplasia with Paneth cell deficiencies. Although patients with collagenous sprue should be given a trial of a gluten-free diet, the prognosis is poor and many patients develop other complications such as ulcerative jejunoileitis and lymphoma (509).

Ulcerative Jejunoileitis

Ulcerative jejunoileitis is an uncommon but serious complication of celiac disease, characterized by multiple chronic small intestinal ulcers. Although this entity has been

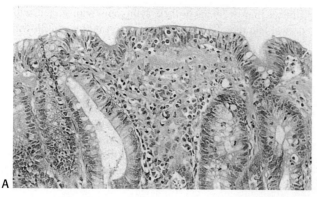

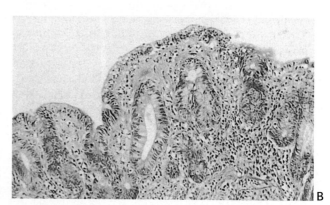

FIG. 6.197. Collagenous sprue. **A:** Histologic appearance demonstrating an acellular eosinophilic band beneath the luminal epithelium. **B:** This band is highlighted by a trichrome stain.

regarded by many as synonymous with lymphoma, ulcerative jejunoileitis without any evidence of lymphoma has been documented in a few cases (538).

The ulcers affect adults, generally after many years of malabsorption. Patients typically present with worsening of their malabsorption symptoms, abdominal pain, and complications including obstruction, perforation, and hemorrhage. Patients are often diagnosed late in the course of the disease. Intestinal perforation and peritonitis may develop.

The linear and shallow ulcers demonstrate a transverse orientation and little surrounding fibrosis but are morphologically nonspecific, usually multiple, and predominantly jejunal in location (Fig. 6.124). Histologically, the bases of the ulcers consist of purulent exudate overlying granulation tissue and fibrosis. The inflammation extends into the submucosa or even the muscle. The serosa may appear edematous and inflamed.

Surgical excision is the most effective therapy. Some patients respond to glucocorticoids and azathioprine.

COW'S MILK INTOLERANCE AND RELATED DISORDERS

Adverse reactions to cow's milk affect approximately 0.1% to 7.5% of children. Infants generally present at 1 week to 3 months of age with protracted vomiting, malabsorption, diarrhea, and dehydration (539). Cow's milk sensitivity is the most frequent cause of this syndrome, but it also occurs with soy, egg, and wheat.

Reactions to cow's milk proteins may be classified clinically as quick onset (symptoms develop within 1 hour of food ingestion) or slow onset (symptoms develop after >1 hour from food ingestion). Quick-onset allergic reactions are IgE mediated and do not result in structural gastrointestinal damage (540). Slow-onset reactions may also be IgE mediated, or they may be the result of T-cell–mediated immune reactions. Such reactions may result in a macrophage influx associated with cytokine release and direct damage to gastrointestinal tissues (540).

Patients develop fever; leukocytosis; cyanosis; vomiting; massive blood-tinged, mucoid diarrhea; dehydration; and metabolic acidosis. Infants with a more insidious onset have diarrhea, protein-losing enteropathy, iron deficiency anemia due to chronic intestinal blood loss, weight loss, and failure to thrive (541). The abnormalities resolve on cow's milk–free diets and recur on cow's milk challenge. Important predisposing factors are age younger than 3, transient IgA immunodeficiency, atopy, and early bottle feeding.

The stool contains occult blood, PMNs, and eosinophils. Typically, the intestinal mucosa appears thin with patchy areas of villous atrophy producing a pattern resembling celiac disease (542). Biopsy specimens reveal flattened villi, edema, a prominent mononuclear cell infiltrate of the epithelium and lamina propria, and an accompanying small number of eosinophils. IELs are usually fewer than seen in celiac disease (542). There is often a large number of IgE-containing plasma cells. The histology becomes normal when milk, soy, or other offending antigens are removed from the diet.

LYMPHOCYTIC AND COLLAGENOUS ENTERITIS

Lymphocytic duodenitis and enteritis are conditions in which the number of intraepithelial lymphocytes is increased in areas away from the lymphoid follicles. IELs are phenotypically heterogeneous. Most are cytotoxic T cells. As already noted, IELs can be increased in a number of disorders, most notably celiac disease (Table 6.40). We use the term *lymphocytic enteritis/duodenitis* when there is an increase in IELs in the absence of what appears to be celiac disease or other known causes for the change. These patients often have chronic diarrhea and/or malabsorption. The lesion may be accompanied by lymphocytic gastritis and lymphocytic colitis. The IELs lack the atypia present in enteropathy-associated T-cell lymphoma. We do state the various entities in which intraepithelial lymphocytosis occurs in an effort to help the gastroenterologist narrow down a specific etiology. Some patients are eventually shown to have celiac disease, but in other cases the cause never becomes evident.

We have also seen rare examples of severe collagenous enteritis accompanied by collagenous gastritis and collagenous colitis in the absence of celiac disease or a history of exposure to NSAIDs. The collagenous gastritis and colitis showed classic features, but the duodenum showed significant epithelial injury, subluminal collagen deposits, and severe fibrosis of the submucosa, a feature not typically seen in collagenous sprue (Fig. 6.198). The etiology of these changes is uncertain and the patients can become severely malnourished, requiring total parenteral nutrition.

MICROVILLOUS INCLUSION DISEASE

Microvillous inclusion disease (MID) occurs worldwide in infants from varying ethnic backgrounds. The disease may have a familial component as it sometimes occurs in multiple siblings (543). A genetic etiology is further supported by the observation that the disease appears to cluster in infants of Navajo descent (544). The mechanism by which microvillous inclusion disease develops is unknown. The underlying defect is thought to represent a genetic alteration that leads to abnormal trafficking of membrane proteins to the apical surface of differentiated epithelial cells (545).

Infants with microvillous inclusion disease present with severe, watery diarrhea. In some cases, the diarrhea can be so watery that it can be mistaken for urine. The volume of stool output in this disease may exceed that seen in association

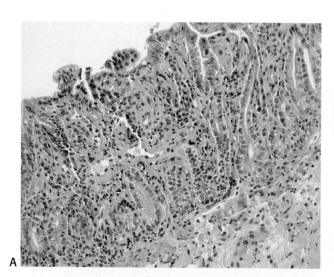
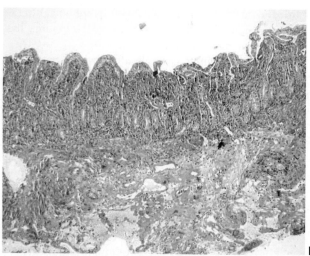

FIG. 6.198. Collagenous duodenitis in a patient who also had collagenous gastritis and collagenous colitis. **A:** There is a prominent eosinophilic band underlying a regenerative-appearing epithelium. In addition, there is fibrosis surrounding mucosal vessels. **B:** Trichrome stain showing extensive mucosal and submucosal fibrosis.

with cholera (545). As a result, affected infants die of dehydration unless adequate fluid replacement is provided.

Both congenital and late-onset forms of MID exist. Patients with late-onset disease have a better prognosis than those with congenital disease. Patients with the congenital form of the disease present with protracted diarrhea from birth and develop mildly hyperplastic villous atrophy (546). The disorder is worsened by oral feeding. The prognosis is extremely poor in infants because they depend completely on total parenteral nutrition. They usually die before the age of 18 months from liver failure, sepsis, and dehydration. All patients experience decreased absorption of water, electrolytes, and nutrients. The only effective therapy is small intestinal or multivisceral transplantation (547).

Small intestinal biopsies show a diffuse villous atrophy with little or no crypt hyperplasia and normal or decreased numbers of inflammatory cells in the lamina propria (Fig. 6.199). Increased mitoses and apoptoses are present in the crypts (548,549). The relatively intact duodenal crypts appear shortened or mildly dilated. Enterocytes usually retain their columnar shape or are only slightly shortened. The epithelium lining the villi appears disorganized with focally piled-up cells. The surface microvilli are either completely absent or appear markedly shortened and disorganized. The apical cytoplasm contains numerous variably sized vesicular bodies and a few lysosomelike inclusions. Other enterocytes contain targetoid intracytoplasmic microvillous inclusions (Fig. 6.200). These have complete brush borders with a microvillous membrane, surface filamentous coat, microfilaments, and terminal webs. The microvillous inclusions lie close to the apical surface or deeper within the supranuclear cytoplasm. Microvillous inclusions occur in the epithelium of the duodenum, jejunum, ileum, colon, gastric antrum, gallbladder, and renal tubules.

The apical cytoplasmic inclusions can be highlighted by PAS, carcinoembryonic antigen (polyclonal), CD10, villin, or alkaline phosphatase staining (548,549). PAS and CD10 stains demonstrate a discontinuous brush border that is most severely disrupted over the atrophic villous apices. Prominent PAS and CD10 staining is seen in the surface

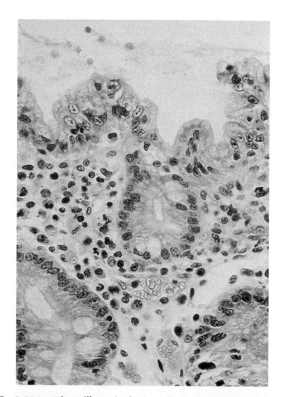

FIG. 6.199. Microvillous inclusion disease. Children with this disorder manifest with microvillous atrophy and crypt hypoplasia. The brush border appears deficient. (Courtesy of E. Cutz, The Hospital for Sick Children, Toronto, Ontario, Canada.)

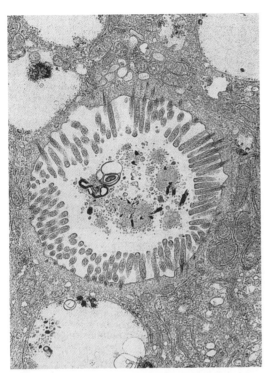

FIG. 6.200. Ultrastructural features of microvillous inclusion disease. (© 1989, reproduced with permission of the author and the Massachusetts Medical Society, all rights reserved: From Cutz E, Rhoads M, Drumm B, et al: Microvillus inclusion disease: an inherited defect of brush-border assembly and differentiation. *N Engl J Med 1989;320:646.*)

enterocytes. Microvillous inclusions are not present in every cell, and sometimes multiple levels on multiple blocks must be examined in order to make the diagnosis.

A definitive diagnosis depends on ultrastructural demonstration of intracytoplasmic microvillous inclusions and poorly developed brush border microvilli of small and large intestinal surface epithelium (Fig. 6.200) (546). Nearby nonenterocytic cells, such as goblet cells and Paneth cells, appear ultrastructurally normal. MID results from defective brush border assembly and differentiation.

TUFTING ENTEROPATHY

Tufting enteropathy is a chronic watery diarrhea syndrome presenting in the first few months of life. Rarely, the disease develops in older patients. Its etiology is unknown. The disease is thought to have a genetic basis since it tends to cluster in certain families (550). Alterations suggestive of abnormal cell–cell and cell–matrix interactions are present. These include an abnormal distribution of $\alpha2\beta1$ integrin along the crypt–villus axis, increased immunohistochemical expression of desmoglein, and ultrastructural alterations in the desmosomes (551,552).

Jejunal biopsies demonstrate partial or total villous atrophy and crypt hyperplasia. There is no increase in inflamma-

tory cells within the lamina propria. Intraepithelial lymphocytes are normal in number. The characteristic feature of the disease is the presence of focal epithelial "tufts" composed of clusters of closely packed enterocytes with rounded, teardrop–shaped projections of their apical cytoplasm.

Patients with tufting enteropathy have a variable prognosis. Most patients require total parenteral nutrition in order to remain adequately nourished for normal growth and development.

AUTOIMMUNE ENTEROPATHY

Autoimmune enteropathy is a life-threatening disorder of infancy that almost exclusively affects males. It is characterized by intractable diarrhea and a constellation of associated autoimmune diseases, including membranous glomerulonephritis, insulin-dependent diabetes, hemolytic or sideroblastic anemia, autoimmune hepatitis, sclerosing cholangitis, and hypothyroidism (553). Infants present with unexplained episodes of protracted diarrhea and no response to dietary therapy. The disease can also occur in adults (553).

Infants with autoimmune enteropathy demonstrate circulating antienterocyte antibodies (554). The autoantigen is a 75-kD protein encoded on chromosome 19p13, with homology to the tumor suppressor gene *MCC*. It has therefore been named *MCC2* (555). A subset of patients suffers from the systemic familial syndrome of autoimmunity: IPEX (immune dysregulation, polyendocrinopathy, and X-linkage) syndrome. This syndrome is also referred to as XLAD (X-linked autoimmunity and allergic dysregulation) (556). All patients with this syndrome develop autoimmune enteropathy. The IPEX syndrome results from germline mutations in the *FOXP3* gene on the X chromosome (557). *FOXP3* controls the development of regulatory CD4+ CD25+ T cells that are essential for maintenance of tolerance to self-tissues. The small intestinal lamina propria normally contains a CD25+ FOXP3+ CD4+ cells (558).

Small bowel biopsies show partial or complete villous atrophy, crypt hypertrophy, mononuclear cell infiltrates in the lamina propria, and increased expression of MHC class II antigens (559). Only a subset of patients has an immunodeficiency, even though the etiology is thought to be related to abnormal T-cell or B-cell regulation. Some patients demonstrate associated IgA deficiencies and T-cell abnormalities. There is a recently described patient with a severe FOXP3+ and CD4+ and CD8+ naïve T-cell lymphopenia who developed a non-IPEX form of autoimmune enteropathy combined with immunodeficiencies and recurrent infections (560).

The histologic features may be surprisingly subtle or they may be severe and involve both the large and small intestines (Fig. 6.201). The changes may be patchy in their distribution. Often, the most consistent feature is a nonspecific increase in lymphocytes involving both the epithelium and the lamina

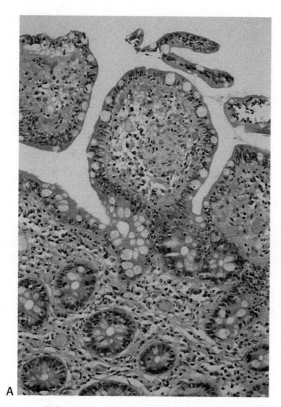
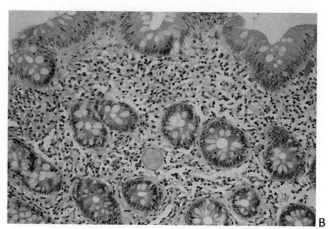

FIG. 6.201. Autoimmune enterocolitis. **A:** Duodenal biopsy demonstrating the presence of mild villous atrophy and a very minimal infiltrate of lymphocytes within the epithelium. **B:** Colonic biopsy in the same patient showing a mild increase in cells in the lamina propria and mild regenerative features with a barely noticeable increase in intraepithelial lymphocytes.

propria (Fig. 6.201). The IELs differ from those present in celiac disease in that they lack γδT-cell receptors and they tend to infiltrate the deep crypts rather than the surface epithelium. There may also be mild villous atrophy and crypt hyperplasia or crypt disorganization and increased apoptoses (561), producing a pattern reminiscent of graft versus host disease. Pyloric metaplasia may be present. Autoimmune enteropathy is often refractory to treatment, and is potentially fatal. Tacrolimus treatment may lead to a partial remission of the disease (562).

INTESTINAL GOBLET CELL AUTOANTIBODY-ASSOCIATED ENTEROPATHY

There is a second form of autoimmune enteropathy that is characterized by the presence of circulating antibodies to goblet cells. These can be demonstrated using the patient's serum applied to sections of normal human intestine that stain the goblet cell mucus. The clinical presentation of these patients is similar to autoimmune enteropathy but the histology is distinctive. Patients with intestinal goblet cell autoantibody-associated enteropathy have a normal intestinal architecture, but the mucosa lacks goblet cells, Paneth cells, and perhaps endocrine cells. The base of the crypts may

contain apoptotic figures and mitoses. The lamina propria often appears hypercellular, infiltrated by mononuclear cells and eosinophils (Fig. 6.202). Similar findings occur in both the small bowel and the colon. There may be an increase in crypt (but not surface) IELs and apoptotic bodies (563).

MALABSORPTIVE DIARRHEA

Malabsorptive diarrhea is a newly discovered autosomal recessive disorder that presents as congenital malabsorptive diarrhea and an almost complete absence of intestinal endocrine cells. The patients present in the first few weeks of life with vomiting, diarrhea, and a severe hyperchloremic metabolic acidosis after the ingestion of standard cow's milk–based formulas. It results from loss of function mutations in the *NEUROG3* gene. The histology of the small intestine shows a normal architecture, but with a severe dysgenesis of the endocrine cells. Enterocytes, Paneth cells, and goblet cells appear normal and there is no intraepithelial or lamina propria infiltration of inflammatory cells. However, there is an almost complete absence of endocrine cells and the rare endocrine cells that are present appear morphologically abnormal. These features can be highlighted using chromogranin immunostains (564).

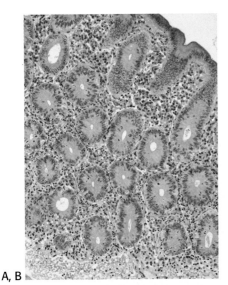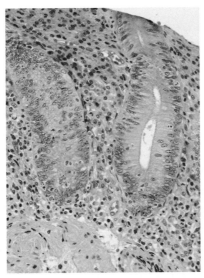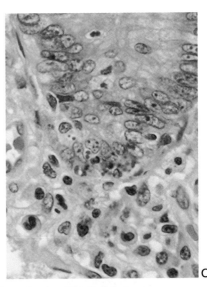

A, B   C

FIG. 6.202. Antigoblet cell antibody enteropathy. The pictures derive from the colon but identical features are seen in the small bowel. **A:** Low magnification of a biopsy that appears reactive with increased cellularity of the lamina propria. Note the complete absence of goblet cells. **B:** Higher magnification showing the details of the lamina propria infiltrate. The crypt contains several apoptotic bodies and mitoses but no goblet cells. **C:** Higher magnification of the base of the crypt showing an absence of endocrine cells and goblet cells along with apoptotic debris. The lamina propria eosinophils are also evident at this magnification.

LIPID MALABSORPTION

The three major forms of lipid malabsorption are abetalipoproteinemia, familial hypobetalipoproteinemia (565), and diabetes. Several other related syndromes result in lipid accumulations in enterocytes producing histologic patterns indistinguishable from abetalipoproteinemia (Table 6.41) (566). The pathogenesis of several lipid malabsorption syndromes is shown in Figure 6.203.

Abetalipoproteinemia

Abetalipoproteinemia is a recessive genetic disease characterized by the virtual absence of apolipoprotein (apo) B and apo B–containing lipoproteins in plasma. Affected patients

TABLE 6.41	Diseases Associated with Fatty Deposits in Enterocytes

Abetalipoproteinemia
Familial hypobetalipoproteinemia
Diabetes
Gluten-sensitive enteropathy
Cow's milk–sensitive enteropathy (and related entities)
Anderson disease (chylomicron retention disease)
Fasting states
Impaired chylomicron metabolism
Juvenile nutritional megaloblastic anemia
Tropical sprue
Following the ingestion of a fatty meal

are usually individuals of Jewish or Mediterranean descent. Approximately one third of cases result from consanguineous marriages, and family studies suggest an autosomal recessive mode of inheritance (567). The sex ratio is 1:1.

In abetalipoproteinemia, chylomicron assembly is defective due to mutations in the microsomal triglyceride transfer protein (MTP) (568). MTP is a resident lipid transfer protein within the endoplasmic reticulum of hepatocytes and enterocytes. The absence of MTP in abetalipoproteinemia results from MTP mutations affecting the large subunit of the protein. The absence of MTP results in an absence of apo B100 and B48 from the plasma, because apo B–containing lipoprotein assembly is disrupted in the liver and intestine.

At birth, infants with abetalipoproteinemia are asymptomatic. Signs and symptoms begin months after birth, once a diet rich in lipids is started. The initial complaints are diarrhea, bloating, vomiting, anemia, weight loss, and failure to thrive. Spinocerebellar degeneration, peripheral neuropathy, and retinitis pigmentosa result from deficiencies in fat-soluble vitamins (vitamin E levels are characteristically extremely low). The gastrointestinal manifestations of the disease often improve with time, in part because affected patients (or their parents) learn to avoid dietary fats.

Acanthocytes are characteristically seen in the peripheral blood. Serum hypolipidemia is present with reduced cholesterol, triglycerides, low-density lipoprotein (LDL), and chylomicrons. Patients have undetectable levels of serum apolipoprotein B.

Small bowel biopsies typically show striking enterocyte vacuolization. Overall, the villous architecture appears normal

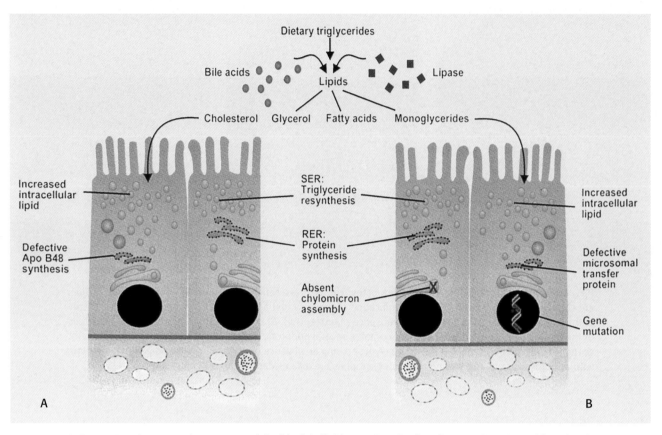

FIG. 6.203. Diagrammatic summary of the block in lipid secretions in abetalipoproteinemia and hypobetal-ipoproteinemia. **A:** Hypobetalipoproteinemia. Lipids accumulate within the cell due to defective apo B48 synthesis. In contrast, in abetalipoproteinemia **(B),** a specific genetic mutation leads to defective microsomal transfer protein and the lack of chylomicron assembly. As a result, intracellular lipids increase. RER, rough endoplasmic reticulum; SER, smooth endoplasmic reticulum.

but the villi are lined by enterocytes containing large amounts of intracellular triglycerides. Enterocyte vacuoliza-tion, although characteristic of abetalipoproteinemia disor-ders (Fig. 6.204), is not entirely diagnostic, since these changes occasionally occur in other settings (Table 6.41) (569). The lipid-engorged, vacuolated enterocytes appear pale and at high magnification contain numerous small, clear, lipid-filled vacuoles that pack the apical and subnu-clear cytoplasm. No lipid droplets are present in the intercel-lular spaces or in the lacteals. The lamina propria appears normal except for the presence of macrophages containing bizarre inclusions. Acanthocytes may be seen in the capillar-ies of the lamina propria.

Chylomicron Retention Disease

Chylomicron retention disease, also known as Anderson disease, is a rare autosomal recessive intestinal lipid trans-port disorder in which apo B48 is absent. Symptoms begin during the first few months of life and include chronic diar-rhea, significant fat malabsorption, and failure to thrive (570). Unlike abetalipoproteinemia, acanthocytosis rarely occurs

and neuromuscular manifestations are much less severe. Fasting triglyceride levels are normal but fat-soluble vita-mins, especially A and E, are severely decreased. Plasma cho-lesterol levels are low but do not reach those seen in abetali-poproteinemia. Apo B, apo AI, and apo IV are decreased. Immunoperoxidase localization of apoprotein B in fasting biopsy specimens shows normal to elevated staining of the lipid-laden intestinal epithelial cells (570).

The enterocytes contain large numbers of fat particles (chylomicrons) in the endoplasmic reticulum and the Golgi complex. The defect appears to be in the translocation of Golgi-derived vesicles to the plasma membrane for excre-tion. Hence, little or no fat is observed in the intercellular spaces and lacteals (570). The ultrastructural features differ from those seen in abetalipoproteinemia in that chylomi-crons and larger lipid vacuoles are seen in the apical entero-cyte cytoplasm (571).

INTERPRETATION OF ILEAL BIOPSIES

Ileal biopsies are commonly taken when patients undergo colonoscopy. As a result, pathologists often have the oppor-

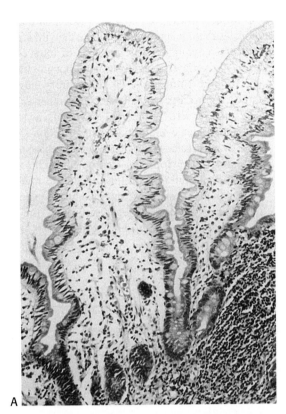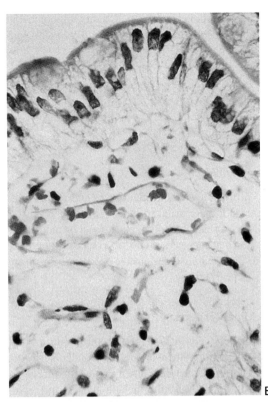

FIG. 6.204. Abetalipoproteinemia. **A:** Moderate-power photograph demonstrating the presence of an essentially intact architecture with normal villous and crypt length. The epithelium appears clear due to the presence of marked lipid accumulations within the epithelium. **B:** Higher magnification showing the displacement of the nuclei upward and the clear nature of the cytoplasm.

tunity to examine changes that may be present in the ileal mucosa. The most common changes include acute inflammation and evidence of chronic disease. Additionally, there may be changes in the Peyer patches. One common mistake that we see is overinterpretation of increased numbers of intraepithelial lymphocytes that are normally present in the follicle-associated epithelium as either lymphocytic enteritis or, worse yet, as evidence of a lymphoma.

In an inflamed ileum, the inflammatory cells might include lymphocytes, plasma cells, neutrophils, eosinophils, mast cells, and/or macrophages with or without surface erosions or ulcers. These may be present in the epithelial compartment or the lamina propria. In addition, granulomas, parasites, viral inclusions, or enterocyte changes may be evident.

Acute ileitis due to bacterial infections causes changes similar to those seen in acute self-limited colitis (see Chapter 13). Thus, there is mucosal edema and a polymorphous inflammatory infiltrate that early on is dominated by neutrophils but becomes replaced by mononuclear cells over time. The neutrophils may cause cryptitis or crypt abscesses as well as lamina propria inflammation. The crypt and villous architecture generally remain normal without significant crypt distortion. The epithelium appears variably degenerated or regenerative depending on the stage of the disease. Some drug-induced damage causes similar changes.

Some bacterial infections cause characteristic granulomatous lesions (Table 6.15). Viral infections often cause prominent lymphoid hyperplasia.

Chronic ileitis is recognized by the presence of crypt and villous distortion and by the presence of pyloric metaplasia. A lymphoplasmacytosis is variably present. The most common etiology for chronic ileitis is Crohn disease (see Chapter 11), but it also can result from chronic infections, drug injury, and chronic ischemia. Additionally, many of the disorders discussed earlier in this chapter may cause chronic ileal damage.

EOSINOPHILIC DISEASES

Food Allergies

Up to 45% of the population report adverse reactions to food (572). Various enteric antigens play a role in the pathogenesis of conditions loosely termed *food allergic diseases*; many conditions associate with food allergies (Table 6.42). Milk and other dairy products are more commonly allergenic among children than among adults. Other common offending agents include nuts, eggs, and soy products (573). The increased susceptibility of young infants to food allergies results from their general immunologic immaturity and the

TABLE 6.42   Diseases Associated with Food Allergies

Systemic anaphylaxis
Rhinitis
Conjunctivitis
Asthma
Allergic alveolitis
Celiac disease
Cow's milk protein enteropathy
Urticaria
Angioedema
Atopic eczema
Dermatitis herpetiformis

overall immaturity of the GI tract (244). There is also a variant of the IPEX syndrome that results in autoimmune enteropathy, hyper-IgE, and severe food allergies that become manifest after weaning. It results from a deletion in the *FOXP3* gene (574). Food allergies affect up to 8% of children. Tissue damage results from either the primary pathologic event or from unavoidable side effects of protective immune responses. A definitive diagnosis of a food allergy requires (a) the demonstration of an unequivocal clinical reaction after a controlled food challenge and (b) elimination of the symptom complex subsequent to removal of the offending food. Thus, one can accept the diagnosis of milk allergy only if (a) symptoms subside with elimination of milk from the diet, (b) symptoms occur within 48 hours after refeeding, (c) three sequential challenges are positive, and (d) symptoms abate after each challenge.

The clinical features of food allergy are extensive and vary in location, severity, and time of onset (575). Clinical findings correlate with the site and extent of mast cell degranulation. The principal organs affected by allergic food reactions are the intestinal tract, skin, and lungs. In some patients, the signs and symptoms of an immediate reaction remain limited to the GI tract, with cramping, bloating, nausea, vomiting, diarrhea, growth failure in children, and weight loss in the adult. Any disease that disrupts mucosal integrity promotes the development of a food allergy by allowing allergens into the lamina propria, facilitating their interaction with immune cells.

Histologically, biopsies show partial villous atrophy with vacuolated cytoplasm, particularly at the surface, and mucosal eosinophilic infiltrates. The eosinophils may aggregate in the lamina propria or extend into the epithelium (Fig. 6.205). Since these infiltrates are usually focal, multiple biopsies are often required to make the diagnosis (576). Also, lymphonodular hyperplasia of the duodenal bulb is present in more than 50% of cases.

Eosinophilic Gastroenteritis

Eosinophilic gastroenteritis is a diagnosis applied to a diverse group of patients who share the following: (a) GI symptoms,

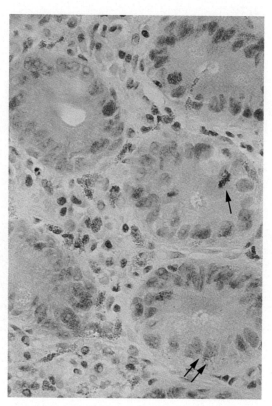

FIG. 6.205. Allergic enteritis. The lamina propria contains an eosinophilic infiltrate. The infiltrate causes subtle epithelial changes including increased mitotic activity (*arrow*), eosinophilic degranulation within the epithelium (*double arrow*), and a lamina propria infiltrate.

(b) gastrointestinal eosinophilic infiltrates, and (c) no demonstrable cause of the eosinophilia such as parasitic infection or a specific allergic response. Nonetheless, many patients have allergic histories, including hay fever, allergic rhinitis, eczema, asthma, drug sensitivities, or elevated IgE levels. Peripheral eosinophilia affects 72% to 90% of patients. Some patients have associated connective tissue diseases, including scleroderma, scleroderma variants, polymyositis, and dermatomyositis. Food intolerance has been postulated as an etiologic factor in eosinophilic gastroenteritis. However, most cases lack a specific allergen that triggers the disease and some patients demonstrate few or no allergic features. The most likely explanation for these discrepancies is that multiple unidentified antigens cause the disease (577).

The clinical presentations vary widely. GI symptoms may include nausea, vomiting, diarrhea, abdominal pain, growth retardation, malabsorption, steatorrhea, protein-losing enteropathy, secondary iron deficiency anemia, hypoalbuminemia, and intestinal obstruction. Patients may also present with an acute abdominal emergency such as acute appendicitis or intestinal perforation. Rare fatalities have been described.

The clinical presentation depends on both the site and extent of the intestinal involvement. Any part of the gut may

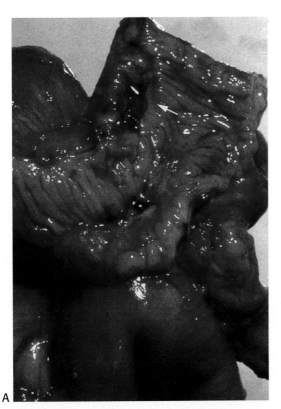

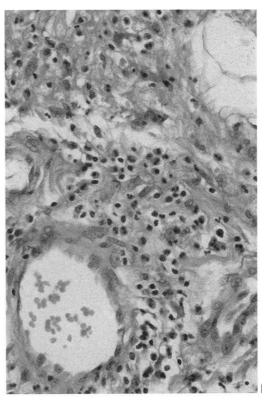

FIG. 6.206. Eosinophilic gastroenteritis. **A:** Resection specimen showing adherent loops of small bowel with fistulae between them. The origin of the fistulae is seen as dark geographic areas. The bowel was resected due to a perforation (*arrow*). Light from the background shows through the perforated site. **B:** Histologic section through an area of the specimen showing the intense eosinophilic infiltrate. (Case courtesy of the Department of Pathology, Tygerberg University, Republic of South Africa.)

be involved, but the stomach and small intestines are the most common sites of involvement. Mucosal disease generally presents with diarrhea, bleeding, malabsorption, and protein-losing enteropathy. Submucosal disease manifests as intestinal obstruction and abdominal pain. Ascites develops when eosinophils infiltrate the serosa or muscularis propria. If the patient develops ascites, the fluid contains eosinophils. Most patients with eosinophilic enteritis show at least partial spontaneous improvement. Patients respond dramatically to a short course of corticosteroid therapy.

The lesions of eosinophilic gastroenteritis tend to be patchy and multiple (Fig. 6.206), and they may be localized or diffuse. Involvement of GI segments measuring up to 50 cm long produces diffuse bowel thickening. The bowel becomes markedly rigid and edematous and contains prominent eosinophilic infiltrates. Increased numbers of eosinophils populate the lamina propria and the epithelium shows variable degrees of damage. The number of eosinophils varies; they often range up to 50 eosinophils per high-powered field (hpf) (Fig. 6.207). However, it should be kept in mind that the presence of eosinophils is nonspecific because they are also seen in other diseases (Table 6.33). Because tissue eosinophils may be increased in other diseases, it is helpful to find the eosinophils extending into the

underlying submucosa or to find associated edema (Fig. 6.208). It is also helpful to find eosinophils within the epithelium of the crypts or villi. The localized eosinophilic infiltrates may cause crypt hyperplasia, epithelial cell necrosis, and villous atrophy. In a minority of cases (approximately 10%), a diffuse enteritis develops with complete villous atrophy producing an appearance identical to that seen in celiac disease. Variable degrees of fibrosis, necrosis, atrophy, and mast cell infiltrates also develop. Often the lesions occupy the submucosa. Submucosal edema is common, and destruction of the wall and fibrosis may also occur. Unexpectedly, large numbers of degranulating mast cells may be present. Contiguous smooth muscle fibers in the muscularis mucosae appear hyperchromatic, enlarged, and irregular with reactive nuclei separated by inflammatory cells. The muscularis propria usually shows some degree of eosinophilic infiltration. Sometimes the mesenteric lymph nodes become hyperplastic and infiltrated with eosinophils. Establishing the diagnosis by endoscopic biopsy can be problematic. In about 10% of cases, mucosal biopsies are nondiagnostic, either because of the sampling error inherent in diagnosing a patchy process or due to mucosal sparing. In these instances, the diagnosis is established by multiple biopsies, full-thickness biopsy, or surgical resection.

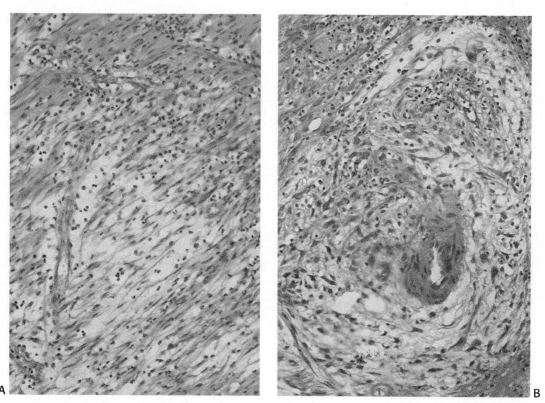

FIG. 6.207. Eosinophilic gastroenteritis. **A:** Medium-power micrograph illustrating the marked eosinophilic infiltrate within the muscularis propria and deep submucosa. The individual fibers of the muscularis propria are separated by the edema. **B:** In some places the infiltrate centers around small vessels and associates with prominent edema.

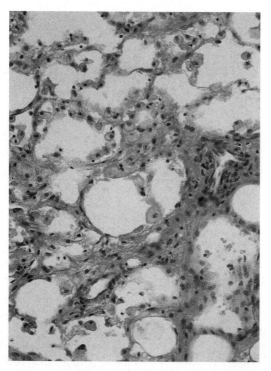

FIG. 6.208. Histiocytic cells surrounding air spaces in pneumatosis intestinalis.

Hypertrophic Eosinophilic Gastroenteropathy

Patients with hypertrophic eosinophilic gastroenteropathy are typically children who present with recurrent bowel obstruction and protein-losing enteropathy. Grossly, ileal and/or jejunal mucosa appears thickened with apparent pseudopolyps. The patients develop massive elongation of the small intestinal villi. This results in a crypt:villus ratio that is two to four times that seen in the normal small bowel. This elongation appears to result from decreased apoptosis. The mucosa may be ulcerated and the inflammatory infiltrate overlying the ulcers as well as the lamina propria is heavily infiltrated by eosinophils. Eosinophils may also be present in the submucosa and muscularis propria (486).

GRANULOMATOUS AND HISTIOCYTIC INFLAMMATORY CONDITIONS

Small intestinal granulomas form in many disorders (Table 6.15). The nature of the granulomas varies significantly from small macrophage collections that may or may not contain foreign material to classic granulomas. Small crypt-associated mucin granulomas complicate mucosal injury. Histiocytes may lie under the free surface or occupy the lamina propria and may

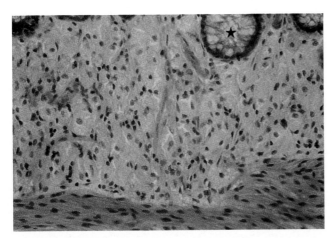

FIG. 6.209. Localized xanthoma. A collection of histiocytes lies beneath the base of the gland (*star*), widening the distance from the gland base to the muscularis mucosae. Special stains for organisms were negative.

contain microorganisms. Vessel-associated histiocytic collections complicate infections, especially CMV (Fig. 6.119). Histiocytic cells also surround the air spaces, characteristic of pneumatosis intestinalis (Fig. 6.208), or they form small mucosal collections in transplant patients without evidence of infection. They also aggregate in the lamina propria (Fig. 6.209) or submucosa in patients with xanthomas. The etiology of granulomas or histiocytic collections differs depending on whether they are compact or loose, are diffuse or localized, contain giant cells or not, and associate with areas of necrosis or not. Peritoneal rosetting microgranulomas may also be encountered in incarcerated small intestinal loops. The rosetted cells are CD68+, distinguishing them from areas of reactive mesothelial hyperplasia (578).

Crohn Disease

The small intestine in Crohn disease often contains granulomas, but the pathology of this disorder is highly variable (see Chapter 11).

Sarcoid

Sarcoid, a systemic granulomatous disease, preferentially affects lymph nodes, but it also involves many other organs, including the gut. Malabsorption, protein-losing enteropathy, and lymphangiectasia may develop secondary to lymphatic obstruction due to the abnormal lymph nodes (579). It is unwise to make a definitive diagnosis of sarcoid in the absence of classic disease in the liver or lungs. The histologic features consist of compact bland granulomas that lack necrosis. These may involve both the bowel wall and the regional lymph nodes. Areas of necrosis suggest the presence of an infection such as tuberculosis or *Yersinia* infection, especially when the granulomas affect the terminal ileum.

Granulomas Associated with Foreign Material

Granulomas develop around foreign material such as talc or sutures. Suture granulomas usually contain a central suture surrounded by palisading histiocytes and foreign body giant cells. Talc granulomas typically contain foreign body–type giant cells and can be distinguished from other granulomas by the use of polarizing lenses, which reveal typical birefringent crystals. Starch-based glove powders also produce granulomas recognizable under polarized light by the presence of a distinctive "Maltese cross." Accidental entry of barium into the intestinal wall during radiologic examinations may provoke barium granulomas. They exhibit distinctive birefringent granular material with a pale green color in the histiocytic collections.

Xanthomas

Small mucosal xanthomas are encountered throughout the GI tract, but they are least common in the small bowel. These represent superficial aggregates of histiocytes in the lamina propria. The lesions are sometimes seen endoscopically as yellowish nodules and may represent vestiges of some prior minor mucosal damage. A more extensive form of xanthomatosis consists of accumulations of lipid-laden macrophages that form mural plaques (Fig. 6.210) or nodules. Generalized or localized xanthomatosis may complicate motility disorders (580). GI xanthomatosis also occurs in patients with hypercholesterolemia and hypertriglyceridemia. An unusual case involved an 85-cm segment of small bowel. The intestinal wall was distorted by regularly spaced nodular accumulations of lipid-laden macrophages expanding the submucosa, muscularis, and serosal surface.

Malakoplakia

Malakoplakia is a distinctive form of a granulomatous process that may form tumorlike masses. This entity is discussed in greater detail in Chapter 13.

NUTRITIONAL DISORDERS

Severe nutritional deficiency can produce marked small intestinal abnormalities. The classic example is kwashiorkor. Malnutrition of this severity seldom occurs in developed countries, but less severe forms may be recognized after gastric surgery or in patients with chronic debilitating diseases. Malnutrition results from a lack of a suitable diet, faulty metabolism, and inadequate absorption of dietary constituents.

Kwashiorkor

Kwashiorkor is one of the most common pediatric illnesses in underdeveloped countries. It affects many African tribes,

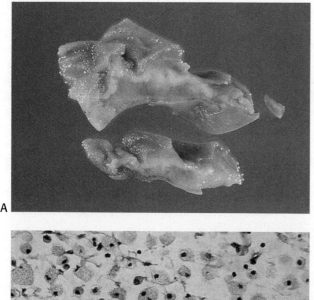

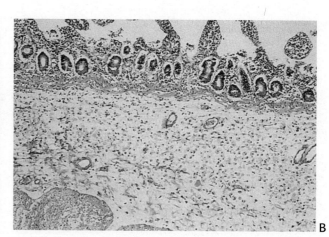

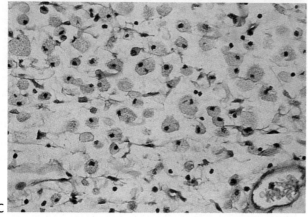

FIG. 6.210. Small intestinal xanthoma. **A:** Gross photograph showing the prominent submucosal expansion by a clear gelatinouslike fluid collection. **B:** Histologic features demonstrating the presence of a diffuse histiocytic infiltrate loosely arranged in the submucosa. **C:** Higher magnification demonstrating the histiocytic cells widely separated from one another.

particularly in eastern and southern Africa, causing high morbidity and mortality. Nutrient malabsorption exacerbates the protein–caloric malnutrition, further damaging the gut, impairing immune competence, and increasing the risk of infections (Fig. 6.211). Diarrheal illnesses are common.

The small intestinal abnormalities may be indistinguishable from untreated celiac disease. Histologically, the mucosa appears flattened. The crypts appear coiled with a relative increase in length and a lower than normal mitotic index. The crypts are not uniformly altered. They may be atrophic in some areas, whereas in others they appear normal or hyperplastic (581). Epithelial cell height decreases and the nuclei are arranged irregularly. The lamina propria becomes infiltrated with mononuclear cells and the basement membrane thickens (582). The presence of neutrophilic infiltrates suggests a coexisting infection. The patients respond to a

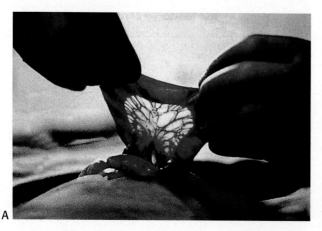

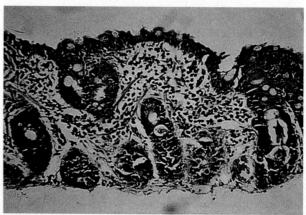

FIG. 6.211. Kwashiorkor. **A:** Hypoplastic bowel in kwashiorkor visualized at the time of surgery. **B:** Severe villous atrophy.

normal diet with concomitant improvement in the appearance of the intestinal mucosa.

Vitamin E Deficiency and Brown Bowel Syndrome

Patients with vitamin E deficiency develop eosinophilic enteritis and brown bowel syndrome. Vitamin E deficiency occurs alone or it complicates other diseases (583,584). Brown bowel syndrome is characterized by lipofuscin deposits in the muscularis propria. Patients range in age from the 20s to the late 70s, with an average age of 51 years. They present with epigastric pain, mild diarrhea, and chronic malabsorption.

Grossly, the bowel is variably orange-brown and is often retrospectively described as being darker than usual by the surgeon. The segmental or diffuse brownish discoloration can be appreciated from the serosal aspect of the GI tract as well as on cut section. The disorder more commonly affects the small intestine and stomach, but it can involve the colon. Occasionally, it involves the entire GI tract. No correlation exists between the degree of pigmentation and the severity of the associated disease.

The mucosa usually appears normal. However, occasionally the villi appear blunted and there may be mild submu-cosal edema. There is usually no inflammation or fibrosis, although eosinophils may populate the submucosa and muscularis propria. A coarsely autofluorescent, granular, golden brown pigment, known as lipofuscin, fills the smooth muscle cells of the muscularis propria, muscularis mucosae, and vascular walls (Fig. 6.212). The pigment appears round to oval, often lying in a perinuclear or central cellular location. Individual pigment granules vary from barely visible to up to 2 to 3 μm in size. In areas of minimal involvement, the pigment is barely visible. In advanced cases, large lipofuscin deposits result in considerable smooth muscle cell loss. Macrophages also contain pigment, especially in the muscular layer. The pigment granules show various tinctorial qualities (Fig. 6.213; Table 6.43). The Fontana-Masson stain is the most sensitive stain for detecting the pigment, especially when the cells contain scant amounts of pigment. The pigments seen in brown bowel syndrome and in melanosis are compared in Table 6.44.

Ultrastructurally, the cytoplasm of the muscle cells contains irregularly shaped, variably electron-dense, intracellular granular aggregates that concentrate centrally in a perinuclear location, sparing the peripheral cytoplasm (Fig. 6.214). Smooth muscle filaments end abruptly or stretch around the pigment. The deposits sometimes assume the shape of myelin figures enveloped by a single unit membrane. Mitochondrial

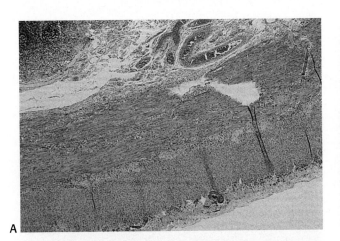

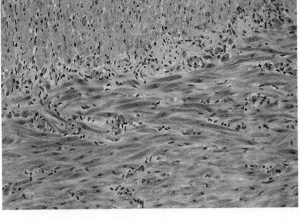

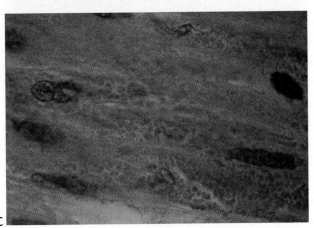

FIG. 6.212. Brown bowel disease. **A:** Low magnification of the lower portion of the mucosa, submucosa, and muscularis propria demonstrating a subtle change in the tinctorial qualities of the muscle cells on hematoxylin and eosin stain. **B:** Higher magnification of the muscularis propria showing a faint brownish tinge. **C:** Very high magnification demonstrating a fine granular golden brownish pigment within the nuclei.

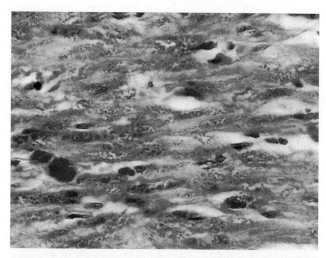

FIG. 6.213. Brown bowel syndrome. Periodic acid–Schiff stain accentuates the granules.

alterations may be the source of the lipofuscin pigment and therefore the term *smooth muscle mitochondrial myopathy* may apply to the disorder (585).

Zinc Deficiencies and Acrodermatitis Enteropathica

Zinc deficiencies can be divided into two groups: A congenital form called acrodermatitis enteropathica and acquired forms. Acrodermatitis enteropathica is a rare autosomal recessive inborn error of metabolism that results in zinc malabsorption and severe zinc deficiency (586). Zinc is a normal constituent of more than 100 enzymes, and therefore zinc deficiencies have an overall detrimental effect on nucleic acid metabolism and protein and amino acid synthesis, eventually leading to growth arrest (587). Diarrhea and anorexia are common, especially in infancy. Growth retardation, alopecia, weight loss, and recurrent infections are prevalent in toddlers and schoolchildren. Without adequate therapy, the disease often leads to death. Biopsies of zinc-deficient individuals demonstrate focal villous shortening with mild crypt hyperplasia and a slight increase in mixed inflammatory cell infiltrates. Electron microscopy of Paneth cells demonstrates

TABLE 6.43	Brown Bowel Tinctorial Features
Stain	Color
None	Golden yellow
H&E	Blue
PAS	Magenta
Sudan black	Black
Fontana-Masson	Brown
Thiazine dye	Intense basophilia
Nile blue sulfate	Blue
Ziehl-Nielson (AFB)	Pink

AFB, acid-fast bacillus; H&E, hematoxylin and eosin; PAS, periodic acid–Schiff.

TABLE 6.44	Brown Bowel Syndrome Versus Melanosis Coli	
Brown Bowel	Syndrome	Melanosis
Location	Small bowel in smooth muscle cells	Macrophages
Associations	Cystic fibrosis, biliary atresia, vitamin E deficiency, hypoalbuminemia	Cathartic abuse
Staining reactions		
PAS	++++	++++
Giemsa	+++	+++
Alcian blue	−	−
Methenamine silver	++++	++++
Acid-fast	++	+−
Fontana	++++	++++
Prussian blue	−	−
Oil red 0	+	−

PAS, periodic acid–Schiff.

characteristic pleomorphic cytoplasmic inclusion bodies typical of acrodermatitis enteropathica. The ultrastructural abnormalities disappear on zinc therapy.

IMMUNODEFICIENCY DISEASES

Patients with immunodeficiency syndromes often present with chronic diarrhea, malabsorption, and other intestinal abnormalities, as well as with the effects of the immunodeficiency,

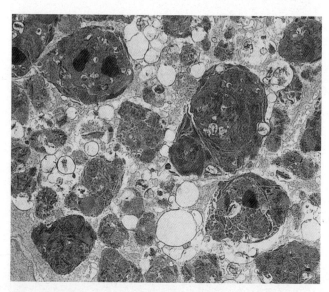

FIG. 6.214. Ultrastructural features of brown bowel disease. Numerous intralysosomal inclusions containing cellular membranes and osmiophilic debris are present.

TABLE 6.45 **Classification of Immunodeficiency Diseases**

Predominantly antibody defects (see Table 6.46)
Predominantly defects of cell-mediated immunity
    Severe combined immunodeficiency
    Chronic mucocutaneous candidiasis
    Nezelof syndrome
    DiGeorge syndrome
    Wiskott-Aldrich syndrome
Immunodeficiency associated with other disorders
    Chronic granulomatous diseases
    Ataxia-telangiectasia
    Transcobalamin II deficiency
    Bare lymphocyte syndrome
    Leukocyte adhesion deficiency
    AIDS

particularly infections. The immunodeficiency syndromes fall into primary and secondary (or acquired) forms (Table 6.45). Primary immunodeficiencies fall into several categories: Those primarily associated with failure to produce antibodies (Table 6.46), those associated with lymphocyte abnormalities, or those involving neutrophils.

Antibody Deficiency Disorders

Selective IgA Deficiency

Selective IgA deficiency is the most common immunodeficiency in Caucasians, being present in about 1 of 600 in the general population as assessed by blood donor screening (588). The incidence varies depending on the population being studied. Published figures range from 1 in 400 in Finland to 1 in 1,500 in Japan (589). IgA deficiency is 10 to 15 times more common in patients with celiac disease than in the general population.

In selective IgA deficiency, IgA, the major mucosal immunoglobulin, is not produced. Patients exhibit an isolated absence or near absence (i.e., <0.10 g/L [<10 mg/dL]) of serum and secretory IgA. In most cases, the cause of the immunodeficiency is unknown. The disease may be congenital or induced by viral infections, leukopenia, and drugs. Unusual cases result from deletion of an IgA gene on chromosome 14 (590). Selective IgA deficiency associates with extended HLA haplotypes that include either a C4A null allele (C4AQ0), 21-hydroxylase gene deletions in the HLA class III region, or rare class IIIC gene haplotypes (591), especially in Caucasians. These haplotypes are rare in Blacks and Asians.

Most patients have defective B-cell maturation with abnormal terminal differentiation of membrane IgA-positive B cells into IgA-secreting plasma cells. A smaller percentage of individuals have a defect in immune regulation of a putative suppressor T cell that selectively inhibits IgA production (592).

Many patients lack clinical abnormalities due to a compensatory increase in IgM. Other patients, especially if deficient in IgG subclasses, present with sinopulmonary disease, diarrhea, malabsorption, autoimmune disease, or bacterial infections, including GI infections (593). Patients with IgA deficiency also frequently have antibodies directed against cow's milk and ruminant serum proteins, immunoglobulins, thyroglobulin, and collagen. Diseases associated with IgA deficiency are listed in Table 6.47.

Biopsies in IgA-deficient patients may appear completely normal with a seemingly full complement of lymphocytes and plasma cells in the lamina propria, especially in adults. Immunohistochemical analysis for immunoglobulins demonstrates that the lamina propria plasma cells produce IgM and IgG but not IgA. Patients may also have evidence of coexisting celiac disease or bacterial infections (Fig. 6.215). Rarely, patients with a selective IgA deficiency will present with a completely flat mucosa (Fig. 6.216) in the

TABLE 6.46 **Antibody Deficiency States**

X-linked infantile agammaglobulinemia
X-linked hypogammaglobulinemia with growth hormone deficiency
Transcobalamin II deficiency and hypogammaglobulinemia
Immunodeficiency with thymoma
Immunodeficiency after a hereditary defective response to Epstein-Barr virus
Common variable immunodeficiency
Immunoglobulin deficiency with normal or increased levels of IgM and IgD
Selective IgA deficiency
Selective IgM deficiency
Selective deficiency of other immunoglobulin isotypes
Light chain deficiency
Immunodeficiency caused by hypercatabolism of immunoglobulin molecules
Immunodeficiency caused by excessive loss of immunoglobulins and lymphocytes

TABLE 6.47 **Conditions Associated with IgA Deficiency**

Pernicious anemia
Addison disease
Thyroiditis
Hemolytic anemia
Idiopathic thrombocytopenic purpura
Systemic lupus erythematosus
Rheumatoid arthritis
Primary biliary cirrhosis
Chronic active hepatitis
Celiac disease
Crohn disease
Nodular lymphoid hyperplasia
Disaccharide deficiency
Antibodies to cow's milk protein

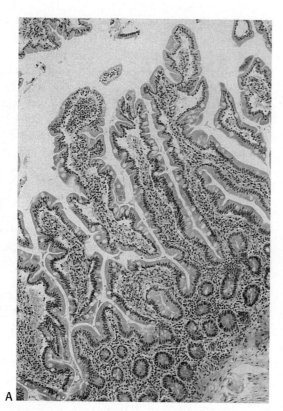
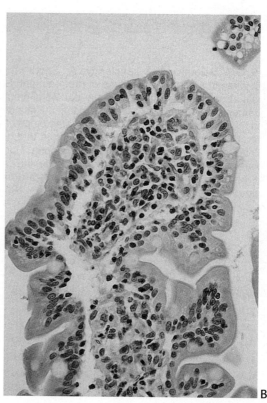

FIG. 6.215. IgA deficiency combined with celiac disease. **A:** There is an essentially normal architecture with a mild increase in the lamina propria infiltrate. **B:** Higher magnification showing intraepithelial lymphocytes. Immunostaining demonstrated a complete absence of IgA-producing plasma cells and the intraepithelial lymphocytes suggested a diagnosis of latent sprue. The patient was put on a gluten-free diet and responded dramatically.

absence of bacterial overgrowth or *Giardia.* Such patients may die from severe malabsorption (594).

Common Variable Immunodeficiency

Common variable immunodeficiency (CVI) is a heterogeneous group of immunoglobulin deficiencies that share the following: (a) low levels of most immunoglobulin isotypes, (b) inability to form antibodies to antigens, (c) absence of a gross defect in cell-mediated immunity, and (d) presence of recurrent bacterial infections. Patients suffer from the effects of their defective antibody production with decreased serum IgG in combination with decreases in serum IgA and IgM (595). Other patients exhibit a different type of CVI that predominantly manifests as a T-cell deficiency and the antibody deficiency is less prominent. The two clinical syndromes tend to be mutually exclusive (595).

CVI is the second most common primary immunodeficiency, following isolated IgA deficiency. It affects 6 to 12 per 1 million live births. The disease is usually sporadic, but familial clustering associated with an autosomal dominant mode of transmission does occur in 20% of patients (596). Haplotype analysis and linkage studies indicate that the HLA-DQ/DR locus is the major site of involvement (597). An association between CVI and homozygosity for genes encoding HLA class II molecules, especially HLA-DQ, has been reported (598). In some patients, there is an association with the TNF-α+488 A allele (599). In one recent study, 4 of 32 patients with adult-onset CVI demonstrated a homozygous deletion of the *ICOS* gene, an inducible costimulator found on activated T cells (600).

The major defect in CVI is a failure of B-cell differentiation with impaired secretion of immunoglobulins, but it is not clear whether this is due to a primary B-cell defect or abnormalities in T cells. B cells in CVI are immature, and show impaired upregulation of markers of activation (601). In some patients, a defect in IgV gene somatic hypermutation is present, an abnormality that would result in production of immunoglobulins with reduced or absent antigen affinities (602). In addition to B-cell abnormalities, CVI patients also show abnormalities in T-cell function. CVI patients exhibit decreased T-cell proliferation and activation, defective antigen-driven responses, and reduced production of cytokines (603).

CVI may clinically resemble X-linked agammaglobulinemia (Fig. 6.217). The major difference is that the patients usually have a later age of onset and somewhat less severe infections. Also, the disorder is almost equally distributed between sexes, contrasting with X-linked agammaglobulinemia, which almost invariably affects boys. Chronic and recurrent sinopulmonary infections are the hallmark of the

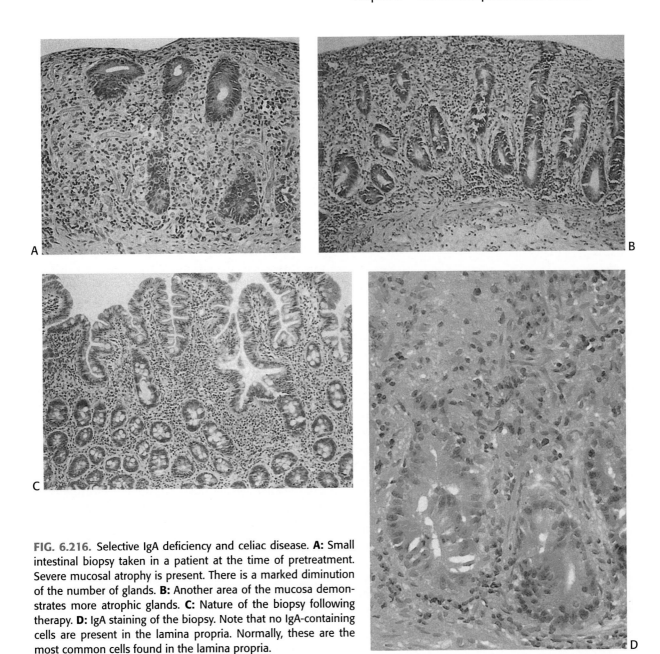

FIG. 6.216. Selective IgA deficiency and celiac disease. **A:** Small intestinal biopsy taken in a patient at the time of pretreatment. Severe mucosal atrophy is present. There is a marked diminution of the number of glands. **B:** Another area of the mucosa demonstrates more atrophic glands. **C:** Nature of the biopsy following therapy. **D:** IgA staining of the biopsy. Note that no IgA-containing cells are present in the lamina propria. Normally, these are the most common cells found in the lamina propria.

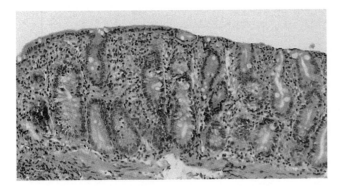

FIG. 6.217. Agammaglobulinemia. The epithelium often becomes flattened and shares features with other causes of villous atrophy.

disease (604). Twenty to thirty percent of patients have mild to moderate malabsorption frequently due to coexisting *Giardia* infections. The enteropathy may also be accompanied by a deficiency in jejunal brush border enzymes (605). Patients with accompanying T-cell abnormalities have fungal or protozoal infections sometimes causing persistent infections, such as with strongyloides. Approximately 33% to 50% of patients have achlorhydria due to a coexisting chronic atrophic gastritis. Patients develop a pernicious anemialike syndrome with intrinsic factor deficiency, gastric atrophy, loss of parietal cells, and low vitamin B_{12} levels. However, unlike classic pernicious anemia, the disease develops at an earlier age, the gastric mucosa lacks a plasma cell infiltrate, and antibodies to parietal cells or intrinsic factor are absent. Coexisting diseases are listed in Table 6.48 (606). Adults are

TABLE 6.48   Disorders Associated with Common Variable Immunodeficiency

Recurrent infections
    Respiratory and sinonasal
    Gastrointestinal
Malabsorption with steatorrhea and villous atrophy
Chronic diarrhea
Cholecystitis
Cholangitis
Pernicious anemia
Protein-losing enteropathy
Giardia infection
Atrophic gastritis
Gastric cancer
Lymphomas
Bronchiectasis

much more likely to develop complications, including lymphomas and small and large intestinal carcinomas. Lactose and gluten intolerance may result from mucosal inflammation and increased mucosal permeability.

The mucosal appearance varies from normal to severe villous atrophy resembling celiac disease (607). Crypt distortion and crypt destruction can be present. Plasma cells are absent. There may also be an intraepithelial lymphocytosis. In contrast to celiac disease, there is only a modest mononuclear cell infiltrate in the lamina propria. Lymphoid aggregates in the lamina propria and between epithelial cells primarily contain T cells rather than immature B cells. Single-cell necrosis (apoptosis) is increased in the crypt bases (608). Biopsies often show an enteritis. Plasma cells are absent. A granulomatous enteropathy is another manifestation of CVI, perhaps due to an underlying infection. Nodular lymphoid hyperplasia consisting of hyperplastic lymphoid follicles with immature B cells may be found throughout the GI tract. Various infections may stimulate the lymphoid hyperplasia.

Cellular and Combined Immunodeficiency Disorders

Nezelof Syndrome

Nezelof syndrome is characterized by lymphopenia, diminished lymphoid tissue, an abnormal thymus, and normal or increased serum immunoglobulin levels. Infants present with recurrent or chronic pulmonary infections, failure to thrive, oral or cutaneous candidiasis, chronic diarrhea, and recurrent infections. Other findings include neutropenia and eosinophilia. Selective IgA deficiency and markedly elevated IgE and IgD levels affect some patients. The disease is usually inherited as an autosomal recessive disorder, but some children exhibit an X-linked mode of inheritance (604). Peripheral lymphoid tissues, including those in the GI tract, appear hypoplastic and demonstrate paracortical lymphocyte depletion. Small intestinal biopsies may show villous

atrophy with increased numbers of plasma cells and neutrophils in the lamina propria. Peyer patches are absent.

Severe Combined Immunodeficiency Disease

The severe combined immunodeficiency disease (SCID) syndromes are characterized by a congenital absence of all adaptive immune functions and by great diversity in the genetic, enzymatic, hematologic, and immunologic features (604). There are multiple variants of SCID, but all of them show a block in T-cell differentiation, which usually requires urgent therapy with allogeneic hematopoietic stem cell transplantation to provide the missing T-cell progenitors. Nine different molecular defects are known to cause SCID as summarized in reference 609. SCID usually is inherited as either an X-linked or an autosomal recessive defect. GI changes include esophageal atresia, imperforate anus, chronic candidiasis, and watery diarrhea. Patients with these disorders have the most severe form of the recognized immune deficiencies.

In one form of SCID, patients lack T cells but have normal numbers of B cells. It associates with a novel defect in the CD 3 gene that results in an early arrest in T-cell development with a nearly complete absence of mature T cells and a complete lack of γ/δ T cells (610). Patients lack T-cell and B-cell immunity and have an increased incidence of viral, fungal, protozoal, and bacterial infections. As a result, children may exhibit serious GI manifestations, including chronic diarrhea, malabsorption, and infections. GI infections result from *Giardia, Salmonella,* enteropathic *E. coli,* rotavirus, candidiasis, coccidiosis, aspergillosis, and cryptosporidiosis. Histologically, Peyer patches are absent or extremely underdeveloped. Biopsies show a partial reduction in intraepithelial T lymphocytes, partial villous atrophy, and numerous vacuolated PAS-positive macrophages in the lamina propria. The intestinal lamina propria is devoid of lymphocytes and plasma cells.

Patients undergoing bone marrow transplantation lack the ability to reject foreign tissue and are therefore at risk for developing GVHD. Some patients develop lactose intolerance. Today complications are rare because most patients receive bone marrow transplants.

Chronic Granulomatous Disease

Chronic granulomatous disease (CGD) is a rare, predominantly male disease with either an X-linked or autosomal recessive inheritance pattern. The neutrophils of patients with X-linked CGD have defective neutrophil cytochrome B, whereas the autosomal recessive form involves abnormalities in the NADPH oxidase system. Leukocytes from these patients fail to show normal oxygen consumption, direct oxidation of glucose, or hydrogen peroxide formation. GI involvement may cause diarrhea, steatorrhea, vitamin B_{12} malabsorption, or intestinal obstruction due to the presence of granulomas. Neutrophils from patients with CGD are defective in their ability to kill catalase-positive bacteria and some fungi such as *Candida* and *Aspergillus,* despite their normal ability to phagocytose the organisms. As a result, patients are prone to severe infections and multiple abscesses. The intestinal wall may contain granulomas, fistulae, fissures, and abscesses, producing a disease resembling Crohn disease. The lamina propria may contain characteristic darkish brown, lipid-filled histiocytes, giant cells, and granulomas (611). These changes affect both the small and large intestines.

SYSTEMIC MASTOCYTOSIS

Systemic mastocytosis is characterized by mast cell proliferation in skin, bones, lymph nodes, and parenchymal organs. Patients usually present with classic dermatologic findings of urticaria pigmentosa. Typical symptoms include pruritus, flushing, tachycardia, asthma, and headache, all thought to result from the release of histamine from the mast cells (612). Fifty to eighty percent of patients have GI symptoms, including peptic ulcers, malabsorption, steatorrhea, nausea, vomiting, copious watery diarrhea, and abdominal pain (613). The clinical features may mimic inflammatory bowel disease. These features occur secondary to gastric hypersecretion or result from the release of histamine and prostaglandins from mast cells. Symptoms are often induced by alcohol consumption. The hyperhistaminemia produces gastric hypersecretion, which can be as marked as that seen in Zollinger-Ellison syndrome (613). Gastric acid levels correlate with the degree of histaminemia and with the presence of acid peptic disease, including peptic duodenitis (613). Mast cell–mediated events include increased intestinal permeability and altered smooth muscle function. Malabsorption occurs secondary to mucosal infiltration.

Histologic changes include mucosal villous atrophy, marked submucosal edema, and clumps of mast cell infiltrates in the lamina propria (Fig. 6.218). Large numbers of mast cells infiltrate the lamina propria, muscularis mucosae,

and submucosa, with aggregates of mast cells within the gland lumens and evidence of glandular destruction. Prominent mast cell degranulation is also present. Eosinophils may also be seen. Toluidine blue or Giemsa stains highlight the presence of the mast cells. Mast cell lesions also stain with antibodies to tryptase and CD68. Neoplastic mast cells have aberrant expression of CD2 and CD25 and have a codon 816 c-kit mutation (614).

GRAFT VERSUS HOST DISEASE

GVHD is an immunologic disorder that results in severe gastrointestinal damage. It represents the response of immunocompetent donor cells to the histocompatibility antigens of the recipient. GVHD follows bone marrow or organ transplantation. Less commonly, it complicates maternal–fetal cell transfer in immunodeficient children (615) or transfusion of nonirradiated cells and blood products (616). GVHD also associates with malignant thymoma.

Basic requirements for GVHD reactions to occur include the following: (a) the graft must contain immunocompetent cells, (b) the host must be sufficiently genetically different from the graft to be perceived as antigenically foreign, and (c) the host must be unable to reject the graft (617). These conditions allow engrafted cells to react to the host through immunologically mediated processes. The incidence of GVHD ranges from <10% to >80%, depending on the degree of incompatibility, the number of T cells in the graft, patient age, and the nature of the immunosuppressive regimen (617). It should be remembered that GVHD may occur even in fully matched MHC donors and recipients due to incompatibilities in minor histocompatibility antigens. The incidence of GVHD is possibly higher in blacks than in other individuals.

CD8+, CD3+, and TiA1+ cytotoxic T cells mediate epithelial cell death in GVHD (619). CD8 cells recognize class II MHC-restricted antigens, producing the lymphokines that lead to the development of the enteropathy associated with

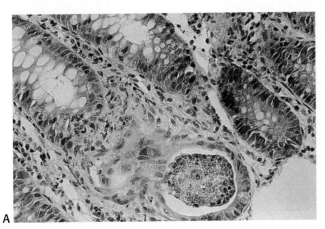
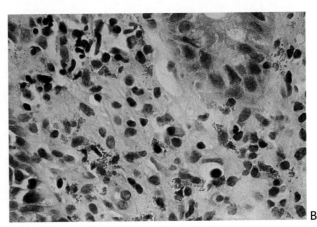

FIG. 6.218. Macrocytosis. **A:** High magnification of an intraluminal collection of mast cells. **B:** High magnification showing the presence of large numbers of degranulating lamina propria mast cells.

GVHD (620). Apoptosis may occur through the Fas/Fas ligand pathway (621).

Acute GVHD occurs within days (7 to 100) in recipients who are not HLA matched or in patients without any prophylaxis. Rarely, acute GVHD occurs later than 100 days posttransplant (618). It is characterized by epithelial cell death mainly in the gastrointestinal tract, liver, and skin, whereas chronic GVHD associates with fibrosis of these and other organs. Clinical features range from mild to intractable diarrhea, malabsorption, abdominal pain, protein-losing enteropathy, and severe malnutrition.

Chronic GVHD is less common than acute GVHD and occurs more than 100 days following transplantation either as an extension of acute GVHD or following a quiescent disease-free interval. It develops up to 400 days following transplantation (615). Fifteen to forty percent of long-term survivors suffer from chronic GVHD. It may result from long-living lymphocytes of donor origin that have become sensitized to unknown antigens, probably minor histocompatibility antigens of the host (622).

The principal target organs of GVHD include skin, GI tract, biliary tree, bone marrow, and lymphoid tissues. These organs have high cell turnover rates and may continually express differentiation antigens, resulting in increased immune surveillance. Alternatively, cells in these organs may harbor latent viruses that could act as targets for donor immune surveillance.

The typical clinical presentation of acute GVHD includes skin rashes, nausea, anorexia, profuse watery diarrhea, intestinal hemorrhage, ileus, crampy abdominal pain, abdominal tenderness, paralytic ileus, malabsorption, and jaundice. The intestine is involved in 70% of cases (623). Intestinal infections account for 13% and acute GVHD for 48% of diarrheal processes in bone marrow transplant

patients. The most common infections are astrovirus, *C. difficile*, adenovirus, and CMV. The degree of diarrhea does not always correspond to the severity of the intestinal inflammation. The severity of intestinal disease varies from grade I to grade IV (Table 6.49). The mortality of moderate to severe acute GVHD is as high as 50%.

Mucosal biopsy provides a sensitive test for detecting GVHD in the intestine. However, the biopsy should not be taken during the first 3 weeks of immunosuppressive therapy because all patients will show some degree of inflammation in the immediate posttransplant period. The lesions of acute GVHD range from necrosis of individual crypt cells to total mucosal loss, with the most severe disease affecting the ileum (Fig. 6.219; Table 6.50). Apoptotic bodies are the sine qua

TABLE 6.49 Clinical Grading of Acute Graft Versus Host Disease

Grade	Organ Involvement
I	Stage I to stage II skin rash; no gut involvement; no liver involvement; no decrease in clinical performance
II	Stage II to stage III skin rash; stage I gut involvement or stage I liver involvement or both; mild decrease in clinical performance
III	Stage II to stage III skin rash; stage II to stage III gut involvement or stage II to stage IV liver involvement or both; marked decrease in clinical performance
IV	Similar to grade III with stage II to stage IV organ involvement and extreme decrease in clinical performance

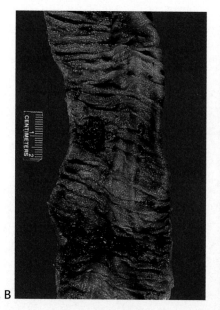
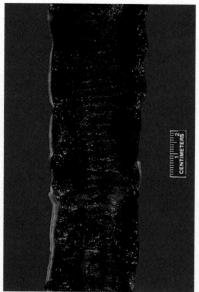
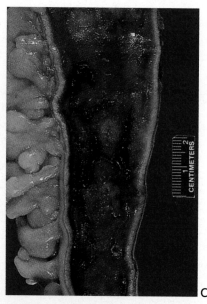

FIG. 6.219. Graft versus host disease. A through C show increasing degrees of severity. **A:** Areas of intestinal ulceration are present in a moderately affected patient. **B:** More diffuse ulceration and marked erythema. **C:** The bowel has been converted to a fibrotic, rigid tube with little residual intervening mucosa.

TABLE 6.50 Histologic Lesions of Graft Versus Host Disease

Grade	Histology
1	Mild necrosis of individual crypts
2	Crypt abscesses and crypt cell flattening
3	Dropout of many crypts
4	Flat mucosa

TABLE 6.51 Situations Associated with Increased Apoptosis

Graft vs. host disease
Rejection
Chemotherapy
Radiation therapy
Zinc deficiency
Fasting
Inflammatory bowel disease
AIDS enteropathy
Thymoma
Certain drugs
Viral infections
Cell-mediated immune reactions
Autoimmune enterocolitis

non of the diagnosis (Fig. 6.220). However, it is important to remember that increased apoptoses or apoptoses located at the crypt bases occur in other settings as well (Table 6.51). These collect at the crypt bases. The necrotic foci in cellular lacunae are sometimes referred to as "popcorn lesions." As the lesions evolve, an entire crypt can drop out of the mucosa, creating single crypt loss. The mucosal architecture is progressively lost with ulceration, mucosal denudation, and submucosal edema. Ulcer healing leads to fibrosis and stricture formation. Ulcers may become infected, particularly by fungi. In chronic GVHD, one sees segmental lamina propria fibrosis and submucosal fibrosis extending to the serosa. These lesions occur throughout the entire length of the GI tract extending from the esophagus to the colon. Occasional patients pass ropy, tan material resembling strands of sloughed mucosal tissue, known as mucosal casts, per rectum (Fig. 6.221). The composition of the material is rarely clear-cut. It usually contains fibrin, PMNs, cellular debris, bacteria, or fungi, and very little identifiable tissue. One confirms the presence of free intestinal epithelium by immunostaining with cytokeratins (624).

SMALL INTESTINAL LESIONS RESEMBLING GRAFT VERSUS HOST DISEASE

Changes similar to those found in GVHD sometimes occur in immunosuppressed or immunodeficient patients, without transplants or transfusions. The lesion affects any portion of the GI tract but it most often involves the intestines. Patients have various associated diseases including lymphoma, leukemia, combined immune deficiency, severe T-cell deficiency, and Hodgkin disease (625,626). The signs and symptoms resemble those developing following bone marrow transplantation but they occur more rapidly and tend to be associated with a higher fatality rate. A novel T-lymphocyte population has been identified in patients with combined immunodeficiency and features of GVHD (627).

Histologically, patients demonstrate subtotal villous atrophy during a period of diarrhea. A marked mixed inflammatory infiltrate develops associated with an unusually high number of neutrophils in the lamina propria. The crypt epithelium shows single-cell necrosis (apoptosis) and numerous intraepithelial neutrophils with crypt abscesses. Lymphoid nodules are also present in the lamina propria. Mast cells may be seen. The vast majority of the cells within the lymphoid nodules manifest the T-cell phenotype and are UCHLI+. A few UCHL1+ cells are also found within the crypt epithelium. Rare B cells are present; plasma cells are absent. Patients, especially those with combined immunodeficiency, show this B-cell absence.

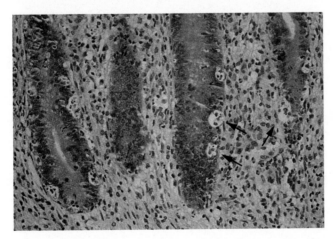

FIG. 6.220. Apoptosis in graft versus host disease. Note the presence of prominent apoptotic bodies in the bases of the crypts (*arrows*).

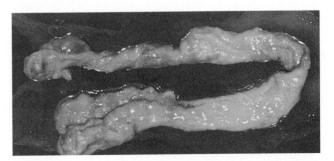

FIG. 6.221. Mucosal cast. Gross photograph of a ropy structure shed from the intestines of a transplant patient. This represented a mucosal cast.

DISEASES ASSOCIATED WITH ABNORMAL DEPOSITS IN THE TISSUES

Hemochromatosis

Hereditary hemochromatosis (HH), an autosomal recessive disease, causes 1 in 7,000 hospital deaths and 1 in 20,000 annual hospital admissions (628). When the disease presents in adults, the patients are usually homozygous for a missense mutation (C282Y) in the *HFE* gene (629). Rare patients with mutations in the gene encoding the *transferrin receptor 2* (TfR2) also present with a clinical phenotype that is similar to that seen in patients with *HFE* mutations. The disease in adults tends to be milder than that seen in children. Most juvenile cases have been mapped to chromosome 1q where the gene *hemojuvelin (HJV)*, previously called *HFE2*, is located. Some children with HH may have mutations in the HAMP gene, which encodes hepcidin, a peptide that plays a key role in iron absorption (630).

Because there is no efficient pathway for iron excretion from the body, it is generally accepted that the main underlying pathophysiology of hereditary hemochromatosis is the excessive absorption of dietary iron in the face of adequate raised body iron stores. However, the mechanism underlying the enhanced iron uptake in HH remains poorly defined and complex, with many biochemical defects being present as summarized in reference 630.

Iron deposits in many organs including the gut (Fig. 6.222), resulting in structural and functional abnormalities. Histologically, one sees mucosal iron deposits throughout the lamina propria in the macrophages, in the epithelium (Fig. 6.222), and in a perivascular distribution.

Hemosiderosis

Hemosiderosis usually follows oral or parenteral iron administration or multiple transfusions. The lamina propria of the villi contains macrophages filled with hemosiderin (Fig. 6.223). The epithelial cells lack iron, contrasting with primary hemochromatosis.

Pseudomelanosis

The presence of spotty brownish or blackish pigmentation in the duodenal mucosa seen at the time of endoscopy is termed *duodenal melanosis* or *pseudomelanosis* (631). Pigmentation is usually maximal in the second part of the duodenum and the duodenal bulb is affected to a lesser extent. The lesion affects AIDS patients and individuals on maintenance hemodialysis. Most patients receive oral iron supplementation. Patients may present with upper abdominal discomfort and anemia, which is the usual reason for the endoscopy. Mucosal pigmentation probably does not cause the symptoms. The macrophages acquire melanin, pseudomelanin, and iron. It is postulated that duodenal pseudomelanosis begins with mucosal iron deposition (631). However, sulfur becomes incorporated into the granules, altering their staining characteristics so that they

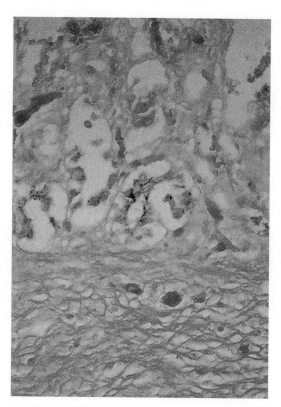

FIG. 6.222. Small bowel in a patient with hemochromatosis (autopsy). An iron stain has been performed and demonstrates the presence of iron within the epithelium. It appears as bluish staining.

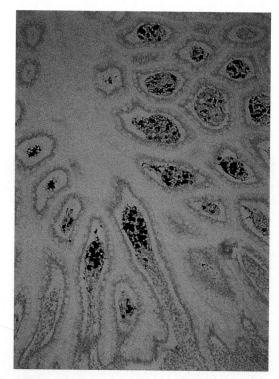

FIG. 6.223. Intestinal hemosiderosis. Iron stain shows the presence of numerous iron-filled intestinal lamina propria macrophages.

TABLE 6.52 Types of Gastrointestinal Amyloid

Disease	Protein
Multiple myeloma and other monoclonal B-cell and plasma cell proliferations	Immunoglobulin light chain (AL)
Secondary amyloidosis associated with chronic disease	Serum amyloid-associated protein (AA)
Hereditary amyloidosis	Mutated transthyretin, prealbumin (AF)
Chronic renal disease	β_2-microglobulin
"Senile" amyloidosis	Normal transthyretin

TABLE 6.53 Forms of Amyloidosis

Primary amyloidosis: Systemic disease associated with plasma cell dyscrasia (deposits in heart, kidney, gut, liver, and spleen), especially around blood vessels and sometimes between muscle fibers (AL amyloid)
Secondary amyloidosis: Systemic chronic disease; amyloid deposits in blood vessels and in the mucosa (AA amyloid)
Hereditary familial amyloidosis: Perireticular deposition throughout muscle fibers and in neural plexuses; single organ amyloid deposition (AF amyloid)

react positively with both iron stains and the Fontana-Masson stain. These pigments include iron, sulfur, and other metallic substances.

Amyloidosis

The gastrointestinal tract is a frequent site of amyloid deposition in patients with systemic or isolated amyloidosis. The term *amyloidosis* includes heterogeneous disorders characterized by extracellular acellular hyaline deposits, known as amyloid. Amyloid consists of β-pleated polypeptides, the components of which vary (Table 6.52). The disease may be localized or systemic, affecting any organ or tissue. All types of amyloidosis (Table 6.53) affect the GI tract (632–634). If one is investigating a patient for amyloidosis, the best places to biopsy are the stomach and the rectum, since these are more likely to be involved than the small intestine.

GI amyloidosis remains asymptomatic or it may present with malabsorption, severe diarrhea, weight loss, abdominal pain, protein-losing enteropathy, ischemia, perforation, or a spectrum of motility disorders (634). Intestinal involve-

ment, in the absence of a chronic inflammatory disease and in the absence of a family history, is most consistent with primary (AL) amyloidosis (Table 6.52). Patients with amyloidosis often have multiple myeloma, plasmacytomas, or Waldenstrom macroglobulinemia.

Amyloid A (AA) produces a coarse mucosal pattern with innumerable fine granular elevations that reflect expansion of the lamina propria by amyloid deposits. Polypoid protrusions and fold thickening occur only in light chain protein, correlating with the presence of massive amyloid deposits in the muscularis mucosae and submucosa. α_2-Microglobulin produces marked delays in transit time and dilation of large and small intestines due to extensive amyloid deposits in the muscularis propria (635).

Macroscopically, amyloidosis is not visible in its early stages, but in advanced disease the small bowel becomes thickened and waxy in appearance. It slowly converts to a rigid tube with walls measuring up to 1 cm in thickness (Fig. 6.224). Rarely, large amyloid deposits, often referred to as tumoral amyloid, cause masses and intestinal obstruction.

Regardless of the specific type of amyloidosis, almost all patients have the so-called linear pattern of distribution in which the amyloid deposits heavily in the submucosal vessels, muscle fibers (Fig. 6.225), and nerve trunks. A much rarer

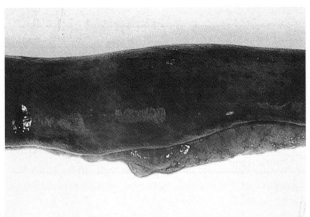
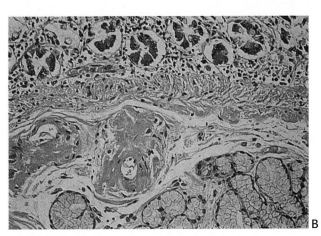

A   B

FIG. 6.224. Amyloidosis. A: Gross appearance of the bowel demonstrates a loss of the usual folds. The bowel is rigid and has lost its distensibility and motility. **B:** Histologic section of small bowel with amyloid as evidenced by the smudgy material in the area surrounding the submucosal blood vessels, as well as in the muscularis mucosae.

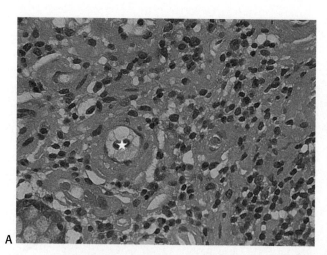
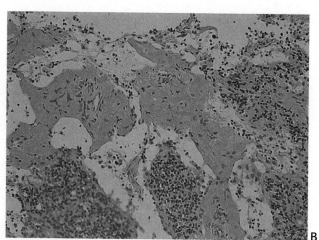

FIG. 6.225. Amyloidosis. **A:** Submucosal changes in amyloidosis. Note the prominent perivascular eosinophilic deposits (*star*). The surrounding tissues contain prominent eosinophils and mast cells. **B:** Submucosal amyloid deposits. They associate with intense mononuclear cell infiltrates.

type of amyloid deposition pattern is the so-called globular form of amyloid that complicates AA and AL amyloidosis (636,637). This form can result in the presence of multiple duodenal and jejunal polyps. Any unusual eosinophilic deposits with a homogenic quality potentially obliterating underlying structural features within the vasculature, muscularis mucosae, or lamina propria should raise the possibility of the diagnosis of amyloid. This would then prompt the use of specialized stains, such as Congo red, coupled with examination with polarizing microscopy to look for its presence. Perivascular deposits (Fig. 6.225) may cause patchy ischemia, infarction, perforation, or bleeding. Because amyloid is usually first detected in submucosal blood vessels, superficial small intestinal biopsies will fail to detect its presence. Lamina propria or submucosal deposits cause malabsorption. The mucosa only becomes infiltrated in cases with massive amyloid deposits, and patients may exhibit partial villous atrophy.

CYSTIC FIBROSIS

Cystic fibrosis (CF) is an autosomal recessive disorder that affects 1 in 100,000 to 200,000 live births. CF results from mutations in the gene encoding the cystic fibrosis transmembrane conductance regulator (CFTR). More than 350 different point mutations in the gene are described (638). These different mutations produce a disease spectrum ranging from malnutrition, chronic bronchitis, asthma, and infertility to fatal pulmonary disease. CFTR is the receptor for *S. typhi* and it is conceivable that heterozygosity of the CFTR allele is selected for in certain populations because it protects against the development of typhoid (639).

CF patients develop a well-defined epithelial abnormality because the mutant protein fails to perform its normal function. The CFTR mutation results in a chloride transport defect with relative chloride impermeability in ductal epithelium and inhibited sodium chloride reabsorption resulting in hypertonic secretions. When secretion falls below a critical minimum, thick mucus develops, blocking the ducts and leading to glandular swelling, cystic degeneration, and atrophy (640). The small intestinal mucosa shows a relatively high expression level of CFTR mRNA with a decreasing gradient of expression along the crypt-to-tip axis. Cells in Brunner glands also express high CFTR levels.

CF has traditionally been diagnosed in the presence of chronic pulmonary disease, pancreatic exocrine insufficiency, and an abnormal sweat test. The clinical features are dominated by respiratory tract involvement. GI involvement affects most patients. The earliest symptom is intrauterine intestinal obstruction due to meconium ileus, which leads to perforation, meconium pseudocysts, meconium peritonitis, intestinal atresia, volvulus, and intussusception. These complications affect 50% of infants with meconium ileus (641). Meconium ileus is seldom seen in the absence of CF. The ileus results from inspissated, protein-rich meconium in the terminal ileum. Uncomplicated meconium ileus demonstrates a narrow terminal ileum with a beaded appearance. The ileal wall appears hypertrophic and becomes distended with extremely sticky, dark green pellets of protein-rich meconium and mucus (Fig. 6.226).

Older patients experience severe anorexia, fecal impaction, rectal prolapse, pneumatosis, bleeding, watery stools, and intussusception (641). Intussusception, usually involving the ileocecal region, results from intestinal obstruction with a tenacious fecal bolus that acts as the lead point. Coexisting GI conditions are listed in Table 6.54. Many patients undergo pancreatic enzyme replacement, which causes colonic complications (see Chapter 13).

The histologic appearance of the mucosa is similar in CF whether or not ileus is present. The villi appear taller than normal (Fig. 6.227). Increased mucus production results in

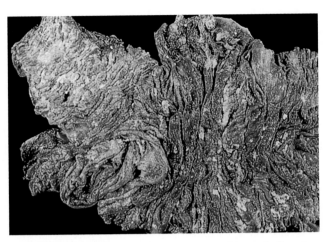

FIG. 6.226. Gross appearance of the bowel in cystic fibrosis.

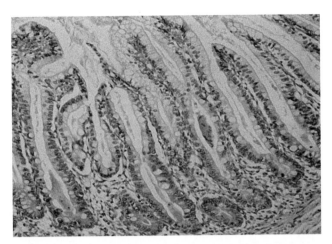

FIG. 6.227. Histologic features of cystic fibrosis. The villi appear elongated. The surface is covered by mucin and the intestinal crypts contain denser mucin accumulations.

enlarged goblet cells and an abundant layer of mucus attached to the luminal surface (Fig. 6.228). Although the goblet mucous cells are often larger than those seen in normal individuals, considerable overlap exists between normal individuals and patients with CF, so that distinguishing among them reliably is difficult at best. Small numbers of inflammatory cells infiltrate the lamina propria.

VASCULAR LESIONS

Vascular lesions include telangiectasias, malformations, dysplasias, and neoplastic proliferations. In this chapter, we will cover malformations and telangiectasias; neoplasms are covered in Chapter 19 and angiodysplasia is covered in Chapter 13.

Hemodialysis-associated Telangiectasias

Patients receiving long-term hemodialysis develop GI telangiectasias involving the stomach, small intestine, and colon (642). (*Telangiectasia* refers to the dilation of preexisting vessels, whereas *angiomatosis* refers to the formation of new vessel growth.) The telangiectatic areas appear small, flattened, and reddish with fernlike margins. The

lesions can be detected endoscopically or angiographically. Several factors predispose to the development of the telangiectasias. Chronic sodium and water overload may cause venous hypertension, thereby dilating submucosal veins. Additionally, dialysis patients receive long-term therapy with aluminum hydroxide gel to control hyperphosphatemia. This compound causes constipation, bowel distention, and cutaneous telangiectasias (642). Hemodialysis

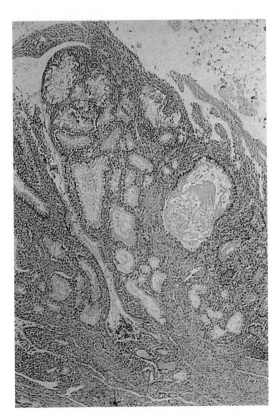

FIG. 6.228. Cystic fibrosis. Microscopic picture demonstrating duodenitis and plump hypertrophic goblet cells.

TABLE 6.54	Conditions Associated with Cystic Fibrosis

Cow's milk intolerance
Celiac disease
Giardiasis
Crohn disease
Rectal prolapse
Rectal stenosis
Pneumatosis intestinalis
Fibrosing colonopathy

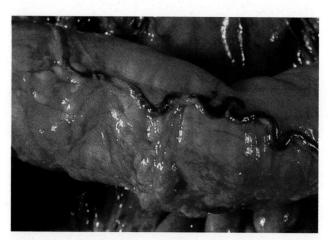

FIG. 6.229. Intestinal varices. Eviscerated organs in a patient with chronic liver disease and chronic heart disease.

patients also develop accelerated atherosclerosis, which may predispose the GI vasculature to develop abnormalities in a manner analogous to the angiodysplasia of the elderly (see Chapter 13).

Varices

Varices occur anywhere in the small or large intestine (Fig. 6.229). They develop in the same settings as esophageal varices, but they are less common and less well known. Varices result from liver disease in approximately 90% of cases. The presence of adhesions, enterostomies, or previous injury (643,644) favors their formation, especially if portal hypertension is present. Intestinal varices may also have a familial basis (644).

Varices develop at sites of portosystemic anastomoses in portal hypertension. The prevalent coronary-azygous system favors the appearance of esophagogastric varices. The development of other areas of communication between the splenic and mesenteric circulation such as rectal, mucosal, umbilical, and periumbilical veins (348) is uncommon, but this sometimes occurs. Grossly, varices appear as discrete, large veins protruding into the lumen, or they may appear as multiple smaller venules occupying the lamina propria. It is unusual for vascular lesions to be biopsied due to fear of bleeding, but they may be resected if significant uncontrolled hemorrhage occurs in the patient. Histologically, vascular lesions resembling esophageal varices or portal gastropathy are present in the submucosa and mucosa.

Vascular Ectasia

Vascular ectasia resembling gastric antral vascular ectasia syndrome (see Chapter 4) may extend from the antrum into the duodenum and jejunum and possibly up to the gastric cardia. It associates with portal hypertension.

LYMPHATIC LESIONS

Lymphangiectasia

Intestinal lymphangiectasia is a rare congenital obstructive defect of the lymphatics primarily affecting children and young adults. It is characterized by protein-losing enteropathy, hypoproteinemia, edema, lymphocytopenia, malabsorption, and dilated lacteals. It is part of a generalized disorder of the lymphatic system. Patients also have chylothorax, chyluria, chylous ascites, or asymmetric lymphedema, singly or in combination, depending on the degree of hypoproteinemia (645). Associations of primary intestinal lymphangiectasia are listed in Table 6.55. Hypoplastic visceral lymphatics obstruct lymph flow, causing increased intestinal lymphatic pressure, thereby dilating lymphatic vessels throughout the small bowel and mesentery. Hypoproteinemia and steatorrhea develop secondary to rupture of the dilated lymphatic vessels with discharge of lymph into the bowel lumen. Loss of major plasma protein components leads to hypoproteinemic edema. Serum levels of albumin, immunoglobulins, and other proteins are decreased. Endoscopically, whitish swollen tips of the villi are fairly characteristic.

The intestinal lumen appears dilated and the valves of Kerckring are swollen and broader than normal due to the presence of the dilated lymphatics. The intestines become edematous with a dusky serosa covered by fibrinous exudates. Serosal lymphatics appear as dilated, yellowish nodules measuring <5 mm in diameter. Villi have enlarged bulblike tips imparting a white pebbly papillary appearance to the mucosal surface (Fig. 6.230). The lymphatic channels are dilated and lined by endothelium, contrasting with the changes seen in its mimics (Whipple disease, pneumatosis, and pseudolipomatosis). The reddish brown pigmentation, characteristic of brown bowel syndrome, is often present. Lymphangiectasia is usually a diffuse process, sometimes involving the colon (646). This contrasts with localized lesions such as lymphangiomas or lymphangitic cysts. The diffuse intestinal involvement precludes surgical intervention.

TABLE 6.55	**Primary Intestinal Lymphangiectasia: Associations**

Disease localized to intestinal lymphatics
    Familial
    Sporadic
Widespread lymphatic disorder
    Milroy disease—congenital hereditary lymphedema
    Widespread lymphatic abnormalities and hypoproteinemia
Association with other diseases
    Nephrotic syndrome
    Noonan syndrome
    DiGeorge syndrome
    Enamel hypoplasia
    Yellow nail syndrome
    Thymic hypoplasia

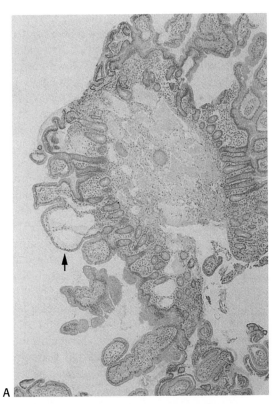
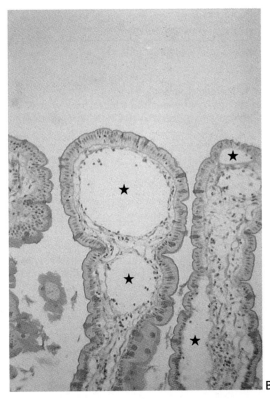

A   B

FIG. 6.230. Lymphangiectasia. **A:** Whole mount section demonstrating the presence of large bulbous villi containing dilated lacteals (*arrow*). **B:** Higher magnification demonstrating the presence of dilated lymphatic spaces (*stars*).

Histologically, lymphangiectatic lesions are microscopic lymphatic hamartomas that preferentially involve the small intestine, where the largest amount of lymphatic tissue is present. Since the lesions can be focal, they often require multiple biopsies to demonstrate their presence. The finding of distended lymphatics in a jejunal biopsy after an overnight fast is diagnostic. The villi appear shortened and broadened. Striking distention of lymphatic channels widens the villi, often causing apparent villous fusion (Fig. 6.230). The lymphatics contain foamy histiocytes; similar cells are seen in the yellowish nodules and lymph nodes. Mesenteric lymphatics are greatly thickened and contain a fragmented elastica interna with medial muscular hypertrophy. Focal acute inflammation may be present. Patients have a reduction in the number of intraepithelial lymphocytes. Lymphangiectasia may be localized to the lamina propria or generalized involving the mucosa, submucosa, serosa, and mesentery. Fat staining of frozen sections may demonstrate the lipid contents of the vacuoles.

Lymphatic Cysts

Single or multiple (Fig. 6.231) lymphatic cysts occur in up to 23% of the small intestines or their mesentery when they are examined at the time of autopsy. Mean patient age is 74, and in one study none was found in individuals younger than 55. The symptomless, submucosal nodules measure up to 1 cm

in diameter and contain thick, yellow, creamy fluid. Mesenteric cysts rarely rupture or cause volvulus or obstruction. The usually unilocular cysts are lined by flattened lymphatic endothelial cells and they contain eosinophilic proteinaceous material (Fig. 6.232).

Lymphatic Dilation

Lymphatic dilation complicates obstructions either of the GI tract or of the lymphatic drainage. The dilated lymphatics present as prominent whitish channels running alongside

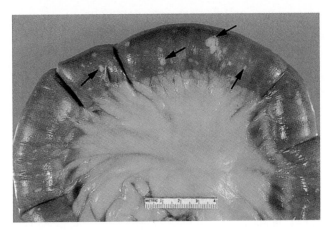

FIG. 6.231. Multiple lymphatic cysts (*arrows*).

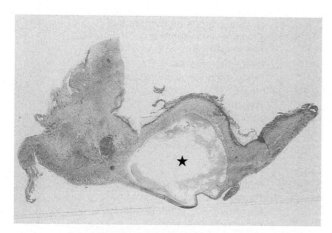

FIG. 6.232. Lymphatic cysts (*star*).

the vascular channels, as illustrated in Figure 6.233. Histologically, one sees diffuse dilation of the lymphatics, which usually is most severe on the serosal surface of the bowel (Fig. 6.234). Secondary causes of lymphangiectasia are listed in Table 6.56.

PNEUMATOSIS INTESTINALIS

Two forms of this relatively rare condition affect the intestines. The most common form affects patients with

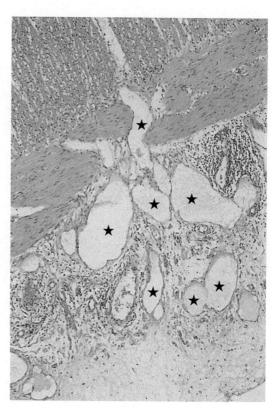

FIG. 6.234. Lymphatic dilation secondary to obstruction. The dilated lymphatic spaces are indicated by *stars.*

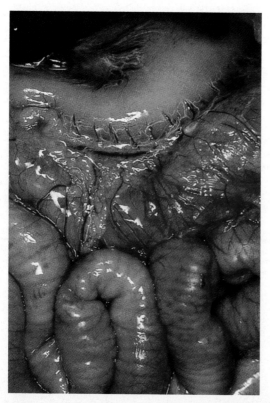

FIG. 6.233. Lymphangiectasia. The blood vessels and lymphatics in this specimen are markedly congested. The lymphatics appear as thin, white structures coursing along the blood vessels, which appear as congested, reddish structures.

obstructive pulmonary disease and results from air dissection through the spaces around the great vessels and their abdominal branches. Patients generally do not have specific intestinal complaints. The second form of the lesion results from the presence of gas-forming bacteria in the bowel wall due to prior mucosal ulceration and secondary bacterial invasion. The second form commonly affects infants suffering from fatal colitis or ileocolitis, or adults with ischemic bowel disease (647). This form often runs a fulminant course. Gas-filled cysts occupy the subserosa, submucosa, or both (Figs. 6.235 and 6.236).

Pneumatosis intestinalis (PI) involves the large and/or the small bowel and affects both infants and adults. The clinical features vary, depending on the underlying condition with which it is associated (647). Symptoms from the underlying disease may dominate the picture. Thus, in infants, coexisting necrotizing enterocolitis dominates the clinical and pathologic features. In adults, symptomatic patients develop diarrhea, flatulence, and excessive mucus in the stool. Other symptoms include constipation, rectal bleeding, passage of mucus via rectum, vague abdominal discomfort, abdominal pain, increased flatulence, urgency, malabsorption, and weight loss (647).

Partial bowel obstruction with luminal narrowing leads to symptoms similar to those seen in inflammatory bowel disease. Complications include volvulus, pneumoperitoneum, intestinal obstruction, intussusception, tension,

TABLE 6.56 **Secondary Causes of Intestinal Lymphangiectasia**

Lymph node obstruction
  Infections
  Filariasis
  Sarcoidosis
  Tuberculosis
  Lymphoma
  Carcinoma
Acute inflammation
  Systemic lupus erythematosus
  Eosinophilic enteritis
  Mesenteric paracolitis
  Infectious enteritis
  Inflammatory bowel disease
Fibrosis
  Radiation
Intraluminal precipitates
  Hypobetalipoproteinemia
Extraluminal compression
  Cancer
  Pregnancy
  Malrotation
  Retractile mesenteritis
  Malignancy in lymph nodes
Lymph node infiltration
  Infection
  Tuberculosis
  Whipple disease
  Inflammation
  Crohn disease
Increased thoracic duct pressure
  Constrictive pericarditis
  Right heart disease
  Cardiomyopathy
  Carcinoid syndrome
  Atrial septal defect
  Pulmonary stenosis
Behçet disease

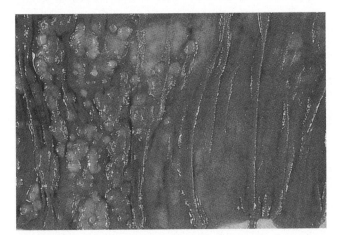

FIG. 6.235. Gross features of small intestinal pneumatosis intestinalis. The air-filled spaces are clustered on the left side of the photograph.

pneumoperitoneum, hemorrhage, and intestinal perforation (647).

There are two major theories to explain PI. The mechanical theory suggests that gas is forced into the bowel by one or more several routes: (a) pulmonary, (b) traumatic, (c) mucosal breaks, (d) anastomoses, (e) obstructive, (f) increased pressure, and (g) increased peristalsis. Obstructive pulmonary disease may associate with PI via coughing and pulmonary hyperinflation with alveolar rupture. Air then dissects along large vessels into the retroperitoneum and along the mesenteric vessels into the bowel serosa. Steroids may play a significant role in the development of PI because corticosteroids induce atrophy of Peyer patches. The resultant mucosal defects allow intraluminal air to dissect into the submucosa or subserosa.

The second theory explains another form of the disease. Microorganisms may enter the bowel wall through mucosal defects caused by a breakdown in the mucosal defenses. Once in the tissue, they proliferate and produce gas. Support for the presence of intestinal infections comes from the documented high levels of hydrogen in the intramural gas. Organisms implicated in PI include *C. perfringens, E. aerogenes,* and *E. coli* (647). Organisms are not usually detectable in the tissues or around the gas-filled cysts.

Usually, when one has the opportunity to study the gross features of PI it is because the PI complicates another disorder that requires resection. Therefore, the gross features are modified by the underlying disease. The gross appearance depends on the location of the cystic spaces and the underlying disease. PI presents as localized or diffuse cysts involving the mucosa, submucosa, and serosa (Fig. 6.237). Examination of the external surface of the bowel discloses the presence of subserosal cysts. They usually lie near the mesenteric border. Cysts often lie on loops of dilated bowel and range in size from a few millimeters to several centimeters. They can occur singly or in clusters, occasionally appearing like serosal bubbles. Predominantly submucosal cysts may not be appreciated on either the serosal or mucosal surfaces and the bowel may feel crepitant on palpation. They may also cause intraluminal mucosal bulging (Fig. 6.236). Cross sections demonstrate a honeycombed appearance of thin-walled, collapsed cysts ranging in size from 1 mm to several centimeters if the bowel is received fresh.

The cysts can be single or multiple, sessile or pedunculated. When the cysts are multiple, they do not intercommunicate. Histologically, PI begins as simple, generally unlined air-filled submucosal spaces (Fig. 6.237). Rarely, the cysts appear to be partially lined by an endothelial layer. Later, inflammatory cells, including leukocytes, eosinophils, plasma cells, lymphocytes, foreign body cells, and macrophages, surround the cysts. Granulomas form around the cyst (Fig. 6.238). The inflammation and giant cell formation most likely represent a reaction to the intestinal intraluminal contents that find their way into the mucosa and submucosa. The mucosa usually appears normal, although it may be thinned over a submucosal cyst. As the lesions fibrose, the cysts decrease in size and eventually disappear.

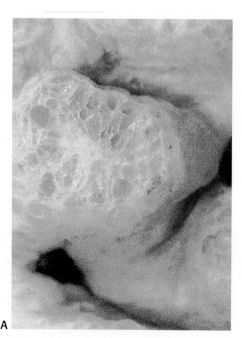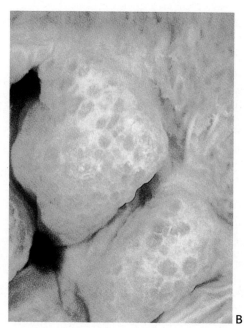

FIG. 6.236. *Pneumatosis intestinalis.* The lacy appearance seen on the cut **(A)** and uncut **(B)** surfaces is secondary to the gas-filled cysts.

BENIGN LESIONS PRESENTING CLINICALLY AS MASSES

Various polyp types occur in the small intestine including lesions normally thought of as polyps, such as adenomas or Peutz-Jeghers polyps, as well as other lesions presenting as polypoid masses (Table 6.57). Most polypoid lesions remain asymptomatic and are detected either endoscopically or radiographically. Symptomatic lesions cause bleeding, obstruction, or intussusception. Uncommonly, the whole GI tract, including the small intestine, is affected by a polyposis syndrome, including juvenile polyposis and Peutz-Jeghers syndrome (see Chapter 12).

Inflammatory polyps assume two major forms: Those associated with inflammatory bowel disease (see Chapter 11) and *inflammatory fibroid polyps* (IFPs). IFPs develop in all age groups and usually arise in the stomach. The small intestine represents the second most common site of origin. Lesions in the small bowel present with intussusception (648), chronic diarrhea, or obstruction. These lesions are inflammatory

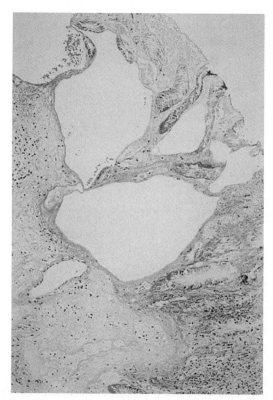

FIG. 6.237. Histology of pneumatosis. Figure shows variably sized, air-filled cysts in a mucosal biopsy.

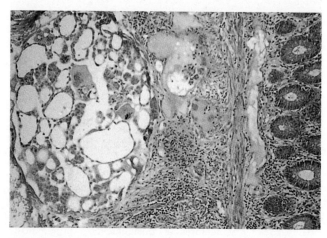

FIG. 6.238. Pneumatosis intestinalis. Typical macrophage and giant cell lining of a cyst.

reactive proliferations of CD34+ perivascular cells (649). The pathologic features (Fig. 6.239) of this lesion are extensively discussed in Chapter 4.

Reactive fibromuscular proliferative lesions consisting of exuberant smooth muscle cell and neural proliferations arise in the small intestinal wall. The smooth muscle fascicles are haphazardly arranged with clusters of ganglion cells, ectatic lymphatic and vascular channels, and fibrous tissues. The smooth muscle bundles merge imperceptibly with the muscularis mucosae. These lesions complicate other disorders, such as inflammatory bowel disease. They produce polypoid lesions covered by smooth, normal-appearing mucosa. They vary in size from several millimeters in diameter to 3 or 4 cm. The lesions arise from a damaged muscularis mucosae to represent an exuberant reparative response. Evidence supporting a reparative process is twofold: (a) the lesion often complicates other diseases and (b) the proliferation involves multiple cell types, including inflammatory cells.

Patients with motility disorders, especially those who have had recurrent intussusceptions, sometimes develop what appear to be polypoid lesions, which, when examined, simulate a papillary adenoma. However, histologic examination discloses the presence of accordionlike folds consisting of the normal mucosal layers. The central core of the fold contains submucosa herniated upward. Often one sees evidence of previous intussusception by examining the muscularis propria or the vessels in the subserosal area.

Inflammatory pseudotumors develop on the serosal surfaces of intestinal sites of transmural inflammation, particularly in Crohn disease, *Yersinia* infections, and tuberculous infections as well as volvulus and intussusception. The presence of a marked inflammatory response protects the bowel from perforation. The reactive proliferations consist of fibroblasts, blood vessels, and variable numbers of inflammatory cells. The overall cellu-

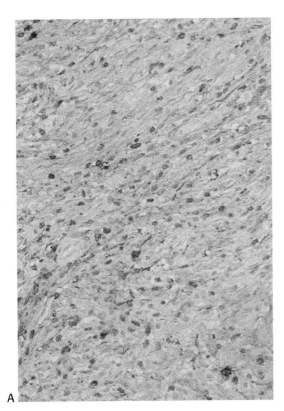
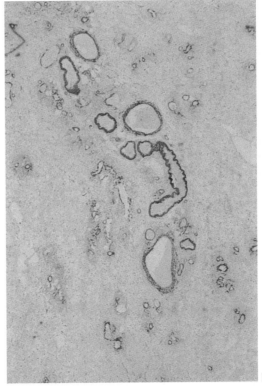

FIG. 6.239. Inflammatory fibroid polyp. **A:** α_1-Antitrypsin immunostain showing the presence of numerous cells with a mesenchymal histiocytic phenotype. **B:** CD34 immunostain showing the presence of numerous vessels.

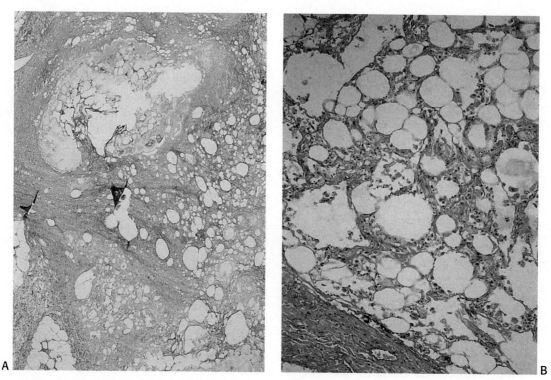

FIG. 6.240. Fat necrosis in the small intestinal serosal fat. **A:** Low magnification showing the presence of lobulated structures demonstrating fat necrosis. **B:** Higher magnification showing the presence of fat cells surrounded by histiocytes and giant cells.

larity of the lesion, its myxoid appearance, its vascularity, and the nature of the inflammatory cells vary depending on the age of the lesion and distinguish the inflammatory process from a neoplasm. Fat necrosis is also often present (Fig. 6.240).

MÜLLERIAN LESIONS

Müllerian lesions may present as mural small intestinal masses. These include endometriosis, which is discussed in detail in Chapter 13, and endocervicosis. Endocervicosis is the presence of benign endocervical glands in ectopic sites. It most typically involves the pelvic peritoneum and lymph nodes but it can present in the small intestine. In this site it presents as a mural nodule that on cut surface consists of variably shaped glands filled with mucin and lined by endocervical-type epithelium. The glands are surrounded by fibrous tissue or the smooth muscle fibers of the muscularis propria. Endometrial-like stroma is not present. The epithelium, which lacks any nuclear atypia, has a CK7+ CK20− phenotype (650).

MISCELLANEOUS LESIONS

Duodenal pseudolipomatosis histologically resembles pseudolipomatosis in the colon and stomach. Numerous clear, rounded, PAS-negative, variably sized vacuoles are present in the lamina propria. These vacuoles can cause expansion of the lamina propria with villous widening and separation of the crypts and Brunner glands (651). The lesion may mimic the fatty deposits seen in Whipple disease or lymphangiectasia. The use of special stains serves to distinguish among these possibilities.

CHANGES OCCURRING IN INTESTINAL TRANSPLANTS

Total intestinal transplantation is used to correct the short gut syndrome. Pediatric candidates for intestinal transplantation are those who undergo extensive intestinal resections for gastroschisis, volvulus, and necrotizing enterocolitis, as well as those with functional disorders such as intestinal pseudo-obstruction, microvillous inclusion disease, and juvenile polyposis (652). The optimum treatment depends on buying time and hoping for maximal intestinal growth and adaptation.

Intestinal transplantation inevitably involves transection of the intestinal wall causing intrinsic and extrinsic denervation, interruption of lymphatic drainage, and preservation-induced injury. Immunologic reactions and immunosuppressive agents may further compromise normal intestinal function. Rejection of the transplant increases intestinal permeability, resulting in bacterial translocation and leading to

TABLE 6.58	**Complications of Transplantation**

Preservation injury
Graft failure
Ischemic damage
Infection
Graft rejection
Graft vs. host disease
Posttransplant lymphoproliferative disorders

sepsis. The large amount of transplanted lymphoid tissue present in the Peyer patches, lamina propria, and mesenteric lymph nodes is responsible for the highly immunogenic character of intestinal allografts. Table 6.58 lists some of the major complications of intestinal transplantation.

Lymphatic regeneration needs to occur following the graft to establish the lymphatic drainage so critical to the nutritional functions of the small bowel, including the absorption of chylomicrons. If this does not occur, lymphedema will develop. Lymphedema reduces absorption of nonlymphatic-dependent proteins and carbohydrates. Impaired gut barrier function may eventually lead to sepsis and multiorgan failure.

Part of the ability of the graft to function normally involves regeneration of the neural components. When failed grafts are evaluated, they demonstrate a lack of extrinsic adrenergic and perivascular fibers in all layers of the bowel wall, but intrinsic neural endocrine transmitters are preserved. Both peptidergic nerves and their receptors are retained following transplantation (653). Patients on cyclosporin therapy may have atypical changes in the bowel wall that do not allow one to detect GVHD or rejection.

A rejected graft demonstrates edema, cellular infiltration of the mucosa and submucosa, and epithelial damage. The number of infiltrating T cells correlates with the extent of tissue damage (654). Lymph nodes in the transplant become totally necrotic by the time of full-thickness intestinal necrosis, perhaps due to host versus graft reaction or therapy with antilymphocyte serum.

Early acute rejection usually occurs within 12 days, although it can occur later. Acute allograft rejection exhibits varying combinations of crypt injury, mucosal infiltration primarily by mononuclear cells, intraepithelial lymphocytes including blastic-appearing lymphocytes, and increased crypt cell apoptoses (>2/10 crypts). The lamina propria appears edematous. CD3+, CD4+, CD8+, and CD25+ T cells are seen along with increased HLA-DR expression by the crypt enterocytes. Rejection presents as a patchy, often ileal-centered process that progresses to mucosal ulceration and eventual fibrosis of the wall (655). Endothelial and crypt damage occurs within 3 days. Cellular infiltrates can be present in the muscle and submucosa in the absence of mucosal changes. In mild rejection, the inflammatory infiltrate surrounds small venules and capillaries in the deep mucosa at the crypt bases (Fig. 6.241). These appear as early as 2 weeks

and as late as 12 months. Other features of rejection include large numbers of lymphocytes between the muscularis mucosae and crypts adjacent to the crypt epithelium. Vessels between the crypts frequently appear activated with enlarged endothelial cells, sometimes with lymphocytes in the lumen. Other inflammatory cells are occasionally present, including plasma cells, eosinophils, and neutrophils. With more substantial involvement, the inflammatory infiltrate becomes more widely dispersed in a patchy or coalescent distribution along with varying degrees of mucosal edema and lymphatic dilation. Markedly enlarged Peyer patches expanded by prominent accumulations of blastic lymphocytes are found in the first month following transplant. This infiltrate consists predominantly of mononuclear cells admixed with lesser numbers of eosinophils and neutrophils. Pronounced mucosal eosinophilia may develop.

When patients exhibit extensive mucosal ulceration, they often have coexisting CMV infections. The patient who survives the episodes of acute graft rejection becomes susceptible to the posttransplantation complications seen in other transplant patients. Chronic graft rejection histologically causes villous atrophy and T-cell infiltration associated with vascular lesions and muscular fibrosis. The lamina propria is infiltrated by CD3+ CD25+ lymphocytes and CD25+ macrophages, abrasion of the cell surface epithelium, and ultimately mucosal sloughing (656). An obliterative arteriopathy is usually present. This occurs in allografts removed up to 660 days posttransplant. The large arteries of the serosa and mesentery are primarily affected, and show patchy luminal narrowing by myointimal hyperplasia and subendothelial accumulation of foamy macrophages and scattered lymphocytes. The mucosa becomes focally necrotic with ulceration and associated granulation tissue and inflammatory exudates. Intact areas show patchy mononuclear infiltrates and distorted mucosal architecture with villous blunting, crypt atrophy and irregularity, and focal lamina propria fibrosis.

Biopsies following treated resolving rejection often demonstrate fibrosis with focal glandular loss, regenerative glands with reparative atypia, and atrophy with a thin mucosa and blunted villi. These changes occur more commonly following severe or persistent rejection, although they are not always present. Patients may develop moderate to severe eosinophilia.

A high incidence of infection complicates small bowel transplantation. These result from both excessive immunosuppression and a compromised barrier function of the native or engrafted small bowel. Small bowel transplant patients who develop rejection or GVHD may have shifts in the intestinal microflora toward potentially pathogenic organisms and bacterial translocation into recipient tissues. Bacterial colony counts are higher in grafts than in the native intestine, and one may see massive bacterial overgrowth in the native intestine in patients developing GVHD.

At least two apoptotic figures in a gland or several single apoptotic cells in the presence of a lymphoid infiltrate with

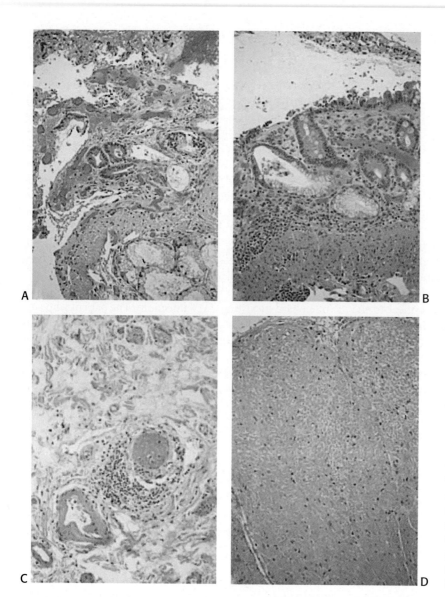

FIG. 6.241. Mild rejection in a patient who underwent a small bowel–pancreatic transplant for diabetes. The transplant failed and the sections come from the duodenal portion of the resected, failed allograft. **A:** The specimen showed evidence of ischemic necrosis presumably as the result of vascular compromise. The specimen demonstrates marked vascular congestion and loss of the epithelial cells on the surface that lies to the left. **B:** Mild regenerative features and an almost inconspicuous infiltrate at the base of the mucosa overlying the muscularis mucosae. **C:** Mild perivascular inflammation. **D:** The muscle shows evidence of denervation injury, presumably the result of the previous surgery.

activated lymphoid follicles and prominent endothelium correlate best with clinical rejection. The patients may develop posttransplant lymphoproliferative disorders, discussed in Chapter 18.

REFERENCES

1. Montgomery RK, Mulberg AE, Grand RJ: Development of the human gastrointestinal tract: twenty years of progress. *Gastroenterology* 1999;116:702.
2. Walters JRF, Howard A, Rumble HEE, et al: Differences in expression of homeobox transcription factors in proximal and distal human intestine. *Gastroenterology* 1997;113:472.
3. Silberg DG, Swain GP, Suh ER, Traber PG: Cdx1 and Cdx 2 expression during intestinal development. *Gastroenterology* 2000;119:961.
4. Sancho E, Batlle E, Clevers H: Live and let die in the intestinal epithelium. *Curr Opin Cell Biol* 2003;15:763.
5. Sancho E, Batlle E, Clevers H: Signaling pathways in intestinal development and cancer. *Annu Rev Cell Biol* 2004;20:695.
6. Gregorieff A, Pinto D, Begthel H, et al: Expression pattern of Wnt signaling components in the adult intestine. *Gastroenterology* 2005;129:626.
7. Fukuda K, Yasugi S: Versatile roles for sonic hedgehog in gut development. *J Gastroenterol* 2002;37:239.
8. Lees C, Howie S, Sartor RB, Satsangi J: The Hedgehog signaling pathway in the gastrointestinal tract: implications for development, homeostasis and disease. *Gastroenterology* 2005;129:1696.
9. Henry GL, Melton DA: Mixer, a homeobox gene required for endoderm development. *Science* 1998;281:91.
10. Kessler DS, Melton DA: Vertebrate embryonic induction: mesodermal and neural patterning. *Science* 1994;266:596.
11. Moore TE, Parson A. The developing human. In: *Clinically Oriented Embryology*, 5th ed. Philadelphia: WB Saunders, 1993, pp 628–644.
12. Henning SJ: Functional development of the gastrointestinal tract. In: Johnson LR (ed). *Physiology of the Gastrointestinal Tract*. New York: Raven Press, 1987, pp 285–293.
13. Colony PC: Successive phases of human fetal intestinal development. In: Kretchmer N, Minkows A (eds). *Nutritional Adaptation of the Gastrointestinal Tract*. Nestle: Vevey/Raven Press, 1983, pp 3–18.
14. Calvert R, Pothier P: Migration of fetal intestinal intervillous cells in neonatal mice. *Anat Rec* 1990;227:199.
15. Sweetser DA, Hauft SM, Hoppe PC, et al: Transgenic mice containing intestinal fatty acid-binding protein-human growth hormone fusion genes exhibit correct regional and cell-specific expression of the reporter gene in their small intestine. *Proc Natl Acad Sci USA* 1988;85:9611.

16. Haffen K, Kedinger M, Simon-Assmann P: Cell contact dependent regulation of enterocyte differentiation. In: Lebenthal E (ed). *Human Gastrointestinal Development.* New York: Raven Press, 1989, pp 19–26.

17. Fang R, Santiago NA, Olds LC, Sibley E: The homeodomain protein Cdx2 regulates lactase gene promoter activity during enterocyte differentiation. *Gastroenterology* 2000;118:115.

18. Yang Q, Bermingham NA, Fiengold MJ, Zoghbi HY: Requirement of Math1 for secretory cell lineage in the mouse intestine. *Science* 2001; 294:2155.

19. Thompson GR, Trexler PC: Gastrointestinal structure and function of germ-free gnotobiotic animals. *Gut* 1971;12:230.

20. Madara J: Regulation of the movement of solutes across tight junctions. *Annu Rev Physiol* 1998;60:143.

21. Clayburgh DR, Shen L, Turner JR: A porous defense: the leaky epithelial barrier in intestinal disease. *Lab Invest* 2004;84:282.

22. Dietschy JM, Sallee VL, Wilson FA: Unstirred water layer and absorption across the intestinal mucosa. *Gastroenterology* 1971;61:932.

23. Perdue MH, McKay DM: Integrative immunophysiology in the intestinal mucosa. *Am J Physiol* 1994;267:G151.

24. Wallace JL, Miller MJS: Nitric oxide in mucosal defense: a little goes a long way. *Gastroenterology* 2000;119:512.

25. Magnusson EK, Sjernstrom I: Mucosal barrier mechanisms. Interplay between secretory IgA, (sIgA), IgG, and mucins on the surface properties and association of salmonellae with intestine and granulocytes. *Immunology* 1982;45:239.

26. Fubara ES, Freter R: Protection against enteric bacterial infection by secretory IgA antibodies. *J Immunol* 1973;111:395.

27. Neutra MR, Phillips TL, Mayer EL, Fishkind DJ: Transport of membrane-bound macromolecules by M cells in follicle-associated epithelium of rabbit Peyer's patch. *Cell Tissue Res* 1987;247:537.

28. Santos LMB, Lider O, Audette J, et al: Characterization of immunomodulatory properties and accessory cell function of small intestine epithelial cells. *Cell Immunol* 1990;127:26.

29. Tagliabue A, Nencioni L, Villa L, et al: Antibody-dependent cell-mediated antibacterial activity of intestinal lymphocytes with secretory IgA. *Nature* 1983;306:184.

30. Tomasi TB, Grey HM: Structure and function of immunoglobulin A. *Prog Allergy* 1972;16:81.

31. Moore R, Carlson S, Madara JL: Rapid barrier restitution in an in vitro model of intestinal epithelial injury. *Lab Invest* 1989;60:237.

32. Habib FI, Corazziari E, Biliotti L, et al: Manometric measurement of human sphincter of Oddi length. *Gut* 1988;29:121.

33. Warwick R, Williams PL: *Gray's Anatomy*, 35th ed. Edinburgh: Longmans, 1973, pp 65–70.

34. Ohtsuka A, Ohtani O, Murakami T: Microvascularization of the alimentary canal as studied by scanning electron microscopy of corrosion casts. In: Motta PM, Fujita H, (eds). *Ultrastructure of the Digestive Tract.* Boston: Martinus Nijhoff, 1988, pp 201–212.

35. Hart TK, Pino RM: Variation in capillary permeability from apex and crypt in the villus of the ileo-jejunum. *Cell Tissue Res* 1985;241:305.

36. Farstad IN, Malavasi F, Haraldsen G, et al: CD38 is a marker of human lacteals. *Virchows Arch* 2002;441:605.

37. Papp M, Rohlich P, Rysmyak I, Toro I: Central chyliferous vessel of intestinal villus. *Fed Proc* 1964;23:T155.

38. Ichikawa S, Okubo M, Uchino S, Hirata Y: The intimate association of nerve terminals with the lacteal endothelium in the canine duodenal villi observed by transmission electron microscopy of serial sections. *Arch Histol Cytol* 1990;53:137.

39. Unthank JL, Bohlen HG: Lymphatic pathways and the role of valves in lymph propulsion from the small intestine. *Am J Physiol* 1988;254:G389.

40. Baker SJ: Geographical variations in the morphology of the small intestinal mucosa in apparently healthy individuals. *Path Microbiol* 1973;39:222.

41. Potten CS, Loeffler M: Stem cells: attributes, cycles, spirals, pitfalls and uncertainties. Lessons for and from the crypt. *Development* 1990; 110:1001.

42. MacDonald WC, Trier JS, Everett NB: Cell proliferation and migration in the stomach, duodenum and rectum of man: radioautographic studies. *Gastroenterology* 1964;46:405.

43. Cheng H, Leblond CP: Origin, differentiation and renewal of the four main epithelial cell types in the mouse small intestine. I. Columnar cells. *Am J Anat* 1974;141:461.

44. Cheng H, Leblond CP: Origin, differentiation and renewal of the four main epithelial cell types in the mouse small intestine. V. Unitarian

theory of the origin of the four epithelial cell types. *Am J Anat* 1974;141:537.

45. Potten CS, Chwalinski S, Swindell R, Palmer M: The spatial organization of the hierarchical proliferative cells of the crypts of the small intestine into clusters of "synchronized" cells. *Cell Tissue Kinet* 1982;15:351.

46. Watson AJ, Wright NA: Morphology and cell kinetics of the jejunal mucosa in untreated patients. In: Cooke WT, Asquith P (eds). *Celiac Disease. Clinics in Gastroenterology,* Vol. 3. Philadelphia: WB Saunders, 1974, pp 20–38.

47. Abreu MT, Palladino AA, Arnold ET, et al: Modulation of barrier function during fas-mediated apoptosis in human intestinal cells. *Gastroenterology* 2000;119:1524.

48. Croitoru K, Riddell RH: Reduce, reuse, and recycle: shedding light on shedding cells. *Gastroenterology* 1993;105:1243.

49. Potten CS: Epithelial cell growth and differentiation. II. Intestinal apoptosis. *Am J Physiol* 1997;273:G253.

50. Mariadason JM, Nicholas C, L'Italien KE, et al: Gene expression profiling of intestinal epithelial cell maturation along the crypt-villus axis. *Gastroenterology* 2005;128:1081.

51. Hubbard AL, Stieger B, Bartles JR: Biogenesis of endogenous plasma membrane proteins in epithelial cells. *Annu Rev Physiol* 1989;51:755.

52. Mooseker MS: Organization, chemistry and assembly of the cytoskeletal apparatus of the intestinal brush border. *Annu Rev Cell Biol* 1985;1:209.

53. Coluccio LM, Bretscher A: Mapping of the microvillar 110K-calmodulin complex (brush border myosin I). Identification of fragments containing the catalytic and F-actin-binding sites and demonstration of a calcium ion dependent conformational change. *Biochemistry* 1990;29:11089.

54. Melligott TF, Beck IT, Dinda PK, Thompson S: Correlation of structural changes at different levels of the jejunal villus with positive net water transport in vivo and in vitro. *Can J Physiol Pharmacol* 1975; 53:439.

55. Farquhar MG, Palade GE: Junctional complexes in various epithelia. *J Cell Biol* 1963;17:375.

56. Madara JL, Dharmsathaphorn K: Occluding junction structure-function relationships in a cultured epithelial monolayer. *J Cell Biol* 1985; 101:2124.

57. Itoh H, Beck PL, Inoue N, et al: Goblet cells make more than just mucus. *J Clin Invest* 1999;104:1539.

58. Plaut AG: Trefoil peptides in the defense of the gastrointestinal tract. *New Engl J Med* 1997;336:506.

59. Madara JL: Cup cells: structure and distribution of a unique class of epithelial cells in guinea pig, rabbit, and monkey small intestine. *Gastroenterology* 1982;83:981.

60. Rossner AJ, Keren DF: Demonstration of M-cells in the specialized follicle-associated epithelium overlying isolated follicles in the gut. *J Leukocyte Biol* 1984;35:397.

61. Pabst R: The anatomical basis for the immune function of the gut. *Anat Embryol* 1987;176:135.

62. Brown D, Cremaschi D, James PS, et al: Brush-border membrane alkaline phosphatase activity in mouse Peyer's patch follicle-associated enterocytes. *J Physiol* 1990;427:81.

63. Sierro F, Pringault E, Assman S, et al: Transient expression of M-cell phenotype by enterocyte–like cells of the follicle-associated epithelium of mouse Peyer's patches. *Gastroenterology* 2000;119:734.

64. Owen RL: M cells—entryways of opportunity for enteropathogens. *J Exp Med* 1994;180:7.

65. Smith MW, James PS, Tivey DR: M cell numbers increase after transfer of SPF mice to a normal animal house environment. *Am J Pathol* 1987;128:385.

66. Gebert A, Rothkotter H, Pabst R: Cytokeratin 18 is an M-cell marker in porcine Peyer's patches. *Cell Tissue Res* 1994;276:213.

67. Kraehenbuhl JP, Neutra MR: Defense of mucosal surfaces: pathogenicity, immunity and vaccines. *Curr Top Microbiol Immunol* 1999;236:1.

68. Allan C, Trier J: Structure and permeability differ in subepithelial villus and Peyer's patch follicle capillaries. *Gastroenterology* 1991;100:1172.

69. Pappo J, Ermak TH: Uptake and translocation of fluorescent latex particles by rabbit Peyer's patch follicle epithelium: a quantitative model for M cell uptake. *Clin Exp Immunol* 1989;76:144.

70. Ermak TH, Steger HJ, Pappo J: Phenotypically distinct subpopulations of T cells in domes and M-cell pockets of rabbit gut-associated lymphoid tissues. *Immunology* 1990;71:530.

71. Wick MJ, Madara JL, Fields BN, Normark SJ: Molecular cross talk between epithelial cells and pathogenic microorganisms. *Cell* 1991; 67:651.

72. Cuvelier CA, Quatacker J, Mielants H, et al: M-cells are damaged and increased in number in inflamed human ileal mucosa. *Histopathology* 1994;24:417.

73. Pappo J, Ermak TH: Uptake and translocation of fluorescent latex particles by rabbit Peyer's patch follicle epithelium: a quantitative model for M cell uptake. *Clin Exp Immunol* 1991;76:144.

74. Cheng H, Bjerknes M: Whole population cell kinetics of mouse duodenal, jejunal, ileal, and colonic epithelia as determined by radioautography and flow cytometry. *Anat Rec* 1982;203:251.

75. Ouellette AJ: Paneth cells and innate immunity in the crypt microenvironment. *Gastroenterology* 1997;113:1779.

76. Marsh MN, Trier JS: Morphology and cell proliferation of subepithelial fibroblasts in adult mouse jejunum. II. Radioautographic studies. *Gastroenterology* 1974;66:636.

77. Kedlinger D, Lefebvre O, Duluc I, et al: Cellular and molecular partners involved in gut morphogenesis and differentiation. *Philos Trans R Soc B Biol Sci* 1998;353:847.

78. Beltinger J, McKaig BC, Makh S, et al: Human colonic subepithelial myofibroblasts modulate transepithelial resistance and secretory response. *Am J Physiol* 1999;277:C271.

79. Mckaig BC, Makh S, Hawkey CJ, et al: Normal human colonic subepithelial myofibroblasts enhance epithelial migration (restitution) via TGFβ3. *Am J Physiol* 1999;276:G1087.

80. Powelll DW, Mifflin RC, Valentich JD, et al: Myofibroblasts. II. Intestinal subepithelial myofibroblasts. *Am J Physiol* 1999;277:C183.

81. Keren DF: Structure and function of the immune system of the gastrointestinal tract. In: Ming SC, Goldman H (eds). *Pathology of the Gastrointestinal Tract*. Philadelphia: Saunders, 1992, pp 69–80.

82. Lundqvist C, Baranov V, Hammarström S, et al: Evidence for regional specialization and extrathymic T cell maturation in human gut epithelium. *Int Immunol* 1995;7:1473.

83. Moghaddami M, Cummins A, Mayrhofer G: Lymphocyte-filled villi: comparison with other lymphoid aggregations in the mucosa of the human small intestine. *Gastroenterology* 1998;115:1414.

84. Cornes JS: Number, size and distribution of Peyer's patches in the human small intestine. *Gut* 1965;6:230.

85. McClugage SG, Low FN, Zimny ML: Porosity of the basement membrane overlying Peyer's patches in rats and monkeys. *Gastroenterology* 1986;91:1128.

86. Spalding DM, Williamson SI, Koopman WJ, McGhee JR: Preferential induction of polyclonal IgA secretion by murine Peyer's patch dendritic cell-T cell mixtures. *J Exp Med* 1984;160:941.

87. Chin Y, Carey GD, Woodruff JJ: Lymphocyte recognition of lymph node high endothelium. *J Immunol* 1982;129:1911.

88. Miura S, Tsuzuki Y, Fukumura D, et al: Intravital demonstration of sequential migration process of lymphocyte subpopulations in rat Peyer's patches. *Gastroenterology* 1995;109:113.

89. Nagata H, Miyairi M, Sekizuka E, et al: In vivo visualization of lymphatic microvessels and lymphocyte migration through rat Peyer's patches. *Gastroenterology* 1994;106:1548.

90. Trejdosiewicz LK: Intestinal intraepithelial lymphocytes in lymphoepithelial interactions in the human gastrointestinal mucosa. *Immunol Lett* 1992;32:13.

91. León F, Roldán E, Sanchez L, et al: Human small-intestinal epithelium contains functional natural killer lymphocytes. *Gastroenterology* 2003;125:345.

92. Giacci C, Mahida YR, Dignass A, et al: Functional interleukin-2 receptor on intestinal epithelial cells. *J Clin Invest* 1993;92:527.

93. Colgan SP, Resnick MB, Parkos CA, et al: IL-4 directly modulates function of a model human intestinal epithelium. *J Immunol* 1994;153:2122.

94. Abreu-Martin MT, Targan DR: Regulation of immune response of the intestinal mucosa. *Crit Rev Immunol* 1996;16:277.

95. Sarnacki S, Begue B, Jarry A, Cerf-Bensussan N: Human intestinal intraepithelial lymphocytes, a distinct population of activated T cells. *Immunol Res* 1991;10:302.

96. Dobbins WO: Human intestinal intraepithelial lymphocytes. *Gut* 1986;27:972.

97. Crowe PT, Marsh MN: Morphometric analysis of intestinal mucosa. VI. Principles in enumerating intra-epithelial lymphocytes. *Virchows Arch* 1994;424:301.

98. Kawabata S, Boyaka PN, Coste M, et al: Intraepithelial lymphocytes from villus tip and crypt portions of the murine small intestine show distinct characteristics. *Gastroenterology* 1998;115:866.

99. Crabbe PA, Heremans JF: The distribution of immunoglobulin-containing cells along the human gastrointestinal tract. *Gastroenterology* 1966;51:305.

100. Maluenda C, Phillips AD, Briddon A, Walker-Smith JA: Quantitative analysis of small intestinal mucosa in cow's milk sensitive enteropathy. *J Pediatr Gastroenterol Nutr* 1984;3:349.

101. Strobel S, Miller HRP, Ferguson A: Human intestinal mast cells: evaluation of fixation and staining techniques. *J Clin Pathol* 1981; 34:851.

102. Sanderson IR, Leung KBP, Pearce FL, Walker-Smith JA: Lamina propria mast cells in biopsies from children with Crohn's disease. *J Clin Pathol* 1986;39:279.

103. Giacosa A: Morphometry of normal duodenal mucosa. *Scand J Gastroenterol* 1989;24:10.

104. Krause WJ: Brunner's glands: a structural, histochemical and pathological profile. *Prog Histochem Cytochem* 2000;35:259.

105. Dott NM: Anomalies of intestinal rotation: their embryology and surgical aspects: report of 5 cases. *Br J Surg* 1923;11:251.

106. Rescorla FJ, Shedd FK, Grosfeld JL, et al: Anomalies of intestinal rotation in childhood: analysis of 447 cases. *Surgery* 1990;108:710.

107. Gilbert HW, Armstrong CP, Thompson MH: The presentation of malrotation of the intestine in adults. *Ann R Coll Surg Engl* 1990; 72:239.

108. Boyd PA, Bhattacharjee A, Gould S, et al: Outcome of prenatally diagnosed anterior abdominal wall defects. *Arch Dis Child Fetal Neonatal Med* 1998;78:F209.

109. Calzolari E, Bianchi F, Dolk H, et al, and EUROCAT Working Group: Are omphalocele and neural tube defects related congenital anomalies? Data from 21 registries in Europe (EUROCAT). *Am J Med Genet* 1997;72:79.

110. Benacerraf BR, Saltzman DH, Estroff JA, et al: Abnormal karyotype of fetuses with omphalocele: prediction based on omphalocele contents. *Obstet Gynecol* 1990;75:317.

111. Hurwitz RS, Manzoni GAM, Ransley PG, Stephens FD: Cloacal exstrophy: a report of 34 cases. *J Urol* 1987;138:1060.

112. Lizcano-Gil LA, Garcia-Cruz D, Sanchez-Corona J: Omphalocele-exstrophy-imperforate-anus-spina bifida (OEIS) complex in a male prenatally exposed to diazepam. *Arch Med Res* 1995;26:95.

113. Nicholls EA, Ford WD, Barnes KH, et al: A decade of gastroschisis in the era of antenatal ultrasound. *Aust N Z J Surg* 1996;66:366.

114. Penman DG, Fisher RM, Noblett HR, Soothill PW: Increase in incidence of gastroschisis in the South West of England in 1995. *Br J Obstet Gynecol* 1998;105:328.

115. Torfs CP, Velie EM, Oechsli FW, et al: A population-based study of gastroschisis: demographic, pregnancy, and lifestyle risk factors. *Teratology* 1994;50:44.

116. Hillebrandt S, Streffer C, Montagutelli X, Balling R: A locus for radiation-induced gastroschisis on mouse chromosome 7. *Mamm Genome* 1998;9:995.

117. Morris-Stiff G, Al-Wafi A, Lari J: Gastroschisis and total intestinal atresia. *Eur J Pediatr Surg* 1998;8:105.

118. Moore T, Khalid N: An international survey of gastroschisis and omphalocele (490 cases). *Pediatr Surg Int* 1986;1:46.

119. Morrison JJ, Klein N, Chitty LS, et al: Intra-amniotic inflammation in human gastroschisis: possible aetiology of postnatal bowel dysfunction. *Br J Obstet Gynecol* 1998;105:1200.

120. Elias S, Simpson JL: *Maternal Serum Screening for Fetal Genetic Disorders*. New York, Edinburgh, Leiden, Melbourne, Toronto: Churchill Livingstone, 1992.

121. Langer JC: Gastroschisis and omphalocele. *Sem Pediatr Surg* 1996; 5:124.

122. Paterson-Brown S, Stalewski H, Brereton RJ: Neonatal small bowel atresia, stenosis and segmental dilatation. *Br J Surg* 1991;78:83.

123. Lambrecht W, Kluth D: Hereditary multiple atresias of the gastrointestinal tract: report of a case and review of the literature. *J Pediatr Surg* 1998;33:794.

124. Louw JH: Congenital intestinal atresia and stenosis in the newborn. Observations on pathogenesis and treatment. *Ann R Coll Surg Engl* 1959;25:109.

125. Halles JA Jr: Atresia of the small intestine. Current concepts in diagnosis and treatment. *Clin Pediatr* 1964;3:257.

126. van der Pol JG, Wolf H, Boer K, et al: Jejunal atresia related to the use of methylene blue in genetic amniocentesis in twins. *Br J Obstet Gynaecol* 1992;99:141.

127. Hoyme HE, Jones KL, Dixon SD, et al: Prenatal cocaine exposure and fetal vascular disruption. *Pediatrics* 1990;85:743.

128. Slee J, Goldblatt J: Further evidence for a syndrome of "apple-peel" intestinal atresia, ocular anomalies and microcephaly. *Clin Genet* 1996;50:260.

129. Fonkalsrud EW, DeLorimier AA, Hays DM: Congenital atresia and stenosis of the duodenum. A review compiled from the members of the Surgical Section of the American Academy of Pediatrics. *Pediatrics* 1968;43:70.

130. Seashore JH, Collins FS, Markowitz RI, Seashore MR: Familial 'apple peel' jejunal atresia: surgical, genetic and radiographic aspects. *Pediatrics* 1987;80:540.

131. Roberts HE, Cragan JD, Cono J, et al: Increased frequency of cystic fibrosis among infants with jejunoileal atresia. *Am J Med Genet* 1998; 78:446.

132. Janik JP, Wayne ER, Janik JS, Price MR: Ileal atresia with total colonic aganglionosis. *J Pediatr Surg* 1997;32:1502.

133. Weinberg AG, Milunsky A, Harrod MJ: Elevated amniotic fluid alpha-fetoprotein and duodenal atresia. *Lancet* 1975;2:496.

134. Kokkonen ML, Kalima T, Jaaskelainen J, Louhimo I: Duodenal atresia: late follow-up. *J Pediatr Surg* 1988;23:216.

135. Puri P, Fujimoto T: New observations on the pathogenesis of multiple intestinal atresias. *J Pediatr Surg* 1988;23:221.

136. Merrill JR, Raffensperger JG: Paediatric annular pancreas twenty years experience. *J Pediatr Surg* 1976;11:921.

137. Dardik H, Klibanoff E: Retroperitoneal enterogenous cyst: report of a case and mechanisms of embryogenesis. *Ann Surg* 1965;162:1084.

138. Gross RE, Holcomb GM Jr, Farber S: Duplications of the alimentary tract. *Pediatrics* 1952;9:449.

139. Vaage S, Knutrud O: Congenital duplications of the alimentary tract with special regard to their embryogenesis. *Prog Pediatr Surg* 1974;7:103.

140. Grosfeld JL, O'Neill JA, Clatworthy HW: Enteric duplications in infancy and childhood: an 18-year review. *Ann Surg* 1970;172:83.

141. Juler JL, List JW, Stemmer EA, Connolly JE: Duodenal diverticulitis. *Arch Surg* 1969;99:572.

142. Lambert MP, Heller DS, Bethel C: Extensive gastric heterotopia of the small intestine resulting in massive gastrointestinal bleeding, bowel perforation, and death: report of a case and review of the literature. *Pediatr Dev Pathol* 2000;3:277.

143. Yoshimitsu K, Yoshida M, Motooka M, et al: Heterotopic gastric mucosa of the duodenum mimicking a duodenal cancer. *Gastrointest Radiol* 1989;14:115.

144. Tanemura H, Uno S, Suzuki M, et al: Heterotopic gastric mucosa accompanied by aberrant pancreas in the duodenum. *Am J Gastroenterol* 1987;82:685.

145. Suda K, Takase M, Shiono S, et al: Duodenal wall cysts may be derived from a ductal component of ectopic pancreatic tissue. *Histopathology* 2002,41:351.

146. Sieck JO, Cowgill R, Larkworthy W: Peritoneal encapsulation and abdominal cocoon. Case report and review of the literature. *Gastroenterology* 1983;84:1597.

147. Localio A, Stahl WM: Diverticular disease of the alimentary tract. Part II: the esophagus, stomach, duodenum and small intestine. *Curr Prob Surg* 1968;5:1.

148. Hagege H, Berson A, Pelletier G, et al: Association of juxtapapillary diverticula with choledocholithiasis but not with cholecystolithiasis. *Endoscopy* 1992;24:248.

149. Eggert A, Teichmann G, Wiltman DH: The pathological implications of duodenal diverticula. *Surg Gynecol Obstet* 1982;154:62.

150. Krishnamurthy S, Kelly MM, Rohrmann CA, Schuffler MD: Jejunal diverticulosis: a heterogeneous disorder caused by a variety of abnormalities of smooth muscle or myenteric plexus. *Gastroenterology* 1983;85:538.

151. Steiner A, Geist A, Scheinfeld A: Non-Meckelian diverticula of the small intestine. *Int Surg* 1967;47:597.

152. Lee FD: Submucosal lipophages in diverticula of the small intestine. *J Pathol Bacteriol* 1966;92:29.

153. Bissett GS 3rd, Kirks DR: Intussusception in infants and children: diagnosis and therapy. *Radiology* 1988;163:141.

154. Stringer MD, Pablot SM, Brereton RJ: Paediatric intussusception. *Br J Surg* 1992;79:867.

155. Kuruvilla TT, Naraynsingh V, Raju GC, Manmohansingh LU: Intussusception in infancy and childhood. *Trop Geogr Med* 1988; 40:342.

156. Schuh S, Wesson DE: Intussusception in children 2 years of age or older. *Can Med Assoc J* 1987;136:269.

157. Reijnen JA, Festen C, Joosten HJ, Van Wieringen PM: Atypical characteristics of a group of children with intussusception. *Acta Paediatr Scand* 1990;79:675.

158. Kurzbart E, Cohen Z, Yerushalmi B, et al: Familial idiopathic intussusception: a report of two families. *J Pediatr Surg* 1999;34:493.

159. Tangi VT, Bear JW, Reid IS, Wright JE: Intussusception in Newcastle in a 25 year period. *Aust NZ J Surg* 1991;61:608.

160. Fanconi S, Berger D, Rickham PP: Acute intussusception: a classic clinical picture. *Helv Paediatr Acta* 1982;37:345.

161. Murphy TV, Gargiullo PM, Massoudi MS, et al: Intussusception among infants given an oral rotavirus vaccine. *N Engl J Med* 2001; 344:564.

162. Wood BJ, Kumar PN, Cooper C, et al: AIDS-associated intussusception in young adults. *J Clin Gastroenterol* 1995;212:158.

163. Ramsden KL, Newman J, Moran A: Florid vascular proliferation in repeated intussusception mimicking primary angiomatous lesion. *J Clin Pathol* 1993;46:91.

164. Frazee RC, Mucha P Jr, Farnell MB, Van Heerden JA: Volvulus of the small intestine. *Ann Surg* 1988;208:565.

165. Gibney EJ: Volvulus of the sigmoid colon. *Surg Gynecol Obstet* 1991; 173:243.

166. Memeo L, Jhang J, Hibshoosh H, et al: Duodenal intraepithelial lymphocytosis with normal villous architecture: common occurrence in H pylori gastritis. *Mod Pathol* 2005;18:1134.

167. Walker MM, Crabtree JE: Helicobacter pylori and the pathogenesis of duodenal ulceration. *Ann NY Acad Sci* 1998;859:96.

168. Nahon S, Patey-Mariaud de Serre N, Lejeune O, et al: Duodenal intraepithelial lymphocytosis during Helicobacter pylori infection is reduced by antibiotic treatment. *Histopathology* 2006;48:417.

169. Starlinger M, Matthews J, Yoon CH, et al: The effect of acid perfusion on mucosal blood flow and intramural pH of rabbit duodenum. *Surgery* 1987;101:433.

170. Whitehead R, Roca M, Meikle DD, et al: The histological classification of duodenitis in fibreoptic biopsy specimens. *Digestion* 1975;13:129.

171. Van de Bovenkamp H, Korteland-van Male AM, Büller HA, et al: Metaplasia of the duodenum shows a Helicobacter pylori-correlated differentiation into gastric-type protein differentiation. *Hum Pathol* 2003;34:156.

172. Frierson HF, Caldwell SH, Marshal B: Duodenal bulb biopsy findings for patients with non-ulcer dyspepsia with or without Campylobacter pylori gastritis. *Mod Pathol* 1990;3:271.

173. Hamlet A, Thoreson A-C, Nilsson H, et al: Duodenal Helicobacter pylori infection differs in cagA genotype between asymptomatic subjects and patients with duodenal ulcers. *Gastroenterology* 1999;116: 259.

174. Rauws EAJ, Tygat GNJ: Cure of duodenal ulcer associated with eradication of Helicobacter pylori. *Lancet* 1990;335:1233.

175. Tan YM, Wong WK: Giant Brunneroma as an unusual cause of upper gastrointestinal hemorrhage: a report of a case. *Surg Today* 2002; 32:910.

176. Sakurai T, Sakashita H, Honjo G, et al: Gastric foveolar metaplasia with dysplastic changes in Brunner gland hyperplasia. Possible precursor lesions for Brunner gland adenocarcinoma. *Am J Surg Pathol* 2005;29:1442.

177. Lu H, Hsu P-I, Graham DY, Yamaoka Y: Duodenal ulcer promoting gene of Helicobacter pylori. *Gastroenterology* 2005;128:833.

178. Marshall BJ, McGechie DB, Rogers PA, Glancy RJ: Pyloric Campylobacter infection and gastroduodenal disease. *Med J Aust* 1985;142:439.

179. Branicki FJ, Boey J, Fok PJ, et al: Bleeding duodenal ulcer, a prospective evaluation of risk factors for rebleeding and death. *Ann Surg* 1990;211:411.

180. Hui W, Lam S: Multiple duodenal ulcer: natural history and pathophysiology. *Gut* 1987;28:1134.

181. Kang JY, Nasiry R, Guan R, et al: Influence of the site of a duodenal ulcer on its mode of presentation. *Gastroenterology* 1986;90:1874.

182. Rhodes RS, DePalma RG: Mitochondrial dysfunction of the liver and hypoglycemia in hemorrhagic shock. *Surg Gynecol Obstet* 1980;150: 347.

183. Bulkley GB, Kvietys PR, Parks DA, et al: Relationship of blood flow and oxygen consumption to ischemic injury in the canine small intestine. *Gastroenterology* 1985;89:852.

184. Granger DN, Hollwarth ME, Parks DA: Ischemia-reperfusion injury: role of oxygen-derived free radicals. *Acta Physiol Scand (Suppl)* 1986;548:47.

185. Park PO, Haglund U, Bulkley GB, Fait K: The sequence of development of intestinal tissue injury following strangulation ischemia and reperfusion. *Surgery* 1990;107:574.

186. Zimmerman BJ, Granger DN: Oxygen free radicals and the gastrointestinal tract: role in ischemia-reperfusion injury. *Hepatogastroenterology* 1994;41:337.

187. Harlan JM: Leukocyte-endothelial interactions. *Blood* 1985;65:513.

188. Haglund U, Bulkley GB, Granger DN: On the pathophysiology of intestinal ischemic injury. Clinical review. *Acta Chir Scand* 1987;153:321.

189. Skinner DB, Zairms I, Moosa AR: Mesenteric vascular disease. *Am J Surg* 1974;128:835.

190. Sitges-Serra A, Mas X, Roqueta F, et al: Mesenteric infarction: an analysis of 83 patients with prognostic studies in 44 cases undergoing a massive small-bowel resection. *Br J Surg* 1988;75:544.

191. Grendell JH, Ockner RK: Mesenteric venous thrombosis. *Gastroenterology* 1982;82:358.

192. Warren S, Eberhard TP: Mesenteric venous thrombosis. *Surg Gynecol Obstet* 1935;61:102.

193. Williams LF Jr: Mesenteric ischemia. *Surg Clin North Am* 1988;68:331.

194. Biedrzycki OJ, Arnaout A, Coppen MJ, Shepherd NA: Isolated intramucosal goblet cells in subacute ischaemic enteritis: mimicry of signet ring cell carcinoma. *Histopathology* 2005;45:460.

195. Park PO, Haglund U: Regeneration of small bowel mucosa after intestinal ischemia. *Crit Care Med* 1992;20:135.

196. Wagner R, Gabbert H, Hohn P: Ischemia and post-ischemic regeneration of the small intestinal mucosa. *Virchows Arch B Cell Pathol* 1979;31:259.

197. Kanto WP Jr, Wilson R, Breart GL, et al: Perinatal events and necrotizing enterocolitis in premature infants. *Am J Dis Child* 1987;141:167.

198. Coutinho HB, da Mota HC Coutinho VB, et al: Absence of lysozyme (muramidase) in the intestinal Paneth cells of newborn infants with inn necrotizing enterocolitis. *J Clin Pathol* 1998;51:512.

199. Crissinger KD, Granger DN: Mucosal injury induced by ischemia and reperfusion in the piglet intestine: influences of age and feeding. *Gastroenterology* 1989;97:920.

200. Lee HC, Huang FY, Hsu CH, et al: Acute segmental obstructing enteritis in children. *J Pediatr Gastroenterol Nutr* 1994;18:1.

201. Flory C: Arterial occlusions produced by emboli from eroded aortic atheromatous plaques. *Am J Pathol* 1945;21:549.

202. Weiser MM, Andres GA, Rentjens JR, et al: Systemic lupus erythematosus and intestinal venulitis. *Gastroenterology* 1981;81:570.

203. Lee RG: The colitis of Behçet's syndrome. *Am J Surg Pathol* 1986;10:888.

204. Stevens SMB, Gue S, Finckh ES: Necrotizing and giant cell granulomatous phlebitis of caecum and ascending colon. *Pathology* 1976;8:259.

205. Saraga EP, Costa J: Idiopathic enterocolic lymphocytic phlebitis. *Am J Surg Pathol* 1989;13:303.

206. Genta RM, Haggitt RC: Idiopathic myointimal hyperplasia of mesenteric vein. *Gastroenterology* 1991;101:533.

207. Bacon PA: Vasculitis, clinical aspects and therapy. *Acta Med Scand* 1988;715:157.

208. Roikjaer O: Perforation and necrosis of the colon complicating polyarteritis nodosa. *Acta Chir Scand* 1987;153:385.

209. Allen DM, Diamond LK, Howell DA: Anaphylactoid purpura in children (Schönlein-Henoch syndrome). *Am J Dis Child* 1960;99:833.

210. Glasier CM, Siegel MJ, McAlister WH, Shackelford GD: Henoch-Schönlein syndrome in children: gastrointestinal manifestations. *AJR Am J Roentgenol* 1981;136:1081.

211. Banerjee B, Rashid S, Singh E, Moore J: Endoscopic findings in Henoch-Schönlein purpura. *Gastrointest Endosc* 1991;37:569.

212. Lie JT: Vasculitis and the gut. *J Rheumatol* 1991;18:647.

213. Leavitt RY, Fauci AS, Bloch DA, et al: The American College of Rheumatology 1990 criteria for the classification of Wegener's granulomatosis. *Arthritis Rheum* 1990;33:1101.

214. Scott DGI, Bacon PA, Tribe CR: Systemic rheumatoid vasculitis: a clinical and laboratory study. *Medicine* 1981;60:288.

215. Klemperer P, Pollack AD, Baehr G: Pathology of disseminated lupus erythematosus. *Arch Pathol* 1941;32:569.

216. Beighton PH, Murdoch JC, Cotteler T: Gastrointestinal complications of the Ehlers-Danos syndrome. *Gut* 1969;10:1004.

217. Kawasaki T, Kosaki F, Okawa S, et al: A new infantile acute mucocutaneous lymph node syndrome prevailing in Japan. *Pediatrics* 1974;54:271.

218. Fishbein VA, Rosen AM, Lack BE, et al: Diffuse hemorrhagic gastroenteropathy: report of a new entity. *Gastroenterology* 1994;106:500.

219. Slavin R, Cafferty L, Cartwright J: Segmental mediolytic arteritis. A clinicopathologic and ultrastructural study of two cases. *Am J Surg Pathol* 1989;13:558.

220. Haber MM, Burrell M, West AB: Enterocolic lymphocytic phlebitis. *J Clin Gastroenterol* 1993;17:327.

221. Flaherty MJ, Lie JT, Haggitt RC: Mesenteric inflammatory venoocclusive disease. *Am J Surg Pathol* 1994;18:779.

222. Perlemuter G, Chaussade S, Soubrane O, et al: Multifocal stenosing ulcerations of the small intestine revealing vasculitis associated with C2 deficiency. *Gastroenterology* 1996;110:1628.

223. Perlemutter G, Guillevin L, Legman P, et al: Cryptogenic multifocal ulcerous stenosing enteritis: an atypical type of vasculitis or a disease mimicking vasculitis. *Gut* 2001;48:333.

224. Olin JW: Thromboangiitis obliterans (Buerger's disease). *N Engl J Med* 2000;343:864.

225. Kempczinski RF, Clark SM, Blebia J, et al: Intestinal ischemia secondary to thromboangiitis obliterans. *Ann Vasc Surg* 1993;7:354.

226. De Las Casas LE, Finley JL: Diabetic microangiopathy in the small bowel. *Histopathology* 1999;35:267.

227. Behçet H: Ber rezidivierende, apthose, durch einen Virus verursachte Geschw re am Mund, am Auge und an den Genitalien. *Deut Wochenschr* 1937;105:1152.

228. Kasahara Y, Tanaka S, Nishino M, et al: Intestinal involvement in Behçet's disease: review of 136 surgical cases in the Japanese literature. *Dis Colon Rectum* 1981;24:103.

229. Akpolat T, Koc Y, Yeniay I, et al: Familial Behçet's disease. *Eur J Med* 1992;1:391.

230. Sun A, Chang JG, Kao CL, et al: Human cytomegalovirus as a potential etiologic agent in recurrent aphthous ulcers and Behçet's disease. *J Oral Pathol Med* 1996;25:212.

231. Hamzaoui K, Kahan A, Hamza M, Ayed K: Suppressive T cell function of Epstein-Barr virus induced activation in active Behçet's disease. *Clin Exp Rheumatol* 1991;9:131.

232. Yamashita S, Suzuki A, Yanagita T, et al: Analysis of neutrophil proteins of patients with Behçet's disease by two-dimensional gel electrophoresis. *Biol Pharm Bull* 2001;24:119.

233. Yamashita S, Suzuki A, Yanagita T, et al: Analysis of a protease responsible for truncated actin increase in neutrophils of patients with Behçet's disease. *Biol Pharm Bull* 2001;23:519.

234. Choi IJ, Kim JS, Cha SD, et al: Long-term clinical course and prognostic factors in intestinal Behçet's disease. *Dis Colon Rectum* 2000;43:692.

235. Kobayashi M, Ito M, Nakagawa A, et al: Neutrophil and endothelial cell activation in the vasa vasorum in vasculo-Behçet disease. *Histopathology* 2000;36:362.

236. Sayek I, Aran O, Uzunalimoglu B, Hersek E: Intestinal Behçet's disease: surgical experience in seven cases. *Hepatogastroenterology* 1991;38:81.

237. Hassard PV, Binder SW, Nelson V, Sasiliauskas EA: Anti-tumor necrosis factor monoclonal antibody therapy for gastrointestinal Behçet's disease: a case report. *Gastroenterology* 2001;120:995.

238. Evereklioglu C: Managing the symptoms of Behçet's disease. *Expert Opin Pharmacother* 2004;5:317.

239. Masi AT, Hunder GG, Lie JT: The American College of Rheumatology 1990 criteria for the classification of Churg-Strauss syndrome (allergic granulomatosis and angitis). *Arthritis Rheum* 1990;33:1094.

240. Solans R, Bosch JA, Perez-Bocanegra C, et al: Churg-Strauss syndrome: outcome and long-term follow-up of 32 patients. *Rheumatology* 2001;40:763.

241. Frankel SK, Sullivan EJ, Brown KK: Vasculitis: Wegner's granulomatosis, Churg-Strauss syndrome, microscopic polyangiitis, polyarteritis nodosa and Takayasu arteritis. *Crit Care Clin* 2002;18:1.

242. Strole WG Jr, Clark WH Jr, Isselbacher KJ: Progressive arterial occlusive disease (Kohlmeier-Degos). *N Engl J Med* 1967;276:195.

243. Oweity T, West AB, Stokes MB: Necrotizing angiitis of the small intestine related to AA-amyloidosis: a novel association. *Int J Surg Pathol* 2001;9:149.

244. Pallesen RM, Rasmussen NR: Malignant atrophic papulosis-Degos' syndrome. *Acta Chir Scand* 1979;145:279.

245. Bick RL, Baker WF: Antiphospholipid and thrombosis syndromes. *Semin Thromb Hemost* 994;20:3.

246. Nachman RL, Silversttein R: Hypercoagulable states. *Ann Intern Med* 1993;19:819.

247. Allaart CF, Poort SR, Rosendaal FR, et al: Increased risk of venous thrombosis in carriers of hereditary protein C defect. *Lancet* 1993; 341:134.

248. Demers C, Ginsberg JS, Hirsch J, et al: Thrombosis in antithrombin III-deficient persons: report of a large kindred and literature review. *Ann Int Med* 1992;116:754.

249. Nilsson IM, Ljungner HM, Tengborn L: Two different mechanisms in patients with venous thrombosis and defective thrombolysis: low concentration of plasminogen activator or increased concentration of plasminogen activator inhibitor *BMJ* 1985;290:1453.

250. Ududa H, Emura I, Naito M: Crystalglobulin-induced vasculopathy accompanying ischemic intestinal lesions of a patient with myeloma. *Pathol Int* 1996;46:165.

251. Jeffries GH, Steinberg H, Sleisenger MH: Chronic ulcerative (non-granulomatous) jejunitis. *Am J Med* 1968;44:47.

252. Canavese G, Villanacci V, Zambelli C, et al: Gastric metaplasia and small bowel ulcerogenesis in a case of ulcerative jejunitis not related to celiac disease. *Int J Surg Pathol* 2004;12:415.

253. Riddell RH: The gastrointestinal tract. In: Riddell RH (ed). *Pathology of Drug-Induced and Toxic Disease*. New York: Churchill Livingstone, 1982, pp 515–531.

254. Ziegler TR, Fernández-Estívariz J, Gu LH, et al: Severe villus atrophy and chronic malabsorption induced by azathioprine. *Gastroenterology* 2003;124:1950.

255. Dinda PK, Buell MG, Morris O, Beck IT: Studies on ethanol-induced subepithelial fluid accumulation and jejunal villus bleb formation. An in vitro video microscopic approach. *Can J Physiol Pharmacol* 1994; 72:1186.

256. Stemmermann GN, Hayashi T: Colchicine intoxication. A reappraisal of its pathology based on a study of three fatal cases. *Hum Pathol* 1971;2:32.

257. Parnes HL, Fung E, Schiffer CA: Chemotherapy-induced lactose intolerance in adults. *Cancer* 1994;74:1629.

258. Clauw DJ, Danshel DJ, Umhau A, Katz P: Tryptophan-associated eosinophilic connective-tissue disease (a new clinical entity?). *JAMA* 1990;263:1502.

259. DeSchryver-Kecskemeti K, Clouse RE: A previously unrecognized group of "eosinophilic gastroenteritis": association with connective tissue diseases. *Am J Surg Pathol* 1984;8:171.

260. Crane PW, Clark C, Sowter C, et al: Cyclosporine toxicity in the small intestine. *Transplant Proc* 1990;22:2432.

261. Wetli CV, Mittleman RE: The "body packer" syndrome: toxicity following ingestion of illicit drugs packed for transportation. *J Forensic Sci* 1981;26:492.

262. Anilkumar TV, Sarraf CE, Hunt T, Alison MR: The nature of cytotoxic drug–induced cell death in murine intestinal crypts. *Br J Cancer* 1992;65:522.

263. Bennett RE, Harrison MW, Bishop CJ, et al: The role of apoptosis in atrophy of the small gut mucosa produced by repeated administration of cytosine arabinoside. *J Pathol* 1984;142:259.

264. Oble DA, Mino-Kenudson M, Goldsmith J, et al: Autoimmune-like panarteritis is associated with the novel cancer adjuvant a-CTLA-4mAb. *Lab Invest* 2007;87:125A.

265. Bjarnason I, Hayllar J, Macpherson AJ, et al: Side effects of non-steroidal anti-inflammatory drugs on the small and large intestine in humans. *Gastroenterology* 1993;104:1832.

266. Laine L, Bombardier C, Hawkey CJ, et al: Stratifying the risk of NSAID-related upper gastrointestinal clinical events: results of a double-blind outcomes study in patients with rheumatoid arthritis. *Gastroenterology* 2002;123:1006.

267. Maiden L, Thjodleifsson B, Theodors A, et al: A quantitative analysis of NSAID-induced small bowel pathology by capsule enteroscopy. *Gastroenterology* 2005;128:1172.

268. Atchison CR, West AB, Balakumaran A, et al: Drug enterocyte adducts: possible causal factor for Diclofenac enteropathy in rats. *Gastroenterology* 2000;119:1537.

269. Davies NM, Saleh JY, Skjodt NM: Detection and prevention of NSAID-induced enteropathy. *J Pharm Pharm Sci* 2000;3:137.

270. Yousfi MM, de Petris G, Leighton JA, et al: Diaphragm disease after use of nonsteroidal anti-inflammatory agents; first report of diagnosis with capsule endoscopy. *J Clin Gastroenterol* 2004;38:686.

271. Roy MJ, Walsh TJ: Histopathologic and immunohistochemical changes in gut-associated lymphoid tissues after treatment of rabbits with dexamethasone. *Lab Invest* 1992;64:437.

272. Tomczok J, Grzybek H, Sliwa W, Panz B: Ultrastructural aspects of the small intestinal lead toxicology. *Exp Pathol* 1988;35:49.

273. Lindhom T, Thysell H, Ljunggren L, et al: Aluminum in patients with uremia and patients with enteropathy. *Nieren-Hochdruckkr* 1983;12: 192.

274. Phillpotts CJ: Histopathological changes in the epithelial cells of rat duodenum following chronic dietary exposure to cadmium, with particular reference to Paneth cells. *Br J Exp Pathol* 1986;67:505.

275. Bosman T, Vonck K, Claeys P, et al: Enterocolitis: an adverse event in refractory epilepsy patients treated with levetiracetam. *Seizure* 2004; 13:76.

276. Keating JP, Neill M, Hill GL: Sclerosing encapsulating peritonitis after intraperitoneal use of povidone iodine. *Aust NZ J Surg* 1997;67:742.

277. Hösli P, Schapira M: Spontaneous duodenal hematoma during oral administration. *N Engl J Med* 2000;343:474.

278. Sukpanichnant S, Srisuthapan N, Kachintorn U, et al: Clofazimine-induced crystal-storing histiocytosis producing chronic abdominal pain in a leprosy patient. *Am J Surg Pathol* 2000;24:129.

279. Miller MJS, Zhang XJ, Gu X, et al: Exaggerated intestinal histamine release by casein and casein hydrolysate but not whey hydrolysate. *Scand J Gastroenterol* 1991;26:379.

280. Jacobson MF: *The Complete Eater's Digest and Nutrition Scoreboard*. Garden City, NY: Anchor Press/Doubleday, 1985.

281. Nagata S, Yamashiro Y, Ohtsuka Y, et al: Quantitative analysis and immunohistochemical studies on small intestinal mucosa of food-sensitive enteropathy. *J Pediatr Gastroenterol Nutr* 1995;20:44.

282. Institute of Medicine: *Naturally Occurring Fish and Shellfish Poisons. Seafood Safety*. Washington, DC: National Academy Press, 1991, p 94.

283. Morrow JD, Margolies GR, Rowald J, et al: Evidence that histamine is the causative toxin of scombroid fish poisoning. *N Eng J Med* 1991; 324:716.

284. Edebo L, Lange S, Li XP, Allenmark S: Toxic mussels and okadaic acid induce rapid hypersecretion in the rat small intestine. *APMIS* 1988; 96:1029.

285. Czaja AJ, McAlbany JC, Pruitt BA: Acute gastroduodenal disease after thermal injury: an endoscopic evaluation of incidence and natural history. *N Engl J Med* 1974;291:925.

286. Berthrong M, Fajardo LF: Radiation injury in surgical pathology. II. Alimentary tract. *Am J Surg Pathol* 1981;5:153.

287. Paris F, Fuks Z, Kang A, et al: Endothelial apoptosis as the primary lesion initiating intestinal radiation damage in mice. *Science* 2001; 293:293.

288. Ruifrok ACC, Mason KA, Lozano G, Thames HD: Spatial and temporal patterns of expression of epidermal growth factor, transforming growth factor alpha and transforming growth factor beta 1-3 and their receptors in mouse jejunum after radiation treatment. *Radiat Res* 1997;1.

289. Wang J, Zheng H, Sung C-C: Cellular sources of transforming growth factor-β isoforms in early and chronic radiation enteropathy. *Am J Pathol* 1998;153:1531.

290. Oya M, Yao T, Tsuneyoshi M: Chronic irradiation enteritis: its correlation with the elapsed time interval and morphological changes. *Hum Pathol* 1996;27:774.

291. Husebye E, Skar V, Høverstad T, et al: Abnormal intestinal motor patterns explain enteric colonization with gram negative bacilli in late radiation enteropathy. *Gastroenterology* 1995;109:1078.

292. Nguyen NP, Antoine JE, Dutta S, et al: Current concepts in radiation enteritis and implications for future clinical trials. *Cancer* 2002;95: 1151.

293. Berlanga J, Prats P, Remirez D, et al: Prophylactic use of epidermal growth factor reduces ischemia/reperfusion intestinal damage. *Am J Pathol* 202;161:373.

294. Falkow S, Isberg RR, Portnoy DA: The interaction of bacteria with mammalian cells. *Annu Rev Cell Biol* 1992;8:333.

295. Abrams GD: Surgical pathology of the infected gut. *Am J Surg Pathol* 1987;11:16.

296. Sansonetti PJ: Bacterial pathogens, from adherence to invasion: comparative strategies. *Med Microbiol Immunol* 1993;182:223.

297. Fields PI, Groisman EA, Heffron F: A Salmonella locus that controls resistance to microbicidal proteins from phagocytic cells. *Science* 1989; 243:1059.

298. Guerrant RL, Bobak DA: Bacterial and protozoal gastroenteritis. *N Engl J Med* 1991;325:327.

299. Neu H: The crisis in antibiotic resistance. *Science* 1992;257:1064.

300. Cohen M: Epidemiology of drug resistance: implications for post-antimicrobial era. *Science* 1992;257:1050.

301. Krause R: The origin of plagues: old and new. *Science* 1992;257:1073.

302. Levine MM: Escherichia coli that cause diarrhea: enterotoxigenic, enteropathogenic, enteroinvasive, enterohemorrhagic, and enteroadherent. *J Infect Dis* 1987;155:377.

303. Drucker MM, Polliack A, Yeivin R, et al: Immunofluorescent demonstration of enteropathogenic E. coli in tissues of infants dying with enteritis. *Pediatrics* 1970;46:855.

304. Sherman P, Drumm B, Karmali M, Cutz E: Adherence of bacteria to the intestine in sporadic cases of enteropathogenic Escherichia coli-associated diarrhea in infants and young children: a prospective study. *Gastroenterology* 1989;96:86.

305. Rothbaum R, McAdams AJ, Giannella R, Partin JC: A clinicopathologic study of enterocyte-adherent Escherichia coli: a cause of protracted diarrhea in infants. *Gastroenterology* 1982;83:441.

306. Sack RB: Human diarrheal disease caused by enterotoxigenic Escherichia coli. *Annu Rev Microbiol* 1975;29:333.

307. Mezoff AG, Giannella RA, Eade MN, Cohen MB: Escherichia-coli enterotoxin (STa) binds to receptors, stimulates guanyl cyclase, and impairs absorption in rat colon. *Gastroenterology* 1992;102:816.

308. Taylor DN, Echeverria P, Sethabutr O, et al: Clinical and microbiologic features of Shigella and enteroinvasive Escherichia coli infections detected by DNA hybridization. *J Clin Microbiol* 1988;26:1362.

309. Knutton S, Shaw RK, Bhan MK, et al: Ability of enteroaggregative Escherichia coli strains to adhere in vitro to human intestinal mucosa. *Infect Immunol* 1992;60:2083.

310. Centers for Disease Control: Salmonella enteritidis infections and shell eggs—United States. *MMWR Morb Mortal Wkly Rep* 1990;39:909.

311. Musher DM, Musher BL: Contagious acute gastrointestinal infections. *N Engl J Med* 2004;351:2417.

312. Olsen SJ, DeBess EE, McGivern TE, et al: A Nosocomial outbreak of fluoroquinolone-resistant salmonella infection. *N Engl J Med* 2001;344:1572.

312a. Reller ME, Olsen SJ, Kressel AB, et al: Sexual transmission of typhoid fever: a multistate outbreak among men having sex with men. *Clin Infect Dis* 2003;37:141.

313. Gay FP: *Typhoid Fever.* New York: Macmillan, 1918.

314. Chuttani HK, Jain K, Misran RC: Small bowel in typhoid fever. *Gut* 1971;12:709.

315. Jones GW, Rabert DK, Svinarich DM, Whitfield HJ: Association of adhesive, invasive, and virulent phenotypes of Salmonella typhimurium with autonomous 60-megadalton plasmids. *Infect Immunol* 1982;38:476.

316. Clark MA, Jepson MA, Simmons NL, Hirst BH: Preferential interaction of Salmonella typhimurium with mouse Peyer's patch M cells. *Res Microbiol* 1994;145:543.

317. Takeuchi A: Electron microscope studies of experimental Salmonella infection. I. Penetration into the intestinal epithelium by Salmonella typhimurium. *Am J Pathol* 1967;50:109.

318. Kraus MD, Amatya B, Kimula Y: Histopathology of typhoid enteritis: morphologic and immunophenotypic findings. *Mod Pathol* 1999;12:949.

319. Bone FJ, Bogie D, Morgan-Jones SC: Staphylococcal food poisoning from sheep milk cheese. *Epidemiol Infect* 1989;103:449.

320. Preliminary FoodNet data on the incidence of foodborne illnesses—selected sites, United States, 2002. *MMWR Morb Mortal Wkly Rep*, 2003;52:340.

321. Riley LW, Finch MJ: Results of the first year of national surveillance of Campylobacter infections in the United States. *J Infect Dis* 1985;151:956.

322. Taylor DN, McDermott KT, Little JR, et al: Campylobacter enteritis from untreated water in the Rocky Mountains. *Ann Intern Med* 1983;99:38.

323. Deming MS, Tauxe RV, Blake PA, et al: Campylobacter enteritis at a university: transmission from eating chicken and from cats. *Am J Epidemiol* 1987;126:525.

324. Skirrown MB: Campylobacter enteritis: a "new" disease. *BMJ* 1977;2:9.

325. Smith GS, Blaser MJ: Fatalities associated with Campylobacter jejuni infections. *JAMA* 1985;253:2873.

326. Sugita K, Ishii M, Takanashi J, et al: Guillain-Barré syndrome associated with IgM anti-G_{M1} antibody following Campylobacter jejuni enteritis. *Eur J Pediatr* 1994;153:181.

327. Florin I, Antillon F: Production of enterotoxin and cytotoxin in Campylobacter jejuni strains isolated in Costa-Rica. *J Med Microbiol* 1992;37:22.

328. Coffin CM, Heureaux PL, Dehner LP: Campylobacter associated enterocolitis in childhood. *Am J Clin Pathol* 1982;78:117.

329. Bode RB, Brayton PR, Colwell RR, et al: A new Vibrio species, Vibrio cincinnatiensis, causing meningitis: successful treatment in an adult. *Ann Intern Med* 1986;104:55.

330. Brenner DJ, Hickman-Brenner FW, Lee JV, et al: Vibrio furnissii (formerly aerogenic biogroup of Vibrio fluvialis), a new species isolated from human feces and the environment. *J Clin Microbiol* 1983;18:816.

331. Davis BR, Fanning GR, Madden JM, et al: Characterization of biochemically atypical Vibrio cholerae strains and designation of a new pathogenic species, Vibrio mimicus. *J Clin Microbiol* 1981;14:631.

332. Hickman FW, Farmer JJ III, Hollis DG, et al: Identification of Vibrio hollisae sp. nov. from patients with diarrhea. *J Clin Microbiol* 1982;15:395.

333. Lee JV, Shread P, Furniss AI, Bryant TN: Taxonomy and description of Vibrio fluvialis sp. nov. (synonym group F vibrios, group EE6). *J Appl Bacteriol* 1981;50:73.

334. Love M, Teebken-Fisher D, Hose JE, et al: Vibrio damsela, a marine bacterium, causes skin ulcers on the damselfish Chromispunctipinnis. *Science* 1981;214:1139.

335. McLaughlin JB, DePaola A, Bopp CA, et al: Outbreak of Vibrio parahaemolyticus gastroenteritis associated with Alaskan oysters. *N Engl J Med* 2005;353:1463.

336. Sommers HM: Infectious diarrhea. In: Youmans GP, Patterson PY, Sommers HM (eds). *Biological and Clinical Basis of Infectious Disease,* 2nd ed. Philadelphia: WB Saunders, 1990, pp 525–529.

337. Mathan M, Chandy G, Mathan VI: Ultrastructural changes in the upper small intestinal mucosa in patients with cholera. *Gastroenterology* 1995;109:422.

338. Kumamoto KS, Vukich DJ: Clinical infections of Vibrio vulnificus: a case report and review of the literature. *J Emerg Med* 1998;16:61.

339. Holmberg SD, Farmer JJ: Aeromonas hydrophila and Plesiomonas shigelloides as causes of intestinal infections. *Rev Infect Dis* 1984;6:633.

340. Zeissler J, Rassfeld-Sternberg L: Enteritis necroticans due to Clostridium welchii type F. *BMJ* 1949;i:267.

341. Gui L, Subramony C, Fratkin J, Hughson MD: Fatal enteritis necroticans (pigbel) in a diabetic adult. *Mod Pathol* 2002;15:66.

342. Hansen K, Jeckeln E, Jochims J, et al: *Darmbrand-Enteritis Necroticans.* Stuttgart: Thieme, 1949.

343. Lawrence G, Walker PD: Pathogenesis of enteritis necroticans in Papua, New Guinea. *Lancet* 1976;1:125.

344. Cover TL, Aber RC: Yersinia enterocolitica. *N Engl J Med* 1989;321:16.

345. Cornelis GR: The Yersinia deadly kiss. *J Bacteriol* 1998;180:5495.

346. Revell PA, Miller VL: Yersinia virulence: more than a plasmid. *FEMS Microbiol Lett* 2001;205:159.

347. Carniel E: The Yersinia high-pathogenicity island. *Int Microbiol* 1999;2:161.

348. Une T: Studies on the pathogenicity of Yersinia enterocolitica. II. Interaction with cultured cells in vitro. *Microbiol Immunol* 1977;21:365.

349. Delorme J, Laverdiere M, Martineau B, et al: Yersiniosis in children. *Can Med Assoc J* 1974;110:281.

350. Simmonds SD, Noble MA, Freeman HJ: Gastrointestinal features of culture-positive Yersinia enterocolitica infection. *Gastroenterology* 1987;92:112.

351. El-Maraghi NR, Mair NS: The histopathology of enteric infection with Yersinia pseudotuberculosis. *Am J Clin Pathol* 1979;71:631.

352. Robins-Browne RM, Prpic JK: Effects of iron desferrioxamine on infections with Yersinia enterocolitica. *Infect Immunol* 1985;47:774.

353. Cantwell MF, Snider DE Jr, Cauthen GM, Onorato IM: Epidemiology of tuberculosis in the United States, 1985 through 1992. *JAMA* 1994;272:535.

354. Division of Tuberculosis Elimination: Surveillance reports: reported tuberculosis in the United States 2000. Atlanta: Centers for Disease Control and Prevention. Available at: http://www.cdc.gov/hchstp/tb/surv/surv2000. Accessed June 1, 2007.

355. Dolin PJ, Raviglione MC, Kochi A: Global tuberculosis incidence and mortality during 1999-2000. *Bull World Health Organ* 2004;72:213.

356. Tuberculosis mortality among US-born and foreign-born populations United States, 2000. *MMWR Morb Mortal Wkly Rep* 2002;51:101.

357. Geiter L (ed): Advancing toward elimination. In: *Ending Neglect; the Elimination of Tuberculosis in the United States.* Washington, DC: National Academy Press, 2000, pp 86–121.

358. McKenna MT, McCray E, Onorato I: The epidemiology of tuberculosis among foreign-born persons in the United States, 1986-1993. *N Engl J Med* 1995;332:1071.

359. Targeted tuberculin skin testing and treatment of latent tuberculosis infection. *Am J Resp Crit Care Med* 2000;161:S221.

360. Stead W, Senner J, Reddick W, Lofgren J: Racial differences in susceptibility to infection by mycobacterium tuberculosis. *N Engl J Med* 1990;322:422.

361. Barnes PF, Cave MD: Molecular epidemiology of tuberculosis. *N Engl J Med* 2003;249:1149.

362. Smith MB, Boyars MC, Veasey S, Woods GL: Generalized tuberculosis in the acquired immune deficiency syndrome. A clinicopathologic analysis based on autopsy findings. *Arch Pathol Lab Med* 2000;124:1267.

363. Anand SS: Hypertrophic ileocaecal tuberculosis in India with a record of fifty hemicolectomies. *Ann R Coll Surg Engl* 1956;19:205.

364. Osaki M, Adachi H, Gomyo Y, et al: Detection of mycobacterial DNA in formalin-fixed, paraffin-embedded tissue specimens by duplex polymerase chain reaction: application to histopathologic diagnosis. *Mod Pathol* 1997;10:78.

365. Horsburgh CR: The pathophysiology of disseminated Mycobacterium avium complex disease in AIDS. *J Infect Dis* 1999;179:S461.

366. Klatt EC, Jensen DF, Meyer PR: Pathology of Mycobacterium avium-intracellulare infection in acquired immunodeficiency syndrome. *Hum Pathol* 1987;18:709.

367. Rotterdam H, Tsang P: Gastrointestinal disease in the immunocompromised patient. *Hum Pathol* 1994;25:1123.

368. Porrecto RP, Haverkamp AD: Brucellosis in pregnancy. *Obstet Gynecol* 1974;44:597.

369. Lubani M, Sharda DC, Helin I: Probable transmission of brucellosis from breast milk to a new born. *Trop Geogr Med* 1988;40:151.

370. Pappas G, Akritidis N, Bosilkovski M, Tsianos E: Brucellosis. *N Engl J Med* 2005;352:2325.

371. Detilleux PG, Deyoe BL, Cheville NF: Effect of endocytic and metabolic inhibitors on the internalization and intracellular growth of Brucella abortus in vero cells. *Am J Vet Res* 1991;52:1658.

372. Akhtar M, Ali A: Pathology of brucellosis: a review of 88 biopsies. *Ann Saudi Med* 1989;9:247.

373. Bojsen-Moller J: Human listeriosis: diagnostic, epidemiological and clinical studies. *Acta Pathol Microbiol Scand* 1972;229:1.

374. Kvenberg JE: Outbreaks of listeriosis/Listeria-contaminated foods. *Microbiol Sci* 1988;5:355.

375. Dalton CB, Austin CC, Sobel J, et al: An outbreak of gastroenteritis and fever due to Listeria monocytogenes in milk. *N Engl J Med* 1997;336:100.

376. Lecuit M, Vandormael-Pournin S, Lefort J, et al: A transgenic model for listeriosis: role of internalin in crossing the intestinal barrier. *Science* 2001;292:1722.

377. Relman DA, Schmidt TM, MacDermott RP, Falkow S: Identification of the uncultured bacillus of Whipple's disease. *N Engl J Med* 1992;327:293.

378. Fenollar F, Puéchal X, Raoult D: Whipple's disease. *N Engl J Med* 2007;356:55.

379. Dobbins WO, Kawanishi H: Bacillary characteristics in Whipple's disease: an electron microscopic study. *Gastroenterology* 1981;80:1468.

380. Enzinger FM, Helwig EB: Whipple's disease—review of the literature and report of 15 patients. *Virchows Arch A Pathol Anat* 1963;336:238.

381. Dobbins WO III: *Whipple's Disease.* Springfield, IL: Charles C Thomas, 1987.

382. von Herbay A, Maiwald M, Ditton HJ, Otto HF: Histology of intestinal Whipple's disease revisited. A study of 48 patients. *Virchows Arch* 1996;429:335.

383. Klipstein FA: Tropical sprue. In: Sleisenger MH, Fordtran JS (eds). *Gastrointestinal Disease,* 4th ed. Philadelphia: WB Saunders, 1989, pp 1281–1286.

384. Hellmig S, Ott S, Musfeldt M, et al: Life-threatening chronic enteritis due to colonization of the small bowel with Stenotrophomonas maltophilia. *Gastroenterology* 2005;129:706.

385. Kotiranta A, Lounatmaa K, Haspasalo M: Epidemiology and pathogenesis of Bacillus cereus infections. *Microbes Infect* 2000;2:189.

386. Kramer JM, Gilbert RJ. In: Doyle MP (ed). Bacillus cereus: *Foodborne Bacterial Pathogens.* New York: Marcel Dekker Inc, 1989, pp 21–70.

387. Andersson A, Granum PE, Rönner U: The adhesion of Bacillus cereus spores to epithelial cells might be an additional virulence mechanism. *Int J Food Microbiol* 1998;39:93.

388. Eras P, Goldskin MJ, Sherlock P: Candida infections of the gastrointestinal tract. *Medicine* 1972;51:367.

389. Wey SB, Mori M, Pfaller MA, et al: Risk factors for hospital-acquired candidemia: a matched case-control study. *Arch Intern Med* 1989;149:2349.

390. Bailey JE, Kliegman RM, Annable WL, et al: T. glabrata sepsis appearing as necrotizing enterocolitis and endophthalmitis. *Am J Dis Child* 1984;183:965.

391. Ahonen P, Myllarniemi M, Sipila I, Perheentupa J: Clinical variation of autoimmune polyendocrinopathy-candidiasis-ectodermal dystrophy (APECED) in a series of 68 patients. *N Engl J Med* 1990;322:29.

392. Walsh TJ, Merz WG: Pathologic features in the human alimentary tract associated with invasiveness of Candida tropicalis. *Am J Clin Pathol* 1986;85:497.

393. Kennedy MJ: Regulation of Candida albicans populations in the gastrointestinal tract: mechanisms and significance in GI and systemic candidiasis. *Curr Top Med Mycol* 1989;3:315.

394. Bullock WE, Wright SD: Role of adherence-promoting receptors, CR3, LFA-1, and p150,95, in binding of Histoplasma capsulatum by human macrophages. *J Exp Biol* 1987;165:195.

395. Long KH, Gomez FJ, Morris RE, Newman SL: Identification of heat shock protein 60 as the ligand on Histoplasma capsulatum that mediates binding to CD18 receptors on human macrophages. *J Immunol* 2003;170:487.

396. Zancope-Oliveira RM, Reiss E, Lott TJ, et al: Molecular cloning, characterization and expression of the M antigen of Histoplasma capsulatum. *Infect Immunol* 1999;67:1047.

397. Schafer MP, Dean GE: Cloning and sequence analysis of an H$^+$-ATPase-encoding gene from the human dimorphic pathogen Histoplasma capsulatum. *Gene* 1993;136:295.

398. Cappell MS, Mandell W, Grimes MM, et al: Gastrointestinal histoplasmosis. *Dig Dis Sci* 1988;33:353.

399. Wheat LJ, Slama TG, Zeckel ML: Histoplasmosis in the acquired immunodeficiency syndrome. *Am J Med* 1985;78:203.

400. Baker RD, Bassert DE, Ferrington E: Mucor mycosis of the digestive tract. *Arch Pathol* 1957;63:176.

401. Rocha N, Suguiama EH, Maia D, et al: Intestinal malakoplakia associated with paracoccidioidomycosis: a new association. *Histopathology* 1997;30:79.

402. Deng Z, Connor DH: Progressive disseminated penicilliosis caused by Penicillium marneffei: report of eight cases and differentiation of the causative organisms from Histoplasma capsulatum. *Am J Clin Pathol* 1985;84:323.

403. Supparatpinyo K, Khamwan C, Baosoung V, et al: Disseminated Penicillium marneffei infection in Southeast Asia. *Lancet* 1994;244:110.

404. Ko C-I, Hung C-C, Chen M-Y, et al: Endoscopic diagnosis of intestinal penicilliosis marneffei: report of three cases and review of the literature. *Gastrointest Endosc* 1999;50:111.

405. Matson DO, Estes MK: Impact of rotavirus infection at a large pediatric hospital. *J Infect Dis* 1990;162:598.

406. Reeves RR, Morrow AL, Bartlett AV, et al: Child day care increases the risk of clinic visits for acute diarrhea and diarrhea due to rotavirus. *Am J Epidemiol* 1993;137:97.

407. Morrison C, Gilson T, Nuovo GJ: Histologic distribution of fatal rotaviral infection: an immunohistochemical and reverse transcriptase in situ polymerase chain reaction analysis. *Hum Pathol* 2001;32:216.

408. Wolf JL, Dambrauskas R, Sharpe AH, Trier JS: Adherence to and penetration of the intestinal epithelium by reovirus type I in neonatal mice. *Gastroenterology* 1987;92:82.

409. Pérez-Schael I, Guntiñas MJ, Pérez M, et al: Efficacy of the rhesus rotavirus-based quadrivalent vaccine in infants and young children in Venezuela. *N Engl J Med* 1997;337:1181.

410. Centers for Disease Control and Prevention: Intussusception among recipients of rotavirus vaccine-United States, 1998-1999. *JAMA* 1999;282:52.

411. Ruiz-Palacios GM, Pérez-Schael I, Velázquez FR, et al: Safety and efficacy of an attenuated vaccine against severe gastroenteritis. *N Engl J Med* 2006;354:11.

412. Mead PS, Slutsker L, Dietz V, et al: Food-related illness and death in the United States. *Emerg Infect Dis* 1999;5:607.

413. Kapikian AZ:. The discovery of the 27nm Norwalk virus: an historic perspective. *J Infect Dis* 2000;181:S295.

414. Fankhauser RL, Monroe SS, Noel JS, et al: Epidemiologic and molecular trends of "Norwalk-like viruses" associated with outbreaks of gastroenteritis in the United States. *J Infect Dis* 2002;186:1.

415. Marionneau S, Ruvoën N, Moullac-Vaidye B, et al: Norwalk virus binds to histo-blood group antigens present on gastroepithelial cells of secretor individuals. *Gastroenterology* 2002;122:1967.

416. Schreiber DS, Blacklow NR, Trier JS: The mucosal lesion of the proximal small intestine in acute infectious nonbacterial gastroenteritis. *N Engl J Med* 1973;288:1318.

417. Blacklow NR, Greenberg HB: Viral gastroenteritis. *N Engl J Med* 1991;325:252.

418. Berho M, Torroella M, Viciana A, et al: Adenovirus enterocolitis in human small bowel transplants. *Pediatr Transpl* 1998;2:277.

419. Konno T, Suzuki H, Ishida N, et al: Astrovirus-associated epidemic gastroenteritis in Japan. *J Med Virol* 1982;9:11.

420. Esahi H, Breback K, Bennet R, et al: Astroviruses as a cause of nosocomial outbreaks of infant diarrhea. *Pediatr Infect Dis J* 1991;10:511.

421. Gray EW, Angus KW, Snodgrass DR: Ultrastructure of the small intestine in astrovirus-infected lambs. *J Gen Virol* 1980;49:71.

422. Manez R, Kusne S, Abu-Elmagd K, et al: Factors associated with recurrent cytomegalovirus disease after small bowel transplantation. *Transplant Proc* 1994;26:1422.

423. Kusne S, Mañez R, Frye B, et al: Use of DNA amplification for diagnosis of cytomegalovirus enteritis after intestinal transplantation. *Gastroenterology* 1997;112:1121.

424. Page MJ, Dreese JC, Poritz LS, Koltun WA: Cytomegalovirus enteritis. A highly lethal condition requiring early detection and intervention. *Dis Colon Rectum* 1998;41:619.

425. Chin J: Current and future dimensions of the HIV/AIDS pandemic in women and children. *Lancet* 1990;336:221.

426. World Health Organization and Centers for Disease Control: Statistics from the World Health Organization and the Centers for Disease Control. *AIDS* 1990;4:605.

427. Center for Disease Control: Update: trends in AIDS incidence, deaths, and prevalence—United States, 1996. *JAMA* 1997;277:874.

428. Cu-Urvin S, Flanigan TP, Rich JD, et al: Human immunodeficiency virus infection and acquired immunodeficiency syndrome among North American women. *Am J Med* 1996;101:316.

429. Monkemuller KE, Wilcox CM: Investigation of diarrhea in AIDS. *Can J Gastroenterol* 2000;14:933.

430. Bonfanti P, Valsecchi L, Parazzini F, et al: Incidence of adverse reactions in HIV patients treated with protease inhibitors: a cohort study. *J Acquir Immune Defic Syndr* 2000;23:236.

431. Farthing MJG, Kelly MP, Veitch AM: Recently recognised microbial enteropathies and HIV infection. *J Antimicrob Chemother* 1996;37:61.

432. Gyorkos T, Meerovitch E, Pritchard R: Estimates of intestinal parasite prevalence in 1984: report of a five year follow-up survey of provincial laboratories. *Can J Public Health* 1984;78:185.

433. Horwitz MA, Hughes JM, Craun GF: Outbreaks of waterborne disease in the United States. The Centers for Disease Control. *J Infect Dis* 1976;133:588.

434. Kean BH, William DC, Luminais SK: Epidemic of amoebiasis and giardiasis in a biased population. *Br J Vener Dis* 1979;55:375.

435. Saha TK, Ghosh TK: Invasion of small intestinal mucosa by Giardia lamblia in man. *Gastroenterology* 1977;72:4027.

436. Wolfe MS: Giardiasis. *N Engl J Med* 1978;298:319.

437. Harter L, Frost F, Grunenfelder G, et al: Giardiasis in infant and toddler swim class. *Am J Public Health* 1984;74:155.

438. Wright SG, Tomkin AM, Ridley DS: Giardiasis: clinical and therapeutic aspects. *Gut* 1977;18:343.

439. Oberhuber G, Stolte M: Giardiasis: analysis of histological changes in biopsy specimens of 80 patients. *J Clin Pathol* 1990;34:641.

440. Chester AC, MacMurray FG, Restifo MD, Mann O: Giardiasis as a chronic disease. *Dig Dis Sci* 1985;30:215.

441. Chen X-M, Keithly JS, Paya CV, LaRusso NF: Cryptosporidiosis. *N Engl J Med* 2002;346:1723.

442. Guerrant RL: Cryptosporidiosis: an emerging, highly infectious threat. *Emerg Infect Dis* 1997;3:51.

443. Mosier DA, Oberst RD: Cryptosporidiosis: a global challenge. *Ann NY Acad Sci* 2000;916:102.

444. Xiao L, Morgan UM, Fayer R, et al: Cryptosporidium systematics and implications for public health. *Parasitol Today* 2000;16:287.

445. Mackenzie WR, Hoxie NJ, Proctor ME, et al: A massive outbreak in Milwaukee of Cryptosporidium infection through the public water supply. *N Engl J Med* 1994;331:161.

446. Morbidity and Mortality Weekly Report: Outbreaks of diarrheal illness associated with Cyanobacteria (blue-green algae), Chicago and Nepal, 1989 and 1990. *MMWR Morb Mortal Wkly Rep* 1991;40:325.

447. Chen X-M, LaRusso NF: Mechanisms of attachment and internalization of Cryptosporidium parvum to biliary and intestinal epithelial cells. *Gastroenterology* 2000;118:368.

448. Siddons CA, Chapman PA, Rush BA: Evaluation of an enzyme immunoassay kit for detecting Cryptosporidium in faeces and environmental samples. *J Clin Pathol* 1992;45:479.

449. Ungar BL, Ward DJ, Fayer R, Quinn CA: Cessation of Cryptosporidium-associated diarrhea in an acquired immunodeficiency syndrome patient after treatment with hyperimmune bovine colostrum. *Gastroenterology* 1990;98:486.

450. Reisner BS, Spring J: Evaluation of a combined acid-fast-trichrome stain for detection of microsporidia and Cryptosporidium parvum. *Arch Pathol Lab Med* 2000;124:777.

451. Bryan RT, Cali A, Owen RL, Spencer HC: Microsporidia: opportunistic pathogens in patients with AIDS. *Prog Clin Parasitol* 1991;2:1.

452. Gumbo T, Sarbah S, Gangaidzo IT, et al: Intestinal parasites in patients with diarrhea and human immunodeficiency virus infection in Zimbabwe. *AIDS* 1999;13:819.

453. Kotler DP, Orenstein JM: Prevalence of intestinal microsporidiosis in HIV-infected individuals referred for gastroenterologic evaluation. *Am J Gastroenterol* 1994;89:1998.

454. Orenstein JM, Dietrich DT, Lew EA, Kotler DP: Albendazole as a treatment for intestinal and disseminated microsporidiosis due to Septata intestinalis in AIDS patients: a report of four patients. *AIDS* 1993;7:S40.

455. Schwartz DA, Sobottka I, Leitch GJ, et al: Pathology of microsporidiosis: emerging parasitic infections in patients with acquired immunodeficiency syndrome. *Arch Pathol Lab Med* 1996;120:173.

456. Molina J-M, Tournieur M, Sarfati C, et al: Fumagillin treatment of intestinal microsporidiosis. *N Engl J Med* 2002;346:1963.

457. Gunnarsson G, Hurlbut D, DeGirolami PC, et al: Multiorgan microsporidiosis: report of five cases and review. *Clin Infect Dis* 1995;21:37.

458. Ma P, Kaufman D: Isospora belli diarrheal infection in homosexual men. *AIDS Res* 1984;1:327.

459. Nahlen BL, Chu SY, Nwanyanwu OC, et al: HIV wasting syndrome in the United States. *AIDS* 1993;7:183.

460. Comin CE, Santucci M: Submicroscopic profile of Isospora belli enteritis in a patient with acquired immune deficiency syndrome. *Ultrastruct Pathol* 1994;18:473.

461. Daszak P, Ball J, Pittilo RM, Norton CC: Ultrastructural observations on caecal epithelial cells invaded by first-generation merozoites of Eimeria tenella in vivo. *Ann Trop Med Parasitol* 1993;87:359.

462. Pape JW, Verdier RI, Boncy M, et al: Cyclospora infection in adults infected with HIV—clinical manifestations, treatment and prophylaxis. *Ann Intern Med* 1994;121:654.

463. Connor B, Shlim D, Scholes J, et al: Pathologic changes in the small bowel in nine patients with diarrhea associated with a coccidia-like body. *Ann Intern Med* 1993;119:377.

464. Bundy DAP, Cooper ES, Thompson DE, et al: Epidemiology and population dynamics of Ascaris lumbricoides and Trichuris trichiura infection in the same community. *Trans R Soc Trop Med Hyg* 1987;81:987.

465. Croese J, Loukas A, Opdebeeck J, et al: Human enteric infection with canine hookworms. *Ann Intern Med* 1994;120:369.

466. Longworth DL, Weller PF: Hyperinfection syndrome with strongyloidiasis. In: Remington JS, Swartz MN (eds). *Current Clinical Topics in Infectious Diseases*. New York: McGraw-Hill, 1986, pp 1–7.

467. Milder JE, Walzer PD, Kilgore G, et al: Clinical features of Strongyloides stercoralis infection in an endemic area of the United States. *Gastroenterology* 1981;80:1481.

468. Scaglia M, Brustia R, Gatti S, et al: Autochthonous strongyloidiasis in Italy: an epidemiological and clinical review of 150 cases. *Bull Soc Pathol Exot Filiales* 1984;77:328.

469. Genta RM, Weesner R, Douce RW, et al: Strongyloidiasis in US veterans of the Vietnam and other wars. *JAMA* 1987;258:49.

470. Vazquez J, Boils P, Sola J, et al: Angiostrongyliasis in a European patient: a rare cause of gangrenous ischemic enterocolitis. *Gastroenterology* 1993;105:1544.

471. Cross JH: Intestinal capillariasis. *Clin Microbiol Rev* 1992;5:120.

472. Canals BD, Cabrera BD, Dauz U: Human intestinal capillariasis. II. Pathological features. *Acta Med Philipp* 1967;4:84.

473. Despommier DD: Tapeworm infection—the long and the short of it. *N Engl J Med* 1992;327:727.

474. Omar MS, Abu-Zeid HA, Mahfouz AA: Intestinal parasitic infections in schoolchildren of Abha (Asir), Saudi Arabia. *Acta Tropica* 1991;48:195.

475. Meyers WM, Neafie RC: Fascioliasis. In: Binford CH, Connor DH (eds). *Pathology of Tropical and Extraordinary Diseases.* Washington, DC: Armed Forces Institute of Pathology, 1976, pp 524–528.

476. Park CI, Ro JY, Kim H, Gutierrez Y: Human ectopic fascioliasis in the cecum. *Am J Surg Pathol* 1984;8:73.

477. Elmes BGT, McAdam IWJ: Helminthic abscesses: surgical complication of oesophagostomes and hookworms. *Ann Trop Med Parasitol* 1954;48:1.

478. Adams ARD, Seaton DR: Oesophagostomiasis. Presentation of a case. *Trans R Soc Trop Med Hyg* 1963;57:3.

479. Steffen R, Rickenbach M, Wilhem U, et al: Health problems after travel to developing countries. *J Infect Dis* 1987;156:84.

480. Ryan ET, Kain KC: Health advice and immunizations for travelers. *N Engl J Med* 2000;342:1716.

481. Wolfe MS: Diseases of travelers. *Clin Symp* 1984;36:1.

482. Ryan ET, Wilson ME, Kain KC: Illness after international travel. *N Engl J Med* 2002;347:505.

483. Mattila L, Siitonen A, Kyronseppa H, et al: Seasonal variation in etiology of travelers' diarrhea. *J Infect Dis* 1992;165:385.

484. Kean BH: The diarrhea of travelers to Mexico: summary of five-year study. *Ann Intern Med* 1963;59:605.

485. Rubin CE, Dobbins WO III: Peroral biopsy of the small intestine. A review of its diagnostic usefulness. *Gastroenterology* 1965;49:676.

486. Cuperus R, Shäppi MG, Shah N, et al: Hypertrophic eosinophilic gastroenteropathy is associated with reduced enterocyte apoptosis. *Histopathology* 2005;46:73.

487. Wilson ID, McClain CJ, Erlandsen SL: Ileal Paneth cells and IgA system in rats with severe zinc deficiency: an immunohistochemical and morphological study. *Histochemistry* 1980;12:457.

488. Wright NA, Pike C, Elia G: Induction of a novel epidermal growth factor secreting lineage by mucosal ulceration in human gastrointestinal stem cells. *Nature* 1990;383:82.

489. Dewar DH, Ciclitra PJ: Clinical features and diagnosis of celiac disease. *Gastroenterology* 2005;128:S19.

490. Kagnoff MF: AGA Institute medical position statement on the diagnosis and management of celiac disease. *Gastroenterology* 2006;131:1977.

491. Maki M, Mustalahti K, Kokkonen J, et al: Prevalence of celiac disease among children in Finland. *N Engl J Med* 2003;348:2517.

492. Catassi C, Ratsch IM, Fabiani E, et al: Coeliac disease in the year 2000: exploring the iceberg. *Lancet* 1994;343:200.

493. Schuppan D: Current concepts of celiac disease pathogenesis. *Gastroenterology* 2000;119:234.

494. Green PH, Shane E, Rotterdam H, et al: Significance of unsuspected celiac disease detected at endoscopy. *Gastrointest Endosc* 2000;51:60.

495. Marsh MN, Bjarnason I, Shaw J, et al: Studies of intestinal lymphoid tissue. XIV-HLA status, mucosal morphology, permeability and epithelial lymphocyte populations in first degree relatives of patients with coeliac disease. *Gut* 1990;31:32.

496. Kumar V, Rajadhyaksha M, Wortsman J: Celiac disease-associated autoimmune endocrinopathies. *Clin Diag Lab Immunol* 2001;8:678.

497. Kagnoff MF: Celiac disease: pathogenesis of a model immunogenetic disease. *J Clin Invest* 2007;117:41.

498. Ciclitra PJ, Ellis HJ: Investigation of cereal toxicity in coeliac disease. *Postgrad Med J* 1987;63:767.

499. Sjostrom H, Friis SU, Noren O, Anthonsen D: Purification and characterisation of antigenic gliadins in coeliac disease. *Clin Chim Acta* 1992;207:227.

500. Shan L, Molberg O, Parrot I, et al: Structural basis for gluten intolerance in celiac sprue. *Science* 2002;297:2275.

501. Kagnoff MF, Paterson YJ, Kumar PJ, et al: Evidence for the role of a human intestinal adenovirus in the pathogenesis of coeliac disease. *Gut* 1987;28:995.

502. Holopainen P, Naluai AT, Moodie S, et al: Candidate gene region 2q33 in European families with coeliac disease. *Tissue Antigens* 2004;63:212.

503. Greco L, Corazza G, Barbon MC, et al: Genome search in celiac disease. *Am J Hum Genet* 1998;62:669.

504. Molberg O, McAdam SN, Korner R, et al: Tissue transglutaminase selectively modifies gliadin peptides that are recognized by gut-derived T cells in celiac disease. *Nature Med* 1998;4:713.

505. Schuppan D, Dieterich W, Riecken EO: Exposing gliadin as a tasty food for lymphocytes. *Nature Med* 1998;4:666.

506. Ráki M, Tollefsen S, Molberg Ø, et al: A unique dendritic cell subset accumulates in the celiac lesion and efficiently activates gluten-reactive T cells. *Gastroenterology* 2006;131:428.

507. Oberhuber G, Schwarzenhofer M, Vogelsang H: In vitro model of the pathogenesis of celiac disease. *Dig Dis* 1998;16:341.

508. Jabri B, deSerre NP, Cellier C, et al: Selective expansion of intraepithelial lymphocytes expressing the HLA-E-specific natural killer receptor CD94 in celiac disease. *Gastroenterology* 2000;118:867.

509. Cellier C, Delabesse E, Helmer C, et al: Refractory sprue, coeliac disease and enteropathy-associated T-cell lymphoma. *Lancet* 2000;356:203.

510. Marsh MN: Studies of intestinal lymphoid tissue: XIII. Immunopathology of the evolving celiac sprue lesion. *Pathol Res Pract* 1989;185:774.

511. Hankey GL, Holmes GK: Coeliac disease in the elderly. *Gut* 1994;35:65.

512. Farrell RJ, Kelly CP: Celiac sprue. *N Engl J Med* 2002;346:180.

513. Ludvigsson JF, Montgomery SC, Ekom A: Celiac disease and risk of adverse fetal outcome: a population-based cohort study. *Gastroenterology* 2005;129:454.

514. Donaldson MR, Zone JJ, Schmidt LA, et al: Epidermal transglutaminase deposits in perilesional and uninvolved skin in patients with dermatitis herpetiformis. *J Invest Derm* 2007;127:1268.

515. Karpati S: Dermatitis herpetiformis: close to unraveling a disease. *J Dermatol Sci* 2004;34:83.

516. Abdo A, Meddings J, Swain M: Liver abnormalities in celiac disease. *Clin Gastroenterol Hepatol* 2004;2:107.

517. Kaukinen K, Halme L, Collin P, et al: Celiac disease in patients with severe liver disease: gluten-free diet may reverse hepatic failure. *Gastroenterology* 2002;122:881.

518. Sjoberg K, Eriksson KF, Bredgerg A, et al: Screening for coeliac disease in adult insulin-dependent diabetes mellitus. *J Intern Med* 1998;243:133.

519. Ventura A, Magazzù G, Greco L, et al: Duration of exposure to gluten and risk for autoimmune disorders in patients with celiac disease. *Gastroenterology* 1999;117:297.

520. Askling J, Linet M, Gridley G, et al: Cancer incidence in a population-based cohort of individuals hospitalized with celiac disease or dermatitis. *Gastroenterology* 2002;123:1428.

521. Corrao G, Corazza GR, Bagnardi V, et al: Mortality in patients with coeliac disease and their relatives: a cohort study. *Lancet* 2001;358:356.

522. Harris OD, Cooke WT, Thompson H, et al: Malignancy in adult coeliac disease and idiopathic steatorrhoea. *Am J Med* 1967;42:899.

523. Mention J-J, Ahmed MB, Begue B, et al: Interleukin 15: a key to disrupted intraepithelial lymphocyte homeostasis and lymphomagenesis in celiac disease. *Gastroenterology* 2003;125:730.

524. Frick EJ, Kralstein JR, Scarlato M, Hoover HC: Somatostatinoma of the ampulla of Vater in celiac sprue. *J Gastroint Surg* 2000;4:388.

525. Maki M: The humoral immune system in coeliac disease. *Baillieres Clin Gastroenterol* 1995;9:231.

526. Kapuscinska A, Zalewski T, Chorzelski TP, et al: Disease specificity and dynamics of changes in IgA class anti-endomysial antibodies in celiac disease. *J Pediatr Gastroenterol Nutr* 1987;6:529.

527. Uibo O, Uibo R, Kleimola V, et al: Serum IgA anti-gliadin antibodies in an adult population sample. High prevalence without celiac disease. *Dig Dis Sci* 1993;38:2034.

528. Shah VH, Rotterdam H, Kotler DP, et al: All that scallops is not celiac disease. *Gastrointest Endosc* 2000;51:717.

529. Goldstein NS, Underhill J: Morphologic features suggestive of gluten sensitivity in architecturally normal duodenal biopsy specimens. *Am J Clin Pathol* 2001;116:63.

530. Ferguson A, Murray D: Quantitation of intraepithelial lymphocytes in human jejunum. *Gut* 1971;12:988.

531. Jarvinen TT, Collin P, Rasmussen M, et al: Villous tip intraepithelial lymphocytes as markers of early-stage coeliac disease. *Scand J Gastroenterol* 1994;39:428.

532. Mino M, Lauwers GY: Role of lymphocytic immunophenotyping in the diagnosis of gluten-sensitive enteropathy with preserved villous architecture. *Am J Surg Pathol* 2003;27:1237.

533. Shaoul R, Marcon MA, Okada Y, et al: Gastric metaplasia: a frequently overlooked feature of duodenal biopsy specimens in untreated celiac disease. *J Pediatr Gastroenterol Nutr* 2000;4:397.

534. Pink IJ, Creamer B: Response to a gluten-free diet of patients with the coeliac syndrome. *Lancet* 1967;1:300.

535. Kolsteren MM, Koopman HM, Schalekamp G, Mearin ML: Health-related quality of life in children with celiac disease. *J Pediatr* 2001; 138:593.

536. Verkarre V, Romana S-P, Cellier C, et al: Recurrent partial trisomy 1q22-144 in clonal intraepithelial lymphocytes in refractory celiac sprue. *Gastroenterology* 2003;125:40.

537. Farstad IN, Johansen F-E, Vlatkovic L, et al: Heterogeneity of intraepithelial lymphocytes in refractory sprue: potential implications of CD30 expression. *Gut* 2002;51:372.

538. Enns R, Lay T, Bridges R: Use of azathioprine for nongranulomatous ulcerative jejunoileitis. *Can J Gastroenterol* 1997;11:503.

539. Parker SL, Leznoff A, Sussman GL, et al: Characteristics of patients with food-related complaints. *J Allergy Clin Immunol* 1990;86:503.

540. Walker-Smith J: Cow's milk allergy: a new understanding from immunology. *Ann Allergy Asthma Immunol* 2003;90:81.

541. Sampson H, Metcalfe D: Food allergies. *JAMA* 1992;268:2840.

542. Phillips AD, Rice SJ, France NE, Walker-Smith JA: Small intestinal intraepithelial lymphocyte levels in cow's milk protein intolerance. *Gut* 1979;20:509.

543. Cutz E, Sherman PM, Davidson GP: Enteropathies associated with protracted diarrhea of infancy: clinicopathological features, cellular and molecular mechanisms. *Pediatr Pathol Lab Med* 1997;17:335.

544. Pohl JF, Shub MD, Trevelline EE, et al: A cluster of microvillus inclusion disease in the Navajo population. *J Pediatr* 1999;134:103.

545. Sherman PM, Mitchell DJ, Cutz E: Neonatal enteropathies: defining the causes of protracted diarrhea of infancy. *J Pediatr Gastroenterol Nutr* 2004;38:16.

546. Cutz E, Rhoads JM, Drumm B, et al: Microvillous inclusion disease: an inherited defect of brush-border assembly and differentiation. *N Engl J Med* 1989;320:646.

547. Oliva M, Perman J, Saavedra J, et al: Successful intestinal transplantation for microvillus inclusion disease. *Gastroenterology* 1994;106:771.

548. Groisman GM, Ben-Izhak O, Schwersenz A, et al: The value of polyclonal carcinoembryonic antigen immunostaining in the diagnosis of microvillus inclusion disease. *Hum Pathol* 1993;24:1232.

549. Groisman GM, Amar M, Livne E: CD10: a valuable tool for the light microscopic diagnosis of microvillous inclusion disease (familial microvillous atrophy). *Am J Surg Pathol* 2002;26:902.

550. Goulet O, Kedinger M, Brousse N, et al: Intractable diarrhea of infancy with epithelial and basement membrane abnormalities. *J Pediatr* 1995;127:212.

551. Reifen RM, Cutz E, Griffiths AM, et al: Tufting enteropathy: a newly recognized clinicopathological entity associated with refractory diarrhea in infants. *J Pediatr Gastroenterol Nutr* 1994;18:379.

552. Patey N, Scoazec JY, Cuenod-Jabri B, et al: Distribution f cell adhesion molecules in infants with intestinal epithelial dysplasia (tufting enteropathy). *Gastroenterology* 1997;113:833.

553. Casis B, Fernandez-Vazquez I, Barnardos E, et al: Autoimmune enteropathy in an adult with autoimmune multisystemic involvement. *Scand J Gastroenterol* 2002;37:1012.

554. Colletti RB, Guillot AP, Rosen S, et al: Autoimmune enteropathy and nephropathy with circulating anti-epithelial cell antibodies. *J Pediatr* 1991;118:858.

555. Ishikawa S, Kobayashi I, Hamada JI, et al: Interaction of MCC2, a novel homologue of MCC tumor suppressor, with PDZ-domain protein AIE-75. *Gene* 2001;267:101.

556. Wildin RS, Smyk-Pearson S, Filipovich AH: Clinical and molecular features of the immunodysregulation, polyendocrinopathy, enteropathy, X-linked (IPEX) syndrome. *J Med Genet* 2002;39:537.

557. Ruemmele FM, Brousse N, Goulet O: Autoimmune enteropathy: molecular concepts. *Curr Opin Gastroenterol* 2004;20:587.

558. Makita S, Kanai T, Oshima S, et al: CD4+cd25 bright T cells in human intestinal lamina propria as regulatory cells. *J Immunol* 2004;173:3119.

559. Martin-Villa JM, Regueiro JR, DeJuan D, et al: T-lymphocyte dysfunctions occurring together with apical gut epithelial cell autoantibodies. *Gastroenterology* 1991;101:390.

560. Zuber J, Viguier M, Lemaitre F, et al: Severe FOXP3+ and naïve T lymphopenia in a non-IPEX form of autoimmune enteropathy combined with an immunodeficiency. *Gastroenterology* 2007;132:1694.

561. Ciccocioppo R, D'Alò S, Di Sabatino A, et al: Mechanisms of villous atrophy in autoimmune enteropathy and coeliac disease. *Clin Exp Immunol* 2002;128:88.

562. Steffen R, Wyllie R, Kay M, et al: Autoimmune enteropathy in a pediatric patient: partial response to tacrolimus therapy. *Clin Pediatr* 1997; 36:295.

563. Hori K, Fukuda Y, Tomita T, et al: Intestinal goblet cell autoantibody associated enteropathy. *J Clin Pathol* 2003;56:629.

564. Wang J, Cortina G, Wu SV, et al: Mutant neurogenin-3 in congenital malabsorptive diarrhea. *N Eng J Med* 2006;355:270.

565. Bouma M-E, Beucler I, Aggerbeck L-P, et al: Hypobetalipoproteinemia with accumulation of an apoprotein B-like protein in intestinal cells: immunoenzymatic and biochemical characterization of seven cases of Anderson's disease. *J Clin Invest* 1986;78:398.

566. Roy CC, Levy E, Green PHR, et al: Malabsorption, hypocholesterolemia and fat-filled enterocytes with increased intestinal apoprotein B: chylomicron retention disease. *Gastroenterology* 1987; 92:390.

567. Berriot-Varoqueaux N, Aggerbeck LP, Samson-Bouma ME, Wetterau JR: The role of the microsomal triglyceride transfer protein in abetalipoproteinemia. *Annu Rev Nutr* 2000;20:663.

568. Ohashi K, Ishibashi S, Osuga JI, et al: Novel mutations in the microsomal triglyceride transfer protein gene causing abetalipoproteinemia. *J Lipid Res* 2000;41:1199.

569. Joshi M, Hyams J, Treem W, Ricci A Jr: Cytoplasmic vacuolization of enterocytes: an unusual histopathologic finding in juvenile megaloblastic anemia. *Mod Pathol* 1991;4:62.

570. Bouma ME, Beucler I, Aggerbeck LP, et al: Hypobetalipoproteinemia with accumulation of an apoprotein B-like protein in intestinal cells: immunoenzymatic and biochemical characterization of seven cases of Anderson's disease. *J Clin Invest* 1986;78:398.

571. Boldrini R, Biselli R, Bosman C: Chylomicron retention disease—the role of ultrastructural examination in differential diagnosis. *Pathol Res Pract* 2001;197:753.

572. Sampson H, Metcalfe D: Food allergies. *JAMA* 1992;268:20.

573. Guarjardo JR, Plotnick LM, Fende JM, et al: Eosinophil-associated gastrointestinal disorders: a world-wide-web based registry. *J Pediatr* 2002;141:576.

574. Torgerson TR, Linane A, Moes N, et al: Severe food allergy as a variant of IPEX syndrome caused by a deletion in a noncoding region of the FOXP3 gene. *Gastroenterology* 2007;132:1703.

575. Parker SL, Leznoff A, Sussman GL, et al: Characteristics of patients with food-related complaints. *J Allergy Clin Immunol* 1990;86:503.

576. Odze RD, Bines J, Leichtner AM, et al: Allergic proctocolitis in infants: a prospective clinicopathologic biopsy study. *Hum Pathol* 1993;24:668.

577. Lee CM, Changchien CS, Chen PC, et al: Eosinophilic gastroenteritis: 10 years experience. *Am J Gastroenterol* 1993;88:70.

578. Lespi PJ, Drut R: Peritoneal rosetting microgranulomas in an incarcerated small bowel loop. *Histopathology* 1999;34:181.

579. Popovi O, Brki S, Boji P, et al: Sarcoidosis and protein losing enteropathy. *Gastroenterology* 1980;78:119.

580. Beutler SM, Fretzin DF, Jao J, Desser R: Xanthomatosis resembling scleroderma in multiple myeloma. *Arch Pathol Lab Med* 1978;102:567.

581. Stanfield JP, Hutt MSR, Tunnicliffe R: Intestinal biopsy in kwashiorkor. *Lancet* 1965;2:802.

582. Cook GC, Lee FD: The jejunum after kwashiorkor. *Lancet* 1966;2:1263.

583. Rapola J, Santavuori P, Savilahi E: Suction biopsy of rectal mucosa in the diagnosis of infantile and juvenile types of neuronal ceroid lipofuscinoses. *Hum Pathol* 1984;15:352.

584. Gersham GA, Cruickshank JA, Valentine JC: Pigmentation of the intestinal muscle in steatorrhea. *Nature* 1958;181:538.

585. Foster CS: The brown bowel syndrome: a possible smooth muscle mitochondrial myopathy. *Histopathology* 1979;3:1.

586. Bohane TD, Cutz E, Hamilton JR, et al: Acrodermatitis enteropathica, zinc, and the Paneth cell. *Gasteroenterology* 1977;73:587.

587. Danbolt N, Closs K: Acrodermatitis enteropathica. *Acta Derm Venereol (Stockh)* 1942;23:12.

588. Schaffer FM, Monteiro RC, Volanakis JE, Cooper MD: IgA deficiency. *Immunodeficiency* 1991;3:15.

589. Cunningham-Rundles C: Selective IgA deficiency. *J Pediatr Gastroenterol Nutr* 1988;7:482.

590. van Loghem E, Zegers BJ, Bast EJ, Kater L: Selective deficiency of immunoglobulin A2. *J Clin Invest* 1983;72:1918.

591. Schaffer FM, Palermos J, Zhu ZB, et al: Individuals with IgA deficiency and common variable immunodeficiency share polymorphisms of major histocompatibility complex class III genes. *Proc Natl Acad Sci USA* 1989;86:8015.

592. Atwater JS, Tomasi TB Jr: Suppressor cells and IgA deficiency. *Clin Immunol Immunopathol* 1978;9:379.

593. Buckley RH: Breakthroughs in the understanding and therapy of primary immunodeficiency. *Clin Immunol* 1994;41:665.

594. WHO Scientific Group: Primary immunodeficiency diseases: report of a WHO sponsored meeting. *Clin Exp Immunol* 1995;99:1.

595. Dawson J, Bryant MG, Bloom SR, Peters TJ: Jejunal mucosal enzyme activities, regulatory peptides and organelle pathology of the enteropathy of common variable immunodeficiency. *Gut* 1986;27:273.

596. Nijenhuis T, Klasen I, Weemaes CM, et al: Common variable immunodeficiency (CVID) in a family: an autosomal dominant mode of inheritance. *Neth J Med* 2001;59:134.

597. Kralovicova J, Hammarstrom L, Plebani A, et al: Fine-scale mapping at IGAD1 and genome-wide genetic linkage analysis implicate HLA-DQ/DR as a major susceptibility locus in selective IgA deficiency and common variable immunodeficiency. *J Immunol* 2003;170:2765.

598. De La Concha EG, Fernandez-Arquero M, Martinez A, et al: HLA class II homozygosity confers susceptibility to common variable immunodeficiency (CVID). *Clin Exp Immunol* 1999;116:516.

599. Mullighan CG, Fanning GC, Chapel HM, Welsh KI: TNF and lymphotoxin-alpha polymorphisms associated with common variable immunodeficiency: role in the pathogenesis of granulomatous disease. *J Immunol* 1997;159:6236.

600. Grimbacher B, Hutloff A, Schlesier M, et al: Homozygous loss of ICOS is associated with adult-onset common variable immunodeficiency. *Nature Immunol* 2003;4:261.

601. Groth C, Drager R, Warnatz K, et al: Impaired up-regulation of CD70 and CD86 in naive (CD27-) B cells from patients with common variable immunodeficiency (CVID). *Clin Exp Immunol* 2002;129:133.

602. Levy Y, Gupta N, Le Deist F, et al: Defect in IgV gene somatic hypermutation in common variable immuno-deficiency syndrome. *Proc Nat Acad Sci USA* 1998;95:13135.

603. North ME, Webster AD, Farrant J: Defects in proliferative responses of T cells from patients with common variable immunodeficiency on direct activation of protein kinase C. *Clin Exp Immunol* 1991;85:198.

604. Leiva LE, Zelazco M, Carniero-Sampaio, et al: Primary immunodeficiencies in Latin America; the second report of the LAGID registry. *J Clin Immunol* 2007;27:101.

605. Dawson J, Bryant MG, Bloom SR, Peters TJ: Jejunal mucosal enzyme activities, regulatory peptides and organelle pathology of the enteropathy of common variable immunodeficiency. *Gut* 1986;27:273.

606. Ament ME: Immunodeficiency syndromes and the gut. *Scand J Gastroenterol* 1985;20:127.

607. Luzi G, Zullo A, Iebba F, et al: Duodenal pathology and clinical-immunological implications in combined variable immunodeficiency patients. *Am J Gastroenterol* 2003;118.

608. Washington K, Stenzel TT, Buckley RH, Gottfried MR: Gastrointestinal pathology in patients with common variable immunodeficiency and X-linked agammaglobulinemia. *Am J Surg Pathol* 1996;20:1240.

609. Fischer A: Have we seen the last variant of severe combined immunodeficiency? *N Engl J Med* 2003;349:1789.

610. Dadi HK, Simon AJ, Roifman CM: Effect of CD3 deficiency on maturation of α/β and γ/δ T-cell lineages in severe combined immunodeficiency. *N Engl J Med* 2003;349:1821.

611. Ament ME, Ochs HD: Gastrointestinal manifestations of chronic granulomatous disease. *N Engl J Med* 1973;288:382.

612. Horan RF, Austen KF: Systemic mastocytosis: retrospective review of a decade's clinical experience at the Brigham and Women's Hospital. *J Invest Dermatol* 1991;96:5S.

613. Keller RT, Roth HP: Hyperchlorhydria and hyperhistaminemia in a patient with systemic mastocytosis. *N Engl J Med* 1979;301:465.

614. Valent P, Horny HP, Escribano L, et al: Diagnostic criteria and classification of mastocytosis: a consensus approach. *Leuk Res* 2001;25:603.

615. Grogan TB, Odom RB, Burgess JH: Graft-v-host reaction in a newborn. *Acta Derm Venereol* 1974;54:133.

616. Anderson KC, Weinstein HJ: Transfusion-associated graft-versus-host disease. *N Engl J Med* 1990;323:315.

617. Billigham RE: The biology of graft-v-host reactions. *Harvey Lect* 1966–1967;62:21.

618. Glucksburg H, Storb R, Fefar A, et al: Clinical manifestations of graft-versus-host disease in human recipients of marrow from HLA-matched sibling donors. *Transplantation* 1984;18:295.

619. Burdick JF, Vogelsang GB, Smith WJ, et al: Severe graft-versus-host disease in a liver-transplant recipient. *N Engl J Med* 1988;318:689.

620. Dolstra H, Preijers F, Van de Wiel-van Kemenade E, et al: Expansion of CD8+CD57+ T cells after allogeneic BMT is related with a low incidence of relapse and with cytomegalovirus infection. *Br J Haematol* 1995;90:300.

621. Nagata S: Apoptotic by death factor. *Cell* 1997;88:355.

622. Graze PR, Gale RP: Chronic graft-versus-host disease: a syndrome of disordered immunity. *Am J Med* 1979;66:611.

623. Cox G, Matsui S, Lo R, et al: Etiology and outcome of diarrhea after marrow transplantation: a prospective study. *Gastroenterology* 1994;107:1398.

624. Silva MR, Henne K, Sale GE: Positive identification of enterocytes by keratin antibody staining of sloughed intestinal tissue in severe GVHD. *Bone Marrow Transplant* 1993;12:35.

625. Lee E, Clouse R, Aliperti G, DeSchryver-Kecskemeti K: Small intestinal lesion resembling graft-vs-host disease. *Arch Pathol Lab Med* 1991;115:529.

626. Betzhold J, Hong R: Fatal graft-versus-host disease after a small leukocyte transfusion in a patient with lymphoma and varicella. *Pediatrics* 1978;62:63.

627. Wirt DP, Brooks EG, Vaidya S, et al: Novel T-lymphocyte population in combined immunodeficiency with features of graft-vs-host disease. *N Engl J Med* 1989;321:370.

628. Finch SC, Finch CA: Idiopathic hemochromatosis, an iron storage disease. *Medicine* 1955;34:381.

629. Feder JN, Gnirke A, Thomas W, et al: A novel MHC class I-like gene is mutated in patients with hereditary haemochromatosis. *Nat Genet* 1996;13:399.

630. Pietrangelo A: Hereditary hemochromatosis – a new look at an old disease. *N Engl J Med* 2004;350:2383.

631. Kang JY, Wu AYT, Chia JLS, et al: Clinical and ultrastructural studies in duodenal pseudomelanosis. *Gut* 1987;28:1673.

632. Gertz MA, Kyle RA, Thibodeau SN: Familial amyloidosis: a study of 52 North American-born patients examined during a 30-year period. *Mayo Clin Proc* 1992;67:428.

633. Yamada M, Hatakeyama S, Tsukagoshi H: Gastrointestinal amyloid deposition in AL (primary or myeloma-associated) and AA (secondary) amyloidosis: diagnostic value of gastric biopsy. *Hum Pathol* 1985;16:1206.

634. Isobe T, Osserman EF: Patterns for amyloidosis and their association with plasma cell dyscrasia, monoclonal immunoglobulins and Bence-Jones proteins. *N Engl J Med* 1974;290:473.

635. Gilat T, Spiro HM: Amyloidosis and the gut. *Am J Dig Dis* 1968;13:619.

636. Hemmer PR, Topazian MD, Gertz MA: Globular amyloid deposits isolated to the small bowel. A rare association with AL amyloidosis. *Am J Surg Pathol* 2007;31:141.

637. Demirhan B, Bilzikei B, Kiyici H, Boyacioglu S: Globular amyloid deposits in the wall of the gastrointestinal tract: report of six cases. *Amyloid* 2002;42.

638. Hearst J, Elliott K: Identifying the killer in cystic fibrosis. Understanding the genetic defects underlying cystic fibrosis is only half the battle. Identifying the specific bacterium infecting CF patients is just as important. *Nature Med* 1995;1:661.

639. Pier GB, Grout M, Zaidi T, et al: Salmonella typhi uses CFTR to enter intestinal epithelial cells. *Nature* 1998;393:79.

640. Collins FS: Cystic fibrosis: molecular biology and therapeutic implications. *Science* 1992;256:774.

641. Littlewood JM: Cystic fibrosis: gastrointestinal complications. *Br Med Bull* 1992;48:847.

642. Dave PB, Romeu J, Antonelli A, Eiser AR: Gastrointestinal telangiectasias. A source of bleeding in patients receiving hemodialysis. *Arch Intern Med* 1984;144:1781.

643. Viggiano TR, Gostout CJ: Portal hypertensive intestinal vasculopathy. A review of the clinical endoscopic, and histopathologic features. *Am J Gastroenterol* 1992;87:944.

644. Morini S, Caruso F, De Angelis P: Familial varices of the small and large bowel. *Endoscopy* 1993;25:188.

645. Waldmann TA, Steinfeld JL, Dtucher TF, et al: The role of the gastrointestinal system in "idiopathic hypoproteinemia." *Gastroenterology* 1961;41:197.

646. Cohen W: Intestinal lymphangiectasia. *Radiology* 1967;89:1080.

647. Galandiuk S, Fazio VW: Pneumatosis cystoides intestinalis. *Dis Colon Rectum* 1986;29:358.

648. Johnstone JM, Morson BC: Inflammatory fibroid polyp of the gastrointestinal tract. *Histopathology* 1978;2:349.

649. Willie P, Borchard F: Fibroid polyps of the intestinal tract are inflammatory-reactive proliferations of CD 34-positive cells. *Histopathology* 1998;32:498.

650. Chen TKC: Endocervicosis of the small intestine. *Int J Surg Pathol* 2002;10:65.

651. Cook DS, Williams GT: Duodenal 'pseudolipomatosis.' *Histopathology* 1998;33:394.

652. Todo S, Tzakis A, Abu-Elmagd K, et al: Clinical intestinal transplantation. *Transplant Proc* 1993;25:2195.

653. Bass B, Sayadi H, Harmon J, et al: VIP receptors and content after bowel transplantation. *J Surg Res* 1989;46:431.

654. Garcia B, Zhong R, Wijsman J, et al: Pathological changes following intestinal transplantation in the rat. *Transplant Proc* 1990;22:2469.

655. Oberhuber G, Schmid T, Thaler W, et al: Increased number of intraepithelial lymphocytes in rejected small-bowel allografts: an analysis of subpopulations involved. *Transplant Proc* 1990;22:2454.

656. Brousse N, Canioni D, Rambaud C, et al: Intestinal transplantation in children: contribution of immunohistochemistry. *Transplant Proc* 1990;22:2495.

Epithelial Tumors of the Small Intestine

GENERAL FEATURES OF SMALL INTESTINAL TUMORS

Benign and malignant small intestinal tumors are uncommon. Most small bowel malignancies are metastases from tumors arising elsewhere (1). Primary small bowel tumors constitute only 1% to 3% of all primary gastrointestinal (GI) malignancies (1–4) and <2% of all human malignancies (1). The major malignant tumors that arise in this location include adenocarcinomas, lymphomas (discussed in Chapter 18), carcinoid tumors (discussed in Chapter 17), and GI stromal tumors (discussed in Chapter 19). Data from the Surveillance, Epidemiology, and End Results (SEER) Program found that small bowel tumors had an annual average incidence rate of 9.9 per million people (5). Carcinoid tumors and adenocarcinomas were the most common histologic types with an average annual incidence rate of 3.8 and 3.7 per million people, respectively, followed by stromal tumors and lymphomas (5). The small intestine also gives rise to a number of benign lesions including Brunner gland lesions, adenomas, and a variety of polyps that are often a component of a polyposis syndrome (see Chapter 12). Table 7.1 shows the World Health Organization (WHO) classification of small intestinal tumors (6).

PROLIFERATIVE BRUNNER GLAND LESIONS

Enlarged Brunner gland lesions present endoscopically as a submucosal mass. The enlargement most commonly results from hyperplasia, although rare neoplastic lesions also develop (Fig. 7.1). Brunner gland hamartomas and true Brunner gland adenomas do exist, but adenomas are much less common than reported in the literature. The lesions generally affect older individuals and arise on the posterior wall of the duodenum. They are usually detected at the time of upper endoscopy, although they occasionally become symptomatic causing vomiting, bleeding, or obstruction. Both hamartomas and adenomas usually retain their lobular architecture (Fig. 7.1). Hamartomas have fibrous septa coursing between the hyperplastic lobules. They may be accompanied by ciliated cysts and prominent adipose tissue

(7). Prominent ducts can be seen as well. The diagnosis of Brunner gland adenomas is based on both architectural and cytologic features. There may be mild architectural distortion and the glands appear more crowded than usual (Fig. 7.2). Cytologically, the nuclei are enlarged and they may be overlapping. These neoplastic cells merge imperceptibly with more normal-appearing epithelial cells. Mitotic figures are rare. This lesion may associate with peptic duodenitis (Fig. 7.2). Rarely, Brunner gland adenomas develop atypical hyperplasia (Fig. 7.2) or undergo malignant transformation (8,9).

NONNEOPLASTIC INTESTINAL EPITHELIAL POLYPS

A number of nonneoplastic polyps develop in the small intestine, including Peutz-Jeghers polyps and juvenile polyps. These are often part of a polyposis syndrome and occasionally these polyps contain areas of malignancy. They are discussed in Chapter 12. Lymphoid polyps can also develop in the small intestine and they are discussed in Chapter 18.

INTESTINAL ADENOMAS

Small intestinal adenomas are rare, constituting <0.05% of all intestinal adenomas (10). Since most adenomas arise near the ampulla of Vater, it is postulated that carcinogens or cocarcinogens present in bile or pancreatic secretions play a role in their development. Bile salts are believed to act as tumor promotors, especially when combined with acid from the stomach (11). However, no specific dietary substance, chemical, or toxin is a demonstrated etiologic agent responsible for adenoma production. The only clear risk factor for developing small intestinal adenomas is the presence of one of the genetically inherited polyposis syndromes (see Chapter 12) or the presence of an underlying condition (Table 7.2). A rare example of fraternal sisters with adult polycystic kidney disease and ampullary adenomas also raises the possibility of a genetic link between autosomal dominant polycystic kidney disease and ampullary adenomas (12).

TABLE 7.1 World Health Organization Classification of Small Intestinal Tumors

Epithelial tumors

Adenoma
    Tubular
    Villous
    Tubulovillous
Intraepithelial neoplasia (dysplasia) associated with chronic
  inflammatory diseases
    Low-grade intraepithelial neoplasia
    High-grade intraepithelial neoplasia
Carcinoma
    Adenocarcinoma
    Mucinous adenocarcinoma
    Signet ring cell carcinoma
    Small cell carcinoma
    Squamous cell carcinoma
    Adenosquamous carcinoma
    Medullary carcinoma
    Undifferentiated carcinoma
Carcinoid (well-differentiated endocrine neoplasm)
    Gastrin cell tumor, functioning (gastrinoma) or
      nonfunctioning
    Somatostatin cell tumor
    EC-cell, serotonin-producing tumor
    L-cell, glucagonlike peptide, and PP/PYY-producing tumor
Mixed carcinoid–adenocarcinoma
Gangliocytic paraganglioma
Others

Nonepithelial tumors

Lipoma
Leiomyoma
Gastrointestinal stromal tumor
Leiomyosarcoma
Angiosarcoma
Kaposi sarcoma
Others

Malignant lymphomas

Immunoproliferative small intestinal disease (includes
  α-heavy chain disease)
Western-type B-cell lymphoma of MALT
Mantle cell lymphoma
Diffuse large B-cell lymphoma
Burkitt lymphoma
Burkitt-like/atypical Burkitt lymphoma
T-cell lymphoma
    Enteropathy associated
    Unspecified
Others

Secondary tumors

Polyps
Hyperplastic
Peutz-Jeghers
Juvenile

MALT, mucosa-associated lymphoid tissue.

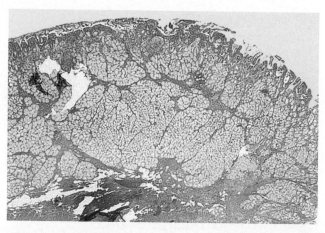

FIG. 7.1. Histologic features of hyperplastic Brunner glands. The lesion presented as a mass lesion. Note the retained lobular architecture with fibrous septa coursing through the lesion. Each of the lobules, especially the deeper ones, appears markedly expanded. The hyperplastic lobules occupy a widened submucosa and extend toward the luminal surface.

Patients with small intestinal adenomas range in age from 30 to 90 years, with a peak incidence in the 7th decade. Patients with adenomas are generally younger than those with carcinomas or adenomas containing carcinoma (13). Adenomas affect both sexes equally. Many small adenomas remain asymptomatic, only to be discovered incidentally at the time of upper endoscopy for other reasons. They may also be found in those undergoing endoscopic surveillance because they have a polyposis syndrome or have a family history of a polyposis syndrome. Large lesions become

TABLE 7.2 Conditions That Predispose Patients to Develop Small Intestinal Epithelial Neoplasms

Celiac disease
α-Chain disease
Crohn disease
Adenomas
Familial polyposis
Peutz-Jeghers syndrome
Multiple cancer syndrome (familial cancer syndrome)
Juvenile polyposis syndrome
Hereditary nonpolyposis colon cancer syndrome
Neurofibromatosis
Congenital abnormalities
    Duplications
    Heterotopic pancreas
    Meckel diverticulum
Longstanding ileostomies
Ileal pouches
Cystic fibrosis
Peptic ulcer disease
Smoking and alcohol use
Previous radiation

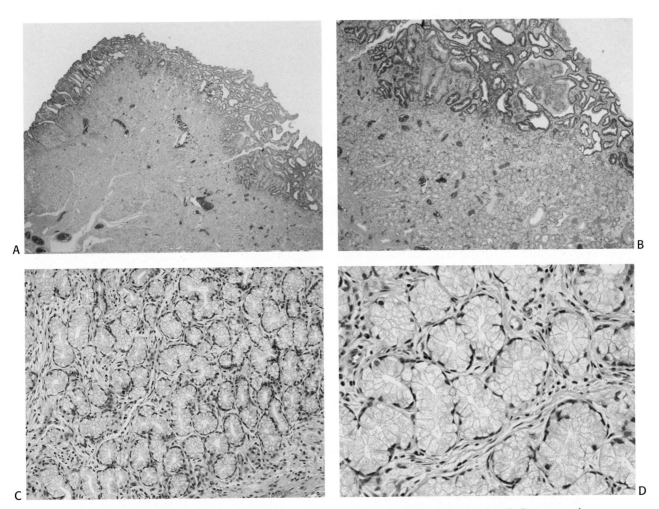

FIG. 7.2. Brunner gland adenoma. **A:** There is a large expansion of the Brunner gland epithelium. Note that the fibrous septa are lacking in some areas. **B:** The lack of the septa is more obvious in this slightly higher power picture. There is no lobulation present in this area. The overlying mucosa is affected by peptic duodenitis. **C:** Some of the glands contain cells with an increased nuclear:cytoplasmic ratio. **D:** Isolated cells lose the semilunar basal shape of the nuclei.

symptomatic. Ampullary adenomas present as biliary colic, biliary obstruction, cholangitis, jaundice, pancreatitis, and/or pain (10). Partial or total intestinal obstruction, low-grade bleeding, cramps, vomiting, nausea, anorexia, weight loss, intussusception, or hemorrhage may also develop depending on adenoma size and location. Villous adenomas tend to be larger and are more likely to become symptomatic than smaller tubular adenomas. Rare patients with secretory villous adenomas present with mucorrhea and electrolyte imbalances (14).

Adenomas appear as soft, lobulated, pedunculated or sessile, single or multiple lesions (Fig. 7.3). The mucosa may have a discolored granular appearance, but without erosions or ulcers (15). Evenness of the granularity helps distinguish adenomas from cancers. Sessile adenomas are more frequent than pedunculated ones. Tubular adenomas vary in size from 0.5 to 3 cm in maximum diameter. Villous adenomas are usually larger and may attain a size of ≥8 cm.

Large villous adenomas may encircle the bowel lumen (1) and appear as a cauliflowerlike lobulated sessile polypoid mass. Villous adenomas may also be encountered in the jejunum. The presence of multiple small intestinal adenomas suggests that the patient has a polyposis syndrome (see Chapter 12) or an underlying disorder such as Crohn disease (16).

Adenomas are benign neoplasms that display varying degrees of dysplasia. They are tubular (Fig. 7.4), tubulovillous, or villous (Fig. 7.5) in nature, resembling their colonic counterparts. Tall, immature columnar, pseudostratified epithelial cells displaying a typical "picket fence" pattern line the neoplastic tubules (Figs. 7.5 to 7.8). Goblet cells that exhibit variable degrees of differentiation lie among the immature enterocytes. Sometimes the goblet cells appear to be dystrophic as evidenced by the presence of signet ring cells. Small intestinal adenomas can also contain endocrine cells (Fig. 7.6), Paneth cells (Fig. 7.7), and squamous cells

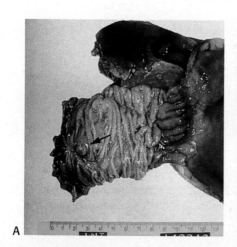
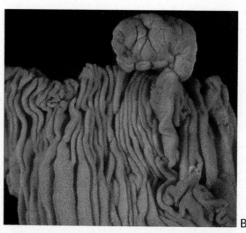

FIG. 7.3. Gross appearance of small intestinal adenomas. **A:** A semisessile polypoid adenoma arising in the second portion of the duodenum (*arrow*). The red tissue to the right of the duodenal mucosa as well as above it represents gastric mucosa that was resected at the same time. It shows severe hemorrhagic gastritis. **B:** Jejunal adenoma presenting as a discrete polypoid mass.

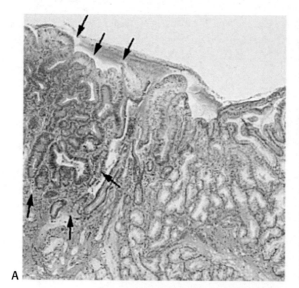
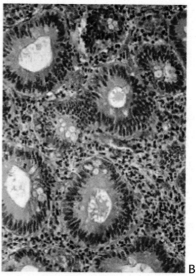

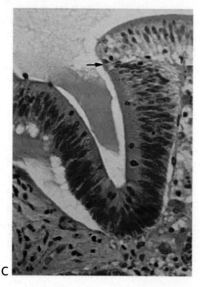

FIG. 7.4. Duodenal adenoma. **A:** Note the focal adenomatous proliferation present in the duodenum (*arrows*). **B:** Tubular adenoma. Note the presence of pseudostratified penicillate nuclei and the paucity of goblet cells. Numerous mitoses are present. **C:** Junction of immature adenomatous epithelium (*below arrow*) with normal small intestinal surface epithelium (*above arrow*). The nuclei appear pseudostratified in a way that produces the characteristic "picket-fence" pattern.

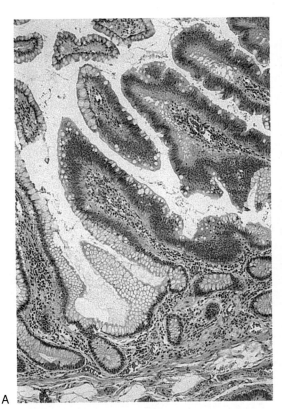
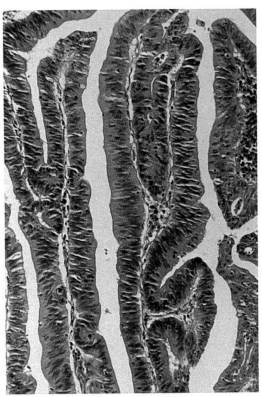

A   B

FIG. 7.5. Sessile villous adenoma. **A:** Adenomatous epithelium extends along the duodenal villi and replaces the pre-existing normal epithelium. **B:** Higher magnification of a different villous lesion demonstrating a slightly higher degree of dysplasia as evidenced by the focal loss of the normal epithelial polarity. Neoplastic cells have completely replaced the normal epithelium.

(Fig. 7.7), attesting to their origin from multipotential crypt stem cells. Paneth cells may be quite numerous, especially in patients with familial polyposis. Variable degrees of nuclear atypia affect all cell types present within adenomas, supporting the concept that each represents an inherent neoplastic component of the lesion and not entrapped normal cells. In

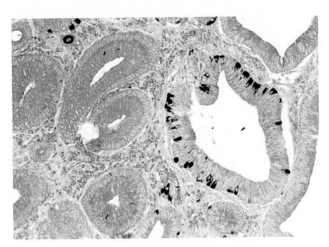

FIG. 7.6. Chromogranin immunostaining of small intestinal adenoma demonstrating the presence of numerous neuroendocrine cells (*dark brown cells*).

small lesions, the adenomatous epithelium may be confined to the surface and not involve the crypts. Normal lamina propria separates the neoplastic glands (Figs. 7.4 to 7.8).

A small villous component may be present on the surface, but most of the lesion should consist of tubules to classify it as a tubular adenoma (Fig. 7.4). Villous adenomas consist of fingerlike villous or papillary processes containing central thin cores of lamina propria lined by a neoplastic epithelium resembling that seen in tubular adenomas (Fig. 7.5). Occasionally one sees mixed tubulovillous adenomas.

A full spectrum of neoplasia can be seen in small intestinal adenomas, ranging from low-grade dysplasia to high-grade dysplasia to invasive carcinoma. The probability of finding areas of carcinoma depends on the size and location of the lesion (17). The larger the tumor, the more likely one is to find invasive cancer and the less likely one is to see residual adenoma. As the dysplasia becomes more severe, the nuclear:cytoplasmic ratio increases, epithelial polarity disappears, and the cells demonstrate increased mitotic activity (Figs. 7.8 and 7.9). The nuclei consistently approach the glandular lumens in high-grade dysplasia. Marked glandular budding with loss of nuclear polarization and variable loss of mucinous differentiation heralds the development of malignancy. If one sees severe dysplasia with unequivocal invasion into the lamina propria, with a back-to-back glandular

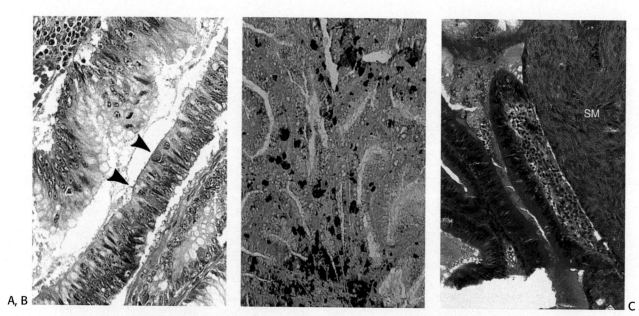

A, B

C

FIG. 7.7. Cell types in adenomas. **A:** Dysplastic Paneth cells (*arrowheads*) in this adenoma appear more eosinophilic and granular than their neighbors. The granules are larger than the smaller subnuclear eosinophilic endocrine cell granules. **B:** Lysozyme immunostain (*dark brown*) highlights the numerous Paneth cells within the lesion. **C:** Squamous morule (SM) in an adenoma. It abuts on the adjacent adenomatous epithelium. The squamous epithelium has a bland histologic appearance.

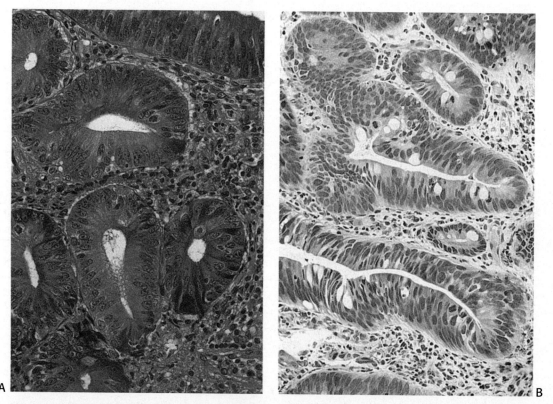

A

B

FIG. 7.8. High-grade dysplasia in a duodenal adenoma. **A:** The cells contain rounded nuclei rather than penicillate nuclei and some lose their polarity. **B:** Note the extreme stratification of the nuclei of the cells lining the glands. Some of the cells have begun to lose their normal polarity. Normal lamina propria separates the neoplastic glands.

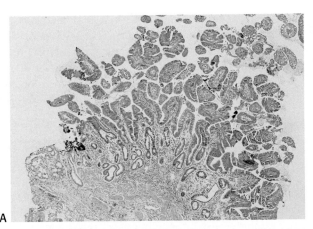 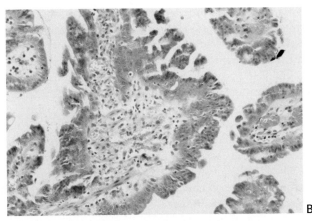

FIG. 7.9. Duodenal villous adenoma. **A:** Low magnification showing the overall architecture of the lesion. **B:** Higher magnification showing the complex surface tufting and multilayering of the epithelium that covers the lamina propria core of the villous structures. High-grade dysplasia is present but there is no invasion into the underlying lamina propria.

configuration and glandular fusion, one can make the diagnosis of intramucosal carcinoma.

SERRATED ADENOMAS

We have encountered occasional examples of serrated duodenal adenomas and there is one reported case of this lesion (18). They resemble their large intestinal counterparts. These adenomas have serrated lumens lined by eosinophilic-appearing cells that contain pseudostratified nuclei with prominent nucleoli (Fig. 7.10). Goblet cells are typically not well developed in these lesions. These lesions are too uncommon in the duodenum to comment on the implications of this histologic variant. However, we have not seen any containing either high-grade dysplasia or carcinoma.

INTERPRETATION OF BIOPSIES WITH AREAS SUSPICIOUS FOR EPITHELIAL NEOPLASIA

Typically, the initial diagnosis of a duodenal neoplasm involves interpretation of small biopsy specimens that yield only a small sample of the superficial parts of the lesion. The deeper parts of an adenoma, where an invasive tumor is most likely to develop, are often not present in the biopsy. For this reason, it is difficult to exclude the presence of an invasive cancer, especially in larger lesions. In one study of duodenal villous adenomas, biopsies missed areas of malignancy in 56% of cases, indicating the poor sensitivity of biopsies in detecting an invasive cancer (19). Generally, the best that one can do is to recognize that the lesion is neoplastic and to provide an accurate assessment of the degree of dysplasia that is present, stating whether there is invasion into the lamina

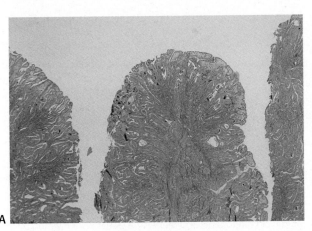 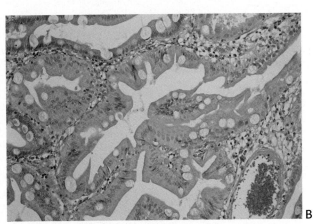

FIG. 7.10. Duodenal serrated adenoma. **A:** Low-power illustration of the lesion that, at this magnification, appears densely crowded but otherwise not unlike other duodenal adenomas. **B:** Higher magnification of the lesion discloses the characteristic eosinophilic epithelium and saw-toothed pattern of a serrated adenoma.

propria and whether one sees lymphovascular invasion or desmoplasia. One can also state whether submucosal tissue is present to be evaluated for the presence of invasion. If severe dysplasia or intramucosal carcinoma is present, consideration should be given to resection of the lesion, because it may harbor an invasive malignancy. The absence of identifiable lamina propria surrounding glands, the presence of large vessels near the tumor cells, a desmoplastic response, and an intravascular or intralymphatic invasion all support a diagnosis of invasive cancer. Tumors with high-grade dysplasia or a villous morphology are more likely to harbor an invasive carcinoma than adenomas lacking these features (19). Larger, ulcerated lesions that are fixed or cause obstruction usually contain invasive cancer.

Special caution must be applied to the evaluation of ampullary lesions because the anatomy of this area is quite complex and numerous small branched submucosal glands normally reside in this region (see Chapter 6). A significant diagnostic dilemma results when carcinoma in situ or intramucosal cancer involves these submucosal glands (Figs. 7.11 and 7.12). It is easy to confuse involvement of ampullary glands with invasive disease, and care needs to be taken not to overdiagnose invasive malignancy in this setting. If one sees a lobular glandular architecture with lamina propria surrounding the glands, invasive malignancy is unlikely. Further, if the glands are round and not angulated, the lesion

is more likely to be benign. The lack of desmoplasia also favors a benign lesion.

It is important not to mistake regenerative atypia present on the eroded surface of an adenoma for high-grade dysplasia or an invasive cancer. Areas of acute inflammation containing prominent capillaries and fibrin deposits, especially when superficial, should alert the examiner to the possibility of reparative atypia in the setting of surface erosion.

Another common area of diagnostic error is the presence of the marked reactive atypia that can be present in the duodenum, especially in the area surrounding the ampulla of Vater in patients with sclerosing papillitis (see Chapter 6). Patients who have had stents or who have had cholelithiasis may exhibit very significant ampullary inflammation, often accompanied by a marked papillary hyperplasia with significant reactive atypia. The papillary hyperplasia can appear polypoid and may even obstruct the ampulla—leading to secondary alterations in the biliary tree or pancreatic ducts. These circumstances lead to the strong clinical impression that the patient has a neoplasm. We see many cases of reactive atypia that were misdiagnosed as adenoma, often as adenoma with high-grade dysplasia. One should exercise caution in making a diagnosis of dysplasia in the presence of acute inflammation. We find that Ki-67 immunostaining can be helpful in distinguishing between a reactive and a neoplastic lesion. In reactive lesions, one usually sees a proliferative

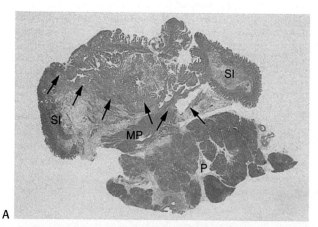

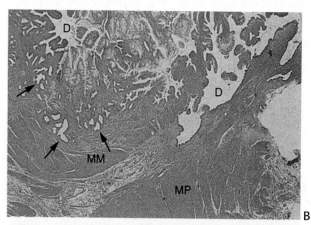

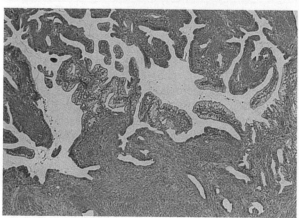

FIG. 7.11. Ampullary tumor. **A:** Whole mount section through the tumor demonstrates the relationship of the pancreas (*P*) to the muscularis propria of the duodenal wall (*MP*) and surrounding normal small intestinal mucosa (*SI*). A complex neoplasm involves the ampullary region and surface of the duodenum (*arrows*). **B:** This figure represents a higher magnification of the lesion illustrated in A. One can see residual normal-appearing ducts (*D*) as well as nonneoplastic glandular epithelium (*arrows*). In other areas, the ductal epithelium is replaced by changes that variously appear papillary, clear, hyperplastic, and dysplastic. Normal-appearing lamina propria and muscle fibers separate the various glandular components and there is no evidence of invasion by the neoplastic epithelium. The muscularis mucosa is indicated by *MM* and the muscularis by *MP*. **C:** The nonneoplastic glands display angular features easily misinterpreted as neoplastic.

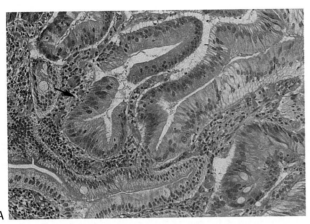
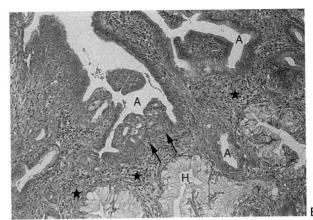

FIG. 7.12. Higher magnification of the lesion illustrated in Figure 7.11. **A:** Stratified epithelium lines the glandular spaces. The glands are separated by normal-appearing lamina propria. In some foci the epithelium appears more dysplastic than in others (*arrow*). These same glands also lack normal mucinous differentiation. **B:** This area of the tumor demonstrates areas of glandular hyperplasia (*H*) as well as foci of adenoma (*A*). One of the adenomatous glands contains an area of intramucosal carcinoma (*arrow*). Normal lamina propria separates the hyperplastic and adenomatous glands (*stars*). Note the absence of desmoplastic stroma. This neoplasm is of the hepatobiliary type.

zone that extends upward from the base of the crypt. Not all cells exhibit positive staining. In contrast, neoplastic lesions often have much stronger Ki-67 staining that is localized superficially and not in the crypt base, especially if the lesion is early. If one is unable to distinguish a reactive from a neoplastic process, a diagnosis of indefinite for dysplasia is appropriate.

MIXED HYPERPLASTIC AND ADENOMATOUS POLYPS OF GASTRIC ORIGIN

Rare polypoid lesions that contain both hyperplastic and adenomatous gastric mucosa arise in areas of heterotopic gastric mucosa. The hyperplastic foci resemble those seen in gastric hyperplastic polyps. These hyperplastic foci intermingle with adenomatous epithelium indistinguishable from small intestinal adenomas (20). The lesions are histologically identical to similar lesions arising in the stomach (see Chapter 4).

CARCINOMAS
Epidemiology

Relative to the length and surface area of the small intestine, adenocarcinomas are quite rare. It was estimated that in 2006 there were approximately 6,000 new cases of small intestinal cancer in the United States (21). Most carcinomas develop in the duodenum and their incidence is increasing slightly due to the increased use of upper endoscopy and enteroscopy. As a result, they are commonly detected early. Small intestinal

carcinomas generally present between the ages of 50 and 70 unless the patient has an underlying inflammatory condition or polyposis syndrome. The median age at presentation is approximately 55 to 67 years. However, these tumors have been described in children as young as 12 (22). The frequency of small bowel cancer roughly parallels the frequency of colon cancer among the participating registries of the International Association of Cancer Registries (23). The U.S. registries for the years 1993–1997 showed the highest rates, followed by Canada and Western Europe, with the lowest rates in Africa and East Asia. Ethnic variations in small bowel cancer in the United States constitute an interesting example of this trend. African-American small bowel cancer rates (male, 2.4; female, 1.8) are double those of U.S. Caucasians (male, 1.2; female, 0.9) and, although the differences are not as large, their large bowel rates are also higher than those of U.S. Caucasians for both sexes. A population-based study of 13 of these registries found 10,946 small bowel cancers among over 4 million first primary cancers (24). There were 4,096 small bowel carcinomas (37.4%), compared to 3,991 carcinoids (36.5%), 1,334 sarcomas (12.2%), 442 lymphomas (4%), and 1,083 unspecified (9.9%). There was a statistically significant increase in the risk of acquiring a second primary cancer. Second primary cancers of the colorectum and the hepatobiliary tree showed the strongest associations between small bowel cancer ($p = 0.01$), followed by pancreas and ovary ($p = 0.02$) and soft part sarcoma ($p = 0.06$). There were similar associations when small bowel cancer followed cancer at another primary site. When assessed by subsite, cancers proximal to the sigmoid colon showed the strongest associations with small bowel cancer. These associations have been attributed to common genetic defects in mismatch or other DNA repair pathways and to common environmental exposures.

Risk factors for small bowel cancer include dietary factors similar to those implicated in large bowel cancer, smoking (25), alcohol intake, and other medical conditions (Table 7.2) (26–28). Adenocarcinomas are four times more common in smokers than in nonsmokers (25). Small intestinal adenocarcinomas develop as sporadic lesions or they arise on a background of chronic inflammation (Crohn disease or celiac disease) or in the setting of a polyposis syndrome. Patients with familial adenomatous polyposis and its variant syndromes have a greatly increased incidence of small intestinal adenomas and carcinomas. In fact, upper GI cancer, especially involving the periampullary region, represents a major cause of death in these patients (29). Patients with hereditary nonpolyposis colon cancer (HNPCC) and germline mutations of *hMSH2* or *hMLH1* have an approximately 4% lifetime risk of small intestinal cancer, which exceeds that in the normal population 100-fold (30). The tumors tend to develop at a younger age than in other polyposis patients, often arising in the jejunum or ileum as well as in the periampullary region.

The risk of developing carcinoma in the setting of Crohn disease is increased up to 18-fold that of the general population (31). The risk of tumor development in Crohn disease may be increased by treatment with 6-mercaptopurine (32). The average age at diagnosis is 48 years and there is a male preponderance. The tumors tend to arise primarily in the ileum but also are seen in the jejunum. The risk of tumor development relates to the disease duration. The tumors are often multifocal and appear to progress through a dysplasia–carcinoma sequence.

Celiac disease also increases the incidence of small bowel adenocarcinoma but adenocarcinomas are not as frequent as enteropathy-associated lymphomas. Celiac disease–associated carcinomas account for approximately 10% of all small intestinal carcinomas (33). These adenocarcinomas predominantly affect the duodenum and upper jejunum, although occasionally they arise in the distal jejunum (34). Multiple synchronous or metachronous tumors may develop in this setting (35).

Adenocarcinomas also arise in ileostomies and ileal conduits, with the time interval between the formation of the ileostomy and carcinoma development usually involving several decades (36). Many develop in patients with inflammatory bowel disease (IBD) who had either antecedent backwash ileitis or dysplasia (36). Ileal pouches fashioned as part of the treatment of adenomatous polyposis, or ulcerative colitis, may develop adenocarcinomas, although the risk is low (37). Ileal carcinomas may also develop in the setting of abetalipoproteinemia (38). Finally, ampullary carcinomas may affect siblings without a known polyposis syndrome, suggesting a possible underlying genetic disorder (39).

Pathogenesis

Adenocarcinomas develop far less frequently in the small intestine than they do in the colon or rectum, despite the fact that the small bowel has a high cellular turnover rate and one of the largest epithelial surfaces in the body. More than 50% to 70% of small intestinal carcinomas arise in the duodenum in the periampullary region, even though it constitutes only 4% of the entire small intestine. The longest small intestinal segment, the ileum, is most resistant to tumor formation unless the patient has Crohn disease.

The preponderance of duodenal carcinomas at the ampulla of Vater may suggest that some component(s) of the biliary or pancreatic secretions play a role in their genesis. Alternatively, the constant influx of alkaline bile and/or acidic pancreatic juice may cause local cell damage. Increased mitotic activity associated with mucosal repair from injury induced by these secretions may predispose to tumor development (40).

The reasons for the relative rarity of small bowel carcinomas in contrast to colon carcinomas remain unknown, but several explanations exist (41–44).

1. The luminal contents are more liquid in the small intestine than in the large intestine and potential luminal carcinogens become diluted, leading to reduced mucosal contact.
2. Small intestinal transit time is rapid as compared to colonic transit time so that potential intraluminal carcinogens have shorter mucosal contact times.
3. The small bowel usually lacks the anaerobic bacteria present in the large bowel that are capable of converting bile salts to potential carcinogens (42). (When bacterial flora is disturbed, as in bacterial overgrowth syndromes, small intestinal carcinomas develop with a higher frequency than expected.) The antibacterial function of Paneth cells may contribute to the relative sterility of the small bowel lumen (43).
4. Large amounts of lymphoid tissue in the lamina propria, and especially in Peyer patches, provide potential intensive immunosurveillance against neoplastic cells as they develop.
5. Large amounts of small intestinal mucosal enzymes, such as benzopyrene hydroxylase, detoxify luminal contents (42).
6. The liquefied chyme induces less mechanical trauma than the harder, better formed stool in the colon.
7. Stem cells located at the crypt base lie deeper in the small intestinal mucosa than in the large intestine because of the presence of both crypts and villi in the former and therefore the stem cells do not come in as close contact with potential luminal carcinogens as do colonic crypt cells.
8. The apoptosis-suppressing protein bcl2 is not expressed in the normal small intestinal mucosa (44) so that cells affected by genotoxic damage can be eliminated by unrestrained apoptosis.

Molecular Biology of Small Intestinal Carcinomas

There is good evidence for the accumulation of molecular abnormalities during the adenoma–carcinoma progression of small intestinal tumors. These alterations involve activating mutations in oncogenes and inactivating mutations in tumor suppressor genes and share many similarities with the alterations found in colon cancers. In addition, there are a series of epigenetic changes that occur, but these are not as well characterized in small bowel tumors as they are in colon cancers. The alterations begin even before the appearance of an adenoma and increase in frequency and number as carcinomas develop and then metastasize.

The molecular features differ depending on whether the tumors arise as part of familial adenomatous polyposis, HNPCC, Peutz-Jeghers syndrome, or juvenile polyposis. Germline mutations in patients with inherited syndromes that predispose to small intestinal malignancy involve the following genes: *APC, hMSH2, hMLH1, LKB1,* and *SMAD 4* (see Chapters 12 and 14).

APC alterations (mutations and deletions) occur in patients with familial adenomatous polyposis (FAP) and sporadic tumors and in Crohn-associated tumors. *APC* and *β-catenin* alterations are common in ampullary and duodenal lesions, whereas microsatellite instability (MSI) is uncommon. *APC* mutations are present in 67% of adenomas and 50% of carcinomas of FAP patients (45); their incidence is much lower in sporadic lesions.

The mutation rate in mismatch repair genes in patients with HNPCC is 81% (46). The tumors show an MSI-high phenotype. They show a decreasing gradient from the duodenum to the ileum, reflecting the distribution of sporadic small bowel cancers (46). The MSI phenotype characteristic of HNPCC patients occurs in approximately 20% of ampullary carcinomas. This finding associates with a lower incidence of *p53* mutations and lymph node metastases and a better survival (47).

The sensitivity of each microsatellite marker is similar to that for colorectal cancer and thus, the recommended marker panel for colon cancer is also suitable for evaluation of high MSI in small bowel cancers (see Chapter 14) (46). The majority of the tumors lose immunohistochemical expression of at least one of the mismatch repair proteins (MLH1, MSH6, or MSH2). There are also commonly secondary mutations in genes containing microsatellite repeat sequences such as TGFRβ2, BAX, MSH3, or MSH6 (46–49).

K-ras mutations occur in sporadic, FAP-associated (50), and Crohn-associated (48,49,51) tumors. These occur early and do not significantly increase in the transition from adenoma to carcinoma. The incidence of *K-ras* mutations differs in ampullary tumors, depending on whether they are of the intestinal phenotype or the pancreaticobiliary phenotype. They are more common in the pancreaticobiliary type (52). Mutations also occur in the *p53* gene (53). p53 proteins are expressed in 30% of adenomas and about 50% of sporadic and Crohn-associated adenocarcinomas (49). Data on the prognostic significance of p53 immunostaining are conflicting (49).

p16 protein is overexpressed in 92% of adenomas and 91% of adenocarcinomas. The increased expression of p16 is paradoxic, since it is a tumor suppressor gene, and this finding remains to be further evaluated. There is also an increased expression of cyclin D, cyclin E, and p21 in both adenomas and carcinomas (49,54). Cyclin D1 overexpression associates with decreased survival (49). It also associates with aberrant *β*-catenin expression and *K-ras* mutation (55). Loss of the p27 protein occurs in 17% of adenomas and 23% of carcinomas. Increased expression of Her2/neu affects 60% of small bowel tumors, a finding associated with a poorer prognosis (56). *DCC* alterations, which are common in colon carcinomas, are uncommon in small intestinal carcinomas (48).

Epigenetic changes also occur in small intestinal tumors. These mainly involve methylation changes in a number of genes. Some methylation changes associate with ras mutations and others associate with high MSI (57). Thus, the MSI phenotype results from mutations in mismatch repair genes (predominantly MLH1 or MLH2) or via epigenetic silencing by hypermethylation of the MLH1 promoter. The latter tends to occur in sporadic tumors, whereas gene mutations occur in HNPCC patients. Inactivation of the gene by either mutation or hypermethylation results in loss of protein expression.

Clinical Features

The clinical features of small intestinal adenocarcinomas differ depending on the size of the lesion and its location and growth pattern. Most malignant small bowel tumors present in a nonspecific way, often resulting in a therapeutic delay. Early symptoms of ileal and jejunal tumors include vague, nonspecific abdominal pain. Later, crampy abdominal pain, nausea, vomiting, and weight loss occur. Gastrointestinal bleeding or anemia can develop. Polypoid lesions, especially those arising in the jejunum or ileum, can cause chronic, intermittent, or acute obstruction by intussusception. (Intussusception does not occur in the duodenum because its retroperitoneal location does not allow free mobility.) Intestinal obstruction resulting from mural infiltration by tumor cells or blockage of the lumen by a bulky tumor (Figs. 7.13 and 7.14) are common presentations in advanced tumors. The bowel proximal to the tumor dilates. Carcinomas may also perforate (58,59).

Duodenal tumors produce nausea, vomiting, anemia, and postprandial distress. Ampullary tumors typically cause jaundice by obstructing the common bile duct or pancreatitis by blocking the pancreatic duct (60). Ampullary tumors generally are smaller than nonampullary lesions because they tend to become symptomatic early. They may also be detected earlier than more distal tumors due to the frequent use of upper gastrointestinal endoscopy. Patients with primary small intestinal cancers have a high incidence of other cancers involving both gastrointestinal and extraintestinal sites. Most of the other primaries are colonic adenocarcinomas, but other primary sites include the prostate, female genital tract, lung, urinary tract, skin, and breast (61,62). Some of these patients will have HNPCC or FAP. The

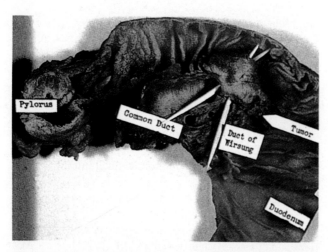

FIG. 7.13. Gross photograph of a polypoid neoplasm protruding into the duodenal lumen. The resection specimen came from a 52-year-old woman who presented with jaundice, abdominal pain, nausea, and vomiting. It shows a carcinoma of the duodenum obstructing the ductal system at the ampulla of Vater. The ducts draining into the ampulla are massively dilated. Note the dilation of the common bile duct.

presence of multiple tumors may also suggest the presence of metastatic cancer.

Gross Features

Small bowel adenocarcinomas most commonly arise in the duodenum (55.2%) followed by the jejunum (17.6%), ileum (13%), and the remainder of the small bowel (1). The location of the tumor often reflects the nature of the associated conditions. Familial adenomatous polyposis, HNPCC (46), and neurofibromatosis (63) predispose to ampullary carcinomas, whereas celiac disease and Crohn disease predispose to more distal tumors.

The gross features of the tumors reflect the site of origin, the presence of an underlying condition, and the stage of the

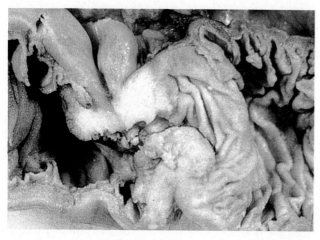

FIG. 7.14. A carcinoma occludes the ileal lumen. Bile stains the mucosa proximal to the obstructing lesion and is absent distally.

lesion. Duodenal carcinomas are typically polypoid rather than ulcerating or infiltrative in their gross appearance. If the tumor arises within the ampulla itself and is small, the duodenal mucosa may appear normal but stretched over what appears to be a submucosal mass. Jejunal and ileal tumors are typically advanced lesions that appear flat, stenosing, ulcerative, infiltrating (Fig. 7.15), or polypoid in their growth patterns. The tumors measure from 1.2 to 15 cm in greatest diameter, with the largest lesions tending to occur distally because they fail to become symptomatic early. The tumors tend to develop in areas of strictures in patients with Crohn disease, making it difficult to detect them, either at the time of the surgery or in pathology specimens, since the gross features of strictures and infiltrating carcinomas may resemble one another. This is further complicated by the fact that the development of enteritis cystica profunda may mimic a neoplasm. Patients with Crohn disease may have multiple tumors. Tumors that develop in ileal pouches and ileostomies show the features of the surgical intervention as well as the tumor.

Histologic Features

Small intestinal carcinomas develop along the same adenoma (dysplasia)–carcinoma sequence as seen in the colon. Therefore, the lesions begin as adenomas (or as areas of dysplasia in Crohn disease) that progressively increase in size and eventually develop into metastasizing carcinomas. As the tumors enlarge, the cytologic features become increasingly abnormal and the architecture becomes increasingly complex. The tumor is considered to be a carcinoma once the neoplastic cells invade into the lamina propria or through the muscularis mucosae into the underlying submucosa (6). This contrasts with colon carcinomas that require invasion into the submucosa to be diagnosed as invasive. The basis for the difference relates to the lymphatic distribution in the small bowel versus the colon. The colon lacks lymphatics in the mucosa except in the area of the muscularis mucosae (64). In contrast, the central lacteal, which is the most superficial part of the small intestinal lymphatic system, lies immediately beneath the luminal epithelium and the lymphatics richly supply the mucosa facilitating absorption of many nutrients.

Ampullary Tumors

Small intestinal carcinomas are divided into ampullary tumors and tumors arising in the remainder of the small bowel. Ampullary tumors include those arising in the duodenal mucosa, the ampulla itself, the common bile ducts, or the pancreatic ducts. In contrast, periampullary carcinomas present as tumors that show a circumferential growth pattern around the ampulla of Vater. The most difficult practical issue is deciding whether a tumor involving the ampulla is primarily ampullary or duodenal or whether it is periampullary extending into the ampulla. Occasionally, it is

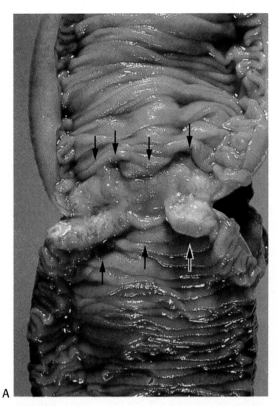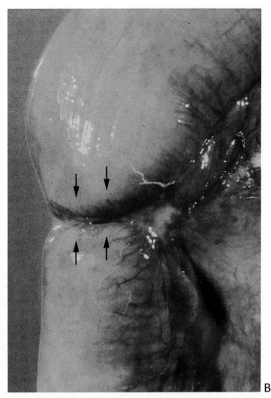

A   B

FIG. 7.15. Gross features of small intestinal cancers. **A:** Opened bowel demonstrating a napkin ring–like lesion (*arrows*). Focal ischemia is present proximally as evidenced by the reddened mucosa. **B:** The unopened specimen with evidence of extension to the serosal surface as noted by the area of indentation and prominent engorgement of the vasculature surrounding the bowel (*arrows*).

difficult to determine the exact site of origin of a cancer arising in this general area. Nonetheless, it is important to try to differentiate among these various lesions, since a significant difference exists between the 5-year survival rates of patients with ampullary carcinomas (20% to 50%) and those with pancreas cancers (15%) and bile duct cancers (17%) (1,65,66). It is also important to try to distinguish among these lesions because stage affects outcome and the staging systems are site dependent (67). Finding residual adenomatous epithelium in the duodenal mucosa allows one to diagnose a primary duodenal carcinoma with certainty. Similarly, finding residual adenomatous epithelium in the bile duct helps identify invasive biliary cancer. Pancreatic intraepithelial neoplasia accompanies both pancreatic and ampullary tumors (68).

Ampullary carcinomas differ from those arising elsewhere in the small bowel in that the ampullary epithelium shows features of the duodenal epithelium as well as that of the associated ducts. Ampullary tumors are divided into several histologic types: an *intestinal type* arising from the covering intestinal mucosa of the papillae (intestinal-type adenocarcinoma of duodenal origin) (Figs. 7.16 and 7.17), a *pancreaticobiliary type* deriving from biliary or pancreatic ductal epithelium that penetrates the duodenal muscularis propria (ampullary carcinoma of pancreatobiliary origin) (Fig. 7.18), a *mixed type* containing both types of epithelium,

and an *undifferentiated type* (69). Intestinal-type tumors outnumber pancreaticobiliary-type tumors. The age distribution and size of the two types of tumors are similar but the intestinal type has a better prognosis than the pancreaticobiliary type (69). Small adenocarcinomas of the intestinal type tend to be much less invasive than tumors of the pancreaticobiliary type. As a result, nodal metastases are much more common in pancreaticobiliary-type tumors. The intestinal type histologically resembles intestinal carcinomas elsewhere, containing a mixture of Paneth and endocrine cells; often residual adenomatous epithelium is present. Intestinal-type adenocarcinomas often develop in large bulky papillary adenomas (1). Ampullary tumors may appear poorly differentiated as they infiltrate the bowel wall but they frequently have a superficial papillary component. The pancreaticobiliary type is characterized by papillary growth with scant fibrous cores. The pancreaticobiliary type lacks Paneth cells and endocrine cells.

When the tumors are small, one may be able to distinguish between these two types of tumors on histologic grounds, but when they are large it may be impossible to distinguish between a duodenal, pancreatic, or biliary neoplasm purely on histologic grounds. However, immunostaining may be helpful (see below). Of interest, ampullary adenomas and adenocarcinomas commonly associate with concurrent pancreatic intraductal neoplasia. The latter is frequently high

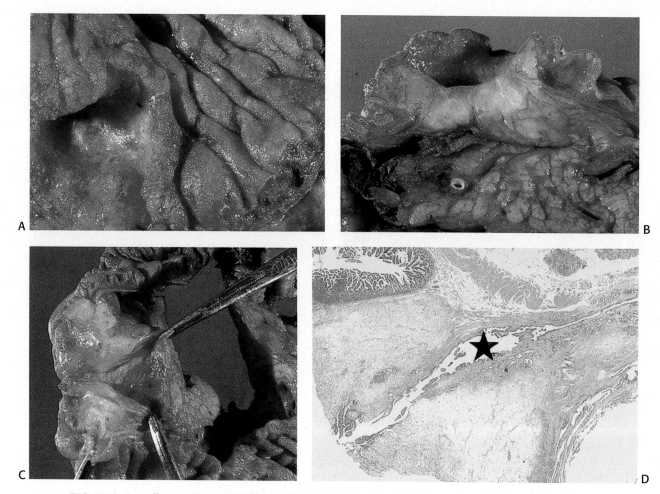

FIG. 7.16. Ampullary carcinoma. **A:** The neoplasm arises from the duodenal surface of the ampulla of Vater. Microscopically residual adenomatous epithelium is present in the heaped-up margins surrounding the ulcer crater. **B:** Cross section through the tumor showing the relationship with the underlying pancreas and pancreatic duct. **C:** Opened common bile duct showing relationship of tumor to other ampullary structures. **D:** Cross section of the common bile duct (*star*) surrounded by a signet ring cell carcinoma.

grade in nature (68). This is true whether the tumors arise in the ampulla itself or in the duodenal mucosa.

Extra-ampullary Carcinomas

Small intestinal tumors arising away from the ampulla resemble large intestinal carcinomas. Extra-ampullary tumors tend to be larger than ampullary ones and therefore the cancer more commonly overgrows the benign component so that no residual adenoma is present by the time the tumors are detected. The adenocarcinomas usually invade lymphatics and nerves and extend through the muscularis propria, often metastasizing to regional lymph nodes (70) by the time they are initially diagnosed.

Features Common to Both Intestinal Ampullary and Extra-Ampullary Tumors

Small intestinal carcinomas usually have a tubular architecture, although some tumors are papillary in nature. The glands are lined by cells with significant cellular and nuclear pleomorphism and loss of epithelial polarity. The tumors show a variable back-to-back, gland-in-gland architecture with invasion into the submucosa and adjacent normal tissues. Most small intestinal adenocarcinomas are moderately well-differentiated tumors with variable mucin production. Neoplastic endocrine cells (Fig. 7.19) and Paneth cells can be present. The tumors may also contain benign or malignant squamous cells (Fig. 7.20). The presence of squamous, endocrine, or Paneth cells has no prognostic significance.

Duodenal carcinomas may also contain areas of adenocarcinoma, squamous cell carcinoma, and small cell carcinoma admixed with one another and attesting to the origin of these various cell types from a common stem cell (71). About 20% of tumors are poorly differentiated, sometimes containing signet ring cells (Fig. 7.21). The use of immunohistochemical stains in these poorly differentiated tumors may help establish the histologic type of tumor that is present.

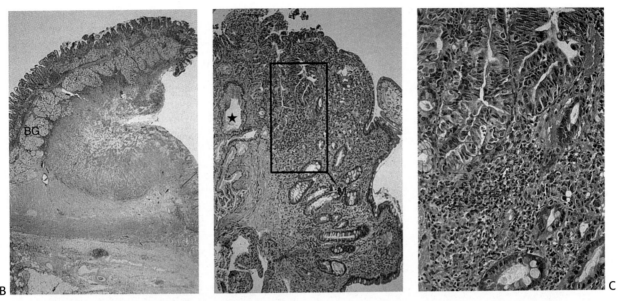

A, B ... C

FIG. 7.17. Duodenal adenocarcinoma. **A:** Moderately differentiated carcinoma invades the underlying tissues in the area of the ampulla of Vater. Parts of the tumor lie superficial to the Brunner glands (*BG*). **B:** Higher magnification of the tumor at its junction with the normal mucosa (*M*). The normal ducts in the ampulla are indicated by the *star*. **C:** The area represents a higher magnification of the area outlined by the box in B. The tumor appears moderately differentiated. Well-defined glands are present. In other areas the tumor is poorly differentiated and grows in more solid nests (*lower left*).

Immunohistochemical Features

Small intestinal adenocarcinomas usually produce carcinoembryonic antigen (CEA) (72), CDX2 (73), and villin. They are also commonly positive for cyclooxygenase-2 (COX-2), SPLA-2, and cPLA2 (74). COX-2 expression may associate with a poor outcome in resected ampullary carcinomas (75). The endocrine components of the adenocarcinomas will be positive for neuroendocrine cell markers and Paneth cells stain with antibodies to lysozyme.

CDX2 helps identify tumors of duodenal origin since this marker is specific for intestinal differentiation (73) and it is

absent in the vast majority of pancreatic and hepatobiliary tumors. Villin is also helpful in this regard, although it is sometimes produced by hepatobiliary tumors. We prefer to use CDX2 and villin to show the intestinal differentiation. However, it must be kept in mind that tumors arising in the small bowel or colon as well as those arising from areas of intestinal metaplasia in the stomach or esophagus will also be positive for these markers. However, tumors arising in the pancreas, hepatobiliary tract, lung, ovaries, and other nonintestinalized sites are generally negative when stained with these antibodies.

Adenocarcinomas in the Setting of Genetically Defined Diseases

The relative risk of developing a duodenal carcinoma in patients with FAP is >300 times that of the normal population (76) and is a major cause of death in these patients. The tumors arising in this setting usually have residual adenoma and they are frequently accompanied by additional adenomas in the second and third parts of the duodenum. These lesions are discussed further in Chapter 11.

Carcinomas also arise in the setting of HNPCC and these tumors may be the first manifestation of the disease. The median age at diagnosis is 39 years (46). The tumors range from well-differentiated to poorly differentiated lesions. The tumors may have expansile rather than infiltrating margins and a high number of peritumoral lymphocytes may be seen creating the pattern of a medullary carcinoma (46). The tumors may also have a prominent mucinous component.

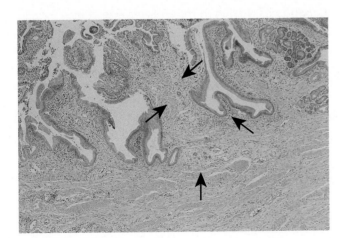

FIG. 7.18. Ampullary carcinoma of the hepatobiliary type. There is a small invasive carcinoma (*arrows*) arising from the epithelium of the ampulla.

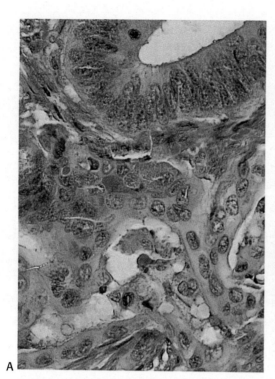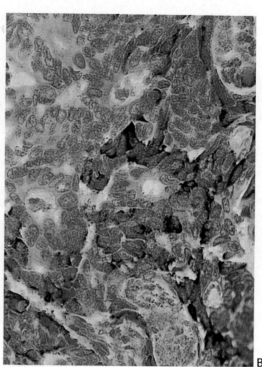

FIG. 7.19. Carcinoma-containing endocrine cells. **A:** The hematoxylin phloxine safranin–stained section shows defined glandular structures. **B:** Demonstrates numerous neurosecretory granules that stain with the Grimelius stain.

Patients are generally diagnosed with localized disease and this is reflected in the excellent overall survival (46).

Carcinomas Arising in Meckel Diverticulum

Meckel diverticulum develops numerous complications (see Chapter 6), including tumor development (77). Patients with carcinomas arising in Meckel diverticulum range in age from 13 to 52. Intermittent colicky abdominal pain represents the most common presenting symptom. Other patients experience milder, nonspecific GI complaints such as

anorexia, nausea, vomiting, and constipation. Sometimes a mass is palpable in the right lower quadrant. The tumors vary in size from 1 to >10 cm. The tumors have been described as medullary, mucinous, papillary, and anaplastic carcinomas. Sometimes they resemble gastric or pancreatic cancers because they arise in heterotopic gastric or pancreatic tissues within the diverticulum (78,79). The tumors metastasize to mesenteric and aortic lymph nodes as well as to the liver. They may also spread diffusely throughout the abdomen. Long-term survival is generally poor.

Carcinomas Arising in Heterotopic Pancreas

Pancreatic heterotopia is a common congenital small intestinal abnormality. It may exist alone or lie within a congenital abnormality such as a duplication or, more commonly, Meckel diverticulum. The full spectrum of pancreatic neoplasms may develop in this heterotopic tissue. Adenocarcinomas usually arise from the ducts and they may metastasize to regional lymph nodes. Intraductal papillary mucinous adenomas may also develop (80), as may islet cell tumors or acinar tumors, although these are very uncommon.

Unusual Histologic Variants

Adenosquamous carcinomas are uncommon small intestinal tumors. They contain both malignant glandular as well as squamous components and they resemble their large intestinal

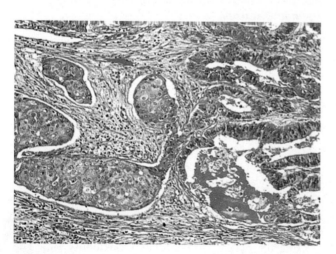

FIG. 7.20. Adenosquamous carcinoma of the small bowel.

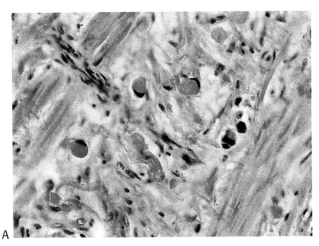
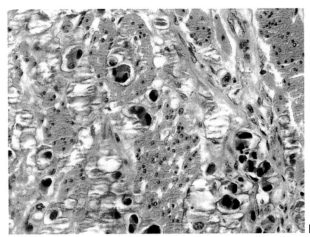

FIG. 7.21. Signet ring cell carcinoma. **A:** Histologic features of the signet ring cell tumor invading the muscularis propria. Individual neoplastic cells filled with mucin displacing the nucleus are present. **B:** Mucicarmine stain demonstrating the presence of intracytoplasmic mucin (*red*) within individual tumor cells.

counterparts. Many patients present with metastatic disease at the time of initial diagnosis (81).

Pure *squamous cell carcinomas* involving the small intestine are rare (82) and usually develop in congenital anomalies such as duplications and Meckel diverticula. They may also develop in ileoanal pouches in patients with ulcerative colitis (83). Most small bowel squamous cell carcinomas represent metastases from other sites such as the cervix or lung.

Mucinous (colloid) adenocarcinomas and *signet ring cell carcinomas* are adenocarcinoma variants characterized by prominent mucus secretion. These tumors may appear gelatinous grossly. Abundant mucus forms pools in the connective tissue. The amount of mucus required to qualify a tumor as mucinous is 50% or more. In mucinous (colloid) tumors the mucin is primarily extracellular in location; in signet ring cell carcinoma the mucin accumulation is intracellular. These tumor types, especially colloid-type tumors, are more common in patients with HNPCC and Crohn disease. Signet ring cell tumors tend to affect younger patients and are aggressive tumors.

Small intestinal carcinomas with *hepatoid differentiation* are rare and they produce unusual tumor markers such as α-fetoprotein (AFP). These tumors are usually moderately to poorly differentiated adenocarcinomas that resemble AFP-producing tumors arising in the stomach (see Chapter 5) (84,85). Histologically, the tumors consist of solid, papillary, and/or tubular proliferations. Clear cell areas can be seen. The glandular areas produce mucin and are strongly CEA-positive (84,85). Most tumor cells react with antibodies to antichymotrypsin, prealbumin, transferrin, and AFP (85). The serum of these patients contains elevated AFP levels. Occasionally, variably sized intracellular, eosinophilic, α_1-antitrypsin immunoreactive hyaline droplets are present. Bile production also occurs. Small bowel metastases from primary liver cell carcinoma or hepatoid gastric cancer should be ruled out before making a diagnosis of this extremely uncommon lesion.

Primary small intestinal *choriocarcinomas* are rare. Grossly, they appear extensively hemorrhagic and necrotic. The tumors consist of standard adenocarcinoma admixed with aggregates of uniform eosinophilic cells containing basophilic vesicular nuclei. Multinucleated syncytial cells with bizarre anaplastic nuclei and irregular cytoplasmic margins cap the more uniform smaller cytotrophoblastic cells. Cytotrophoblastic cells also intermingle with knots of multinucleated syncytial cells. Vascular invasion is common. The tumor produces both human chorionic gonadotropin (hCG) and human placental lactogen (hPL). hCG immunoreactivity is restricted to syncytiotrophoblasts and hPL positivity localizes to syncytial cells and to focal collections of cytotrophoblasts (86). This tumor is distinguished from giant cell variants of adenocarcinoma by the presence of the dual-cell population (syncytio- and cytotrophoblasts) and by its positivity for hPL. A metastasis from a primary intrauterine, ovarian, or testicular choriocarcinoma should be excluded (Fig. 7.22). The presence of adjacent adenocarcinoma or anaplastic large cell carcinoma and the absence of other germ cell elements suggest that the tumors arise from multipotential stem cells.

Sarcomatoid small intestinal carcinomas are biphasic with evidence of a spindle cell or sarcomatoid morphology admixed with areas of more conventional adenocarcinoma. The sarcomatoid areas are usually positive for both cytokeratin and vimentin and may produce mucin. These lesions may have a herringbone or storiform pattern and they may resemble unusual GI stromal tumors. The tumors may also show rhabdoid (87) or osteoclastic (88) differentiation. The prognosis of these lesions is poor. The few tumors that the authors have seen have behaved in a very aggressive fashion with prominent lymphatic involvement and metastases present at the time of diagnosis. The differential diagnosis of the lesion includes GI stromal tumors, pleomorphic carcinoma, sarcoma, and amelanotic malignant melanoma. Some tumors exhibit *neuroendocrine differentiation*. These are discussed in Chapter 17.

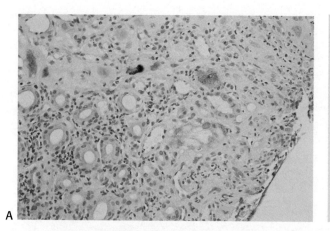
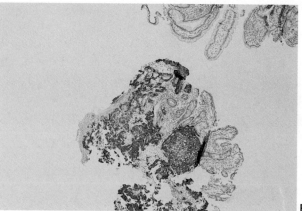

FIG. 7.22. Metastatic choriocarcinoma from the testis. **A:** Hematoxylin and eosin–stained section showing both syncytiotrophoblast and cytotrophoblast. **B:** Tumor stained with an antibody to CK7. The metastatic tumor is positive, whereas the surrounding small intestine is negative.

Staging Small Intestinal Carcinomas

The spread of small intestinal carcinomas resembles that of colonic carcinomas. Direct invasion occurs into other loops of the small bowel, stomach, colon, pancreas, omentum, mesentery, and retroperitoneum. Because lymphatic invasion is common, regional nodal metastases are frequently present. The regional lymph nodes for the duodenum are the pancreaticoduodenal, pyloric, hepatic (pericholedochal), cystic duct, hilar, and superior mesenteric nodes. The regional lymph nodes for the jejunum and ileum are the mesenteric nodes including the superior mesenteric nodes. Lesions arising in the distal ileum may also metastasize to the ileocolic nodes including the posterior cecal nodes. Hematogenous and intraperitoneal spread also commonly occurs. The staging of small intestinal tumors only applies to carcinomas and not other tumor types. The staging classifications are shown in Tables 7.3 and Table 7.4.

Prognosis

The overall prognosis of small intestinal carcinomas relates to a number of factors, including patient age, tumor location, tumor size, stage, resectability, histologic type and grade, and the presence or absence of lymphovascular invasion (22). With the exception of ampullary tumors, the prognosis of patients with small intestinal carcinoma remains uniformly poor due to the fact that patients often present late in the course of their disease and metastases are commonly present at the time of diagnosis. An exception to the generally poor prognosis of small intestinal tumors may be the cancers that arise in the setting of HNPCC because these tumors tend to be diploid and display less aggressive growth characteristics. Early carcinomas arising at the area of the ampulla of Vater have an excellent prognosis when the

TABLE 7.3 TNM Classification of Small Intestinal Tumors

TNM classification

T—Primary tumor

TX	Primary tumor cannot be assessed
T0	No evidence of primary tumor
Tis	Carcinoma in situ
T1	Tumor invades lamina propria or submucosa
T2	Tumor invades the muscularis propria
T3	Tumor invades through the muscularis propria into subserosa or into the nonperitonealized perimuscular tissue (mesentery or retroperitoneum with extension 2 cm or less)
T4	Tumor perforates visceral peritoneum or directly invades other organs or structures (includes loops of small intestine, mesentery, or retroperitoneum more than 2 cm and abdominal by way of serosa; for duodenum only, invasion of the pancreas)

N—Regional nodes

NX	Regional nodes cannot be assessed
N0	No regional node metastases
N1	Regional node metastases

M—Distant metastases

MX	Distant metastases cannot be assessed
M0	No distant metastases
M1	Distant metastases

Stage grouping

Stage	T	N	M
Stage 0	Tis	N0	M0
Stage I	T1	N0	M0
	T2	N0	M0
Stage II	T3	N0	M0
	T4	N0	M0
Stage III	Any T	N1	M0
Stage IV	Any T	Any N	M1

TABLE 7.4   TNM Classification: Ampulla of Vater

TNM classification

T—Primary tumor

TX	Primary tumor cannot be assessed
T0	No evidence of primary tumor
Tis	Carcinoma in situ
T1	Tumor limited to the ampulla of Vater or sphincter of Oddi
T2	Tumor invades the duodenal wall
T3	Tumor invades pancreas
T4	Tumor invades peripancreatic tissues or other adjacent organs or structures

N—Regional nodes

NX	Regional nodes cannot be assessed
N0	No regional node metastases
N1	Regional node metastases

M—Distant metastases

MX	Distant metastases cannot be assessed
M0	No distant metastases
M1	Distant metastases

Stage grouping

Stage 0	Tis	N0	M0
Stage I A	T1	N0	M0
Stage IB	T2	N0	M0
Stage IIA	T3	N0	M0
Stage IIB	T1, T2, T3	N1	M0
Stage III	T4	Any N	M0
Stage IV	Any T	Any N	M1

growth is confined to the wall of the ampulla or the common duct, or immediately surrounding tissues, and does not infiltrate either the lymph nodes or the pancreas (89). Patients with node-negative ampullary cancers enjoy a 5-year survival of up to 50% following radical resection (89). One of the reasons for the good prognosis of ampullary carcinomas is their more expansive rather than infiltrative growth pattern. These are less likely to show lymphatic or venous invasion than are bile duct or pancreatic carcinomas of the same stage (90,91). Today, these lesions also tend to be detected early due to the widespread use of upper endoscopy.

However, ampullary carcinomas extending beyond the sphincter of Oddi have as poor a prognosis as tumors arising in other parts of the small bowel (92). The prognosis may actually be even worse since the patients require a Whipple procedure rather than a mere intestinal resection (22). Ampullary tumors arising in the pancreas or distal bile ducts have a worse prognosis than those arising in the duodenum (93,94).

Polypoid tumors tend to have a better prognosis than infiltrative ones. Patients with well-differentiated carcinomas (90,95) or papillary lesions (92) enjoy a better prognosis than patients with moderately or poorly differentiated tumors. Tumor proliferative rate may also serve as a useful prognostic indicator. Independent adverse prognostic factors include involvement of resection margins, presence of metastases, small blood vessel invasion, and perineural infil-

tration by tumor cells (90,92,94–96). Tumors that invade into the pancreas or those with nodal metastases display a particularly poor prognosis. The median overall survival time is 20 months. The overall 5-year survival rate is 22% to 28% for adenocarcinoma (22). The prognosis is particularly poor when the mesenteric lymph nodes are involved. In a recent study, 4% of patients had stage I, 20% had stage II, 39% had stage III, and 35% had stage IV disease (22). The liver is the most common site of metastasis.

Small intestinal carcinomas recur both locally and at distant sites. The most common sites of tumor recurrence include the tumor bed, regional lymph nodes, and liver. Most recurrences become evident within 2 years of curative resection, but one also sees relapses 5 years or more following the initial surgery (97,98). Peritoneal carcinomatosis is a common recurrence pattern and associates with a very poor prognosis (99).

Treatment

Surgery remains the mainstay of treatment, but there is a significant increase in the use of adjuvant therapy in the last 5 or 6 years (99,100). Overall, only approximately 50% to 60% of patients can undergo curative resections and 50% of patients die within a year of diagnosis. Patients with peritoneal carcinomatosis are very resistant to standard chemoradiation (100). Treatment is usually palliative. However, more recently, cytoreductive surgery and intraperitoneal hyperthermic chemotherapy have become treatment options (101), and can significantly improve patient prognosis (102). Thus, the surgical pathologist may encounter multiple specimens from the cytoreductive surgical procedure. In this setting it may be impossible to recognize that the tumor arose in the small bowel rather than the appendix or colon.

SECONDARY TUMORS

Metastatic tumors and tumors extending into the duodenum from adjacent organs are the most common tumors to involve the small intestine (1). These may closely mimic primary small intestinal carcinomas both grossly and microscopically. No specific histologic features distinguish a small intestinal adenocarcinoma from other gastrointestinal carcinomas unless one sees residual adenoma. Clues for distinguishing primary from secondary tumors are listed in Table 7.5.

Tumors arising in the mesentery, pancreas, stomach, or colon spread contiguously into the small bowel. Well-differentiated pancreatic cancer grows in irregular tubular and glandular patterns. The glands are lined by cylindric to cuboidal cells that produce variable amounts of mucin. As the tumor becomes more undifferentiated, the glandular pattern becomes more bizarre, epithelial anaplasia increases, and mucin production decreases. The tumors induce a marked desmoplastic response (103) and are often associated with multiple areas of pancreatic intraepithelial neoplasia.

TABLE 7.5 Clues for Distinguishing Primary from Secondary Small Intestinal Carcinomas

Primary Cancer	Secondary Cancer
Association with adenomatous epithelium	No evidence of premalignancy
Small lesion confined to the mucosa or upper submucosa	Large lesion appearing to come from the external surface of the bowel
Radiologic evidence that the lesion is solitary	Evidence of cancer histologically identical elsewhere
	Primarily intramural mass
	Multiple lesions
	Radiologic evidence of extension from another site
	Presence of extensive lymphatic involvement

We have seen secondary cancers, especially pancreatic cancer (Fig. 7.23), induce a hyperplastic epithelial response in the duodenal mucosa that resembles premalignant changes adjacent to primary small intestinal carcinomas. Very atypical cells line the villi. The cells demonstrate cytologic features suggestive of malignancy. The cells often appear more disorderly than does adenomatous epithelium and the characteristic pseudostratified nuclei of adenomatous epithelium are absent. It is unclear whether the atypia represents an unusual hyperplastic response, transformation of the native intestinal mucosa, or pagetoid spread of the tumor.

Some types of tumors (such as ovarian carcinomas or pseudomyxoma peritonei) characteristically seed the serosal surfaces of the small bowel (Fig. 7.24). Metastases may also present as intramural masses forming submucosal nodules or plaques. These eventually bulge into the intestinal lumen producing polypoid structures or sessile lesions that can present as an acute obstruction, intussusception, or perforation. They may also ulcerate. Napkin ring–like circumferential stenotic lesions also develop, leading to localized serosal retraction and intestinal kinking. When a linitis plastica–type of infiltration of the bowel wall occurs, the metastatic malignancy simulates Crohn disease or an ischemic stricture.

Metastases from melanoma (Fig. 7.25) and carcinomas of the lung, testes, adrenal, ovary, stomach, breast, large intestine, uterus, cervix, liver (104), and kidney to the small intestine have all been reported. Of these, melanomas and ovarian tumors are the most common. Melanoma, perhaps the most common tumor to metastasize to the small intestine, accounts for approximately one third of all small intestinal metastases (105). Metastatic malignant melanomas may mimic primary GI malignancies. They may be carcinomalike, carcinoidlike,

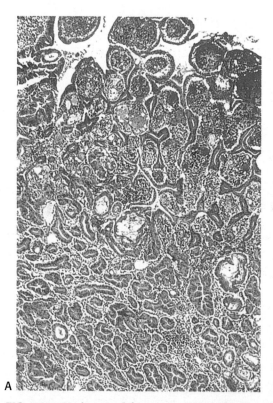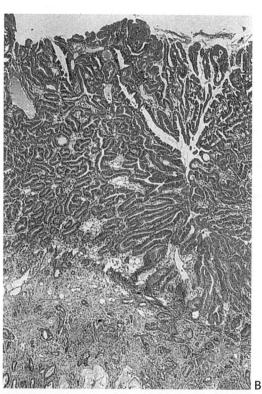

FIG. 7.23. Carcinoma of the pancreas extending into the small intestine. This case was published in the first edition of this book as primary adenocarcinoma. Subsequently, it became apparent that the patient had a pancreatic primary. **A:** The mucosa demonstrates hyperplastic features that somewhat resemble adenomatous epithelium. **B:** Carcinoma is seen dropping off the bottom of the mucosa.

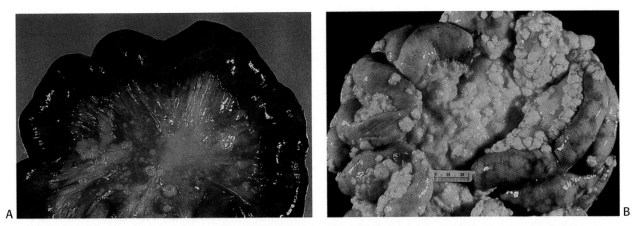

FIG. 7.24. Metastatic carcinoma to the small bowel. **A:** The metastases are clustered at the mesenteric border as well as in the mesentery itself. **B:** Multiple metastases are present throughout the mesentery as well as on the serosal surfaces of the bowel. Both patients had primary gynecologic malignancies.

or sarcomalike. The lesion may also resemble a pleomorphic neuroendocrine cell carcinoma but special stains allow one to diagnose the lesions correctly. Multiple metastatic melanotic or amelanotic lesions involve the serosal surfaces of the bowel wall. The diagnosis is generally straightforward if one has a previous history of melanoma or if the tumor cells contain melanin pigment. In amelanotic melanoma, the diagnosis may be more difficult. Tumor

color and consistency rarely indicate the primary site of the metastases, except in the case of malignant melanoma when the lesion may appear jet black (Fig. 7.25). If the metastases demonstrate a fish flesh consistency, then a lymphoma may be suspected.

Approximately 5% of testicular tumors, usually embryonal carcinomas and choriocarcinomas, involve the GI tract. These patients usually also have extensive retroperitoneal

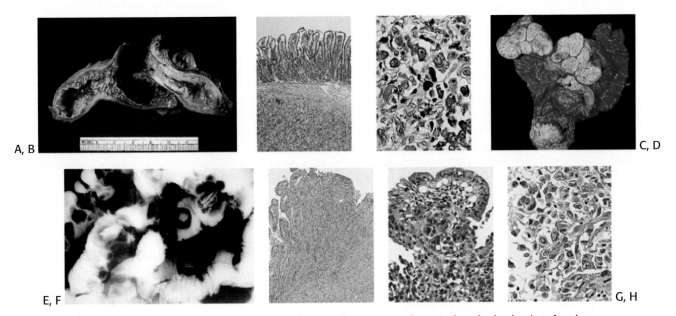

FIG. 7.25. Metastatic melanoma. **A:** Large submucosal metastases that acted as the lead point of an intussusception. **B:** Low-power examination shows the submucosal tumor. **C:** Higher magnification showing the pleomorphic pigmented cells accounting for the black gross appearance seen in A. **D:** Numerous nodules of metastatic melanoma involving mesentery and bowel wall. **E:** Single-contrast examination of the small bowel shows numerous target lesions representing ulcerated metastases from malignant melanoma. **F:** A low-power photograph demonstrating extensive replacement of the small intestinal mucosa by tumor cells. **G:** One sees diffuse involvement of the mucosa by highly pleomorphic cells, both within the lamina propria of the villous and within the lymphatic channels. **H:** A higher magnification of the tumor demonstrating the highly anaplastic appearance of the individual cells along with the prominent amphophilic cytoplasm. This tumor was positive for HMB45, negative for cytokeratin, and negative for neuroendocrine markers.

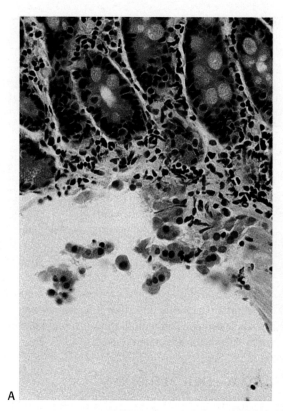

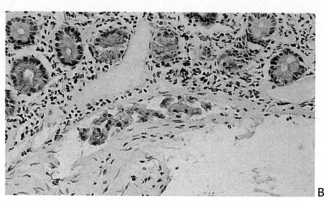

FIG. 7.26. Metastatic gastric carcinoma involving small intestinal lymphatics. **A:** Biopsy that was removed in a patient with epigastric distress. Highly atypical cells lie at the base of the mucosa in the area where the muscularis mucosae has been stripped off by the biopsy procedure. **B:** In a deeper level that was used to perform immunostains, one can see the presence of cytokeratin-positive cells within the lymphatics. The immunostain was ordered because of the atypia of the cells at the base of the mucosa seen in A. The patient subsequently was shown to have a gastric cancer.

node involvement (106). GI metastases occur via direct tumor infiltration from affected lymph nodes or via lymphatic (Fig. 7.26) or hematogenous spread. If the site is in the small intestine, the duodenum is most commonly affected.

Retrograde lymphatic metastases cause another pattern of metastasis. This occurs most often with gastric, pancreatic, or colon cancers. Subserosal lymphangitic spread appears as small nodules associated with a delicate grayish network of lymphatic channels. Colon cancers may also preferentially metastasize to the duodenum since the lymphatics from the right colon drain into the paraduodenal lymph nodes. When this occurs, the duodenal loop enlarges, ulcerates, and becomes distorted with eventual mucosal erosion.

Hematogenous spread to the small intestine occurs more commonly in tumors originating outside of the digestive tract, such as melanomas. Occasionally one sees intravenous tumor associated with areas of thrombosis, suggesting either secondary venous involvement by an intraintestinal metastasis or retrograde dissemination due to venous invasion and thrombosis of a large mesenteric vein.

Metastatic lung tumors, particularly of the spindle cell squamous cell variant, may grossly and histologically simulate a sarcoma, requiring the use of special stains to arrive at the appropriate diagnosis. Lung cancers, particularly squa-

mous cell carcinoma, appear to preferentially localize to the proximal jejunum (1). Finally, sarcomas rarely metastasize to the small bowel (1).

Use of antibodies to CDX2, villin, CK7, CK20, CEA, HAM56, HMB45, MELAN-A, and TTF-1 help separate primary small intestinal tumors from metastatic nongastrointestinal carcinomas.

HANDLING THE SPECIMENS FROM PATIENTS WITH SMALL BOWEL CARCINOMAS

Pancreaticoduodenectomy (Whipple)

Patients with invasive duodenal adenocarcinomas are often treated with a pancreaticoduodenectomy (i.e., Whipple resection: A resection of the distal stomach, duodenum, distal biliary tree, and head of pancreas). The stomach and duodenum should first be placed in a fixative, preferably formalin, to allow for deep fixation. Inserting a probe from the cut surface of the common bile duct through the biliary tree and into the duodenal lumen is not recommended. Metal probes damage and distort the lining cells of these ducts and subsequent sections will often show complete loss of the epithelial lining. Neoplasms involving the ampulla and distal bile ducts should be blocked in their entirety. Sections should be taken parallel to the long axis of the bile duct and pancreatic ducts as they enter the ampullary area. In this manner, the entire distal duct system can be followed and reconstructed, as the ducts will appear on more than one slide. In addition, the entire mucosal surface surrounding the ampulla should be examined. In many cases, residual adenomatous epithelium can be found involving the adjacent duodenal mucosa, the ampulla, or the biliary and/or pancreatic ducts.

If, on gross examination, a tumor grossly involves the serosal surface or the adjacent pancreas, sections should be taken in these areas to document the extent of local invasion. Sections should be taken of the pancreas, including the surgical line of resection, to examine the pancreatic ductal system. Carcinomas arising in the duodenum and ampulla will infrequently be associated with atypical changes within pancreatic ducts away from the ampulla, and usually not at the line of resection. In contrast, carcinomas arising in the head of the pancreas are often associated areas of pancreatic intraepithelial neoplasia. Similarly, one should examine the resected end of the common bile duct to look for atypia of the lining cells. Again, as for the pancreatic ducts, one usually will not find dysplastic or neoplastic changes in the lining cells of the common bile duct at the line of resection when the tumor originates in the duodenum. However, an invasive carcinoma that has extended from a primary site may be found in the wall of the bile duct. The connective tissue between the duodenum and pancreas should be examined carefully for lymph nodes. Adenocarcinomas arising in the duodenum or ampulla metastasize first to these pancreaticoduodenal nodes and then more distantly (1). The College of American Pathologists' suggested protocol for examining and reporting these specimens is found in reference 107.

Other Small Intestinal Resections

Carcinomas arising in the distal duodenum, jejunum, or ileum are often treated by segmental resection. The resected segment of bowel should be opened and fixed, preferably in formalin. Sections should show the relationship of the tumor to the adjacent mucosa and to the underlying serosa. If the resection margins are closer than 5 cm to the tumor, they should be examined. The mesentery should be examined for lymph nodes.

Invasive carcinomas arising in Crohn disease may also produce grossly apparent lesions that resemble other small bowel carcinomas. However, the carcinomas may also produce stenotic areas or diffuse thickening of the bowel wall, mimicking the gross appearance of the underlying Crohn disease. In this setting, the carcinomas may not be recognized at the time of surgery or even when the pathologist examines the gross specimen. In many cases, the diagnosis of carcinoma is made at the time of histologic examination.

Because carcinomas arising in intestines affected by inflammatory bowel disease may be difficult to identify by gross examination, we recommend that many sections be obtained of the resection specimens from patients with long-standing Crohn disease. Ideally, sections should be taken along the entire length of the grossly abnormal bowel, but this may not be practical, especially when long segments of bowel are involved. At least one section should be taken for every 5 cm of inflamed bowel, but in the relatively short resection specimens often obtained in Crohn disease cases, the entire length of the grossly diseased bowel should be sectioned.

REFERENCES

1. Fenoglio-Preiser CM, Perzin K, Pascal RR: *Tumors of the Large and Small Intestine, AFIP Fascicle,* 2nd Series. Washington, DC: AFIP, 1990, pp 175–187.
2. Mittal VK, Bodzin JH: Primary malignant tumors of the small bowel. *Am J Surg* 1980;140:396.
3. Treadwell TA, White RR III: Primary tumors of the small bowel. *Am J Surg* 1975;130:749.
4. Weiss NS, Yang CP: Incidence of histological types of cancer of the small intestine. *J Nat Cancer Inst* 1987;78:653.
5. Chow JS, Chen CC, Ahsan H, Neugut AI: A population-based study of the incidence of malignant small bowel tumours: SEER, 1973-1990. *Int J Epidemiol* 1996;25:722.
6. Wright NH, Howe JR, Rossini FP, et al: Carcinoma of the small intestine. In: Hamilton SR, Aaltonen J (eds). *Pathology and Genetics of Tumors of the Digestive System, World Health Organization Classification of Tumors.* Lyon, France: IARC Press, 2000, pp 71–76.
7. Chatelain D, Maillet E, Boyer L, et al: Brunner gland hamartomas with predominant adipose tissue and ciliated cysts. *Arch Pathol Lab Med* 2002;126:734.
8. Zanetti G, Casadei G: Brunner's gland hamartoma with incipient ductal malignancy. Report of a case. *Tumori* 1981;67:75.
9. Cortese AF, McDivitt RW: Carcinoma of the duodenum arising in Brunner's glands. *NY State J Med* 1973;73:1687.
10. Perzin KH, Bridge MF: Adenomas of the small intestine: a clinicopathologic review of 51 cases and a study of their relationship to carcinoma. *Cancer* 1981;48:799.
11. Scates DK, Spigelman AD, Phillips RK, Venitt S: DNA adducts detected by 32P-postlabelling, in the intestine of rats given bile from patients with familial adenomatous polyposis and from unaffected controls. *Carcinogenesis* 1992;13:731.
12. Norton ID, Pokorny CS, Painter DM, et al: Fraternal sisters with adult polycystic kidney disease and adenoma of the ampulla of Vater. *Gastroenterology* 1995;109:2007.
13. Sellner F: Investigations on the significance of the adenoma-carcinoma sequence in the small bowel. *Cancer* 1990;66:702.
14. Reddy RR, Schuman BM, Priest RJ: Duodenal polyps: diagnosis and management. *J Clin Gastroenterol* 1981;3:139.
15. Kim MH, Lee SK, Seo DW, et al: Tumors of the major duodenal papilla. *Gastrointest Endosc* 2001;54:609.
16. Burt RW, Berenson MM, Lee RG, et al: Upper gastrointestinal polyps in Gardner's syndrome. *Gastroenterology* 1984;86:295.
17. Baczako K, Buchler M, Beger HG, et al: Morphogenesis and possible precursor lesions of invasive carcinoma of the papilla of Vater: epithelial dysplasia and adenoma. *Hum Pathol* 1985;16:305.
18. Rubio CA: Serrated adenoma of the duodenum. *J Clin Pathol* 2004;57:1219.
19. Attanoos R, Williams GT: Epithelial and neuroendocrine tumors of the duodenum. *Semin Diagn Pathol* 1991;8:149.
20. Russin V, Krevsky B, Caroline DF, et al: Mixed hyperplastic and adenomatous polyp arising from ectopic gastric mucosa of the duodenum. *Arch Pathol Lab Med* 1986;110:556.
21. Jemal A, Siegel R, Ward E, et al: Cancer statistics, 2006. *CA Cancer J Clin* 2006;56:106.

22. Dabaja BS, Suki D, Pro B, et al: Adenocarcinoma of the small bowel: presentation, prognostic factors, and outcome of 217 patients. *Cancer* 2004;101:518.

23. Parkin DM, Whelan SL, Ferlay J, et al: *Cancer Incidence in Five Continents.* Vol. VIII. Lyons, France: IARC, 2002, pp 549–551.

24. Scelo G, Boffeta P, Hemminki K, et al: Associations between small intestine cancer and other primary cancers: an international population-based study. *Int J Cancer* 2006;118:189.

25. Chen CC, Neugut AI, Rotterdam H: Risk factors for adenocarcinomas and malignant carcinoids of the small intestine: preliminary findings. *Cancer Epidemiol Biomarkers Prev* 1994;3:205.

26. Selby WS, Gallagher ND: Malignancy in a 19-year experience of adult coeliac disease. *Dig Dis Sci* 1979;24:684.

27. Neugut AI, Jacobson JS, Suh S, et al: The epidemiology of cancer of the small bowel. *Cancer Epidemiol Biomarkers Prev* 1998;7:243.

28. Heiskanen I, Kellokumpu I, Jarvinen H: Management of duodenal adenomas in 98 patients with familial adenomatous polyposis. *Endoscopy* 1999;31:412.

29. Pauli RM, Pauli ME, Hall JG: Gardner syndrome and periampullary malignancy. *Am J Med Genet* 1980;6:205.

30. Vasen HF, Wijinen JT, Menko FH, et al: Cancer risk in families with hereditary nonpolyposis colorectal cancer diagnosed by mutation analysis. *Gastroenterology* 1996;110:1020.

31. Gillen CD, Andrews HA, Prior P, Allan RN: Crohn's disease and colorectal cancer. *Gut* 1994;35:651.

32. Lashner BA: Risk factors for small bowel cancer in Crohn's disease. *Dig Dis Sci* 1992;37:1179.

33. Bruno CJ, Batts KP, Ahlquist DA: Evidence against flat dysplasia as a regional field defect in small bowel adenocarcinoma associated with celiac sprue. *Mayo Clin Proc* 1997;72:320.

34. Nielsen SNJ, Wold LE: Adenocarcinoma of jejunum in association with nontropical sprue. *Arch Pathol Lab Med* 1986;110:822.

35. Begos DG, Kuan S, Dobbins J, Ravikumar TS: Metachronous small bowel adenocarcinoma in celiac sprue. *J Clin Gastroenterol* 1995;20:233.

36. Roberts PL, Veidenheimer MC, Cassidy S, Silverman ML: Adenocarcinoma arising in an ileostomy. *Arch Surg* 1989;124:497.

37. Borjesson L, Willen R, Haboubi R, et al: The risk of dysplasia and cancer in the ileal pouch mucosa after restorative protocolectomy for ulcerative proctocolitis is low: a long term follow-up study. *Colorectal Dis* 2004;6:494.

38. Al-Shali K, Wang J, Rosen F, et al: Ileal adenocarcinoma in a mild phenotype of abetalipoproteinemia. *Clin Genet* 2003;63:135.

39. Austin JC, Organ CH, Williams GR: Vaterian cancer in siblings. *Ann Surg* 1988;207:655.

40. Ross RK, Harnett NM, Bernstein L, Henderson BE: Epidemiology of adenocarcinomas of the small intestine: is bile a small bowel carcinogen? *Br J Cancer* 1991;63:143.

41. Lowenfeld AB: Why are small bowel tumors so rare? *Lancet* 1973;1:24.

42. Wattenberg LW: Studies of polycyclic hydrocarbon hydroxylase of the intestine possibly related to cancer. *Cancer* 1971;28:99.

43. Salzman NH, Chou MM, de Jong H, et al: Protection against salmonellosis in transgenic mice expressing human intestinal defensin. *Nature* 2003;422:478.

44. Potten CS: Stem cells in gastrointestinal epithelium: numbers, characteristics and death. *Philos Trans R Soc Lond B Biol Sci* 1998;353:821.

45. Toyooka M, Konishi M, Kikuchi-Yanoshita R, et al: Somatic mutations of the adenomatous polyposis coli gene in gastroduodenal tumors from patients with familial adenomatous polyposis. *Cancer Res* 1995;55:3165.

46. Schulmann K, Brasch FE, Kunstmann E, et al: The German HNPCC Consortium. HNPCC-associated small bowel cancer: clinical and molecular characteristics. *Gastroenterology* 2005;128:590.

47. Achille A, Baron A, Zamboni G, et al: Molecular pathogenesis of sporadic duodenal cancer. *Br J Cancer* 1998;77:760.

48. Rashid A, Hamilton SR: Genetic alterations in sporadic and Crohn's-associated adenocarcinomas of the small intestine. *Gastroenterology* 1997;113:127.

49. Arber N, Hibshoosh H, Yasui W, et al: Abnormalities in the expression of cell cycle-related proteins in tumors of the small bowel. *Cancer Epidemiol Biomarkers Prev* 1999;8:1101.

50. Scarpa A, Zamboni G, Achille A, et al: ras-Family gene mutations in neoplasia of the ampulla of Vater. *Exp Biol Med* 1994;59:39.

51. Arber N, Shapira I, Ratan J, et al: Activation of c-K-ras mutations in human gastrointestinal tumors. *Gastroenterology* 2000;118:1045.

52. Matsubayashi H, Watanabe H, Yamaguchi T, et al: Differences in mucus and K-ras mutation in relation to phenotypes of tumors of the papilla of Vater. *Cancer* 1999;86:596.

53. Scarpa A, Capelli P, Zamboni G, et al: Neoplasia of the ampulla of Vater. *Am J Pathol* 1993;142:1163.

54. Takashima M, Ueki T, Nagai E, et al: Carcinoma of the ampulla of Vater associated with or without adenoma: a clinicopathologic analysis of 198 cases with reference to p53 and Ki-67 immunohistochemical expressions. *Mod Pathol* 2000;13:1300.

55. Yamazaki K, Hanami K, Nagao T, et al: Increased cyclin D1 expression in cancer of the ampulla of Vater: relevance to nuclear beta catenin accumulation and k-ras gene mutation. *Mol Pathol* 2003;56:336.

56. Zhu L, Kim K, Domenico DR, et al: Adenocarcinoma of duodenum and ampulla of Vater: clinicopathology study and expression of p53, c-neu, TGF-alpha, CEA, and EMA. *J Surg Oncol* 1996;61:100.

57. Kim SG, Chan AO, Wu TT, et al: Epigenetic and genetic alterations in duodenal carcinomas are distinct from biliary and ampullary carcinomas. *Gastroenterology* 2003;124:1300.

58. Ostermiller W, Joergenson EJ, Weibel L: A clinical review of tumors of the small bowel. *Am J Surg* 1966;111:403.

59. Darling RC, Welch CE: Tumors of the small intestine. *N Engl J Med* 1959;260:397.

60. Burt RW, Rikkers LF, Gardner EJ, et al: Villous adenoma of the duodenal papilla presenting as necrotizing pancreatitis in a patient with Gardner's syndrome. *Gastroenterology* 1987;92:532.

61. Ripley D, Weinerman BH: Increased incidence of second malignancies associated with small bowel adenocarcinoma. *Can J Gastroenterol* 1997;11:65.

62. Stemmermann GN, Goodman MT, Nomura AMY: Adenocarcinoma of the proximal small intestine—a marker for familial and multicentric cancer. *Cancer* 1992;70:2766.

63. Costi R, Caruana P, Sarli L, et al: Ampullary adenocarcinoma in neurofibromatosis type 1. Case report and literature review. *Mod Pathol,* 2001;14:1169.

64. Fenoglio CM, Kaye GI, Lane N: Distribution of human colonic lymphatics in normal, hyperplastic and adenomatous tissue. Its relationship to metastasis from small carcinomas in pedunculated adenomas with two case reports. *Gastroenterology* 1973;64:926.

65. Yeo CJ, Sohn TA, Cameron JL, et al: Periampullary adenocarcinoma: analysis of 5-year survivors. *Ann Surg* 1998;227:821.

66. Howe JR, Klimstra DS, Moccia RD, et al: Factors predictive of survival in ampullary carcinoma. *Ann Surg* 1998;228:87.

67. Sobin LH, Wittekind CH (eds). *TNM Classification of Malignant Tumors,* 6th ed. New York: Wiley, 2002, pp 69–71, 90–92.

68. Agoff SN, Crispin DA, Bronner MP, et al: Neoplasms of the ampulla of Vater with concurrent pancreatic intraductal neoplasia: a histological and molecular study. *Mod Pathol* 2001;14:139.

69. Kimura W, Futakawa N, Yamagata S, et al: Different clinicopathologic findings in two histologic types of carcinoma of papilla of Vater. *Jpn J Cancer Res* 1994;85:161.

70. Bridge MF, Perzin KH: Primary adenocarcinoma of the jejunum and ileum. A clinicopathologic study. *Cancer* 1975;36:1876.

71. Barnhill M, Hess E, Guccion JG, et al: Tripartite differentiation in a carcinoma of the duodenum. *Cancer* 1994;73:266.

72. Blackman E, Nash SV: Diagnosis of duodenal and ampullary epithelial neoplasms by endoscopic biopsy. A clinicopathological and immunohistochemical study. *Hum Pathol* 1985;16:901.

73. Werling RW, Yaziji H, Bacchi CE, Gown AM: CDX2, a highly sensitive and specific marker of adenocarcinomas of intestinal origin: an immunohistochemical survey of 476 primary and metastatic carcinomas. *Am J Surg Pathol* 2003;27:303.

74. Wendum D, Svrcek M, Rigau NV, et al: COX-2, inflammatory secreted PLA2 and cytoplasmic PL2 protein expression in small bowel adenocarcinomas compared to colorectal adenocarcinomas. *Mod Pathol* 2003;16:130.

75. Santini D, Vincenzi B, Tonini G, et al: Cyclooxygenase-2 overexpression is associated with a poor outcome in resected ampullary cancer patients. *Clin Cancer Res* 2005;11:3784.

76. Offerhaus GJ, Giardello FM, Krush AJ, et al: The risk of upper gastrointestinal cancer in familial adenomatous polyposis. *Gastroenterology* 1991;102:1980.

77. Weinstein EC, Dockety MB, Waugh L: Neoplasms of Meckel's diverticulum. *Int Abstr Surg* 1963;116:503.

78. Gray HK, Kernohan JW: Meckel's diverticulum associated with intussusception and adenocarcinoma of ectopic gastric mucosa; report of a case. *JAMA* 1937;108:1480.

79. Brotman SJ, Pan W, Pozner J, et al: Ductal adenocarcinoma arising in duodeno-pyloric heterotopic pancreas. *Int J Surg Pathol* 1994;2:37.

80. Cates JM, Williams TL, Suriawinata AA: Intraductal papillary mucinous adenoma that arises from pancreatic heterotopia within a Meckel diverticulum. *Arch Pathol Lab Med* 2005;129:e67.

81. Ngo N, Villamil C, Macauley W, Cole SR: Adenosquamous carcinoma of the small intestine. Report of a case and review of the literature. *Arch Pathol Lab Med* 1999;123:739.

82. Viamonte M, Viamonte M: Primary squamous-cell carcinoma of the small bowel. Report of a case. *Dis Colon Rectum* 1992;35:806.

83. Schaffzin DM, Smith LE: Squamous-cell carcinoma developing after an ileoanal pouch procedure: report of a case. *Dis Colon Rectum* 2005; 48:1086.

84. Sato Y, Tominaga H, Tangoku A, et al: Alpha-fetoprotein-producing cancer of the ampulla of Vater. *Hepatogastroenterology* 1992;39: 566.

85. Gardiner GW, Lajoie G, Keith R: Hepatoid adenocarcinoma of the papilla of Vater. *Histopathology* 1992;20:541.

86. Matthews TH, Heaton GE, Christopherson WM: Primary duodenal choriocarcinoma. *Arch Pathol Lab Med* 1986;110:550.

87. Chen Y, Jung SM, Chao TC: Malignant rhabdoid tumor of the small intestine in an adult: a case report with immunohistochemical and ultrastructural findings. *Dig Dis Sci* 1998;43:975.

88. Odeh M, Misselevich I, Oliven A, Boss JH: Small intestinal carcinoma with osteoclast-like giant cells. *Am J Gastroenterol* 1995;90:1177.

89. Talbot IC, Neoptolemos JP, Shaw DE, Carr-Locke D: The histopathology and staging of carcinoma of the ampulla of Vater. *Histopathology* 1988;12:155.

90. Martin FM, Rossi RL, Dorrucci V, et al: Clinical and pathologic correlations in patients with periampullary tumors. *Arch Surg* 1990;125: 723.

91. Yamaguchi K, Enjoji M, Tsuneyoshi M: Pancreatoduodenal carcinoma: a clinicopathologic study of 304 patients and immunohistochemical observation for CEA and CA19-9. *J Surg Oncol* 1991;47:148.

92. Neoptolemos JP, Talbot IC, Carr-Locke DL, et al: Treatment and outcome in 52 consecutive cases of ampullary carcinoma. *Br J Surg* 1987;74:957.

93. Yamaguchi K, Enjoji M: Carcinoma of the ampulla of Vater. A clinicopathologic study and pathologic staging of 109 cases of carcinoma and 5 cases of adenoma. *Cancer* 1987;59:506.

94. Dawson PJ, Connolly MM: Influence of site of origin and mucin production on survival in ampullary carcinoma. *Ann Surg* 1989;210:173.

95. Bakkevold KE, Kambestad B: Staging of carcinoma of the pancreas and ampulla of Vater. Tumor (T), lymph node (N), and distant metastasis (M) as prognostic factors. *Int J Pancreatol* 1995;17:249.

96. Sperti C, Pasquali C, Piccoli A, et al: Radical resection for ampullary carcinoma: long-term results. *Br J Surg* 1994;81:668.

97. Willett CG, Warshaw AL, Convery K, Compton CC: Patterns of failure after pancreaticoduodenectomy for ampullary carcinoma. *Surg Gynecol Obstet* 1993;176:33.

98. Pyke CM, Donohue JH, Lewis JE: Late anastomotic recurrence after radical resection of carcinoma of the ampulla of Vater. *Surgery* 1992; 111:714.

99. Pilati P, Rossi CR, Mocellin S, et al: Multimodal treatment of peritoneal carcinomatosis and sarcomatosis. *Eur J Surg Oncol* 2001;27:125.

100. Howe JR, Karnell LH, Menck HR, Scott-Conner C: The American College of Surgeons Commission on Cancer and the American Cancer Society. Adenocarcinoma of the small bowel: review of the National Cancer Data Base, 1985-1995. *Cancer* 1999;86:2693.

101. Sugarbaker PH: Cytoreductive surgery and peri-operative intraperitoneal chemotherapy as a curative approach to pseudomyxoma peritonei syndrome. *Eur J Surg Oncol* 2001;27:239.

102. Jacks SP, Hundley JC, Shen P, et al: Cytoreductive surgery and intraperitoneal hyperthermic chemotherapy for peritoneal carcinomatosis from small bowel adenocarcinoma. *J Surg Oncol* 2005;91:112.

103. Kloppel G, Maillet B: Histological typing of pancreatic and periampullary carcinoma. *Eur J Surg Oncol* 1991;17:139.

104. Narita T, Nakazawa H, Hizawa Y, et al: Hepatocellular carcinoma with unusual metastasis to the small intestine. *Acta Pathol Jap* 1993;43:779.

105. Patel JK, Dodolar MS, Pickrin JW, Moore RH: Metastatic pattern of malignant melanoma. *Am J Surg* 1978;135:808.

106. Chait M, Kurtz RC, Hajdu SI: Gastrointestinal tract metastases in patients with germ cell tumor of the testis. *Am J Dig Dis* 1978;23:925.

107. Compton CC: Protocol for the examination of specimens from patients with carcinoma of the ampulla of Vater: a basis for checklists. Cancer Committee, College of American Pathologists. *Arch Pathol Lab Med* 1997;121:673.

Nonneoplastic Diseases of the Appendix

NORMAL EMBRYONIC DEVELOPMENT

The cecum appears during the fifth fetal week, arising as a diverticulum from the distal primitive intestinal loop before it differentiates into the small and large intestine. The appendix develops from the cecum and matures in the second trimester (1). As the appendix lengthens, the junction between the appendix and the cecum becomes increasingly more distinct. Longitudinal folds and ridges form, producing a segmented appearance; villi form (Fig. 8.1) that eventually involute. The epithelium appears clear due to large amounts of intracytoplasmic glycogen. Endocrine cells develop in the subepithelial connective tissue around the ninth fetal week when the epithelial basement membrane is not fully formed and the muscularis mucosae has not yet developed.

Lymphoid stem cells migrate into the appendiceal mesenchyme. Mature lymphocytes appear when the fetus measures approximately 100 mm in length (2); lymphoid aggregates appear by the 17th week. The apical poles of incipient lymphoid follicles impinge on the surface epithelium by the time the fetus reaches 150 mm in length and lymphoid cells invade the epithelium. Germinal centers develop between the third and sixth postnatal weeks after the introduction of foreign protein (by eating) into the gut. Macrophages appear shortly after the lymphocytes (3). Primitive neural structures develop in the first trimester.

NORMAL GROSS ANATOMY

The appendix usually arises from the posteromedial cecal wall, 2.5 to 3 cm below the ileocecal valve at the convergence of the taeniae coli (Fig. 8.2). The adult appendix averages 7 cm in length; lengths up to 20 cm have been reported. The appendix is longer in adults than in children. Its external diameter ranges from 0.3 to 0.8 cm. The appendiceal lumen measures from 1 to 2 mm in diameter appearing round, oval, irregular, or slitlike. The distal tip obliterates in adults. The appendix is suspended from the mesoappendix, and attaches to the cecum in several ways (4). In 65% of adults, the appendix lies behind the cecum with its orifice opening into the cecum near the ileocecal valve. It may also lie to the side of the ascending colon, in front of, or behind, the ileum, lying

on the psoas muscle or hanging over the pelvic brim (4). The appendix receives its blood supply from a branch of the posterior cecal artery; its venous drainage is to the portal system, explaining the coexistence of hepatic inflammation in the setting of appendicitis. The lymphatics first drain into the nodes of the mesoappendix and then to the right pericolic lymph nodes as well as to the ileocecal lymph nodes.

HISTOLOGY OF THE APPENDIX

The appendiceal mucosa resembles that of the large intestine, except for the prominent circumferential arrangement of lymphoid follicles known as Peyer patches. Peyer patches (Fig 8.3) are most prominent in children, decreasing in size with age. They are markedly diminished or absent in the elderly. The appendiceal epithelium is modified over the dome of each lymphoid follicle to form M cells with a structure similar to that seen in the small intestine (see Chapter 6). Nonbranching crypts are lined by tall mucus-secreting goblet cells that extend from the luminal surface to the crypt bases. The crypts also contain endocrine cells, Paneth cells, and small numbers of intraepithelial lymphocytes. The muscularis mucosae is often absent; it is sometimes difficult to determine the mucosal–submucosal boundary.

The regularly arranged Peyer patches lie at the mucosal–submucosal junction (Fig. 8.3), and a well-defined lymphatic sinus surrounds both the lateral and basal parts of the follicle. These lymphatic sinuses empty into the submucosal-collecting lymphatics. Lymphocytes that proliferate in the gut-associated lymphoid tissues migrate into the surrounding lymphatic sinus or capillaries and enter the systemic circulation to be redistributed to other lymphoid tissues and organs. The endocrine cell population is discussed in Chapter 17.

CONGENITAL ABNORMALITIES OF THE APPENDIX

Congenital appendiceal anomalies are rare (5). They include appendiceal agenesis (6), hypoplasia, duplications, horseshoe shape (7), heterotopia, and diverticula. These

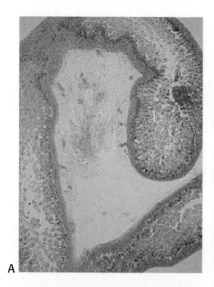 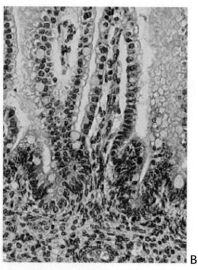

FIG. 8.1. Fetal appendix. **A:** Differentiation of the ileum, cecum, and appendix is not easy at this time since villi are present in all three areas. **B:** Higher magnification of the fetal villi showing a glycogenated epithelium, proliferating crypts, and villi. The section comes from the blind distal end of the specimen shown in A.

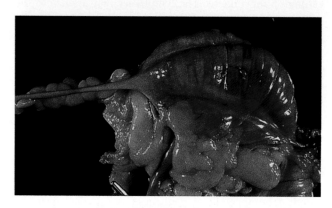

FIG. 8.2. The normal appendix arises at the junction of the three taenia coli.

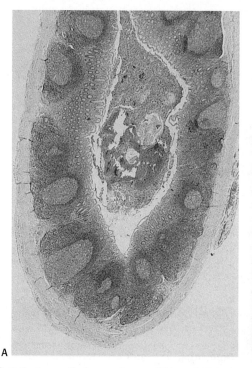 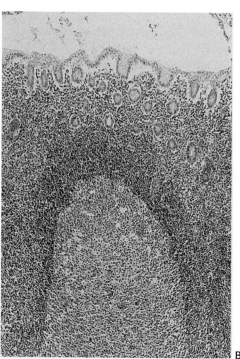

FIG. 8.3. Appendix from a 1-year-old boy. **A:** Low-power magnification showing the regular arrangement of the lymphoid follicles and the straight tubular crypts. **B:** Higher magnification showing a single follicle.

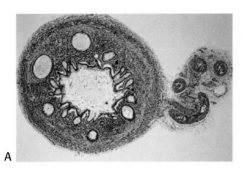
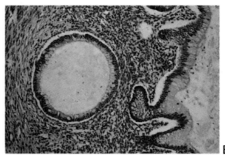

FIG. 8.4. Hypoplastic appendix. **A:** The lamina propria blends into the underlying submucosa and muscularis propria. No muscularis mucosae is present. Numerous cystically dilated glands are present in the submucosa. **B:** Higher magnification showing the lack of a distinction between the lamina propria and the underlying submucosa.

occur in the presence of either a normal cecum or with cecal dysgenesis.

Appendiceal Agenesis

Appendiceal agenesis (or absence) differs from appendiceal hypoplasia in that in the latter condition, the appendix is present but underdeveloped with a simplified structure and with mucosal cysts (Fig. 8.4). There are five types of appendiceal agenesis (Fig. 8.5) (6). All result from failure of the primitive cecal diverticulum to differentiate into the appendix, except for the fourth type. The fourth type results from intrauterine atrophy of a previously well-formed appendix. Appendiceal agenesis sometimes accompanies ileal atresia (8), thalidomide ingestion (9), or trisomy 18. Patients with trisomy 18 usually have multiple gastrointestinal and extra-gastrointestinal congenital abnormalities (6).

Positional Abnormalities

The appendix may lie in unusual locations, usually because of the cecal mobility, excessive appendiceal length, situs inversus, or intestinal malrotation. This may cause an otherwise typical appendicitis to present in atypical ways.

Duplications

Three patterns of appendiceal duplication exist: Double barreled, paired, and accessory (10). In "double-barrel" appendix, two separate tubes, each lined by a mucosa and separated by a submucosa, lie within a single muscular coat. Two symmetrically placed appendices lie on either side of the ileocecal valve in the paired form of duplication. This only occurs in infants with multiple congenital anomalies. A normal-appearing appendix lying in its usual position and a second rudimentary appendix arising from the cecum represents the accessory type of duplication. Triplication of the appendix can also occur (11).

Heterotopias

Heterotopic tissues rarely affect the appendix. However, heterotopic gastric, esophageal, ileal, and pancreatic tissues can all occur in this location.

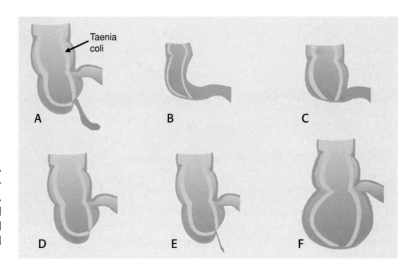

FIG. 8.5. Forms of appendiceal agenesis. **A:** Normal appendix. **B:** Absent cecum and appendix. **C:** Rudimentary cecum and absent appendix. **D:** Normal cecum and absent appendix. **E:** Normal cecum and rudimentary appendix. **F:** Enlarged deformed cecum distal to the ileocecal valve and absent appendix.

DIVERTICULOSIS

Diverticula affect 0.004% to 2.8% of histologically examined appendices (5,12). They can be congenital or acquired; both types may be single or multiple. Congenital diverticula present as antimesenteric outpouchings with complete muscular walls, contrasting with acquired diverticula that lack the muscularis propria (Fig. 8.6). Some congenital diverticula are attached to the umbilicus by a fibrous band, resembling Meckel diverticulum.

Acquired diverticula are ten times more frequent than their congenital counterparts (5). They affect both sexes equally and develop along the area of the penetrating arteries, often secondary to inflammation or tumors. Associated neoplasms, particularly low-grade mucinous neoplasms, are present in many patients (Fig. 8.6) (13). Diverticula develop due to the increased pressure of the accumulated intraluminal mucin. A similar mechanism may be responsible for the relatively high incidence (14%) of appendiceal diverticula in patients with cystic fibrosis.

Acquired diverticula are commonly multiple (Fig. 8.6), lying along the mesenteric and antimesenteric borders. They usually involve the distal appendix, giving the appendix a beaded appearance. Their size varies from 2 to 5 mm. Like colonic diverticula, they are subject to inflammation or perforation. Inflammation may distort, obliterate, or disrupt a diverticulum. When the inflammatory process spreads into the periappendiceal tissues, an abscess results.

APPENDICEAL INTUSSUSCEPTION, AUTOAMPUTATION, AND INVERTED APPENDICEAL STUMP

Appendiceal intussusception is rare, usually affecting young boys (14). Patients range in age from 8 months to 75 years. Predispositions to intussusception include the presence of a fetal cone-shaped appendix, an unusually thin mesoappendix, or the presence of mass lesions, most typically

TABLE 8.1	Types of Appendiceal Intussusception
Intussusception	Intussuscipiens
Appendix tip	Proximal appendix
Appendix base	Cecum
Proximal appendix	Distal appendix
Complete inversion (inside-out appendix)	

endometriosis, adenomas, carcinoid tumors, or the lymphoid hyperplasia associated with viral infections. The presenting signs and symptoms resemble those of acute appendicitis. The lesions may also remain asymptomatic only to be discovered incidentally.

There are four types of appendiceal intussusceptions (Table 8.1). In some cases, the distal appendix intussuscepts into the proximal appendix; in other cases, the proximal appendix intussuscepts into the cecoappendicular opening or the whole appendix intussuscepts into the cecum (Fig. 8.7), presenting as an edematous or infarcted cecal "polyp." Intussusception can also appear as an umbilicated area at the junction of the taeniae coli on the cecal serosal surface. The mucosa may appear normal, hyperplastic, inflamed, eroded, or ischemic. The latter occurs if the vascular supply has been compromised. If there have been recurrent intussusceptions, the mucosa and muscular layers may become hyperplastic. In intussusception, the histology may also appear to be reversed from normal, with the epithelium lying on the external surface of tissue and the submucosa and muscularis propria lying inside the mucosa (Fig. 8.8). The submucosa becomes edematous and the muscularis propria may appear

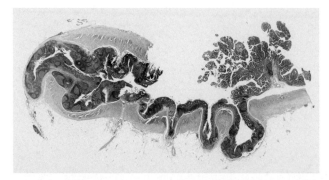

FIG. 8.6. Appendiceal diverticulosis associated with an appendiceal adenoma. There are multiple diverticula extending through the appendiceal wall. They lack the muscularis propria as is typical of acquired diverticula.

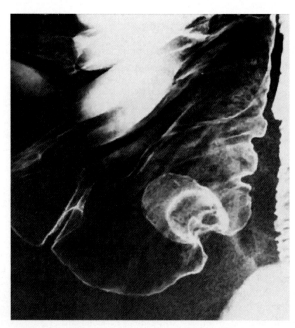

FIG. 8.7. Appendiceal intussusception. Double-contrast barium examination demonstrating inverted appendiceal stump.

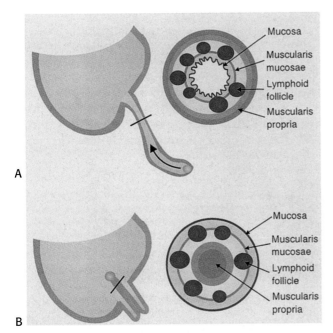

A

B

FIG. 8.8. Diagram of appendiceal intussusception. **A:** The tip of the appendix begins to move toward the junction of the appendix with the cecum. A section taken through the appendix (indicated by the *black line*) demonstrates essentially normal histologic features. **B:** Once the appendix intussuscepts into the cecum, it may produce a small polyp. A cross section through the lesion taken at the level of the black line shows the inverted histology.

hyperplastic, fibrotic, or splayed (Fig. 8.9). The muscular layers maintain a normal relationship with one another and with the submucosa and mucosa. Sometimes the bowel wall appears to have two muscularis propriae. It is important that the appendix be examined carefully in this setting to exclude the presence of an underlying neoplasm or other lesion such as endometriosis that may have been the lead point for the intussusception. Treatment of the intussusception is surgical resection.

Occasionally, the appendix autoamputates following intussusception or volvulus. The presence of cecal scarring and hemosiderin in the absence of other cecal abnormalities provides clues that the appendix was present at birth. Inverted appendiceal stump follows appendiceal autoamputation, and may appear as a cecal polyp grossly or endoscopically. One of the complications of an appendiceal stump is a vascular malformation. Patients may present with massive bleeding from cecal ulcerations. Histologically, massively dilated vessels are present.

TORSION

Appendiceal torsion is rare, and when it occurs it causes ischemic appendicitis (Fig. 8.10). Histologically, one sees distal inflammation with areas of hemorrhage and necrosis. As with intussusceptions, a careful examination for the presence of an underlying neoplasm, as well as the assessment of the adequacy of the resection of the appendix if a neoplasm is present, is important.

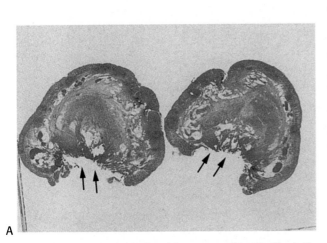

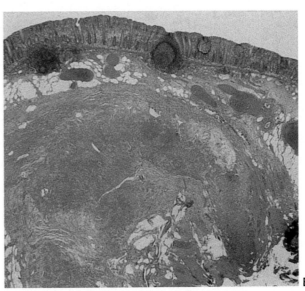

A   B

FIG. 8.9. Appendiceal intussusception. **A:** The lesion presented as a cecal polyp. One can see the cautery margin (*arrows*) of the "polypectomy" specimen. The center of the "polyp" consists of hyperplastic muscularis propria. External to this is an edematous submucosa. The surface of the polyp is covered by appendiceal-type mucosa with prominent lymphoid follicles. **B:** Higher magnification showing the presence of the submucosal edema and marked lymphatic dilation.

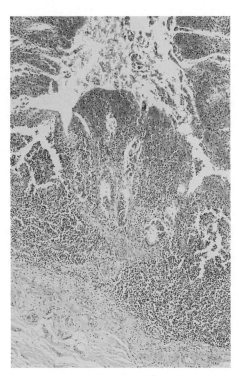

FIG 8.10. Appendices that undergo torsion usually show some evidence of ischemia.

SEPTATED APPENDIX

Single or multiple, complete or incomplete septa consisting of mucosa and submucosa may divide in the appendiceal lumen into compartments (Fig. 8.11), predisposing the appendix to develop appendicitis. The inflammation usually remains confined to one compartment of the septated lumen. These lesions present most often in the 15- to 19-year age group with a clear-cut male predominance. They represent residual fetal septations.

"ABSENT APPENDIX"

The appendix may appear to be absent for several reasons: (a) agenesis; (b) previous resection; (c) obliteration from previous episodes of acute appendicitis, intussusception, or torsion; or (d) its presence in unusual locations. Retrocecal, retrocolic, and retroileal appendices are uncommon but can cause clinical confusion, especially in the individual who presents with acute abdominal pain. Acute appendicitis can resolve, leaving only a thin fibrous cord. Resection of the appendix should be suspected in individuals who have undergone previous surgical procedures. The confluence of the three cecal taeniae is the only consistent landmark for the appendiceal origin.

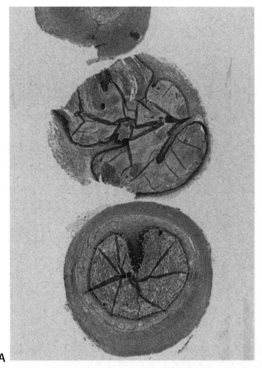

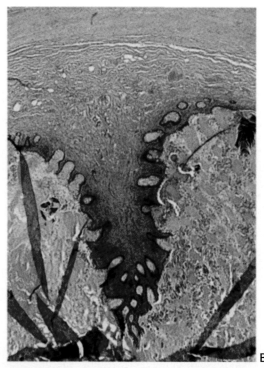

A   B

FIG. 8.11. Septated appendix. **A:** Several cross sections through areas showing incomplete septa. The lumen contains projections of tissue covered by atrophic appendiceal mucosa. Extensions of the submucosa form the core of the septum. **B:** Higher magnification of the septum.

APPENDICITIS

Demographic Features

Appendicitis develops at any age, with a peak incidence in the 2nd and 3rd decades. However, it also affects neonates and the very elderly. Between 7% and 12% of the U.S. population develop appendicitis. Appendicitis occurs more commonly in Western cultures than in Eastern cultures, likely due to dietary differences between these populations (15). Heredity may also play a role in the pathogenesis of appendicitis (16). Appendicitis affects males more commonly than females, particularly during early childhood (17).

Acute appendicitis may also develop in neonates. Although this is rare, it associates with high morbidity and mortality rates (18,19). Neonatal appendicitis usually results from the presence of neonatal necrotizing enterocolitis, cystic fibrosis, Hirschsprung disease, or the bacteremia associated with maternal chorioamnionitis (18).

Despite the proclivity of appendicitis to involve younger individuals, it also affects the elderly and other age groups. The incidence of appendicitis in the elderly may be increasing due to their longer life expectancies. Appendicitis in the elderly also has a high mortality and complication rate (20), perhaps due to concomitant nonsteroidal anti-inflammatory drug (NSAID) use. NSAIDs may impair the inflammatory processes and suppress white cell responses increasing the risk of developing appendicitis (20). Additionally, NSAIDs mask the symptoms so that patients present with late-stage disease.

Pathophysiology

The etiology of appendicitis is multifactorial. It may involve obstruction, ischemia, infections, and hereditary factors. A common scenario in the pathogenesis of the disease involves a sequential series of events that begins with luminal obstruction due to any of the factors listed in Table 8.2. The obstruction is followed by loss of mucosal integrity, ischemia, and bacterial invasion. Secretions accumulate under pressure behind the obstruction. The mucosa can also be primarily involved by infections, as in the rest of the intestines without antecedent obstruction, or it may be

TABLE 8.2   **Causes of Appendiceal Obstruction Leading to Appendicitis**

Stones (fecaliths)
Food
Mucus—most often in cystic fibrosis
Kinks (angulated appendix)
Parasites
Tumors in the appendix or cecum
Endometriosis
Foreign objects
Lymphoid hyperplasia—usually secondary to viral infection

affected by inflammatory bowel disease (IBD). Bacterial, viral, fungal, and parasitic diseases may all cause specific forms of acute appendicitis. However, microbiologic studies generally show that no single organ is identified; rather, a mixed aerobic and anaerobic bacterial population is present in most cases. The most commonly isolated bacteria are *Bacteroides fragilis* and *Escherichia coli* (21). *Streptococcus milleri* can also be detected (22). *S. milleri* may be more important than some of the other bacterial species, since these have a sevenfold increased risk for abscess formation (22). *Campylobacter jejuni* is also an important cause of acute appendicitis (23).

Once an infection becomes established, pressure from inflammation and edema predisposes to the rapid development of gangrene, perforation, and peritonitis. Infections may also cause fibrin thrombi, which can block the small appendiceal vessels, causing secondary ischemia. The appendix is particularly prone to ischemia, since the appendiceal artery is an end artery. The enteric nervous system may also play a role in the pathogenesis of acute appendicitis. Increased numbers of nerve fibers, Schwann cells, and enlarged ganglia have all been found in patients with acute appendicitis (24).

Clinical Features

The diagnosis of appendicitis is straightforward when it presents classically with right lower quadrant abdominal pain of short duration, abdominal rigidity, and anorexia. Appendicitis also causes acute periumbilical, colicky pain or vomiting. Fever and leukocytosis develop early. However, there are many examples of appendices that are removed for suspected acute appendicitis in which histologic evidence of an acute appendicitis is lacking.

Pathologic Features

Normally, the appendiceal mucosa appears smooth, light yellow-tan; the serosa appears pink-tan, smooth, and glistening. When the inflammation is restricted to the mucosa, the exterior of the appendix may grossly appear normal. Dilation and congestion of serosal vessels produce localized or generalized hyperemia and constitute the earliest visible external changes (Figs. 8.12 to 8.14). Well-developed acute appendicitis shows marked congestion with a dull (rather than glistening) serosal surface or there may be a serosal granular, fibrinous, or purulent coating and vascular engorgement reflecting severe necrosis and inflammation. The mesoappendix appears edematous and contiguous structures may become inflamed. The appendix often exudes purulent material from the cut surface; one may sometimes identify an impacted intraluminal fecalith. Mucosal necrosis and ulceration are usually present. The acute inflammation can localize to one segment of the organ or the entire appendix may be affected. There may be the appearance of a mucocele. If so, the appendix should be well sampled to exclude the presence of a coexisting mucinous neoplasm.

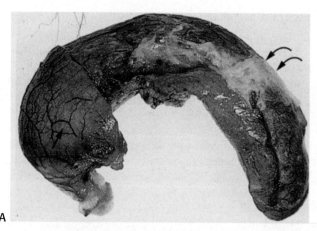

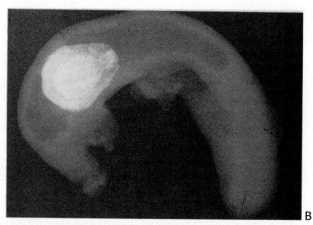

FIG. 8.12. Fecalith and acute appendicitis. **A:** Gross photograph. The proximal bulge is due to the presence of an intraluminal fecalith. Marked vascular engorgement is seen and a fibropurulent exudate covers the appendix (*curved arrows*). **B:** Specimen radiograph showing a radiopaque fecalith.

By the time full-blown gangrenous appendicitis develops, the organ appears soft, purplish, and hemorrhagic or even greenish black, sometimes with visible thrombi in the mesoappendix. These may spread along the ileocecal and upper mesenteric veins. Perforation may be present. In complicated cases, abscesses may form around a site of perforation and inflammation may extend into the mesoappendix (Fig. 8.15).

Histologic changes associated with appendicitis reflect disease duration and severity, and some changes may not reflect clinical disease at all. The term *acute intraluminal appendicitis* has been used when there are neutrophils in the appendiceal lumen but they have not yet infiltrated the mucosa (25). This may not be of any significance since this finding can be seen in incidental appendectomy specimens. Other minimal changes may consist of focal neutrophilic collections in the lumen and lamina propria. This is sometimes referred to as *mucosal* or *early* appendicitis. The term *mucosal appendicitis* has been used both in the presence and the absence of ulcers if the inflammation is restricted to the mucosa (26–28). The clinical significance of pure mucosal inflammation in the absence of ulcers is uncertain. Since these changes may reflect sampling error, more sections should be taken of the appendix to be certain that there is not more extensive inflammation elsewhere in the appendix.

In better-developed disease, focal erosions, cryptitis, and crypt abscesses develop. The inflammation then extends to the submucosa. After the inflammatory process reaches the submucosa, it spreads quickly to involve the remaining appendix. Eventually, the mucosa erodes, the wall becomes necrotic, and the vessels may thrombose. Submucosal abscesses, edema, and congestion follow. Some appendices contain prominent eosinophilic infiltrates. Extravasated mucin in the bowel wall may induce a foreign body reaction or even small mucin granulomas.

Gangrenous appendicitis shows extensive suppuration, often extending deep into or through the appendiceal wall with complete mural destruction (Figs. 8.16 and 8.17) with or without rupture. If perforation occurs, an intense nonspecific

FIG. 8.13. Acute appendicitis showing vascular engorgement and serosal erythema. A white purulent membrane covers the serosal surface.

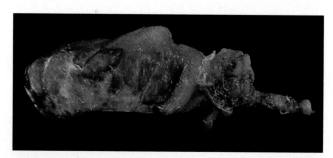

FIG. 8.14. Gangrenous appendicitis. The external surface of the appendix is hemorrhagic and reddened with a well-developed fibropurulent membrane.

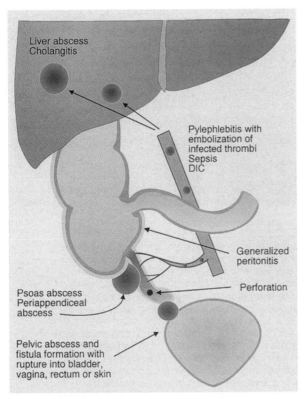

FIG. 8.15. Diagram illustrating the complications of acute appendicitis. DIC, disseminated intravascular coagulation.

inflammatory process ensues. Perforation may be suspected clinically, but it is sometimes difficult to see in the resected specimen due to the extensive inflammation. Resolving appendicitis is characterized by the presence of a predominantly lymphocytic infiltrate involving the subserosa and muscularis propria or the subserosa. When appendicitis heals, it assumes one of two basic patterns: The "usual" pattern, sometimes with an intraluminal cord of granulation tissue, and a xanthogranulomatous pattern (29). Fibrosis may develop.

Although full-blown appendicitis is histologically easily identified by mucosal ulceration and neutrophilic infiltrates extending through the appendix wall to the peritoneal serosa, occasionally minimal inflammation can be difficult to diagnose due to inconspicuous pathologies. Staining with E-selectin, the first inducible cell adhesion molecule, expressed in early appendicitis, may help detect minimal or less obvious disease (30), although correlation between clinical findings and pathologic abnormalities may be speculative at best.

Complications

The most common complication of appendicitis is perforation, which can lead to generalized peritonitis, subdiaphragmatic and periappendiceal abscesses, serosal pneumatosis, and suppurative pylephlebitis (Fig. 8.15). Infected thrombi may involve the serosal and mesoappendiceal small vessels and may extend or embolize to distant sites such as the liver,

where they can establish secondary bacterial infections, cholangitis, and hepatic abscesses (31). Fistulae may form between the appendix and the rest of the gastrointestinal tract, vagina, or bladder.

If a perforation occurs slowly, the inflammation often walls itself off, producing a *periappendiceal abscess* that typically localizes in the right iliac fossa lateral to the cecum. One may find little in the way of residual appendix and only a mass of granulation or xanthomatous tissue surrounding the abscess. This can progress to larger masses of chronic fibrous tissue containing granulomas. Extensive granulomatous reactions may raise the clinical suspicion of a cecal carcinoma. These granulomas often contain foreign material including feces. In some cases, the inflammatory reaction results in mesothelial entrapment that eventually becomes cystic, simulating a benign cystic mesothelioma, particularly if the mesothelial lining appears reactive and atypical.

SPECIFIC FORMS OF INFECTIOUS APPENDICITIS

Any infection affecting the large or small intestine may also affect the appendix. The features of specific bacterial infections resemble those seen in the rest of the intestines (see Chapters 6 and 13). Some of the more common appendiceal infections are discussed briefly here.

Actinomyces israelii is part of the normal oral flora. Yet, the same organism can become pathogenic. When it survives passage through gastric acid and reaches the appendix, it usually lodges there without causing disease or inflammation. Sometimes, however, one sees inflammation surrounding organisms in the appendix and one assumes that the *Actinomyces* caused the appendicitis. Actinomycotic appendicitis is rare, but it is important to diagnosis, since it can cause a chronic suppurative appendicitis, periappendicitis, or periappendicular mass. The infection can lead to a granulomatous mass with multiple sinus tracts draining to the overlying skin, or leading to pelvic abscesses. The infection can also spread to the liver via the portal system, creating hepatic abscesses. Fluid draining from the sinuses usually contains characteristic "sulfur granules" (Fig. 8.18). Examination of hematoxylin and eosin (H&E)-stained sections reveals collections of long dark blue filamentous organisms, often associated with characteristic sulphur granules. Acute inflammation is often present. A dense fibrous connective tissue mass may surround the actinomycotic mycelia. The diagnosis should be suspected in any patient who develops sinus tracts and/or fistulas following appendectomy. *Actinomyces turicensis* can also be found in patients with appendicitis (32).

Tubercular appendicitis may complicate tubercular infections in other parts of the gastrointestinal tract or may develop as an isolated disorder. The appendix is frequently involved in this setting due to the abundant lymphoid tissues that are present in this location. The disease is more progressive in children than in adults. Individuals who perforate are likely to

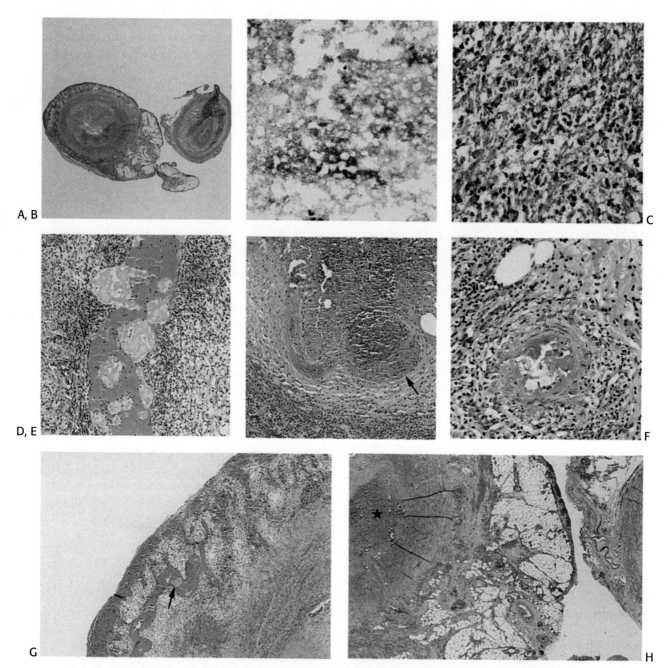

FIG. 8.16. Acute appendicitis. **A:** Cross section through the appendix showing the transmural inflammation. **B:** High magnification of the surface exudate that contains necrotic debris and bacteria. **C:** Below the surface of the debris shown in B there is acute and chronic inflammation. **D:** Acute and chronic inflammation with small thrombi within the dilated and congested veins. **E:** Cross section through a larger vessel containing an organizing thrombus at the base of the vessel (*arrow*). Overlying the vessel is necrotic and inflammatory debris. Under the vessel is a zone of acute and chronic inflammation. **F:** Cross section through a small vessel demonstrating with fibrinoid necrosis and acute and chronic inflammation. **G:** The serosa shows marked vascular engorgement and small thrombi in the dilated vessels (*arrow*). **H:** Lower magnification showing the extension of fibrosing stands of tissue extending into the mesoappendiceal fat. The vessels on the serosal surface are markedly engorged. The lumen of the appendix at this level is completely necrotic (*star*).

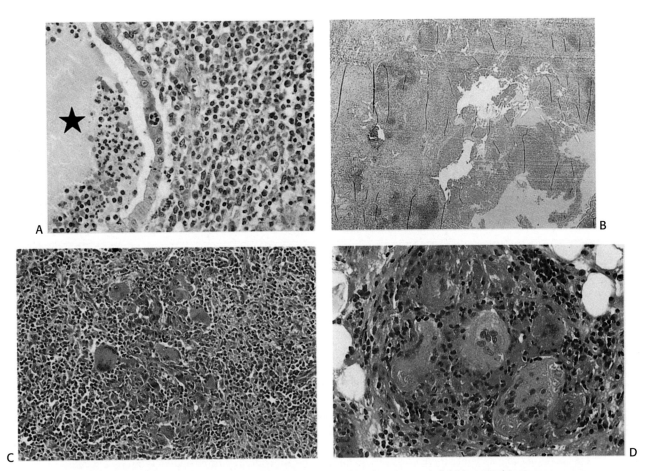

FIG. 8.17. Appendicitis (A and B, acute appendicitis; C and D, chronic appendicitis). **A:** At this stage, one sees acute inflammation involving the appendiceal epithelium. The epithelium lining the crypt becomes flattened and cuboidal in shape. An intense inflammatory process is present in the luminal side of the crypt (*star*). Cryptitis appears. The inflammatory cells present on the opposite side of the epithelium represent the normal lamina propria. **B:** Necrosis. The entire epithelium has become denuded and replaced by hemorrhage and exudate. **C:** Higher power magnification of the inflammatory process showing chronic inflammation and giant cells. **D:** Higher power magnification of the giant cells.

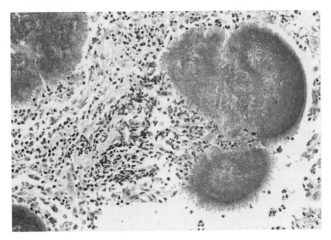

FIG. 8.18. Actinomycosis. Multiple sulfur granules are present.

develop generalized peritonitis (33). The histologic features resemble those described in the intestines (see Chapter 13).

Yersinia infections may localize to the appendix producing a granulomatous appendicitis. The infections affect both children and adults. Both *Yersinia enterocolitica* (*YE*) and *Yersinia pseudotuberculosis* (*YP*) cause gastrointestinal disease. These two forms of *Yersinia* infection can coexist in the same patient. The granulomas are predominantly epithelioid and noncaseating in nature with striking lymphoid cuffing. Prominent microabscesses in the center of the granulomas may be seen in *YP* infections. The granulomas may be located in all layers of the appendiceal wall, or they may be restricted to the mucosa and submucosa. The number of granulomas varies from 1 to >15/4× objective field (Fig. 8.19). There is usually an accompanying transmural mixed inflammatory infiltrate associated with the prominent lymphoid aggregates.

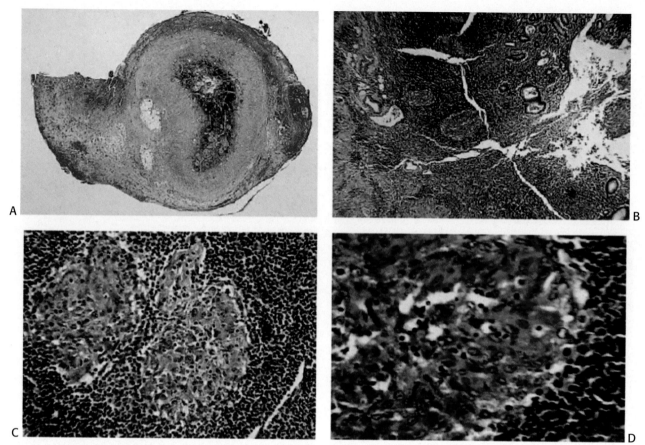

FIG. 8.19. *Yersinia* appendicitis. **A:** Cross section through the appendix in *Yersinia* appendicitis demonstrates the presence of a thickened wall and small nonconfluent granulomas. **B:** Low-power magnification photograph showing the prominent lymphoid follicles within the Peyer patches and inflammation extending from the lumen to the submucosa. Areas of ulceration overlying the lymphoid tissue are evident. In addition, granulomas are present. **C, D:** Progressively higher power magnifications of the granulomatous process.

This inflammation may extend into the mesoappendix. Other features that may be present include marked lymphoid hyperplasia, giant cells, mucosal ulceration, focal architectural distortion, and crypt abscesses (34).

The appendix is seldom removed in patients with viral appendicitis since the disease remains self-limited and the appendicitis resolves once the viral infection resolves. Viral infections frequently localize to the lymphoid tissue of Peyer patches, inducing lymphoid hyperplasia. The enlarged follicles may temporarily block the egress of luminal secretions, producing the characteristic symptoms of acute appendicitis.

Viral infections commonly associated with transient appendicitis include *measles* and *adenovirus* infections. Finding huge, multinucleated giant lymphoreticular cells known as *Warthin-Finkeldey* cells in the lymphoid tissues of Peyer patches suggests the diagnosis of measles (Fig. 8.20). However, similar cells may also occur in other viral infections as well. Furthermore, Warthin-Finkeldey cells may not be specific for viral infections, since they have been seen in patients with systemic lupus erythematous. Thus, they may merely indicate reactive lymphocytic lesions (35).

The appendix of patients with *adenovirus* infections appears normal or demonstrates marked lymphoid hyperplasia, unless an intussusception has occurred. The most common site of the intussusception is at the ileocecal valve with focal lymphoid hyperplasia acting as the lead point (see Chapter 6). The epithelium overlying the lymphoid hyperplasia appears tattered and necrotic when an intussusception develops. Clues to the presence of the virus include focally necrotic-appearing epithelium showing loss of nuclear polarity. Affected cells may have an eosinophilic appearance due to mucin depletion. The intranuclear inclusions of adenovirus are typically Cowdry type B, consisting of nuclear smudging (Fig. 8.20). Cowdry A inclusions featuring sharply demarcated globules surrounded by a clear zone can also be found. Histologically, the intranuclear inclusions appear as reddish globules surrounded by halos or a poorly demarcated purple smudge in otherwise well-preserved cells. If one wishes to confirm that a specific virus is present, one can use antibodies to the virus or perform in situ hybridization with an appropriate genetic probe.

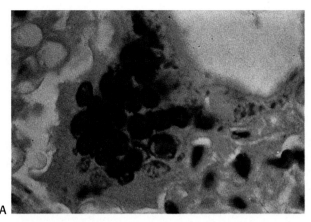 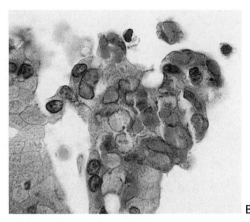

A   B

FIG. 8.20. Viral infections. **A:** Warthin-Finkeldey cell in the lymphoid tissue in a patient with a known measles infection. The figure demonstrates the characteristic multinucleated giant cells seen in this disorder. **B:** Adenovirus infection. The cells are fused together in a syncytium and contain characteristic intranuclear inclusions. (B courtesy of Dr. Renate Reif, "Assaf Harofe" Medical Center, Tel Aviv Medical School, Zrifin, Israel.)

Cytomegalovirus (CMV) infections also represent a possible etiologic agent for appendicitis, particularly in immunocompromised individuals. The changes resemble those seen in the large and small intestines.

Acute abdominal pain from abdominal lymphadenopathy, hepatitis, splenic involvement, or involvement of the gut-associated lymphoid tissues in the intestine and appendix may be the presenting feature of *infectious mononucleosis* (36). One sees intense lymphoid hyperplasia with marked expansion of the interfollicular lamina propria by a mixed diffuse proliferation of immunoblasts including Reed-Sternberg–like cells admixed with large and small lymphocytes. Mitoses are absent and the glands appear to be reduced in number because of the extensive lymphoid hyperplasia. The lymphoid infiltrate extends deep into the underlying submucosa. The predominant cell type is an atypical lymphocyte, many of which lie around vessels, producing a vasculitislike pattern. In fatal forms of the disease, the mucosa becomes ulcerated.

Appendiceal *fungal infections* resemble similar infections in the intestines. They include mucormycoses (Fig. 8.21), histoplasmosis, South American blastomycosis, aspergillosis, and candidiasis.

Enterobius vermicularis (pinworm) is one of the most common parasites seen in the appendiceal lumen with the incidence varying from 0.2% to 75% worldwide (37,38). The organism occurs more frequently in temperate and cold climates than in the tropics and the disease is common in developed countries of the northern hemisphere. In the United States about 3% of appendix specimens contain *E. vermicularis* (39). Children are especially susceptible to the infection, with the most common method of transmission being the anus–finger–mouth route (Fig. 8.22). Ingested ova hatch in the duodenum where the larvae molt twice and

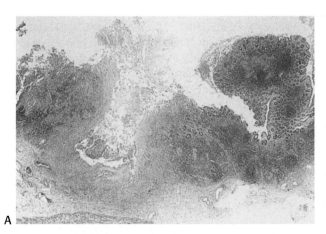 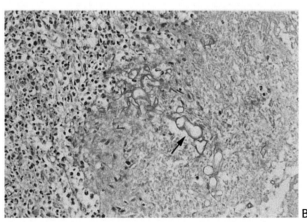

A   B

FIG 8.21. Mucor appendicitis. **A:** Focal ulceration in the appendix of a severely malnourished 10-year-old child. **B:** High magnification of necrotic debris in the center of the area of ulceration showing the presence of irregularly branched hyphae of mucor *(arrow)*.

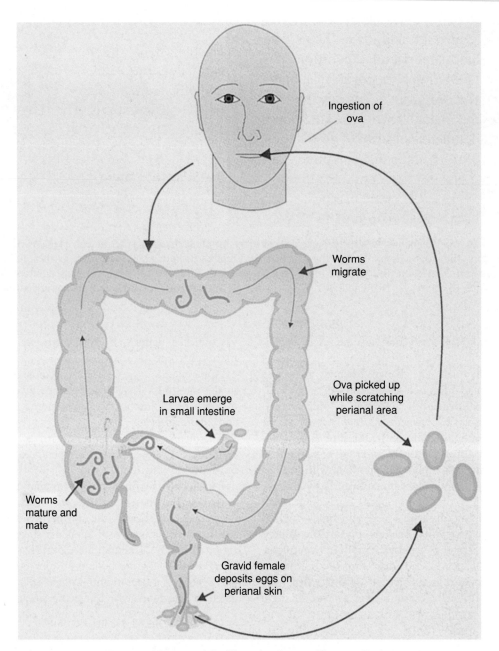

Ingestion of
ova

Worms
migrate

Ova picked up
while scratching
perianal area

Larvae emerge
in small intestine

Worms
mature and
mate

Gravid female
deposits eggs on
perianal skin

FIG. 8.22. Diagram of the life cycle of *Enterobius vermicularis.*

become sexually mature. Infrequent bathing, use of soiled underwear, crowded habitation, and lack of exposure to sunshine all favor disease transmission. Autoinfection results in repeated infections and a heavy worm burden. Symptoms include perineal or perianal pain and itching. *E. vermicularis* may also represent an incidental finding in an asymptomatic patient (40).

Adult female worms measure 6 to 12 mm and males 2 to 5 mm in length. Because of their gross appearance, they are commonly called pinworms or thread worms (Fig. 8.23). There are three labia in adult females and a lateral pair of cephalic winglike alae; the muscular esophagus terminates in a bulb and the posterior tip is attenuated. The reproductive system is T-shaped in cross section and characteristic eggs are present within the uteri. Adult males possess a ventrally curved tail with caudal alae and a single large copulatory spicule. Adult worms live in the colon and appendix, where they mate. The males die soon after copulation; females migrate to the perianal and perineal regions to lay eggs and die after oviposition. About 11,000 ovoid, asymmetrically flattened, and almost colorless eggs are produced by a gravid female. The asymmetric eggs measure 50 to 60 microns and contain fully developed larvae when they are detected in stools. The eggs of *Enterobius* species are highly contagious because they are infectious at body temperature about 6 hours after deposition and require no intermediate host. The ova

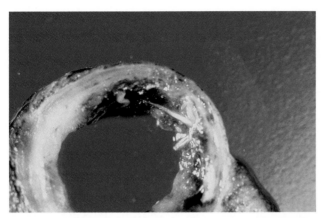

FIG. 8.23. Enterobius. Cross section of an appendix of a 9-year-old girl who presented with acute appendicitis. The appendix contains several worms attached to the wall. (Picture courtesy of Dr. Lida Crooks, Laboratory Services, Albuquerque VA Medical Center, Albuquerque, NM.)

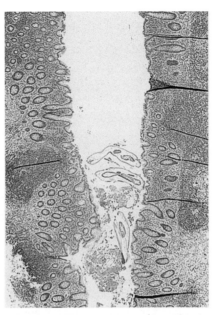

FIG. 8.25. *Enterobius vermicularis.* Cross section through the appendix showing worms in the lumen. Note that the underlying mucosa appears essentially normal except for a mild increase in the number of eosinophils.

are also highly resistant to commonly used disinfectants and can survive as long as 2 weeks in the environment. Identification of adult worms in the tissue depends on demonstrating a pair of cuticular crests (Fig. 8.24), typical eggs in the parasitic uterus, or the characteristic narrow meromyarian type of musculature, which consists of two or three muscle layers per quarter section divided by four cords.

Often worms lying in the appendiceal lumen fail to elicit an inflammatory response, except for mild mucosal eosinophilia (Fig. 8.25). However, when the worms obstruct the appendiceal lumen, acute appendicitis develops. Severe infestations cause lesions in the colon, cecum, appendix, and lower ileum. The usual manifestations include superficial ulceration, petechial hemorrhages, and sometimes mucosal or submucosal abscesses. When mucosal inflammation is

present, it usually surrounds parasitic ova and not the organism itself. The parasite only rarely invades the mucosa, but when it does, granulomas known as *Oxyuris nodules* form. Severe mucosal eosinophilia occurs in approximately 2% of infections. A rim of granulation tissue enclosed by a fibrous capsule surrounds an eosinophilic center. In addition, one can see eosinophils, lymphocytes, giant cells, and Charcot-Leyden crystals in the nodules. The nodules eventually fibrose and hyalinize, forming obstructive masses that lead to secondary obstruction followed by acute appendicitis. In some cases, the adult worms migrate into the peritoneum and omentum, where they induce a foreign body inflammatory reaction.

Schistosomiasis, a water-borne trematode infection, represents one of the most widespread parasitic diseases; an estimated 300 million people are affected worldwide (41). In endemic areas, schistosomes are found in 1% to 15% of appendiceal resections (42). Not all infected individuals become symptomatic. Granulomatous appendicitis develops in younger patients in the early phase of egg laying in the appendix when an acute granulomatous inflammation surrounds viable ova. Concomitant tissue necrosis, tissue eosinophilia, and neutrophil exudation ensue. Obstructive appendicitis may develop as a result of fibrosis of the appendiceal wall, secondary to a longstanding inflammatory reaction to the schistosomal eggs, which may appear calcified in tissue sections. Ova can also be impacted within vascular lumens, sometimes causing hemorrhagic ischemic necrosis (43).

Ascaris (Fig. 8.26), fascioliasis, sparganosis, various types of amoebae, *Balantidium coli* (44), *Toxocara* species, *Trichuris*

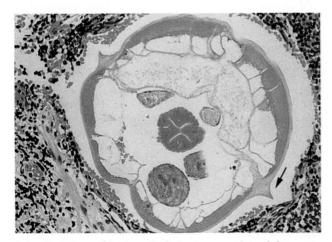

FIG. 8.24. *Enterobius vermicularis.* Cross section of the worm in the appendiceal lumen. Note the characteristic cuticular crests (*arrow*).

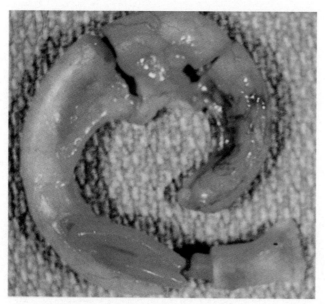

FIG. 8.26. Ascaris adult worm present within the appendiceal lumen.

trichiura, *Trichuris vulpis* (45), Reticularis (46), Strongyloides, and *Capillaria hepatica* all can infect the appendix, either alone or in conjunction with infestation of other parts of the intestine. The histologic features of these infections are described in Chapters 6 and 13.

Consumption of food contaminated with bovine spongiform encephalopathy is believed to cause *variant Creutzfeldt-Jakob disease* (vCJD) (47). The infection requires normal numbers of Peyer patches to be present in the small intestine and appendix (48). Immunoreactivity for prion proteins, particularly in the germinal centers of the lymphoid follicles in the appendix, can be seen before the clinical onset of the vCJD. The appendix does not show evidence of acute appendicitis. The presence of the prion proteins in the appendix during the incubation period of vCJD potentially offers the opportunity for screening for the disease in patients undergoing appendectomy (49). However, it should be noted that the abnormal prion protein is not present in all cases of vCJD (50).

"IDIOPATHIC" GRANULOMATOUS APPENDICITIS

Idiopathic appendicitis is a poorly understood disease that is seen in 0.1% to 2% of appendectomy specimens (51,52). It may represent an early manifestation of other granuloma-associated diseases, such as Crohn disease, sarcoidosis, or parasitic or bacterial infections (53). In this setting, appendiceal involvement occurs before other disease manifestations become evident, and therefore the etiology of the granuloma is unclear. In other cases, idiopathic granulomatous appendicitis may in fact be just that. However, the histologic features alone may

have very low sensitivity in differentiating among these various etiologies.

It has been suggested that, when up to 20 granulomas per tissue section of the appendix are found, this most likely represents isolated idiopathic granulomatous appendicitis (54). However, others have found that patients with 21 granulomas per cross section later developed Crohn disease elsewhere in their gastrointestinal tract, suggesting that the number of granulomas present is not a reliable criterion for separate Crohn disease and idiopathic granulomatous appendicitis (55,56). When neural hyperplasia is present in addition to the granulomas, this may represent early Crohn disease.

Lamps et al confirmed that *Yersinia* infections are an important cause of granulomatous appendicitis by using a combination of histologic evaluation and molecular techniques to demonstrate *Yersinia* DNA sequences in tissues. There were no reliable histologic features (described in an earlier section) that distinguished between *Yersinia*-negative and *Yersinia*-positive cases. *Yersinia* infections could only be reliably diagnosed using the polymerase chain reaction (PCR) analysis (53).

When granulomas are found, an effort should be made to determine their etiology by correlation with other findings. In cases suspicious for *Yersinia*, an attempt should be made to rule in (or rule out) this as the etiology of the granulomas, either by serologic tests or PCR analysis on the tissues in order to facilitate appropriate treatment. If no etiology can be established, the diagnosis of idiopathic granulomatous appendicitis can be made until some other etiology (such as Crohn disease) becomes clear. The provisional nature of the diagnosis can be reflected in a comment.

APPENDICEAL CHANGES IN IMMUNOCOMPROMISED PATIENTS

Immunocompromised individuals develop the usual form of appendicitis as well as involvement by the same infections seen in the remainder of the gastrointestinal tract. In addition, the appendix may be involved by neutropenic enterocolitis. The clue to the diagnosis is the absence of acute inflammation in the presence of ulcers as would be expected in nonneutropenic patients. The histologic features of this entity are described in detail in Chapter 13. One may also see the side effects of drugs used in the transplant setting (see Chapter 13) or increased apoptotic activity in AIDS patients. Lymphoid hyperplasia is also very common in the setting of AIDS.

INFLAMMATORY BOWEL DISEASE

Both ulcerative colitis (UC) and Crohn disease (CD) affect the appendix, although appendiceal involvement occurs more commonly in CD than in UC. The diagnosis of appendiceal UC and CD relies on a combination of clinical, radiologic, and morphologic findings. Examination of an appendectomy specimen may provide the first clue to the presence of IBD,

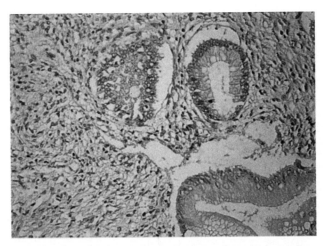

FIG. 8.27. Appendix in patient on long-term cancer chemotherapy. The architecture is markedly distorted secondary to fibrosis. The lamina propria is severely depleted of its normal immune cells.

TABLE 8.3	Causes of Inflammation in Periappendicitis
Abdominal aortic aneurysm	
Appendicitis in another appendiceal segment	
Colitis	
Diverticulitis	
Inflammation associated with colonic neoplasms	
Inflammatory bowel disease	
Pelvic inflammatory disease	
Urologic diseases	
Unknown causes	
Intestinal infections	

especially when the disease remains confined to the appendix. The histologic changes resemble those seen in the remainder of the intestines. The histologic features of appendiceal involvement by IBD are discussed in Chapter 11.

DRUG EFFECTS

The appendix is affected by drugs in much the same way as the small intestine and large intestine (see Chapters 6 and 13); however, there are some unique features that affect the appendix. *Chemotherapy* severely depletes the normal lymphoid tissues, producing a hypocellular lamina propria and loss of Peyer patches (Fig. 8.27). The epithelial cells may appear necrotic or megaloblastic. There is an increased incidence of appendicitis during locoregional chemoradiation for patients treated for rectal and cervical cancers. *Thalidomide* has been connected with appendiceal agenesis.

The introduction of *highly active antiretroviral therapy* (HAART) has revolutionized the management of HIV-infected individuals and its use is usually followed by immune restoration and clinical improvement. While this therapy has changed the profile of HIV-related morbidity, there have been several reports linking HAART with acute inflammatory or infective conditions, including possibly acute appendicitis (57). This may result from the so-called immune restoration inflammatory syndrome. Appendicitis may be precipitated by local lymphatic hyperplasia or by an infectious process in the appendix during the restoration. Another possibility is that the antiretroviral therapy itself may cause appendicitis.

PERIAPPENDICITIS

Periappendicitis is defined as appendiceal serosal inflammation without mucosal involvement (Fig. 8.28). Periappendicitis

most commonly affects boys below the age of 12 years and females between the ages of 17 and 21. Periappendicitis can be classified into two types, juvenile and secondary. In the juvenile form, the inflammation reaches the submucosa but there is a gradient in the severity of the process. It is slight in the submucosa and increases as the serosa is approached. This form is believed to result from previous episodes of appendicitis with resolution of the mucosal inflammation. Secondary periappendicitis complicates concurrent intra-abdominal infections or other inflammatory conditions. Common causes of periappendicitis are listed in Table 8.3. Salpingitis caused by *Chlamydia trachomatis* is especially prone to produce periappendicitis (58). Serious complications develop in a large percentage of patients with periappendicitis, suggesting that establishing a diagnosis of periappendicitis has clinical significance (59).

The histologic findings reflect the duration of the inflammatory process. Most commonly one sees acute inflammation and edema limited to the serosa and muscularis propria. There may be accompanying mesothelial hyperplasia. (If one only sees scattered neutrophils on the serosal surface of the appendix with actively marginating neutrophils, it is likely that these changes reflect surgical handling of the appendix and not true periappendicitis.) In some cases there is a prominent fibrinous exudate without much in the way of inflammation. As the process resolves, fibrous tissue and chronic inflammatory cells replace the acute inflammation and edema and fibrosing strands penetrate the mesoappendix (Fig. 8.28).

PROGRESSIVE FIBROUS OCCLUSION

Fibrous occlusion (fibrous obliteration) of the distal tip of the appendix occurs as part of the natural aging process. The fibrosing process starts distally and progresses proximally (Fig. 8.29), eventually resulting in the loss of the normal appendiceal mucosa and Peyer patches. During the initial stages of fibrosis, the mast cell density in the lamina propria increases, accompanied by neural hyperplasia.

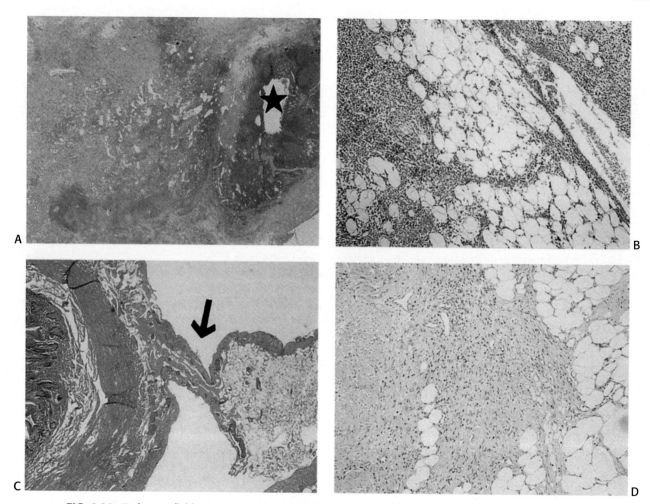

FIG. 8.28. Periappendicitis. **A:** Acute periappendicitis. The appendiceal lumen is indicated by the *star*. The majority of the inflammation surrounds the appendix. This patient had diverticulitis with a ruptured diverticulum. **B:** Higher power magnification of the inflammatory process involving the periappendiceal fat. **C:** The end result of periappendiceal inflammation is the formation of adhesions between the appendix and adjacent structures. A periappendiceal adhesion is indicated by the *arrow*. **D:** Periappendicitis at a later stage in its evolution demonstrating the presence of proliferating fibroblasts and chronic inflammatory cells.

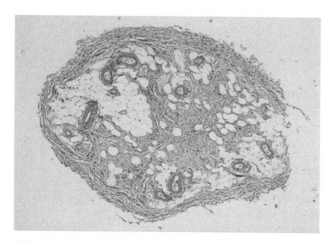

FIG. 8.29. Appendiceal atrophy with fibrous obliteration demonstrating the loss of the epithelium as well as its surrounding lamina propria and lymphoid follicles. Fatty infiltration and ingrowth of fibrous tissue has occurred. The muscularis propria appears atrophic.

NEURAL HYPERPLASIA

As noted above, distal fibrous occlusion may be accompanied by *neural hyperplasia*. The incidence of neural hyperplasia varies geographically, occurring more commonly in countries with a high incidence of appendicitis. The finding of increased numbers of nerve fibers, Schwann cells, and enlarged ganglia in patients with acute appendicitis suggests that not all neural hyperplasias seen in appendices represent a physiologic aging phenomenon as has been postulated. Rather, it may result from previous episodes of inflammation followed by neural remodeling. The neural proliferation may be augmented by mast cells that produce nerve growth factors.

Three types of neural proliferations are seen: One accompanying distal fibrous occlusions, one arising from the plexuses, and one involving the lamina propria. In the form associated with distal fibrous occlusion, one sees small nodules of Schwann cells with spindled comma-shaped nuclei

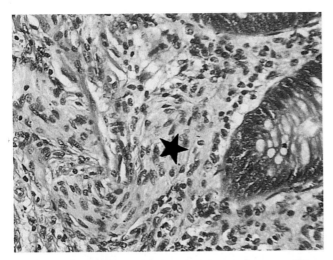

FIG. 8.30. Neural hyperplasia. Hyperplastic Schwann cells are present involving the lamina propria between the crypts of Lieberkühn (*star*).

and scant indistinct cytoplasm aggregated in onionskinlike lamellae in a myxoid stroma, producing a vaguely whorled pattern (Fig. 8.30). These features may be best appreciated using immunostains for neural markers such as S100, PGP 9.5, or Leu-7. In the mucosal form, one sees focal collections of pale spindle cells in the lamina propria or in an obliterated appendix (60). S100, PGP 9.5, Leu-7, or synaptophysin highlights the neuronal or the perineuronal Schwann cells. Neural hyperplasia arising from the mucosal nerve plexuses tends to involve Meissner and Auerbach plexuses, and can extend into the periappendiceal fat.

RETENTION MUCOCELE

Retention mucoceles (simple mucoceles, retention cysts) result from luminal obstruction with distention of part or all of the appendiceal lumen by mucus accumulations (Fig. 8.31). We recommend that the term *mucocele* be reserved solely for appendices that are dilated and contain inspissated mucin in which there are no mucin-secreting neoplasms. Mucoceles have an equal sex distribution and most typically affect the middle-aged. They usually follow acute appendicitis with postinflammatory fibrosis, obstruction, and progressive mucin accumulations. Usually mucoceles are small and symptomless, but they may enlarge and contain a thick, gelatinous mucin that can result in abdominal pain, with or without a palpable mass.

Retention mucoceles are usually unilocular, thin walled, and lined by flattened, atrophic epithelium. The lining may also contain normal-appearing goblet cells. The appendiceal wall may appear focally fibrotic and chronically inflamed. Rupture of a retention mucocele produces localized periappendiceal mucin accumulations that are easily resectable and the mucin does not reaccumulate. However, a careful search should be made for neoplastic epithelium to rule out the presence of an underlying neoplasm. A granulomatous response may develop (Fig. 8.32).

MYXOGLOBULOSIS

Myxoglobulosis, a variant of appendiceal mucocele, is characterized by the presence of mucinous, occasionally calcified pearl- or caviarlike globules in a usually dilated appendiceal lumen. The distinctive features of the globules give rise to terms such as "fish-egg" or "caviar" appendix (Fig. 8.33). Myxoglobulosis constitutes 0.35% to 8.0% of mucoceles (61,62).

The lesions can present clinically as an acute abdomen or may represent an incidental finding at the time of laparotomy or autopsy. Grossly, the characteristic finding is that of a group of opaque white globules consisting of calcified amorphous material (Fig. 8.33) without an underlying architecture. Perforation represents an infrequent complication,

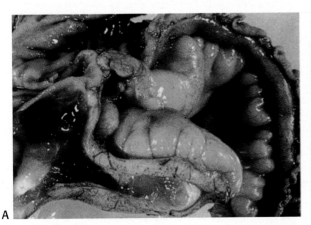

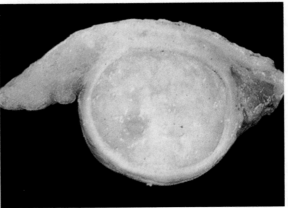

A   B

FIG. 8.31. Mucocele. **A:** The appendix is opened lengthwise to show the presence of gelatinous material within the appendix. The proximal portion of the appendix is more dilated than the distal portion. **B:** Cross section through the appendix of a patient with a mucocele. The appendiceal lumen is completely filled with gelatinous mucoid material. No neoplasms were present.

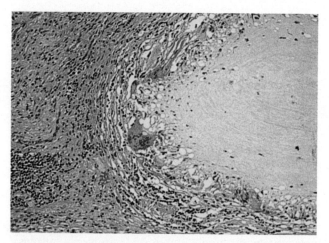

FIG. 8.32. Mucocele. The lumen contains mucus and collections of giant cells and inflammatory cells. This form of granulomatous reaction is often seen in mucoceles of various etiologies.

with the usual consequence being peritonitis. In the case of perforation, the white globules may become walled off by fibrous adhesions in a pericecal collection. An occlusive membrane in the proximal appendix may lead to the development of this lesion (63).

Histologically, the "pearls" or "caviar" consist of concentrically layered mucous and cell debris. Factors that lead to the transformation of mucin into globular masses are unknown. Hypotheses include the formation of a tissue core that acts as a nidus for concentric mucin deposition. The core may represent an organizing mass of mucin and granulation tissue that originates in the appendiceal wall, breaks off, and undergoes necrosis.

BENIGN NONNEOPLASTIC POLYPS

Small, localized hyperplastic polyps resembling those in the colorectum develop in the appendix (Fig. 8.34). The glands have serrated lumens lined by benign epithelium demonstrating an orderly progression of cellular maturation. The collagen table appears thickened and cytologic atypia is absent. Peutz-Jeghers and juvenile polyps also affect the appendix as part of a more generalized syndrome. They resemble Peutz-Jeghers and juvenile polyps arising elsewhere (see Chapter 12). These lesions should be distinguished from serrated adenomas and sessile serrated polyps (see Chapter 14).

LYMPHOID HYPERPLASIA

Lymphoid hyperplasia usually affects younger individuals (Fig. 8.35), producing obstruction and secondary appendicitis. Viral infections often induce the lymphoid hyperplasia. Appendices with virally induced lymphoid hyperplasias

are seldom removed unless a secondary acute appendicitis ensues, since the process remains self-limited and the lymphoid hyperplasia eventually regresses. The process is characterized by the presence of enlarged lymphoid follicles containing prominent germinal centers and a mantle of surrounding benign-appearing lymphocytes. The germinal centers may contain numerous tingible body macrophages.

GRAFT VERSUS HOST DISEASE

Graft versus host disease (GVHD) affects the appendix as part of a more generalized gastrointestinal involvement. In GVHD, the lamina propria appears extremely acellular with loss of Peyer patches due to the pretransplant conditioning. The characteristic apoptotic lesions develop as elsewhere in the gut (Fig. 8.36). Because of the setting in which this lesion occurs, concomitant CMV infections may be present.

VASCULAR DISEASES

Vascular disorders that affect the appendix include varices, vascular malformations, vascular neoplasms, angiodysplasia, and vasculitis (Fig. 8.37). Appendiceal necrotizing arteritis varies in incidence from 0.89% to 1.9% of patients (64,65). It results in mucosal ulceration or infarction. Often the vasculitis exists in the absence of appendicitis. The disorder represents part of the clinicopathologic spectrum of systemic polyarteritis nodosa. It may be diagnosed first in the appendix due to the frequency of appendectomies that are performed annually. The features of these vascular lesions are discussed elsewhere in this book.

GYNECOLOGIC ABNORMALITIES SEEN IN THE APPENDIX
Endometriosis

Endometriosis affects 1% to 8% of examined appendices (66,67). Most patients are between the ages of 20 and 40. Endometriosis usually involves the serosal surface or the muscular layers (Fig. 8.38). Only rarely does it involve the mucosa. It can present as appendicitis, especially when bleeding occurs in the endometriotic tissue, or as an intussusception. Grossly, endometriosis may appear as discrete brownish foci, although more often it is an incidental histologic finding, not having been appreciated grossly. Both endometrial glands and stroma associate with variable amounts of fibrosis and hemosiderin deposits.

Appendiceal endometriosis occurs alone or coexists with other conditions such as appendiceal inversion. The latter results from muscular hyperplasia, which stimulates appendiceal peristalsis, causing complete inversion and

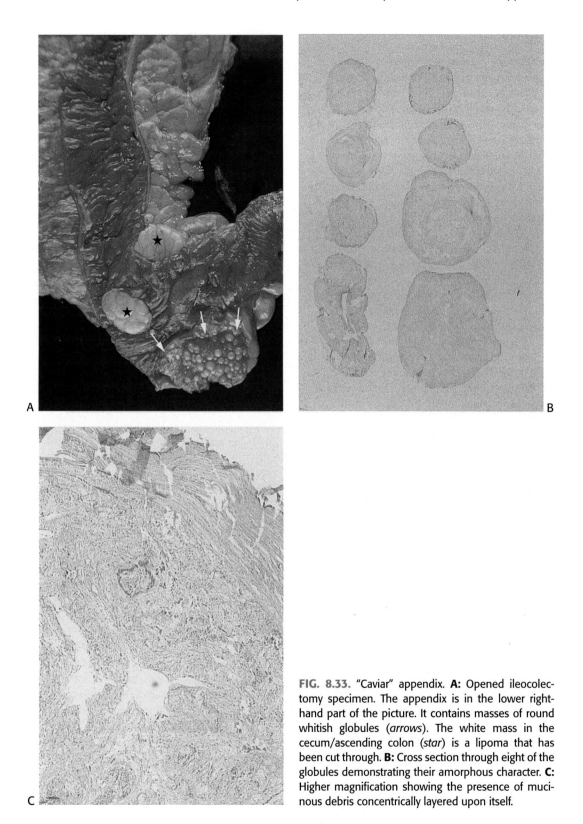

FIG. 8.33. "Caviar" appendix. **A:** Opened ileocolectomy specimen. The appendix is in the lower right-hand part of the picture. It contains masses of round whitish globules (*arrows*). The white mass in the cecum/ascending colon (*star*) is a lipoma that has been cut through. **B:** Cross section through eight of the globules demonstrating their amorphous character. **C:** Higher magnification showing the presence of mucinous debris concentrically layered upon itself.

intussusception of the appendix into the cecum. There is a rare case of mucinous metaplasia with epithelial dysplasia occurring in the endometriotic epithelium of the appendix (66). The endometrial glands display extensive areas of mucinous epithelium and Paneth cells. Focally, the mucinous epithelium demonstrate low-grade epithelial dysplasia. Both the intestinal and endometrial epithelium are surrounded by typical endometrial stroma, showing strong positivity for estrogen receptor proteins. Support for a metaplastic origin of the mucinous epithelium was the

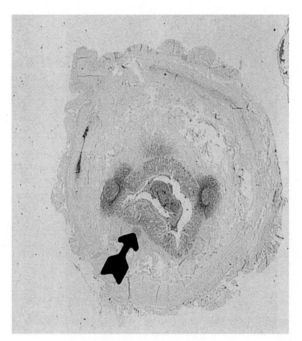

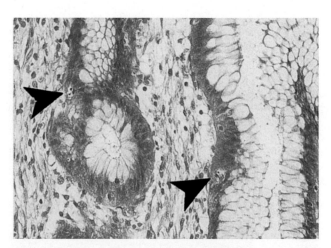

FIG. 8.36. Graft versus host disease. The glands are separated by a hypocellular lamina propria. Single-cell necrosis typical of graft versus host disease (*arrowheads*) is present. (Case courtesy of Drs. Shulman, Sale, and Myerson, Fred Hutchinson Cancer Center, Seattle, WA.)

FIG. 8.34. Hyperplastic polyp of the appendix. The *arrow* indicates an area where the mucosa is focally thicker than the surrounding areas. The lesion is histologically identical to similar lesions that more commonly arise in the colon.

presence of glands containing mixtures of mucinous cells, goblet cells, Paneth cells, ciliated cells and nonciliated endometrial cells, and ciliated and nonciliated mucinous cells, all showing estrogen receptor positivity (67).

Endosalpingiosis

Endosalpingiosis, the ectopic location of benign epithelium resembling that lining the normal fallopian tube, often involves the peritoneal and gastrointestinal serosal surfaces. It likely results from metaplasia of the peritoneal surface (68). The lesion consists of papillary, multiglandular structures that may be complex in nature but do not demonstrate cytologic atypia. Psammoma bodies may be present.

The distinction of this lesion from endometriosis is relatively straightforward since endometrial epithelium and stroma, areas of periglandular hemorrhage, and hemosiderin-laden macrophages are absent in endosalpingiosis. The identification of müllerian-type cells differentiates this lesion from mesonephric remnants and mesothelial inclusion cysts. The absence of goblet cells also precludes a gastrointestinal origin. Furthermore, the lesion is positive for CA-125 and estrogen receptors (ER) (Fig. 8.39), further confirming its müllerian origin (69).

Endosalpingiosis causes diagnostic difficulty since it may be difficult to distinguish from serosal implants of low-grade (borderline) ovarian cancer. The diagnosis of endosalpingiosis is favored when the following factors are absent: (a) past or present ovarian surface borderline peritoneal masses; (b) stromal desmoplasia, a destructive infiltrative pattern with disrupted or interrupted glandular basement membranes; and (c) nuclear atypia and mitoses (68). A mesothelial lesion is also in the differential diagnosis but immunostains with antibodies to calretinin and ER, progesterone receptors (PR), and CA-125 can easily distinguish between these two entities.

Decidual Islands

Decidual islands may stud the appendiceal serosa (Fig. 8.40) in the appendices of pregnant women. They can also be found in the mucosa or muscularis propria. These islands contain sheets of large polyhedral decidual cells. Unlike endometriosis, glands are absent. This change may be mistaken for some form of neoplasm, but immunostains for keratin, S100, carcinoembryonic antigen (CEA), and EMA are

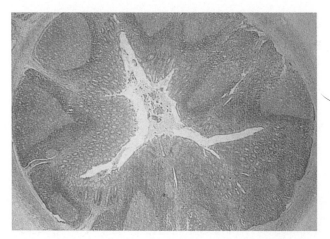

FIG. 8.35. Lymphoid hyperplasia. Cross section of an adult appendix demonstrating confluent hyperplastic lymphoid follicles.

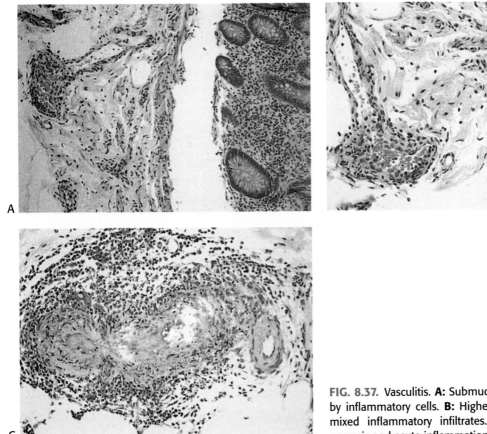

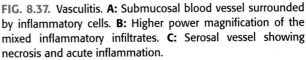

FIG. 8.37. Vasculitis. **A:** Submucosal blood vessel surrounded by inflammatory cells. **B:** Higher power magnification of the mixed inflammatory infiltrates. **C:** Serosal vessel showing necrosis and acute inflammation.

usually negative. The decidual cells may express vimentin, desmin, and/or smooth muscle actin.

MESOTHELIAL CYSTS

Mesothelial cysts frequently involve the tip of the appendix (Fig. 8.41) or they develop in association with periappendiceal

inflammatory pseudotumors. They are often multiple and lined by cuboidal or flattened mesothelium, depending on how much pressure atrophy of the epithelium has occurred. Mesothelial cells contain abundant cytoplasm and a small centrally placed nucleus. They lie above a submesothelial mesenchyme. Mesothelial cells can appear quite reactive, normal, or flattened in the cysts. These cells are periodic acid–Schiff (PAS), CEA, and EMA negative and are cytokeratin and calretinin positive.

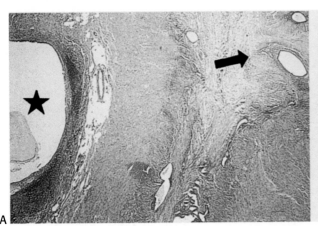

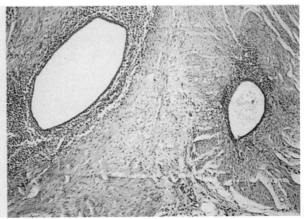

FIG. 8.38. Endometriosis. **A:** Cross section through the appendix demonstrating the lumen (*star*). Endometrial glands and stroma are present in the wall (*arrow*). **B:** Higher power magnification of two endometrial glands surrounded by endometrial stroma in muscularis propria.

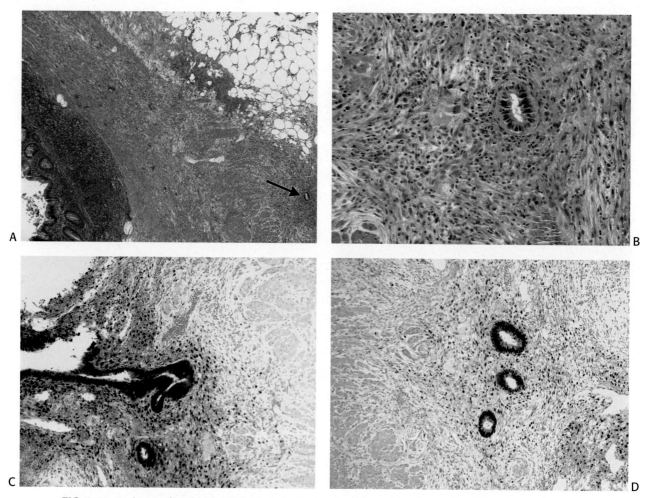

FIG. 8.39. Periappendiceal endosalpingiosis. **A:** Low-power picture showing a gland surrounded by a peculiar stroma in the periappendiceal tissues (*arrow*). **B:** Higher magnification of the gland. **C:** The nuclei of the glands and stroma are strongly positive with an antibody to the estrogen receptor. **D:** Some of these cells are also positive for the progesterone receptor.

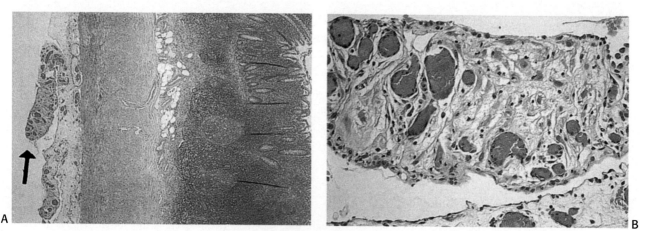

FIG. 8.40. Decidual nodules. **A:** Cross section of appendix with serosal decidual nodules (*arrow*). **B:** Higher power view demonstrating the details of the decidual cells.

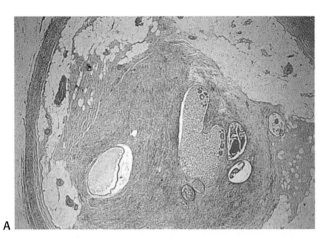
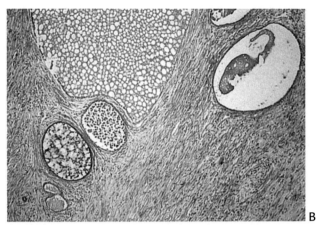

FIG. 8.41. Mesothelial cysts. **A:** Cross section through the tip of the appendix demonstrating multiple cystic cavities. **B:** The cysts contain mucin and are lined by mesothelium.

CYSTIC FIBROSIS

Cystic fibrosis (CF) represents the most common hereditary disease in Caucasians. The common denominator for the gastrointestinal abnormalities seen in the setting of CF is abnormal mucus production. Mucus viscosity depends on the structure of the glycogen protein, the concentration of hydrogen and calcium ions, and water content. These are abnormal in CF. CF may be diagnosed based on the presence of appendiceal changes (Fig. 8.42). Increased numbers of hyperdistended goblet cells line the entire length of the crypts. These goblet cells release their abnormal mucin content and the appendix swells and becomes hyperdistended with inspissated eosinophilic secretions. Appendicitis results when the lumen is obstructed by the thick secretions. Diverticula may develop due to accumulations of thick mucin and increased intraluminal presence. Patients may develop appendicocutaneous fistula (69).

MELANOSIS

Melanosis is defined as the accumulation of lipofuscin granules within mucosal macrophages. These granules are composed of membrane-bound intracytoplasmic bodies with electron-dense lipid material (70). These cells are seen predominantly in the mucosa, although submucosal collections can also be seen. Melanosis is present in 7.4% to 46% of appendices (71,72). Melanosis is also present in a large percentage of pediatric patients, suggesting that it is a common nonspecific alteration (72). It is currently thought that it results from increased apoptosis (72) due to many different causes, including infections (71) and laxative ingestion.

The intensity of the change varies significantly from scanty solitary histiocytic cells to large aggregates of heavily pigmented macrophages (Fig. 8.43). The latter are particularly prominent in patients with an associated melanosis coli. The melanosis is most prominent in the proximal portion of the appendix with minimal or no involvement of the distal tip.

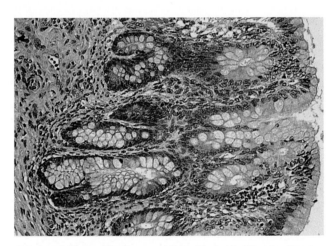

FIG. 8.42. Appendix from a child with cystic fibrosis showing enlarged goblet cells and the regenerated mucous membrane.

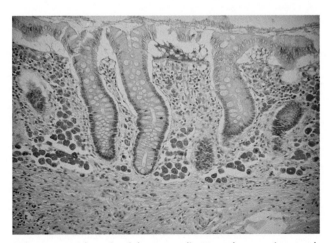

FIG. 8.43. Melanosis of the appendix. Note the prominent collections of pigmented macrophages deep in the lamina propria. This was associated with extensive melanosis coli.

MISCELLANEOUS CHANGES

Patients who have undergone appendectomies may have residual alterations that are identifiable endoscopically as well as microscopically. The most common change is *appendiceal stump inversion*, which may present as a cecal polyp. Patients who have had previous gynecologic surgeries may show ovarian tissue adherent to the appendiceal mesoappendix. *Gastrointestinal sarcoid* is rare (73) and is best diagnosed in the presence of a positive Kveim test or clinical and histologic evidence of a disseminated disease. Appendiceal sarcoid may present as an acute appendicitis. Infiltrative diseases such as *eosinophilic granuloma, amyloidosis, malacoplakia* (74), *Whipple disease* (75), and *inflammatory pseudotumor* can all involve the appendix. The pathologic features of these entities resemble those described elsewhere in the text.

FOREIGN BODIES

Foreign bodies are present in 5.5% of the appendectomy specimens (12). They lodge there and may cause localized appendicitis, with fecaliths representing the most common foreign body. Other common foreign materials include barium and parasites. However, almost every other type of conceivable foreign body may be present, such as pins, nails, bubble gum, teeth, and seeds. Foreign bodies may cause mucosal atrophy and foreign body granulomas.

REFERENCES

1. Malas MA, Sulak O, Gokcimen A, Sari A: Development of the vermiform appendix during the fetal period. *Surg Radiol Anat* 2004;26:202.
2. Horowitz E: Zur Histogenese des Colon und der Appendix beim Menschen. *Z Anat Entwickl* 1933;101:679.
3. Bockman DE: Functional histology of appendix. *Arch Histol Jpn* 1983; 46:271.
4. Wakeley CPG, Gladstone RF: The relative frequency of the various positions of the vermiform appendix as ascertained by an analysis of 5000 cases. *Lancet* 1928;1:178.
5. Collins D: A study of 50,000 specimens of the human vermiform appendix. *Surg Gynecol Obstet* 1955;101:437.
6. Collins DC: Agenesis of the vermiform appendix. *Am J Surg* 1951;82:689.
7. Mesko TW, Lugo R, Breitholtz T: Horseshow anomaly of the appendix: a previously undescribed entity. *Surgery* 1989;106:563.
8. Yokose Y, Maruyama H, Tsutsumi M, et al: Ileal atresia and absence of appendix. *Acta Pathol Jpn* 1986;36:1403.
9. Bremner DN, Mooney G: Agenesis of appendix; a further thalidomide anomaly. *Lancet* 1978;i:826.
10. Narula IM, Pendse AK, Dandia SD: Appendix duplex. *Int Surg* 1974;59:173.
11. Tinckler LF: Triple appendix vermiformis: a unique case. *Br J Surg* 1968; 55:79.
12. Collins DC: 71,000 Human appendix specimens, a final report summarizing forty years' study. *Am J Proctol* 1963;14:65.
13. Lamps LW, Gray GF Jr, Dilday BR, Washington MK: The coexistence of low-grade mucinous neoplasms of the appendix and appendiceal diverticula: a possible role in the pathogenesis of pseudomyxoma peritonei. *Mod Pathol* 2000;13:495.
14. Forshall I: Intussusception of the vermiform appendix with a report of seven cases in children. *Br J Surg* 1953;40:305.
15. Rode J, Dhillon AP, Hutt MSR: Appendicitis revisited: a comparative study of Malawian and English appendices. *J Pathol* 1987;153:357.
16. Basta M, Morton NE, Mulvihill JJ, et al: Inheritance of acute appendicitis: familial aggregation and evidence of polygenic transmission. *Am J Hum Genet* 1990;46:377.
17. Gamal R, Moore TC: Appendicitis in children aged 13 years and younger. *Am J Surg* 1990;159:589.
18. Pressman A, Kawar B, Abend M, et al: Acute perforated neonatal appendicitis associated with chorioamnionitis. *Eur J Pediatr Surg* 2001;11:204.
19. Beluffi G, Alberici E: Acute appendicitis in a premature baby. *Eur Radiol* 2002;12:S152.
20. Campbell KL, Debeaux AC: Non-steroidal anti-inflammatory drugs and appendicitis in patients aged over 50 years. *Br J Surg* 1992;79:967.
21. Rautio M, Saxen H, Siitonen A, et al: Bacteriology of histopathologically defined appendicitis in children. *Pediatr Infect Dis J* 2000;19:1078.
22. Hardwick RH, Taylor A, Thompson MH, et al: Association between Streptococcus milleri and abscess formation after appendicitis. *Ann R Coll Surg Engl* 2000;82:24.
23. Campbell LK, Havens JM, Scott MA, Lamps L: Molecular detection of Campylobacter jejuni in archival cases of acute appendicitis. *Mod Pathol* 2006;19:1042.
24. Xiong S, Puri P, Nemeth L, et al: Neuronal hypertrophy in acute appendicitis. *Arch Pathol Lab Med* 2000;124:1429.
25. Stephenson J, Snoddy WT: Appendiceal lesions: observation in 4000 appendectomies. *Arch Surg* 1961;83:661.
26. Pieper R, Kager L, Nasman P: Clinical significance of mucosal inflammation of the vermiform appendix. *Ann Surg* 1983;197:368.
27. Herd ME, Cross PA, Dutt S: Histological audit of acute appendicitis. *J Clin Pathol* 1992;45:456.
28. Butler C: Surgical pathology of acute appendicitis. *Hum Pathol* 1981; 12:870.
29. Birch PJ, Richmond I, Bennett MK: Xanthogranulomatous appendicitis. *Histopathology* 1993;22:597.
30. Bittinger F, Brochhausen C, Kohler H, et al: Differential expression of cell adhesion molecules in inflamed appendix: correlation with clinical stage. *J Pathol* 1998;186:422.
31. Milliken NT, Stryker HB Jr: Suppurative pylothrombophlebitis and multiple liver abscesses following acute appendicitis. Report of case with recovery. *N Engl J Med* 1951;244:52.
32. Sabbe LJ, Van De Merwe D, Schouls L, et al: Clinical spectrum of infections due to the newly described Actinomyces species A. turicensis, A. radingae, and A. europaeus. *J Clin Microbiol* 1999;37:8.
33. Rabenandrasana HA, Ahmad A, Samison LH, et al: Child primary tubercular appendicitis. *Ped Int* 2004;46:374.
34. Lamps LW, Madhusudhan KT, Greenson J, et al: The role of Yersinia enterocolitica and Yersinia pseudotuberculosis in granulomatous appendicitis. *Am J Surg Pathol* 2001;25:505.
35. Kubota K, Tamura J, Kurabayashi H, et al: Warthin-Finkeldey-like giant cells in a patient with systemic lupus erythematosus. *Hum Pathol* 1988;19:1358.
36. O'Brien A, O'Briain S: Infectious mononucleosis: appendiceal lymphoid tissue involvement parallels characteristic lymph node changes. *Arch Pathol Lab Med* 1985;109:680.
37. Gatti S, Lopes R, Cevini C, et al: Intestinal parasitic infections in an institution for the mentally retarded. *Ann Trop Med Parasitol* 2000; 94:453.
38. Yoon HJ, Choi YJ, Lee SU: Enterobius vermicularis egg positive rate of preschool children in Chunchon, Korea. *Korean J Pathol* 1999;38:279.
39. Arca MJ, Gates RL, Groner JI, et al: Clinical manifestations of appendiceal pinworms in children: an institutional experience and a review of the literature. *Pediatr Surg Int* 2004;20:372.
40. Williams DJ, Dixon MF: Sex, Enterobius vermicularis and the appendix. *Br J Surg* 1988;75:1225.
41. Jordan P, Webbe G (eds): *Schistosomiasis: Epidemiology Treatment and Control*. London: Heinemann Medical Books, 1982.
42. Al-Kraida A, Giangreco A, Shaikh MU, Al-Shehri A: Appendicitis and schistosomiasis. *Br J Surg* 1988;75:58.
43. Ramdial PK, Madiba TE, Kharwa S, et al: Isolated amoebic appendicitis. *Virchows Arch* 2002;441:63.
44. Arean VM, Echevarria R: Balantidiasis. In: Marcial-Rojas PA (ed). *Pathology of Protozoal and Helminthic Diseases with Clinical Correlation*. Baltimore: Williams & Wilkins, 1971, p 238.
45. Kenney M, Yermakov V: Infection of man with Trichuris vulpis, the whipworm of dogs. *Am J Trop Med Hyg* 1980;29:1205.
46. Kenney M, Eveland LK, Yermakov V, Kassouny DY: A case of rictularia infection of man in New York. *Am J Trop Med Hyg* 1975;24:596.

47. Aguzzi A, Montrasio F, Kaesar PS: Prions: health scare and biological challenge. *Nat Rev Mol Cell Biol* 2001;2:118.

48. Prinz M, Huber G, Macpherson AJS, et al: Prion infection requires normal numbers of Peyer's patches but not of enteric lymphocytes. *Am J Pathol* 2003;162:1103.

49. Hilton DA, Fathers E, Edwards P, et al: Prion immunoreactivity in appendix before clinical onset of variant Creutzfeldt-Jakob disease. *Lancet* 1998;352:703.

50. Joiner S, Linehan J, Brandner S, et al: Irregular presence of abnormal prion protein in appendix in variant Creutzfeldt-Jakob disease. *J Neurol Neurosurg Psychiatry* 2002;73:597.

51. Lindhagen T, Ekelund G, Leandoer L, et al: Crohn's disease confined to the appendix. *Dis Colon Rectum* 1982;25:805.

52. Naschitz JE, Yeshurun D, Rosner I, et al: Idiopathic granulomatous appendicitis. *J Clin Gastroenterol* 1995;2:290.

53. Lamps LW, Madhusudhan KT, Greenson JK, et al: The role of Yersinia enterocolitica and Yersinia pseudo-tuberculosis in granulomatous appendicitis: a histologic and molecular study. *Am J Surg Pathol* 2001;25:508.

54. Dudley TH Jr, Dean PJ: Idiopathic granulomatous appendicitis, or Crohn's disease of the appendix revisited. *Hum Pathol* 1993;24:595.

55. Richards ML, Aberger FJ, Landercasper J: Granulomatous appendicitis: Crohn's disease, atypical Crohn's or not Crohn's at all? *J Am Coll Surg* 1997;185:13.

56. Huang JC, Appelman HD: Another look at chronic appendicitis resembling Crohn's disease. *Mod Pathol* 1996;9:975.

57. Aldeen T, Horgan M, Macallan DC, et al: Is acute appendicitis another inflammatory condition associated with highly active antiretroviral therapy (HAART)? *HIV Med* 2000;1:252.

58. Mardh PA, Wolner-Hanssen P: Periappendicitis and chlamydia salpingitis. *Surg Gynecol Obstet* 1985;160:304.

59. Fink AS, Kosakowski CA, Hiatt JR, Cochran AJ: Periappendicitis is a significant clinical finding. *Am J Surg* 1990;159:564.

60. Franke C, Gerharz CD, Bohner H, et al: Neurogenic appendicopathy: a clinical disease entity? *Int J Colorectal Dis* 2002;17:185.

61. Gonzalez JEG, Hann SE, Trujillo YP: Myxoglobulosis of the appendix. *Am J Surg Pathol* 1988;12:962.

62. Viswanath YK, Griffiths CD, Shipsey D, et al: Myxoglobulosis, a rare variant of appendiceal mucocele, occurring secondary to an occlusive membrane. *J R Coll Surg Edinb* 1998;43:204.

63. Moyana TN: Necrotizing arteritis of the vermiform appendix. A clinicopathologic study of 12 cases. *Arch Pathol Lab Med* 1988;112:738.

64. Gordon BS: Necrotizing arteritis of the appendix. *Arch Surg* 1951;62:92.

65. Clement PB: Endometriosis, lesions of the secondary muellerian system, and pelvic mesothelial proliferations. In: Kurman RJ (ed). *Blaustein's Pathology of the Female Genital Tract.* New York: Springer Verlag, 1987.

66. Mai KT, Burns BF: Development of dysplastic mucinous epithelium from endometriosis of the appendix. *Histopathology* 1999;35:368.

67. Cajigas A, Axiotis CA: Endosalpingiosis of the vermiform appendix. *Int J Gynecol Pathol* 1990;9:291.

68. McCluggage WG, Clements WD: Endosalpingiosis of the colon and appendix. *Histopathology* 2001;39:465.

69. Rogers TN, Joseph C, Bowley DM, Pitcher GJ: Appendico-cutaneous fistula in cystic fibrosis. *Pediatr Surg Int* 2004;20:151.

70. Rutty GN, Shaw PA: Melanosis of the appendix: prevalence, distribution and review of the pathogenesis of 47 cases. *Histopathology* 1997;30:319.

71. Graf NS, Arbuckle S: Melanosis of the appendix: common in the paediatric age group. *Histopathology* 2001;39:243.

72. Byers RJ, Marsh P, Parkinson D, Haboubi NY: Melanosis coli is associated with an increase in colonic epithelial apoptosis and not with laxative use. *Histopathology* 1997;2:160.

73. Clarke H, Pollett W, Chittal S, Ra M: Sarcoidosis with involvement of the appendix. *Arch Intern Med* 1983;143:1603.

74. Gray GF Jr, Wackym PA: Surgical pathology of the vermiform appendix. *Pathol Annu* 1986;21:111.

75. Misra PS, Lebwohl P, Laufer H: Hepatic and appendiceal Whipple's disease with negative jejunal biopsies. *Am J Gastroenterol* 1981;75:302.

The Neoplastic Appendix

Appendiceal tumors constitute <0.4% of all intestinal neoplasms. They pathologically resemble their small and large intestinal counterparts. The most significant difference between appendiceal and intestinal neoplasms is in the frequency of specific tumor types arising in these sites, with the appendix giving rise to a higher incidence of carcinoid tumors than carcinomas (1). Small appendiceal tumors may obstruct the appendiceal lumen, often causing appendicitis. Nevertheless, because many tumors remain asymptomatic, a diagnosis of neoplasia is seldom made prior to pathologic examination of the resected specimen. The World Health Organization (WHO) classification of appendiceal tumors is shown in Table 9.1 (2). Table 9.2 lists mucinous lesions that may be encountered with appendiceal lesions.

ADENOMAS

Several types of adenomas develop in the appendix. By far, the most common involve the appendiceal mucosa in a circumferential fashion creating a mucinous cystadenoma (Fig. 9.1); less commonly they grow as a localized lesion resembling their more common colonic counterparts (Fig. 9.2). Both types of adenomas may exhibit tubular, tubulovillous, or villous architectures and the degree of dysplasia can be low grade or high grade. Invasive carcinomas can develop in both. Appendiceal adenomas commonly associate with synchronous colorectal neoplasia (3,4). The molecular features of appendiceal neoplasia are similar to those found in colorectal neoplasms (5).

Mucinous Cystadenomas

Mucinous cystadenomas (also sometimes referred to as *low-grade appendiceal mucinous neoplasms*) (6) arise in both males and females, with many series reporting a higher incidence in females. Patients range in age from 27 to 77 years, with an average age of 53 years and a median age of 64 years (7). Approximately 20% of patients have a metachronous or synchronous colonic adenocarcinoma (8). The tumors are usually sporadic lesions but they may complicate longstanding ulcerative colitis. Some patients develop acute appendicitis because

the mucin accumulation obstructs the appendiceal lumen (Fig. 9.3). Patients also develop abdominal pain, nausea and vomiting, and, sometimes, a palpable right lower quadrant mass, perforation, or intussusception (Fig. 9.4). Other patients present with pseudomyxoma peritonei or with what appears to be an ovarian tumor.

Mucinous cystadenomas can produce large amounts of mucus converting the appendix into a sausage-shaped, cystic or spherical, mucus-filled mass (Fig. 9.3); the average diameter is 2.2 cm with a range of 0.3 to 9 cm (6). Diverticula are often present and there may be areas of rupture. There may also be grossly visible mucus on the serosal surface of the appendix. Mural calcification may produce the gross pattern of a "porcelain appendix" or the obstruction can produce myxoglobulosis, a lesion discussed in Chapter 8.

A circumferential proliferation of neoplastic mucinous epithelium replaces the normal epithelium. This neoplastic epithelium may exhibit a full range of neoplasia including low-grade dysplasia, high-grade dysplasia, and invasive carcinoma. Usually a single layer of tall crowded columnar adenomatous epithelium with basally located hyperchromatic, pseudostratified nuclei and clear to eosinophilic cytoplasm lines the neoplastic glands (Fig. 9.5). The elongated nuclei lack nucleoli. Mitotic activity is usually low and usually limited to the base of the glands (7). The glands may be tubular, although a villous architecture may be present. More often the epithelial proliferation produces an undulating pattern. Most mucinous cystadenomas show minimal cytologic atypia, qualifying for a diagnosis of low-grade dysplasia. However, some cases contain moderate to marked atypia and abundant mitotic activity. Areas of high-grade dysplasia (including carcinoma in situ) appear as a disorderly proliferation of cells that lose their polarity (Fig. 9.6) and may exhibit a back-to-back glandular pattern that obliterates the intervening lamina propria. As in the colon, these changes remain confined to the area above the muscularis mucosae. Since the likelihood of an invasive carcinoma increases with the degree of dysplasia, these areas should be well sampled to rule out an invasive process.

The nonneoplastic mucosa often appears atrophic and the usually prominent Peyer patches are often absent. Mucosal denudation is common (Fig. 9.7), either from compression by the intraluminal mucin or by ulceration due to a

TABLE 9.1 World Health Organization Classification of Epithelial Nonendocrine Appendiceal Tumors

Adenoma
  Tubular
  Villous
  Tubulovillous
  Serrated
Carcinoma
  Adenocarcinoma
  Mucinous adenocarcinoma
  Signet ring cell carcinoma
  Undifferentiated carcinoma

coexisting appendicitis. The mucosal ulcers may produce a granulomatous reaction with subsequent mural fibrosis. The intraluminal mucin may compress the lining epithelium in such a way that the flattened epithelium may not be easily recognizable as being neoplastic. A feature that should increase one's suspicion that an underlying neoplasm is present is the diameter of the appendix. Benign mucoceles seldom measure more than a centimeter in diameter; larger lesions almost always result from an underlying neoplasm. Therefore, these larger mucoceles should be well sampled to rule out the presence of a tumor, if one was not identified in the original sections.

Epithelial or mucinous displacement is common in mucinous cystadenomas due to the pressure from the intraluminal mucin or from a coexisting appendicitis. Increased intraluminal pressure from the mucin can also cause diverticula, ruptures, or fistulae. The wall of the appendix may be fibrotic and significantly attenuated at the rupture site. Mucin with or without epithelial cells may be present in the perforation site and extend to the serosal surface (Fig. 9.8). The serosa itself may show an acute or chronic serositis with inflammation and mesothelial hyperplasia. It is important to search these areas carefully for the presence of both mucin and epithelial cells and to report their presence if they are seen. The histologic features of mucinous cystadenomas with and without extra-appendiceal spread are identical (with the exception of the identification of a breach in the appendiceal wall in the former) (6). The mucus extravasation can be limited to the periappendiceal area or it can spread over large areas of the peritoneal surface (see below). Noninvasive lesions that exhibit marked cytologic atypia or complex intraepithelial proliferations tend to have a higher proliferative rate than low-grade tumors, and if these lesions gain access to the peritoneal cavity, they tend to behave more aggressively than low-grade lesions. We have found that the proliferative rate of the primary tumor as well as its extra-appendiceal extensions is an important prognostic factor.

Neoplastic epithelium can also extend into diverticula (Fig. 9.9), but this does not constitute an invasive carcinoma as evidenced by the presence of lamina propria surrounding the

TABLE 9.2 Mucinous Lesions of the Appendix and Peritoneum

Lesion	Features
Mucocele	Gross term for a dilated appendix filled with mucus secondary to a either a neoplastic or nonneoplastic obstruction
Mucinous cystadenoma (low-grade mucinous tumor)	Benign tumor that often circumferentially surrounds the appendiceal lumen. It may produce the gross appearance of a mucocele. The lesion may contain either low-grade or high-grade dysplasia
Mucinous tumor of uncertain malignant potential	Mucinous tumor with areas of questionable invasive carcinoma
Mucinous adenocarcinoma	Mucin-producing carcinoma that typically arises in a mucinous cystadenoma and invades through the muscularis mucosae into the submucosa. The invasive foci are surrounded by a desmoplastic response and the cells are cytologically malignant
Mucinous cystadenoma with mucus dissection	Low-grade or high-grade cystadenoma with mucin dissection into but not through the appendiceal wall
Pseudomyxoma peritonei	The presence of mucin collections in the abdomen and/or pelvis. Histologically it may show mucinosis, low-grade mucinous tumor, or a mucinous adenocarcinoma
Mucinosis	Presence of mucin in the peritoneal cavity, including on the surface of the appendix. No cells are present in the mucin. This lesion usually complicates a mucinous cystadenoma
Low-grade peritoneal mucinous tumor	These lesions also complicate mucinous cystadenoma. The peritoneal mucinous deposits contain neoplastic cells with the cytologic features of a low-grade or high-grade adenoma
Mucinous peritoneal adenocarcinoma	The mucin accumulations contain cytologically malignant cells. The cells often invade the underlying tissues

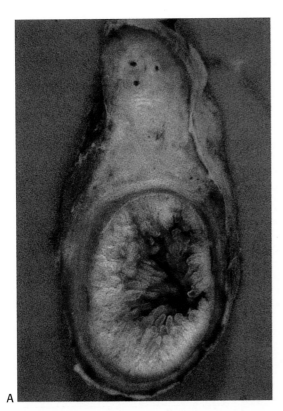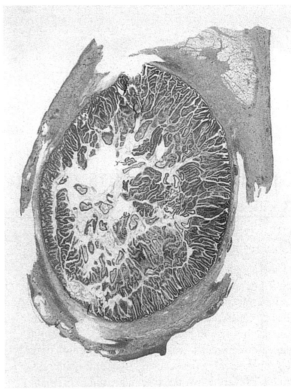

A

B

FIG. 9.1. Circumferential adenoma. **A:** Gross appearance of a cross section of a circumferential appendiceal villous adenoma. Note the long fingerlike villiform structures in the center of the photograph. **B:** Low-power histologic features of the lesion demonstrated in A showing the villous architecture. The lesion is confined to the mucosa and no evidence of invasive malignancy was seen in this lesion.

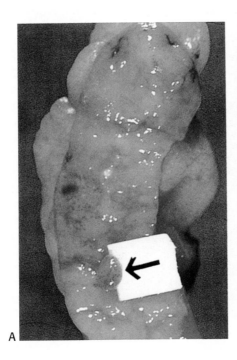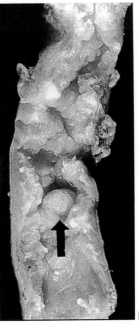

FIG. 9.2. Adenoma. **A:** Polyp within the lumen of the appendix (*arrow*). A piece of paper has been slipped under the polyp to distinguish it from the surrounding normal mucosa. **B:** Small whitish adenomatous polyp (*arrow*) in the appendix of a patient who underwent an ileocolectomy for a carcinoma of the cecum.

A

B

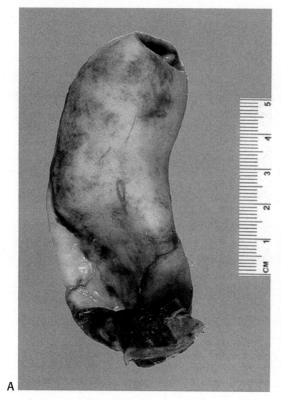

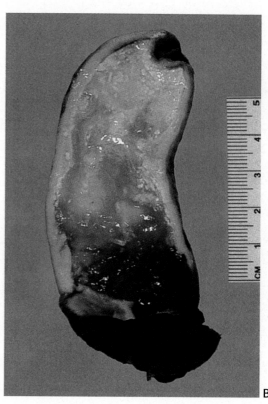

FIG. 9.3. Mucinous cystadenoma with secondary appendicitis. **A:** Gross appearance of the unopened specimen with appendicitis as indicated by the serosal erythema and adhesions. **B:** Opened specimen demonstrating a mass at the base of the appendix. The distal portion of the appendix is filled with inspissated mucinous secretions. The dusky color at the base of the specimen in A and B correlates with the presence of acute appendicitis.

neoplastic glands. It does not carry the same prognostic significance as serosal mucin extension by dissection or rupture, provided the diverticulum has not ruptured.

Mucinous cystadenomas are often not appreciated when the appendix is grossed in, especially if there is a coexisting

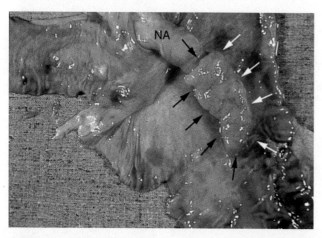

FIG. 9.4. Ileocolectomy specimen from a patient with a large sessile nonmucinous adenoma of the distal appendix. The appendix has intussuscepted into the cecum. The *arrows* delineate the areas of the appendiceal adenoma. Normal-appearing appendix (*NA*) is present proximally.

acute appendicitis. Therefore, if a tumor is found, the pathologist should carefully re-examine the appendix for areas of perforation, serosal mucin accumulations, and invasive carcinoma, since these modify the patient's prognosis and treatment if identified. Perforation sites and serosal mucin deposits should be sampled; the entire tumor should be submitted to rule out invasion. The proximal margin of resection should be identified and submitted for histologic examination. It has also become our practice to obtain a Ki-67 immunostain on the tumor and to report the proliferative rate in the most mitotically active part of the tumor.

The pathology report should indicate the degree of dysplasia in the cystadenoma and whether there is invasive cancer or perforation, whether tumor or mucin is seen outside of the appendix, and the status of the proximal margin. These factors are important because even benign neoplasms that escape the appendix may give rise to subsequent pseudomyxoma peritonei. The prognosis of patients with peritoneal spread is guarded, with just over half of the patients dying after 10 years. Because of the differences in the prognosis, some have proposed the term *mucinous borderline tumor of the appendix* to reflect the uncertain biology of the lesions (9). These lesions may also be diagnosed as *mucinous cystadenoma with mucinosis* or *cystadenoma with low-grade peritoneal mucinous tumor* depending on whether epithelial

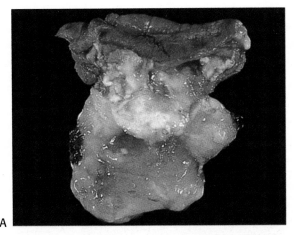

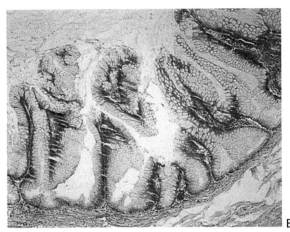

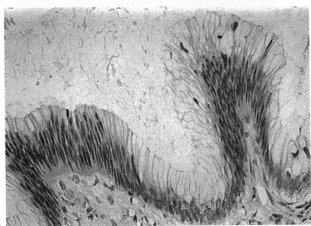

FIG. 9.5. Mucinous cystadenoma of the appendix. **A:** Gross photograph showing the presence of whitish papillary excrescences within the lumen of the appendix. Abundant mucoid material is present. **B:** A microscopic section through this lesion. The appendix is lined circumferentially by papillary proliferations of appendiceal cells resembling a hypersecretory papillary adenoma of the large bowel. **C:** A cystadenoma of the appendix. The prominent pencil-shaped nuclei characteristic of adenomatous epithelium are evident. Some of the cells contain abundant mucus, whereas others do not.

cells are identified in the mucin deposits (see below). We, unlike others (3,10), do not believe that cystadenomas with extra-appendiceal extension should be called appendiceal adenocarcinomas, since these patients have a better prognosis than patients with peritoneal carcinomatosis (6,11). Some tumors without evidence of extra-appendiceal extension

may also go on to develop pseudomyxoma peritonei. In these cases failure to adequately sample the appendix to detect the tumor extension is the likely explanation.

Mucinous Cystadenoma Coexisting with Carcinoid Tumor

Occasionally one sees an appendiceal mucinous cystadenoma coexisting with an appendiceal carcinoid tumor. The carcinoid and the epithelial components may lie side by side or may arise in different parts of the appendix. Carr et al used the term *dual carcinoid epithelial neoplasia* to describe this phenomenon (12). One usually does not see intermediate histologies between the epithelial and neuroendocrine tumors. The carcinoid tumor may have the histologic features of any appendiceal carcinoid (see Chapter 17). Therefore, they may be trabecular, tubular, or goblet cell in type. The prognosis is determined by the histologic features of each of the components.

Localized Adenomas

Isolated sessile or pedunculated adenomas resembling their colonic counterparts occur, but it is difficult to assess their incidence because these lesions tend to remain asymptomatic and most pathologists do not open the appendix along its long axis.

FIG. 9.6. High-grade dysplasia (carcinoma in situ). The neoplastic cells have lost their polarity and in this area mucin production is reduced.

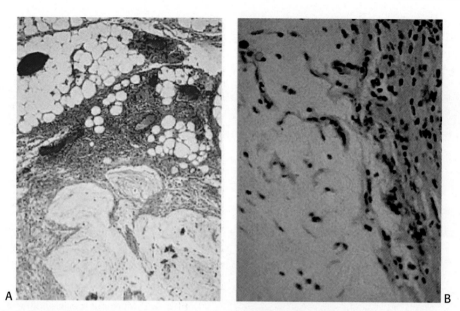

FIG. 9.7. Wall of a ruptured mucinous cystadenoma. **A:** Mucinous lakes dissect into the periappendiceal tissues. A prominent inflammatory infiltrate surrounds the edge of the mucinous lakes in the appendiceal fat. **B:** Higher magnification of the edge of the lesion showing fibrous tissue; benign, flattened epithelium; and inflammatory cells. Finding an area such as this in an appendix should prompt a search for a mucinous tumor in the remainder of the appendix.

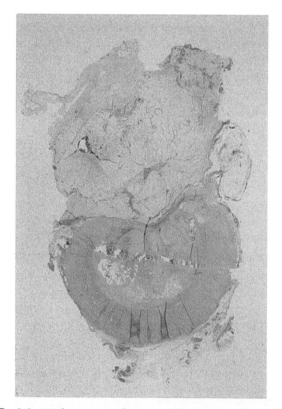

FIG. 9.8. Mucinous cystadenoma with rupture. Low-power magnification demonstrating a cross section of the appendix distal to the tumor. The appendix shows central fibrous obliteration of the lumen. External to the appendiceal wall is a collection of mucin.

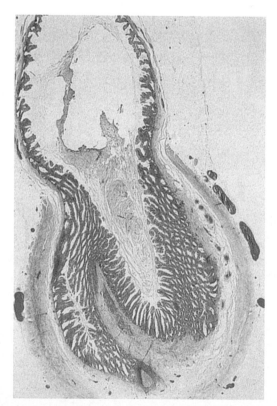

FIG. 9.9. Appendiceal mucinous cystadenoma with secondary diverticulum formation. A villiform mucin-secreting epithelium lines the appendiceal lumen as well as the diverticulum. The wall of the appendix on the left-hand side of the picture has become markedly thinned due to dilation.

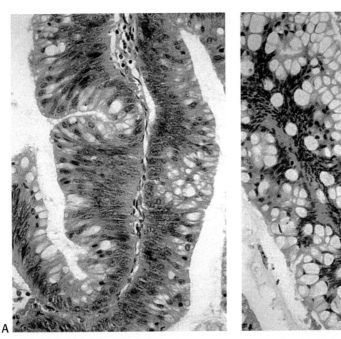

FIG. 9.10. Adenoma of the appendix. **A:** The epithelium resembles that seen in colonic adenomas. The adenomatous epithelium demonstrates the typical picket fence–arranged nuclei and the presence of immature goblet cells as evidenced by the small goblet cell collections. **B:** Another area of the tumor demonstrating marked goblet cell dystrophy.

The adenomas affect patients of all ages, including children (13); median patient age is the mid-50s (14). Adenomas occur in younger individuals in patients with familial polyposis. It is important to remember that patients with appendiceal adenomas often have additional primary tumors at other sites including the colon, breast, kidney, ovary, and gallbladder (14–16).

Isolated adenomas are generally discovered incidentally in appendices removed for other reasons. They may also be detected at the time of colonoscopy if they prolapse through the appendiceal orifice into the cecum. Larger sessile adenomas produce appendicitis by obstructing the appendiceal lumen. They may also produce diverticula (Fig. 8.6). These adenomas histologically resemble colorectal adenomas (see Chapter 14); the evolution of an adenoma into a carcinoma follows the same sequence. Sporadic adenomas may be tubular, tubulovillous, or villous in architecture and contain varying degrees of dysplasia (Fig. 9.10). Grossly invisible tubular adenomas occur in patients with familial polyposis. As in the colon, a tumor must invade through the muscularis mucosae into the underlying submucosa in order to diagnose an invasive cancer. Simple appendectomy represents adequate treatment for patients with adenomas that do not contain an invasive cancer.

Mixed Hyperplastic–Adenomatous Polyps, Serrated Adenomas, and Sessile Serrated Polyps

Mixed hyperplastic–adenomatous polyps, serrated adenomas, and sessile serrated polyps can develop in the appendix.

As with traditional adenomas, the histologic features of these lesions resemble their colonic counterparts, and the features of the mixed lesions are discussed in Chapter 14.

Serrated adenomas represent a distinctive form of adenomatous polyp with a tendency to develop in the appendix and right colon (17). The polyp architecture reminds one of a hyperplastic polyp because of the presence of serrated lumens (Fig. 9.11), but the cytologic features differ from those seen in hyperplastic polyps in that the often eosinophilic cells appear immature and the hyperdistended goblet cells and thickened collagen table typically present in hyperplastic polyps are absent. The epithelium usually contains more mucin than seen in typical adenomas but less than one sees in mucinous cystadenomas. The nuclei appear pseudostratified and elongated in comparison to the basally located, rounder nuclei typical of hyperplastic polyps. Mitotic activity is increased over that seen in hyperplastic polyps and mitoses can be identified at the free surface in serrated adenomas (17). The lesion may exhibit a high level of microsatellite instability (18).

Sessile serrated polyps also develop in the appendix, although they are seldom reported as such, especially in the older literature. The lesions described by Younes et al are an example of this lesion (19). Sessile serrated polyps superficially resemble hyperplastic polyps but they tend to be larger than the usual hyperplastic polyp, sometimes covering extensive areas of the mucosa. Typically, the glands appear serrated and the serrations extend deeper into the crypt than the usual hyperplastic polyp. The base of the glands tends to

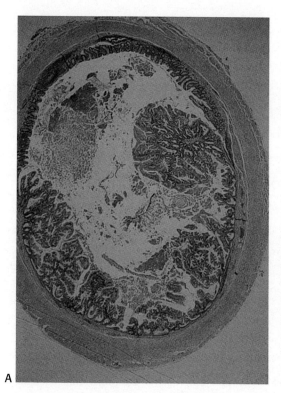

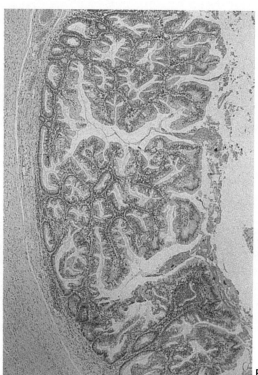

A   B

FIG. 9.11. Serrated adenoma **A:** Low-power magnification demonstrating the presence of an almost completely circumferential serrated adenoma. **B:** Higher magnification demonstrating the presence of glands with a serrated architecture. Closer examination of the lesion shows the presence of serrated glandular lumens lined by cells that have histologic features between those of a classic adenoma or hyperplastic polyp.

extend sideways above the muscularis mucosae and the proliferative zone is asymmetric in appearance. The cells lining the glands do not appear to be obviously adenomatous, but they are crowded and contain variable amounts of mucin. These appendiceal lesions have a high association with right-sided colonic carcinomas (19). These three lesions are discussed in greater detail in Chapter 14.

ADENOCARCINOMAS

Appendiceal adenocarcinomas occur far less commonly than carcinoid tumors or mucinous cystadenomas. They are found in only 0.1% to 1.35% of appendectomy specimens (1,8) and represent only 0.5% of all gastrointestinal neoplasms (19,20). Patients with these cancers have an average age of 51.4 to 60 years and show a male:female ratio of 3:1 (8,10,14). However, incidence rates reported by Surveillance, Epidemiology, and End Results (SEER) registries suggest that the tumors affect both sexes equally (21). The age of presentation is significantly older than that of patients with appendiceal carcinoid tumors (22). Patients with familial polyposis may develop appendiceal carcinomas at a young age. Appendiceal carcinomas also develop in patients with underlying inflammatory bowel disease (23). A minority of appendiceal mucinous carcinomas may arise via a defective

mismatch repair pathway (24) in a manner analogous to a subset of colorectal carcinomas that frequently have a mucinous histology (see Chapter 14).

Clinical presentations include acute appendicitis, the presence of an abdominal mass, or obstruction. Carcinomas that masquerade as acute appendicitis often have clinical clues suggesting that a more serious condition is present, including a prolonged history, weight loss, anemia, or the presence of a palpable mass. Some patients have widespread abdominal carcinomatosis at the time of diagnosis. Mucinous tumors tend to present with pseudomyxoma peritonei, whereas nonmucinous carcinomas present with appendicitis. The tumors may also cause appendiceal intussusception. The tumors develop in mucinous cystadenomas, in localized adenomas, and exceptionally from goblet cell carcinoids (see Chapter 17) (12). The TNM classification of appendiceal tumors is shown in Table 9.3.

Grossly, most appendiceal carcinomas appear as a polypoid, ulcerating, or infiltrative mass at the base of the appendix (Fig. 9.12), contrasting with carcinoid tumors that usually develop in the tip (11). They often produce abundant mucin (Fig. 9.13). The presence of diffuse appendiceal induration may suggest the diagnosis. Mean tumor diameter is larger than that of mucinous cystadenomas (2.9 cm) (6). Perforation or diverticula may be present. Perforations of appendiceal adenocarcinomas develop in 50% to 62% of

TABLE 9.3	**TNM Classification of Appendiceal Tumors**

T—Primary Tumor

TX Primary tumor cannot be assessed
T0 No evidence of primary tumor
Tis Carcinoma in situ: Intraepithelial or invasion of
      lamina propria
T1 Tumor invades submucosa
T2 Tumor invades muscularis propria
T3 Tumor invades through the muscularis propria into
      subserosa or into nonperitonealized periappendiceal
      tissue
T4 Tumor directly invades other organs or structures
      and/or perforates visceral peritoneum

N—Regional Lymph Nodes

NX Regional lymph nodes cannot be assessed
N0 No evidence of nodal metastases
N1 Metastases in one to three regional lymph nodes
N2 Metastases in four or more regional lymph nodes

M—Distant Metastases

MX Distant metastases cannot be assessed
M0 No distant metastases
M1 Distant metastases

Stage Grouping

Stage 0	Tis	N0	M0
Stage I	T1 or T2	N0	M0
Stage II	T3 or T4	N0	M0
Stage III	Any T	N1 or N2	M0
Stage IV	Any T	Any N	M

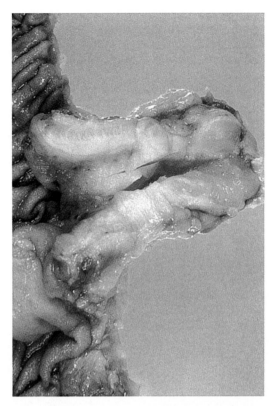

FIG. 9.12. Carcinoma of the appendix. The appendix shows obliteration of the appendiceal wall by an infiltrating white process. At the tip of the appendix one notices the gelatinous appearance of the tumor.

tumors (20,25), allowing the tumor to disseminate into the peritoneum. Advanced lesions may appear as a mass enveloping or obliterating the appendix. Cecal extension may make it difficult to determine the exact site of the origin. If the major part of the mass lies in the appendix, or if one finds areas of residual adenoma in the appendix, one can be confident that the tumor is a primary appendiceal lesion.

There are three major histologic patterns of appendiceal carcinoma: Those resembling ordinary colorectal carcinoma (Fig. 9.14), mucinous (colloid) carcinomas (Fig. 9.15), and signet ring carcinomas (Fig. 9.16). Mucinous adenocarcinomas account for approximately 85% of appendiceal carcinomas. By

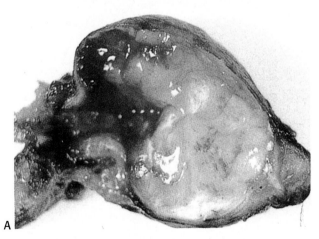

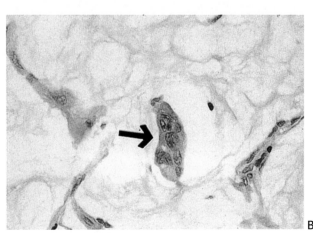

FIG. 9.13. Mucinous cystadenocarcinoma. **A:** Mucus is seen within the opened appendiceal lumen. **B:** Cytologically malignant cells (*arrow*) are present floating within the lumen and were present in other parts of the lining epithelium of this appendix.

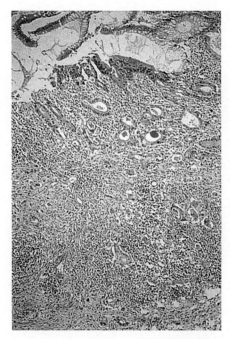

FIG. 9.14. Carcinoma infiltrating the appendiceal wall. Carcinoma shown in the upper portion of the photograph demonstrates the histologic features of a typical colorectal carcinoma. Prominent mucin differentiation is not seen.

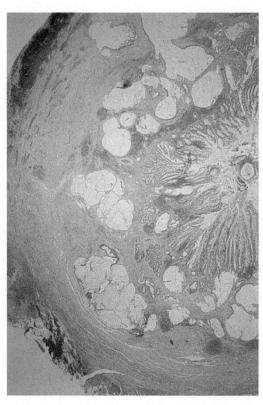

FIG. 9.15. Colloid carcinoma. Cross section of the appendix demonstrating the presence of mucinous cysts lined by malignant glands. Large mucus collections extend through the appendix wall.

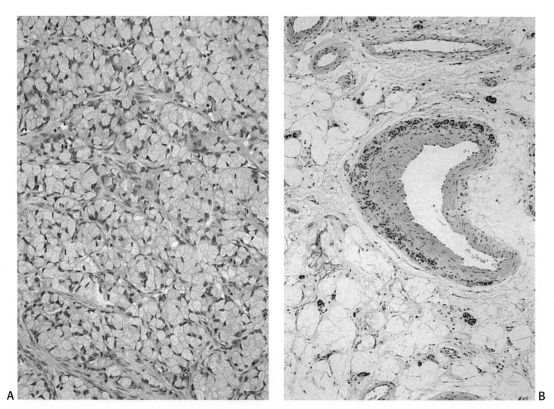

FIG. 9.16. Signet ring cell carcinoma arising in the appendix. This tumor obliterated the appendix and became widely metastatic throughout the peritoneal cavity. **A:** There's back-to-back arrangement of the signet ring cells. **B:** Prominent perivascular lymphatic invasion is evident.

definition, at least 50% of the tumor is mucinous in nature (2). The tumors arise from mucinous cystadenomas and they produce copious amounts of mucin, leading to the presence of a mucocele as well as mucinous cysts within the appendiceal wall (Fig. 9.15). Depending on when the lesion is detected, one may identify an underlying cystadenoma with areas of invasion. In more advanced tumors the precursor lesion is absent, replaced by tumor or eroded away by the accompanying appendicitis. Mucinous tumors tend to be well differentiated and to produce pseudomyxoma peritonei. Papillary projections of adenocarcinoma may line the appendiceal lumen. The epithelium appears cuboidal to columnar in shape and contains enlarged nuclei with prominent nucleoli. The wall of the appendix contains irregular infiltrating glands associated with desmoplasia and extracellular mucin pools lined by very atypical mucinous epithelium. Small infiltrating glands and even single cells may be present. Carcinomatous glands differ from their benign counterparts in that they have features of malignancy, including a large nuclear:cytoplasmic ratio; submucosal, vascular, or lymphatic invasion; desmoplasia; and the absence of lamina propria around the invading glands. Their destructive invasion leads to extra-appendiceal spread of the tumor. However, it should be kept in mind that well-differentiated tumors that invade in a broad front may lack a desmoplastic response. If one is uncertain whether a tumor is invasive or not, the tumor may be diagnosed as a *mucinous tumor of uncertain malignant potential.*

Non–mucin-producing appendiceal adenocarcinomas occur less frequently than mucinous tumors (see Fig. 9.14). These lesions arise in pre-existing adenomas, and because they resemble their large intestinal counterparts, they are referred to as colonic-type adenocarcinomas. These lesions tend not to produce pseudomyxoma peritonei. They exhibit the full range of histologies that can be seen in tumors arising in the colon and rectum, including tumors that may contain areas of small cell carcinoma (see Chapters 14 and 17).

Appendiceal *signet ring cell carcinomas* are rare and often develop in young people in their 30s. The tumors are frequently detected at an advanced stage; as a result, many patients die of their disease within a year or two of their original diagnosis. At least 50% of the tumor should consist of signet ring cells to classify the tumor as such. The tumors consist of proliferations of signet ring cells diffusely invading the bowel wall, usually in the absence of an associated adenoma. The signet ring cells form solid tumor sheets, or they insinuate themselves through the bowel wall. Focal larger colloid lakes may coexist with the sheets of signet ring cells. The latter tend to involve lymphatics early (Fig. 9.16) and they tend to spread beyond the appendix by the time they are detected (22). The presence of signet ring cells raises the possibility of an adenocarcinoid tumor (see Chapter 17), but the latter contains large numbers of endocrine cells and the cells are not as malignant appearing as in signet ring cell carcinomas.

The biology of well-differentiated mucinous tumors differs significantly from that of appendiceal colonic-type carcinomas in that nearly all of the patients have peritoneal

dissemination at the time of diagnosis (26) and disease progression mainly affects the peritoneum. Only 2% of patients have lymph node or liver metastases at the time of diagnosis (27,28). In contrast, colonic-type carcinomas behave like ordinary colorectal tumors, metastasizing to the regional lymph nodes, including the ileocolic, infraduodenal, and para-aortic chains, or to the liver rather than presenting with peritoneal-based disease. Nodal metastases are present in approximately 25% of resection specimens and the patients experience an overall 5-year survival rate of 46% to 60% (29,30).

It is unclear whether the colonic and mucinous types differ with respect to survival. Some reports show better survival for patients with mucinous adenocarcinoma, while others have found better survival for the colonic type (29,31,32); a more recent study found that the survival was the same in both types (22). The overall 5-year survival rate in ones series of tumors was 60% (30). Patients with signet ring cell carcinoma have a significantly worse prognosis than patients with either mucinous or colonic-type tumors. Fifty-four percent of patients with signet ring cell tumors have lymph node involvement (22), contrasting with approximately 25% of tumors without a signet ring cell morphology (30).

The extent of disease at the time of diagnosis is one of the most important predictors of survival. Patients with stage IV lesions usually succumb to their disease within 5 years. Hemicolectomy is recommended for patients diagnosed with stage II or higher stage appendiceal cancers that have been initially treated with appendectomy. The value of hemicolectomy in patients with T1 lesions is less clear. Significantly better 5-year survivals follow a successful right hemicolectomy and lymph node dissection (73%) when compared with patients undergoing only appendectomy (34%) (25,29,30).

PSEUDOMYXOMA PERITONEI

The term *pseudomyxoma peritonei* (PMP) refers to any condition in which the peritoneal cavity becomes filled with extracellular mucin. PMP complicates both benign and malignant appendiceal neoplasms, as well as carcinomas of other sites, including the ovary, colon, or gallbladder and pancreas (33,34). Additionally, it is possible that the peritoneal lesions arise from a mucinous metaplasia of the peritoneal lining (35). Since the term PMP is nonspecific, one cannot determine whether the lesions are benign or malignant. Some have suggested that the definition of PMP be restricted to histologically benign peritoneal tumors arising from appendiceal adenomas. These authors favor the term *disseminated peritoneal adenomucinosis* to distinguish less aggressive lesions from overtly malignant *peritoneal carcinomatosis* arising from true carcinomas (27,34). As will be seen below, we utilize a different terminology to diagnose these lesions.

Patients range in age from 23 to 83, with an average age of 49 years. The condition affects both males and females.

Patients with PMP present with increasing abdominal girth, mucinous ascites, appendicitis, appendiceal abscess, obstruction, an inguinal hernia, or an ovarian tumor. Intestinal obstruction is caused by extensive tumor accumulation within the pelvis, causing pelvic outlet obstruction surrounding the gastric antrum, causing gastric outlet obstruction, or occluding the ileocecal valve region. As intestinal obstruction develops, fistulas become more common.

PMP is usually a locally persistent cancer that is non-metastasizing and is characterized by a redistribution mechanism in which large volumes of tenacious, semisolid, mucinous tumor deposits are present in the undersurface of the right and left hemidiaphragm, abdominal gutters, and pelvis, but are relatively absent from the peritoneal surfaces of the gastrointestinal tract. The primary tumor constitutes only a minor part of the abdominopelvic cancer. Despite the low-grade biology of most of the lesions and the absence of metastases, progressive disease may cause death by a mass effect in the abdominal and pelvic cavities.

The gross appearance of the tumor is characteristic and depends in part on whether the primary lesion is benign or malignant. The hallmark of the disease is an omental cake. The tumor implants appear as glistening, mucinous globules attached to the peritoneal surfaces, the intestinal serosa, and other abdominal organs, including the spleen. In advanced disease, a mucinous mass admixed with fibrous tissue surrounds and obstructs all of the intra-abdominal organs, filling the entire abdominal cavity, giving rise to the term "jelly belly." All intestinal surfaces are relatively spared; they are not as extensively involved as the rest of the peritoneum unless there have been multiple prior surgical procedures or unless the disease is very advanced with debilitating impacted mucinous ascites throughout the abdominal cavity. Invasion into the peritoneum and abdominal viscera does not occur unless the tumor is malignant.

Pedunculated surface PMP polyps develop in patients with benign tumors, usually on the small bowel, the small bowel mesentery, and occasionally the anterior surface of the stomach. Most patients have multiple polyps that measure up to 20 mm in diameter (35). It is believed that the polyps result from the motion of the bowel so that eventually, an elongated stalk is created. This bowel motion not only creates the polyps, but also repeatedly clears the mucinous tumors from the small bowel surfaces (35).

The histologic features of PMP vary (Table 9.2). Some authors divide PMPs into *adenomucinosis, adenomucinosis hybrid,* and *mucinous adenocarcinoma.* Adenomucinosis includes mainly aggressive peritoneal tumors that produce large volumes of mucous ascites. The lesions typically arise from benign appendiceal cystadenomas (34). Hybrid malignancies show adenomucinosis combined with mucinous adenocarcinomas. Mucinous adenocarcinomas show obvious cytologic features of malignancy and the cells may even have a signet ring morphology. The features can be recognized in both histologic and cytologic preparations. The cytologic features accurately reflect the histology (36). Cytologic

preparations often contain abundant mucin, reactive mesothelial cells, variable numbers of epithelial cells and fibroblasts, and chronic inflammation. The epithelium may be completely absent in mucinosis. In low-grade mucinous tumors, one may see strips of epithelial cells with basal located nuclei, single cells, or tight three-dimensional cell clusters (37). We prefer to use a different terminology that we believe more specifically describes the histologic features of the lesions that are present. It is described below.

Peritoneal Mucinosis (Adenomucinosis)

This lesion is characterized by the presence of acellular mucin collections that coat the surfaces of the peritoneum and the abdominal contents. No neoplastic epithelial cells are found after a diligent examination of multiple sections. The lack of cells reflects a sampling problem in a paucicellular lesion and does not indicate that the tumors lack the ability to grow. Mesothelial hyperplasia may be present. The lesion typically complicates appendiceal mucinous cystadenomas. These lesions have a much better prognosis than mucin accumulations that contain neoplastic cells.

Low-Grade Peritoneal Mucinous Neoplasm

The defining features of this diagnosis are the presence of neoplastic cells (unlike the situation in mucinosis) and benign cytologic features (Fig. 9.17) (in contrast to mucinous adenocarcinomas). The diagnosis is made whether the epithelial cells are very sparse in number or are quite numerous. Usually, the cells lie at the periphery of the mucin deposits on various tissue surfaces. In classic cases, more than 90% of the globular masses are composed of mucin rather than cells. These lesions consist of uniform, scant to moderately cellular low-grade adenomatous mucinous epithelium within abundant extracellular mucin accumulations. The epithelium appears as epithelial strips or undulating glands. These are lined by a single layer of cytologically bland adenomatous epithelium and they cover the surfaces of various sites. The epithelium may appear flattened in some areas and focal tufting may be present. Areas of calcification may develop. The cells display minimal cytologic atypia and mitotic activity. There is no evidence of invasion into the underlying tissues. Hyalinization, fibrosis, vascularization, mesothelial hyperplasia (Fig. 9.18), and chronic inflammation may all accompany the tumor. The fibroblastic and vascular proliferation associated with the mucin may impart a myxomatous appearance to the lesion. PMP is a disease of MUC2-expressing goblet cells (38) and the extracellular mucin accumulates because the number of MUC2-secreting cells increases and the mucin has no place to drain. These low-grade lesions may progress to frank mucinous adenocarcinoma in patients who fail reductive surgery and intraperitoneal chemotherapy (39). Appendiceal lesions are nearly always confined to the peritoneal surfaces and only

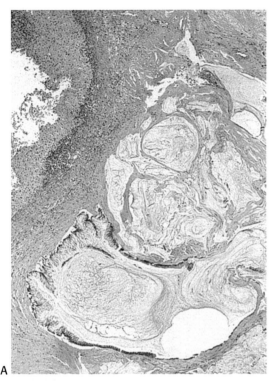
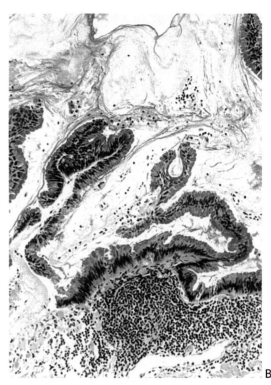

FIG. 9.17. Low-grade mucinous neoplasm. **A:** Note the implantation of neoplastic epithelium on the peritoneal surfaces. Neoplastic epithelium lines the large colloid-filled space at the lower portion of the picture. **B:** Mucicarmine stain demonstrating the presence of prominent apical mucin within the neoplastic cells.

rarely are the lesions identified within lymph nodes or invading the parenchyma of abdominal or pelvic organs.

Pedunculated PMP polyps contain a head, stalk, and base resembling the pattern seen in adenomas. Histologically, the head contains pools of acellular mucin associated with blunt fibrous trabeculae. A few adenomatous epithelial cells may be identified by repeated searching. Their presence can be

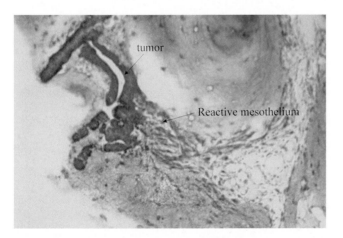

FIG. 9.18. Low-grade mucinous neoplasm associated with mesothelial hyperplasia. The specimen is stained with Alcian blue (*blue*) highlighting the mucin, cytokeratin immunostain highlighting the mucinous neoplasm (*red*), and calretinin immunostain (*brown*) highlighting the mesothelial hyperplasia.

appreciated by immunostaining surfaces devoid of an epithelial layer. Mesothelial cells often cover these lesions (35).

Peritoneal Mucinous Adenocarcinoma

In peritoneal mucinous adenocarcinoma, the mucin deposits frequently contain abundant proliferative epithelium that may be arranged in nests, irregularly shaped glands, or even single cells, all demonstrating significant cytologic atypia (Fig. 9.19). Multiple layers of neoplastic cells may be present. The cells line the surfaces of the mucin deposits, float in the middle of the mucin, or invade into the parenchyma of the organs and surfaces that the tumor coats. These surfaces include the mesentery, peritoneum, spleen, liver, and stomach. The glandular architectural complexity is greater than that seen in low-grade mucinous tumors. The tumors often demonstrate atypical mitoses, marked nuclear hyperchromasia, and loss of polarity (Fig. 9.19). Occasional signet ring cells may be seen. These lesions associate with an identifiable primary mucinous adenocarcinoma of the appendix or colon. In general, appendiceal carcinomas show lower proliferative rates as measured by Ki-67, lower M30 counts, and lower CD44 expression than their colonic counterparts. This may relate to their more indolent behavior compared to adenocarcinomas of the colon and rectum (40). The tumors strongly express epithelial growth factor receptor (EGFR), making the use of anti-EGFR targeted therapy an attractive option.

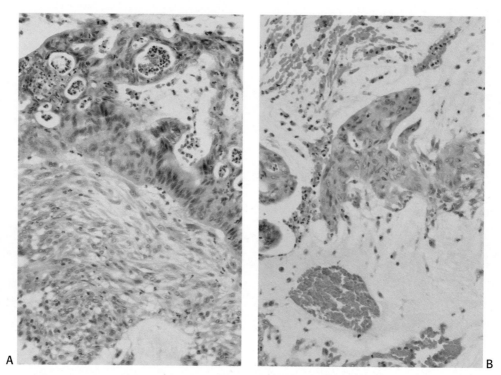

A   B

FIG. 9.19. Mucinous adenocarcinoma. **A:** The tumor cells are cytologically malignant with loss of nuclear polarity. There is associated desmoplasia. **B:** Cytologically malignant cells lie free in mucinous pools.

It should be kept in mind that the appearance of the epithelium in the mucus can be deceptively benign, even when the lesion in the appendix is an obvious carcinoma. Therefore, one should try to examine the appendix if it is available, and if a carcinoma is present, the peritoneal lesion should be diagnosed as a well-differentiated carcinoma.

Patients with peritoneal carcinomatosis are sometimes treated with intraperitoneal chemotherapy, and the therapy may alter the histologic features. Intraperitoneal chemotherapy with 5-fluorouracil and mitomycin C induces a marked reduction in the number of foci of atypical epithelium lining the mucin globules and in atrophy and degeneration of atypical neoplastic lining epithelium (41).

Secondary involvement of the ovaries by mucinous carcinomas of gastrointestinal origin (Fig. 9.20) simulates primary ovarian tumors clinically and histologically. In this situation, the question arises as to whether the patient has two primary lesions or whether the findings represent spread of the disease from the appendix to the ovary or vice versa. Table 9.4 compares primary and secondary ovarian mucinous tumors. The synchronous presence or history of an appendiceal tumor always suggests that the ovarian involvement is secondary in nature. In this setting, the histologic features of the tumors usually resemble one another. Today, most people believe that ovarian involvement represents secondary spread from an appendiceal lesion (9,34,38,42).

Some patients have an excellent survival, despite the presence of massive peritoneal and omental mucin accumulations

(28,43). The long-term survival relates to the slowly progressive nature of the neoplastic process, which rarely metastasizes to the liver or lymph nodes. Patient survival differs depending on whether the patient has mucinosis, a low-grade peritoneal mucinous tumor, or a peritoneal mucinous adenocarcinoma (11,44). Extension, metastasis, or death usually does not follow PMP localized to the right lower quadrant, as may occur in some patients with low-grade mucinous cystadenoma that has escaped into the peritoneal cavity. In contrast, if the underlying lesion is malignant, diffuse progressive peritoneal involvement results, with obliteration of the entire

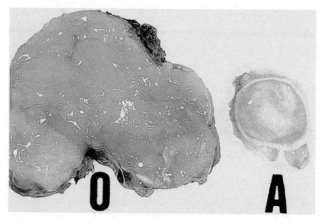

FIG. 9.20. Pseudomyxoma peritonei. Patient with ovarian cystadenoma (*O*) and an appendiceal mucinous cystadenoma (*A*).

TABLE 9.4   **Comparison of Appendiceal and Ovarian Mucinous Tumors**

Feature	Appendiceal Origin	Ovarian Origin
Ovarian involvement	Surface involvement with or without superficial stromal involvement; frequently bilateral. When the ovarian tumor is unilateral, it is usually right sided	Predominantly stromal involvement. May be bilateral
Signet ring cells	May be present	Usually not present
Tumor present in the appendix	Yes	No
Mucin:cell ratio	10:1	1:1
CDX-2	Usually positive	Often negative
CK20	Usually positive	Positive in approximately 50%
CK7	Positive in approximately one third of cases	Usually positive
MUC2	Positive	Negative

abdominal cavity and recurrent bouts of intestinal obstruction, infection, or invasion of contiguous structures. The 3-year survival rates are 77% for patients with mucinosis and low-grade tumors versus 35% for mucinous adenocarcinomas (44). It also relates to patient age at presentation, the time between the diagnosis and the treatment, the extent of the peritoneal disease, the resection status, and the length of the chemoperfusion (44). Patients with tissue invasion have a significantly worse survival than those without invasion (47% vs. 80% at 3 years).

Currently these lesions are treated with cytoreductive surgery and intraperitoneal hyperthermic chemotherapy (11). Peritonectomy can be used to clear mucinous tumor from parietal and visceral peritoneal surfaces. The peritonectomy procedures include greater omentectomy and splenectomy, stripping of the left hemidiaphragm, stripping of the right hemidiaphragm, lesser omentectomy/polycystectomy, antrectomy, and pelvic peritonectomy with or without sigmoid colon resection. Not all of the procedures are performed in all patients, only if deemed necessary. Typically the pathologist receives specimens from all of these sites and more. We average about 20 specimens per initial procedure. Each of these should be diagnosed separately. Patients with mucinosis fare better than those with high-grade adenocarcinomas, and minimal peritoneal surface residual disease is treated more successfully than large volume residual disease in the abdomen (11,44). Medical treatment failure results from a generalized recurrence due to resistance to the chemotherapy and/or from nonuniform chemotherapy distribution. Surgical treatment failure results from the inability to surgically clear the abdomen of tumor.

NEUROMAS

Appendiceal neuromas occur relatively commonly; their frequency increases with age. Some develop in patients with neurofibromatosis. Controversy exists as to whether they are true neoplasms or merely a nonneoplastic proliferation, possibly induced by previous episodes of appendicitis (see Chapter 8) (45,46). Some neuromas coexist with carcinoids, particularly microcarcinoidosis, suggesting that some neuromas give rise to some carcinoid tumors. Ganglioneuromas have also been reported in this location (47). The tumors may be single or multiple.

Grossly, neuromas may be invisible. Alternatively, the appendix may appear firm, light tan or gray, frequently with a glistening fibrous myxoid appearance. Microscopically, appendiceal neuromas show three architectural patterns. The most common pattern is a *central obliterative neuroma* (Fig. 9.21) that consists of loosely arranged spindle cell aggregates on a background network of fine eosinophilic cell processes. The muscularis mucosae between the mucosa and the adjacent appendiceal neuroma varies, being normal or completely absent. *Intramucosal appendiceal neuromas* represent another microscopic pattern (Fig. 9.21). Pale-staining, ill-defined, lamina propria expansions of neural tissue separate the crypts from one another. S100-stained sections show intensely positive focal areas in the lamina propria. The third histologic pattern consists of a localized but nonencapsulated nodular accentuation of the central obliterative process. The spindled Schwann cells form rounded laminated swirls that are uniformly S100 and neuron-specific enolase (NSE) positive. Occasionally, serotonin-positive cells intermingle with the spindle cell proliferation. The presence of neuroendocrine cells in appendiceal neuromas suggests that they represent an integral part of the neuronal proliferation (45).

OTHER TUMORS

The appendix may also become involved by direct extension of tumors arising in adjacent organs such as the cecum, and

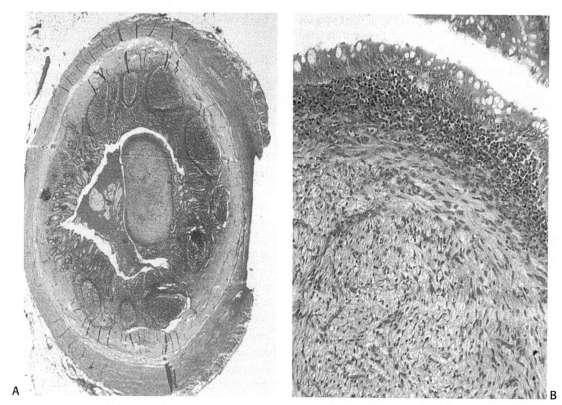

FIG. 9.21. Intramucosal neural proliferation demonstrating the presence of a focal neuromatous growth. **A:** Low-power cross section demonstrating the relationship of this lesion to the remainder of the appendix. **B:** Higher magnification demonstrating the typical Schwann cell histology of the proliferation surrounded by normal-appearing lamina propria and covered by an intact appendiceal epithelium.

in advanced cancer one may not be able to determine the exact site of origin of a given tumor. Metastases also affect the appendix. Tumors that metastasize to the appendix include ovary (Fig. 9.22), breast, stomach, cervix, and lung cancer (48,49). Leukemic infiltrates can also secondarily involve the appendix and may even present as appendicitis (50).

Mesenchymal tumors and lymphomas can originate in the appendix. They resemble similar tumors occurring elsewhere and are discussed in Chapters 18 and 19. Appendiceal mesenchymal tumors include leiomyosarcomas, leiomyomatosis peritonealis disseminata, Kaposi sarcoma, and granular cell tumors.

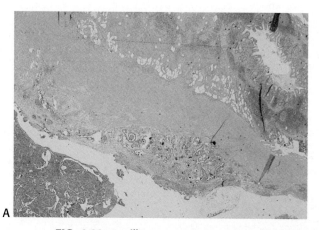
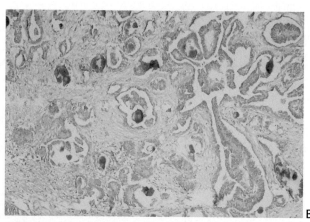

FIG. 9.22. Papillary serous tumor of ovarian origin metastatic to the appendix. **A:** The tumor lies on the serosal surface of the appendix. **B:** Higher power showing the psammoma bodies.

REFERENCES

1. Collins DC: 71,000 Human appendix specimens, a final report summarizing forty years' study. *Am J Proctol* 1963;4:265.

2. Carr NJ, Arends MJ, Deans GT, et al: Adenocarcinoma of the appendix. In: Hamilton SR, Aaltonen LA (eds). *World Health Organization Classification of Tumours; Pathology and Genetics of Tumours of the Digestive System.* Lyon, France: IARC Press, 2000, pp 94–98.

3. Carr NJ, McCarthy WF, Sobin LH: Epithelial noncarcinoid tumors and tumor-like lesions of the appendix: a clinicopathologic study of 184 patients with a multivariate analysis of prognostic factors. *Cancer* 1995;75:757.

4. Deans GT, Spence RAJ: Neoplastic lesions of the appendix. *Br J Surg* 1995;82:299.

5. Szych C, Staebler A, Connolly D, et al: Molecular genetic evidence supporting the clonality and appendiceal origin of pseudomyxoma peritonei in women. *Am J Pathol* 1999;154:1849.

6. Misdraji J, Yantiss RK, Graeme-Cook FM, et al: Appendiceal mucinous neoplasms. A clinicopathologic analysis of 107 cases. *Am J Surg Pathol* 2003;27:1089.

7. Williams GR, Du Boulay CEH, Roche WR: Benign epithelial neoplasms of the appendix: classification and clinical associations. *Histopathology* 1992;21:447.

8. Wolff M, Ahmed N: Epithelial neoplasms of the vermiform appendix (exclusive of carcinoid). I. Adenocarcinoma of the appendix. *Cancer* 1976;37:2493.

9. Young RH, Gilks CB, Scully RE: Mucinous tumors of the appendix associated with mucinous tumors of the ovary and pseudomyxoma peritonei. A clinicopathological analysis of 22 cases supporting an origin in the appendix. *Am J Surg Pathol* 1991;15:415.

10. Higa E, Rosai J, Pizzimbono CA, Wise L: Mucosal hyperplasia, mucinous cystadenoma, and mucinous cystadenocarcinoma of the appendix. A re-evaluation of appendiceal "mucocele." *Cancer* 1973;32:1525.

11. Ronnett BM, Yan H, Kurman RJ, et al: Patients with pseudomyxoma peritonei associated with disseminated peritoneal adenomucinosis have a significantly more favorable prognosis than patients with peritoneal mucinous carcinomatosis. *Cancer* 2001;92:85.

12. Carr NJ, Remotti H, Sobin LH: Dual carcinoid/epithelial neoplasia of the appendix. *Histopathology* 1995;27:557.

13. Shnitka TK, Sherbaniuk RW: Adenomatous polyps of the appendix in children. *Gastroenterology* 1957;32:462.

14. Appelman HD: Epithelial neoplasia of the appendix. In: Norris HT (ed). *Pathology of the Colon, Small Intestine, and Anus.* New York: Churchill Livingstone, 1983, p 233.

15. Wolff M, Ahmed N: Epithelial neoplasms of the vermiform appendix (exclusive of carcinoid). II. Cystadenomas, papillary adenomas and adenomatous polyps of the appendix. *Cancer* 1976;37:2511.

16. Qizilbash AH: Primary adenocarcinoma of the appendix. *Arch Pathol* 1975;99:556.

17. Longacre TA, Fenoglio-Preiser CM: Mixed hyperplastic adenomatous polyps. A distinctive form of colorectal neoplasia. *Am J Surg Pathol* 1990;14:524.

18. Rudzki Z, Zazula M, Bialas M, et al: Synchronous serrated adenoma of the appendix and high grade ovarian carcinoma: a case demonstrating different origin of the two neoplasms. *Pol J Pathol* 2002;53:29.

19. Younes M, Katikaneni PR, Lechago J: Association between mucosal hyperplasia of the appendix and adenocarcinoma of the colon. *Histopathology* 1995;26:33.

20. Chang P, Attiyeh F: Adenocarcinoma of the appendix. *Dis Colon Rectum* 1981;24:176.

21. *Surveillance, Epidemiology, and End Results: Incidence and Mortality Data, 1973–77: National Cancer Institute Monograph 57.* NIH Publication No. 81-2330. Bethesda, MD: U.S. Department of Health and Human Services, 1981.

22. McCusker ME, Cote TR, Clegg LX, Sobin LH: Primary malignant neoplasms of the appendix: a population-based study from the surveillance, epidemiology and end-results program, 1973-1998. *Cancer* 2002; 94:3307.

23. Sonwalkar SA, Denyer ME, Verbeke CS, Guillou PJ: Cancer of appendix as a presenting feature of Crohn's disease. *Eur J Gastroenterol Hepatol* 2002;14:1029.

24. Misdraji J, Burgart LJ, Lauwers GY: Defective mismatch repair in the pathogenesis of low grade appendiceal mucinous neoplasms and adenocarcinomas. *Mod Pathol* 2004;17:1447.

25. Lenriot JP, Huguier M: Adenocarcinoma of the appendix. *Am J Surg* 1988;155:470.

26. Sugarbaker PH: Are there surgical options to peritoneal carcinomatosis. *Ann Surg* 2005;242:748.

27. Sugarbaker PH: New standard of care for appendiceal epithelial neoplasms and pseudomyxoma peritonei syndrome? *Lancet Oncol* 2006;769.

28. Sugarbaker PH, Alderman R, Edwards G, et al: Prospective morbidity and mortality assessment of cytoreductive surgery plus perioperative intraperitoneal chemotherapy to treat peritoneal dissemination of appendiceal mucinous malignancy. *Ann Surg Oncol* 2006;13:635.

29. Nitecki SS, Wolff BG, Schlinkert R, Starr MG: The natural history of surgically treated primary adenocarcinoma of the appendix. *Ann Surg* 1994;219:51.

30. Hesketh K: The management of primary adenocarcinoma of the vermiform appendix. *Gut* 1963;4:158.

31. Cortina R, McCormick J, Kolm P, Perry RR: Management and prognosis of adenocarcinoma of the appendix. *Dis Colon Rectum* 1995;38:848.

32. Lyss AP: Appendiceal malignancies. *Semin Oncol* 1988;15:129.

33. Seidman JD, Elsayed AM, Sobin LH, et al: Association of mucinous tumors of the ovary and appendix. A clinicopathologic study of 25 cases. *Am J Surg Pathol* 1993;17:22.

34. Ronnett BM, Kurman RJ, Zahn CM, et al: Pseudomyxoma peritonei in women: a clinicopathologic analysis of 30 cases with emphasis on site of origin, prognosis, and relationship to ovarian mucinous tumors of low malignant potential. *Hum Pathol* 1995;26:509.

35. Sugarbaker PH, Yan H, Shmookler B: Pedunculated peritoneal surface polyps in pseudomyxoma peritonei syndrome. *Histopathology* 2001;39:525.

36. Jackson SL, Fleming RA, Loggie BW, Geisinger KR: Gelatinous ascites: a cytohistologic study of pseudomyxoma peritonei in 67 patients. *Mod Pathol* 2001;14:664.

37. Shin HJ, Sneige N: Epithelial cells and the cytologic features of pseudomyxoma peritonei in patients with ovarian and/or appendiceal mucinous neoplasms. A study of 12 patients including 5 men. *Cancer* 2000;90:1.

38. O'Connell JT, Tomlinson JS, Roberts AA, et al: Pseudomyxoma peritonei is a disease of MUC2-expressing goblet cells. *Am J Pathol* 2002; 161:551.

39. Yan H, Pestieau SR, Shmookler BM, Sugarbaker PH: Histopathologic analysis in 46 patients with pseudomyxoma peritonei syndrome: failure versus success with a second look operation. *Mod Pathol* 2001;14:164.

40. Carr NJ, Emory TS, Sobin LH: Epithelial neoplasms of the appendix and colorectum: an analysis of cell proliferation, apoptosis, and expression of p53, CD44, bcl-2. *Arch Pathol Lab Med* 2002;126:837.

41. Sugarbaker PH, Landy D, Jaffe G, Pascal R: Histologic changes induced by intraperitoneal chemotherapy with 5-fluorouracil and mitomycin C in patients with peritoneal carcinomatosis from cystadenocarcinoma of the colon or appendix. *Cancer* 1990;65:1495.

42. Guerrieri C, Franlund B, Boeryd B: Expression of cytokeratin 7 in simultaneous mucinous tumors of the ovary and appendix. *Mod Pathol* 1995;8:573.

43. Smith JW, Kemeny N, Caldwell C, et al: Pseudomyxoma peritonei of appendiceal origin. *Cancer* 1992;70:396.

44. Stewart JH, Shen P, Russell GB, et al: Appendiceal neoplasms with peritoneal dissemination: outcomes after cytoreductive surgery and intraperitoneal hyperthermic chemotherapy. *Ann Surg Oncol* 2006;13:624.

45. Olsen BS, Holck S: Neurogenous hyperplasia leading to appendiceal obliteration: an immunohistochemical study of 237 cases. *Histopathology* 1987;11:843.

46. Stanley MW, Cherwitz D, Hagen K, Snover DC: Neuromas of the appendix. *Am J Surg Pathol* 1986;10:801.

47. Zarabi M, LaBach JP: Ganglioneuromas causing acute appendicitis. *Hum Pathol* 1998 ;13:1143.

48. Latchis KS, Canter JW: Acute appendicitis secondary to metastatic carcinoma. *Am J Surg* 1966;111:220.

49. Dieter RA Jr: Carcinomas metastatic to the vermiform appendix: report of three cases. *Dis Colon Rectum* 1970;13:336.

50. Toubai T, Kondo Y, Ogawa T, et al: A case of leukemia of the appendix presenting as acute appendicitis. *Acta Haematol* 2003;109:199.

CHAPTER 10

Motility Disorders

INTRODUCTORY COMMENTS

Normal gastrointestinal (GI) motility depends on intact neuromuscular functions that consist of both intrinsic and extrinsic innervation. Extrinsic control of peristalsis includes the sympathetic (thoracolumbar) and parasympathetic (vagal) innervation in the ganglionated plexuses. Intrinsic control includes the enteric nervous system (ENS), smooth muscle cells, and interstitial cells of Cajal (ICCs), with the latter serving as both pacemaker cells and as intermediaries of enteric innervation (1,2). Motility disturbances constitute a complex array of clinical and pathologic disorders that result from neural, muscular, neuromuscular, or ICC abnormalities (Tables 10.1 to 10.4). Intestinal neuropathies appear to be more common than intestinal myopathies. Motility disorders occur at any age and may be primary or may complicate systemic diseases. Primary motility diseases more typically affect children than adults. Conversely, secondary conditions, such as scleroderma-associated myopathy, diabetic neuropathy, drug-induced damage, or viral infections, more frequently affect adults. Primary motility disorders may be familial or sporadic. They may remain limited to the gut, as in Hirschsprung disease (HD), or they may be part of a generalized peripheral autonomic neuropathy, as in familial visceral neuropathy. Familial disorders are inherited as both autosomal recessive and autosomal dominant diseases.

The clinical and/or pathologic findings of gastrointestinal motility disorders may be subtle or dramatic. They can present as dysphagia, nausea, vomiting, diffuse esophageal spasm, gastroparesis, intestinal pseudo-obstruction, constipation, or intestinal diverticulosis. *Intestinal pseudoobstruction* is defined as a rare, severe disabling disorder characterized by repetitive episodes or continuous symptoms and signs of bowel obstruction, including radiographic documentation of a dilated bowel with air–fluid levels in the absence of a fixed, lumen-occluding lesion (3). In contrast, *Ogilvie syndrome* is a term used synonymously with *acute* colonic pseudo-obstruction. The terms *megaesophagus*, *megaduodenum, megajejunum, megacolon,* and *megarectum* describe visceral enlargement of each of these anatomic sites. There is no agreement on the criteria for the minimum diameters of the dilated gastrointestinal segments.

Small intestinal pseudo-obstruction leads to diarrhea, malabsorption, and steatorrhea secondary to bacterial overgrowth. Some patients become malnourished with extreme weight loss.

Extraintestinal manifestations depend on the nature of the underlying disease; some help define specific syndromes. Features suggesting autonomic dysfunction include postural dizziness, difficulties in visual accommodation to bright light, and sweating abnormalities. Recurrent urinary infections and difficulty emptying the urinary bladder suggest a general visceral neuromyopathic disorder. Patients should also be questioned about drug use. Bedridden patients, such as those with dementia, stroke, and spinal cord injuries, are particularly prone to developing megacolon and a chronic pseudo-obstruction.

Motility disorders are clinically diagnosed using specific physiologic measurements of gastrointestinal motor function, including scintigraphy, gastroduodenojejunal manometry, and surface electrogastrography. The clinician will also often seek the pathologist's assistance to rule out the presence of infiltrative lesions, such as amyloidosis or connective tissue diseases, or to document the presence of neuromuscular abnormalities.

Even though the clinical or gross findings may be dramatic, the histologic features are often inconspicuous, and they may also overlap with nonspecific neural and/or muscular histologic abnormalities accompanying other conditions, such as carcinoma or previous surgery. Additionally, some patients with clinically evident motility disorders may have histologic abnormalities that have not been well described or placed into specific syndromes. In other patients, there may be neurotransmitter alteration that may or may not associate with morphologic abnormalities. These most commonly involve alterations in the nitrergic neural system or changes in vasoactive intestinal polypeptide (VIP) or substance P (SP)-containing nerves. Changes may also be present in the muscle cells or ICCs.

Histologic examination using conventional hematoxylin and eosin (H&E) stains is usually augmented with the use of special stains or ultrastructural examination (Table 10.5). Some histologic changes are so subtle that they require precise neuronal counting to document their presence. However, this is fraught with problems, since the number of

TABLE 10.1 Gastrointestinal Neural Disorders

Developmental abnormalities
Hirschsprung disease and its variants
   Hypoganglionosis (intestinal neuronal dysplasia [IND]
     type A)
   Hyperganglionosis (IND type B)
   Hyperganglionosis associated with ganglioneuromatosis
   Neuronal immaturity
   Absent enteric nervous system
   Neuropathies currently difficult to classify
Familial visceral neuropathies (see Table 10.12)
Sporadic visceral neuropathies
   Type I
   Type II
Paraneoplastic pseudo-obstruction
Isolated ganglionitis
Eosinophilic ganglionitis
Granulomatous visceral neuropathy
Megacystis–microcolon and intestinal hypoperistalsis
Severe idiopathic constipation
Acquired hypoganglionosis
Neurotransmitter disorders
   Chronic slow transit constipation
   Internal anal sphincter achalasia
   Achalasia
   Allgrove syndrome
   Infantile hypertrophic pyloric stenosis
Associated with systemic neurological diseases
   Polio
   Multiple sclerosis
   Friedreich ataxia
   Parkinson disease
   Wallenberg syndrome
   Amyotrophic lateral sclerosis
   Shy-Drager syndrome
Infections
   Herpes zoster
   Cytomegalovirus
   Epstein-Barr virus
   Chagas disease
   Lyme disease
Drugs and toxins
   Opiates and methadone
   Tricyclic antidepressants
   Clonidine
   Ganglionic blockers
   Phenothiazines
   Antineoplastics
   Theophylline
   Antiretroviral drugs
   Amanita poisoning

TABLE 10.2 Gastrointestinal Muscular Disorders

Megacystis–microcolon and intestinal hypoperistalsis
Developmental defects in the intestinal musculature
Familial visceral myopathies
Autosomal dominant
   Autosomal recessive with total gastrointestinal
     dilatation
   Autosomal recessive with ptosis and external
     ophthalmoplegia
Sporadic visceral myopathies
Mitochondrial myopathies
Autoimmune enteral leiomyositis
Hereditary internal anal sphincter myopathy
Disorders affecting the skeletal muscles
   Myotonic dystrophy
   Progressive muscular dystrophy

Treatment of motility disorders ranges from dietary changes or pharmacologic treatment to surgery or intestinal transplantation. Prokinetic drugs such as cisapride, metoclopramide, and octreotide benefit some patients. Patients with acute colonic pseudo-obstruction may benefit from neostigmine treatment (5). Bowel decompression through gastrostomy and jejunostomy may help some patients. Small bowel transplantation is the only definitive cure for patients with chronic pseudo-obstruction. Candidates for transplantation include those receiving total parenteral nutrition with frequent episodes of sepsis, limited intravenous access to nutritional support, or impending liver failure. However, small bowel transplantation tends to be challenging in this clinical setting.

NORMAL NEUROMUSCULAR STRUCTURE

Muscles

The muscularis propria is a continuous structure composed of two smooth muscle layers that extend from the upper esophagus to the anal canal (Fig. 10.1). The only exception to this occurs in the stomach, where three muscle layers are

TABLE 10.3 Disorders Involving the Interstitial Cells of Cajal

Hirschsprung disease
Intestinal neuronal dysplasia type A
Intestinal neuronal dysplasia type B
Congenital hyperplasia of interstitial cells of Cajal
Neurofibromatosis
Internal anal sphincter achalasia
Achalasia
Infantile hypertrophic pyloric stenosis
Visceral myopathies
Diabetic gastroparesis

nerves and ganglia vary with age, location, other disease processes, and section thickness. A method for rapidly assessing enteric ICCs and neuronal morphology has been developed using antibodies to c-kit and NF 68. The procedure takes approximately an hour to perform (4). It remains to be seen whether it will be widely adopted.

TABLE 10.4 Secondary Neuromuscular Disorders

Scleroderma and other connective tissue disorders
Diabetes
Amyloidosis
Radiation
Cytomegalovirus infections
Chagas disease

present. At the junctions between adjacent organs, the muscular coat rearranges to form sphincters including the pharyngoesophageal, esophagogastric, pyloric, ileocecal, and anal sphincters. The function of these sphincters is based on physiologic and pharmacologic characteristics of the musculature and on their innervation. The muscle fibers are usually arranged in a concentric circular fashion in the inner muscular layer (the *circular layer*), whereas the outer muscle fibers are arranged longitudinally (the *longitudinal layer*). In the cecum and in parts of the colon, the longitudinal muscle is extremely attenuated except in the regions where it forms thick cords (i.e., the taeniae coli).

Circular muscle, from the esophagus to the internal anal sphincter, behaves as an electrical syncytium resulting from nexuses between the plasma membranes of contiguous muscle fibers. These nexuses function as intracellular pathways for excitation conduction between adjacent cells. Even in the absence of neural influences, these syncytial properties allow three-dimensional spread of excitation (6). Smooth muscle cells also contain gap junctions or nexuses that electrically couple adjacent cells (6). The musculature also contains the

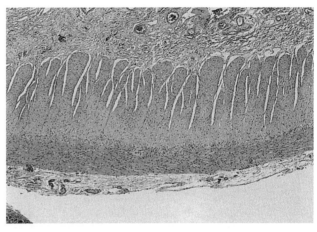

FIG. 10.1. Hematoxylin and eosin–stained section demonstrating the circular and longitudinal smooth muscle layers of the muscularis propria. This layer is present throughout the gastrointestinal tract.

ICCs, which act as pacemakers for the GI muscle (see below) and facilitate active propagation of electrical events.

The cells of the muscularis contain numerous receptors, allowing them to respond to neural signals, as well as other stimulatory and inhibitory signals during the digestive process. Contraction of the circular layer constricts the lumen; contraction of the longitudinal layer shortens the digestive tube. When the bowel becomes obstructed or the intestinal lumen distends on a persistent basis, the muscle increases in volume through both hypertrophy and hyperplasia. Smooth muscle hyperplasia also follows myenteric ablation. Obstruction results in a number of changes to both the muscular and neural layers.

Innervation

The ENS is the most complex portion of the peripheral nervous system. Three divisions of the nervous system (sympathetic, parasympathetic, and enteric) contribute to the neural control of at least four physiologic effector systems: The visceral smooth muscle responsible for motility and sphincteric functions, the mucosa responsible for gastric acid secretion and intestinal fluid and electrolyte homeostasis, the immune cells responsible for mucosal immunity, and the vasculature. Complex reflex activities involving GI motility, ion transport, and mucosal blood flow all occur in the absence of extrinsic autonomic and sensory input.

Functionally, neurons of the ENS fall into five types: (a) motor neurons, efferent or effector neurons acting to control smooth muscle tone in the wall of the gut; (b) vasomotor neurons, which control vascular muscle tone; (c) secretory neurons, other effector neurons regulating exocrine and endocrine secretion; (d) sensory neurons, which carry sensory information to the central nervous system; and (e) interneurons, which provide communication between neurons and the gut wall (Fig. 10.2). These intermingle in the myenteric and submucosal ganglia.

TABLE 10.5 Markers Useful in Evaluating Intestinal Motility Disorders

Marker	
PGP 9.5	Stains nerves
NSE	Stains nerves, ganglia
MAP-2	Stains nerves
NCAM	Stains nerves
Nerve growth factor	Stains nerves
Neuropeptide Y	Stains nerves
Neurofilament protein	Stains nerves
Synaptophysin	Stains nerves
Ret	Stains ganglia
Acetylcholinesterase activity	Stains cholinergic nerves
c-kit	Stains interstitial cells of Cajal
VIP	Stains VIP-containing nerves
Substance P	Stains substance P–containing nerves
S100	Stains Schwann cells and glia
GFAP	Stains glia
actin	Stains smooth muscle cells

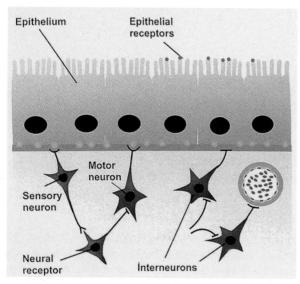

FIG. 10.2. Diagram showing the interactions of sensory neurons and motor neurons with interneurons, epithelial cells, blood vessels, and portions of the muscularis mucosae.

The ENS consists of three ganglionated plexuses in the gut wall: The myenteric (Auerbach) plexus located between the longitudinal and circular muscle layers of the muscularis propria and the submucosal (Meissner) plexus found in the submucosa. A third plexus, which derives from extrinsic nerves, occurs in the inner quarter of the circular muscle coat adjacent to the submucosa and is rich in ICCs (7). These plexuses extend uninterrupted from the esophagus to the anus, innervating the mucosa, muscle layers, and blood vessels. Interconnections between submucosal and myenteric plexuses coordinate motility and ion transport. Intramural ganglia contain nerve cells, glia (Fig. 10.3), and a neuropil formed by neuronal processes (some of extrinsic origin and others issued by intrinsic neurons) and glial processes. Since neural fibers from many different origins exist within the neuropil, the neuronal organization is extremely complex with controls coming from both the intramural and extramural ganglia.

Generally, the longitudinal musculature is poorly innervated (6). The innervation of the musculature is particularly dense at the level of the sphincters. The anal sphincter has the densest adrenergic innervation found in the GI tract. Most of its fibers originate from the superior mesenteric ganglion, but some derive from ganglionic neurons of the sacral sympathetic chain. Adrenergic fibers are also plentiful in the sphincter of Oddi. Nerve fibers containing VIP are numerous in the musculature of the gastroesophageal junction, the pylorus, and the sphincter of Oddi.

It is estimated that there are more neurons in the GI tract than there are in the spinal cord (8). Neurons of the ENS may be classified by their transmitters. Utilizing this classification, there are at least five types of neurons: (a) cholinergic (acetylcholine containing); (b) adrenergic (norepinephrine containing); (c) GABAergic (γ-aminobutyric acid containing); (d) peptidergic (peptide containing); and (e) nitrergic. The intrinsic nerve fibers are nonadrenergic noncholinergic (NANC) peptidergic nerves. The myenteric plexus neurons may also be viewed as argyrophilic and argyophobic cells based on their silver staining characteristics. Argyrophilic cells are often multiaxonal. The argyophobic cells are cholinergic nerve fibers that may directly contact the muscle cells; argyrophilic neurons do not commonly contact muscle cells. Myenteric nerve trunks consist of both extrinsic (sympathetic and parasympathetic) and intrinsic nerve fibers. In most GI regions, the ENS independently regulates many gut functions including motility, vascular tone, secretion, and release of hormones, although the central nervous system modulates the reflexes (9,10).

Normal bolus propagation depends on both cephalic excitation of gut segments producing propulsive pressure and on caudal relaxation and reduction in flow resistance.

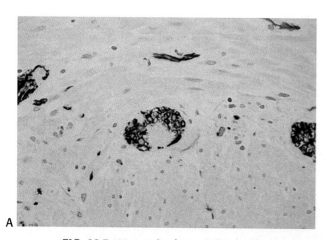
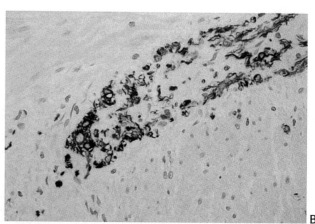

FIG. 10.3. Myenteric plexus stained with an antibody to glial fibrillary acidic protein showing the large glial component. **A:** The plexus in cross section. The central unstained area corresponds to a ganglion cell. **B:** Longitudinal section of plexus. The unstained portions correspond to neurons.

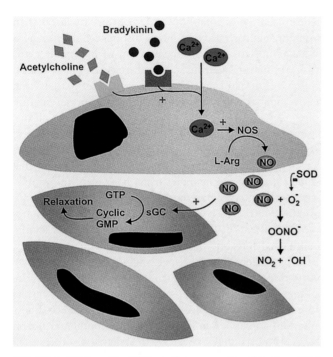

FIG. 10.4. Nitric oxide (NO) mediates vascular relaxation. NO is produced in endothelial cells by the action of calcium-dependent nitric oxide synthase (NOS). Mediators such as acetylcholine and bradykinin stimulate its production. NO acts on smooth muscle cells through a process involving conversion of guanosine triphosphate (GTP) to cyclic guanosine monophosphate (GMP), affecting relaxation. NO released into the interstitium may produce damaging free radicals after interacting with superoxide molecules.

Further, active relaxation of the sphincters is critical to prevent functional obstruction of these regions. Motor neurons of the myenteric plexus, which can be excitatory or inhibitory in nature, are responsible for the immediate neural control of gut tone. The major excitatory motor pathway involves acetylcholine, enkephalin, and tachykinins such as substance P and neurokinin A, whereas the main inhibitory transmitters are nitric oxide (NO), VIP, and adenosine triphosphate. Neural NO is produced by neural nitric oxide synthase (nNOS) (11). VIP and NO are cotransmitters in the NANC nerve–mediated smooth muscle relaxation, and part of VIP actions may be mediated by NO (Fig. 10.4) (12). The nitrergic neurons lie within the myenteric plexus. NO is also produced by the smooth muscle cells (13). The pyloric sphincter has the highest nNOS levels (13). The internal anal sphincter also contains high levels of the enzyme (13).

Interstitial Cells of Cajal

ICCs act as the pacemaker cells controlling smooth muscle contractions (14). They also act as spatial coordinators (15) and intermediaries in the neural control of gut muscular activity (16). ICCs are present in the esophagus, stomach, small and large intestine, and anorectum (17,18). There are distinct subpopulations of ICCs including intramuscular ICCs, myenteric plexus ICCs, and submucosal ICCs (19). In the esophagus, gastric cardia, and fundus, they are present in the muscularis propria but not in the myenteric plexus or submucosa. In the gastric nonfundic corpus and pylorus and in the intestines, they are present in the myenteric plexus. Submucosal ICCs are seen in the small and large intestines. ICCs express the proto-oncogene c-kit (1), making them easy to visualize with immunohistochemical stains. ICCs have long cell processes and show bipolar or multipolar configurations.

DEVELOPMENT OF THE ENTERIC NERVOUS SYSTEM

The ENS derives from vagal and sacral regions of the neural crest (10). Crest-derived cells migrate to the gut at a stage when they are morphologically indistinguishable from surrounding mesenchymal cells. Interactions of the neural crest cells with components of the extracellular matrix play a role in specifying where crest-derived cells migrate. Precursors arriving in the gut are multipotential and the enteric microenvironment to which they migrate dictates the phenotypic differentiation of developing enteric ganglion cells.

Enteric neuronal migration and differentiation involves complex interactions of lineage-determined microenvironmental elements, including transcription factors, tyrosine kinase receptor oncogenes and their ligands, the extracellular matrix, and specific adhesion molecules (10,20–22). Among some of the more important ligands of the tyrosine kinase receptor ligands are the neurotrophin family of growth factors that promote the differentiation, growth, and survival of various neurons (23). Glial cell line–derived neurotrophic factor (GDNF) and neurturin play an important role in the migration of enteric neuron precursors into and along the small and large intestines and the esophagus, a process that is RET dependent (24,25). GDNF, which acts as a chemoattractant for enteric neural cells, promotes migration of neural crest cells throughout the gastrointestinal tract, attracting them to this site and preventing them from straying out of the gut (26). Analysis of animal models (transgenic and knockout mice) has played an important role in identifying the genes critical for ENS development (21,27–29) (Table 10.6).

Vagal nerve trunks can be found in the upper esophagus by the fifth fetal week. Nerve trunks extend on the outer surface of the gut wall and neuroblasts are found along the gastric cardia by the sixth week, the cephalic limb of the midgut by the seventh week, and the entire gut up to the distal half of the colon and rectum by the eighth week. By the 12th week, they have migrated as far as the rectum. The myenteric plexus forms just outside the circular muscle coat, which then develops its longitudinal muscle coat (30). Neuroblasts migrate from the myenteric plexus to form the submucosal plexus; this is completed during the third and fourth months (30). Following neural crest cell migration, the cells proliferate and the neurons

TABLE 10.6	**Genes Involved in Enteric Nervous System (ENS) Development**

Gene	Intestinal Phenotype after Genetic Manipulation
Ednrb (endothelin receptor B) Growth factor receptor	Neural crest cells in Ednrb knockouts fail to colonize the hindgut
Hox-4 Homeobox transcription factor expressed in the foregut	Transgenic animals show abnormal ganglia in the colon and short segment hypoganglionosis in the distal colon
Mash-1 Encodes a transcription factor required for development of the autonomic nervous system	Knockout leads to aganglionosis of the esophagus and gastric cardia; absence of early lineage of enteric neurons in the rest of the bowel
NCX1 Homeobox transcription factor expressed by ENS after midgestation in the distal gut	Homozygous-targeted disruption animals show neural hyperplasia and hyperganglionosis
Phox2P Homeodomain-containing transcription factor expressed by neural crest cells as they invade foregut mesenchyme	Phox2 knockout mice die in utero. There is an absence of foregut and midgut ENS
ret/gdnf/gfrd1 Encodes Ret, a receptor tyrosine kinase expressed by neural crest-derived cells that colonize the gut. Ret is the functional receptor for glial cell line–derived neurotrophic factor (GDNF)	Knockout leads to complete failure of enteric neurons and glia to develop in the entire bowel below the foregut
Sox 10 Encodes a transcription factor expressed by ENS precursors before and after colonization of gut mesenchyme	Sox transgenics develop distal intestinal aganglionosis and die shortly after birth

mature (Fig. 10.5), developing processes and synapses that allow for communication within ganglia, between ganglia, and between ganglia and smooth muscle cells. Interruption of this process at different stages produces various myenteric plexus abnormalities ranging from agenesis to incomplete maturation. Interruption of the orderly cranial–caudal migration of nerves and neuroblasts explains the variable length of aganglionic segments in Hirschsprung disease.

At birth, normal enteric ganglia contain both mature and immature neurons. Premature infants have more immature neurons than term infants. Mature neurons are larger than immature neurons and they have a distinct cell membrane, a vesicular nucleus, and a large amount of basophilic cytoplasm. Immature neurons are small cells with dark nuclei, clumped chromatin, and scant cytoplasm (Fig. 10.6). Neural stains highlight immature neurons. The normal mature colon contains 7 ganglion cells/mm of myenteric plexus, 3.6/mm in the jejunum, and 4.3/mm in the ileum in 3 micron sections (31). Ganglion cells lie approximately 1 mm apart; they may occur in clusters of from one to five cells in normal adults (32). Normal neonates often have plentiful, prominent ganglion cells, but they appear small when they are immature (30).

Most patients with congenital myenteric plexus abnormalities fall into one of five categories: (a) aganglionosis, (b) hypoganglionosis, (c) hyperganglionosis, (d) ganglionic immaturity, and (e) poorly classified abnormalities. The pathogenesis of developmental disorders of the ENS results from genetic defects, failed neural crest migration or differentiation, anoxia, or inflammation. Developmental neural diseases occur alone or coexist with systemic disorders such as neurofibromatosis.

HIRSCHSPRUNG DISEASE

Synonyms for Hirschsprung disease include aganglionic megacolon, congenital megacolon, and aganglionosis.

HD is a congenital disorder characterized by intestinal megacolon, neural hyperplasia, and aganglionosis. Several forms of the disease are recognized.

- **Classic form:** The aganglionic segment begins in the distal colorectum and extends proximally for variable distances into the adjoining proximally dilated bowel (Fig. 10.7).
- **Short segment form:** The aganglionic segment involves several centimeters of the rectum and rectosigmoid. The aganglionic segment may be as short as 3 cm, so that this variant may be missed if the biopsy is taken too high above the pectinate line. This form affects 67% to 90% of patients.
- **Long segment form:** The aganglionic segment extends beyond the sigmoid and involves a variable length of colon but does not extend beyond the cecum. This form affects <10% of patients (33).
- **Total colonic aganglionosis:** The entire colon is involved along with variable lengths of ileum, jejunum, and even the stomach. This form affects 2.6% to 14.9% of cases. This form almost always presents in the first weeks of life.
- **Zonal colonic aganglionosis** (synonym: Skip segment HD): A short bowel segment is involved in this form of HD (Fig. 10.8). Ganglion cells are present, both proximal and distal to the aganglionic segment. (This form of the disease may in fact not be HD, but the result of intrauterine injury.)

HD affects 1 in every 5,000 to 30,000 live births; 80% of patients are male (34). Approximately 4% to 6% of cases

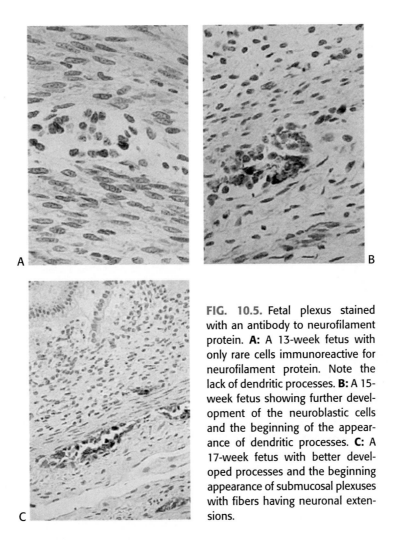

FIG. 10.5. Fetal plexus stained with an antibody to neurofilament protein. **A:** A 13-week fetus with only rare cells immunoreactive for neurofilament protein. Note the lack of dendritic processes. **B:** A 15-week fetus showing further development of the neuroblastic cells and the beginning of the appearance of dendritic processes. **C:** A 17-week fetus with better developed processes and the beginning appearance of submucosal plexuses with fibers having neuronal extensions.

are familial (34), especially when the megacolon extends to the cecum. Five percent of patients have an affected sibling (35).

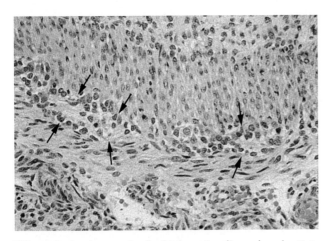

FIG. 10.6. Fetal gut stained with hematoxylin and eosin. Note the presence of immature neuroblastlike cells without clearly identifiable ganglia (*arrows*).

Etiology and Pathophysiology of the Disease

HD is a heterogeneous genetic disorder with autosomal dominant, autosomal recessive, and polygenic forms of inheritance. Current etiologic hypotheses revolve around two major schools of thought: Arrested neuroblast migration and intestinal microenvironmental abnormalities that cause failed neuronal differentiation. Specific genetic mutations are present in about 50% of cases. Much of the phenotypic variability of the disease relates to the biologic complexity underlying the normal development of the ENS and the diversity of the molecular alterations that have been identified. Thus, no single genetic abnormality accounts for the development of the disease.

There are several susceptibility genes for HD (Table 10.7) (36–44). Other genes that may be abnormal include *endothelin-converting enzyme* and the transcription factor *Sox 10* (40,41). Several genes may modify the severity of the HD phenotype in patients with or without coexisting intestinal neuronal dysplasia. These may lie near 21q22 (43) and may account for the prevalence of HD among patients with trisomy 21 (43). The nerves in HD also fail to express the trkC tyrosine receptor and its ligand neurotrophin, suggesting

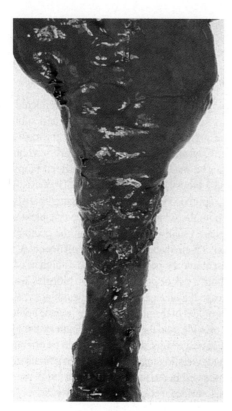

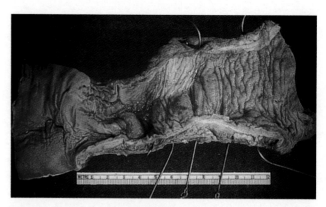

FIG. 10.8. Zonal aganglionosis. The distal bowel lies to the right of the photograph and the proximal bowel to the left. The aganglionic segment is the contracted segment in the middle. The proximal bowel appears dilated and featureless, with loss of the mucosal markings.

FIG. 10.7. Gross specimen of a patient with Hirschsprung disease. Note the contracted distal bowel, which tapers distally. The proximal bowel is dilated.

that neurotrophic factors that are critical for cellular survival and differentiation may play a role in the pathogenesis of HD (45).

The ret protein is a tyrosine kinase receptor with extracellular cadherinlike and cysteine-rich domains, a transmembrane domain, and an intracellular tyrosine kinase domain (46). Point mutations in the *RET* gene give rise to HD, multiple endocrine

neoplasia (MEN) types IIA and IIB, and familial medullary thyroid carcinoma (47). In the case of MEN-II, the RET mutations are activating, enhancing the function of the encoded protein, whereas in HD, the mutations are inactivating, leading to loss of its function (48). A ret codon 618 ser mutation could predispose patients with MEN-IIA to HD (49).

More than 50 *RET* mutations, including missense, nonsense, deletion, and insertion mutations, have been described in HD. These mutations occur throughout the gene, without any mutational hot spots (50). They fall loosely into two groups: Frame shift or missense mutations that disrupt the structure of the intracellular tyrosine kinase domains and missense mutations in exons 2, 3, 5, or 6 of the extracellular domain (51). Patients with mutations of the intracellular domain have either short segment or long segment HD, whereas those with mutations in the extracellular domain all have long segment HD. *RET* mutations are more

TABLE 10.7   **Mutations Present in Hirschsprung Disease (HD)**

Mutated Gene	Function	Disease
ret (intracellular tyrosine kinase domain)	Tyrosine kinase receptor	Short segment HD Long segment HD
ret (extracellular domain)	Tyrosine kinase receptor	Long segment HD
Endothelin B receptor (EDNRB)	Growth factor receptor	Short segment HD
EDN3	Ligand for EDNRB	Shah-Waardenburg syndrome
Glial cell line–derived neurotropic factor (GDNF)	Ligand for ret	Serves as HD modifier
Neurturin	Ligand for ret	Serves as HD modifier
SMADIP1	Transcription factor	Syndromic HD with microcephaly, facial dysmorphism, and mental retardation

common among familial cases (50%) than among sporadic cases (15% to 33%) (50). Immunohistochemically, the bowels of patients with HD show reduced ret protein expression.

In addition to the presence of specific *RET* mutations that may lead to the development of HD, there are also *RET* intragenic polymorphisms that lead to various clinical phenotypes (52). The *c*135G/A polymorphism or sequence variations in linkage disequilibrium with this polymorphism modulate the phenotypic influences of *RET* germline mutations. The *c*135A variant associates more commonly with short segment disease when it is on the same chromosome with the germline mutation (52).

Alterations in the intrinsic gastrointestinal innervation contribute to the clinical and pathologic features of HD. VIP and NO, components of the NANC system that relax smooth muscle and form part of the inhibitory component of the peristaltic reflex, are absent (53–55). However, extrinsic parasympathetic, cholinergic, and sympathetic adrenergic innervation persist. As a result, the distal aganglionic bowel is under constant, unopposed extramural stimulation so that it becomes narrowed, spastic, and unable to support peristalsis. There are also conflicting reports on the ICCs in HD. Some authors find normal numbers of ICCs, whereas others suggest that they are decreased in number.

The pathogenesis of the enterocolitis, which affects some patients, is not well understood. It is likely to result from the toxemia due to bacterial stasis in the dilated colonic lumen. Risk factors for enterocolitis include a delayed diagnosis of HD, long segment disease, family history for HD, female gender, and trisomy 21 (56).

Clinical Features

HD is the most common form of congenital intestinal obstruction, often presenting within the first 24 to 48 hours of life. Up to 80% of cases are diagnosed during the first year of life; 10% first present in adults. Typically, the lack of propulsive movements and inhibitory reflexes in an intestinal segment leads to abdominal distension, vomiting, severe constipation, and marked dilation of the proximal ganglionic segment. Infants with obstruction but without megacolon should be suspected of having HD involving the entire colon. Reduced food intake and malabsorption result in failure to thrive. As the nutritional status deteriorates, infections may worsen the underlying motility problem. Some patients develop mucosal prolapse at the junction of the ganglionic and aganglionic bowel due to differential luminal pressures in these bowel segments. Mucosal prolapse is more prominent in older patients and correlates with disease duration. HD patients may also present in the neonatal period with perforation due to a coexisting necrotizing enterocolitis. The enterocolitis has an ischemic basis and is characterized by mucosal ulceration, colonic bleeding, perforation, sepsis, and toxemia. Patients with trisomy 21 exhibit an increased incidence of HD-associated enterocolitis (56).

Ten to fifteen percent of patients have associated congenital anomalies or other diseases (Table 10.8). Ten percent of patients have Down syndrome; 5% have other serious neurologic abnormalities (57).

Pathologic Findings

The widely dilated, fluid-filled, hypertrophic colon empties into a funnel-shaped transitional zone extending to the anus (Fig. 10.7). Plain abdominal films may show air–fluid levels. The anal canal and rectum are small and empty, and the anal sphincter is tight. In adults, an abrupt, smooth rectal transition zone with proximal colonic dilation, in the setting of an appropriate clinical history, suggests the diagnosis.

A diagnosis of HD is usually made on a suction rectal biopsy containing both the mucosa and submucosa since the aganglionosis coincides closely in both the submucosal and myenteric plexuses. Biopsies are usually taken 2 cm from the pectinate line and at about a 5-cm distance. In very small neonates, the biopsy is taken just above the pectinate line and as high as can be taken safely without risking perforation. Two biopsies are preferred to increase the chances of an adequate biopsy, to overcome the possibility of a hypoganglionic segment, and to provide guidance as to the length of the aganglionic segment. Full-thickness rectal biopsy is reserved for patients in whom the diagnosis cannot be made with a more superficial biopsy.

TABLE 10.8 **Other Abnormalities Affecting Patients with Hirschsprung Disease**

Genetic abnormalities
  Down syndrome
  Tetrasomy 9p
  Tetrasomy 9q
Congenital abnormalities
  Deafness
  Intestinal malrotation
  Esophageal and intestinal atresia
  Hypothalamic hamartoblastoma
  Cartilage–hair hypoplasia
  Dandy-Walker cysts
  Brachydactyly and polydactyly
  Congenital hypoventilation
  Holoprosencephaly
  Imperforate anus
  Congenital muscular dystrophy
  Infantile osteopetrosis
Tumors
  Neuroblastoma
  Neurofibromatosis
  Medullary carcinoma of the thyroid
  Pheochromocytoma
Other syndromes
  Pallister-Hall syndrome
  Jaw winking syndrome
  Haddad syndrome
  Goldberg-Shprintzen syndrome
  Achalasia
  Multiple endocrine neoplasia type IIB
  Waardenburg-Shah

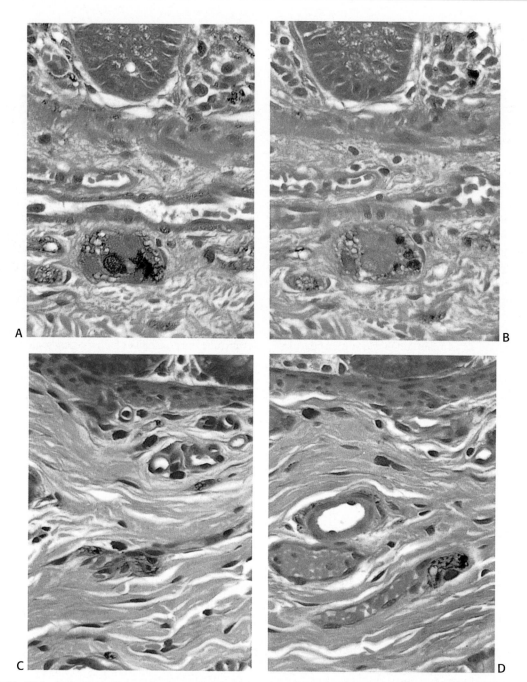

FIG. 10.9. **A:** Section of normal colon stained with anti–neuron-specific enolase (NSE) to highlight the submucosal ganglion. **B:** Serial section stained with anti-S100. The ganglion cells are negative. **C:** Hirschsprung disease stained with anti-NSE. Ganglion cells are absent, and there is nerve fiber proliferation. This is seen better at higher power magnification. **D:** Serial section stained with anti-S100. Nerve fibers are positive.

Typical features of HD include aganglionosis (Fig. 10.9) and increased numbers of hypertrophic, nonmyelinated, submucosal, and myenteric plexus cholinergic nerves (part of the extrinsic parasympathetic innervation) (Fig. 10.10). While neural hyperplasia is characteristic of HD, it should be noted that neural hyperplasia is present in other disorders (Table 10.9). Ganglion cells are absent from both plexuses in the distal narrowed bowel and are decreased in number in the first few centimeters of the transitional zone. An increase in the number of ganglion cells occurs as one progresses proximally into the funnel-shaped transitional zone and into the normally innervated bowel. The transitional zone usually occurs over a short distance with ganglia appearing almost simultaneously in both the myenteric and submucosal

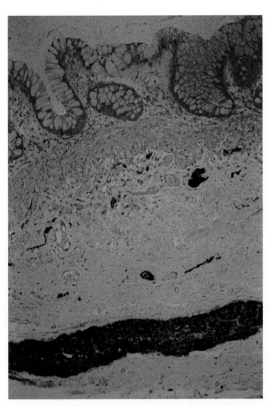

FIG. 10.10. Hypertrophic nerve in Hirschsprung disease stained with an antibody to S100.

plexuses. Some patients have longer transitional zones than others; prominent nerve trunks may be present for several centimeters. The transitional zone may contain abnormally shaped ganglia. Some transition zones show features of colonic neuronal dysplasia (see below).

In premature infants it may be difficult to recognize the immature ganglion cells due to their small size and inconspicuous nuclei (Fig. 10.6). They form rosettelike structures arranged around a central neuropil-type matrix producing a horseshoelike structure. The immature ganglia may mimic macrophages, smooth muscle cells, and Schwann cells. The ganglia may be highlighted with special stains. However, it should be kept in mind that immature ganglia may fail to stain with ganglionic markers. These patients also have decreased numbers of synaptophysin-positive synapses in the circular and longitudinal muscle layers in the transitional

TABLE 10.9	**Conditions Associated with Hyperplasia of the Myenteric Plexus**

Hirschsprung disease
Neurofibromatosis
Multiple endocrine neoplasia type IIB
Crohn disease
Neuronal dysplasia
Hyperganglionosis with ganglioneuromatosis
Hyperplastic response to many forms of injury

segments and in aganglionic segments (58) and the adrenergic and peptidergic innervation of aganglionic gut is abnormal. Patients also have a relative loss of ICCs (59), although this finding is not present in all studies (60). Increased numbers of mast cells, often in direct contact with the hypertrophic nerves, are present. These produce nerve growth factor, which stimulates neural growth.

Frequently, the bowel wall proximal to the aganglionic segment is biopsied at the time of surgery to ensure that the proximal resection margin is normal. Submucosal nerve trunks >40 μm in diameter or abnormal-appearing ganglia strongly correlate with abnormal innervation and aganglionosis (Fig. 10.11) (61). If hypertrophic nerve trunks or abnormal ganglion cells are present in frozen sections, the surgeon should extend the resection proximally and monitor it with additional frozen sections to identify a region that contains completely normal neural structures in order to prevent recurrent disease. Once resection specimens are received, the extent of the aganglionosis should be determined and the status of the proximal margin should be ascertained, if this was not done intraoperatively. Patients who develop postoperative symptoms may have either a retained portion of the transitional zone with neuronal dysplasia or an aganglionic segment or they may have developed an acquired disorder secondary to postoperative ischemia or infection.

If enterocolitis develops, the histology may include crypt dilation with mucin depletion, cryptitis, crypt abscesses, mucosal ulcers, transmural necrosis, and perforation. Enterocolitis affects both ganglionic and aganglionic intestinal segments, and resembles other forms of enterocolitis. Pneumatosis intestinalis may be present. One occasionally sees abnormal submucosal blood vessels in HD. The abnormal arteries are most conspicuous in the transitional zone, where they appear thickened and may show bizarre microscopic changes. Adventitial fibromuscular dysplasia, as evidenced by increased collagen around the internal elastic lamina, marked hypertrophy of the media, and obliterative endarteritis, also develops (62). The vascular changes predispose to ischemic injury.

Histologic Variants

There are several histologic variants of HD. One associates with intestinal neuronal dysplasia. Generally, there is a hypoganglionic transitional zone at the cranial end of the aganglionic segment, but hyperganglionic segments can also be found.

Total colonic aganglionosis can be divided into two groups based on the histologic findings. Some cases are histologically similar to short segment and long segment disease, whereas in others, the bowel is aganglionic but there is little or no neural hyperplasia. The latter finding can lead to a false-negative diagnosis.

In *HD with coexisting intestinal neuronal dysplasia (IND)*, the IND lies within, or just proximal to, the aganglionic

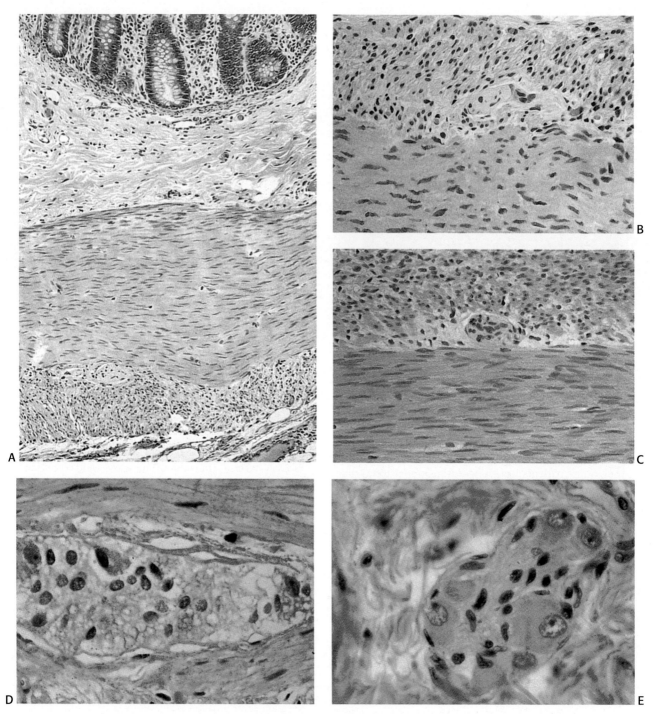

FIG. 10.11. Hirschsprung disease. **A:** Full-thickness section through the wall demonstrates the usual layers, but no ganglion cells. **B:** High-power magnification of the myenteric plexus shows abnormal small ganglion cell in the transitional area. **C:** A higher power magnification of another abnormal-appearing ganglion cell. **D:** Abnormal ganglion compared to a normal ganglion **(E).**

transitional zone. Patients have also been described with aganglionosis involving the entire colon and terminal ileum and coexisting jejunal and gastric IND. The IND accounts for residual symptoms in HD patients following pullthrough operations (63).

Zonal aganglionosis, or skip segment HD, may affect some patients with total colonic aganglionosis (64). In this setting, one sees variable lengths of hypoganglionic or normoganglionic transverse or ascending colon resulting in a segmental aganglionic colon. Normal distal innervation or a skip area containing some ganglia is present within an area of aganglionosis (64). Such cases are thought to have an ischemic origin. If biopsies are performed on the unaffected segments, the diagnosis will be missed.

Special Techniques for Evaluating Hirschsprung Disease Specimens

Acetylcholinesterase (ACE) enzymatic staining (Fig. 10.12) demonstrates an increased network of coarse, thickened, irregular, cholinergic nerve fibers within the muscularis mucosae and lower mucosa. The lamina propria fibers travel in a plane parallel to the mucosal surface. Numerous submucosal small nerve fibers and smaller and larger nerve trunks

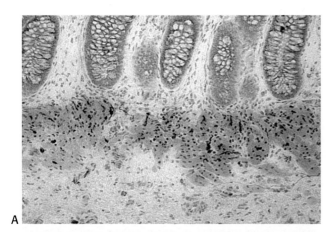

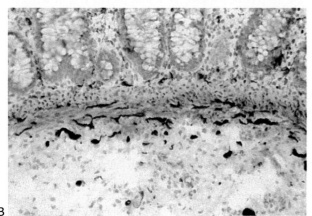

FIG. 10.12. Acetylcholinesterase staining reactions. The positive reaction is shown by the blackish brown color. **A:** Normal bowel characterized by the presence of thin, wispy, acetylcholinesterase-positive nerve fibers within the muscularis mucosa. None is present in the overlying lamina propria of the mucosa. **B:** Patient with Hirschsprung disease demonstrating thick, irregular fibers both within the muscularis mucosae and extending up into the lamina propria and around the glands. (Pictures courtesy of Dr. Kevin Bove, Cincinnati Children's Hospital.)

may also be present. This pattern is evident even in the most distal biopsies, including those from the mucocutaneous junction. Increased ACE nerve fibers are consistently present in short and long segment HD, but they may be absent in total colonic aganglionosis. ACE staining patterns are also less dramatic in neonates than in older individuals, possibly leading to false-negative diagnoses.

The common procedure for the ACE staining is as follows: Two mucosal suction biopsies are obtained 3 to 4 cm above the pectinate line. One is snap-frozen at the bedside. The other is placed in formalin for paraffin embedding. Delayed freezing after specimen delivery may cause false-negative results due to enzyme degradation. The frozen sample is cut in a plane perpendicular to the mucosal surface. Several paraffin sections are used to complement the evaluation of acetylcholinesterase activity. The special stains listed in Table 10.5 help delineate specific structures.

Treatment and Prognosis

Surgery is invariably necessary to treat symptomatic HD and the HD-associated enterocolitis. Persistent constipation is the most important long-term problem in patients operated on for HD. Inadequate resection, anastomotic strictures, coexisting IND, or achalasia of the internal anal sphincter may also cause these sequelae.

INTESTINAL NEURONAL DYSPLASIA

IND, another developmental abnormality involving the ENS, occurs in two forms: Type A is characterized by decreased or immature gastrointestinal sympathetic innervation, and type B is characterized by increased numbers of ganglion cells, a dysplastic submucosal plexus, and defective neuronal nerve fiber differentiation (65,66). IND type A is also known as *hypoganglionosis*. IND type B is also known as *hyperganglionosis*. The entity known as *oligoneuronal disease*, which is sometimes called the *hypogenetic type of dysganglionosis* (67), may also be a form of intestinal neuronal dysplasia type A. These diseases are poorly understood and widely used consensus definitions for each entity are not available.

Intestinal Neuronal Dysplasia Type A

IND type A is very rare, and the symptoms caused by hypoganglionosis resemble those seen in HD. In newborns, there may be delayed meconium discharge; affected infants and small children have rare bowel evacuations that respond to enemas. With increasing age, fecal masses can be palpated through the abdominal wall. The colon becomes dilated and contains fecalomas. Distension causes intermittent colicky pain, often relieved by massive flatulence. Some children experience overflow discharge of sometimes bloody stool.

The diagnosis of hypoganglionosis is usually difficult to establish. X-ray studies, determination of transit times, and anorectal manometry are unreliable indicators of the disease.

The disorder is characterized by an immaturity or hypoplasia of the extrinsic sympathetic nerves supplying the gut (68). Hypoganglionosis occurs in three forms: (a) an isolated form occurring as a segmental or even disseminated disease, (b) hypoganglionosis of variable length adjacent to an aganglionic HD, and (c) hypoganglionosis in combination with IND type B of a proximal segment. *Hypoganglionosis* may result from a developmental hypoplasia of the myenteric plexus (65), possibly due to the absence or abnormal expression of neurotrophic factors.

Patients with IND type A have reduced numbers of myenteric ganglia and myenteric plexus neurons, no or low colonic mucosal ACE levels, and secondary hypertrophy of the muscularis mucosae and the circular muscle of the muscularis propria. Absent or small submucosal and myenteric ganglia containing only one or two ganglia and immature neuroblastlike cells extend throughout the affected parts of the gut. Some patients have irreversible neuronal degeneration. Patients with IND type A may also have reduced numbers of ICCs, perhaps contributing to the dysmotility (69).

There is no consensus of how few ganglion cells there should be to make a diagnosis of hypoganglionosis. Meier-Ruge suggests that a 10-fold decrease in the number of ganglion cells per centimeter of bowel as compared to normal bowel is diagnostic (66). The distance between the ganglia in hypoganglionosis is nearly double that of the normal bowel. The treatment of hypoganglionosis (IND type A) is resection of the affected bowel and a pullthrough operation.

Intestinal Neuronal Dysplasia Type B

In contrast to IND type A, the incidence of IND type B varies from 0.3% to 40% of rectal suction biopsies (65,66). The mean age at diagnosis is 1.5 years. It occurs as an isolated disorder or it complicates many disorders (Table 10.10) (68,70). Patients with MEN-IIB and IND type B have RET mutations. In some cases, IND and neurofibromatosis are familial and associate with a tandem duplication in the *NFI* gene and a reciprocal translocation (t15;16) (q26.3;q12.1) (71). IND may also be one component of a complex malformation pattern.

IND type B clinically both mimics and complicates HD, as discussed in an earlier section. Patients present with nausea/vomiting, diarrhea, constipation, intestinal obstruction, intussusception, and volvulus. Symptoms develop insidiously, with progressive development of severe constipation that results in overflow incontinence (66). Many patients eventually spontaneously develop normal colonic motility (66). A significant number of patients develop severe intra-abdominal complications during the perinatal period, including necrotizing enterocolitis (NEC), meconium ileus,

TABLE 10.10 Conditions That May Be Associated with Intestinal Neuronal Dysplasia

Tumors
  Carcinoid tumors
  Familial gastrointestinal stromal tumors
  Lipoblastomatosis
  Medullary carcinoma of the thyroid
  Neurofibromatosis
  Pheochromocytoma
Paraneoplastic syndromes
Cystic fibrosis
Other gastrointestinal abnormalities
  Anal atresia
  Choleduodenal cyst
  Congenital hyperplasia of the interstitial cells of Cajal
  Esophageal atresia
  Hirschsprung disease
  Intestinal duplication
  Intestinal malrotation
  Microvillous atrophy
  Persistent urachus
  Pyloric stenosis
  Rectal or sigmoid stenosis
  Short bowel syndrome
Extra-abdominal malformations
  Aortic stenosis
  Congenital diaphragmatic hernia

or bowel perforations. Such complications are especially common in premature neonates.

Neuronal dysplasia can be diffuse, involving both the small and large intestine, or it may remain confined to a single intestinal segment. Extensive disease may involve the stomach and esophagus. The bowel grossly appears either normal or variably dilated.

Controversy exists over the diagnostic criteria of IND type B. The diagnostic controversy is best exemplified by a study in which three pathologists agreed on the diagnosis in only 14% of children without aganglionosis (72). Smith also found that according to the criteria described by Borchard, only 11% of patients with megacolon had the obligatory criteria (hyperplasia of the submucosal plexus, an increase in ACE-positive nerve fibers around submucosal blood vessels, and ACE activity in the lamina propria) (73). The diagnosis of IND type B is also complicated by the fact that the density of ganglion cells in the myenteric plexus decreases significantly with age during the first 3 to 4 years of life and estimates of nerve cell density are influenced by section thickness (74).

The diagnostic criteria of IND type B have included prominent hyperplasia of the parasympathetic myenteric and submucosal plexuses characterized by increased numbers of neurons and ganglia (Fig. 10.13); giant submucosal ganglia containing 7 to 15 ganglion cells; hypertrophic nerve bundles containing increased numbers of thickened, beaded, and disorganized axons (Fig. 10.13); increased ACE activity

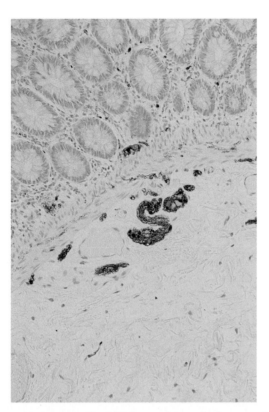

FIG. 10.13. Four-month-old infant with intestinal dysplasia type B. The hypertrophic nerves are accentuated by an S100 immunostain.

in mucosal, submucosal, and arterial adventitial nerves (66); a proliferation of fine nerve fibers in the lamina propria and circular muscle; and the presence of isolated ganglion cells in the submucosa, muscularis mucosae, or lower mucosa (Fig. 10.14) (65–68,72,73). The myenteric ganglia may be large and almost continuous with numerous readily identifiable neurons. The finding of giant ganglia, while almost always seen in IND type B, is not specific for it and this feature may be present in the proximal colon in patients with HD and in some patients with hypoganglionosis. Many neurons contain bizarre nuclei and poorly defined cytoplasm. Hypertrophic nerve bundles contain an increased number of thickened, beaded, and disorganized axons. These nerves may show an absence of NCAM and nicotinamide adenine dinucleotide phosphate (NADPH) diaphorase activity (75).

Inflammatory changes, as might be seen in visceral myopathies or neuropathies, are absent. Prominent hypertrophy of the circular and longitudinal muscle layers also occurs.

Only about 5% of the ganglia in IND are giant ganglia (74). The specificity of giant ganglia as a marker for IND type B has been questioned, since occasional giant ganglia can be found in individuals without constipation. The presence of giant ganglia may be age-independent changes, whereas hyperplasia of the submucosal plexus and increases in ACE activity in the nerve fibers of the lamina propria appear to be age-dependent findings that disappear with maturation of the enteric nervous system. Therefore, neural

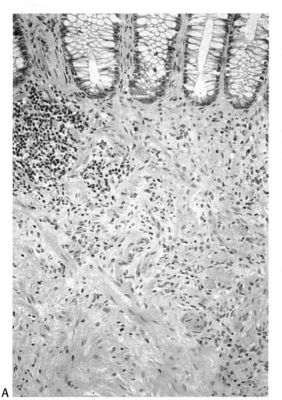

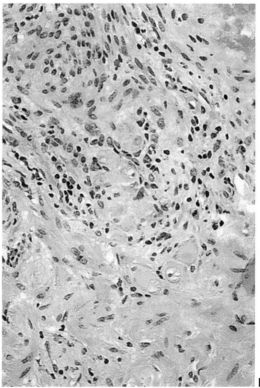

A   B

FIG. 10.14. Area of hyperganglionosis in the same specimen illustrated in Figure 10.13. **A:** Low magnification showing a large collection of ganglion cells lying in the hypertrophic muscle and in the lower portion of the mucosa. **B:** Higher magnification showing the large numbers of ganglion cells.

hyperplasia is significantly more common in neonates <4 weeks of age than in older individuals (76). This may explain our experience that one often sees hyperganglionosis in the absence of neural hyperplasia in young children with a history of chronic constipation.

Patients with IND may also exhibit ICC hyperplasia (77). When it is marked, it can be visible grossly as a thick, white, fibrous band between the inner circular and outer longitudinal muscle layers throughout the full length of the resected bowel, especially in children with neurofibromatosis type 1 (NF-1). Microscopically, this bandlike layer consists of haphazardly arranged spindled to oval-shaped cells. The nuclei are long and oval in shape with slightly tapered ends and possess hyperchromatic or clumped chromatin and occasional small nucleoli. The cells have a moderate amount of eosinophilic cytoplasm; mitotic figures are rare. The muscle layers are partially replaced by these hyperplastic spindle cells and focally the full thickness of the inner muscular layer can be involved. Residual myenteric plexus can be identified in the midst of the hyperplastic cells. The hyperplastic cells are c-kit positive.

Patients with IND often have large numbers of mast cells in the bowel wall compared to the normal colon. Mast cells produce nerve growth factors that support the development and functional maintenance of the sympathetic and cholinergic neurons, and they may be important in the neuronal hyperplasia seen in this condition (78). We have also seen endocrine cell hyperplasia associated with hyperganglionosis in the neonate.

Individuals with IND also often have secondary changes in the muscularis propria. There may be areas of significant muscle atrophy in one or another layer of the muscularis propria. Alternatively, there may be hyperplasia of either the circular or longitudinal layer of the muscularis propria or these two changes may both be present. These changes may be focal or diffuse in nature and they may be present in the circular layer in some parts of the gut and in the longitudinal layer in others. These secondary changes undoubtedly reflect abnormal innervation of the muscle layers and the neuromuscular junction.

Overall, it would be desirable to have better quantitative diagnostic criteria of IND to distinguish normal variants from pathologic conditions, particularly in very young children. Moore et al introduced a morphologic scoring system based on the finding of hyperganglionosis, giant ganglia, neuronal maturity, heterotopic neuronal cells, and ACE activity in the lamina propria, muscularis mucosae, or adventitia of submucosal blood vessels. Hyperganglionosis and increased ACE activity of nerve fibers in the lamina propria had major importance in this scoring system (79). The best diagnostic indicator of IND in adults may be the detection of six to ten giant ganglia with more than seven nerve cells in 15 biopsy sections (80).

Some patients, especially those with IND type B, outgrow their disease as the ENS matures. Patients with persistent symptoms are managed medically with prokinetic agents, colonic irrigations, and cathartics. If bowel symptoms persist after 6 months of conservative treatment, surgery is often considered. Resection and pullthrough operations may be indicated in extensive IND.

HYPERGANGLIONOSIS AND GANGLIONEUROMATOSIS

Patients with hyperganglionosis and diffuse ganglioneuromatosis (Fig. 10.15) almost always have MEN-IIB and a mutation in the *RET* oncogene. The changes may associate with or be a form of IND type B.

NEURONAL IMMATURITY

Neuronal immaturity, also known as *neuronal maturational arrest syndrome,* is characterized by the failure of neural elements to mature properly so that the ganglia appear immature and the patients present with clinical features resembling HD and IND. There may be overlap with IND. The underlying cause of failed neuronal maturation is unknown. Pathogenetic mechanisms may include (a) failure of normal numbers of neural crest cells to migrate into the gut, (b) inadequate neural proliferation in the gut, or (c) lack of growth or death of neuroblasts once they arrive in the gut due to the failure of the local microenvironment to support normal neuronal development during fetal life. There may also be a lack of neurotrophins since the latter are known to be important in neuronal development, differentiation maturation, survival, and maintenance. There may also be absence or delayed maturation of the ICCs, contributing to pseudo-obstruction in neonates.

The histologic features differ depending on the stage at which myenteric plexus development ceased. Patients exhibit several major histologic abnormalities: (a) no myenteric plexus seen in either H&E or specially stained sections, (b) small numbers of neuronal structures (ganglia and nerve trunks), or (c) an apparently normal myenteric plexus seen on H&E-stained sections but a neural deficiency shown by silver or immunohistochemical staining. The immature neurons lack neurofilaments. The ganglion cells may also line up at the periphery of the ganglia (ring-shaped ganglia) as occurs in premature infants (Figs. 10.16 and 10.17). There is no inflammation or neural degeneration. These findings contrast with those seen in patients with HD or IND type B in that there is no neural hyperplasia, but as noted there may be overlap with IND.

Neuronal immaturity often spontaneously improves with conservative therapy and the normal development of the child unless it occurs as part of IND. In other patients the changes persist.

CONGENITAL HYPERPLASIA OF INTERSTITIAL CELLS OF CAJAL

As noted earlier, ICCs are the pacemaker cells of the GI tract that initiate peristalsis in the stomach and the intestines.

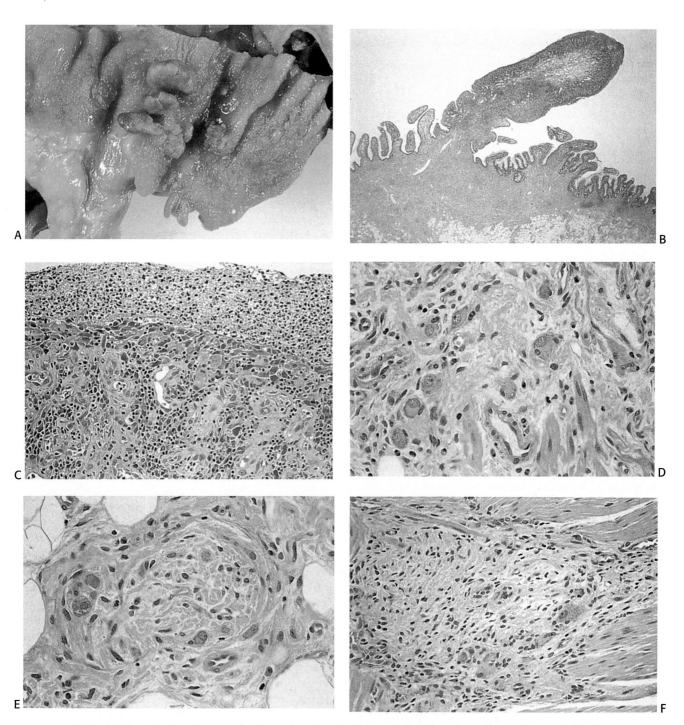

FIG. 10.15. Patient with pseudo-obstruction, intestinal neuronal dysplasia, and ganglioneuromatosis. **A:** Gross appearance of the bowel lumen demonstrates numerous polyps. **B:** Histologic examination shows a cellular proliferation that obliterates the normal mucosal–submucosal junction. **C:** Section through the base of the polyp showing a ganglioneuroma. **D:** Higher power magnification shows the neural tissue and ganglion cells. **E:** Submucosal ganglion demonstrating peripheral fibrosis and abnormal architecture. **F:** The architecture of the myenteric plexus is abnormal and there are numerous inflammatory cells within the myenteric plexus. (Case courtesy of Dr. E. Foucar, Albuquerque, NM.)

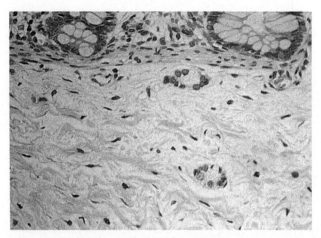

FIG. 10.16. Infant with pseudo-obstruction and neuronal immaturity. The submucosa contains ring-shaped ganglia.

They are better known to pathologists as the cells of origin of gastrointestinal stromal tumors (see Chapter 19). These cells may be congenitally hyperplastic, presenting clinically as a pediatric motility disorder. A recent case of a 2-year-old girl was reported who had had scanty stool from birth. Radiographically, the distal colon was rigid and narrowed. The proximal colon was dilated and atonic. She underwent an ileocolectomy and the specimen showed a continuous proliferation of spindle cells located between the layers of the muscularis propria throughout the right colon. The spindle cells were positive for c-kit and CD34 but were negative for neural markers. In addition, the submucosa showed the changes characteristic of IND type B as discussed in an earlier section (77).

ABSENT ENTERIC NERVOUS SYSTEM

The absence of nerves and ganglia from the stomach to the colon characterizes the absent enteric nervous system. This

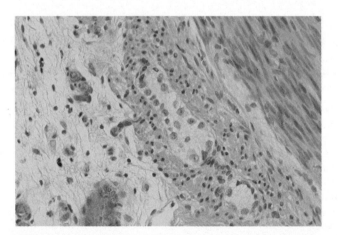

FIG. 10.17. Infant with pseudo-obstruction and neuronal immaturity. This picture of the myenteric plexus is from the same case that is shown in Figure 10.16. A number of immature ganglion cells line up at the periphery of the myenteric plexus.

very rare disorder presents as severe perinatal pseudo-obstruction. No nerves or ganglia are present in either the submucosal or myenteric plexus, or in the muscularis propria. S100 and ACE staining confirm the absence of enteric neural structures. Sparse PGP 9.5–positive extrinsic nerve fibers are present in the submucosa. Prominent ICCs are present in the area between the circular and longitudinal muscle layers in a normal distribution in some parts of the gut. In other parts they are absent or in various stages of destruction. The overall prognosis is poor (81).

PEDIATRIC MOTILITY DISORDERS NOT FITTING SPECIFIC DIAGNOSTIC CRITERIA

Damage to the ENS results in enteric neuropathies, the best characterized of which is HD. However, a number of children present clinically with pseudo-obstruction syndromes in the first few weeks, months, or years of life who lack the classic features of either HD or IND (type A or B). These cases are challenging for clinicians to manage and they often look to the pathologist for help in establishing a diagnosis that will guide them into the appropriate therapy for the affected children. Pathologic features are not readily associated with clinical findings and vice versa.

The cases that we see in consultation are challenging in this regard since they often lack features that allow them to be easily categorized (Fig. 10.18). We have seen examples of neuronal immaturity with variable numbers of ganglia and with or without obvious neural disorganization in the bowel wall. Increased, thickened nerve fibers with or without giant ganglia or aganglionosis cases are also encountered. There may be cases with neural degeneration, variable inflammation, and increased apoptosis. We have also seen some cases associated with myenteric plexus loss and cases of hypo- or aganglionosis with shriveled ganglia and dense submucosal fibrosis that may be the equivalent of what has been described as zonal HD. Often in these cases there is a history of intestinal atresia, and we have interpreted such cases as representing prenatal neural injury rather than HD. This injury is likely to be ischemic in nature, complicating the complex series of intestinal twists and turns that associate with fetal intestinal development. Ischemia secondary to malrotational or other events may damage the neuromuscular structures of the gut, especially in the intestines.

The development of the gastrointestinal tract is in some ways more complex than other organ systems with marked lengthenings, rotations, and a cranial–caudal differentiation gradient. Additionally, as noted in earlier sections of this chapter, ENS development is a complex process that is governed by the interactions of numerous proteins that are responsible for neural migration, growth, differentiation, and survival. Alterations in any of these proteins can presumably result in disorders that present clinically like HD but fail to

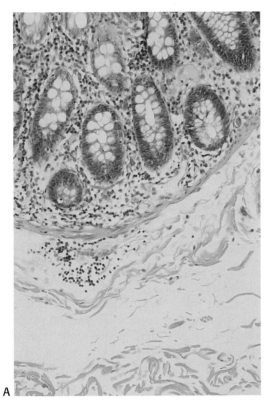

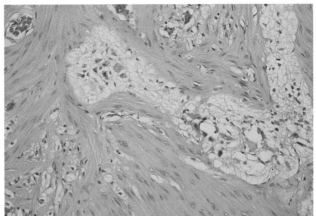

FIG. 10.18. Example of a neuropathy in a 1-month-old with pseudo-obstruction that is difficult to classify into currently recognized disorders. Ganglia are present in both the submucosal **(A)** and myenteric plexus **(B)**. They are neither increased nor decreased in number but they appear small and shriveled. There is no neural hyperplasia.

meet the diagnostic criteria for that disease. Lastly, the developing ENS may be negatively influenced by other fetal events such as intrauterine infections that may lead to ganglionic loss or other neural abnormalities.

A specific patient with a motility disorder may show one or more of the following abnormalities: Aganglionosis, hypoganglionosis, intestinal neuronal dysplasia, neural hyperplasia including ganglioneuromas, neural intranuclear inclusions, inflammatory changes, neural degeneration or apoptosis, or alterations in the ICC. Hypoganglionosis occurring in the pediatric population may represent one of several entities. It may be a finding in the transitional zone of patients with HD or represent IND type A, or it could be a finding associated with neuronal immaturity. It may also be unrelated to any of these diseases and represent a failure of the cells to migrate or grow in the gut or represent the loss of cells once neuroblastic migration has occurred.

Given the confusion surrounding the diagnosis of pediatric motility disorders, the question arises how to best diagnose the changes present. Our current practice is to diagnose HD, IND, or neural immaturity if classic features of these diseases are present. In cases in which the pathologic findings do not fit a specific diagnostic entity we tend to be descriptive, listing the major findings that are present and stating whether these findings could account for the clinical findings. Perhaps a standardized template approach to reporting these cases could lead to a better understanding of pediatric motility disorders in general. Once such approach is shown in Table 10.11. If one does not have tissue for ACE staining,

the abnormal neural proliferations can be highlighted by silver stains or antibodies to synaptophysin, S100, neuron-specific enolase (NSE), PGP 9.5, NPY, or neurofilament protein.

TABLE 10.11 **Possible Template for Reporting Pediatric Motility Disorders That Fail to Meet the Diagnostic Criteria of Hirschsprung Disease or Intestinal Neuronal Dysplasia**

Ganglia
  Present
  Absent
  Reduced in number
  Giant ganglia present (highest number of ganglion cells in a single ganglion)
  No giant ganglia present
  Inflammation: Present or not
  Mature or immature
  Ectopic ganglion cells in the muscularis mucosae or lower mucosa: Present or absent
  Histologically normal or shriveled
  Staining characteristics with special stains: State the stains that are positive and negative
Neural hyperplasia (present or absent)
  Seen on hematoxylin and eosin
  Acetylcholinesterase stains
Interstitial cells of Cajal
  Normal numbers
  Hyperplasia
  Reduced in number

These makers will only identify the neural hyperplasia and will not allow one to determine whether or not the nerves are cholinergic.

FAMILIAL VISCERAL NEUROPATHIES

Hereditary familial visceral neuropathies are a rare group of genetic diseases characterized by pseudo-obstruction (Fig. 10.19) and by myenteric plexus abnormalities with variable inheritance patterns and characteristic clinical and extraintestinal manifestations (Table 10.12). The nerves often appear vacuolated (Fig. 10.20). Silver stains or immunostains highlight both the number and the shape of the myenteric plexus neurons and nerve fibers.

Neuronal Intranuclear Inclusion Disease

This disease presents with symptoms of intestinal pseudo-obstruction, diffuse neurologic abnormalities, evidence of mild autonomic insufficiency, and denervation hypersensitivity of the smooth muscles (82,83). Patients characteristically pass less than one stool per week despite the use of laxatives and enemas (82), and they exhibit abnormal esophageal, small intestinal, and colonic motility. Patients

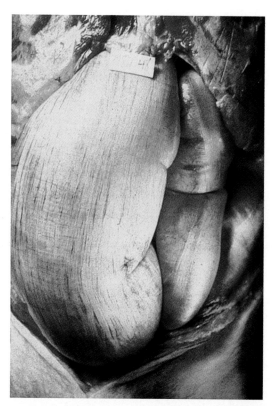

FIG. 10.19. Gross appearance of the dilated colon in a patient with pseudo-obstruction at the time of autopsy. Note the markedly dilated colon, which bulges out through the abdominal incision.

also develop gastroparesis, neurogenic bladders, and atrophy in other organs. The abnormalities are restricted to the myenteric plexus with a significant reduction in the number of neurons, a third of which contain a round, eosinophilic intranuclear inclusion (82). Most remaining neurons are misshapen with reduced numbers of nerve fibers in the nerve tracts. Ultrastructural examination in this autosomal recessive visceral neuropathy shows intranuclear neuronal inclusions consisting of a random array of straight or slightly curving filaments. They have a characteristic beaded pattern with a periodicity of 15 to 30 nm and measure 17 to 27 nm in diameter.

Autosomal Recessive Disease with Mental Retardation and Calcification of Basal Ganglia

Some mentally retarded individuals present with episodes of pseudo-obstruction and malabsorption. The intestinal smooth muscle layers appear normal or reduced in thickness. The variably sized neurons are decreased in the colon but normal in the esophagus, stomach, and small intestine and they appear degenerated with misshapen pyknotic nuclei. The brain shows extensive foci of calcification within the subcortical white matter and a striking reduction of neurons in the basal ganglia (83).

Autosomal Dominant Visceral Neuropathies

Some patients have intestinal pseudo-obstruction predominantly affecting the small intestine, without evidence of central, autonomic, or peripheral nervous system involvement. Special stains show decreased numbers of degenerated neurons and axons and many ganglia contain only one or two neurons with decreased argyrophilia. These appear swollen, distorted, and vacuolated and they lack inclusions. Nerve fibers appear hypertrophic with swellings or beading. Inflammation is absent but muscular hyperplasia may be present (83).

SPORADIC VISCERAL NEUROPATHIES

Sporadic visceral neuropathies include at least two distinct morphologic diseases affecting the myenteric plexus of any part of the GI tract. The changes are not familial and do not affect extragastrointestinal structures. The disorders typically affect adults.

Type I Sporadic Visceral Neuropathy

In *type I sporadic visceral neuropathy*, the number of myenteric plexus neurons is reduced and they are swollen and fragmented with neuronal dropout. Neurons appear irregular and have slightly concave shapes. Their cell boundaries are sharply defined and have a number of distinct tapering processes emanating from the nerve bodies. Remaining

TABLE 10.12 Findings in Visceral Neuropathies

Disease and Genetic Transmission	Clinical Findings	Gastrointestinal Lesions	Microscopic Lesions	Silver Stains	Extraintestinal Lesions
Familial Forms					
Autosomal recessive with mental retardation and basal ganglia calcification	CIIP Mental retardation	Megaduodenum Generalized dilation of small intestine; redundant colon	Atrophy of smooth muscle in all gastrointestinal tissues	Argyrophilic neurons decrease in number; remaining neurons appear misshapen and pyknotic	Extensive focal calcification of basal ganglia and subcortical white matter
Neuronal intranuclear inclusion disease (autosomal recessive)	CIIP Diffuse neurologic abnormalities Mild autonomic insufficiency Denervation hypersensitivity of pupillary and esophageal smooth muscle Progressive spasticity Ataxia Absent deep tendon reflexes Dysarthria Gastroparesis Neurogenic bladder	Dilation and nonperistaltic hypoactivity involving the esophagus, stomach, and small intestine Extensive colonic diverticulosis	Reduction and degeneration of myenteric plexus neurons Eosinophilic neurofilament containing intranuclear inclusions in myenteric and submucosal plexus neurons	Decreased neurons in myenteric plexus; remaining argyrophilic neurons are misshapen with only a few processes	Neural inclusions in central and peripheral nervous systems
Autosomal dominant visceral neuropathy type I	Patients present at any age with intestinal pseudo-obstruction Symptom onset at any age Postprandial abdominal pain Distension Diarrhea Gastroparesis Constipation	Abnormal gastric emptying Dominant segmental dilation of jejunum and ileum Small intestinal diverticulosis Proximal small intestine always involved	Hypertrophy of smooth muscle Reduction and degeneration of myenteric plexus Argyrophilic neurons	Decreased number of degenerated neurons with poorly defined cell borders and decreased silver staining; some neurons appear vacuolated or beaded	None
Autosomal recessive visceral neuropathy type II	Symptoms start in infancy	Hypertrophic pyloric stenosis Short dilated small intestine Intestinal malrotation	Neural abnormalities Neuroblasts present Hypertrophy of muscularis propria No muscle degeneration	Deficiency of argyrophilic cells No visible intrinsic neurons or processes	CNS malformations with heterotopia and absence of operculum temporale Patent ductus arteriosus

(continued)

TABLE 10.12 Findings in Visceral Neuropathies (Continued)

Disease and Genetic Transmission	Clinical Findings	Gastrointestinal Lesions	Microscopic Lesions	Silver Stains	Extraintestinal Lesions
Sporadic Visceral Neuropathy					
Type I sporadic	Similar to other forms of CIIP		Reduced myenteric neurons No inflammation Neuronal swelling Gliosis No inclusions	Neuronal swelling, fragmentation, and dropout Eventually neurons disappear	None
Type II sporadic	Similar to other forms of CIIP	Affects both the large and small intestine	Degenerated argyrophilic and argyophobic neurons Loss of antral staining producing signet ring cell appearance No inflammation	Axonal disorganization and degeneration	None

CIIP, chronic idiopathic intestinal pseudo-obstruction; CNS, central nervous system.

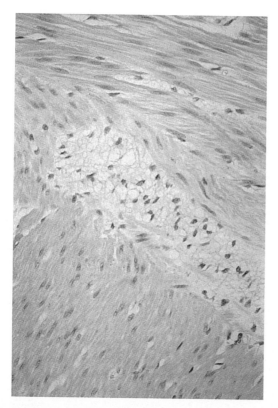

FIG. 10.20. Sporadic visceral neuropathy. Note the extensive vacuolization of the neural elements in the myenteric plexus with the cells simulating signet ring cells.

neuronal processes may appear thickened and haphazardly arranged. Some neurons swell two to three times their normal size, causing their cell boundaries to become rounded and indistinct with fewer processes than normal. Gliosis replaces the plexus. These areas are devoid of neurons and only a few axons remain within the glial scar. The changes are difficult to appreciate without the use of silver or immunohistochemical stains. The disorder differs from neuronal intranuclear inclusion disease by the absence of intranuclear inclusions and clubbed dendrites, the presence of swollen neurons with degenerated cytoplasm, and the presence of gliosis (83).

Type II Sporadic Visceral Neuropathy

Type II sporadic visceral neuropathy affects both the small and large intestines, and is characterized by neural degeneration. Neurons within individual ganglia vary in a continuum from near-normal to having a central loss of staining when stained with silver stains. Only a peripheral rim of cytoplasm remains, providing a pattern somewhat resembling signet ring cells. Axonal disorganization and degeneration are also present, but no dendritic swelling or glial cell proliferation is noted. Nuclear inclusions and inflammatory cells are absent. Some ganglia show neuronal dropout, producing intercellular spaces containing only traces of neuronal cytoplasm (83).

SLOW TRANSIT CHRONIC CONSTIPATION

Slow transit constipation, also referred to as *chronic severe idiopathic constipation* or *colonic inertia,* is a distinctive clinical syndrome affecting adults. This poorly understood disease has many potential causes (82,84,85–93). Most often the changes are thought to result from a visceral motor neuropathy. A complicating feature is the fact that many adults use antidepressants and narcotics for abdominal pain and related disorders, making it unclear whether the disease is a primary myenteric plexus disorder or the result of long-term cathartic, antidepressant, or narcotic use (abuse) (94). If there is any history of use of these drugs, the cases should be classified as drug-induced motility disorders and not an idiopathic disorder. Some postulate that the abnormalities are developmental in origin, rather than an acquired destructive lesion, since frank axonal degeneration, Schwann cell hyperplasia, and inflammation are absent (94).

This disease typically affects two major groups of patients: Adult women with severe chronic constipation or children with a similar presentation. Patients present with chronic constipation. Symptoms vary in their severity. Adults with severe disease may have no more than one bowel movement per week, despite laxative use. Patients may also develop abdominal pain, bloating, and nausea, and may require manual disimpaction. Rarely, marked ileus and large intestinal pseudo-obstruction develop (94). Complications include stercoral ulceration, intestinal ischemia, GI bleeding, bowel perforation, and peritonitis. Patients may also exhibit abnormal gastric emptying and gastroparesis.

Despite the fact that patients experience severe constipation, the degree of intestinal dilation is seldom sufficient to warrant a diagnosis of megacolon or megarectum. If the bowel is resected, the intestinal wall may appear contracted, thickened, and markedly stenotic. Alternatively, the bowel may appear dilated and thinned (Fig. 10.21). Diverticula, prolapsing mucosal folds, and/or stercoral ulcers (Fig. 10.22) may be present.

Pathologists typically encounter specimens from these patients if the patient develops pseudo-obstruction or stercoral ulcers severe enough to warrant a resection. Some surgeons will also resect the bowel in patients with severe, recurrent stool impactions. At this time, any of the abnormalities listed in Table 10.13 may be present. These include decreased, small, irregular neurons; decreased neuronal processes; and clusters of variably sized intraganglionic nuclei, which represent glia, Schwann cells, or immature neurons (94–96). There is also a notable decrease in ganglionic density and size. In other patients, there may be an increase in neuronal supporting tissues demonstrable by S100 staining. There are also increased numbers of PGP 9.5–immunoreactive nerve fibers in the muscularis propria. Melanosis coli is frequently present.

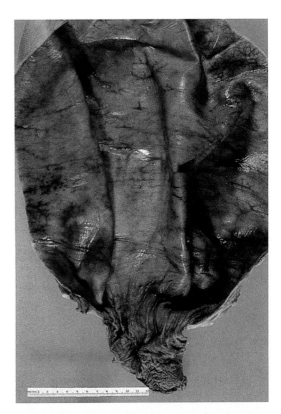

FIG. 10.21. Idiopathic constipation. Note the shrunken, contracted distal anorectum and the massively dilated megarectum.

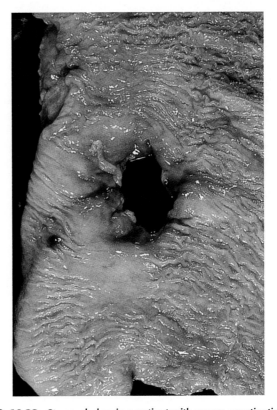

FIG. 10.22. Stercoral ulcer in a patient with severe constipation.

TABLE 10.13	Changes That May Be Present in Slow Transit Constipation

Decreased numbers of ganglia, neurons, and/or axons
Abnormal-appearing neurons or ganglia
Decreased nerve density in the myenteric plexus
Increased numbers of nerves in the muscularis propria
Gliosis of the myenteric plexus
Decreased or increased VIPergic nerves
Decreased or increased substance P nerves
Increased nitrergic nerves
Increased galanin
Increased neuropeptide Y
Decreased enkephalin
Decreased neurofilament staining in the myenteric plexus
Decreased numbers of interstitial cells of Cajal

VIP, vasoactive intestinal peptide.

PARANEOPLASTIC PSEUDO-OBSTRUCTION

Paraneoplastic pseudo-obstruction develops in patients with neuroendocrine or neural neoplasms (small cell carcinoma of the lung [97], carcinoid tumors, medulloblastomas, oligodendrogliomas, and ganglioneuroblastoma [97–99]) due to the production of autoantibodies that cross-react with neural tissues, destroying them (100,101). Patients develop distinctive antineuronal autoantibodies (Table 10.14) (97–101). The most common antineuronal antibody is anti-Hu, which recognizes a group of nervous system–specific RNA-binding proteins with molecular weights in the range of 35 to 40 kilodaltons expressed by both neurons and neoplastic cells. The antibodies induce neuronal apoptosis, contributing to the enteric neural disorder (102).

Patients present with GI dysmotility and autonomic dysfunction, often before the diagnosis of the underlying malignancy. They experience weight loss; pseudo-obstruction affecting the stomach, small intestine, and colon; constipation; gastroparesis; gastroesophageal reflux; esophageal spasm or achalasia; intractable dysphagia; postprandial fullness; nausea; vomiting; diarrhea; incontinence; and/or bloating (97,100). They also develop associated peripheral, sensory, and motor neuropathies; neurogenic bladders; ataxia; encephalopathy; orthostatic hypotension; and decreased deep tendon reflexes (97), giving a clue to the likely etiology of this motility disorder.

Myenteric neurons, from the esophagus to the colon, are reduced in number and the myenteric plexus is infiltrated with plasma cells, lymphocytes, and eosinophils (Fig. 10.23). Remaining neurons appear vacuolated and display cytoplasmic irregularities and decreased cellular processes. Axons swell, become fragmented, and drop out. The damage leads to gliosis, sometimes completely replacing the neural tissues. Only a few normal-appearing neurons remain. *The key finding that should alert one to the possibility of this diagnosis is the presence of numerous lymphoid cells and plasma cells within the myenteric plexus.* Serologic testing for the Hu antibody offers a simple means of identifying the majority of patients with paraneoplastic gut dysmotility syndromes (101).

The differential diagnosis includes toxic neural damage from drugs, infection, an autoimmune neuropathy, or aganglionosis in the absence of a tumor. Treatment of the underlying tumor does not necessarily reverse the intestinal manifestations, which require symptomatic and supportive therapy.

IDIOPATHIC GANGLIONITIS

Ganglionitis can be primary or secondary to a wide array of disorders. When it is primary, it is referred to as idiopathic ganglionitis. This motility disorder is associated with chronic inflammation of the gastrointestinal ganglia in the absence of a known cause for the inflammation. Idiopathic ganglionitis often affects young women with an average age of 25 years. Its etiology is poorly understood. Potential mechanisms of injury include viral antigen expression in the enteric neural environment, molecular mimicry of onconeural antigens, and cellular and humoral autoimmunity (103). The disease may result from circulating autoantibodies directed against the ENS in the absence of cancer. Some patients have antineuronal autoantibodies, especially anti-Hu and -Yo proteins; antibodies against neurotransmitter receptors; and ion channels (103).

The clinical symptoms reflect the involved gastrointestinal segment (achalasia, gastroparesis, pseudo-obstruction,

TABLE 10.14	Antibodies Identified in Paraneoplastic Pseudo-obstruction

Antibody	Target
Type I Anti-Hu	Neurons
Type II anti-Ri	Neurons
Anti-Yo	Anti–Purkinje cell cytoplasmic antibodies
N-type voltage-gated calcium channel antibodies	N-type voltage-gated calcium channels
P/Q-type calcium channel antibodies	P/Q-type calcium channel
Ganglionic and muscle-type nicotinic acetylcholine receptor antibodies	Nicotinic acetylcholine receptors

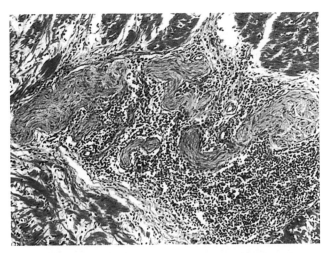

FIG. 10.23. Pseudo-obstruction in a patient with a carcinoid tumor of the ovary. Note the inflammation of the myenteric plexus.

and megacolon). Patients present with severe constipation and abdominal pain late in childhood. Some may have associated mental retardation or psychiatric disorders. Initially, the motility disorder remains limited to the colon. Later it involves the entire gut. Other patients present with abdominal pain, nausea, vomiting, malnutrition, diarrhea, weight loss, and hypergammaglobulinemia (104). The rectum tends to be full of stool; fecal impaction is not unusual. A rectal diameter >6.5 cm at the pelvic brim on lateral radiograph view is common, as is a cecal diameter in excess of 12 cm.

The gastrointestinal tract may show extensive inflammation of the ganglia (ganglionitis) with neuronal vacuolization and destruction. The diffuse lymphoplasmacytic infiltrate may affect all layers of the intestinal wall, but it tends to center around the neural microenvironment, extensively damaging the submucosal and myenteric nerve plexuses and resulting in a marked reduction in the number of myenteric nerve fibers. The nerves may show increased apoptosis. CD3+ and CD4+ T lymphocytes surround the altered ganglia and nerves. However, it should be noted that neural degeneration does not occur in all patients. There may also be a reduction in a specific subset of nerves, most commonly substance P–containing nerves (68). The histology of the musculature varies, appearing hypertrophic or atrophic, probably secondary to the neural abnormalities (104). The differential diagnosis includes paraneoplastic ganglionitis, drug injury, and infectious injury to the ganglia most commonly from viruses or Chagas disease.

EOSINOPHILIC GANGLIONITIS

Eosinophilic ganglionitis is a very rare form of ganglionitis, and it is characterized by an eosinophilic infiltrate in the myenteric plexus in the absence of neural degeneration. It affects both children and adults who present with pseudo-obstruction (68,105).

GRANULOMATOUS VISCERAL NEUROPATHY

Granulomatous visceral neuropathy affects the intestines and complicates non–small cell carcinoma of the lung (106).

ACQUIRED HYPOGANGLIONOSIS IN ADULTS

Hypoganglionosis is both a congenital and an acquired disease (Table 10.15). It may be part of both HD and IND. Hypoganglionosis also develops secondary to the inflammation as seen in patients with inflammatory bowel disease, Chagas disease, HIV, or cytomegalovirus infections and paraneoplastic syndromes.

INTERNAL ANAL SPHINCTER ACHALASIA

Internal anal sphincter achalasia is a disorder characterized by the failure of the internal anal sphincter to relax in the presence of ganglion cells in rectal suction biopsies (107). This disorder used to be referred to as the *ultrashort form of HD* but is now recognized as a separate and distinct entity. It results from abnormal innervation of the internal anal sphincter. Normal relaxation of the internal anal sphincter occurs secondary to activation of the intramural NANC nerves (108) via NO, the transmitter involved in NANC signaling (109). In anal sphincter achalasia, there is loss of NANC function in the anal sphincter due to abnormalities in NOS and NADPH-diaphorase. There is also a reduction in ICCs (110). The diagnosis is established by anorectal manometry, which shows the absence of the rectosphincteric reflex. Patients are treated by internal sphincter myotomy or botulinum toxin injections.

TABLE 10.15 **Causes of Hypoganglionosis**

Congenital
Failed migration
Failed differentiation
Loss from inadequate microenvironment

Acquired
Infections
Drugs
Inflammatory bowel disease
Necrotizing enterocolitis
Status postsurgery
Status postradiotherapy
Prenatal ischemia

ACHALASIA

Achalasia is a rare disorder that results in neural degeneration and esophageal aperistalsis, impaired esophageal motility, and failed relaxation of the lower esophageal sphincter. It is sometimes referred to as *cardiospasm* or megaesophagus. The disorder affects about 7 to 13 per 100,000 population in Europe and the United States. Patients are usually adults between the ages of 21 and 60, affecting both sexes equally (111). Approximately one third of patients are newly diagnosed after age 60. Some cases are sporadic; others are familial (112–114).

Achalasia probably results from a combination of genetic, autoimmune, and infectious factors. Familial achalasia may result from a common exposure to an infection or environmental toxin or it may represent a genetically transmitted disease. Implicated environmental factors include bacteria, viruses (115,116), esophageal trauma, and fetal ischemic esophageal damage resulting from gastrointestinal malrotations (117–119).

An autoimmune etiology is suspected because of achalasia's association with the class II human leukocyte antigen (HLA) antigen DQw1 and evidence of circulating antibodies against the myenteric plexus. A significant association exists between idiopathic achalasia and the DQB1*0602 allele and the DRB1*15 allele in whites. In blacks, there is no association between these two alleles and achalasia but a trend is

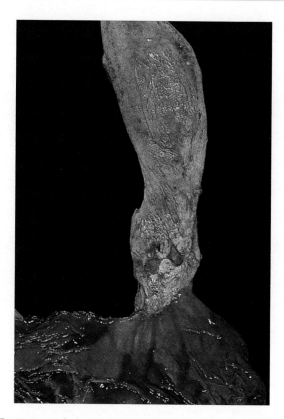

FIG. 10.25. Achalasia with esophagitis and squamous hyperplasia. The distal esophagus shows prominent whitish patchy squamous hyperplasia and two ulcers. This patient had had a sphincterotomy for the treatment of the achalasia and developed subsequent reflux esophagitis.

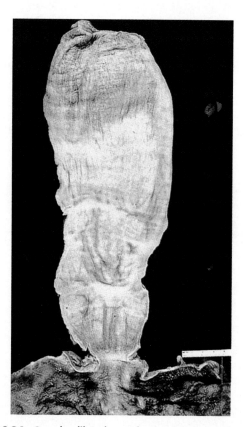

FIG. 10.24. Grossly dilated esophagus from a patient with achalasia.

present with DRB1*12, suggesting that idiopathic achalasia associates with HLA alleles in a race-specific manner (113). The expression of HLA antigens on ganglion cells could initiate their autoimmune destruction by T lymphocytes (113). An unknown factor may trigger the expression of the DQw1 class II HLA antigen on myenteric ganglia. This antigen is then recognized as foreign by T lymphocytes, which initiate an autoimmune attack, destroying neurons and ganglion cells. The degenerative process preferentially affects NO producing inhibitory neurons that affect the relaxation in the esophageal smooth muscle. There is also loss of inhibitory VIP-containing nerve fibers that results in a hypertonic lower esophageal sphincter (LES).

Since the esophagus never completely empties, it dilates (Fig. 10.24) and a column of swallowed food builds up within it (120), presenting clinically as recurrent, progressive dysphagia; pain; regurgitation; dyspepsia; retrosternal fullness; aspiration; and weight loss (121). As the esophagus dilates, it may compress the bronchi. Erosive esophagitis (Fig. 10.25) complicates achalasia when acid reflux develops, but it may also occur secondary to bacterial fermentation in a stagnant esophageal pool. Manometry is the most sensitive test for the disease (122). Some patients have an increased

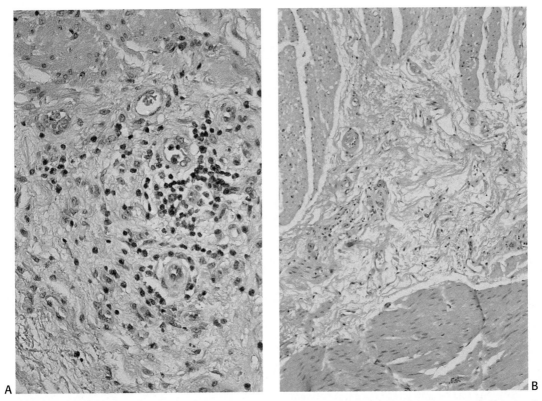

FIG. 10.26. Achalasia. **A:** Chronic inflammation in the myenteric plexus. **B:** Chronic disease with fibrosis of the myenteric plexus.

incidence of constipation and abnormal anorectal function, suggesting that there may be a variant esophagorectal syndrome (123).

The characteristic gross features of achalasia consist of an enormously dilated, lengthened esophagus that tapers into a shortened narrowed tube at the esophagogastric junction (Fig. 10.24). The changes may also extend into the proximal stomach. In advanced disease, diverticula form, sometimes attaining a diameter of 10 cm or more. Some patients develop esophagobronchial fistulas.

Histologic abnormalities affect the esophageal myenteric plexus, dorsal vagal nucleus, and vagal trunks. The earliest changes consist of myenteric inflammation with injury to, and subsequent loss of, neurons and ganglia and subsequent fibrosis of the myenteric plexus (124). Lewy bodies identical to those seen in Parkinson disease may be found in the ganglion cells in the myenteric plexus. Ganglionitis consisting of a mixture of lymphocytes and eosinophils with a less conspicuous population of plasma cells and mast cells develops. The lymphocytic infiltrate is also present along nerve fascicles (125). The majority of the myenteric lymphocytes are CD3+, CD8+ T cells (125). They also express TIA-1, indicating that these cells are cytotoxic T cells. The TIA-1 cells appear to decrease in number as the disease progresses (126).

In late-stage disease, the infiltrate becomes more patchy and located in and around myenteric nerves (Fig. 10.26).

Occasionally, one sees marked eosinophilia of the muscularis propria. Presumably, the eosinophils contribute to neuronal loss by activation and/or liberation of toxic proteins. The Auerbach plexus widens as scar tissue and small infiltrating inflammatory cells replace dying neurons (Fig. 10.26) (124,126). Satellite cells increase in number and may be difficult to distinguish from the lymphocytes. Sometimes the muscularis propria becomes markedly thickened as a result of a combination of smooth muscle fiber hypertrophy and fibrosis. Small leiomyomas may develop (Fig. 10.27). Patients with disease severe enough to necessitate esophageal resection may completely lack myenteric ganglia, especially in the dilated segment (122,124). Some patients have residual ganglion cells in the proximal esophagus and a few randomly distributed ganglion cells in the mid- and distal esophagus. There may also be reduced numbers of ganglion cells in the proximal stomach. In the most severe cases, there is an almost total loss of the myenteric ganglion cells in the distal third of the esophagus. The remaining ganglion cells appear degenerated. There may also be a reduced number of contacts between the ICCs and the nerves (127). The muscularis propria appears atrophic, hypertrophic, or normal depending on disease severity; the changes preferentially involve the inner circular layer, especially distally (124,128). The muscle fibers may be infiltrated with eosinophils. There may also be degeneration and vacuolation of the muscle fibers. These changes are secondary to the neural and ganglionic

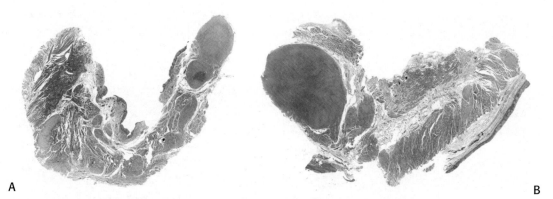

FIG. 10.27. Microleiomyoma in chronic achalasia. **A:** Low-power magnification of a cross section of the esophageal wall. **B:** Higher power magnification of the leiomyoma.

alterations. Occasionally there is dystrophic calcification. Neural fibers in the vagal trunk degenerate and become fragmented. The esophageal vagal branches demonstrate myelin sheath abnormalities, disruption of axonal membranes, and changes typical of wallerian degeneration.

Mucosal abnormalities include a diffuse marked squamous hyperplasia with papillomatosis and basal cell hyperplasia and intraepithelial lymphocytosis (lymphocytic esophagitis) (129). The CD3+ and CD20 (to a lesser extent) lymphocytes infiltrate the lamina propria and submucosa, surrounding submucosal ductal glands with the formation of prominent germinal centers. With the passage of time, chronic inflammation and ulceration result in fibrosis and stricture formation. The mucosa also shows an increased frequency of p53 immunostaining, which may be related to the increased incidence of squamous cell carcinoma seen in achalasic patients (129).

The clinical features are mimicked by Chagas disease and by diffuse esophageal leiomyomatosis. The histologic features are mimicked by Chagas disease, autoimmune ganglionitis, drug injury, and paraneoplastic pseudo-obstruction.

No therapy can reverse or halt the enteric neuronal degeneration. Therefore, treatment is aimed at decreasing the resting LES pressure by pharmacologic or mechanical means to the point that the sphincter no longer poses a substantial barrier to the passage of ingested material. Esophagomyotomy and pneumatic dilation remain the major treatment modalities. Patients who are poor operative risks can be given a trial of medical therapy with nitrates or calcium channel blockers. Intrasphincteric injection with botulinum toxin is gaining widespread appeal, particularly in the elderly. Most patients need repeated injections to maintain remission.

Patients who have undergone a previous esophagomyotomy and who experience esophageal reflux show all the changes and complications associated with reflux disease (see Chapter 2), including Barrett esophagus and adenocarcinomas (124). Squamous cell carcinomas may also develop in longstanding achalasia. This risk is estimated to be increased 33-fold in patients who have had the disease for decades (111). The tumors can arise at all levels of the esophagus, but they are most common in its middle third (111). Small cell carcinomas also develop (130).

ACHALASIA OF THE CARDIA IN ALLGROVE SYNDROME

Allgrove syndrome (achalasia, Addison disease, and alacrima syndrome [AAAS]) is a rare autosomal recessive disorder seen in children. It associates with mutations in the AAAS gene on chromosome 12q13. The gene encodes the protein known as aladin or adracalin.

AAAS develops in the first 6 months of life and differs from achalasia in adults in that the achalasia is part of a multisystemic disorder. Children often present with vomiting undigested food, failure to thrive, and recurrent chest infections. They also develop chest pain, progressive dysphagia, nocturnal regurgitation, chest infections, and weight loss. Other abnormalities include an autonomic and motor neuropathy, short stature, microcephaly, nerve deafness, and prominent ophthalmic symptoms (131).

All patients with AAAS show a striking fibrosis of the myenteric plexus. Myenteric ganglia and ICCs are absent or markedly decreased. Numerous CD3+ lymphocytes surround the myenteric ganglia. The nerves fail to stain for nNOS, a finding that may be related to the failure of the lower esophageal sphincter to relax (132).

SECONDARY ACHALASIA

Secondary achalasia, also known as pseudoachalasia, causes 2% to 4% of esophageal motor abnormalities. The symptoms result from neoplasms or benign disorders or diseases that interfere with its innervation (133). The most frequent cause is an adenocarcinoma involving the gastric cardia. Secondary achalasia also complicates vagal involvement by tumor. Megaesophagus also follows stenosis induced by acid or alkali burns and it complicates amyloid deposition. Achalasia may also complicate inflammatory disorders including Chagas disease. Some suggest that achalasia complicates neurologic and psychiatric diseases, including Parkinson disease, depression, hereditary cerebellar ataxia, and neurofibromatosis.

INFANTILE HYPERTROPHIC PYLORIC STENOSIS (CONGENITAL PYLORIC STENOSIS)

Infantile hypertrophic pyloric stenosis (IHPS) ranges in incidence from 0.28% to 0.4% of all live births (134), commonly affects Anglo-Saxons, and rarely develops in Latin Americans or blacks (135). The disorder usually affects the firstborn child, with a male:female ratio of approximately 4:1. The incidence of this disorder is decreasing in some countries such as Denmark and Canada and increasing in others such as Great Britain (136). Other anomalies coexist with IHPS in 6% to 12% of infants (137). Some children manifest the Brachman de Lange syndrome. Pyloric stenosis also associates with chromosome 9q duplications (138).

The etiology of this disorder is unclear and genetic and environmental causes have been postulated including the use of prenatal antibiotics (139). Pylorospasm has also been a postulated etiology, although this may reflect underlying neuromuscular abnormalities. Excessive gastrin production (140) abnormalities in somatostatin (140) ENS immaturity (141), lack of ICCs (142), inherent submucosal peptidergic nerve fiber abnormalities, or a lack of nitric oxide (NO) synthetase (143) may all play a role in its development. Indeed, transgenic mice carrying an inactivating gene for NOS develop pyloric hypertrophy (144).

Some infants become symptomatic at birth, but most remain well during the first few weeks of life, only to return to the hospital at about a month of age with abdominal distension and projectile nonbilious vomiting. The circular muscle of the pylorus becomes hypertrophic and hyperplastic (Fig. 10.28). The muscular hypertrophy is usually absent at birth but starts to develop during the first few weeks of life; growth continues into the third month. As the muscle mass enlarges, pyloric channel narrowing and lengthening develop. The pyloric channel appears two to four times its normal length, and its thickness exceeds 1 cm (normal is 4 to 8 mm) and an epigastric mass may be present. Pyloric luminal narrowing causes gastric outlet obstruction.

Grossly, a concentric bulbous pyloric thickening, with the consistency of cartilage, abruptly terminates at the duodenum. The inner circular muscle increases up to four times

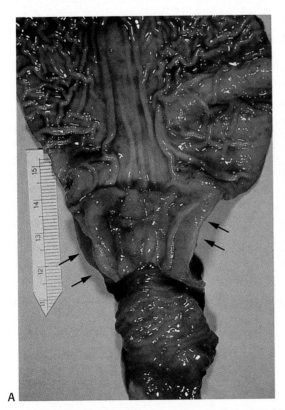
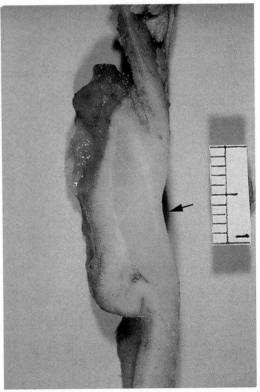

FIG. 10.28. Gross features of idiopathic hypertrophic pyloric stenosis. **A:** The stomach has been opened along the greater curvature. Note the prominent pyloric ring indicated by the *arrows*. **B:** Cross section through the gastric pylorus showing the marked thickening and hypertrophy of the muscularis propria (*arrow*). (Picture courtesy of Dr. K. Bove, Children's Hospital Medical Center, Cincinnati, OH.)

the normal thickness. The hyperplastic and hypertrophic muscle fibers often appear disorganized and there may be a mild lymphocytic infiltrate. The outer longitudinal muscle coat often appears thinner than normal. The myenteric plexus may appear hypertrophic with increased Schwann cells. Myenteric ganglion cells and glial cells degenerate and become reduced in number. ICCs are also reduced. The mucosa and submucosa appear mildly edematous. Since patients usually undergo pyloromyotomy without tissue removal, pathologists rarely see this entity, except at the time of autopsy. Following therapy, children recover completely.

NONSPHINCTERIC NEUROTRANSMITTER DISORDERS

The best characterized neurotransmitter disorders involve sphincters (achalasia, anal sphincter achalasia, and congenital hypertrophic pyloric stenosis). These associate with loss of intrinsic inhibitory neurons (NO, VIP, and somatostatin) (145). However, there are cases of acquired megacolon–megarectum and severe chronic constipation that also show abnormalities in neurotransmitters. These disorders tend to affect adults and often there are prolapsing mucosal folds suggesting that a motility disorder is present. There is a significant decrease in VIP concentrations and decreased acetylcholinesterase activity in the muscularis propria. The VIP-containing nerve fibers are diminished in the circular and longitudinal muscle and the immunostaining of nerve cell bodies in the plexus is also diminished. An increase or decrease in substance P– and NO-containing nerve fibers can also be seen (84,89,90,92). Histologically, the muscularis propria appears variably hypertrophic, atrophic, or normal.

MUSCLE DISORDERS

Intestinal muscle diseases occur either as a primary disorder or secondary to muscular dystrophy or a variety of collagen vascular disorders. Adults commonly have intestinal muscular motility disorders as part of the manifestations of an underlying systemic disease, whereas children typically have a primary intestinal myopathy that usually presents clinically as pseudo-obstruction.

Megacystis–Microcolon and Intestinal Hypoperistalsis Syndrome (MMIHS)

Megacystis–microcolon and intestinal hypoperistalsis syndrome (MMIHS), a rare (<100 reported cases), generally fatal, congenital disorder affecting newborns, is characterized by intestinal and urinary bladder distension; an atonic, short, dilated small intestine; a displaced or malrotated microcolon; and widespread gastrointestinal hypoperistalsis, hydronephrosis, and hydroureters (146). It is also referred to

TABLE 10.16	Megacystis–Microcolon–associated Gastrointestinal Conditions
Anal atresia	
Colonic atresia	
Esophageal atresia	
Imperforate anus	
Intestinal malrotation	
Intestinal stenosis	
Mesenteric anomalies	
Omphalocele	
Pyloric hypertrophy	

as *neonatal small left colon syndrome, adynamic bowel disease, non-Hirschsprung megacolon,* and *neonatal hollow visceral myopathy.* It predominantly affects girls (female:male ratio 4:1) (146). *Prune belly syndrome* may be the male equivalent of the disease. An autosomal recessive mode of inheritance is present (146). More than 50% of affected infants are born to diabetic mothers. Recent evidence suggests that the disorder results from the absence of the $\alpha 3$ nicotinic acetylcholine receptor subunit (146).

MMIHS invariably presents during the first week of infancy. All patients develop intestinal and urinary bladder pseudo-obstruction. The most common gross abnormalities include megacystis, bilateral hydronephrosis, megaureters, short bowel, microileum, microcolon, and intestinal malrotation. A megaesophagus resembling achalasia may develop. Uterine ganglioneuromas may be present. Other associated gastrointestinal changes are listed in Table 10.16 (146).

The major pathologic abnormalities involve the intestinal musculature. The longitudinal muscle coat is thinned, with abundant connective tissue lying between the muscle fibers. The smooth muscle cells of the bowel and bladder appear vacuolated and degenerated (146). Ultrastructurally, the smooth muscle cells show myofilament disorganization, cytoplasmic central core degeneration, and abundant interstitial connective tissue proliferation. Excessive intracytoplasmic glycogen displaces contractile fibers to the cell periphery, suggesting defective glycogen energy utilization (147). Neural abnormalities are absent.

Patient prognosis is generally poor. Most patients die in the first few days of life from intestinal pseudo-obstruction and sepsis (146). Some patients live up to 4 years, but they usually need to be maintained on total parenteral nutrition and they may also require renal transplantation for renal failure.

Developmental Defects of the Intestinal Musculature

Some patients completely lack a muscularis propria (Fig. 10.29), making the affected areas vulnerable to spontaneous rupture. In other patients, developmental abnormalities in the arrangement of the muscle coats occur, and patients may

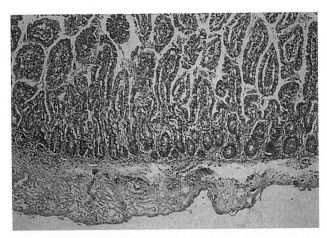

FIG. 10.29. Congenital absence of muscularis propria. The small intestinal wall is markedly thinned. A muscularis mucosae is present, as well as a submucosa and serosa.

present with chronic constipation and intestinal pseudo-obstruction (148). Deficiencies in α-smooth muscle actin in the circular muscle coat suggest that contractile protein abnormalities may contribute to the motility disorder. No other significant morphologic changes are identified histologically or ultrastructurally (148).

Hollow Visceral Myopathies

Hollow visceral myopathies are muscle disorders that affect the gastrointestinal tract or they may affect all the hollow viscera, including the entire gastrointestinal tract, urinary tract,

and gallbladder. They are characterized by degeneration, thinning, and fibrous replacement of the gastrointestinal smooth muscle. They affect both children and adults, and 75% of symptomatic patients are females (83,149–158). Some cases are sporadic; others are familial in nature. Among the familial cases, the genetic mode of transmission differs (Table 10.17). Other cases may have a relationship with glycogenosis type IV (154), polysaccharidosis (142), or the dysplastic nevus syndrome (143).

The morphologic abnormalities are identical in all families, but the pattern of gut and bladder involvement and the mode of genetic transmission differ, and include autosomal dominant, autosomal recessive, and possibly X-linked dominant forms (83). *Type I familial visceral myopathy* is transmitted as an autosomal dominant trait (156). It is characterized by esophageal dilation, megaduodenum, redundant colon, and megalocystis. The stomach and distal small intestine are usually normal, although the jejunum may appear distended.

Type II familial visceral myopathy is transmitted as an autosomal recessive trait and is characterized by gastric and small intestinal dilation and small intestinal diverticulosis of the entire small intestine. Patients have ptosis and external ophthalmoplegia, but they do not have a megacystis or megaduodenum.

Type III familial visceral myopathy was reported in a family with marked dilation of the entire GI tract from the esophagus to the rectum (83). No extraintestinal manifestations were observed and an autosomal recessive inheritance was probable.

Type IV familial visceral myopathy was described in two siblings with gastroparesis, a tubular narrow small intestine

TABLE 10.17 Classification of Familial Visceral Myopathies

	Type I	Type II	Type III
Genetic transmission	Autosomal dominant	Autosomal recessive	Autosomal recessive?
Age at onset	After the 1st decade of life	Teenagers	Middle age
Percentage of symptomatic cases	<50%	>75%	100%
Symptoms	Varies from dysphagia and constipation to intestinal pseudo-obstruction	Severe abdominal pain; intestinal pseudo-obstruction	Intestinal pseudo-obstruction
Extragastrointestinal manifestation	Megacystis; uterine inertia; mydriasis	Ptosis and external ophthalmoplegia; mild degeneration of striated muscle	None
Gross findings	Esophageal dilation, megaduodenum, redundant colon, and megalocystis	Gastric dilation, slight dilation of the entire small intestine; small intestinal diverticulosis	Marked dilation of the entire digestive tract from the esophagus to the rectum
Histologic features	Degeneration and fibrosis of both muscle layers of digestive tract	Resembles type I	Resembles type I

without diverticula, and a normal esophagus and colon. Severe vacuolar degeneration and atrophy of the longitudinal muscle of the small intestine was associated with a striking hypertrophy of the circular muscle in both cases. The hypertrophy probably caused the small intestinal tubular narrowing and it was likely that the disorder was transmitted as an autosomal recessive trait.

Clinical Features of Visceral Myopathies

Symptoms usually develop after menarche and persist with recurrences of varying intensity and chronicity (83,149). Other forms only become evident in middle age. Symptoms include dysphagia, heartburn, bloating, pain, distension, nausea, vomiting, constipation, and alternating diarrhea and constipation. Patients are usually short, underweight, and malnourished with postprandial abdominal pain, leading to decreased food intake. Sigmoid or cecal volvulus results from a redundant colon. Patients with bacterial overgrowth in a dilated duodenum develop malabsorption and diarrhea, which often improve when treated with antibiotics. Severe constipation may occur during pregnancy. In some women, spontaneous labor does not occur and may need to be induced. Intestinal pseudo-obstruction characterized by gastric and small intestinal dilation and diffuse small intestinal diverticulosis complicates most symptomatic cases (149,150). Small intestinal diverticula may perforate leading to peritonitis and intra-abdominal abscesses (83). Extragastrointestinal manifestations, if present, include megacystis and microscopic hematuria. The clinical differential diagnosis includes other causes of megacolon, including metabolic causes such as hypothyroidism, hypercalcemia, and systemic disorders such as amyloidosis, progressive systemic sclerosis, and diabetes.

Pathologic Findings

Typically, patients develop an atonic dilated esophagus, megaduodenum, small intestinal diverticulosis, redundant colon, and megacystis. The stomach and distal small intestine usually appear normal, although the jejunum may become distended. Areas of dilation vary considerably in length (153).

The morphologic abnormalities in all of the familial myopathies resemble one another and are easily recognizable by routine light microscopy. The changes that are present predominantly affect the muscularis propria (153,154), but some patients also have abnormalities in smooth muscle cells of the muscularis mucosae and/or the blood vessels. In the muscularis propria the changes may preferentially affect the inner circular or outer longitudinal layer or both layers may be equally affected. The smooth muscle fibers show various changes (Table 10.18). The may appear smudgy with indistinct boundaries (Fig. 10.30). Other muscle fibers appear densely eosinophilic or fragmented and have a threadlike appearance. Myocyte degeneration and dropout lead to fibrosis of the muscularis propria (Fig. 10.31). The muscularis propria may also show muscular hyperplasia and

TABLE 10.18	**Muscle Changes in Intestinal Familial Myopathies**
Smudgy appearance	
Loss of staining intensity	
Cellular eosinophilia	
Indistinct cell boundaries	
Fragmentation	
Vacuolar degeneration	
Cellular dropout and apoptosis	
Fibrosis of the muscularis propria	
Cytoplasmic inclusions	

hypertrophy, especially in early stages of the disease. This may represent a compensatory response to muscularis propria degeneration. The muscle cells of the muscularis propria and muscularis mucosae may contain numerous ovoid, translucent gray, cytoplasmic inclusions, which may be easily visualized in routine H&E-stained sections, but are enhanced by their strong periodic acid–Schiff (PAS) positivity. Ultrastructurally, the muscle cells appear very abnormal. The inclusions stain at the periphery with antibodies to muscle-specific actin and appear to result from progressive myofibrillar degeneration (Fig. 10.32).

In late-stage disease, a severe reduction in cell numbers is accompanied by extensive patchy fibrosis, a change easily highlighted with trichrome stains. Collagen sometimes deposits around degenerating muscle cells producing a honeycombed appearance. In the most advanced stages, the muscle layers are completely replaced by collagen with extreme thinning of the intestinal wall (158). Neurons, nerve processes, nerve terminals, and the myenteric plexus all appear normal. However, ICCs may be absent (159). There is no inflammation or vasculitis.

Patients with a malabsorption syndrome due to luminal stasis develop a patchy chronic mucosal inflammatory cell infiltrate in the superficial lamina propria. A myopathy may be suspected when the bowel appears polypoid due to mucosal prolapse (Fig. 10.33). In late-stage disease, the muscle lesions mimic those seen in scleroderma or diabetes, but these two disorders can be distinguished clinically.

Nonfamilial Myopathies

Pathologically, sporadic visceral myopathies are heterogeneous, although the clinical features resemble one another. Unlike the familial forms, which show segmental GI dilation, the nonfamilial form shows more extensive involvement, usually involving both the GI tract and urinary bladder with concomitant megacystis and megaloureters. As a result, patients are often very ill and there is little that surgery or medical therapy can do to alleviate the disease. Patients present at all ages. Infants present within the first few months of life with pseudo-obstruction and involvement of the entire

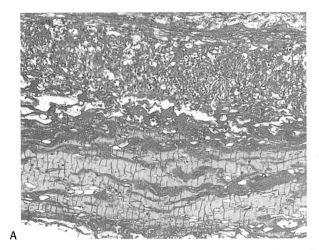
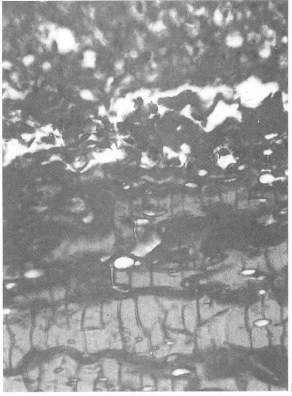

FIG. 10.30. Primary visceral myopathy in a patient presenting with intestinal pseudo-obstruction. **A:** The muscularis propria appears distinctly abnormal. The muscle fibers in both the circular and longitudinal layers are disorderly and edematous. **B:** Higher power magnification of the junction of the circular and longitudinal layers demonstrates prominent contraction bands. The entire muscular layer has acquired a smudgy appearance. (Courtesy of Dr. Michael Schuffler, University of Washington, Seattle, WA.)

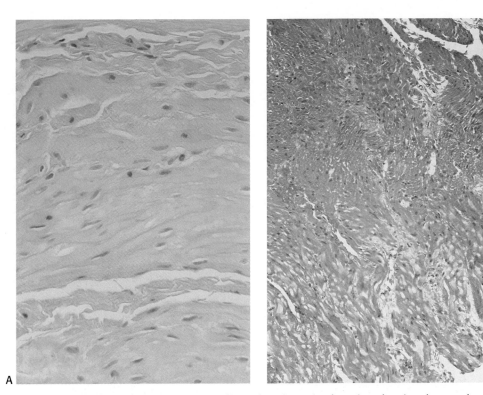

FIG. 10.31. Intestinal myopathy. **A:** Hematoxylin and eosin–stained section showing the smudgy, almost syncytial-like appearance of the smooth muscle cells in the lamina propria. **B:** Trichrome-stained section of a different area of the same bowel showing the fibrosis of the muscularis propria.

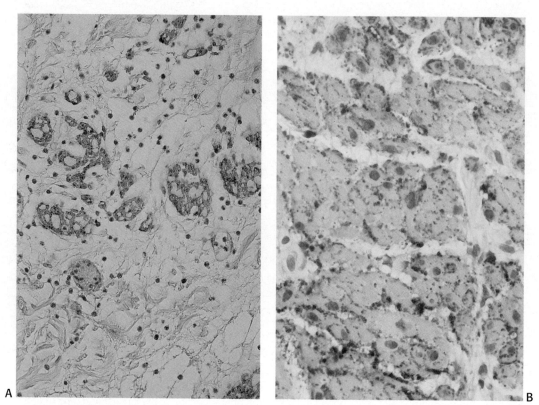

FIG. 10.32. Intestinal myopathy stained with anti–smooth muscle actin antibody. **A:** The immunostain serves to highlight the atrophy and vacuolar degeneration of the smooth muscle cells. **B:** In some patients the distribution of actin filaments in the cells is abnormal with clearing of the cytoplasm and a peripheral localization of the actin filaments.

GI system. Adults experience recurrent or persistent bowel obstruction as well as dysphagia, nausea, vomiting, post-prandial abdominal pain, and bloating. Bowel habits are erratic and alternate between constipation and diarrhea. Severe bowel dysfunction may occur with impaction, stercoral ulcerations, or colonic perforation. The perforation usually results from ischemia secondary to vascular obstruction during volvulus, torsion, or intussusception.

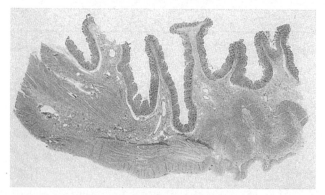

FIG. 10.33. Some patients with motility disorders show mucosal prolapse as recognized by the presence of multiple mucosal polypoidlike extensions containing a core of submucosal tissue.

The gross features resemble other forms of chronic intestinal pseudo-obstruction. The histologic abnormalities involve the smooth muscle cells and include edema, fragmentation and degeneration, marked nuclear enlargement and irregularity, interstitial fibrosis, and perinuclear cytoplasmic vacuolization (Fig. 10.34). Smooth muscle hypertrophy with hyperplasia develops. Unlike the familial form of visceral myopathy, which lacks inflammation, nonfamilial visceral myopathies often have a moderate increase of polymorphonuclear leukocytes and mononuclear cells scattered throughout both muscle layers. These changes are most severe in the muscularis propria, but similar changes develop in the muscularis mucosae and blood vessels. In its most advanced stages, fibrosis replaces the muscularis propria, causing extreme thinning of the intestinal wall. The mucosa sometimes exhibits polypoid projections typical of the redundant mucosal folds that can be present in any motility disorder. These folds consist of upward submucosal extensions covered by an essentially normal mucosa.

Diffuse Lymphoid Infiltration without Neuronal Damage

Patients with this disorder present with diarrhea, malabsorption, and intestinal pseudo-obstruction. Grossly, the bowel

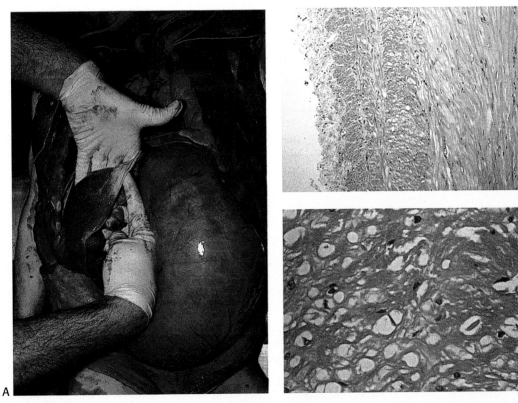

FIG. 10.34. Sporadic visceral myopathy. **A:** The most dramatic changes in this patient affected the stomach, which is massively dilated. The liver is being held to the side. The vessels along the greater curvature are easily visualized. **B:** Low magnification of the muscularis propria demonstrating the presence of vacuolar degeneration involving the external longitudinal cell layer of the stomach. **C:** Higher magnification showing the presence of extensive vacuolar damage.

appears dilated and thickened. Diffuse lymphocytic infiltrates involve the lamina propria, submucosa, serosa, and muscularis propria. The muscle cells appear hyperplastic and hypertrophic along with muscle cell dropout and there is fibrosis of the muscularis propria. There are no neuronal or axonal morphologic abnormalities. The loss of muscle cells in the vicinity of the lymphoid infiltrates may account for the pseudo-obstruction. Alternatively, the lymphocytes may secrete cytokines that inhibit smooth muscle contractility.

Mitochondrial Neurogastrointestinal Encephalomyopathies

Mitochondrial encephalomyopathies are a heterogeneous group of diseases characterized by the presence of defective mitochondrial DNA and various neuromuscular abnormalities (Table 10.19) (160,161). These disorders result from structural, biochemical, or genetic mitochondrial derangements and they are usually maternally inherited.

Mitochondria contain DNA known as mitochondrial DNA, or mtDNA (162), which differs from nuclear DNA in that it is maternally inherited, demonstrates DNA heteroplasmy and mitotic segregation, and is more susceptible to mutation than nuclear DNA (163). (Heteroplasmy refers

to the fact that cells harbor both wild-type and mutant mtDNA.) Point mutations in mitochondrial structural genes result in impaired mitochondrial protein synthesis (163), disruption of oxidative phosphorylation and the respiratory chain, and decreased mitochondrial protein synthesis (164). There is no relationship between the site of mutation and the clinical phenotype (163). The presence of heteroplasmy allows different tissues harboring the same mtDNA mutation to be affected to different degrees, resulting in tremendous symptom variation.

TABLE 10.19 **Mitochondrial Myopathies Affecting the Gastrointestinal Tract**

Kearns-Sayre syndrome
OGIMD (oculogastrointestinal muscular dystrophy) syndrome
MINGE (mitochondrial neurogastrointestinal encephalomyopathy) syndrome
MEPOPL (mitochondrial encephalopathy, sensorimotor polyneuropathy, ophthalmoplegia, pseudo-obstruction) syndrome
POLIP (polyneuropathy, ophthalmoplegia, leuko-encephalopathy, intestinal pseudo-obstruction) syndrome

Mitochondrial neurogastroencephalomyopathy (MINGE) is an autosomal recessive disease caused by mutations in the thymidine phosphorylase (TP) gene. This results in markedly increased concentrations of thymine and deoxyuridine (160), which in turn causes mtDNA defects (depletion, multiple deletions, and point mutations) (165). Patients with MINGE show multiple deletions and site-specific point mutations in mtDNA (166). *Kearns-Sayre syndrome* (KSS) is a sporadic condition that almost invariably associates with large-scale mtDNA rearrangements (deletions and more rarely duplications) (167). A deletion flanked by a 13-bp direct repeat is the most common molecular defect (164).

Mitochondrial disorders should always be considered when patients exhibit unexplained neuromuscular, gastrointestinal, and nonneuromuscular symptoms. These multisystem mitochondrial diseases are characterized by gastrointestinal dysmotility with pseudo-obstruction, abdominal pain and persistent vomiting, gastric and duodenal dilation, and duodenal diverticulosis, ophthalmoplegia, and peripheral neuropathy. The gastrointestinal manifestations of mitochondrial myopathies may present at any age: In the neonate with hepatomegaly or hepatic failure, in infancy with failure to thrive and diarrhea, and in childhood and early adulthood with hepatic failure and chronic intestinal pseudo-obstruction. Patients may appear chronically malnourished and exhibit severe growth failure. Muscle biopsies show a mitochondrial myopathy usually with ragged red fibers (166). Patients with some of the mitochondrial myopathies, particularly those with *oculogastrointestinal muscular dystrophy* (OGIMD), are sometimes included under the familial visceral myopathies type II (chronic intestinal pseudo-obstruction with ophthalmoplegia). Mitochondrial myopathies can be diagnosed based on biochemical respiratory chain analysis or by mitochondrial DNA analysis.

The external layer of the muscularis propria becomes atrophic, and increased numbers of abnormal-appearing mitochondria are present in ganglia and smooth muscle cells, especially in the small intestine (165). Megamitochondria manifest as round, brightly eosinophilic, refractile, cytoplasmic inclusions in submucosal ganglion cells (167). The smooth muscle cells show a marked depletion of mtDNA (165). Microvesicular steatosis affects the liver, skeletal, and gastrointestinal smooth muscle and Schwann cells of the peripheral nerves. Other changes that occur include increased numbers of mitochondria within endothelial and vascular smooth muscle cells (163).

Therapy is largely supportive, including total parenteral nutrition and treatment of complications, such as perforated diverticula and bacterial overgrowth. The prognosis of MINGE is poor and prior to the availability of long-term parenteral nutrition, the average patient died around age 30 (166). Therapy with coenzyme Q, riboflavin, and other vitamins, cofactors, and oxygen scavengers may be useful (161,162). These therapies are used with the aim of mitigating, postponing, or preventing damage to the respiratory chain (163).

Autoimmune Enteric Myositis

This rare motility disorder combines intestinal pseudo-obstruction with a diffuse transmural lymphoid infiltrate in the absence of neural damage (168). It may follow an attack of acute gastroenteritis (168) or chronic active hepatitis. The latter is of interest because immune responses to hepatitis viruses may result in the production of smooth muscle antibodies through molecular mimicry (169). Hepatitis B virus shows sequence homology with myosin and caldesmon and hepatitis C virus shares sequence homologies with vimentin and myosin.

Several autoantibodies can be found in these patients, including antineutrophil cytoplasmic antibody (ANCA) antinuclear antibodies, anti-DNA antibodies, and anti–smooth muscle antibodies, supporting an autoimmune etiology. Patients present in the same way as other patients with chronic intestinal pseudo-obstruction.

Lymphocytes infiltrate the lamina propria, submucosa, muscularis propria, and serosa of the ileum and colon. This infiltrate, which largely consists of CD3+ and CD8+ positive cells with some CD3– and CD4+ cells and occasional B cells, is especially dense in the muscularis propria around blood vessels. The infiltration of the muscularis propria can be intense enough to obscure the circular muscle coat. There is loss of smooth muscle actin immunoreactivity in the inner circular muscle. As the disease progresses, myonecrosis occurs in the circular muscle layer. Although there are scattered lymphocytes in the myenteric plexus, there are no neural abnormalities. Both layers of the muscularis propria become thickened secondary to muscular hyperplasia, hypertrophy, and collagen deposition (168).

Treatment with immunosuppressive drugs may alleviate the pseudo-obstruction. Following treatment with immunosuppressive agents, the infiltrates decrease, although some lymphocytic infiltrates may remain. Some patients require parenteral nutrition (168).

Hereditary Internal Sphincter Myopathy

Patients with hereditary internal sphincter myopathy present with proctalgia fugax usually in the 3rd to 5th decades of life. Proctalgia fugax is characterized by sudden episodes of severe pain in the anorectum that lasts for several seconds or a few minutes and then spontaneously resolves, leaving the patient asymptomatic until the next episode. Patients experience severe pain intermittently during the day and hourly during the night. They also experience constipation and difficulty with rectal evacuation (84). The disease is inherited in an autosomal dominant fashion (170).

The internal anal sphincter appears thickened and has decreased compliance. Histologically, the hypertrophic muscle demonstrates unique myopathic changes consisting of vacuolar damage and PAS-positive polyglycosan bodies in the smooth muscle fibers (170), as well as an increased endomysial fibrosis.

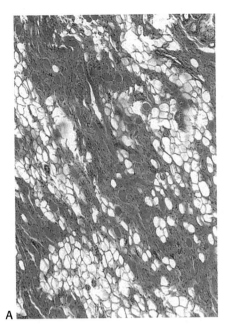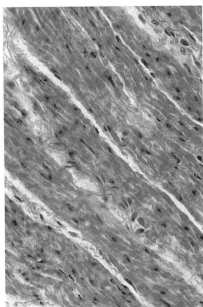

FIG. 10.35. Muscular dystrophy involving the proximal esophagus. **A:** The upper esophageal skeletal muscle demonstrates marked fatty infiltration. **B:** Skeletal muscle fibers in an area away from the fatty infiltration show marked variations in the staining quality with eosin.

Muscular Dystrophy

Esophageal motor dysfunction complicates several types of muscular dystrophy (myotonic, oculopharyngeal, oropharyngeal, and Duchenne). Myotonic dystrophy is a slowly progressive illness, inherited as an autosomal dominant disorder that affects smooth muscles in any part of the gut (171). Duchenne muscular dystrophy is a fatal X-linked recessive disease. Patients complain of dysphagia (171). The dysphagia may become so severe that the patients starve themselves. Patients also frequently aspirate. The most severe changes affect the upper esophageal sphincter, which demonstrates weak pharyngeal contractions and diminished sphincter pressure. Grossly, the esophageal musculature appears pale. Histologically, the abnormalities remain restricted to the skeletal muscle cells and they vary in their severity from cell to cell. The caliber of the striated muscle fibers varies due to the presence of necrosis and regeneration, and the fibers contain internalized pyknotic nuclei. The muscle fibers contain excessive amounts of lipofuscin and multinucleated fibers are present. Myosin immunostains highlight the variability of the muscle fibers. Fatty infiltrates separate the muscle fibers (Fig. 10.35). There is usually little or no inflammation and the neural structures are normal in appearance.

Acute gastric dilation and intestinal pseudo-obstruction can be fatal in these patients. The gastric dilation results from a lack of dystrophin in the smooth muscle cells. Significant motor abnormalities (hypomotility with delayed transit) affect the esophagus, stomach, small intestine, large bowel, and anal sphincters. The changes are most prominent in the esophagus, stomach, and colon. Occasionally, intestinal symptoms dominate the clinical picture and these may appear before the typical musculoskeletal features become apparent. Megacolon may also develop.

Generally, the nerves appear normal. Smooth muscle atrophy and fibrosis all develop, with the histologic changes being most marked in the esophagus and stomach and less apparent in the small and large intestines (171). Some smooth muscle cells appear swollen, partially destroyed, and replaced by fat (Fig 10.35). The muscle fibers in the circular and longitudinal layer of the muscularis propria become thinned, disordered, and wavy and vary in size. Edema, smooth muscle hypereosinophilia, nuclear pyknosis, and cell fragmentation occur. In longstanding disease, the intestinal smooth muscle can be replaced by collagen. Inflammation is generally absent.

INFECTIOUS CAUSES OF MOTILITY DISORDERS

Secondary gastrointestinal neuropathies and pseudo-obstruction can result from infections that damage the nerves, muscles, or both. Infections with neurotrophic viruses may damage the myenteric plexus. These viruses include herpes zoster (172), Epstein-Barr virus (EBV) (173), and cytomegalovirus (CMV) (174). Other infections result in autoimmune attacks on neural structures due to the presence of cross-reacting antigens, such as those present in some *Campylobacter* infections. Transient delayed gastric emptying occurs as a consequence of acute viral gastroenteritis, due to CMV (174), rotaviruses (175), or Norwalk or Hawaii virus infections (176). Motility returns to normal after the patient recovers from the viral infection. However, patients have been described in whom pseudo-obstruction and abdominal pain persist following treatment. Patients with Lyme disease may develop pseudo-obstruction (177). Chagas disease is discussed on p. 580.

Gastrointestinal CMV neuropathy is rare. Viral inclusions may be identifiable in the myenteric plexus neurons or in the muscle fibers (Fig. 10.36). These may be accompanied by inflammation and gliosis. Axons degenerate, resulting in extensive axonal dropout. The remaining axons appear hypertrophic and disorganized, with evidence of sprouting. Neuronal injury and dropout also occur. The process is patchy in nature; not all ganglia are affected. In patients without obvious inclusions, the enteric nerves may harbor either latent virus or residual inflammation without significant mucosal alterations. Ultrastructural examination, immunohistochemistry, or in situ hybridization can demonstrate the presence of the virus in cases that are not obvious in H&E-stained sections.

Chagas Disease

Chagas disease affects approximately 18 to 20 million people in Central and South America. Moreover, 25% of the populations living in these areas are under a high transmission risk (178). The disease is caused by the parasite *Trypanosoma cruzi*, which is transmitted to humans by blood-sucking triatomine bugs and by blood transfusions. The organism can also be acquired by accidental contamination with infected blood or cultures in laboratories, and congenitally by transplacental passage of parasites (178). Adult bugs ingest trypanosomes when sucking blood from infected animals. Trypanosomes multiply and develop in the insect's gut to be deposited in the feces on the skin when a person is bitten (Fig. 10.37). The parasites penetrate the skin, enter the bloodstream, and invade smooth muscles and the myocardium. The organisms lie in pseudocysts in the circular and longitudinal muscles of the gut in the acute phase of the disease. Following pseudocyst rupture, organisms penetrate the bloodstream, repeating the process. Neurotoxin release induces inflammation and damages the ganglia and myenteric plexus. The organism also elicits a cellular

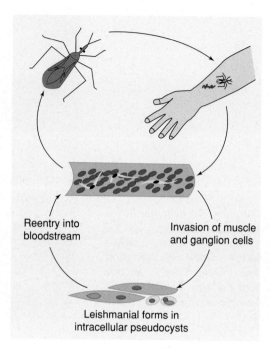

FIG. 10.37. Life cycle of Chagas disease.

immune response, further damaging the plexus. The prevailing view is that Chagas disease results from autoimmune injury long after the parasites are apparently absent from the tissues (179). An alternative view postulates that the damage results from the failure of the host to clear the infection, resulting in infection-induced immune damage (180).

The disease has two successive phases, acute and chronic. The acute phase lasts 6 to 8 weeks. After several years of starting the chronic phase, 20% to 35% of infected individuals develop irreversible lesions in the heart and gastrointestinal system (181). The infection leads to GI motility disorders, including pseudo-obstruction. Patients present with cardiac manifestations and a dilated esophagus and colon (182). The esophageal changes resemble those seen in achalasia. Intestinal involvement manifests as a motility disorder and pseudo-obstruction. Chagasic megacolon may evolve into toxic megacolon and enterocolitis, often resulting in death (182).

The histologic features reflect the stage of the disease. In the acute infection, the organism is found in and around the myenteric plexus (Fig. 10.38). However, the acute disease is rarely seen. More commonly, patients present with complications of the myenteric plexus involvement. Early on, there is marked degeneration of the muscularis propria and the myenteric plexus, with decreased nerves in Auerbach plexus. Motor functions and aperistalsis develop when >90% of ganglion cells are lost (183). The autonomic innervation becomes destroyed, probably via the combined action of the parasitic toxins and the production of various cytokines and other inflammatory mediators and ischemia secondary to changes induced in the cardiovascular system. ICCs are severely reduced in numbers (184). Because of the severe neural changes, the smooth muscle becomes hypertrophic.

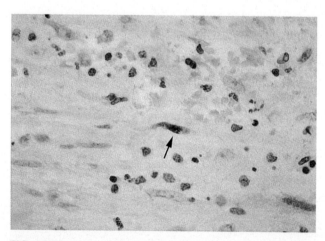

FIG. 10.36. Cytomegalovirus immunoreactivity in the muscularis propria. One of the muscle fibers (*arrow*) shows this reactivity. The surrounding tissues appear inflamed.

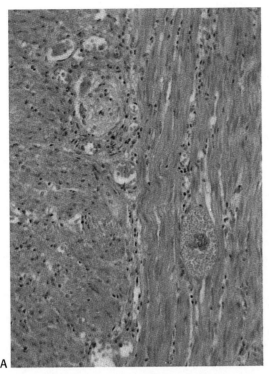
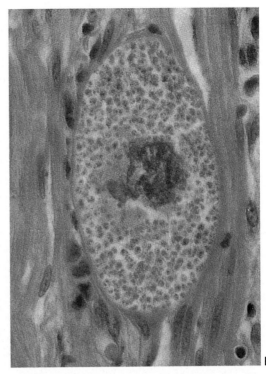

FIG. 10.38. Acute Chagas disease involving the intestine. **A:** An organism is seen within the myenteric plexus. **B:** Higher power magnification of the trypanosomes. (Courtesy of Dr. Gilles Landman, Brazil.)

Eventually, the infected sites become fibrotic (Fig. 10.39). At the time that tissues involved by chronic disease are examined, the parasites are usually no longer evident. However, the organisms are detectable by more sensitive techniques such as polymerase chain reaction (PCR) (180). In cases where the diagnosis is in doubt, tissue can be analyzed by a PCR test for the organism.

Patients with chagasic achalasia have an up to 20% possibility of developing esophageal squamous cell carcinoma. Of interest is the finding that the achalasic esophagus without cancer shows evidence of multiple chromosomal aneuploidies and loss of the p53 gene in up to 60% of specimens. The tumors arising in these esophagi show multiple chromosomal aneuploidies and p53 deletions in 100% of the tumors (185).

MOTILITY DISORDERS ACCOMPANYING SYSTEMIC DISEASES

Scleroderma

Scleroderma is a generalized autoimmune connective tissue disorder characterized by fibrosis and degenerative changes of the skin and multiple internal organs including the gastrointestinal tract. By definition, esophageal scleroderma is part of the CREST syndrome (calcinosis acutus, Raynaud, esophageal sclerosis, sclerodactyly, and telangiectasia).

It is the most common connective tissue disease causing generalized GI dysmotility. Scleroderma has a worldwide distribution and it is more common in women than in men, usually affecting them in their 3rd to 5th decades. Ethnic origin plays a role in disease susceptibility. The disease is significantly more likely in black than white women. There are also differences in genetic backgrounds for the various HLA types in various ethnic groups.

Scleroderma associates with an increased frequency of class I and class II major histocompatibility complex (MHC) alleles. Autoantibody associations divide patients into two groups: Those with anticentromere antibodies (ACAs) that are associated with limited scleroderma, and those with anti-topoisomerase-1 (SCL-70) with the diffuse form. In some patients, antibodies specifically inhibiting M3-muscarinic receptor–mediated enteric cholinergic neurotransmission may account for the gastrointestinal dysfunction seen in patients with scleroderma.

Pathogenesis

The pathogenesis of scleroderma involves vascular, immunologic, and fibrosing processes. Progressive fibrosis of various organs, including the gastrointestinal tract, is the pathologic hallmark of scleroderma. The fibrosis disrupts the normal architecture of the affected organs, ultimately leading to their dysfunction and failure; the extent and rate of progression of the fibrosis determine the patients' clinical course and prognosis. Fibrosis of the walls of medium- and small-sized arterioles also plays a critical role in many manifestations of the disease.

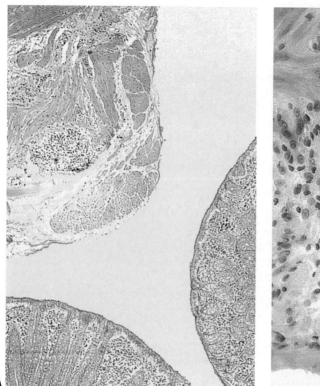
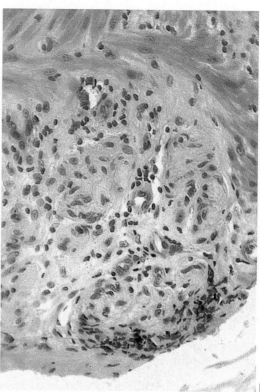

FIG. 10.39. Chronic Chagas disease. **A:** The myenteric plexus is fibrotic, and nerves and ganglia are destroyed. **B:** Higher power magnification demonstrates the fibrosing process. Organisms are not demonstrable.

The microvascular system is one of the first targets to be involved in the disease (186). Vascular changes affect small arteries and consist of arteritis and myointimal proliferation with luminal narrowing and irregularity, intimal fibrosis, and disruption of the internal elastic lamina. Capillary basement membranes thicken. Vessels of vessels (vasa vasora) and of nerves (vasa nervosa) are altered early in the disease. Vasoconstriction occurs secondary to increased levels of the vasoconstrictor endothelin-1 and decreased NO resulting in ischemia and neural and muscular dysfunction (186). Neural atrophy and collagen deposition occur before smooth muscle contractility is impaired (187). Complete denervation releases the intestinal smooth muscle from its customary inhibitory factors, resulting in loss of normal peristalsis.

Clinical Features

Scleroderma presents either as a localized disease or as a systemic disorder. The localized form remains confined to the skin; GI involvement complicates systemic disease. The esophagus, small intestine, colon, and stomach are affected in a decreasing order of frequency (188). The clinical features differ depending on the site of involvement. Up to 90% of patients show esophageal disease with ineffective peristalsis resulting in delayed esophageal emptying. LES pressure progressively diminishes until no high-pressure zone lies between the esophagus and stomach, and gastroesophageal reflux

(GER) develops. Peptic esophagitis, with all of its complications, ensues. GER results from three major physiologic defects: Decreased LES pressure; failure to clear acid in the esophagus, due to poor peristalsis; and delayed gastric emptying. All of the complications of GER as discussed in Chapter 2 develop. The patients also develop lower mucosal rings at the esophagogastric junction (189). Some patients with Raynaud phenomenon have cold-induced vasospasm of the esophageal vessels (esophageal Raynaud).

Gastric dysmotility and gastroparesis affect more than 50% of patients (190) causing dyspepsia. Gastric involvement may also present with bleeding secondary to the development of vascular abnormalities, including gastric antral vascular ectasia (191). Forty percent of patients with generalized scleroderma develop intestinal symptoms in their 4th to 6th decades of life (188). Patients with small intestinal involvement present with anorexia, early satiety, nausea, vomiting, intestinal pseudo-obstruction, abdominal pain, weight loss, impaired motility, malabsorption, steatorrhea, diarrhea, constipation, and intestinal perforation. Patients also develop multiple diverticula or megaduodenum (192). Colonic involvement affects 10% to 50% of patients. Patients with large intestinal disease develop colonic or rectal diverticula, pseudo-obstruction, constipation, diarrhea, fecal incontinence, rectal prolapse, spontaneous perforation, and infarction. They also develop wide-mouthed diverticula. Anorectal involvement is almost as common as esophageal involvement. It leads to fecal incontinence or rectal prolapse (182).

Specific serologic tests help identify the exact collagen vascular disease that is present. Antinuclear antibody (ANA) profiles are particularly helpful. ANAs are usually positive in scleroderma patients. Nuclear ribonucleoprotein (RNP) and centromere antibodies are more specific but not very sensitive. Patients with CREST have ANA restricted to the centromeric DNA. ANA with anti-SS-A/Ro specificity associates with vasculitis and nephritis and ANA with anti-SS-dLA and anti-nRNP specificity associated with milder clinical disease (193).

Pathologic Findings

The early changes of well-developed scleroderma are seldom seen because tissue is not removed until complications develop. A mild inflammatory infiltrate may affect the neural plexuses, but the myenteric plexus generally appears histologically normal unless it has become entrapped by fibrous tissue. Smooth muscle atrophy follows the neural damage (Fig. 10.40) and progressive fibrosis develops (Fig. 10.41). The changes affect the circular layer of the muscularis propria more than the longitudinal layer. At this stage the muscle fibers appear atrophic, fragmented, and fibrotic, often completely disappearing. Initially, the damage appears patchy, but with time it becomes more extensive. These changes are superimposed on neural damage. The submucosa and muscularis propria become progressively atrophic and replaced by fibrous tissue. The fibrosis may mimic amyloidosis.

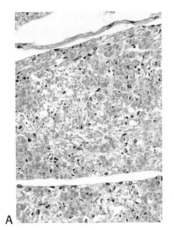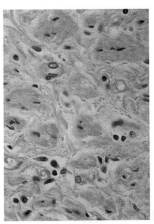

FIG. 10.40. Comparison of scleroderma with primary visceral myopathy. **A:** Note that in the case of the primary visceral myopathy, marked atrophy is present as evidenced by variation in the size of the muscle fibers. The tissues have dropped out but they are not surrounded by fibrosis. This particular example does not show much in the way of vacuolar degeneration. **B:** In contrast, the atrophic muscle fibers in scleroderma are surrounded by fibrous tissue.

Ceroid pigment granules may deposit in degenerating muscle cells. Intimal fibrosis and elastosis affects smaller arteries and blood vessels may be markedly thickened with perivascular collagen deposition. Degranulating mast cells, macrophages, and activated lymphocytes infiltrate the perivascular tissue.

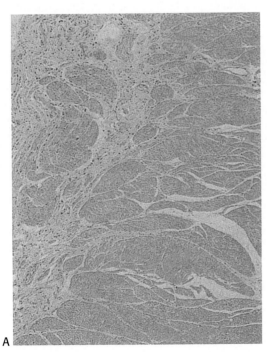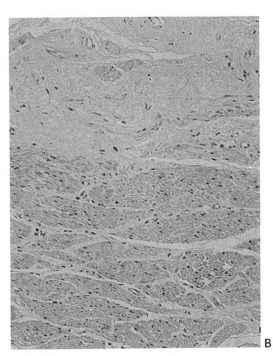

FIG. 10.41. Scleroderma. **A:** Smooth muscle layers of the esophageal wall are being replaced by fibrous tissue. **B:** Higher power view shows encroachment on the muscle by fibrous tissue. The muscle fibers appear atrophic.

In uncomplicated cases, the mucosa appears normal. At most, there may be edema and mild chronic inflammation in the lamina propria. Mucosal erosions and ulcerations may occur, especially in patients with reflux esophagitis. Gastric alterations may include gastric mucosal atrophy. Duodenal Brunner glands may develop periglandular fibrosis (194). The intestinal mucosa may also show a nonspecific increase in the mononuclear cells in the lamina propria. This is often a manifestation of the decreased motility and a change in the bacterial flora. Patients with scleroderma may also develop eosinophilic gastroenteritis. The eosinophilic infiltrate often localizes in the basal mucosa and the muscularis propria, resulting in myonecrosis (Fig. 10.42).

Pathologists may receive GI biopsies to rule out the diagnosis of scleroderma. Unfortunately, this is usually not possible because the biopsies are generally too superficial, sampling mainly the mucosa and rarely sampling the submucosa. The muscularis propria is virtually never biopsied. The biopsied tissues either appear normal or may show evidence of mild nonspecific mucosal inflammation or fibrosis. Patients with malabsorption may show evidence of mild atrophy or inflammation secondary to bacterial overgrowth.

Differential Diagnosis

Early scleroderma can usually be differentiated from a visceral myopathy by the presence of fibrosis of the intestinal smooth muscle and the absence of a vacuolated honeycombed appearance. Remaining muscle cells appear normal or atrophic. The changes in scleroderma are patchier than those found in patients with primary myopathies. In severe disease, it may be impossible to distinguish between a primary myopathy and scleroderma based solely on histologic examination. However, the clinical features serve to separate the two disorders, as does serologic testing.

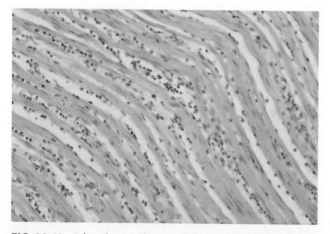

FIG. 10.42. Scleroderma. The muscle layers may demonstrate a prominent eosinophilic infiltrate between the smooth muscle cells.

Treatment and Prognosis

Since there is no effective treatment for scleroderma, therapy is directed at supportive symptomatic treatment. Antireflux measures help alleviate the symptoms of reflux esophagitis and are important in preventing its complications. Early muscle dysfunction is partially reversible with prokinetic drugs. In addition, prokinetic drugs decrease the acidity of the refluxate, increase lower esophageal sphincter pressure, and increase gastric emptying. Patients with end-stage disease (characterized by severe muscle fibrosis) are not amenable to pharmacologic functional restoration. The main therapeutic options for bacterial overgrowth consist of antibiotics and nutritional supplementation. Approximately 19% of patients require total parenteral or enteral nutrition.

Diabetes Mellitus

Diabetic neuropathies encompass a group of clinical syndromes affecting both somatic and autonomic peripheral nerves (195). The term *diabetic gastroenteropathy* describes a generalized diabetes-associated gastrointestinal motility disorder. *Diabetic gastroparesis* is diabetes-associated delayed gastric emptying occurring in the absence of mechanical obstruction (Fig. 10.43) (195). Diabetic gastroparesis affects as many as 20% to 50% of diabetics, especially those with longstanding, poorly controlled disease.

Gastrointestinal diabetes-related alterations occur via several mechanisms: A visceral neuropathy involving the parasympathetic or sympathetic nervous system; a microangiopathy; abnormal plasma glucose and electrolyte levels; increased susceptibility to infections and bacterial overgrowth; altered production of insulin, motilin, pancreatic polypeptide, somatostatin, gastrin, and glucagon; and ischemic effects (195,196). The predisposition to accelerated atherosclerosis is a risk factor for developing mesenteric ischemia and intestinal infarction. The most important underlying condition appears to be the visceral autonomic neuropathy that causes decreased motility, hypotonia, and diminished secretions. Diabetic gastroparesis involves a neuropathy, a myopathy, and decreased ICCs. The latter may result from reduced insulin/insulinlike growth factor (IGF)-I signaling, which may also result in smooth muscle atrophy and reduced stem cell factor production (197).

The gastrointestinal effects of diabetes are not commonly appreciated. Many diabetics, especially patients with type I diabetes, develop gastrointestinal problems, including gastroparesis, diarrhea, constipation, delayed esophageal and intestinal transit, megacolon, chronic nausea, weight loss, and fecal incontinence (195–199). Diabetic gastroparesis manifests as postprandial fullness, vague epigastric pain, nausea, vomiting, heartburn, bloating, early satiety, excessive eructation, and anorexia. Symptom onset is usually insidious. Bezoar formation and pulmonary aspiration may be complications. Additionally, small intestinal stasis and bacterial overgrowth lead to fat malabsorption, steatorrhea, and diarrhea. Incontinence affects up to 24% of diabetics (195).

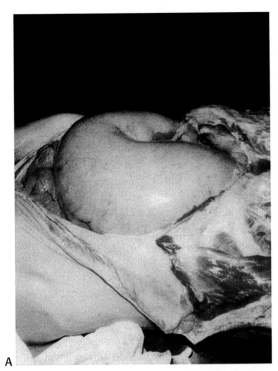
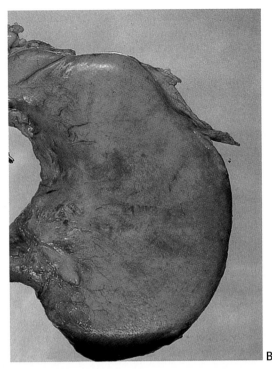

FIG. 10.43. Diabetic gastropathy. **A:** The stomach in situ in a patient with severe diabetic gastroparesis. The stomach appears massively distended. **B:** Even when the stomach is removed, it appears to be massively enlarged.

Pathologic Findings

Patients with diabetic diarrhea have vagal and sympathetic neural degenerative changes. Several types of neural changes occur, including hydropic neural degeneration resulting in giant sympathetic neurons, dendritic swelling of postganglionic neurons, and perineural fibrosis (Fig. 10.44). These changes do not consistently affect the intestinal neural plexuses. The stomach often shows a severe reduction in the density of unmyelinated axons. Glycosylation abnormalities result in abnormal collagen deposits with diffuse basement membrane thickening affecting vessels and nerves throughout the gut. The capillary basement membranes are widened by a homogeneous, multilayered, eosinophilic substance. The vasculopathy causes variable ischemia. "M" bodies, which represent scattered necrobiotic smooth muscle cells, appear as homogeneous round eosinophilic bodies scattered among areas of smooth muscle atrophy and fibrosis. Fibrosis and "M" bodies are characteristic of end-stage diabetic GI neuropathies. ICCs may be reduced to 40% of the normal population (200).

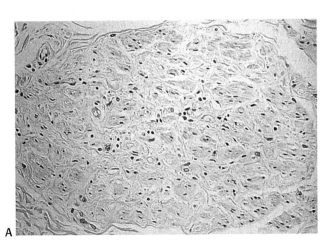
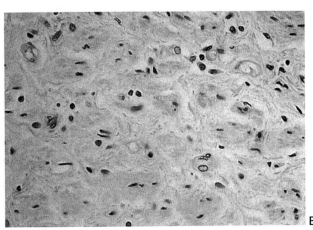

FIG. 10.44. Diabetes. Mesenteric nerve in a patient with diabetes demonstrates the presence of marked fibrosis **(A)** and nerve atrophy **(B)**.

AMYLOIDOSIS

Amyloidosis consists of acellular eosinophilic proteinaceous tissue deposits. The deposited proteins have a characteristic β-pleated structure, ultrastructural appearance, and tinctorial qualities. The prevalence of amyloidosis increases with age. All known types of amyloid affect the gastrointestinal tract, including amyloid A (AA), amyloid of lambda or kappa light chain origin, transthyretin amyloid (ATTR), and β2-microglobulin-A (β2M). The chemical type of amyloid often determines the dominant clinical features (Table 10.20). Two mechanisms explain the intestinal motor dysfunction present in patients with amyloidosis: Amyloid deposition in gastrointestinal smooth muscle and amyloid-induced neural damage.

Patients with primary and secondary amyloidosis show gastrointestinal involvement anywhere from the esophagus to the anus (201). In the esophagus, amyloid deposits in both striated and smooth muscles, leading to a weakening of both the proximal and distal esophageal sphincters (201). Neural abnormalities also develop. Esophageal involvement mimics achalasia. Intestinal pseudo-obstruction results from a myopathy or a neuropathy (202). Intestinal amyloid neuropathy leads to diarrhea, steatorrhea, or constipation (201). Gastric amyloidosis presents as hematemesis or prolonged nausea and vomiting associated with weight loss, gastroparesis, gastric amyloid tumors, or gastric outlet obstruction. Grossly, the bowel may appear normal. Alternatively, intramural amyloid deposits cause mural thickening and rigidity. Bowels with β2M amyloid deposits exhibit a distinctive rippled serosal appearance. Amyloid tumors produce firm, bulky, intramural masses.

Eosinophilic, homogeneous, hyaline amyloid deposits around the muscle fibers and blood vessels in the lamina propria and in the myenteric plexus. The primary site of deposition varies depending on the type of amyloid present. Amyloid of light chains and β2M deposit throughout the gastrointestinal tract, especially in the small intestine in the muscularis propria. The outline of the muscle layers is preserved but most muscle fibers are encircled by the amyloid deposits.

They then become atrophic and disappear. Because the changes affect the deeper layers of the intestinal wall, they are hard to demonstrate on biopsy. The esophagus is less involved than the rest of the gastrointestinal tract in this form of amyloidosis. AA protein preferentially deposits in the myenteric plexus without appreciable muscle infiltration. Patients with familial amyloidosis show a severe reduction in the number of ganglion cells or degeneration of ganglion cells without extensive deposition of amyloid in the enteric plexus.

Amyloidosis is usually diagnosed on H&E-stained sections and its presence is confirmed with a Congo red stain and the presence of a characteristic apple-green birefringence when examined under polarized light. It can also be confirmed ultrastructurally, in which case the amyloid fibers exhibit their characteristic periodicity. The different forms of amyloid may be distinguished using immunostains for the specific protein.

DRUG-INDUCED MOTILITY DISORDERS

A number of drugs affect gastrointestinal motility, causing neural and/or muscular injury (Figs. 10.45 and 10.46). The most common drugs that cause motility problems include tricyclic antidepressants, phenothiazines, anticholinergic drugs, opiates, methadone (203), theophylline (204), and antineoplastic drugs. All of these drugs can cause severe constipation, ileus, and pseudo-obstruction. It is unclear whether the drugs cause the symptoms or unmask an underlying gastrointestinal motility disorder.

Laxative-Induced Injury

Cathartic colon is an end-stage colon that no longer effectively contracts, presumably due to extensive myenteric plexus damage induced by long-term cathartic use (abuse). Motility disorders, chronic constipation, and pseudo-obstruction all complicate chronic laxative use. Patients with

TABLE 10.20	Gastrointestinal Amyloidosis		
Protein	**Associated Disease**	**Forms of Amyloidosis**
Immunoglobulin light chain (AL)	Multiple myeloma and other monoclonal B-cell and plasma cell proliferations	Primary amyloidosis: Systemic disease associated with plasma cell dyscrasia (deposits in heart, kidney, gut, liver, and spleen), especially around blood vessels and sometimes between muscle fibers; gastrointestinal involvement is common with massive submucosal involvement
Serum amyloid-associated protein (AA)	Associated with chronic disease	Secondary amyloidosis: Systemic chronic disease; amyloid deposits in blood vessels and in the mucosa; lamina propria deposits cause mucosal nodularity
Transthyretin, AA prealbumin (AF)	Hereditary amyloidosis	Hereditary familial amyloidosis: Small intestine commonly involved; perireticular deposition throughout muscle fibers and in neural plexuses; single organ amyloid deposition

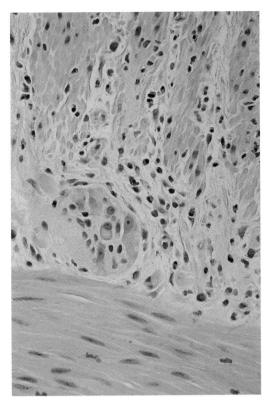

FIG. 10.45. Specimen from a patient on long-term morphine showing inflammation and degeneration of the myenteric plexus.

cathartic colon tend to present with chronic constipation, abdominal bloating or distension, pseudo-obstruction, abdominal pain, and incomplete evacuation. These result from toxic effects of the drugs on neural structures in the bowel wall with secondary muscle damage. Narcotic use

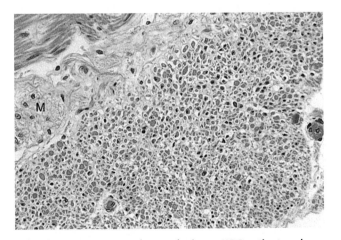

FIG. 10.46. Severe muscle atrophy in an AIDS patient on long-term azidothymidine (AZT). The fibers of the external layer of the muscularis propria show marked variations in the size of individual muscle fibers. Many are surrounded by fibrous tissue. The myenteric plexus (*M*) appears more or less normal and the small portion of inner circular muscle that is seen is histologically normal.

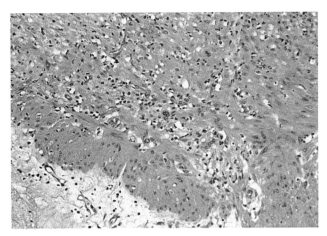

FIG. 10.47. Patients with toxic neural damage due to laxative abuse show inflammatory cells in the myenteric plexus.

often aggravates the symptoms. Severe constipation leads to the formation of hard fecaliths that can cause local chronic inflammation, acute inflammation, stercoral ulceration, bleeding, and perforation. Concomitant medication use and previous intestinal surgeries complicate the clinical picture.

In early cases of cathartic colon the mucosa appears mildly inflamed and glandular atrophy may develop. Eosinophilia and mucosal ulcers may be present. Myenteric plexus abnormalities include neuronal swelling and pallor. Later, there is neuronal loss, axonal fragmentation, gliosis of the myenteric plexus, and ganglionic vacuolization. Remaining neurons appear shrunken, with clubbed, swollen processes. Often the myenteric plexus becomes inflamed (Fig. 10.47). Degenerative changes also involve the submucosal plexus and include axonal ballooning and neural degeneration. Atrophy or hyperplasia of the muscularis propria develops secondary to denervation injury following neural damage. Although these changes have been ascribed to laxatives, it is possible that they represent a primary disorder of the enteric plexuses that causes the initial constipation and subsequent laxative ingestion.

RADIATION EFFECTS

Intestinal pseudo-obstruction, gastroparesis, or esophageal motility disorders may be induced by previous radiation. Histologically, there is evidence of vascular ectasia and sclerosis, serosal fibrosis, neuronal proliferation within the submucosa, and degeneration of the myenteric plexus and muscle fibers of the muscularis propria.

REFERENCES

1. Huizinga JD: Gastrointestinal peristalsis: joint action of enteric nerves, smooth muscle, and interstitial cells of Cajal. *Microsc Res Tech* 1999;47:239.
2. Ward SM: Interstitial cells of Cajal in enteric neurotransmission. *Gut* 2000;47:40.

3. Rudolph CD, Hyman PE, Altschuler SM, et al: Diagnosis and treatment of chronic intestinal pseudo-obstruction in children: report of consensus workshop. *J Pediatr Gastroenterol Nutr* 1997;24:102.

4. Bettolli M, Rubin SZ, Staines W, et al: The use of rapid assessment of enteric ICC and neuronal morphology may improve patient management in pediatric surgery: a new clinical pathological protocol. *Pediatr Surg Int* 2006;22:78.

5. Ponec RJ, Saunders MD, Kimmey MB: Neostigmine for the treatment of acute colonic pseudo-obstruction. *N Engl J Med* 1999;341:37.

6. Gabella G: Structure of muscles and nerves in the gastrointestinal tract. In: Johnson LE (ed). *Physiology of the Gastrointestinal Tract*, 2nd ed. New York: Raven Press, 1987, p 335.

7. Rumessen JJ, Peters S, Thuneberg L: Light and electron microscopical studies of interstitial cells of Cajal and muscle cells at the submucosal border of human colon. *Lab Invest* 1993;68:481.

8. Karaosmanoglu T, Aygun B, Wade PR, Gershon MD: Regional differences in the number of neurons in the myenteric plexus of the guinea pig small intestine and colon: an evaluation of markers used to count neurons. *Anat Rec* 1996;244:470.

9. Furness JB: Types of neurons in the enteric nervous system. *J Auton Nerv Syst* 2000;81:87.

10. Gershon MD: *The Second Brain.* Harper Collins, London: 1998.

11. Mashimo H, Goyal RK: Lessons from genetically engineered animal models. IV. Nitric oxide synthase gene knockout mice. *Am J Physiol* 1999;277:G745.

12. Rattan S, Chakder S: Role of nitric oxide as a mediator of internal anal sphincter relaxation. *Am J Physiol* 1992;262:G107.

13. Chakder S, Bandyopadhyay A, Rattan S: Neuronal NOS gene expression in gastrointestinal myenteric neurons and smooth muscle cells. *Am J Physiol* 1997;273:C1868.

14. Thuneberg L: Interstitial cells of Cajal: intestinal pacemaker cells? *Adv Anat Embryol Cell Biol* 1982;71:1.

15. Farraway L, Ball AK, Hunzinga JD: Intercellular metabolic coupling in canine colon musculature. *Am J Physiol* 1995;268:C1492.

16. Daniel EE, Posey-Daniel V: Neuromuscular structures in opossum esophagus: role of interstitial cells of Cajal. *Am J Physiol* 1984;246:G305.

17. Faussone-Pellegrini MS: Histogenesis, structure and relationships of interstitial cells of Cajal (ICC): from morphology to functional interpretation. *Eur J Morphol* 1992;30:137.

18. Hagger R, Gharaie S, Finlayson C, Kumar D: Distribution of interstitial cells of Cajal in the human anorectum. *J Auton Nerv Syst* 1998;73:75.

19. Burns AJ, Herbert TM, Ward SM, Sanders KM: Interstitial cells of Cajal in the guinea pig gastrointestinal tract as revealed by c-Kit immunohistochemistry. *Cell Tissue Res* 1997;290:11.

20. Meijers JH, Tibboel D, van der Kamp AW, et al: A model for aganglionosis in the chicken embryo. *J Pediatr Surg* 1989;6:557.

21. Gariepy CE: Intestinal motility disorders and development of the enteric nervous system. *Pediatr Res* 2001;49:605.

22. Gershon MD, Chalazonitis A, Rothman TP: From neural crest to bowel: development of the enteric nervous system. *J Neurobiol* 1993;24:199.

23. Tsaur ML, Wan YC, Lai FP, Cheng HF: Expression of B-type endothelin receptor gene during neural development. *FESB Lett* 1997;417:208.

24. Eide FF, Lowenstein DH, Reichardt LF: Neurotrophins and their receptors. *Exp Neurol* 1993;121:200.

25. Yan H, Bergner AJ, Enomoto H, et al: Neural cells in the esophagus respond to glial cell line-derived neurotrophic factor and neurturin and are RET-dependent. *Dev Biol* 2004;272:118.

26. Young HM: GDNF is a chemoattractant for enteric neural cells. *Dev Biol* 2001;229:503.

27. Baynash A, Hosoda K, Giaid A, et al: Integration of endothelin-3 with endothelin-B receptor is essential for development of epidermal melanocytes and enteric neurons. *Cell* 1994;179:1277.

28. Hosoda K, Hammer RE, Richardson JA, et al: Targeted and natural (piebald-lethal) mutations of endothelin-B receptor gene produce megacolon associated with spotted coat color in mice. *Cell* 1994;79:1267.

29. Shirasawa S, Yunker AM, Roth KA, et al: Enx (Hox11L1)-deficient mice develop myenteric neuronal hyperplasia and megacolon. *Nat Med* 1997;3:646.

30. Lake BD: Hirschsprung's disease and related diseases. In: Whitehead R (ed). *Gastrointestinal and Esophageal Pathology*. New York: Churchill Livingstone, 1995, p 327.

31. Smith B: Pre- and post-natal development of the ganglion cells of the rectum and its surgical implications. *J Pediatr Surg* 1968;3:386.

32. Aldridge RT, Campbell PE: Ganglion cell distribution in the normal rectum and anal canal. A basis for the diagnosis of Hirschsprung's disease by anorectal biopsy. *J Pediatr Surg* 1968;3:475.

33. Fekete CN, Ricour C, Martelli H, et al: Total colonic aganglionosis (with or without ileal involvement). A review of 27 cases. *J Pediatr Surg* 1986;21:251.

34. Rescorla FJ, Morrison AM, Engles D, et al: Hirschsprung's disease: evaluation of mortality and long-term function in 260 cases. *Arch Surg* 1992;127:934.

35. Russell MB, Russell CA, Fenger K, Niebuhr E: Familial occurrence of Hirschsprung's disease. *Clin Genet* 1994;45:231.

36. Coventry S, Yost C, Palmiter RD, Kaupr RP: Migration of ganglion cell precursors in the ileoceca of normal and lethal spotted embryos, a murine model for Hirschsprung's disease. *Lab Invest* 1994;71:82.

37. Kusafuka T, Puri P: Mutations of the endothelin-β receptor and endothelin-3 genes in Hirschsprung's disease. *Pediatr Surg Int* 1997;12:19.

38. Doray B, Salomon R, Amiel J, et al: Mutation of the RET ligand, neurturin supports multigenic inheritance in Hirschsprung disease. *Hum Mol Genet* 1998;7:1449.

39. Puffenberger E, Hosoda K, Washington S, et al: A missense mutation of the endothelin-B receptor gene in multigenic Hirschsprung's disease. *Cell* 1994;79:1257.

40. Camilleri M: Enteric nervous system disorders: genetic and molecular insights for the neurogastroenterologist. *Neurogastroenterol Motil* 2001;13:277.

41. Pingault V, Bondurand N, Kuhlbrodt K, et al: Sox 10 mutations in patients with Waardenberg-Hirschsprung disease. *Nat Genet* 1998;18:171.

42. Amiel J, Espinosa-Parilla Y, Steffan J, et al: Large scale deletions and SMADIP1 truncating mutations in syndromic Hirschsprung's disease with involvement of midline structures. *Am J Hum Genet* 2001;69:1370.

43. Sarnacki S, Goulet O, Ricour C, et al: Germline mutations of the RET ligand GDNF are not sufficient to cause Hirschsprung disease. *Nat Genet* 1996;14:345.

44. Treanor J, Goodman L, de Sauvage F, et al: Characterization of a multicomponent receptor for GDNF. *Nature* 1996;382:80.

45. Hoehner JC, Wester T, Pahlman S, Olsen L: Alterations in neurotrophin and neurotrophin-receptor localization in Hirschsprung's disease. *J Ped Surg* 1996;31:1524.

46. Schneider R: The human protooncogene ret: a communicative cadherin? *Trends Biochem Sci* 1992;17:468.

47. Romeo G, Ronchetto P, Luo Y, et al: Point mutations affecting the tyrosine kinase domain of the RET photo-oncogene in Hirschsprung's disease. *Nature* 1994;367:377.

48. Eng C: The RET proto-oncogene in multiple endocrine neoplasia type 2 and Hirschsprung's disease. *N Engl J Med* 1996;335:943.

49. Borst MJ, VanCamp JM, Peacock ML, Decker RA: Mutational analysis of multiple endocrine neoplasia type 2A associated with Hirschsprung's disease. *Surgery* 1995;117:386.

50. Attie T, Pelet A, Edery P, et al: Diversity of RET proto-oncogene mutations in familial and sporadic Hirschsprung disease. *Hum Mol Genet* 1995;4:1381.

51. Edery P, Pelet A, Mulligan LM, et al: Hirschsprung's disease: variable clinical expression at the RET locus. *J Med Genet* 1994;31:602.

52. Fitze G, Cramer J, Ziegler A, et al: Association between c135/A genotype and RET proto-oncogene germline mutations and phenotype of Hirschsprung's disease. *Lancet* 2002;359:1200.

53. Kusafuka T, Puri P: Altered mRNA expression of the neuronal nitric oxide synthase gene in Hirschsprung's disease. *Pediatr Surg Int* 1997;32:1054.

54. Tsuto T, Obata-Tsuto HL, Iwai N, et al: Fine structure of neurons synthesizing vasoactive intestinal peptide in the human colon from patients with Hirschsprung's disease. *Histochemistry* 1989;93:1.

55. Koch T, Schulte-Bockholt A, Telford G, et al: Acquired megacolon is associated with alteration of vasoactive intestinal peptide levels and acetylcholinesterase activity. *Regul Pept* 1993;48:309.

56. Teitelbaum DH, Caniano DA, Qualman SJ: The pathophysiology of Hirschsprung's associated enterocolitis: importance of histologic correlates. *J Pediatr Surg* 1989;24:1271.

57. Caniano DA, Teitelbaum DH, Qualman SJ: Management of Hirschsprung's disease in children with trisomy 21. *Am J Surg* 1990;159:402.

58. Kobayashi H, Miyano T, Yamataka A, et al: Use of synaptophysin polyclonal antibody for the rapid intra-operative immunohistochemical evaluation of functional bowel disorders. *J Pediatr Surg* 1997;32:38.

59. Rolle U, Piotrowska AP, Nemeth L, Puri P: Altered distribution of interstitial cells of Cajal in Hirschsprung's disease. *Arch Pathol Lab Med* 2002;126:928.

60. Newman CJ, Laurini RN, Lesbros Y, et al: Interstitial cells of Cajal are normally distributed in both ganglionated and aganglionic bowel in Hirschsprung' disease. *Pediatr Surg Int* 2003;19:662.

61. Monforte-Munoz H, Gonzalez-Gomez I, Rowland JM, Landing BH: Increased submucosal nerve trunk caliber in aganglionosis: a "positive" and objective finding in suction biopsies and segmental resections in Hirschsprung's disease. *Arch Pathol Lab Med* 1998;122:721.

62. Taguchi T, Tanaka K, Ikeda K: Fibromuscular dysplasia of arteries in Hirschsprung's disease. *Gastroenterology* 1985;88:1099.

63. Kobayashi H, Hirakawa H, Surana R, et al: Intestinal neuronal dysplasia is a possible cause of persistent bowel symptoms after pull-through operation for Hirschsprung's disease. *J Pediatr Surg* 1995;30:253.

64. Yunis E, Sieber WK, Akers DR: Does zonal aganglionosis really exist? Report of a rare variety of Hirschsprung's disease and a review of the literature. *Pediatr Pathol* 1983;1:33.

65. Kobayashi H, Hirakawa H, Puri P: What are the diagnostic criteria for intestinal neuronal dysplasia? *Pediatr Surg Int* 1995;10:459.

66. Meier-Ruge W, Gambazzi F, Käufeler RE, et al: The neuropathological diagnosis of neuronal intestinal dysplasia (NIB). *Eur J Pediatr Surg* 1994;4:267.

67. Schärli AF, Sossai R: Hypoganglionosis. *Sem Pediatr Surg* 1998;7:187.

68. DiGiorgio L, Camilleri M: Human enteric neuropathies: morphology and molecular pathology. *Neurogastroenterol Motil* 2004;16:515.

69. Rolle U, Yoneda A, Solari V, et al: Abnormalities of c-kit positive cellular network in isolated hypoganglionosis. *Pediatr Surg* 2002;37:709.

70. Holschneider AM, Meier-Ruge W, Ure BM: Hirschsprung's disease and allied disorders—a review. *Eur J Pediatr Surg* 1994;4:260.

71. Bahuau M, Laurendeau I, Pelet A, et al: Tandem duplication within the neurofibromatosis type I gene (NF1) and reciprocal t(15;16)(q26.3; q12.1) translocation in familial association of NF1 with intestinal neuronal dysplasia type B (IND B). *J Med Genet* 2000;37:146.

72. Koletzko S, Ballauff A, Hadziselimovic F, Enck P: Is histological diagnosis of neuronal intestinal dysplasia related to clinical and manometric findings in constipated children. Results of a pilot study. *J Pediatr Gastroenterol Nutr* 1993;17:59.

73. Smith VV: Isolated intestinal neuronal dysplasia: a descriptive pattern or a distinct clinicopathological entity? In: Hadziselimomic F, Herzog B (eds). *Inflammatory Bowel Disease and Morbus Hirschsprung.* Dordrecht, The Netherlands: Kluwer Academic, 1992, pp 203–214.

74. Wester T, O'Briain DS, Puri P: Notable postnatal alterations in the myenteric plexus of normal human bowel. *Gut* 1999;44:666.

75. Kobayashi H, Hirakawa H, Puri P: Abnormal internal anal sphincter innervation in patients with Hirschsprung's disease and allied disorders. *J Pediatr Surg* 1996;31:794.

76. Meier-Ruge WA, Bronnimann PB, Gambazzi F, et al: Histopathological criteria for intestinal neuronal dysplasia of the submucosal plexus (type B). *Virchows Arch* 1995;426:549.

77. Jeng YM, Mao TL, Hsu WM, et al: Congenital interstitial cell of Cajal hyperplasia with neuronal intestinal dysplasia. *Am J Surg Pathol* 2000;24:1568.

78. Kobayashi H, Yamataka A, Fujimoto T, et al: Mast cells and gut nerve development: implications for Hirschsprung's disease and intestinal neuronal dysplasia. *J Pediatr Surg* 1999;34:543.

79. Moore SW, Laing D, Kaschula ROC, et al: A histological grading system for the evaluation of co-existing NID with Hirschsprung's disease. *Eur J Pediatr Surg* 1994;4:293.

80. Ammann K, Stoss F, Meier-Ruge W: Intestinale neuronale dysplasia des erwachsenen als ursache der chronischen obstipation. Morphometrische charakterisierung der coloninnervation. *Chirurg* 1999;70:771.

81. Huizinga JD, Thuneberg L, Kluppel M, et al: c-kit gene required for interstitial cells of Cajal and for intestinal pacemaker activity. *Nature* 1995;373:347.

82. Krishnamurthy S, Shuffler MD, Rorman CA, Pope CE: Severe idiopathic constipation is associated with a distinctive abnormality of the colonic myenteric plexus. *Gastroenterology* 1985;88:26.

83. Anuras S: Intestinal pseudoobstruction syndrome. *Ann Rev Med* 1988;30:1.

84. Cortesini C, Cianchi F, Infantino A, Lise M: Nitric oxide synthase and VIP distribution in the enteric nervous system in idiopathic chronic constipation. *Dig Dis Sci* 1995;40:2450.

85. Koch TR, Carney JA, Go L, Go VL: Idiopathic chronic constipation is associated with decreased colonic vasoactive intestinal polypeptide. *Gastroenterology* 1988;94:300.

86. Shouten WR, ten Kate FJ, de Graaf EJ, et al: Visceral neuropathy in slow transit constipation: an immunohistochemical investigation with monoclonal antibodies against neurofilament. *Dis Colon Rectum* 1993; 36:1112.

87. Park HJ, Kamm MA, Abbasi AM, Talbot IC: Immunohistochemical study of the colonic muscle innervation in idiopathic chronic constipation. *Dis Colon Rectum* 1995;38:509.

88. Hutson JM, Chow CW, Hurley MR, et al: Deficiency of substance P immunoreactive nerve fibres in children with intractable constipation: a form of intestinal neuronal dysplasia. *J Paediatr Child Health* 1997; 33:187.

89. Tzavella K, Riepl RL, Klause AG, et al: Decreased substance P levels in rectal biopsies from patients with slow transit constipation. *Eur J Gastroenterol Hepatol* 1996;8:1207.

90. Sjolund K, Fasth S, Ekman R, et al: Neuropeptides in chronic constipation (slow transit constipation). *Neurogastrenterol Motil* 1997; 9:143.

91. Porter AJ, Wattchow DA, Hunter A, Costa M: Abnormalities of nerve fibers in the circular muscle of patients with slow transit constipation. *Int J Colorectal Dis* 1998;13:208.

92. Faussone-Pellegrini MS, Infantino A, Matini P, et al: Neuronal anomalies and normal muscle morphology in patients with idiopathic chronic constipation. *Histol Histopathol* 1999;14:1119.

93. He C-L, Burgart L, Wang L, et al: Decreased interstitial cell of Cajal volume in patients with slow-transit constipation. *Gastroenterology* 2000;118:14.

94. Krishnamurthy S, Heng Y, Schuffler MD: Chronic intestinal pseudoobstruction in infants and children caused by diverse abnormalities of the myenteric plexus. *Gastroenterology* 1993;104:1398.

95. Wedel T, Spiegler J, Soellner S, et al: Enteric nerves and interstitial cells of Cajal are altered in patients with slow-transit constipation and megacolon. *Gastroenterology* 2002;123:1459.

96. Wedel T, Roblick UJ, Ott V, et al: Oligoneuronal hypoganglionosis in patients with idiopathic slow-transit constipation. *Dis Colon Rectum* 2002;45:54.

97. Chinn JS, Schuffler MD: Paraneoplastic visceral neuropathy as a cause of severe gastrointestinal motor dysfunction. *Gastroenterology* 1988;95: 1279.

98. Gultekin SH, Dalmau J, Graus Y, et al: Anti-Hu immunolabeling as an index of neuronal differentiation in human brain tumors. *Am J Surg Pathol* 1998;22:195.

99. Schobinger-Clement S, Gerber HA, Stallmach T: Autoaggressive inflammation of the myenteric plexus resulting in intestinal pseudoobstruction. *Am J Surg Pathol* 1999;23:602.

100. Lennon VA, Sas DF, Busk MF, et al: Enteric neuronal autoantibodies in pseudoobstruction with small-cell lung carcinoma. *Gastroenterology* 1991;100:137.

101. Condom E, Vidal A, Rota R, et al: Paraneoplastic intestinal pseudoobstruction associated with high titres of Hu autoantibodies. *Virchows Arch A Pathol Anat* 1993;423:507.

102. Sutton I, Winer JB: The immunopathogenesis of paraneoplastic neurological syndromes. *Clin Sci* 2002;102:475.

103. DiGiorgio R, Bovara M, Barbara G, et al: Anti-HuD-induced neuronal apoptosis underlying paraneoplastic gut dysmotility. *Gastroenterology* 2003;125:70.

104. Smith V, Gregson N, Foggensteiner L, et al: Acquired intestinal aganglionosis and circulating autoantibodies without neoplasia or other neural involvement. *Gastroenterology* 1997;112:1366.

105. Schappi MG, Smith VV, Milla PJ, Lindley KJ: Eosinophilic myenteric ganglionitis is associated with functional obstruction. *Gut* 2003; 52:752.

106. Roberts PF, Stebbings WS, Kennedy HJ: Granulomatous visceral neuropathy of the colon associated with non small cell lung carcinoma. *Histopathology* 1997;30:588.

107. Fujimoto T, Puri P, Miyano T: Abnormal peptidergic innervation in internal sphincter achalasia. *Pediatr Surg Int* 1992;7:12.

108. O'Kelly T, Brading A, Mortensen N: Nerve mediated relaxation of the human internal anal sphincter: the role of nitric oxide. *Gut* 1993; 34:689.

109. Burleigh DE, D'Mello A: Neural and pharmacologic factors affecting motility of the internal anal sphincter. *Gastroenterology* 1983;84:409.

110. Piotrowska AP, Solari V, Puri P: Distribution of interstitial cells of Cajal in the internal sphincter of patients with internal anal sphincter achalasia and Hirschsprung's disease. *Arch Pathol Lab Med* 2003; 127:1192.

111. Meijssen MAC, Tilanus HW, van Blankenstein M, et al: Achalasia complicated by oesophageal squamous cell carcinoma: a prospective study in 195 patients. *Gut* 1992;33:155.

112. Nihoul-Fekete C, Bawab F, Lortat-Jacob S, Arhan P: Achalasia of the esophagus in childhood. Surgical treatment in 35 cases, with special reference to familial cases and glucocorticoid deficiency association. *Hepatogastroenterology* 1991;38:510.

113. Verne GN, Hahn AB, Pineau BC, et al: Association of HLA-DR and -DG alleles with idiopathic achalasia. *Gastroenterology* 1999;117:26.

114. Mayberry JF, Rhodes J: Achalasia in the city of Cardiff from 1926 to 1977. *Digestion* 1980;20:248.

115. Berquist WE, Byrne WJ, Ament ME: Achalasia: diagnosis, management, and clinical course in 16 children. *Pediatrics* 1983;71:798.

116. Smith B: The neurologic lesion in achalasia of the cardia. *Gut* 1970;11:388.

117. Barrett NR: Achalasia of the cardia. Reflections on a clinical study of over 100 cases. *BMJ* 1964;i:1135.

118. Dumars KW, Williams JJ, Steele-Sandlin C: Achalasia and microcephaly. *Am J Med Genet* 1980;6:309.

119. Spiess AE, Kahritas PJ: Treating achalasia: from whalebone to laparoscope. *JAMA* 1998;280:638.

120. Couturier D, Samama J: Clinical aspects and manometric criteria in achalasia. *Hepatogastroenterology* 1991;38:481.

121. Ali GN, Hunt DR, Jorgensen JO, et al: Esophageal achalasia and coexistent upper esophageal sphincter relaxation disorder presenting with airway obstruction. *Gastroenterology* 1995;109:1328.

122. Marshall JB, Diaz-Arias AA, Bochna GS, Vogele KA: Achalasia due to diffuse esophageal leiomyomatosis and inherited as an autosomal dominant disorder. Report of a family study. *Gastroenterology* 1990; 98:1358.

123. Shafik A: Anorectal motility in patients with achalasia of the esophagus: recognition of an esophago-rectal syndrome. *BMC Gastroenterol* 2003;17:28.

124. Goldblum JR, Whyte RI, Orringer MB, et al: Achalasia: a morphologic study of 42 resected specimens. *Am J Surg Pathol* 1994;18:327.

125. Raymond L, Lach B, Shamji FM: Inflammatory aetiology of primary oesophageal achalasia: an immunohistochemical and ultrastructural study of Auerbach's plexus. *Histopathology* 1999;35:445.

126. Clouse RE, Abramson BK, Todorczuk JR: Achalasia in the elderly. Effects of aging on clinical presentation and outcome. *Dig Dis Sci* 1991;36:225.

127. Faussone-Pellegrini MS, Cortesini C: The muscle coat of the lower esophageal sphincter in patients with achalasia and hypertensive sphincter. *J Submicrosc Cytol* 1985;17:673.

128. Goldblum JR, Rice TW, Richter JE: Histopathologic features in esophagomyotomy specimens from patients with achalasia. *Gastroenterology* 1996;111:648.

129. Lehman MB, Clark SB, Ormsby AH, et al: Squamous mucosal alterations in esophagectomy specimens from patients with end stage achalasia. *Am J Surg Pathol* 2001;25:1413.

130. Procter DD, Faser JL, Mangano MM, et al: Small cell carcinoma of the esophagus in a patent with longstanding primary achalasia. *Am J Gastroenterol* 1992;87:664.

131. Brooks BP, Kleta R, Caruso RC, et al: Triple–A syndrome with prominent ophthalmic features and a novel mutation in the AAAS gene: a case report. *BMC Ophthalmol* 2004;4:7.

132. Khelif K, de Laet M-H, Chaouachi B, et al: Achalasia of the cardia in Allgrove's (triple A) syndrome. *Am J Surg Pathol* 2003;25:667.

133. Sandler RS, Bozymski EM, Orlando RC: Failure of clinical criteria to distinguish between primary achalasia and achalasia secondary to tumor. *Dig Dis Sci* 1982;27:209.

134. Swann TT: Congenital pyloric stenosis in the African infant. *BMJ* 1961;i:545.

135. Scharli A, Sieber WK, Keisewetter WB: Hypertrophic pyloric stenosis at the Children's Hospital of Pittsburgh from 1912 to 1967: a critical review of current problems and complications. *J Pediatr Surg* 1969;4:108.

136. Nielson JP, Haahr P, Haaahr J: Infantile hypertrophic pyloric stenosis. Decreasing incidence. *Dan Med Bull* 2000;47:223.

137. Hulka F, Harrison MW, Campbell TJ, Campbell JR: Complications of pyloromyotomy for infantile hypertrophic pyloric stenosis. *Am J Surg* 1997;173:450.

138. Yamamoto Y, Oguro N, Nara T, et al: Duplication of part of 9q due to maternal 12;9 inverted insertion associated with pyloric stenosis. *Am J Med Genet* 1988;31:379.

139. Cooper WO, Griffin MR, Arbogast P, et al: Very early exposure of erythromycin and infantile hypertrophic pyloric stenosis. *Arch Pediatr Adolesc Med* 2002;156:647.

140. Dick AC, Ardill J, Potts SR, et al: Gastrin, somatostatin and infantile hypertrophic pyloric stenosis. *Acta Pediatr* 2001;90:879.

141. Guarino N, Shima H, One T, et al: Glial derived growth factor signaling pathway in infantile hypertrophic pyloric stenosis. *J Pediatr Surg* 2001;36:1468.

142. Vanderwinden JM, Liu H, De laet MH, et al: Study of the interstitial cells of Cajal in infantile hypertrophic pyloric stenosis. *Gastroenterology* 1996;111:279.

143. Vanderwinden J-M, Mailleux P, Schiffmann SN, et al: Nitric oxide synthase activity in infantile hypertrophic pyloric stenosis. *N Engl J Med* 1992;327:511.

144. Huang PL, Dawson TM, Bredt DS, et al: Targeted disruption of the neuronal nitric oxide synthase gene. *Cell* 1993;75:1273.

145. Saur D, Seidler B, Paehge H, et al: Complex regulation of human neuronal nitric-oxide synthase exon 1c gene transcription. *J Biol Chem* 2002;277:25798.

146. Granata C, Puri P: Megacystis-microcolon-intestinal hypoperistalsis syndrome. *J Pediatr Gastroenterol Nutr* 1997;25:12.

147. Ciftci AO, Cook RC, van Velzen D: Megacystis microcolon intestinal hypoperistalsis syndrome: evidence of a primary myocellular defect of contractile fiber synthesis. *J Pediatr Surg* 1996;31:1706.

148. Smith V, Lake B, Kamm M, Nicholls R: Intestinal pseudo-obstruction with deficient smooth muscle a-actin. *Histopathology* 1999; 221:535.

149. Ionasescu V, Thompson SH, Ionasescu R, et al: Inherited ophthalmoplegia with intestinal pseudo-obstruction. *J Neurol Sci* 1983;59:215.

150. Igarashi M, MacRae D, O-Uchi T, Alford BR: Cochleo-saccular degeneration in one of three sisters with hereditary deafness, absent gastric motility, small bowel diverticulosis and progressive sensory neuropathy. *Ann Otol Rhinol Laryngol* 1981;43:4.

151. Jones SC, Dixon MF, Lintott DJ, Axon ATR: Familial visceral myopathy: a family with involvement of four generations. *Dig Dis Sci* 1992;37:464.

152. McMaster KR, Powers JM, Hennigar GR Jr, et al: Nervous system involvement in type IV glycogenosis. *Arch Pathol Lab Med* 1979;103: 105.

153. Mitros FA, Schuffler MD, Teja K, Anuras S: Pathologic features of familial visceral myopathy. *Hum Pathol* 1982;13:825.

154. Nonaka M, Goulet O, Arahan P, et al: Primary intestinal myopathy, a cause of chronic idiopathic intestinal pseudo-obstruction syndrome (CIPS): clinicopathological studies of seven cases in children. *Pediatr Pathol* 1989;9:409.

155. Rodrigues CA, Shepherd NA, Lennard-Jones JE, et al: Familial visceral myopathy: a family with at least 6 involved members. *Gut* 1989; 30:1285.

156. Schuffler MD, Lowe MC, Bill AH: Studies of idiopathic intestinal pseudoobstruction. I. Hereditary hollow visceral myopathy: clinical and pathological studies. *Gastroenterology* 1977;73:327.

157. Goebel HH, Shin YS, Gullotta F, et al: Adult polyglycosan body myopathy. *J Neuropathol Exp Neurol* 1992;51:24.

158. Foucar E, Lindholm J, Anuras S, et al: A kindred with dysplastic nevus syndrome associated with visceral myopathy and multiple basal cell carcinomas. *Lab Invest* 1985;52:32A.

159. Kubota M, Ksnda E, Ida K, et al: Severe gastrointestinal dysmotility in a patient with congenital myopathy: causal relationship to decrease of interstitial cells of Cajal. *Brain Dev* 2005;27:447.

160. Mueller LA, Camilleri M, Emslie-Smith AM: Mitochondrial neurogastrointestinal encephalopathy: manometric and diagnostic features. *Gastroenterology* 1999;116:959.

161. Peterson PL: The treatment of mitochondrial myopathies and encephalomyopathies. *Biochim Biophys Acta* 1995;1271:275.

162. Grossman LI, Shoubridge EA: Mitochondrial genetics and human disease. *Bioessays* 1996;18:983.

163. DiMauro S, Schon EA: Mitochondrial respiratory-chain diseases. *N Engl J Med* 2003;348:2656.

164. Moraes CT: Mitochondrial disorders. *Curr Opin Neurol* 1996;9:369.

165. Giordano C, Sebastiani M, Plazzi G, et al: Mitochondrial neurogastrointestinal encephalomyopathy: evidence of mitochondrial DNA depletion in small intestine. *Gastroenterology* 2006;130:893.

166. Hirano M, Silvestri G, Blake DM, et al: Mitochondrial neurogastrointestinal encephalomyopathy (MNGIE): clinical, biochemical, and genetic features of an autosomal recessive mitochondrial disorder. *Neurology* 1994;44:721.

167. Perez-Atayde AR, Fox V, Teitelbaum JE, et al: Mitochondrial neurogastrointestinal encephalomyopathy. Diagnosis by rectal biopsy. *Am J Surg Pathol* 1998;22:1141.

168. Ruuska TH, Karikoski R, Smith VV, Milla PJ: Acquired myopathic intestinal pseudo-obstruction may be due to autoimmune enteric leiomyositis. *Gastroenterology* 2002;122:1133.

169. Bogdanos DP, Choudhuri K, Vergani D: Molecular mimicry and autoimmune liver disease: virtuous intentions, malignant consequences. *Liver* 2001;21:225.

170. Martin JE, Swash M, Kamm MA, et al: Myopathy of internal anal sphincter with polyglucosal inclusion. *J Pathol* 1990;161:221.

171. Pierce JW, Creamer B, MacDermot V: Pharynx and oesophagus in dystrophica myotonica. *Gut* 1965;6:392.

172. Kebede D, Barthel JS, Singh A: Transient gastroparesis associated with cutaneous herpes zoster. *Dig Dis Sci* 1987;32:318.

173. Vassallo M, Camilleri M, Caron BL, Low PA: Gastrointestinal motor dysfunction in acquired selective cholinergic dysautonomia associated with infectious mononucleosis. *Gastroenterology* 1991;100:252.

174. Nowak TV, Goddard M, Batteiger B, Cummings OW: Evolution of acute cytomegalovirus gastritis to chronic gastrointestinal motility in a nonimmunocompromised adult. *Gastroenterology* 1999;116:953.

175. Bardhan PK, Salam MA, Molla AM: Gastric emptying of liquid in children suffering from acute rotaviral gastroenteritis. *Gut* 1992;3:26.

176. Meeroff JC, Schreiber DS, Trier JS, Blacklow NR: Abnormal gastric motor function in viral gastroenteritis. *Ann Intern Med* 1980;92:370.

177. Chatila R, Kapadia CR: Intestinal pseudoobstruction in acute Lyme disease. A case report. *Am J Gastroenterol* 1998;93:1179.

178. World Health Organization. *Chagas Disease. Thirteenth Programme Report UNDP/WB/TDR.* Geneva, Switzerland: World Health Organization, 1997, pp 112–123.

179. Kalil J, Cunha-Neto E: Autoimmunity in Chagas disease cardiomyopathy fulfilling the criteria at last? *Parasitol Today* 1996;12:396.

180. Tarleton RL, Zhang L: Chagas disease etiology: autoimmunity or parasite persistence? *Parasitol Today* 1999;15:94.

181. Moncayo A: Chagas disease: current epidemiological trends after the interruption of vectorial and transfusional transmission in the Southern cone countries. *Mem Inst Oswaldo Cruz, Rio de Janeiro* 2003;98:577.

182. Edgcomb JH, Johnson CM: American trypanosomiasis (Chagas' disease). In: Binford CH, Connor DH (eds). *Pathology of Tropical and Extraordinary Diseases.* Washington, DC: AFIP, 1976, p 244.

183. Koberle F: Enteromegaly and cardiomegaly in Chagas' disease. *Gut* 1964;34:399.

184. Geraldino RS, Ferreira AJ, Lima MA, et al: Interstitial cells of Cajal in patients with Chagastic megacolon originating from a region of old endemicity. *Pathophysiology* 2006;13:71.

185. Manoel-Caetano FDA, Borim AA, Caetano A, et al: Cytogenetic alterations in chagastic achalasia compared to esophageal carcinoma. *Cancer Genet Cytogenet* 2004;149:17.

186. Pearson JD: The endothelium: its role in scleroderma. *Ann Rheum Dis* 1991;50:866.

187. Jimenez SA, Saitta B: Alterations in the regulation of expression of the alpha 1(I) collagen gene (COL1A1) in systemic sclerosis (scleroderma). *Semin Immunopathol* 1999;21:397.

188. Sjogren RW: Gastrointestinal features of scleroderma. *Curr Opin Rheumatol* 1996;8:569.

189. Lovy MR, Levine JS, Steigerald JC: Lower esophageal rings as a cause of dysphagia in progressive systemic sclerosis–coincidence or consequence? *Dig Dis Sci* 1983;28:780.

190. Wegener M, Adamek RJ, Wedmann J, et al: Gastrointestinal transit through esophagus, stomach, small and large intestine in patients with progressive systemic sclerosis. *Dig Dis Sci* 1994;39:2209.

191. Manolios N, Eliades C, Duncombe V, Spencer D: Scleroderma and watermelon stomach. *J Rheumatol* 1996;23:776.

192. Lock G, Holstege A, Lang B, Scholmerich J: Gastrointestinal manifestations of progressive systemic sclerosis. *Am J Gastroenterol* 1997; 92:763.

193. Hang LM, Nakamura RM: Current concepts and advances in clinical laboratory testing for autoimmune diseases. *Crit Rev Clin Lab Sci* 1997;34:275.

194. Rosson RS, Yesner R: Peroral duodenal biopsy in progressive systemic sclerosis. *N Engl J Med* 1965;272:391.

195. Nilsson PH: Diabetic gastroparesis: a review. *J Diabetes Complications* 1996;10:113.

196. Quigley EMM: The pathophysiology of diabetic gastroenteropathy: more vague than vagal? *Gastroenterology* 1997;113:1790.

197. Horvath VJ, Vittal H, Lorincz A, et al: Reduced stem cell factor links smooth muscle myopathy and loss of interstitial cells of Cajal in murine diabetic gastroparesis. *Gastroenterology* 2006;130:759.

198. Katz LA, Spiro H: Gastrointestinal manifestation of diabetes. *N Engl J Med* 1966;275:1350.

199. Koch KL: Diabetic gastropathy: gastric neuromuscular dysfunction in diabetes mellitus: a review of symptoms, pathophysiology, and treatment. *Dig Dis Sci* 1999;44:1061.

200. Nakahara M, Isozaki K, Hirota S, et al: Deficiency of KIT-positive cells in the colon of patients with diabetes mellitus. *Gastroenterol Hepatol* 2002;17:666.

201. Menke D, Kyle R, Fleming R, et al: Symptomatic gastric amyloidosis in patients with primary systemic amyloidosis. *Mayo Clin Proc* 1993;68:763.

202. Koppelman RN, Stollman NH, Baigorri F, Rogers AI: Acute small bowel pseudo-obstruction due to AL amyloidosis. *Am J Gastroenterol* 2000;95:294.

203. Yuan C-S, Foss JF, O'Connor M, et al: Methylnaltrexone for reversal of constipation due to chronic methadone use. *JAMA* 2000; 283:367.

204. Brubacher JR, Levine B, Hoffman RS: Intestinal pseudo-obstruction (Ogilivie's syndrome) in theophylline overdose. *Vet Human Toxicol* 1996;38:368.

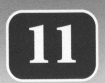

Inflammatory Bowel Disease

hronic idiopathic inflammatory bowel disease (IBD) includes two chronic gastrointestinal disorders of unknown etiology: Ulcerative colitis (UC) and Crohn disease (CD). The natural history of IBD differs from patient to patient. Disease severity at its onset, disease extent, and patient age at the time of diagnosis, along with other variables, determine overall disease severity and the likelihood of subsequent morbidity and mortality. Once established, IBD patients suffer episodic acute attacks that become superimposed on chronic disease. As a result, the patient is likely to suffer from disabling disease for decades.

GENERAL CLINICAL AND EPIDEMIOLOGIC FEATURES OF INFLAMMATORY BOWEL DISEASE

The annual incidence of IBD in the United States is approximately 6 cases per 100,000 persons (1). Both CD and UC are predominantly diseases of young adults, with a peak incidence occurring between 15 and 30 years of age. Age-specific incidence rates by sex are slightly greater for males with UC and for females with CD (2). At age 10, both diseases rapidly increase in incidence. Overall, both UC and CD show three peaks in incidence rates. The first and highest peak occurs between ages 20 and 24, the second at ages 40 to 44, and the third at ages 60 to 64 years. In females, the first peak appears at ages 15 to 19, 5 years younger than in males (3). By age 60, the incidence of UC exceeds that of CD.

Ethnicity

Epidemiologic studies show that the incidence and prevalence of IBD vary significantly depending on geographic location and patients' racial or ethnic backgrounds. IBD occurs worldwide and exhibits a relatively low incidence in Asian, Mediterranean, and Middle Eastern countries and a higher incidence in European countries, the United States, Canada, Australia, and New Zealand. This may reflect racial, ethnic, and genetic factors. Prevalence rates for IBD among non-Caucasians in the United States are lower than rates for Caucasians. In one study, the prevalence of Crohn disease was 43.6 per 100,000 population for Caucasians, 29.8 per

100,000 for African Americans, 5.6 per 100,000 for Asians, and 4.1 per 100,000 for Hispanics (4). A study of African-American children reported a Crohn disease incidence of 7 to 12 cases per 100,000 (5). However, recent data indicate that the incidence of IBD among African Americans and second-generation South Asians is increasing (6). Among ethnic groups, Jews in the United States have the greatest risk for developing IBD compared with non-Jewish Caucasians. The incidence rate is two to four times greater and the prevalence two to nine times greater in this group. Ashkenazi Jews exhibit a particularly high IBD risk, especially those originating in Middle Europe, Poland, or Russia.

Etiology

Chronic IBD is a common inflammatory disorder of unknown etiology. The intrinsic complexity of IBD and its variable manifestations hampers progress in understanding its pathogenesis. However, currently favored theories implicate genetically determined, immunologically mediated mechanisms of injury. The fundamental pathogenic question could be: Does the chronic recurring inflammatory activity in IBD reflect an appropriate response to a persistently abnormal stimulus (a structural alteration of the intestine or causative agent in the environment) or an abnormally prolonged response to a normal stimulus (aberrant regulation of immune responses) (Fig. 11.1)? It is conceivable that some factors initiate the disease, whereas others sustain the inflammatory process or possibly even reactivate it.

Genetic Factors

There is considerable evidence that the development of both CD and UC is determined, at least in part, by genetic factors. Overwhelming evidence exists that both ulcerative colitis and Crohn disease cluster within families. In population-based studies, 5% to 10% of individuals with IBD report having an affected family member (7). In fact, having a family member with IBD represents the greatest risk factor for developing the disease. Individuals with a first-degree relative with IBD have a 10- to 15-fold increased risk of also developing the disease compared with those without an affected family member (8). Approximately 75% of families

593

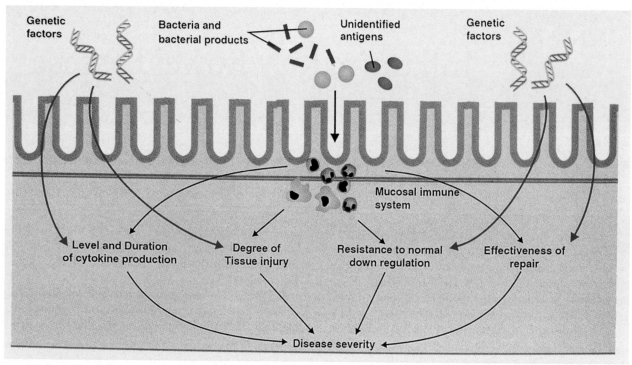

FIG. 11.1. Inflammatory bowel disease (IBD) likely results from a combination of genetic predisposition, cellular alterations, and up-regulated immunity. The genetic influences affect both the predisposition to injury and the nature of the response to the injury.

with multiple affected members show concordance for disease type (i.e., all affected family members have CD disease or all have UC). In the remaining 25%, some members have CD while others have UC (9). This finding suggests that UC and CD may have some common, as well as distinct, susceptibility genes. Twin studies show that monozygotic twin concordance for CD ranges from 42% to 58% (10). In contrast, concordance in dizygotic twins is only 4% (11). Monozygotic twin concordances are significantly lower for UC (10). These findings suggest that although there is a strong genetic component that determines susceptibility to inflammatory bowel disease, there are also environmental factors that play an important role in disease development.

Susceptibility Genes

Genetic linkage studies have identified a number of potential genetic susceptibility loci for inflammatory bowel disease. Some of these genes appear to confer a general risk for development of IBD, while others confer specific risk for either UC or CD. These are listed in Table 11-1.

IBD1

The IBD1 locus is located in the pericentromeric region of chromosome 16 and shows disease linkage only for CD, not for UC. This locus contains the gene NOD2/CARD15 that has now been definitively identified as the gene responsible

for disease linkage to this chromosomal region. The family of Nod proteins includes NOD2/CARD15 as well as several additional regulatory proteins. The Nod proteins contain a central nucleotide-binding domain and an N-terminal caspase recruitment domain (12). In addition, they possess a C-terminal leucine-rich repeat (LRR) region that bears a high degree of homology with plant genes known to be involved in disease resistance. This finding suggests that Nod proteins may play a similar role in mammals (12).

NOD2 is expressed in monocytes, intestinal epithelial cells, and intestinal Paneth cells. This protein recognizes and binds muramyl dipeptide, the biologically active moiety of bacterial peptidoglycan, resulting in activation of the proinflammatory cytokine NF-κB (13). It is the leucine-rich repeat region of the protein that functions in peptidoglycan recognition. Human mutations in NOD2 occur in both the LLR and in the central nucleotide-binding domain. Three major mutations have been described in the LRR, all of which are associated with Crohn disease (14,15). Interestingly, these mutations occur predominantly in Caucasian populations and are extremely rare in Asian and African-American populations (16,17). Mutations in the nucleotide-binding domain result in Blau syndrome, a rare disease characterized by early-onset granulomatous arthritis, uveitis, and skin rash.

Patients who have one defective copy of NOD2 demonstrate a two- to fourfold increased risk for the development of Crohn disease, while homozygous mutants show a 20- to

TABLE 11.1 **Major Susceptibility Loci for Inflammatory Bowel Disease (IBD)**

Locus Designation	Chromosomal Location	IBD Type	Candidate Genes
IBD1	16q12	CD	NOD2
IBD2	12q13	UC	VDR, IFN-γ
IBD3	6p13	CD, UC	MHC I, MHC II, TNF-α
IBD4	14q11	CD	TCR α/δ complex
IBD5	5q31-33	CD	IL-3, IL-4, IL-5, IL-13, CSF-2
IBD6	19p13	CD, UC	ICAM-1, C3, TBXA2R, LTB4H
IBD7	1p36	CD, UC	TNF-R family, CASP9
IBD8	16p	CD	Unknown
IBD9	3p26	CD, UC	CCR5, CCR9, nMLH1
Other	7q	CD, UC	Multidrug resistance 1
Other	10q23	CD	Drosophila discs large homolog 5
Other	9q32-33	CD, UC	Toll-like receptor-4
Other	1q41-42	CD	Toll-like receptor-5
Other	7p14	CD, UC	NOD1/CARD4

CD, Crohn disease; IFN, interferon; IL, interleukin; MHC, major histocompatibility complex; UC, ulcerative colitis.

40-fold increased risk (15,18). Approximately 8% to 17% of CD patients carry two mutant NOD2 alleles. NOD2 mutations are associated with disease onset at a young age, disease located in the small intestine, and stricturing and fistulizing forms of the disease (14,15,19,20). The Crohn disease–associated mutations in the LRR of NOD2 all result in inactivation of the protein with a resultant defect in the cellular response to peptidoglycan (16). This abnormality on monocytes could result in an inability of the innate immune system to recognize bacterial products and a subsequent overreaction to bacteria by the adaptive immune system. In addition, defective NOD2 function in intestinal epithelial and Paneth cells may result in an abnormal immunologic response to normal commensal bacteria within the gut (21).

IBD2

The IBD2 gene locus lies on chromosome 12 and appears to be more closely linked to the development of UC than CD (22). A number of possible candidate genes are located in this region, but investigation of several of these has yielded negative results.

IBD3

Several studies have linked the IBD3 locus, located on chromosome 6, to both ulcerative colitis and Crohn disease (22,23). Recent data suggest that this region may be specific to men (24). This region contains the major histocompatability complex (MHC), as well as the tumor necrosis factor (TNF) gene. Several human leukocyte antigen (HLA) associations with IBD are well known. Among Caucasians, susceptibility to ulcerative colitis has been convincingly linked to the HLADRB1*0103 allele. In addition, this allele is associated with severe colitis and extraintestinal manifestations of

UC. In Japanese and Jewish populations, susceptibility to UC has been linked to the HLADRB1*1052 allele. Polymorphisms in TNF-α and their relationship to Crohn disease risk are also under current investigation.

IBD5

The IBD5 locus resides on chromosome 5q31-q33. It was identified by a genomewide scan of Canadian families with early-onset CD. Heterozygous carriage of the risk alleles increased the risk for developing CD twofold, while homozygous carriage increases this risk by sixfold (25). IBD5 may also be associated with risk for development of UC (25). The specific causative gene has not yet been identified. Candidate genes include organic cation transporter genes 1 and 2, interferon regulatory factor isoform 1, PDZ and LIM domain protein (PDLIM4), and prolyl 4-hydroxylase (P4HA2).

Immunologic Factors

Both CD and UC represent, at least in part, disorders of both innate (macrophage, neutrophil) and acquired (T and B cell) immunity. It is currently believed that the main abnormality responsible for the development of inflammation in these disorders is a loss of tolerance to enteric commensal bacteria or other pathogens (26). In normal individuals, tolerance is mediated by regulatory T cells, B cells, natural killer T cells, and dendritic cells that produce transforming growth factor beta (TGF-β), interleukin (IL)-10, interferons, and prostaglandin J2. In IBD, lamina propria macrophages and dendritic cells are increased in number, demonstrate an activated phenotype, and express many proinflammatory cytokines and chemokines. In addition, expression of costimulatory molecules and adhesion molecules, vital to the extravasation of macrophages

TABLE 11.2	Cytokine Production in Inflammatory Bowel Disease	
Cytokine	Crohn Disease	Ulcerative Colitis
Innate immune response		
IL-1β	Increased	Increased
TNF	Markedly increased	Increased
IL-6	Increased	Increased
IL-8	Increased	Increased
IL-12	Increased	Normal
IL-18	Increased	Increased
IL-23	Increased	Normal
IL-27	Increased	Normal
Acquired (T cell) response		
IFN-γ	Increased	Normal
IL-5	Normal	Increased
IL-13	Normal	Increased
IL-17	Increased	Normal
IL-21	Increased	Normal

IFN, interferon; IL, interleukin; TNF, tumor necrosis factor.

and neutrophils from the vasculature, is also increased in both CD and UC (27).

Crohn disease is associated predominantly with T_H1 cytokine production (28). Ulcerative colitis, on the other hand, does not fit clearly into either the T_H1 or T_H2 category, although an atypical or modified T_H2 response seems to occur in established UC (26). Although the types of cytokines produced in UC and CD differ somewhat (Table 11.2), both diseases are associated with abnormal immune responses to nonpathogenic commensal bacteria within the gut. Cross-reactivity of peripheral blood and colonic lamina propria CD4+ T cells with indigenous flora in patients with UC and CD suggests that abnormal T cell–specific immune responses to the normal flora of the host are important in the pathogenesis of both diseases (29).

In normal individuals, pathogens are recognized by germline encoded pattern recognition receptors on epithelial cells, neutrophils, macrophages, and dendritic cells. These pattern recognition receptors include lectins, mannose receptors, complement receptors, scavenger receptors, Nod proteins, and toll-like receptors (TLRs). At least ten different TLRs have been described, each of which recognizes a different bacterial factor. Activation of TLRs ultimately results in expression and activation of NF-κB (30). NF-κB is activated in the tissues of IBD patients, where it is thought to have proinflammatory activity. NF-κB stimulates expression of many molecules that likely play a role in IBD including IL-1β, TNF, IL-6, IL-8 and other chemokines, ICAM1 and other adhesion molecules, CD40, CD80, CD86, and the T-cell stimulator ICOS (31). NF-κB also stimulates expression of protective molecules including TNF-induced protein 3,

CARD15, cyclo-oxygenase 2, β defensins, and peroxisome proliferator-activated receptor (PPAR)-γ(31).

Activated T lymphocytes are regulated by both effector and regulator T-cell subpopulations in healthy gut mucosa. Effector T cells are capable of inducing intestinal inflammation, while regulator T cells are able to control or prevent inflammation. The immunosuppressive function of the regulator cells is mediated through production of IL-10 and TGF-β. These regulator cells are thought to play pivotal roles in mediating tolerance toward luminal antigens. Genetically engineered IL-10–deficient mice develop severe transmural inflammation of the small and large intestine reminiscent of CD (32). In addition, studies suggest that defects in the IL-10 and TGF-β regulatory signaling pathway may exist in humans with UC (33).

Activation of effector cytotoxic T cells and cytokine release result in generation of activated matrix metalloproteinases, enzymes that are mediators of tissue destruction. In addition, cytokines act directly on the microvasculature, upregulate adhesion molecules, and enhance recruitment of additional effector cells including neutrophils and macrophages, which amplify and perpetuate the inflammatory response and contribute to additional tissue injury.

As a result of these immunologic events, the mucosa becomes heavily infiltrated by inflammatory cells. Soluble inflammatory mediators produced by neutrophils, lymphocytes, monocytes, fibroblasts, mast cells, neuroendocrine cells, and nerves generate many of the functional and histologic changes that characterize the disease (Fig. 11.2). One sees a large number of activated T and B cells, increased immunoglobulin secretion, the presence of anticolon antibodies (34), and aberrant expression of class II HLA molecules (35).

T-cell profiles differ between patients with Crohn disease and those with ulcerative colitis. As previously mentioned, CD is characterized primarily by a T_H1 response. T_H1 responses are mediated by IFN-γ, the production of which is stimulated by IL-12. Patients with CD also exhibit a T_H17 response, associated with IL-17 production. IL-17 expression is stimulated by IL-6, TGF-β, and IL-23. In patients with ulcerative colitis, the T-cell profile has been more difficult to characterize, but may represent an atypical T_H2-type response. This atypical T_H2 response may be mediated by natural killer T cells that secrete IL-13 (36).

Autoantibodies

Populations of mucosal B cells and plasma cells increase in UC, a finding that initially suggested that the disease was antibody mediated and complement dependent. In addition, patients with UC demonstrate circulating autoantibodies including those directed against human intestinal tropomyosin isoform as well as anticolonocyte antibodies (34,37). This production of antiself antibodies is now thought to represent a phenomenon that is a secondary protective response aimed at clearing apoptotic cells.

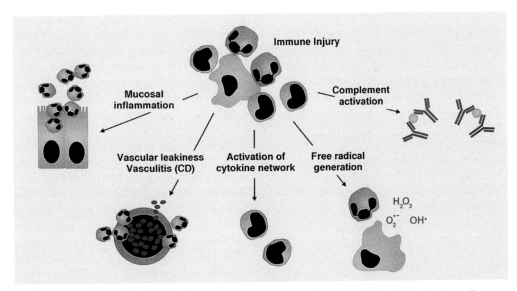

FIG. 11.2. Immune reactions in inflammatory bowel disease (IBD). Immune reactivity is generally up-regulated in many immune cellular subsets, leading to the synthesis and release of cytokines, reactive oxygen molecules, and immunoglobulins. The release of these products and interactions between the various cell types eventually result in the phenotypes that we recognize clinically and pathologically as IBD. CD, Crohn disease.

Patients with UC also commonly demonstrate the presence of circulating antineutrophil cytoplasmic antibodies (ANCAs) (38,39). Antineutrophil cytoplasmic antibodies were initially described as sensitive and specific markers for active Wegener granulomatosis but are now known to occur in a wide range of diseases. The antigens recognized by ANCAs are by definition cytoplasmic, predominantly localizing to the primary granules of neutrophils. ANCAs exhibit two distinct patterns on ethanol-fixed human neutrophils: (a) a coarse granular cytoplasmic staining (C-ANCA) or (b) a perinuclear staining pattern (P-ANCA). The perinuclear staining pattern results from redistribution of the cytoplasmic antigen to the nucleus. Serine proteinase 3, cathepsin G, and elastase are the antigens to which C-ANCAs react and myeloperoxidase is the usual antigen to which P-ANCAs react in patients with vasculitis. In contrast, a unique subset of P-ANCAs characterizes UC patients. The identity of the antigen is unclear.

The prevalence of a positive P-ANCA in UC patients ranges from 49% to 86% (40,41). The perinuclear ANCA pattern is 93% to 97% specific (39), but only 46% to 60% sensitive for the diagnosis (42). P-ANCAs are also found in up to 25% of patients with CD (40,43). Titers of these antibodies, however, do not correlate with the degree of severity of the associated colitis, and although they may serve as a convenient clinical marker for UC, their role in the pathogenesis of the disease is unclear. Interestingly, a recent report suggests that P-ANCA in UC may represent a cross-reacting antibody to an antigenic target on *Escherichia coli* and *Bacteroides* bacterial strains (44).

The absence of P-ANCAs in the serum defines one population of CD patients, whereas a smaller number of patients are positive for P-ANCA. CD patients with serum P-ANCA expression exhibit a UC-like clinical phenotype (45). One hundred percent of CD patients with P-ANCA have symptoms of left-sided colitis with clinical and histopathologic features of UC. The patients also express a rare allele (R241) of the intercellular adhesion molecule-1 (ICAM1) gene, suggesting the possibility that R241 is a marker for a CD–UC overlap syndrome (46).

Apoptosis

In normal mucosa, the inflammatory response is terminated by induction of apoptosis in activated T cells once the pathogen has been eliminated. However, in CD, mucosal T lymphocytes are resistant to apoptosis, leading to their accumulation and persistence of the inflammatory response (19,47). In UC patients, T cells are more susceptible to Fas-mediated apoptosis. In addition, Fas ligand is strongly expressed by T cells in active UC, but not in CD, suggesting the Fas-Fas ligand-induced apoptosis contributes to mucosal damage in UC (48).

Exogenous Agents

Numerous data suggest that environmental factors play a role in the development and progression of both forms of IBD. Susceptibility genes for both UC and CD are known to demonstrate incomplete penetrance. As noted earlier, concordance rates for monozygotic twins are >50% for Crohn disease and <10% for UC. This finding suggests that factors other than genotype must be involved in the pathogenesis of IBD. In addition, the incidence of IBD has increased in the developed parts of the world over the last 50 years, and is now becoming increasingly common in less developed countries as they become more industrialized and the standard of living improves. Environmental changes that might affect development of the mucosal immune system or the indigenous enteric flora include improved hygiene, consumption of sterile or at least noncontaminated foods, childhood vaccinations, and increased age at first exposure to a variety of intestinal pathogens.

Exogenous agents, including diet, infections, smoking, and other environmental factors, all may play an etiologic role in IBD. Environmental influences related to certain forms of industrial pollution may also account for the recent increase in CD incidence in certain countries.

Food Antigens

Numerous studies have demonstrated that exposure to food-associated antigens plays an important role in the gastrointestinal inflammation that occurs in patients with CD. In addition, patients treated with simplified or elemental diets containing proteins in the form of amino acids or small peptide fragments improve symptomatically and show decreased endoscopic or serologic evidence of inflammation (49). Rectal exposure of CD patients to a series of food antigens resulted in increased rectal blood flow and lymphocyte proliferation in comparison to non-CD control patients (50), a finding that suggests that patients with CD show gut-specific sensitization to food antigens. Reactions were seen with yeast and citrus antigens, although individual patients reacted also to other antigen groups. Although it is possible that this sensitivity to food antigens is merely a reflection of exposure to antigens through mucosal defects, the absence of similar sensitivities in patients with UC makes this possibility unlikely (50). It is not likely, however, that exposure to food-associated antigens represents the primary abnormality in patients with CD. Instead, exposure to food in the proximal gastrointestinal tract may lead to sensitization and stimulation of the immune system in genetically susceptible individuals.

Infectious Agents

For many years investigators have been suspicious that IBD may have an infectious etiology. These suspicions are based on several observations. First, CD patients have an increased incidence of childhood infections including pharyngitis, tonsillitis, and rhinitis (51). In addition, gastroenteritis in early infancy has been linked to later development of CD (52). Furthermore, studies have shown that patients with CD tend to have increased serum levels of antibodies directed against nonpathogenic as well as pathogenic enteric organisms (53). Many studies have attempted to link IBD to infections with *Mycobacteria*, *Yersinia*, and several viruses. However, no definitive link with any one infectious agent has ever been made.

Current evidence, instead, suggests that the resident bacterial flora of the gut may be a factor in initiating and propagating the inflammation in IBD. In CD patients, T lymphocytes are hyperreactive to bacterial antigens, a factor that suggests that local bacterial tolerance mechanisms may be abnormal in these individuals (54). Patients with both UC and CD show higher numbers of bacteria attached to their intestinal mucosa than do unaffected individuals (55). In addition, bacterial invasion of the mucosa has been reported in both UC and CD patients (56). IBD patients also have increased mucosal production of IgG antibodies directed against a wide range of commensal organisms (57). The clinical observation that, in some patients, disease flares may be ameliorated by antibiotic administration is supportive of a bacterial role. Finally, recent evidence suggests that the NOD2 CD susceptibility gene is involved in regulation of host responses to bacterial organisms (12). Overall, many view inflammatory bowel disease as a disease initiated by a general loss of tolerance for the commensal bacteria of the gut.

Tobacco Use and Exposure

The association between tobacco use and development of IBD is well established. Smoking decreases the risk for the development of UC, but exacerbates and aggravates Crohn disease (58,59). Former smokers have a lower risk of UC than do those who never smoked. In addition, exposure to passive smoke also appears to confer a lessened risk of developing UC relative to nonexposed nonsmokers (60). Overall, the effect of smoking appears to be dose dependent (61). Interestingly, nicotine has been shown to have an inhibitory effect on T_H2 lymphocyte function, the type of cells most implicated in UC (62). Indeed, nicotine-based enemas have been demonstrated to be beneficial in patients with milder forms of distal colitis. Nicotine has no effect on T_H1 cells characteristic of the Crohn inflammatory response. Tobacco use is also associated with protection against sclerosing cholangitis and pouchitis in UC patients (61,63).

Intestinal Permeability

Increased intestinal permeability may play a role in the pathogenesis of CD. Increased permeability not only occurs in the intestines of patients affected by the disease, but also in their unaffected first-degree relatives (64). It has been suggested that this increased permeability may represent a predisposing factor to the development of CD because a leaky intestinal barrier may intensify antigen absorption, leading to exaggerated systemic immune stimulation.

Appendectomy

Appendectomy early in life (before the age of 20) has been shown in several studies to decrease the risk of developing UC (65,66). Interestingly, the risk for UC is reduced only in patients who undergo appendectomy for acute appendicitis, and not in those whose appendices are removed because of nonspecific abdominal pain or incidentally during surgery for other causes. This finding suggests that the appendicitis that results in appendectomy, rather than appendectomy itself, is protective. Alternatively, there may be other factors among patients destined to develop UC that prevent those individuals from developing appendicitis. A recent report suggests that the risk for Crohn disease may also be decreased in patients who have undergone appendectomy (67).

Other Environmental Factors

Epidemiologic data suggest that use of nonsteroidal anti-inflammatory drugs (NSAIDs) can exacerbate existing UC, and may even induce it de novo (68). This effect was initially attributed to the cyclooxygenase (COX)-1 inhibitory effect of the drugs, but recent reports suggest that even COX-2–specific inhibitors also demonstrate this effect (69). Possible mechanisms by which NSAIDs exert these effects include inhibition of protective mucosal prostaglandin production and increased leukocyte migration and adherence. It has been estimated that NSAID use increases the risk of IBD exacerbation by as much as 30%.

As many as 40% of UC patients report that psychological stress represents a trigger for their disease (70). There is evidence to link psychological stress with increased susceptibility to infection and illness through stress-related impairment of the immune system. Some animal models suggest that stress may play a role in the development of colitis. Cotton-top tamarins, primates that spontaneously develop colitis and serve as a model for human IBD, develop colitis only in long-term captivity (71).

Occupation

Differences in IBD incidence exist among individuals with different occupations. Occupations involving work in the open air and physical exercise appear to protect against development of IBD, whereas exposure to air-conditioned, artificial working conditions or extended and irregular shifts can confer an increased IBD risk (72).

CROHN DISEASE

Incidence

As noted previously, there has been a steady rise in the incidence and prevalence of CD in Western Europe, Canada, and the United States over the past several decades. The incidence of CD ranges from 3.4 to as many as 14.6 per 100,000 in differing Western countries (1,73). CD affects all ages and both sexes, but its incidence peaks in the 2nd and 3rd decades of life. A second minor peak in incidence occurs in patients aged 50 to 70 years. Crohn disease is more common among Caucasians than among other racial groups, and is more frequent in Jewish than non-Jewish populations (4,5).

Multiple Forms of Crohn Disease

Recent epidemiologic evidence suggests that there are two forms of CD: One *inherently indolent* (nonperforating), which tends to recur slowly, and another *inherently aggressive* (perforating), which tends to evolve more rapidly. Patients with the relatively aggressive "perforating" type of CD are more prone to develop fistulae and abscesses, whereas the more indolent "nonperforating" type tends to lead to stenotic obstruction. The latter associates with an exaggerated inflammatory response and an exaggerated proinflammatory cytokine response (74). Host responses determine which form of CD becomes manifest in any individual, and differences in cytokine expression between the two forms of CD might have diagnostic, investigative, and therapeutic implications (74).

Clinical Features

The signs and symptoms of CD are often subtle, frequently resulting in a delay in diagnosis until months, or sometimes years, after symptom onset. However, the diagnosis can usually be made on the basis of a careful clinical history, physical examination, and diagnostic testing. The presentation of a patient with CD depends in large part on the location, extent, and severity of gastrointestinal involvement. Crohn disease most frequently affects the ileocecal region, followed (in decreasing order of frequency) by the terminal ileum alone, diffuse involvement of the small bowel, and isolated colonic disease (75). Because the clinical manifestations of CD are very diverse, both in the sites of tissue involvement and in the severity of the inflammation, a wide spectrum of clinical manifestations results (Table 11.3).

TABLE 11.3 Clinical Features of Crohn Disease Related to Site of Bowel Involvement

Isolated small intestinal involvement
  Anorexia
  Weight loss
  Early satiety
  Abdominal pain
  Postprandial cramping
  Variable diarrhea
  Lactase deficiency
  Zinc deficiency
Ileal disease (or resection)
  Vitamin B12 malabsorption
  Fat-soluble vitamin malabsorption
Colonic involvement
  Diarrhea
  Cramping
  Urgency
  Bleeding
Ileocecal involvement
  Presentation mimicking appendicitis
  Obstruction, especially with transmural inflammation

Patients with ileocolonic disease experience intermittent episodes of crampy, often postprandial, abdominal pain. Pain may be referred to the periumbilical region, especially in children (75). The abdominal discomfort may be accompanied by loose stools. Stools are small, frequent at night, loose to watery, but not usually overtly bloody. Such symptoms are often attributed to dietary factors or irritable bowel disease. The past history commonly includes perirectal or perianal abscesses and fistulae. Physical examination may localize tenderness to the right lower quadrant. Occasionally, an inflammatory mass may be palpable. Patients with diffuse small intestinal Crohn disease present with diffuse abdominal pain, diarrhea, anorexia, and weight loss. Malabsorption may also occur. These patients demonstrate diffuse abdominal tenderness on physical examination. Colonic CD may mimic ulcerative colitis. Patients complain of diarrhea often containing blood and/or mucus and crampy lower abdominal pain that may be relieved with defecation. Crohn colitis is characterized by more extensive bleeding, more perianal disease, and less pain than Crohn ileitis.

Growth retardation occurs in many pediatric patients with CD, and may occur before other disease signs or symptoms develop. The growth failure and malnutrition result from inadequate dietary intake, malabsorption, and increased nutritional requirements, and, in treated patients, from drug therapy, particularly corticosteroids.

Progressive transmural inflammation with scarring and deep ulceration may ultimately lead to symptoms associated with intestinal obstruction, perforation, bleeding, or fistula formation. When obstruction develops, it usually does so in the distal ileum. Extensive mucosal ulceration predisposes the patient to bacterial translocation with all of its complications, including a predisposition to bacterial endocarditis (76). Patients also demonstrate altered small intestinal motility with abnormal receptor-mediated small intestinal contraction (77). Deep linear ulcers or fistulae may sometimes give rise to profound lower GI bleeding.

A sudden worsening of clinical symptoms and/or an unusual disease presentation should alert one to the possibility of ischemia or viral infection superimposed on pre-existing CD. Ischemia may develop secondary to vasculitis, or may occur because of endothelialitis resulting from infection with cytomegalovirus (CMV), particularly if immunosuppressive therapy has been utilized.

Anorectal Disease

Anorectal complications are common in patients with CD. In some patients, these anorectal symptoms may be the most troubling aspect of their disease. Approximately one quarter of patients with CD involving the small bowel and three quarters of individuals with colonic CD will have an anal lesion sometime during the course of their disease (78). Anorectal complications are more likely to occur during severe attacks when the colon is extensively involved. Perianal involvement may predate, postdate, or develop concurrently with primary intestinal CD.

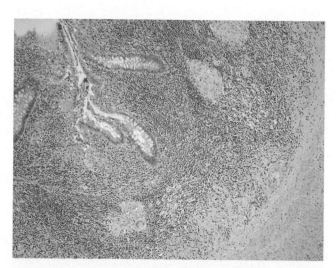

FIG. 11.3. Granulomatous appendicitis. Numerous compact granulomas lie in the submucosa of the appendix of a child with symptoms of acute appendicitis. This finding sometimes represents the initial presentation of a child with Crohn disease.

Perianal disease consists of thickened, indurated, perianal skin with tags, scarring, erosions, superficial ulcers, cavitating ulcers, excoriation, fissures, fistulae, abscesses, and blind sinus tracts (79). Perianal abscesses affect about 25% of patients with CD. Persistence or healing of perianal lesions does not correlate with intestinal activity. Of the various perianal lesions, those that tend to persist are the anal skin tags. Persistent fistulae may remain asymptomatic but many also heal spontaneously. New fistulae may also form (79).

Jejunal Disease

The term *regional jejunitis* is used to describe a variant of CD that manifests initially or predominantly as jejunal disease. It rarely coexists with duodenal CD. More often it occurs as part of diffuse jejunoileitis. It also manifests as a particularly devastating and sometimes fatal pattern of CD recurrence following surgery for ileitis. The lesion may be confused with ulcerating jejunitis.

Appendiceal Disease

Sometimes CD initially presents in the appendix (Fig. 11.3), making it very difficult to differentiate from ordinary appendicitis because of the similarity of the clinical symptoms. The distinction between these two entities is most easily made if granulomas are found in the appendix.

Esophageal Disease

Esophageal CD occurs, although it is rarer than oral, pharyngeal, or laryngeal involvement. Esophageal disease affects 6% of CD patients (80). Esophageal lesions include aphthous ulcers measuring 2 to 3 mm in size, strictures, esophagitis,

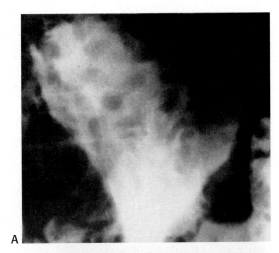
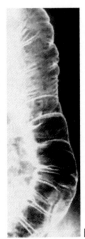
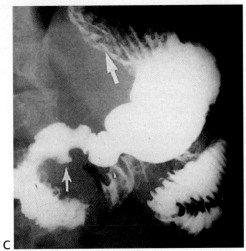

FIG. 11.4. Crohn disease. **A:** Single-contrast examination of duodenal bulb demonstrates numerous aphthous ulcerations. **B:** Double-contrast enema of left colon demonstrates tiny discrete aphthous ulcerations with intervening normal mucosa. **C:** Upper gastrointestinal series demonstrates duodenal ulcer (*smaller arrow*). There is also thickening of the mucosal folds in the remainder of the duodenum and proximal jejunum in this patient with Crohn disease (*larger arrow*).

esophageal ulcers, and granulomas. The diagnosis should not be made unless typical lesions are found elsewhere in the gut.

Gastric Disease

Gastric CD typically involves the distal stomach producing thickening and granulomatous inflammation of the gastric wall, which results in pyloric obstruction and vomiting. Patients often have concomitant duodenal disease. Gastric CD may antedate small bowel involvement, and some of the reported cases of isolated granulomatous gastritis may actually represent early gastric CD. The diagnosis can only be made with certainty if there is associated CD in the small bowel or colon.

Endoscopy exhibits antral stenosis and rigidity; aphthous ulcers; nodules; thickening and blunting of the gastric folds associated with mucosal cobblestoning and denudation; fibrosis; and ultimately stricture formation. Antral stenosis is the most characteristic feature of gastric involvement. Gastric fistulae usually originate from the intestine with direct extension to the stomach (81). Features of gastric CD grossly and radiologically mimic gastric carcinoma or other inflammatory conditions.

Duodenal Disease

CD produces pathologically and radiologically typical lesions in the duodenum in approximately 0.5% to 4% of patients (81). Duodenocolic or duodenoileal fistulae develop, originating in the diseased duodenum or from previous ileocolic anastomoses. Duodenal–enteric fistulae also complicate CD arising in other parts of the gastrointestinal (GI) tract. Usually, but not invariably, duodenal CD coexists with ileal involvement and the duodenal lesions frequently extend proximally to involve the gastric antrum or distally into the jejunum (Fig. 11.4). The clinical features include symptoms of duodenal obstruction and/or ulceration. Duodenal CD predisposes patients to develop pancreatitis. Rare patients with duodenal disease develop massive upper GI hemorrhage.

Crohn Disease in the Elderly

About 5% of patients develop CD after age 60 (82). Older patients range in age from 64 to 85, tend to have a longer delay in diagnosis, have more hematochezia, and have a higher incidence of coexisting diverticular and vascular disease. Elderly patients often have less pain, a palpable abdominal mass, less

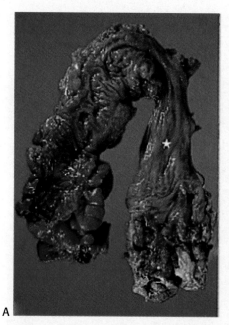
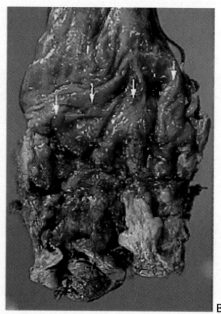

A

B

FIG. 11.5. Proctocolectomy specimen in an elderly individual with Crohn disease. **A:** The sigmoid has become relatively featureless and atrophic, as indicated by the *star*. The most distal portion of the rectosigmoid is involved by active disease. **B:** Higher magnification showing the prominent severe distal disease. The *arrows* indicate the boundary of the normal and the involved portion by active disease, as verified by histologic examination. Significant anorectal disease is present.

small bowel disease, less drug treatment, and no family history of IBD; elderly patients are also less likely to have small intestinal disease. In some series, nearly all patients presenting with CD after age 60 have large bowel involvement (83). Older individuals may have more distal Crohn colitis (Fig. 11.5) than younger patients, who tend to have more extensive colonic involvement. Coexisting anorectal disease may clinically masquerade as diverticulitis. The most reliable hallmarks of CD in older persons include the presence of anorectal disease, rectal bleeding, and fistulae. The anal area may show edematous skin tags, ulcers, fissures, and fistulae. Elderly patients require total colectomy more frequently than those in the younger age groups (84).

Patient Misdiagnosis

Some patients are diagnosed with CD who do not have the disease. Two major reasons account for such a mistaken diagnosis: (a) diseases in organs adjacent to the ileocecum produce a clinical syndrome of acute right lower quadrant pain and inflammation, which could suggest the diagnosis; and (b) neoplastic, vascular, infectious, or other small intestinal diseases mimic CD. Table 11.4 lists diseases that can mimic CD clinically.

Association with Other Diseases

CD associates with extraintestinal diseases that represent part of the inherent disease process (see Extraintestinal Manifestations). Additionally, CD associates with other diseases as listed in Table 11.5.

Extraintestinal Manifestations

Approximately 25% of patients with known CD have a history of at least one extraintestinal manifestation. Multiple

TABLE 11.4   Diseases Clinically Mimicking Crohn Disease

Ulcerative colitis
Yersinia infections of the ileum, appendix, and cecum
Tuberculous infections of the ileum, appendix, and cecum
Acute appendicitis
Appendiceal abscess
Appendiceal mucocele
Meckel diverticulitis
Pelvic inflammatory disease
Ectopic pregnancy
Ovarian cysts and tumors
Cecal diverticulitis
Carcinoma of the cecum spreading to ileum
Ileal carcinoid
Ileal lymphomas, plasmacytoma, and Hodgkin disease
Metastatic carcinoma
Acute terminal ileitis
Ischemic ileitis
Systemic vasculitis
Radiation enteritis
Ileocecal tuberculosis
Amebiasis

TABLE 11.5	Crohn Disease: Associations

Turner syndrome
Autosomal recessive Hermansky-Pudlak syndrome
Cystic fibrosis
Hereditary neutrophilic defects
Glycogen storage type IB
Autoimmune diseases
   Ankylosing spondylitis
   Behçet disease
   Sclerosing cholangitis
   Psoriasis
   Thrombocytopenic purpura
   Systemic lupus erythematosus
   Autoimmune thyroiditis
   Pernicious anemia
   Insulin-dependent diabetes mellitus
   Alopecia areata
   Multiple sclerosis
   Myasthenia gravis
   Scleroderma

extraintestinal manifestations occur in the same patient more frequently than would be expected by chance. Large bowel involvement and longer disease duration predispose the patient to extraintestinal manifestations.

Need for Surgical Intervention

The majority of patients with CD undergo surgery at some time during their lives. Approximately 42% of children with CD require surgical intervention as compared with only 5% of those with UC (85), and approximately 20% require surgical intervention within the first year of diagnosis (86). The remainder undergo surgery at a rate of 5% per year (87). CD patients typically require repeated operations, with 63% of patients undergoing a repeat operation by the 15th postoperative year.

In general, radical resection does not decrease the recurrence rate of the disease, and repeated resections place patients at risk for the development of short bowel syndrome. Therefore, conservative surgical techniques have evolved in recent times to treat patients with CD-associated complications not amenable or responsive to medical therapy. Surgery in CD patients is indicated for treatment of abdominal abscesses, internal or external fistulae, bleeding, and bowel obstruction secondary to strictures, and in patients with medically intractable disease. Many patients experience recurrence of their disease, but many also report an overall improvement in their quality of life following surgery.

Recurrence of Crohn Disease

CD is a recurring chronic illness, with 94% of patients experiencing recurrent disease. Nearly all patients have a recurrence within 10 years of their initial diagnosis. Recurrence occurs most commonly in patients with ileocecal disease (53%) compared with isolated colonic disease (45%) or isolated small bowel disease (44%) (88). Patients who have undergone surgical procedures are particularly prone to recurrent disease. Ileal recurrence is determined in part by the retrograde reflux of the colonic fecal stream, microvascular injury, and ischemia (89,90). Additionally, increased use of acetaminophen and other nonnarcotic analgesics and increased consumption of simple sugars sometimes heralds the development of recurrent disease. For patients whose original disease was ileitis, recurrent disease almost invariably appears just proximal to the ileocolonic anastomosis. For those with an initial colitis or ileocolitis, recurrence develops on either side or both sides of the anastomosis.

Patient Survival

Patients with Crohn disease develop a large number of complications, some of which impact patient survival. Patient survival is not influenced by disease extent at the time of diagnosis. Patients die both from their underlying IBD as well as from associated diseases, including GI cancer, respiratory diseases, and other GI diseases.

Gross Features

The gross features of the bowel reflect the stage of the disease, with the most severe lesions being seen in advanced transmural disease. Patients with severe disease are those most likely to come to resection. Thus, the pathologist is only likely to see the gross pathology of advanced disease.

Lesion Distribution

CD classically involves the distal 15 to 25 cm of the terminal ileum, often in association with disease involving the right colon, but any part of the GI tract may become involved (Table 11.6). Thus, CD can involve the mouth, esophagus, stomach, duodenum, proximal jejunum, ileum, large intestine, and anus. Ileocolic, small intestinal, and upper gastrointestinal CD occurs in approximately 30% to 50%, 25% to 50%, and 5% to 30% of all cases, respectively. Disease limited

TABLE 11.6	Gastrointestinal Forms of Crohn Disease

Acute ileitis
Chronic regional ileitis
Localized disease of small bowel, not in terminal ileum
Extensive small intestinal disease
Ileocolitis with skip lesions
Crohn colitis
Anorectal Crohn disease
Gastric, esophageal, and duodenal Crohn disease

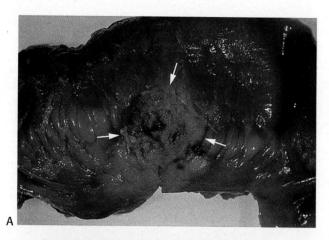

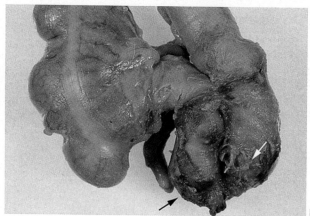

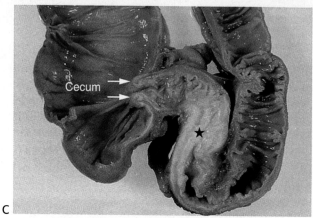

FIG. 11.6. Crohn disease. **A:** Serosal surface of Crohn disease demonstrating the presence of numerous fine adhesions and erythema on the entire serosal aspect. A portion of a fistulous tract was transected in the removal of the specimen from the patient (*arrows*). **B:** Unopened ileocolectomy specimen in patient with Crohn disease. The colon lies to the left and shows prominent taenia coli. The appendix coils around the specimen. The distal ileum is covered with shaggy exudates and portions of transected adhesions (*arrows*). This process extends into the cecum. In the area of the ileocecal valve there is an abscess. **C:** The specimen shown in B has been opened, and the ileocecal valve is cut in cross section (*arrows*). The cecum and ascending colon are present on the left-hand side of the photograph and the terminal ileum is on the right. The portion immediately adjacent to the cecum is markedly stenotic and the terminal ileum lumen is almost completely occluded by the disease (*star*).

to the colon affects 15% to 30% of patients (91,92). The terminal ileum is involved in about 5% of Crohn colitis patients. The involved segments of small intestine vary from 5 to 76 cm in length with an average of 20 cm. Transition from involved to uninvolved areas is usually abrupt in the small bowel, but is less well defined in the large intestine.

Grossly, colonic CD shows three major patterns: (a) diffuse (almost total involvement), (b) stricture formation, and (c) disease mainly confined to the rectum. Any of these forms can exist in isolation or can coexist with other gastrointestinal lesions, especially those involving the terminal ileum. In the colon, diffuse mucosal disease with relatively less involvement of deeper structures can produce an inflammatory pseudopolypoid mucosal pattern indistinguishable from UC, except for its patchy distribution. Patients with CD have a normal rectum in approximately 50% of cases.

External Gross Features

The external surface of the bowel appears reddened, hyperemic, and covered with serosal exudates producing serositis (Fig. 11.6). Areas of serositis appear rough and nodular, often coexisting with dense fibrous adhesions between bowel loops or fixation of the bowel to other abdominal organs, pelvic organs, or the abdominal wall. Fat encircles the antimesenteric serosal surface, producing a pattern known as "creeping fat" (Figs. 11.7 and 11.8). Miliary serosal lesions, the macroscopic equivalent of granulomas, may be seen. The miliary lesions appear as multiple, minute, white nodules resembling peritoneal seeding by carcinoma or the serosal tubercles characteristic of tuberculosis. They are usually distributed along the serosal lymphatics and may be seen on the surface of the adjacent mesentery and peritoneum. These may represent an early stage of the disease. Initially, the area of the distal ileum at the area of the ileocecal valve (Fig. 11.6). Large inflammatory pseudotumors may form at this site, simulating a carcinoma (Fig. 11.6). Granulomata within the lymph nodes are grossly visible as tiny gray-white specks (Fig. 11.9).

Internal Gross Features

The earliest grossly visible mucosal change consists of the formation of an aphthous ulcer overlying lymphoid tissue. As these ulcers enlarge, they may develop a hemorrhagic rim that makes them visible. In their early stages, aphthous ulcers are most easily seen in the colon (Fig. 11.10) because villi tend to obscure their presence in the small intestine. It is important to note that aphthous ulcers are not specific for CD, but may also occur in infectious enterocolitis (see Chapters 6 and 13). In some patients, these tiny ulcers are the only or predominant sign of the disease, whereas in other patients they associate with more severe changes elsewhere in the bowel. Recognition of discrete ulcers in areas of otherwise normal mucosa may precede the development of more flagrant changes of CD by weeks or years.

The small, stellate, aphthous ulcers enlarge into discontinuous, serpiginous, or linear ulcers that then enlarge to form wide-based ulcers (Fig. 11.11). At this stage the mucosa appears reddened and swollen. The ulcers ultimately coalesce longitudinally and transversely. Grossly, the disorder is characterized by segmentally or diffusely arranged serpiginous or longitudinal furrowed ulcers with areas of intervening normal-appearing mucosa. The deep fissuring ulcers of CD differ from the superficial ulcers present in UC. The mucosa demonstrates islands of nonulcerated mucosa interspersed among ulcerated areas (Fig. 11.11), producing a cobblestoned appearance. This feature is also not specific for CD because it occurs in other conditions, such as ischemia.

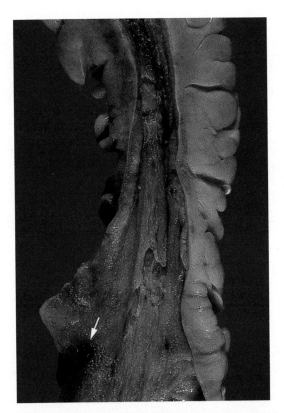

FIG. 11.7. Crohn disease. High power of creeping fat. The figure shows the prominent creeping fat and an area of stenosis. The mucosa appears irregular with shaggy ulcerations. An area of perforation was present, as indicated by the *arrow*. The perforation is surrounded by numerous aphthous ulcers.

intestinal wall remains pliable, even though it may appear slightly thickened (Figs. 11.7 and 11.8). With disease progression, the bowel becomes increasingly fibrotic and rigid (Fig. 11.8). Eventually, strictures may develop, usually in the

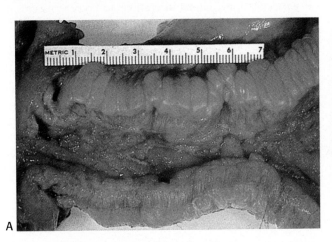
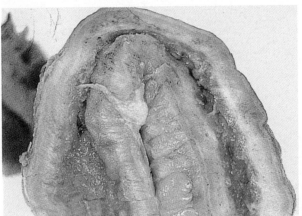

FIG. 11.8. Mucosal thickening in Crohn disease. **A:** Opened small bowel in a patient with Crohn disease. In the central portion of the photograph the bowel wall is markedly thickened and edematous. Creeping fat is seen at the margin of the cut. At both the right- and left-hand margins the bowel widens out and is more normal. **B:** Opened ileal segment in Crohn disease. The bowel wall is markedly thickened. The thickening predominantly is due to dense fibrous tissue. The bowel lumen is almost totally occluded by the scarring process.

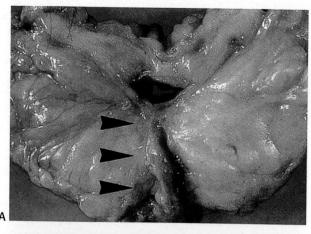

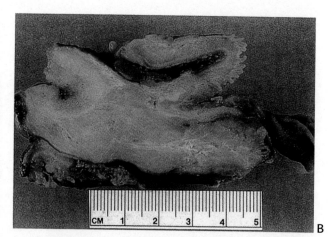

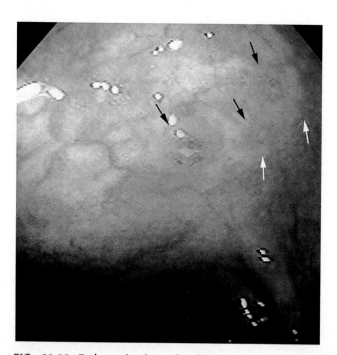

FIG. 11.9. Crohn disease. **A:** The mucosa is at the top of the photo. A fistulous track (*arrowheads*) extends from an abscess coursing through the mesenteric fat. **B:** Cross section through a fixed specimen of ileum in Crohn disease. The loops of bowel are adherent to one another as a result of scarring and fibrosis. **C:** The bowel wall appears markedly thickened with irregular linear ulcers covered by hemorrhagic exudate. Numerous pseudopolyps are present. In addition, a lymph node containing white specks corresponding to granulomas is present (*arrowhead*).

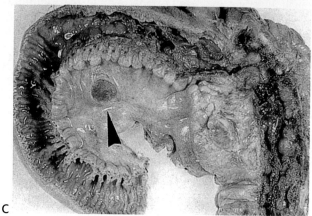

FIG. 11.10. Endoscopic view of aphthous ulcers. Aphthous ulcers appear as erythematous "pimplelike" mucosal lesions. The aphthous ulcers are outlined by the *arrows*.

When the linear ulcers heal, long railroad track–like scars remain (Fig. 11.12). Ulcers often lie close to the resection margins of the specimen and, if left in the patient, may form the basis of recurrent disease. Transmural inflammation predisposes the longitudinal ulcerations to become fissures or fistulae secondarily involving adjacent organs or the abdominal wall. Eventually, dense adhesions form.

With disease progression, the cut surface of the bowel demonstrates full-thickness inflammation, scarring, and fibrosis of the submucosa, muscularis propria, and serosa. The fibrosis is superimposed on other macroscopic features. Intervening normal bowel separates diseased bowel segments, creating skip areas. This patchy pattern of inflammation contrasts with the continuous pattern of inflammation and prominent rectal involvement seen in UC. The mucosa may even become atrophic in longstanding disease.

Abscesses, Fissures, and Fistulae

Fistulae and adhesions (see Figs. 11.9 and 11.13) occur less commonly in patients with colonic involvement than in those with small intestinal disease. Internal and external fistulae form in up to 60% of patients (93). Fistulae occur spontaneously, and are more frequent in patients who have

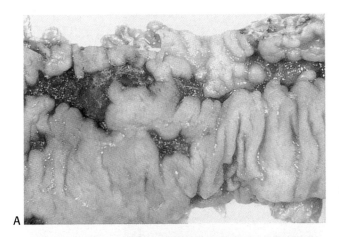

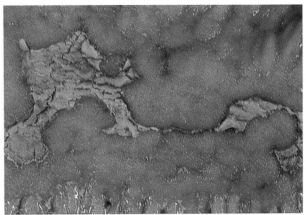

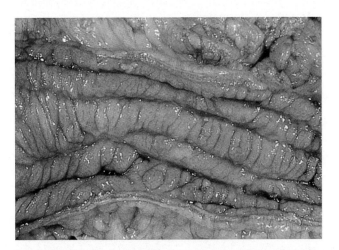

FIG. 11.11. Crohn disease. **A:** Large serpiginous ulcers are present. The ulcers contain granulation tissue and a fibropurulent exudate. The ulcerations extend deep into the bowel wall. The remaining mucosa appears edematous. **B:** Numerous geographic ulcers are present surrounded by mural edema. **C:** Closer magnification picture demonstrating the presence of sharp punched-out ulcers with clean, pearly bases.

had previous surgery and who had residual diseased bowel. If the process remains localized, an abscess forms (Fig. 11.14). Vaginal fistulae commonly occur because of the anatomic proximity of the diseased rectal mucosa to the vagina. They may also result from extension of perirectal abscesses.

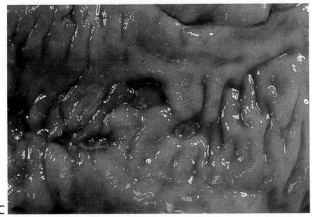

FIG. 11.12. Crohn disease. The bowel is opened. Prominent linear ulcers are present. The combination of ulceration and edema produces long linear ulcers, which produce "railroad tracks" when they heal. Since both linear and transverse ulcers are present, the mucosa has a cobblestone appearance.

Intra-abdominal abscesses develop in patients with CD. These abscesses may be intraperitoneal or, less commonly, retroperitoneal. There is marked preponderance of males in the retroperitoneal abscess group (93).

Perforation only affects 1.5% of CD patients (see Fig. 11.13) (94) because the inflammatory process penetrates the tissues slowly, causing loops of inflamed bowel to adhere to one another, thereby walling off any free perforation that might occur. Perforations result from deep penetration of fissures or fistulae through the bowel wall, from ingestion of some medicines, or from complicating ischemia (Fig. 11.15) or superimposed infection. Patients may also undergo spontaneous free rupture of an abscess into the peritoneal cavity.

Strictures

CD is characterized by strictures in the small and large intestine and in the anorectum. These strictures commonly lead to partial, intermittent obstruction. Strictures and fistulae are more common with ileitis, ileocolitis, and perianal disease than with disease predominating in the colon. The nature of the obstructive symptoms depends on the part of the bowel that is affected. The most severe stenosis usually affects the ileocecal valve. Multiple strictures may be present (Fig. 11.16). The strictures result

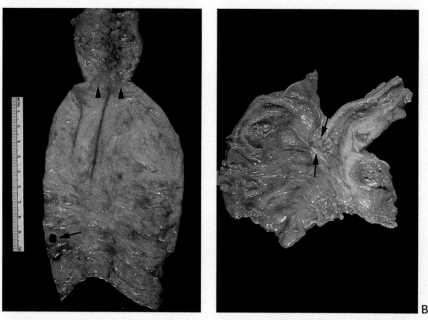

FIG. 11.13. Crohn disease. **A:** Ileum with area of stenosis (*arrowheads*). The proximal bowel became dilated and ruptured (*arrow*). **B:** Portion of ileocolectomy with fistula communicating between the small bowel and the colon (*arrows*). The colon is densely adherent to the small intestine. The small intestine lies to the right of the photograph and shows prominent thickening of the wall. The colon nearby is dilated.

from transmural inflammation, fibrosis, scarring, and fibromuscular proliferation. Rectal strictures are not unique to CD because they also complicate other disorders (Table 11.7).

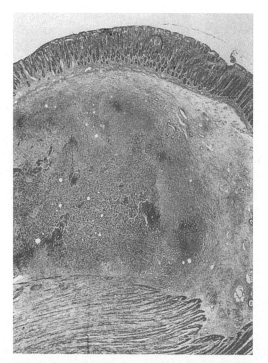

FIG. 11.14. Colonic abscess in a patient with Crohn disease. A large submucosal abscess is present. It expands and occupies the majority of the submucosa on the left-hand and middle portions of the photograph.

Pseudopolyps

Pseudopolyps develop in CD. Many of these are inflammatory in nature, whereas others represent residual mucosal islands (Fig. 11.17). Giant pseudopolyps sometimes form in the colon. These large polyps measure up to 5 cm in height and 2 cm in diameter, and project into the colonic lumen. The lesions have a predilection to involve the transverse colon and splenic flexure, but they occur anywhere in the large intestine. The surfaces exhibit a cribriform appearance and may contain inspissated feces. In addition to the presence of bulky, lobulated polyps, one may also see narrow, tall, filiform polyps.

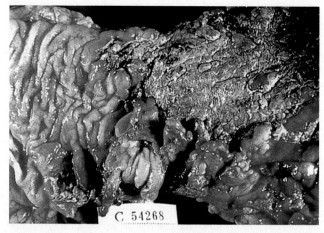

FIG. 11.15. Crohn disease complicated by ischemic colitis. The ischemic area is in the upper right-hand portion of the mucosa and is covered by a fibrinous pseudomembranous exudate.

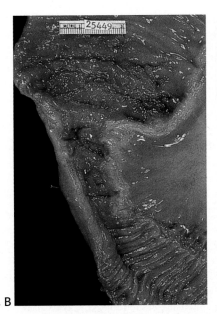
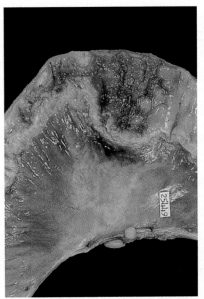
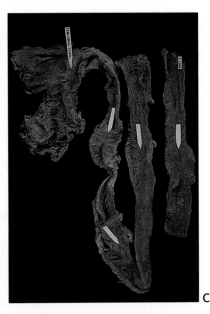

A, B   C

FIG. 11.16. Strictures in Crohn disease. **A:** A several-inch-long strictured area is present in the ileum. The lumen immediately proximal to it is markedly dilated. **B:** This is the same specimen shown in A after fixation highlighting extension of the disease into the surrounding fat. **C:** Numerous strictures are present in the small intestine of this patient. The area just above the ileocecal valve shows several inches of stenosis marked by focal dilation (*upper white arrow* in the middle of the photograph). Immediately beneath this is another area of stricturing. The remaining arrows indicate the presence of fistulous tracts.

HISTOLOGIC FEATURES

General Comments

The ease of making the diagnosis of CD depends on whether one examines biopsy or resection specimens. Resection specimens are more likely to exhibit all of the classic changes of CD, especially those that typically affect the deeper layers of the bowel wall (Table 11.8). The features of CD were originally described in the landmark article published by Crohn and Ginsberg in 1932 (95). Irregularly distributed aphthous-type ulcers, nodular lymphoid aggregates, irregular hypertrophy of the muscularis mucosae, proliferation of submucosal nerves, and loosely organized granulomas occur in various combinations within the mucosa and the submucosa (Fig. 11.18). The biopsy diagnosis of CD remains more problematic because only the mucosa and superficial submucosa are available for examination. In addition, many of the histologic features, including the presence of granulomas, are relatively nonspecific. The pattern and distribution of changes in biopsies are frequently characteristic enough to allow one

to suggest that CD is present and/or enable one to exclude other diagnoses that might be in the differential diagnosis.

Epithelial and Mucosal Changes

The patchy distribution of CD results in an epithelium that exhibits a range of changes, depending on whether or not the tissues are examined early or late in the course of the disease and whether the tissues come from more normal or more diseased parts of the bowel. The epithelium ranges in appearance from completely normal, to acutely damaged, to regenerative

TABLE 11.7 Rectal Strictures: Etiology
Crohn disease
Ulcerative colitis
Ischemic colitis
Chlamydial infections
Syphilis
Status postradiotherapy

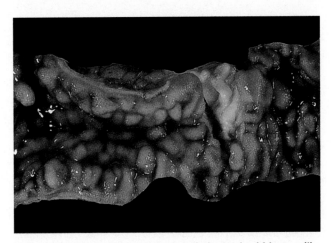

FIG. 11.17. Mucosal polyposis. Irregularly sized cobblestonelike structures are present. They represent residual islands of mucosa. The clefts between them represent linear ulcers.

TABLE 11.8	Resection Features That Suggest a Diagnosis of Crohn Disease

Transmural inflammation

Focal or segmental ulceration

Deep fissures with knifelike clefts passing into the bowel wall

Deep sinus tracts that extend into or through the muscularis propria

Focal lymphocyte collections (lymphoid nodules) in all bowel layers, including the serosal fat

Submucosal widening

Lymphangiectasia, especially in submucosa

Confluent linear ulcers

Perivascular inflammation along the perforating vessels (vascular tracking)

Intestinal wall thickening secondary to fibrosis

Inflammation of the superficial muscularis propria strongly suggests the presence of Crohn disease

Neuronal hyperplasia

Increased vasoactive intestinal polypeptide content in nerves

Serosal inflammation (sometimes including granulomas and lymphoid nodules)

Absence of known etiology (i.e., infection or ischemia)

(Fig. 11.19). In longstanding CD, the crypts and villi show marked distortion of the normal architecture. Distorted glandular architecture is characterized by areas of glandular irregularity and branching (Figs. 11.20 and 11.21). This feature is best appreciated in sections of crypts cut in a plane perpendicular to the muscularis mucosae. In sections cut parallel to the muscularis mucosae, regenerated crypts can be recognized by the presence of cross sections of glands that show variable diameters (Fig. 11.22) and an uneven distribution.

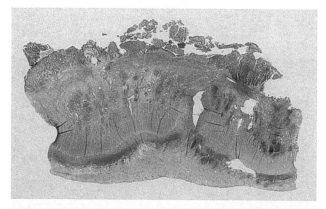

FIG. 11.18. Whole mount sections of Crohn disease. The mucosal surface demonstrates thickening with areas of ulceration and denudation. The submucosa is considerably thickened and contains numerous prominent lymphoid aggregates as evidenced by the darker circular areas. The muscularis propria appears hypertrophic. There is a prominent serosal exudate. Lymphoid aggregates are also seen on the serosal surface. This photograph demonstrates transmural inflammation.

Distorted glands often show epithelial hyperplasia (Fig. 11.23), crypt abscesses, epithelial cell degeneration, and ulceration (Figs. 11.24 and 11.25). In the small intestine, villi become distorted or atrophic and one commonly sees pyloric metaplasia, especially in the ileum. The presence of distorted villi and/or crypts and areas of pyloric metaplasia or increased numbers of Paneth cells, especially in the left colon, indicates that the disease is chronic in nature.

The mucosa often appears cobblestoned and mildly polypoid, but not to the extent seen in UC. Although focal crypt abscesses affect patients with CD, they are often not as numerous as in UC. Regenerative changes occur at ulcer margins, but the mucosa away from ulcers may appear normal except for a lymphoplasmacytic infiltrate in the basal part of the lamina propria. Goblet cell depletion and reactive epithelial cells are present only in areas of severe inflammation. Active apoptosis affects the deeper parts of the glands. Areas of mucosal fibrosis may be predictive for CD. In patients with chronic disease, the mucosa may exhibit localized areas of hyperplasia lined by prominent and hyperplastic goblet cells (Fig. 11.23).

Aphthous and Other Ulcers

Two distinctive types of ulceration affect both the small and large intestines. The first is the histologic equivalent of the grossly evident aphthous ulcer. This lesion develops even before inflammatory cells diffusely infiltrate the lamina propria.

Antigen entry into M cells might lead to the proliferation of antigen-sensitized cells and granuloma formation. The underlying lymphoid nodule may contain giant cells or granulomas. As the lesion progresses, it superficially ulcerates, obliterating its associated lymphoid follicle (Figs. 11.24 and 11.25). A thin stream of mucus, neutrophils, and inflammatory debris exudes from the ulcer mouth and empties into the bowel lumen (Figs. 11.24 and 11.25). The ulcers progressively enlarge, forming a continuum with the larger ulcers normally seen in CD (Fig. 11.26). Larger ulcers may eventually become lined by a single layer of atrophic cuboidal epithelial cells. There is an associated reduction in the number of crypts and loss of villi in the small bowel.

The second type of ulcer is the knifelike fissure, which occurs at right angles to the long axis of the bowel (Fig. 11.27). These may extend through the bowel wall and are likely the basis for fistula formation. Fissures branch and penetrate deeply into the underlying bowel wall, producing adhesions, fistulae, abscesses, and peri-intestinal inflammatory pseudotumors (Fig. 11.28). Fissures contain acute inflammatory cells and a granulation tissue lining with conspicuous pale, plump histiocytic cells. The latter resemble the epithelioid histiocytes seen in granulomas. Giant cells may also be present.

Healed ulcers result in architectural distortion, pyloric metaplasia (Fig. 11.29), and a thickened or duplicated muscularis mucosae often associated with a marked dense sub-

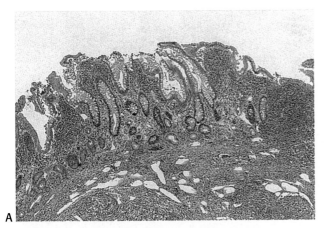

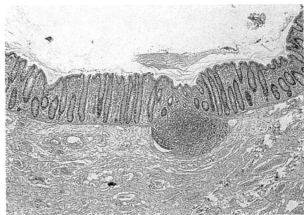

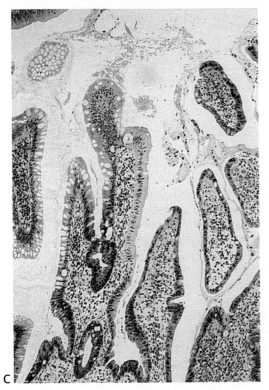

FIG. 11.19. Variable histologic features of Crohn disease (CD). **A:** This picture is from a resection specimen and shows prominent mucosal and submucosal inflammation with marked lymphangiectasia. Areas of re-epithelializing ulceration are present at the right-hand portion of the photograph. **B:** Portion of colonic mucosa in a patient with CD showing essentially normal histologic features. **C:** Portion of small bowel showing marked regenerative changes at the bases of the crypt and extension of the proliferative zone up along the sides of the crypt. Focal chronic inflammation is present, particularly at the right-hand side of the photograph. The villi are fused, hyperplastic, and irregularly shaped.

mucosal fibrosis. As a result, it is often impossible to distinguish the muscularis mucosae from the submucosa or underlying muscularis propria. Fibroblasts and myofibroblasts proliferate in these areas of fibrosis, usually with accompanying chronic inflammatory cells. Fibrosis extends from the bowel wall to involve adjacent structures and traps within it lobules of fat that may demonstrate variable degrees of fat necrosis.

Mucosal Metaplasia

Patients with chronic disease often develop pyloric metaplasia (Fig. 11.29), especially in the ileum. The large intestine often develops Paneth cell metaplasia. In the small bowel, the number of Paneth cells may increase, although they are normally present in this location.

The cells in pyloric metaplasia, also known as aberrant pyloric glands, have also come to be known as ulcer-associated cell lineage (UACL) cells (96). This distinctive cell lineage typically arises in sites of enteric ulceration, most notably in the ulcerated gut in CD. The pyloric glands usually occur singly or in clusters in the mucosa adjacent to ulcer margins. They are also found near single discrete ulcers in the edematous segments away from involved mucosal areas.

These cells share many features of pyloric and Brunner glands, although they do not extend deeper than the muscularis mucosae, a feature that distinguishes them from Brunner glands. The regular acinar glands have a coiled tubular neck and therefore the entire neck is rarely seen in a single section. They extend down to, but usually not through, the muscularis mucosae and have a number of terminal branches that are given off at right angles to the neck,

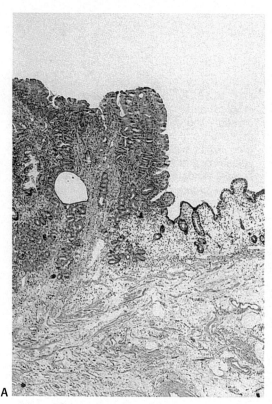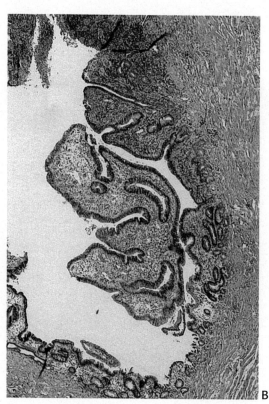

FIG. 11.20. Histologic features of Crohn disease. **A:** A portion of small intestine from a resection specimen showing the focality of the changes. The epithelium on the right-hand side of the photograph is greatly simplified and edematous. On the left-hand side of the photograph, one sees an expansion of the mucosal thickness due to the presence of large numbers of pyloric glands. The villi appear atrophic and the lamina propria is infiltrated with mononuclear cells. The underlying muscularis mucosae appears markedly distorted. **B:** Crohn colitis from a resection specimen. The mucosa demonstrates variable inflammation. The epithelium appears markedly regenerative and mucin depleted. The underlying muscularis mucosae is fused with the muscularis propria.

so that they are usually seen in cross section. The glands are lined by clear or pale-staining columnar cells containing indistinct neutral mucin granules. The nuclei appear oval or round and are located near the base of the cell. The glandu-

lar structures have a looser architectural pattern than either pyloric or Brunner glands (96).

Lymphatic Dilation (Lymphangiectasia)

Another notable feature of CD is submucosal lymphatic dilation (Fig. 11.30), which commonly coexists with edema and lymphoid hyperplasia. Plasma cells, eosinophils, and neutrophils may infiltrate along the dilated vessels. In more advanced stages of the disease, fibrous tissue replaces the edema.

Nature of the Inflammatory Infiltrate

Early morphologic lesions include increased numbers of mucosal plasma cells, lymphocytes, macrophages, mast cells, eosinophils, and neutrophils in all layers of the bowel wall. A basal lymphocytic–plasmacytic infiltrate occupies the lower part of the mucosa (Fig. 11.31). In active IBD, one sees a constant emigration of neutrophils and monocytes from the circulation into the inflamed mucosa and through the epithelium into the intestinal lumen. Neutrophils infiltrate the intestinal epithelium, forming the lesion known as cryptitis.

FIG. 11.21. Crohn disease. Portion of colonic mucosa showing marked glandular distortion with relative preservation of the mucinous content within the glands.

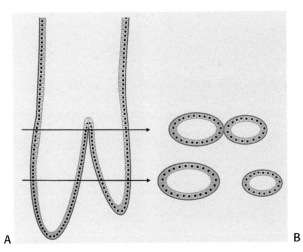

FIG. 11.22. Diagrammatic representation of the appearance of regenerative crypts. **A:** Regenerative branched crypts are relatively easy to recognize when they are cut in a plane perpendicular to the muscularis mucosae. One sees crypt after crypt demonstrating irregular branching often with other features of chronicity, such as Paneth cell metaplasia or pyloric metaplasia. One must be careful in making the diagnosis of regeneration based on the finding of a single "branched crypt," since the edges of mucosal territories may appear branched. For this reason, one would like to see several branched crypts in a row to make the diagnosis. **B:** Crypts cut in cross section are more difficult to recognize as being regenerative. Clues to their regenerative nature include variability in crypt diameter when one measures each through an equatorial plane. Additionally, the presence of back-to-back glands in the absence of significant cytologic atypia also suggests regeneration.

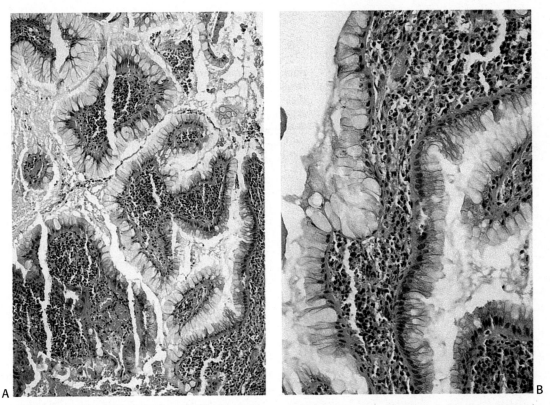

FIG. 11.23. Mucosal hyperplasia in Crohn disease. **A:** Low-power magnification photograph of a portion of the terminal ileum showing complex glandular structures cut in cross section. These represent sections through villi. The villi are lined by cells containing hyperplastic goblet cells. The cores of the villi contain dense mononuclear cell infiltrates. **B:** Higher magnification in an area of junction between the hyperplastic goblet cells (*left*) and more normal-appearing goblet cells (*right*).

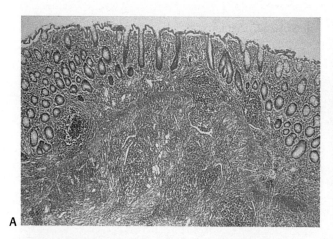

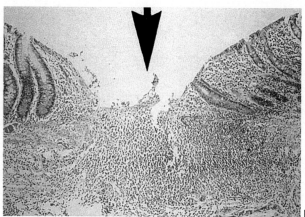

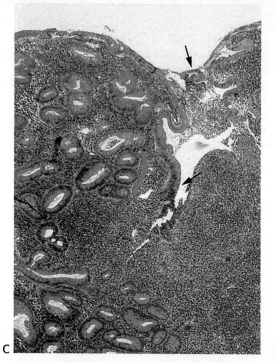

FIG. 11.24. Progression of aphthous ulcers in Crohn disease. **A:** The colonic mucosa and submucosa contain prominent lymphoid aggregates. The lamina propria is infiltrated with mononuclear cells. Mild regenerative features are present. The goblet cell population is still intact. **B:** Wider-based aphthous ulcer (*arrow*). **C:** Aphthous ulcer. An area of ulceration is noted over a lymphoid aggregate. Inflammatory debris is present in the ulcer tract overlying the lymphoid aggregate (*arrow*). The epithelium on both sides of the ulceration is regenerative (*arrow*).

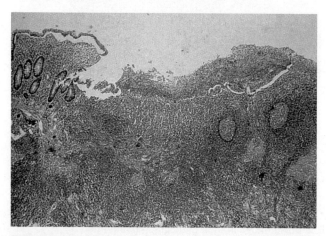

FIG. 11.25. Crohn disease. Further extension of the aphthous ulcer. There is more extensive inflammation and wider area of ulceration extending from the aphthous ulcer than one sees in Figure 11.24.

Collections of granulocytes within the crypt lumens are called crypt abscesses (Fig. 11.32). Variable edema and/or fibrosis are present, depending on the stage of the disease (see Fig. 11.18). The inflammatory infiltrate often also surrounds submucosal and serosal lymphatics and blood vessels, where they penetrate the muscularis propria. Denser lymphocytic aggregates also lie in the submucosa away from the lymphatics or they may appear scattered throughout all layers of the bowel wall (see Fig. 11.18).

An early but nonspecific finding of CD is an increased number of eosinophils and macrophages (Fig. 11.33) in the lamina propria beneath the surface epithelium. Eosinophils degranulate in ulcerated areas, leading to deposition of eosinophil cationic protein and cathepsin G. These proteins contribute to the inflammatory process (97).

Mucosal and submucosal mast cell hyperplasia and degranulation also represent constant features of both UC and CD. Mucosal mast cells maintain a direct association with substance

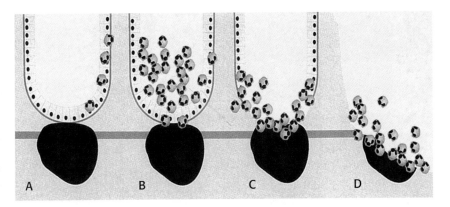

FIG. 11.26. Diagrammatic summary of the development of aphthous ulcers. **A:** Neutrophils infiltrate the epithelium at the base of the crypt. **B:** Larger numbers of neutrophils accumulate. **C:** The proteolytic enzymes released by the neutrophilic infiltrate destroy the epithelium in the crypt overlying the lymphoid follicle. **D:** Areas of microulceration develop, eventually destroying the crypt.

P (SP)-containing nerves, as well as with capillaries, blood vessels, Schwann cells, nerve fibers, myofibroblasts, and collagen fibers. They also lie along epithelial cells, providing an anatomic basis for communication between nerves and the immune system. Inflammatory mediators released from mast cells contribute to the pathophysiology of CD due to the release of preformed and newly generated inflammatory mediators (98). The bowel develops focal edema and inflammation in the lamina propria, submucosa, and deeper layers, even in the presence of a more or less normal-appearing mucosa.

Dendritic cells lie adjacent to granulomas and fissures. The number of macrophages in the lamina propria increases. They are arranged in bandlike zones at the bottom of ulcers or fissures, perhaps playing a scavenging role directed against microbial agents or dietary substances penetrating the GI wall through the mucosal defects. Aggregates of macrophages lead to the formation of noncaseating granulomas.

Lymphoid Aggregates

Lymphoid aggregates, which may contain germinal centers, generally lie at the mucosal–submucosal junction. Lymphoid aggregates form even in the absence of granulomas, and they may be more helpful than granulomas in establishing the diagnosis of CD (Figs. 11.18 and 11.34). Lymphoid aggregates occur in both CD and UC; however, when they lie in the submucosa or deeper in the bowel and are separated from the muscularis mucosae, and when the lymphoid aggregates coexist with submucosal edema or fibrosis in the presence of an intact mucosa, the diagnosis is more likely to be CD than UC. Prominent lymphoid aggregates also commonly affect the serosal fat in CD. Finally, the lymphoid tissue of the terminal ileum may become hyperplastic, forming multiple lymphoid polyps.

Granulomas

Compact sarcoidlike granulomas are the sine qua non for the diagnosis of CD (Figs. 11.35 and 11.36) and, when present, are a reliable histopathologic criterion for differentiating CD from UC. Granulomas assume particular diagnostic significance when seen in tissues remote from areas of ulceration in situations where foreign body granulomas are unlikely. Although the presence of granulomas represents a useful diagnostic feature for CD, they can be seen in various other conditions (see Table 11.9).

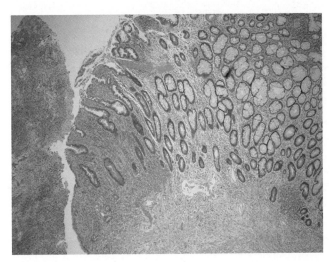

FIG. 11.27. Ulceration in Crohn disease. A deep knifelike ulcer is present.

TABLE 11.9 Differential Diagnosis of Granulomas in the Intestine

Mucin granuloma	Fungal infections
Bacterial infections	Chlamydial infections
Campylobacter	Sarcoid
Yersinia	Crohn disease
Salmonella	Hermansky-Pudlak syndrome
Shigella	Diverticulosis
Escherichia coli	
Mycobacterium	
tuberculosis	
Neisseria	
gonorrhoeae	
Clostridium difficile	
Treponema pallidum	

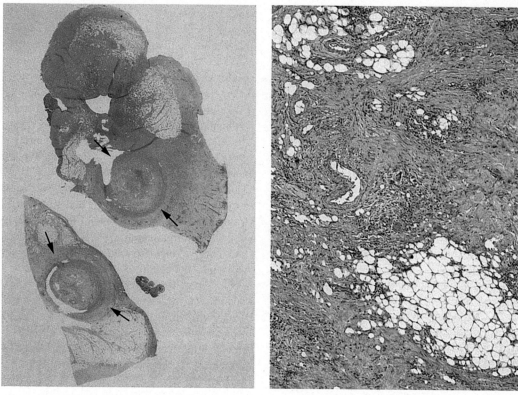

FIG. 11.28. Transmural inflammation in Crohn disease. **A:** Cross section through the area of the appendix showing marked periappendiceal inflammation. The patient presented with a right lower quadrant mass (an inflammatory pseudotumor). The appendix is outlined by the *arrows*. **B:** Prominent submucosal inflammation with cicatrizing fibrosis.

Pathologists should be cautious when diagnosing a granuloma in biopsy material. Ruptured crypts release mucin into the lamina propria, stimulating the formation of mucin granulomas (Fig. 11.37). Such mucin granulomas may include mature macrophages and foreign body–type giant cells. They can be recognized because of the predominance of giant cells, their association with and orientation around perforated crypts (Fig. 11.37), and their positivity for mucin stains. Mucin granulomas are not specific for CD because they occur in any situation that results in crypt destruction with epithelial cell loss, including UC.

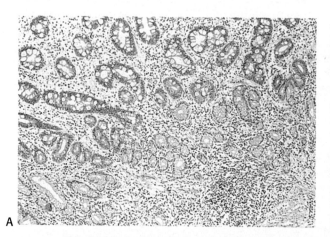

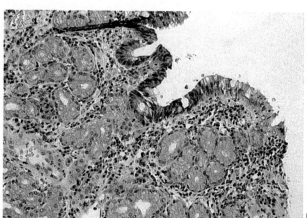

FIG. 11.29. Ileal pyloric metaplasia. **A:** Low power of the basal portion of the mucosa showing expansion of the mucosal thickness. Prominent pylori glands lie beneath the intestinal epithelium and above the muscularis mucosae. **B:** Higher magnification of pyloric metaplasia in a different case showing the presence of pyloric glandular collections in the basal mucosa. In the center of the photograph, it connects with an actively regenerating crypt.

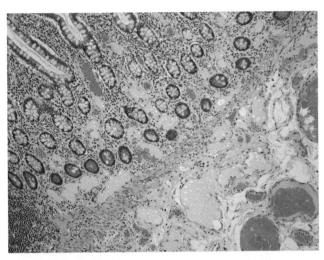

FIG. 11.30. Lymphangiectasia in Crohn disease. This section from the ileum of a patient with Crohn disease shows prominent dilation of the lymphatics in the submucosa and deep mucosa.

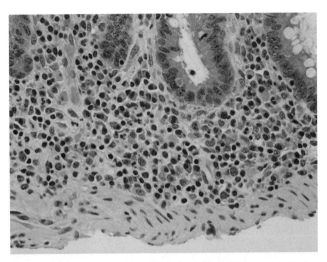

FIG. 11.31. Basal plasmacytosis in inflammatory bowel disease. The lamina propria of the deep mucosa contains numerous plasma cells. Scattered lymphocytes and eosinophils are also present.

The reported frequency with which granulomas are identified in CD varies markedly between studies. Possible explanations for this include the criteria used to diagnose granulomas; whether or not isolated giant cells are included among granulomas; the number of biopsies obtained; and the number of sections examined. Granulomas are found in the bowel wall in 50% to 87% of colectomy specimens, in 15% to 36% of colonoscopic biopsies, and in 20% to 38% of regional lymph nodes (87,99,100). CD granulomas do not usually affect the regional lymph nodes when they are absent in the bowel wall.

Sometimes the granulomas are quite small (microgranulomas). Microgranulomas consist of only a few histiocytes, and are easily overlooked (Fig. 11.36). In one study, 16% of granulomas were so small as to be seen in only 6 of 90 serial sections. Isolated mucosal or submucosal giant cells are seen in 13% of patients (99).

Fewer granulomas occur in the ileum than in the colon. Granulomas progressively increase in number from the ileum to a maximum number in the rectum (101). The granulomas also occur in various other tissues and organs, including the lymph nodes, pancreas, mesentery,

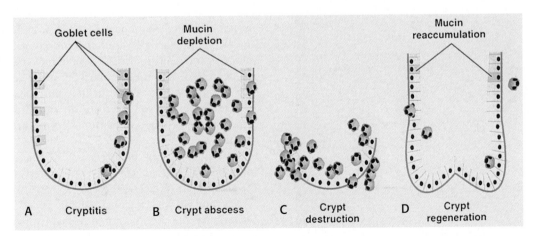

FIG. 11.32. Diagrammatic representation of the different forms acute inflammation takes in inflammatory bowel disease. **A:** When neutrophils infiltrate the epithelium without causing destruction, the lesion is termed cryptitis. **B:** When a large number of neutrophils infiltrate the glandular lumen, the lesion is referred to as a crypt abscess. **C:** Because the neutrophils contain large numbers of lysosomal enzymes, they destroy the underlying crypt and the acute inflammation extends into the surrounding lamina propria. This is sometimes referred to as crypt herniation. **D:** In time, these changes resolve with new epithelium repopulating the crypt. Epithelial cells migrate upward and again reaccumulate mucin within them. Variable numbers of neutrophils may be present at this stage.

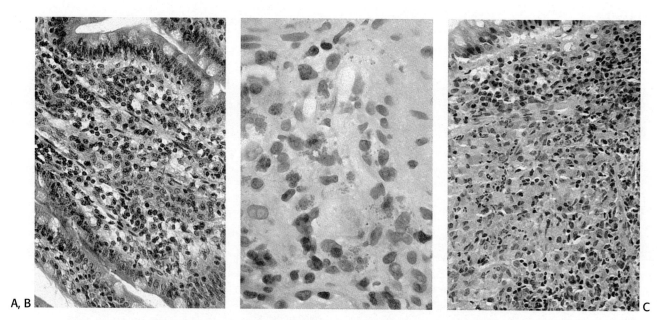

FIG. 11.33. Inflammation in Crohn disease. **A:** Prominent mononuclear cell infiltrate consisting mainly of lymphocytes and plasma cells. There is a mild increase in intraepithelial lymphocytes. **B:** The lamina propria contains a large number of eosinophils and mast cells recognizable by their prominent reddish granules. These cells are actively degranulating. **C:** Localized histiocytic collection surrounded by lymphocytes, plasma cells, and eosinophils.

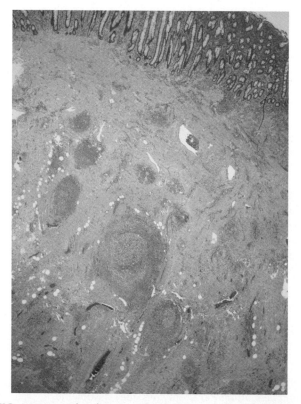

FIG. 11.34. Crohn disease. Inflammation extends through the full thickness of the bowel wall. Prominent lymphoid aggregates are present within the submucosa and muscularis propria.

peritoneum, liver, lung, kidney, and, occasionally, bones, joints, and skeletal muscle. The presence of granulomas does not indicate disease activity, nor does it affect the postoperative recurrence rate.

The granulomas consist of small, localized, well-formed, loose or more compact aggregates of epithelioid histiocytes with or without Langerhans giant cells, often with a surrounding cuff of lymphocytes (see Figs. 11.35 and 11.36). Nodal granulomas also contain centrally located T lymphocytes and dendritic cells. Older lesions may show varying degrees of hyalinization and fibrosis. The granulomas may be numerous or very difficult to find. Granulomas that have definite foci of necrosis or suppuration, or are restricted to the edges of ruptured crypts, are not specific for CD.

Granulomas may be observed anywhere within the intestinal wall and along blood vessels or nerves, especially in the submucosa (Fig. 11.35), mucosa (Fig. 11.36), and subserosa, and in the regional lymph nodes (Fig. 11.38). Granulomas may lie adjacent to dilated lymphatics, causing compression of the lymphatic wall or projecting within the lumen of lymphatic spaces (Fig. 11.39). Sometimes granulomas are present in the lamina propria or in the wall of microabscesses of aphthoid ulcers.

On those rare occasions when microorganisms are found within the granulomas, they probably represent secondary invaders.

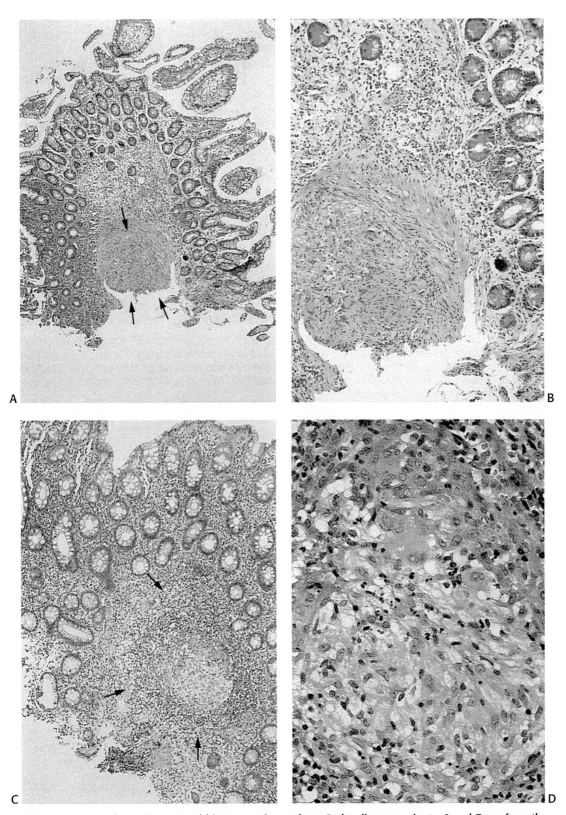

FIG. 11.35. Granulomas in mucosal biopsy specimens from Crohn disease patients. **A** and **B** are from the terminal ileum, and show the presence of a prominent granuloma just beneath the muscularis mucosae. Figure A provides a low-power magnification overview showing the prominence and nodular arrangement of the granuloma (*arrows*). The lower left-hand corner of the specimen is more intensely infiltrated with mononuclear cells when compared with the rest of the specimen. **B:** Higher magnification of the granuloma in the basal epithelium. **C** and **D** represent a colonic mucosal biopsy showing a prominent granuloma. The overlying epithelium in C appears regenerative. The granuloma is surrounded by a dense cuff of lymphocytes (*arrows*). **D:** Higher magnification of the granuloma.

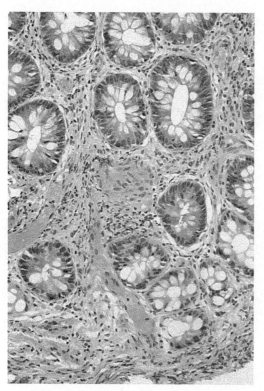

FIG. 11.36. Microgranuloma in a colonic biopsy from a patient with Crohn disease. Note the presence of a compact histiocytic granuloma in the basal portion of the mucosa. The glands surrounding the lesion appear mildly regenerative.

Vascular Lesions

Some postulate that CD results from an underlying vascular disease. The changes appear primarily degenerative or inflammatory in nature. Obliterating endarteritis, chronic phlebitis, and other vascular lesions affect approximately 5% of patients (Figs. 11.40 and 11.41). Obliterative changes include intimal proliferation, subintimal fibrosis, medial hypertrophy, medial fibrosis, and adventitial fibrosis, all without a significant inflammatory cell component. Degenerative arterial lesions may narrow the vascular lumen due to duplication of the internal elastic lamina with medial hypertrophy. Venous lesions feature an irregular vascular sclerosis with thickening of the wall due to hyperplasia of fibrous, elastic, and muscular tissues.

The inflammatory lesions consist of perivascular inflammation and chronic inflammatory and/or granulomatous cell infiltrates associated with an obliterative vasculopathy. Lymphocytes and plasma cells infiltrate one or more layers of small arteries or arterioles, leading to interruption of the internal elastic fibers. Areas of thrombosis are rare.

The vascular changes seen in CD must be distinguished from a primary systemic vasculitis involving the GI tract. When a primary vasculitis affects a patient with CD, extraintestinal manifestations of the disorder are usually evident.

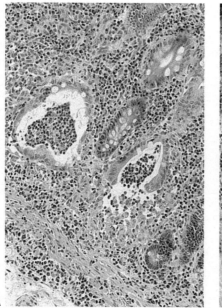
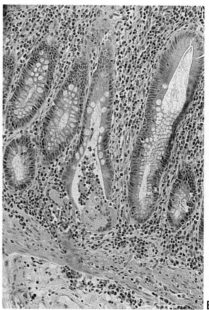

A

B

FIG. 11.37. Early mucin granuloma in a mucosal biopsy from a patient with ulcerative colitis. This specimen shows evidence of basal plasmacytosis, which is most evident in B. **A:** One sees several crypt abscesses. The right one has ruptured and herniated with extension into the surrounding lamina propria. Histiocytic cells collect at the area of herniation. **B:** A crypt that has ruptured and is associated with two giant cells intermingling with apoptotic cell fragments and with extravasating inflammatory cells. These lesions have a completely different appearance than the microgranulomas associated with Crohn disease. Compare this photograph with Figure 11.36.

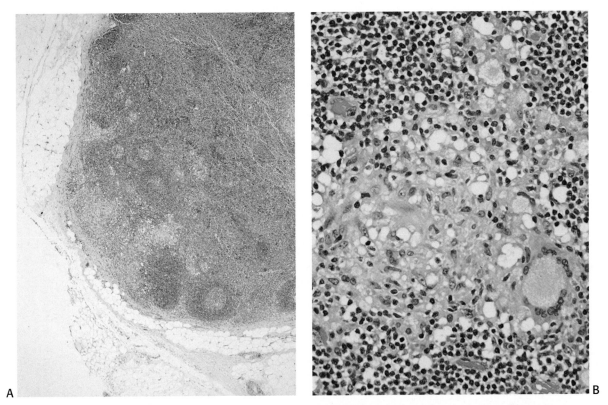

FIG. 11.38. Granulomatous lymphadenitis in Crohn disease. **A:** Numerous compact, nonnecrotizing granulomas are present in this peri-intestinal lymph node from a patient with Crohn disease. **B:** Higher magnification showing the compact sarcoidlike granulomas. A multinucleated giant cell is present in the upper right.

Neural Changes

The autonomic neural plexuses often appear hypertrophic in CD. Large, abnormal, irregular, fusiform nerve bundles and nerve trunks are present throughout the mucosa, submucosa,

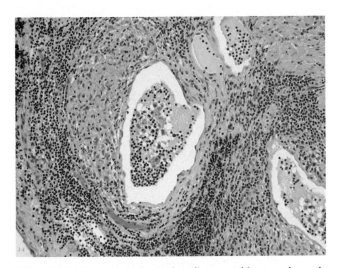

FIG. 11.39. Granuloma in Crohn disease. This granuloma is arising in association with a dilated submucosal lymphatic. Granulomas in Crohn disease are commonly located adjacent to lymphatics.

and muscularis propria (Figs. 11.42 and 11.43). These often contain increased numbers of ganglion cells. Occasionally, striking plexiform neuromatous proliferations associate with tortuous thick-walled arterioles. The nerve fibers contain increased amounts of vasoactive intestinal peptide (VIP) and substance P (102). They express MHC class I antigens (103) and thus the abnormal nerves become infiltrated with mast cells, lymphocytes, and plasma cells (Figs. 11.42 and 11.43). The nerves also show evidence of extensive axonal and dendritic swelling and degeneration.

Strictures

Stricture formation characterizes CD, especially in the small bowel. These strictures result from fibroblast proliferation and increased collagen deposition in the bowel wall (Fig. 11.44). The fibrosis extends along lymphatics and vascular planes and also involves the serosa and pericolonic tissues. Sclerosing lymphangitis, proliferative endophlebitis, and endarteritis are the end result of many of the inflammatory and fibrosing processes.

Some CD patients develop distinctive polypoid lesions in stricturing areas. These consist of proliferations of vessels, nerves, and muscular tissue, sometimes referred to as neuromuscular hamartomas. Grossly, one sees a cluster of sessile polyps covering normal mucosa. Although the lesions have

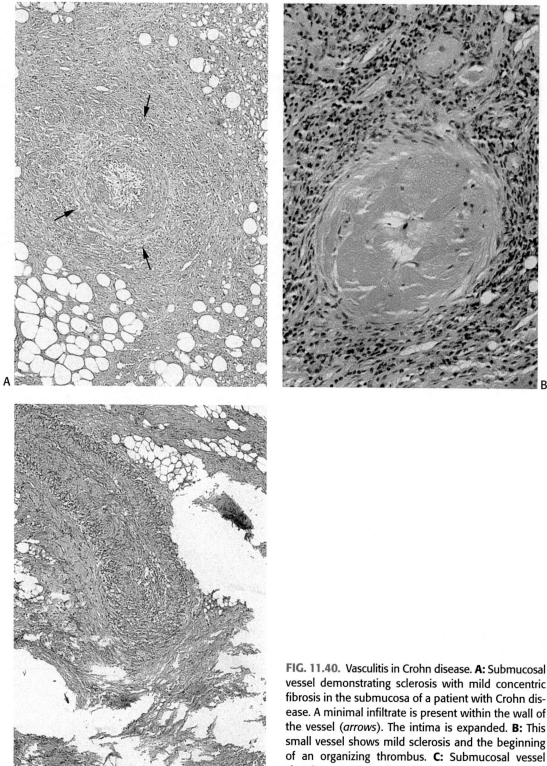

FIG. 11.40. Vasculitis in Crohn disease. **A:** Submucosal vessel demonstrating sclerosis with mild concentric fibrosis in the submucosa of a patient with Crohn disease. A minimal infiltrate is present within the wall of the vessel (*arrows*). The intima is expanded. **B:** This small vessel shows mild sclerosis and the beginning of an organizing thrombus. **C:** Submucosal vessel showing prominent chronic vasculitis. The entire wall of the vessel is infiltrated by mononuclear cells.

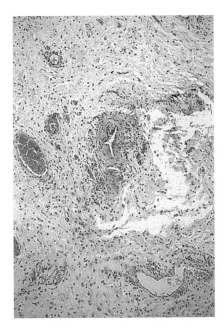

FIG. 11.41. Vasculitis in Crohn disease. Not all cases of vasculitis are as dramatic as those illustrated in Figure 11.40. This patient with CD had only minimal vascular inflammation. Such changes might be seen in a patient with severe ulcerative colitis, so that these features may show histologic overlap.

been described as hamartomas, it is more likely that they represent reparative lesions (Fig. 11.45).

Pseudopolyps

Several types of polypoid lesions develop in CD. One type consists solely of inflammatory and regenerative tissues (Figs. 11.46 and 11.47). These fingerlike polyps arise in both the small and the large bowel. They contain granulation tis-

sue and variable degrees of inflammation, sometimes covered by regenerating surface epithelium. Sometimes pseudopolyps are removed endoscopically. Other polyps contain mucosa, muscularis mucosae, edematous submucosa, submucosal fibrosis, and smooth muscle hyperplasia. These represent residual mucosal islands.

Histologically, giant pseudopolyps consist of complex processes that branch and fuse to form a honeycomb pattern (Fig. 11.48). They contain an inflamed mucosa with intramucosal hemorrhage and fibrosis (Fig. 11.48). The lamina propria and surface epithelium become heavily infiltrated by plasma cells, eosinophils, lymphocytes, and neutrophils. The latter sometimes form crypt abscesses. Granulomas may also be present. Erosions, granulation tissue, and pyloric gland metaplasia can also be present. The lamina propria consists of small blood vessels, loose fibrous tissues, and smooth muscle fibers derived from the muscularis mucosae.

Displaced Epithelium

It is not uncommon to encounter displaced epithelium in resection specimens of CD patients. This entity is referred to as enteritis cystica profunda or colitis cystica profunda when it affects the small bowel or colon, respectively (Fig. 11.49). Enteritis cystica profunda occurs less commonly than its colonic counterpart, colitis cystica profunda. Displaced epithelium results from epithelial implantation into the submucosa, muscularis propria, or serosa following mucosal ulceration or the formation of mucosal microdiverticula, a common event in CD patients. Mucosal repair following regeneration of an ulcer leaves the detached epithelium buried in the submucosa. It eventually becomes covered by an intact mucosa (Fig. 11.49). Displaced epithelium also results from epithelialization of fissures or fistulous tracts. The displaced epithelium often becomes cystically dilated, containing large mucin accumulations.

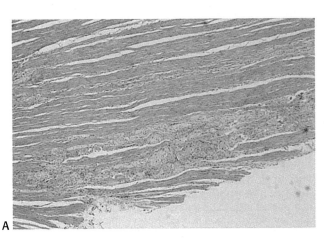
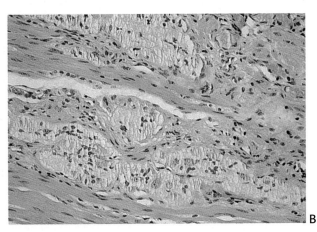

FIG. 11.42. Neural hyperplasia in Crohn disease. **A:** Low magnification showing the presence of prominent ganglia and supporting neural elements in this muscularis propria. **B:** Higher magnification.

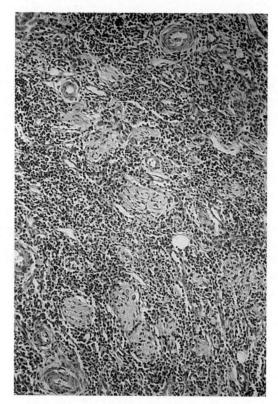

FIG. 11.43. Submucosal inflammation in Crohn disease. The photograph is taken at the midportion of the submucosa and shows an intense mononuclear infiltrate and cross sections of numerous hyperplastic neural structures.

Grossly, the bowel wall appears thickened. The cut surface of the bowel discloses the presence of numerous cystic submucosal spaces. These are often quite prominent and glisten because of their mucinous content. The mucosa overlying such lesions usually demonstrates histologic evidence of active or healed CD. Histologically, one sees mucus-filled cysts in the submucosa, muscularis propria, and serosa. These are lined by cuboidal to columnar epithelium containing numerous goblet cells, enterocytes, and Paneth cells, all supported by a normal lamina propria. Sometimes the cyst lining disappears due to pressure atrophy from large intracystic mucinous accumulations.

Sometimes it is difficult to determine whether the displaced epithelium represents an invasive mucinous carcinoma or merely displaced epithelium, especially when lamina propria does not surround the glands or when the benign epithelium produces excessive amounts of mucin, resulting in large mucinous cysts containing scant epithelial elements (Fig. 11.50). Features that help to rule out malignancy include the absence of desmoplasia, the presence of surrounding lamina propria, and an absence of cytologic atypia within the displaced glands. Cytologic atypia and areas of desmoplasia around angular, irregularly shaped glands characterize invasive cancers, particularly of the nonmucinous type.

In some cases, it may be impossible to determine whether one is dealing with displaced epithelium or an invasive cancer. Sometimes careful sampling and examination of the surface epithelium helps resolve the diagnostic dilemma. If the surface epithelium appears dysplastic, the possibility of an invasive lesion increases.

Serosal and Mesenteric Changes

The subserosa becomes considerably thickened, often as the result of hyperplasia of the subserosal fatty tissues, edema, fibrosis, acute and chronic inflammation, and granuloma formation. Nodular lymphoid aggregates are very common, and these may resemble serosal miliary granulomas grossly. The serosa may also become covered with a fibrinous precipitate or a fibropurulent exudate. The mesenteric changes closely parallel those seen in the serosa. The draining lymph nodes often become enlarged and frequently contain lipogranulomas.

Superficial Crohn Disease

The microscopic features of superficial CD are those of classic CD with aphthous ulcers, fissures, hypertrophy of the muscularis mucosae, and submucosal nerves with associated nodular lymphoid aggregates and granulomas in skip areas. However, the Crohn-type inflammatory changes remain limited to the mucosa and submucosa. Microscopically, there is no or minimal transmural inflammation and no fissures extend below the submucosa. Rare lymphoid nodules are present in the subserosa adjacent to the muscularis propria. The diagnosis is based on the association with classic CD in other segments of the same resection specimen.

Patients with both long and short segment superficial CD may have watery diarrhea. Obstructive symptoms and evidence of a stricture affect a small number of such patients, and these patients typically have transmural CD elsewhere in the surgical specimen. The gross mucosal appearance of superficial CD consists of a cobblestoned pattern that is more diffuse and more finely nodular than that seen in classic CD. The bowel wall tends to be thin and pliable rather than thick and rigid.

Histologic Features of Proximal Gastrointestinal Lesions

The villous architecture in the proximal small intestine varies from normal to a complete loss of villi and a flattened mucosa covered by an abnormal surface epithelium infiltrated by large numbers of neutrophils. Areas of flattening may lie adjacent to more normal-appearing tissues. In the duodenum, the most severe damage occurs proximal to the ligament of Treitz. The mucosa may contain crypt abscesses, erosions, granulation tissue, pyloric metaplasia, increased numbers of plasma cells, and neutrophils, often in the

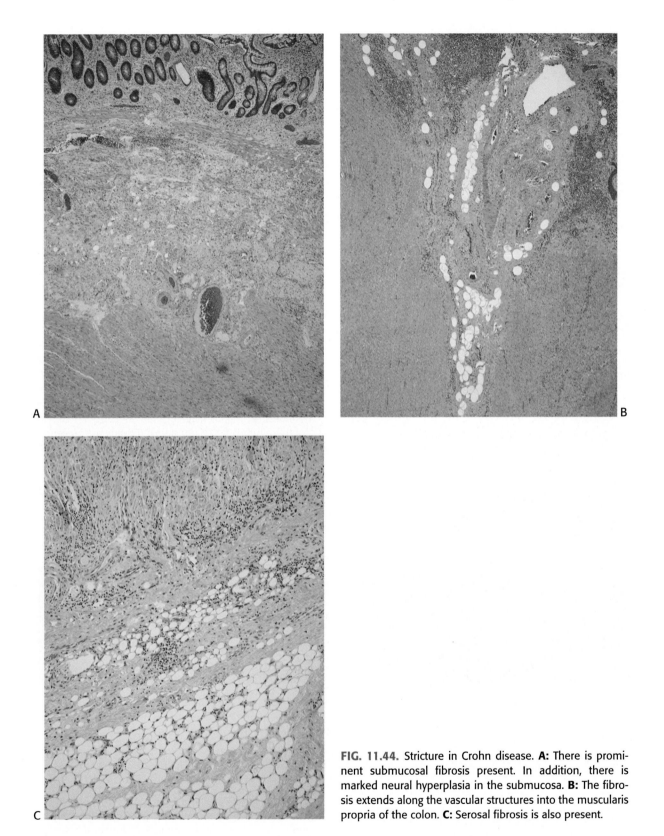

FIG. 11.44. Stricture in Crohn disease. **A:** There is prominent submucosal fibrosis present. In addition, there is marked neural hyperplasia in the submucosa. **B:** The fibrosis extends along the vascular structures into the muscularis propria of the colon. **C:** Serosal fibrosis is also present.

absence of granulomas. When only minimal changes are present, one sees acute inflammation consisting of focal neutrophilic collections in the lamina propria and surface epithelium. Surface cells vary from normal, to cuboidal, to completely flattened. Some appear vacuolated and others are

frankly megaloblastic, presumably due to coexisting vitamin deficiencies. Intraepithelial lymphocytes may be mildly increased, but are not present in the number typically seen in celiac disease. Neutrophils often infiltrate the epithelium in large numbers. Noncaseating granulomas are sometimes

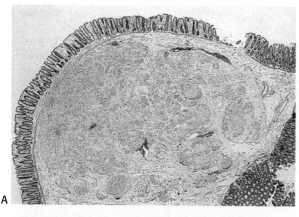

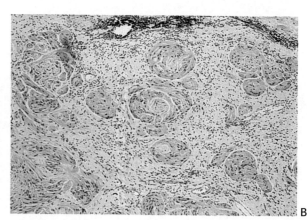

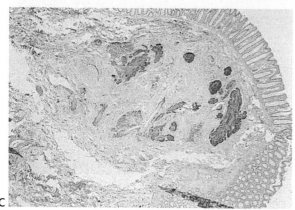

FIG. 11.45. Reactive neural hyperplasia in Crohn disease (CD). **A:** Low magnification of a polypoid lesion in the colon of a patient with CD demonstrating the presence of a prominent proliferation consisting of nerve fibers and fibroblasts. These are arranged in prominent swirling bundles. **B:** Higher magnification showing the structure of these bundles. **C:** S100 stain indicating the presence of neural elements.

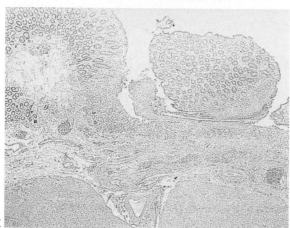

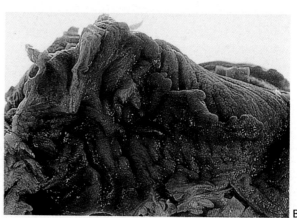

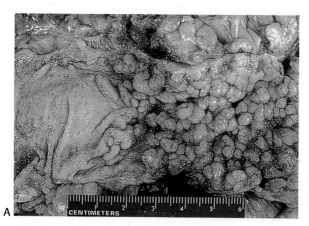

FIG. 11.46. Crohn disease. **A:** Multiple inflammatory pseudopolyps. The mucosa immediately adjacent is essentially normal. **B:** Filiform polyposis. The mucosa has multiple fingerlike extensions measuring several centimeters in length and extending from the surface. When these fuse, mucosal bridges are produced. **C:** Pseudopolyp composed essentially of residual, more or less normal colonic mucosa covering an area of ulceration.

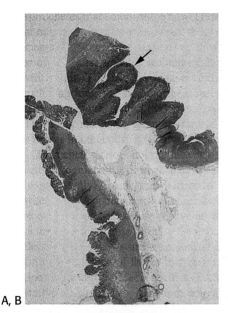
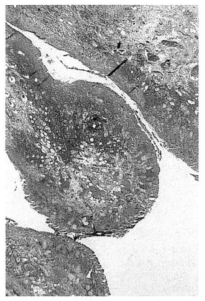
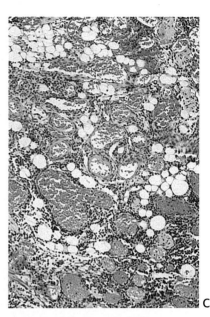

A, B   C

FIG. 11.47. Inflammatory pseudopolyps. **A:** The inflammatory pseudopolyps present in this photograph differ from those shown in Figure 11.46, in that they represent residual islands of mucosa and submucosa. They contain a prominent submucosal core. The surrounding tissues are ulcerated down to the level of the muscularis propria. **B:** Higher magnification of the pedunculated lesion indicated by the *arrow* in A. One can see the central fibrovascular submucosal core with a covering of granulation tissue and extravasated red cells. **C:** Higher magnification of the lesion.

seen, and are often present on a background of lymphocytic and plasmacytic inflammation. A normal biopsy does not exclude the possibility of involvement by CD, since the inflammation is usually patchy.

Gastric biopsies show some degree of abnormality in as many as 75% of patients with CD (104,105). The most commonly identified alteration is focal infiltration of the gastric pits and glands by inflammatory cells (Fig. 11.51). These infiltrates may include neutrophils, T lymphocytes,

and histiocytes in variable numbers. This focal inflammation affects both the neck region and deep aspects of the gastric glands, and is more commonly seen in the antrum than in the body of the stomach. In addition, granulomas may be seen in from 9% to 16% of patients (104,105) (Fig. 11.51).

The major differential diagnosis is with *Helicobacter pylori* gastritis. *H. pylori* gastritis may also demonstrate chronic active inflammation, but the infiltrates are almost entirely neutrophilic, and localize to the neck region of the glands. The presence of deep active inflammation should alert the pathologist to the possibility of CD. However, the possibility of *H. pylori* infection should be ruled out with the use of special stains in all patients demonstrating any form of chronic active gastritis. It is important to note that some patients with CD may have superimposed *H. pylori* infection.

Crohn disease may affect the esophagus, and when it does, it may be difficult to separate the lesions from other forms of granulomatous esophagitis, especially if one is unaware that the patient has known Crohn disease (Fig. 11.52). Clinically, severe forms of esophageal Crohn disease may simulate carcinoma because of the presence of an irregular, stenotic esophageal segment.

Crohn Disease of the Orogenital System

Oral vesicular lesions and aphthous ulcers affect 49% of patients with CD. Typical CD is usually present in the gut,

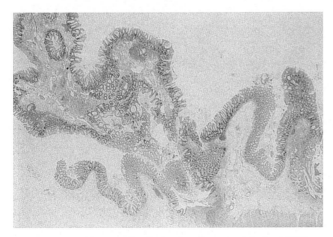

FIG. 11.48. Filiform polyp in Crohn disease. This long filiform polyp was one of dozens present in the colon. They are characterized by long submucosal extensions covered by regenerative mucosa.

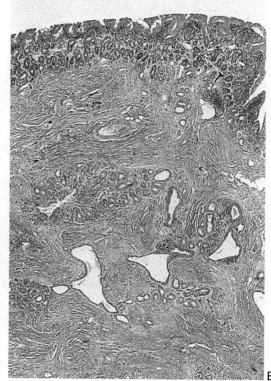

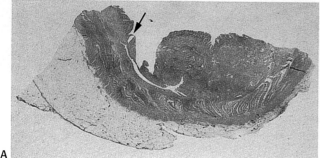

FIG. 11.49. Epithelial misplacement in Crohn disease. **A:** Whole mount section showing a large knifelike fissure, the mouth of which is indicated by the *arrow*. The thickened bowel wall contains submucosal islands of glands surrounded by lamina propria. **B:** Higher magnification of the misplaced epithelium. Many of the glands are surrounded by residual lamina propria.

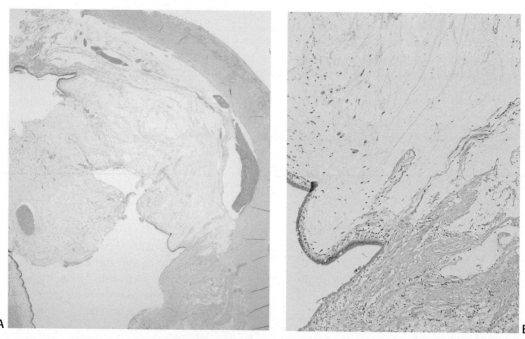

FIG. 11.50. Epithelial misplacement in Crohn disease. **A:** The displaced glands in this photo are filled with large amounts of mucin, some of which have extravasated into the wall of the small intestine. **B:** Higher magnification demonstrating the residual epithelium lining the gland. There is no cytologic atypia present, a feature that distinguishes this lesion from invasive carcinoma.

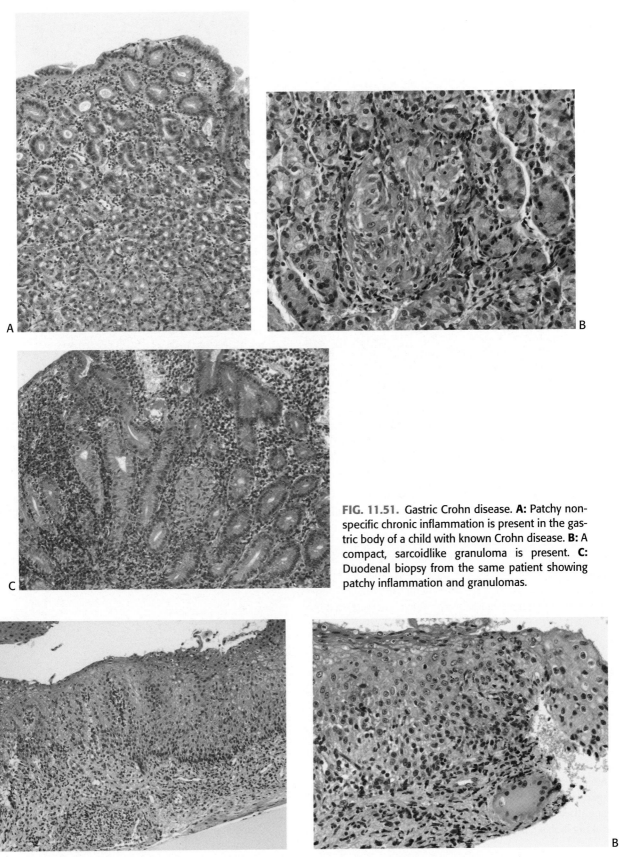

FIG. 11.51. Gastric Crohn disease. **A:** Patchy non-specific chronic inflammation is present in the gastric body of a child with known Crohn disease. **B:** A compact, sarcoidlike granuloma is present. **C:** Duodenal biopsy from the same patient showing patchy inflammation and granulomas.

FIG. 11.52. Esophageal Crohn disease. Figures A and B are from the esophagus of the child whose stomach is depicted in Figure 11.51. **A:** The esophageal squamous mucosa shows nonspecific inflammation and regenerative changes. **B:** Although no granulomas were present in this biopsy, a multinucleated giant cell is present in the submucosa.

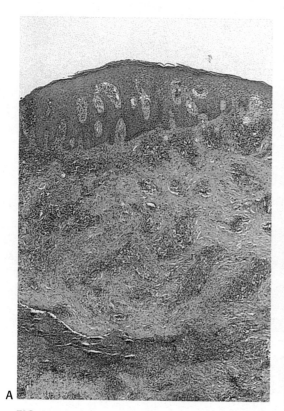
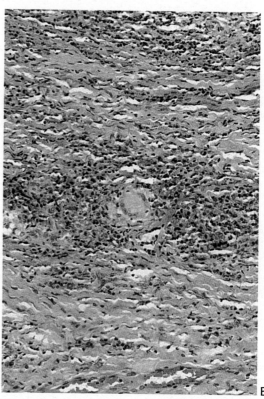

FIG. 11.53. Vulvar Crohn disease. **A:** Low magnification showing the presence of prominent acanthosis. The underlying submucosa contains numerous collections of lymphocytes and plasma cells. A small fissure containing large numbers of acute inflammatory cells passes through the lower portion of the photograph. **B:** Higher magnification of one of the areas of inflammation showing the presence of a giant cell.

but occasionally CD first presents as oral lesions. Lesions may develop in the lips, epiglottis, and aryepiglottic folds.

Oral lesions appear nodular and firm. Biopsy demonstrates the presence of chronic inflammatory cells and granulation tissue. Numerous large, well-formed, noncaseating granulomas containing epithelioid cells, giant cells, and peripheral lymphocytes may also be present. Patients with anal or perianal disease often have vaginal involvement characterized by the presence of nonspecific inflammation, fissures, and fistulae. Occasionally, granulomas are present (Fig. 11.53).

Evaluation of Resection Margins in Crohn Disease

Frozen sections of resection margins are unnecessary and should be avoided (280). This is because the rate of recurrence in CD following surgical resection is not influenced by the status of the resection margins (106). Factors that do affect the risk of postoperative recurrence of CD include extent of disease at the time of surgery and the indication for surgery, with those who failed medical therapy or had perforating disease having a higher risk of recurrence (106,107). Smoking is also a factor affecting disease recurrence (108).

Complications

The complications of CD are listed in Table 11.10. The extraintestinal and neoplastic manifestations are discussed

TABLE 11.10	Complications of Crohn Disease

Local intestinal
  Perforation
  Hemorrhage
  Fistulas to adjacent bowel
  Fistulas to urinary bladder (pneumaturia)
  Fistulas to vagina
  Intestinal obstruction
  Enterolith production
  Malabsorption
  Lactose deficiency
  Zinc deficiency
  Enteritis cystica profunda
  Toxic megacolon
  Psoas abscesses
Respiratory
  Bronchitis
  Emphysema
  Asthma
Amyloid
Tumors
  Small bowel carcinoma
  Large intestinal carcinoma
  Cholangiocarcinoma
  Renal oncocytoma
  Lymphoma, leukemia, and Hodgkin disease
  Carcinoid
  Squamous cell carcinoma, anus and vagina

later in this chapter. Complications also result from therapy. These include steroid-related osteonecrosis often affecting the hip or knee, as well as secondary viral or bacterial infections.

ULCERATIVE COLITIS

Incidence

In recent decades, the incidence of UC in the United States and in Europe has risen, whereas in other countries the incidence has plateaued (2,87,109). It is likely that two factors have contributed to this increase: (a) improved survival of incident cases and (b) diagnosis of milder cases due to increased use of sigmoidoscopy and fecal occult blood testing in the community. UC mostly affects young white people, but there is an increasing recognition that the disease affects many ages and many ethnic groups (2). The incidence of UC inversely correlates with smoking and clinical relapses have been associated with smoking cessation (110).

Clinical Features

UC demonstrates a wide clinical spectrum affecting all age groups, with a predominance of the disease in young and middle-aged persons. The peak age of incidence is the 3rd decade. Women are more commonly affected than men. Mean age at diagnosis is 32 years (111). The disorder is less common in black persons than white persons. Fifty to sixty percent of patients present with an insidious onset of vague abdominal discomfort. Symptoms vary from those of mild rectal irritation to an acute severe colitis. In children, growth failure, characterized by decreased linear growth and delayed sexual maturation, often represents the first sign of disease. Patients with UC develop this complication less commonly than CD patients (112).

Diarrhea, hematochezia, urgency of defecation, attacks of crampy abdominal pain, and perianal soreness are common in early stages of the disease. Abdominal pain is usually less severe than in CD. Approximately 10% of patients initially present with severe colitis characterized by abdominal pain, more than 40 bloody stools per day, fever, tachycardia, weight loss, and hypoalbuminemia. When UC remains limited to the left colon, constipation rather than diarrhea may result because colonic spasm results in stool retention in the right colon where the normal absorptive capacity is unimpaired.

Disease onset is abrupt in approximately 30% of patients. The disease may be explosive, with a sudden onset of acute diarrhea, frequent bloody stools, continuous abdominal pain, anorexia, rapid weight loss, chronic iron deficiency anemia, and a persistent fever. Acute and massive rectal bleeding affects up to 3% of patients (111). The bleeding originates from large denuded areas of the mucosa in the face of widespread telangiectatic lamina propria vessels. In contrast, the bleeding seen in CD usually originates from a localized source such as an eroded blood vessel in the submucosa or deeper layers.

Characteristically, UC is a chronic mucosal disease with relapses and spontaneous remissions. It usually starts in the rectum and then spreads more proximally. Most patients have distal disease at the time of first attack, but some have more proximal disease, including total colonic involvement. There are several major clinical presentations: (a) acute fulminating colitis, in which the whole colon and rectum are affected with extensive and deep ulcerations; (b) continuous colitis, in which the symptoms persist from the onset and vary in severity (usually only affecting the left side of the colon); and (c) recurrent colitis, in which the attacks are limited and separated by varying periods of remission. Disease distribution usually remains relatively constant, with about 50% of patients in clinical remission in any one time. Relapses are unpredictable except that the disease activity in foregoing years indicates a 70% to 80% probability that the disease will continue the following year (113). The cumulative probability of having a relapsing course is 90% after 25 years of disease. Activity in the first 2 years of diagnosis significantly correlates with having an increased probability of 5 consecutive years of disease activity. The probability of maintaining work capacity after 10 years is 92.8%, with a range of 90.8% to 94.8%.

UC progresses to a more serious form in 53.8% of patients. Factors associated with disease progression include toxic colitis, extent of disease at diagnosis, presence of joint symptoms, younger age at diagnosis, and severe bleeding (111). Various infections (CMV, *Salmonella,* and *Clostridium difficile*), medications, and intervening ischemic disease also exacerbate UC (Table 11.11).

Toxic Megacolon

Acute toxic megacolon is a potentially lethal complication that affects between 1.6% and 6% of all UC patients and 17% of severe attacks of UC (114). Toxic megacolon usually affects patients with pancolitis, and is characterized by total or segmental colonic dilation, loss of contractile ability, and rapid clinical deterioration. The colonic wall progressively thins until perforation occurs. A distended, tender, silent abdomen suggests that the bowel is about to perforate. An

TABLE 11.11 Factors Associated with Relapse or Exacerbation of Ulcerative Colitis Symptoms

Infections	Medications
Viral	Antibiotics
Cytomegalovirus	Sulfasalazine
Upper respiratory viruses	5-Aminosalicylic acid
Enteroviruses	Azodisalicylate
Bacterial	Ischemia
Salmonella	Neoplasia
Clostridium difficile	
Other enteric pathogens	
Mycoplasma pneumoniae	
Entamoeba histolytica	

abdominal mass is rarely present, although a distended colon may become palpable in toxic megacolon. Rarely, air leaks from the toxic megacolon produce pneumomediastinum or subcutaneous emphysema. Disturbed motility with loss of contractility results from extension of the inflammation into muscularis propria, serosa, and visceral peritoneum. The hypertrophic muscle loses its muscular tone with stretching and the pressure of the intraluminal contents. Damage to the myenteric plexus results in atony. Hypokalemia aggravates the already weakened peristalsis and hypoproteinemia augments the bowel wall edema. The mortality associated with toxic megacolon is high. Other complications include massive hemorrhage and pulmonary embolism.

Toxic megacolon not only complicates UC, but can also develop in association with any inflammatory condition of the colon including Crohn disease, infectious colitis (*C. difficile, Salmonella, Shigella, Campylobacter,* and amoeba), and ischemic colitis.

Ileitis

Inflammation in the terminal ileum occurs in 5% to 17% of patients with ulcerative colitis (115,116). The ileal inflammation, known as *backwash ileitis,* occurs in continuity with cecal inflammation, and is thought to result from incompetence of the ileocecal valve and reflux of intestinal contents across it. Grossly, the ileal mucosa appears diffusely abnormal, contrasting with the aphthous ulcers and discontinuous and serpiginous ulcerations of Crohn disease. The involved ileum shows inflammation, erosions, and sometimes ulcerations. The ileitis usually resolves following colectomy.

Ileitis may develop after colectomy in preanastomotic portions of the small bowel. The disease develops following various types of reconstruction, including ileorectal and ileoanal, with or without a pouch. Patients remain asymptomatic or experience severe pain and diarrhea.

Perianal Disease

Some patients first seek medical advice because of the presence of extraintestinal manifestations, such as arthritis or perianal disease. Perianal disease is usually limited to hemorrhoids, anal excoriations, and fissures. Perianal or ischiorectal abscesses, fistulae, and rectovaginal fistulae rarely develop. The complications of UC in the anus are acute and superficial, contrasting with those seen in CD.

Role of Surgery

Surgical therapy for ulcerative colitis may be used either for emergencies or as elective treatment. Indications for urgent surgery include failed medical treatment in patients with acute severe colitis, toxic megacolon, perforation, or severe bleeding. There are essentially three indications for elective colectomy for UC: Failed medical treatment, growth retardation in a child with UC, and the development, or concern for,

neoplastic transformation in a patient with longstanding disease. Failed medical treatment includes chronic disease, recurrent acute exacerbations, severe symptoms in an otherwise systemically well patient, suboptimal quality of life, steroid dependence, or extraintestinal manifestations of the disease.

In patients undergoing emergency surgery, the most common procedure is colectomy with ileostomy and preservation of the rectosigmoid stump. Under the conditions of elective surgery, several surgical options exist including conventional proctocolectomy, colectomy with ileorectal anastomosis, and restorative proctocolectomy with ileal reservoir.

Patient Survival

Since the introduction of effective medical and surgical treatments in the early 1960s, UC has a surprisingly low mortality. Patients with ulcerative colitis have a normal life expectancy compared with persons in the general population (117,118). Severe acute attacks, usually occurring during the first 2 years of disease, are the major killer, especially in patients over 50 years of age (119). Patients with longstanding extensive disease have an increased risk for the development of dysplasia or colorectal carcinoma.

Gross Features

Since patients usually undergo resection when they have extensive chronic colitis involving at least the rectum and left side of the colon, or when neoplastic alterations develop in the bowel, most of the described gross features are those that characterize severe forms of the disease. Table 11.12 compares the gross features of UC and CD.

Disease Location

Disease extent and involvement vary with the clinical severity of the disease. The distal bowel is always involved, with variable proximal continuous extension. Among patients with UC, approximately 45% have proctosigmoiditis, 20% to 62% have pancolitis, and 17% to 22% have left-sided colitis from the dentate line to the splenic flexure. There is a greater tendency for extension proximal to the descending colon in children than in adults.

External Features

UC is primarily a mucosal colonic disease characterized by an inflammatory reaction that remains limited to the mucosa and the superficial portion of the submucosa. For this reason, the external surface of the bowel appears normal unless cancer or toxic megacolon has developed. In chronic disease, the overall length of the bowel may appear contracted. In the case of toxic megacolon, the bowel appears massively dilated and the wall appears paper thin. The extremely thin, friable wall tends to fall apart with the

TABLE 11.12 Gross Features of Crohn Disease Versus Ulcerative Colitis

Feature	Crohn Disease	Ulcerative Colitis
Distribution	Segmental; 50% have normal rectum	Diffuse; circumferential continuous with rectum[a]
Rectal involvement	+	+ + +
Terminal ileum	Often thickened, ulcerated, and stenosed; creeping mesenteric fat; terminal 15–25 cm	Involved 10%; short segment; backwash ileitis
Mucosal surface	Aphthous ulcers; linear ulcers; cobblestone appearance; fissures	Granular; ulcers
Mucosal atrophy	Minimal	Marked
Serosa	Inflamed, creeping fat, adhesions	Usually normal
Colonic involvement	Predominantly right sided; granulomata	Usually left sided and continuous to right
Colon shortening	Due to fibrosis	Due to muscle hypertrophy
Strictures	Common	Rare
Fistulas	10% with enteroenteric or enterocutaneous	Rare
Free perforation	Very rare	Occurs with toxic megacolon
Pseudopolyps	Occurs	Common
Oral lesions	Common	Uncommon
Malignancy	Increased frequency over control population	Increased frequency over control population
Anal disease	+ +	+ +

[a]The appendix can also be involved in the absence of right-sided disease.

gentlest handling. Frequently, one sees peritonitis as well as fibrinous or fibrinopurulent exudates on the peritoneal surfaces. The descending and sigmoid colon show the most severe acute lesions. Edema widely separates the fibers of the muscularis propria, leading to incipient perforation. Rarely, perforation is seen in patients without megacolon.

Determination of Disease Extent

Typically, when one opens a resected UC colon, blood oozes diffusely from the congested vasculature of the mucosal surface. The disease usually involves the rectum and extends proximally in a contiguous fashion affecting each successive segment of the bowel with a symmetric inflammatory response (Fig. 11.54). The length of the proximal extension varies. UC manifests as proctitis, proctosigmoiditis, left-sided proctocolitis, subtotal proctocolitis, or total involvement of the large bowel (pancolitis). The disease stops abruptly either at the ileocecal valve or in more distal portions of the colon. Variations in the intensity of inflammation may give a false impression of discontinuous focal or skip lesions, particularly in acute UC with patchy full-thickness mucosal loss (Fig. 11.55). One may see ulcerated areas with intervening mucosa that looks macroscopically normal. Additionally, treatment with steroid enemas and mucosal healing may lead to the false gross impression of rectal sparing (Fig. 11.56). However, grossly apparent skip areas or rec-

tal sparing always show histologic evidence of architectural abnormalities characteristic of healed colitis. The only exceptions to this statement are the presence of appendiceal disease in a patient without pancolitis and patients with toxic colitis and a normal right colon who may develop ileal disease.

Similarly, the exact extent of mucosal involvement is not always easy to determine in the excised specimen because microscopic evidence of disease may be found in a macroscopically normal mucosa. Sometimes inflammatory changes of rectal UC go into spontaneous remission, while the proximal colonic inflammation remains active. This gives the gross impression of right-sided disease with rectal sparing. However, again, histologic examination discloses the presence of an abnormal rectal mucosa with regeneration in areas of resolved previous damage. The exact extent of disease in UC can only be accurately judged histologically.

Ulcers

In active UC the mucosa acquires a diffuse, uniformly granular, and erythematous, hemorrhagic appearance (Fig. 11.57). When ulcerations are present, the intervening intact mucosa appears granular and hemorrhagic. Ulcers undermine adjacent intact mucosa to form polypoid mucosal tags or inflammatory pseudopolyps (Fig. 11.58). The presence of broad areas of superficial ulceration covered by an overlying

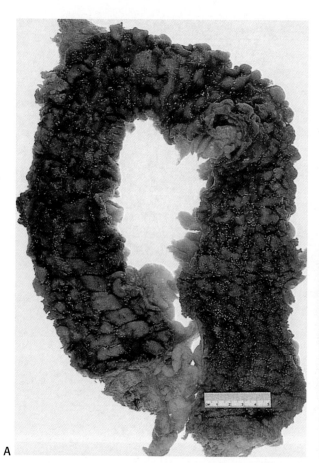

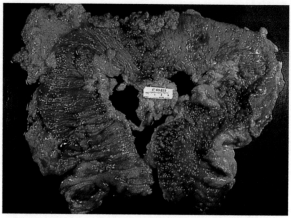

A   B

FIG. 11.54. Acute ulcerative colitis. **A:** Pancolitis with ulceration and numerous pseudopolyps throughout the entire length of the specimen. **B:** Ulcerative colitis demonstrating the presence of mucosal changes throughout the length of resected bowel. These changes are much more marked in the distal portion of the bowel and decrease in severity as one goes proximally. There are not as many pseudopolyps as seen in A.

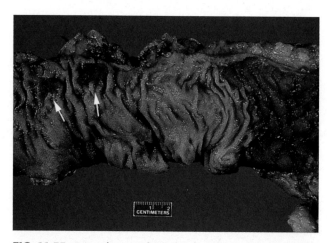

FIG. 11.55. Resection specimen in ulcerative colitis. Superficial examination of this bowel suggests that the patient has Crohn disease because grossly skip lesions appear to be present. The *arrows* indicate two reddened areas that are separated from the main hemorrhagic and erythematous portion of the bowel at the right of the photograph. However, histologic examination disclosed significant colitis in the intervening, apparently grossly normal mucosa.

mucopurulent exudate results in partial or complete loss of the mucosa. The ulcers exhibit a linear distribution (Fig. 11.59), particularly in relation to the attachment of the taeniae coli. The ulcers lay bare the underlying muscularis propria (Fig. 11.58) and penetrate it only in fulminant UC. Extensive longitudinal ulcers, especially if connected by transverse ulcers, are not a feature of UC but rather of CD. Perforation occurs when the ulceration penetrates the muscularis completely.

UC patients who also have diverticulosis may have extension of their mucosal disease into a diverticulum, perhaps obliterating the underlying architecture, resulting in an appearance of a primary fistula and creating changes that mimic CD.

Chronic Colitis

In chronic continuous UC the mucosa appears granular with or without inflammatory polyps and the hemorrhagic component is muted or absent. When UC goes into remission, it is possible for the mucosa to return to a normal gross

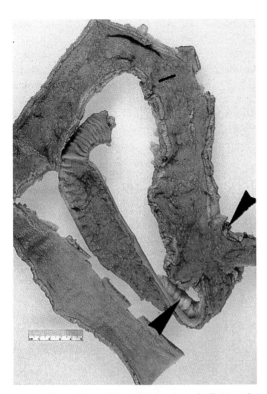

FIG. 11.56. Ulcerative colitis with backwash ileitis. The distal bowel has become completely atrophic. The more proximal portions still contain evidence of active inflammation. The ileocecal valve (*arrowheads*) is incompetent, and inflammation extends into the terminal ileum. In the middle of the specimen extensive ulceration is present.

appearance; however, usually microscopic signs of former active disease remain with the mucosa appearing smooth and atrophic, or showing variable granularity.

Sometimes the most striking gross feature is intestinal shortening with loss of the haustral folds, which produces an appearance of a contracted, stiff, thickened bowel (Fig. 11.60). This shortening results from muscular abnormalities and is most obvious in the distal colon and rectum. Fibrosis may cause the mucosa to lose its mobility over the underlying muscularis propria.

Pseudopolyps

Pseudopolyps represent discrete areas of mucosal inflammation and regeneration. They complicate various forms of colitis but are most common in UC. These pseudopolyps do not correlate with the disease severity and are not precancerous. Their distribution depends on the extent of the primary disorder. Both localized and diffuse forms of polyposis complicate UC (Fig. 11.58, 11.59, and 11.61 to 11.63). Pseudopolyps are numerous only in a minority of cases and are usually present in patients with severe chronic disease.

The pseudopolyps are typically short, measuring <1.5 cm in height. They result from full-thickness mucosal ulceration and almost always represent either the surviving mucosal islands between areas of ulceration (Fig. 11.59) or heaped-up granulation tissue that becomes covered with epithelium. Once formed, pseudopolyps tend to persist and may serve as an indicator of previous episodes of colitis.

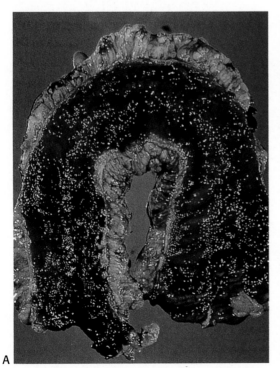
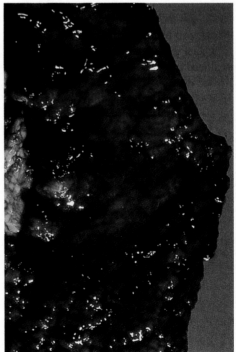

FIG. 11.57. Hemorrhagic ulcerative colitis. **A:** The entire resection specimen demonstrates the presence of a diffusely reddened, oozing mucosa that appears essentially the same throughout the entire length of the large bowel. **B:** Higher magnification showing the diffuse oozing and redness of the mucosal surface.

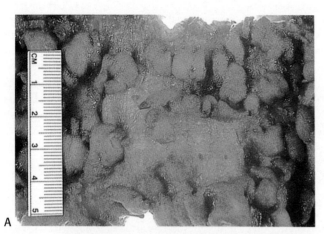

FIG. 11.58. Pseudopolyps. **A:** Higher power magnification of the bowel shown in Figure 11.6B. The mucosa is ulcerated all the way down to the level of the muscularis propria, leaving pseudopolypoid islands of mucosa. **B:** Cross section demonstrating the pseudopolyps. Ulcerations can be seen extending all the way to the muscularis propria. In these areas no residual submucosa is evident.

Pseudopolyps are more prominent in the colon than in the rectum; they can completely spare the distal large bowel. Polyp fusion results from the approximation of two adjacent polyps that become superficially ulcerated. Fibroblasts grow into the granulation tissue between the polyp surfaces. Fused polyps create a labyrinthine appearance and mucosal bridging (Fig. 11.63). The polyps often lie in the direction of the fecal stream, as if accentuated by it (Fig. 11.62).

There are also unusual polyps that attain a large size or have a bizarre architecture. These form a continuum with the more ordinary pseudopolyps but because of their unusual features are separated from them. Pseudopolyps (especially large ones) may produce acute obstruction or intussusception or may mimic carcinomas.

Filiform polyposis, which represents an exaggerated form of pseudopolyps, usually coexists with chronic IBD, especially

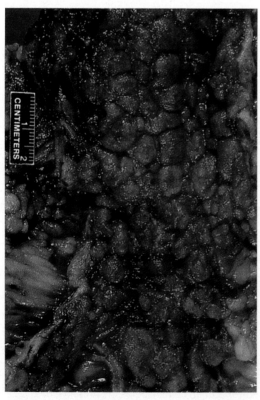

FIG. 11.59. Cobblestoned mucosa that results from loss of the intervening mucosal surface, showing mucosal ulceration.

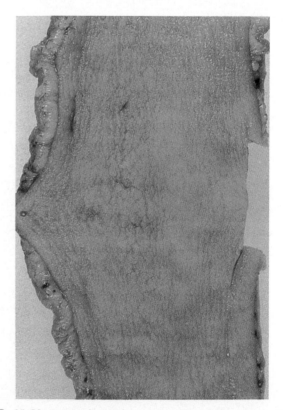

FIG. 11.60. Mucosal atrophy in ulcerative colitis. This patient shows an atrophic foreshortened bowel due to muscular contraction. Active disease was present histologically.

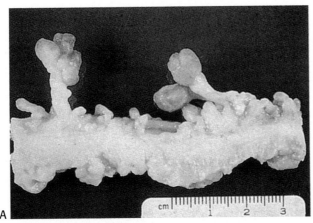
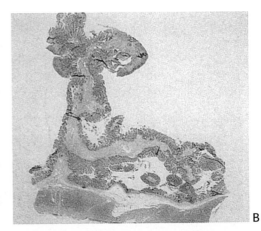

FIG. 11.61. **A:** Cross section of the bowel demonstrating the presence of multiple filiform pseudopolyps. **B:** Cross section through a filiform pseudopolyp demonstrating the presence of a prominent fibroblastic core. The epithelium is inflamed and regenerated.

CD and UC. It is characterized by numerous wormy, densely packed, villiform colonic polyps associated with a moderate degree of inflammation and edema. These may grossly resemble villous adenomas (Fig. 11.61) (see Chapter 20). Arborization is a striking feature. The polyps are found anywhere in the colon. Filiform polyps reach heights of 2 to 3 cm. Filiform polyposis frequently spares the rectum.

Toxic Megacolon

The internal features of toxic megacolon reflect the external ones, with marked dilation of the bowel lumen and thinning of the intestinal wall (Fig. 11.64). Severe extensive mucosal ulcers lead to almost complete mucosal denudation. Deeper ulcers that penetrate the mucosa lay the muscularis propria bare. The latter may become covered by only a very thin layer of granulation tissue.

Ileal Disease

The terminal ileum becomes involved only in continuity with total colitis in 5% to 20% of specimens, and no more than 10 to 25 cm proximal to the ileocecal valve is involved by the disease. Macroscopically, the ileal mucosa appears diffusely abnormal (see Fig. 11.56), contrasting with the terminal ileitis of CD, which shows aphthous ulcers and discontinuous and serpiginous ulcerations. The diseased ileum shows inflammation, erosions, ulcerations, and sometimes strictures.

Inflammation occurring in the setting of colectomy followed by ileostomy is usually not due to the UC per se but is secondary to the ileostomy. It is called *prestomal ileitis*. In this disorder, one sees ulcers scattered throughout the ileum and jejunum with the intervening mucosa appearing normal or edematous. Because these ulcers have a tendency to

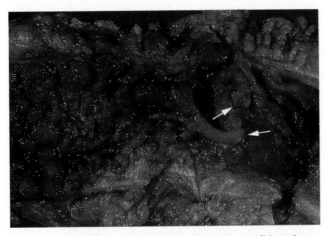

FIG. 11.62. Filiform polyposis in ulcerative colitis. Picture demonstrating a thickened, contracted bowel and numerous filiform polyps (*arrows*). They all line up in the direction of the fecal flow. The distal rectum is to the right-hand portion of the picture.

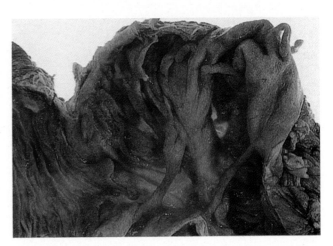

FIG. 11.63. Mucosal bridge in ulcerative colitis. Gross specimen demonstrating the presence of pseudopolyps, filiform polyposis, and mucosal bridging resulting from fusion of pseudopolyps.

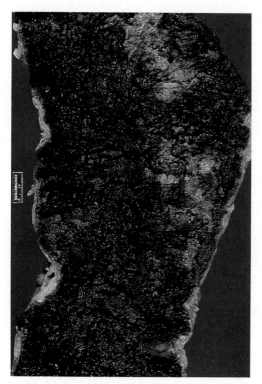

FIG. 11.64. Toxic megacolon. A shaggy hemorrhagic mucosa and colonic dilation as evidenced by the increased width of the specimen.

perforate, peritonitis and fistulae develop, and the lesions may prove fatal.

Histologic Features

The histologic appearance varies with the clinical phase of the disease, allowing one to classify UC into three stages: Active colitis, UC going into remission (resolving colitis), and colitis in remission. UC is characteristically a mucosal and submucosal disease. Table 11.13 compares the histologic features of UC and CD. Table 11.14 compares the major changes seen in acute, resolving, and chronic colitis.

Features of Active Colitis

Cryptitis, Crypt Abscesses, and Ulcers

The mucosa in active UC is characterized by an intense inflammatory cell infiltrate, crypt abscesses, mucin depletion, and surface ulceration. The hallmark of acute activity in UC is the presence of neutrophils infiltrating the lamina propria and crypt epithelium. The term *chronic active colitis* serves to indicate the presence of acute activity superimposed on a background of chronic changes.

An early feature of active colitis is the formation of cryptitis, which evolves to crypt abscesses and crypt ulcers (Fig. 11.65).

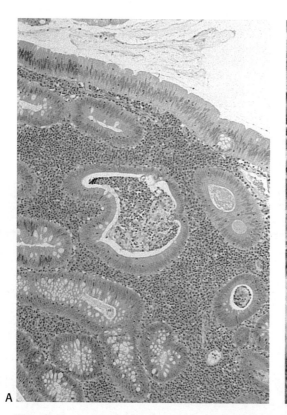

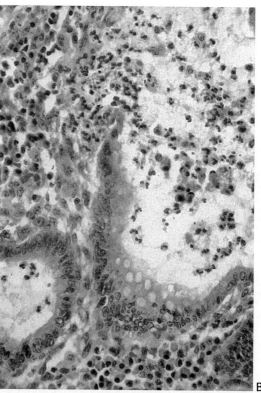

FIG. 11.65. Active chronic ulcerative colitis. **A:** The lamina propria shows an intense infiltrate of lymphocytes and plasma cells. There is evidence of glandular distortion. A prominent crypt abscess is seen. **B:** Crypt herniation. The crypt at the right-hand side of the photograph has ruptured and is spewing its contents into the surrounding lamina propria.

TABLE 11.13 **Microscopic Features of Ulcerative Colitis Versus Crohn Colitis**

Feature	Crohn Colitis	Ulcerative Colitis
Inflammation	Skip lesions; transmural	Diffuse; mucosal and submucosal; 20% transmural including toxic megacolon
Submucosa	Normal, inflamed, or reduced width	Normal or reduced width
Hyperemia	Seldom prominent	Prominent
Lymphoid hyperplasia	Common; separated from muscularis mucosae; transmural and pericolonic tissue; associated with submucosal edema and fibrosis	Rare; mucosa and submucosa; not associated with submucosa, edema, and fibrosis
Neuromatous hyperplasia	Common	Rare
Edema	Marked	Minimal
Crypt abscess	Uncommon; when present, few in number	Common
Cytoplasmic mucin	Slightly reduced	Mucin depleted; greatly reduced
Paneth cell metaplasia	Occurs	Common
Granulomas (sarcoidlike)	Common	Rare
Fissures and sinuses	Common	Absent
Focal lymphoid aggregates in submucosa	Presence suggests Crohn, especially when deep	Usually absent
Lymph nodes	Granulomas	Reactive hyperplasia
Ileal lesions	More than half	Minimal, not more than 10 cm
Anal lesions	Granulomas	Nonspecific
Dysplasia and cancer	Increased	Increased
Aphthous ulcers	Common	Rare
Inflammatory pseudopolyps	Less common than in ulcerative colitis	Common
Filiform polyposis, giant polyps	Occurs	Occurs
Accuracy rate of rectal biopsy	40%	70%

As in CD, cryptitis reflects migration of neutrophils into crypt epithelium. A collection of neutrophils in the crypt lumen represents a crypt abscess (see Fig. 11.32). Crypt abscesses may be relatively isolated and present in a background of intense infiltration by mononuclear cells (Fig. 11.65) or they may be part of a more diffuse process (Fig. 11.66). Crypt ulcers represent areas of crypt destruction from the inflammation. Once the crypt ruptures (crypt herniation) (Figs. 11.65 and 11.67), the luminal contents and mucus extravasate into the surrounding lamina propria, sometimes creating histiocytic collections around the area of rupture. Such histiocytic collections may simulate or suggest a diagnosis of CD. However, these histiocytic collections lack the typical features of compact granulomas more characteristic of CD (compare Figs. 11.35 and 11.37). The presence of acute inflammation, primarily based in the epithelium rather than the lamina propria, and the presence of changes

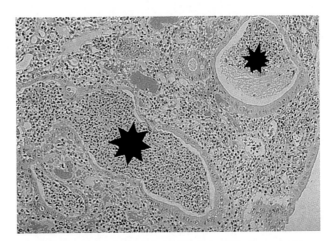

FIG. 11.66. Crypt changes in ulcerative colitis. A crypt abscess (*small star*) and herniating crypt abscess (*large star*) are both present in this example of active ulcerative colitis.

TABLE 11.14 Histologic Features of Ulcerative Colitis[a]

Acute (active) stage
   Vascular congestion
   Mucin depletion
   Cryptitis, crypt abscesses
   Epithelial loss and ulcers
   PMNs, eosinophil and mast cell infiltrates
   Luminal pus
   Basal plasma cells
   Vascular congestion
Resolving stage
   Less vascular congestion than seen in the active phase
   Gradual disappearance of PMNs
   Gradual disappearance of crypt abscesses
   Continued basal plasma cells
   Epithelial regeneration
   Expansion of the mitotically active cells
Chronic healed stage
   Architectural distortion
      Atrophy
      Branching
      Crypt shortening
      Villous transformation
   Metaplasia
      Pyloric
      Paneth cell
   Lymphoid hyperplasia
   Filiform polyposis
   Epithelial displacement
   Increased mononuclear cells in the lamina propria
   Endocrine cell hyperplasia
   Squamous metaplasia

PMNs, polymorphonuclear leukocytes.
[a] An individual patient may have all three stages present in the same specimen.

associated with chronic injury serve to distinguish UC from acute self-limited colitis.

The diagnosis of UC primarily based on the presence of crypt abscesses is hazardous because crypt abscesses occur as part of acute inflammation associated with many disorders, including CD or acute self-limited colitis. Although crypt abscesses are not specific for UC, when they are very prominent and involve nearly all the crypts, the disease is much more likely to represent UC than CD. In contrast, the presence of isolated crypt abscesses with chronic inflammation and completely uninvolved crypts, particularly with neutrophils in the lamina propria, is more common in CD (100).

The crypt abscesses play a role in the generation of the ulcerations that occur in severe disease because when they burst into the surrounding tissues, they spread laterally and beneath the mucosa, which then sloughs, leaving an ulcer. Ulcers may also spread into the submucosa and undermine adjacent, relatively intact mucosa. Except in severe colitis, these ulcers tend to be grossly small and generally shallow. When severe, the ulcers extend to the muscularis propria (Fig. 11.68), but deep penetration of the muscular layer or serosa only occurs in toxic megacolon. The crypt abscesses also contain mucous debris and bacteria. Because the crypt abscesses rupture into the bowel lumen, one finds white cells in the feces. Secondary infection of an already damaged mucosa by organisms present in the fecal stream further extends the damage.

The microscopic findings also include mucin depletion from goblet cells (Figs. 11.65 to 11.67), epithelial cell necrosis and regeneration, reduced goblet cell numbers, Paneth cell metaplasia, and dense infiltration of the lamina propria by neutrophils, plasma cells, and other acute and chronic inflammatory cells. At the height of a severe attack, goblet cells disappear completely. Because of the mucosal loss, the epithelium actively regenerates and the proliferative fraction of cells in the crypts increases to compensate for the cell loss. Patients with active disease show expansion of the proliferative compartment as demonstrated by Ki-67 immunostaining (Fig. 11.69) (120) as well as by flow cytometric analysis.

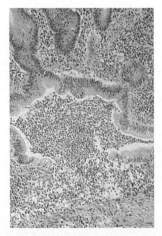

FIG. 11.67. Crypt herniation in ulcerative colitis. Low magnification showing the herniation of a crypt at its bottom. It is spewing out its inflammatory contents into the surrounding lamina propria.

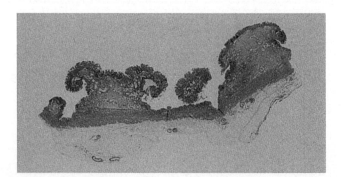

FIG. 11.68. Fulminant colitis. In fulminant colitis, the ulceration may extend down to the level of the muscularis propria leaving residual mucosal and submucosal islands forming pseudopolyps.

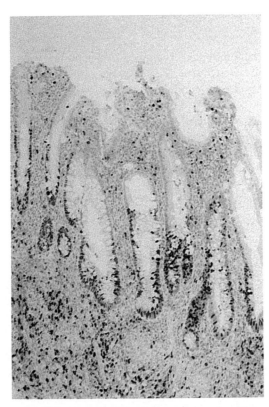

FIG. 11.69. Ki-67 immunoreactivity in active ulcerative colitis. Note the expansion of the proliferative zone along the lengths of the crypts in the actively regenerating mucosa. The intense stromal staining corresponds to the proliferation of lymphocytes.

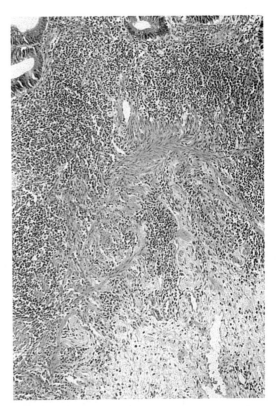

FIG. 11.70. Biopsy specimen from a patient with ulcerative colitis. The patient shows basal plasmacytosis. There is mild widening of the distance between the base of the crypts and the muscularis mucosae. The muscularis mucosae appears frayed. The inflammation spills into the upper submucosa. Some inflammation is diffusely present in the muscularis mucosae.

Inflammatory and Stromal Changes

Basal accumulations of lymphocytes and plasma cells (referred to as basal lymphoplasmacytosis) (Fig. 11.70), together with hyperplasia of lymphoid tissue, probably represents an early immunologic manifestation of the underlying disease process. The chronic inflammatory cells may also infiltrate the superficial mucosa (see Fig. 11.65). A subset of patients with predominantly rectal disease has a high number of IgE-bearing plasma cells (121). Dendritic cells lie in a bandlike infiltrate under the mucosal surface and near lymphoid follicles, if present. Hyperplastic mucosal lymphoid follicles may be quite prominent, especially in the rectum. The inflammation remains superficial and primarily mucosal (Fig. 11.71). Occasionally, this inflammation extends into the superficial submucosa (Fig. 11.71). Deeper inflammation may occur in areas adjacent to or underlying ulcers. The lamina propria contains a dense infiltrate of lymphocytes and plasma cells (Fig. 11.72). Mast cells and eosinophils increase in number, and the tissue histamine content rises (122). Both mast cells and eosinophils degranulate in areas of active inflammation, suggesting that inflammatory mediators released from them contribute to the pathophysiology of the disorder (122). Mast cells also release heparin and proteolytic enzymes, thereby exaggerating and facilitating the spread of the inflammation and necrosis. As the intensity of inflammation increases, the mucosa becomes extensively superficially ulcerated. The mucosal contour becomes irregular and covered with pus, blood, and exfoliated cells.

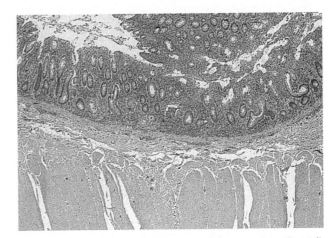

FIG. 11.71. Regenerating colonic epithelium in ulcerative colitis. The epithelium appears mucin depleted. Much of the acute inflammation has subsided, but one sees an intense mononuclear cell infiltrate in the mucosa. The cells at the base of the crypt appear more hyperchromatic and more immature than those higher up in the crypt.

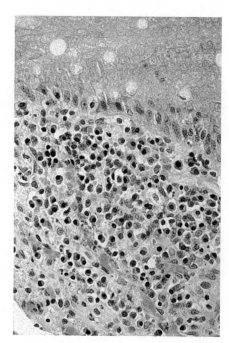

FIG. 11.72. Inflammatory infiltrate in ulcerative colitis. The lamina propria contains a dense infiltrate of lymphocytes and prominent plasma cells.

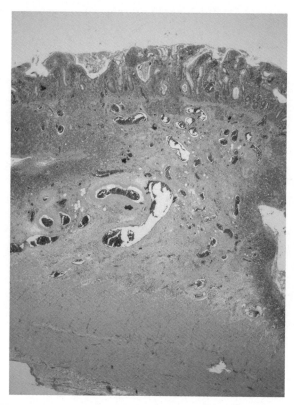

FIG. 11.73. Telangiectasia in ulcerative colitis. There is prominent dilation of both submucosal and mucosal blood vessels.

Mucosal capillary congestion and vascular ectasia with intramucosal hemorrhages are common, especially in severe disease (Fig. 11.73). The entire intestinal vasculature becomes congested, but this feature is most prominent in the mucosa. The vascular changes associate with varying degrees of epithelial necrosis and regeneration.

Neural Changes

The nerves may show mild hyperplasia, but never to the extent seen in CD. In contrast to the situation that occurs with CD, the mucosa of patients with UC shows a deficit of substance P–containing and VIP-containing nerves. They are decreased (sometimes almost completely absent) in the areas of severe inflammation (123,124). The loss of VIP correlates with the degree of inflammation.

Features of Resolving Colitis

Active disease resolves spontaneously or in response to therapy. Initially, one sees a reduction in the vascular dilation and disappearance of the active inflammation and crypt abscesses (Figs. 11.74 and 11.75). During the healing phase, the epithelium actively regenerates, epithelial continuity is restored (Fig. 11.75), the inflammatory infiltrate and abscesses begin to resolve, and the epithelial mucin content begins to be restored. Epithelial regeneration extends from the base of the crypts (Fig. 11.76) and from the edge of the ulcers (Fig. 11.77). As the cells regenerate, they exhibit syncytial-like qualities with large amounts of cytoplasm. They may

appear flattened at first and then they generally increase in height, first becoming cuboidal and then eventually columnar in shape. During these phases, the epithelium is devoid of mucinous secretions. As the epithelium matures and the inflammation subsides, the columnar epithelium begins to produce mucins again. The crypts begin to appear branched (Fig. 11.78).

Lymphocytes and plasma cells decrease in number and tend to become more focal as the inflammation subsides. Variable numbers of acute and chronic inflammatory cells, Paneth cells (Fig. 11.79), and endocrine cells are also present during this phase. Some patients develop endocrine cell hyperplasia. The mucosal inflammation is confined to the increased lymphocytic and plasma cell content of the lamina propria and occasional crypt abscesses in an intact mucosa. Mucosal lymphoid follicles increase in number, particularly distally. Resolution of the chronic inflammation may produce a patchy infiltrate that can resemble CD in biopsy specimens.

It takes weeks to months for active disease to become quiescent. If the resolution is complete and if the initial damage was minimal, complete architectural restoration occurs. More commonly, permanent architectural abnormalities persist, which represent useful signs of former active disease (Fig. 11.80). Histologic recovery, however, is often incomplete and microscopic evidence of inflammation is common (Fig. 11.80) even in patients with clinically and sigmoidoscopically quiescent colitis.

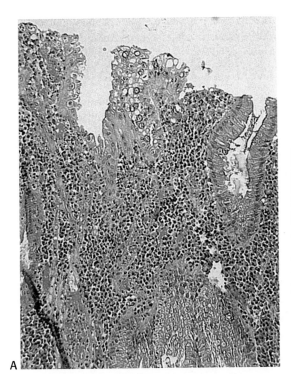

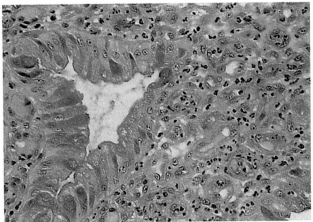

FIG. 11.74. Resolving colitis. **A:** Prominent epithelial regeneration is almost complete. The lamina propria is still acutely inflamed, and large numbers of proliferating blood vessels are present. **B:** A prominent regenerating gland is present. The surrounding mucosa is inflamed.

Prominent crypt branching, surface villiform transformation, and persistence of mucus-depleted epithelial cells with nuclear changes may lead to confusion with dysplasia in the setting of UC. Early regenerative features can be readily distinguished from dysplasia when the number of epithelial cells is not increased. The cytoplasm appears attenuated, the nuclear chromatin appears relatively sparse and finely distributed, and the nuclear-to-cytoplasmic ratio favors the cytoplasm (Figs. 11.75 to 11.77). The use of proliferation markers may help to distinguish between the lesions. Other reparative lesions are more difficult to differentiate from dysplasia.

Features of Fulminant Colitis

Patients with fulminant colitis usually have pancolitis. Microscopic examination shows mucosal denudation; highly vascular granulation tissue; heavy infiltration by histiocytes,

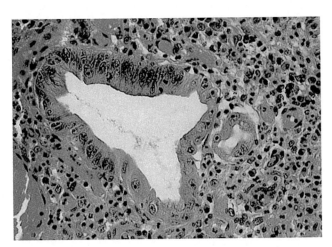

FIG. 11.75. Regeneration in ulcerative colitis. A gland is present in which one half is intensely hyperchromatic. The remainder of the gland is more typically regenerative.

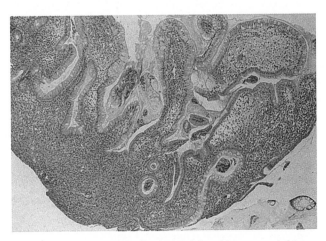

FIG. 11.76. Resolving ulcerative colitis. This mucosal biopsy shows resolving inflammation with transition toward a villiform pattern. The bases of the crypts appear regenerative. The epithelium at the surface contains mucin and some appear hyperplastic.

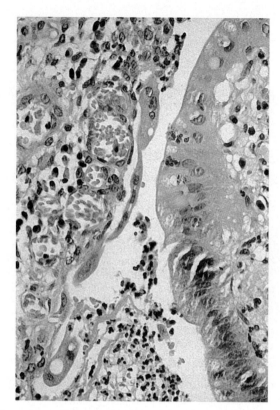

FIG. 11.77. Active regeneration. The epithelium covering the lamina propria on the right-hand portion of the specimen shows a gradient of differentiation from the bottom of the picture to the top. The cells toward the base of the crypt (*bottom*) appear much more hyperchromatic and immature. The cells at the free surface have a large amount of cytoplasm. Several apoptotic bodies are present within the epithelium. Immediately opposite the more mature eosinophilic epithelium on the right-hand side are elongated, multinucleated, syncytial-like epithelial cells covering an area of previous ulceration. A small gland abscess is in the lower middle of the photograph.

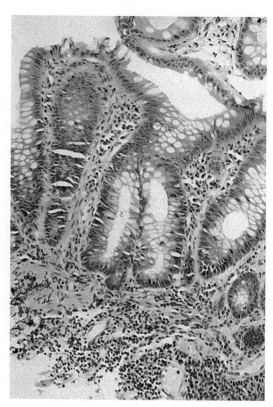

FIG. 11.78. Chronic ulcerative colitis. The crypts appear branched, a sign of previous injury.

plasma cells, lymphocytes, and neutrophils; and marked submucosal edema. The inflammation extends to the circular and longitudinal layers of the muscularis propria with varying degrees of muscle degeneration and necrosis. Often, individual muscle fibers appear shortened and rounded with aggregates of eosinophilic staining cytoplasm within the myofibrils. The myenteric plexuses may be distorted and edematous, particularly in the areas adjacent to extensive mucosal ulceration. The bowel wall lacks fibrosis or the prominent lymphocytic aggregates seen in CD. Prominent lymphoid follicles can be seen in the submucosa in UC in this setting, but they should not be present in areas away from the ulceration.

Features of Inactive (Quiescent) and Chronic Healed Colitis

The changes that characterize active colitis, including superficial ulceration, diffuse acute and chronic inflammation of the mucosa and superficial submucosa, goblet cell depletion, and telangiectasia, disappear during the resolving or quiescent phases of the disease. In quiescent disease, the mucosa becomes diffusely atrophic with architectural changes resulting from damage that occurred during active disease. Mucosal atrophy (Fig. 11.81) takes the form of loss of crypt parallelism with branching or a severe reduction in the number of crypts per unit area. The crypts characteristically shorten and the space between the base of the crypts and the

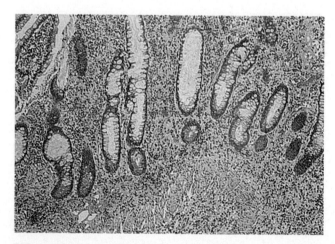

FIG. 11.79. Regenerated mucosa. The glands are almost completely restored. Prominent Paneth cells are present at the band of the crypts.

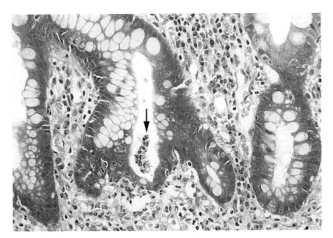

FIG. 11.80. Chronic ulcerative colitis in relapse. The mucosa has a regenerated architectural appearance. Evidence of cryptitis with early crypt abscess is seen within the central branched crypt (*arrow*). In addition, the lamina propria is infiltrated with a large number of eosinophils.

luminal surface of the muscularis mucosae widens (Fig. 11.81). The atrophy may become so extreme that the mucosa consists of little more than a single layer of surface columnar epithelium with only a few very short crypts. Because of the repeated episodes of ulceration followed by periods of healing, glands become embedded in the submucosa (Fig. 11.82). This epithelial herniation into the submucosa may represent a consequence of sustained contractions of the muscularis mucosae. This change affects as many as 40% of patients. The muscularis mucosae thickens and frays (Fig. 11.81) due to previous ulceration and muscular regeneration. Paneth cell metaplasia distal to the hepatic flexure, pyloric metaplasia (Fig. 11.81), and endocrine cell hyperplasia often indicate a long history of colitis.

The atrophic mucosa exhibits a variably increased inflammatory cell infiltrate, sometimes associated with focal accumulations of lymphocytes and plasma cells. In some cases, the mucosa shows no increase in inflammatory cells. Bizarre multinucleated stromal giant cells derived from fibroblasts sometimes appear in the colonic mucosa in biopsy specimens from patients with longstanding quiescent UC (125). The changes are most marked distally, but they may affect the entire bowel, with the proximal changes usually being less severe than the distal ones unless the patient has been given steroid enemas to treat the disease.

Ileitis

Backwash ileitis shows acute and chronic inflammation resembling that seen in the cecum. Crypt abscesses may be present (Fig. 11.83). Histologically, any areas of ulceration are shallow, contrasting with the deep, fissuring ulcers seen in Crohn disease. Characteristically, skip lesions are absent and all contiguous uninvolved segments are unaffected by the inflammatory response.

Strictures

Disagreement exists concerning the frequency of benign strictures in chronic UC. UC-associated strictures develop as a result of muscular hypertrophy and thickening of the muscularis mucosae and muscularis propria rather than from fibrosis. The hypertrophic muscle remains in a spastic or contracted state, resulting in intestinal hypomotility. In addition, there are secondary changes that occur in the muscle that lead to motility abnormalities, shortening, and contraction of the large intestine and loss of the haustral folds. When fibrosis does develop in the setting of UC, it never develops

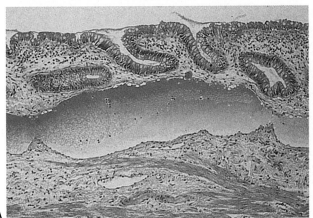 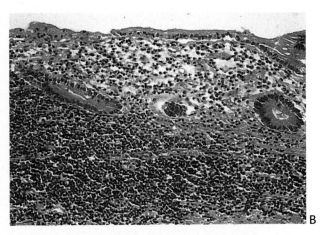

FIG. 11.81. Quiescent colitis. **A:** The mucosa has regenerated. An enlarged telangiectatic vessel is present in the lower portion of the mucosa. In addition, one of the crypts runs parallel to the level of the muscularis mucosae rather than perpendicularly. The overall architecture is simplified. **B:** Subtotal rectal atrophy with diminished numbers of glands and a thinned mucosa. A prominent lymphoplasmacytic infiltrate is also seen straddling both sides of the muscularis mucosae.

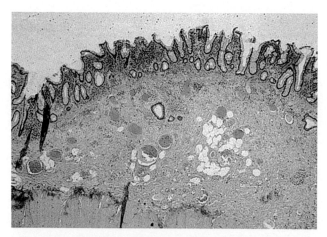

FIG. 11.82. Ulcerative colitis with regenerative mucosa and epithelial displacement. Both sections are from a resection specimen. The overlying mucosa appears regenerative and intensely infiltrated with mononuclear cells. Several glands can be seen in the superficial submucosa. There is a group of three glands just to the left of center and another gland just at the right edge of the photograph.

to the same extent as seen in CD, even when there is deep ulceration with destruction of the muscularis mucosae.

Other strictures form in UC, but these have an ischemic origin. Ischemic strictures show extensive fibrosis, and the mucosa and submucosa become replaced by dense cicatriz-

ing granulation tissue. Ischemia may complicate concurrent CMV infection.

Pseudopolyps

Inflammatory pseudopolyps are typically covered by normal or at least nondysplastic colonic epithelium. The histologic features of the pseudopolyps vary, depending on whether or not they represent residual islands of mucosa separated by wide-based ulcerations, as illustrated in Figure 11.81. In this situation, one sees all of the normal structures of the bowel wall (Fig. 11.84). In other situations, one may see localized expansions of the mucosa with marked infiltrates of mononuclear cells expanding the lamina propria and creating a polypoid elevation of the mucosa, as illustrated in Figure 11.85. In still other cases, the mucosa may exhibit exuberant regeneration with exophytic, highly branched, filiform polyps composed of regenerated glands, as illustrated in Figure 11.85. Finally, the polyps may represent polypoid collections of granulation tissue that extend upward into the gastrointestinal lumen.

Toxic Megacolon

When patients develop toxic megacolon, the most striking histologic feature is the relative lack of involvement of the mucosa by acute inflammation and the very marked expansion of the submucosa by edema. Deep ulcers may be present

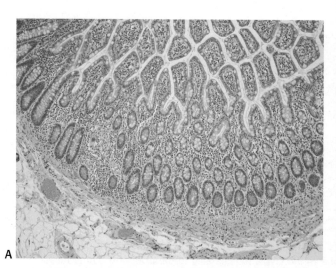

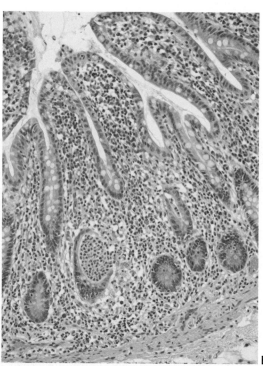

FIG. 11.83. Backwash ileitis in ulcerative colitis. **A:** Low-power photomicrograph showing preservation of the normal villous architecture of the small bowel. There is patchy active inflammation present. **B:** A crypt abscess is seen on higher magnification. Features of chronic injury, however, are not present.

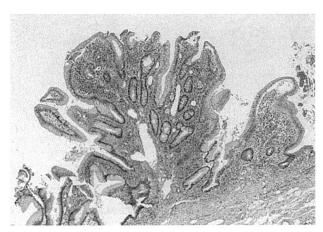

FIG. 11.84. Pseudopolyp. Protuberant mucosal masses that extend above the original height of the mucosa. The lamina propria is expanded by a mononuclear cell infiltrate.

in other portions of the bowel wall and perforations may be present as well (Fig. 11.86).

Ulcerative Appendicitis

Ulcerative appendicitis, the appendiceal counterpart of UC, is present in 50% to 87% of colectomy specimens from patients with pancolitis due to UC. Appendiceal involvement represents part of the continuous inflamma-

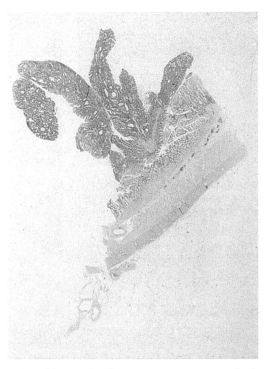

FIG. 11.85. This pseudopolyp represents a more marked extension of the process seen in Figure 11.84, with large numbers of regenerative glands. Such lesions must be examined carefully for the presence of dysplasia, particularly when they appear so cellular.

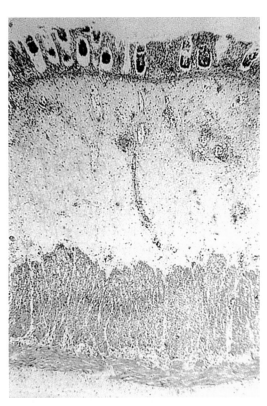

FIG. 11.86. Toxic megacolon with transmural inflammation, marked edema, and inflammation of the overlying mucosa.

tory process that characterizes UC. Appendiceal inflammation also affects 15% to 86% of patients without pancolitis (126–128). Additionally, some patients demonstrate patchy cecal inflammation or appendiceal orifice inflammation associated with left-sided colitis (128). Studies suggest that such "skip lesions" are of no clinical significance, and should not be misinterpreted as features of Crohn disease in patients with otherwise typical ulcerative colitis. Additionally, some patients have what is known as a cecal patch that may represent the cecal equivalent of the appendiceal disease. In some patients, the appendiceal disease appears more active than the cecal disease. One should not be deterred from rendering an unequivocal diagnosis of UC when encountering ulcerative appendicitis as the skip lesion or a more severe lesion in a colectomy specimen that is otherwise absolutely characteristic for UC. The histologic features of ulcerative appendicitis are illustrated in Figure 11.87.

Upper Gastrointestinal Involvement

Rare cases of chronic active duodenal or gastric inflammation have been reported in association with ulcerative colitis (129–131). It is as yet unclear whether these cases represent an unusual manifestation of ulcerative colitis or a separate associated disorder. Longer follow-up of the reported cases is required before such a determination can be made.

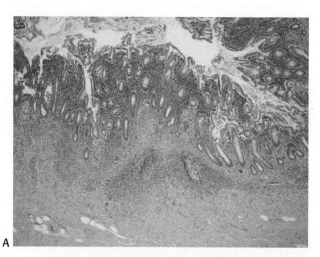
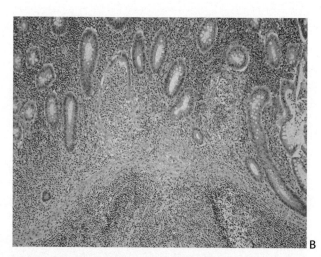

FIG. 11.87. Ulcerative appendicitis. **A:** The appendix shows changes similar to those that were present in the colon in this patient. There is prominent crypt architectural distortion present and active inflammation involving the mucosa. **B:** Higher magnification showing active inflammation and numerous crypt abscesses.

Ulcerative Colitis with Superimposed Infections

UC patients experience a significantly higher incidence of infections than control patients. These may induce a relapse of the UC or a superimposed ischemic colitis. Common infections include CMV and *C. difficile*. If a patient unexpectedly experiences a relapse of the disease, stool cultures or toxin assays may detect a complicating infection. The pseudomembranous characteristics of *C. difficile* infection in the noncolitic patient do not occur in UC (Fig. 11.88). CMV infections cause endothelialitis, formation of small intravascular thrombi, and ischemic necrosis. Biopsies taken from such patients exhibit deeper inflammation than usually characterizes UC (because of

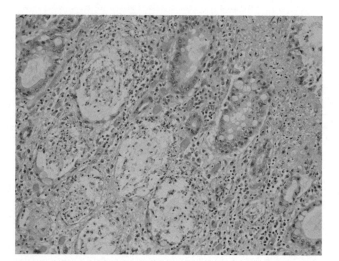

FIG. 11.88. *Clostridium difficile* colitis superimposed on ulcerative colitis. There is patchy withering of the colonic crypts and other features reminiscent of ischemic injury. The patient had documented *C. difficile* colitis. The typical volcanolike eruptions of neutrophils from the eroded mucosal surface and pseudomembranes were not present in this case.

the ischemia), and chronic changes when severe may obscure the underlying UC. This is particularly problematic when a biopsy is seen for the first time in an emergent setting because of sudden worsening of the disease and previous biopsies are unavailable for review. In this setting, one must decide whether the clinical diagnosis of UC is correct, whether other changes are superimposed on the pre-existing disease, or whether the patient has CD or some other disorder. This distinction is of more than academic interest because the clinician often faces a critical clinical treatment decision as to whether to increase immunosuppressive therapy to control the UC. If the diagnosis of UC is made without recognizing a coexisting CMV infection, the clinician is likely to increase the dose of steroids or azathioprine, drugs that will only worsen the infection. In contrast, if one makes a diagnosis of CMV, the patient may receive ganciclovir or a related drug. Failure to recognize a CMV infection may eventually lead to more generalized ischemic damage and even perforation (Figs. 11.89 to 11.92). The diagnosis of CMV infection is made by detecting the presence of viral inclusions within the endothelium, macrophages, or epithelium. Most typically, the viral inclusions are in the stromal cells, particularly the endothelial cells. Fibrin thrombi and endothelialitis are often present. When thrombi occur, features of ischemia are superimposed on the ulcerative colitis.

Effects of Therapy

Various therapies used to treat IBD, whether they be local instillation of corticosteroid enemas or systemically administered anti-inflammatory agents, may suppress some of the more classic gross or histologic features associated with the diagnosis of UC. Suppression of rectal inflammation can lead to the false impression of a rectal-sparing disease such as CD. Therapy may also predispose the intestine to develop

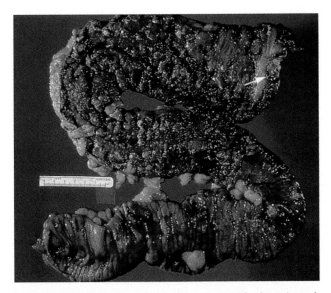

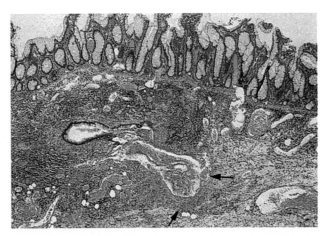

FIG. 11.89. Resection specimen in a patient with ulcerative colitis, a cytomegalovirus infection, ischemia, and perforation. The area of perforation lies adjacent to the ileocecal valve (*arrow*). In this patient, it appears as though the disease is more severe on the right side of the colon than on the left. This is due to the fact that ischemic injury was present from the ileocecal valve to the midtransverse colon and to the fact that the distal disease was more quiescent in nature.

FIG. 11.90. Histologic features from the resection specimen shown in Figure 11.88. One sees misplaced glandular epithelium within the submucosa. Barium (the greenish material indicated by the *arrows*) lies near the misplaced epithelium. Note the prominent irregular submucosal inflammation and the submucosal telangiectasia.

secondary complicating features, such as a CMV infection, with or without secondary endotheliitis, and ischemia. Patients who undergo steroid withdrawal may develop an acute ileus simulating intestinal obstruction (132).

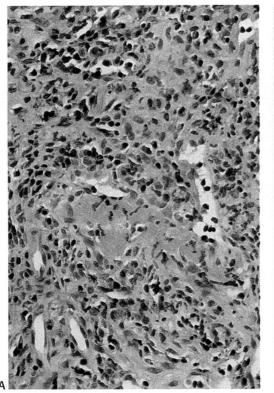

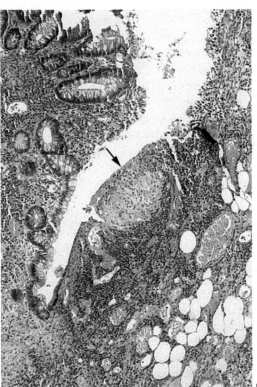

FIG. 11.91. Histologic features from the colectomy specimen shown in Figure 11.88. **A:** Small fibrin thrombus in a capillary. **B:** A portion of an ulcer in which a granulomalike response centers around a small capillary (*arrow*). This presumably resulted from the cytomegalovirus endotheliitis.

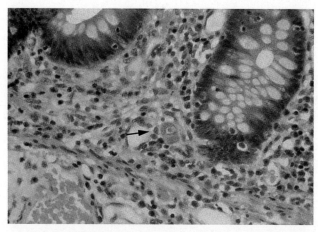

FIG. 11.92. Inclusion-bearing cell in the lamina propria of the patient whose colectomy is illustrated in Figure 11.88 (*arrow*).

INDETERMINATE COLITIS AND COMBINED CROHN DISEASE AND ULCERATIVE COLITIS IN THE SAME PATIENT

Only about 5% to 20% of IBD patients exhibit overlapping features falling into the category of "indeterminate" or "mixed" colitis. Judging from material seen in consultation, the diagnosis of indeterminant colitis is overused and generally reflects inadequate clinical information on the extent and distribution of the disease, information from radiographic or endoscopic studies, or unfamiliarity with some of the nuances of both diseases or the effects of intercurrent infections of therapy (Table 11.15). UC and CD may coexist. As noted in a previous section, CD patients with serum P-ANCA expression exhibit UC-like phenotypes, and this may account for the presence of both histologic features in the same patient.

TABLE 11.15 Difficulties in Differentiating Ulcerative Colitis (UC) from Crohn Disease (CD)

Limited morphologic expression in the colon
Incomplete expression of the disease
Occurrence of indeterminate colitis with features of both UC and CD
Clinical mimicry of UC and CD by other inflammatory diseases
Absence of rectal involvement in otherwise classic UC
Simultaneous occurrence of both CD and UC
Modification of the pathologic features by therapy
Presence of second complicating disease, such as ischemia or infection
Lack of adequate clinical information
Small biopsy size
Inadequate number of biopsies to evaluate disease distribution and extent
Unfamiliarity of the pathologist with the full range of morphologic findings in both diseases

DIAGNOSIS OF INFLAMMATORY BOWEL DISEASE IN ENDOSCOPIC BIOPSIES

Some of the most common biopsies seen in a surgical pathology practice involve the histologic assessment of colonic inflammatory conditions. Often the surgical pathology requisition states, "Rule out acute self-limited colitis (ASLC), rule out UC, rule out ischemia." Alternatively, the requisition may request one to distinguish UC from CD. The diagnosis of IBD is best distinguished from the other forms of colitis by a systematic approach (Tables 11.16 and 11.17). It is always helpful if one examines biopsies in a standardized way in order to assess each diagnostic feature. In this way, one is unlikely to miss a helpful parameter that might be present. Such a systematic approach involves evaluation of several parameters, including epithelial alterations (whether acute or chronic), changes in the lamina propria, vascular changes, and changes in the muscularis mucosae. Signs of chronicity include architectural alterations with prominent crypt branching or atrophy, a villiform structure, Paneth cell or pyloric metaplasia, lymphoid follicles, or prominent plasma cells above the muscularis mucosae. The diagnosis of

TABLE 11.16 Features To Be Consistently Evaluated in Biopsies for the Diagnosis of Inflammatory Bowel Disease

Architectural changes
Architectural parameters focus on the crypt architecture evaluating the following:
Crypt orientation (distortion)
Crypt length
Distance of crypt bases from muscularis mucosae
Intercryptal distance
Crypt branching
Villiform transformation of crypt surface
Ratio crypt surface/lamina propria surface
Epithelial changes
Mucus content
Presence of Paneth or pyloric cells
Presence or absence of intraepithelial lymphocytes or eosinophils
Cryptitis
Endocrine cell hyperplasia
Presence or absence of specific microorganism
Lamina propria changes
Presence or absence of inflammation
Nature of inflammation: Acute or chronic
Distribution of inflammation:
Focal or diffuse
Superficial or basal
Within crypts or in lamina propria
Mucosal or extension beyond mucosa
Presence or absence of specific microorganism
Presence or absence of fibrosis
Presence or absence of granulomas
Characteristics and location of granulomas, if present

TABLE 11.17 Differences in Biopsy Appearances of Ulcerative Colitis and Crohn Disease

	Ulcerative Colitis	Crohn Disease
Distribution of inflammation or mucosal atrophy		
Diffuse or segmental	Diffuse	Segmental, especially among several biopsies
Most marked distally	Typical	Uncommon
Proximal change with distal sparing	No[a]	Sometimes
Inflammation		
Uniform intensity in each biopsy	Typical	Occasional
Marked focality within and between biopsies[b]	Uncommon	Usual
Neutrophils diffusely attack crypts	Typical	Sometimes
Neutrophils free in the lamina propria, crypt sparing	Very uncommon	Typical, focal
Disproportionate submucosal inflammation	No	Typical but uncommon
Granulomas[c]	Only to foreign material	Characteristic when present (maximum 50%)
Submucosal inflammation	Rare—continuous	Common, often patchy
Muscularis mucosae	If present is continuous	No
Noncaseating, compact	No	Typical
Focal ulceration with minimal adjacent inflammation	Fulminant disease only	Typical
Mucosa sinus tracts	No	Common
Epithelial features		
Villous	Common	Occasional presence favors ulcerative colitis
Diffuse mucin depletion in active disease	Usual	Occasional
Paneth cell metaplasia	Common	Occasional
Pyloric metaplasia in the ileum	Absent	Typical but uncommon
Stromal changes		
Vasculitis	Absent unless concomitant cytomegalovirus	Occasional
Telangiectasia	Common	Absent
Neural hyperplasia	Rare	Common

[a] The use of rectal steroid-containing enemas may create the appearance of rectal sparing.

[b] A false impression of focal disease can be obtained from biopsies of inflammatory polyps and biopsies of granulation tissue at anastomotic lines.

[c] The absence of granulomas does not exclude the diagnosis. The presence of loose mucin granulomas does not establish the diagnosis.

different forms of colitis does not rely solely on the histologic features that are present. Knowledge of the endoscopic appearance, the clinical features, and the disease distribution are essential. Such a diagnostic approach facilitates distinction of UC from the diseases that mimic it (Table 11.18).

Patients with UC and CD share many similarities, but there are also significant differences that create the need to distinguish between them. Different surgical approaches are used to treat IBD patients depending on the nature of the underlying disease. Surgical techniques for continent ileostomy or ileoanal anastomosis with construction of a pouch reservoir allow one to avoid an ileostomy following colectomy. The operation is designed to improve the quality of life in UC patients by preserving fecal continence. However, this procedure is not generally used to treat CD patients. Total proctocolectomy in a UC patient with backwash ileitis allows the ileum to heal, but the same operation in a patient with CD ileocolitis may leave residual disease or

TABLE 11.18 Diseases Clinically Mimicking Colonic Inflammatory Bowel Disease

Bacterial infection
  Escherichia coli 0157:H
  Salmonella
  Shigellosis
  Tuberculosis
  Clostridium
  Campylobacter
  Gonorrhea
  Syphilis
  Staphylococcal enteritis
  Yersinia
  Lymphogranuloma venereum
Fungal infection
  Histoplasmosis
Chlamydial infection
  Chlamydial colitis–proctitis
Viral infection
  Cytomegalovirus
  Herpes simplex
Protozoan infection
  Amebiasis
  Schistosomiasis
  Anisakiasis
Ischemic colitis
  Polyarteritis
  Large vessel disease
  Drugs digitalis (contraceptives, potassium salts)
  Colitis-complicating obstruction
Other specific diseases
  Eosinophilic gastroenteritis
  Pseudomembranous colitis
  Behçet syndrome
  Uremic colitis
  Immunodeficiency syndromes
  Collagenous colitis
  Radiation colitis
Diverticulitis
Solitary ulcer syndrome
Inflammation due to therapeutic interventions
  Enemas and laxatives
  Drug-induced colitis
  Colitis in graft vs. host disease
  Antibiotic-associated colitis

may be followed by a high incidence of stomal dysfunction and recurrent ileitis. As a result, pathologists are under great pressure to distinguish UC from CD on biopsies before the patients undergo surgical intervention.

When the diseases are well developed, UC and CD have unique and distinguishing features that allow their separation from one another (see Tables 11.12 and 11.13). Because no one feature is invariably present, and because the features change with disease evolution, all of the pathologic features need to be assessed in aggregate. Reasons for difficulty in differentiating UC from CD are summarized in Table 11.15.

Separating IBD from other causes of enterocolitis can also be quite difficult due to the significant overlap that may exist in the clinical, radiologic, endoscopic, and pathologic manifestations of the inflamed intestine (see Table 11.14).

The presence of several specific histologic features correlates with a high predictive probability of diagnosing IBD. The confidence ratio is 87% to 100% when the histologic findings include distorted crypt architecture (Fig. 11.93), increased numbers of both round cells and neutrophils in the lamina propria (Fig. 11.93), a villous surface (Fig. 11.76), crypt atrophy, basal lymphoid aggregates, and basally located isolated giant cells (Fig. 11.35). The presence of villous surface, basal lymphoid aggregates, crypt atrophy, and surface erosions all favor the diagnosis of UC, whereas the presence of granulomas favors the diagnosis of CD. Because CD is a focal disease, it is important to note that a patient with CD may have biopsy specimens that show a completely normal mucosa, a focal or diffuse colitis, or granulomas. Giant cells occur as often in ASLC as in IBD.

When a series of biopsies shows a consistent pattern of focal inflammation (Fig. 11.94) or when the biopsy shows an ulcer, erosion, or crypt destruction with crypt abscess formation in one focus and relatively normal adjacent mucosa, the possibility of UC is essentially ruled out and the diagnosis of CD is confirmed. However, it should be emphasized that many biopsies from CD patients show diffuse inflammation indistinguishable from UC.

Preservation of colonic mucin is a common feature of CD (Fig. 11.94), but it may only represent a manifestation of an essentially focal disorder, and it may not distinguish CD from UC. Its main value is to distinguish a normal biopsy from specimens showing IBD.

The prototypic biopsy for UC comes from a patient with classic endoscopic features (and this information has been transmitted to the pathologist) who has evidence of diffuse colonic mucosal damage that may straddle the muscularis mucosae to involve the upper submucosa. The diagnosis of UC is easiest when one finds increased numbers of lymphocytes and plasma cells within the lamina propria and a basal plasmacytosis in association with characteristic cryptitis or crypt abscesses. Some patients with UC show an inflammatory infiltrate that crosses the muscularis mucosae to involve the upper submucosa. This inflammation occurs in a band-like fashion and is continuous with the overlying mucosal inflammation (Fig. 11.95). If there is a gap between the mucosal and submucosal inflammation or if the submucosal inflammation is focal in nature (Figs. 11.94 and 11.96), the more likely diagnosis is CD. The presence of focal fibrosis in a setting that otherwise suggests inflammatory bowel disease is consistent with CD.

The presence of any significant ileal disease establishes the diagnosis of CD rather than UC with backwash ileitis. Ileocecal valve incompetency in UC can produce ileal changes (backwash ileitis), but the involved ileal segment should be short and the bowel should lack other characteristic features of CD.

FIG. 11.93. Mucosal biopsy in a patient with Crohn colitis. **A:** A biopsy specimen with mild glandular irregularity and an intense infiltrate in the submucosa. The inflammation is more or less diffuse. The amount of submucosal inflammation is out of proportion for what would be seen in ulcerative colitis unless one were in the area of a lymphoid follicle in which follicular structures should be seen. The arrows indicate the muscularis mucosae, the boundary between the mucosa and the submucosa. **B:** Histiocytic cells in the lamina propria adjacent to the glands. The upper lamina propria contains large numbers of mononuclear cells.

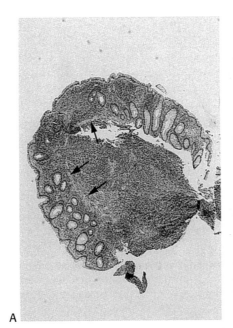
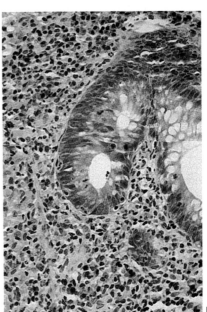

A   B

The diagnostic value of rectal biopsies in CD is proportional to the distance of the diseased segment from the anal margin. When disease is distal to the splenic flexure, 50% of biopsies will be diagnostic. When primarily ileal disease is present, the rectal biopsy is diagnostic in only 12% of patients. The diagnostic accuracy rate of rectal biopsies for CD ranges from 15% to 40% as compared to 70% for UC (133,134). The low diagnostic accuracy rate for CD relates to the sampling error inherent in diagnosing a patchy disorder with discontinuous pathologic features (133). The yield of a positive diagnostic finding directly relates to the presence of sigmoidoscopic or radiologic abnormalities in the distal colon and rectum.

In some studies, the presence of lymphoid aggregates discriminates patients with IBD (135). On average, one lymphoglandular complex occurs approximately every 2 cm in normal subjects and one every 0.7 cm in patients with colitis (136). However, Theodossi et al found that lymphoid follicles had a similar frequency in patients with CD, in patients with UC, and in normal individuals (137).

The range of agreement over the final diagnosis of UC versus CD ranges from 40% to 76% (133,137). The low accuracy rate for diagnosing CD is attributed to the sampling error inherent in the diagnosis of a patchy disease. There is good agreement in discriminating between normal mucosa and IBD. However, for normal slides, the term "nonspecific

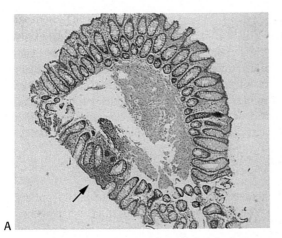
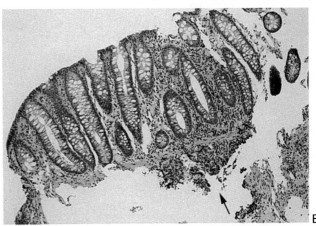

A   B

FIG. 11.94. Mucosal biopsy in Crohn colitis. **A:** This mucosal biopsy shows mild glandular irregularity suggestive of mild previous damage and an area of focal inflammation that extends into the underlying submucosa (*arrow*). **B:** Another biopsy from the same patient showing patchy muscular inflammation (*arrow*). The patchiness of the inflammation in the mucosa and involvement of the muscularis mucosae suggests a focal process. This distinguishes the lesion from ulcerative colitis but does not rule out other entities, such as ischemia. A knowledge of the clinical context in which the biopsy was taken would be critical to its interpretation.

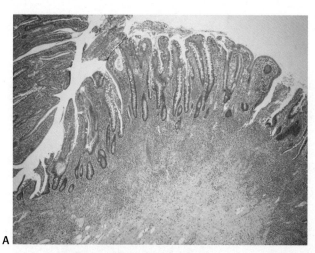
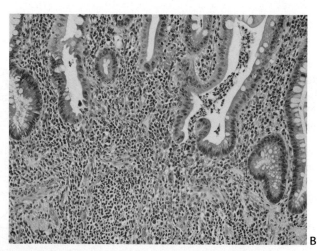

A   B

FIG. 11.95. Submucosal inflammation in ulcerative colitis. **A:** Some patients with ulcerative colitis demonstrate prominent superficial submucosal inflammation that could be misinterpreted as representing Crohn disease. This patient had longstanding disease with a distribution pattern of ulcerative colitis. **B:** Higher power magnification. The muscularis mucosae appears discontinuous in this area.

inflammation" is often applied without any consistency. In addition, true CD is often thought to be UC. Frei and Morson concluded that in practical terms an accuracy rate in CD of 40% is probably adequate. The rate of false-positive diagnoses was 5% (133).

There will be some circumstances in which it is not possible to distinguish between UC and CD.

EXTRAINTESTINAL COMPLICATIONS OF INFLAMMATORY BOWEL DISEASE

A large percentage of IBD patients suffer from one or more extraintestinal complications at some time during the course of their disease. These complications affect many organ sys-

tems and may be of little clinical consequence or they may be severe, disabling, and critical determinants in directing the patient therapy (Fig. 11.97).

Musculoskeletal Complications

Table 11.19 lists the musculoskeletal complications of IBD. The most common extraintestinal manifestation of IBD is arthritis, the incidence of which ranges from 7% to 25% (138–140). The incidence varies, depending on whether the

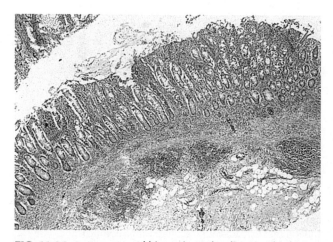

FIG. 11.96. Large mucosal biopsy in Crohn disease. This biopsy is deeper than many and contains superficial submucosa. In this setting, it is possible to see the prominent lymphoid aggregates and also the lack of mucin depletion.

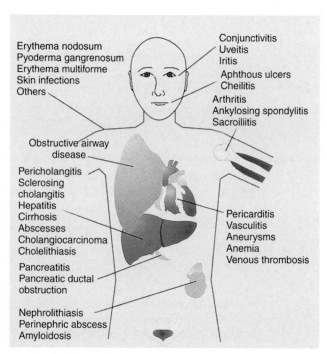

FIG. 11.97. Diagram of the extraintestinal manifestations of inflammatory bowel disease.

TABLE 11.19	Musculoskeletal Complications of Inflammatory Bowel Disease
Peripheral arthritis, arthralgia	Granulomatous myositis (rare)
Sacroiliitis	Septic arthritis
Ankylosing spondylitis	Osteomyelitis
Finger clubbing	

TABLE 11.20	Hepatobiliary Diseases Complicating Inflammatory Bowel Disease

Liver
  Fatty liver (steatosis)
  Pericholangitis
  Chronic active hepatitis
  Liver abscesses
  Fibrosis and cirrhosis
  Hepatic granulomas
  Amyloidosis
  Nodular regenerative hyperplasia
  Abscesses and pylephlebitis
Biliary tract
  Pericholangitis
  Primary sclerosing cholangitis
  Bile duct carcinoma
  Cholelithiasis
Miscellaneous
  Portal vein thrombosis
  Occlusion of hepatic acini

diagnosis is made only in patients with objective findings and abnormal radiographs diagnostic of arthritis, or whether it also includes patients with symptomatic arthralgias. Musculoskeletal complaints may predate the onset of intestinal symptoms. Peripheral arthritis occurs with greater frequency in patients with CD than with UC, and it affects patients with colonic CD more frequently than those with only small intestinal involvement. The joint manifestations of CD cannot be distinguished from those associated with UC. Arthritis usually does not affect patients with quiescent disease, but it does accompany disease exacerbations and frequently associates with aphthous ulcers, skin lesions, and iritis. The peripheral arthritis affects the hips, ankles, wrists, and elbows in decreasing order of frequency. Small joints of the hands and feet are less commonly involved. Synovial biopsies demonstrate a nonspecific synovitis with changes including loss of synovial cells and inflammation.

The major manifestations of sacroiliitis include narrowing of the joint space, erosions, and sclerosis of the sacroiliac joints. There is a high incidence of silent IBD in patients with spondyloarthropathy. Twenty-five percent of patients have early features of CD (141). An increase in intraepithelial T cells suggests that augmented mucosal antigen handling and involvement of the MHC plays a role in the pathogenesis of spondyloarthropathy-related gut inflammation in CD (141).

It is well established that IBD associates with osteoporosis in from 2% to 30% of cases (142). Osteopenia occurs in an even larger number of patients. Many factors play a role in IBD-associated bone loss, including malnutrition, calcium, and vitamin D deficiency attributable to small bowel disease or surgical resection. Steroid therapy is also a contributing factor.

Hepatobiliary Disorders

Up to 50% of patients with IBD have minor liver and biliary tract abnormalities or elevated liver enzymes, but probably no more than 5% to 10% have clinically significant liver disease (143). Hepatobiliary complications overall occur with comparable frequency in UC and CD patients, even though different frequencies exist for specific complications. The frequency and severity of hepatobiliary diseases correlates with the extent, duration, and severity of the underlying IBD. Table 11.20 lists the major IBD-associated liver diseases.

Steatosis

Steatosis affects approximately 30% of IBD patients (144). Extensive fatty infiltration usually affects seriously ill patients and resolves with patient recovery. The fat is of the macrovesicular type with large lipid droplets in liver cells. The fat exhibits a diffuse, centrilobular, and periportal distribution. The pathogenesis is unknown, but it may result from malabsorption or a generally poor nutritional status. It may also result from bacterial metabolites released when bacteria gain access to the portal system secondary to the mucosal ulcerations. Other etiologic factors may include anemia, drugs, toxins, or other "toxic" substances absorbed through an eroded inflamed intestinal mucosal surface.

Pericholangitis

Pericholangitis is the most common bile duct lesion complicating IBD (Fig. 11.98); it affects both children and adults (145). The disorder represents a variant of primary sclerosing cholangitis that involves the smaller intrahepatic bile ducts. Pericholangitis affects patients with extensive colonic involvement and develops in three phases: (a) an acute phase, (b) a subacute phase with early periportal fibrosis, and (c) a chronic lesion with circumductal fibrosis. When the disease first presents, patients may have minimal signs and symptoms of liver disease.

Histologically, one sees portal triad enlargement, edema, bile ductular proliferation, and an inflammatory cell infiltrate, usually consisting of lymphocytes, plasma cells, occasional neutrophils, and eosinophils (Fig. 11.98). The heaviest infiltrate surrounds the interlobular bile ducts, but it may also be evenly distributed throughout the portal spaces. A loose proliferation of fibroblasts surrounds the interlobular

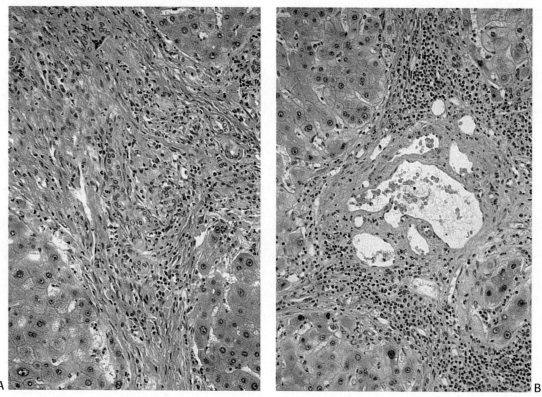

FIG. 11.98. Pericholangitis in inflammatory bowel disease. **A:** The portal tracts are widened with beginning bridging fibrosis and prominent chronic inflammatory cells surround proliferating bile ductules, which are inconspicuous and difficult to see. **B:** As the lesions progress, increasing amounts of fibrosis surround the ductal structures and the portal tracts because pericholangitis and sclerosing cholangitis often go hand in hand. The expanded portal tracts also show a heavy infiltration of chronic inflammatory cells around the sclerotic portal tracts.

bile ducts and dense circumductal fibrosis becomes more marked as the disease progresses. In many patients harmless periductal fibrosis replaces the inflammation. In others, the lesion progresses to chronic liver disease, even to biliary cirrhosis.

Patients with cholangitis develop heavily thickened bile duct basement membranes and translucent areas containing bilelike material. The extravasated bile enhances the development of periductal fibrosis progressing to sclerosing cholangitis (146). Intracanalicular bile thrombi and bile inclusions may develop in the hepatocytes.

Primary Sclerosing Cholangitis

Primary sclerosing cholangitis (PSC), a serious chronic progressive cholestatic liver disease characterized by inflammation and fibrosis of the bile ducts, strongly associates with a diagnosis of UC. PSC affects 2% to 7% of UC patients (63,147). Conversely, most patients with PSC have UC (70% to 80%). The risk of PSC is higher in patients with pancolitis and is greater for UC than CD (148). The converse association is much stronger, with up to 80% of individuals with PSC having UC (149). PSC primarily affects young males who usually present with progressive fatigue, pruritus, jaun-

dice, and a cholestatic biochemical profile. The lesion is most easily demonstrated by cholangiography.

An immunologic abnormality might underlie the development of the lesion. The association of sclerosing cholangitis with Riedel thyroiditis, retroperitoneal fibrosis, mediastinal fibrosis, and pernicious anemia is cited as indirect evidence for an immune-mediated etiology (150). Additionally, a colitis-associated immunoglobulin antibody cross-reacts with an antigen on colonic and biliary epithelium (151), and an ANCA occurs in both UC and PSC (152). ANCAs may serve as a prognostic indicator for the development of PSC (153).

The familial occurrence of PSC and UC suggests that genetic factors also play a role in the etiology of the disease, especially because it associates with a high incidence of B8 and DRW3 haplotypes of the major histocompatibility system (154). Liver biopsies often fail to diagnose the lesion but are useful for staging once the disease is diagnosed.

PSC is characterized by a progressively sclerosing obliterative process involving the extrahepatic bile ducts and, occasionally, the intrahepatic bile ducts (Fig. 11.99). The liver may appear normal or reveal acute, subacute, and chronic pericholangitis, cholestasis, or cirrhosis (Fig. 11.100. Histologically the fibrotic thickening of the bile duct wall contains a diffuse mononuclear infiltrate, which is predominantly lymphocytic

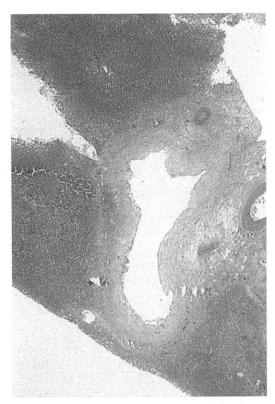

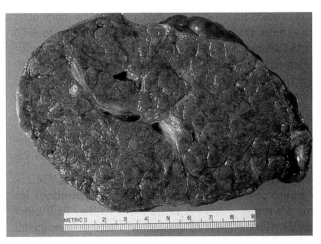

FIG. 11.100. Irregular cirrhosis in a patient with sclerosing cholangitis.

Biliary Carcinoma

Carcinoma of the biliary tract affects 1% to 4% of IBD patients, an incidence ten times greater than that seen in the normal population. Males are affected more commonly than females. IBD patients usually present with their tumors in the 4th and 5th decades, whereas such tumors usually present in the 7th decade in the general population (156). Most patients have a long history of extensive colonic disease. Biliary cancer predominantly affects UC patients, but it may also affect those with CD. The mean duration of colonic symptoms prior to cancer development is 15 years. Patients have often undergone colectomy, sometimes decades earlier. The most common clinical presentation is painless obstructive jaundice (Fig. 11.101). Carcinomas develop in all parts of the biliary tree, but the extrahepatic ducts are more commonly affected than the intrahepatic ducts or the gallbladder. The tumors are usually adenocarcinomas and are often multicentric in origin.

FIG. 11.99. Sclerosing cholangitis. A dense onion-skinning fibrosis surrounds the large bile duct. The amount of inflammation is minimal.

in nature. A lesion classified as small duct primary sclerosing cholangitis consists of hepatobiliary lesions within the intrahepatic bile ducts. The histologic features resemble those of large duct sclerosing cholangitis. Some patients go on to develop cirrhosis.

PSC serves as a marker for the development of colorectal cancer in UC. UC patients with PSC are five times more likely to develop dysplasia than those without it (63,155).

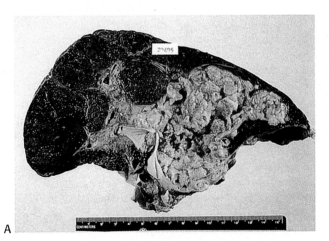

A

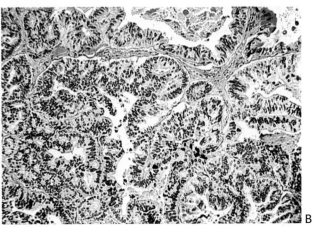

B

FIG. 11.101. Cholangiocarcinoma arising in a patient with biliary cirrhosis secondary to longstanding ulcerative colitis and sclerosing cholangitis with pericholangitis. **A:** As can be seen from the photograph, the patient had been markedly jaundiced. The patient died of ulcerative colitis and its complications. **B:** Histologic features of cholangiocarcinoma shown in A.

Cholelithiasis

Gallstones affect IBD patients more frequently than those in the general population (140). Distal ileal dysfunction may predispose to the secretion of lithogenic bile.

Pancreatic Abnormalities

Pancreatic abnormalities occur with increased frequency in IBD, complicating either the disease itself or sometimes the drug therapy. Clinically significant and non–drug-related pancreatitis affects two subgroups of IBD patients: (a) patients with duodenal CD who develop reflux of duodenal contents into the pancreatic duct through an incompetent ampulla or through direct ampullary involvement (157), and (b) UC patients with sclerosing cholangitis or pericholangitis who develop pancreatitis on the basis of ductal inflammation. Occasionally, patients with CD present with acute relapsing pancreatitis (157). Also, some patients with CD have evidence of compact sarcoidlike granulomas in the pancreatic tissue.

Amyloid

Secondary amyloidosis is a rare complication of IBD, most often affecting CD patients (158). The amyloid deposits in multiple organs, including the liver and kidneys. Some patients may die of renal failure. The amyloid that develops in patients with UC may resolve, making this form of amyloid unique (159).

Skin Lesions

Many mucocutaneous lesions complicate IBD. Cutaneous lesions affect 10% of patients at the time of IBD diagnosis, and up to 20% throughout the course of their disease (138). IBD-associated cutaneous manifestations may be divided into three types: Granulomatous, reactive, and secondary to nutritional deficiency (140).

Erythema Nodosum

Erythema nodosum affects about 3% to 8% of patients with IBD and 1% to 2% of patients with CD limited to the small bowel (138). It represents the most common extracolonic manifestation of IBD in children. Women are affected three or four times more frequently than men. The lesions may appear before the diagnosis of IBD and their presence often correlates with activity of the bowel disease. The characteristic lesions present as raised, red or reddish-blue, warm, tender nodules, predominantly distributed on the lower legs, especially on the anterior surfaces (Fig. 11.102). They may also be present on the lateral or posterior surfaces of the legs and occasionally on the arms. Some lesions ulcerate. Erythema nodosum is thought to result from hypersensitivity reactions but the specific inciting antigens are unknown.

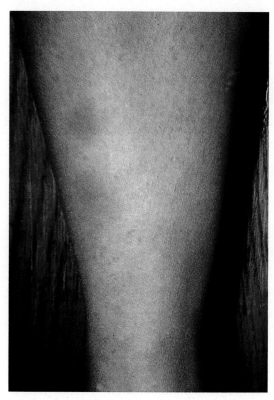

FIG. 11.102. Erythema nodosa on the forearm.

Histologically, erythema nodosum may undergo endothelial cell necrosis, thrombus formation, and ulceration. Oral aphthous ulcers, iritis, and peripheral arthritis sometimes accompany the erythema nodosum.

Pyoderma Gangrenosum

Pyoderma gangrenosum is a serious lesion that occurs exclusively in IBD patients. Pyoderma gangrenosum affects approximately 1% to 5% of patients with UC and is roughly three times more common in UC patients than CD patients (160). The presence of the lesions correlates with the presence of active disease. Eighty-five percent of patients with pyoderma gangrenosum have pancolitis. Symptoms usually occur before the diagnosis of IBD is made. The lesions may recur after initially responding to medical treatment and are rare following colectomy. Patients usually give a history of preceding minor trauma. The lesion most commonly involves the pretibial region, although it may be seen on any part of the body, including the face and scalp. Patients also develop peristomal pyoderma gangrenosum.

The skin lesions are macroscopically described as single or multiple deep discrete ulcerations with a necrotic center, an undermined border, and violaceous skin surrounding the lesion. Individual lesions evolve from small pustules that coalesce into painful ulcers, frequently in a few days.

Histologic features are not characteristic and include necrosis, suppuration, angiitis with fibrinoid necrosis, thrombosis, and sometimes granulomas. The lesions are sterile and contain a dense dermal neutrophilic infiltrate. If left untreated, the lesions may penetrate deeply causing osteomyelitis, even necessitating amputation of an extremity.

Pyoderma Vegetans

The presence of pyoderma vegetans is highly suggestive of IBD (161). Patients may have associated sclerosing cholangitis (162). Pyodermatitis–pyostomatitis vegetans is an annular, pustular eruption that involves the oral mucosa, groin, axillae, face, scalp, lower trunk, and limbs. The oral lesions are the most easily recognizable on clinical examination and are virtually pathognomonic (161). Pyoderma vegetans initially begins in intertriginous areas with vegetating plaques and vesicular pustules that resolve with postinflammatory hyperpigmentation. Multiple pustules occur on an erythematous base and may coalesce and undergo necrosis to form a characteristic snail-track appearance. Patients typically demonstrate peripheral eosinophilia. Histologically, the main features include pseudoepitheliomatous hyperplasia with intraepidermal abscesses containing neutrophils and eosinophils. Pyoderma vegetans may represent an incomplete form of pyoderma gangrenosum.

Cutaneous Crohn Disease

Ulceration of the skin around colostomies or ileostomies usually represents a reoccurrence of the CD and can be cured by resection or revision of the ostomy. Cutaneous disease also results from direct extension of IBD from the perianal area onto the perianal skin. Granulomas separated from the GI tract by normal skin are called distant cutaneous CD. This uncommon cutaneous manifestation of CD presents as subcutaneous nodules, plaques with or without ulceration, ulcerated patches, lichenoid papules, or intertriginous ulcerations and erysipelaslike lesions (163). Histologically, one sees dermal and sometimes subcutaneous noncaseating granulomas that may be perivascular in location. As with other extraintestinal cutaneous manifestations, distant cutaneous CD affects patients whose CD involves the colon.

Vesiculopustular Eruptions

Localized or generalized vesiculopustular eruptions affect some UC patients (164). The lesions consist of grouped erythematous vesiculopustules (3 to 5 mm) that sequentially crust and heal with postinflammatory hyperpigmentation. Some consider this to represent an abortive form of pyoderma gangrenosum. Histologic examination reveals intraepidermal neutrophilic abscesses with mixed inflammatory dermal infiltrates.

Other Cutaneous Lesions

Zinc deficiencies in CD lead to acrodermatitis enteropathica, a psoriasislike lesion that responds to zinc therapy. Alopecia

areata associates with UC, has a familial aggregation, and has an HLA association common to both disorders (165). Cutaneous vasculitic gangrene affects IBD patients and differs in appearance from pyoderma gangrenosum. The underlying cause of the vasculitis often remains unclear.

Mucosal Lesions

Oral lesions, both symptomatic and asymptomatic, affect 6% to 20% of CD patients (166). Similar lesions in UC are less well documented. Most oropharyngeal manifestations of IBD occur in patients with active intestinal disease and their presence frequently correlates with disease activity.

Recurrent aphthous ulcers are the most common oral manifestation of IBD (Fig. 11.103). The cause of oral aphthous ulcers is multifactorial. They may result from nutritional deficiencies of iron, folic acid, and vitamin B_{12}. Discrete punched-out superficial ulcers begin shortly before or during acute exacerbations of the IBD and may associate with other extraintestinal complications, including arthritis, erythema nodosum, and iritis. In patients prone to develop aphthous ulcers, the development of a new crop of oral ulcers often heralds flare-up of the bowel disease. The ulcers may be painful, interfering with eating and drinking. These lesions must be differentiated from oral candidiasis, which also complicates severe IBD, particularly in a patient treated with steroids and antibiotics.

CD patients develop diffuse swelling of the lips and cheeks, inflammatory hyperplasias of the oral mucosa, indurated polypoid taglike lesions in the vestibular and retromolar mucosa, persistent deep linear ulcerations with hyperplastic margins, and indurated fissuring in the midline of the lower lip. CD patients may also develop the oropharyngeal lesions and lesions of the epiglottis and aryepiglottic folds characterized by palatal submucosal edema, lymphatic dilation, and nonspecific perivascular chronic inflammatory cell infiltrates. Lymphoid nodules and microgranulomas consisting of clusters of histiocytes and occasional multinucleated

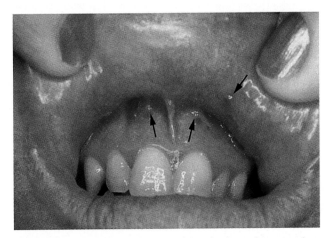

FIG. 11.103. Aphthous ulcers involving the buccal mucosa in a patient with Crohn disease.

TABLE 11.21	Eye Lesions in Inflammatory Bowel Disease Patients
Uveitis	Chorioretinitis
Conjunctivitis	Keratitis
Iritis	Blepharitis
Cataracts	Retinal detachment
Marginal corneal ulcers	Uveitis
Antral serous retinopathy	Scleromalacia
Episcleritis	Ischemic optic neuropathy
Orbital myositis	

TABLE 11.23	Vasculitides Associated with Inflammatory Bowel Disease.
Thromboembolism	
Polyarteritis nodosa	
Takayasu disease	
Giant cell arteritis	
Large vessel disease with aneurysm formation	
Gastrointestinal vasculitis	
Cutaneous vasculitis	

giant cells also develop. Oral findings in UC patients include ulcers analogous to pyoderma gangrenosum of the skin and pyostomatitis vegetans.

Some patients develop ulcerative tracheobronchitis years after colectomy for UC (167), and severe upper airway stenosis affects some UC patients (168). UC patients also develop oral hairy leukoplakia (169), a lesion more commonly associated with AIDS. The lesion may serve as a marker of severe immunosuppression.

Eye Lesions

Approximately 10% of IBD patients develop ocular complications (140). The most common eye lesions are listed in Table 11.21. Eye lesions often appear early in acute episodes or relapses of the bowel disease, and they subside as the disease goes into remission. Orbital myositis, a nonspecific inflammation involving the ocular muscles, develops in some patients.

Gynecologic Features

CD patients have a number of gynecologic problems (Table 11.22). The lesions are typified by chronic granulomatous inflammation with exudation and marked tissue destruction (see Fig. 11.53). Special stains for acid-fast bacilli, fungi, and Donovan bodies are negative in vulvar CD. Vulvovaginal disease has also been complicated by the development of Bowen disease in the area of CD (170). CD involving the labia may present as unilateral labial hypertrophy, especially in young children.

TABLE 11.22	Gynecologic Problems of Inflammatory Bowel Disease Patients
Vulvar, vaginal, perineal, or labial lesions	
Ulcers	
Granulomas	
Fistulas	
Bowen disease	
Infertility	
Adnexal masses	
Preterm deliveries	

IBD patients also sometimes present with an acute abdomen or with an adnexal or pelvic mass that may be incorrectly diagnosed as pelvic inflammatory disease, as acute appendicitis, or even as an ovarian cyst. Pregnant patients may have an increased incidence of preterm delivery (171), and 30% to 50% of pregnant women have an exacerbation of their IBD during their pregnancy and postpartum period.

Vasculitis

Vasculitis (Table 11.23) affects different parts of the body in patients with different forms of IBD. Some believe that vascular lesions represent a universal intestinal finding in CD, playing an important role in the development of the pathologic features of the disease (172). Cutaneous, systemic, and cerebral circulations are affected. No specific clinical features distinguish patients with vascular involvement from those without this phenomenon.

Cutaneous Vasculitis

Both necrotizing (leukocytoclastic) vasculitis and benign cutaneous polyarteritis nodosa occur in IBD patients (173). Cutaneous or systemic polyarteritis nodosa associates with CD. The vasculitis results from deposition of immune complexes in blood vessel walls, and presents as purpuric skin lesions or as visceral disease. The usual sites of involvement are the legs and acral areas. Mixed cryoglobulinemia may be demonstrated in some patients. Histologic examination shows a typical necrotizing panarteritis with granulomatous features when associated with CD, and leukocytoclasia, hemorrhage, and vessel wall damage.

Large Vessel Disease

Large vessel disease leads to aneurysm development, often affecting the major intestinal vasculature, including the superior mesenteric artery. Aneurysms also develop in the iliac and brachiocephalic vessels and in the aortic arch. Histologic examination shows the presence of intimal and medial fibrosis, extensive degeneration of the medial elastomuscular lamellae, and adventitial inflammation, predominantly consisting of a mononuclear cell infiltrate.

Takayasu Arteritis

Takayasu arteritis, an inflammatory and stenotic disease of medium-sized and large arteries with a strong predilection for involvement of the aortic arch and its branches, the pulmonary artery, and cerebral arteries, affects a small number of UC patients (174).

Giant Cell Arteritis

Giant cell arteritis has also been described complicating IBD (175). The disease presents as recurrent erythematous, tender, painful cords and subcutaneous nodules that tend to ulcerate, involving the skin of the lower and upper extremities. Most patients are in their 20s, with patients ranging in age from 13 to 31 years. Histologically, one sees granulomatous panarteritis involving the muscular arteries of the subcutis and adjacent dermis, as well as vessels of peripheral nerves and skeletal muscle.

Genitourinary Complications

Genitourinary (GU) complications affect 4% to 23% of IBD patients (176). The three most common GU complications are urinary tract calculi, ureteral obstruction, and vesicle fistulae (176). These most commonly affect patients with severe, longstanding CD. Nephrolithiasis affects 2% to 10% of patients (177), contrasting with an incidence of <1 per 1,000 in the general population. Frequently implicated lithogenic factors include oliguria, diminished water absorption, urinary tract obstruction, infection, abnormal urate excretion, alterations in oxalate absorption and excretion, steroid administration, hypercalcemia, prolonged bedrest, and decreased intestinal sodium absorption with concomitant decreased urinary sodium (177). Proctocolectomy with ileal pouch–anal anastomosis increases the risk of stone formation. Severe diarrhea or profuse ileostomy discharge following colectomy leads to a low volume of concentrated urine, often with a low pH secondary to intestinal bicarbonate loss. These factors contribute to the formation of urate stones. In addition, ileal resections or extensive ileal disease, as occurs in CD, often causes hyperoxaluria.

Obstructive hydronephrosis affects CD patients; it results from ureteral compression by abscesses or inflammatory masses, retroperitoneal extension of intestinal inflammatory processes originating as perforations or fistulae.

Bladder involvement by CD results from direct extension of the inflammatory process from a contiguous segment of inflamed bowel, with or without intervening abscess formation. When fistulae develop, patients may experience pneumaturia and urinalysis may reveal pyuria and infection.

Thromboembolic Complications

Thromboembolic complications affect 1.3% to 6.4% of CD and UC patients (Fig. 11.104) (178). Both venous throm-

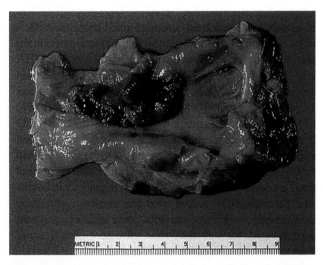

FIG. 11.104. Portal vein thrombosis in a patient with a hypercoagulable state and inflammatory bowel disease.

boembolism and arterial thrombosis develop. Arterial thrombosis, however, is rare, occurring most commonly following surgery. Extensive arterial thrombosis (179) occasionally occurs in UC patients. Portal vein, mesenteric vein, and hepatic vein thrombosis also associate with a high mortality.

Cerebral venous thrombosis is an extremely rare complication of IBD with only a small number of cases reported in the literature. When it develops, the outcome is poor (180). In most instances, permanent neurologic sequelae or death results (179). Even young infants may develop central nervous system thrombosis (180). Thromboembolic episodes more commonly affect the deep peripheral veins or result in pulmonary emboli. The risk of thrombotic complications increases with disease activity or other precipitating events. In some series, 64% of patients have active disease at the time of thrombosis (172).

The thrombosis in IBD is generally considered to result from the presence of a hypercoagulable state. Other contributing factors include bedrest, toxemia, and surgical procedures. Hemostatic abnormalities include thrombocytosis, elevated fibrinogen, factors V and VII, vitamin K, and decreased protein C and S, factor XIII, and antithrombin III levels (172,181,182). Sixty-three percent of CD and 25% of UC patients demonstrate free protein S deficiency. Protein C deficiency also occurs. Protein C activity may return to normal on disease remission or following subtotal colectomy (183). Other abnormalities include the presence of fibrin microclots. Platelets circulate in an activated state in IBD, and the increased platelet activation and aggregation found in this disorder may contribute to the risk of systemic thromboembolism and mucosal inflammation secondary to ischemia. Circulating immune complexes contribute to the development of vasculitis (184), which then predisposes to thrombosis. Additionally, patients might have CMV infections that can precipitate localized clotting secondary to an endothelialitis.

Pulmonary Complications

Respiratory disorders complicating IBD include pulmonary vasculitis, localized interstitial fibrosis, apical fibrosis, panbronchiolitis, chronic suppurative bronchitis, and bronchiectasis involving both large and small airways. The lung may also represent a latent site of involvement by CD based on the demonstration of a lymphocytic alveolitis and granulomatous lung disease (185). Patients also develop sulfasalazine pneumonitis (186).

Hematologic Abnormalities

Hematologic abnormalities affect many IBD patients, with iron deficiency anemia due to GI blood loss representing the most common abnormality. As many as one third of IBD patients have hemoglobin levels <12 g/dL (187). Macrocytic anemia develops as the result of folate deficiency during sulfasalazine therapy or with impaired B_{12} absorption in patients with terminal ileal CD (188). CD patients also produce inadequate amounts of erythropoietin because cytokines, such as interleukin-6, suppress erythropoietin production (189). Patients also spontaneously develop autoantibodies directed against red cells or develop Coombs-positive autoimmune hemolytic anemias as a result of sulfasalazine therapy (190). Azathioprine therapy causes bone marrow toxicity with thrombocytopenia and leukopenia (191). IBD patients also present with refractory anemia and myelodysplasia (192).

Other Lesions

Perineuritis resulting in a peripheral neuropathy may represent an autoimmune manifestation of the disease (193). Patients with pericarditis develop asymptomatic pericardial effusions and cardiac tamponade (194). The pericarditis associated with IBD may represent an adverse drug effect. Some patients also develop hyperthyroidism (195). A rare patient has also been described who had selective IgA deficiency, UC, and celiac disease (196).

COMPLICATIONS OF INFLAMMATORY BOWEL DISEASE THERAPY
COMPLICATIONS OF DRUG THERAPY

Because patients with UC and CD often have lifelong problems associated with their inflammation, they are treated with many drugs to reduce the inflammatory response. This can predispose patients to infections, including *C. difficile* and CMV. Sulfasalazine treatment results in pneumonitis or a Coombs-positive autoimmune hemolytic anemia (190). Mesalazine causes interstitial nephritis (197). Long-term steroid therapy leads to all of the well-known problems associated with steroid use, including osteonecrosis. Therapy may also mask the usual histologic features of IBD.

Changes Seen with Fecal Stream Diversion

Fecal stream diversion induces inflammation in the defunctionalized intestinal segment. The changes are predominantly mucosal and they may generate histologic confusion, especially when granulomas develop. Rectal stumps typically show such features as follicular hyperplasia (which may sometimes be quite extensive), transmural inflammation, granulomas, fissures, and changes akin to ischemia with pseudomembranous colitis (Fig. 11.105). Even though the patient's underlying disease may be UC, the changes may mimic CD.

Changes in Ileostomies

Ileostomies are prone to develop pathologic lesions, including inflammatory polyps and adenocarcinomas (Fig. 11.106).

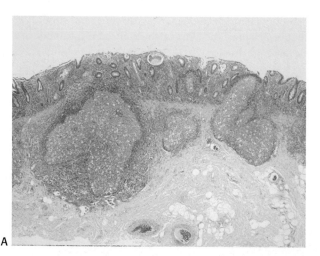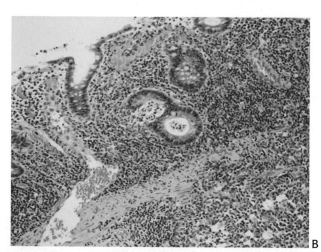

FIG. 11.105. Diversion colitis in a patient who underwent previous total abdominal colectomy for ulcerative colitis. **A:** Low-power view showing marked lymphoid hyperplasia in the rectal pouch. **B:** Higher magnification demonstrating scattered foci of active inflammation including crypt abscesses.

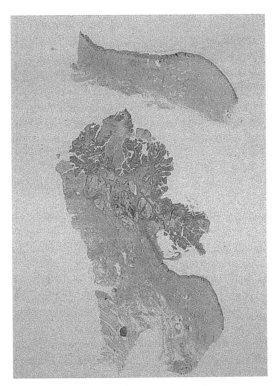

FIG. 11.106. Carcinoma arising in ileostomy. These two figures represent different patients with cancers developing in their ileostomies. The cancer remains relatively superficial and the part lying on the right-hand portion of the specimen shows a dense cellular infiltrate corresponding to an area of poorly differentiated carcinoma.

Additionally, a small percentage of patients will require ileostomy revision because of prolapse, tightening of the stoma, or localized sepsis. Histologic evaluation of the resected ileostomy shows variable mucosal atrophy and inflammation. The mucosa may also appear ulcerated. When carcinomas develop, they are sometimes surrounded by large intestinal mucosa.

Complications of Restorative Proctocolectomy (Pouchitis)

Abdominal colectomy with ileal pouch–anal anastomosis has become the surgical treatment of choice for most patients with uncontrollable UC. This procedure removes all of the diseased mucosa while preserving continence and transanal defecation. With the creation of ileal pouches, the primary function of the terminal ileum changes from absorption to fecal storage. The most common long-term complication of the procedure is nonspecific inflammation of the ileal reservoir, commonly known as pouchitis. This complication affects 15% to 47% of patients (198,199) and becomes chronic in 5% (200). Complications of pouchitis are likely to be much more severe if patients had histologic evidence of CD. Pouchitis is also more common in patients with primary sclerosing cholangitis, with a cumulative prob-

ability of developing the condition of 79% at 10 years (201). Smoking appears to be protective against pouchitis in patients with UC (202).

Bacterial overgrowth resulting from stasis is thought to play a major role in the development of pouchitis (203). Anaerobic bacterial concentrations in ileal pouchitis correlate with the presence of nonspecific histologic changes, including villous atrophy and chronic inflammation. Fecal stasis and aerobic and anaerobic bacterial overgrowth may contribute to the development of colonic metaplasia. Other factors that may play a role in the development of pouchitis include the presence of volatile fatty acids, fecal bile acids, oxygen-free radicals, ischemia, platelet-activating factor, and hormonal factors (199,203,204).

Definition

In some centers, pouchitis is defined clinically as the following: (a) a syndrome of frequent watery and often bloody stools associated with fecal urgency, incontinence, abdominal cramps, malaise, and fever; and (b) symptoms present for 2 or more days that respond promptly to metronidazole (199,205). At St. Mark's Hospital, pouchitis is defined as the triad consisting of (a) diarrhea, (b) endoscopic features of inflammation in the pouch, and (c) histologic evidence of active inflammation (204).

Sandborn et al developed a pouchitis disease activity index (PDAI) (198). The PDAI was significantly greater in patients with clinical features of pouchitis than it was for patients who did not have pouchitis. Such a pouchitis disease activity index may be useful in prospective studies to facilitate valid comparisons between medical centers and to objectively measure the response in therapeutic trials.

Clinical Features

Clinical symptoms of pouchitis include diarrhea, rectal bleeding, abdominal cramps, urgency, tenesmus, and malaise. In severe cases, these symptoms may be accompanied by incontinence and fever (198). Endoscopic findings include edema, mucosal erythema, granularity, friability, bleeding, loss of the vascular pattern, and the presence of a mucus exudate with small superficial areas of ulceration (204). Generally, a significant relationship exists between the endoscopic and the histologic features.

The endoscopic findings are also similar to those in UC including edema, granularity, friability, bleeding, loss of the vascular pattern, and the presence of a mucus exudate with a trend toward mucosal ulceration (206).

Mucosal Adaptation

Three basic patterns of mucosal adaptation develop in pelvic ileal pouches: (a) normal mucosa or mild villous atrophy with no or mild inflammation, (b) transient atrophy with temporary moderate or severe villous atrophy followed by normalization of architecture, and (c) constant atrophy with permanent subtotal or total villous atrophy and severe pouchitis (Fig. 11.107). The pouch mucosa converts to one with a colonic phenotype in 80% of cases (207) and pouchitis most commonly affects those in whom metaplasia has developed (200). The greater the degree of colonic metaplasia in the pouch mucosa, the more likely one is to see histologic pouchitis (200). The metaplasia is detected in a manner similar to its detection in ileostomies.

Histologic Features

Patients with pouchitis have a pattern of mucosal inflammation similar to that seen in UC. Early changes consist of neutrophilic and eosinophilic inflammation with architectural distortion, Paneth cell metaplasia, and a partial transition to the colonic mucinous phenotype, as well as an increased proliferative index (208). These features remain relatively stable after 6 months, except for a greater degree of mononuclear

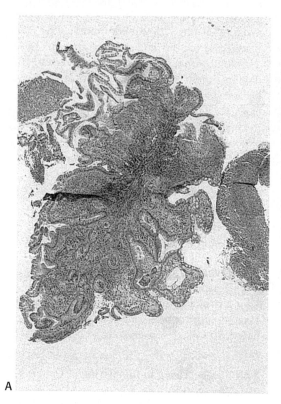

A

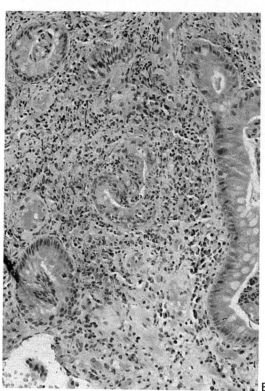

B

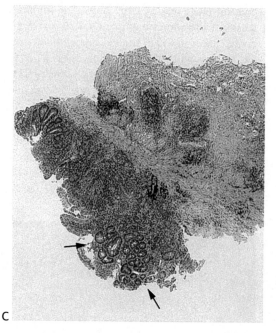

C

FIG. 11.107. Pouchitis. **A** and **B** show a low and high magnification of a biopsy from a patient with pouchitis. The villi appear distorted and broadened with beginning colonic metaplasia. The mucosa is infiltrated with acute and chronic inflammatory cells. Cryptitis is present and is shown at higher magnification in the center of B. This patient had undergone an ileoanal anastomosis following resection for ulcerative colitis. The changes resemble those seen in active ulcerative colitis. In contrast, **C** shows mucosal biopsies from another patient who underwent an ileoanal anastomosis and who developed severe pouchitis. Here the changes more closely resemble those seen in Crohn disease because of the nodular lymphoid aggregates found in the submucosa. Review of the original specimens in the patient confirmed that the previous disease was ulcerative colitis.

infiltration and a progressive increase in eosinophilic inflammation. Additionally, various infections may be present, including *Candida.*

Refractory chronic pouchitis may resemble Crohn disease. However, review of the colectomy specimen usually shows unequivocal UC, and the patients do not have any other clinical, radiologic, or pathologic evidence to support a diagnosis of CD. However, because of the histologic resemblance to CD, one should exclude the presence of transmural inflammation, granulomas, fibrosis, or strictures in areas distant from the anastomosis. Review of previous biopsy material also proves helpful in delineating the true nature of the inflammatory process. Sometimes, an analysis of serologic markers may also be useful in difficult-to-distinguish cases. A correlation exists between pouchitis, primary sclerosing cholangitis, and extraintestinal manifestations of IBD (198,199).

Aphthous ulcerations are one of the earliest lesions affecting the neoileum in CD. They develop in approximately 80% of patients within 1 year of ileal resection (209). Fistulae also develop as a result of previously unrecognized CD. These usually extend from the pouch to other sites such as the vagina or bladder.

CANCER COMPLICATING INFLAMMATORY BOWEL DISEASE

General Comments

Patients with IBD, including both UC and CD, are at increased risk for the development of gastrointestinal carcinoma, particularly colorectal adenocarcinoma (210–212). The incidence of carcinoma is estimated to be 10 to 20 times greater for the small bowel and 4 to 20 times greater for the large bowel than in the general population. Cancer affects 4.8% of patients with CD and 11.2% with UC. The cancer risk positively correlates with disease duration and the anatomic extent of the colitis. Patients with left-sided colitis develop both their colitis and their cancers about a decade later than those with extensive disease, and the mean duration of the colitis before a cancer diagnosis ranges from 17 to 21 years (213–215).

The cancer incidence is greater in persons with extensive UC (i.e., those in whom the disease extends proximally to the midtransverse colon). Multiple carcinomas develop with equal frequently in CD and UC (11% and 12%, respectively) (215). Patients also develop carcinomas outside of the GI tract.

Relationship to Disease Duration and Age at Diagnosis

The median duration of disease to diagnosis of cancer is long (CD 15 years and UC 18 years). Most cancers develop after more than 8 years of disease (CD 75%, UC 90%). The average age at the time of diagnosis of carcinoma is approximately 10 to 20 years earlier than carcinomas arising in patients without IBD. The median age at diagnosis of colorectal cancer in IBD patients is 54.5 years for CD and 43 to 45 years for UC patients (215,216). The risk is 20 to 30 times higher in individuals with pancolitis of 10 or more years' duration than in a control population. The risk of cancer complicating colitis is 0.5% per year for 10 to 20 years after diagnosis and 0.9% for 20 to 30 years, and 1.5% thereafter (217). Some data suggest that an increased risk exists for patients who develop IBD at an early age, although this remains controversial (218).

Cancer Arising in the Setting of Ulcerative Colitis

UC associates with an increased colon cancer risk. Carcinoma in UC affects young patients and is associated with a high incidence of multicentricity. Among 1,248 UC patients seen at the Cleveland Clinic and followed for a mean duration of 14.4 to 21 years (216), 66.5% developed colorectal cancer and 3.8% had extracolonic malignancies (216). Most cancer patients are men (2:1) with extensive (90%) and long-lasting (20 years or more) colitis. The colitis was inactive before the diagnosis of cancer in 48% of patients. The cumulative risk of colorectal cancer is significantly higher in patients with extensive colitis than in those with left-sided disease (11.9% vs. 1.8% at 20 years, and 25.3% vs. 3.7% at 30 years) (215). Although the carcinomas arise predominantly in the left side of the colon and in the rectum, there may be a higher incidence of right-sided colon cancer than in the noncolitis population. The diagnosis was suspected clinically in 64% of cases (215).

Among those with extracolonic malignancy, the incidence of bile duct carcinoma, leukemia, bone tumors, and endometrial cancer is significantly greater than expected, whereas that of lung cancer is significantly lower.

PSC patients represent a subset of UC patients who exhibit a markedly increased incidence of colonic neoplasia. Patients with both PSC and colitis, but not cholangitis alone, have a 10-fold elevated colorectal cancer risk (219). DNA aneuploidy in nonneoplastic mucosa in UC patients predicts a high risk for future development of neoplasia (220). Patients with both PSC and UC are six times more likely to exhibit mucosal aneuploidy than patients with UC alone (155).

Cancer Arising in the Setting of Crohn Disease

Patients with longstanding CD (>7 years) have an increased incidence of large bowel carcinomas (221,222); these are sometimes multiple (223). The risk of developing cancer in CD is similar in magnitude to that found in UC patients with left-sided colitis but is much less than that found in UC patients overall. As in UC, the cancers tend to develop in patients with longstanding disease and in patients who are younger, on the average, than those with intestinal carcinoma

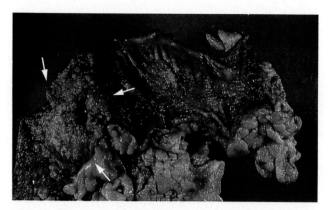

FIG. 11.108. Gross features of dysplasia in inflammatory bowel disease. Portion of the transverse and descending colon from a patient with ulcerative colitis. Note the presence of a large plaquelike lesion (*arrows*) occupying much of the left-hand side of the photograph. Several smaller plaquelike lesions are present. All of these were dysplastic histologically.

in the general population (224). Cancers develop in the large intestine, small intestine (Fig. 11.108 and 11.109), and anus.

The relative risk for developing colorectal cancer in CD patients overall is 3.4. Patients with extensive colitis exhibit a relative risk of 18.2 (225). Patients with CD also evidence an excess number of cancers of the upper GI tract, mainly rep-

resented by an increased number of small intestinal cancers. Risk factors for developing small intestinal carcinoma include surgically excluded small bowel loops, chronic fistulous disease, and male sex. A relationship also exists between cancer development and certain occupations, particularly those that involve exposure to halogenated aromatic compounds, aliphatic amines, asbestos, cutting oils, solvents, and abrasives (214).

Unlike sporadic small intestinal carcinomas that commonly involve the duodenum, small intestinal carcinomas complicating CD arise in the distal small bowel in areas involved by CD. The distribution of GI cancers in CD is 25% in the small bowel (30% in the jejunum, 70% in the ileum), 70% in the large bowel, and 5% in the remaining sites (223). Crohn disease patients also develop carcinomas within their ileostomy stomas (226).

Patients who develop anorectal carcinomas have longstanding severe CD. There is also an increased incidence of urinary bladder carcinoma (227).

Risk Factors and Pathophysiology of Cancer Development

There is considerable interest in the relationship between oxidant stress and the development of cancer. As noted previously, both UC and CD are associated with increased reactive

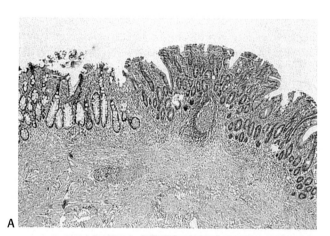

A

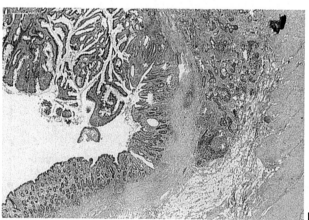

B

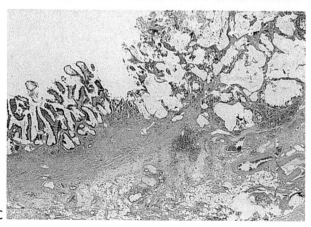

C

FIG. 11.109. Carcinoma arising in the small intestine of a patient with Crohn disease. A and B come from the same patient; C comes from a second patient. In **A,** one sees a large area of dysplasia on the right-hand portion of the mucosa. In **B,** one can see a polypoid exophytic lesion with a carcinoma invading into the underlying submucosa. In both A and B, the epithelium has become so atrophic that it resembles colonic mucosa. **C:** Dysplasia and invasive carcinoma. The dysplastic epithelium to the left of the photograph replaces the normal villous structure of the small bowel. A mucinous carcinoma has developed in the right-hand side of the photograph. It invades the superficial portion of the submucosa.

oxygen metabolites (ROMs). ROMs can cause oxidative DNA damage leading to base changes, strand breaks, and enhanced protooncogene expression; oxidative stress can induce malignant transformation (228). Factors such as the rate of damage, the status of antioxidant defenses, DNA repair mechanisms, and the necessity for multiple steps (initiation, promotion, and progression) all play a role in whether or not cancer develops.

Dysplasia as a Marker for Cancer Risk

Dysplasia was first postulated to be a precursor of carcinoma in UC by Warren and Sommers in 1949 (229); its histologic appearance in polypoid lesions was described in detail by Dawson and Pryse-Davies in 1959 (230), and in 1967 Morson and Pang (231) demonstrated that dysplasia could be detected on biopsy, thereby identifying patients who are likely either to have or to develop carcinoma.

The evidence supporting the concept of dysplasia as an indicator of malignancy in UC derives largely from two types of observations. First, retrospective analyses of resected colons harboring carcinomas from patients with UC almost uniformly disclose coexisting dysplasia, either adjacent to, or remote from, the carcinomas. The relationship between colon cancer and dysplasia is stronger when the dysplasia is adjacent to the cancer and when the dysplasia is high grade (232). Second, studies of patients who have undergone colectomy following biopsy demonstration of dysplasia often have a coexisting suspected (or unsuspected) carcinoma in the colectomy specimen (233).

Patients with CD also develop dysplasia resembling that seen in UC. Precancers in CD histologically resemble those seen in patients with UC (Fig. 11.110). One often finds multifocal precancer characterized by epithelial dysplasia, adenomatous growth patterns, and villiform transformation of the mucosa. These signs are identical to those associated with UC and are present both adjacent to and distant from infiltrating cancers. The dysplasia ranges from widespread multifocal disease to focal dysplasia (234). The more severe the dysplasia, the closer a lesion is to becoming an invasive carcinoma. However, carcinomas may rarely arise from areas of low-grade dysplasia. The finding of low-grade or high-grade dysplasia indicates that the colon is at high risk for malignant changes, although the time frame between the onset of dysplasia and malignant transformation may vary. Dysplasia-associated lesions or masses (DALMs) (Figs. 11.108 and 11.111) are the most consistent indicator of carcinoma (232,235).

Despite the usefulness of dysplasia in predicting neoplastic transformation and cancer development, the concept of dysplasia predicting cancer development has the following drawbacks: (a) it involves a certain degree of subjectivity and skill to make the diagnosis and to grade the dysplasia; (b) the dysplasia has a patchy mucosal distribution, so that a negative rectal biopsy does not exclude large bowel neoplasia; (c) dysplasia is not always grossly visible or the gross features may be atypical; (d) a proportion of IBD patients develop cancers in the absence of demonstrable dysplasia; and (e) not all patients with dysplasia develop cancer.

Options for Reducing the Cancer Risk

The recognition that IBD has a malignant potential places the responsibility on clinicians to minimize or eliminate the risk that these patients will die from colonic cancer. Although most agree that patients with high-grade dysplasia have a strong risk for either concomitant cancer or the development of cancer, not all agree on the management of such patients.

Endoscopic Surveillance

Surveillance programs have been accepted as the standard of care for UC patients. Carcinomas detected in surveillance programs tend to be of lower stage than those occurring in patients not undergoing surveillance (236). Surveillance increases life expectancy due to earlier cancer detection (214). The death rates in patients with cancers detected in and out of surveillance programs are 11% and 60%, respectively (236).

Patients who develop colorectal carcinoma when under surveillance develop them mainly in the left colon (237,238). Most failures in surveillance programs, as evidenced by the presence of extensive cancer, usually develop in individuals who are referred for the first time for colonoscopic surveillance screening. Such patients have often been lost to follow-up before they were eligible for surveillance or had been remote from the medical system (214).

Since areas of dysplasia and cancer are equally distributed throughout the colon, total colonoscopy is required to detect their presence. The best method of surveillance involves regular colonoscopy, allowing visualization and biopsy of the entire colon. A recent consensus statement provides guidelines for surveillance in patients with IBD (239). In patients with UC, an initial screening colonoscopy should be performed 8 to 10 years after the onset of symptoms, following which a regular program of surveillance should begin. Patients with extensive colitis or left-sided colitis who have a negative screening colonoscopy should be seen within 1 to 2 years. With two negative examinations, the screening interval may be increased to up to 3 years until the disease duration reaches 20 years. At this time the surveillance interval should be decreased to every 1 to 2 years since the risk for colon cancer increases with long duration of colitis (240). Patients with primary sclerosing cholangitis should undergo initial screening colonoscopy at the time of diagnosis of PSC, and then should have annual surveillance colonoscopy thereafter. Individuals with only ulcerative proctitis (no macro- or microscopic disease proximal to 35 cm) may be screened according to the guidelines for colorectal screening for the general population.

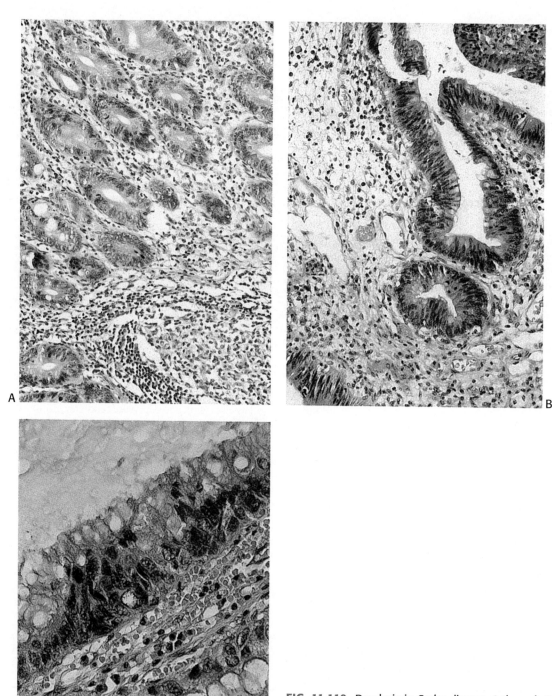

FIG. 11.110. Dysplasia in Crohn disease. A through C represent different areas of dysplasia in patients with Crohn disease. All figures come from the small bowel. **A:** A mixture of both high-grade and low-grade dysplasia in the basal portion of the mucosa. **B:** Stratified epithelium resembling that found in adenomas. **C:** Note the loss of nuclear polarity and the marked hyperchromasia of the cells lining this villous projection.

Abnormal findings on surveillance colonoscopy are followed up in a variety of ways depending on the degree of dysplasia present. All diagnoses of dysplasia should be confirmed by an experienced gastrointestinal pathologist.

Indefinite for Dysplasia

Patients with confirmed diagnoses indefinite for dysplasia should be followed up with repeat surveillance colonoscopy in 3 to 6 months.

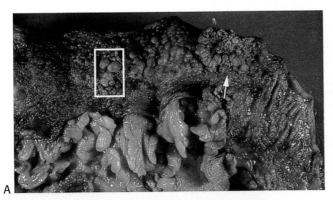

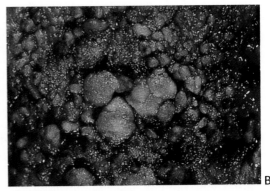

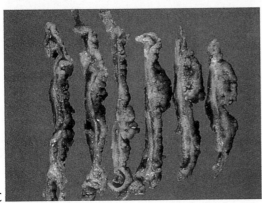

FIG. 11.111. Carcinoma and dysplasia in inflammatory bowel disease. **A:** Portion of the transverse and descending colon demonstrating diffuse mucosal abnormalities. A dysplasia-associated lesion or mass is indicated by the *arrow*. The *box* highlights a series of nodular lesions that do not appear more worrisome than other parts of the mucosa. These are shown at higher magnification in **B** and in cross section in **C,** and represent an early invasive carcinoma.

Flat Low-grade Dysplasia

Controversy exists about the management of low-grade dysplasia because the natural history of this lesion is unknown. For patients complying with a strict surveillance program, finding flat low-grade dysplasia during surveillance may not carry the same high risk of progression to high-grade dysplasia or cancer as finding flat low-grade dysplasia on initial screening examination (241,242). There is evidence that with low-grade dysplasia as the worst histologic diagnosis at colonoscopy, an unrecognized synchronous colorectal cancer may already be present in up to 20% of individuals (241,243). Therefore, competing options should be discussed with each patient. A prophylactic colectomy should be offered given the possibility of a synchronous adenocarcinoma, particularly if the number of colonoscopic biopsies is insufficient.

A patient confirmed to have *multifocal* flat low-grade dysplasia (two or more biopsies from a single surveillance examination) or *repetitive* flat low-grade dysplasia (two or more examinations with at least a single focus of low-grade dysplasia) should be strongly encouraged to undergo prophylactic total proctocolectomy.

Regardless of the focality of flat low-grade dysplasia, if colectomy is deferred and the patient elects to continue with surveillance, a repeat examination should be performed within 3 months and no later than 6 months from the discovery of the low-grade dysplasia. Repeat examinations should include sufficient sampling so that there is no error in the histologic diagnosis. A subsequent negative examination is not sufficiently reassuring to return to routine surveillance (242,243). Therefore, continued examinations at 6-month or shorter intervals should be pursued.

High-grade Dysplasia in Flat Mucosa

Patients with high-grade dysplasia should undergo total proctocolectomy given the high rate of synchronous and metachronous adenocarcinoma associated with this diagnosis (241,244).

Raised Lesions (Polyps) with Dysplasia

Raised lesions encountered within areas of colitis may include one or more polyps that visually resemble sporadic adenomas and may be amenable to complete polypectomy (245). If polypectomy is complete and biopsies of surrounding mucosa (four biopsies taken immediately adjacent to the raised lesion and submitted separately) are negative for dysplasia and there is no dysplasia elsewhere in the colon, a follow-up examination should be performed within 6 months, with regular surveillance resumed if no dysplasia is found. However, if dysplasia is present in the surrounding mucosa, or if the dysplastic polypoid lesion is unresectable or does not resemble a typical adenoma, a high risk of associated synchronous colorectal cancer would justify recommending complete proctocolectomy.

The surveillance approach to patients with colonic CD is similar to that of patients with UC (239). Patients with CD confined to the small intestine are not considered to have an increased risk for colorectal cancer, and as such may be followed using the general guidelines for colorectal cancer surveillance in the general population.

Pathologic Identification of Dysplasia

In recent years, attention has focused on the identification of precancerous epithelial dysplasia in the large bowel as a histologic marker for identifying individuals at increased cancer risk and as a potential indicator for patients who should undergo colectomy. However, diagnosing dysplasia is a complex process due to the fact that its diagnosis is not straightforward and even experienced pathologists may disagree as to whether a change represents dysplasia or not. The diagnosis of dysplasia is difficult due to the recurrent and persistent inflammatory changes associated with the underlying IBD.

In 1983, the Inflammatory Bowel Disease—Dysplasia Morphology Study Group focused its attention on (a) developing standardized definitions of terms pertaining to IBD and dysplasia, (b) establishing criteria for diagnosing dysplasia and for differentiating it from other epithelial changes occurring in IBD, (c) developing a system for grading and classifying dysplasia, (d) assessing the accuracy and precision of the grading system for dysplasia, and (e) formulating guidelines for the clinical management of IBD patients (234). The classification scheme developed by this group is still in use today, with some modifications.

The classification system contains three major categories: Negative for dysplasia, indefinite for dysplasia, and positive

TABLE 11.24 Biopsy Classification of Dysplasia in Inflammatory Bowel Disease	
Negative for dysplasia	Positive for dysplasia
Normal mucosa	Low-grade dysplasia
Inactive (quiescent) colitis	High-grade dysplasia
Active colitis	

for dysplasia (Table 11.24). The study group defined dysplasia as an unequivocal neoplastic alteration of the intestinal epithelium (Fig. 11.110). Dysplasia presents with various gross appearances, including (a) a flat mucosa that is unremarkable except for loss of mucosal folds (Fig. 11.108), or that has a granular or pebbly appearance (Fig. 11.108); (b) a velvety appearance due to mucosal villiform transformation (Fig. 11.112); and (c) a spectrum of plaques (Fig. 11.111), nodules, and other polypoid excrescences that may resemble adenomas (Fig. 11.113). The dysplasia is itself neoplastic and may coexist with an invasive malignancy.

Histologically, one bases the diagnosis of dysplasia on a combination of microscopic features, including architectural alterations that exceed those resulting from reparative processes and cytologic abnormalities (Fig. 11.110). The architectural alterations often result in glandular arrangements that may resemble adenomas. The cytologic abnormalities principally consist of cellular and nuclear pleomorphism, nuclear hyperchromatism, loss of nuclear polarity, and marked nuclear stratification (Fig. 11.110) (234). Epithelium negative for dysplasia appears completely normal

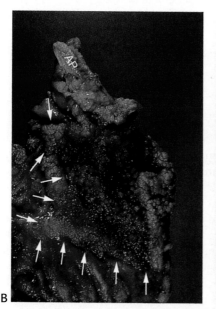
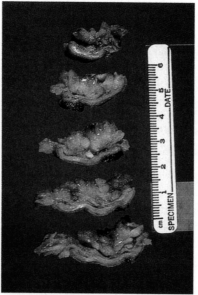
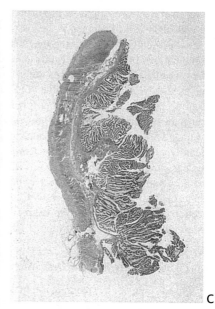

FIG. 11.112. Appendiceal cystadenoma in inflammatory bowel disease. **A:** Note the large, plaquelike cecal lesion, which represents a dysplasia-associated lesion or mass. Its borders are indicated by the *arrows*. The extension to the left of the photograph represents the appendix (AP). The AP contained a papillary noninvasive neoplasm, which is seen best in B when it is cut in cross section. **B:** Several serial cross sections of this papillary lesion are shown. **C:** Histologic features of this papillary cystadenoma.

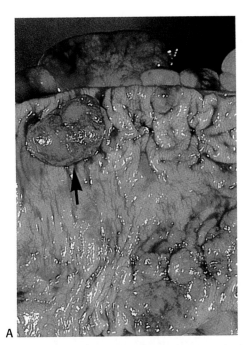
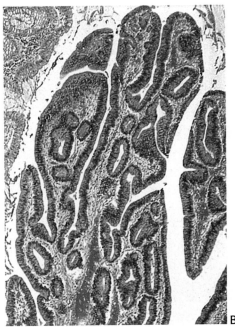

FIG. 11.113. Adenomatous polyp occurring on the background of ulcerative colitis. **A:** The gross specimen demonstrates the presence of areas of scarring, pseudopolyp formation, and adenomatous growth, which is indicated by the *arrow*. **B:** Histologic sections through the adenoma show the presence of typical adenomatous epithelium. In addition, there were areas of dysplasia in the surrounding bowel mucosa.

or it exhibits a range of destructive or regenerative changes. These result from the recurrent episodes of ulceration and repair characteristic of both forms of IBD.

Mucosa Indefinite for Dysplasia

Various factors alter the mucosa, making it impossible to classify some epithelial changes as unequivocally positive or negative for dysplasia. Odd growth patterns and unusually florid areas of active inflammation and/or regeneration may be classified as equivocal for dysplasia. In other cases, the use of picric acid– or mercury-based fixatives that enhance nuclear details creates worrisome nuclear hyperchromasia (234). The diagnosis of "indefinite for dysplasia" is made when the cytologic changes appear to exceed what one would expect to see in an active colitis but are insufficient for a definitive diagnosis of dysplasia.

When the reparative processes associated with active colitis reach the point where the epithelium appears columnar, the chance of confusing regenerative atypia with dysplasia increases. At this stage the nuclei tend to acquire more chromatin, particularly around the nuclear membranes; they become elongated and may retain large eosinophilic nucleoli. (Mitoses can be found in both regenerating and dysplastic mucosa and they do not distinguish between regeneration and dysplasia.) If the nuclei are increased in number and are markedly stratified, the appearance may be so similar to dysplastic epithelium that a part of a single crypt examined in isolation, as in biopsy material, may be difficult to distinguish from true dysplasia (Fig. 11.114). In large biopsies, one

might be able to evaluate the overall histologic context in which the changes are occurring. In such biopsies, one often observes a junction between the regenerating epithelium and the nonulcerated epithelium in the same or adjacent crypts,

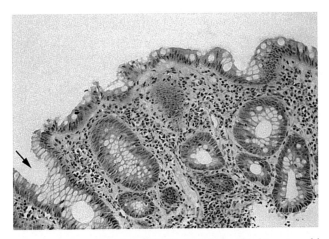

FIG. 11.114. Mucosa indefinite for dysplasia. This biopsy could be interpreted as indefinite for dysplasia, probably reactive. The gland at the far left (*arrow*) contains more mucin than the glands immediately to its right. In addition, it exhibits much less nuclear stratification at the same level in the mucosa. For this reason, the glands to the right of the one indicated by the arrow might be interpreted as indefinite for dysplasia, probably reactive, because the nuclear features are not atypical, and yet the epithelium shows more nuclear stratification and less mucin production than the gland to its left in the absence of any evidence of active inflammation.

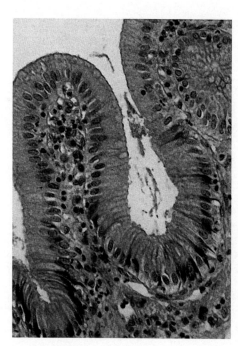

FIG. 11.115. Indefinite for dysplasia. Incomplete differentiation. The epithelium lacks differentiation to mature absorptive cells and mature goblet cells.

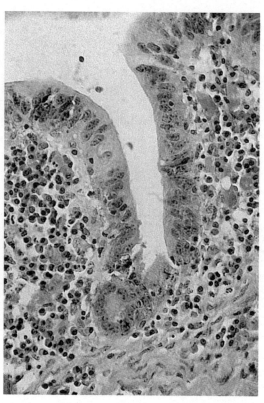

FIG. 11.116. Indefinite for dysplasia. This epithelium, like that in Figure 11.115, shows no evidence of glandular maturation. In contrast to Figure 11.115, the nuclei appear more hyperchromatic and they contain enlarged, prominent nucleoli. One cannot be certain that this does not represent the end part of a regenerative process.

allowing one to diagnose such areas as reactive. In small biopsies, this may be impossible. Reparative changes may be particularly exuberant in children and young adults (234).

Unusual growth patterns may also cause concern because they are commonly observed in colons harboring definite areas of carcinoma or dysplasia, but they have not been observed to give rise directly to invasive carcinoma. In one of the patterns, the crypts fail to differentiate into normal mature cell types and the nuclei appear uniformly enlarged. This pattern is recognized by the presence of columnar epithelium and a marked reduction in the number of goblet cells (Figs. 11.115 and 11.116) (234). Whether such crypts contain absorptive cells only or only relatively undifferentiated intermediate cells is unknown. In one variant of this pattern, every cell contains small mucin droplets. In another variant, goblet cells become rounded and displaced from the luminal aspect of the crypt. As a result, they resemble signet ring cells. Such cells are called dystrophic goblet cells. Dystrophic goblet cells may occasionally be found in nondysplastic mucosa, but when they are numerous they should alert one to the possibility of the presence of dysplasia.

In other specimens, the superficial parts of the crypts contain a serrated or saw-toothed pattern similar to that seen in sessile serrated and hyperplastic polyps, or they may acquire a villous architecture but lack the classic changes seen in villous adenomas. A complete spectrum of epithelial alterations exists in these serrated lesions, ranging from negative for dysplasia (Fig. 11.117) to clear-cut dysplasia (Fig. 11.118). The dysplasia is often confined to the basal portion of the crypts, with the upper part containing more

mature cells and a serrated pattern, but the entire thickness of the mucosa may be involved. Villous lesions are likely to be dysplastic. As with other unusual growth patterns, the presence and the degree of dysplasia should be determined principally on the basis of the nuclear features. These lesions often resemble serrated adenomas.

Another pattern that sometimes causes difficulty and places lesions in the "indefinite for dysplasia" category is the presence of unusual lesions covering prominent lymphoid follicles (Fig. 11.119), usually in the rectum. Often, the crypts overlying these follicles appear markedly distorted and exuberant regeneration of the surface epithelium is present. This complex arrangement may mimic dysplasia.

Finally, in other cases, the epithelium shows features of dysplasia, but because they are associated with prominent active inflammation in a background of a regenerating mucosa or because the nuclear features do not cross a person's threshold for neoplasia (Fig. 11.120), one is not completely certain that the lesion is not reactive. Although it may be possible to diagnose dysplasia in the presence of acute inflammation and ulceration, one should exercise extra caution under these circumstances and be absolutely certain that dysplasia is present before making the diagnosis.

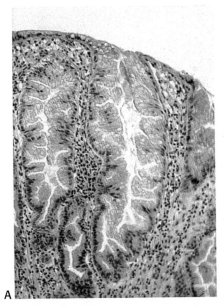
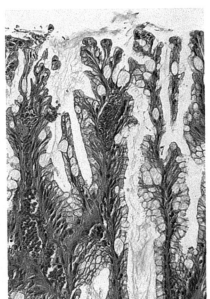

FIG. 11.117. Indefinite for dysplasia, serrated glandular pattern. A and B represent two separate lesions with glandular serration. **A:** The epithelium mostly resembles that seen in hyperplastic polyps and is probably not dysplastic. **B:** The serrated pattern is more prominent with glandular hyperplasia and occasionally dystrophic goblet cells. This pattern represents an area truly indefinite for dysplasia.

Mucosa Positive for Dysplasia

By definition, the category "positive for dysplasia" includes mucosa that is unequivocally neoplastic. This diagnosis therefore indicates that a lesion may be associated with, or may subsequently give rise to, an invasive adenocarcinoma. Although invasive carcinoma is probably more common in cases with severe or high-grade dysplasia, it may also be found in colons containing lesser degrees of dysplasia. Operationally, dysplasia is divided into low-grade and high-

grade forms based on its degree of deviation from normal colonic epithelium.

Low-grade Dysplasia Low-grade dysplasia is characterized by mucosal changes resembling those found in adenomas (Figs. 11.120 and 11.121). The involved crypts usually appear uniformly lined by tall epithelial cells with elongated hyperchromatic pseudostratified nuclei that evidence failure to differentiate into normal goblet cells and absorptive cells at

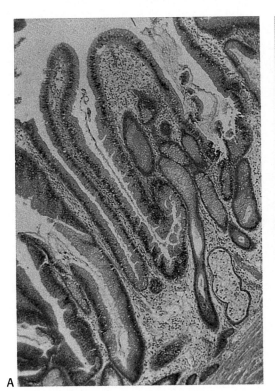
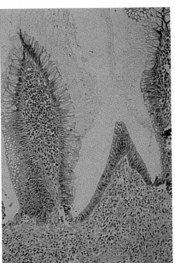
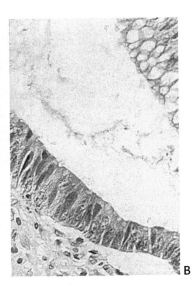

FIG. 11.118. Villiform changes. **A:** Ulcerative colitis with an area of villous dysplasia resembling a villous adenoma. This was one of multiple areas of low-grade dysplasia in the bowel of this patient with a long history of pancolitis. **B:** Area of unusual villiform transformation (*left*) with atypia at the basal part of the mucosa (*right*) and evidence of maturation toward the surface. It is indefinite for dysplasia, probably positive.

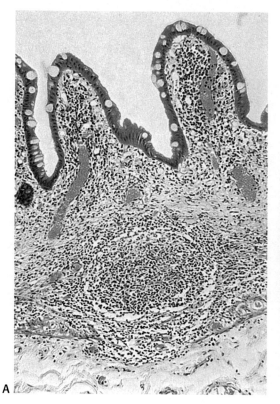

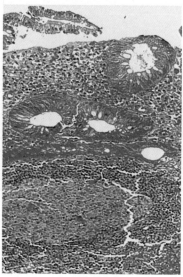

FIG. 11.119. Follicular proctitis. **A:** The epithelium overlying the lymphoid follicle is simplified. It has some resemblance to the incomplete maturation shown in Figure 11.52. However, evidence of goblet cell differentiation is seen. This does not represent a dysplastic change. **B:** A prominent hyperplastic lymphoid follicle is seen at the junction of the mucosa and submucosa (*left*). Overlying this is a mucin-depleted gland with some nuclear stratification (*right*). This lesion is probably reactive in nature.

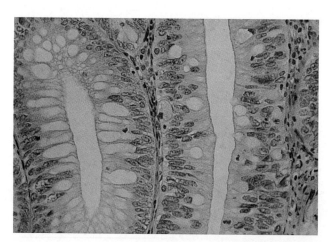

the free surface. Some mucin may be produced by the neoplastic cells, but it is usually reduced in amount. Dystrophic goblet cells may be present. The surface of low-grade dysplasia may be villous or flat (Fig. 11.121). Mitotic activity is unrestricted and is found at all levels of the low-grade and high-grade dysplastic crypt. However, some basal polarity of the nuclei is maintained in low-grade lesions. Low-grade dysplasia can be accompanied by endocrine cell hyperplasia and Paneth cell metaplasia. Acute inflammation should be minimal.

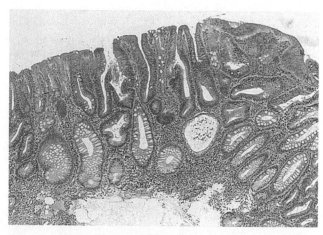

FIG. 11.120. Low-grade dysplasia. Sections of two glands are seen along their longitudinal axis. The epithelium becomes progressively cytologically more atypical as one proceeds from the left-hand portion of the photograph to the right-hand part. The nuclear changes increase as one progresses in this direction, as does the degree of nuclear disorganization. The gland on the left does not contain any definite dysplasia despite the presence of occasional enlarged nuclei with irregular chromatin. The right-hand gland shows changes on its left side that could be diagnosed as indefinite for dysplasia, probably dysplasia, due to the nuclear stratification and the irregularity. The right-hand portion of this gland is definitely a low-grade dysplasia, as evidenced by the jumbled architectural arrangement of the nuclei, the presence of dystrophic goblet cells, nuclear stratification, and the increased nuclear:cytoplasmic ratios.

FIG. 11.121. Low-grade dysplasia. The dysplastic epithelium lies at the superficial portions of the mucosa, resembling that seen in an ordinary tubular adenoma.

When the dysplastic epithelium is restricted to the upper portion of the mucosa, one sees a disturbed pattern of cellular maturation as evidenced by the presence of large numbers of mitotically active cells near the free surface (Fig. 11.121). Crypt architecture tends to be preserved, and distortion, if present, is mild; the nuclei may be stratified, particularly near the base of the crypts, but this stratification does not reach the crypt lumen; nuclei are crowded and hyperchromatic (234).

Most examples of low-grade dysplasia pose few diagnostic problems because they bear a strong histologic resemblance to tubular adenomas (Fig. 11.121). Potential problems in diagnosing low-grade dysplasia exist at either end of the spectrum. It may be difficult to decide whether a biopsy specimen should be classified as "indefinite for dysplasia" or as "low-grade dysplasia." However, this is of no consequence since both diagnoses require an early repeat biopsy. At the other end of the spectrum are specimens that contain areas of both low- and high-grade dysplasia; in these it is best to rate the lesion according to the higher grade (234).

High-grade Dysplasia In most cases, the diagnosis of high-grade dysplasia is relatively straightforward. The distinction from low-grade dysplasia depends primarily on the degree of cytologic atypia present. High-grade dysplasia shows true nuclear stratification. The level of the nuclei in the epithelium helps distinguish low-grade from high-grade lesions (Fig. 11.122). In contrast to low-grade dysplasia, in which fairly regular nuclei are confined to the basal halves of the cells, most cases of high-grade dysplasia show nuclear stratification that extends beyond the midportion of the cells.

High-grade dysplasia also evidences a greater degree of cytologic variability (Figs. 11.122 and 11.123), nuclear hyperchromasia, and pleomorphism, and the epithelium more resembles the cells seen in invasive cancers than the regular tall cells of adenomas. In high-grade dysplasia, the nuclei lose their polarity, and instead of being elongated with the long axis of the nucleus perpendicular to the basement membrane, the nuclei round out and develop prominent nucleoli. High-grade dysplasia often coexists with low-grade dysplasia, and there is a tendency for the cells to form expansile nests that appear to push the cells with an adenomatous appearance to the side. In some patients villous dysplasia is present (234). The category "high-grade dysplasia" includes carcinoma in situ. One recognizes carcinoma in situ by the presence of a cribriform glandular pattern (Fig. 11.123). DALMs usually contain high-grade dysplasia (Fig. 11.123).

One judges the severity of the dysplasia based on the worst changes present and not the predominant ones. However, the appearance of high-grade features in just one or two crypts probably does not justify upgrading the dysplasia into a higher category if this is all that is present (234). As a general rule of thumb, evidence of dysplasia in three crypts or more is sufficient for the diagnosis.

Polyploid Areas of Dysplasia and Adenomas in Inflammatory Bowel Disease (Dysplasia-associated Lesions or Masses)

By convention, the dysplastic tissue that precedes the development of carcinomas in sporadic colon cancer is referred to

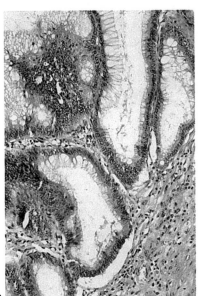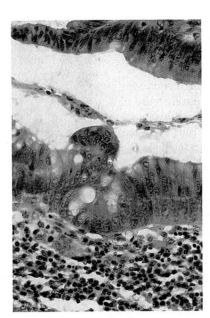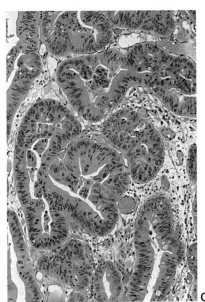

A, B   C

FIG. 11.122. Dysplasia. A: Low-grade dysplasia. The hyperchromatic nuclei occupy less than one half of the distance of the epithelial height. **B:** High-grade dysplasia with nuclei extending all the way to the lumen of the gland and early glandular budding. **C:** High-grade dysplasia with nuclear irregularity and a back-to-back cribriform pattern.

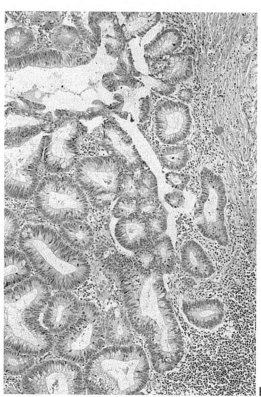

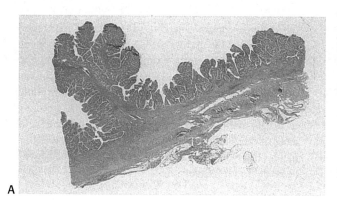

FIG. 11.123. High-grade dysplasia. **A:** A whole mount section of the lesion. The entire surface of the colon is replaced by dysplastic epithelium. It is seen in higher magnification in B. **B:** Portion of the mucosa as it joins the submucosa, indicating that this back-to-back configuration remains confined to the area above the muscularis mucosae.

as an adenoma, whereas polypoid areas of dysplasia occurring in the setting of IBD are diagnosed as DALMs.

True adenomas similar to those seen in non-IBD patients may be encountered in IBD patients, particularly in patients over age 40 (Fig. 11.124). The incidence of adenomas increases in this age group, just as it does in the normal population, and the presence of an adenoma may have nothing to do with the underlying IBD. However, the significance of isolated polypoid adenomas in patients with UC remains controversial. The major difficulty concerns patient management and follow-up. The options are to treat IBD patients with adenomas found in the setting of IBD as polypoid areas of dysplasia, and interpret them as signals for the presence of synchronous or subsequent carcinoma. Alternatively, they could be regarded as having a significance no greater than that of the sporadic adenoma in the general population. In such patients it is important to determine whether additional dysplasia is present in the nonpolypoid mucosa. If the dysplasia is confined to the polypoid lesion in a well-sampled colon, then it may be possible to treat the patient as one would treat a noncolitic patient with an adenoma. If the dysplasia is present in the adenoma and in the surrounding mucosa or elsewhere in the bowel, then the case must be considered as dysplasia in the IBD setting (Fig. 11.125).

Dysplasia in Inflammatory Pseudopolyps

Dysplasia in inflammatory pseudopolyps is rare, but it does occur. As with the nonpolypoid mucosa, an entire spectrum of features, ranging from inflammatory changes to high-grade dysplasia, may exist in inflammatory pseudopolyps. The major problem is that the polyps frequently have areas of residual regeneration that may be difficult to distinguish from true dysplasia. When dysplasia is suspected in what appears to be an inflammatory pseudopolyp, additional specimens obtained from the surrounding flat mucosa should be examined to determine whether the polyp is part of a larger area of dysplasia (234).

Agreement on the Diagnosis of Dysplasia

The degree of observer variation in detecting and grading dysplasia in the setting of UC, even among experienced pathologists, is poor. The best agreement is for slides that show no dysplasia. The level of agreement in the diagnosis of dysplasia varies depending on how it is assessed. The agreement between whether dysplasia is present or absent is better than agreement among various degrees of dysplasia; it ranges from 68% to 84%. The level of agreement for "atypia present" (including reactive atypia and low- and high-grade

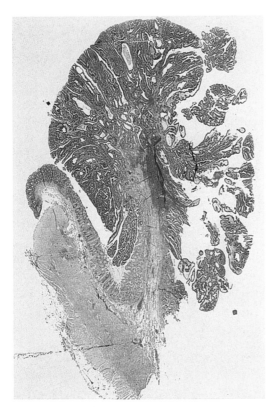

FIG. 11.124. Portion of a polypoid mass in a patient who underwent resection for dysplasia and ulcerative colitis. The patient had numerous other areas of dysplasia. The lesion resembles a sporadic adenoma.

dysplasia) versus "no atypia" achieves a consensus of >90%. Agreement on the diagnosis of high-grade dysplasia ranges from 100% to as low as 33% (246). Nonetheless, dysplasia does represent a successful marker in clinical practice. Pathologists should have access to previous slides from the

same patient and adequate clinical information before reporting biopsies as positive for dysplasia because of the clinical implications of the diagnosis.

Ancillary Tools for Diagnosing Dysplasia

Because of the difficulty in reliably diagnosing dysplasia, various alternative approaches have been employed to make the diagnosis more objective. These techniques have included the use of enzyme assays, immunophenotypic markers, ultrastructural examination, immunohistochemistry, flow cytometry, genetic probes, and mucin and lectin staining. Markers such as carcinoembryonic antigen, secretory component, and epithelial IgA are not useful in distinguishing regenerative from dysplastic lesions (246). To date, of the markers that predict subsequent cancer development, clearly histologic identification of dysplasia continues to be the best predictor.

Mucin Stains

Mucins have also been used to distinguish dysplastic from regenerative changes. Sialomucins increase in UC and dysplasia (247,248). However, since sialomucins increase in both inflammatory dysplasia and cancer, they are not specific for a diagnosis of neoplasia.

Flow Cytometric Analysis

Cellular aneuploidy represents a common development in the pathway to dysplasia and cancer in UC. The degree of DNA aneuploidy correlates well with the presence and grade of dysplasia (249–253). Detailed mapping studies carried out on colectomy specimens show that as many as 14 or 15 different and overlapping regions of aneuploidy may be present in

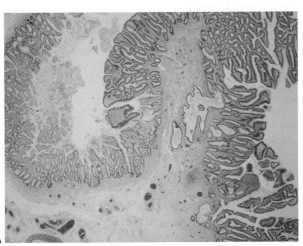

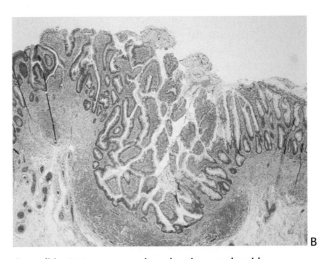

FIG. 11.125. Polypoid dysplasia in a patient with ulcerative colitis. **A:** Low-power view showing a polypoid area of dysplasia resembling somewhat an adenomatous polyp. **B:** The adjacent flat mucosa, however, also shows low-grade dysplasia. This finding confirms that the polypoid dysplasia is inflammatory bowel disease associated and not a sporadic adenoma.

the colonic mucosa (253). The presence of multiple aneu-ploid stem cell lines suggests that a high level of genomic instability is present and that the patient probably has a higher risk of progressing to colorectal carcinoma (253). Although dysplasia correlates closely topographically with DNA aneuploidy, aneuploidy also occurs without concomitant dysplasia. Changes in nuclear DNA content occur earlier than dysplasia and malignant transformation of the colorectal mucosa in UC. Aneuploidy also occurs in 2% of biopsies from mucosa classified as normal (252) and in 10% to 42% of biopsies with inflammation, hyperplasia, or atrophy; in 20% to 100% of polyps and in biopsies with dysplasia; and in the majority of adenocarcinomas. The presence of aneuploidy in nonneoplastic mucosa may help select patients who should undergo surveillance colonoscopies. Approximately 32 biopsies are required to achieve a 90% confidence that a histologic abnormality is detected or about 55 biopsies for a 95% confidence. Similarly, a total of 20 biopsies analyzed flow cytometrically are required for a 90% confidence that aneuploidy will be detected if present, and 30 biopsies for a 95% confidence (220). These levels are clearly not within the realm of what can be done for standard diagnostic purposes.

Proliferative Markers

We have found that because cell proliferation is abnormally regulated in neoplastic lesions, immunostaining in problematic areas with MIB-1 immunostains helps to delineate areas of dysplasia from a regenerative mucosa. Statistically significant differences in the pattern of MIB-1 immunoreactivity occur between nonneoplastic and neoplastic lesions. In regenerative mucosa, MIB-1 immunoreactivity localizes to the bases of crypts and the proliferative zone appears expanded. In dysplasia, immunoreactivity is prominent in the cells in the superficial mucosa as well as in the crypt base. In some dysplasias and all invasive carcinomas, MIB-1 staining is diffusely distributed throughout the crypts, suggesting complete deregulation of normal cell proliferation. Additionally, the intensity of the staining and the percentage of cells staining positively tend to be greater in areas of dysplasia (120,254,255).

Carcinomas

Carcinoma in UC commonly arises throughout the colon. It may develop in multiple sites, and it often does not produce clear-cut symptoms before advanced disease has developed. Cancer may also arise in the retained rectum after colectomy. Patients with cancer or dysplasia in the colon at the time of colectomy are at increased risk for the later development of rectal cancer (256).

Gross Features

Most carcinomas develop in areas of macroscopic disease. The gross appearance of the neoplasms may resemble ordi-

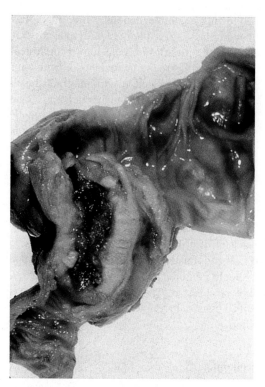

FIG. 11.126. Carcinoma arising in inflammatory bowel disease. Carcinoma of the terminal ileum arising in patient with long-standing Crohn disease.

nary intestinal carcinomas arising on an atrophic but grossly more or less normal bowel (Fig. 11.126). Often the tumors are flat or slightly depressed, poorly circumscribed, and spreading, and can be more easily felt than seen (Figs. 11.127 and 11.128). In this regard, they resemble gastric cancer of the diffuse type. In some instances, the lesions appear somewhat raised.

Histologic Features

Intestinal stem cells may become hyperstimulated due to the inflammation inherent in IBD, which leads to hyperplasia or neoplastic transformation. Such a process could explain the broad spectrum of tumor types that arise in IBD, including adenocarcinomas, small cell carcinomas, and carcinoid tumors (257–260). It can also explain the presence of widespread dysplasia and the occurrence of multiple carcinomas and multiple carcinoid tumors that one sees in the setting of IBD. Intramucosal carcinoma falls within the realm of high-grade dysplasia. Intramucosal carcinomas may represent focal lesions or may be present diffusely in large patchlike areas. Very exceptionally, one encounters a form of intramucosal carcinoma analogous to that seen in the stomach, in which signet ring cells infiltrate the lamina propria but do not extend beyond the muscularis mucosae (Fig. 11.129). The metastasizing potential of this lesion is unknown.

Adenocarcinomas arising in a setting of UC may show any degree of histologic differentiation (Figs. 11.130 to

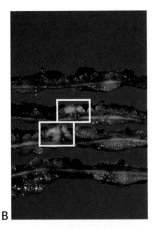
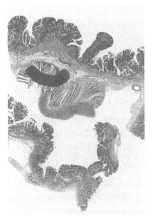
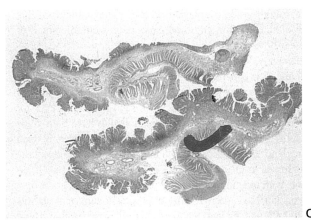

A, B   C

FIG. 11.127. Superficially invasive carcinoma developing in ulcerative colitis. **A:** This carcinoma would have been impossible to find had one not palpated the bowel and/or examined cross sections of it. The specimen was bread-loafed. These serial, several-millimeter cross sections demonstrate an area of whitish discoloration that extends into the underlying submucosa corresponding to the invasive cancer **(B). C:** A section from a second slice from the lesion showing the invasive carcinoma. This bowel had four other invasive carcinomas. The pen marks on the slide in B and C indicate the area of cancer. Carcinoma extends into the submucosa in both of these areas. Dysplasia surrounds the invasive cancer.

11.133), but there is a higher proportion of poorly differentiated and mucinous tumors in IBD patients as compared to sporadic colon cancers. In one study, 54% of tumors had mucinous features and 27% had signet ring cells (216). Mucinous and signet ring cell features are as common in CD as in UC (Fig. 11.134). In CD, dysplasia and cancer may be exclusively located in the small bowel, whereas other cases may be found in the colon.

Carcinoid tumors affect both sexes equally. Patients also develop single (257) or multiple microcarcinoids, sometimes in association with synchronous carcinomas (258). The neoplasms tend to occur in inflamed areas or in tissues that show evidence of previous damage. Microcarcinoids measure <2 mm in diameter and are not generally grossly visible. These

resemble gastric microcarcinoids seen in patients with autoimmune gastritis and pernicious anemia (258).

The coexistence of an intestinal carcinoid (incidence 1 to 1.3 per 100,000) and UC incidence (2 to 10 per 100,000) or CD (1 to 6 per 100,000) could be fortuitous (261) because the clinical profile of patients resembles that of patients with sporadic carcinoid tumors. Some patients have a long history of CD or UC with extensive involvement of their bowels when their carcinoid is first described and others have a relatively short history (618). Adenocarcinoid tumors also arise in pre-existing UC (261).

Role of Cytology in Ulcerative Colitis

Brush cytology of the colon and rectum may aid in cancer detection in IBD patients (262), especially in patients with strictures or in whom there is widespread neoplasia. The malignant cells show marked anisocytosis, pleomorphism, and nuclear hyperchromasia, and appear in loosely cohesive clusters or in single forms in an inflammatory and necrotic background. In some cases, moderate or severe atypia is found in brushing specimens when biopsies only reveal mildly reactive changes. The two diagnostic techniques are complementary to one another (263).

Prognosis

Some have said that cancers arising in the setting of UC behave more aggressively than sporadic colon cancers. Poor prognosis results in part due to the difficulty of early diagnosis of cancer in these patients and because the patients are often young and the cancers are highly malignant. Others have shown that there is no significant difference in 5-year survival among colitis and noncolitis patients with colorectal

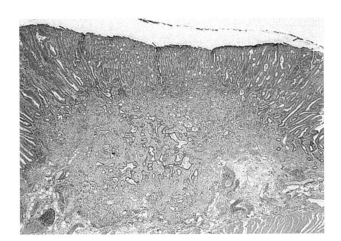

FIG. 11.128. Carcinoma extending into the submucosa. Note that the surface is covered by a broad area of dysplasia. An invasive carcinoma underlies the dysplasia. No dysplasia-associated lesion or mass is present in this area.

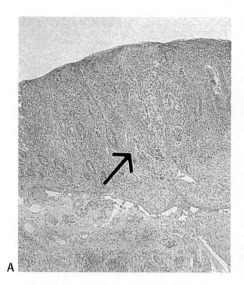

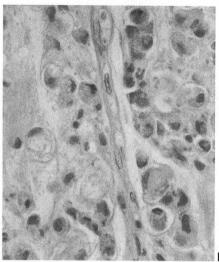

FIG. 11.129. Intramucosal carcinoma in a patient with a 17-year history of ulcerative colitis who underwent a colectomy following the diagnosis of dysplasia. An intramucosal signet ring cell carcinoma was present (**A,** *arrow*). The tumor was composed exclusively of signet ring cells (**B**).

carcinoma when matched for stage (262). Multivariate analysis shows that the stage is the best prognostic indicator, followed by tumor differentiation and DNA ploidy status. Tumor location, number of cancers, duration of disease, age, and sex do not correlate with prognosis (216). Other factors associated with significantly poorer prognosis include larger tumor size, infiltrating and ulcerating configuration, and higher mucin content.

Extraintestinal Cancers

Patients with IBD have an increased incidence of extraintestinal carcinomas. The extraintestinal neoplasms may coexist with intestinal carcinomas. The proportion of extraintestinal cancers is greater in CD than UC, 43% versus 12%. The incidence of gastrointestinal cancer increases with duration of disease in both CD and UC, but extraintestinal cancers show less correlation with increasing disease duration. Extraintestinal cancers include cancers of the breast, thyroid, bladder, brain, skin, stomach, hepatobiliary system, lymph nodes, larynx, and uterus, and Kaposi sarcoma (264–266).

Patients with IBD show an increased risk of reticuloendothelial neoplasms with an excess of leukemias in UC and an excess of lymphomas in both UC and CD. Additionally, there is an increased incidence of squamous cell cancers of the perianal region, an incidence 30 times greater than expected, as well as an increased incidence of squamous cell cancers of the vagina. Lymphomas, leukemia, squamous cell carcinomas, and Kaposi sarcoma all occur in excess in immunosuppressed or irradiated patients. Thus, one can speculate that the increased incidence of these neoplasms in patients with ileitis and colitis may result from underlying immunologic deficiencies associated with IBD, or to the long-term administration of steroids or other immunosuppressive medications.

Atypical lymphoid lesions and true lymphomas complicate both UC and CD (265,267–269). Lymphomas range in

incidence from 0.43% in UC to 0.27% in CD. UC patients sometimes develop gastrointestinal and extraintestinal non-Hodgkin lymphoma. These tumors represent a heterogeneous group with tumors displaying both B-cell and T-cell phenotypes, although lymphomas complicating UC are usually B-cell lesions.

Squamous cell carcinoma in situ (Fig. 11.135) and invasive squamous carcinoma arise in both CD and UC, but they are more common in the setting of CD (270). Most commonly, they associate with fistulae or they occur in the anal region.

Molecular Changes Associated with Cancer Development

Cancer development in IBD is a multistep process and the molecular abnormalities have been better defined in UC than in CD. Numerous genetic alterations exist in dysplasias and carcinomas arising in IBD patients. Molecular abnormalities also exist in mucosa that is not obviously dysplastic, suggesting that their identification may serve as an aid to predicting increased cancer risk in IBD patients. These involve many of the same genes that are abnormal in sporadic colorectal tumors. These include multiple sites of allelic deletion, microsatellite instability (271–277), telomere shortening (278,279), and mutations of SMAD2, SMAD4 (280), and p53 genes (281–283). Ras, APC, and DPC4 mutations are more common in IBD-associated neoplasia than in sporadic colorectal cancers (284,285). The frequency and order of genetic alterations in UC-associated colon carcinomas may differ from those seen in sporadic tumors, suggesting that neoplastic progression in UC might proceed by different mechanisms than in sporadic cancer.

Chromosomal Instability

Chromosomal instability in IBD occurs at many sites. Fluorescence in situ hybridization (FISH) has demonstrated

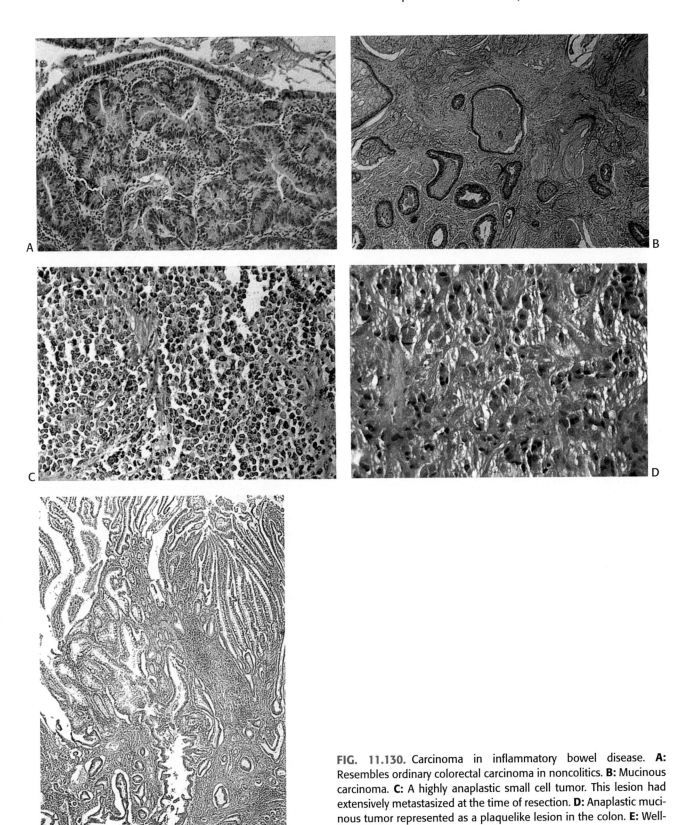

FIG. 11.130. Carcinoma in inflammatory bowel disease. **A:** Resembles ordinary colorectal carcinoma in noncolitics. **B:** Mucinous carcinoma. **C:** A highly anaplastic small cell tumor. This lesion had extensively metastasized at the time of resection. **D:** Anaplastic mucinous tumor represented as a plaquelike lesion in the colon. **E:** Well-differentiated ileal adenocarcinoma.

losses or gains on chromosomes 8, 11, 17, and 18 in patients with IBD-associated dysplasia or cancer. These chromosomal changes precede the development of histologically identifiable dysplasia, supporting the concept of a large field effect with a mutator phenotype in these patients. Comparative genomic hybridization studies also show widespread chromosomal instability in patients with IBD-associated neoplasia. Such studies have also shown loss on chromosome 18q,

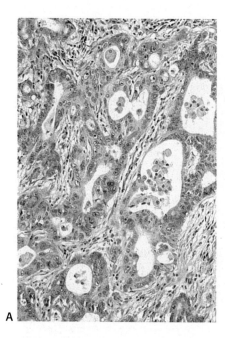

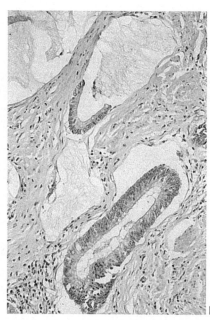

A

B

FIG. 11.131. Histologic features of two different carcinomas arising in the setting of ulcerative colitis. **A:** Histologic features closely resembling those seen in ordinary colorectal carcinomas. **B:** Mucinous carcinoma admixed with well-differentiated tubular carcinoma.

the site of the deleted in colon cancer (DCC) gene, SMAD2, and SMAD4 (273,286).

Chromosomal instability in colonic mucosa from UC patients has also associated with telomere shortening (279). Telomere alterations are also seen in nondysplastic mucosa from patients who ultimately progressed to develop dysplasia or carcinoma (278).

p53 Alterations

Numerous studies have shown that p53 overexpression and/or mutation occur in various colonic lesions in patients with ulcerative colitis (281–283,287). p53 mutations occur in from 0% to 29% of nonneoplastic colonic mucosa, 3% to 41% of lesions indefinite for dysplasia, 30% to 75% of dysplasias, and 41% to 100% of carcinomas (282,283,288,289). p53 overexpression is reported with a somewhat higher frequency than p53 mutation. Interestingly, increased levels of p53 have recently been reported in the serum of UC patients (290). The significance of this finding is not yet clear.

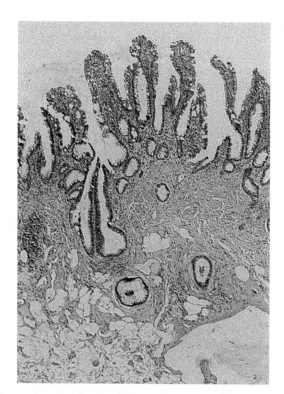

FIG. 11.132. Carcinoma arising in ulcerative colitis. Some carcinomas appear to drop off the mucosa and invade the underlying submucosa. In this photograph, the overlying epithelium appears villiform without significant dysplasia. A microinvasive carcinoma extends into the underlying submucosa. The invading glands appear neoplastic.

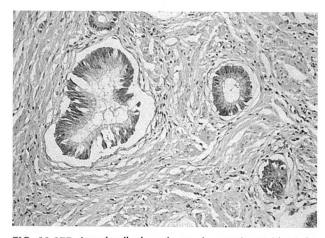

FIG. 11.133. Invasive ileal carcinoma in a patient with Crohn disease. The tumor appears so well differentiated that it might be difficult to distinguish from displaced epithelium. This tumor had infiltrated the entire ileal wall and had metastasized to the regional lymph nodes.

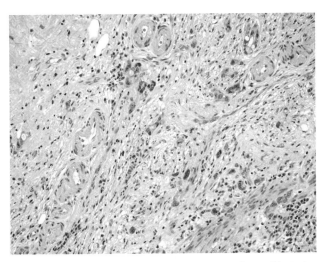

FIG. 11.134. Colonic adenocarcinoma in a patient with Crohn disease. The tumor cells are poorly differentiated and infiltrate as single cells, some of which have a signet ring appearance.

Microsatellite Instability

Studies of microsatellite instability (MSI) in IBD have shown variable and even discordant results. These studies are difficult to compare, as the types of patients studied, the methods used, and the samples analyzed vary tremendously among studies. In addition, the microsatellite markers used and criteria defining MSI are also highly variable among studies.

Overall, it appears that MSI does play some role in IBD-associated neoplasia, but this role is probably not the same as that associated with sporadic colorectal cancers. Ulcerative colitis cancers may not display as high a level of MSI as is seen in sporadic colon cancers, and sites of MSI in IBD versus sporadic colonic neoplasia appear to differ. For example, transforming growth factor-β receptor II mutations are common in sporadic MSI-high colon cancers, while islet cell autoantigen 1 (ICA1) mutations are more frequent in UC

(274). In addition, the underlying causes of instability in IBD may be different. In sporadic colorectal cancers, MSI results most commonly from hMLH1 promoter hypermethylation. In contrast, hMLH1 methylation is less common in MSI-positive tissues from IBD patients (291).

Finally, MSI in ulcerative colitis is commonly of the low type (MSI-L). Interestingly, studies have shown that oxidative injury may inactivate the mismatch repair system in a dose-dependent fashion, providing an explanation for the higher frequency of MSI-L in UC (292).

Methylation

An increasing number of genes are being described whose silencing through promotor methylation occurs in IBD-associated neoplasia. High levels of methylation occur in the estrogen receptor, MyoD, p16, p14, E-cadherin, and CSPG2 genes in IBD-associated dysplasia (293–299). In addition, some of these genes are hypermethylated in nondysplastic tissues from IBD-related cancer patients. Methylation abnormalities are not observed in the colonic tissues of UC patients without dysplasia or cancer, raising the possibility that some of these markers could be useful for IBD surveillance.

SPECIMEN HANDLING

Resection specimens are received for one of two major reasons: (a) the bowel has developed acute complications as a result of the inflammatory process, including obstruction, perforation, fistula formation, toxic megacolon, or concomitant ischemia or infection; or (b) the development of carcinoma or dysplasia. The approach to handing the specimen varies, depending on the reason for the resection. Those specimens removed for inflammatory complications that demonstrate perforations or changes out of proportion to

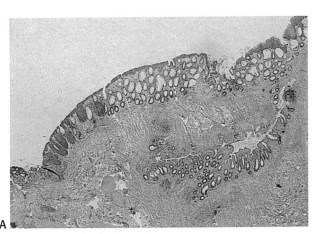
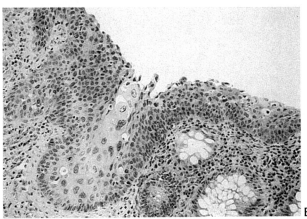

FIG. 11.135. Anal intraepithelial neoplasia in Crohn disease. This patient underwent an ileocolectomy. No evidence of other areas of dysplasia was found in the patient. **A:** Low magnification showing the presence of multiple glands replaced by neoplastic squamous epithelium. **B:** Another area demonstrating the presence of moderate to severe dysplasia within the anal epithelium.

the rest of the disease should be searched for evidence of ischemia and/or viral infections.

In resections that are done in patients with longstanding disease who harbor areas of dysplasia or carcinomas, it is helpful to record and photograph all of the pertinent features present in the mucosa and to extensively sample unusual lesions, particularly those that are polypoid or firm. Because cancers develop in multiple sites and because they are hard to detect, it is helpful to divide the bowel into quarters and then to remove the pericolonic or peri-intestinal fat and dissect the groups of lymph nodes individually from each of the quarters. In this way, one can accurately stage individual carcinomas should more than one be present. Once the pericolonic or peri-intestinal fat has been removed from the specimen, it is helpful to palpate the intestine because carcinomas may be more easily felt than seen and all firm areas should be sampled. Although it is a tedious process, each quadrant of the bowel should be bread-loafed into several-millimeter sections and the cut surfaces examined for unusual areas of whitish discoloration that extend below the muscularis mucosae. These areas usually turn out to be carcinoma. If there are no definable lesions in the bowel, then sections should be taken approximately every 10 cm in progressive order from the right side of the bowel to the left.

The presence of dysplasia in intestinal biopsies of patients with CD should arouse the suspicion of a carcinoma and force one to take multiple sections of strictures and polypoid lesions. Detection of tumors arising in CD is difficult due to the fact that CD typically is a transmural process. Diffuse thickening of the bowel wall makes cancer detection more difficult. Additionally, neoplasms in CD patients may develop at sites remote from the bowel in fistulae and fissures.

REFERENCES

1. Loftus EV Jr, Silverstein MD, Sandborn WJ, et al: Crohn's disease in Olmsted County, Minnesota, 1940-1993: incidence, prevalence, and survival. *Gastroenterology* 1998;114:1161.
2. Ekbom A, Helmick C, Zack M, Adami HO: The epidemiology of inflammatory bowel disease: a large, population-based study in Sweden. *Gastroenterology* 1991;100:350.
3. Yoshida Y, Murata Y: Inflammatory bowel disease in Japan: studies of epidemiology and etiopathogenesis. *Med Clin North Am* 1990;74:67.
4. Kurata JH, Kantor-Fish S, Frankl H, et al: Crohn's disease among ethnic groups in a large health maintenance organization. *Gastroenterology* 1992;102:1940.
5. Ogunbi SO, Ransom JA, Sullivan K, et al: Inflammatory bowel disease in African-American children living in Georgia. *Pediatrics* 1998;133:103.
6. Loftus EV Jr, Sandborn WJ: Epidemiology of inflammatory bowel disease. *Gastroenterol Clin North Am* 2003;31:1.
7. Russell MG, Pastoor CJ, Janssen KM, et al: Familial aggregation of inflammatory bowel disease: a population-based study in South Limburg, The Netherlands. The South Limburg IBD Study Group. *Scand J Gastroenterol Suppl* 1997;223:88.
8. Peeters M, Nevens H, Baert F, et al: Familial aggregation in Crohn's disease; increased age-adjusted risk and concordance in clinical characteristics. *Gastroenterology* 1996;111:597.
9. Binder V: Genetic epidemiology in inflammatory bowel disease. *Dig Dis* 1998;16:351.
10. Tysk C, Lindberg E, Jarnerot G, Floderus-Myrhed B: Ulcerative colitis and Crohn's disease in an unselected population of monozygotic and dizygotic twins. A study of heritability and the influence of smoking. *Gut* 1988;29:990.
11. Russell RK, Satsangi J: IBD: a family affair. *Best Pract Res Clin Gastroenterol* 2004;18:525.
12. Inohara N, Nunez G: The NOD: a signaling module that regulates apoptosis and host defense against pathogens. *Oncogene* 2001;20:6473.
13. Girardin SE, Boneca IG, Viala J, et al: Nod2 is a general sensor of peptidoglycan through muramyl dipeptide (MDP) detection. *J Biol Chem* 2003;278:8869.
14. Ahmad T, Armuzzi A, Bunce M, et al: The molecular classification of the clinical manifestations of Crohn's disease. *Gastroenterology* 2002;122:854.
15. Cuthbert AP, Fisher SA, Mirza MM, et al: The contribution of NOD2 gene mutations to the risk and site of disease in inflammatory bowel disease. *Gastroenterology* 2002;122:867.
16. Bonen DK, Nicolae DL, Moran T, et al: Racial differences in NOD2 variation: characterization of NOD2 in African-Americans with Crohn's disease. *Gastroenterology* 2002;122:A29.
17. Inoue N, Tamura K, Kinouchi Y, et al: Lack of common NOD2 variants in Japanese patients with Crohn's disease. *Gastroenterology* 2002;123:86.
18. van der Linde K, Boor PPC, Houwing-Duistermaat JJ, et al: CARD15 and Crohn's disease: healthy homozygous carriers of the 3020insC frameshift mutation. *Am J Gastroenterol* 2003;98:613.
19. Abreu MT, Taylor KD, Lin YC, et al: Mutations in NOD2 are associated with fibrostenosing disease in patients with Crohn's disease. *Gastroenterology* 2002;123:679.
20. Radlmayr M, Torok HP, Martin K, Folwaczny C: The c-insertion mutation of the NOD2 gene is associated with fistulizing and fibrostenotic phenotypes in Crohn's disease. *Gastroenterology* 2002;122:2091.
21. Gaya DR, Russell RK, Nimmo ER, Satsangi J: New genes in inflammatory bowel disease: lessons for complex diseases? *Lancet* 2006;367:1271.
22. Barmada MM, Brant SR, Nicolae DL, et al: A genome scan in 260 inflammatory bowel disease-affected relative pairs. *Inflamm Bowel Dis* 2004;10:15.
23. Hampe J, Schreiber S, Shaw SH, et al: A genomewide analysis provides evidence for novel linkages in inflammatory bowel disease in a large European cohort. *Am J Hum Genet* 1999;64:808.
24. Fisher SA, Hampe J, Macpherson AJ, et al: Sex stratification of an inflammatory bowel disease genome search shows male specific linkage to the HLA region on chromosome 6. *Eur J Hum Genet* 2002;10:259.
25. Rioux JD, Silverberg MS, Daly MJ, et al: Genomewide search in Canadian families with inflammatory bowel disease reveals two novel susceptibility loci. *Am J Hum Genet* 2000;66:1863.
26. Farrell JR, Peppercorn MA: Ulcerative colitis. *Lancet* 2002;359:331.
27. Sartor RB, Hoentjen F: Proinflammatory cytokines and signaling pathways in intestinal innate immune cells. In: Mestecky J, (ed). *Mucosal Immunology*. Philadelphia: Elsevier, 2005, pp 681–701.
28. Niessner M, Volk BA: Altered Th1/Th2 cytokine profiles in the intestinal mucosa of patients with inflammatory bowel disease as assessed by quantitative reverse transcribed polymerase chain reaction (RT-PCR). *Clin Exp Immunol* 1995;101:428.
29. Duchmann R, May E, Heike M, et al: T cell specificity and cross reactivity towards enterobacteria, bacteroides, bifidobacterium, and antigens from resident intestinal flora in humans. *Gut* 1999;44:812.
30. Neurath MF, Pettersson S, Meyer zum Buschenfelde KH, Strober W: Local administration of antisense phosphorothioate oligonucleotides to the p65 subunit of NF-κB a abrogates established experimental colitis in mice. *Nat Med* 1996;2:998.
31. Sartor RB: Mechanisms of disease: pathogenesis of Crohn's disease and ulcerative colitis. *Nat Clin Pract Gastroenterol Hepatol* 2006;3:390.
32. Kuhn R, Lohler J, Rennick D, et al: Interleukin-10-deficient mice develop chronic enterocolitis. *Cell* 1993;75:263.
33. Melgar S, Yeung MM, Bas A, et al: Over-expression of interleukin 10 in mucosal T cells of patients with active ulcerative colitis. *Clin Exp Immunol* 2003;134:127.
34. Marcussen H: Anti-colon antibodies in ulcerative colitis. A clinical study. *Scand J Gastroenterol* 1976;11:763.
35. Kobayashi K, Atoh M, Konoeda Y, et al: HLA-DR, DQ and T cell antigen receptor constant beta genes in Japanese patients with ulcerative colitis. *Clin Exp Immunol* 1990;80:400.

36. Fuss IJ, Heller F, Boirivant M, et al: Nonclassical CD1d-restricted NK T cells that produce IL-13 characterize and atypical T_H2 response in ulcerative colitis. *J Clin Invest* 2004;113:1490.

37. Onuma EK, Amenta PS, Ramaswamy K, et al: Autoimmunity in ulcerative colitis (UC): a predominant colonic mucosal B cell response against human tropomyosin isoform 5. *Clin Exp Immunol* 2000;121:466.

38. Proujansky R, Fawcett PT, Gibney KM, et al: Examination of anti-neutrophil cytoplasmic antibodies in childhood inflammatory bowel disease. *J Pediatr Gastroenterol Nutr* 1993;2:193.

39. Winter HS, Lander CJ, Winkelstein A, et al: Anti-neutrophil cytoplasmic antibodies in children with ulcerative colitis. *J Pediatr* 1994;5:707.

40. Oudkerk-Pool M, Ellerbroek PM, Ridwan BU, et al: Serum antineutrophil cytoplasmic autoantibodies in inflammatory bowel disease are mainly associated with ulcerative colitis: a correlation study between perinuclear antineutrophil cytoplasmic autoantibodies and clinical parameters, medical and surgical treatment. *Gut* 1993;34:46.

41. Duerr RH, Targan SR, Landers CJ, et al: Anti-neutrophil cytoplasmic antibodies in ulcerative colitis: comparison with other colitides/diarrheal illnesses. *Gastroenterology* 1991;100:1590.

42. Colombel JF, Reumaux D, Duthilleul P, et al: Antineutrophil cytoplasmic autoantibodies in inflammatory bowel diseases. *Gastroenterol Clin Biol* 1992;16:656.

43. Satsangi J, Landers CJ, Welsh KI, et al: The presence of anti-neutrophil antibodies reflects clinical and genetic heterogeneity within inflammatory bowel disease. *Inflamm Bowel Dis* 1998;4:18.

44. Cohavy O, Bruckner D, Cordon LK, et al: Colonic bacteria express an ulcerative colitis pANCA-related protein epitope. *Infect Immun* 2000;68:1542.

45. Vasiliauskas E, Plevy S, Landers C, et al: Perinuclear antineutrophil cytoplasmic antibodies in patients with Crohn's disease define a clinical subgroup. *Gastroenterology* 1996;110:1810.

46. Yang H, Rotter J, Toyoda H, et al: Ulcerative colitis—a genetically heterogeneous disorder defined by genetic (HLA class-II) and subclinical (antineutrophil cytoplasmic antibodies) markers. *J Clin Invest* 1993;92:1080.

47. Boirivant M, Marini M, Di Felice G, et al: Lamina propria T cells in Crohn's disease and other gastrointestinal inflammation show defective CD2 pathway-induced apoptosis. *Gastroenterology* 1999;116:557.

48. Yukawa M, Iizuka M, Horie Y, et al: Systemic and local evidence of increased Fas-mediated apoptosis in ulcerative colitis. *Int J Colorectal Dis* 2002;17:70.

49. Mansfield JC, Giaffer MH, Holdsworth CD: Controlled trial of oligopeptide versus amino acid diet in treatment of active Crohn's disease. *Gut* 1995;36:60.

50. van den Bogaerde J, Cahill J, Emmanuel AV, et al: Gut mucosal response to food antigens in Crohn's disease. *Aliment Pharmacol Ther* 2003;16:1903.

51. Wurzelman JI, Lyles CM, Sandler RS: Childhood infection and the risk of inflammatory bowel disease. *Dig Dis Sci* 1994;39:555.

52. Persson PG, Leijonmarck CE, Bernell O, et al: Risk indicators for inflammatory bowel disease. *Int J Epidemiol* 1993;22:268.

53. Ibbotson JP, Pease PE, Allan RN: Serological studies in Crohn's disease. *Eur J Clin Microbiol* 1987;6:286.

54. Pirzer U, Schonhaar A, Fleischer B, et al: Reactivity of infiltrating T lymphocytes with microbial antigens in Crohn's disease. *Lancet* 1991;338:1238.

55. Swidsinski A, Ladhoff A, Pernthaler A, et al: Mucosal flora in inflammatory bowel disease. *Gastroenterology* 2002;122:44.

56. Kleessen B, Kroesen AJ, Buhr HJ, Blaut M: Mucosal and invading bacteria in patients with inflammatory bowel disease compared with controls. *Scand J Gastroenterol* 2002;37:1034.

57. Macpherson A, Khoo UY, Forgacs I, et al: Mucosal antibodies in inflammatory bowel disease are directed against intestinal bacteria. *Gut* 1996;38:365.

58. Boyko EJ, Koepsell TD, Perera DR, Inui TS: Risk of ulcerative colitis among former and current cigarette smokers. *N Engl J Med* 1987;316:707.

59. Sutherland LR, Ramcharan S, Bryant H, Fick G: Effect of cigarette smoking on recurrence of Crohn's disease. *Gastroenterology* 1990;98:1123.

60. Sandler RS, Sandler DP, McDonnell CW, Wurzelmann JI: Childhood exposure to environmental tobacco smoke and the risk of ulcerative colitis. *Am J Epidemiol* 1992;135:603.

61. Lindberg E, Tysk C, Andersson K, et al: Smoking and inflammatory bowel disease: a case control study. *Gut* 1988;29:352.

62. Madretsma S, Wolters LM, van Dijk JP: In-vivo effect of nicotine on cytokine production by human non-adherent mononuclear cells. *Eur J Gastroenterol Hepatol* 1996;8:1017.

63. Loftus EV Jr, Sandborn WJ, Tremaine WJ, et al: Primary sclerosing cholangitis is associated with nonsmoking: a case-control study. *Gastroenterology* 1996;110:1496.

64. Hollander D, Vadheim C, Brettholz E, et al: Increased intestinal permeability in patients with Crohn's disease and their relatives: a possible etiologic factor. *Ann Intern Med* 1986;105:883.

65. Anderson RE, Olaison G, Tysk C, Ekbom A: Appendicectomy and protection against ulcerative colitis. *N Engl J Med* 2001;344:808.

66. Koutroubakis IE, Blachonikolis IG: Appendicectomy and the development of ulcerative colitis: results of a metanalysis of published case-control studies. *Am J Gastroenterol* 2000;95:171.

67. Andersson RE, Olaison G, Tysk C, Ekbom A: Appendectomy is followed by increased risk of Crohn's disease. *Gastroenterology* 2003;124:40.

68. Evans JM, McMahon AD, Murray FE, et al: Non-steroidal anti-inflammatory drugs were associated with emergency admission to hospital for colitis due to inflammatory bowel disease. *Gut* 1997;40:619.

69. McCartney SA, Mitchell JA, Fairclough PD, et al: Selective COX-2 inhibitors and human inflammatory bowel disease. *Aliment Pharmacol Ther* 1999;13:1115.

70. Levenstein S, Prantera C, Varvo V: Stress and exacerbation in ulcerative colitis: a prospective study of patients enrolled in remission. *Am J Gastroenterol* 2000;95:1213.

71. Madara JL, Podolsky DK, King NW, et al: Characterization of spontaneous colitis in cotton-top tamarins (*Sanguinus oedipus*) and its response to sulfasalazine. *Gastroenterology* 1985;88:13.

72. Sonnenberg A: Occupational distribution of inflammatory bowel disease among German employees. *Gut* 1990;31:1037.

73. Trallori G, Palli D, Saieva C, et al: A population-based study of inflammatory bowel disease in Florence over 15 years (1978-92). *Scand J Gastroenterol* 1996;31:892.

74. Gilberts ECAM, Greenstein AJ, Katsel P, et al: Molecular evidence for two forms of Crohn disease. *Proc Natl Acad Sci USA* 1994;91:12721.

75. Hendrickson BA, Gokhale R, Cho JH: Clinical aspects and pathophysiology of inflammatory bowel disease. *Clin Microbiol Rev* 2002;15:79.

76. Kreuzpaintner G, Horstkotte D, Heyll A, et al: Increased risk of bacterial endocarditis in inflammatory bowel disease. *Am J Med* 1992;92:391.

77. Vermillion DL, Huizinga JD, Riddell RH, Collins SM: Altered small intestinal smooth muscle function in Crohn's disease. *Gastroenterology* 1993;104:1692.

78. Statter MB, Hirschl RB, Coran AC: Inflammatory bowel disease. *Pediatr Surg* 1993;40:1213.

79. Buchmann P, Keighley MRB, Allan R, et al: Natural history of perianal Crohn's disease. Ten year follow-up: a plea for conservatism. *Am J Surg* 1980;140:642.

80. Lenaerts C, Roy CC, Vaillancourt M, et al: High incidence of upper gastrointestinal tract involvement in children with Crohn's disease. *Pediatrics* 1989;83:777.

81. Jones GW Jr, Dooley MR, Schoenfield LJ: Regional enteritis with involvement of the duodenum. *Gastroenterology* 1966;51:1018.

82. Harper P, McAuliffe T, Beeken W: Crohn's disease in the elderly. A statistical comparison with younger patients matched for sex and duration of disease. *Arch Intern Med* 1986;146:753.

83. Alexander-Williams J: Late-onset Crohn's disease. In: Weterman IT, Pena AS, Booth CC (eds). *The Management of Crohn's Disease*. Amsterdam: Excerpta Medica, 1976, p 43.

84. Fabricius PJ, Gyde SN, Shouler P, et al: Crohn's disease in the elderly. *Gut* 1985;26:461.

85. Gryboski JD: Ulcerative colitis in children ten years old or younger. *J Pediatr Gastroentol Nutr* 1993;17:24.

86. de Boer Visser N, Bryant HE, Hershfield NB: Predictors of hospitalization early in the course of Crohn's disease. *Gastroenterology* 1990;99:380.

87. Podolsky DK: Inflammatory bowel disease. *N Engl J Med* 1991;325:928.

88. Whelan G, Farmer RG, Fazio VW, Goormastic M: Recurrence after surgery in Crohn's disease. Relationship to location of disease (clinical pattern) and surgical indication. *Gastroenterology* 1985;88:1826.

89. Cameron JL, Hamilton SR, Coleman J, et al: Patterns of ileal recurrence in Crohn's disease—a prospective randomized study. *Ann Surg* 1992;215:546.

90. Osborne MJ, Hudson M, Piasecki C, et al: Crohn's disease and anastomotic recurrence—microvascular ischaemia and anastomotic healing in an animal model. *Br J Surg* 1993;80:266.

91. Higgens CS, Allan RN: Crohn's disease of the distal ileum. *Gut* 1980;21:933.

92. Okada M, Yao T, Fuchigami T, et al: Anatomical involvement and clinical features in 91 Japanese patients with Crohn's disease. *J Clin Gastroenterol* 1987;9:165.

93. Ribeiro M, Greenstein A, Yamazaki Y, Aufses AH Jr: Intra-abdominal abscess in regional enteritis. *Ann Surg* 1991;213:32.

94. Greenstein AJ, Sachar DB, Mann D, et al: Spontaneous free perforation and perforated abscess in 30 patients with Crohn's disease. *Ann Surg* 1987;205:72.

95. Crohn BB, Ginzburg L, Oppenheimer GD: Regional ileitis: a pathologic and clinical entity. *JAMA* 1932;99:1323.

96. Hanby AM, Wright NA: The ulcer-associated cell lineage: the gastrointestinal repair kit? *J Pathol* 1993;171:3.

97. Hallgren R, Colombel J, Dahl R, et al: Neutrophil and eosinophil involvement of the small bowel in patients with celiac disease and Crohn's disease: studies on the secretion rate and immunohistochemical localization of granulocyte granule constituents. *Am J Med* 1989;86:56.

98. Fox CC, Lazenby AJ, Moore WC, et al: Enhancement of human intestinal mast cell mediator release in active ulcerative colitis. *Gastroenterology* 1990;99:119.

99. Surawicz CM, Meisel JL, Ylvisaker T, et al: Rectal biopsy in the diagnosis of Crohn's disease: value of multiple biopsies and serial sectioning. *Gastroenterology* 1981;81:66.

100. Petri M, Poulsen SS, Christensen K, Jarnum S: The incidence of granulomas in serial sections of rectal biopsies from patients with Crohn's disease. *Acta Pathol Microbiol Immunol Scand [A]* 1982;90:145.

101. Chambers TJ, Morson BC: Large bowel biopsy in the differential diagnosis of inflammatory bowel disease. *Invest Cell Pathol* 1980;3:159.

102. O'Morain C, Bishop A, McGregor GP, et al: Vasoactive intestinal peptide concentrations and immunocytochemical studies in rectal biopsies from patients with inflammatory bowel disease. *Gut* 1984;25:57.

103. Geboes K, Rutgeerts P, Ectors N, et al: Major histocompatibility class II expression on the small intestinal nervous system in Crohn's disease. *Gastroenterology* 1992;103:439.

104. Oberhuber G, Hirsch M, Stolte M: High incidence of upper gastrointestinal tract involvement in Crohn's disease. *Virchows Arch* 1998;432:49.

105. Wright CL, Riddell RH: Histology of the stomach and duodenum in Crohn's disease. *Am J Surg Pathol* 1998;22:383.

106. Yamamoto T: Factors affecting recurrence after surgery for Crohn's disease. *World J Gastroenterol* 2005;11:3971.

107. Penner RM, Madsen KL, Fedorak RN: Postoperative Crohn's disease. *Inflamm Bowel Dis* 2005;11:765.

108. Ryan WR, Allan RN, Yamamoto T, Keighley MR: Crohn's disease patients who quit smoking have a reduced risk of reoperation for recurrence. *Am J Surg* 2004;187:219.

109. Gilat T: Incidence of inflammatory bowel disease: going up or down? *Gastroenterology* 1983;85:196.

110. Smith MB, Lashner BA, Hanauer SB: Smoking and inflammatory bowel disease in families. *Am J Gastroenterol* 1988;83:407.

111. Farmer RG, Easley KA, Rankin GB: Clinical patterns, natural history, and progression of ulcerative colitis: a long-term follow-up of 1116 patients. *Dig Dis Sci* 1993;38:1137.

112. Rosenthal SR, Snyder JD, Hendricks KM, et al: Growth failure and inflammatory bowel disease: approach to treatment of a complicated adolescent problem. *Pediatrics* 1983;72:481.

113. Langholz E, Munkholm P, Davidsen M, Binder V: Course of ulcerative colitis: analysis of changes in disease activity over years. *Gastroenterology* 1994;107:3.

114. Caprilli R, Latella G, Vernia P, et al: Multiple organ dysfunction in ulcerative colitis. *Am J Gastroenterol* 2000;95:1258.

115. Goldstein N, Dulai M: Contemporary morphologic definition of backwash ileitis in ulcerative colitis and features that distinguish it from Crohn disease. *Am J Clin Pathol* 2006;126:365.

116. Haskell H, Andrews CW, Reddy SI, et al: Pathologic features and clinical significance of "backwash" ileitis in ulcerative colitis. *Am J Surg Pathol* 2005;29:1472.

117. Farrokhyar F, Swarbrick ET, Crace RH, et al: Low mortality in ulcerative colitis and Crohn's disease in three regional centers in England. *Am J Gastroenterol* 2001;96:501.

118. Palli D, Trallori G, Saieva C, et al: General and cancer specific mortality of a population based cohort of patients with inflammatory bowel disease: the Florence study. *Gut* 1998;42:175.

119. Winther KV, Jess T, Langholz E, et al: Survival and cause-specific mortality in ulcerative colitis: follow-up of a population-based cohort in Copenhagen County. *Gastroenterology* 2003;125:1576.

120. Noffsinger AE, Miller MA, Cusi MV, Fenoglio-Preiser CM: The pattern of cell proliferation in neoplastic and nonneoplastic lesions of ulcerative colitis. *Cancer* 1996;78:2307.

121. Heatley RV, James PD: Eosinophils in rectal mucosa. A simple method of predicting the outcome of ulcerative proctocolitis? *Gut* 1978;20:787.

122. Fox CC, Lichtenstein LM, Roche JK: Intestinal mast cell responses in idiopathic inflammatory bowel disease: histamine release from human intestinal mast cells in response to gut epithelial proteins. *Dig Dis Sci* 1993;38:1105.

123. Kimura M, Masuda T, Hiwatashi N, et al: Changes in neuropeptide-containing nerves in human colonic mucosa with inflammatory bowel disease. *Pathol Int* 1994;44:624.

124. Surrenti C, Renzi D, Garcea MR, et al: Colonic vasoactive intestinal polypeptide in ulcerative colitis. *J Physiol* 1993;87:307.

125. Pitt MA, Knox WF, Haboubi NY: Multinucleated stromal giant cells of the colonic lamina propria in ulcerative colitis. *J Clin Pathol* 1993;46:874.

126. Goldblum JR, Appelman HD: Appendiceal involvement in ulcerative colitis. *Mod Pathol* 1992;5:607.

127. Groisman GM, George J, Harpaz N: Ulcerative appendicitis in universal and nonuniversal ulcerative colitis. *Mod Pathol* 1994;7:322.

128. Kroft SH, Stryker SJ, Rao MS: Appendiceal involvement as a skip lesion in ulcerative colitis. *Mod Pathol* 1994;7:912.

129. Mitomi H, Atari E, Uesugi H, et al: Distinctive diffuse duodenitis associated with ulcerative colitis. *Dig Dis Sci* 1997;42:684.

130. Sasaki M, Okada K, Koyama S, et al: Ulcerative colitis complicated by gastroduodenal lesions. *J Gastroenterol* 1996;31:585.

131. Valdez R, Appelman HD, Bronner MP, Greenson JK: Diffuse duodenitis associated with ulcerative colitis. *Am J Surg Pathol* 2000;24:1407.

132. Stelzner M, Phillips JD, Fonkalsrud EW: Acute ileus from steroid withdrawal simulating intestinal obstruction after surgery for ulcerative colitis. *Arch Surg* 1990;125:914.

133. Frei JV, Morson BC: Medical audit of rectal biopsy diagnosis of inflammatory bowel disease. *J Clin Pathol* 1982;35:341.

134. Hill R, Kent T, Hansen R: Clinical usefulness of rectal biopsy in Crohn's disease. *Gastroenterology* 1979;77:938.

135. Allison MC, Hamilton-Dutoit SJ, Dhillon AP, Pounder RE: The value of rectal biopsy in distinguishing self-limited colitis from early inflammatory bowel disease. *Q J Med* 1987;65:985.

136. O'Leary AD, Sweeney EC: Lymphoglandular complexes of the colon; structure and distribution. *Histopathology* 1986;10:267.

137. Theodossi A, Spiegelhalter DJ, Jass J, et al: Observer variation and discriminatory value of biopsy features in inflammatory bowel disease. *Gut* 1994;35:961.

138. Veloso FT, Carvalho J, Magro F: Immune-related systemic manifestations of inflammatory bowel disease. A prospective study of 792 patients. *J Clin Gastroenterol* 1996;23:29.

139. De Vos M: Review article: joint involvement in inflammatory bowel disease. *Aliment Pharmacol Ther* 2004;20:36.

140. Danese S, Semeraro S, Papa A, et al: Extraintestinal manifestations in inflammatory bowel disease. *World J Gastroenterol* 2005;11:7227.

141. Leirisalo-Repo M, Turunen U, Stenman S, et al: High frequency of silent inflammatory bowel disease in spondyloarthropathy. *Arthritis Rheum* 1994;37:23.

142. Compston JE, Judd D, Crawley EO, et al: Osteoporosis in patients with inflammatory bowel disease. *Gut* 1987;28:410.

143. Desmet VJ, Geboes K: Liver lesions in inflammatory bowel disorders. *J Pathol* 1987;151:247.

144. Bargiggia S, Maconi G, Elli M, et al: Sonographic prevalence of liver steatosis and biliary tract stones in patients with inflammatory bowel disease: study of 511 subjects at a single center. *J Clin Gastroenterol* 2003;36:417.

145. Ong JC, O'Loughlin EV, Kamath KR, et al: Sclerosing cholangitis in children with inflammatory bowel disease. *Aust NZ J Med* 1994;24:149.

146. Ludwig J: Small-duct primary sclerosing cholangitis. *Semin Liver Dis* 1991;11:11.
147. Schrumpf E, Fausa O, Elgjo K, Kolmannskog F: Hepatobiliary complications of inflammatory bowel disease. *Semin Liver Dis* 1988;8:201.
148. Aadland E, Schrumpf E, Fausa O, et al: Primary sclerosing cholangitis: a long-term follow up study. *Scand J Gastroenterol* 1987;22:655.
149. Broome U, Bergquist A: Primary sclerosing cholangitis, inflammatory bowel disease, and colon cancer. *Semin Liver Dis* 2006;26:31.
150. Wee A, Ludwig J: Pericholangitis in chronic ulcerative colitis: primary sclerosing cholangitis of the small bile ducts? *Ann Intern Med* 1991; 102:581.
151. Das KM, Vecchi M, Sakamaki S: A shared and unique epitope(s) on human colon, skin and biliary epithelium detected by a monoclonal antibody. *Gastroenterology* 1990;98:464.
152. Duerr RH, Targan SR, Landers CJ, et al: Neutrophil cytoplasmic antibodies: a link between primary sclerosing cholangitis and ulcerative colitis. *Gastroenterology* 1991;100:1385.
153. Pokorny CS, Norton ID, McCaughan GW, Selby WS: Anti-neutrophil cytoplasmic antibody: a prognostic indicator in primary sclerosing cholangitis. *J Gastroenterol Hepatol* 1994;9:40.
154. Chapman RW, Varghese Z, Gaul R: Association of primary sclerosing cholangitis with HLA-B8. *Gut* 1983;24:38.
155. Brentnall T, Haggitt R, Rabinovitch P, et al: Risk and natural history of colonic neoplasia in patients with primary sclerosing cholangitis and ulcerative colitis. *Gastroenterology* 1996;110:331.
156. Mir-Madjlessi SH, Farmer RG, Sivak MV Jr: Bile duct carcinoma in patients with ulcerative colitis. *Dig Dis Sci* 1987;32:145.
157. Malka D, Levy P, Chemtob A, Bernades P: Acute relapsing pancreatitis revealing Crohn's disease. *Gastroenterol Clin Biol* 1994;18:892.
158. Gitkind M, Wright S: Amyloidosis complicating inflammatory bowel disease. A case report and review of the literature. *Dig Dis Sci* 1990; 35:906.
159. Edwards P, Cooper DA, Turner J, et al: Resolution of amyloidosis (AA type) complicating chronic ulcerative colitis. *Gastroenterology* 1988; 95:810.
160. Mir-Madjlessi SH, Taylor JS, Farmer RG: Clinical course and evolution of erythema nodosum and pyoderma gangrenosum in chronic ulcerative colitis: a study of 42 patients. *Am J Gastroenterol* 1985;80: 615.
161. VanHale HM, Rogers RS, Zone JJ, Greipp PR: Pyostomatitis vegetans: a reactive mucosal marker for inflammatory disease of the gut. *Arch Dermatol* 1985;121:94.
162. Philpot H, Elewski B, Banwell J, Gramlich T: Pyostomatitis vegetans and primary sclerosing cholangitis: markers of inflammatory bowel disease. *Gastroenterology* 1992;103:668.
163. Taverela Veloso F: Review article: skin complications associated with inflammatory bowel disease. *Aliment Pharmacol Ther* 2004;20:50.
164. Fenske NA, Gern JE, Pierce D, Vasey FB: Vesiculopustular eruption of ulcerative colitis. *Arch Dermatol* 1983;119:664.
165. Treem W, Veligati L, Rotter J, et al: Ulcerative colitis and total alopecia in a mother and her son. *Gastroenterology* 1993;104:1187.
166. Basu MK, Asquith P: Oral manifestations of inflammatory bowel disease. *Clin Gastroenterol* 1980;9:307.
167. Vasishta S, Wood JB, McGinty F: Ulcerative tracheobronchitis years after colectomy for ulcerative colitis. *Chest* 1994;106:1279.
168. Rickli H, Fretz C, Hoffman M, et al: Severe inflammatory upper airway stenosis in ulcerative colitis. *Eur Res J* 1994;7:1899.
169. Fluckiger R, Laifer G, Itin P, et al: Oral hairy leukoplakia in a patient with ulcerative colitis. *Gastroenterology* 1994;106:506.
170. Prezyna AP, Kalyanaraman U: Bowen's carcinoma in vulvovaginal Crohn's disease (regional enterocolitis): report of first case. *Am J Obstet Gynecol* 1977;128:914.
171. Donaldson RM Jr: Management of medical problems in pregnancy—inflammatory bowel disease. *N Engl J Med* 1985;312:616.
172. Talbot RW, Heppell J, Dozois RR, Beart RW: Vascular complications of inflammatory bowel disease. *Mayo Clin Proc* 1986;61:140.
173. Kahn EI, Daum F, Aiges HW, et al: Cutaneous polyarteritis nodosa associated with Crohn's disease. *Dis Colon Rectum* 1980;23:258.
174. Bansal R, Aggarwal A, Handa R, et al: Ulcerative colitis associated with Takayasu arteritis. *Int J Cardiol* 2003;88:91.
175. Teja K, Crum C, Friedman C: Giant cell arteritis and Crohn's disease. *Gastroenterology* 1980;78:796.
176. Manganiotis AN, Banner MP, Malkowicz SB: Urologic complications of Crohn's disease. *Surg Clin North Am* 2001;81:197.
177. Shield DE, Lytton B, Weiss RM, Schiff M Jr: Urologic complications of inflammatory bowel disease. *J Urol* 1976;115:701.
178. Hudson M, Chitolie A, Hutton RA, et al: Thrombotic vascular risk factors in inflammatory bowel disease. *Gut* 1996;38:733.
179. Jain S, Bhatt P, Muralikrishna GK, et al: Extensive arterial and venous thrombosis in a patient with ulcerative colitis—a case report. *Med Gen Med* 2005;7:10.
180. Mezoff AG, Cohen MB, Maisel SK, Farrell MK: Crohn disease in an infant with central nervous system thrombosis and protein-losing enteropathy. *J Pediatrics* 1990;117:436.
181. Aadland E, Odegaard OR, Roseth A, Try K: Free protein-S deficiency in patients with chronic inflammatory bowel disease. *Scand J Gastroenterol* 1992;27:957.
182. Wisen O, Gardlund B: Hemostasis in Crohn's disease: low factor XIII levels in active disease. *Scand J Gastroenterol* 1988;23:961.
183. Korsten S, Reis HE: Acquired protein-C deficiency in ulcerative colitis as a cause of thromboembolic complications. *Dtsch Med Wochenschr* 1992;117:419.
184. Conlan M, Haire W, Burnett D: Prothrombotic abnormalities in inflammatory bowel disease. *Dig Dis Sci* 1989;34:1089.
185. Calder CJ, Lacy D, Raafat F, et al: Crohn's disease with pulmonary involvement in a 3-year-old boy. *Gut* 1993;34:1636.
186. Mayer L, Janowitz HD: Extra-intestinal manifestations of ulcerative colitis including reference to Crohn's disease. In: Allan RN, Keighley MRB, Alexander-Williams J, et al (eds). *Inflammatory Bowel Disease*. London: Churchill Livingstone, 1983.
187. Oldenburg B, Koningsberger JC, Van Berge Henegouwen GP, et al: Iron and inflammatory bowel disease. *Aliment Pharmacol Ther* 2001;15:429.
188. Elsborg L, Larsen L: Folate deficiency in chronic inflammatory bowel disease. *Scand J Gastroenterol* 1979;14:1019.
189. Gasche C, Reinisch W, Lochs H, et al: Anemia in Crohn's disease—importance of inadequate erythropoietin production and iron deficiency. *Dig Dis Sci* 1994;39:1930.
190. Ramakrishna R, Manoharan A: Autoimmune haemolytic anaemia in ulcerative colitis. *Acta Haematol* 1994;91:99.
191. Connell WR, Kamm MA, Ritchie JK, Lennard-Jones JE: Bone marrow toxicity caused by azathioprine in inflammatory bowel disease—27 years of experience. *Gut* 1993;34:1081.
192. Sahay R, Prangnell DR, Scott BB: Inflammatory bowel disease and refractory anaemia (myelodysplasia). *Gut* 1993;34:1630.
193. Chad DA, Smith TW, DeGirolami U, Hammar K: Perineuritis and ulcerative colitis. *Neurology* 1986;36:1377.
194. Sarrouj BJ, Zampino DJ, Cilursu AM: Pericarditis as the initial manifestation of inflammatory bowel disease. *Chest* 1994;106:1911.
195. Triantafillidis JK, Cherakakis P, Zervakakis A, Theodorou M: Coexistence of hyperthyroidism and ulcerative colitis: report of 4 cases and a review of the literature. *Ital J Gastroenterol* 1992;24:494.
196. Falchuk KR, Falchuk ZM: Selective immunoglobulin A deficiency, ulcerative colitis, and gluten-sensitive enteropathy—a unique association. *Gastroenterology* 1975;69:503.
197. Philipson BM, Kock NG, Jagenburg R, et al: Functional and structural studies of ileal reservoirs used for continent urostomy and ileostomy. *Gut* 1983;24:392.
198. Sandborn WJ, Tremaine WJ, Batts KP, et al: Pouchitis after ileal pouch-anal anastomosis: a pouchitis disease activity index. *Mayo Clin Proc* 1994;69:409.
199. Lohmuller JL, Pemberton JH, Dozois RR, et al: Pouchitis and extraintestinal manifestations of inflammatory bowel disease after ileal pouch-anal anastomosis. *Ann Surg* 1990;211:622.
200. Luukkonen P, Jarvinen H, Tanskanen M, Kahri A: Pouchitis—recurrence of the inflammatory bowel disease? *Gut* 1994;35:243.
201. Penna C, Dozois R, Tremaine W, et al: Pouchitis after ileal pouch-anal anastomosis for ulcerative colitis occurs with increased frequency in patients with associated primary sclerosing cholangitis. *Gut* 1996; 38:234.
202. Stahlberg D, Gullberg K, Liljeqvist L, et al: Pouchitis following pelvic pouch operation for ulcerative colitis. Incidence, cumulative risk, and risk factors. *Dis Colon Rectum* 1996;39:1012.
203. Ruseler-van Embden JG, Schouten WR, van Lieshout LM: Pouchitis: result of microbial imbalance? *Gut* 1994;35:658.
204. Madden MV, Farthing MJ, Nicholls RJ: Inflammation in the ileal reservoir: pouchitis. *Gut* 1990;31:247.
205. Pemberton JH, Kelly KA, Beart RW, et al: Ileal pouch-anal anastomosis for chronic ulcerative colitis: long-term results. *Ann Surg* 1987;206:504.

206. Bach SP, Mortensen NJM: Revolution and evolution: 30 years of ileoanal pouch surgery. *Inflamm Bowel Dis* 2006;12:131.

207. De Silva HJ, Millard PR, Kettlewell M, et al: Mucosal characteristics of pelvic ileal pouches. *Gut* 1991;32:61.

208. Apel R, Cohen Z, Andrews CW Jr, et al: Prospective evaluation of early morphological changes in pelvic ileal pouches. *Gastroenterology* 1994;107:435.

209. Rutgeerts P, vanTrappen G, Geboes K: Endoscopy in inflammatory bowel disease. *Scand J Gastroenterol* 1989;170:12.

210. Ekbom A, Helmick C, Zack M, Adami HO: Ulcerative colitis and colorectal cancer: a population-based study. *N Engl J Med* 1990;323:1228.

211. Ekbom A, Helmick C, Zack M, Adami HO: Increased risk of large-bowel cancer in Crohn's disease with colonic involvement. *Lancet* 1990;336:357.

212. Langholz E, Munkholm P, Davidsen M, Binder V: Colorectal cancer risk and mortality in patients with ulcerative colitis. *Gastroenterology* 1992;103:1444.

213. Sugita A, Sachar DB, Bodian C, et al: Colorectal cancer in ulcerative colitis. Influence of anatomical extent and age at onset on colitis-cancer interval. *Gut* 1991;32:167.

214. Lashner B, Silverstein M, Hanauer S: Hazard rates for dysplasia and cancer in ulcerative colitis. *Dig Dis Sci* 1989;34:1536.

215. Choi PM, Nugent FW, Schoetz DJ, et al: Colonoscopic surveillance reduces mortality from colorectal cancer in ulcerative colitis. *Gastroenterology* 1993;105:418.

216. Heimann TM, Oh SC, Martinelli G, et al: Colorectal carcinoma associated with ulcerative colitis: a study of prognostic indicators. *Am J Surg* 1992;164:13.

217. Lennard-Jones J: Colitic cancer: supervision, surveillance, or surgery? *Gastroenterology* 1995;109:1388.

218. Eaden J, Abrams KR, Mayberry JF: The risk of colorectal cancer in ulcerative colitis: a meta-analysis. *Gut* 2001;48:526.

219. Broome U, Lindberg G, Lofberg R: Primary sclerosing cholangitis in ulcerative colitis—a risk factor for the development of dysplasia and DNA aneuploidy? *Gastroenterology* 1992;102:1877.

220. Rubin C, Haggitt R, Burmer G, et al: DNA aneuploidy in colonic biopsies predicts future development of dysplasia in ulcerative colitis. *Gastroenterology* 1992;103:1611.

221. Cuvelier C, Bekaert E, Potter C, et al: Crohn's disease with adenocarcinoma and dysplasia. *Am J Surg Pathol* 1989;13:187.

222. Greenstein AJ, Meyers S, Azporn A, et al: Colorectal cancer in regional ileitis. *Q J Med* 1987;62:33.

223. Petras RE, Mir-Madjlessi SH, Farmer RG: Crohn's disease and intestinal carcinoma. A report of 11 cases with emphasis on associated epithelial dysplasia. *Gastroenterology* 1987;93:1307.

224. Connell WR, Sheffield JP, Kamm MA, et al: Lower gastrointestinal malignancy in Crohn's disease. *Gut* 1994;35:347.

225. Gillen CD, Andrews HA, Prior P, Allan RN: Crohn's disease and colorectal cancer. *Gut* 1994;35:651.

226. Sherlock DJ, Suarez V, Gray JG: Stomal adenocarcinoma in Crohn's disease. *Gut* 1990;31:1329.

227. Persson PG, Karlen P, Bernell O, et al: Crohn's disease and cancer: a population-based cohort study. *Gastroenterology* 1994;107:1675.

228. Halliwell B, Aruoma OI: DNA damage by oxygen-derived species. Its mechanism and measurement in mammalian systems. *FEBS Lett* 1991;281:9.

229. Warren S, Sommers SC: Pathogenesis of ulcerative colitis. *Am J Pathol* 1949;25:657.

230. Dawson IM, Pryse-Davies J: The development of carcinoma of the large intestine in ulcerative colitis. *Br J Surg* 1959;47:113.

231. Morson BC, Pang LS: Rectal biopsy as an aid to cancer control in ulcerative colitis. *Gut* 1967;8:423.

232. Blackstone MO, Riddell RH, Rogers BHG, Levin B: Dysplasia-associated lesion or mass (DALM) detected by colonoscopy in long-standing ulcerative colitis: an indication for colectomy. *Gastroenterology* 1981; 80:366.

233. Lynch DA, Lobo AJ, Sobala GM, et al: Failure of colonoscopic surveillance in ulcerative colitis. *Gut* 1993;34:1075.

234. Riddell RH, Goldman H, Ransohoff DF, et al: Dysplasia in inflammatory bowel disease: standardized classification with provisional clinical applications. *Hum Pathol* 1983;14:931.

235. Jess T, Loftus EV Jr, Velayos FS, et al: Incidence and prognosis of colorectal dysplasia in inflammatory bowel disease: a population-based study from Olmsted County, Minnesota. *Inflamm Bowel Dis* 2006;12:669.

236. Provenzale D, Kowdley KV Arora S, Wong JB: Prophylactic colectomy or surveillance for chronic ulcerative colitis? A decision analysis. *Gastroenterology* 1995;109:1188.

237. Jonsson B, Ahsgren L, Andersson LO, et al: Colorectal cancer surveillance in patients with ulcerative colitis. *Br J Surg* 1994;81:689.

238. Connell WR, Talbot IC, Harpaz N, et al: Clinicopathological characteristics of colorectal carcinoma complicating ulcerative colitis. *Gut* 1994;35:1419.

239. Itzkowitz SH, Present DH: Consensus conference: colorectal cancer screening and surveillance in inflammatory bowel disease. *Inflamm Bowel Dis* 2005;11:314.

240. Lashner BA, Provencher KS, Bozdech JM, et al: Worsening risk for the development of dysplasia or cancer in patients with chronic ulcerative colitis. *Am J Gastroenterol* 1995;90:377.

241. Bernstein CN, Shanahan F, Weinstein WM: Are we telling patients the truth about surveillance colonoscopy in ulcerative colitis? *Lancet* 1994;343:71.

242. Woolrich AJ, DaSilva MD, Korelitz BI: Surveillance in the routine management of ulcerative colitis: the predictive value of low-grade dysplasia. *Gastroenterology* 1992;103:431.

243. Ullman TA, Croog T, Harpaz N, et al: Progression of flat low-grade dysplasia to advanced neoplasia in patients with ulcerative colitis. *Gastroenterology* 2003;125:1311.

244. Connell WR, Lennard-Jones JE, Williams CB, et al: Factors affecting the outcome of endoscopic surveillance for cancer in ulcerative colitis. *Gastroenterology* 1994;107:934.

245. Odze RD, Farraye FA, Hecht JL, et al: Long-term follow-up after polypectomy treatment for adenoma-like dysplastic lesions in ulcerative colitis. *Clin Gastroenterol Hepatol* 2004;2:534.

246. Rognum TO, Elgjo K, Fausa O, Brandtzaeg P: Immunohistochemical evaluation of carcinoembryonic antigen, secretory component and epithelial IgA in ulcerative colitis with dysplasia. *Gut* 1982;23:123.

247. Ehsanullah M, Naunton Morgan M, Filipe MI, Gazzard B: Sialomucins in the assessment of dysplasia and cancer-risk patients with ulcerative colitis treated with colectomy and ileo-rectal anastomosis. *Histopathology* 1985;9:223.

248. Ehsanullah M, Filipe MI, Gazzard B: Mucin secretion in inflammatory bowel disease: correlation with disease activity and dysplasia. *Gut* 1982;23:485.

249. Burmer GC, Rabinovitch PS, Haggitt RC, et al: Neoplastic progression in ulcerative colitis: histology, DNA content and loss of a p53 allele. *Gastroenterology* 1992;103:1602.

250. Hammarberg C, Rubio C, Slezak P, et al: Flow-cytometric DNA analysis as a means for early detection of malignancy in patients with chronic ulcerative colitis. *Gut* 1984;25:905.

251. Fozard JB, Quirke P, Dixon MF, et al: DNA aneuploidy in ulcerative colitis. *Gut* 1986;27:1414.

252. Lofberg R, Brostrom O, Karlen P, et al: DNA aneuploidy in ulcerative colitis: reproducibility, topographic distribution and relation to dysplasia. *Gastroenterology* 1992;102:1149.

253. Levine DS, Rabinovitch PS, Haggitt RC, et al: Distribution of aneuploid cell populations in ulcerative colitis with dysplasia or cancer. *Gastroenterology* 1991;101:1198.

254. Shinozaki M, Watanabe T, Kubota Y, et al: High proliferative activity is associated with dysplasia in ulcerative colitis. *Dis Colon Rectum* 2000;43:S34.

255. Sjoqvist U, Ost A, Lofberg R: Increased expression of proliferative Ki-67 nuclear antigen is correlated with dysplastic colorectal epithelium in ulcerative colitis. *Int J Colorectal Dis* 1999;14:107.

256. Grundfest SF, Fazio V, Weiss RA, et al: The risk of cancer following colectomy and ileorectal anastomosis for extensive mucosal ulcerative colitis. *Ann Surg* 1981;193:9.

257. Haidar A, Dixon MF: Solitary microcarcinoid in ulcerative colitis. *Histopathology* 1992;21:487.

258. McNeely B, Owen DA, Pezim M: Multiple microcarcinoids arising in chronic ulcerative colitis. *Am J Clin Pathol* 1992;98:112.

259. Levy PJ, Lebenthal A, Pappo O, Caine YG: The coexistence of Crohn's disease and a nongastrointestinal carcinoid tumor. *Am J Gastroenterol* 1993;88:1120.

260. Hock YL, Scott KW, Grace RH: Mixed adenocarcinoma carcinoid tumour of large bowel in a patient with Crohn's disease. *J Clin Pathol* 1993;46:183.

261. Dayal Y: Critical commentary to "Carcinoid tumor complicating inflammatory bowel disease." *Pathol Res Pract* 1995;191:1193.

262. Sugita A, Greenstein AJ, Ribeiro MB, et al: Survival with colorectal cancer in ulcerative colitis—a study of 102 cases. *Ann Surg* 1993;218:189.

263. Melville DM, Richman PI, Shepherd NA, et al: Brush cytology of the colon and rectum in ulcerative colitis: an aid to cancer diagnosis. *J Clin Pathol* 1988;41:1180.

264. Mellemkjaer L, Olsen JH, Frisch M, et al: Cancer in patients with ulcerative colitis. *Int J Cancer* 1995;60:330.

265. Barki Y, Boult I: Two uncommon malignancies complicating chronic ulcerative colitis. *J Can Assoc Radiol* 1981;32:136.

266. Adlersberg R: Kaposi's sarcoma complicating ulcerative colitis: report of a case. *Am J Clin Pathol* 1970;54:143.

267. Kini SU, Pai PK, Rao PK, Kini AU: Primary gastric lymphomas associated with Crohn's disease of the stomach. *Am J Gastroenterol* 1986; 81:23.

268. Lenzen R, Borchard F, Lubke H, Strohmeyer G: Colitis ulcerosa complicated by malignant lymphoma: case report and analysis of published works. *Gut* 1995;36:306.

269. Vanbockrijck M, Cabooter M, Casselman J, et al: Primary Hodgkin's disease of ileum complicating Crohn's disease. *Cancer* 1993;72:1784.

270. Church JM, Weakley FL, Fazio VW, et al: The relationship between fistulas in Crohn's disease and associated carcinoma. Report of four cases and review of the literature. *Dis Colon Rectum* 1985;28:361.

271. Suzuki H, Harpaz N, Tarmin L, et al: Microsatellite instability in ulcerative colitis-associated colorectal dysplasias and cancers. *Cancer Res* 1994;54:4841.

272. Heinen CD, Noffsinger AE, Straughen J, et al: Regenerative lesions in ulcerative colitis are characterized by microsatellite mutation. *Genes Chromosomes Cancer* 1997;19:170.

273. Willenbucher RF, Aust DE, Chang CG, et al: Genomic instability is an early event during the progression pathway of ulcerative-colitis-related neoplasia. *Am J Pathol* 1999;154:1825.

274. Schulmann K, Mori Y, Croog V, et al: Molecular phenotype of inflammatory bowel disease-associated neoplasms with microsatellite instability. *Gastroenterology* 2005;129:74.

275. Noffsinger A, Kretschmer S, Belli J, Fenoglio-Preiser CM: Microsatellite instability is uncommon in Crohn's colitis and ileitis. *Dig Dis Sci* 2000;45:378.

276. Park WS, Pham T, Wang C, et al: Loss of heterozygosity and microsatellite instability in non-neoplastic mucosa from patients with chronic ulcerative colitis. *Int J Mol Med* 1998;2:221.

277. Brentnall TA, Crispin DA, Bronner MA, et al: Microsatellite instability in nonneoplastic mucosa from patients with chronic ulcerative colitis. *Cancer Res* 1996;56:1237.

278. Kinouchi Y, Hiwatashi N, Chida M, et al: Telomere shortening in the colonic mucosa of patients with ulcerative colitis. *J Gastroenterol* 1998;33:343.

279. O'Sullivan JN, Bronner MP, Brentnall TA, et al: Chromosomal instability in ulcerative colitis is related to telomere shortening. *Nat Genet* 2002;32:280.

280. Terdiman JP, Aust DE, Chang CG, et al: High resolution analysis of chromosome 18 alterations in ulcerative colitis-related colorectal cancer. *Cancer Genet Cytogenet* 2002;136:129.

281. Noffsinger AE, Belli JM, Kretschmer S, et al: A unique basal pattern of p53 expression is associated with mutation in colonic mucosa of patients with ulcerative colitis. *Histopathology* 2001;39:482.

282. Yin J, Harpaz N, Tong Y, et al: p53 mutations in dysplastic and cancerous ulcerative colitis lesions. *Gastroenterology* 1993;104:1633.

283. Brentnall TA, Crispin DA, Rabinovitch PS, et al: Mutations in the p53 gene: an early marker of neoplastic progression in ulcerative colitis. *Gastroenterology* 1994;107:369.

284. Burmer GC, Levine DS, Kulander BG, et al: C-Ki-ras mutations in chronic ulcerative colitis and sporadic colon carcinoma. *Gastroenterology* 1990;99:416.

285. Aust DE, Terdiman JP, Willenbucher RF, et al: The APC/beta-catenin pathway in ulcerative colitis-related colorectal carcinomas: a mutational analysis. *Cancer* 2002;94:1421.

286. Willenbucher RF, Zelman SJ, Ferrell LD, et al: Chromosomal alterations in ulcerative colitis-related neoplastic progression. *Gastroenterology* 1997;113:791.

287. Harpaz N, Peck AL, Yin J, et al: p53 protein expression in ulcerative colitis-associated colorectal dysplasia and carcinoma. *Hum Pathol* 1994;25:1069.

288. Holzmann K, Klump B, Borchard F, et al: Comparative analysis of histology, DNA content, p53 and Ki-ras mutations in colectomy specimens with long-standing ulcerative colitis. *Int J Cancer* 1998;76:1.

289. Taylor HW, Boyle M, Smith SC, et al: Expression of p53 in colorectal cancer and dysplasia complicating ulcerative colitis. *Br J Surg* 1993;80:442.

290. Rosman-Urbach M, Niv Y, Birk Y, et al: A high degree of aneuploidy, loss of p53 gene, and low soluble p53 protein serum levels are detected in ulcerative colitis patients. *Dis Colon Rectum* 2004;47:304.

291. Fleisher AS, Esteller M, Harpaz N, et al: Microsatellite instability in inflammatory bowel disease-associated neoplastic lesions is associated with hypermethylation and diminished expression of the DNA mismatch repair gene, hMLH1. *Cancer Res* 2000;60:4864.

292. Chang CL, Marra G, Chauhan DP, et al: Oxidative stress inactivates the human DNA mismatch repair system. *Am J Physiol Cell Physiol* 2002;283:C148.

293. Issa JP, Ahuja N, Toyota M, et al: Accelerated age-related CpG island methylation in ulcerative colitis. *Cancer Res* 2001;61:3573.

294. Fujii S, Tominaga K, Kitajima K, et al: Methylation of the oestrogen receptor gene in non-neoplastic epithelium as a marker of colorectal neoplasia risk in longstanding and extensive ulcerative colitis. *Gut* 2005;54:1287.

295. Tominaga K, Fujii S, Mukawa K, et al: Prediction of colorectal neoplasia by quantitative methylation analysis of estrogen receptor gene in nonneoplastic epithelium from patients with ulcerative colitis. *Clin Cancer Res* 2005;11:8800.

296. Hsieh CJ, Klump B, Holzmann K, et al: Hypermethylation of the p16INK4a promoter in colectomy specimens of patients with long-standing and extensive ulcerative colitis. *Cancer Res* 1998;58:3942.

297. Sato F, Harpaz N, Shibata D, et al: Hypermethylation of the p14(ARF) gene in ulcerative colitis-associated colorectal carcinogenesis. *Cancer Res* 2002;62:1148.

298. Wheeler JM, Kim HC, Efstathiou JA, et al: Hypermethylation of the promoter region of the E-cadherin gene (CDH1) in sporadic and ulcerative colitis associated colorectal cancer. *Gut* 2001;48:367.

299. Azarschab P, Porschen R, Gregor M, et al: Epigenetic control of the E-cadherin gene (CDH1) by CpG methylation in colectomy samples of patients with ulcerative colitis. *Genes Chromosomes Cancer* 2002;35:121.

12 Polyposis and Hereditary Cancer Syndromes

POLYPOSIS SYNDROMES

Introduction

Polyps develop throughout the gastrointestinal (GI) system either as sporadic lesions or as part of a polyposis or hereditary cancer syndrome. The most common syndromes are those that involve neoplastic intestinal adenomas. These include familial adenomatous polyposis, MYH polyposis, and hereditary nonpolyposis colorectal cancer syndrome. Less common polyposis syndromes involve development of hamartomas and include Peutz-Jeghers, juvenile polyposis, Bannayan-Riley-Ruvalcaba, neurofibromatosis 1, and Cowden syndromes. Another hamartomatous polyposis syndrome, Cronkhite-Canada syndrome, is nonfamilial. Other syndromes, such as hyperplastic polyposis and hereditary mixed polyposis, include both adenomatous and nonadenomatous polyps. Some rare forms of polyposis involve proliferations of lymphoid or mesenchymal tissues and are discussed elsewhere in this text.

Less than 1% of all GI malignancies result from intestinal polyposis syndromes. One classification scheme of polyposis syndromes is shown in Table 12.1. In order to diagnose a specific polyposis syndrome, one must be aware of (a) the number of polyps a patient has and their location, (b) the patient's age, (c) the family history, and (d) other clinical information that identifies a patient as having a specific syndrome. Overlap exists between several syndromes.

HEREDITARY ADENOMATOUS POLYPOSIS SYNDROMES

Familial Adenomatous Polyposis and Its Variants

General Comments

Familial adenomatous polyposis (FAP) (OMIM entry #175100) is a generalized growth disorder that includes intestinal polyposis as well as numerous extracolonic manifestations. Overlap exists among the different adenomatous polyposis syndromes, and the varied extraintestinal manifestations of FAP have led to confusion in their nomenclature.

Gardner syndrome was the term applied to patients with colonic polyposis, epidermoid cysts, osteomas, and desmoids. *Turcot syndrome* was diagnosed if the patient had colonic polyposis with brain tumors. However, our current understanding of these disorders indicates that FAP, Gardner syndrome, and Turcot syndrome all represent variations of the same disease rather than distinct entities, and result from defects in a single pleiotropic gene with variable expressivity.

Genetic Features

The FAP-associated gene is located on chromosome 5, and is called *APC* for adenomatous polyposis coli (1–4). *APC* has 15 exons (Fig. 12.1) and encodes a protein of 2,843 amino acids (2,4). The large size of the gene may account for the high frequency of new mutations that occur in it. Germline mutations in *APC* account for most cases of FAP (2,3,5). Every cell in an FAP patient contains one inactive *APC* allele; an alteration in the other allele gives rise to intestinal tumors. Inactivation of the second allele occurs in the earliest recognizable phase of the tumors, including some lesions containing as few as two adenomatous crypts, confirming that inactivation of the second *APC* allele occurs early in neoplastic development.

APC germline mutations are notable in that they are almost exclusively single base pair (bp) changes leading to termination codons, or small (one to four bp) deletions, insertions, or splicing mutations causing translational frame shifts and subsequent downstream stop codons (2,3,6). Even though 45% of patients have detectable germline defects in exon 15, mutations are located throughout the length of the *APC* gene. Most mutations disrupt the coding sequence in the 5' half of the FAP open reading frame (7).

The first clue to the function of the APC protein came when immunoprecipitation experiments showed that anti-APC antibodies precipitated β-catenin (8). APC and β-catenin are part of a complex signaling pathway, the Wnt pathway, that controls many cellular processes including proliferation, differentiation, apoptosis, and body patterning during development (Fig 12.2). In addition to its role in mediating β-catenin degradation, APC also plays a part in controlling the cell cycle, inhibiting progression from the G_0/G_1 phase of the cycle to the S phase (9). APC also

TABLE 12.1   **Classification of Intestinal Polyposes**

Familial Disorders		Nonfamilial Disorders	
Adenomatous	Nonadenomatous	Adenomatous	Nonadenomatous
Familial adenomatous polyposis and its variants	Peutz-Jeghers syndrome	Multiple adenomas	Cronkhite-Canada syndrome
MYH polyposis	Juvenile polyposis	? Hyperplastic polyposis	Lymphoid polyposis
Multiple adenomas	Bannayan-Riley-Ruvalcaba syndrome		Lymphomatous polyposis
Hereditary nonpolyposis colorectal cancer syndrome	Cowden disease		
Muir-Torre syndrome	Basal cell nevus syndrome		
Hereditary mixed polyposis	Multiple endocrine neoplasia IIB		
? Hyperplastic polyposis	Neurofibromatosis 1		

stabilizes microtubules, promoting chromosomal stability. Loss of APC function results in defective mitotic spindle formation and abnormal chromosomal segregation (10).

Disease Expression

Patients with FAP exhibit considerable phenotypic variability of their colonic and extracolonic lesions, even within the same family. This suggests that the nature of the inherited genetic defect is only one parameter determining patient phenotype. Inactivation of APC may provide affected cells with a proliferative growth advantage (6), allowing the colon to then acquire additional genetic abnormalities, thereby facilitating disease progression. Environmental factors may also be important. Bile from FAP patients appears to be more mutagenic than that from non-FAP patients (11), perhaps inducing secondary changes both in APC and other genes in the adenoma–carcinoma sequence (see Chapter 14). Many manifestations of FAP may be partially controlled by hormonal status and other genetic factors. Data supporting such

a postulate include (a) stimulation of polyp growth during puberty, (b) adenoma inhibition by sulindac (12), (c) the preponderant development of thyroid carcinomas in women (13), and (d) the association of repeated trauma with the development of desmoid tumors (see Chapter19).

Relationship of APC Mutations to Disease Expression

Mutations in specific regions of APC produce different clinical phenotypes, and the length of the truncated gene product influences the severity of the colonic disease and the presence of eye lesions or desmoid tumors (Fig. 12.1). Patients with mutations toward the 3' end of exon 15 who produce longer protein products have a more severe phenotype than patients with mutations toward the 5' end of the gene (exons 3 and 4). Patients with less severe forms of the disease are referred to as having attenuated adenomatous polyposis (discussed below). Patients with the severe form of the disease tend to have large numbers of polyps that arise early in life (14–16). The commonly observed deletion of five

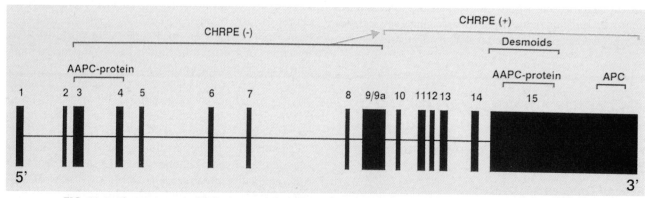

FIG. 12.1. The *APC* gene with its 15 exons shown as *blue boxes.* Mutations occurring within the part of the gene designated by the red line result in a congenital hypertrophy of the retinal pigment epithelium (CHRPE)-negative phenotype. Those occurring in the area designated by the *yellow line* are associated with CHRPE lesions. The *yellow arrow* indicates the region of the gene in which mutations begin to result in the appearance of CHRPE lesions. The *orange area* of the gene is associated with formation of desmoid tumors. Mutations in the *green* and *purple areas* result in the attenuated APC and full-blown APC phenotypes, respectively. AAPC, attenuated adenomatous polyposis coli.

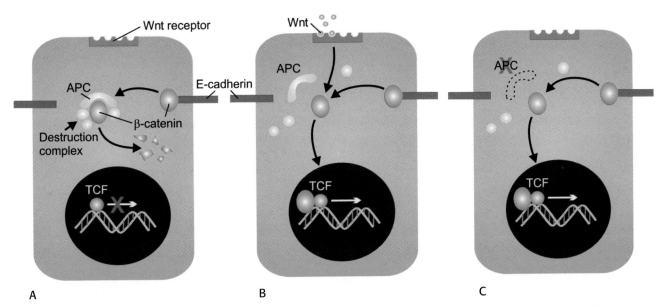

FIG. 12.2. Diagram of the Wnt signaling pathway. **A:** In normal cells, most endogenous β-catenin is bound to the intercellular adhesion molecule E-cadherin on the cell membrane. Any unbound, cytoplasmic β-catenin is quickly targeted for degradation by a protein complex that includes the proteins Axin, protein phosphatase 2A, protein kinases GSK3β and CK1α, and APC. Phosphorylation of β-catenin by this complex targets it for ubiquitin-mediated destruction. **B:** Stimulation of the wnt receptor by its ligand results in the destruction protein complex, which is inactivated, allowing cytoplasmic β-catenin to enter the nucleus and interact with the Tcf family of transcription factors. The result is expression of WNT target proteins and increased cell proliferation. **C:** In patients with familial adenomatous polyposis, the dysfunctional APC protein disrupts the activity of the multisubunit destruction complex, and results in accumulation of free β-catenin in the cell. β-Catenin is free to enter the nucleus of the cell where it interacts with Tcf, resulting in sustained expression of c-Myc, cyclin D1, and other Wnt target proteins.

bp at codon 1309 within exon 15 associates with early onset of colon cancer (1) and the early development of colonic adenomas.

Attenuated Adenomatous Polyposis

A less severe form of FAP, known as attenuated adenomatous polyposis coli (AAPC), is characterized by a relatively low number of adenomas (15). AAPC is associated with a germline *APC* mutation in approximately 10% of affected patients (17). This syndrome differs significantly from classic FAP in that affected individuals have fewer adenomas that tend to cluster on the right side of the colon where they appear flat rather than polypoid. The number of adenomas varies among family members, ranging from 1 or 2 to 100. Upper gastrointestinal lesions, particularly fundic gland polyps, are almost invariably present. In addition, affected patients exhibit a reduced risk for colorectal cancer compared with those with classic FAP.

The lifetime penetrance of colon cancer is high in AAPC families, however, even among members with relatively few adenomas. When colorectal cancers do develop, they arise later than in classic FAP. The average age of colon cancer onset in AAPC patients is approximately 15 years later than that of patients with classic FAP and approximately 10 years

earlier than individuals with sporadic colorectal cancer. Table 12.2 compares classic FAP and AAPC.

Clinical Features

FAP is the most frequent genetic polyposis syndrome, affecting 1 in 6,850 to 29,000 live births. It is transmitted as an autosomal dominant disorder with up to 90% penetrance. Fifty percent of the children of an affected individual and a normal individual will inherit the polyposis gene and will develop the disease. Ten to thirty percent of patients with FAP have no familial history and represent spontaneous new mutations. FAP patients develop at least a few adenomas by age 21. The adenomas almost always involve the rectosigmoid, where they tend to develop rapidly and in large numbers. Males and females are equally affected (18).

As noted above, variation in the expression of the FAP phenotype within families exists, and may result from dietary or environmental factors. Even more variation exists between families, presumably due to the fact that *APC* mutations occur at multiple sites in the gene and that different mutations confer different phenotypes.

Adenomas are not present at birth in FAP patients. Most affected individuals remain asymptomatic until puberty, at which time the polyps begin to appear (19). In untreated,

TABLE 12.2 Comparison of FAP and AAPC Colorectal Cancer Syndromes

Classic FAP	AAPC
Number of colonic adenomas	
Usually thousands; usually more than 100	Usually 1–50; seldom more than 100
Gross features	
Invisible to polypoid adenomas	Flat or slightly elevated plaques
Histology	
Polypoid or sessile	Flat adenomas
Location of colonic adenomas	
Throughout the colon	Predominantly located proximal to splenic flexure
Location of colon cancer	
Throughout the colon	Predominantly located proximal to splenic flexure
Average age of cancer onset	
39	55
Fundic gland polyps	
Present	Almost invariably present
Extracolonic cancers	
Periampullary carcinoma, papillary thyroid carcinoma, sarcomas, brain tumors, small bowel cancer	Periampullary carcinoma

AAPC, attenuated familial adenomatous polyposis; FAP, familial adenomatous polyposis.

unscreened patients, the mean age of polyp development is 24.5 years, symptom onset is 33 years, polyp diagnosis is 35.8 years, cancer diagnosis is at 39.2 years, and death from cancer averages a mean of 42 years (19). Young patients present with a small number of polyps, the number of which progressively increases with time. Eventually, the entire length of the colon becomes carpeted with adenomas. By the time a patient comes to colectomy, he or she may have hundreds to tens of thousands of polyps. Progression to cancer is inevitable; by age 30, approximately 75% of FAP patients will have developed colon carcinoma unless a prophylactic colectomy is performed. Most untreated patients die of cancer by the 5th decade of life.

Adenomas also develop in extracolonic sites, most commonly in the duodenum around the ampulla of Vater. Patients less frequently develop adenomas in the stomach or in other portions of the small intestine. Carcinomas may subsequently arise in these sites, but are relatively rare. Gastric cancers are more common in FAP patients living in parts of the world where gastric cancer rates are high. Fifty percent of Japanese FAP patients develop gastric adenomas, and gastric carcinoma is more common in these patients than ampullary cancers. In contrast, Western gene carriers exhibit a higher rate of ampullary than gastric neoplasms (20).

Colonic adenomas are often present for years before giving rise to symptoms including rectal bleeding, colicky abdominal pain, diarrhea, and mucous discharge (19). Seventy-five percent of polyposis patients without cancer have rectal bleeding, and 63% have diarrhea (19). When symptoms are severe enough to cause concern, two thirds of the patients have already developed a carcinoma. Very rarely, patients develop severe electrolyte depletion as a result of diffuse polyposis (21). Acute pancreatitis develops secondary to obstruction of the pancreatic duct at the ampulla of Vater by adenomas. Intussusception due to the adenomas may also occur.

Diagnosis of Familial Adenomatous Polyposis

The diagnosis of symptomatic patients is usually not difficult because they present with bleeding, diarrhea, or abdominal pain. Surveillance of children in affected kindreds results in earlier adenoma detection and in a lower cancer incidence. Today the tendency is to diagnose the presymptomatic individual by genetic testing and then confirm the diagnosis by sigmoidoscopy. Some advocate beginning flexible sigmoidoscopy by age 10 to 12 and continued yearly examinations until age 35 (22). Upper GI endoscopy should begin once the diagnosis of FAP is made and should be continued every 3 years thereafter in the absence of gastroduodenal adenomas (23). Genetic techniques will detect 50% of carriers of APC mutations (24).

The child of an FAP patient has a 50% likelihood of inheriting the genetic mutation. Prescreening strategies can be designed to detect mutations at the 12 most commonly mutated loci, which account for nearly 40% of germline mutations in FAP patients (25). The use of DNA extracted from archival specimens of affected available FAP patients increases the number of at-risk individuals who can be diagnosed presymptomatically (25). The association of the DNA markers and the presence of congenital hypertrophy of the retinal pigment epithelium (CHRPE) make it possible to identify gene carriers even in the absence of rectal polyps. CHRPEs affect up to 90% of classic FAP patients, especially those with both upper gastrointestinal and extraintestinal manifestations (26). They may be single or multiple, bilateral or unilateral, and are easily identified on funduscopic exam-

ination. These congenital lesions are observed in very young or even preterm infants, and represent the earliest diagnostic stigma of FAP. If one family member has CHRPE, all family members with the disease will have CHRPE. Similarly, other kindreds exist in which no family members have the retinal lesions.

Cancer Development

Carcinoma invariably develops in FAP patients if the colon is not resected by age 40 or 50. Indeed, FAP is the "experiment of nature" that provides support for the colonic adenoma–carcinoma sequence (Fig. 12.3). Adenomas also represent the precursor for small intestinal cancer, but small intestinal adenomas are less likely to become malignant than are colonic lesions. Adenomas and carcinomas also develop in the retained rectum following colectomy.

Carcinomas develop approximately 6 years after symptom onset. The incidence of carcinoma is approximately 10% in

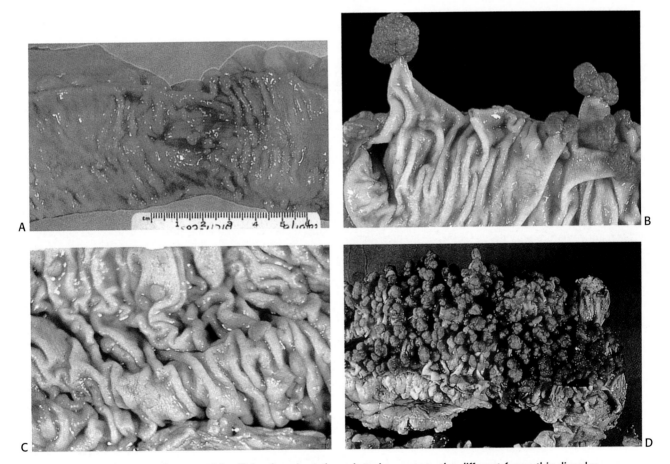

FIG. 12.3. Gross features of familial polyposis. A through D demonstrate the different forms this disorder may take. **A:** Numerous sessile, small rounded polypoid lesions are present, often on the mucosal folds. Large intervening areas of apparently normal colon are present. **B:** Clusters of pedunculated adenomatous polyps, larger than those seen in A, are present. They tend to pull up the mucosal folds into stalks. **C:** Numerous sessile and pedunculated polyps are scattered over the mucosal surface. **D:** The bowel is carpeted by numerous larger raspberrylike pedunculated polyps.

patients observed for 5 years and 50% in those observed for 20 years. Each 10-year age group has a 2.4-fold increase in cancer risk (27). Multiple cancers are frequent, with synchronous lesions affecting 41% of patients and metachronous lesions affecting 70%. Polyp count and patient age, but not sex, predict cancer risk. Patients with >1,000 polyps have a 2.3 times greater risk of cancer than those with <1,000 polyps.

Patients who undergo prophylactic colectomy may still die of other tumors, including ampullary cancers, brain tumors, hepatoblastomas, and desmoid tumors (28).

Treatment

Because of the high cancer risk, FAP patients undergo prophylactic total colectomy once the diagnosis is established. The procedure is timed so as not to interfere with psychosocial development, if the individual is a teenager or younger. It is recommended that the procedure be performed by age 20 to 25 (29). Patients have four surgical options: Total proctocolectomy, continent ileostomy (Koch pouch), total abdominal colectomy with ileorectal anastomosis, and ileoanal reservoir procedure. Total proctocolectomy with ileostomy eliminates the possibility of rectal carcinoma, but this procedure is unacceptable to many patients. The ileoanal reservoir procedure removes the bulk of the colorectal mucosa at risk for developing cancer while preserving the anal sphincter, but the cancer risk continues in the retained rectum. Rectal preservation is an ideal therapy for patients with relatively few rectal polyps because such patients are less likely to develop rectal carcinoma than those with numerous rectal adenomas (30). Patients with a retained rectum undergo semiannual screening with removal of all polyps that develop. According to some, more than 50% of patients will develop carcinoma in the rectal stump despite semiannual sigmoidoscopic surveillance and removal of all polyps (30).

A trend is emerging to treat FAP patients with nonsteroidal anti-inflammatory drugs (NSAIDs), as these drugs associate with disappearance of rectal polyps (31). However, sulindac treatment does not prevent the development of adenocarcinomas in the rectal segment (32).

Adenoma and Carcinoma Distribution

Adenomas develop throughout the entire colon (Fig. 12.4) and appendix. They are fairly evenly distributed throughout the large intestine, with a tendency for them to be larger in the sigmoid and the rectum, thereby making the density appear greater in this region (19). Rarely, the rectum is spared, especially in AAPC. When extensive, the entire large bowel becomes carpeted with adenomas (Fig. 12.3). Adenomas show gradations in size and shape from pedunculated tumors 1 cm or more in diameter, to smaller, broader-based nodules, to tiny lesions 1 mm or less in size. Adenomas tend to be larger in propositi (Figs. 12.3 to 12.5) than in patients undergoing screening surveillance (Fig. 12.5). In classic FAP, the number of polyps ranges from <100 (Fig. 12.3) to >5,000

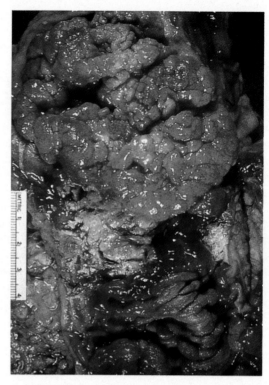

FIG. 12.4. Resection specimen in a familial adenomatous polyposis patient. There is a large fungating tumor present that represented an invasive carcinoma. Numerous pedunculated adenomas are seen in the surrounding mucosa.

with an average of 1,000, depending on when one sees the patient (19). Colorectal carcinomas may be multifocal and more frequently develop on the left side of the colon (33). Patients with AAPC develop flatter, nonpolypoid adenomas than are seen in classic FAP. They arise throughout the colon, with preferential involvement of the right colon. They also originate in the retained rectum following colectomy.

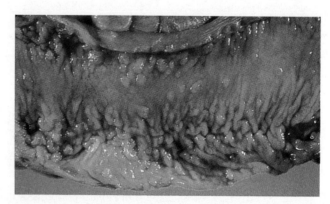

FIG. 12.5. Resection specimen from a patient who was part of a surveillance program. The patient has numerous small nodular lesions only mildly elevated over the mucosal surface. The lesions are smaller in patients undergoing surveillance than those who are not part of surveillance programs.

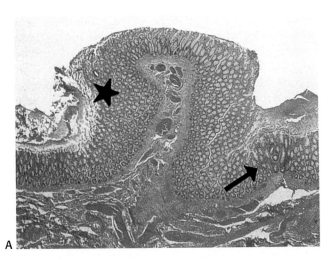
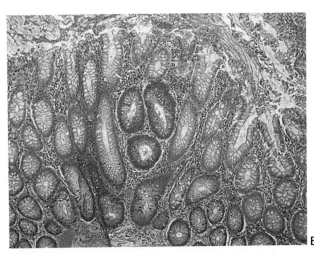

FIG. 12.6. Cross sections of the grossly apparently normal mucosa in patients with familial polyposis. **A:** Low-power picture showing two foci containing adenomatous glands. A unicryptal adenoma is present above the *star*. A tricryptal adenoma is illustrated by the *arrow*. **B:** A tricryptal adenoma is illustrated.

Pathologic Features of Adenomas

Adenomas and carcinomas in FAP patients grossly resemble their sporadic counterparts. Endoscopically, very small adenomas resemble hyperplastic polyps (Figs. 12.3 and 12.5). It is only when they become larger that the typical raspberrylike configuration of an adenoma becomes evident. As in sporadic colon cancer, the incidence of malignancy relates to adenoma size.

In the early stages, adenomas consist of small groups of adenomatous tubules. They range from unicryptal, bicryptal, or tricryptal lesions in grossly normal-appearing mucosa (Figs. 12.6 and 12.7) to the more typical multicryptal grossly visible polyps seen in patients without FAP (Fig. 12.8). The presence of unicryptal, bicryptal, and tricryptal adenomas strongly suggests the diagnosis of FAP. Even in unicryptal adenomas, the entire tubule is completely lined by neoplastic epithelium (Fig. 12.7). Proliferation throughout the entire length of the adenomatous crypt leads to branching, budding, infolding, and mucosal elevation. As the lesions enlarge to a grossly visible size, they become tubulovillous. Pure villous adenomas are rare in FAP patients.

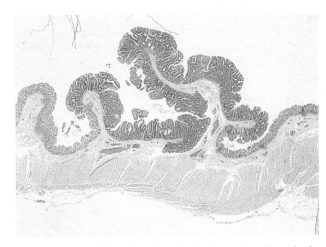

FIG. 12.7. Longitudinal section of the mucosa showing the presence of a unicryptal adenoma (*arrow*). Even the single adenomatous crypts are easily visible.

FIG. 12.8. Familial polyposis. Histologic section through the mucosa demonstrating the presence of multiple adenomatous polyps arising on the surface of the mucosa.

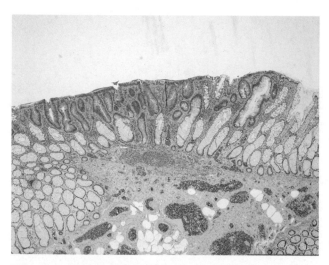

FIG. 12.9. Flat adenoma in a patient with attenuated adenomatous polyposis coli. Note that the adenomatous glands (*center*) lie at or below the level of the normal mucosa.

FAP patients develop depressed, flat, or polypoid adenomas (34), with AAPC patients showing a tendency to develop flat lesions. In contrast to pedunculated adenomas, the whole surface of flat or depressed adenomas lies at or below the level of the normal mucosa (Fig. 12.9). Polypoid adenomas are those with convex surfaces. Flat adenomas differ endoscopically and histologically from the usual adenoma. They present as slightly elevated plaques of adenomatous mucosa, not more than twice as thick as the adjacent normal mucosa. Further growth is by radial extension of adenomatous epithelium so that the lesions remain flat. When cancer develops, then one sees a reddish depression surrounded by marginal elevations (35). Occasionally, patients with FAP develop serrated polyps (see Chapter 14) or, more rarely, they develop juvenile polyps.

Upper Gastrointestinal Lesions

Nearly all FAP patients have polyps in the upper GI tract, with as many as 90% of patients developing gastric or duodenal adenomas by age 70 (36). Adenomas develop in the gastric antrum, duodenum, periampullary region, and ileum. However, it is the periampullary region that is most commonly involved, and adenomas tend to cluster at this site. More than 50% of FAP patients who undergo upper endoscopy have a grossly polypoid lesion, 90% of which arise in the periampullary region (37), suggesting that bile plays a role in their growth (38). The bile of FAP patients has a greater proportion of chenodeoxycholic and a lower proportion of deoxycholic acid than does the bile of patients without polyposis (38) and is more mutagenic. Patients also exhibit fecal flora abnormalities resulting in the possible production of carcinogenic compounds.

Periampullary carcinoma is a major cause of death in FAP patients (39), affecting from 2.9% to 12% of all FAP patients

(19,39,40) and causing death in 22.2% of patients following colectomy (40).

Duodenal Lesions

Duodenal adenomas develop in as many as 100% of patients in Japanese series (40,41) and in 50% in Western countries (19,42,43). Duodenal adenomas develop when patients are in their 2nd to 5th decades of life. The average age of FAP patients with adenomas involving the ampulla of Vater is 31.7 years, compared with 59.6 years in those without FAP. Duodenal adenomas vary in size and appearance from microadenomas in a normal-appearing ampulla to sessile polyps measuring 3 cm in diameter (43). Duodenal adenomas are generally small in screened populations. Over 90% of duodenal adenomas are tubular lesions. Large lesions become tubulovillous with dysplasia ranging from mild to moderate in degree. FAP-associated duodenal adenomas show a significant increase in the number of Paneth cells (Fig. 12.10) and endocrine cells per crypt compared to controls. This specialized cell hyperplasia affects the flat mucosa of FAP patients, regardless of the presence or absence of adenomas, and may represent a primary defect in the regulation of duodenal stem cell differentiation in FAP patients (44).

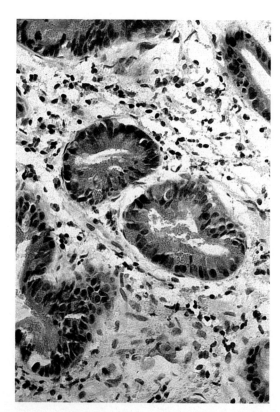

FIG. 12.10. Duodenal adenoma in familial adenomatous polyposis patient showing the presence of adenomatous epithelium and a large number of Paneth cells, as evidenced by the eosinophilic granules within the cytoplasm.

Ileal and Jejunal Lesions

Adenomas also develop in the ileum and jejunum, but to a lesser extent than in the duodenum. As many as 82% of FAP patients develop ileal adenomas (45). Ileorectal anastomoses, ileostomies, and ileal pouches predispose the ileal mucosa to become neoplastic (32,46,47). The ileal mucosa undergoes colonic metaplasia, which then gives rise to adenomas. Ileal adenomas resemble duodenal, gastric, and large intestinal adenomas. Ileal adenomas tend to be sessile, measuring 1 to 5 mm in size. Multiple lymphoid polyps also develop in the terminal ileum in FAP patients.

Gastric Lesions

Gastric polyps develop in approximately two thirds of FAP patients (23). Two different types of polyps arise in the stomach. Antral polyps are usually adenomas, whereas the small polyps arising in the fundus and body are usually fundic gland polyps (see Chapter 4) (48). Fundic gland polyps affect 25% to 60% of FAP patients.

Fundic gland polyps occur earlier than gastric adenomas, presumably because they originate in the existing fundic mucosa without the requirement for intervening intestinal metaplasia. Most patients with fundic polyps are under age 20. Fundic gland polyps are often multiple and small in diameter, appearing sessile or semi-sessile. They are identical to sporadic fundic gland polyps (see Chapter 4) (Fig. 12.11).

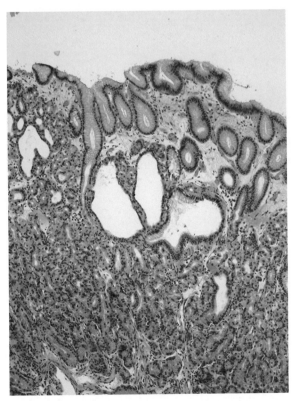

FIG 12.11. Fundic gland polyp in a patient with attenuated familial adenomatous polyposis. The lesion is similar in appearance to a sporadic fundic gland polyp.

The gastric mucosa may be studded with numerous small, sometimes eroded polyps that may increase in number and size over a several-year period. Alternately, they may decrease, or even disappear. Lesions that decrease or disappear may be followed by the appearance of a new crop of polyps (48). The fundic gland lesions are generally considered to be benign with little or no malignant potential, yet dysplasias and carcinomas have been described in FAP-associated fundic gland polyps (49,50). Superimposed gastric adenomas may give the false impression of dysplasia arising in a fundic gland polyp.

In Western countries, FAP-associated gastric adenomas and carcinomas are rare, contrasting with the Japanese experience, and supporting the role of environmental or other genetic factors in gastric cancer development. Gastric adenomas develop in the antrum in areas of intestinal metaplasia, a histologic requirement for the formation of gastric adenomas. When one compares gastric adenomas with colonic adenomas, the gastric lesions tend to be smaller and more sparsely distributed. In addition, gastric adenomas occur later in life than colonic adenomas. Gastric adenocarcinomas develop in the adenomas. Finally, FAP patients may develop gastric microcarcinoid tumors (48).

Adenomas and Carcinomas in the Rectal Remnant

Overall, the cumulative risk of developing cancer in the retained rectum ranges from 4% to 59% during a period of 10 to 30 years following surgery (51,52). The cancers may be small, depressed, and restricted to the mucosa. The age of the patient at the time of colectomy, the length of the retained colon, the tendency for spontaneous regression of polyps in the retained rectum, and the presence of carcinoma in the excised colon all influence the subsequent development of rectal cancer. Carcinomas and adenomas can develop, even in patients who are closely followed (32).

Kinetic and Other Biologic Abnormalities

FAP patients have a generalized abnormality of DNA synthesis that eventually results in uncontrolled cellular replication in the GI tract and in extragastrointestinal sites. FAP patients often exhibit increased ornithine decarboxylase activity, an enzyme that is essential for intestinal mucosal proliferation (53). As a result, FAP patients demonstrate increased cell proliferation in the adenomatous epithelium as well in the nonneoplastic crypts, on the luminal surface, and in the mucosa between adenomatous polyps (54). The markedly increased replication rate and the large number of adenomatous cells available for mutation and malignant transformation increase the likelihood of cancer developing.

APC mutation is a requisite initiating event for the formation of adenomas and provides a permissive environment for the subsequent development of carcinomas. Further steps in the neoplastic progression, including severe dysplasia and invasive carcinoma, associate with somatic mutations in K-*ras* and *p53* (55,56). In addition to mutations, losses of the *APC*, *p53*, and *DCC* also occur (56–58). Additionally, c-myc is frequently overexpressed (59). Some patients also develop microsatellite instability (60).

Extraintestinal Manifestations

FAP patients have a high incidence of extraintestinal manifestations, including dental and skin abnormalities and the development of various types of neoplasms (Fig. 12.12). The dental abnormalities include unerupted teeth, supernumerary teeth, dentigerous cysts, and mandibular cysts. Subcutaneous lesions include epidermoid cysts, lipomas, fibromas, neurofibromas, and trichoepitheliomas. The latter appear at an early age, even before polyps appear. Those that occur in prepubertal years are strong indicators for the presence of a polyposis syndrome, and to some represent an indicator for regular sigmoidoscopy, even without a history of polyposis. Epidermal inclusion cysts are often multiple. The epidermoid cysts occur anywhere on the body but most are located on the arms, buttocks, legs, and face, and occasionally in the testis.

Not surprisingly, patients who carry germline mutations in a tumor suppressor gene exhibit tumors in sites other than the GI tract. These are summarized in Figure 12.12.

Osteomas commonly occur in the skull or jaw, although they can affect any bone. These benign tumors rarely become malignant. FAP associates with nasopharyngeal angiofibromas (61). The lesion occurs 25 times more commonly in FAP patients when compared with the general population.

FAP patients also develop a number of endocrine and other neoplasms. Thyroid carcinomas, which occur with increased frequency in FAP patients, are all follicular neoplasms, sometimes containing papillary, cribriform, solid, and spindle cell components. FAP-associated thyroid cancers are commonly multifocal and predominantly affect young women. Since multicentricity is unusual for follicular thyroid tumors, it should alert the pathologist to the possibility of FAP (62). Soft tissue lesions include fibromas, lipomas, and desmoid tumors.

Desmoid tumors are a locally invasive form of fibromatosis (see Chapter 19) that affects 9% to 32% of FAP patients (63,64), particularly women (3:1). Affected patients are often young, with a mean age of 29.8 years (65). The overall prevalence of these lesions in FAP is 15%, a risk approximately 850 times greater than that of the general population (65,66).

Desmoid tumors tend to involve members of the same family and associate with mutations in exon 15 of *APC* (Fig. 12.1). Most patients have undergone a previous colec-

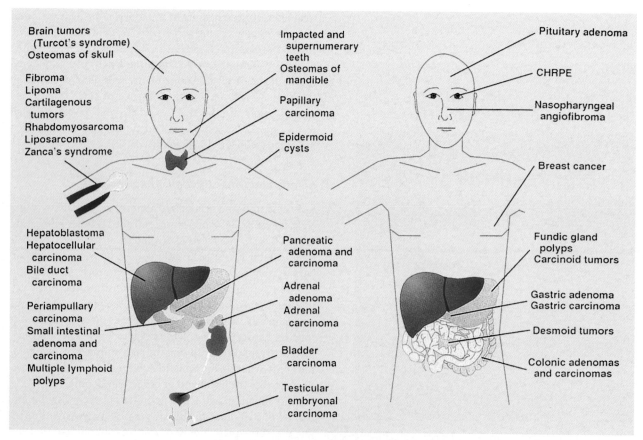

FIG. 12.12. Diagram of the various manifestations of familial adenomatous polyposis, which is essentially a systemic disorder. CHRPE, congenital hypertrophy of the retinal pigment epithelium.

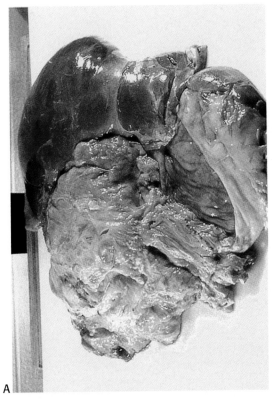
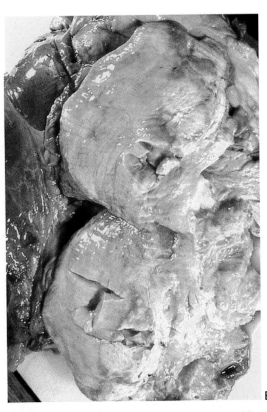

FIG. 12.13. Desmoid tumor in a patient who died of complications from the desmoid. **A:** Autopsy en bloc resection of the liver, spleen, intestines, and desmoid tumor. One can see that the tumor diffusely infiltrates the abdominal contents and extends up to the liver. Numerous organs were entrapped within this neoplasm, including the biliary tree, large numbers of vessels, and loops of bowel. **B:** Higher magnification of the neoplasm showing the presence of a fleshy mass with areas of ischemic necrosis.

tomy (86%). Hormonal factors such as pregnancy and estrogen use may also play etiologic roles in desmoid development. Although the desmoids can develop on the shoulder girdle, buttocks, groin, and abdominal wall, the majority arise within the small intestinal mesentery.

Desmoid tumors represent an adverse prognostic factor in FAP patients because they associate with a high frequency of complications and tumor recurrence. These nonencapsulated, irregular, infiltrative (Fig. 12.13), locally aggressive lesions do not metastasize, but they can cause significant intestinal obstruction, ureteral or vascular compression, or other local problems. Extensive mesenteric or retroperitoneal involvement leads to recurrent small bowel obstruction. Many patients die from these lesions. In one center, desmoid tumors were second only to colorectal cancer as a cause of death in FAP patients (39). Death results from vascular compromise, small bowel gangrene, perforation, or intra-abdominal sepsis.

Surgery is usually reserved for a specific indication, such as relief of intestinal or ureteric obstruction. Surgery on these lesions is extremely difficult because it is rare for the tumors to be small enough or sufficiently localized to allow resection without sacrificing vital structures. In most cases, attempts at surgical resection are followed by tumor recurrence. The recurrence rate after wide surgical resection is 81% (63). As a result, some have abandoned surgical procedures in favor of other therapies.

Other therapies have been tried including radiotherapy and various chemotherapies. Radiotherapy slows or reverses abdominal wall and mesenteric tumor growth, but the dose is limited by the need to preserve underlying intraperitoneal structures. Hormonal therapy, especially with antiestrogens, has met with minimal success. Tamoxifen has been effective in some patients (67), as has progesterone (68). Recently, NSAIDs have been used to halt the tumor growth, presumably by interfering with prostaglandin metabolism. Treatment with sulindac has resulted in a reduction in tumor size in some patients, but the response is inconsistent (67).

Histologically, desmoids consist of uniform, mature fibroblasts arranged in intertwining bundles. Mitoses are infrequent and never atypical. The extent of vascularization varies and may be prominent (Fig. 12.14). This prominent vascular ectasia, which sometimes occurs in FAP patients, is not a feature in non-FAP individuals and may account for intraoperative hemorrhagic complications. The tumor infiltrates the intestinal loops and peritoneum. The arteries and veins become surrounded by tumor but it does not infiltrate them (Fig. 12.14). The tumor cells actively produce collagen fibers.

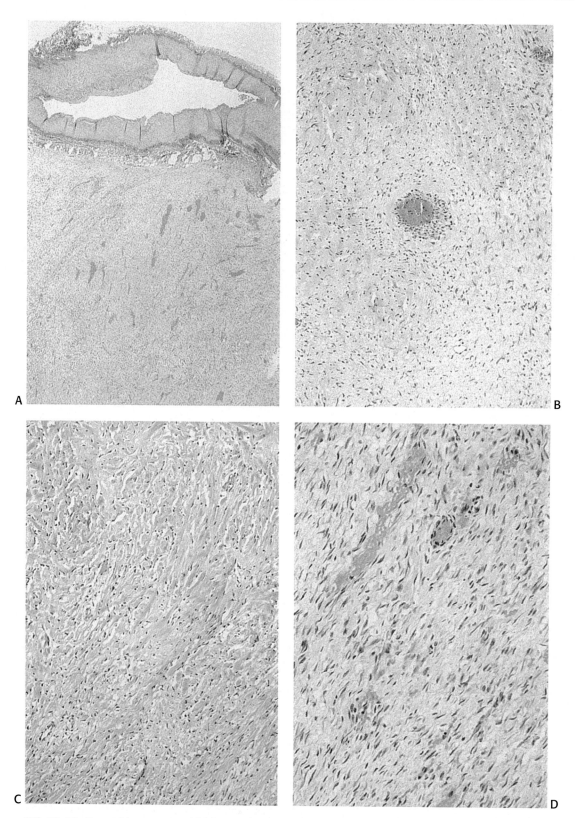

FIG. 12.14. Desmoid tumor. **A:** A highly vascular spindled cell mass is present, which extends up to a large sclerotic vessel but does not invade it. **B:** Higher magnification showing the haphazard arrangement of the spindled cells. **C:** A more hyalinized area of the tumor. **D:** A more vascular portion of the tumor.

TABLE 12.3	Central Nervous System Lesions in Turcot Syndrome

Medulloblastoma
Glioblastoma
Cavernous hemangioma
Astrocytoma
Arteriovenous malformation
Spongioblastoma
Lymphoma
Glioma
Ependymoma
Craniopharyngioma

Desmoids in FAP patients contain both germline and somatic *APC* mutations, suggesting that inactivation of this gene plays a role in the development of the lesions (69). Desmoid tumors also demonstrate deletion of 5q (70).

Turcot Syndrome

Turcot syndrome is the association of FAP with malignant tumors of the central nervous system. Central nervous system tumors arise around the time of puberty, often before the diagnosis of FAP (Table 12.3). The brain tumors are often lethal (71). Both familial and nonfamilial cases occur, resulting in a controversy concerning its mode of inheritance. Some suggest an autosomal recessive inheritance pattern (72,73). However, patients often die before having children, making it difficult to test the inheritance pattern. Lewis et al proposed classifying Turcot syndrome based on a study of family pedigrees (74) (Table 12.4).

Patients with Turcot syndrome fall into three groups based on their intestinal lesions: (a) those with a low number of colonic polyps (20 to 200), (b) those with large polyps measuring over 3 cm in diameter, and (c) those with colonic carcinoma developing during the 2nd to 3rd decades. Patients in the second group often have very few polyps. The gastrointestinal adenomas predominantly arise in the colon and rectum, but small intestinal and gastric lesions also develop.

Turcot syndrome is linked to the *APC* locus. Hamilton et al detected genetic abnormalities in 13 of 14 registry families (75). Germline *APC* mutations were detected in ten. The glioblastomas and colorectal tumors in three of the families

TABLE 12.4	Lewis Classifications of Turcot Patients
Group I	Patients who have siblings with the disease
Group II	Patients in families in which colonic polyps are found in several generations
Group III	Isolated nonfamilial cases

and in the original family studied by Turcot also had replication errors characteristic of hereditary nonpolyposis colorectal cancer (HNPCC). In addition, germline mutations in mismatch repair genes *MLH1* or *PMS2* were found in two families. Thus, the association between the brain tumors and multiple colorectal adenomas can result from two distinct types of germline defects (i.e., mutation of *APC* or a mismatch repair gene) (75).

Somatic *p53* mutations are found in both the brain and colon tumors in Turcot syndrome, although the mutations are not the same in the two sites (76). Gliomas also exhibit allelic deletions of chromosome 17p (77). K-*ras* mutations are also found (77).

MYH Adenomatous Polyposis

In 2002, Al-Tassan et al reported a Welsh family in which three members had multiple colorectal adenomas and carcinoma with an autosomal recessive pattern of inheritance (78). Their tumors demonstrated an excess of somatic mutations in *APC*, all of which represented G:C to T:A substitutions. The authors observed that such mutations are frequently the result of oxidative injury to DNA and, therefore, tested oxidative repair genes for germline changes in these patients. They found that affected patients carried two missense mutations (Y165C and G382D) in the human base excision repair gene *MYH*, located on chromosome 1. Subsequent studies by others have confirmed the association between multiple adenomatous polyps, early-onset adenocarcinoma, and biallelic germline mutations in *MYH* (79,80). Besides the two originally described *MYH* mutations, other mutations have now been observed including truncating, missense, in-frame insertions and putative splice site mutations (78,80,81).

The *MYH* protein functions as a base excision repair DNA glycosylase that excises adenines incorrectly incorporated opposite 8-oxo-7,8-dihydro-2'-deoxyguanosine, one of the most stable products of oxidative DNA damage (82). Adenomas and carcinomas from patients with inherited defects in *MYH* demonstrate an excess of G:C to T:A transversions in both the *APC* and *ras* genes (78,83).

Germline abnormalities in both *MYH* alleles correlate with the number of polyps observed clinically. The likelihood of *MYH* mutations increases with increasing numbers of polyps (80). However, bilallelic germline *MYH* mutations may occur in patients with early-onset colorectal carcinoma without polyposis (81,84). Some data suggest that heterozygous *MYH* mutations may also associate with an increased risk for carcinoma, and may act in an autosomal dominant mode of inheritance with relatively low penetrance (84). In fact, 47% of colorectal carcinomas arising in patients with monoallelic *MYH* mutation show loss of heterozygosity at the *MYH* locus, a finding that suggests that *MYH* may be an important factor in cancer development in this group of patients. In addition, patients with monoallelic *MYH* mutation more commonly report a family history of colorectal cancer (84). Loss of heterozygosity at *MYH* has been observed in sporadic colon carcinomas (85).

NONHEREDITARY ADENOMATOUS POLYPOSIS SYNDROMES

Multiple Colonic Adenomas

The presence of multiple adenomas (<100 in the colorectum) defines a group of patients without a clear genetic disorder, but who exhibit an increased risk for developing colon carcinoma. Morson surveyed patients with intestinal neoplasia at St. Mark's Hospital and found 1,846 individuals who had multiple adenomas (86). Of these, 27.9% had more than one adenoma; 4.5% had more than five adenomas. In this series, the patients with familial polyposis had a minimum of 200 polyps, whereas the nonfamilial group had a maximum of 48. The percentage of patients with associated carcinoma increased with increasing numbers of adenomas; 80% of patients with 6 to 48 polyps had a carcinoma (86). Many of these patients may in actuality have AAPC or *MYH* polyposis.

Hyperplastic Polyposis

Hyperplastic polyposis (HP) is a rare syndrome first described in 1980 as "metaplastic polyposis" (87). In the original series, seven patients were described, each with more than 50 colonic hyperplastic polyps. None of the patients in the group developed colonic adenocarcinoma. However, numerous reports have subsequently described the occurrence of colorectal cancers in HP patients (88–90), suggesting that patients with this syndrome are at increased risk for colon cancer development. Familial aggregation of the disorder has been observed in some patients, but a definite genetic association has not been demonstrated (91).

Patients with hyperplastic polyposis develop not only hyperplastic polyps, but also sessile serrated polyps, serrated adenomas, classic adenomas, and mixed serrated and adenomatous polyps (Fig. 12.15). The World Health Organization (WHO) criteria for diagnosis of the syndrome are summarized in Table 12.5 (92). The mean age at diagnosis is 52 to 61 years (90), although the disease has also been reported in younger patients. Both sexes appear to be affected equally. Most patients have more than 30 but fewer than 100 polyps.

Molecular studies suggest that at least some patients with hyperplastic polyposis have an underlying defect in DNA methylation, leading to hypermethylation of CpG islands throughout the genome (93).

HEREDITARY MIXED POLYPOSIS SYNDROME

As the name implies, hereditary mixed polyposis syndrome (OMIM entry #601228) is characterized by a variety of colorectal tumor types including atypical juvenile polyps, serrated polyps including serrated adenomas, classic adenomas,

and carcinomas (94). This disease appears to affect the colon only; no other gastrointestinal or extraintestinal manifestations have been described. Two forms of hereditary mixed polyposis syndrome appear to exist. The first is linked to a genetic locus mapped to chromosome 15 (95,96), and the second to the BMPR1 locus on 10q23 (97).

HEREDITARY HAMARTOMATOUS POLYPOSIS SYNDROMES

Peutz-Jeghers Syndrome

Clinical Features

The Peutz-Jeghers syndrome (PJS) (OMIM entry #175200) is inherited in an autosomal dominant disorder with pleiotropic inheritance and variable penetrance. PJS has an estimated incidence of 1 in 120,000 births (98). Approximately 50% of cases are familial; the remaining 50% are new mutations. The incidence of PJS is roughly one tenth that of familial adenomatous polyposis (99). The syndrome consists of two major components: (a) gastrointestinal hamartomatous polyps and (b) pigmented macules involving mucous membranes and skin (Fig. 12.16). The pigmentation affects 90% of patients, and polyps may occasionally be absent. Conversely, some family members have only the intestinal polyps. The disease affects males and females equally. The diagnostic criteria for PJS are listed in Table 12.6.

A diagnosis of PJS has been made in an individual as young as 15 days (100). Jejunal and ileal hamartomatous polyps often produce intussusception, leading to abdominal pain, partial or complete intestinal obstruction, or bleeding (99). As a result, most patients have recurrent attacks of crampy abdominal pain. Infants or older patients may present with anal extrusion when large rectal polyps prolapse. Polyps that autoamputate or undergo torsion, intussusception, or prolapse become ischemic, leading to bleeding, anemia, or massive hemorrhage. The polyposis progresses by the intermittent growth of polyps and with new "crops" of polyps appearing simultaneously in different parts of the bowel.

Pigmented lesions generally develop by age 2 years. Pigmented macules involve the mucous membranes of the lips and oral cavity. Macular lesions tend to cluster around the mouth, eyes, and nostrils. They also occur on the gums, palate, and oropharynx, or the skin of the face, forearms, hands, feet, and perianal area. The pigmented spots on the skin may fade or disappear as the patient ages, often at the time of puberty. This feature may make diagnosis difficult, especially in patients with no symptoms attributable to gastrointestinal polyps.

Buccal pigmentation presents as ill-defined, bluish areas. Histologically, these lesions resemble freckles, with hyperpigmentation along the basal epithelial layer due to increased numbers of melanocytes. Although the pigmentation is characteristic for PJS, acquired pigmentation simulating PJS

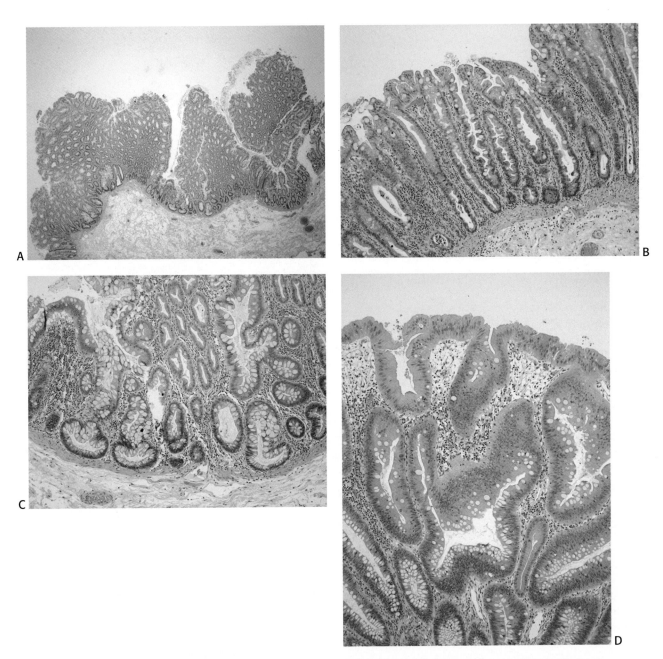

FIG 12.15. Hyperplastic polyposis. A: Low-power view showing areas of serrated-appearing glands in a patient with hyperplastic polyposis. **B:** Some polyps resemble typical hyperplastic polyps, while others show features of sessile serrated polyps **(C). D:** Occasional foci of dysplasia or adenomatous change are present in some polyps.

may also affect non-PJS patients with colon cancers (101). A number of other nonneoplastic conditions affect PJS patients (Fig. 12.17). Whether these lesions should be considered part of PJS or merely coincidental findings remains to be determined.

Genetic Features

The PJS gene lies on chromosome 19p13.3 and encodes the serine/threonine kinase STK11/LKB1 (102,103). Germline mutations or loss of heterozygosity in the *STK11* gene

TABLE 12.5	World Health Organization Working Definition of Hyperplastic Polyposis

1. At least five histologically diagnosed hyperplastic polyps proximal to the sigmoid colon, of which two are >10 mm in diameter, or
2. Any number of hyperplastic polyps occurring proximal to the sigmoid colon in an individual with a first degree relative with hyperplastic polyposis, or
3. Greater than 30 hyperplastic polyps distributed throughout the colon

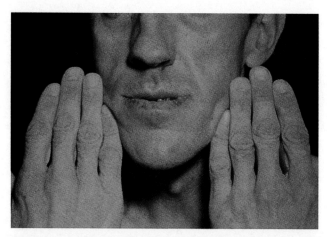

FIG. 12.16. Photograph of a patient with Peutz-Jeghers syndrome demonstrating the characteristic mucosal pigmentation.

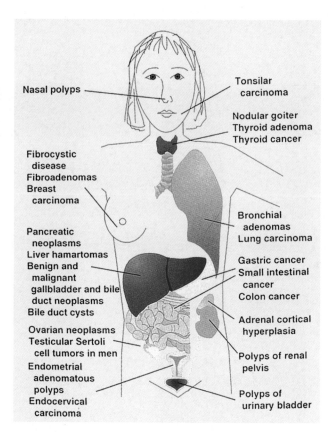

FIG. 12.17. Diagrammatic representation of many of the intestinal and extraintestinal lesions found in patients with Peutz-Jeghers syndrome.

account for most PJS cases (103). PJS kindreds inherit mutations in *STK11* as a single hit on one allele corresponding to the autosomal dominant inheritance pattern. The second hit then occurs in affected PJS tissues. Germline mutations are usually truncating, but missense mutations also occur. Approximately 70% of familial and 30% to 70% of sporadic PJS patients have *STK11* mutations (104).

STK11 is a tumor suppressor gene, consisting of nine exons. It is ubiquitously expressed in adults (103). The *STK11* gene product localizes to both the nucleus and cytoplasm and is a substrate of cyclic adenosine monophosphate (AMP)-dependent protein kinase (105). The encoded protein, LKB1, interacts with p53 and regulates specific p53-dependent apoptotic pathways (106). Restoring LKB1 activity to cancer cell lines defective for its expression results in G1 cell cycle arrest and induction of the CDK1 inhibitor p21 (107).

Identification of the PJS gene makes genetic screening possible for affected families. Mutation testing is done by full sequencing of the gene. Patients with neoplasia in their hamartomas exhibit 19p LOH, β-catenin mutations, or mutations or LOH at the *p53* locus. These findings suggest that mutations of β-catenin gene and/or *p53* may help convert hamartomatous polyps into adenomas and carcinomas (108).

TABLE 12.6 **Diagnostic Criteria for Peutz-Jeghers Syndrome (PJS)**

1. Three or more histologically confirmed Peutz-Jeghers polyps, or
2. Any number of Peutz-Jeghers polyps with a family history of PJS, or
3. Characteristic prominent mucocutaneous pigmentation with a family history of PJS, or
4. Any number of Peutz-Jeghers polyps and characteristic prominent mucocutaneous pigmentation

---

Gross Features

Hamartomatous polyps occur throughout the intestinal tract affecting the jejunum, ileum, colon, stomach, duodenum, and appendix in decreasing order of frequency. The distribution of the polyps depends on the patient population. Intestinal PJS polyps usually number in the dozens rather than in the hundreds, and may be sessile or pedunculated with a smooth lobulated outer surface. They range in size from a few millimeters to 6 or 7 cm in greatest dimension (Figs. 12.18 and 12.19), but most measure 0.5 to 1 cm in diameter. Patients who present predominantly with jejunal and ileal polyps most likely have PJS because the other polyposis syndromes do not usually produce multiple polyps in these sites.

Gastric PJS polyps usually arise in the antrum, and are often larger than the gastric polyps associated with juvenile polyposis, Cowden disease, or Cronkhite-Canada syndrome. They often resemble gastric adenomas grossly.

Histologic Features

Intestinal hamartomas of the PJS type have a fairly distinctive histologic appearance, although grossly they are not easily differentiated from other gastrointestinal polyps. The

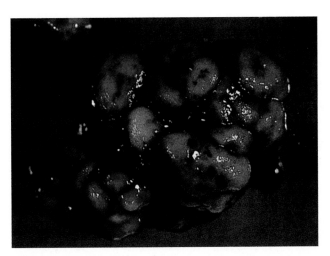

FIG. 12.18. Peutz-Jeghers syndrome. Gross photograph of a Peutz-Jeghers polyp.

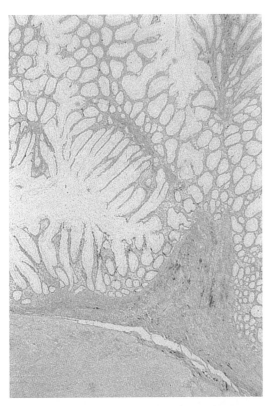

epithelial component of the polyp resembles the normal epithelium indigenous to its site of origin. Small intestinal polyps consist of crypts and villi of varying lengths divided by arborizing muscle bundles. The muscle fibers branch out from the center of the lesion like branches of a tree (Figs. 12.19 and 12.20). The smooth muscle bands span out into the head of the polyp and become progressively thinner as they project toward the surface of the polyp. Each branch is covered by mucosa (Fig. 12.20). Unlike juvenile polyps, the lamina propria appears normal. Some crypts become cystically dilated, whereas others may show intraluminal papillary projections, producing a serrated pattern reminiscent of that found in hyperplastic polyps or serrated adenomas. Cells of the normal small bowel mucosa, including goblet cells, absorptive cells, enteroendocrine cells, and Paneth cells, line the crypts and villi of small intestinal PJS polyps.

FIG. 12.19. Low-power magnification of a Peutz-Jeghers polyp showing the treelike arborizing pattern of the musculature covered by branched glands.

Duodenal lesions contain Brunner glands. These cells retain their normal relationships with each other. However, in some foci, one cell type may predominate. The surfaces of PJS polyps often appear acutely inflamed and superficially eroded, with evidence of regeneration. As a result, abnormally long rows of darkly staining replicating cells of the expanded regenerative zone may line elongated crypts.

FIG. 12.20. Colonic Peutz-Jeghers polyp. **A:** Low magnification showing the presence of a branching polypoid structure containing the normal elements from the rectum where this polyp arose. One sees a central muscular core, lymphoid follicles, and essentially normal colonic mucosa covering the central cores. **B:** Higher magnification showing the details of the central muscular cores and the covering colonic epithelium.

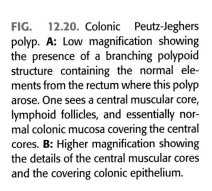

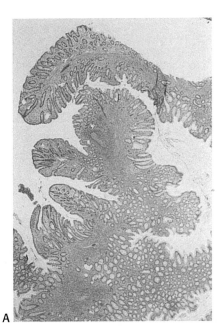

A

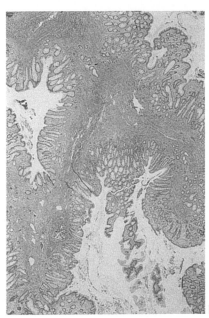

B

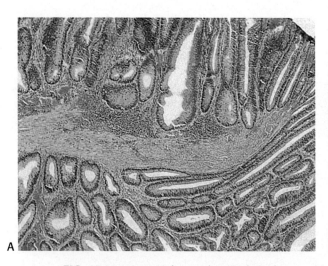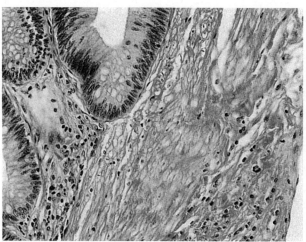

FIG. 12.21. Peutz-Jeghers polyps in the colon. **A:** This lesion has undergone adenomatous transformation. **B:** Wide, smooth muscle bands course through the lesion.

Mitotic figures usually can be identified in these regenerative areas. Rare polyps contain areas of osseous metaplasia.

Colonic PJS polyps demonstrate similar, but less complex, features than small intestinal polyps. They contain elongated, occasionally branching crypts (Fig. 12.21). The surface may have a villous architecture. Absorptive and goblet cells line the crypts, with goblet cells predominating in most cases (Figs. 12.19 and 12.20). Elongated zones of immature epithelium and mitoses occur in eroded polyps. Interlacing smooth muscle bands occur less frequently in colonic lesions than in small bowel polyps, and may be absent, especially in small lesions.

Gastric PJS polyps consist of foveolar or pyloric glandular cells intermingled with endocrine cells. Like their counterparts in the colon, gastric PJS polyps may lack the arborizing smooth muscle bundles typical of small intestinal PJS lesions. When the smooth muscle bundles are absent, gastric PJS polyps may resemble gastric hyperplastic polyps.

Benign glands lie within the submucosa, the muscularis propria, or even the serosa in 10% of small intestinal PJS polyps (Figs. 12.22 and 12.23). Such epithelial misplacement does not usually affect gastric or large intestinal lesions. Sometimes the deep glands appear to be connected to the more superficial glands; in other cases, they lack continuity with the superficial part of the lesion. Such lesions may show prominent mucinous cysts at the base (Fig. 12.23). Infoldings of columnar epithelium and dystrophic calcification can be seen in the mucinous pools. The benign appearance of the epithelium differentiates these areas from invasive carcinoma.

Rarely, one encounters glands deep in the bowel wall or in the serosa in the absence of a surface polyp. Grossly, these

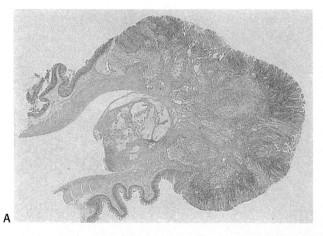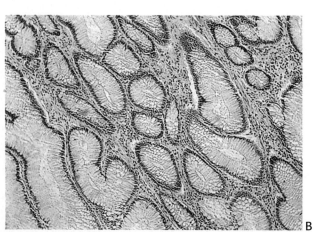

FIG. 12.22. Histologic features of Peutz-Jeghers polyps (PJP). **A** represents PJP of the small intestine; **B** represents PJP of the colon. Both are distinctive for their irregular architecture and the intimate admixture of glandular epithelium native to the site of origin with bundles of smooth muscle fibers. The small intestinal PJP also contains enterogenous cysts.

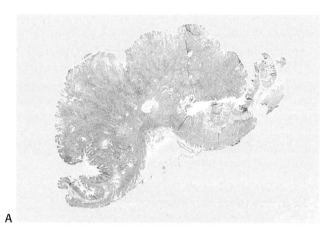 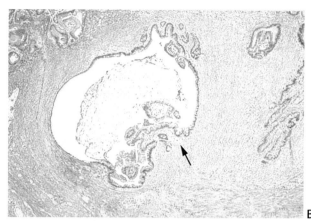

A

B

FIG. 12.23. A small intestinal Peutz-Jeghers polyp. **A:** Low-power magnification showing the presence of a broad-based, semi-pedunculated, semi-sessile polyp. A series of glands are entrapped within the proliferative muscle. The central portion of the lesion contains a large cystic area, shown better in B. **B:** One sees a mucinous collection in the center of the cyst. Much of the cyst is lined by hyperplastic-appearing glandular epithelium, sometimes in association with its lamina propria (*arrow*). In some places, the mucosa becomes attenuated or almost completely unrecognizable.

lesions appear as intramural nodules. Histologically, they may be partially or totally lined by normal goblet cells, columnar absorptive cells, endocrine cells, and/or Paneth cells. Alternatively, the mucinous cysts may lack an epithelial lining. This entity has been termed *enteritis cystica profunda* (Figs. 12.22 and 12.23). The presence of displaced glands deep in the bowel wall results from one of two processes. First, they may occur as part of the development of these hamartomatous intestinal lesions, or second, they may result from glandular entrapment due to previous trauma, perhaps secondary to episodes of intussusception.

One may also see circumscribed foci of signet ring cells in PJS polyps as a result of intestinal intussusception or polyp stretching or torsion. These events cause focal mucosal ischemia and epithelial sloughing. The sloughed epithelial cells, including the goblet cells, accumulate in mucosal folds in which the surface openings are obstructed. The sloughed goblet cells assume a round shape and signet ring appearance. These benign signet ring cell aggregates superficially simulate signet ring cell carcinomas, but they lack the usual cytologic features necessary to make a diagnosis of cancer.

Extraintestinal Tumors

Patients with PJS exhibit an increased incidence of extraintestinal hamartomas and malignancies (Fig. 12.17). Hamartomatous polyps may occur in the ureter, bladder, renal pelvis, bronchus, and nose. Extraintestinal carcinomas arising in association with PJS most commonly develop in the reproductive organs and breast. Adenoma malignum of the uterine cervix, mucinous ovarian neoplasms, and ovarian sex cord tumors with annular tubules (SCTATs) occur frequently in the reproductive organs of women with PJS (109). SCTATs are an almost constant finding in women and

are considered to be a phenotypic expression of the syndrome. The tumors usually occur alone, although all three tumor types may rarely coexist in a single patient (110). Patients also develop bilateral breast cancers (111).

The morphologic features of SCTATs are intermediate between those of a granulosa cell tumor and a Sertoli cell tumor (Fig. 12.24). SCTATs are usually benign, typically bilateral, multifocal, very small, even microscopic in size, calcified, and almost always an incidental finding at the time of surgery in ovaries removed for reasons. SCTATs are characterized by ring-shaped tubules encircling hyaline masses (Fig. 12.24).

Other stromal tumors cause sexual precocity or menstrual irregularities due to hyperestrogenism. These tumors differ from SCTATs in that they are large (112) and have a

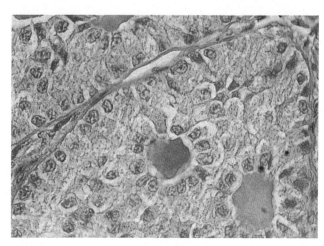

FIG. 12.24. Ovarian sex cord tumor with annular tubules in a young girl with Peutz-Jeghers syndrome.

complex histologic appearance, featuring diffuse areas and foci of hollow tubular differentiation, microcysts, and papillae. They contain two predominant epithelial cell types, one with scant and the other with abundant cytoplasm. The combination of patterns and cell types is unique and only occurs in PJS patients (113).

Adenoma malignum is an extremely well-differentiated adenocarcinoma or a minimal deviation endocervical adenocarcinoma. Histopathologically, the tumor consists of benign-looking, irregularly shaped endocervical glands. The tumor invades cervical stroma, nerves, and vessels. Some patients with PJS and adenoma malignum also exhibit mucinous epithelium in the endometrium and fallopian tubes (114), representing direct spread from the adenoma malignum (115). Other types of mucinous lesions affect the fallopian tube, including mucinous metaplasia, in the absence of other ovarian or uterine mucinous lesions, mucinous adenocarcinoma in situ, and mucinous cystadenomas (116).

Male PJS patients develop testicular tumors. The patients are usually children who overproduce estrogen and develop gynecomastia, the equivalent of the ovarian SCTATs. Feminizing Sertoli tumors in boys microscopically consist of greatly enlarged seminiferous tubules packed with ovoid Sertoli-like cells. Prominent eosinophilic basement membranes surround the tubules and intersect between the cells forming hyalinized ovoid globules and microcalcifications. They result in increased estrogen synthesis due to the presence of increased transcription of the aromatase cytochrome P450 gene (117).

PJS patients may develop intra-abdominal desmoplastic small cell tumors (118). In the single case described, the widely disseminated intra-abdominal desmoplastic small cell tumor showed evidence of divergent differentiation. Histologically, the tumor consisted of solid cell nests composed of medium-sized cells demarcated by desmoplastic stroma. Glandlike spaces were found within many cell nests (118).

Gastrointestinal Carcinomas

Gastrointestinal tumors developing in the setting of PJS include colonic, gastric, pancreatic, small intestinal, gallbladder, and biliary carcinomas. There is also a report of a sarcoma that arose in a small intestinal PJS polyp and then metastasized to the liver (119). The Polyposis Registry at Johns Hopkins University reported a 48% incidence of cancer, with 73% of the tumors arising in the GI tract (110). Spigelman et al reported an overall incidence of carcinoma of 22% (120). In this series, slightly more than half the tumors were of gastrointestinal origin. Carcinomas develop from adenomatous foci within the PJS polyps, usually located near the luminal surfaces of the polyps (Fig. 12.25).

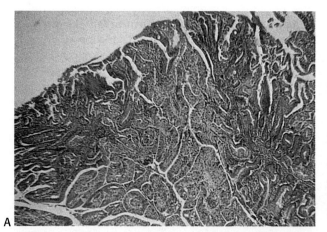

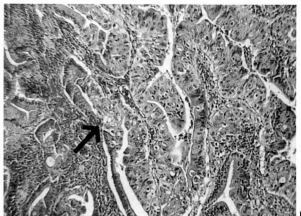

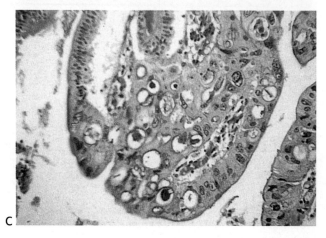

FIG. 12.25. Peutz-Jeghers polyps in the small intestine containing foci of adenomatous epithelium as well as intramucosal carcinoma. **A:** The lesion shows disorganization of the underlying structures as well as adenomatous glands. **B:** Transitional area between the adenomatous epithelium and intramucosal malignancy is seen just above the *arrow.* **C:** This figure represents a higher power magnification of the intramucosal carcinoma. The cells are obviously cytologically malignant. A small amount of residual normal epithelium is also present.

TABLE 12.7 Classifications of Juvenile Polyps

Type of Polyp	Location of Polyps	Familial History
Solitary juvenile polyp	Colon and rectum only	Absent
Juvenile polyposis coli	Colon and rectum, few in small bowel	Present in approximately 40%
Juvenile gastrointestinal polyposis	Stomach to rectum	Present
Familial juvenile polyposis of stomach	Stomach only	Present

The cancers histologically resemble other carcinomas arising in these sites. The tumors contain irregular glands that vary in size and shape and lie within a desmoplastic stroma. The epithelium appears hyperchromatic and pleomorphic, containing numerous mitoses. An unusually large number of PJS patients develop their carcinomas at an early age (110), sometimes in the 2nd or 3rd decade of life. In addition, the carcinomas often arise in the gastroduodenal area, a site not usually prone to cancer development in the general population. Both patient age and the anatomic distribution of the carcinomas suggest that the cancers result from the syndrome and do not occur as random, independent events.

Treatment

Because of the increased risk for cancer, patients suspected of having PJS undergo regular screening. The screening recommendations for gastrointestinal malignancies include colonoscopy beginning with symptoms or in late teens if no symptoms occur (121). The interval is determined by the number of polyps, but it is at least once every 3 years. If multiple polyps are found on initial screening, endoscopy should be performed at least annually until all of the polyps have been removed. Screening for gastric neoplasia consists of upper GI endoscopy every 2 years starting in the midteens (122). Screening for small bowel neoplasms occurs via annual small bowel radiography or capsule endoscopy. Screening for pancreatic cancer involves endoscopic or abdominal ultrasound or computed tomography (CT) every 1 to 2 years after age 30 (122,123). Annual breast examinations and mammography every 2 to 3 years beginning at age 25 are performed to detect breast cancers. Screening for gynecologic neoplasms by annual pelvic examination and Pap smear begins at age 20, and screening for testicular tumors begins at age 10.

Juvenile Polyposis

Juvenile polyps are the most common pediatric gastrointestinal polyps, affecting an estimated 1% of children (124). In the past, juvenile polyps were considered inflammatory lesions, but today they are viewed as hamartomas. Most juvenile polyps are solitary lesions that are not part of a generalized polyposis syndrome. They are usually discovered between the ages of 1 and 10 with a peak incidence between 2 and 4 years of age. A second peak incidence occurs around age 25. Isolated polyps occur with equal frequency in males and females, but there is a male predominance when multiple polyps develop (124). When multiple juvenile polyps are present, the entity is termed *generalized juvenile polyposis, multiple juvenile polyposis, familial juvenile polyposis,* or *juvenile polyposis coli* (Table 12.7). Multiple juvenile polyps may also be encountered in patients with Cowden disease or Bannayan-Riley-Ruvalcaba syndrome, but these patients have other abnormalities in addition to juvenile polyps.

Juvenile intestinal polyposis (polyposis, juvenile intestinal [PJI], OMIM entry #174900) occurs in both familial and sporadic forms. It is an autosomal dominant condition, with 20% to 50% of patients reporting a family history of polyps. The disorder is rare, occurring in an estimated 1 per 100,000 births, an incidence 10-fold lower than that of FAP (125). Patients with PJI present with multiple juvenile polyps, which are not limited to the colon, but also occur in the small intestine and stomach. Rare patients demonstrate polyps limited to the stomach, and were at one time considered to have a separate form of polyposis. Familial gastric juvenile polyposis is now considered to be a variant of PJI per OMIM. The criteria for establishing the diagnosis of juvenile polyposis are shown in Table 12.8.

Clinical Features

The clinical course of PJI varies depending on polyp number and location. Eighty-eight percent of polyps lie within 20 cm of the anal verge and are easily detectable by sigmoidoscopy. Patients with gastric involvement exhibit a gastric coating of polyps on upper endoscopy. Patients with PJI become symptomatic during childhood, contrasting with children with FAP

TABLE 12.8 Diagnostic Criteria for Juvenile Polyposis

No extraintestinal manifestations of either Cowden disease or Bannayan-Riley-Ruvalcaba syndrome are present, and one or more of the following:

1. Five or more juvenile polyps are present in the colon.
2. Any number of hamartomatous polyps are present in a patient with a family history of juvenile polyposis.
3. Extracolonic juvenile polyps are present.

who rarely become symptomatic before puberty. Juvenile polyposis may be divided into several different subtypes based on clinical presentation and disease course (126). Three subtypes are recognized: Juvenile polyposis of infancy, juvenile polyposis coli, and generalized juvenile polyposis. Juvenile polyposis of infancy (also referred to as infantile Cronkhite-Canada syndrome) is characterized by bloody diarrhea, protein-losing enteropathy, hypoproteinemia, anemia, anasarca, failure to thrive, and death prior to 1 year of age. An autosomal recessive pattern of inheritance has been suggested for this form of juvenile polyposis (127).

Patients with juvenile polyposis coli have polyps limited to the colon, while those with generalized juvenile polyposis develop polyps throughout the gastrointestinal tract. Presentation of both of these subtypes usually occurs in the 1st or 2nd decade of life. The most common clinical presentation is painless rectal bleeding, a finding that affects nearly all patients. A minority of patients present with other clinical manifestations including rectal prolapse or polyp extrusion, abdominal pain, anal pruritus, diarrhea, constipation, or hemorrhage. Intussusception, protein-losing enteropathy, malabsorption, and diarrhea may be observed in patients with extensive polyposis. Autoamputation of polyps with passage of tissue also occurs.

Patients with juvenile polyposis may exhibit extracolonic manifestations including digital clubbing, failure to thrive, hypertelorism, and macrocephaly. Fifteen percent of patients, usually those without a family history of polyposis, show associated congenital birth defects including malrotation of the midgut, cardiac and cranial abnormalities, cleft palate, polydactyly, genitourinary defects, pulmonary arteriovenous malformations, pulmonary stenosis, and telangiectasias (128) (Table 12.9). Juvenile polyposis patients have an increased risk

for the development of colorectal adenocarcinoma, as well as for cancers of the stomach, duodenum, and pancreas (129,130).

Several families have been described in which an autosomal dominant juvenile polyposis syndrome occurs with pulmonary and/or cerebral arteriovenous malformations, cutaneous telangiectasia, subarachnoid hemorrhage, hypertrophic pulmonary osteoarthropathy, and digital clubbing (OMIM entry #175050). Many of these patients present in childhood or adolescence with polyps located mainly in the colon and small intestine (126). It is currently unclear whether this entity represents a single gene abnormality distinct from juvenile polyposis or represents coincidental juvenile polyposis and Osler-Rendu-Weber disease.

Genetic Features

Approximately one half of families with juvenile polyposis have germline mutations in one of two genes, the dysfunction of which interrupts the transforming growth factor-β (TGF-β) signaling pathway: *SMAD-4* and the bone morphogenic protein receptor 1A (*BMPR1A*) (131–133). Mutations in *SMAD-4* and *BMPR1A* occur with equal frequency, with abnormalities in each being identified in approximately 20% of juvenile polyposis patients (134).

SMAD-4 (also known as *MADH4* or *DPC4*) is located on chromosome 18q21.1. Somatic mutations in this gene occur in 15% of colorectal carcinomas and as many as 50% of pancreatic ductal carcinomas (131,132). The most common mutation is a 4 base deletion in exon 9, but numerous other mutations have been reported (133,134). *SMAD-4* encodes a 60.4 kDa protein that acts as a cytoplasmic mediator in the TGF-β signaling pathway. Upon activation of TGF-β or related ligands, serine and threonine kinase receptors phosphorylate proteins of the SMAD family, which then form heteromeric complexes with *SMAD-4*. These complexes are then transported to the nucleus where they interact with DNA, resulting in growth inhibition and initiation of apoptosis.

BMPR1A is the gene upstream from *SMAD-4* in the TGF-β pathway. It encodes a serine/threonine kinase receptor that, when activated through phosphorylation, phosphorylates SMAD protein family members. Many different mutations in *BMPR1A* have been identified to date in PJI families (134). Mutations usually result in a receptor lacking its intracellular serine–threonine kinase domain, an alteration that results in loss of signaling through *SMAD-4*.

Some clinicopathologic differences may be observed in *SMAD-4* mutation–positive versus *BMPR1A* mutation–positive patients. Those with *SMAD-4* mutations have a higher frequency of upper gastrointestinal polyps and are more likely to have a family history of juvenile polyps than are patients with *BMPR1A* mutations (135,136).

Gross and Endoscopic Features

Patients with juvenile polyposis usually have 50 to hundreds of polyps (137). Juvenile polyps are relatively small lesions,

---

TABLE 12.9 **Abnormalities Associated with Juvenile Polyposis**

Congenital lesions
Intestinal malrotation
Meckel diverticulum
Umbilical fistula
Mesenteric lymphangioma
Hydrocephalus
Ganglioneuromas
Cardiac lesions
Hydrocephalus
Amyotonia congenitum
Hypertelorism
Porphyria
Undescended testis
Supernumerary toes
Other lesions
Pulmonary arteriovenous malformation
Hypertrophic osteoarthropathies
Retroperitoneal fibrosis
Villous adenomas

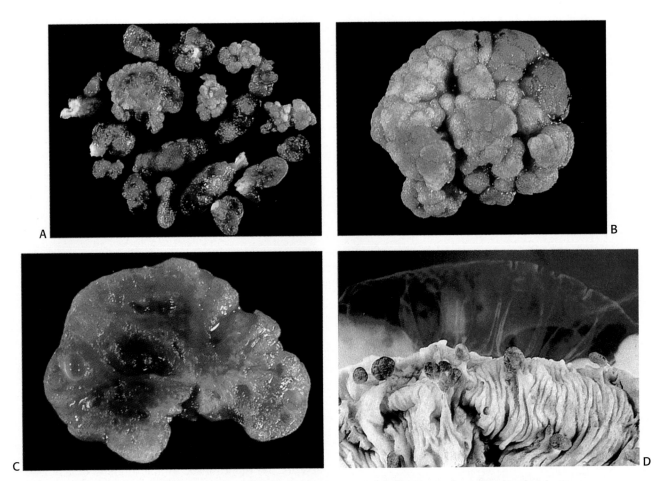

FIG. 12.26. Juvenile polyposis. **A:** Collection of polyps removed during one endoscopic procedure in a young boy. **B:** Higher power magnification showing the surface, which is granular and divided into territories. **C:** Cut surface of one of these polyps showing the characteristic presence of areas of hemorrhage as well as numerous cystic spaces. **D:** Radiograph of same patient with the resected bowel specimen superimposed on it. Numerous pedunculated lesions are obvious.

ranging in size from <1 mm to 5 cm, with most measuring 1 to 1.5 cm in diameter. The colonic mucosa between polyps is normal in appearance. The majority of polyps appear pedunculated; only about 25% are sessile. Polyps developing in different parts of the GI tract grossly resemble one another. Large lesions present as grayish-pink-red, spherical, mushroomlike, lobulated lesions. The lobulation results from secondary inflammation and ulceration. If the polyps are received fresh, they often exhibit small white patches due to the presence of underlying cysts filled with mucin. Small lesions have a more rounded shape with a smooth surface. The external gross features of juvenile polyps are often indistinguishable from those of adenomas (Fig. 12.26). However, their cut surfaces display variably sized mucus-containing cysts embedded in a gray fibrous stroma (137) (Fig. 12.26).

Histologic Features

Juvenile polyps histologically fall into several categories, including typical juvenile polyps or juvenile polyps contain-

ing hyperplastic, metaplastic, ganglioneuromatous, adenomatous, or adenocarcinomatous foci. Typical juvenile polyps consist of gastrointestinal glands indigenous to the site of origin, surrounded by a prominent stroma (Figs. 12.27 to 12.29). The large amount of stroma surrounds branched, sometimes cystically dilated, tortuous glands (Figs. 12.27 and 12.28). The glands demonstrate considerable variation in size and shape, and may occasionally demonstrate a serrated pattern (Fig. 12.29) resembling that seen in hyperplastic polyps, serrated adenomas, or sessile serrated polyps. The serrated pattern results from epithelial hyperplasia. The epithelial-lined cysts are empty or filled with mucus or inflammatory cells (Figs. 12.27 and 12.28). Cystically dilated glands herniate, resulting in extension of mucus, inflammatory cells, and debris into the surrounding lamina propria (Fig. 12.30). The lining epithelium appears columnar, cuboidal, or flattened depending on the degree of pressure atrophy present. Sometimes the epithelial lining disappears completely (Fig. 12.30). Paneth cells may be quite prominent. The polyp surface may be covered by a single layer of

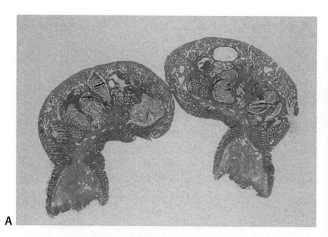

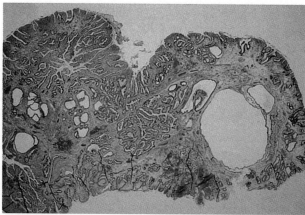

FIG. 12.27. Polypectomy specimens of juvenile polyps. **A:** A pedunculated colonic lesion that was removed by electrocautery. It contains a proliferation of epithelium and large cystic spaces. **B:** A different specimen containing large amounts of congested stroma and large cystic spaces.

cuboidal or columnar epithelial cells. Goblet cells are often interspersed between these cells. When the polyps become ulcerated, capillaries proliferate in the superficial lamina propria, forming a granulation tissue cap. With additional ulceration, the glands become more dilated, capillaries show greater degrees of cellular proliferation, and the number of inflammatory cells increases.

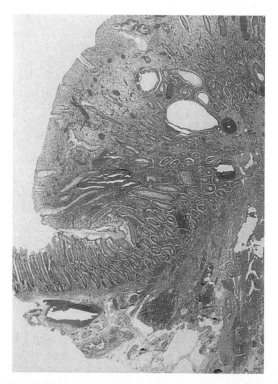

FIG. 12.28. Resection specimen from a patient with juvenile polyps. One can see the marked congestion present within the polyp, as well as a cystic dilation of glands. The specimen contains a disproportionate amount of stroma and an underrepresentation of glands.

Smooth muscle fibers are usually absent except in the center of the lesion. These fibers are more abundant in the neck of the polyp than in the head. In pedunculated polyps, the neck region may contain dense intertwined smooth muscle cells. However, the bundles of smooth muscle cells are much less dense than those found in Peutz-Jeghers polyps (Fig. 12.31).

An edematous, often inflamed stroma separates the glands of the polyp. As a result, the crypts appear widely separated from one another. The amount of stroma usually appears disproportionate to the amount of epithelium. Juvenile polyps contain comparatively more stroma than either Peutz-Jeghers polyps or adenomas. The stroma often contains dilated vessels, areas of hemorrhage or hemosiderin deposition, and variable numbers of inflammatory cells (Fig. 12.32). Neutrophils are particularly prominent around ulcerated edges and dilated telangiectatic vessels (Fig. 12.32). The stroma may also contain prominent lymphoid follicles. When the stalk twists, the polyp undergoes torsion with hemorrhage and ulceration. Metaplastic stromal changes include the presence of ectopic bone or cartilage (Fig. 12.32).

Gastric juvenile polyps consist of hyperplastic foveolae and edematous stroma with inflammatory cells, resembling the more common gastric hyperplastic polyps. They also resemble the polyps seen in Cronkhite-Canada syndrome. A definitive diagnosis requires knowledge of the clinical background of the patient, including patient age, symptoms, distribution of the polyps, the number of polyps, and associated extraintestinal manifestations. Dysplasia and carcinoma may develop in colonic or gastric lesions.

Ganglioneuromas in Juvenile Polyps

The ganglioneuromatous proliferation seen in juvenile polyps is characterized by clusters of mature ganglion cells and hypertrophic nerve fiber bundles in the lamina propria and submucosa (Fig. 12.33). The patients usually do not have a history of neurofibromatosis or multiple endocrine

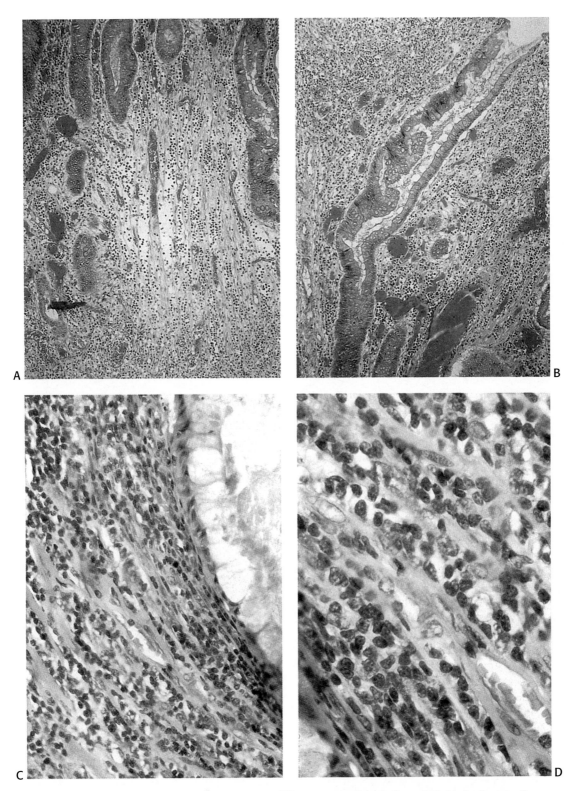

FIG. 12.29. Juvenile polyp. A through D represent different areas of the lesions. **A, B:** Marked congestion as well as an infiltration of the lamina propria with large numbers of mononuclear cells. In B, the epithelium has become hyperplastic, giving the glands a somewhat tortuous appearance. **C:** The edge of hyperplastic colonic epithelium and prominent mucin within the gland. The nuclei are pushed to the base of the cell. The surrounding lamina propria contains an intense infiltrate of mononuclear cells. **D:** Higher magnification of the mononuclear cell infiltrate.

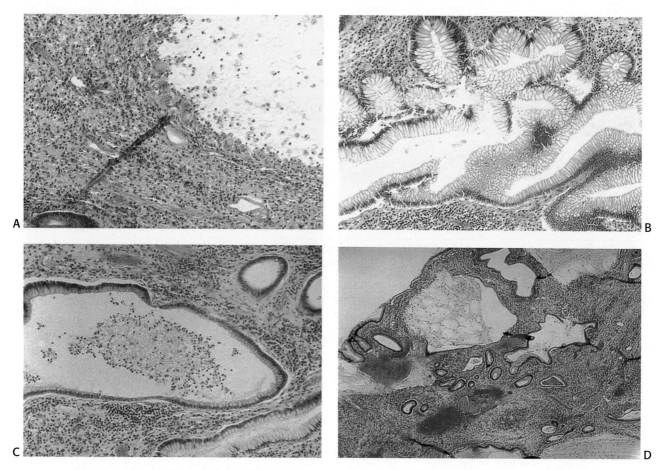

FIG. 12.30. Sections of juvenile polyps demonstrating various aspects of histologic features. **A** represents an area in which the mucus-filled gland has disintegrated. The lining epithelium is no longer evident. **B** shows the marked tortuosity that the glands can achieve. **C** represents a small crypt abscess in an otherwise atrophic gland. In **D**, marked disorganization of the tissue is evident.

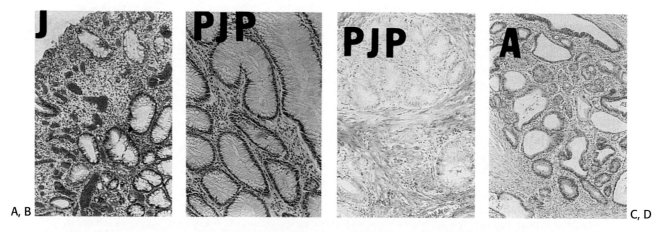

FIG. 12.31. Comparison of juvenile polyps, Peutz-Jeghers polyps, and adenomatous polyps. As can be seen, the juvenile polyp **(A)** shows far more congestion and a greater percentage of stroma than other polyps **(B, C)**. The Peutz-Jeghers polyps show large numbers of glands with variable amounts of smooth muscle. The epithelia in A through C appear benign, whereas the epithelium in **D** is hyperchromatic and some of the glands have a back-to-back configuration.

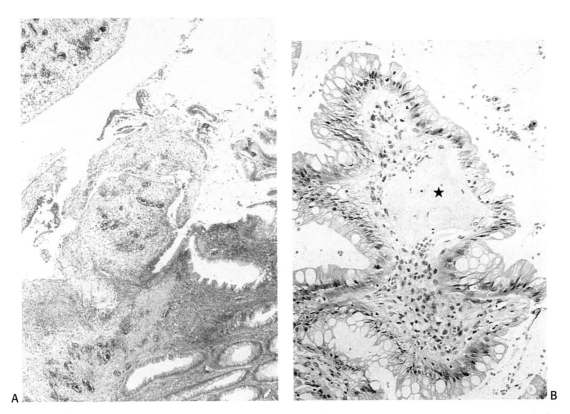

FIG. 12.32. Stromal changes in juvenile polyps. **A:** The surfaces of juvenile polyps frequently become eroded and ulcerated, as in this case. **B:** Some polyps undergo osseous or cartilaginous metaplasia, as illustrated in this figure (*star*).

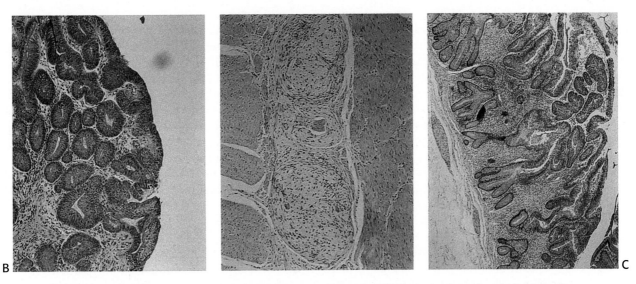

FIG. 12.33. Juvenile polyp combined with ganglioneuromatous proliferation. A through C derive from the same polyp. **A:** Note the presence of atypical epithelium within the polyp. **B:** Marked hyperplasia and neuromatous proliferation of the myenteric plexus are seen. **C:** A more typical area of a juvenile polyp with proliferation of neural tissue within the lamina propria, causing the lamina propria to appear more cellular than normal.

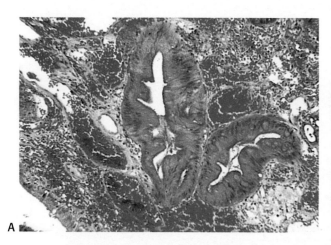
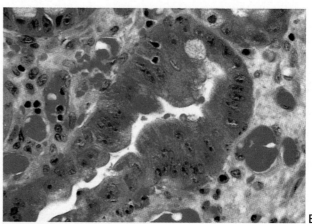

FIG. 12.34. Juvenile polyps. **A** represents mixed hyperplastic adenomatous-type epithelium, in which stratified nuclei are evident, as are serrated lumens. **B** represents a gland with mild dysplasia.

neoplasia type IIB (138), but may have Bannayan-Riley-Ruvalcaba syndrome (macrocephaly, multiple lipomas, and hemangiomata syndrome), one of the PTEN hamartoma syndromes (139). It is unclear whether the ganglioneuromatous proliferation represents a reactive or neoplastic process.

Relationship of Juvenile Polyps to Dysplasia and Carcinoma

Relatives of patients with juvenile polyposis, as well as the patients themselves, are at increased risk for developing gastrointestinal carcinoma (140,141). In contrast, patients with solitary juvenile polyps rarely develop colon cancer (140). Coburn et al found a total of 218 PJI patients who developed cancer (140). A family history of polyps was present in 50% of the patients, and 15% had associated congenital malformations. The mean age at diagnosis of carcinoma was 35.5 with a range of 4 to 60 years. Most malignancies were located in the distal colon and rectum with isolated cases of gastric and duodenal carcinoma. Tumor stage at diagnosis was usually advanced, with poor patient survival (140). Bentley found that 8% to 20% of PJI patients have either juvenile polyps containing adenomatous (dysplastic) areas or have both juvenile polyps and adenomas. Approximately 20% to 30% of these patients had cancer (142). Dysplasia is more common in larger polyps (>1 cm in size) (137).

Dysplasia or adenomatous foci occur in two forms: (a) as a focus of adenomatous change in a juvenile polyp or (b) as an adenoma showing no residual juvenile features. Adenomatous changes occur as early as age 3. Carcinomas arise in the dysplastic adenomatous areas. The histologic features suggest a sequence of early hyperplasia passing through dysplasia to carcinoma (Fig. 12.34). The adenomas and adenomatous foci develop in the colon as well as in the stomach, duodenum, jejunum, and ileum. Carcinoma may also develop in polyps at gastrojejunostomy sites (143). Cancers that develop at an early age have a poor prognosis.

Colonic biopsies are warranted in patients with large lesions and multiple juvenile polyps to exclude the presence of neoplasia. The terminology used to describe these lesions is inconsistent, but it is important to make the distinction between regenerative and dysplastic changes, because the implications for clinical follow-up are different. The diagnosis of dysplasia is often straightforward, especially when the lesions consist exclusively of adenomatous epithelium. However, in mixed lesions it is sometimes extremely difficult to distinguish dysplastic areas from the epithelial atypia associated with reparative responses (Fig. 12.35). One may find small, somewhat eosinophilic, irregular glands lined by mucin-depleted, pseudostratified, columnar epithelium. The cells often exhibit large hyperchromatic nuclei with prominent nucleoli and increased mitotic figures, therefore resembling adenomas.

The dysplasia found in juvenile polyps is usually low grade. The frequency and severity of the dysplasia correlates with greater polyp diameter in individuals with generalized polyposis (144). Dysplasia is much more likely to be present in villous areas. Jass et al reported a dysplasia incidence of 46.7% in lesions showing a villous architecture, contrasting with only 9% in typical juvenile polyps (144). The dysplasia often resembles that seen in ulcerative colitis (see Chapter 16) or in sporadic or hereditary polyposis syndromes.

Lesions that should be examined closely for the presence of dysplasia include those that at first glance do not look like typical juvenile polyps. Often, atypical juvenile polyps contain relatively less lamina propria and more epithelium than are found in typical juvenile polyps (Fig. 12.36). Epithelial dysplasias affect both typical and atypical polyps, but the frequency varies considerably in the two types of lesions.

Patients with single juvenile polyps are treated conservatively. Polypectomy is performed and patients are then discharged from care. Patients with multiple polyps, juvenile polyposis, or polyps containing dysplasia or adenomatous transformation require more rigorous follow-up. Genetic

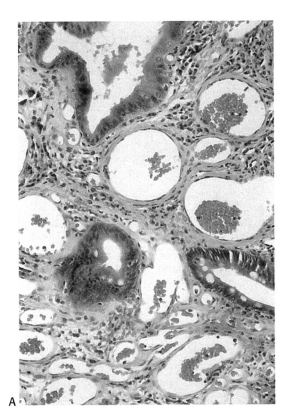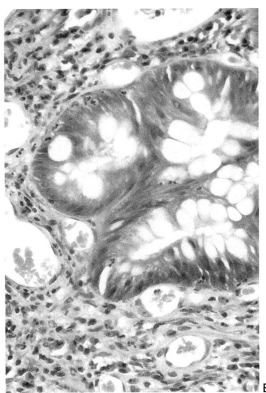

A   B

FIG. 12.35. Atypical epithelium in juvenile polyp. **A:** One sees the darkly staining epithelium surrounded by a markedly congested stroma. Acute inflammation is absent. Such areas can be designated as atypical. **B:** Higher magnification of another area in this polyp showing an apparent back-to-back configuration of glands that are difficult to distinguish between a regenerative process and early low-grade dysplasia. Such lesions can be classified as atypical epithelium. The presence of the neutrophils suggests that this is in an area of resolving inflammation.

testing is available for juvenile polyposis. Patients with PJI should begin upper endoscopy and colonoscopy in adolescence. If multiple polyps are identified, they should all be removed. Annual surveillance is then indicated. All polyps should be examined by a pathologist to rule out the presence of dysplasia or invasive carcinoma. If no polyps are identified on initial endoscopy, screening should be performed at 3-year intervals. Colectomy may be necessary if polyps are too numerous to be removed, or if dysplasia or carcinoma are identified.

Familial Gastric Polyposis

Familial gastric polyposis may represent a new autosomal dominant syndrome. Cases without a family history may result from new mutations. Patients show a high incidence of cutaneous psoriasis. Gastric hyperplastic polyposis patients have numerous hyperplastic polyps that average 1 cm in size with most lesions measuring <1.5 cm in diameter. The multiple polyps generally appear uniform in shape and size. When more than 50 polyps are present, the term *hyperplastic polyposis* is applied. Gastric polyps develop in 34% to 60% of affected patients (145).

Histologically, the polyps resemble atypical juvenile colonic polyps, fundic gland polyps, or hyperplastic polyps. They are scattered throughout the gastric fundus and body with less frequent involvement of the cardia and antrum. These polyps tend to remain asymptomatic and there appears to be only a slightly increased risk for the development of gastric cancer over that seen in the general population. Carcinoma develops in the hyperplastic polyps.

Cowden Disease (PTEN Hamartomatous Tumor Syndrome)

Cowden disease (OMIM entry #158350) is a rare disorder named after the family in which it occurred. Synonyms for this syndrome include Lhermitte-Duclos disease and the recently proposed term *PTEN hamartomatous tumor syndrome.*

Cowden disease results from mutations in the *PTEN* gene. *PTEN* encodes a dual specificity phosphatase that affects apoptosis and inhibits cell spreading via the focal adhesion kinase pathway. Mutations include missense and nonsense point mutations, deletions, insertions, and splice site mutations, and occur scattered over the entire length of the gene

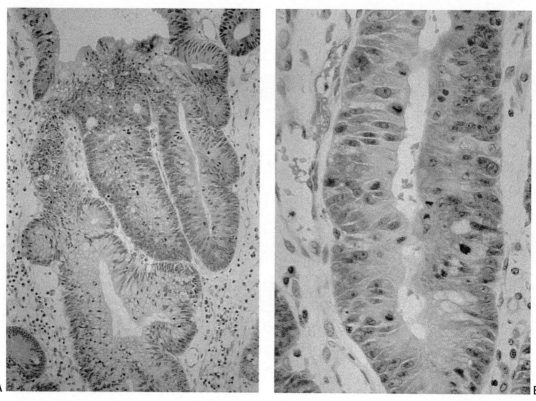

FIG. 12.36. True dysplasia within a juvenile polyp. **A:** A medium magnification of the dysplastic area that resembles adenomatous epithelium. One sees nuclear stratification and an increased number of mitotic figures. In addition, there is a complex glandular branching imparting a back-to-back architectural pattern. **B:** Higher magnification showing the nuclear stratification and the increased number of mitotic figures.

with the exception of the first, fourth, and last exons (146). Approximately two thirds of the mutations occur in exons 5, 7, and 8, with 40% affecting exon 5.

Clinical Features

Cowden disease is characterized by hamartomatous neoplasms of ectodermal, mesodermal, and endodermal origin. The estimated incidence of the disorder is 1 per 200,000. Ten to fifty percent of cases are familial, with as many as 90% of patients manifesting signs or symptoms of the disease by age 20 (147). By age 30, 99% of patients demonstrate at least the mucocutaneous features of the disease. The disease affects males and females equally.

Most tumors arising in Cowden disease are benign and commonly develop on the face and in the thyroid gland, breast, or GI tract. Gastrointestinal polyps occur in 60% of patients, and may be histologically indistinguishable from juvenile polyps. However, Cowden disease can be distinguished from juvenile polyposis with knowledge of the extraintestinal manifestations in the affected patient. Other gastrointestinal polyps that occur in Cowden disease patients include ganglioneuromas, lipomatous lesions, and inflammatory polyps.

Facial tricholemmomas are considered pathognomonic for Cowden disease, but affected patients present with other facial abnormalities as well (Fig. 12.37). The skin lesions typically develop between ages 20 and 30. Thyroid disease is the most common extracutaneous abnormality, occurring in 68% of patients (147). The benign lesions are usually goiters or adenomas. Skeletal abnormalities affect 33% of patients. Bone cysts, syndactyly, and other digit abnormalities have been described. Breast carcinoma is the most common malignancy occurring in patients with Cowden syndrome. It affects 36% to 50% of females with the disease (148). Nonmalignant breast lesions are also common and are often bilateral.

Gastrointestinal Lesions

Patients may have coexisting gastrointestinal polyps, ganglioneuromatosis of the colon, and glycogen acanthosis of the esophagus (147). Polyps affect 71% of patients who undergo evaluation of the alimentary tract (149). These occur anywhere from the esophagus to the rectum, but the distal colon is the preferentially involved site. Intestinal polyps in this syndrome include juvenile polyps (Fig. 12.38), Peutz-Jeghers-type polyps, lipomas, inflammatory polyps,

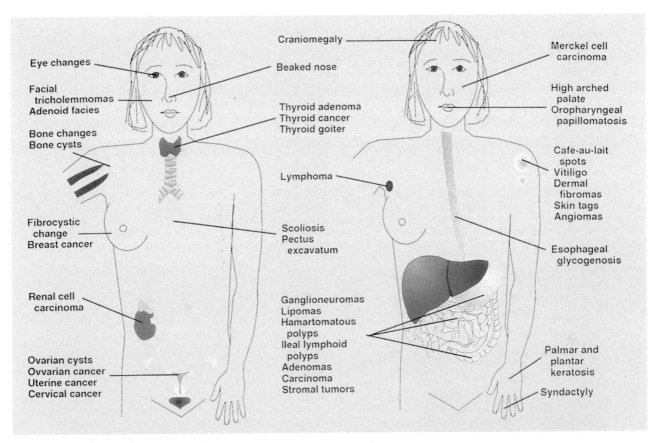

FIG. 12.37. Diagrammatic representation of many of the intestinal and extraintestinal lesions found in patients with Cowden syndrome.

lymphoid polyps, hyperplastic polyps, epithelioid leiomyomas, and ganglioneuromas. The lesions are usually small and asymptomatic, and grossly resemble hyperplastic polyps.

Microscopically, the polyps contain a mixture of cell types, including fibroblasts and adipose tissue (Fig. 12.39).

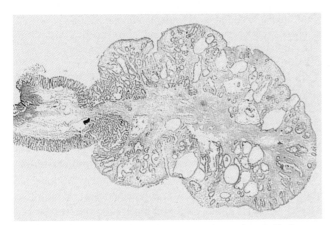

FIG. 12.38. Polyp in Cowden syndrome. Note the similarity to a juvenile polyp. Only the presence of the extraintestinal lesions allowed the classification of this polyp.

The most common colonic polyp in Cowden disease contains elongated, irregular, regenerative-appearing crypt epithelium with cystic dilation, mild lamina propria edema, inflammation, and variable fibrosis. Cellular pleomorphism or atypia are absent. One may also see thickening of the collagen table underlying the luminal surface as occurs in patients with hyperplastic polyps or collagenous colitis. Biopsies of the polyps may show only mild glandular architectural distortion with variable fibrosis and inflammation of the lamina propria predominantly consisting of plasma cells, lymphocytes, and eosinophils. Fat cells may be present in the lamina propria. Dysplasia and adenomas are rare.

Polyps may also be found in the stomach. Gastric lesions show foveolar hyperplasia or show a resemblance to Peutz-Jeghers or hyperplastic-type lesions. The polyps in the stomach may also contain neural elements. Other gastrointestinal lesions include duodenal lymphoid polyps, duodenal lymphangiectasia, and jejunal lymphangiomas.

Treatment and Prognosis

There does not appear to be a significantly increased risk of gastrointestinal cancer in Cowden disease. As a result, many believe that gastrointestinal examinations are unnecessary

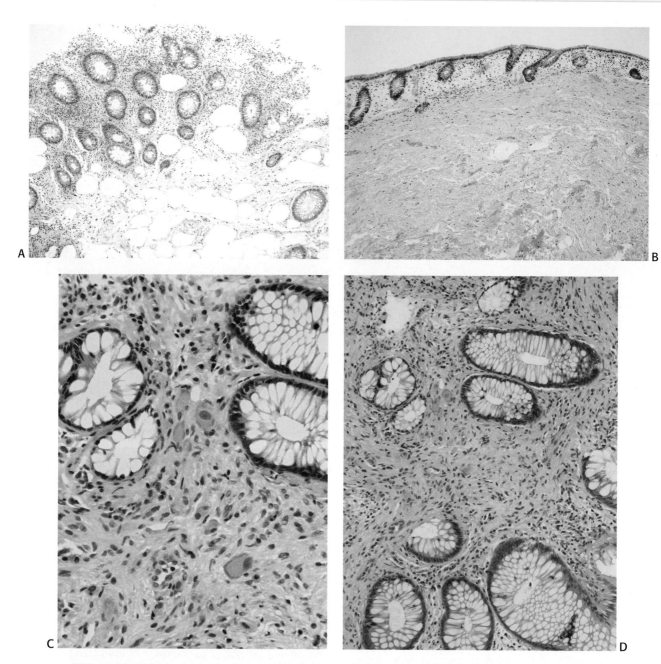

FIG. 12.39. Colonic polyps in Cowden disease. **A:** Colonic polyp containing abundant adipose tissue. **B:** Another polyp in the same patient showing a fibrous proliferation underlying the mucosa. **C:** Ganglioneuroma in another patient with Cowden disease. The colonic glands are separated by a spindle cell proliferation. **D:** On higher power, scattered ganglion cells are seen within the mucosal spindle cell areas.

unless GI symptoms are present. Screening strategies for extraintestinal tumors should be undertaken, however, since 74% of patients develop some form of malignant disease, most commonly invasive ductal breast carcinomas and thyroid tumors. The mean age at diagnosis of breast cancer is 10 years earlier than that of breast cancer in the general population. Men with Cowden disease are also at risk for development of breast cancers. The risk of thyroid cancer (predominantly follicular carcinoma) may be as high as 10% (147). Patients also have an increased risk of endometrial cancer. Other tumors that develop include brain tumors, mucocutaneous basal cell and squamous cell carcinomas, melanomas, lymphomas, Merkel cell carcinomas, non–small cell lung cancers, ovarian cancers, renal cell carcinomas, transitional cell carcinomas of the bladder, and osteosarcomas. Rarely, gastric, colorectal, hepatocellular, or pancreatic carcinomas develop (147,148).

Bannayan-Riley-Ruvalcaba Syndrome

Another rare hamartomatous syndrome is Bannayan-Riley-Ruvalcaba syndrome (BRRS) (OMIM entry #153480) (Fig. 12.40), also known as the Ruvalcaba-Myhre-Smith syndrome, Bannayan-Zonana syndrome, and Riley-Smith syndrome. This is a generalized hamartomatous syndrome that mainly affects men, and overlaps with Cowden disease. It is inherited as an autosomal dominant disorder and, like Cowden disease, has been associated in 60% of cases with inherited mutations in the PTEN gene (150,151). Unlike Cowden disease, the PTEN mutations found in BRRS do not occur in the PTPase core motif of the gene. Some BRRS patients have PTEN gene deletions (152).

BRRS is noted at birth or shortly thereafter and is characterized by delayed psychomotor development, ileal and colonic juvenile polyps, lingual lesions, subcutaneous and visceral lipomas and hemangiomas, multiple variable congenital anomalies, mental retardation, ocular abnormalities, skeletal abnormalities, thyroid tumors, and pigmented penile macules (Fig. 12.40) (153). The hamartomatous gastrointestinal lesions resemble juvenile polyps, and may occasionally contain areas of dysplasia (154). A definite association with cancer development has not been demonstrated among patients with BRRS.

Neurofibromatosis 1

Neurofibromatosis 1 (NF1), or von Recklinghausen disease (OMIM entry #162200), is not classically considered a hamartomatous polyposis syndrome, but affected patients may develop multiple submucosal gastrointestinal neurofibromas. This entity is discussed in Chapter 19.

NONHEREDITARY HAMARTOMATOUS POLYPOSIS SYNDROMES

Cronkhite-Canada Syndrome

Clinical Features

Cronkhite-Canada syndrome (CCS) is a rare, nonhereditary, adult gastrointestinal polyposis syndrome that occurs worldwide. It affects both sexes equally, with patients ranging in age from 31 to 83 years at the time of diagnosis (155). Eighty percent of patients present after the age of 50. All cases are sporadic, and CCS is not considered a genetic disease. Proposed etiologic theories include nutritional deficiency states, disaccharidase deficiency accompanied by bacterial overgrowth, infection, disturbances of intestinal mucin secretion, or some form of immunologic disorder (156,157).

CCS associates with skin hyperpigmentation, patchy vitiligo, alopecia, onychodystrophy, marked edema, tetany, glossitis, and cataracts (Fig. 12.41). The most common symptoms include diarrhea, protein-losing enteropathy, weight loss, abdominal pain, anorexia, weakness, hematochezia, vomiting, paresthesias, and xerostomia. The diarrhea usually consists of loose, watery bowel movements

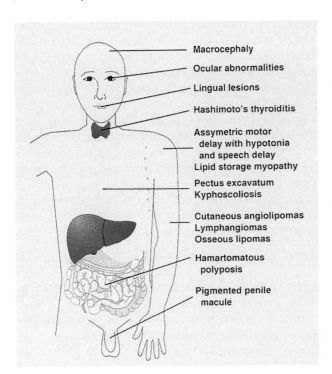

FIG. 12.40. Diagrammatic representation of many of the intestinal and extraintestinal lesions found in patients with Bannayan-Riley-Ruvalcaba syndrome.

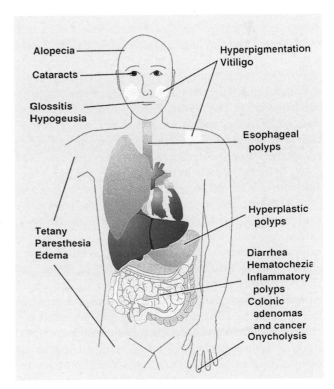

FIG. 12.41. Diagrammatic representation of many of the intestinal and extraintestinal lesions found in patients with Cronkhite-Canada syndrome.

occurring five to seven times per day. They may be grossly bloody, and the blood loss may be significant enough that the patient requires transfusions. Malabsorption invariably develops, probably due to diffuse small intestinal mucosal injury. Laboratory findings include hypoproteinemia, particularly hypoalbuminemia, hypocalcemia, hypomagnesemia, anemia, occult blood in the stool, and electrolyte deficiencies.

Symptom onset may be acute and the course rapidly progressive. The major clinical problem in these patients results from protein loss from the damaged mucosa and variable malabsorption. Profound malnutrition may occur and is a major cause of morbidity and mortality. Aggressive supportive therapy with nutritional supplementation, fluid and electrolyte replacement, and transfusion of blood components is warranted to correct the existing or impending deficiencies. The use of total parenteral nutrition is successful in some patients. The mortality rate is 50% to 60%. While spontaneous remissions may occur, survival beyond 2 years for symptomatic patients is uncommon. Other therapies have included corticosteroids, antibiotics, and surgery, but results are unpredictable.

Since as many as 20% of CCS patients develop an adenoma or carcinoma, colonoscopic surveillance is indicated (155). The neoplasms develop primarily in the colon and less frequently in the stomach. Colonic lesions tend to occur in a proximal location. Surgery is recommended when complications such as bleeding, intussusception, bowel obstruction, malignancy, or prolapse develop.

Pathologic Features

Polyps develop throughout the GI tract, sometimes occupying the entire mucosal surface of affected sites. Polyp density is greatest in the stomach and colon, followed by the duodenum, ileum, and jejunum. The polyps vary in color from tan to red, sometimes demonstrating areas of surface ulceration and hemorrhage. Their gross appearance varies from diffuse mucosal micronodularity or granularity to gelatinous-appearing pedunculated polyps. The gelatinous appearance results from the presence of large mucosal cysts (Fig. 12.42).

Polyp morphology reflects the site of origin. The polyps resemble colonic juvenile polyps or gastric hyperplastic polyps. Gastric polyps are broad-based sessile lesions that contain corkscrew-shaped glands. Smooth muscle fibers extend up into the mucosa. The polyps contain an expanded, edematous lamina propria and distended, cystic glands lined by flattened epithelium, variable edema, and chronic inflammation. Gastric polyps tend to occur in the antrum forming hyperplastic gastric folds, some of which mimic Menetrier disease. The lesions can spontaneously regress. Adenomatous changes may be present, as can coexisting colorectal carcinomas. Small intestinal lesions are essentially similar, although the degree of inflammation and edema tends to be greater than in the stomach and the lesions tend to involve the entire bowel wall thickness. Villi and crypts decrease in number. Goblet cells increase in the remaining crypts.

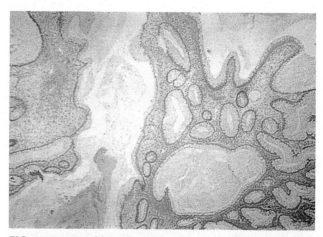

FIG. 12.42. Cronkhite-Canada syndrome. Sessile pedunculated lesion in a patient with numerous other polyps. Large mucus-filled cysts distort the architecture.

The only reliable distinction between CCS and colonic juvenile polyposis is the pedunculated growth of the latter. However, it is important to note that pedunculation is not always present in juvenile polyps. The diagnosis of CCS polyps, especially when located in the stomach, requires knowledge of the clinical context.

Other Polyposis Syndromes

There are other syndromes associated with the development of gastrointestinal polyps. *Ganglioneurofibromatosis* may associate with juvenile polyposis or multiple endocrine neoplasia syndrome. The pathologic features of ganglioneurofibromatosis are discussed in Chapter 19. Patients with the *basal cell nevus syndrome* may develop multiple gastric polyps. *Multiple recurrent inflammatory fibroid polyps* of the stomach and intestine have been reported in families (158). Affected patients present with repeated bouts of intussusception and the polyps range in size from 0.5 to 8 cm. Multiple inflammatory polyps also complicate various infectious diseases or idiopathic inflammatory bowel disease. These polyps are discussed in Chapters 13 and 11, respectively. Multiple lipomatosis is discussed in Chapter 19. Multiple lymphoid polyps and lymphomatosis are discussed in Chapter 18. Patients with hereditary angiomatoses may present as a polyposis syndrome. These lesions are discussed more fully in Chapter 19.

HEREDITARY GASTROINTESTINAL CANCER SYNDROMES WITHOUT POLYPOSIS

Hereditary Nonpolyposis Colorectal Cancer Syndrome

HNPCC, or Lynch syndrome, is the colon cancer family syndrome not classically associated with large numbers of colonic adenomas. The features of HNPCC are listed in

TABLE 12.10 **Features of Hereditary Nonpolyposis Colorectal Cancer**

Autosomal dominant inheritance pattern

Patients develop cancer at a young age (peak age 45 years) as compared with sporadic colon cancer

Tumors tend to originate proximal to the splenic flexure

Tendency to develop multiple tumors

Abundant mucin secretion by the tumor (in 20% of cases)

Tumors tend to be diploid

Tumors tend to be surrounded by prominent lymphoid infiltrates

Small intestinal cancers arising at sites other than the periampullary region

Frequent association with tumors of other sites, especially the endometrium, urothelium, and stomach

Table 12.10 HNPCC-associated lesions are summarized in Figure 12.43. Several international diagnostic criteria have been established for the diagnosis of HNPCC (Table 12.11) (159,160). The Amsterdam criteria were developed to ensure international uniformity and to facilitate comparison of clinical, pathologic, and molecular genetic data in these patients (159). The Bethesda guidelines, and the revised Bethesda guidelines, introduced molecular genetic considerations, and provided criteria to be used to determine which individuals' tumors should undergo microsatellite instability and/or genetic testing (160,161).

Overall, HNPCC-associated colorectal cancers account for only a small percentage of the total colorectal cancer burden (6% to 15.8%), but they represent the most common form of inherited colorectal cancer (162). HNPCC is five times more common than FAP. It is estimated that the prevalence of HNPCC-associated mutations in the general population in Western countries is between 1 in 200 and 1 in 2,000 (162). HNPCC affects many races, including Europeans, Native Americans, Australians, Asians, and South Americans. First-degree relatives of patients with HNPCC have a sevenfold increased colon cancer incidence compared with the general population. HNPCC patients develop cancer at a younger age than patients with sporadic cancer, with a mean age of 39 years for men and 37 years for women.

One difficulty in recognizing an HNPCC patient is that the syndrome gives no hint of its existence in the individual patient unless an increased family incidence of colon cancer has already become evident. In the past, identification of the syndrome required examination of family pedigrees. Today, the use of genetic testing for specific mutations allows the diagnosis of individual cases of HNPCC.

Genetics of Hereditary Nonpolyposis Colorectal Cancer

HNPCC is inherited as an autosomal dominant condition, with affected patients carrying germline mutations in a DNA

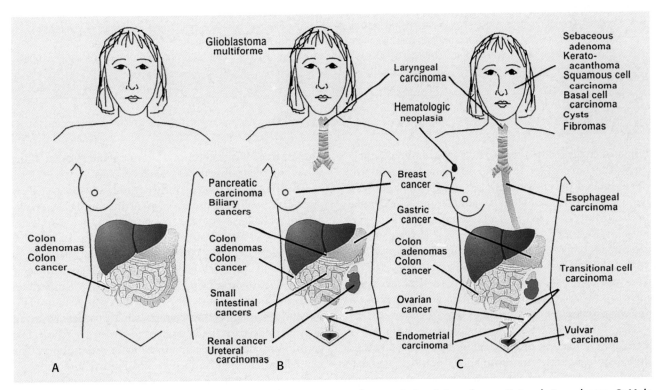

FIG. 12.43. Neoplasms arising in patients with hereditary cancer syndromes. **A:** Lynch I syndrome. **B:** Lynch II syndrome. **C:** Muir-Torre syndrome.

TABLE 12.11 Clinical and Molecular Criteria for Diagnosis of Hereditary Nonpolyposis Colorectal Cancer (HNPCC)

Amsterdam I Criteria

At least three relatives with histologically verified colorectal cancer:
1. One is a first-degree relative of the other two
2. At least two successive generations are affected
3. At least one relative is diagnosed with colorectal cancer before the age of 50
4. Familial adenomatous polyposis has been excluded

Amsterdam II Criteria

At least three relatives with an HNPCC-associated cancer (colorectal, endometrial, stomach, ovary, ureter/renal pelvis, brain, small intestine, hepatobiliary tract, or sebaceous tumor of skin):
1. One is a first-degree relative of the other two
2. At least two successive generations are affected
3. At least one relative is diagnosed with an HNPCC-associated cancer before the age of 50
4. Familial adenomatous polyposis has been excluded

Bethesda Guidelines for Testing Colorectal Neoplasms for Microsatellite Instability

1. Individuals with cancer in families that meet Amsterdam criteria
2. Individuals with two HNPCC-related cancers including synchronous or metachronous colorectal or extracolonic tumors
3. Individuals with colorectal cancer and a first-degree relative with colorectal cancer, and/or HNPCC-related extracolonic cancer, and/or a colorectal adenoma; one of the cancers diagnosed at age <45 years, or adenoma diagnosed at <40 years of age
4. Individuals with colorectal cancer or endometrial cancer diagnosed at age <45 years
5. Individuals with right-sided colorectal cancer with an undifferentiated pattern (solid/cribriform) on histopathology diagnosed at <45 years of age
6. Individuals with signet ring cell–type colorectal cancer diagnosed at <45 years of age
7. Individuals with adenomas diagnosed at <40 years of age

Revised Bethesda Guidelines

1. Colorectal cancer diagnosed in a patient < 50 years of age
2. Presence of synchronous, metachronous colorectal or other HNPCC-associated tumors (colorectal, endometrial, stomach, ovarian, pancreas, ureter and renal pelvis, biliary tract, small bowel, brain, and sebaceous adenomas and keratoacanthomas) regardless of age
3. Colorectal cancer with microsatellite instability-high histology (tumor infiltrating lymphocytes, Crohn-like lymphocytic reaction, mucinous/signet ring cell differentiation, or medullary growth pattern) diagnosed in a patient <60 years of age
4. Colorectal cancer diagnosed in one or more first-degree relatives with an HNPCC-related tumor, with one of the cancers being diagnosed under age 50
5. Colorectal cancer diagnosed in two or more first- or second-degree relatives with HNPCC-related tumors, regardless of age

mismatch repair (MMR) gene. The most commonly implicated genes are *MLH1* located on chromosome 3p and *MSH2* located on chromosome 2p. *MLH1* mutations are found in 43% to 63% of HNPCC families, and *MSH2* mutations in 25% to 45% (163,164). Less commonly, mutations in other MMR genes occur. Patients carrying HNPCC-associated mutations exhibit a 40% to 80% lifetime risk of developing colorectal cancer (165–167). Because the HNPCC genes are not 100% penetrant, one may see the cancer phenotype in the maternal or paternal lineages but not in the patient's parents.

The MMR genes act as tumor suppressors, with loss of both copies of the gene resulting in unrestrained growth and ultimately neoplastic transformation. HNPCC patients inherit one defective copy of an MMR gene, and the second copy is lost or inactivated as a somatic event. Loss of the second MMR gene often occurs as a result of methylation of the gene promoter rather than through deletion.

The DNA MMR proteins form heterodimers that recognize and repair small sequence errors occurring during DNA replication, including base–base mispairings and insertion/deletion loops or slipped strand mispairings (Fig. 12.44). One result of defective DNA MMR is a phenomenon referred to as microsatellite instability (MSI). MSI occurs in approximately 90% to 95% of cancers in HNPCC (168,169). Microsatellites represent short repetitive DNA sequences scattered throughout the genome. Microsatellite instability is defined as an increase or decrease in the number of nucleotide repeats in a given microsatellite allele in normal tissue versus tumor. The new alleles that are identified in MSI-positive tumors represent small insertions or deletions that occur as a consequence of uncorrected errors in DNA replication.

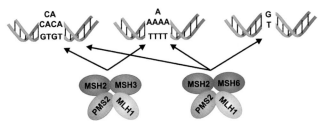

FIG. 12.44. DNA mismatch repair mechanism. The mismatch repair proteins form tetrameric complexes to repair DNA mismatches. The components of the repair complexes differ depending on the type of DNA mispairing that occurs.

When MSI is assessed in the laboratory, it is divided into three groups depending on the number of markers showing alterations in microsatellite length: MSI-High (MSI-H), MSI-Low (MSI-L), and MS-Stable (MS-S) (170). A National Institutes of Health (NIH) consensus panel convened in 1997 recommended testing a standard panel of five microsatellite repeat markers to ensure uniform interpretation of MSI in colorectal cancers (170). These five markers are BAT25, BAT26, D2S123, D5S346, and D17S250. Instability at two or more of these markers is considered to be MSI-H, while one out of five markers defines MSI-L. A complete lack of instability characterizes MS-S. In clinical practice, most molecular diagnostic laboratories now use as many as ten markers to distinguish these groups, with instability at <10% of markers representing MS-S, instability at 10% to 30% of markers defining MSI-L, and instability at >30% of markers defining MSI-H . MSI analysis has a sensitivity of 93% in detecting MMR deficiency in carriers of pathogenic MMR gene mutations (171,172). The clinical phenotype of MSI-L and MS-S colorectal cancers is essentially indistinguishable, whereas MSI-H tumors are diagnostic of defective mismatch repair and often have a characteristic pathologic appearance (see below).

Antibodies to many of the mismatch repair proteins are now commercially available and are useful for identifying tumors that are likely to be MSI-H and to help target future genetic testing for affected patients (173). The use of immunohistochemistry for recognizing the heterodimeric partners MSH2-MSH6 and MLH1-PMS2 helps identify the causal mutations in HNPCC patients (Fig. 12.45).

Extracolonic Cancers in Hereditary Nonpolyposis Colorectal Cancer

Endometrial carcinoma is the most common extracolonic cancer observed in HNPCC families (174). The cumulative incidence is 9% to 45% by age 75 compared with 3% in the general population. The rate of developing endometrial cancer is greater in patients with an abnormal *MSH2* gene compared with individuals carrying *MLH1* mutations (6% vs. 42%). A very high relative risk of developing small bowel

cancer (>100) affects carriers of either *MSH2* or *MLH1* mutations. Carriers of *MSH2* mutations also have a significantly increased risk of renal and ureteral cancers (relative risk of 75.3), gastric cancer (relative risk 19.9), and ovarian cancer (relative risk 8.0) (159). One phenotypic variation of HNPCC associates with desmoid tumors, a feature more classically associated with FAP (see Chapter 19). Another HNPCC variant associates with glioblastoma multiforme (175). Genetic analyses have shown that patients with Turcot syndrome have mutations in either MMR genes or in the *APC* gene. These different mutations result in different brain tumors.

Adenomas in Hereditary Nonpolyposis Colorectal Cancer Patients

Despite the name *hereditary nonpolyposis colorectal cancer,* adenomas do develop in HNPCC patients. Overall, adenomas in HNPCC patients tend to be large (>10 mm), show a villous architecture, contain high-grade dysplasia (176) with a right-sided predominance, develop at an earlier age than sporadic adenomas, and exhibit mucinous differentiation. A high proportion of HNPCC adenomas become malignant (177), and the rate of progression to cancer may be higher than that seen in sporadic adenomas (177). This contrasts with the large numbers of low-grade dysplastic adenomas found in FAP patients (Table 12.12).

In addition to traditional tubular adenomas, HNPCC patients also develop hyperplastic polyps, serrated adenomas, and mixed polyps comprising both serrated and adenomatous components (178). Mixed lesions are larger than adenomas and tend to show pseudoinvasion. They may demonstrate a number of bizarre cytologic features, including multinucleation, atypical mitoses, and chromatin aggregation into coarse clumps.

Colorectal Cancers Arising in Hereditary Nonpolyposis Colorectal Cancer Patients

The average age of onset of colon cancer in HNPCC patients is 45 years (179), contrasting with age 65 in the general population (180). Average age at presentation varies with the genetic defect that is present; patients with *MLH1* mutations present earlier than those with *MSH2* alterations (181). Patients with *MSH6* mutations present latest, with an average age at presentation of 49 years. Eighty percent of colorectal tumors develop before age 50, with 12% developing before age 30. Patients tend to develop multiple tumors. Synchronous and metachronous cancers affect 18% and 24.2% of HNPCC patients, respectively (180). HNPCC cancers occur proximal to the splenic flexure in 60% to 69% of patients (180).

HNPCC-associated malignancies are relatively nonaggressive, despite their tendency to be poorly differentiated and mucinous. Stage for stage, the prognosis for HNPCC-

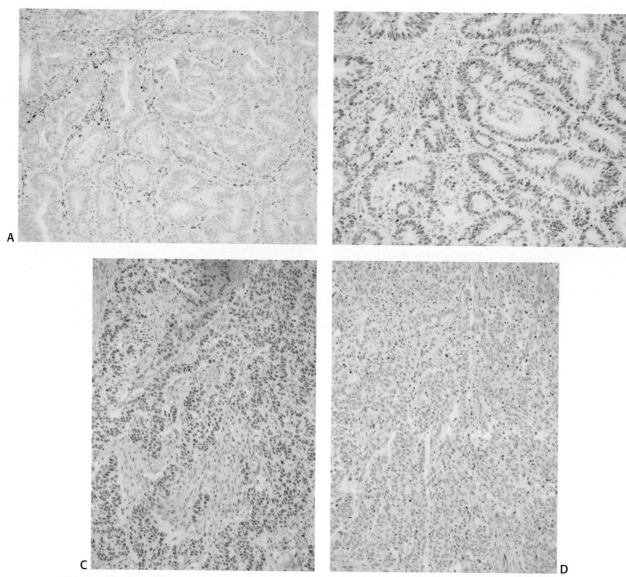

FIG. 12.45. Mismatch repair protein expression in colon cancer. **A:** MLH-1 immunostain shows an absence of immunoreactivity in this moderately differentiated colonic adenocarcinoma. **B:** MSH-2 staining is preserved in the same tumor. **C:** A different adenocarcinoma shows retention of MLH-1 staining. Note the poor differentiation in this tumor. **D:** MSH-2 staining is lost in the tumor illustrated in C.

TABLE 12.12   Comparison of HNPCC and FAP

	HNPCC	FAP
Onset	Early	Early
Adenoma number	<10	>100
Adenoma histology	Tubular adenomas	Tubular adenomas
Polyp distribution	Mainly right side	Left or total
Degree of dysplasia in adenoma	High grade	Low grade
Cancer distribution	Mainly right side	Random or mostly rectal
Other cancers	See Figure 12.12	See Figure 12.43
Proportion of adenomas becoming malignant	High	Low
Types of polyps	Adenomas, serrated polyps, mixed hyperplastic–adenomatous polyps	Adenomas

FAP, familial adenomatous polyposis; HNPCC, hereditary nonpolyposis colon cancer.

associated carcinomas is better than that for sporadic colon cancer (167). Survival rates are better among patients with localized and nonlocalized tumors, discounting the notion that the more favorable prognosis is based on a more favorable stage at diagnosis. The overall 5-year survival rate is 65% in patients with HNPCC compared with 44% with sporadic carcinomas (182). Their better survival rates may be caused by the heavy mutation burden affecting MMR-deficient tumor cells. This heavy burden may decrease the overall viability of the individual tumor cells.

Pathologic Features

HNPCC-associated colorectal tumors usually arise in the right colon, and may be small, measuring as little as 4 mm in size (182). Many of the colorectal cancers arising in patients with HNPCC demonstrate a solid growth pattern, a feature that accounts for the high proportion of poorly differentiated cancers in these patients. In addition, there is an excess of mucinous and signet ring cell tumors among these patients. The tumors often show an expansile or well-circumscribed tumor border (as compared with infiltrating growth) with marked peritumoral lymphocytic infiltrates (182,183) (Fig. 12.46). In addition, colorectal cancers in these patients often demonstrate large numbers of tumor infiltrating lymphocytes. Some tumors show a "Crohn-like

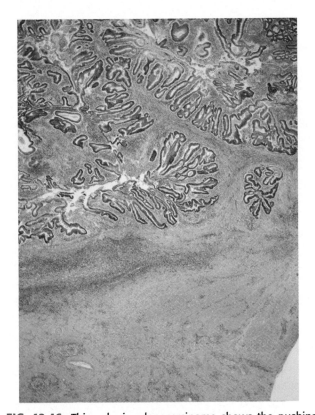

FIG. 12.46. This colonic adenocarcinoma shows the pushing border and prominent lymphocytic reaction typically seen in tumors arising in association with hereditary nonpolyposis colorectal cancer.

reaction" in which lymphoid aggregates, often with germinal centers, ring the periphery of the invasive carcinoma (Fig. 12.47).

Treatment and Surveillance

Patients with a definitive or suspected diagnosis of HNPCC should undergo surveillance for colorectal cancer and other HNPCC-associated cancers. Colonoscopy should be performed every 2 years beginning at age 20 to 25 years until 40 years of age, at which time screening should be undertaken annually (184). It is important that the colon be well prepped, and any polyps that are present should be completely resected. Patients who develop advanced adenomas can be offered the option of prophylactic subtotal colectomy followed by annual proctoscopy.

Annual endometrial cancer screening is recommended for women after age 25 to 35. Screening for other HNPCC-associated malignancies is more controversial (185). Some experts recommend screening for ovarian cancer with transvaginal ultrasound and serum CA-125 measurements, as well as screening for gastric cancer in high-risk geographic regions (e.g., Japan) or in families with a known history of gastric cancer (186). Urine cytology and renal ultrasound may also be used to detect lesions in families with histories of genitourinary neoplasms (186).

As in other autosomal dominant conditions, the affected patient should undergo genetic testing to allow for directed testing later in other family members at risk. This should be performed in patients meeting the Amsterdam criteria, or in those who are suspected of having HNPCC and fit the Bethesda guidelines. The affected patient's tumor should first be tested for MSI, as well as for MSH2 or MLH1 expression by immunohistochemistry. If MSI is not found, then sequencing of MMR genes is not warranted. If the tumor is MSI positive or loss of protein expression is found, then sequencing of the mismatch repair genes is indicated. An algorithm for genetic testing and patient follow-up is outlined in Figure 12.48.

Muir-Torre Syndrome

Muir-Torre syndrome is a rare autosomal dominant disorder in which affected patients develop skin and other tumors, and exhibit a strong family history of cancer. The tumor spectrum in Muir-Torre syndrome resembles that seen in patients with HNPCC (Lynch II syndrome). Muir-Torre syndrome patients develop colon cancer at an early age. The cancers show a right-sided predominance and have a better prognosis than sporadic colonic cancers. Muir-Torre patients also develop skin tumors associated with their internal malignancies (187). The patients develop sebaceous adenomas and isolated or multiple keratoacanthomas, as well as other skin lesions including benign keratoses, squamous cell carcinoma, basal cell carcinoma, cysts, and fibromas. Sebaceous tumors represent a marker for internal malig-

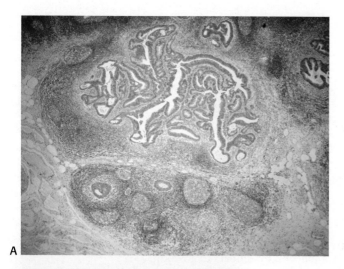

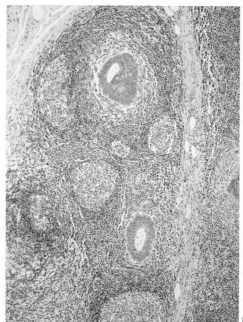

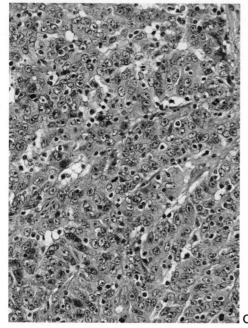

FIG. 12.47. Crohn-like reaction in hereditary nonpolyposis colorectal cancer. **A:** Low-power view of a colonic adenocarcinoma showing a prominent lymphocytic reaction to the tumor. Large germinal centers are seen reminiscent of those occurring in association with Crohn disease. **B:** Higher power view demonstrating the lymphocytic infiltrate around individual infiltrating glands. **C:** Numerous intratumoral lymphocytes are present in this poorly differentiated adenocarcinoma. The tumor showed loss of MSH-2 staining by immunohistochemistry.

nancy and should prompt a search for occult cancer in individual patients and their family members (188).

Like tumors arising in association with HNPCC, those arising in Muir-Torre syndrome are MSI-H. This finding is observed in both skin tumors and visceral malignancies in these patients (189). Based on this finding, some suggest that the syndrome may represent a variant of HNPCC (190). However, a subset of Muir-Torre patients does exist in which no deficiency in mismatch repair can be identified (191).

Inherited Susceptibility to Colonic Adenomas and Colorectal Cancer

An autosomal dominant inheritance pattern affects some patients with discrete colorectal polyps and colorectal can-

cer. A large Utah kindred that lacked the natural history characteristic of typical hereditary colorectal cancer syndromes was described (192). The patients had an increased colon cancer incidence. The cancers developed at an early age and were frequently multiple, with both synchronous and metachronous colorectal cancers. Patients also developed extracolonic malignancies. The disorder is inherited as a unique syndrome.

Familial Aggregation of Neuroectodermal and Gastrointestinal Tumors

Sorensen et al (193) reported a family with multiple tumors, many of which were childhood neoplasms derived from the neuroectoderm. An early onset of colonic cancer was also noted.

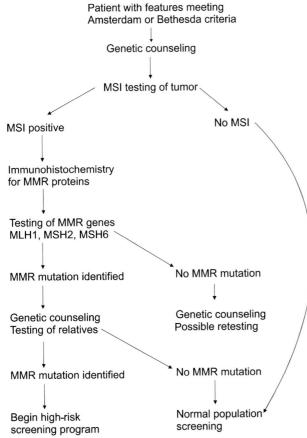

FIG. 12.48. Algorithm for genetic testing and follow-up for patients suspected of having hereditary nonpolyposis colorectal cancer. MMR, mismatch repair; MSI, microsatellite instability.

REFERENCES

1. Bodmer WF, Bailey CJ, Bodmer J, et al: Localisation of the gene for familial adenomatous polyposis on chromosome 5. *Nature* 1987;328:614.
2. Groden J, Thliveris A, Samowitz W, et al: Identification and characterization of the familial adenomatous polyposis coli gene. *Cell* 1991;66:589.
3. Nishisho I, Nakamura Y, Miyoshi Y, et al: Mutations of the chromosome 5q21 genes in FAP and colorectal cancer patients. *Science* 1991;253:665.
4. Kinzler KW, Nilbert MC, Su L-K, et al: Identification of FAP locus genes from chromosome 5q21. *Science* 1991;253:661.
5. Fodde R, Van der Luijt R, Wijnen J, et al: Eight novel inactivating germ line mutations at the APC gene identified by denaturing gradient gel electrophoresis. *Genomics* 1992;13:1162.
6. Vogelstein B, Fearon ER, Hamilton SR, et al: Genetic alterations during colorectal-tumor development. *N Engl J Med* 1988;319:525.
7. Olschwang S, Laurent-Puig P, Groden J, et al: Germ-line mutations in the first 14 exons of the adenomatous polyposis coli (APC) gene. *Am J Hum Genet* 1993;52:273.
8. Rubinfeld B, Souza B, Albert I, et al: Association of the APC gene product with beta-catenin. *Science* 1993;262:1731.
9. Goss KH, Groden J: Biology of the adenomatous polyposis coli tumor suppressor. *J Clin Oncol* 2000;18:1967.
10. Nathke I: APC at a glance. *J Cell Sci* 2004;117:4873.
11. Scates DK, Spigelman AD, Phillips RKS, Venitt S: DNA adducts detected by 32P-postlabelling, in the intestine of rats given bile from patients with familial adenomatous polyposis and from unaffected controls. *Carcinogenesis* 1992;13:731.
12. Giardiello FM, Hamilton SR, Krush AJ, et al: Treatment of colonic and rectal adenomas with sulindac in familial adenomatous polyposis. *N Engl J Med* 1993;398:1313.
13. Bell B, Mazzaferri EL: Familial adenomatous polyposis (Gardner's syndrome) and thyroid carcinoma. *Dig Dis Sci* 1993;38:185.
14. Caspari R, Friedl W, Mandl M, et al: Familial adenomatous polyposis: mutation at codon 1309 and early onset of colon cancer. *Lancet* 1994;343:629.
15. Spirio L, Olschwang S, Groden J, et al: Alleles of the APC gene: Attenuated form of familial polyposis. *Cell* 1993;75:951.
16. Nagase H, Miyoshi Y, Horii A, et al: Correlation between the location of germ-line mutations in the APC gene and the number of colorectal polyps in familial adenomatous polyposis patients. *Cancer Res* 1992;52:4055.
17. Lynch HT, Smyrk T, McGinn T, et al: Attenuated familial adenomatous polyposis (FAP): a phenotypically and genotypically distinctive variant of FAP. *Cancer* 1995;76:2427.
18. Petersen GM, Slack J, Nakamura Y: Screening guidelines and premorbid diagnosis of familial adenomatous polyposis using linkage analysis. *Gastroenterology* 1991;100:1658.
19. Bussey HJR: *Familial Polyposis Coli: Family Studies, Histopathology, Differential Diagnosis, and Results of Treatment.* Baltimore: Johns Hopkins University Press, 1975, pp 73–90.
20. Jagelman DG, DeCosse JJ, Busey HJR, et al: Upper gastrointestinal cancer in familial adenomatous polyposis. *Lancet* 1988;1:1149.
21. Sanner RF: Diffuse polyposis of the colon with severe electrolyte depletion. *Arch Surg* 1973;107:903.
22. Lynch HT, Smyrk T, Watson P, et al: Hereditary colorectal cancer. *Semin Oncol* 1991;18:337.
23. Burt RW, Berenson MM, Lee RG, et al: Upper gastrointestinal polyps in Gardner's syndrome. *Gastroenterology* 1984;86:295.
24. Koorey DJ, McCaughan GW, Trent RJ, Gallagher ND: Risk estimation in familial adenomatous polyposis using DNA probes linked to the familial adenomatous polyposis gene. *Gut* 1992;33:530.
25. Ando H, Miyoshi Y, Nagase H, et al: Detection of 12 germ-line mutations in the adenomatous polyposis coli gene by polymerase chain reaction. *Gastroenterology* 1993;104:989.
26. Iwama T, Mishima Y, Okamoto N, Inoue J: Association of congenital hypertrophy of the retinal pigment epithelium with familial adenomatous polyposis. *Br J Surg* 1990;77:273.
27. Debinski HS, Love S, Spigelman AD, et al: Colorectal polyp counts and cancer risk in familial adenomatous polyposis. *Gastroenterology* 1996;110:1028.
28. Iwama T, Mishima Y: Mortality in young first-degree relatives of patients with familial adenomatous polyposis. *Cancer* 1994;73:2065.
29. Jarvinen HJ: Time and type of prophylactic surgery for familial adenomatosis coli. *Ann Surg* 1985;202:93.
30. Moertel CG, Hill JR, Adson MA: Management of multiple polyposis of the large bowel. *Cancer* 1971;28:160.
31. Labayle D, Fischer D, Vielh P, et al: Sulindac causes regression of rectal polyp in familial adenomatous polyposis. *Gastroenterology* 1991;101:635.
32. Niv Y, Fraser G: Adenocarcinoma in the rectal segment in familial polyposis coli is not prevented by sulindac therapy. *Gastroenterology* 1994;107:854.
33. Bjork J, Akerbrant H, Iselius L, et al: Epidemiology of familial adenomatous polyposis in Sweden: changes over time and differences in phenotype between males and females. *Scand J Gastroenterol* 1999;34:1230.
34. Kubota O, Kino I: Depressed adenomas of the colon in familial adenomatous polyposis: histology, immunohistochemical detection of proliferating cell nuclear antigen (PCNA), and analysis of the background mucosa. *Am J Surg Pathol* 1995;19:318.
35. Matsumoto T, Iida M, Tada S, et al: Early detection of nonpolypoid cancers in the rectal remnant in patients with familial adenomatous polyposis/Gardner's syndrome. *Cancer* 1994;74:12.
36. Bülow S, Björk J, Christensen IJ, et al: Duodenal adenomatosis in familial adenomatous polyposis. The DAF Study Group. *Gut* 2004;53:381.
37. Domizio P, Talbot IC, Spigelman AD, et al: Upper gastrointestinal pathology in familial adenomatous polyposis: results from a prospective study of 102 patients. *J Clin Pathol* 1990;43:738.
38. Spigelman AD, Owen RW, Hill MJ, Phillips RKS: Biliary bile acid profiles in familial adenomatous polyposis. *Br J Surg* 1991;78:321.
39. Arvanitis ML, Jagelman DG, Fazio VW, et al: Mortality in patients with familial adenomatous polyposis. *Dis Colon Rectum* 1990;33:639.
40. Sugihara K, Muto T, Kamiya J, et al: Gardner's syndrome associated with periampullary carcinoma, duodenal and gastric adenomatosis. *Dis Colon Rectum* 1982;25:766.
41. Yao T, Iida M, Watanabe H, et al: Duodenal lesions in familial polyposis of the colon. *Gastroenterology* 1977;73:1086.

42. Jarvinen H, Nyberg M, Peltokallio P: Upper gastrointestinal tract polyps in familial adenomatosis coli. *Gut* 1983;24:333.

43. Alexander JR, Andrews JM, Buchi KN, et al: High prevalence of adenomatous polyps of the duodenal papilla in familial adenomatous polyposis. *Dig Dis Sci* 1989;34:167.

44. Odze RD: Epithelial proliferation and differentiation in flat duodenal mucosa of patients with familial adenomatous polyposis. *Mod Pathol* 1995;8:648.

45. Bertoni G, Sassatelli R, Nigrisoli E, et al: First observation of microadenomas in the ileal mucosa of patients with familial adenomatous polyposis and colectomies. *Gastroenterology* 1995;109:374.

46. Shepherd NA, Jass JR, Duval I, et al: Restorative proctocolectomy with ileal reservoir; pathological and histochemical study of mucosal biopsy specimens. *J Clin Pathol* 1987;40:601.

47. Stryker SJ, Carney JA, Dozois RR: Multiple adenomatous polyps arising in a continent reservoir ileostomy. *Int J Colorect Dis* 1987;2:43.

48. Iida M, Yao T, Itoh H, et al: Natural history of fundic gland polyposis in patients with familial adenomatosis coli Gardner's syndrome. *Gastroenterology* 1985;89:1021.

49. Hofgärtner WT, Thorp M, Ramus MW, et al. Gastric adenocarcinoma associated with fundic gland polyps in a patient with attenuated familial adenomatous polyposis. *Am J Gastroenterol* 1999;94:2276.

50. Zwick A, Munit M, Ryan CK, et al: Gastric adenocarcinoma and dysplasia in fundic gland polyps of a patient with attenuated adenomatous polyposis coli. *Gastroenterology* 1997;113:659.

51. Bülow S: The risk of developing rectal cancer after colectomy and ileorectal anastomosis in Danish patients with polyposis coli. *Dis Colon Rectum* 1984;227:726.

52. Watne AL, Carrier JM, Durham JP, et al: The occurrence of carcinoma of the rectum following ileoproctostomy for familial polyposis. *Ann Surg* 1983;197:550.

53. Luk GD, Baylin SB: Ornithine decarboxylase as a biologic marker in familial colonic polyposis. *N Engl J Med* 1984;311:80.

54. Potten CS, Kellett M, Rew DA, Roberts SA: Proliferation in human gastrointestinal epithelium using bromodeoxyuridine in vivo—data for different sites, proximity to a tumour, and polyposis-coli. *Gut* 1992;33:524.

55. Sasaki M, Sugio K, Sasazuki T: K-ras activation in colorectal tumours from patients with familial polyposis coli. *Cancer* 1990;65:2576.

56. Sasaki M, Okamoto M, Sato C, et al: Loss of constitutional heterozygosity in colorectal tumors from patients with familial polyposis coli and those with nonpolyposis colorectal carcinoma. *Cancer Res* 1989;49:4402.

57. Kikuchi-Yanoshita R, Konishi M, Fukunari H, et al: Loss of expression of DCC gene during progression of colorectal carcinomas in familial adenomatous polyposis and non-familial adenomatous polyposis patients. *Cancer Res* 1992;52:3801.

58. Kikuchi-Yanoshita R, Konishi M, Ito S, et al: Genetic changes of both p53 alleles associated with the conversion from colorectal adenoma to early carcinoma in familial adenomatous polyposis and non-familial adenomatous polyposis patients. *Cancer Res* 1992;52:3965.

59. Sugio K, Kurata S, Sasaki M, et al: Differential expression of c-myc gene and c-fos gene in premalignant and malignant tissues from patients with familial polyposis coli. *Cancer Res* 1988;48:4855.

60. Konishi M, Kikuchi-Yanoshita R, Tanaka K, et al: Molecular nature of colon tumors in hereditary nonpolyposis colon cancer, familial polyposis, and sporadic colon cancer. *Gastroenterology* 1996;111:307.

61. Giardiello FM, Hamilton SR, Krush AJ, et al: Nasopharyngeal angiofibroma in patients with familial adenomatous polyposis. *Gastroenterology* 1993;105:1550.

62. Harach HR, Williams GT, Williams ED: Familial adenomatous polyposis associated thyroid carcinoma: a distinct type of follicular cell neoplasm. *Histopathology* 1994;25:549.

63. Jones IT, Jagelman DG, Fazio VW, et al: Desmoid tumors in familial polyposis coli. *Ann Surg* 1986;204:94.

64. Richards RC, Rogers SW, Gardner EJ: Spontaneous mesenteric fibromatosis in Gardner's syndrome. *Cancer* 1981;47:597.

65. Lynch HT, Fitzgibbons R Jr: Surgery, desmoid tumors, and familial adenomatous polyposis: case report and literature review. *Am J Gastroenterol* 1996;91:2598.

66. Sturt NJ, Gallagher MC, Bassett P, et al: Evidence for genetic predisposition to desmoid tumours in familial adenomatous polyposis independent of the germline APC mutation. *Gut* 2004;53:1832.

67. Klein WA, Miller HH, Anderson M, DeCosse JJ: The use of indomethacin, sulindac, and tamoxifen for the treatment of desmoid tumors associated with familial polyposis. *Cancer* 1987;12:2863.

68. Lanari A: Effect of progesterone on desmoid tumors (aggressive fibromatosis). *N Engl J Med* 1983;309:1523.

69. Sen-Gupta S, Van der Luijt RB, Bowles LV, et al: Somatic mutation of APC gene in desmoid tumor in familial adenomatous polyposis. *Lancet* 1993;342:552.

70. Dangel A, Meloni AM, Lynch HT, Sandberg AA: Deletion (5q) in a desmoid tumor of a patient with Gardner's syndrome. *Cancer Genet Cytogenet* 1994;78:94.

71. Kropilak M, Jagelman DH, Fazio VW, et al: Brain tumors in familial adenomatous polyposis. *Dis Colon Rectum* 1989;32:778.

72. Jarvis L, Bathurst N, Mohan D, Beckly D: Turcot's syndrome—a review. *Dis Colon Rectum* 1988;31:907.

73. Lasser DM, Devivo, DC, Garvin J, Wilhelmsen KC: Turcot's syndrome: evidence for linkage to the adenomatous polyposis coli (APC) locus. *Neurology* 1994;44:1083.

74. Lewis J, Ginsberg A, Toomey K: Turcot's syndrome. Evidence for autosomal dominant inheritance. *Cancer* 1983;51:524.

75. Hamilton SR, Liu B, Parsons RE: The molecular basis of Turcot's syndrome. *N Engl J Med* 1995;332:839.

76. Rochlitz CF, Heide I, de Kant E, et al: Molecular alterations in a patient with Turcot's syndrome. *Br J Cancer* 1993;68:519.

77. Bigner SH, Mark J, Burger PC, et al: Specific chromosomal abnormalities in malignant human gliomas. *Cancer Res* 1988;48:405.

78. Al-Tassan N, Chmiel HN, Maynard J, et al: Inherited variants of MYH associated with somatic G:C → T:A mutations in colorectal tumors. *Nat Genet* 2002;30:227.

79. Isidro G, Laranjeira F, Pires A, et al: Germline MUTYH (MYH) mutations in Portuguese individuals with multiple colorectal adenomas. *Hum Mutat* 2004;24:353.

80. Sieber OM, Lipton L, Crabtree M, et al: Multiple colorectal adenomas, classic adenomatous polyposis, and germ-line mutations in MYH. *N Engl J Med* 2003;348:791.

81. Bai H, Jones S, Guan X, et al: Functional characterization of two human MutY homolog (hMYH) missense mutations (R227W and V232F) that lie within the putative hMSH6 binding domain and are associated with hMYH polyposis. *Nucleic Acids Res* 2005;33:597.

82. Slupska MM, Baikalov C, Luther WM, et al: Cloning and sequencing a human homolog (hMYH) of the Escherichia coli mutY gene whose function is required for the repair of oxidative DNA damage. *J Bacteriol* 1996;178:3885.

83. Jones S, Lambert S, Williams GT, et al: Increased frequency of the k-ras G12C mutation in MYH polyposis colorectal adenomas. *Br J Cancer* 2004;90:1591.

84. Chiotoru ME, Cleary SP, Di Nicola N, et al: Association between biallelic and monoallelic germline MYH gene mutations and colorectal cancer risk. *J Natl Cancer Inst* 2004;96:1631.

85. Kambara T, Whitehall VL, Spring KJ, et al: Role of inherited defects of MYH in the development of sporadic colorectal cancer. *Genes Chromosomes Cancer* 2004;40:1.

86. Morson BC: *The Pathogenesis of Colorectal Cancer*. Philadelphia: WB Saunders, 1978.

87. Williams GT, Arthur JF, Bussey HJ, Morson BC: Metaplastic polyps and polyposis of the colorectum. *Histopathology* 1980;4:155.

88. Abeyasundara H, Hampshire P: Hyperplastic polyposis associated with synchronous adenocarcinomas of the transverse colon. *ANZ J Surg* 2001;71:686.

89. Hyman NH, Anderson P, Blasyk H: Hyperplastic polyposis and the risk of colorectal cancer. *Dis Colon Rectum* 2004;47:2101.

90. Leggett BA, Devereaux, B, Biden K, et al: Hyperplastic polyposis: association with colorectal cancer. *Am J Surg Pathol* 2001;25:177.

91. Ferrandez A, Samowitz W, DiSario JA, Burt RW: Phenotypic characteristics and risk of cancer development in hyperplastic polyposis: case series and literature review. *Am J Gastroenterol* 2004;99:2012.

92. Burt R, Jass JR: Hyperplastic polyposis. In: Hamilton SR, Aaltonen LA (eds). *Pathology and Genetics of Tumours of the Digestive System. World Health Organization Classification of Tumours*, Vol. 2. Lyon, France: IARC Press, 2000, p 135.

93. Chan AO, Issa JP, Morris JS, et al: Concordant CpG island methylation in hyperplastic polyposis. *Am J Pathol* 2002;160:529.

94. Whitelaw SC, Murday VA, Tomlinson IP, et al: Clinical and molecular features of the hereditary mixed polyposis syndrome. *Gastroenterology* 1997;112:327.

95. Jaeger EE, Woodford-Richens KL, Lockett M, et al: An ancestral Ashkenazi haplotype at the HMPS/CRAC1 locus on 15q13-q14 is associated with hereditary mixed polyposis syndrome. *Am J Hum Genet* 2003;72:1261.

96. Park WS, Park JY, Oh RR, et al: A distinct tumor suppressor gene locus on chromosome 15q21.1 in sporadic form of colorectal cancer. *Cancer Res* 2000;60:70.

97. Cao X, Eu KW, Kumarasinghe MP, et al: Mapping of hereditary mixed polyposis syndrome (HMPS) to chromosome 10q23 by genomewide high-density single nucleotide polymorphism (SNP) scan and identification of BMPR1A loss of function. *J Med Genet* 2006;43:e13.

98. Wirtzfeld DA, Petrelli NJ, Rodriguez-Bigas MA: Hamartomatous polyposis syndromes: molecular genetics, neoplastic risk, and surveillance recommendations. *Ann Surg Oncol* 2001;8:319.

99. Aaltonen LA, Jarvinen H, Gruber SB, et al: Peutz-Jeghers syndrome. In: Hamilton SR, Aaltonen LA (eds). *WHO International Classification of Tumors: Pathology and Genetics of Tumours of the Digestive System,* 3rd ed. Berlin: Springer-Verlag, 2000, pp 74–76.

100. Fernandez Seara MJ, Martinez Soto MI, Fernandez Lorenzo JR, et al: Peutz-Jeghers syndrome in a neonate. *J Pediatr* 1995;126:965.

101. Gass J, Glatzer R: Acquired pigmentation simulating Peutz-Jeghers syndrome: initial manifestation of diffuse uveal melanocytic proliferation. *Br J Ophthalmol* 1991;75:693.

102. Hemminki A, Tomlinson I, Markie D, et al: Localization of a susceptibility locus for Peutz-Jeghers syndrome to 19p using comparative genomic hybridization and targeted linkage analysis. *Nature Genet* 1997;15:87.

103. Jenne DE, Reimann H, Nezu J, et al: Peutz-Jeghers syndrome is caused by mutations in a novel serine threonine kinase. *Nature Genet* 1998;18:38.

104. Trojan J, Brieger A, Raedle J, et al: Peutz-Jeghers syndrome: molecular analysis of a three-generation kindred with a novel defect in the serine threonine kinase gene STK11. *Am J Gastroenterol* 1999;94:257.

105. Collins SP, Reoma JL, Gamm DM, Ohler MD: LKB1, a novel serine/threonine protein kinase and potential tumour suppressor, is phosphorylated by cAMP-dependent protein kinase (PKA) and prenylated in vivo. *Biochemistry* 2000;345:673.

106. Karuman P, Gozani O, Odze RD, et al: The Peutz-Jegher gene product LKB1 is a mediator of p53-dependent cell death. *Molec Cell* 2001;7:1307.

107. Tiainen M, Vaahtomeri K, Ylikorkala Y, Makela TP: Growth arrest by the LKBI tumor suppressor: induction of p21(WAF1/CIP1). *Hum Molec Genet* 2002;11:1497.

108. Miyaki M, Iijima T, Hosono K, et al: Somatic mutations of *LKB1* and β-catenin genes in gastrointestinal polyps from patients with Peutz-Jeghers syndrome. *Cancer Res* 2000;60:6311.

109. Young RH, Welch WR, Dickersin GR, Scully SE: Ovarian sex-cord tumor with annular tubules. Review of 74 cases including 27 with Peutz-Jeghers syndrome and four with adenoma malignum of the cervix. *Cancer* 1982;50:1384.

110. Giardiello FM, Welsh SB, Hamilton SR, et al: Increased risk of cancer in the Peutz-Jeghers syndrome. *N Engl J Med* 1987;316:1511.

111. Trau H, Schewach-Millet M, Fisher BK, Tsur H: Peutz-Jeghers syndrome and bilateral breast carcinoma. *Cancer* 1982;50:788.

112. Clement S, Efrusy ME, Dobbins WO, Palmer RN: Pelvic neoplasia in Peutz-Jeghers syndrome. *J Clin Gastroenterol* 1979;1:341.

113. Young R, Dickerson G, Scully R: A distinctive ovarian sex cord-stromal tumor causing sexual precocity in the Peutz-Jeghers syndrome. *Am J Surg Pathol* 1983;7:233.

114. Chen KTK: Female genital tract tumors in Peutz-Jeghers syndrome. *Hum Pathol* 1986;17:858.

115. Gilks CB, Young RH, Aguirre P, et al: Adenoma malignum (minimal deviation adenocarcinoma) of the uterine cervix: a clinicopathological and immunohistochemical analysis of 26 cases. *Am J Surg Pathol* 1989;13:717.

116. Seidman JD: Mucinous lesions of the fallopian tube—a report of seven cases. *Am J Surg Pathol* 1994;18:1205.

117. Young S, Gooneratne S, Straus F, et al: Feminizing Sertoli cell tumors in boys with Peutz-Jeghers syndrome. *Am J Surg Pathol* 1995;19:50.

118. Shintaku M, Baba Y, Fujiwara T: Intra-abdominal desmoplastic small cell tumour in a patient with Peutz-Jeghers syndrome: a pathologic anatomy and histopathology. *Virchows Arch A Pathol Anat Histol* 1994;425:211.

119. Morson BC: Some peculiarities in the histology of intestinal polyps. *Dis Colon Rectum* 1962;5:337.

120. Spigelman AD, Murday V, Phillips RKS: Cancer and the Peutz-Jeghers syndrome. *Gut* 1989;30:1588.

121. Dunlop MG: Guidance on large bowel surveillance for hereditary nonpolyposis colorectal cancer, familial adenomatous polyposis, juvenile polyposis, and Peutz-Jeghers syndrome. *Gut* 2002;51:V21.

122. Hemminki A: The molecular basis and clinical aspects of Peutz-Jeghers syndrome and sporadic colon cancer. *Cancer Res* 1998;58:4799.

123. Ballhausen WG, Gunther K: Genetic screening for Peutz-Jeghers syndrome. *Expert Rev Mol Diagn* 2003;3:471.

124. Lowichik A, Jackson WD, Coffin CM: Gastrointestinal polyposis in childhood: clinicopathologic and genetic features. *Pediatr Devel Pathol* 2003;6:371.

125. Schreibman IR, Baker M, Amos C, McGarrity TJ: The hamartomatous polyposis syndromes: a clinical and molecular review. *Am J Gastroenterol* 2005;100:476.

126. Corredor J, Wambach J, Barnard J: Gastrointestinal polyps in children: advances in molecular genetics, diagnosis, and management. *J Pediatr* 2001;138:621.

127. Scharf GM, Becker JH, Laage NJ: Juvenile gastrointestinal polyposis or the infantile Cronkhite-Canada syndrome. *J Pediatr Surg* 1986;21:953.

128. Desai DC, Murday V, Phillips RK, et al: A survey of phenotypic features of juvenile polyposis. *J Med Genet* 1998;35:476.

129. Agnifili A, Verzaro R, Gola P, et al: Juvenile polyposis: case report and assessment of the neoplastic risk in 271 patients reported in the literature. *Dig Surg* 1999;16:161.

130. Rozen P, Samuel Z, Brazowski E, et al: An audit of familial juvenile polyposis at the Tel Aviv Medical Center: demographic, genetic and clinical features. *Familial Cancer* 2003;2:1.

131. Friedl W, Kruse R, Uhlhaas S: Frequent 4-bp deletion in exon 9 of the SMAD4/MADH4 gene in familial juvenile polyposis patients. *Genes Chromosomes Cancer* 1999;25:403.

132. Zhou XP, Woodford-Richens K, Lehtonen R: Germline mutations in BMPR1A/ALK3 cause a subset of cases of juvenile polyposis syndrome and of Cowden and Bannayan-Riley-Ruvalcaba syndromes. *Am J Hum Genet* 2001;69:704.

133. Howe JR, Shellnut J, Wagner B, et al: Common deletion of SMAD4 in juvenile polyposis is a mutational hotspot. *Am J Hum Genet* 2002;70:1357.

134. Howe JR, Ahmed AF, Ringold J, et al: The prevalence of MADH4 and BMPR1A mutations in juvenile polyposis and absence of BMPR2, BMPR1B, and ACVR1 mutations. *J Med Genet* 2004;41:484.

135. Friedl W, Uhlhaas S, Schulmann K, et al: Juvenile polyposis: massive gastric polyposis is more common in MADH4 mutation carriers than in BMPR1A mutation carriers. *Hum Genet* 2002;111:108.

136. Howe JR, Roth S, Ringold JC, et al: Mutations in the SMAD4/DPC4 gene in juvenile polyposis. *Science* 1998;280:1086.

137. Coffin C, Dehner L: What is a juvenile polyp? An analysis based on 21 patients with solitary and multiple polyps. *Arch Pathol Lab Med* 1996;120:1032.

138. Pham BN, Villanueva RP: Ganglioneuromatous proliferation associated with juvenile polyposis coli. *Arch Pathol Lab Med* 1989;113:91.

139. Lowichik A, White FV, Timmons CF: Bannayan-Riley-Ruvalcaba syndrome: spectrum of intestinal pathology including juvenile polyps. *Pediatr Dev Pathol* 2000;3:155.

140. Coburn MC, Pricolo VE, DeLuca FG, Bland KI: Malignant potential in intestinal juvenile polyposis syndromes. *Ann Surg Oncol* 1995;2:386.

141. Heiss KF, Schaffner D, Ricketts RR, Winn K: Malignant risk in juvenile polyposis coli: increasing documentation in the pediatric age group. *J Pediatr Surg* 1993;28:118.

142. Bentley E, Chandrasoma P, Radin R, Cohen H: Generalized juvenile polyposis with carcinoma. *Am J Gastroenterol* 1989;11:1456.

143. Saul S, Raffensperger E: Juvenile polyposis: intramucosal signet-cell adenocarcinoma arising in a polyp at a gastrojejunostomy site. *Surg Pathol* 1988;1:2.

144. Jass JR, Williams CB, Bussey HJR, Morson BC: Juvenile polyposis—a precancerous condition. *Histopathology* 1988;13:619.

145. Sener SF, Miller HH, DeCosse JJ: The spectrum of polyposis. *Surg Gynecol Obstet* 1984;159:525.

146. Tsou HC, Ping XL, Xie XX, et al: The genetic basis of Cowden's syndrome: three novel mutations in PTEN/MMAC1/TEP1. *Hum Genet* 1998;102:467.

147. Starink TM, van der Veen JPW, Arwert F, et al: The Cowden syndrome: A clinical and genetic study in 21 patients. *Clin Genet* 1986;29:222.

148. Salem OS, Steck WD: Cowden's disease (multiple hamartoma and neoplasia syndrome): a case report and review of the English literature. *J Am Acad Dermatol* 1983;8:686.

149. Chen YM, Ott DJ, Wu WC, Gelfand DW: Cowden's disease: a case report and literature review. *Gastrointest Radiol* 1987;12:325.

150. Celebi JT, Tsou HC, Chen FF, et al: Phenotypic findings of Cowden syndrome and Bannayan-Zonana syndrome in a family associated with a single germline mutation in PTEN. *J Med Genet* 1999;36:360.

151. Marsh DJ, Kum JB, Lunetta KL, et al: PTEN mutation spectrum and genotype-phenotype correlations in Bannayan-Riley-Ruvalcaba syndrome suggest a single entity with Cowden syndrome. *Hum Molec Genet* 1999;8:1461.

152. Zhou XP, Waite KA, Pilarski R, et al: Germline PTEN promoter mutations and deletions in Cowden/Bannayan-Riley-Ruvalcaba syndrome result in aberrant PTEN protein and dysregulation of the phosphoinositol-3-kinase/Akt pathway. *Am J Hum Genet* 2003;73:404.

153. Gorlin R, Cohen M, Condon L, Burke B: Bannayan-Riley-Ruvalcaba Syndrome. *Am J Med Genet* 1992;44:307.

154. Lowichik A, White FV, Timmons CF, et al: Bannayan-Riley-Ruvalcaba syndrome: spectrum of intestinal pathology including juvenile polyps. *Pediatr Dev Pathol* 2000;3:155.

155. Katayama Y, Kimura M, Konn M: Cronkhite-Canada syndrome associated with a rectal cancer and adenomatous changes in colonic polyps. *Am J Surg Pathol* 1985;9:65.

156. Daniel ES, Ludwig SL, Lewin KJ, et al: The Cronkhite-Canada syndrome: an analysis of clinical and pathologic features and therapy in 55 patients. *Medicine* 1982;61:293.

157. Burke A, Sobin L: The pathology of Cronkhite-Canada polyps. *Am J Surg Pathol* 1989;13:940.

158. Allibone RO, Nanson JK, Anthony PP: Multiple and recurrent inflammatory fibroid polyps in a Devon family ("Devon polyposis syndrome"): an update. *Gut* 1992;33:1004.

159. Vasen HF, Mecklin JP, Khan P, Lynch HT: The International Collaborative Group on Hereditary Nonpolyposis Colorectal Cancer (ICG-HNPCC). *Dis Colon Rectum* 1991;34:424.

160. Rodriguez-Bigas MA, Boland CR, Hamilton SR, et al: A National Cancer Institute Workshop on Hereditary Nonpolyposis Colorectal Cancer Syndrome: meeting highlights and Bethesda guidelines. *J Natl Cancer Inst* 1997;89:1758.

161. Umar A, Boland CR, Terdiman JP, et al: Revised Bethesda guidelines for hereditary nonpolyposis colorectal cancer (Lynch syndrome) and microsatellite instability. *J Natl Cancer Inst* 2004;96:261.

162. Samowitz WS, Curtin K, Lin HH, et al: The colon cancer burden of genetically defined hereditary nonpolyposis colon cancer. *Gastroenterology* 2001;121:830.

163. Wagner A, Barrows A, Wijnen JT, et al: Molecular analysis of hereditary nonpolyposis colorectal cancer in the United States high mutation detection rate among clinically selected families and characterization of an American founder genomic deletion of the MSH2 gene. *Am J Hum Genet* 2003;72:1088.

164. Merg A, Lynch HT, Lynch JF, Howe JR: Hereditary colorectal cancer—part II. *Curr Probl Surg* 2005;42:267.

165. Hampel H, Stephens JA, Pukkala E, et al: Cancer risk in hereditary nonpolyposis colorectal cancer syndrome: later age of onset. *Gastroenterology* 2005;129:415.

166. Jenkins MA, Baglietto L, Dowty JG, et al: Cancer risks for mismatch repair gene mutation carriers: a population-based early onset case-family study. *Clin Gastroenterol Hepatol* 2006;4:489.

167. Lorenzo Bermejo JL, Eng C, Hemminki K: Cancer characteristics in Swedish families fulfilling criteria for hereditary nonpolyposis colorectal cancer. *Gastroenterology* 2005;129:1889.

168. Aaltonen LA, Peltomaki P, Mecklin JP, et al: Replication errors in benign and malignant tumors from hereditary nonpolyposis colorectal cancer patients. *Cancer Res* 1994;54:1645.

169. Lothe RA, Peltomaki P, Meling GI, et al: Genomic instability in colorectal cancer: relationship to clinicopathological variables and family history. *Cancer Res* 1993;53:5849.

170. Boland CR, Thibodeau SN, Hamilton SR, et al: A National Cancer Institute workshop on microsatellite instability for cancer detection and familial predisposition: development of international criteria for the determination of microsatellite instability in colorectal cancer. *Cancer Res* 1998;58:5248.

171. Rigau V, Sebbagh N, Olschwang S, et al: Microsatellite instability in colorectal carcinoma: the comparison of immunohistochemistry and molecular biology suggests role for hMLH6 immunostaining. *Arch Pathol Lab Med* 2003;127:694.

172. Hampel H, Frankel WL, Martin E, et al: Screening for the Lynch syndrome (hereditary nonpolyposis colorectal cancer). *N Eng J Med* 2005;352:1851.

173. Thibodeau SN, French AJ, Roche PC, et al: Altered expression of hMSH2 and hMLH1 in tumors with microsatellite instability and genetic alterations in mismatch repair genes. *Cancer Res* 1996;56:4836.

174. Watson P, Vasen HF, Mecklin JP, et al: The risk of endometrial cancer in hereditary nonpolyposis colorectal cancer. *Am J Med* 1994;96:516.

175. Hamilton SR, Liu B, Parson RE, et al: The molecular basis of Turcot's syndrome. *N Engl J Med* 1995;332:839.

176. De Jong AE, Morreau H, Van Puijenbroek, M, et al: The role of mismatch repair gene defects in the development of adenomas in patients with HNPCC. *Gastroenterology* 2004;126:42.

177. Jass JR, Stewart SM: Evolution of hereditary non-polyposis colorectal cancer. *Gut* 1992;33:783.

178. Jass JR, Cottier DS, Pokos V, et al: Mixed epithelial polyps in association with hereditary non-polyposis colorectal cancer providing an alternative pathway of cancer histogenesis. *Pathology* 1997;29:28.

179. Svendsen LB, Bulow S, Mellemgaard A: Metachronous colorectal cancer in young patients: expression of the hereditary non-polyposis colorectal cancer syndrome? *Dis Colon Rectum* 1991;34:790.

180. Lynch HT, de la Chapelle A: Genetic susceptibility to non-polyposis colorectal cancer. *J Med Genet* 1999;36:801.

181. Barnetson RA, Tenesa A, Farrington SM, et al: Identification and survival of carriers of mutations in DNA mismatch-repair genes in colon cancer. *N Engl J Med* 2006;354:2815.

182. Jass JR: Colorectal adenomas in surgical specimens from subjects with hereditary non-polyposis colorectal cancer. *Histopathology* 1995;27:263.

183. Yearsley M, Hampel H, Lehman A, et al: Histologic features distinguish microsatellite-high from microsatellite-low and microsatellite-stable colorectal carcinomas, but do not differentiate germline mutations from methylation of the MLH1 promoter. *Hum Pathol* 2006;37:831.

184. Winawer SJ, Zauber AG, Fletcher RH, et al: Guidelines for colonoscopy surveillance after polypectomy: a consensus update by the US multisociety task force on colorectal cancer and the American Cancer Society. *Gastroenterology* 2006;130:1872.

185. Burke W, Petersen G, Lynch P, et al: Recommendations of follow-up care of individuals with an inherited predisposition to cancer. I. Hereditary nonpolyposis colon cancer. Cancer Genetic Studies Consortium. *JAMA* 1997;277:915.

186. Lynch HT, Lynch J: Lynch syndrome: genetics, natural history, genetic counseling, and prevention. *J Clin Oncol* 2000;18:19S.

187. Alessi E, Brambilla L, Luporini G, et al: Multiple sebaceous tumors and carcinomas of the colon. Torre syndrome. *Cancer* 1985;55:2566.

188. Paraf F, Sasseville D, Watters AK, et al: Clinicopathological relevance of the association between gastrointestinal and sebaceous neoplasms: the Muir-Torre syndrome. *Hum Pathol* 1995;26:422.

189. Machin P, Catasus L, Pons C, et al: Microsatellite instability and immunostaining for MSH-2 and MLH1 in cutaneous and internal tumors from patients with Muir-Torre syndrome. *J Cutan Pathol* 2002;29:415.

190. Mangold E, Pagenstecher C, Leister M, et al: A genotype-phenotype correlation in HNPCC: strong predominance of MSH2 mutations in 41 patients with Muir-Torre syndrome. *J Med Genet* 2004;41:567.

191. Ponti G, Ponz de Leon M: Muir-Torre syndrome. *Lancet Oncol* 2005;6:980.

192. Cannon-Albright LA, Thomas A, Goldgar DE, et al: Familiality of cancer in Utah. *Cancer Res* 1994;54:2378.

193. Sorensen SA, Jensen OA, Klinken L: Familial aggregation of neuroectodermal and gastrointestinal tumors. *Cancer* 1983;52:1977.

The Nonneoplastic Colon

The large intestine is divided into the appendix; the cecum; the ascending, transverse, descending, and sigmoid colon; and the rectum (Fig. 13.1). Since both the appendix and the anus are distinctive and their diseases differ from the remainder of the large intestine, they are treated separately.

The colon functions as a reservoir, and it also moves its contents caudally toward the anus. As the intestinal contents travel distally, water and electrolytes are absorbed, and some substances are secreted into the lumen. The histologic organization of the colon reflects its functions (i.e., resorption of water and elimination of undigested material, feces). Elimination is facilitated by the secretion of mucus that lubricates and protects the mucosa from the luminal contents. Like the small intestine, the large intestine has immune and endocrine functions. The immune functions are served by the prominent lymphoid follicles in the appendix and rectum and by immune cells in the lamina propria. Endocrine functions are served by a heterogeneous population of endocrine cells.

EMBRYOLOGY

The embryologic midgut gives rise to the proximal colon, including the cecum, the ascending colon, and the first two thirds of the transverse colon. The rest of the colon and rectum derive from the embryologic hindgut. The colon comes to lie in its final position in the abdominal cavity through a complex series of rotations (Fig. 13.2). Early in development, midgut lengthening results in the formation of a dorsal mesentery that suspends the developing intestine from the posterior abdominal wall. Rapid elongation of the midgut results in formation of the primary intestinal loop, which communicates with the yolk sac via the vitellointestinal duct. Concurrent rapid hepatic growth decreases the space in the abdominal cavity, causing the midgut to herniate into the umbilical coelom during the sixth embryonic week. The cecum becomes recognizable as a small diverticulum of the caudal limb of the midgut at approximately 6 weeks' gestation. The midgut returns to the abdominal cavity during the third fetal month. The small intestine enters the abdomen first, followed by the cecum. During re-entry,

the gut rotates an additional 180 degrees, so that the cecum comes to lie in the right upper quadrant. Later, elongation of this portion of the gut results in cecal descent to the right lower quadrant and formation of the ascending colon. The postsplenic colon is pushed to the left side and lies anterior to the small intestine.

Upper hindgut development follows that of the midgut. The hindgut develops into the left transverse colon, descending colon, sigmoid colon, rectum, and upper anal canal. The descending colon becomes fixed. The sigmoid retains a mesocolon that reduces in length as other hindgut derivatives become fixed in the abdomen. The distal hindgut enters the cloaca, the structure that ultimately forms the anal canal and some of the urogenital structures.

At the 20-mm developmental stage the colon is lined by villi resembling those in the small bowel. As the fetus continues to grow, they thicken, shorten, and then disappear until the mucosa resembles that found in the adult.

GROSS FEATURES

The large intestine is a hollow muscular organ that begins at the ileocecal valve and ends at the anus (Fig. 13.1). It includes the cecum, with the attached vermiform appendix; the ascending, transverse, descending, and sigmoid colon; and the rectum. It measures approximately 150 cm (5 feet) in length. The diameter of the large intestine is greater than the small intestine. The cecum has the largest diameter and is nestled in the right iliac fossa. The diameter of the colon decreases as it proceeds distally so that the lumen of the sigmoid is considerably smaller than that of the cecum. In the rectum, the diameter widens again slightly.

The junction of the colon with the rectum is not a precise anatomic point, and it is loosely described as the *rectosigmoid*. This area lies just below the sacral promontory, approximately 15 cm from the anal verge. The rectum is divided into two parts: An upper part that extends from the third sacral vertebrae to the pelvic diaphragm, and a lower part, or anal canal, that continues down to the anus. The latter is discussed further in Chapter 15.

The ascending colon extends from the cecum to the hepatic flexure and lies retroperitoneally against the right

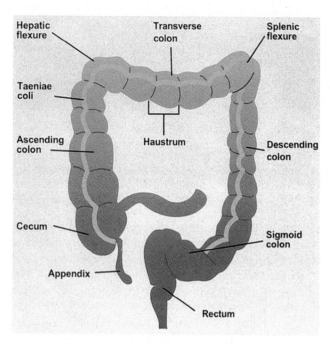

FIG. 13.1. Anatomy of the large intestine.

and may have a partial mesentery as it approaches the sigmoid colon in the left iliac fossa. The sigmoid colon lies within the peritoneal cavity and possesses a mesentery that is sometimes called the mesosigmoid or sigmoid mesocolon. The sigmoid colon may rest on the urinary bladder or uterus. As it passes through the peritoneal reflection, the sigmoid colon becomes the rectum. The rectum curves gently downward and anteriorly along the sacrococcygeal concavity onto the pelvic diaphragm, for a distance of about 12 cm. It abuts the prostate or the vagina inferiorly before turning posteriorly and caudad through the pelvic floor to become the anal canal at the dentate line. For most of its path, the colon lies against the posterior abdominal wall, forming a frame around the loops of small intestine.

The muscularis propria consists of longitudinal and circularly arranged smooth muscle fibers (Fig. 13.3). The outer longitudinal layer forms a continuous coat, which thickens into three flat bands called taenia coli. These run from the base of the appendix to the rectum, where the fibers fan out to form a continuous longitudinal coat (Fig. 13.4). Because the taeniae coli are not as long as the colon, they gather the wall into sacculations or haustra. Taenia are absent from the appendix and rectum. The circular muscle layer is continuous from the cecum to the anal canal, where it increases in thickness to form the internal anal sphincter. The circular muscle and taenia are thinner in the cecum than in other parts of the colon.

Between the sacculations, the mucosa and submucosa are thrown into crescenteric folds (plicae semilunares) (Fig. 13.5) that project into the lumen. The ileocecal valve consists of two of these folds. The submucosa resembles the submucosa of the rest of the gut. Lymphoid nodules straddle the boundary between the mucosa and the submucosa (Fig. 13.6) and may

posterior abdominal wall. It abuts the right lobe of the liver at the hepatic flexure and lies lateral to the gallbladder. The transverse colon is the longest segment of the large intestine, extending across the abdomen from the hepatic flexure to the splenic flexure. It attaches to the stomach by the gastrocolic ligament and contacts the second part of the duodenum, the pancreas, and the spleen. The omentum is attached to its anterior. The descending colon begins at the splenic flexure and lies retroperitoneally along the left posterior abdominal wall, abuts the lateral border of the left kidney,

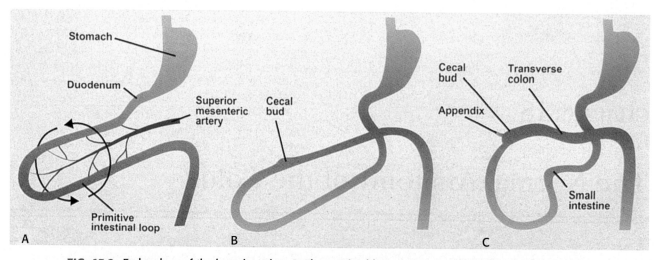

FIG. 13.2. Embryology of the large intestine. **A:** The proximal large intestine derives from the embryologic midgut, which herniates into the umbilical coelom during the sixth fetal week. The midgut loop then rotates around the axis of the superior mesenteric artery to lie in the position illustrated in **B. C:** Relative positions of the developing small and large intestines after return of the midgut loop to the abdominal cavity in the third month of gestation.

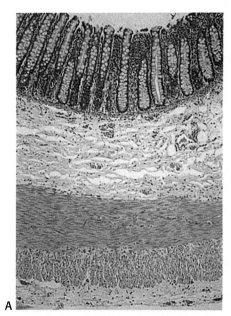
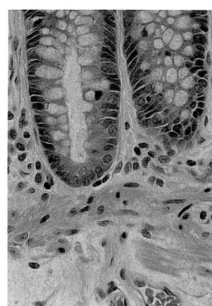

FIG. 13.3. Normal colon. **A:** The four layers of the colonic wall, including the mucosa, submucosa, muscularis propria, and serosa, are present. **B:** Lower portion of a normal crypt and the underlying muscularis mucosae.

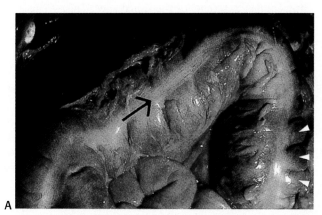
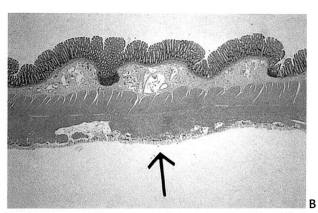

FIG. 13.4. Taeniae coli. **A:** Colon showing a longitudinal band that corresponds to a single taenia coli (*arrow*). Haustra are also identifiable (*arrowheads*). **B:** The whole mount section shows thickenings of the muscularis propria that correspond to the taenia coli (*arrow*).

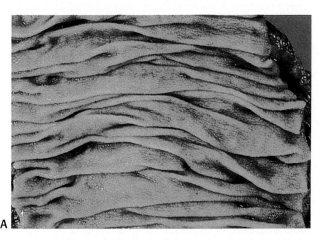
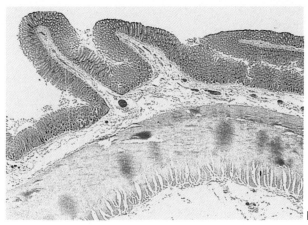

FIG. 13.5. Plicae semilunares. **A:** The colon is thrown into grossly visible folds. **B:** Histologically, these folds contain mucosa and submucosal extensions.

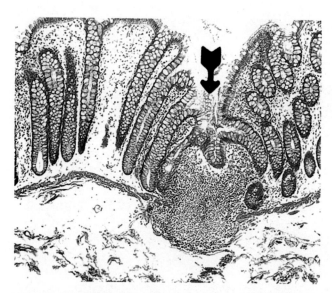

FIG. 13.6. A lymphoid follicle (*arrow*) spans the muscularis mucosae and extends into the submucosa. A normal mucosal cleft with nonparallel crypts lies above it. Trichrome stain.

be quite prominent, especially in children, producing a diffusely nodular mucosa.

The serosal surface is incomplete since the ascending and descending colon are retroperitoneal in location. The distal part of the rectum is not covered by peritoneum since it is below the peritoneal reflection. The serosa can contain lobules of fat that form pendulous projections called *appendices epiploicae* (Fig. 13.7).

INNERVATION

Like other portions of the gut, the large bowel is innervated by the autonomic nervous system. Parasympathetic nerves stimulate colonic motor activity, whereas sympathetic nerves inhibit motility and decrease blood flow to the mucosa. The cecum and the ascending and transverse portions of the colon are innervated by the vagus nerve, and the descending and sigmoid regions are innervated by pelvic postganglionic parasympathetic nerves. Sympathetic nerves emerge from the superior mesenteric ganglion to innervate the proximal two thirds of the colon. The remainder is innervated by sympathetic fibers derived from the inferior mesenteric ganglion. Sympathetic fibers innervating the distal rectum and anus derive from the hypogastric ganglion.

In the right colon and transverse colon the preganglionic cell bodies of the sympathetic supply lie in the lateral columns of the lower thoracic segments of the spinal cord. Axons from these bodies synapse in the celiac, preaortic, and superior mesenteric plexuses. Postganglionic fibers pass to the right and transverse colon along the superior mesenteric artery. The cell bodies for the parasympathetic system are in the vagal nuclei. Long preganglionic fibers synapse with the cells in the submucosal and myenteric plexuses. Afferent fibers arise from sensory endings in the colon wall that are sensitive to stretching and spasm. Sympathetic nerves supplying the distal colon lie in the lateral columns of the first three lumbar segments of the spinal cord. They synapse in the ganglia of the inferior mesenteric plexus. The postganglionic fibers then pass to the left colon and rectum via the inferior mesenteric vessels. Parasympathetic nerves arise from the second to the fourth sacral segments and they proceed to the left colon, rectum, and internal anal sphincter, where they anastomose with the intramural cell bodies.

Axons of the parasympathetic, sympathetic, and sensory enteric plexuses contribute to the fiber network and form connections with the intrinsic neurons. Many types of nerves are present and are ultrastructurally differentiated by the types of vesicles seen in the nerve endings. The types of nerves and their functions are discussed further in Chapter 10.

BLOOD SUPPLY

The cecum, ascending colon, and right part of the transverse colon (midgut-derived structures) are supplied by the superior mesenteric artery via the ileocolic, right colic, and middle colic arteries (Fig. 13.8). The left half of the transverse colon, the descending and sigmoid colon, and most of the rectum (hindgut-derived structures) receive their blood supply from the inferior mesenteric artery through the left colic, sigmoid, and superior rectal arteries (Fig. 13.8). The rectum is supplied by the superior rectal branch of the inferior mesenteric artery. Middle rectal arteries arise from the internal iliac vessels and the inferior rectal arteries come from the internal pudendal vessels. Anastomoses exist between the superior and inferior mesenteric arteries. Major branches of the ileocolic, right colic, left colic, and sigmoid arteries anastomose, forming a series of arches. These joined arches form a single continuous artery, referred to as the marginal artery of Drummond. The vasa recta, which supply the length of the colon, derive from this marginal artery. It is fed by

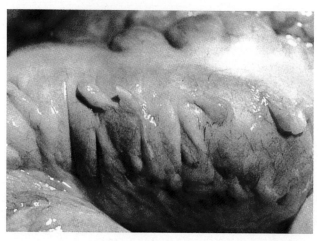

FIG. 13.7. The appendices epiploicae appear as fatty dewdrops on the external surface of the colon.

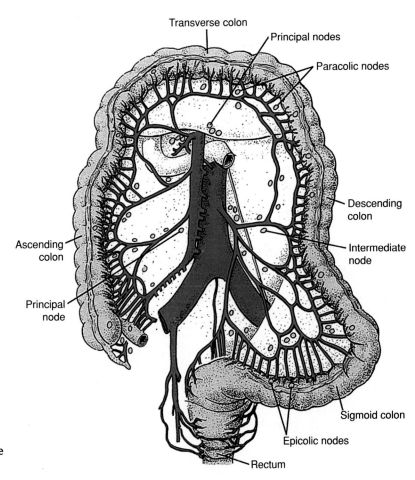

FIG. 13.8. Blood supply and lymphatic drainage of the large intestine.

branches of the superior mesenteric artery, the inferior mesenteric artery, and the hypogastric artery. The point of junction between superior mesenteric and inferior mesenteric arteries is known as the Griffith point. The junction between the inferior mesenteric artery and the hypogastric vessels is called the critical point of Sudeck. The colon is most vulnerable to ischemia at these two regions (1). In addition, the marginal artery is often small at the area of the splenic flexure, making this area particularly vulnerable to the consequences of reduced blood flow. There is a well-defined capillary network beneath the absorptive cells of the surface epithelium (Fig. 13.9).

Veins draining blood from the colon arise from a well-developed submucosal plexus and from a second less well-developed plexus outside the muscularis propria. The main veins correspond to the major arteries and are tributaries of the portal system. The venous drainage of the cecum, ascending colon, and part of the transverse colon is via the superior mesenteric vein. The left colon drains into the inferior mesenteric vein. These veins form part of the portal system with drainage from the gut going directly to the liver. The proximal rectum is drained by the superior hemorrhoidal vein that flows to the portal system via the inferior mesenteric vein. The middle and distal rectum are drained by the middle and inferior hemorrhoidal veins.

LYMPHATIC DRAINAGE

The lymphatics begin as a capillary plexus that wraps around the muscularis mucosae (Fig. 13.10). This plexus sends small branches into the mucosa to reach no higher than the bases of the crypts of Lieberkühn (2). These vessels pass into and through the submucosa and form another plexus around the muscularis propria. The efferent lymphatics from this system form increasingly larger channels, which eventually join lymphatic vessels in the mesocolon. There are generally four groups of external lymphatics: (a) epicolic, which lie on the colon; (b) paracolic, located along the marginal artery; (c) intermediate, located along the main colic vessels and their branches; and (d) principal, located along the superior and inferior mesenteric arteries.

The subserosal lymphatics unite, forming collecting lymphatic trunks in the mesentery proceeding centrally toward the paracolic lymph nodes along the marginal vascular arcades. The serosa also contains small foci of lymphocytes. Efferent collecting lymphatic trunks proceed from the paracolic lymph nodes to the intermediate lymph nodes in the midmesentery, near the bifurcations of colic vessels. From the intermediate group, large efferents reach the central or principal lymph node at the root of the mesentery draining next to the inferior and superior mesenteric lymph nodes

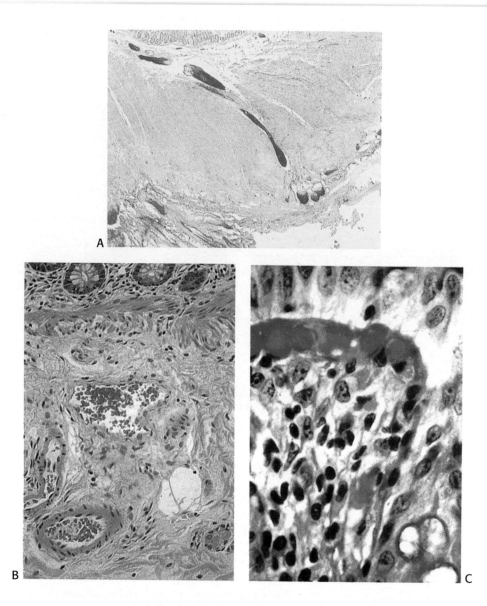

FIG. 13.9. Colonic blood supply. **A:** A penetrating artery extends from the serosa through the muscularis propria into the submucosa. **B:** Large vessels are present in the submucosa. **C:** A proliferation of capillaries is seen immediately beneath the luminal surface.

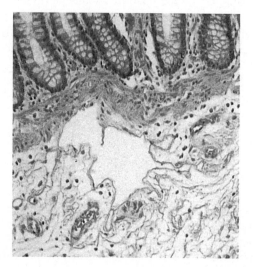

FIG. 13.10. A dilated lymphatic is seen immediately beneath the muscularis mucosae.

and then into the cisterna chyli. The rectosigmoid mesentery is the most richly supplied with lymphatics and lymph nodes.

HISTOLOGIC FEATURES

The mucosa is smooth and without folds except distally in the rectum. There are no villi. The mucosal surface is flat and regular with interconnected territories containing 10 to 100 parallel crypt mouths measuring 25 to 50 μm in diameter, separated by deep clefts (3). The orifices of the crypts appear as regularly arranged and spaced round depressions that have a uniform size and diameter. The clefts are known as the innominate grooves and they appear as small depressions surrounded by elevations of luminal cells. Visualization of the normal surface pattern has become more important with the increasing use of chromoendoscopy and magnifying

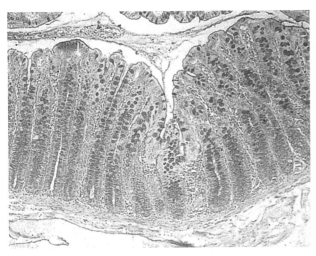

FIG. 13.11. Periodic acid–Schiff–stained section of colon demonstrating mucin secretion. Fine strands of mucoproteins cover the surface.

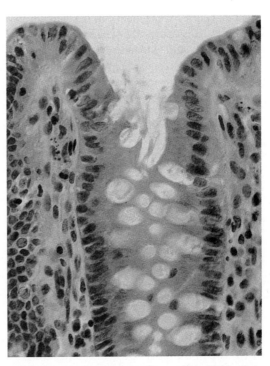

FIG. 13.12. Numerous goblet cells are identifiable lining the crypt. Goblet cells contain abundant mucin granules that are discharged into the colonic lumen by exocytosis.

endoscopy to detect neoplastic and preneoplastic lesions at the time of colonoscopy.

The crypts are straight tubular structures that lie absolutely parallel to one another and measure approximately 0.5 mm in length. They are unbranched, and extend from the lumen to the muscularis mucosae. However, sections through the crypts making up the innominate grooves demonstrate a branching or cloverleaf pattern. The epithelial lining is columnar in shape and contains an abundance of enterocytes and goblet cells and a small number of endocrine cells. Mucin flows from the crypt openings and covers the mucosal surface (Figs. 13.11 and 13.12) (3).

The colonic epithelium contains undifferentiated cells, goblet cells, absorptive cells, tuft cells, and endocrine cells (4). An orderly pattern of differentiation proceeds from the crypt base to the luminal surface (5). Undifferentiated stem cells in the crypt bases resemble those in the small intestine. The crypt sides are lined by mucus-secreting cells, immature absorptive cells, and rare endocrine cells. Most of the cells lining the middle and upper crypt are in the second replicative zone (i.e., the zone in which partially differentiated cells can still undergo mitosis). The surface epithelium contains goblet cells and mature absorptive cells (5). Cells in the upper 25% of the crypt do not divide but continue to differentiate to form mature absorptive or goblet cells. In addition, M cells are present in the epithelium overlying lymphoid follicles, and intraepithelial T lymphocytes lie scattered within the colonic epithelium.

Absorptive Cells

Absorptive cells outnumber goblet cells 3:1 (Fig 13.13) (6). Mature absorptive cells absorb water and electrolytes; have numerous short, regularly spaced microvilli; and are joined by junctional complexes and lateral desmosomes. The intercellular spaces are variably dilated depending on the physiologic

activity of the colon (5). A glycocalyx covers the microvilli on the luminal surface of the epithelial cells. Microvilli increase in number and elongate as the cells mature. Hairlike, loosely packed projections extend perpendicularly from the plasma membrane into the lumen and radiate from the microvilli. Small, round, 30- to 100-nm vesicles, called C bodies, are embedded among the filaments (7). Similar bodies are seen in the apical cytoplasm of mature absorptive cells. These are called R bodies and measure 106 to 250 nm in diameter. As the cells mature, there is a concomitant migration of the R bodies to the apex of the cell. The cytoplasmic microfilaments form a loose, stratified network that retains the same basic organization as that found in the small intestine (8). The apical cytoplasm contains a terminal web composed of microfilaments and core rootlets. Mitochondria, lipid droplets, lysosomes, apical vesicles, and round basally located nuclei are present in the cytoplasm (5). These cells secrete secretory component, which participates in the epithelial translocation of IgA as discussed in Chapter 6.

Goblet Cells

There are more goblet cells in the large intestine than in the small intestine. They are most abundant in the sigmoid colon and rectum, with approximately one goblet cell for every four columnar cells (Figs. 13.12 and 13.13). Their broad shape creates the false impression that they constitute the majority of the cells. As they differentiate, they migrate toward the mucosal surface and become progressively filled

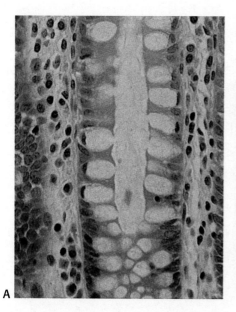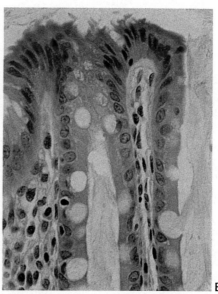

A   B

FIG. 13.13. Normal colon. **A:** Midportion of the crypt showing maturing goblet cells and absorptive cells. **B:** Free surface demonstrating the paucity of goblet cells and the presence of well-differentiated absorptive cells.

with mucus granules. The nucleus is compressed into a small dense structure in the basal region of the cell. Mucus secretion occurs throughout the life span of the cell. The membrane-bound mucin granules migrate toward the apical surface of the cell, where they are released by exocytosis. As the cells become more distended with mucin, the microvilli become sparser. The lateral cell surfaces are interlocked by cytoplasmic processes. Junctional complexes are present at the cell apices, and desmosomes are located at various points along the lateral surfaces.

The goblet cell secretes mucin derived from the carbohydrate–protein complex synthesized in the rough endoplasmic reticulum, which is then glycosylated, sulfated, and packaged in the Golgi. These mucins react strongly with Alcian blue at pH 2.5 and 1.0 (9). Sulfomucins predominate in the lower parts of the crypts, whereas carboxymucins are found in the upper crypts and surface epithelium (10).

Gastrointestinal mucins have been extensively studied in recent years, largely facilitated by the large number of immunohistochemical reagents that have become available to characterize them (11). Mucins are glycoproteins that are formed by the sequential addition of monosaccharides into chains attached to polypeptide backbones. Goblet cells secrete MUC1, MUC2, MUC3, and MUC4. Columnar cells secrete MUC1, MUC3, and MUC4 (12).

Other Cells

Tuft cells constitute approximately 1% to 2% of the colonic epithelium. They are characterized by an apical tuft of long, thick microvilli that project into the colonic lumen. The cores of these microvilli extend deep into the cytoplasm, sometimes reaching the basally located nucleus. The function of the tuft cells is unknown, but some speculate that they have a sensory or chemoreceptive function (13). The

colon has the least number of *endocrine cells* of any region of the gastrointestinal (GI) tract. This cell population is discussed further in Chapter 17. Scattered *Paneth cells* are present in the cecum and proximal ascending colon (Fig. 13.14). They are absent from the remainder of the normal large intestine.

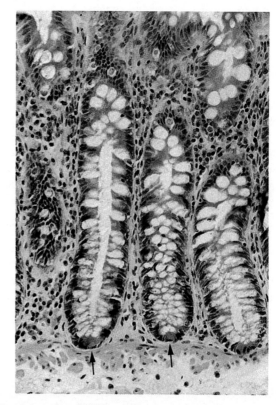

FIG. 13.14. Paneth cells (*arrows*) occur in the cecum, particularly in the area of the ileocecal valve. They are not found in other parts of the large intestine.

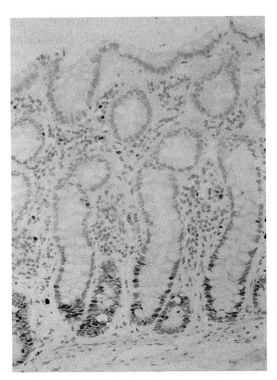

FIG. 13.15. Ki-67–immunostained section shows that the proliferating cells are restricted to the lower part of the crypts.

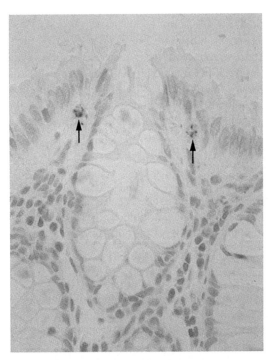

FIG. 13.16. Scattered apoptotic bodies lie in the superficial mucosa. They appear brown in this TUNEL assay (*arrows*).

Cell Renewal and Differentiation

Intestinal epithelial cells are one of the most actively replicating populations in the body. The process of intestinal cell renewal involves their proliferation, migration, differentiation, and sloughing or death. The clonogenic compartment consists of a pool of pluripotent GI stem cells and early undifferentiated progenitors that possess a multilineage clonogenic potential (14). Dividing cells lie in the proliferative compartment of the crypts, which is larger than that seen in the small intestine (Fig. 13.15) and involves the lowest two thirds of the crypts. Cells migrate from the proliferative zone toward the gut lumen. This migration takes 3 to 8 days (15). Normal colonic epithelium turns over approximately every 3 to 4 days. Undifferentiated stem cells in the crypt bases give rise to daughter cells committed to differentiate into columnar, goblet, endocrine, and tuft cells. Columnar, goblet, and tuft cells migrate with one another up the crypt wall onto the flat mucosal surface and they are sloughed into the lumen or undergo apoptosis (Fig. 13.16). Epithelial cells synthesize type IV collagen and laminin, contributing to the formation of the underlying basal lamina.

Pericryptal Myofibroblast Sheath

A pericryptal myofibroblast sheath invests the crypts, maintaining the normal morphology and cellular dynamics of the colonic mucosa (Figs. 13.17). The cells are a unique group of smooth musclelike fibroblasts. They arise by mitosis in the crypt base and migrate toward the mucosal surface. Platelet-derived growth factor and stem cell factor are responsible for

differentiating myofibroblasts from stem cells. Myofibroblasts play an important role in organogenesis, oncogenesis, inflammation repair, and fibrosis and they secrete extracellular matrix molecules, cytokines, and growth factors (16). The myofibroblast sheath maintains a state of differentiation similar to that of the adjacent epithelium and there is synchronized proliferation in the sheath and the epithelium (17).

These cells were originally thought to invest the crypts, but it is now clear that they form a syncytium throughout the lamina propria, merging with pericytes surrounding blood vessels that course through the tissues. In the crypts they are oval and scaphoid in appearance and overlap like shingles on

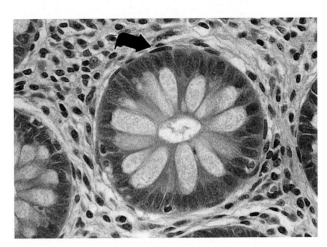

FIG. 13.17. Pericryptal myofibroblast sheath investing a cross section of the crypt of Lieberkühn (*arrow*).

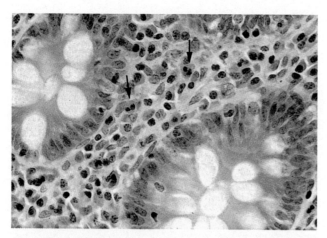

FIG. 13.18. Eosinophils occur scattered throughout the lamina propria (*arrows*).

a roof (18). At the surface they become stellate and appear like octopi sending cytoplasmic processes toward the basal lamina. Eventually these cells enter the lamina propria (18). There are close contacts between these cells and nerve terminals.

Lamina Propria

The lamina propria separates the crypts of Lieberkühn and consists of loose connective tissue containing reticulin fibers, fibroblasts, capillaries, and mononuclear cells, including macrophages, plasma cells, lymphocytes, and scattered mast cells (15). The lymphocytes are predominantly T cells; the plasma cells mainly produce IgA, but IgG- and IgM-producing cells are present as well. The area immediately under the epithelium primarily contains fibroblasts, myofibroblasts, and macrophages. Macrophages are predominantly located in the upper mucosa. They have abundant cytoplasmic vacuoles, lysosomes, and irregular nuclei. Mast cells are round with pleomorphic inclusions containing histamine. Eosinophils (Fig. 13.18), when present, can be recognized by their eosinophilic granules. Significant geographic and seasonal variation exists in the number of eosinophils present (19). Few if any neutrophils are seen. Isolated smooth muscle fibers may be seen in the lamina propria, and their presence may be highlighted by staining them with antibodies to actin and desmin.

The lamina propria contains solitary lymphoid nodules that may be large enough to displace the crypts and extend into the submucosa (Fig. 13.19). They may splay apart the fibers of the muscularis mucosae, or the muscularis mucosae may be discontinuous. These follicles have a ring of lymphocytes surrounding a central germinal center. Their size varies with age, being largest in young children and adolescents. The abundance of lymphoid cells and nodules reflects the presence of hundreds of bacterial species that inhabit the large intestine of healthy humans.

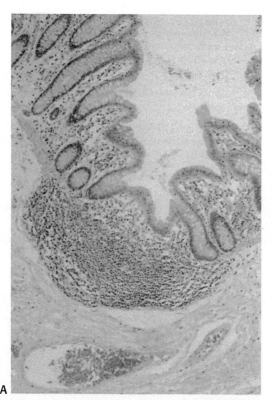

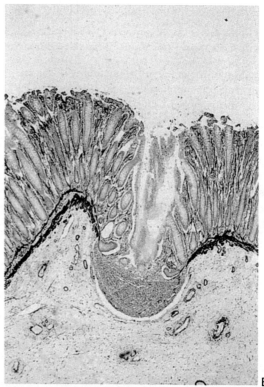

A

B

FIG. 13.19. A: Lymphoid follicles span the muscularis mucosae occupying both the mucosa and superficial submucosa. The overlying crypts are shortened, and the architecture is mildly distorted to accommodate the underlying lymphoid tissue. **B:** The muscularis mucosae is discontinuous near lymphoid follicles as demonstrated by an actin immunostain.

Lymphoglandular Complexes

Foci of lymphoid tissue straddle the muscularis mucosae, causing the fibers to splay around them. These domelike aggregates of gut-associated lymphoid tissue have been termed lymphoepithelial complexes or lymphoglandular complexes. They associate with a specialized surface and crypt epithelium referred to as dome epithelium, which participates in the translocation of antigens from the colonic lumen into the mucosa. The dome epithelium contains M cells. M cells are discussed in detail in Chapter 6. The structure of the lymphoid follicles is discussed further in Chapters 6 and 18.

Submucosa

The submucosa contains collagen, reticulin fibers, elastic tissue, nerves, fat, blood vessels, lymphatics, and small groups of ganglion cells located immediately below the muscularis mucosae and above the muscularis propria.

Muscularis Propria

The muscularis propria contains bands of smooth muscle fibers separated by connective tissue, including elastic and collagen fibers. The smooth muscle cells have a spindle cell shape and have pinocytotic vesicles along the cell membrane. The cells contain actin, myosin, and desmin filaments. Nerves penetrate throughout the muscular layers. The circular muscle is an expanding meshwork of interlinked bands. The muscle of the longitudinal layer, particularly the taeniae coli, is very tough and contains more collagen and elastic tissue than the circular muscle. The muscularis propria is pierced at regular intervals by the main arterial supply and venous drainage. Between the inner and outer muscle layers are the myenteric plexus and the CD34 and c-kit–positive interstitial cells of Cajal. Abundant connective tissue is present inside the inner circular layer and between it and the outer layer.

Serosa

The serosa is located just outside the muscle coat and contains blood vessels and lymphatics in a thin, connective tissue layer covered in many places by peritoneum. A well-defined elastic lamina exists beneath the peritoneal lining cells.

CONGENITAL ABNORMALITIES

Cecal Agenesis

Intestinal agenesis is the failure of a portion of the enteric tube to form. This disorder is rare, occurring in 1 in 50,000 pregnancies. Males are more commonly affected than females. It can affect the rectosigmoid (where it associates

with other major caudal anomalies) or the cecum. Cecal agenesis may result from misexpression of the endoderm-specific homeodomain gene *IDX-1* (20). IDX-1 binds to CDX-2, the caudal homeodomain factor important in intestinal differentiation (21).

Malrotations

Most large intestinal malpositions (Fig. 13.20) accompany small intestinal malrotations that occur when the contents of the physiologic abdominal hernia return to the abdominal cavity (see Chapter 6). In malrotations, the cecum usually fails to rotate and lies in the left iliac fossa, in the midline of the pelvis, or in the upper abdomen. The ascending colon retains its mesentery and runs upward, just to the left of the midline, to lie below the gastric curvature, where a loop of transverse colon connects to a normally situated descending colon. When rotation occurs beyond 180 degrees, the colon crowds into the left side of the abdomen or the cecum assumes an unfixed position in the right upper quadrant. The transverse colon and splenic flexure may lie posterior to the stomach and anterior to all or part of the pancreas, a location known as pancreatic interposition. They may also lie in a retrosplenic location (22). The entire malpositioned bowel remains unanchored, supported by a single mesentery with a very narrow base that predisposes it to undergo intestinal volvulus (22). The body attempts to correct the unstable state of the malpositioned intestine by forming fibrous bands or adhesions between abdominal

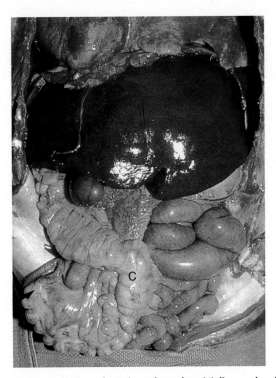

FIG. 13.20. Colonic malrotation. The colon (C) lies to the right of the midline and the small bowel lies to the left.

structures. These bands and adhesions become sources of future problems.

Atresia and Stenosis

Large intestinal atresias and stenoses (Fig. 13.21) occur far less commonly than esophageal, small intestinal, or anal atresias. Atresias of the ascending and transverse colon develop more commonly than distal ones. Colonic atresia may coexist with other gastrointestinal or laryngeal atresias, gastroschisis (23), and Hirschsprung disease (24).

Hereditary multiple gastrointestinal atresias affect the gut from the pylorus to the rectum. Patients with multiple intestinal atresias may also have biliary atresia (23) or immunodeficiency syndromes (25). Cardiovascular and other gastrointestinal malformations constitute the most common associated major abnormalities; these are a major cause of morbidity and mortality. Skeletal and limb defects account for the most common minor anomalies. Atresias and stenoses are described in detail in Chapter 6.

Duplications, Congenital Diverticula, and Enterogenous Cysts

Large intestinal duplications (Fig. 13.22), congenital diverticula, and enterogenous cysts are related defects (Fig. 13.23) that affect both children and adults. They resemble their small intestinal counterparts described in Chapter 6. There is partial or complete formation of a second luminal structure with its own mucosa and submucosa and incomplete separation of the muscular walls of the two tubes. The duplication always lies on the antimesenteric aspect of the bowel.

The extent of the duplicated bowel varies from an entire GI duplication to more segmental duplications. These uncommon lesions affect the cecum, transverse colon, and rectum. Hindgut duplications are rarer than other gastrointestinal duplications. As in the small bowel, duplications communicate with the main intestinal lumen in various ways as discussed in Chapter 6. Distal large intestinal duplications fall into two categories: Those associated with

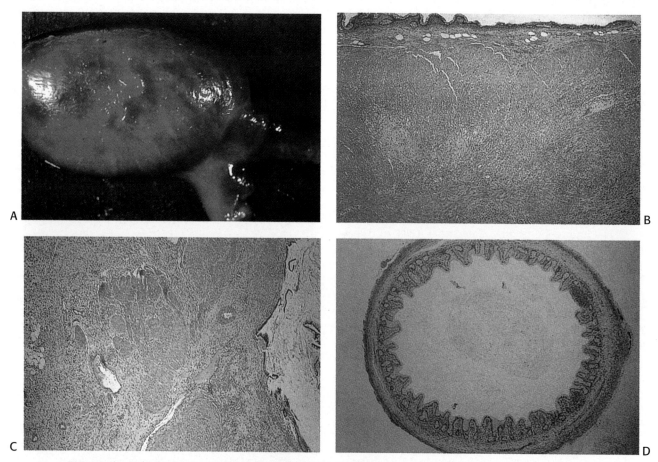

FIG. 13.21. Colonic atresia. **A:** The atresia is immediately adjacent to a colonic duplication. The bowel proximal to the duplication is massively dilated. **B:** Histologic section through an area of duplication showing the architectural abnormalities of the wall. **C:** At the right a small portion of the lumen is identified. It contains a vastly simplified colonic mucosa. **D:** Section through one of the duplicated segments of the bowel. The crypts are simplified, although the basic structure is preserved. Lymphoid follicles are present. The muscular coats are incomplete.

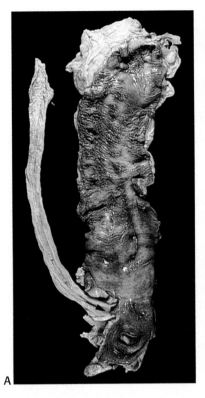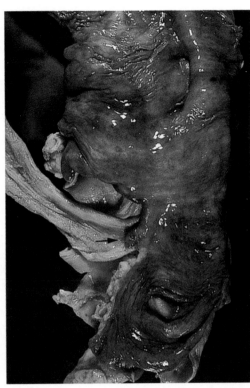

FIG. 13.22. Colonic duplication. **A** and **B** derive from an 81-year-old man who was autopsied and died of a myocardial infarction. He had a duplicated intestinal segment that emptied into the rectum *(arrow)*; it ended blindly proximally. B represents a higher magnification of A showing the junction with the rectum.

urinary bladder, urethral, or anorectal abnormalities and those that occur alone. Cystic rectal duplications are rare and may cause neonatal intestinal obstruction or rectal prolapse (26). Rarely carcinomas develop within them (27). Anorectal abnormalities are discussed in detail in Chapter 15. Most duplications present in the newborn period, although occasionally the lesions remain asymptomatic, only to be detected in adults.

Eighty percent of solitary congenital cecal diverticula occur within 2.5 cm of the ileocecal valve (28). Patients present with one of three distinct clinical syndromes: (a) distension, pressure, pain, and possibly perforation due to diverticulitis; (b) ulceration and bleeding, usually from the presence of acid-secreting heterotopic gastric mucosa; or (c) intussusception leading to sudden pain and bleeding.

Large intestinal enterogenous cysts resemble their small intestinal counterparts (see Chapter 6) and often project into the colonic lumen (Fig. 13.23). They are generally lined by normal colonic epithelium but may contain heterotopic tissues (usually gastric or pancreatic), and are prone to undergo intussusception.

Heterotopias

Heterotopic Gastric Mucosa

Large intestinal heterotopias are rare and usually complicate malformations, especially duplications. Ectopic gastric tissue is the most common large intestinal heterotopia

(Fig. 13.24) (29). When it contains acid-secreting epithelium, peptic ulceration develops in the adjacent colonic mucosa (29). Rectal heterotopic gastric mucosa may cause significant rectal bleeding or present as a polyp (30), a mass, or hemorrhoids. Symptoms include proctitis, pain, mild rectal bleeding, and proctalgia. Rarely, heterotopic gastric mucosa causes hematochezia and perianal or retrovesical fistulae (31). It usually associates with other congenital anomalies, including incomplete colonic rotation and vertebral body defects, Meckel diverticulum, rectal duplication, rectal diverticula, scoliosis, and megacolon (29–31).

Gastric heterotopias more or less recapitulate the normal fundic gastric architecture. The gastric epithelium usually contains chief cells, parietal cells, and foveolar cells (Fig. 13.24). Gastric endocrine cells are often absent, but when present reflect their gastric origin (32). Gastric heterotopia may coexist with ectopic respiratory epithelium, presumably representing the equivalent of heterotopic foregut (Fig. 13.24). It differs from the pyloric metaplasia in that it is an acquired lesion that develops in the setting of chronic inflammation. The "pyloric" tissue does not exhibit normal architectural patterns of the gastric antropyloric region.

Heterotopic Pancreas

Large intestinal heterotopic pancreatic tissue resembles gastric heterotopic pancreas seen elsewhere (see Chapter 4).

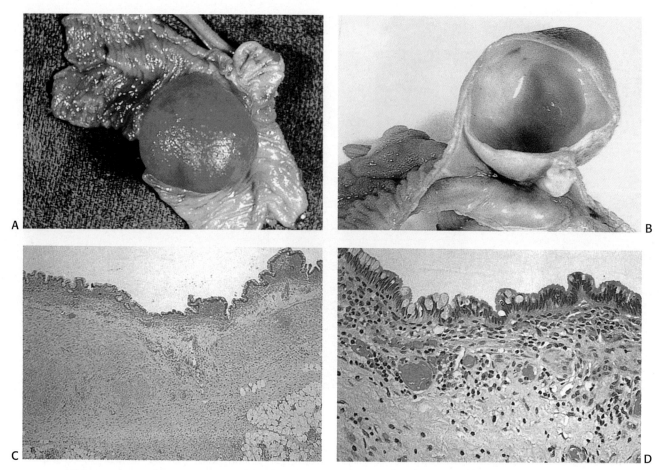

FIG. 13.23. Cecal enterogenous cyst. **A:** The cyst appears as an intraluminal polyp. The reddish color is due to the fact that the duplication caused a terminal ileal intussusception. **B:** Opened cyst. **C:** Lining of the cyst shows a thickened muscularis and a simplified mucosa. **D:** The cyst is lined by a simple layer of colonic epithelial cells. Crypts are absent.

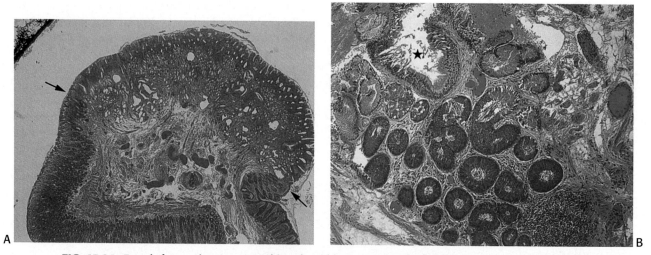

FIG. 13.24. Ectopic foregut in rectum. **A:** This polypoid lesion presented clinically as a hemorrhoid. The left and right sides of the photograph are lined by normal colorectal mucosa. The junction of the colorectal mucosa with gastric mucosa is indicated by *arrows*. The gastric epithelium consists of shortened pits without colonic crypts. It contains a glandular expansion; some of the glands are cystically dilated. **B:** Ciliated respiratory epithelium (*star*) is present along with the dark staining gastric glands. Prominent parietal cells are present. The clear cells are either antral or Brunner glands.

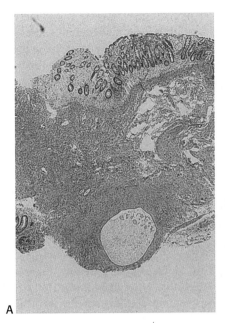 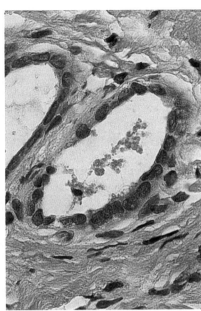

FIG. 13.25. Ectopic müllerian tissue in the rectum. **A:** The lesion presented as a submucosal mass. The majority of the lesion consists of a proliferation of fibromuscular tissue and a cyst. **B:** Higher magnification of the cysts shows a flattened ciliated epithelium surrounded by smooth muscle.

A

B

Seromucinous Heterotopia

Seromucinous tissue resembling salivary glands can occur in the rectal wall, either alone or associated with retrorectal cystic hamartomas. The lesions usually contain both serous and mucinous glands, although pure mucinous lesions have been described (33). The lesions may arise from vestiges of the postanal gut (34).

Innervation Abnormalities

A number of congenital innervation abnormalities affect the large intestine, usually presenting with intestinal pseudo-obstruction. These are discussed in detail in Chapter 10.

Cloacal Dysgenesis

In cloacal dysgenesis, the bladder and rectum fail to separate into distinct and separate structures. As a result, the common cloacal cavity is lined on one side by transitional epithelium and on the other by rectal mucosa. Infants who exhibit this anomaly often have dilated small intestinal segments that contain calcified concretions.

Embryonic Rests

Occasionally one receives a rectal biopsy or resection specimen in which residual nests of müllerian or mesonephric ducts that failed to involute lie scattered deep in the rectal wall. These embryologic remnants represent morphologic curiosities without any clinical significance (Fig. 13.25). Usually these lesions are clinically silent, but they may become symptomatic when secondary changes such as abscesses develop (35). Nephrogenic rests may also be present and these may be part of a multiple congenital anomaly syndrome (36).

ACQUIRED ABNORMALITIES

Diverticular Disease

Etiology

Colonic diverticular disease has become increasingly prevalent in the United States and other economically developed countries. Its incidence varies with national origin, cultural background, and diet, and its frequency increases with advancing age. In Western societies, it affects approximately 5% to 10% of the population over 45 years old and almost 80% of those over age 85 (37). The increased incidence of diverticular disease seen in Japan (38), South Africa (39), and Israel (40) in the last few decades results from incorporation of Western-type foods into the diet in these geographic regions.

Three major forms of diverticular disease exist: (a) one that is associated with classic intestinal muscle abnormalities; (b) a form that complicates connective tissue diseases (41); and (c) forms that complicate neural abnormalities (41). In the most common form of the disease, aging; elevated colonic intraluminal pressure; decreased dietary fiber consumption; consumption of beef, beef fat, and salt; lack of physical activity; and the presence of constipation correlate with its development (42,43). The prevalence of diverticular disease in Western countries increased abruptly 30 years after the introduction of grain milling factories, which decreased the fiber content in grain (44). Decreased luminal fiber and lower stool volume require more colonic segmentation to propel feces forward. The increased segmentation generates greater intraluminal pressures predisposing to diverticula formation. The colonic wall is weakest where penetrating arteries pierce the muscularis propria; this is where the diverticula typically form. Genetic factors may also play a role in the development of diverticular disease since diverticula arise in the right colon in Asians (45) and young patients, contrasting with sigmoid and left colonic involvement among Occidentals and older individuals (46,47). Alternatively, right-sided diverticulosis is a different disease than left-sided predominant diverticulosis. Some patients with solitary rectal diverticula have scleroderma (48). Children with colonic diverticulosis often have underlying Marfan or Ehlers-Danlos syndrome or an association with polycystic kidney disease (49).

Clinical Features

Most people with diverticulosis remain asymptomatic, only to be diagnosed incidentally (Fig. 13.26). Ten to twenty-five percent of patients become symptomatic (49), usually due to development of diverticular inflammation (diverticulitis). Diverticulosis affects both sexes equally (45), although complicated diverticulosis more frequently affects obese males (50). Children with diverticulosis often have an underlying connective tissue disease or polycystic renal disease (49). Acute diverticulitis varies in severity. Clinical features include lower abdominal pain, made worse by defecation, and signs of peritoneal irritation, including muscle spasm, guarding, rebound tenderness, fever, and leukocytosis. Symptom duration may be short and rectal examination may reveal the presence of a tender mass. Patients developing diverticulitis at an early age appear to have a more virulent form of the disease than other individuals (50).

Rectal bleeding, usually microscopic, affects 25% of patients. Significant bleeding occurs in 3% to 5%. Diverticular bleeding can be sudden in onset, painless, massive, and not accompanied by signs or symptoms of diverticulitis. Bleeding is more common in patients with diverticulosis complicating an underlying connective tissue disease. Although most diverticula arise on the left side, most diverticular bleeds complicate right-sided diverticula (51). The reason for this is unclear. One explanation may be that right-sided diverticula have wider necks than left-sided ones (51). The blood appears bright red, maroon, or melanic, especially if it comes from the right colon. Bleeding most often occurs from a single diverticulum and it stops spontaneously in 80% to 90% of patients (52). Some patients develop recurrent, left lower quadrant, colicky pain without clinical or pathologic evidence of acute diverticulitis. Alternating bouts of constipation and diarrhea result from muscle spasm. Most patients have elevated white blood cell counts, erythrocyte sedimentation rates, and C-reactive protein. When diverticulitis develops, the clinical features reflect host defenses and bacterial virulence.

Complications of diverticular disease are shown in Figure 13.27. They are more common among individuals ingesting nonsteroidal anti-inflammatory drugs (NSAIDs) (53), perhaps

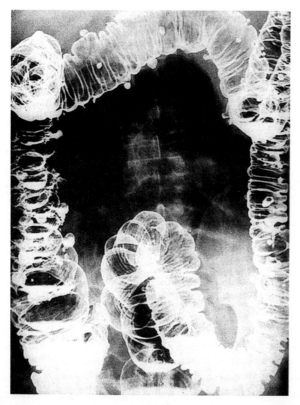

FIG. 13.26. Diverticulosis. Double-contrast barium enema demonstrates numerous small outpouchings representing colonic diverticula.

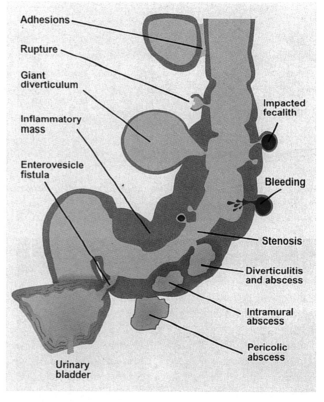

FIG. 13.27. Complications of diverticular disease (see text).

because the drugs mask the symptoms of earlier disease or because the NSAIDs interfere with natural mucosal defenses. Life-threatening complications are more common among patients with chronic renal failure or on high-dose steroid therapy (54,55). Complications include bleeding, perforation, fistula formation, peritonitis, obstruction, and peridiverticular abscesses. Fistulae complicate transmural inflammation. When fistulae develop, diverticular disease resembles Crohn disease (CD). Pseudodiverticula result from partial drainage of an abscess cavity into the colon. Patients may die from recurrent pericolic abscesses, peritonitis, fecal peritonitis, bleeding, or bowel obstruction (56).

Giant colonic diverticula are rare complications of diverticular disease. They are characterized by the formation of large, unilocular, gas-filled cysts measuring 7 cm or more in diameter (Fig. 13.28). Rare lesions measure over 27 cm in diameter. Giant diverticula typically develop on the mesenteric border of the sigmoid colon. Patients range in age from their mid-30s to their 80s. The lesions mimic enterogenous cysts (57).

Barium enema often establishes the diagnosis of diverticulosis. Early changes consist of the presence of fine mural serrations known as the *prediverticular state* or *myochosis*. "Saw tooth" luminal irregularities reflect associated muscle spasm. A contracted haustral pattern may also be seen. The sigmoid becomes shortened and distorted, causing it to acquire a concertinalike appearance with bunched, redundant mucosal folds. These can significantly narrow the colonic lumen and may cause obstruction with dilation proximal to the area of obstruction.

Pathologic Features

Diverticula are flask-shaped mucosal outpouchings that develop anywhere in the colon. In the Western world, 90% of

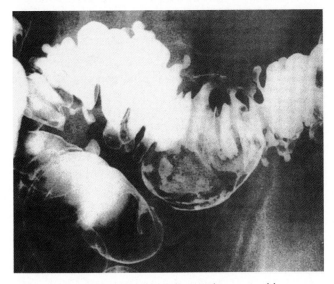

FIG. 13.28. Giant sigmoid diverticulum. Double-contrast enema of the sigmoid shows a large air-filled, barium-coated defect projecting from midsigmoid colon that represents a giant sigmoid diverticulum.

patients have involvement of the sigmoid colon and 20% of patients have pancolonic involvement. In contrast, Asians with diverticular disease develop multiple diverticula in the right colon (45). Diverticula usually form where the penetrating arteries pierce the muscular wall. Because the penetrating arteries enter on the mesenteric side of the two lateral taeniae coli, diverticula commonly appear as two parallel rows of beaded outpouchings along the bowel wall (Fig. 13.29). Appendices epiploicae also lie in this location and they may cover diverticula beneath them. The presence of pronounced muscular hypertrophy provides a clue to the presence of the diverticula, since the muscle thickening is the most consistent and striking abnormality. The taeniae coli appear thickened, developing an almost cartilaginous quality; the circular muscle becomes corrugated (Figs. 13.30 and 13.31) (58). The mouths of the diverticula lie between the muscular corrugations as they penetrate the muscularis propria (Fig. 13.32).

Because the diverticula often lack the muscular layer, secretions and fecal material easily enter them where they accumulate because they cannot be expelled (Fig. 13.29). Feces in the diverticular orifice block the outflow of secretions. The resulting obstruction and ulceration (with bacterial invasion) leads to diverticulitis via mechanisms resembling those seen in appendicitis (see Chapter 8). Mucosal ulceration by a fecalith leads to infection, diverticulitis, and bleeding.

Bleeding usually comes from uninflamed diverticula (Fig. 13.33) and the exact bleeding point is often difficult to identify. Occasionally, one is lucky enough to see a bleeding point or to obtain a histologic section through a diverticulum that identifies the bleeding source. Arteriolar rupture involves small vessels measuring <1 mm in diameter and always occurs on the side of the vessel facing the bowel lumen (Fig. 13.34) (59). The colonic wall may be thickened by pericolic fibrosis, grossly simulating a neoplasm or inflammatory bowel disease.

Tonic muscular contractions produce redundant, accordionlike, mucosal folds (Fig. 13.35), which appear as exaggerations of the mucosal folds or as larger, leaflike, smooth-surfaced "polyps" with broad bases (60). When multiple, they form two rows between the diverticula. Repeated trauma to the folds causes mucosal erosion and bleeding.

Colonoscopic examination in patients with diverticulosis-associated colitis shows confluent granularity and friability affecting the sigmoid colon surrounding the diverticular ostia. The colonic mucosa proximal and distal to the area of diverticulosis appears endoscopically normal. Not uncommonly, a diagnosis of Crohn disease is entertained due to the segmental nature of the colonoscopic findings. The biopsy can often be differentiated between the two entities if the pathologist is made aware of the presence of diverticulosis in the segment of interest.

The histologic features depend on whether one is dealing with simple diverticulosis or with its complications. The major pathologic features of uncomplicated diverticulosis

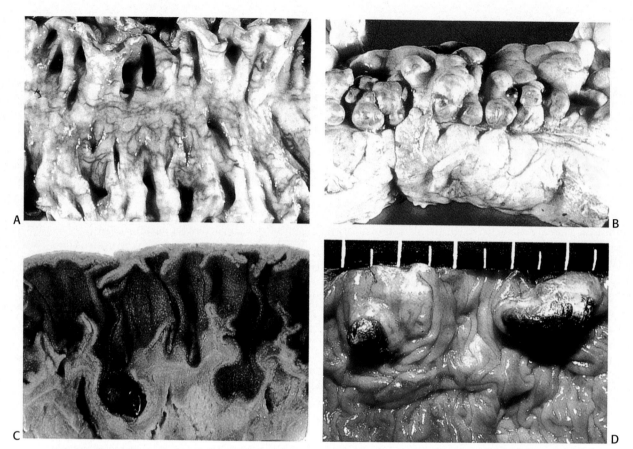

FIG. 13.29. Colonic diverticulosis. **A:** Opened bowel. Two parallel rows of numerous diverticular openings are easily visualized. **B:** The serosal aspect of the specimen in A. Numerous diverticular outpouchings are present. Their relationship with the appendices epiploica is also seen. **C:** Cross section of diverticulosis demonstrating the flasklike outpouchings extending into the colonic fat. **D:** Luminal surface showing two diverticula filled with feces.

include a thickened muscularis propria and the diverticular outpouchings (Fig. 13.32), usually lined by mucosa, muscularis mucosae, submucosa, and variable amounts of muscularis propria (Figs. 13.31 and 13.32). Early diverticula may still possess an outer lining of attenuated muscle. This disappears as the diverticula extend beyond the colonic wall. The mucosa appears normal or may show marked chronic inflammation, with or without acute inflammation producing a pattern sometimes referred to as "isolated sigmoiditis" (Fig. 13.36). Trauma within a diverticulum may induce asymmetric intimal proliferations and scarring of the associated vessels, predisposing them to rupture and bleeding (59). The arterial wall exhibits duplication of the internal elastic lamina and eccentric medial thinning, especially on its luminal side (Fig. 13.34). Some have suggested that the thick-walled vessels are angiodysplastic and that there is an association between angiodysplasia and diverticular disease (61). The myenteric plexus may become abnormal and disorganized (Fig. 13.37), a change leading to secondary motility disturbances.

When diverticulitis develops, the diverticulum becomes infiltrated with acute inflammatory cells, followed by chronic inflammation. As the inflammation extends, the mucosa ulcerates and abscesses or fistulae form. Granulomas may also be present. Sometimes one receives tissues thought to represent a "serosal mass." It results from the walling-off of an abscess or a diverticulum in which the fibrosis produces a localized, serosal, interlacing matrix of connective tissue surrounding fecal material (Fig. 13.38).

Redundant mucosal folds appear polypoid with increased mucosal height, crypt elongation, mucosal distortion, edema, vascular congestion, and hemorrhage, possibly associated with thrombi, hemosiderin deposits, erosions, granulation tissue, and fibrosis (Fig. 13.35). Fibers of the muscularis mucosae extend high into the lamina propria, producing changes resembling those seen in mucosal prolapse.

In *isolated sigmoiditis, crescenteric colitis,* or *diverticular disease–associated colitis* (these are all synonyms), the histologic changes may exactly mimic those found in inflammatory bowel disease (IBD). Changes include a lymphoplasmacytic and eosinophilic expansion of the lamina propria with cryptitis, crypt abscesses, basal lymphoplasmacytosis, lymphoid aggregates, distorted crypt architecture, surface

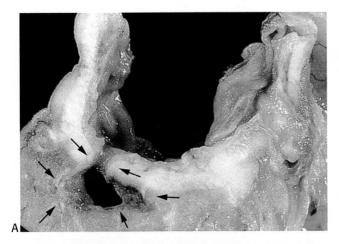

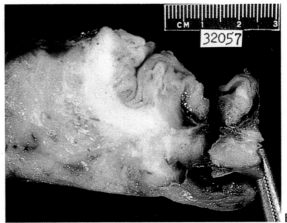

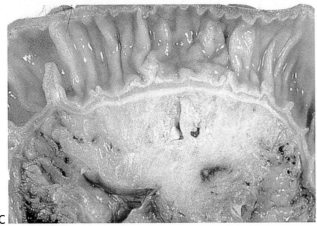

FIG. 13.30. Complications of diverticulosis. **A:** A diverticulum at approximately 7 o'clock has ruptured and produced a pericolonic abscess (*arrows*). **B:** Cross section through the bowel demonstrating the marked muscular thickening in the area of perforation. **C:** An area of diverticulosis with a secondary separated abscess in the mesocolon. (Courtesy of Dr. D. B. Herring, Department of Pathology, Presbyterian Hospital, Albuquerque, NM.)

epithelial sloughing, focal Paneth cell metaplasia, and granulomatous cryptitis (62). The only way to distinguish this entity from IBD is to interpret the finding in the context of the entire clinical, gross, and endoscopic picture. All of these changes lie near the diverticula and are not present away from the diverticula, distinguishing the changes from ulcerative colitis and Crohn disease (Figs. 13.36 and 13.39). In some cases it may be impossible to distinguish between these entities. The mucosa may also appear hyperplastic or it may appear to have a thickened collagen table mimicking collagenous colitis. This resemblance may be further accentuated if there is associated mild colitis.

Isolated sigmoiditis tends not to cause diagnostic dilemmas when one receives a resection specimen in a patient with obvious diverticulosis or diverticulitis. However, given the frequency with which diverticulosis is encountered in the population and the frequency of colonic biopsies, isolated sigmoiditis may cause diagnostic difficulties in biopsy specimens. This is particularly problematic because the chronic colitis of diverticular disease shows the same distribution as ulcerative colitis (UC). If the endoscopist biopsies both the area around diverticula and areas remote from them, the biopsies will show a patchy distribution of the inflammation, allowing one to distinguish sigmoiditis from UC but not from Crohn disease. However, if the biopsies only come from

the areas surrounding a diverticulum, a misdiagnosis of IBD may be made. Finally, because diverticulosis occurs commonly in the Western world, it often coexists with other diseases, including adenomas and carcinomas, idiopathic IBD, and other forms of colitis. Occasionally, the carcinomas appear to arise within the diverticulum and tumors may exhibit differing histologic patterns.

It is important to distinguish between congenital and acquired diverticula, since the latter often result from underlying pathology either in the bowel itself or in a structure outside the bowel. The most important feature distinguishing the two is the absence of an intact muscularis propria in acquired diverticula.

When diverticular disease ruptures forming abscesses and peridiverticulitis, it has features that overlap with those seen in CD. Features that suggest the presence of CD complicating diverticular disease include the presence of ulcers away from the diverticulum, fissures, and internal fistulae other than colovesical or colovaginal fistula. If acute inflammatory masses are present in diverticular disease, they may grossly resemble a carcinoma. Additionally, the colonic wall may become thickened by pericolonic, postinflammatory fibrosis, also grossly simulating a neoplasm or inflammatory bowel disease. To further complicate the matter, patients may have both IBD and diverticular disease. UC patients who also have

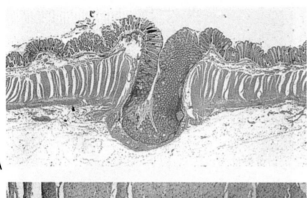

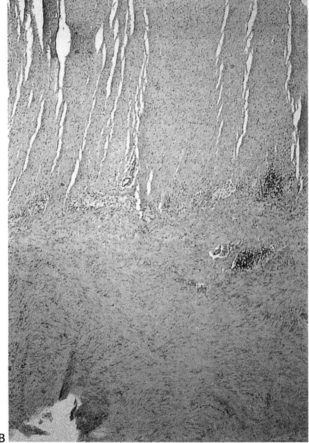

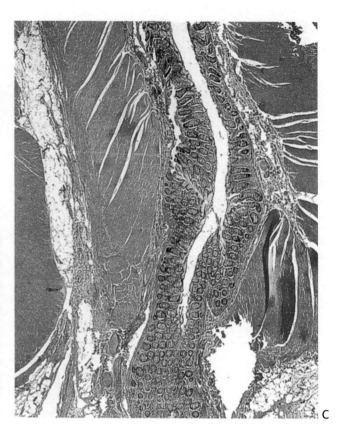

FIG. 13.31. Muscular hypertrophy in diverticulosis. **A:** The corrugated nature of the muscularis propria, particularly the inner circular muscle, is evident. **B:** The mucosa shows a mild increase in mononuclear cells in the lamina propria. A hyperplastic muscularis abuts the diverticulum and shows a "fish flesh" cracking. **C:** Myenteric hypertrophy. Both the circular and longitudinal muscles are hypertrophic and thickened.

diverticulosis may have extension of their mucosal disease into a diverticulum, perhaps obliterating the underlying architecture, resulting in an appearance of a primary fistula and creating changes that mimic CD.

Torsion and Volvulus

A volvulus is an axial twist of a portion of the gastrointestinal tract around its mesentery. The rotation causes a partial or complete bowel obstruction and variable degrees of arterial and venous obstruction. Colonic volvulus affects both children and adults. Sigmoid volvulus accounts for 40% to 80% of colonic volvulus; volvulus of the transverse colon accounts for only 4% to 9% (63,64). The splenic flexure is the least common site of volvulus since it is fixed in position

by the gastrocolic, phrenocolic, and splenocolic ligaments. Cecal volvulus usually complicates inadequate colonic fixation, which allows the colon to freely rotate around its axis. *Primary volvulus* develops in patients lacking a predisposing anatomic abnormality. *Secondary volvulus* affects patients with an acquired or congenital abnormality that predisposes the bowel to rotate.

Colonic volvulus occurs more frequently in countries where the population consumes a diet high in fiber. In the Western world it is the third most common cause of large bowel obstruction (following cancer and diverticular disease) (65). The high fiber content results in bulky stools with a volume that leads to a persistently loaded, elongated colon. As the sigmoid elongates, its two ends tend to approximate one another, producing a narrower mesenteric attachment,

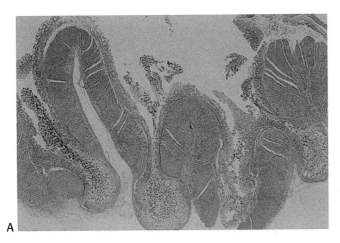

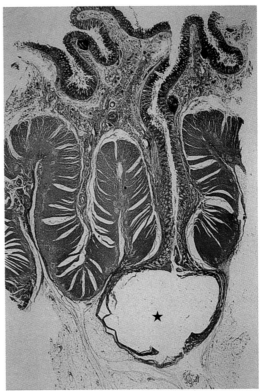

FIG. 13.32. Diverticulosis. A: There is prominent muscular hypertrophy and four diverticula extend through the wall of the bowel. **B:** This trichrome-stained section illustrates the prominent muscular hypertrophy seen in red at the middle portion of the photograph. A long diverticular neck passes through the bowel wall in the area of the penetrating artery and ends in a dilated sac that protrudes into the pericolonic fat (*star*).

predisposing to volvulus. The actual precipitating cause is often a minor event, such as straining at stool or coughing.

Before age 60, cecal volvulus and sigmoid volvulus have the same incidence; after age 60, the incidence of sigmoid volvulus increases. Elderly individuals, especially those given psychotropic drugs or those with chronic constipation (66), previous surgery (64,67), pelvic tumors or cysts that displace the intestine, and neuromuscular disorders (68), acquire an enlarged, redundant sigmoid colon predisposing to volvulus.

In its early stages, a volvulus produces a check valve effect allowing flatus and fecal material to enter the loop but preventing them from leaving, resulting in rapid bowel distension. As the volvulus tightens, a complete closed loop obstruction develops with vascular compression and ischemic necrosis. The muscle often appears hypertrophic and hyperplastic and the bowel wall contains thick-walled blood vessels. The mucosa is variably inflamed and there may be coexisting melanosis coli or even pneumatosis coli.

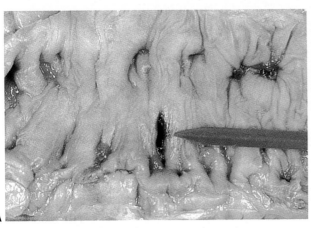

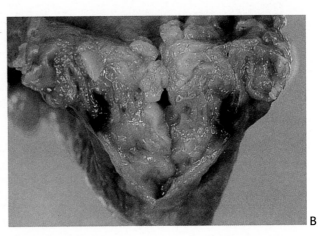

FIG. 13.33. Bleeding diverticulum. This relatively unimpressive specimen derives from a patient who bled out several units of blood and required an emergency colectomy. The only bleeding site that was identified is indicated by the tip of the pointer in **A.** The other diverticular orifices that contain bloody material represent blood that extended into the diverticula. **B:** Cross section shows the presence of a diverticulum filled with blood.

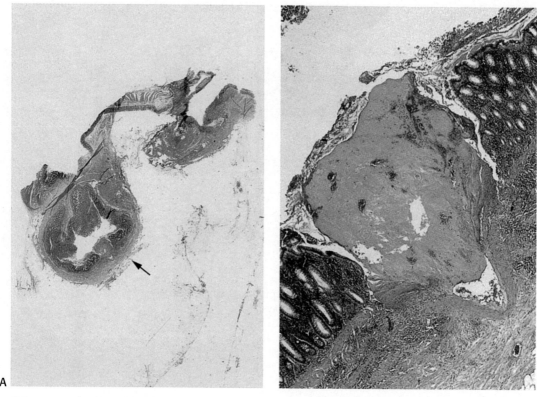

FIG. 13.34. Bleeding site in the diverticulum illustrated in Figure 13.33. **A:** The bleeding site is highlighted by the *arrow.* **B:** Higher magnification of this site shows an eroded artery with a blood clot on the surface.

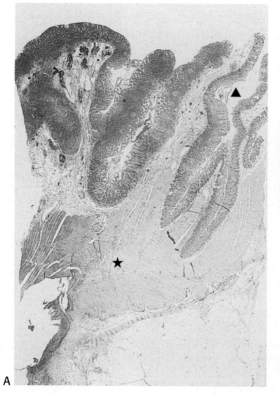

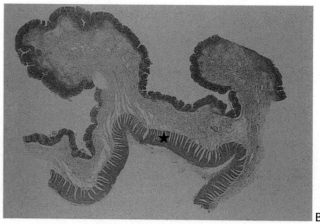

FIG. 13.35. Prolapsing mucosal folds. **A:** Redundant mucosal folds and a branched diverticulum in the right colon. Note the marked hypertrophy of the muscularis propria (*star*) and the accordion-pleated–like mucosal folds. The diverticulum (*triangle*) has the branched shape characteristic of right-sided diverticula. **B:** Patients often exhibit redundant mucosal folds with marked hypertrophy of the muscularis mucosae and almost total obliteration of the submucosal space. The muscularis propria (*star*) shows a typical fish-flesh artifact seen in patients with diverticulosis.

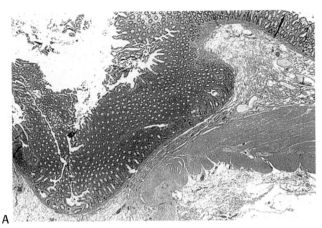 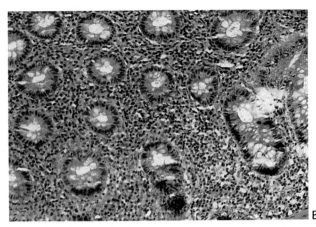

FIG. 13.36. Diverticular sigmoiditis. **A:** Low magnification shows a hypercellular lamina propria. **B:** Note the increased number of mononuclear cells in the lamina propria.

Variable degrees of acute or chronic ischemia may also be present.

A rare type of sigmoid volvulus is referred to as *ileosigmoid knotting*. It is best known in Africa, Finland, and Eastern Europe. A loop of ileum knots around the base of a sigmoid volvulus resulting in gangrenous necrosis of both loops.

Redundant Sigmoid

An elongated redundant sigmoid colon predisposes to volvulus formation, intussusception, and focal ischemia (Fig. 13.40). Patients with redundant sigmoid colons often also have associated diverticular disease and the dysmotility may further contribute to the pathologic features. The muscularis propria and muscularis mucosae may fuse, producing redundant mucosal folds. The mucosa appears chronically damaged. Acute inflammation may be superimposed on chronic changes. The submucosal vessels become prominently dilated and collections of chronic inflammatory cells infiltrate the submucosa (Fig. 13.41). The tissue may display profound eosinophilia as in any other chronic forms of colitis.

Intussusception

Intussusceptions occur throughout the large intestine. Specimens obtained from patients with intussusceptions fall

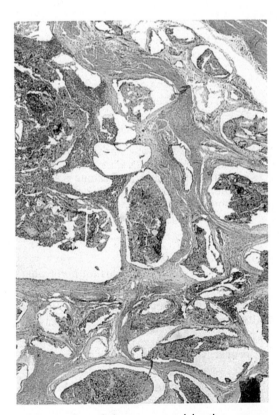

FIG. 13.38. Portion of tissue removed by the surgeon as a "serosal implant." The patient had extensive diverticulosis. The "implant" appeared multiloculated and contained fecal material. Individual fecal collections were walled off by a fibrous inflammatory reaction.

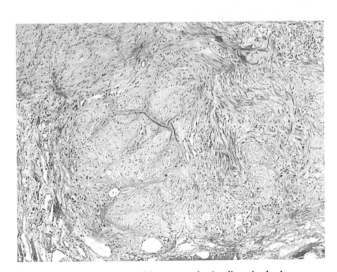

FIG. 13.37. Neural hypertrophy in diverticulosis.

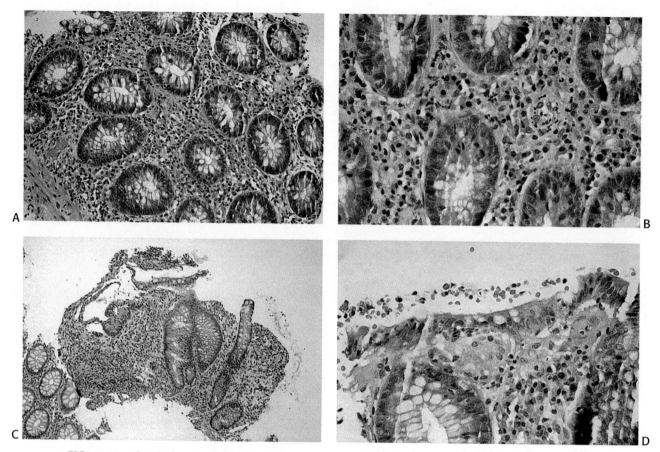

FIG. 13.39. Diverticular sigmoiditis. **A:** Mildly regenerative crypts are separated by a lamina propria containing large numbers of mononuclear cells. **B:** Higher magnification of the mononuclear cell. **C:** Other areas demonstrate obvious regenerative changes with branched glands and even early fibrosis. **D:** Superficial collections of lamina propria macrophages are present.

into several groups: (a) intussusception associated with segmental ischemic necrosis (Fig. 13.42) occurring in patients with neoplasms or other lesions that act as lead points (Fig. 13.43); (b) appendiceal intussusception, a disorder that presents as a cecal "polyp"; the lesion results from retrograde

appendiceal intussusception into the cecal wall; (c) rectal intussusception, which occurs 6 to 8 cm above the anal verge, usually involving the entire rectal circumference, and often developing in connection with straining; and (d) intussusceptions in which underlying motility disturbances cause

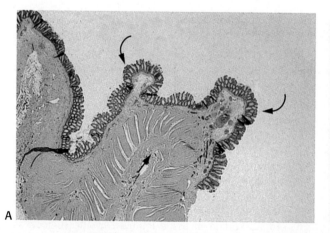
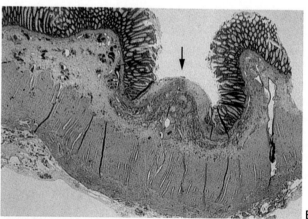

FIG. 13.40. Redundant sigmoid. **A:** Low-magnification photograph showing the presence of a buckled muscularis propria (*arrow*) with the muscularis propria showing a typical fish-flesh separation of the outer muscular layer. The *curved arrows* indicate mucosal protrusions presenting as polyps. **B:** Another area from the same resection specimen showing an isolated ischemic ulcer (*arrow*).

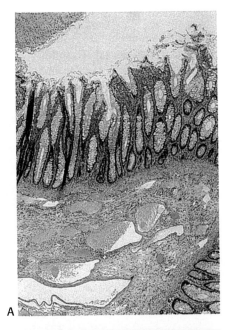

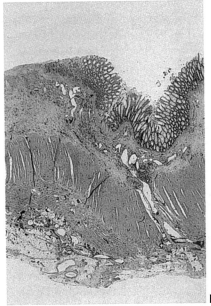

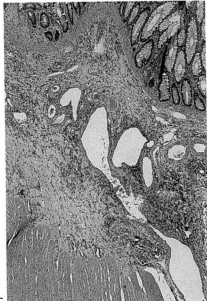

FIG. 13.41. Redundant sigmoid. **A:** The mucosa shows evidence of chronic injury. The submucosal vessels are markedly dilated. **B:** There is marked thickening of the muscularis propria and perivascular inflammation. **C:** Higher magnification of the perivascular inflammation and perivascular hemosiderin-laden macrophages.

portions of the bowel to intussuscept into one another. Viral infections are important causes of ileal intussusception into the cecum in children. Adenovirus infections are the most common cause, but acute primary infections with human herpesvirus (HHV)-6, HHV-7, and Ebstein-Barr virus (EBV) are etiologic factors (69). The pathologic features of an acute intussusception are usually dominated by those of ischemic injury as described later.

Diagnosing a resected, unreduced intussusception is not difficult. However, recurrent or past intussusceptions that spontaneously reduce may be more difficult to recognize. Histologic clues that point to recurrent intussusception include (a) marked disorganization of the muscularis propria, sometimes showing features of peristaltic drag; (b) fusion of

the muscularis mucosae with the muscularis propria; (c) focal submucosal fibrosis; (d) marked telangiectasia; (e) evidence of healed serosal disease, including adhesions; and (f) localized mucosal hyperplasia. Sometimes the bowel wall kinks on itself with only the muscularis propria demonstrating the twisted appearance of the previous intussusception (Fig. 13.44).

Intussusceptions can produce a florid vascular proliferation that can be exuberant enough to raise the possibility of an angiosarcoma. The lesion consists of a lobular proliferation of small vascular channels that extend from the submucosa through the entire thickness of the bowel wall (70). The endothelial cells have minimal cytologic atypia, mitoses are rare, and the vascular channels are not interanastomosing as seen in angiosarcomas (see Chapter 19).

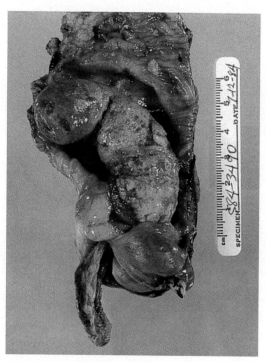

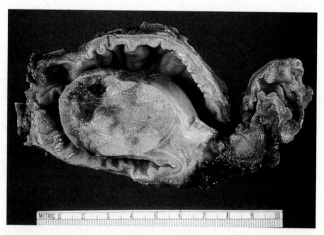

FIG. 13.43. Lipoma serving as a lead point for an intussusception.

FIG. 13.42. A large intestinal intussusception. The bowel has herniated within itself and has become necrotic.

Mucosal Prolapse Syndromes

The different entities in the mucosal prolapse syndrome include rectal prolapse, solitary rectal ulcer syndrome (SRUS), proctitis cystica profunda (PCP), and inflammatory cloacogenic polyp. They show overlapping features, and the relationships among the four entities are confusing. We advocate that these entities be all lumped together under the term *mucosal prolapse* because the changes often coexist and overlap with one another. Prolapse affects 85%

to 90% of patients with SRUS (71) and 54% of patients with PCP (72). Perhaps the easiest way to view this spectrum of diseases is that an ulcer develops first. As the mucosa regenerates, a polypoid lesion develops. At the same time, some of the glands become displaced into the underlying submucosa.

Patients present with signs and symptoms of anorectal disease, usually in their 3rd or 4th decades of life. Symptoms include rectal bleeding, diarrhea, anorectal pain, abdominal cramps, and difficulty defecating. The latter presents as constipation, straining, rectal prolapse, or incomplete rectal evacuation necessitating digital manipulation. Fifty percent of patients have incontinence. Ulcerated and indurated areas are often present on the anterior or anterolateral wall. The ulcers often straddle a rectal fold and vary in size from a few millimeters to several centimeters in diameter. Not all patients have ulcers, and in some the only abnormality is an

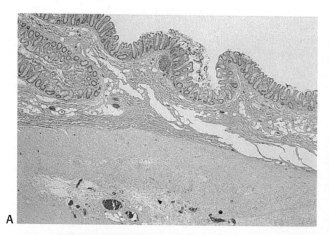

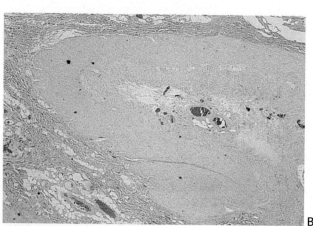

FIG. 13.44. Features of chronic intussusception. **A** and **B** are from a colonic resection. The most impressive portions of the resection specimen are not shown but consisted of a pericolonic inflammatory pseudotumor. The only clue as to the underlying etiology of the changes was the curved nature of the muscularis propria and the marked hypertrophy and distortion of the myenteric plexus associated with the specimen. The patient has had a long history of recurrent abdominal problems.

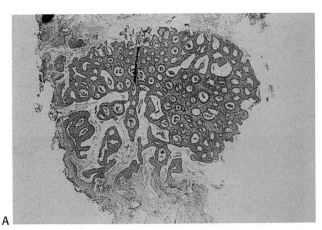
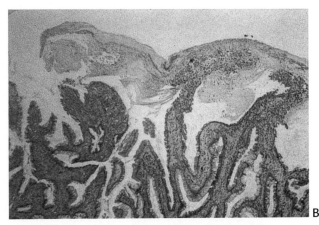

FIG. 13.45. Early mucosal prolapse. **A:** An inflammatory polyp is present. **B:** Higher magnification of the lesion shows the marked villiform hyperplasia. A "cap" of fibrin, inflammatory cells, and debris covers the surface.

erythematous area, sometimes associated with polypoid projections (73). Rare patients present with an acute abdomen secondary to perforation.

Rectal Prolapse

Rectal prolapse is defined as anal protrusion of some or all rectal wall layers. Prolapse first occurs in infants; it becomes uncommon in childhood and early adulthood, only to increase in frequency after age 40. Prolapse is more common in women. The problem in children usually corrects itself as they grow (74). Rectal prolapse is either complete or incomplete (71). Complete rectal prolapse remains concealed (not externally visible at rest), externally visible with straining, or externally visible without straining. The prolapse involves all of the layers of the rectum, essentially creating a rectal wall intussusception (71). It may complicate other disorders such as underlying neoplasms, lymphoid hyperplasia (75) or malacoplakia (76), severe disabling diarrheal diseases, or anorexia nervosa (77). Patients with underlying mass lesions sometimes suffer from recurrent prolapse.

Presenting symptoms include straining during defecation, a sense of obstruction, defecatory pain, fecal incontinence, mucous discharge, pruritus, rectal bleeding, a sense of incomplete rectal evacuation, perineal or intervaginal pressure, and the need to digitally disimpact the rectum (71). Patients may have a palpable mass on digital examination. Endoscopically, there is mucosal reddening, ulceration, and edema (71). Typical features of SRUS and localized PCP may also be present.

The earliest manifestation of rectal prolapse may consist of nothing more than mucosal erosions or ulcers, or just nonspecific inflammation with thickening of the collagen table mimicking collagenous colitis. Ulceration is heralded by capillary dilation and congestion beneath the surface epithelium. Ulcers covered by a fibrous exudate erupt from the surface mucosa in a volcanolike fashion (Fig. 13.45),

reminiscent of pseudomembranous colitis. The ulcers never penetrate deeply into the submucosa. Later, the lamina propria becomes replaced by smooth muscle cells and fibroblasts arranged at right angles to the muscularis mucosae (Fig. 13.46) (78). The overlying epithelium appears regenerative with mucin depletion, branching, and hyperplasia. These features overlap with those found in inflammatory cloacogenic polyps (see Chapter 15). Ulceration and healing can also lead to the presence of cysts deep in the submucosa (73). Inflammatory polyps also develop.

Solitary Rectal Ulcer Syndrome

SRUS results from inappropriate anal sphincter contraction during defecation. Repeated straining during defecation, possibly associated with muscular spasm, may create a shear on the rectal mucosa causing traumatic ulceration. Excessive straining also facilitates mild mucosal redundancy in the anterior rectal wall. The term *solitary rectal ulcer syndrome* is a misnomer because ulceration is a late feature of the disease and the ulcers may be multiple.

Some of the histologic changes result from an impaired mucosal blood supply during the prolapse. In acute phases, the crypts appear elongated and lined by immature basophilic epithelial cells (Fig. 13.47). Fibrovascular and fibromuscular components proliferate in the lamina propria; telangiectasia is common. The mucosa may become extremely hyperplastic and polypoid, and may even resemble hyperplastic polyps or adenomas, especially if the mucosa acquires a villiform appearance. The submucosal vessels may become ectatic or hyalinized. Smooth muscle fibers extend from the muscularis mucosae toward the lumen. The presence of the diffuse mucosal fibrosis is a reliable and discriminating feature between SRUS (Fig. 13.46), UC, and other forms of acute colitis. The fibrosis can be accentuated using trichrome stains. Unfortunately, fibrosis is a late event. Surface ulcers and erosions are present. The ulcers typically do not extend into the submucosa. There may be features of ischemia along with

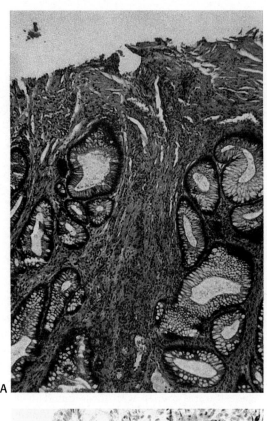

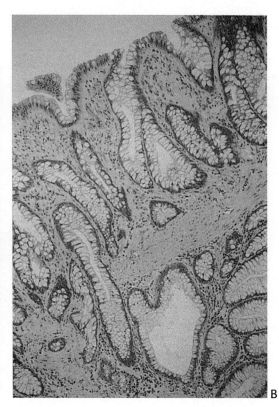

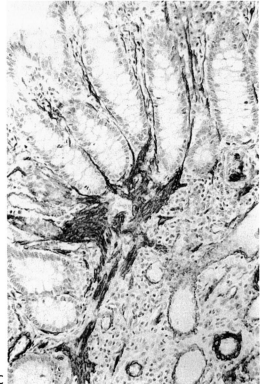

FIG. 13.46. Mucosal prolapse. The mucosa in the various prolapse syndromes share the features of glandular dilation and branching with variable degrees of fibrous and smooth muscle proliferations. Early on, the lesions appear inflamed, as shown in **A. B:** Later, the muscle bands course through the highly branched glands with less inflammation. **C:** Medium magnification showing the presence of the hyperplastic fibers of the muscularis mucosae extending upward into the lamina propria (actin immunostain).

pseudomembranes. These result from vascular compromise during the mucosal prolapse. Inflammatory cap polyps may develop. The lesion may develop in patients with an associated rectal malignancy (79); when this happens the underlying tumor may go unrecognized.

Proctitis Cystica Profunda

Rectal mucosa displaced into the submucosa is termed *proctitis cystica profunda*. PCP is a benign condition that may mimic a colloid carcinoma (Table 13.1). Patients often present

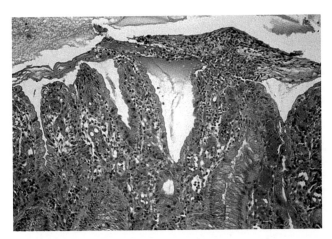

FIG. 13.47. Mucosal prolapse showing flat hyperplasia covered by a fibrinous membrane.

with blood and mucus in the stools. PCP often, but not invariably, associates with rectal mucosal prolapse and disordered puborectalis function (73). PCP may complicate SRUS, developing as the crypts become trapped by reactive fibromuscular proliferations.

Patients who develop PCP show mucosal edema; erythema; a lumpy-bumpy mucosa with increased folds; obvious cysts, polyps, or pseudopolyps; mucosal friability; oval, linear, stellate, or serpiginous ulcers; or a cauliflower-shaped mass measuring up to 5 cm in size (Fig. 13.48). Thick mucus may exude from the cysts when compressed. Surface ulceration is uncommon, but loss of superficial lining cells occurs frequently. Tracts extending from the mucosa toward the mucinous cysts are sometimes visible. The remaining mucosa frequently appears scarred, with glandular loss. Strictures or stenosis may develop. Sections through the cysts demonstrate gelatinous or mucinous secretions. The histologic features of PCP resemble those of colitis cystica profunda (see below). Other histologic findings reflect ischemia secondary to vascular compression, especially when the prolapse becomes impacted in the upper end of the anal canal.

Colitis Cystica Profunda

Colitis cystica profunda (CCP) presents either as a localized lesion or diffusely as multiple lesions. Diffuse CCP involving the entire colon along with enteritis cystic profunda are exceptionally rare, and they may coexist (80). Patients with CCP range in age from 4 to 68 years, with a mean of 33 years. Males outnumber females 7:1. Mucus submucosal retention cysts may follow episodes of bacillary dysentery. The epithelium becomes displaced during mucosal ulceration in the acute phase of the disease (81). Areas near lymphoid follicles may create points of weakness in the muscularis mucosae, facilitating the mucosal herniation (82).

Symptoms include rectal bleeding, passage of mucus and blood, diarrhea, tenesmus, and crampy abdominal pain. Endoscopy may demonstrate a nodular mucosa (73). Associated diseases include IBD (82), Peutz-Jeghers syndrome (PJS), and congenital anomalies. The patients develop innumerable prominent, circumferential, polypoid mucosal elevations and submucosal cysts measuring up to 2 cm in diameter. The ascending and transverse colon are diffusely involved (83).

Microscopically, flattened epithelium incompletely lines the submucosal, mucin-filled cysts. Complete or incomplete cuboidal columnar epithelium resembling normal colonic mucosa lines newly formed cysts (Fig. 13.49). Serial sections may demonstrate a communication between the cysts and the mucosal surface. Older cysts often lack an epithelial lining and are surrounded by fibrous tissue and/or a polymorphic inflammatory infiltrate, hemosiderin, or foreign body giant cells. The material in the cysts may calcify or ossify. The degree of fibrosis is usually moderate but it can be significant, extending into the muscularis propria or even into the serosa. The cyst lining appears benign, lacking cytologic atypia so that confusion with a malignant process is generally not a problem. However, low-grade dysplasia may be present in the displaced epithelium in patients with longstanding ulcerative colitis (83).

A lesion that may superficially resemble colitis cystica profunda causing localized cystic masses with variable degrees of inflammation is endometriosis (Fig. 13.50). However, the endometrial epithelial lining should not contain mucin and the stroma surrounding the glands should be the denser endometrial stroma rather than the looser lamina propria typical of the intestinal mucosa.

Colitis Cystica Superficialis

Colitis cystica superficialis is a condition in which mucinous cysts remain confined to the intestinal mucosa (Fig. 13.51). These are seen in pellagra and following healing of chronic inflammation, as in UC.

TABLE 13.1 Colitis Cystica Profunda Versus Colloid Carcinoma

Histologic Feature	Colitis Cystica Profunda	Carcinoma
Surface mucosa	Features of mucosal prolapse	Neoplastic epithelium
Mucin pools	Rounded	Irregular
Lamina propria	Often present	Absent
Hemosiderin deposits	May be present	Absent
Desmoplasia	Absent	Present
Dysplasia	Absent	Present

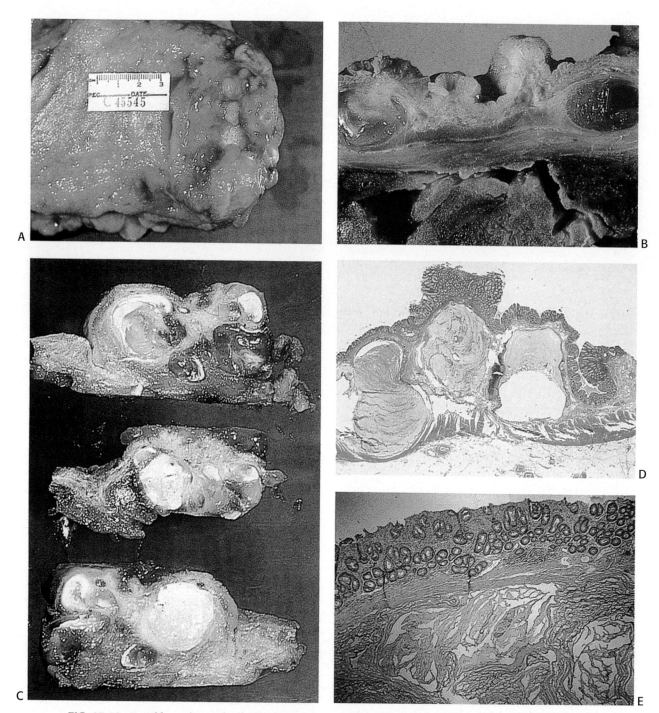

FIG. 13.48. Proctitis cystica profunda. **A:** Nodular area of colitis cystica profunda in a proctectomy specimen. The proximal mucosa is uninvolved. **B:** Cross section shows numerous mucin-filled submucosal cysts surrounded by fibrosis. **C:** In this Bouin-fixed specimen the mucosa is highlighted (*yellow*). **D:** Whole mount of lesion illustrated in C demonstrates the presence of multiple mucus-filled cysts. **E:** High-power magnification of the lesion illustrated in B. Numerous submucosal cysts are seen. The overlying mucosa is not neoplastic.

Stercoral Ulcers

Stercoral perforation generally develops in the rectosigmoid. Reasons for this include (a) local pressure from structures surrounding the rectosigmoid that keep it from distending; (b) the presence of hard feces in this area; and (c) the presence of a relatively narrow intestinal lumen. Stercoral ulceration with perforation is an uncommon but frequently fatal condition because patients often develop peritonitis. Perforation often occurs during difficult bowel

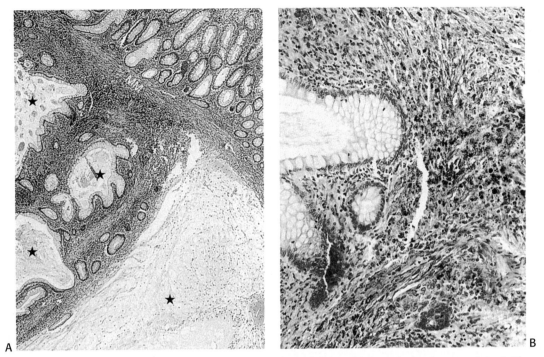

FIG. 13.49. Colitis cystica profunda. **A:** Cross sections through four submucosal cysts are seen (*stars*). They are lined by variably flattened nonneoplastic colorectal epithelium. The epithelium appears regenerative. **B:** Higher magnification of the central cysts showing prominent hemosiderin deposition with resulting fibrosis. Lamina propria surrounds the cysts.

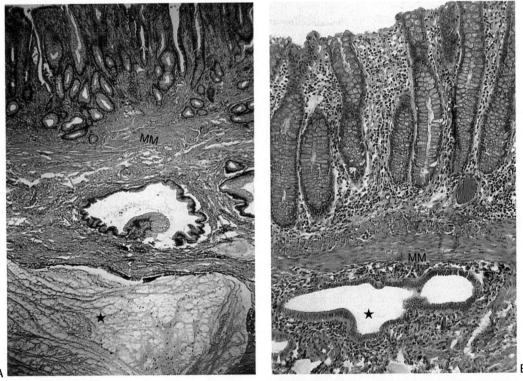

FIG. 13.50. Comparison of colitis cystica profunda and endometriosis. **A:** Colitis cystic profunda. A nonneoplastic mucosa lies above the muscularis mucosae (*MM*). The submucosa contains glands lined by mucin-secreting epithelium with mucin in the cyst lumen. The lower cyst (*star*) has a large accumulation of mucus within it. **B:** Endometriosis. The endometriotic focus lies in the submucosa. It is surrounded by dense stroma and lined by non–mucin-secreting epithelium (*star*). The stroma surrounding the endometrial gland is much denser than the lamina propria surrounding the displaced epithelial glands seen in A.

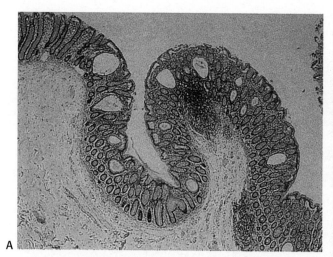

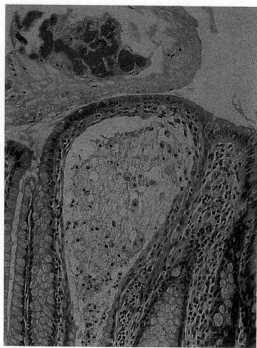

FIG. 13.51. Colitis cystica superficialis. Multiple mucosal cysts are present. These are seen at low and high power in **A** and **B**.

movements. Many patients are renal patients with severe constipation due to ingestion of nonabsorbable antacids, particularly magnesium and aluminum hydroxide gels, and cation exchange resins used to treat their hyperkalemia (84). The inspissated stool causes local pressure, ischemia, necrosis, and perforation. The situation is made worse by loss of normal mucosal barrier function due to coexisting uremia.

Grossly, stercoral ulcers are characterized by the presence of longitudinal tears or perforations (Figs. 13.52 and 13.53). One often finds hard feces corresponding in size to the perforation site. Sometimes the hard feces protrude through the perforation site. Histologically, the intestinal wall is acutely and chronically inflamed (Fig. 13.53).

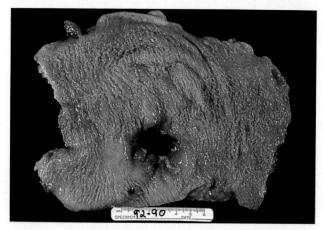

FIG. 13.52. Stercoral ulcer.

INTERPRETATION OF COLONIC BIOPSIES

The ability to endoscopically visualize the entire mucosal surface of the large bowel and to biopsy or cytologically sample normal- and abnormal-appearing areas allows clinicians to diagnose and manage colorectal diseases. Biopsies yield information concerning disease patterns, distribution, extent and/or severity, acuity versus chronicity, clinical state of remission or relapse, and complications. In one study, interpretation of mucosal biopsies yielded a positive diagnosis in 31% of patients with chronic diarrhea who did not have a definitive diagnosis prior to the biopsy (85). The most common diagnoses were IBD and microscopic colitis, although cases of ischemia and infection were also first diagnosed on the biopsy (85).

Optimal biopsy evaluation can only occur when careful consideration is given to the clinical, historical, endoscopic, radiographic, microbiologic, and other available patient data. Once tissue has been removed, it may be cultured, examined histologically or ultrastructurally, or submitted for biochemical analysis. Not only can it be examined in routine hematoxylin and eosin (H&E) sections, but it may also be submitted to a battery of histochemical and immunocytochemical stains as well as molecular biologic techniques, many of which can be performed on formalin-fixed, paraffin-embedded materials. One may also re-embed colonic biopsies in which there is a discrepancy between the clinical impression and the histologic findings. In so doing new diagnoses can be made in up to 31% of biopsies (86). In our opinion, this is not likely to be cost effective, especially since in most cases the new diagnosis was that of a small hyperplastic polyp (86), a lesion of little clinical consequence.

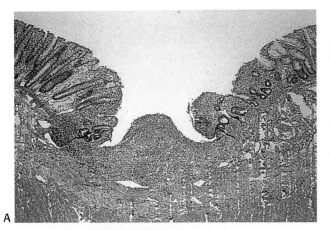

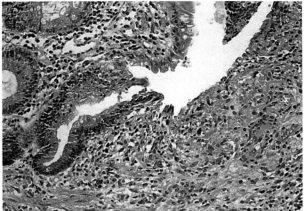

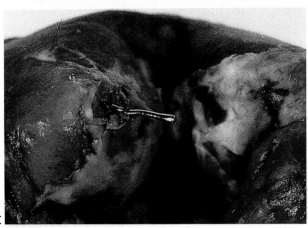

FIG. 13.53. Stercoral ulcers and erosions. **A:** An isolated erosion only into the superficial submucosa. **B:** There is acute and chronic inflammation and glandular regeneration. **C:** Gross appearance of a perforated stercoral ulcer viewed from the outside. Note the serosal adhesions.

One of the most common uses of the colorectal biopsy is to determine the etiology of a colitis or proctitis, which may share overlapping clinical, radiologic, or pathologic features with other disorders (Table 13.2). In the best of circumstances, analysis of the biopsy specimen, in conjunction with an interpretation of the clinical data (Table 13.3), will yield a definitive diagnosis. More often, however, the biopsy does not provide a specific diagnosis, but rather narrows down the differential diagnosis. The histologic features may suggest an inflammatory condition and provide knowledge concerning the severity of the underlying lesion or the extent of disease, allowing one to correlate the clinical impression with the histologic findings. One may also be able to diagnose the presence of specific neoplasms or the presence of a treatable organism.

Mucosal biopsy interpretation can be difficult due to normal architectural variants, effects of the biopsy procedure, and lack of knowledge of the dynamic mucosal events accompanying mucosal repair. Some of the mucosa features that are often unappreciated are the following:

- Crypt branching is normal in the area of the innominate groves.
- There is normally a mononuclear cell infiltrate in the upper mucosa that is sometimes referred to as a *physiologic infiltrate*. It is densest in the cecum (a site of bacterial stasis) and least in the rectum. The crypts are normal (87).

- In general, the lamina propria cellularity is greatest in the cecum and ascending colon and it decreases distally.
- Mild crypt irregularity in the rectum is not considered to be clinically significant.
- While there are normally five intraepithelial lymphocytes per 100 colonocytes, the number is increased in the cecum (perhaps secondary to the stasis that occurs there) and there are abundant intraepithelial lymphocytes in the epithelium overlying lymphoid follicles.
- A previously inflamed bowel may return to a histologically normal appearance. This is especially important in evaluating biopsies from patients with ulcerative colitis.

It is important to examine mucosal biopsies in a standardized way in order to determine that they are abnormal and to establish a probable diagnosis. A systemic analysis should include evaluation of the features listed in Table 13.4. The most common pattern one sees when evaluating a biopsy for colitis are diffuse and focal active colitis or proctitis without other specific features. The pathology report should indicate whether features are acute, chronic, or chronic active and whether the changes are focal or diffuse. Specific features such as the presence of microorganisms, granulomas, or abnormal infiltrates should be noted. An attempt should be made to establish the etiology of the changes since "diagnoses" such as nonspecific colitis are of little help to the

TABLE 13.2 **Differential Diagnosis of Colitis**

Features	Infectious	Antibiotic Associated	Ischemic	Ulcerative Colitis	Crohn Disease
Clinical	Acute onset Fever Constitutional symptoms Watery/bloody diarrhea Positive cultures and/or serology Travel to high-risk areas	Recent antibiotic use ± abdominal pain Diarrhea *Clostridium difficile* organism or toxin detected Membranes seen at endoscopy	Concurrent ischemia elsewhere; Poor cardiovascular status Segmental distribution of disease Older age	Bloody diarrhea Toxic megacolon Extraintestinal symptoms Diffusely ulcerated rectal mucosa decreasing in severity as one progresses proximally; extraintestinal disease	Perianal disease Fissures Fistulae Associated small bowel disease Skip lesions Extraintestinal disease Rectal sparing
Radiographic	May resemble ulcerative colitis	Segmental or limited colitis with or without pseudomembranes Edema	Segmental distribution Thumbprinting with reversion to normal or progression to stricture Rectal involvement rare	Backwash ileitis Pseudopolyps Diffuse involvement starting in rectum and progressing proximally with decreasing severity	Segmental disease with skip lesions Small bowel involved Fistulae/fissures Ulcers/cobblestoned appearance Strictures
Pathologic	Edema prominent Polymorphonuclear leukocytes Crypt inflammation No crypt distortion No basal plasmacytosis ± granulomas Low degree of vascularity	Acute inflammation ± pseudomembranes Superficial erosions Focal lesions can resemble ischemia "Volcanic" eruptions of exudates	Focal lesion Mucosal necrosis ± pseudomembranes Hemosiderin deposits in lamina propria Submucosal involvement (acute granulation tissue, scarring) Strictures No granulomas Highly vascular Glandular ghosts	Continuous involvement Edema rare Inflammation limited to mucosa and submucosa Crypt abscesses Basal plasmacytosis No granulomas Pseudopolyps Goblet cell dysplasia High degree of vascularity Abnormal mucosal architecture	Segmental disease with skip lesions Fissures, fistulae Granulomas Transmural inflammation Aphthous ulcers Pseudopolyps Gland distortion Basal plasmacytosis Focal inflammation

TABLE 13.3 Information That Aids Pathologists Interpreting Colorectal Biopsies

Patient age
Patient sex
Ethnicity
Endoscopic findings
Country of domicile
Travel history
Reason for the biopsy
Drug use
History of associated diseases
    AIDS
    Neoplasias
    Infections
    Metabolic diseases
    Immune deficiencies
    Prior surgery
    Cardiovascular disease
    Allergies
    Diverticulosis
    Polyposis syndromes

TABLE 13.4 Evaluation of the Colonic Mucosal Biopsies

1. What is the overall architecture?
2. Is there inflammation?
   • Is there architectural distortion?
       ?Branched crypts
       ?Atrophy
       ?Loss of parallel arrangement of the crypts
       ?Metaplasia
       ?Widening between the crypt bases and the muscularis mucosae
   • Are there granulomas?
   • Is there an invasive neoplasm?
   • Is the inflammation acute or chronic?
   • Is the inflammation diffuse or focal?
   • Does the inflammation preferentially affect any part of the mucosa?
       ?Surface
       ?Basal mucosa
       ?Superficial mucosa
       ?Lamina propria
       ?Crypts
3. What is the appearance of the epithelium?
   • Is it ulcerated?
   • Are there microorganisms attached to its surface?
   • Does it contain viral inclusions?
   • Is it covered by a pseudomembrane?
   • Is there cryptitis?
   • Is there intraepithelial lymphocytosis?
   • Are there unusual cell types?
       Paneth cells?
       Increased endocrine cells?
       Pyloric metaplasia?
   • Is there increased apoptosis?
   • Is there macrocytosis?
   • Is there separation from the basement membrane?
   • Is their subepithelial collagenization?
   • Is there dysplasia?
   • Is there surface injury?
4. What is the appearance of the lamina propria?
   • Is the cellularity normal? (If not, what cell types are present?)
   • Are there abnormal deposits?
   • Are the vessels normal?
   • Are there viral inclusions?
   • Are there parasites?
   • Are there granulomas or histiocytic collections?
       Caseating or noncaseating?
       Any organism present?
       Is there a storage disease?
   • What is the appearance of the submucosa (if present)?
       Are the vessels normal?
       Are there infiltrates?
       Are there neoplasms or endometriosis?
       Is there amyloid present?
       Is there displaced epithelium?

clinicians who already know that the patient has some form of colitis.

One study suggests that most colonic biopsies from patients with nonneoplastic disease are inflamed, that in most cases a specific diagnosis can be made, and that pathologists tend to overdiagnose the mild chronic inflammation that may be present, especially in the right colon (88).

Definition of Terms and Description of Changes that May Be Present

The following are some definitions that can be used in describing the patterns of inflammation that may be present. *Acute colitis* is an inflammatory colonic condition with an acute clinical onset that lacks histologic features of chronicity including architectural distortion and Paneth cell metaplasia. There are neutrophilic infiltrates in the lamina propria and/or the crypts (*cryptitis*) or in the glandular lumens (*crypt abscesses*). There may be degeneration of the surface or crypt epithelium. Less obvious changes include mild surface damage, red cell extravasation into the lamina propria, and mucosal edema. These more subtle changes often accompany toxic injury and some infections (Fig. 13.54). At the other end of the spectrum, severe acute or active disease results in erosions and ulcers. *Chronic colitis* is characterized by architectural distortion (crypt branching and budding, loss of their parallel arrangement, or villiform transformation) with variable degrees of mucosal atrophy. The crypts may appear shortened and the distance between the base of the crypts and the muscularis mucosae may be increased. Paneth cell metaplasia may be present in the transverse and distal colon (Fig. 13.55). There is often a marked increase in the number of mononuclear inflammatory cells and/or eosinophils in the lamina propria. One may also see endocrine

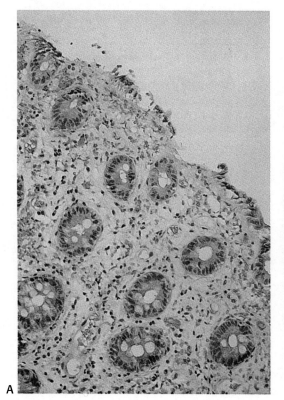 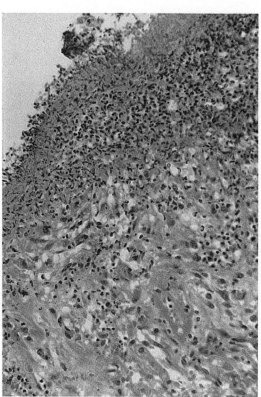

A   B

FIG. 13.54. Mild versus severe injury. **A:** Biopsy from a patient with toxigenic *Escherichia coli* infection shows only mild edema and mild superficial epithelial loss. These changes contrast with those seen in **B** in *Clostridium difficile* infection with marked epithelial necrosis, acute inflammatory infiltration, and fibrin thrombi.

cell hyperplasia. *Chronic active colitis* is present when both mononuclear cells (lymphocytes and plasma cells) and neutrophils infiltrate the mucosa (Fig. 13.56). The term *active inflammation* implies acute inflammation. The terms *inactive* or *quiescent* indicate chronic conditions that are in remission.

Other architectural abnormalities include *crypt atrophy* when the crypts appear shortened and more widely spaced (Fig. 13.57) and sometimes at a greater distance from the

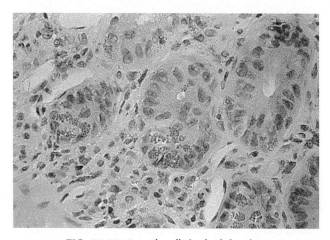

FIG. 13.55. Paneth cells in the left colon.

muscularis mucosae than normal, and when villiform transformation has occurred at the surface. *Branched crypts* are usually defined as the presence of two or more bifurcated crypts in an otherwise well-oriented section (Fig. 13.58). *Superficial inflammation* is defined as inflammation limited to the upper third of the mucosa, whereas *basal plasmacytosis* consists of lymphocytes and plasma cells limited to the lower third of the mucosa (Fig. 13.59). *Nodular lymphoid hyperplasia* is present when there are collections of lymphocytes, with or without germinal centers located between the muscularis mucosae and the crypts (Fig. 13.60). Usually at least two aggregates should be present to be considered abnormal. *Basal lymphoid hyperplasia* is defined as an increased number of lymphocytes at the crypt bases without a nodular configuration (Fig. 13.59). *Isolated giant cells* contain multiple nuclei and homogeneous fine granular cytoplasm. These occur singly without associated epithelioid cells. When a focus of granulomatous inflammation or giant cells is detected, serial sections can be cut to determine whether they are in continuity or proximity with a disrupted crypt and therefore represent a *mucin granuloma*. *Epithelioid granulomas* are defined as discrete collections of epithelioid cells with or without accompanying giant cells and without caseating necrosis or foreign bodies. They should not be in continuity with or proximity to a perforated crypt (Fig. 13.61). A *microgranuloma* is defined as a collection

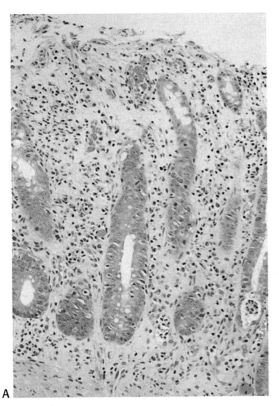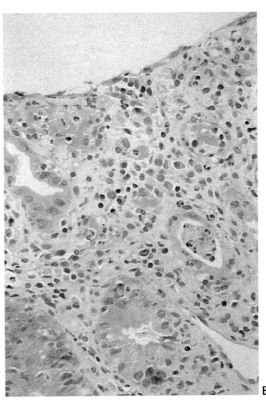

FIG. 13.56. Mixed cell infiltrates in a *Salmonella* infection. **A:** Neutrophils infiltrate the crypts and lamina propria. There are also increased numbers of mononuclear cells in the edematous lamina propria. **B:** Higher magnification showing a crypt abscess and increased mononuclear cells.

of epithelioid cells small enough to be interposed between two crypts without distorting their architecture, without giant cells (Fig. 13.61). *Goblet cell mucus depletion* is defined as marked reduction or absence of goblet cell mucus (Fig. 13.62). *Reactive epithelial hyperplasia* is defined by the presence of elongated, crowded, stratified nuclei or by markedly enlarged, hyperchromatic, vesicular nuclei. The crypts appear bluer than normal.

Focal active colitis (FAC) is a term used to describe the isolated finding of focal infiltration of the colonic epithelium by neutrophils. This can vary from one focus of cryptitis in a single colonic biopsy to multiple foci of cryptitis scattered throughout multiple colonic biopsies (89). Often

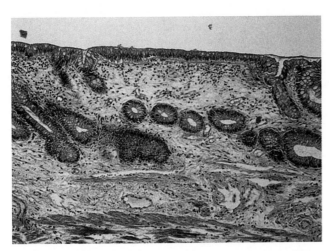

FIG. 13.57. Colonic atrophy. The glands are widely spaced and differ in diameter. The distance from the base of the glands to the muscularis mucosae is widened.

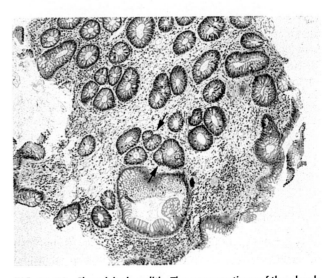

FIG. 13.58. Chronicity in colitis. The cross sections of the glands show marked variability in their diameters. Several of the crypts have glandular budding (*arrows*) with smaller cross-sectional lumens lying adjacent to larger ones without intervening lamina propria.

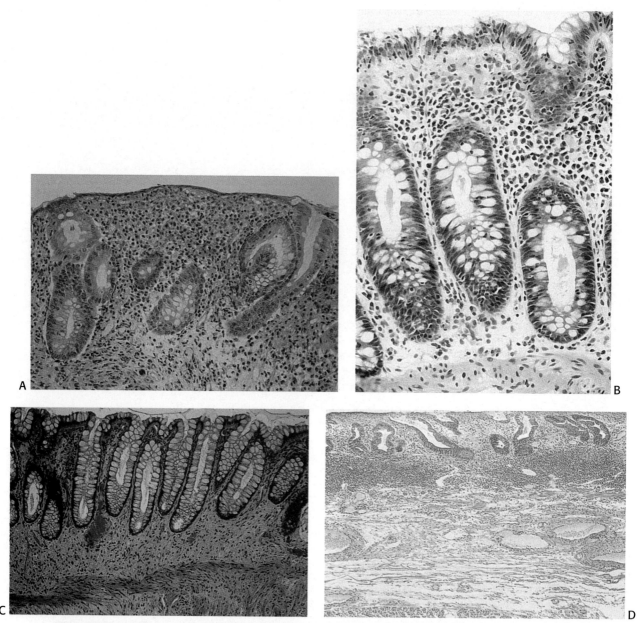

FIG. 13.59. Superficial versus basal inflammation. A and B show inflammation that is more prominent in the superficial mucosa. **A:** The inflammation is acute in nature and is superimposed on branched glands. **B:** The patient has collagenous colitis with a mild increase in the lamina propria mononuclear cells in the upper one half of the mucosa and an increased collagen table. Inflammatory cells are also present within the epithelium. **C:** Collections of histiocytes separate the bases of the colonic glands from the underlying muscularis mucosae. **D:** From a patient with ulcerative colitis. A bandlike infiltrate of mononuclear cells separates the bases of the glands from the underlying muscularis mucosae.

there is increased inflammation in the lamina propria surrounding the inflamed crypts. Up to 13% of patients are ultimately found to have Crohn disease. Nearly half the patients have infectious colitis and in about a quarter of cases the finding had no clinical significance (90,91). Those cases without any clinical significance may have focal inflammation secondary to the bowel prep. However, children with FAC have a higher likelihood of subsequently developing Crohn disease (27.6%) compared with adults.

FAC in children may also be the result of infectious colitis and rare patients have ulcerative colitis, allergic colitis, or Hirschsprung disease. Patients with FAC that does not correlate with symptoms or the ultimate clinical diagnosis are said to have idiopathic focal active colitis, a finding in 27.6% of patients in one study (89). Unfortunately, one cannot predict which patients will fall into the idiopathic category and which will be ultimately diagnosed with IBD or some other process (89).

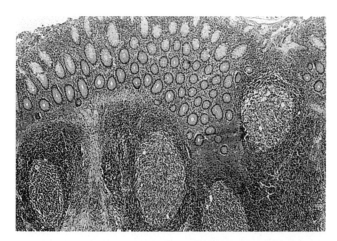

FIG. 13.60. Nodular inflammation. Follicular proctitis. Note the presence of prominent lymphoid follicles both in the mucosa and the underlying submucosa. The epithelium overlying the nodule of lymphoid hyperplasia becomes attenuated and somewhat distorted.

Changes Induced by Bowel Preparations, Instrumentation, and Biopsy

In order to effectively interpret diagnostic large intestinal biopsies, one must be aware of the changes that result from the bowel preparation and/or the biopsy procedure.

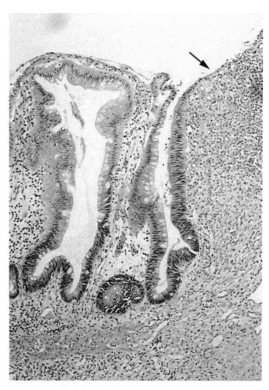

FIG. 13.62. Mucin depletion. A regenerating branched gland is present. The epithelium at the base of the gland is hyperchromatic. The mucin droplets are small. The *arrow* indicates an area of denuded mucosa.

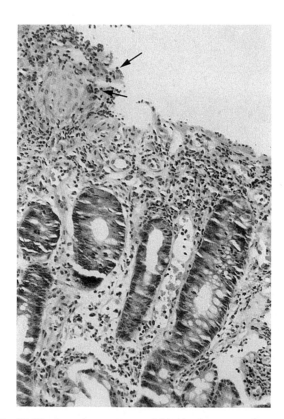

FIG. 13.61. Granuloma. Mucosal biopsy from a patient with Crohn disease showing the presence of a small, compact, sarcoidlike granuloma (*arrows*).

Preparatory procedures may flatten the surface epithelium, decrease the number of goblet cells, deplete the goblet cell mucus, slightly increase the number of neutrophils in the superficial lamina propria, or cause edema (Figs. 13.63 and 13.64) and focal hemorrhage. Hypertonic phosphate enemas, such as Fleet enemas and bisacodyl laxatives, may mimic mild colitis with surface epithelial vacuolization, subepithelial neutrophilic infiltration (92), sloughing, goblet cell mucin depletion, increased crypt mitoses, marginated polymorphonuclear cells, lamina propria edema, and erythrocytic extravasation into the lamina propria (92,93). These changes resolve within a week (94). Crypt abscesses or inflammation rarely extend to more than the superficial zones of the lamina propria.

Today most gastroenterologists use osmotic enema preparations, which cause lamina propria edema without inflammation (Fig. 13.64) (95). The crypts appear more widely separated than normal and the distance from the base of the crypts to the muscularis mucosae widens. The endoscopy and biopsy also sometimes cause focal red cell extravasation into the lamina propria.

Artifacts, including crushing, glandular telescoping, and cautery artifacts in biopsy specimens, can interfere with one's ability to interpret certain lesions (Fig. 13.65). Sometimes the cautery artifact may be so severe that it may render the biopsy impossible to read. Conversely, the presence of cautery artifact

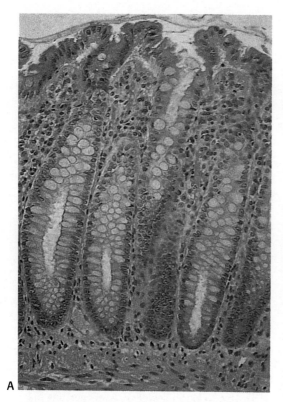

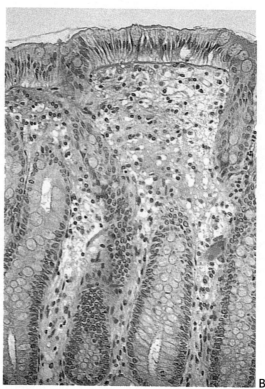

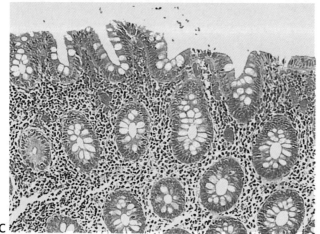

FIG. 13.63. Enema effects. **A:** Mild changes consist of mucin depletion. **B:** The lamina propria is edematous. **C:** Telangiectasia and mild local mucosal hemorrhage.

can be useful in recognizing the resection margin of polypectomy specimens, particularly when the polyps are adenomas containing carcinoma.

ISCHEMIC COLITIS

General Comments

Acute ischemia results from an acute reduction in the blood flow resulting from an acute occlusive event or as a result of a decreased blood flow. It can result from either arterial or venous impairment. Ischemic colitis affects patients of all ages including infants, but it preferentially affects elderly patients with a history of arteriosclerosis, diabetes, hypertension, renal insufficiency, and/or cardiovascular disease. The

mesenteric arteries become atherosclerotic with either gradual arterial occlusion or acute blockage by a thrombus. It is also more common in patients with a thrombophilic state including the presence of factor V Leiden mutations (96). Ischemia developing in a younger person without a history of drug use and in a patient without apparent predisposing factors, such as cardiac failure or arrhythmia, should be investigated for one of the vascular lesions listed in Table 6.8 or for a primary clotting abnormality. In women, the use of hormones or oral contraceptives should be investigated. Ischemia also complicates many other disorders, including some infections, especially cytomegalovirus (CMV). Common causes of low flow states include cardiac failure, arrhythmias, digitalis toxicity, shock resulting from a marked reduction in left ventricular output, and sepsis. Occlusive causes of acute ischemia include arteriolar or venous obstruction

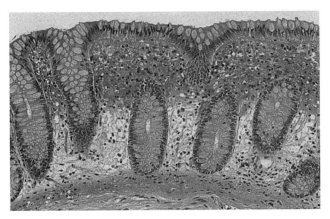

FIG. 13.64. The effects of bowel preps include mucosal edema and red cell extravasation.

(Table 13.5) as the consequence of thromboembolism (Fig. 13.66), dissecting aneurysm, vascular spasm, or vascular compression during prolapse, intussusception, etc. Colonic ischemia also complicates major surgery, infections, drug use (see below), retroperitoneal fibrosis (97), and cocaine abuse. Marathon runners may also develop colonic ischemia (98). Large intestinal ischemia exhibits a spectrum of changes ranging from fatal infarctions with gangrene (Fig. 13.67) to reversible ischemia.

Clinical Features

The clinical signs and symptoms vary according to the underlying etiology, duration and linear extent, and depth of mural involvement. In elderly individuals with generalized cardiovascular disease, a rapidly developing syndrome that starts with mild to moderate abdominal pain and quickly evolves with nausea, vomiting, diarrhea, rectal bleeding, and abdominal distention suggests the presence of ischemia (99). Such patients often have a predisposing hypotensive period.

TABLE 13.5	Causes of Intestinal Venous Compromise

Mesenteric venous thrombosis
Venulitis associated with systemic diseases
  Behçet disease
  Systemic lupus erythematosus
  Necrotizing giant cell granulomatous phlebitis
  Crohn disease
Enterocolic lymphocytic phlebitis (mesenteric inflammatory veno-occlusive disease)
Idiopathic myointimal hyperplasia of mesenteric veins

Reversible colonic ischemia manifests as crampy, usually left-sided, lower abdominal pain, associated with tenesmus, fever, and leukocytosis. Severe pain, fever, leukocytosis, peritoneal irritation, and/or profound ileus indicates extensive, and probably irreversible, ischemic damage (100). Anorexia, nausea or vomiting, abdominal distention from ileus, an altered sensorium, and clinical signs or symptoms of sepsis or shock can also develop. When ischemia extends to the muscularis propria, motility problems develop.

Three types of colonic ischemia develop: (a) a transient reversible form that usually remains confined to the mucosa or submucosa; (b) a chronic form that extends into the bowel wall and lasts for months; and (c) an acute fulminant form that progressively destroys all layers of the bowel wall, usually with catastrophic consequences, including transmural necrosis and perforation. Complete recovery often follows mild ischemia. More severe disease undergoes partial resolution complicated by fibrosis and stricture formation.

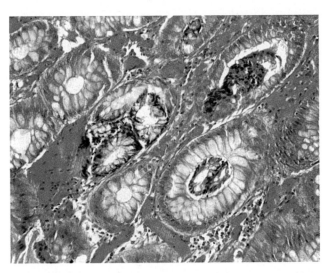

FIG. 13.65. Biopsy artifact. The glands have intussuscepted into one another, appearing as glands lying within the lumen of other glands.

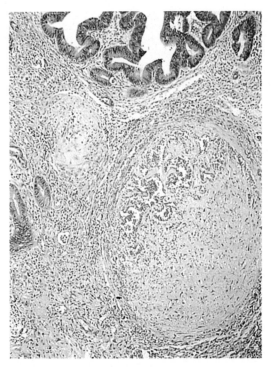

FIG. 13.66. A recanalized thrombus is present in a submucosal vessel. The overlying mucosa is neoplastic.

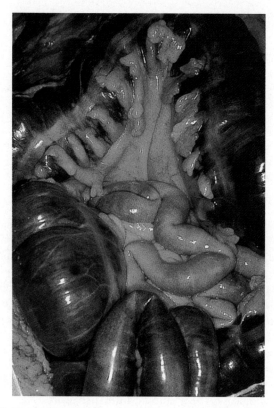

FIG. 13.67. Massive infarction of the small and large intestine.

The most severe form of injury, transmural infarction, requires resection of the affected segment; otherwise, perforation or death will ensue. Almost half of patients with colonic ischemia have a transient, reversible form of the disease; 20% to 25% have chronic colitis or deep colonic infarction; and more than 10% to 15% develop late ischemic strictures (100–102). Approximately 15% to 20% of patients develop gangrene or perforation, either as an initial presentation of the disease or within a variable time following symptom onset. Sigmoidoscopic findings can include striking mucosal edema, ulceration, nodularity, hypervascularity, friability, and pseudomembranes. Ulcers may or may not be present. These features evolve rapidly from one examination to the next.

Pathophysiology of Ischemic Injury

As in the small intestine, the physiology of the circulation is such that a countercurrent exchange mechanism shunts oxygen into the lower mucosa at the expense of its upper portion (103). Consequently, the normally relatively hypoxic upper mucosa, which is particularly vulnerable to the effects of hypoperfusion, becomes necrotic, while the lower mucosa remains intact (Fig. 13.68). The degree of ischemic damage depends on the adequacy of the collateral circulation, on vascular autoregulatory mechanisms, and on tissue resistance to hypoxia. The extent and pattern of disease also depends on the anatomy of the blood supply, duration of the hypoxic episode, and bacte-

rial population within the bowel lumen. The mildest lesions affect only the mucosa, and one sees superficial necrosis and hemorrhage. If reflow occurs, neutrophils infiltrate the tissues (see Chapter 6). There are three phases in the colonic reaction to ischemia: (a) acute with hemorrhage and necrosis, (b) repair with the formation of granulation tissue and fibrosis, and (c) the formation of structures and other complications. A number of disorders and damaging agents cause colonic injury via an ischemic mechanism (Table 13.6).

Large Vessel Occlusion Versus Small Vessel Occlusion

The severity of the lesions varies from microscopic focal damage to involvement of the entire colon. The size of the lesion correlates directly with the size of the affected vessels. Colonic ischemia results from occlusion of large vessels such as the mesenteric arteries or diseases or thromboemboli, which affect the intramural circulation with its smaller vasculature. Obstruction or diffuse vasospasm involving the major arterial supply of the large intestine results in severe ischemia to extensive regions of the colon or rectum. More distal obstruction of the colonic blood supply results in segmental ischemia or infarction. Only rarely does one see complete vascular occlusion. The superior branch of the mesenteric artery is more prone to undergo embolization than the inferior mesenteric artery due to the smaller caliber and more acute angle of take-off of the inferior mesenteric artery (103). The ostium may undergo thrombosis at its origin from the aorta due to aortic atherosclerosis, but the presence of a collateral circulation often maintains an adequate perfusion (104). Small vessel disease results from microangiopathies as seen in patients with hypertension, arteriolosclerosis, diabetes, vasculitis, radiation injury, or coagulation diatheses. Vascular obstruction also results from nonocclusive factors or obstruction of the vessels by external forces, as discussed in Chapter 6.

Sites of Injury

Ischemia affects the colon more commonly than it affects the small bowel, probably because of the vast collateral vascular network that exists in the small bowel (105). Colonic regions with poor collateral circulation, particularly around the splenic flexure and the rectosigmoid, are especially vulnerable (106). The superior and inferior mesenteric arteries communicate via the left branch of the middle colic artery and the ascending branch of the left colic artery at the arc of Riolan (marginal artery of Drummond). Approximately 5% of individuals have underdeveloped or absent connections between the two arterial systems at the splenic flexure, making them susceptible to ischemic damage (107).

Gross Features

The gross features of large intestinal ischemia resemble those of small intestinal ischemia. The changes vary depending on

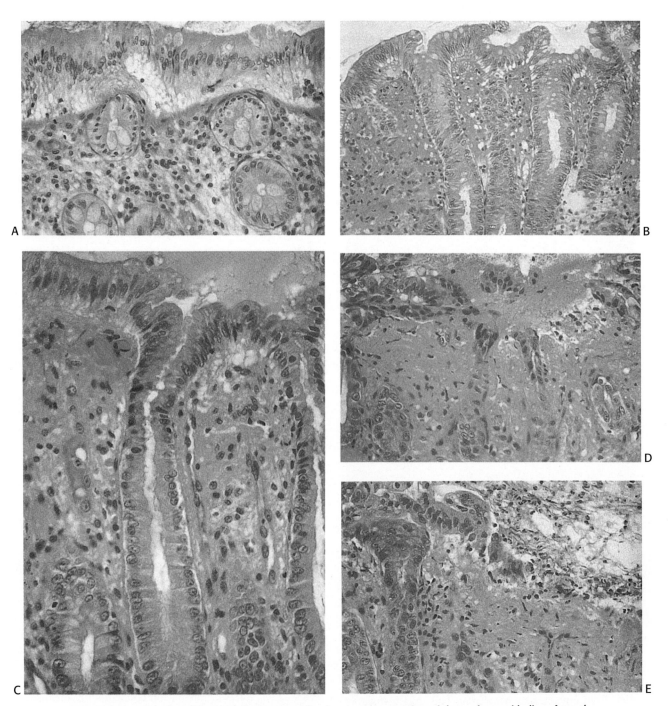

FIG. 13.68. Ischemic colitis. **A:** Early change with edema and separation of the surface epithelium from the underlying basement membrane. **B:** Epithelial regeneration and mucin depletion are present. The intervening lamina propria is hemorrhagic and edematous. **C:** High-power magnification of the mucin depletion. The lamina propria is hypocellular in this particular area. **D:** Active regeneration from the crypt bases in a patient with repeated ischemic episodes. The lamina propria is fibrotic. **E:** Surface re-epithelialization. A pseudomembrane overlies the surface epithelium.

the severity and depth of the ischemic process, whether the event is acute or chronic, and the stage of healing that may have occurred (Figs. 13.69 to 13.71). In early ischemia (usually seen during endoscopic procedures), the mucosa appears paler than normal but an increased vascular pattern with patchy, granular, swollen areas may be present. Bowels

with transmural infarction may either appear pale or hemorrhagic depending on the circumstances. If hemorrhage has occurred, the bowel appears darkish blue or purple with blood in the bowel lumen. The wall may appear thinner than normal. As the disease becomes more severe, it extends into the submucosa causing edema and hemorrhage. Eventually,

TABLE 13.6 **Disorders with an Ischemic Basis**

Small vessel disease
Arteritis/venulitis
Rheumatoid arthritis
Diabetes mellitus
Systemic lupus erythematosus
Scleroderma
Polyarteritis nodosa
Wegener granulomatosis
Amyloidosis
Drug-associated colitis
Antibiotic-associated colitis
Oral contraceptives
Potassium salts
Cocaine
Immunosuppressive agents
Digitalis
Uremia
Hemolytic uremic syndrome
Radiation
Collagen vascular diseases
Venoms and toxins
Disseminated intravascular coagulation
Colitis complicating obstruction
Infections
Staphylococcal enterocolitis
Necrotizing enterocolitis of the newborn
Polycythemia vera
Trauma to mesenteric vasculature during abdominal
   surgery
Pheochromocytoma-associated colitis

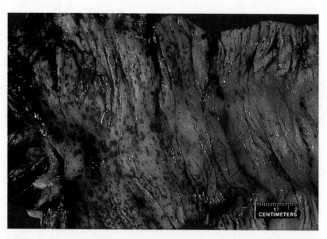

FIG. 13.69. Numerous mucosal petechial hemorrhages are present in this early area of ischemia.

the mucosa sloughs and areas of grayish green necrosis develop, producing pseudomembranes. Ulcers may be present. These may be only superficial or they may be deep and linear. Occasionally the ulceration is extensive and confluent. Perforation may occur. The features may mimic fulminant UC or toxic megacolon. The ischemic changes exhibit a geographic distribution, often with a sharp line of demarcation between the involved and uninvolved mucosa (Fig. 13.70).

In patients who survive the acute event, the wall will appear thickened, fibrotic, and contracted. Strictures covered either by an ulcerated granular-appearing mucosa or by a re-epithelialized mucosa may be present. The gross features of chronic disease may mimic Crohn disease or a neoplasm.

Resection specimens for ischemia should be handled in a regular way so as to evaluate the extent of the ischemic damage, the viability of the margins, and, if possible, the etiology. The vessels should be examined both macroscopically and microscopically to detect evidence of thrombosis or vascular occlusion. Handling an intestinal resection specimen is discussed in detail in Chapter 6.

Transitory Ischemia

There is a form of ischemia that is transient and reversible. Usually the patients present with mild GI complaints and no

obvious cardiovascular event precedes or appears to precipitate the ischemia. The patients may also have crampy abdominal pain and rectal bleeding. The diagnosis is usually a clinical one. Therefore, the lesion is not typically resected or biopsied because the bowel will heal if the damage is minimal. However, sometimes biopsies are performed to elucidate the cause of the pain or the bleeding. The biopsies may show the acute ischemic changes described below or they may show evidence of mucosal regeneration.

Acute Ischemia

The earliest ischemic lesions vary in their histologic appearance depending on the size of the occluded vessel. If the vessel is small and the degree of ischemia is minimal, the first changes affect the superficial parts of crypts and spare all but the superficial lamina propria. With continuing injury the damage progressively involves more of the crypts, eventually reaching the base. Biopsies in the acute stage show variable mucosal necrosis with loss of surface epithelium (Figs. 13.68 and 13.72 to 13.74), dilated capillaries and lymphatics, mucosal edema with hemorrhage and fibrin deposition (Fig. 13.72), and crypt dropout. In severe cases, the crypts appear to be bursting, dilated, and lined by an attenuated epithelium (Fig. 13.73). The crypts become filled with mucus and inflammatory debris. One may also see crypt abscesses. The epithelial loss leaves dilated, ghostlike, bare crypts supported by a congested lamina propria (Fig. 13.73). Goblet cells become mucin depleted and neutrophils infiltrate the mucosa. The muscularis mucosae becomes frayed. Early in the process neutrophils are relatively sparse.

In patients with more extensive lesions, the submucosa becomes markedly edematous with concomitant capillary and lymphatic dilation. The submucosa contains inflammatory cells and it appears edematous, congested, and hemorrhagic (Fig. 13.74). Red cells sludge in the vessels, causing further thrombosis and hemorrhage. The mucosa becomes necrotic. Ulcers develop. The depth of the ulcers varies

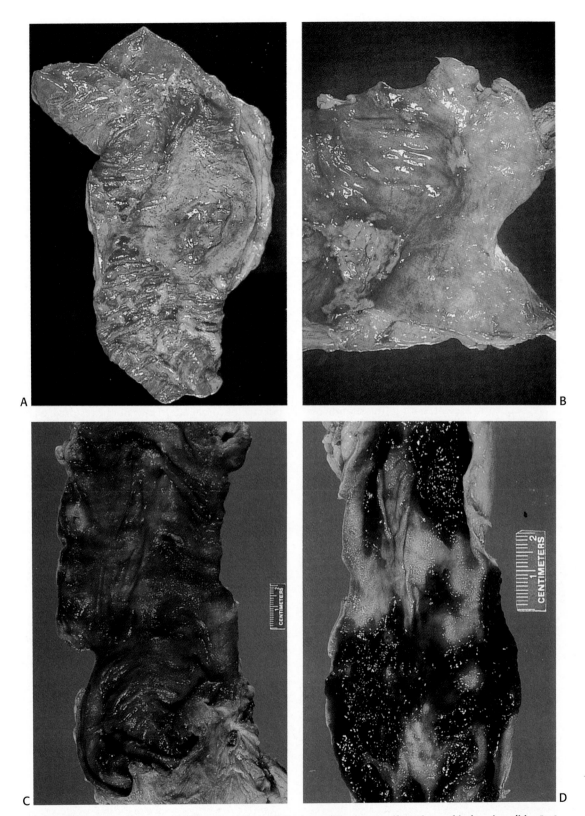

FIG. 13.70. Gross features of ischemia. A through D show different manifestations of ischemic colitis. **A:** A discrete, patchy pseudomembrane covers a geographic mucosal area. The region immediately surrounding it is hyperemic. **B:** An atrophic mucosa with diffuse mucosal hyperemia and a small, triangular, pseudomembranous patch. **C:** Diffuse mucosal hyperemia without patches. **D:** Patchy involvement of the mucosa without pseudomembranes.

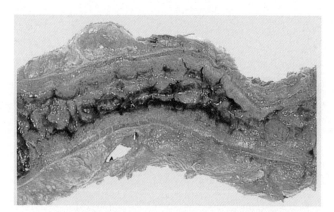

FIG. 13.71. Stricture complicating ischemic colitis.

depending on the extent of the anoxic injury. They may be mucosal, extend into the submucosa or muscularis propria, or be transmural (Fig. 13.75). Transmural ulcers lead to perforation and these perforation sites may appear well demarcated and punched-out.

Once the mucosa breaks down, bacteria may invade, eliciting a neutrophilic infiltration. Neutrophils also infiltrate the bowel as a result of reperfusion injury. At this stage, fibrin thrombi are frequently present, both in the submucosa and mucosa. Because the damage is typically patchy, normal mucosa is present between the involved areas. As the disease becomes more severe and the duration of the ischemia continues, the anoxia causes deeper injury to the bowel wall, possibly with transmural necrosis. Often there is an endophlebitis beneath the ulcers. This is present in the

mucosa and submucosa and in severe cases it may extend along the veins, involving the extramural vessels. In this situation it may be difficult to tell whether the phlebitis is the cause or the effect of the ischemia.

Reparative Phase

If the patient survives the acute injury, a reparative phase will follow. The ulcer bases are replaced by granulation tissue and fibrosis. The granulation tissue response may be quite extensive. Large numbers of infiltrating neutrophils are present initially; these are gradually replaced by chronic inflammatory cells, including lymphocytes, plasma cells, and histiocytes. Fibroblasts proliferate in the lamina propria, obliterating the normal cell population and leading to mucosal fibrosis. If the hypoxic damage remains superficial and spares the crypt bases, regeneration ensues with increased mitotic activity in the crypt bases. If the injury was minor with only mild crypt dropout, the epithelium will regenerate using the pericryptal myofibroblast sheath as a scaffold and the architecture may return to a completely normal state (Fig. 13.76). Ulcers re-epithelialize from residual viable cells at the base of the crypts and from ingrowth of surface epithelium. The regenerating epithelium forms crypts, but a normal mucosal pattern may not be restored. Glandular distortion persists and the new lamina propria consists of fibrous tissue containing hemosiderin-filled histiocytes. At this time, very prominent submucosal collections of chronic inflammatory cells may be present. These may present as bandlike infiltrates that are populated by large numbers of plasma cells, and the changes may mimic CD. The resemblance to CD

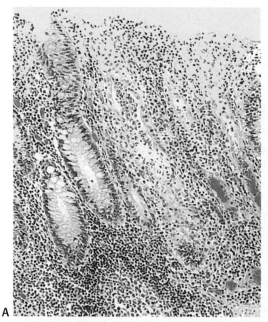
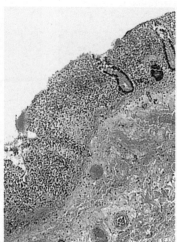
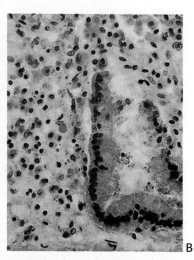

FIG. 13.72. Ischemic colitis. **A:** Focal crypt dropout. Two relatively normal crypts overlie the lymphoid follicle. The crypts to the right are partially necrotic. **B:** The *left panel* shows extensive ischemic damage. Only a few residual crypts remain. One of these is shown at higher magnification in the *right panel.*

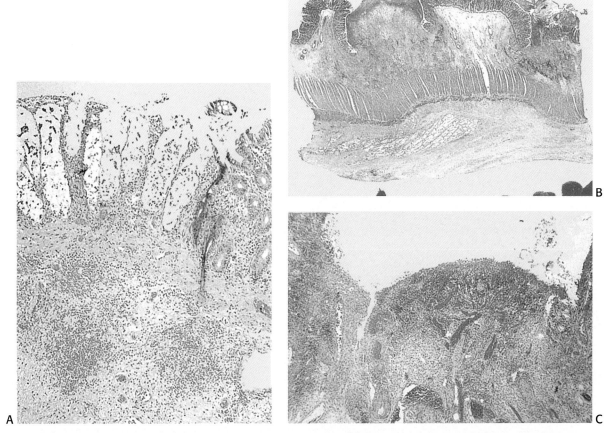

FIG. 13.73. Ischemic colitis. **A:** Crypt dropout is present in the left side of the picture. **B:** Ischemic colitis is a patchy process that affects some areas and leaves adjacent ones more or less normal. **C:** An ischemic ulcer.

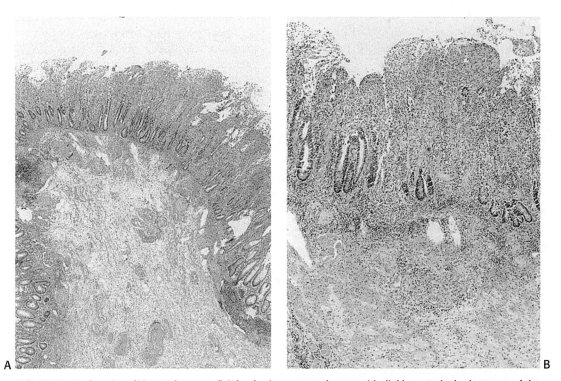

FIG. 13.74. Ischemic colitis. **A:** The superficial colonic mucosa shows epithelial loss. Only the bottoms of the crypts are left. The submucosa is markedly edematous. **B:** Higher magnification of the damaged crypts with residual epithelium at the crypt base (*left*). The mucosa is infiltrated with acute and chronic inflammatory cells. The submucosa is congested, edematous, and inflamed.

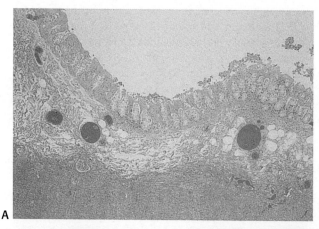

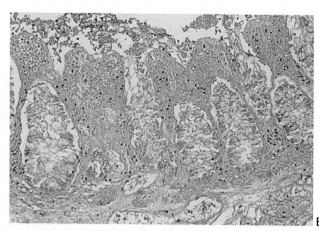

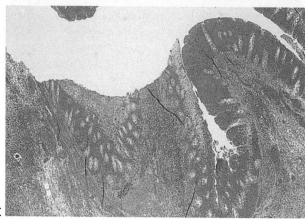

FIG. 13.75. Severe acute ischemia. **A:** Low-magnification photograph demonstrating the transmural coagulative necrosis with marked vascular congestion and no inflammation. **B:** Higher magnification showing the details of the mucosal necrosis. **C:** Portion of another case showing a marked mucosal hemorrhage.

is enhanced if mild acute injury continues. Large ulcers may heal, leaving only an area of re-epithelialized flat surface without crypts. Patients with resolved ischemic injury may develop strictures, glandular irregularities, architectural distortions, and areas of pyloric gland; Paneth cell metaplasia; or colitis cystica profunda. Additionally, endocrine cell hyperplasia may develop. Acute changes may persist with continuing ischemia or resolve with fibrosis, scarring, and stricture formation (Fig. 13.71).

Regenerating crypts often appear hyperchromatic and disorganized and the hyperchromatic epithelium may mimic dysplasia. However, because the hyperchromasia occurs in the setting of other histologic features of ischemia, including lamina propria fibrosis, inflammation, and sometimes hemosiderin deposits, a misdiagnosis of dysplasia is seldom made.

Fibrosis and Stricture Formation

The features of the strictures involve all layers of the bowel wall. The mucosa architecture is typically distorted and may show any of the features typically associated with chronic colitis. It may exhibit a range of changes that include continuing acute inflammation, ulceration, granulation tissue, variable degrees of repair, and fibrosis. The muscularis mucosae is often hyperplastic, frayed, and fibrotic. Initially the submucosa is chronically inflamed and edematous. This is replaced by increasing fibrosis that extends into the muscularis propria.

Biopsy Findings of Ischemia

The major clinical differential diagnosis in patients presenting with colitis is IBD, infection, ischemia, and microscopic

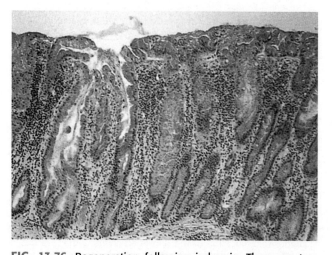

FIG. 13.76. Regeneration following ischemia. There are two regenerative crypts surrounded by a more normal mucosa.

colitis. The biopsy features of ischemic colitis may overlap those seen in other diseases, particularly clostridial and enterohemorrhagic *Escherichia coli* infections. Clues to the diagnosis of ischemia are listed in Table 13.7. The biopsy features reflect the stage in the evolution of the injury. Early ischemic lesions consist of mucosal necrosis and hemorrhage with minimal or no inflammation if reperfusion injury has not occurred. These changes are usually restricted to the superficial mucosa. The more severe the ischemia, the more severe the changes are. The epithelium appears flattened with mild crypt dropout. As the lesions evolve, one may see erosions and areas of acute inflammation (Figs. 13.77 and 13.78) and reactive epithelial hyperplasia. The lamina propria appears variably cellular and there may be eosinophils in addition to mononuclear cells and

TABLE 13.7	Clues to the Biopsy Diagnosis of Ischemia

Features present

Glandular dropout
Injury preferentially affecting the glands
Injury preferentially affecting the superficial parts of the glands
Presence of thrombi
Presence of a vasculitis
Hemosiderin in the lamina propria
Presence of abnormal vessels

Features absent

Granulomas

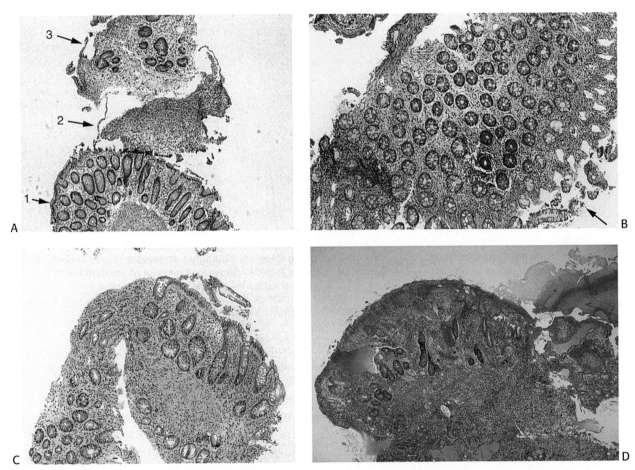

FIG. 13.77. Mucosal biopsies in ischemic colitis. **A:** Three tissue fragments are present. These are labeled *1, 2,* and *3.* Number 1 shows mild inflammation in the lamina propria and mild glandular irregularity. Specimen 2 is a portion of a pseudomembrane or ulcer bed, and specimen 3 is a piece of mucosa demonstrating severe damage with focal glandular loss and regeneration as seen by fused glands and glands of differing sizes. Such features are typical of ischemia, which is a focal disease. **B:** Patchy chronic inflammation in an otherwise more or less normal-appearing mucosa. There is crypt dropout at the surface (*arrow*). This patient had known circulatory disturbances and previous documented ischemic bowel. **C:** A portion of colonic mucosa with focal fibrosis and glandular loss. The mucosa appears fibrotic. **D:** A biopsy from a patient who had significant rectal bleeding. The biopsy shows severe ischemic injury with marked hemorrhage and dilation of the vasculature, loss of the individual crypts, and dropout at the superficial portion. These acute changes are superimposed on chronic damage as evidenced by the presence of the branched crypt bases. The inflammation extends to the underlying submucosa.

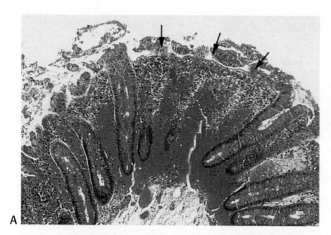
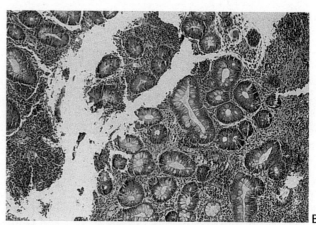

FIG. 13.78. Mucosal biopsies in ischemia. **A:** Acute ischemia with hemorrhagic necrosis. The *arrows* indicate three crypts that have dropped out of the mucosa. The *right-hand arrow* shows where an entire crypt has been lost. The *middle arrow* indicates a crypt with a small amount of residual basal epithelium in the base of the crypt. The *left-hand arrow* shows another crypt in which the base has a larger number of cells. **B:** Multiple irregularly shaped glands and focal chronic inflammation are present. This patient had known multiple past episodes of ischemia.

neutrophils. The crypts may appear distorted with variable atrophy and fibrosis of the lamina propria. A pseudomembrane may cover the mucosal surface and the lesions may resemble those seen in *Clostridium difficile*–associated colitis described later in this chapter. Biopsies in individuals with clinically evident disease may have injury extending into the underlying submucosa or deeper portions of the wall.

The changes may also overlap with Crohn disease because of the focal nature of the inflammation (Fig. 13.78). However, unlike CD, some patients lack features of chronicity as evidenced by architectural distortion. In contrast, patients with severe chronic ischemic disease may develop chronic damage, with marked architectural distortion, fibrosis, and strictures. In this setting, the presence of hemosiderin-laden macrophages in the lamina propria helps to establish a diagnosis of ischemia rather than CD. The presence of what appears to be a transmural infiltrate in a biopsy may also mimic CD. However, in ischemia, cryptitis and crypt abscesses are usually absent and the adjacent colonic epithelium does not usually appear mucus depleted. Additionally, in ischemia one does not have the compact granulomas typical of CD.

The biopsy features also overlap with pseudomembranous colitis. Both *C. difficile* enterocolitis and ischemic enterocolitis produce pseudomembranes. Hyalinization of the lamina propria is highly predictive of the presence of ischemic injury, as are atrophic microcrypts. Additionally, lamina propria hemorrhage, full-thickness mucosal necrosis, and diffuse microscopic distribution of the pseudomembranes are more common in ischemia than in *C. difficile* colitis. In contrast, endoscopic identification of diffuse pseudomembranes favors the diagnosis of *C. difficile* (108). Ischemia may also be the result of some of the entities in the differential diagnosis.

Ischemic Enterocolitis (Necrotizing Enterocolitis)

Necrotizing enterocolitis represents a type of ischemic injury. Ischemic enterocolitis, also known as pseudomembranous enterocolitis, usually produces massive necrosis of the small intestine and colon, often as a terminal event following an episode of shock. The disease also affects newborns (see Chapter 6). Some patients develop toxic megacolon (109). The severity of the lesion depends on (a) the severity of the ischemia, (b) the virulence of the luminal microbial flora, and (c) the overall general health of the patient at the time of the episode. It differs from segmental forms of ischemia, which remain localized to a small area of the colon. Perforation, peritonitis, and sepsis contribute to its high mortality rate.

In the acute stage, the infarcted area shows mucosal necrosis, submucosal hemorrhage, and edema with congested capillaries often containing fibrin plugs. As the mucosa sloughs, ulcers develop and their bases become covered by fibrin, neutrophils, and necrotic debris. Bacterial and fungal invasion occur as a result of the loss of the mucosal integrity. The ulcer margins and the edges of the ulcer base show ischemic injury and vascular congestion. The adjacent nonulcerated mucosa appears erythematous. A pseudomembrane containing fibrin and white blood cells covers the surface. As the lesions evolve, plasma cells, lymphocytes, and macrophages infiltrate the area and the capillaries proliferate, forming granulation tissue. The macrophages may contain hemosiderin. Capillary endothelium may become swollen and appear atypical. The nerves and muscle cells may become vacuolated and degenerate. As these lesions evolve, they are replaced by granulation tissue and then fibrosis. Often, a well-demarcated zone of neutrophilic infiltration forms between the necrotic and viable bowel wall. Pneumatosis intestinalis may also develop. The differential

TABLE 13.8 Diseases Associated with Formation of Pseudomembranes

Antibiotic-associated colitis
Ischemia
Hemolytic uremic syndrome
Heavy metal toxicity
Chemotherapy-induced intestinal damage
Neutropenic enterocolitis
Shigellosis
Colitis complicating obstruction
Amebiasis
Mucosal prolapse
Microscopic colitis (rare)

diagnosis of pseudomembranous colitis is listed in Table 13.8. If the patient recovers, prominent submucosal fibrosis may develop, leading to stricture formation. Morphologically, one may see all stages of injury and repair in the specimen. When a stricture develops, the lesion may mimic colonic carcinoma.

Enterocolitis in Hirschsprung Disease

Enterocolitis is the most severe, potentially life-threatening complication of Hirschsprung disease. It is estimated that 5% of patients with Hirschsprung disease will die of enterocolitis. The enterocolitis develops any time during the disease course irrespective of age, sex, or method of management. It is characterized by abdominal distention, diarrhea, fever, and hypovolemic shock. The diagnosis is made clinically and confirmed radiologically. Radiography demonstrates colonic dilation, mucosal ulceration, GI hypomotility, and sometimes pneumatosis coli. Several factors contribute to its pathogenesis, including proximal colonic dilation with resultant mucosal ischemia and bacterial invasion, and hypersensitivity to bacterial antigens. More recently, *C. difficile* and its toxin have been implicated in its development (110).

Tropical Enterocolitis

Tropical enterocolitis, a distinct form of necrotizing enterocolitis, differs from neonatal enterocolitis discussed in Chapter 6. It presents as an acute abdomen with pain, bilious vomiting, constipation, or bloody diarrhea due to the presence of a segmental jejunitis, ileitis, or colitis and, rarely, duodenitis. The pathology appears to involve a local hyperimmune reaction in the affected bowel segment. Changes range from punctate hemorrhages in the muscular layer of the bowel to a generalized fiery red appearance and possible perforation secondary to mucosal ulceration. Whatever the causative agent, the pathogenesis involves a local vasculitis leading to variable ischemic damage (111).

Obstructive Colitis

The term *obstructive colitis* refers to ulceroinflammatory lesions measuring 0.5 to 2.5 cm in length that occur proximal to obstructing lesions including tumors, diverticular disease, volvulus, torsion, hernias, strictures, or atresias (112). The diseased bowel is separated from the obstruction by a variable length (2.5 to 35 cm) of normal mucosa. The patients are typically female and elderly with a mean age of 73 years. They usually have coexisting hypertension, diabetes, or other prior chronic illnesses. This lesion likely results from vascular compromise by the obstructing lesion. An altered intestinal flora may exert a synergistic effect (112).

The changes vary depending on whether the obstruction developed over a long time or acutely. Slowly developing lesions result in chronic superficial ulceration with evidence of both acute and chronic injury. Ulcers and pseudopolyps may be present and the overall architecture may appear cobblestoned. The changes are patchy in nature, distinguishing the lesion from ulcerative colitis, which it grossly resembles. In contrast, rapidly developing lesions resemble necrotizing enterocolitis. Loss of individual muscle fibers in the muscularis propria results in "vanishing muscle." This disorder often develops in the right colon.

The lesions range in severity from discrete ulcers to extensive areas of fulminant colitis with necrosis, diffuse ulceration, and fibrosis (113). Endoscopically, the involved colon usually appears mildly to massively dilated and exhibits moderate intramural thickening with a granular luminal surface accentuated by deeper longitudinal transverse ulcers. Perforation and peritonitis may develop. Because the biopsy features of obstructive colitis are nonspecific, it may be impossible to distinguish this entity from other disorders, particularly ischemia, due to other causes. The mucosa distal to the obstructing lesion usually appears normal, but this may not allow one to make a diagnosis of obstructive colitis unless one has been informed that an obstruction was present. These histologic changes are those of ischemic colitis.

Ischemic Colitis Complicating Chronic Renal Disease

Renal transplant patients develop various gastrointestinal complications. Half of posttransplant deaths result from GI complications (114). Large doses of corticosteroids, azathioprine, and other immunosuppressive drugs deplete the gut of its lymphoid tissue and depress cellular immune responses to noxious agents, predisposing the bowel to infection. Additionally, epithelial cell turnover is delayed, impeding mucosal repair. Several drugs, especially cyclosporine, induce vascular damage.

Systemic calciphylaxis is an uncommon complication of chronic renal failure characterized by disseminated intravascular calcification and progressive vascular compromise that may involve many parts of the body including the GI tract. Mural calcification of medium and large vessels leads to severe ischemic necrosis (115). Parathyroidectomy may lead to clinical improvement.

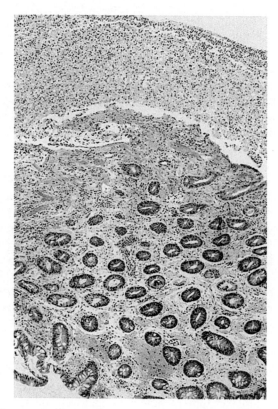

FIG. 13.79. Biopsy from a renal transplant patient with hemolytic uremic syndrome. The changes show features typical of ischemia with loss of the superficial epithelium, focal glandular dropout, mucosal congestion, and a pseudomembrane overlying the surface.

Hemolytic Uremia Syndrome

Hemolytic uremic syndrome (HUS) usually affects children under 7 years of age following a prodromal period of bloody diarrhea caused by the Shiga toxin from *E. coli* 0157:H or renal transplant patients of any age. It consists of the triad of microangiopathic hemolytic anemia, thrombocytopenia, and oliguric renal failure. Neurologic manifestations may also occur. GI involvement is seen in 75% of children with HUS (116). GI symptoms include bloody diarrhea, vomiting, abdominal pain and tenderness, peritonitis, and hepatomegaly. Proctoscopy demonstrates a friable rectal mucosa with rectal ulcers and mucosal pseudomembranes (Fig. 13.79). Patients may present with segmental colonic gangrene (117). The illness may be clinically misdiagnosed as ulcerative colitis, pseudomembranous colitis, or intussusception. Endoscopic appearances vary and include normal, mild patchy colitis with edema, focal mucosal hemorrhage, aphthous ulcers, and erythema anywhere from the ileocecal valve to the rectum.

In most cases no causative agent is identified but a genetic predisposition (118); certain viruses, especially enteroviruses (119); Shiga toxin–producing, Gram-negative enteric bacteria (120); estrogens; and postpartum and postrenal transplant oliguria all associate with HUS. Endothelial damage underlies the injury. Bacterial enzymes, endotoxins, and immune injury mediate the endothelial damage initiating the coagulation cascade (121). Patients develop localized Schwartzman-type reactions with fibrin and platelet thrombi formation.

Histologically, colonic submucosal vessels show perivascular mononuclear infiltrates, focal mural necrosis, and thrombi in various stages of organization. The latter cause secondary ischemic necrosis. Neutrophils infiltrate the lamina propria and crypts. The inflammatory changes vary from mild and patchy to a more widespread diffuse cryptitis with crypt abscesses. The focal nature of the infiltrate and absence of chronic damage distinguish the disorder from ulcerative colitis. Apoptoses are present in the superficial epithelium and lamina propria. Pseudomembranes develop as the ischemia progresses.

Vasculitis

The diagnosis of vasculitis involving the colon is more easily made in a resection specimen than in a biopsy. Vasculitis may affect both the small and large intestines and causes either localized or more widespread ischemic disease that may appear as areas of ulceration, hemorrhage, or wider gastrointestinal infarction. In order to make a diagnosis of vasculitis, the tissue specimen must include the submucosa. In its absence, all one can say is that ischemic damage is present. Some of the vasculitides are discussed below. The remainder are discussed in Chapter 6.

Phlebosclerotic Colitis

Colonic phlebosclerosis is a rare disease characterized by a thickening of the colonic wall with fibrosis, hyalinization, and calcification of the affected veins (122,123). These cause a unique form of ischemic colitis. The lesion occurs sporadically or in association with colonic adenomas (122). Radiographic studies demonstrate linear calcifications in the intestinal wall. The right colon is preferentially affected and there are no skip lesions. Grossly the mucosa may appear discolored with ulcers. Histologically there is a mucosal fibrosis, hyalinization, and calcification diffusely involving the colon. The mucosa shows architectural distortion and mild lymphoplasmacytic infiltrates, all features of chronic ischemia. The fibrosis often centers around the veins. The mesenteric vasculature appears calcified.

The differential diagnosis includes amyloidosis, but a negative Congo red stain rules out this as an etiology of the histologic alterations. Diabetic colonopathy, also in the differential diagnosis, is unlikely given the fibrosis that affects the veins and randomly involves the lamina propria. Collagenous colitis involves superficial fibrosis and it does not center around the veins.

Idiopathic Myointimal Hyperplasia of Mesenteric Veins

Idiopathic myointimal hyperplasia of mesenteric veins (IMHMV) is a rare cause of intestinal ischemia secondary to venous compromise that typically affects the sigmoid area. The disorder affects males who present with lower abdominal pain, diarrhea, and rectal bleeding (124). Colonoscopic mucosal biopsies may show the presence of many dilated thick-walled, eosinophilic, hyalinized blood vessels lined by plump endothelial cells. Depending on the stage of the disease, the mucosa exhibits varying degrees of ischemic damage. Some vessels may contain fibrin thrombi. In resection specimens similar vessels are present in the submucosa, adventitia, and mesocolon. There is a marked myointimal hyperplasia of the vessels, reducing their luminal caliber to small slitlike spaces. The abnormal veins appear more prominent than the arteries. The veins also show increased deposition of Alcian blue material and collagen type IV. There is no inflammation of the veins (124). Patients do well following surgical resection of the affected segment.

Mesenteric Inflammatory Veno-occlusive Disorder (Enterocolic Lymphocytic Phlebitis)

Mesenteric inflammatory veno-occlusive disease, also known as enterocolic lymphocytic phlebitis, is a rare disease involving small veins of the large and less frequently the small intestine. The colon, distal ileum, and appendix may be affected (125). The disease occurs twice as frequently in males than in females and patients range in age from 24 to 78 years (126). It results from an isolated vasculitis involving mesenteric veins and their intramural tributaries that leads to intestinal ischemia and produces changes that may mimic IBD (127). It presents with the insidious onset of abdominal pain, bloody or nonbloody diarrhea, nausea, and a tumorlike mass. The pathogenesis of this disorder is unknown, although it has been suggested that there may be an etiologic relationship with the drugs rutoside or flutamide (125). A predominantly lymphocytic infiltration surrounds intramural tributaries of the mesenteric veins, sometimes with the formation of perivenous lymphocytic cuffs. Giant cells may be present (128). In some areas the phlebitis does not compromise the vascular lumens, but in others there are subintimal fibroproliferative lesions that are focally occlusive (129). It is thought that the myointimal hyperplasia is a reactive vasculopathy secondary to chronic vasculitis, perhaps related to mesenteric thrombosis from hypercoagulable states, trauma, or sepsis. The vascular changes lead to the typical features of colonic ischemia

The lymphocytic infiltrate consists of both B and T cells. Some have shown a zonal arrangement of the T and B cells, but this has not been found by all (129). The T cells are of a cytotoxic lineage and express TIA-1 (T cell–restricted intracellular antigen-1) (129), a protein found in cytotoxic granules of T cells. These findings suggest that the vascular damage is lymphocyte mediated.

At the present time it is unclear whether myointimal hyperplasia of mesenteric veins and enterocolic lymphocytic phlebitis are different stages of the same disease or two separate but interrelated diseases (128). The other disease that

may be interrelated with both myointimal hyperplasia of mesenteric veins and enterocolic lymphocytic phlebitis is necrotizing giant cell granulomatosis. The rarity of all of these disorders makes it impossible to sort out these possibilities at the present time. These patients do well after surgical resection.

Collagen Vascular Diseases

Colonic ischemia may complicate collagen vascular diseases such as systemic lupus erythematosus. Patients may develop massive intestinal hemorrhage, total colonic necrosis, or limited infarctions and perforations (130,131). Patients often have concurrent renal failure. They develop a vasculitis involving smaller arteries and veins due to deposition of circulating immune complexes in the vessel walls (131). The vascular changes are worsened by the presence of uremia, coagulopathy, and medications.

Behçet Syndrome

Behçet syndrome and its associated vasculitis typically affect the terminal ileum and cecum. Its histologic features are discussed in Chapter 6.

CHANGES INDUCED BY DRUGS AND TOXINS

The etiology of drug-induced colitis varies significantly, as does the underlying pathophysiologic disturbance that results from the drug ingestion. Since drug-induced colitis is likely underrecognized, its true incidence is unknown, especially since the changes induced are usually nonspecific and they mimic many other conditions. Drug-induced injury can cause acute diarrhea soon after the drug is started. Alternatively, chronic diarrhea may appear long after the drug administration. The histologic changes range from a normal-appearing colon to fulminant colitis and extensive necrosis. Drugs can induce ischemia, eosinophilic colitis, necrotizing colitis, microscopic colitis, IBD-like changes, and infectious colitis (Table 13.9).

Laxatives

Melanosis coli results from chronic ingestion of anthraquinones and laxatives derived from plants, including cascara sagrada, aloes, senna, frangula, and rhubarb. Evidence is beginning to emerge that melanosis coli does not result solely from laxative use. It can also occur in patients with IBD (both Crohn disease and ulcerative colitis) who have not used laxatives (132) and in individuals with diarrhea unrelated to IBD who have not used laxatives.

Anthraquinones concentrate in the colon, particularly in the right colon, where they are potent cellular poisons causing apoptosis, even when taken in small doses (133). The

TABLE 13.9	Examples of Colonic Toxicity Due to Medications

Cause ischemia

Cocaine
Estrogen
Ergotamine
Amphetamines
Digitalis
Vasopressin
Methysergide
Cyclosporine

Cause pseudo-obstruction

Anticholinergics
Phenothiazines
Amitriptyline hydrochloride
Antineoplastic drugs, especially vincristine
Tranquilizers
Clonidine
Ganglionic blockers
Narcotics
Cimetidine

Cause infectious or necrotizing enterocolitis

Antibiotics
Chemotherapy
Deferoxamine
Loperamide
Steroids
Immunosuppressants

Cause allergic, cytotoxic, or inflammatory injury

Nonsteroidal anti-inflammatory drugs
Gold salts
Potassium chloride
Mycophenolate
α-Methyldopa
Methotrexate

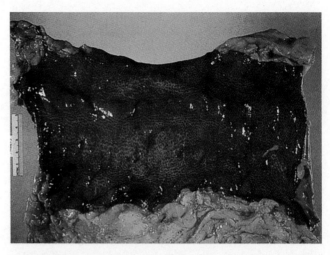

FIG. 13.80. Severe melanosis coli. The bowel is dilated, has lost its haustral folds, and appears darkly pigmented.

Many patients are symptomless only to be diagnosed following endoscopic examination for other reasons. Individuals with surreptitious laxative abuse typically present with unexplained chronic diarrhea. Some patients may have an obsession regarding their need to have a bowel "cleansing."

The colon in patients with melanosis appears dark brownish (Figs. 13.80 and 13.81). Melanosis primarily affects the right colon, but in severe cases the discoloration extends to the left colon or diffusely involves the entire large intestine.

apoptotic bodies are phagocytosed by macrophages and transformed into lipofuscin pigment by lysosomal enzymes (134). The mean apoptotic count is significantly increased in those with melanosis coli compared with a control population. It is said that it takes 4 to 12 months for melanosis coli to be visible and the same amount of time for it to disappear. It is possible that any condition associated with increased apoptosis may result in melanosis coli (135). When present in small quantities, anthraquinones probably stimulate neural tissues leading to their purgative actions. Anthraquinones and other laxatives also damage the myenteric plexus causing neuronal loss, Schwann cell proliferation (133), axonal fragmentation, axonal and dendritic swelling, and smooth muscle damage. This eventually leads to cathartic colon. Bisacodyl, anthraquinone purgatives, phenolphthalein, castor oil, and other agents also cause cathartic colon.

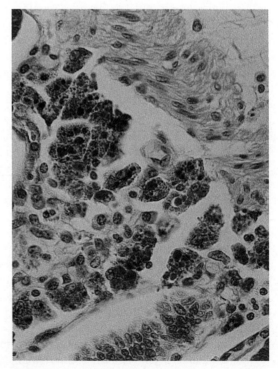

FIG. 13.81. High-power melanosis coli showing macrophages containing prominent brown pigment.

The appendix and terminal ileum may also become affected. Abnormal mucosal proliferations, such as adenomas or colon cancers, arising in a mucosa affected by melanosis coli retain their normal mucosal color rather than becoming pigmented. In severe cases, the entire lamina propria, the submucosa, and even the draining mesenteric lymph nodes contain pigmented macrophages. Migration of pigmented macrophages to regional lymph nodes results in sequential loss of the pigment from the superficial and deep lamina propria (134).

The histologic features of laxative use range from mild melanosis coli to severe cathartic colon. Because the autofluorescent pigment of melanosis coli contains melanin as well as glycoconjugates, it has been suggested that the pigment be termed *melanized ceroid* (136). The ceroid pigment develops from the abundant apoptotic epithelial cells, whereas the precursors of the melanic substance may derive from the anthranoids (136). Autofluorescent, refractile, golden brown, pigmented macrophages populate the lamina propria (Fig. 13.81). Occasionally, one also sees inflammation in the lamina propria, increased apoptotic bodies in the lining epithelium, superficial collections of apoptotic debris, and thickening of the muscularis mucosae. The associated inflammation probably represents a nonspecific response to an underlying injury or to stasis that may have been the cause for the laxative ingestion, rather than a direct effect of the laxative consumption. Subluminal microgranulomas often containing pigment may form (Fig. 13.82).

The pigment stains positively with periodic acid–Schiff (PAS), acid-fast, aniline blue sulfate, and Schmorl stains, but it is negative with the Perl reaction. The brown pigment may be confused with hemosiderin, which usually appears larger and more refractile than melanosis. Special stains for iron can be used in questionable cases.

Mucosal laceration or perforation with mucosal hemorrhage can complicate enema tube insertion. Devices other than the usual enema nozzle used to administer home enemas may cause erosions, mucosal tears, ulcers, or perforations. Patients utilizing enema solutions with various cleansing agents, including *ethyl alcohol* and *hydrogen peroxide,* may develop a severe proctitis (137,138). Hydrogen peroxide enemas, as used by some naturopaths, may induce a clinical picture resembling ischemic colitis, ulcerative colitis, or pseudomembranous colitis (137). The mucosal damage may result from ischemia secondary to the explosive entrance of the generated gases into the bowel wall. Histologically, one may see pneumatosis intestinalis, intense mucosal congestion, hemorrhage, or frank gangrenous necrosis.

Patients sometimes receive *formalin enemas* to cleanse the rectum either for health reasons or to sterilize the bowel wall during cancer surgery. Fortunately, this practice is very rarely used because 10% formalin causes severe, sharp pain and rectal bleeding within a few minutes of instillation. Within a week, the colonic mucosa becomes edematous, with multiple petechiae and superficial erosions. Histologically, one sees a nonspecific chronic colitis

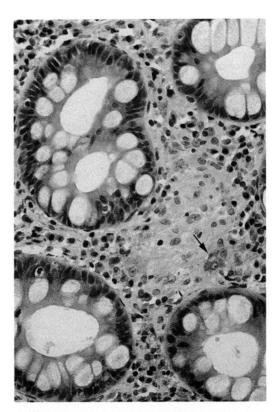

FIG. 13.82. Melanosis coli with granuloma formation. Some of the epithelioid cells contain evidence of brown pigment (*arrow*).

with superficial erosions. The lesions usually heal with a severe fibrosing process that progresses to stricture formation (139).

Kayexalate-Sorbitol Enemas

Kayexalate-sorbitol enemas, used to treat hyperkalemia after renal transplantation, cause intestinal necrosis. Since Kayexalate causes severe constipation, it is administered along with sorbitol, which acts as an osmotic laxative. The osmotic load from the sorbitol causes vascular shunting, resulting in mild colonic ischemia. Patients treated with Kayexalate-sorbitol enemas always have underlying renal disease and many are renal transplant patients (140,141). The colonic damage is potentiated by the presence of uremia. Patients present with an abrupt onset of severe abdominal pain within hours of enema administration. In some cases, elimination of the Kayexalate enemas causes resolution of the colonic manifestations.

At the time of resection, long segments of (or even the entire) colon and rectum may appear necrotic. Histologically, one sees transmural necrosis as seen in acute ischemic injury without reperfusion. The lesion mimics autolysis, although a mild neutrophilic infiltrate may be present. The presence of dark purple crystals that are PAS positive and stain with acid-fast stains establishes the diagnosis (140,141).

TABLE 13.10 Colonic Effects of Nonsteroidal Anti-inflammatory Drugs

Colitis
  Colonic ulcers
  Nonspecific
  Acute eosinophilic colitis
  Ulcerating colitis
  Pseudomembranous colitis
  Eosinophilic colitis
  Collagenous colitis
  Lymphocytic colitis
  Ischemic colitis
Chronic bleeding and perforation
Relapse of inflammatory bowel disease
Strictures
? Diverticula formation
Complicated diverticular disease

Drugs that Damage the Myenteric Plexus and Cause Stercoral Ulceration

Many drugs (in addition to laxatives) damage the myenteric plexus and cause severe chronic constipation, pseudo-obstruction, and stercoral ulceration (Table 13.9). Severe constipation leads to formation of hard fecaliths that can cause local chronic inflammation, acute inflammation, ulceration, bleeding, perforation, and abnormal Schwann cell proliferation.

Nonsteroidal Anti-inflammatory Drugs

NSAIDs exhibit diverse gastrointestinal effects; their pathogenesis is discussed in Chapter 6. The drugs cause a nonspecific colitis and they exacerbate pre-existing colonic diseases including IBD and diverticulitis. IBD patients may undergo reactivation of their disease, especially those who are allergic to salicylates (142). Colonic complications include those listed in Table 13.10. It is difficult to estimate the exact incidence of NSAID-induced colonic injury. Elderly patients, or those with long-term or high-dose NSAID use, exhibit the highest risk of NSAID-associated complications including large intestinal ulcers, bleeding, and perforation. If one is unaware that the patient is taking NSAIDs, the diagnosis may be difficult.

Several forms of colitis associate with NSAID use. The most common is nonspecific in nature and difficult to distinguish from ulcerative colitis early in its natural history. Fenamates are a common cause for this pattern (143). The likelihood of a drug association increases if there is prominent apoptosis (144) and increased intraepithelial lymphocyte counts (microscopic colitis). The apoptotic biopsies are often seen in the crypt bases and in lymphocytes and monocytes under the luminal surface. Collagenous colitis, eosinophilic colitis, and pseudomembranous colitis can also be seen (Fig. 13.83). The changes may also mimic Crohn disease or ischemia. There may be extensive damage, particularly in the proximal colon, and mucosal bridges or diaphragms or strictures may develop (145). Diclofenac can cause granulomatous colonic injury (146).

Patients taking NSAID-containing suppositories develop localized anorectal erosions, ulcers, and stenosis. The abnormalities usually resolve following cessation of NSAID therapy.

Immunosuppressive Agents

Immunosuppressive agents including steroids, indomethacin, mycophenolate, azathioprine, tacrolimus, and cyclosporine all damage the gastrointestinal tract. Immunosuppressive drugs lead to mucosal erosions and ulcerations. Steroid-associated ulcers are usually superficial but deeper ulcerations may lead to perforation. Endoscopically, the mucosa appears edematous with a decreased vascular pattern. Patchy erythema and erosive changes are common. Ulcerative lesions, if present, may be discrete and require biopsy to exclude ischemia, CMV, or other opportunistic infections.

Corticosteroids and azathioprine deplete lymphoid tissues, including gut-associated lymphoid tissues (147), causing a decrease in the size of lymphoid follicles and focal small erosions with M-cell necrosis. This predisposes to bacterial invasion and subsequent perforation. The follicular regions become severely B-cell depleted. Steroids also cause inflammation and cellular necrosis. They slow mucosal cell renewal and decrease the reparative activity of fibroblasts, further predisposing to perforation. Patients on steroids are also prone to develop CMV infections, which may result in an acute colitis.

Mycophenolate mofetil is a relatively new immunosuppressive drug that inhibits inosine monophosphate dehydrogenase, a key enzyme in the de novo pathway of purine synthesis. It causes lymphocyte-selective immunosuppression. It is used to prevent allograft rejection and is usually administered together with cyclosporine or tacrolimus and corticosteroids. Its major adverse effects are on the gastrointestinal tract (149). Mycophenolate causes colonic necrosis and secondary regenerative changes (Fig. 13.84) and intestinal changes that mimic graft versus host disease (GVHD) (148). High doses of mycophenolate also inhibit the proliferation of the stem cells in the intestinal tract (149). The drug may also cause a higher rate of CMV reactivation than is seen in control populations (150).

Cyclosporine causes generalized intestinal microvascular injury (151). Tacrolimus, a potent immunosuppressive drug, decreases mitochondrial adenosine triphosphate (ATP) production, increases intestinal permeability by a mechanism similar to that seen with NSAIDs, and predisposes patients to endotoxemia and impaired intestinal absorption (152). Recipients of organ allografts may develop a GVHD-like condition when receiving tapering doses of cyclosporine, a phenomenon possibly related to an autoimmune reaction. Colonic perforation also complicates high-dose interleukin-2 (IL-2) therapy (153).

Heavy Metal–induced Enterocolitis

Heavy metal therapy with arsenic, mercury, silver, and gold causes colitis. Gold salt therapy causes most heavy metal–induced enterocolitis (154,155), a disease associated with mortality rates as high as 42% (155). The enterocolitis

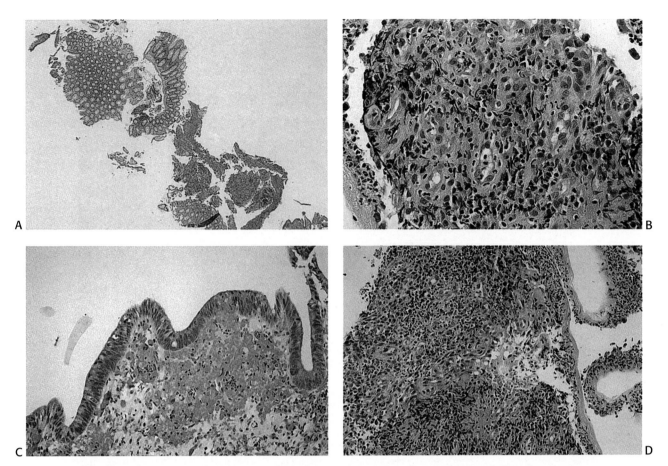

FIG. 13.83. Nonsteroidal anti-inflammatory drug (NSAID) injury. **A:** Low magnification of a mucosal biopsy in a patient with heavy NSAID ingestion. **B:** High magnification showing a portion of the mucosa demonstrating nothing more than granulation tissue. **C:** A portion of gastrointestinal mucosa with red cell extravasation into the lamina propria and regenerative superficial lining cells. **D:** Medium magnification demonstrating the presence of a marked mononuclear cell infiltrate and prominent capillaries.

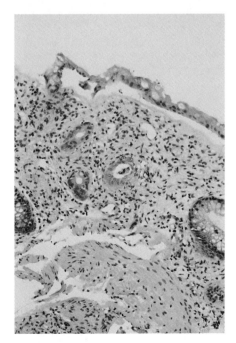

FIG. 13.84. Mycophenolate injury in a renal transplant patient. The lamina propria is hypocellular and there is crypt destruction.

usually starts within several weeks of beginning the drug. Patients present with nausea, vomiting, profuse diarrhea, abdominal pain, fever, proteinuria, maculopapular rashes, and hypogammaglobulinemia. Some patients develop toxic megacolon and perforation (154). Twenty-five percent of patients develop peripheral eosinophilia. The enterocolitis results from either a direct toxic mucosal effect or an immune-mediated hypersensitivity reaction (156). Endoscopically and grossly, petechial hemorrhages, focal ulcers, toxic megacolon, or pseudomembranes may be present (157).

Patients with gold-induced colitis usually have a more or less preserved glandular architecture, although individual crypts may drop out. Diffuse chronic inflammation, often with a prominent eosinophilic component, infiltrates the mucosa (Fig. 13.85). Patients may also develop pseudomembranous colitis and ulcers.

Chemotherapeutic Agents

Some of the most severe drug-induced colitis results from chemotherapeutic agents. Mucosal toxicity varies depending on the type and number of drugs used, their dosage, complicating

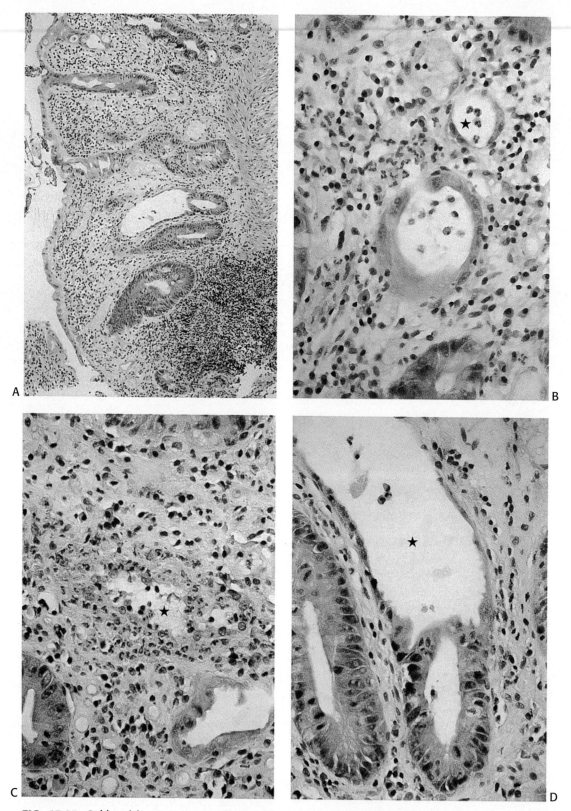

FIG. 13.85. Gold toxicity. **A:** Low-magnification biopsy in a patient with gold toxicity. Note the chronic mucosal damage as evidenced by focal neutrophilic infiltrates, a disorganized muscularis mucosae, and mild glandular distortion. **B:** Higher magnification demonstrating the presence of acute inflammatory cells, including numerous eosinophils and crypts that appear to be disappearing and are difficult to distinguish from capillaries (*star*). Flattened epithelial cells still line the residual gland. **C:** A gland has completely disappeared (*star*) and is only surrounded by acute inflammatory cells. The adjacent glands appear abnormal and the lamina propria appears inflamed. **D:** Regeneration begins at the base of the damaged glands lined by flattened epithelium (*star*). The regenerative epithelium appears hyperchromatic and contains mitotic figures.

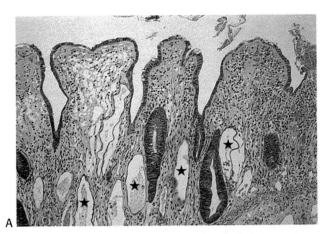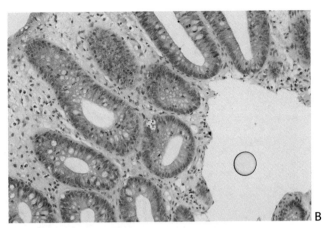

FIG. 13.86. Chemotherapeutic injury. **A:** The mucosa is severely damaged with crypt dropout intermingled with regenerating glands. The cystically dilated glands superficially resemble either lymphatics or blood vessels. These are lined by flattened epithelial cells and represent damaged crypts (*stars*). **B:** Cytoxan injury with prominent apoptosis in the crypt bases.

effects of surgery, extent of tumor involvement, and concomitant radiotherapy. Chemotherapeutic agents primarily affect mitotically active cells, inducing massive cell death. As a result, the mucosa becomes ulcerated and inflamed. The most marked effects result from 5-fluorouracil (5-FU) therapy (158). Additionally, 5-FU, a drug commonly used as an adjuvant in colon cancer therapy, impairs colonic healing, possibly due to reduced collagen synthesis, potentially adversely affecting the integrity of colonic anastomoses following colon cancer surgery. Mucosal injury begins 4 to 9 days after therapy onset. The nuclei in the crypt bases become pyknotic, lose their polarity, and become karyorrhectic (159). Eventually, the damage progresses toward the lumen, resulting in upper mucosal necrosis. Both the crypt epithelium and the lamina propria become inflamed. During the resolution phase, the crypt epithelium appears hyperplastic or the crypts appear disorganized and cystically dilated and lined by bizarre, sometimes flattened epithelial cells (Fig. 13.86). Increased apoptoses may be seen in the crypt bases (Fig. 13.86). Histiocytic cell infiltrates may become quite prominent. Often, colonic biopsies show only nonspecific colitis with cryptitis, ulcers, and acute and chronic inflammation mimicking other forms of acute colitis. Collections of apoptotic cells in the crypt bases, cytologic atypia, and glandular dilation suggest the diagnosis.

Chemotherapy also predisposes the mucosa to infections, ischemia, hemolytic uremic syndrome, and pseudomembranous colitis. The neutrophilic infiltrate may be less than one would ordinarily expect if the patient has significant bone marrow suppression. Severe cases may progress to neutropenic enterocolitis, which is discussed in a later section. Intestinal trefoil factor plays a major role in the mucosal recovery following the injury (160). Irinotecan induces epithelial apoptosis in the surface and crypt neck cells (161).

Drugs Causing Vasculitis or Ischemic Injury

Colonic ischemia complicates high-dose IL-2 and α-interferon immunotherapy (162) and treatment with immunosuppressive agents, neuroleptics (163), ergotamine, and contraceptives (Fig. 13.87) (164). Rutoside, used in Europe to treat varicose veins, associates with a lymphocytic phlebitis. Estrogen and progesterone cause intravascular thrombi and ischemic colitis (165). Alosetron, a drug used to treat irritable bowel syndrome, also can cause ischemic colitis (166). Ischemic colitis also complicates cocaine leakage into the intestines of cocaine body packers. Potassium salts cause venous spasm leading to ischemic ulceration.

Pancreatic Enzyme Supplements and Fibrosing Colonopathy

Fibrosing colonopathy affects young children with cystic fibrosis, most of whom take high-strength pancreatic enzyme

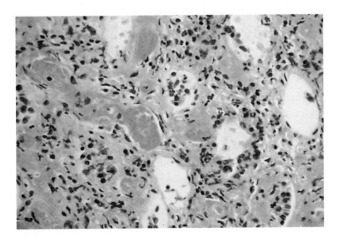

FIG. 13.87. Colonic biopsy in a 24-year-old female on contraceptives showing numerous fibrin thrombi in the vessels. The colon showed ischemic colitis.

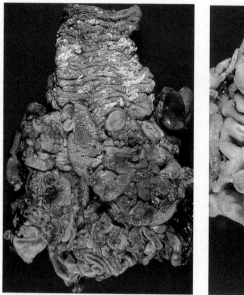
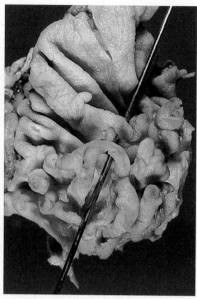
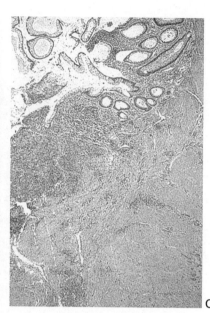

A, B   C

FIG. 13.88. Fibrosing colonopathy. These three figures are from the same specimen in a child with cystic fibrosis treated with enzyme supplements. **A:** Gross photograph of the bowel demonstrating the tenacious mucoid material on the colonic lumen (*upper*). The lower portion of the photograph shows a cecum that appears deformed and has large numbers of pseudopolyps. **B:** Higher magnification of the pseudopolyps. A probe has been passed under one of these. **C:** Portions of the colonic mucosa that are ulcerated and regenerated. Note the dense fibrosis in the underlying submucosa and obliteration of the submucosa and other landmarks. (Photographs courtesy of Dr. Kevin Bove, Department of Pathology, Children's Hospital Medical Center, Cincinnati, OH.)

supplements to control intestinal malabsorption. Use of H_2 blockers, corticosteroids, or recombinant human DNAse increases the risk of developing the disease. Patients present with abdominal distention due to intestinal dilation or ascites, frequent passage of watery stools, and severe anorexia. The changes may be restricted to one intestinal segment, or they may affect the entire colon (167). An intense perianal pruritus affects infants. Prolonged colonic mucosal contact with either the enzymes or the enteric coating or the combination of the two leads to the ulcers and inflammation (167). The toxicity may also result from the underlying gastrointestinal abnormalities from the cystic fibrosis. The pH in the small intestine is abnormally low in patients with cystic fibrosis. As a result, the dissolution of the enteric coatings occurs in the terminal ileum or colon leading to injury in these sites (168).

Rectal exploration shows rectal stenosis; the rest of the colon shows widespread, firm thickening, with narrowing at the flexures. The colon develops a cobblestoned appearance, submucosal fibrosis, thickening of the muscularis propria, and subserosal hemorrhages. Biopsies show acute or chronic inflammation (Fig. 13.88). Moderate to severe eosinophil and mast cell infiltrations develop. Active cryptitis is present in some patients. Dense mature collagen occupies the submucosa and thick, nearly hyalinized collagen bands with a keloidal appearance may be present. Changes in the muscularis mucosae range from focal fraying of the muscle fibers to complete disintegration with loss of the normal demarcation between the mucosa and submucosa. Ganglion cells are unusually prominent and can be found in the deep mucosa near crypt bases. The muscularis propria becomes widened and fibrotic with the process preferentially affecting the inner circular layer. In rare patients, the muscle becomes completely attenuated with disappearance of both layers of the muscularis propria (167). Patients also occasionally demonstrate ischemic changes.

Antimicrobials

Penicillin, ampicillin, tetracycline, isoniazid, and chloramphenicol all can cause a vasculitis. Penicillin, ampicillin, tetracycline, and erythromycin can all cause Henoch-Schönlein purpura secondary to a drug hypersensitivity reaction. Flucytosine causes an ulcerative enterocolitis due to direct mucosal toxicity. Antibiotics are the major cause of *C. difficile*–associated colitis (described in a later section). Antibiotics may also exacerbate symptoms associated with ulcerative colitis. A proximal colitis presenting with bloody diarrhea beginning 2 to 7 days following administration of penicillin and ampicillin has also been described.

Injury by Other Therapeutic Agents

Numerous other drugs cause colon alterations. Most produce nonspecific histologic changes that are easily confused with idiopathic IBD, ischemia, or infectious colitis, depending on lesion distribution and the clinical presentation. Localized nonspecific proctitis results from suppository insertion (169). Sulfasalazine enemas cause nonspecific proctitis. Methyldopa and penicillamine cause a diffuse colitis (170). Hematomas complicate anticoagulation therapy. *Isotretinoin* (Accutane) precipitates IBD (171). Isotretinoin and acyclovir cause allergic colitis (171), and toxic megacolon complicates methotrexate. *Ergotamine tartrate* sometimes causes solitary rectal ulcer formation (172). The phlebotonic drug C3-FORT causes lymphocytic colitis.

CHANGES INDUCED BY RADIOGRAPHIC SUBSTANCES

Barium causes three types of gastrointestinal problems: (a) barium granulomas, (b) bolus obstruction, and (c) an allergic or anaphylactic reaction from the carboxymethylcellulose component of the barium sulfate suspension. Barium granulomas are nodules of histiocytes containing barium sulfate, usually localized to the gastrointestinal submucosa. Allergic reactions to barium sulfate affect less than two individuals per million (173). Perforation is an uncommon complication. When perforation occurs, it does so in several settings: (a) perforation following damage caused by previous mucosal disease, such as active colitis or diverticulitis (173,174); (b) mechanical damage caused by introduction of enema tips, balloons, and catheters; and (c) perforation in those with pre-existing diseases.

By far the most common radiographic substance to cause alterations in the gastrointestinal tract is barium. Barium granulomas develop when barium contrast extravasates during *barium enemas* via mucosal tears, abrasions, or diverticula. Barium incites an inflammatory reaction that is polymorphic and includes histiocytes and foreign body giant cells. Water-soluble radiographic contrast media may also cause an acute colitis (175). Gastrografin may produce a severe colitis, probably due to TWEEN-80, which is used as a wetting agent.

The gross appearance of barium injury differs depending on whether an allergic reaction is present or whether barium has extravasated into the surrounding tissues. Barium granulomas produce brownish-green tumorous masses, fibrosis, and stricturing that may grossly resemble a carcinoma. Most barium granulomas develop in the rectum approximately 10 cm proximal to the anal verge, often on the anterior wall. They vary in size, ranging up to 10 cm in diameter, usually lying in the submucosa. Larger lesions may become centrally umbilicated. Sometimes, the barium forms hard concretions in the bowel lumen. In patients with allergic changes, one may see only the mildest of mucosal changes.

Barium sulfate is sometimes seen in the gastrointestinal lumen, appearing as fine, greenish, nonrefringent granules or as larger, birefringent, rhomboid crystals, sometimes located in granulation tissue (Fig. 13.89). These findings merely indicate prior use of barium in the patient and do not qualify for a diagnosis of a barium granuloma. Barium granulomas consist of collections of macrophages containing brownish-greenish-gray barium sulfate crystals, surrounded by typical foreign body giant cells. There is surprisingly little inflammation due to the inert nature of the barium. Small granular crystals may be found in clusters. The barium sulfate does not bend polarized light but it is refractile and easily seen when the microscope condenser is lowered. Allergic reactions tend to resemble other forms of allergic gastrointestinal diseases. Eosinophils tend to dominate the histologic picture. The mucosa may also appear mildly edematous. When barium gains access to the submucosa, it elicits a granulomatous response (Fig. 13.89).

Gastrografin does not elicit an inflammatory response. Morphologically one sees large rectangular or rhomboid light tan-yellow crystals in the bowel lumen, sometimes associated with an occasional giant cell.

COLITIS DUE TO VENOMS

Most scorpion and snake venoms contain a mixture of toxic proteins and enzymes that induce circulatory collapse, hemolysis, coagulation abnormalities, and changes in vascular resistance. All of these may lead to ischemic colitis (Fig. 13.90) (176).

RADIATION INJURY

Radiation injury causes two types of gastrointestinal damage. The first is the radiation damage itself; the second is the long-term consequence of radiation (i.e., ischemic changes or cancer development). Even though the colon and rectum are relatively radioresistant, they have a high incidence of radiation damage due to both the large radiation doses used to treat tumors arising in the pelvic area and the fixed position of the sigmoid colon. Many patients receiving radiotherapy also receive drugs with radiosensitizing effects. These drugs are directly toxic to the mucosa, predisposing it to further radiation damage. Between 75% and 90% of all intestinal complications affect the distal colon (177), with the rectum being most commonly involved (178,179).

Recent evidence suggests that microvascular endothelial apoptosis represents the primary lesion in gastrointestinal radiation damage (180,181). A single large dose of radiation preferentially damages the endothelial cells and epithelial cells die following the endothelial damage. The pathophysiology of radiation injury is discussed in detail in Chapter 6.

About 75% of patients develop clinical symptoms, usually by the middle of the second week of therapy. These include diarrhea, a mucoid discharge, tenesmus, abdominal distention, and abdominal pain. Mucosal edema, duskiness, and loss of the normal vascular pattern develop. Severe proctosigmoiditis follows radiation therapy in 2.4% to 5% of

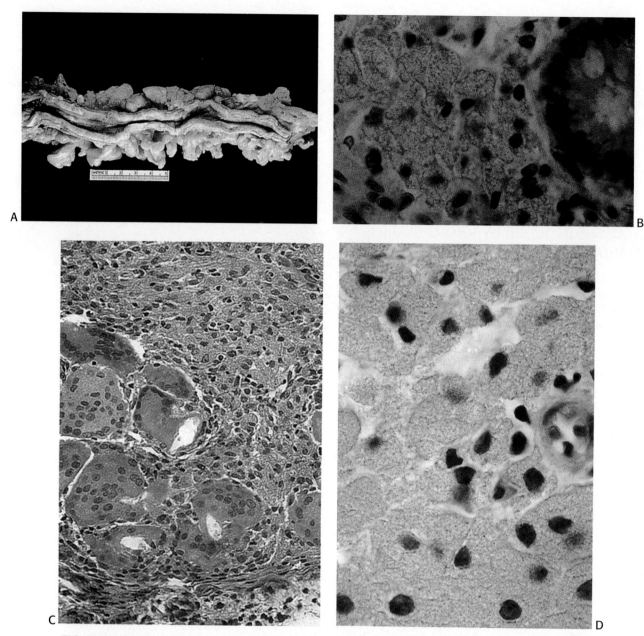

FIG. 13.89. Barium granuloma. **A:** Multiple small barium granulomas are present within this bowel, causing mural inflammation and luminal narrowing. **B:** Barium particles in macrophages. **C:** Histologic section through a barium granuloma demonstrates the presence of numerous epithelioid cells as well as multinucleated giant cells containing birefringent foreign material as seen under polarized light. **D:** Histiocytic cells containing refractile material.

patients; it is more common in patients treated with >6,000 rads over 6 weeks. Diffuse pancolitis may develop, as may ulcerations, stenosis, necrosis, and fistulas, all caused by progressive intramural vasculitis with submucosal and subserosal fibrosis. Delayed lesions include strictures, perforation, intestinal pseudo-obstruction, vascular obliteration, and mural fibrosis. Delayed proctosigmoiditis with intermittent bleeding of mild to moderate severity occurs 6 months to 5 years following therapy but can be delayed for as many as 30 years.

Early colorectal changes include mucosal edema (Fig. 13.91), mucosal discoloration or duskiness, and loss of the normal mucosal vascular patterns. Pallor, loss of mucosal folds, and irregular shallow ulcers, fistulae, and abscesses may also be present. Chronic radiation-induced colitis often manifests as strictures that may be long or short and generally have tapered and smooth margins.

During acute injury, characteristic changes usually remain confined to the mucosa. They include crypt cell damage, crypt abscesses, inflammatory cell infiltrates, nuclear

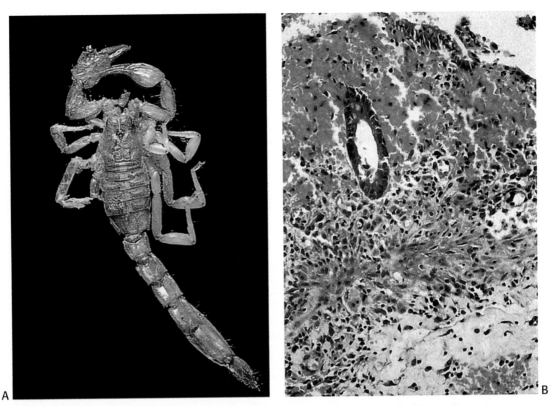

FIG. 13.90. Injury by toxins. **A:** Scorpion indigenous to the southwestern United States. Bites may cause severe hemorrhagic ischemic colitis. **B:** Histologic section from a patient who died from a rattlesnake bite. The acute hemorrhagic colitis is indistinguishable from ischemic colitis.

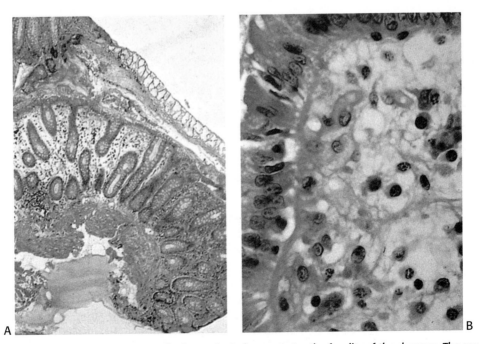

FIG. 13.91. Acute radiation damage. The image in **A** demonstrates the focality of the damage. The mucosa is edematous, and the crypts are separated by edema. At higher power magnification **(B)**, one sees the presence of hemosiderin-laden macrophages.

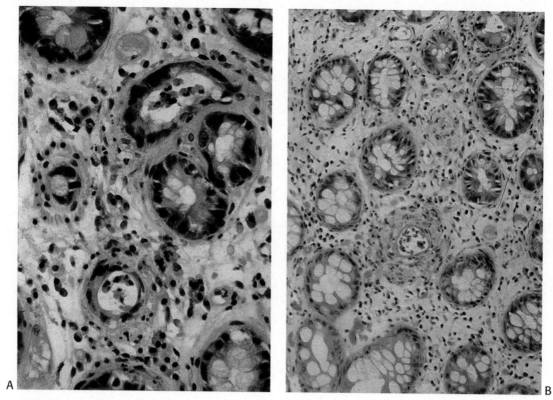

FIG. 13.92. Acute radiation colitis. **A:** High-power magnification demonstrating the presence of degenerating glands lying within an edematous stroma and surrounded by acute inflammatory cells, including eosinophils. **B:** Mucosal vessels demonstrate mild vascular fibrosis.

atypia, reduced mitotic activity, loss of nuclear polarity, crypt loss, and mucosal sloughing. Eosinophils are often prominent (Fig. 13.92). Other acute effects consist of prominent submucosal edema often with a myxoid appearance, ulcers, inflammatory polyps, mucosal telangiectasia, and sometimes ischemia. There may be glandular proliferation with mild cellular atypia. The changes may simulate dysplasia. Most of the changes resolve within a month, although mild atrophy and inflammatory cells may remain and be present at 3 months following treatment cessation (182), but they eventually regress.

Mucosal lesions that develop in the delayed period include erosions, ulcers, perforations, fistulas, atypia, and neoplasia. Carcinomas, sarcomas, and malakoplakia develop in previous radiation fields. The neoplasms follow exposure to both low and medium radiation doses, and they develop after a long latency period (183). Vascular changes include petechiae, hemorrhages, hyalinized arterioles, areas of healed necrosis in the vessels, thrombi, and fibrous intimal plaques. Stromal changes include strictures, submucosal fibrosis, interstitial fibrosis of the muscularis propria, serosal fibrosis, and loss of sphincter control. The strictures and fibrosis result from up-regulation of the multifunctional cytokine transforming growth factor-β, which is a major regulator of epithelial and mesenchymal proliferation, inflammation, extracellular matrix deposition, and angiogenesis (184,185).

More chronic features include architectural distortion with variable atrophy; goblet cell loss; shortened crypts; a thickened, distorted muscularis mucosa; epithelial atypia; intestinal wall fibrosis; serosal thickening; vascular sclerosis (Figs. 13.93 and 13.94); lymphangiectasia; and thickening of the collagen layer beneath the surface and crypt epithelium (186), which may mimic collagenous colitis. The large intestine may show Paneth cell metaplasia. Marked hyalinization of the submucosal vessels may mimic amyloidosis. Variable distortion of the intestinal wall results in glandular entrapment deep in the bowel wall, causing colitis cystica profunda, focal discontinuity of the muscularis mucosa, mucosal erosions, deep ulcers, vascular ectasia, and serosal thickening (186). The atypical nuclei in the displaced glands may simulate an invasive carcinoma. Submucosal neuronal proliferations and muscular degeneration also develop.

Biopsy features that suggest a diagnosis of radiation damage include the patchy nature of the process, marked telangiectasia, enlarged nuclei in either the epithelium or the stroma, and, if one is lucky enough to have submucosa in the biopsy, typical vascular changes sometimes associated with characteristic radiation fibroblasts. In other cases, the tissue appears nonspecifically chronically damaged. The lamina propria also contains excessive numbers of chronic inflammatory cells. The fibroblasts have enlarged nuclei and the cytoplasm tends to become basophilic. The cells may acquire

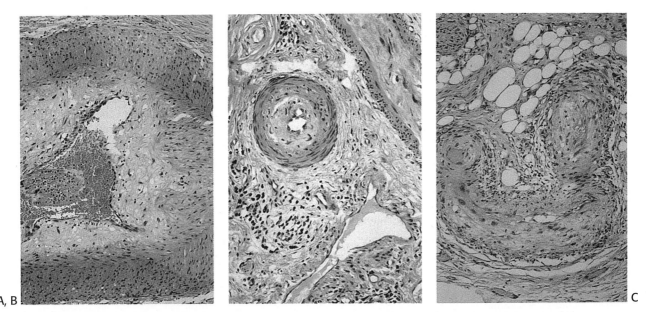

FIG. 13.93. Vascular damage in radiation injury. **A:** A vascular cross section showing foamy histiocytes lying just beneath the endothelium. **B:** A vessel in which the intima has become fibrotic, narrowing the lumen. **C:** A similar vessel seen longitudinally.

a swallow-tailed appearance. The arterioles often show intimal proliferation, sometimes with foamy endothelial cells, particularly earlier in the disease. Biopsies of the strictures typically show portions of distorted colorectal mucosa with fibrosis in the lamina propria and vascular dilation.

The gross appearance of chronic radiation damage may resemble that of Crohn disease but without fissures and without the creeping growth of the mesenteric fat. The gross appearance can also mimic a carcinoma. Microscopically, radiation colitis mimics other large intestinal colitides, including infectious, microscopic, ischemic, drug-induced colitis, allergic/eosinophilic, and IBD, particularly if only a superficial biopsy is examined. The presence of eosinophilic crypt abscesses is highly suggestive of radiation injury (187).

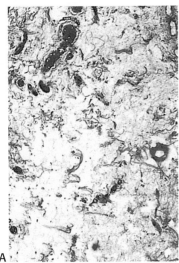
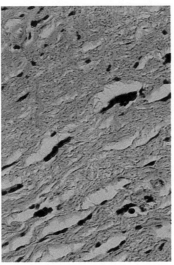

FIG. 13.94. Radiation effects (late). **A:** Chronic radiation damage (*right*) versus acute damage (*left*). Both sections are taken from the submucosa of the bowel. On the right side, one sees that the submucosa has become fibrotic and atypical fibroblasts are present. This contrasts with the acute stage in which the submucosa appears edematous and the vessels are telangiectatic. **B:** Stricture involving the colon in a patient who received radiation.

The vascular damage with myointimal hyperplasia and subintimal collections of foamy macrophages may be seen in radiation damage, chronic allograft cellular rejection with medial sclerosis, fibrinoid necrosis, and thrombosis in varying degrees and combinations (186). Because the mechanisms of radiation injury resemble those seen in ischemia and reperfusion injury, it is not surprising that the histologic features of both ischemia and acute radiation injury resemble one another and overlap.

Increasingly neoadjuvant therapies are used to treat rectal cancer, including preoperative chemotherapy, radiation therapy, or chemoradiation. This is followed by the resection of the tumor a few days or weeks later. Short-term preoperative irradiation induces severe diffuse, transmural inflammation and increased cellularity of the lamina propria. The inflammation consists of a mixture of eosinophils, lymphocytes, and plasma cells. The eosinophils are present in the lamina propria and/or crypts and/or surface epithelium and within crypt abscesses. Some patients have collections of muciphages in the lower mucosa. Neutrophils are present in proximity to ulcers and erosions, but they do not contribute to the crypt abscesses (188). Crypt disarray, surface and crypt epithelial damage, nuclear abnormalities, and apoptotic bodies in the crypt epithelium all develop (188). The crypts show a slitlike or dilated lumen lined by flattened epithelium mimicking the changes induced by chemotherapy. The epithelium may appear intensely eosinophilic and may contain bizarre nuclear atypia. The crypts appear elongated and the distance between the base of the crypts and the muscularis mucosae is increased. Decreased crypt numbers or small residual crypts may be present in severely inflamed areas. In less inflamed areas there is mild crypt distortion. It is important to recognize that the changes induced by the short-term irradiation can spontaneously completely resolve (188).

Sometimes one receives tissues that have had radon needles inserted into them to deliver localized radiation therapy. In such cases, an abscesslike inflammatory infiltrate surrounds a central empty cavity that corresponds to the site where the needle was. The vessels in proximity to the abscesses often show degenerative and fibrinoid changes.

Perirectal seeds used for brachytherapy of prostate cancer may cause localized gastrointestinal toxicity, although this is usually mild in nature (189).

TRAUMA

Most severe colonic trauma results from surgical or endoscopic interventions, accidents, and penetrating wounds. More than 95% of colonic injuries are penetrating (190) due to gunshot and stab wounds, iatrogenic injuries, automobile accidents, war wounds, and miscellaneous sexual injuries, in decreasing order of incidence. Trauma may also result from the insertion of enema tubes. The extent of the damage varies with the cause. The pathologic spectrum ranges from

hematomas to full-thickness lacerations that, if not repaired, lead to perforation and peritonitis. Intramural hematomas complicate blunt abdominal trauma and bleeding diatheses, such as hemophilia. Blunt abdominal trauma in child abuse syndromes associates with significant morbidity and mortality. The midabdomen is particularly vulnerable to the direct blows and results in compression injuries to anatomically fixed viscera against the spine (191). Colonic trauma accounts for only 3% to 5% of blunt abdominal injuries (192) and most affect the descending colon, ascending colon, or cecum (192,193). The clinical features depend on the size of the hematoma and can include acute or chronic pain, obstruction, rectal bleeding, anemia, and hemoperitoneum (194,195).

Histologic changes associated with trauma depend on whether the mucosa is examined during an acute phase or whether a biopsy is taken after repeated traumatic episodes. Acutely, one sees acute inflammation and hemorrhage. If repeated trauma has occurred, mucosal distortion and chronic inflammation may be present. Hemosiderin deposits may be present in the tissues. The tissue along the path of bullet wounds demonstrates coagulation necrosis.

INFECTIOUS COLITIS
General Comments

The indigenous colonic flora and an intact mucosal barrier represent vital components of the body's defenses against invasion by pathogens. Disruption of these defenses facilitates bacterial translocation and contributes to disease severity. Colonic injury results from the presence of bacteria or their toxins. Pathogenic mechanisms of mucosal injury include bacterial adherence, invasion, and toxin production (see Chapter 6). The pathogens typically hijack the host cell cytoskeleton. Altering the cytoskeleton is crucial for mediating pathogen adherence, invasion, and intracellular locomotion, especially for *E coli*, *Salmonella*, and *Shigella* (196).

The risk of developing infectious colitis varies considerably throughout the world and depends on local conditions. Populations inhabiting developing countries often live in ramshackle housing without good sanitation. Enteric infections, particularly bacterial, are readily transmitted in this setting. In contrast, most inhabitants of industrialized countries live in a sanitary environment that generally discourages transmission of enteric pathogens. However, in industrialized countries, other practices facilitate bacterial transmission, including large-scale food production, distribution, and retailing practices, which create opportunities for widespread and extensive outbreaks of food-borne enteric infections (fast-food chains) (197). Infants in daycare centers, patients hospitalized in chronic care facilities, AIDS patients, travelers, and military personnel all have an increased risk of infection. Communication with the clinicians regarding patients' travel, immune status, sexual practices, and food intake facilitates the detection of many infections.

Many gastrointestinal infections are acquired through the ingestion of contaminated food and water. The globalization of the food supply makes the effect of an accidental contamination or deliberate attack on it more widespread. If a bioterrorist attack occurs, pathologists could play a critical role in its identification. Table 13.11 lists factors that should trigger a suspicion of widespread food contamination.

Gastrointestinal changes vary from minimal changes to the classic pattern of acute self-limited colitis, or the production of nonspecific features or a necrotizing enterocolitis. Organisms that produce toxins tend to cause less severe morphologic changes than organisms that invade the mucosa (Fig. 13.95) (see Chapter 6). With the exception of enterohemorrhagic *E. coli* (EHEC), colitis-causing bacteria are invasive and include

TABLE 13.11	**Factors Suggesting Widespread Microbial Food Contamination**

Odd age distributions for common gastrointestinal (GI) diseases
Increased in usual and unusual types of food-borne illnesses
Increased incidence of organisms not typically seen in a geographic area
Unusual temporal clustering of infectious disease
Presence of microbial illness not common to a specific geographic locale
Unusual numbers of patients with signs and symptoms suggesting a GI infectious disease

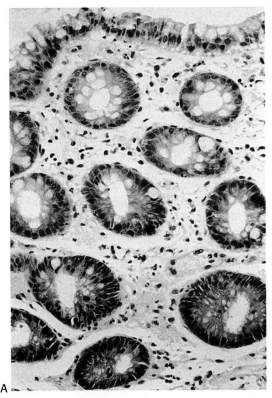

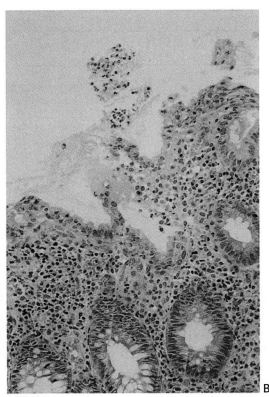

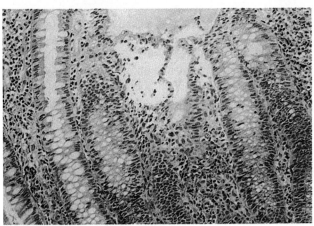

FIG. 13.95. Bacterial colitis. **A:** There is marked mucosal edema without obvious inflammation in a patient with a toxigenic *Escherichia coli* infection. **B:** Area of superficial ulceration and lamina propria inflammation. **C:** A small bulla has formed underlying the surface epithelium. B and C are from patients with two different types of invasive bacterial infections.

TABLE 13.12   Location of Colonic Infections

Attachment to epithelial luminal surfaces
  Cryptosporidia
  Spirochetes
  Enteroadherent *Escherichia coli*
Cytoplasmic localization
  Isospora
  Microsporidia
  Cytomegalovirus (CMV)
  Herpes simplex virus
  Adenovirus
  Histoplasma
Lamina propria localization
  CMV
  Strongyloides
  Mycobacteria
  Histoplasma
  Microsporidia
  Schistosomiasis
Submucosal localization
  Schistosomiasis
Muscularis propria or myenteric plexus localization
  Chagas disease
  CMV

TABLE 13.13   Histologic Features of Acute Self-limited Colitis

1. Edema that is most marked in the superficial two thirds of the mucosa
2. Superficial mucosal ulcers with a thin surface exudate containing neutrophils
3. Cryptitis, crypt ulcers, and crypt abscesses
4. Variable mucin depletion
5. Lamina propria inflammation consisting of neutrophils, lymphocytes, plasma cells, and eosinophils, depending on the stage of the disease (see Table 13.10)
6. Absence of basal plasmacytosis
7. Absence of signs of chronicity

Gram stains or Giemsa stains, and acid-fast bacillus (AFB) stains are useful in identifying tuberculosis or *Mycobacterium avium*. Trichrome stains may help identify amoebae. Ultrastructural examination also aids in the identification of microsporidia and some protozoans. Cultures are often useful, as are stool analyses for the detection of specific toxins or the genes encoding those toxins. Increasing numbers of immunohistochemical stains are becoming available, as are probes for in situ reactions and other molecular methodologies.

General Histologic Features of Bacterial Colitis (Acute Self-limited Colitis)

Histologic features of acute self-limited colitis (ASLC) include the features listed in Table 13.13 (Fig. 13.95). Table 13.14 lists the histologic characteristics at different times in the infection (200). The features of resolving colitis involve a shift from an acute inflammatory response to one that is more chronic in nature. The chronic changes of resolving infections may be more difficult to distinguish from other forms of colitis.

Shigella, Salmonella, Campylobacter, and *Yersinia.* EHEC causes enterocyte damage via a secreted toxin. EHEC is the third most common bacterial pathogen isolated from stool samples from diarrheal patients, trailing only *Salmonella* and *Campylobacter* infections (198,199). Infective colitis also results from *Yersinia enterocolitica* (46% of cases), *Campylobacter jejuni* (20%), *Salmonella* (13%), and *Shigella* (9%) infections (199). Amebiasis and cytomegalovirus infections account for another 11% of cases (199). Of these infections, *Salmonella* and amebiasis mimic ulcerative colitis, whereas the other pathogens cause a focal colitis resembling Crohn colitis (199).

The diagnosis of various forms of infectious colitis is based on a combination of clinical findings, histologic features, and response to therapy. The pathologic diagnosis of gastrointestinal infection depends on the recognition of several factors, including specific pathogens, specific tissue reactions, and specific cytopathic effects of the infection. The recognition of specific pathogens results from their localization to specific tissue sites, including the epithelial apical surfaces, the intestinal lumen, the lamina propria, the submucosa, the muscularis propria, or the myenteric plexus (Table 13.12). Special studies help identify specific pathogens. H&E stains often allow one to diagnose viral inclusions, but these may not always be obvious and the use of immunohistochemical reagents or even in situ hybridization reactions for a particular viral genetic sequence may prove informative. Special stains, particularly fungal stains, are often utilized to confirm the presence of infections, particularly in the setting of diffuse histiocytic infiltrates. Fungi may be highlighted with either Gomori or PAS stains. Microsporidia are highlighted by

TABLE 13.14   Evolving Features of Acute Self-limited Colitis

	Days 0 to 4	Days 6 to 9	Days 9+
Mucosal edema	+ +	+/−	−
Surface exudate	+	−	−
Ulcers	+	−	−
Crypt inflammation	+ + +	+ focal	−
Inflammation lamina propria			
Neutrophils	+ + +	+/−	−
Lymphocytes	+/−	+	+/−
Plasma cells			
Mucin depletion	+	+ +	+/−
Epithelial regeneration	+/−	+ +	+
Epithelial mitoses	−	+	+/−
Crypt distortion	−	−	+/−
Basal plasmacytosis	−	−	−
Granulomas	−	+/−	+/−

TABLE 13.15 Comparison of Acute Self-limited Colitis (ASLC) and Inflammatory Bowel Disease (IBD)

Feature	IBD	ASLC
Distorted architecture	++	−
Villous surface	+	−
Granulomas	+	+/−
Crypt atrophy	+	−
Basal lymphoid aggregates	++	−
Basal plasmacytosis	++	−
Basal giant cells	+	−
Mixed acute and chronic inflammatory cells	+	+/−
Edema	−	+
Pure neutrophilic infiltrate	−	+

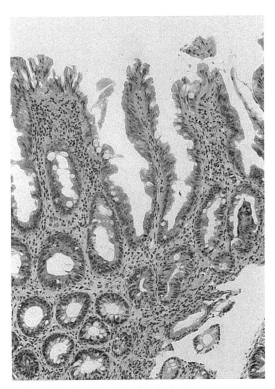

FIG. 13.96. Villiform transformation of the mucosa.

In early infections the mucosa appears expanded by edema and patchy inflammation. Neutrophils are typically prominent in the lamina propria, often near dilated capillaries or alongside the crypts. Marginating neutrophils may be seen in the capillaries. Neutrophils also infiltrate the crypt epithelium, causing cryptitis. Crypt abscesses are not prominent at this stage of many infections. Neutrophils outnumber lymphocytes and plasma cells. The epithelium often appears ragged and degenerating, sometimes with syncytial tufts. The crypt lining may appear mucin depleted, flattened, or reactive. The crypts are arranged in parallel to one another and the upper halves may appear dilated. The lamina propria may contain fresh hemorrhage.

Since ASLC is clinically and endoscopically similar to active idiopathic IBD, pathologists are often asked to distinguish between these two entities (Table 13.15) (see also Chapter 11). *An important histologic feature that distinguishes IBD from ASLC is the crypt architecture. When the architecture is normal, ASLC is likely* (Fig. 13.5) *and IBD is unlikely.* Conversely, a distorted crypt architecture strongly correlates with IBD. The ability to correctly diagnose IBD is very high when the histologic findings include a distorted crypt architecture (branched or forked glands not caused by glands bending around lymphoid follicles), increased numbers of round cells and neutrophils in the lamina propria, a villous architecture, epithelioid granulomas, crypt atrophy (shortening and scarcity of glands), basal lymphoid aggregates, plasmacytosis, Paneth cell metaplasia, and basally located isolated giant cells. Villiform surface configurations usually occur in UC (Fig. 13.96). However, they are relatively uncommon and therefore have limited diagnostic value. One caveat with regard to the foregoing is that when ASLC occurs in populations with a high incidence of infectious disease, the patients may develop crypt distortion. This disorder is sometimes referred to as *tropical colonopathy.* Such patients may show effects of previous infection with organisms known to destroy crypt architecture, such as amoeba, superimposed on an acute bacterial infection.

The nature of the inflammation in the lamina propria also helps differentiate ASLC from acute-onset IBD. *The presence of a pure acute neutrophilic inflammatory infiltrate suggests ASLC because this never occurs in IBD.* However, a mixed acute and chronic infiltrate occurs in both diseases. Inflammatory changes in the basal lamina propria strongly suggest IBD. One reason for this is that the crypt bases are normally relatively acellular, and when plasma cells are increased in this area, they are easily detected. *Both basal lymphoid hyperplasia and basal lymphoid aggregates highly discriminate for IBD because they are more common in IBD patients than in patients with ASLC.* The basal lymphoplasmacytosis affects the lower 20% of the mucosa. Mononuclear cells, including lymphocytes and plasma cells, may increase in ASLC but they are usually not present to the degree found in IBD unless the IBD patients have been treated.

The *resolving form of an acute self-limited colitis* is particularly difficult to distinguish from IBD. Inflammation limited to the superficial one half or two thirds of the lamina propria occurs more frequently in patients with ASLC, but this feature is not always present. The inflammation may form bandlike inflammatory infiltrates preferentially lying in the upper or midzonal parts of the mucosa and sparing the lower mucosa. The inflammation occupies the lamina propria rather than the crypt epithelium as in idiopathic IBD. Edema and hemorrhage, other hallmarks of infectious colitis, are absent or inconspicuous in idiopathic IBD. Focal inflammation occurs more commonly in patients with ASLC than in patients with UC.

TABLE 13.16	Granulomas in Bacterial Colitis
Epithelioid Granulomas	Microgranulomas
Tuberculosis	*Salmonella*
Yersinia	*Campylobacter*
Gonorrhea	
Syphilis	

Some infections produce epithelioid granulomas similar to those seen in CD. Others elicit microgranulomas or histiocytic collections lacking giant cells (Table 13.16). Inconspicuous microgranulomas may be seen in ASLC, particularly with *Campylobacter* and *Salmonella* infections, although these are rare. Granulomas are more frequent in *Yersinia enterocolitica* and *Mycobacterium tuberculosis* infections.

Specific Bacterial Infections

Escherichia coli

As indicated in Chapter 6, humans develop several types of *E. coli* infection. Toxigenic strains tend to cause minimal injury (Fig. 13.97). EHEC infections are discussed here; the remaining *E. coli* infections are covered in Chapter 6.

Enterohemorrhagic colitis results from infections due to Shiga toxin–producing *E. coli*. *E. coli* 0157:H7 is one strain of Shiga toxin–producing *E. coli* (201–203) and the one most commonly associated with HUS in the United States. Other strains cause HUS in other parts of the world. Two similar but distinct bacterial cytotoxins (Shiga-like toxins I and II)

contribute to the pathogenicity of enterohemorrhagic *E. coli* infections. These toxins have two units that are almost identical in structure to Shiga toxin and cholera toxin. Both toxins interact with the same membrane receptor (202). A unique plasmid-encoded fimbrial adhesin facilitates adherence of *E. coli* 0157:H7 to the intestinal mucosa (203). The organism targets Peyer patches, where it creates an attaching/effacing lesion (204). As a result, EHEC does not invade the epithelium but rather adheres to the luminal surface, where it elaborates a toxin. The absorbed toxins interfere with protein synthesis, causing epithelial and endothelial damage (205). These toxins damage the vascular endothelium of the kidneys and intestines and mediate bacillary dysentery, hemorrhagic colitis, HUS, and thrombotic thrombocytic purpura (TTP) in infected patients (206). The damaged endothelium fails to secrete anticoagulants, initiating microvascular thrombosis. Because of the underlying endothelial damage, the tissues often exhibit morphologic changes indistinguishable from ischemic colitis. Not all EHEC strains carry a risk for the development of HUS. HUS develops in 5% to 8% of patients with EHEC infection. High white blood cell counts, elevated C-reactive protein, and fever early in the course of the disease may be indicators of risk for development of HUS (207,208).

The mean annual rates of *E. coli* 0157:H7 infection range from 2 per 100,000 to 12.1 per 100,000 in two different parts of the world (209). In the United States, *E. coli* 0157:H7 infections are widespread, as shown by the number of outbreaks and sporadic cases, severe illnesses, and deaths. In one study, *E. coli* 0157:H7 was the fourth most common bacterial

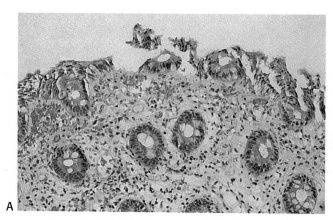

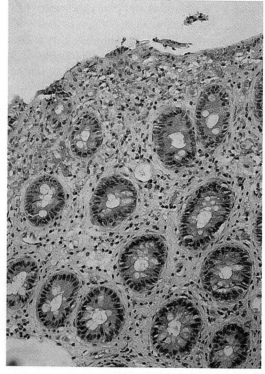

FIG. 13.97. Toxigenic *Escherichia coli* infection. **A** and **B** are from two different areas of the colon. A shows less damage than B, which is almost completely denuded. Both figures demonstrate superficial edema with extravasation of red blood cells. The biopsy is from a 17-year-old boy who ate a hamburger at a picnic and whose stool was positive for the *E. coli* toxin.

stool pathogen (210). Another study by the Centers for Disease Control and Prevention showed that 8% of routine cultures were positive for this organism, with an infection rate higher than that seen for *Shigella* (211). The infection occurs nationwide, although infection rates in the South are lower than those in the rest of the country. Patients range in age from 1 to 80 years, with a median age of 14 years. Populations most susceptible to the infection are the very young and the very old.

The incidence of the infection is highest in the summer, with most cases occurring between May and September (212). *E. coli* 0157:H7 outbreaks usually occur in communities, nursing homes, daycare centers, kindergartens, and children's wading pools (213). *E. coli* 0157:H7 can survive in drinking water and associate with water-borne disease outbreaks (214). The infectious dose of EHEC has been estimated to be fewer than 100 organisms. *Shiga* toxin–producing *E. coli* also associates with the consumption of hamburgers, other beef products, unpasteurized milk, cheese, pork, poultry, lamb, vegetables, and fruits (215,216). Ground beef represents an especially important vehicle of disease transmission (217). The *E. coli* 0157:H7 in ground beef is more sensitive to heat than other bacteria, but it survives for months at −20°C (218). For this reason, proper cooking is the preventive measure of choice. Person-to-person transmission is also possible, as is transmission by environmental contamination (219).

Currently, many laboratories do not routinely perform surveillance cultures for *E. coli* 0157:H7 unless the stool specimen is bloody or a specific request is made for it. Therefore, the infection often goes undetected (220). Screening for *E. coli* 0157:H7 is performed with the use of sorbitol MacConkey agar (218).

The mean incubation period is approximately 3 to 4 days and the illness usually lasts for 2 to 9 days. Asymptomatic infections are common, as is a self-limited, nonbloody, afebrile diarrhea. Other patients develop ileocolitis. Young children, the elderly, and immunosuppressed individuals are more susceptible to HUS and TTP. Antimicrobial treatment does not influence symptom duration, nor does it alter the risk of developing HUS or TTP. Patients with colitis develop bloody diarrhea, severe crampy abdominal pain, and low-grade fever. Fecal leukocytes are absent. Complications include thrombocytopenic purpura, end-stage renal disease, and neurologic damage, including strokes (221).

Endoscopy demonstrates the presence of a normal mucosa with oozing of blood. Other changes include mucosal edema and congestion, erosions, ulcers, erythema, a friable mucosa, and the presence of exudates or pseudomembranes. The submucosa appears swollen. The edema may be so marked that obstruction develops, requiring surgical resection. Resection is also used to control bleeding. The lesions often localize to the right colon but pancolitis may develop, particularly in children.

The histologic features demonstrate overlapping ischemic and infectious patterns due to the presence of both epithelial and endothelial injury (Fig. 13.98). Features associated with

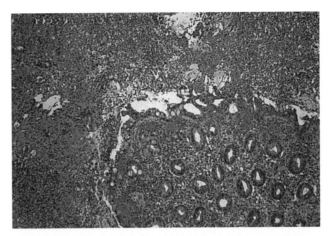

FIG. 13.98. *Escherichia coli* 0157:H7. This patient had a hemorrhagic colitis with pseudomembrane formation.

the ischemic damage include focal marked submucosal edema, hemorrhage, pseudomembranes (221), bland mucosal necrosis, ulceration associated with fibrin thrombi in the mucosal and submucosal capillaries, and abundant intramural fibrin deposits. The ischemia leads to extensive areas of mucosal necrosis, leaving ghosts of crypts with underlying neutrophilic infiltrates. The necrosis may extend to the submucosa or transmurally with an overlying serosal exudate. The intervening mucosa remains minimally affected with mild mucus depletion and occasional neutrophils and capillary platelet thrombi. The intervening mucosa may also exhibit epithelial dropout, fibrin deposition, and adjacent hemorrhage.

Histologic features associated with an infectious histologic pattern include a prominent neutrophilic infiltrate within the crypts, lamina propria, and adherent pseudomembranes. The neutrophilic infiltrate may be mild and patchy, or it may infiltrate the crypt epithelium, producing cryptitis or incipient crypt abscesses. Cryptitis occurs more commonly than crypt abscesses, and in all cases the neutrophilic infiltrate is focally accentuated rather than uniform in appearance, and may even appear as solitary inflammatory foci. Patients often exhibit extreme submucosal edema with hemorrhage and fibrin exudation. The focal nature of the neutrophilic infiltrate, along with the predominance of cryptitis over well-formed crypt abscesses, resembles the histologic changes seen in *Campylobacter*, *Salmonella*, and early amebic infections. Its focal distribution and the presence of fibrin thrombi distinguish the infection from acute UC. The changes may resemble those present in *C. difficile* colitis. A disproportionate amount of lamina propria hemorrhage is often present when compared to the degree of inflammation. Glandular distortion, architectural abnormalities, granulomas, and giant cells are usually absent unless there is underlying pre-existing IBD (222). Because the disease is patchy, biopsies may appear normal or only exhibit a focal, mild, nonspecific increase in lamina propria lymphocytes or plasma cells. The histology does not correlate with either disease duration or the course of the illness. Advanced lesions display regenerative mucosal changes and heavy submucosal plasmacytic infiltrates.

The differential diagnosis includes *C. difficile* colitis and ischemic colitis, which share overlapping features with the *E. coli* infection. The *C. difficile* antigen test may be very helpful in excluding *C. difficile* infections. Culture and serotyping are the mainstays of the diagnosis. Immunohistochemical stains and molecular assays for EHEC exist, but they are not widely available.

Campylobacter *Infections*

Campylobacter infections affect both the large and small intestines. Occasionally, *C. jejuni* is responsible for an acute focal colitis (223). Severe cases may present as an acute toxic ulcerative colitis with pancolitis, toxic megacolon, and colonic perforation. These infections are discussed further in Chapter 6.

Salmonella *Infections*

As discussed in Chapter 6, *Salmonella* infections cause five clinical syndromes. In this chapter, we will focus on *Salmonella* infections that present as colitis. *Salmonella* gastroenteritis results from infection by *Salmonella enteritidis, Salmonella typhimurium, Salmonella argona, Salmonella javiana, Salmonella poona, Salmonella oranienburg* and *Salmonella newport*. It varies from a mild to a severe infection, occasionally associated with bacteremia or bacteriuria. *Salmonella* gastroenteritis is acquired by ingestion of infected foods or drinks accounting for up to 80% of food poisonings. Most outbreaks occur through June and July and associate with consumption of contaminated fish, shellfish, cheese, and poultry (224–227). There is also a high prevalence of *Salmonella* in livestock. The practice of feeding subtherapeutic amounts of antibiotics to improve animal growth has resulted in the emergence of multiple antibiotic-resistant *Salmonella* strains in the animals and an increased incidence of antimicrobial-resistant organisms causing serious human disease. Food handlers who may become human carriers are occasionally implicated in spread of the infection.

The northeastern portion of the United States and parts of Europe has experienced a marked increase in food poisoning due to *S. enteritidis*. *S. enteritidis* is also increasing in South America and Africa (228). The increase relates to increased consumption of infected eggs and poultry. Approximately 400 cases of salmonellosis are reported annually in the United States, with fatality rates ranging from 1.3% to 8.4% (229).

Salmonellosis usually causes a mild self-limited disease that develops 8 to 48 hours following organism ingestion. Signs and symptoms of *Salmonella* gastroenteritis vary widely, but most patients present with nausea, vomiting, abdominal cramps, fever, pain, and diarrhea, which sometimes becomes bloody. Symptoms last for 3 to 12 days. *Salmonella* infections in the elderly have a poorer prognosis than when they occur in younger individuals. This is because the patients are more likely to become septic. Rarely, life-

threatening, massive lower GI bleeding occurs. Bleeding usually arises in the small intestine but large intestinal bleeding also occurs (230). Patients not only develop GI symptoms, but also may develop erythema nodosum, reactive arthropathy, and rectal prolapse, particularly those with massive diarrhea. A pseudoappendicitis or ileocecitis may occur and may be complicated by perforation or toxic megacolon. Infections are particularly virulent in individuals with sickle cell disease or those with HIV infections. Diffuse or patchy mucosal hyperemia, friability, and inflammation may be seen at the time of colonoscopy.

Salmonella bacteria are intracellular parasites that enter the host by penetrating intestinal epithelial barriers, usually in the area of Peyer patches in the M cells. Once they are in close contact with the epithelium, the bacteria induce degeneration of the enterocyte microvilli (231), which is followed by profound membrane ruffling in the area of the bacterial host cell contact. Profuse micropinocytosis leads to bacterial internalization (232). *Salmonella* entry into the epithelium requires several chromosomal genes (*inv/spa*) clustered in a pathogenicity island termed SPI1 (salmonella pathogenicity island 1) (233). Additional pathogenicity factors are summarized in the Armed Forces Institute of Pathology (AFIP) fascicle (234). Bacteria enter membrane-bound vacuoles (phagosomes) inside epithelial cells and macrophages where they replicate (235). Replication also occurs in macrophages of the lymphoid follicles leading to bacteremia, reinfection of additional macrophages, and seeding of distant sites. As a result, the lymphoid follicles become hyperplastic, swollen, congested, and ulcerated, often resulting in typical longitudinally oriented ulcers and areas of hemorrhage. Edema, fibrinous exudation, and vascular thrombosis precede the ulceration. Aphthous ulcers sometimes develop.

Histologically mild cases show nonspecific patchy changes consisting of edema, congestion, and focal inflammation (Fig. 13.99). More severe cases show crypt abscesses with prominent neutrophilic infiltrates in degenerating crypts. The neutrophilic infiltration is more intense in the lamina propria than in the glands. Areas of hemorrhage and ulceration are also present. Crypt abscesses may be present in the nonulcerated areas. There may also be extensive areas of mucosal necrosis and hemorrhage with punched-out mucosal ulcers or erosions with elevated borders, crypt abscesses in the nonulcerated areas, and extensive mucosal and submucosal necrosis and hemorrhage (Fig. 13.100). These changes differ from IBD by the relative scarcity of chronic inflammatory cells. Microthrombi fill small mucosal and submucosal venules, creating a picture resembling that seen in acute ischemia. In severe cases, giant cells may populate the inflamed tissues, which, if transmural inflammation is present, might suggest the presence of CD. However, the giant cells do not form compact granulomas, as seen in CD. Occasional patients will show mild crypt distortion and branching, especially in those with persistent diarrhea.

There is sometimes a concurrence between salmonellosis and IBD (236), creating diagnostic and treatment dilemmas.

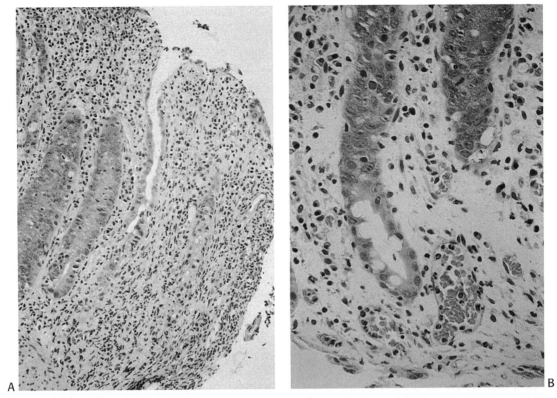

FIG. 13.99. *Salmonella* colitis. **A:** The mucosa is inflamed and there is glandular destruction. There are apoptoses in one of the crypt bases mimicking drug injury and graft versus host disease. **B:** The base of several crypts show increased mitotic activity. The surrounding lamina propria appears edematous and the vessels are congested.

Rectal biopsies show the active inflammation typical of UC (237). The immunosuppression used to treat the IBD may predispose to the infection.

Shigellosis

Shigella is a nonmotile, Gram-negative bacillus that is among the more virulent human enteropathogens. *Shigella* infections are an important cause of morbidity and mortality in developing countries, particularly in tropical areas. It causes approximately 10,000 cases of gastroenteritis each year in the United States (238). *Shigella* infections are more common in AIDS patients. They have a more virulent course and the infection is difficult to treat so that recurrences are common. Outbreaks of shigellosis among men who have sex with men result from direct or indirect oral–anal contact and are usually cause by *Shigella flexneri*. However, there was an outbreak of *Shigella sonnei* in California in 2000–2001 among men having sex with men (239). Person-to-person transmission and ingestion of contaminated food and water also cause the disease (240,241). *Shigella* infections associate with poor hygiene and overcrowding, and are a significant problem among children in nurseries and mental hospitals. Several *Shigella* species (*dysenteriae, flexneri, boydii,* and *sonnei*) cause colitis, with diminishing severity from the first

organism to the last (242). *S. sonnei,* which produces a mild colitis, is the most common cause of bacillary dysentery in the Western world. Shigellosis results from release of bacterial toxins into the bowel lumen, as well as from direct bacterial invasion of the colonic mucosa (243). *Shigella* produces a potent toxin that inhibits protein synthesis and has cytotoxic, neurotoxic, and enterotoxic effects (244).

Children are the main victims of *Shigella* infections. The two major clinical presentations include watery diarrhea and dysenteric syndromes. The watery diarrhea has a short duration before hospitalization. The dysenteric form presents with bloody mucoid stools (27%), intense crampy abdominal pain (94%), diarrhea (98%), fever (87%), and nausea and vomiting (78%). It has a longer illness duration prior to hospitalization (245). Septicemia, hyponatremia, and hypoglycemia are common (246). The small volumes of dysenteric stool contain blood and pus. Patients with longer symptom duration may develop relative vascular insufficiency, activated lymphocytes, eosinophilic and mast cell degranulation, and antibody-mediated damage.

The severity of *Shigella* infections depends on many factors, including previous exposure to the organism and the infecting dose. The infections are usually self-limited, but dysentery can be a life-threatening illness in infants, the elderly, or malnourished individuals. The usual incubation

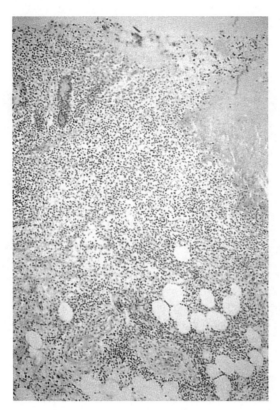

FIG. 13.100. Typhoid ulcer extending into the submucosa. The mucosa is inflamed and necrotic.

period ranges from 1 to 3 days. Watery diarrhea, with or without vomiting, is the initial symptom. After 24 hours, the stool becomes mucoid and grossly bloody. Low abdominal pain is common. Severe disease clinically mimics toxic megacolon, with hemorrhage, paralytic ileus, and perforation. Anal or perianal disease, including fissures, fistulae, hemorrhoids, or prolapse (245), complicates severe diarrhea. Serious complications are rare, especially in infections by *S. flexneri* and *S. sonnei*. However, patients with *Shigella dysenteriae* infection may develop bacteremia, sepsis, paralytic ileus, toxic megacolon, disseminated intravascular coagulation, and renal cortical necrosis severe enough to require hemodialysis (247). Shigellosis also causes hemolytic uremic syndrome, a condition associated with a high mortality (248). Circulating endotoxins cause the coagulopathy, renal microangiopathy, and hemolytic anemia. Other complications include toxic megacolon, intestinal perforation, sepsis, encephalopathy, pneumonia, conjunctivitis, and arthritis (249).

Shigella organisms pass from the mouth to colonize the colon. Small intestinal infections do not occur unless the patient has a motility disturbance. Once they reach the colon, the bacteria penetrate the intestinal mucous layer and invade the epithelium. Multiple genes control epithelial entry (250). The preferential site of entry is through the dome of the lymphoid follicles. An adhesive or invasive phenotype is required for efficient colonization of the M cells of

the follicle-associated epithelium. The invasive phenotype causes major inflammation-mediated tissue destruction, whereas the adhesive phenotype causes alterations in the M cells, which become stretched over large pockets containing aggregates of mononuclear cells. The M cells progressively occupy larger surface areas of the follicle-associated epithelium, causing the enterocytes to come off the epithelial surface (251). The organisms that invade the epithelium reorganize the cell cytoskeleton, a process that requires *Shigella* Ipa proteins. Once inside the cells, bacteria lie within membrane-bound vesicles. Here they multiply, causing mucus secretion and goblet cell depletion and inducing luminal neutrophilic infiltrates. The neutrophils loosen the intercellular barriers, further facilitating *Shigella* invasion (252).

Shigella bacteria direct their own uptake into the colonic mucosa through membrane ruffling and macropinocytosis in a manner similar to *Salmonella* uptake (253). After engulfment, the bacteria are surrounded by a membrane-bound vacuole within the host cell. *Shigella* rapidly lyses the surrounding vacuole and it is released into the cytosol where it grows and divides (251). Once it escapes from the vacuole it is quickly coated with filamentous actin and ultimately forms an actin tail at one pole of the bacterium (254). This actin polymerization propels the bacterium through the cell cytoplasm (255) and when the pathogen reaches the plasma membrane, it forms a long protrusion into the neighboring cell, which subsequently internalizes the microbe (256). The bacterium again breaks out of the vacuole starting a new cycle of infection in a new host cell (257). The cycle of intracellular and intercellular infection allows colonization of large epithelial surfaces while the bacterium is protected from immune host surveillance mechanisms. Bacilli penetrate the intestinal epithelium and pass through the mucosa in a period of several hours (251). The organism induces apoptosis in macrophages, which in agony release mature IL-1β. The IL-1β attracts neutrophils to the site of infection resulting in the massive colonic inflammation characteristic of the disease (258).

The *Shigella* cytotoxin rapidly reduces epithelial protein synthesis. An endotoxin damages mitochondria, leading to further destruction of cellular organelles, cell death, extrusion, and the formation of microulcers in the surface epithelium. Inflammation results in focal abscess and ulcer formation and, when severe enough, ileus, toxic megacolon, gross hemorrhage, and perforation. Endotoxin absorption in the lumen also leads to thrombosis, hemorrhage, and vascular insufficiency, causing further crypt damage.

Endoscopically, the mucosa appears edematous, friable, hyperemic, and ulcerated. All patients have inflammation in the rectosigmoid area. In most patients, the lesions are continuous and diffuse with the intensity of inflammation decreasing as one moves proximally. In severe cases there is a pancolitis with backwash ileitis, which can extend as far as 50 cm from the ileocecal valve (246). There may also be coexisting appendicitis. Serpiginous ulcers develop on the free edge of the mucosal folds oriented transversely to the long axis.

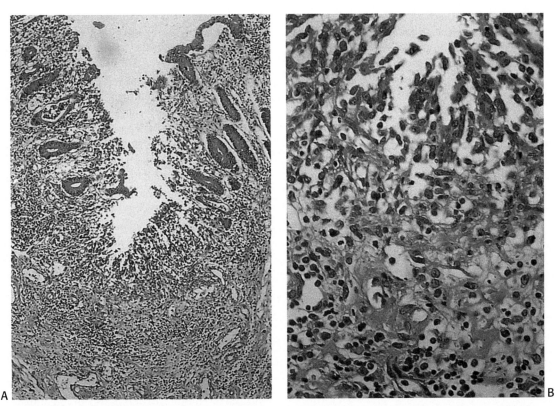

FIG. 13.101. Shigellosis. **A:** Mucosal ulceration and transmural inflammation. **B:** Higher power magnification of fibrinonecrotic debris.

The intervening mucosa appears granular and hemorrhagic. Aphthous erosions may be present (Fig. 13.101). Other causes of aphthous ulcers are listed in Table 13.17. In fatal infections a gray mucopurulent exudate covers the mucosa. Because the findings resemble those seen in *Campylobacter* and *Salmonella* infections and IBD, definitive diagnosis requires stool culture.

Histologic changes in *Shigella* infections include patchy hyperemia and edema with mucosal friability or ragged ulcerations, sometimes associated with pseudomembrane formation. Biopsies of early-stage disease show a surface epithelium that is reduced in height and infiltrated by neutrophils. The epithelial cells then detach from an edematous lamina propria forming microulcers. Neutrophils frequently lie below the microulcers. Detached epithelial cells, neutrophils, and red blood cells form a layer of purulent exudate on the surface. Microulcers and erosions are present in 85% of biopsy samples taken during the acute stage of the disease

(246). Small aphthous ulcers also form. These always arise over the lymphoid follicles because the follicles with their M cells are the portal of entry (Fig. 13.101). Other changes consist of acute inflammation with neutrophilic emigration, superficial crypt abscess formation, early goblet cell depletion, edema, erythema, and mild plasma cell infiltrates (224). *Shigella* bacteria are numerous in the epithelial cells and in the lamina propria of early lesions. Dilated vessels accompany marked edema. As the lesions become more advanced, epithelial necrosis occurs and purulent exudates cover the damaged mucosa. Frank ulceration develops, disturbing the crypt architecture and causing pseudopolyp formation. The changes may remain confined to the mucosa, although they can extend into the submucosa. Patients may show mild crypt distortion and branching. Cellular regeneration progresses from the base of the crypts toward the mucosal surface. Even in the case of extensive mucosal damage, recovery is usually very rapid.

In autopsy cases, chronic ulcers of variable size and depth are present in 100% of cases. The ulcers may be superficial, involving only the upper quarter of the mucosa, but they may extend down to the muscularis mucosae. Some patients have wide areas of mucosal denudation and pseudomembranes. Crypt abscesses may be present along with architectural distortion and thrombosis of small vessels in the mucosa or submucosa. Colitis cystica profunda develops in about a quarter of the cases (246).

TABLE 13.17	**Disorders Associated with Aphthous Ulcers**
Crohn disease	Ileocolic candidiasis
Yersinia infections	Ulcerative colitis (rare)
Behçet syndrome	*Campylobacter* infections
Shigellosis	Ischemia

Convalescent stage biopsies show residual small superficial ulcers and marked inflammation of the lamina propria. The intensity of the lymphocytic and plasmocytic infiltrate is greater than that of the neutrophils.

Clostridium difficile

C. difficile is a well-known cause of epidemics and is the most common cause of nosocomial diarrhea. There are four groups of risk factors for the development of the disease: Patient risks, treatment risks, environmental risks, and the *C. difficile* strain (Table 13.18) (259,260). Infants, children, and adults may acquire *C. difficile* infections when they are hospitalized (261,262). The patients often receive antibiotic therapy in a setting where environmental contamination with *C. difficile* spores is commonplace (263). In one study, 21% of patients acquired *C. difficile* during their hospitalizations. Of these, 63% remained asymptomatic; 37% developed diarrhea. Among patients in the community who are treated with oral antimicrobial agents, only 1 to 3 individuals per 100,000 develop *C. difficile* colitis compared with as many as 1 per 100 hospitalized patients treated with similar drugs (263). Immunodeficient patients are particularly susceptible to developing *C. difficile* infections (264).

C. difficile spores are heat resistant and may persist in the environment for months. The organism may spread person to person by hands, via fomites, or by general contamination (265). The organism can be cultured from hospital floors, toilets, bedding, and furniture, especially in areas where patients with diarrhea from *C. difficile* infection have been recently treated. Features that determine whether or not a patient develops a *C. difficile* infection include the nature of the fecal flora, the size of the *C. difficile* population, produc-

tion of the requisite cytotoxins, and the presence of other organisms that affect toxin expression or activity. Host risk factors include advanced age, severe underlying illness, and prolonged hospital stay. Recent studies suggest that immunologic susceptibility has a role in *C. difficile* infection. The presence of an IgG antibody against toxin A protects against the clinical expression of a *C. difficile* infection and against relapse (266,267).

Toxigenic strains of *C. difficile* release two large protein exotoxins, toxin A and toxin B. Both toxins possess cytotoxic activities inducing the disaggregation of actin microfilaments and cell rounding (268). Binding and internalization of toxin A into cells elicits an acute inflammatory cascade via a sequence of activation signals involving the release of substance P and other neuropeptides from sensory nerves (269). Release of IL-8 and other proinflammatory cytokines from immune cells and enterocytes also occurs. The release of IL-8 depends on an oxidative burst originating from mitochondria and is transduced via the NF-$\kappa\beta$ pathway (270). This is followed by up-regulation of leukocyte adhesion molecules on the vascular endothelium and local infiltration of the lamina propria with acute inflammatory cells (269). The end result is a severe necroinflammatory lesion (pseudomembranous colitis) accompanied by massive fluid secretion and mucosal ulceration. Toxin B is also an inflammatory enterotoxin (271). A previously uncommon strain of *C. difficile* with variations in toxin genes has become more resistant to fluoroquinolones and has emerged as a cause of geographically dispersed outbreaks of *C. difficile*–associated disease (272,273).

C. difficile infections account for 10% to 25% of cases of antibiotic-associated diarrhea and virtually all cases of antibiotic-associated pseudomembranous colitis. The type of antibiotic and the route of its administration influence disease incidence. More cases occur when the drug is given orally than when it is administered parenterally. Clindamycin, ampicillin, and the cephalosporins are most commonly associated with antibiotic-associated pseudomembranous colitis, but virtually any antibiotic may produce the disorder. *C. difficile*–associated diarrhea also complicates the use of chemotherapy.

The laboratory diagnosis of *C. difficile* is based on isolation or detection of components or products of the organism. Stool cultures and assays for *C. difficile* toxin (the preferred method for establishing the diagnosis) are positive in >95% of patients. Cultures performed properly on selected media are the most sensitive method for the detection of *C. difficile,* whereas cell cytotoxin assay for detection of toxin B is the most specific. *C. difficile* may be cultured anaerobically on special antibiotic-containing media selective for it. The organism is readily identified based on colony morphology and microscopic features. Unfortunately, it takes up to 5 days to grow the organism. Additionally, culture detects all *C. difficile* colonies irrespective of their pathogenicity so that colonies that are isolated must be tested for their ability to produce the toxin (274).

TABLE 13.18   **Risk Factors for Acquiring *Clostridium difficile* Infections**

Patient risks
  Older age
  Severity of the diarrhea
  Previous gastrointestinal disease or surgery
  Failure to mount a sufficient IgG antibody response to toxin A
Treatment risks
  Predominantly antibiotics
  Chemotherapy
Environmental risks
  Hospitals
  Chronic care facilities
C. difficile strain
  Production of a binary toxin in addition to toxins A and B
  Presence of a deletion leading to increased production of toxins A and B
  Resistance to broad spectrum quinolones

The cytotoxic assay diagnostic method exploits the cytotoxic feature of *C. difficile* toxins. In this test, the patient's specimen is added to a cell culture line. Cells are examined for cytotoxic changes after an incubation period. Then, to verify that the cytotoxicity was due to the presence of the toxin, the assay is performed with a neutralizing antibody against the *C. difficile* toxin added to the specimen. This assay is the gold standard because of its high sensitivity (94% to 100%) and specificity (99%) (274). Because there is no clinical correlation between stool levels of the toxins and the severity of the disease, the culture is simply reported as positive or negative.

Enzyme immunoassays are used to diagnose *C. difficile* infections. These assays are designed to detect either toxin A alone or both toxins A and B. They have the advantage of being very rapid to perform (<4 hours) and have a sensitivity of 69% to 87% and a specificity of 99% to 100% (275). *C. difficile* toxin can also be identified by the polymerase chain reaction (PCR). The PCR primers amplify a repetitive sequence of the enterotoxin gene, thereby generating a distinctive ladder pattern. This detection technique is more sensitive than standard culture and has a sensitivity similar to cytotoxin testing (276).

The clinical presentations of *C. difficile* infections, in increasing order of severity, include asymptomatic carriage, antibiotic-associated colitis without pseudomembrane formation, pseudomembranous colitis, and fulminant colitis with catastrophic transmural inflammation and myonecrosis. The most severe forms are the least common. Over 50% of healthy neonates are asymptomatic carriers of *C. difficile*. However, even though children are relatively resistant, they can develop pseudomembranous colitis in the presence of *C. difficile* cytotoxin (277). Children with fatal disease usually have underlying Hirschsprung disease or a hematologic malignancy. Less than 1% of healthy adults are carriers, but approximately 25% of adults recently treated with antibiotics are colonized by the organism. The majority of hospital inpatients infected with *C. difficile* remain asymptomatic (261).

When *C. difficile* infection presents as diarrhea, it is usually mild to moderate in severity, sometimes accompanied by lower abdominal cramps. Symptoms usually begin during or shortly after antibiotic therapy; occasionally, they are delayed for several weeks. *C. difficile* toxins are present in the stool at this time but endoscopic and histologic features are frequently almost normal in patients with mild disease. The diarrhea often subsides when antibiotics are stopped.

Severe colitis without pseudomembrane formation presents as a profuse debilitating diarrhea, abdominal pain, and abdominal distention. Common systemic manifestations include fever, nausea, anorexia, malaise, and dehydration. Peripheral blood polymorphonuclear leukocytosis and increased numbers of fecal leukocytes are common. Patients may experience occult colonic bleeding; rarely, they develop frank hematochezia.

The most dramatic form of the disease, pseudomembranous colitis, clinically resembles *C. difficile* colitis without pseudomembranes except for the fact that the diarrhea, abdominal tenderness, and systemic manifestations are more severe. As colonic muscular tone is lost, toxic dilation or megacolon develops. The development of the paralytic ileus or the colonic dilation results in a paradoxic decrease in the diarrhea. Endoscopy should be avoided in such patients because of the risk of perforation. When severe, pseudomembranous colitis requires surgical resection to avoid perforation.

Patients with early pseudomembranous colitis have focal or confluent yellow-white, raised 2- to 10-mm plaques with erythematous bases and a centrally adherent yellow plaque. Small lesions can be mistaken for mucus or an aphthous ulcer. The intervening mucosa typically appears normal or only mildly erythematous or congested. Patients with severe disease may have plaques that coalesce to cover large mucosal areas. The rectum and sigmoid are typically involved, but in approximately 10% of cases the colitis is confined to the proximal colon (278). Edema, blurring of the vascular pattern, and thickening and blunting of the haustral folds are also present. The lesions are most prominent in the large intestine but the distal small bowel occasionally becomes involved. If pseudomembranes are identified endoscopically, stool specimens should be sent to confirm the presence of the *C. difficile* toxin and biopsies should be obtained in order to confirm the diagnosis because other disorders may produce pseudomembranes (Fig. 13.102).

The earliest lesions (type I lesions) consist of focal areas of epithelial necrosis with neutrophils and nuclear dust in an edematous lamina propria. A shower of fibrin and neutrophils erupts from the mucosal surface (Fig. 13.103). The early lesions reflect local epithelial damage occurring on the luminal surface. Plaque formation is initiated by epithelial breakdown with eruption of an exudate into the lumen. The linear deposition of neutrophils and Gram-positive sporulating bacilli within fibrin strands and mucus represents an almost pathognomonic appearance.

Later lesions (type II lesions) consist of a well-demarcated group of disrupted crypts that lose their superficial lining and are distended by mucin, neutrophils, and eosinophils. Later, epithelial damage extends downward to involve the lower parts of the crypts. The epithelium of affected crypts becomes flattened and progressively lost. Occasional fibrin thrombi are found in superficial mucosal capillaries at this stage (Fig. 13.104). Focal mushroom-shaped or focal volcanic eruptions of a pseudomembrane attach to the necrotic mucosa. The pseudomembranes contain epithelial debris, red blood cells, fibrin, mucus, and polymorphs. The adjacent mucosa appears normal.

Type III lesions consist of complete structural mucosal necrosis with only a few surviving glands covered by cellular inflammatory debris, mucin, and fibrin (Fig. 13.105). The lamina propria becomes edematous and bulges into the lumen. Focal congestion and hemorrhage in the lamina

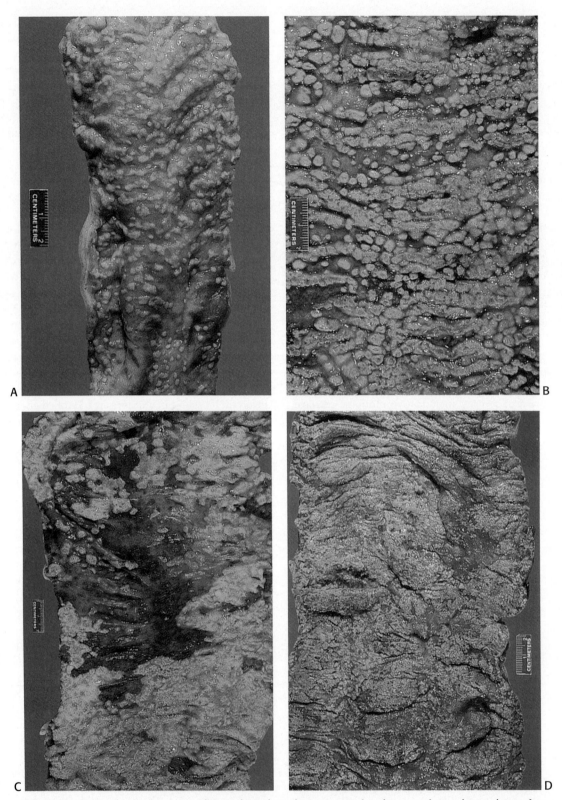

FIG. 13.102. Pseudomembranous colitis. A through D show progressive degrees of pseudomembrane formation. **A:** Discrete separated pseudomembranous lesions are present. **B:** One sees beginning coalescence of the lesions with little intervening normal mucosa. **C:** Represents further progression of the disease. Some areas of the mucosa are spared. **D:** Shows a mucosa that is virtually completely covered by pseudomembrane.

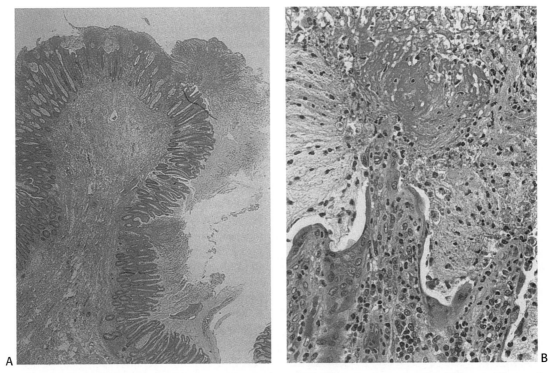

FIG. 13.103. Histologic features of pseudomembranous colitis. **A:** Several volcaniclike eruptions of pseudomembranes overlie the colonic epithelium. **B:** Higher magnification of one of the eruptions demonstrating central fibrin deposition and showers of inflammatory cells expanding from this in a star-burst pattern.

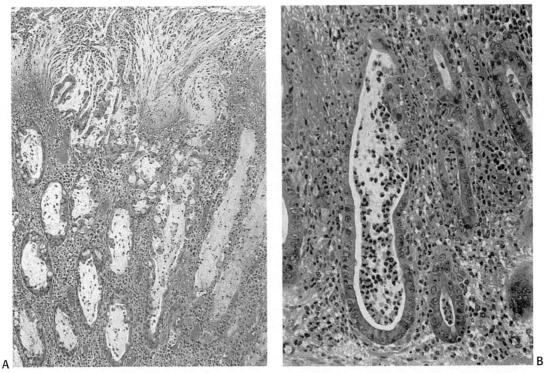

FIG. 13.104. Pseudomembranous colitis due to *Clostridium difficile.* The patient had a positive toxin assay. **A:** The superficial lesion with desquamating epithelium and the beginning of ghostlike structures. A pseudomembrane covers a vast area of the surface and there is evidence of intramural red cell extravasation. **B:** The base of the crypts demonstrates crypt abscesses resembling those seen in some infectious disorders, such as *Salmonella.*

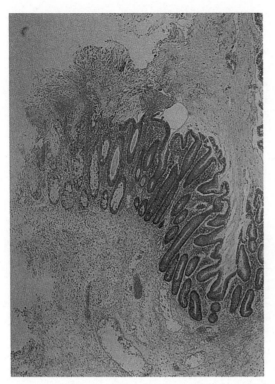

FIG. 13.105. Type III *Clostridium difficile* lesion demonstrating transmural necrosis on the left-hand portion of the mucosa.

propria explain extravasation of blood into the intestinal lumen. In addition to the characteristic mucosal lesions, the colonic specimens show characteristic, marked diffuse mural edema that extends to the muscularis propria (279). When

mucosal necrosis becomes confluent, it may be impossible to distinguish *C. difficile*–induced disease from other forms of severe colitis, especially ischemic colitis or severe idiopathic IBD. In fatal cases, organisms can be found in the colon, necrotic mesenteric lymph nodes, and other organs.

Mucosal biopsies of patients with *C. difficile* are often taken in the area of the pseudomembranes. They may show nonspecific findings demonstrating only evidence of a focal colitis and an inflammatory exudate (Fig. 13.106). Patients who present with a necrotizing enterocolitis pose a diagnostic dilemma because this pathologic picture results from both bacterial and ischemic colitis. Often secondary infections complicate ischemic injury and conversely, bacterial toxins may cause thrombosis and secondary ischemic damage so that it may be impossible to differentiate between ischemia versus a bacterial toxin–induced injury. Areas of focal fibrosis are more likely to associate with ischemia (108), whereas endoscopically visible continuous pseudomembranes are more likely to be associated with *C. difficile* infections (108). Table 13.19 compares the histologic features of three common forms of focal colitis.

Signet ring cells occur in up to 28% of patients with pseudomembranous colitis (280,281), potentially suggesting the diagnosis of carcinoma. However, the cells are confined within the basement membranes, a feature that can be highlighted by cytokeratin immunostains. Furthermore, the nuclei of the signet ring cells are not enlarged and have uniform chromatin and inconspicuous nucleoli, making the diagnosis of carcinoma unlikely. The cells of signet ring cells are negative for p53 and Ki-67 and positive for E-cadherin. In contrast, signet ring cell carcinomas are strongly positive

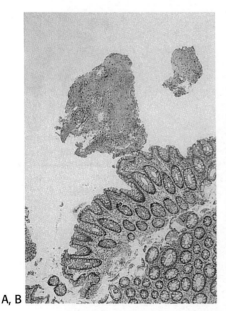
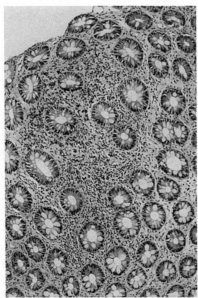
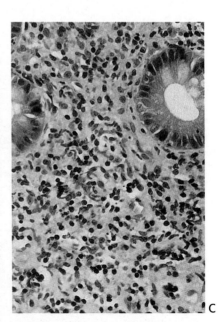

A, B   C

FIG. 13.106. Biopsy of *Clostridium difficile.* **A:** Low-magnification photograph demonstrating the various biopsy fragments of a patient who was toxin positive for *C. difficile.* **B:** Higher magnification shows what appears to be a chronic colitis in the absence of an overlying pseudomembrane. This region comes from a portion of the biopsy not associated with the pseudomembrane. **C:** Higher magnification of the lamina propria demonstrating the acute inflammation.

TABLE 13.19 Comparison of the Histologic Features of Ischemia, *Clostridium difficile*, and Crohn Disease

	Ischemia	C. difficile	Crohn Disease
Focal process	+	+	+
Pseudomembranes	+	+	−[a]
Mucosal changes of chronicity	+/−	−	+
Hemosiderin-laden macrophages in lamina propria	+	−	−
Inflammation extending into submucosa	+	+	+
Crypt abscesses	−	+	+
Glandular ghosts	+	+	−
Granulomas	−	−	+
Atrophic microcysts	+	+	+/−
Lamina propria fibrosis	+	−	+
Basal plasmacytosis	−	−	+

[a] Unless there is coexisting ischemia.

for p53, have a high proliferative rate, and have no or weak positivity for E-cadherin (281).

Patients are generally treated with metronidazole (282). A *C. difficile* toxoid vaccine also has shown promise in treating the disease (283).

Clostridium Septicum

Clostridium septicum, an unusual inhabitant of the human gut, plays a role in the development of neutropenic enterocolitis, an entity discussed in a later section. The organism is a rod-shaped, spore-forming, saprophytic, anaerobic, Gram-positive bacterium that occurs as an opportunistic infection in immunocompromised hosts. Others especially prone to *C. septicum* infections are those with diabetes or malignancies (284). Devitalized tissues or tumors with a low pH offer a perfect environment for germination of the clostridial spores (285). Severe ulcerating intestinal lesions allow organisms to seed the bloodstream and to penetrate the pericolonic tissues and then pass into the psoas and fascial planes. This results in *C. septicum* bacteremia, gas gangrene, or gangrenous myonecrosis (286). When the spores germinate, they produce liquefaction necrosis in both normal and neoplastic tissues. An infection by this organism should be considered in patients harboring malignancies, especially those with colitis.

Clostridium Perfringens

Ingestion of food contaminated by large numbers of vegetative cells of enterotoxigenic strains of *Clostridium perfringens*

produces an unpleasant, self-limited form of diarrhea (287). Rarely, it produces a more serious, often fatal form of disease known as enteritis necroticans (see Chapter 6). The bacteria multiply in the intestine and sporulate, releasing *C. perfringens* enterotoxin. DNA probes are available for the detection of enterotoxin produced by *C. perfringens*.

Mycobacteria

Tuberculosis (TB) is a segmental disease that most commonly involves the ileocecal region or rectum, but the remainder of the colon may also be involved. Perirectal TB often presents as anorectal fissures and fistulae containing giant cells, not always associated with granuloma formation. Stenotic areas measuring several centimeters in length develop in both the rectum and the cecum. Endoscopy reveals nonspecific mucosal friability with nodular changes. In order to establish the diagnosis, multiple deep biopsies of the ulcer bed and its margins must be performed. The differential diagnosis of cecal tuberculous colitis always includes CD and *Yersinia* infection because all three diseases tend to concentrate around the ileocecal valve and all produce granulomatous colitis with strictures, aphthous ulcers, tumorlike lesions, and fistulae. Rarely, tuberculosis associates with a vasculitis (288). Features that distinguish between these three entities are compared in Table 13.20. The clinical and pathologic features of tuberculosis are covered in Chapter 6. *Mycobacterium avium-intracellulare* (MAI) infections rarely exist alone and are seen predominantly in AIDS patients. These infections are also discussed in Chapter 6.

Yersinia

Yersinia enterocolitica causes an ileocolitis and can affect other parts of the colon as well, where it typically causes patchy disease. The rectosigmoid area is frequently spared. The histologic features of colonic disease tend to lack the granulomas that typically associate with the ileocolitis. The histologic features show a focal nonspecific inflammatory response. This infection is discussed in greater detail in Chapter 6.

Gonorrhea

Gonorrheal infections are common in men who have sex with men but in females it may result from spread from the vagina. Perhaps the most common cause of proctitis in individuals who engage in anal intercourse is *Neisseria gonorrhoeae* (289). In a recent study the four most prevalent infectious causes of proctitis among men having sex with men were gonorrhea, herpes simplex, chlamydia, and syphilis, in a decreasing order of frequency (290). Patients may present with anorectal discomfort, mucopurulent rectal discharge, or tenesmus; however, many anorectal gonococcal infections remain asymptomatic. Biopsy findings are nonspecific. Depending on the host's immune response, neutrophils,

TABLE 13.20 Ileocecal Tuberculosis Versus Crohn Disease and *Yersinia* Infection

Feature	Tuberculosis	Crohn Disease	*Yersinia*
Positive chest x-ray	+	−	−
Change in bowel habits	+	+	+
Ileocecal x-ray	Abnormal	Abnormal	Abnormal
Ileal involvement	Tends to be short	Tends to be long	Tends to be short
Stool culture	30% + Tbc	−	Often positive
PPD	−	−	−
Ulcers	Tend to be circumferential	Tend to be linear	Present
Fistulae	+	+	+/−
Lymphadenopathy	+	+	+
Thickened mesentery	+	+	+
Transverse fissures	+	+	−
Edema	+	+	+
Pseudopolyps, rectal bleeding	+	+	+
Vasculitis	Very rare	May be present	−
AFB stain	+	−	−
Granulomas	Usually present in cecum, also commonly present in rectum	Present in 33%–50% of cases	Intramural granulomas with stellate abscesses
Number	Many	Few	Multiple
Size	Large	Small	Large
Nature	Caseating	Noncaseating	
Organism demonstrated	+	−	−
Nodal involvement	Independent of mural involvement	Only present if the wall is involved	Sometimes
Anal lesion	Rare	Frequent	No
Fibrosis muscularis propria	Common	Rare	Rare
Strictures	Usually <3 cm	Generally long	+
Transmural follicular hyperplasia	Usually absent	Usually present	Usually absent
Serology of *Yersinia*	−	−	+

AFB, acid-fast bacillus; PPD, purified protein derivative.

plasma cells, or lymphocytes infiltrate the lamina propria. The diagnosis is best made by Gram stain and culture of a distal rectal mucosal swab, rather than by biopsy. However, biopsies may serve to exclude the presence of other gastrointestinal pathogens. This infection is discussed further in Chapter 15.

Syphilis

Syphilitic proctitis results from direct bacterial inoculation of the anorectum. The spirochetes penetrate the epithelium, inciting a focal inflammatory reaction with ulceration and chancre formation that can mimic a carcinoma, solitary rectal ulcer syndrome polyps, or anal fistulae. Unless secondarily infected, the lesions usually remain painless. Patients may have coexisting sexually transmitted rectal infections, including herpes, gonorrhea, or *Chlamydia trachomatis*. Proctitis may be present in secondary syphilis as well.

The histologic features are characteristic and include an obliterative endarteritis with a mixed inflammatory infiltrate containing numerous plasma cells. Crypt abscesses and granulomas may also be present. Warthin-Starry silver or immunofluorescent stains identify the organism, but the diagnosis is usually established by conventional serologic

tests. The histologic features are described further in Chapter 15. Table 13.21 compares the features of various bacterial forms of colitis.

Intestinal Spirochetosis

Spirochetosis occurs relatively commonly in men having sex with men, especially those who have an HIV infection. However, spirochetosis also affects up to 7% of healthy individuals who do not engage in anal intercourse and up to 30% of homosexual men without evidence of immunodeficiency. The most common organisms are *Brachyspira aalborgi* and *Serpulina pilosicoli*. Both adults and children may be infected. Patients may remain asymptomatic or they may develop nonspecific symptoms including diarrhea (291). There is no difference in the presence or type of intestinal symptoms, sigmoidoscopic appearance of the mucosa, types of sexual practices, or antibiotic use in men with and without spirochetosis. Debate exists as to whether the spirochetes that colonize the bowel represent true pathogens or not. It has been suggested that they represent enteric commensals that become opportunistic pathogens due to unknown factors. The bacteria may cause various GI disturbances, including longstanding diarrhea, rectal bleeding, constipation,

TABLE 13.21 Differential Histologic Features of Bacterial Colitis

Organism	Location in Colon	Ulcers	Granulomas	Pseudomembrane Formation	Blood Vessels	Nature of Cellular Infiltrate
Salmonella	Mostly right sided	Longitudinal	Microgranuloma (rare)	–	Congested, thrombosed	Neutrophilic
Shigella	Distal distribution: mimics ulcerative colitis	Free edges of mucosal folds	No	–	Normal	Neutrophilic
Yersinia	Ileocecal region	Aphthous	Necrotizing	–	Normal	Histiocytic with granuloma formation
Campylobacter	Ileum and colon	Aphthous	Microgranulomas	–	Acute vasculitis	Neutrophilic
Enterohemorrhagic *Escherichia coli*	Patchy	Superficial	No	+/–	Congested	Neutrophilic
Staphylococcus	Anywhere	Superficial	No	–	Normal	Neutrophilic
Clostridium	Patchy	Superficial or deep	No	+	Congested	Neutrophilic
Tuberculosis	Anywhere, but preferentially affects ileocolic and rectal region	Circumferential, aphthous, fissures, fistulae	Necrotizing granulomas, intestines, and lymph nodes	–	Normal	Granulomatous
Mycobacteria avium	Anywhere	Unusual	No	–	Normal	Histiocytic collections
Neisseria gonorrhoeae	Anorectal	Superficial	No	–	Normal	Neutrophilic
Syphilis	Anorectal	Superficial	Chancre	–	Obliterative endarteritis	Lymphocytes and plasma cells
Toxigenic *E. coli*	Anywhere	None	No	–	Congested	None, lamina propria edematous and hemorrhagic
E. coli 0157	Anywhere	Superficial or deep	No	+/–	Congested	Neutrophilic

purulent discharge, abdominal pain, and perianal pain. The infection may also be found in asymptomatic individuals. Treatment results in symptom remission in some patients, whereas in others therapy fails to induce any changes.

Spirochetosis does not produce any grossly or endoscopically recognizable lesions, so that it is first diagnosed histologically. Spirochetes adhere to the mucosal surface, where they appear as a luminal blue fringe (Fig. 13.107). They attach to both neoplastic (292) and nonneoplastic epithelia. The surface epithelium appears unremarkable, as does the underlying lamina propria. One can confirm the presence of the spirochetes by staining tissue sections with PAS or Warthin-Starry stains or by using immunohistochemical stains for *Treponema pallidum* since the antibody cross-reacts with spirochetosis (293). Sometimes the spirochetes are found within epithelial cells or macrophages of the intact mucosa (294).

Aeromonas

Aeromonas hydrophilia causes severe and persistent procto-colitis in children and HIV-infected individuals (295,296) and it superinfects patients with idiopathic IBD. It is easy to confuse this infection with ulcerative colitis (295). *Aeromonas sorbia* may also cause a left-sided segmental coli-tis (297). *Aeromonas* is an oxidase positive, Gram-negative bacillus. Sigmoidoscopy reveals a friable mucosa with ulcers consistent with an acute colitis. Biopsy or resection speci-mens show acute and chronic inflammatory cells in the lam-ina propria together with abscesses (Fig. 13.108). Cultures from the tissues usually yield abundant organisms. The infection is discussed further in Chapter 6.

Actinomyces

The appendix and ileocecal regions are the most common sites of infection, whereas colonic and rectal infections are rare (298). Rectal lesions present as areas of induration with or without ulceration, fistulae, or strictures, mimicking Crohn disease. *Actinomyces* can also cause suppurative cecal lesions. The latter may present as a palpable mass with drain-ing sinuses to the abdominal wall. Most cases of invasive abdominal actinomycosis result from appendiceal or colonic perforations following acute appendicitis, diverticulitis, or

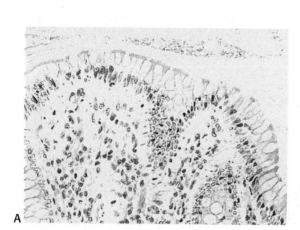
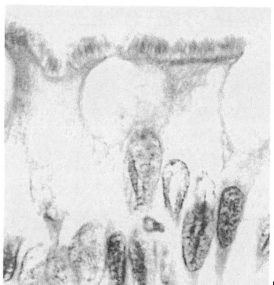

FIG. 13.107. Spirochetosis. **A:** Low-magnification picture showing a prominent blue fringe along the epithelial surface. **B:** Higher magnification shows this apical fringe.

abdominal trauma. These infections are more common in patients with impaired immune defenses. Granulomas that form at anastomotic lines following colonic resection may contain *Actinomyces* (299).

Histologically, the organisms produce rounded masses of faintly discernible branching filaments readily seen on Gram or H&E stains. A radial corona of eosinophilic material called Splendore-Hoepple fibers surrounds the bacterial mass producing the characteristic sulfur granules (Fig. 13.109). The periphery of the Gram-positive bacterial colonies has a club-shaped Gram-negative edge.

Chlamydial Infections

The clinical manifestations and histopathologic features of chlamydial infections depend on the organism's serotype, prior immunity, and the presence or absence of concurrent infections. Both lymphogranuloma venereum (LGV) and non-LGV serotypes cause GI disease. The spectrum of intestinal infection ranges from an asymptomatic infection to severe granulomatous proctocolitis. Infection usually results from direct anal inoculation by infected partners or secondary to lymphatic spread from a penile lesion or from infected vaginal secretions.

Chlamydia bacteria are small bacteria that cannot grow outside a living cell because they cannot synthesize their own ATP. Colonization of chlamydia persists at sites that are inaccessible to phagocytes and immune cells. Additionally, the surface of the *Chlamydia* does not contain proteins that are distinctive enough to induce a full immune response, allowing the infection to persist (300). The life cycle has two stages: The elementary body and the reticulate body. The elementary body is analogous to a spore and it germinates into the reticulate body.

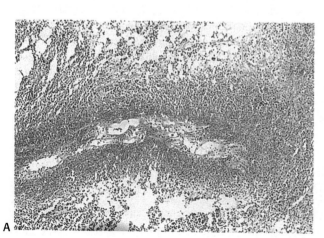
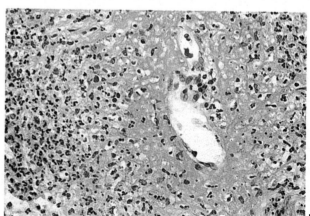

FIG. 13.108. *Aeromonas* colitis. **A:** An abscess is present. **B:** A higher magnification of the inflammation.

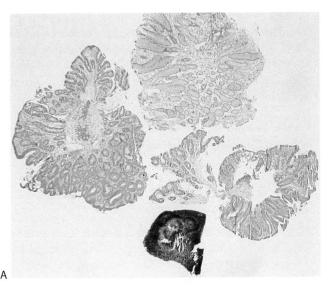
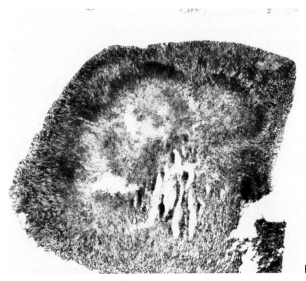

A   B

FIG. 13.109. Colonic actinomyces. **A:** Several tissue fragments are present in this biopsy. The very dark fragment at the bottom of the photo is a "sulfur granule." It is seen at higher magnification in **B.**

Lymphogranuloma Venereum

LGV has a worldwide distribution and its prevalence varies from country to country. The disease develops most commonly in tropical and subtropical countries. It is endemic in Africa, the Indian subcontinent, Southeast Asia, and parts of Central and South America. It occurs sporadically in North America, Europe, and Australia and until recently most cases in these areas were linked to travel in endemic areas (300). The disease is caused by the L1, L2, and L3 serotypes of *C. trachomatis.* However, in the recent past there have been clustered cases of LGV proctitis in men who have sex with men in an outbreak that appears to be centered in the Netherlands but has spread to other cities in Europe and to the United States (301). The patients characteristically have a high rate of concomitant sexually transmitted diseases and the organism has a predominance of the L2 serotype (302).

In countries where the disease is uncommon, it often goes unrecognized (303). Men tend to develop genital lesions followed by suppurative inflammatory reactions, known as buboes, in the inguinal lymph nodes. Women develop rectal disease secondary to lymphatic spread of the organism from the vagina.

Clinically, LGV is divided into three stages. Primary lesions develop 3 to 30 days after the initial infection. In males, the most common lesions involve the penis, often the glans. In women, LGV affects the vaginal wall, labia, or cervix. The primary lesion is transient, often imperceptible, and painless. No specific histopathologic findings identify the early lesion. The primary lesion may heal quite rapidly and scars develop. The second stage begins 10 to 30 days after the primary lesion as the obligate intracellular parasite travels through the lymphatics and into the draining lymph nodes, leading to the development of lymphadenitis. Proctitis is common at this stage. A fluctuant mass in the rec-

tum may lead to the development of abscesses, fistulae, and sinus tracts. If the disease is untreated, it progresses to the third stage, which is marked by fibrosis and the formation of strictures (303) or even the late development of adenocarcinoma or squamous carcinoma (304). The changes may extend proximally as far as to the transverse colon, although the disease tends to remain confined to the distal bowel (Fig. 13.110).

LGV proctitis causes diarrhea, a bloody or mucopurulent discharge, fever, and inguinal and perirectal lymphadenopathy. The disease mimics idiopathic IBD because of the presence of proctitis associated with fibrosis, strictures, deep fissures, ulcers, and granulomas. The disease also mimics herpetic proctitis. However, unlike herpes, the lesions tend to be painless. The diagnosis of LGV is supported by a positive complement fixation test, although 17% of patients have a negative serology. The diagnosis is established by isolation of the organism in

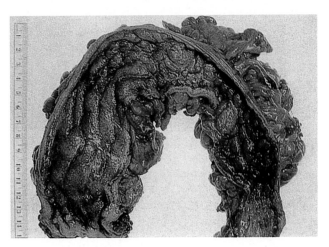

FIG. 13.110. Lymphogranuloma venereum. The bowel wall is irregularly thickened and distorted by the inflammatory process.

culture, direct immunofluorescence testing of biopsies or rectal swabs, or application of gene probes to the tissues.

The rectal mucosa appears ulcerated, friable, granular, nodular, hemorrhagic, and edematous with fibrosis of the underlying tissues. The degree of each of these reactions depends on the disease stage. Early changes show surface injury with an inflammatory exudate and extensive crypt injury, lamina propria inflammation, and cryptitis. The lamina propria contains lymphocytes, plasma cells, and neutrophils. The neutrophils are especially prominent around the crypts with cryptitis and crypt abscesses, crypt injury, and crypt loss (300). Granulomas are not present early. When the inflammatory response is exuberant, pseudomembranes form. The rectal wall appears thickened, rigid, and severely ulcerated. Rectal strictures are usually tubular in nature, with an abrupt line of demarcation with the noninvolved, more proximal large intestine. The mucosa may also become hypertrophic and granular. Severe rectal LGV shows a complete mucosal loss that becomes replaced by granulation tissue. After a short time, the inflammatory response changes to a mixed and even predominantly mononuclear cell response. Macrophages are particularly common in LGV. The infections often induce lymphoid follicle formation. Late-stage disease associates with granulomas, fistulae, and marked fibrosis. Infections restricted to lymph nodes show marked lymphoid hyperplasia and transformation of the macrophages into epithelioid cells.

Nonlymphogranuloma Venereum Chlamydial Infections

Non-LGV strains of *C. trachomatis* occasionally cause mild proctitis (305). The clinical and histologic features resemble anorectal gonorrhea. Endoscopically, one sees a mucopurulent discharge, mucosal friability, and diffuse erythema. Rectal biopsy demonstrates a lamina propria–based pericryptal neutrophilic cell infiltrate. Small erosions, mild inflammation, or prominent lymphoid follicles affect the distal rectum. The infections may also involve anorectal crypts, but these may be difficult to visualize histologically because of the unwillingness of most clinicians to take deep biopsies in the area near the anal sphincter.

Anthrax

Bacillus anthracis is a large Gram-positive bacillus that resides as a spore in the soil and causes fatal disease in livestock (306). Humans become incidentally infected when contacting spores on dead animals or their meat, hides hair, or wool. The most common form of the disease is cutaneous, but gastrointestinal disease may develop if raw or undercooked infected meat is consumed. This mostly occurs in tropical Africa and Asia. The other two forms of the disease are oral-oropharyngeal and inhalational (306). Today there is renewed interest in this disease because of possible terrorist use of the organism.

Patients with gastrointestinal anthrax present with fever, anorexia, nausea, vomiting, and later severe abdominal pain (307). The portal of entry for the gastrointestinal form of the disease is believed to be the distal ileum or cecum where the pathologic findings are a solitary hemorrhagic, necrotic, edematous mucosal lesion and hemorrhagic mesenteric lymphadenitis (308). At least 50% of cases are fatal with septicemic toxemia and in some cases hemorrhagic, bacillus-laden ascites or gastrointestinal hemorrhage (306).

Viral Infections

Cytomegalovirus Infections

CMV infection represents the single most common pathogen identified in autopsy series among AIDS patients. Most patients with GI involvement have disease in the esophagus, stomach, and colon. CMV infections in immunosuppressed and immunocompetent patients fall into primary infections, reactivation infections, and superinfections. CMV is usually not eliminated from the body after a primary infection. Rather, it persists as a low-grade chronic infection or remains in a latent state allowing reactivation at a later time and further viral transmission to new hosts. The macrophage serves as the infection reservoir during latent periods (309).

A number of host and viral factors determine the outcome of a CMV infection. The determinants of CMV infection vary among newborns, organ or bone marrow transplant recipients, HIV-infected persons, or blood transfusion recipients. CMV is transmitted to neonates transplacentally, by passage through a contaminated birth canal, or by ingestion of infected breast milk. In adults, CMV is sexually transmitted or transmitted via infected organs, blood, or needles (310).

Immunocompromised individuals tend to develop CMV viremia, endothelial viral infection (Fig. 13.111) followed by endothelialitis, submucosal ischemia, and secondary ulceration. CMV-associated vasculitis (Fig. 13.112) in the GI

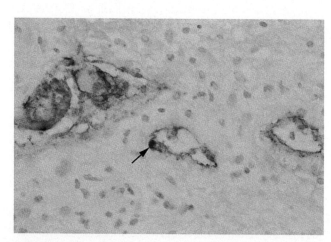

FIG. 13.111. Cytomegalovirus (CMV) endothelialitis. This picture represents a dual immunostain for endothelium (*brown*) and CMV (*red*) (*arrow*).

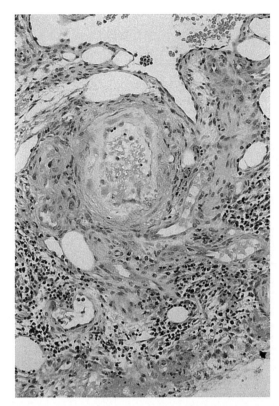

FIG. 13.112. Cytomegalovirus (CMV) vasculitis. Often patients with CMV have moderately occlusive vascular lesions without obvious viral inclusions. These cause secondary ischemic necrosis. Careful examination of the tissues, either by histologic examination or by immunostained preparations, demonstrates the presence of CMV in adjacent portions of the mucosa.

tract is especially well documented in the AIDS population, where it preferentially involves the colon in up to 67% of patients. The affected vessels include arteries and veins that undergo segmental necrosis, perivascular hemorrhage, and possible thrombosis (311). Treatment with ganciclovir is capable of reversing many of these effects and hence emphasizes the critical need to diagnose CMV infections in these patients.

The incidence of symptomatic disease differs in the three forms of CMV infection. At least 66%, <20%, and as many as 40% of patients with primary infections, reactivated latent infections, and superinfections become symptomatic, respectively. Clinically evident CMV infections most commonly affect immunosuppressed patients, including renal transplant patients and those with AIDS. CMV colonic infections also complicate ulcerative colitis (see Chapter 11), nonspecific ulcer disease, or adenocarcinomas. CMV infections have a special predilection for pre-existing inflammation (312), explaining in part the enhanced susceptibility of UC patients to CMV infections. The infection may also affect immunocompetent hosts, sometimes developing in a hospital setting.

CMV colitis presents with abdominal pain; watery, bloody diarrhea; colonic hemorrhage; perforation; and peri-

tonitis. Patients may die following a major GI bleed. The organism characteristically causes colonic ulcers, which tend to localize in the ileocecal region. Rare patients develop CMV pancolitis (313). Infection in the myenteric plexus leads to intestinal pseudo-obstruction (314). CMV colitis develops as part of disseminated disease.

Pathologic features of CMV colitis range from discrete ulcers to more diffuse inflammatory changes characterized by edema, erythema, mucosal erosions, pseudomembranous colitis, or perforations (Fig. 13.113). A mildly abnormal intervening mucosa separates discrete ulcers in many patients. In its severest form, multiple ulcers and perforations occur throughout the length of the gut. The gross appearance may resemble ischemic colitis.

The diagnosis of CMV infection in mucosal biopsies is often not difficult. In severely immunosuppressed patients, numerous CMV-infected cells are identified. CMV-infected cells often appear enlarged (cytomegalic) and they contain eosinophilic intranuclear inclusions surrounded by a halo and granular basophilic cytoplasm. Nuclear and cytoplasmic inclusions often coexist. Inclusion-bearing cells are most numerous in areas of ulceration, especially in the ulcer bases and in the endothelium. They also occur in granulation tissue, pseudopolyps, and intervening mucosa. CMV infects epithelium, endothelial cells (Fig. 13.114), smooth muscle cells, fibroblasts, histiocytes, and ganglion cells. CMV exhibits a wide variation in the intensity of inflammation and associated necrosis. It ranges from a relatively bland lesion to extensive acute and chronic inflammation with widespread necrosis and perforation. The number of inclusions generally parallels the severity of the inflammatory response, although occasional cases show numerous inclusions in the absence of significant inflammation. The accompanying inflammatory infiltrate consists of lymphocytes, histiocytes, plasma cells, and polymorphonuclear leukocytes (PMNs). More subtle infections require an awareness of, or high suspicion for, the possibility that the infection might exist so that multiple sections and/or levels should be carefully examined to find the characteristic cells.

In severe infections, ischemia causes many of the gross features. Some intestinal lesions exhibit a severe CMV-related occlusive vasculitis. Cytomegalic inclusions occur within endothelial cells of medium-sized arteries and veins, arterioles, venules, and capillaries. The affected endothelial cells appear markedly enlarged and crowded, leading to partial or complete vascular occlusion with occasional thrombus formation. In addition, a leukocytoclastic vasculitis and lymphoplasmacytic perivascular infiltrate develop, leading to a loss of vascular integrity with complete or segmental necrosis. As a result, the patient develops ischemia, intestinal ulceration, and perforation. The vasculitis may associate with exuberant fibroblastic reactions (315) that are especially prominent in ulcer bases. The lesions may represent a peculiar reaction of the immunologically compromised host to CMV in the intestinal blood vessels (Fig. 13.112). The ischemia causes localized edema,

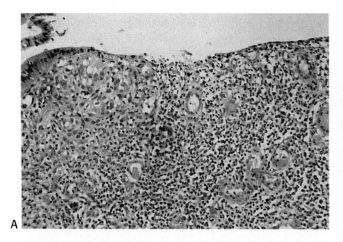

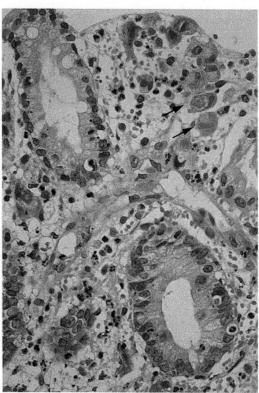

FIG. 13.113. Cytomegalovirus (CMV). **A:** CMV colitis with chronic inflammation, prominent granulation tissue, and an ulcer. **B:** Higher magnification of this specimen demonstrating the presence of CMV inclusions in many of the mononuclear cells (*arrows*).

inflammation, thrombosis, necrosis, and frank perforation. Stromal cells surrounding the infected vessels are also commonly infected in patients with vasocentric infections. When the virus localizes to the myenteric plexus, the myenteric plexus becomes inflamed and contains neuronal intranuclear inclusions surrounded by a halo, axonal dilation with pyknotic axons, and glial cell hyperplasia. The absence of viral inclusions does not exclude a diagnosis of CMV. Immunohistochemical stains or genetic probes aid in detecting the infection (Fig. 13.115).

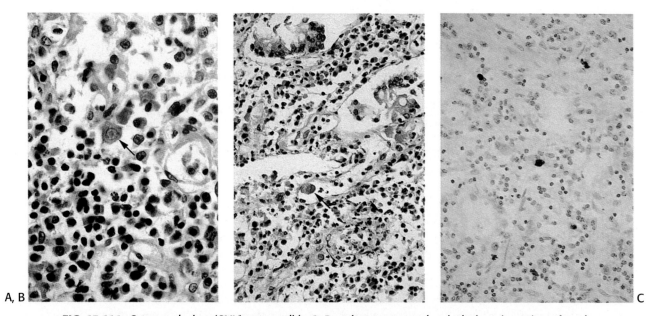

FIG. 13.114. Cytomegalovirus (CMV) enterocolitis. **A:** Prominent mononuclear inclusions (*arrow*) are found in the lamina propria. **B:** Lower magnification shows a detaching endothelial cell containing a CMV inclusion (*arrow.*) **C:** Immunostain demonstrating several immunopositive cells. The infected cells are not all cytomegalic and might have been overlooked in standard hematoxylin–eosin preparations.

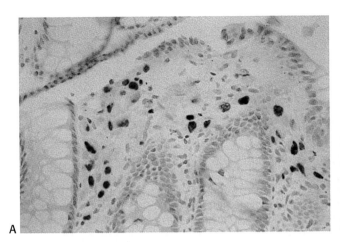

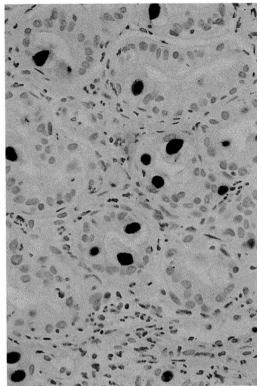

FIG. 13.115. Immunostains of cytomegalovirus infection. **A:** Large numbers of mononuclear cells in the lamina propria. **B:** A large number of immunoreactive epithelial cells.

Herpes Infections

Large intestinal herpetic infections arise in the same clinical settings as herpes infection affecting other parts of the GI tract (see Chapters 2 and 15). Herpes simplex virus (HSV) infections, usually HSV type II, and herpesvirus hominis type I (HHV-I) affect the anorectum. Disease transmission requires direct contact with infectious lesions or secretions. Anorectal infections usually occur 2 to 7 days following sexual contact (316). The virus penetrates the epithelium, causing cytolysis and a localized inflammatory reaction. Patients present with localized paresthesias, tenesmus, pruritus, anorectal pain, change in bowel habits, and anal discharge (317). Abdominal pain can simulate a bowel obstruction. Herpesviruses usually infect squamous mucosa, although they can infect colonocytes as well. The diagnosis is often made clinically and confirmed by cultures or biopsy of the ulcer. Biopsies of the ulcer edges optimize viral detection. Rectal biopsy in HSV and HHV infection usually shows only nonspecific acute inflammation, but in some cases typical Cowdry type A inclusions and multinucleated cells are present.

Adenovirus Infections

Adenoviruses may cause colitis, particularly in immunosuppressed patients. The histologic features resemble those seen in the appendix or small bowel (see Chapters 6 and 8). The viral inclusions are found in the epithelium of the upper parts of the crypts or along the luminal surface, and are recognizable by smudgy nuclear enlargement.

Fungal Infections

Various fungi infect the large intestine. *Candida* infections occur relatively commonly (Fig. 13.116), particularly as superinfections involving necrotic tissues. The clinical settings in which *Candida* infections are found and their pathologic features are discussed further in Chapter 6.

Blastomycosis

Blastomycosis (North American blastomycosis, Gilchrist disease) is a chronic mycosis caused by the dimorphic fungus *Blastomyces dermatitidis*. It grows in tissues as a thick-walled round cell measuring 8 to 15 μm in diameter; it reproduces by broad-based budding. The organism spreads in the intestine by invading submucosal lymphoid tissue and by subsequent erosion into the mucosa and lumen. The typical histologic picture consists of granulomatous inflammation with superimposed pyogenic inflammation. Lesions without secondary infections resemble the epithelioid granulomas of sarcoidosis.

Paracoccidioidomycosis (South American Blastomycosis)

Paracoccidioidomycosis (South American blastomycosis) is a chronic mycosis caused by the dimorphic fungus *Paracoccidioides brasiliensis*. This fungus is an important public health problem in South America, but it does not usually extend further north than Central America and Mexico. This rare fungal disease usually infects the lungs, but it may

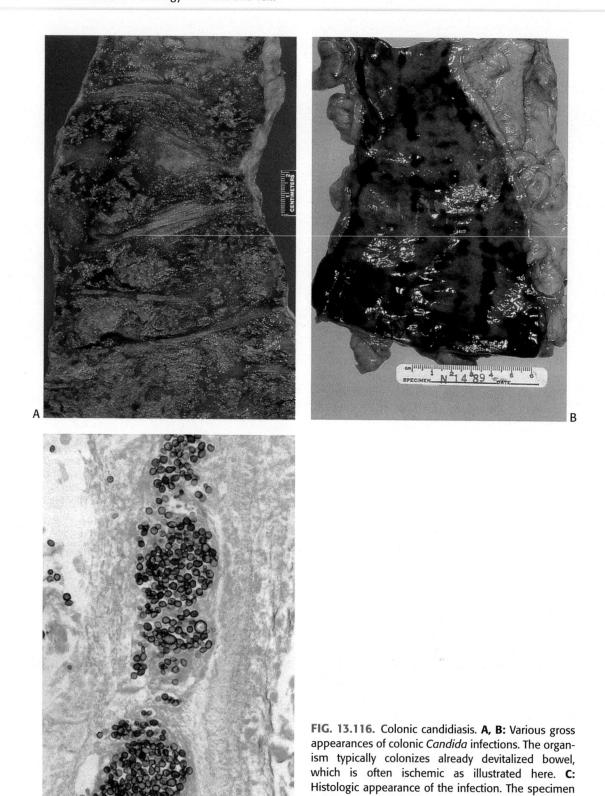

FIG. 13.116. Colonic candidiasis. **A, B:** Various gross appearances of colonic *Candida* infections. The organism typically colonizes already devitalized bowel, which is often ischemic as illustrated here. **C:** Histologic appearance of the infection. The specimen has been stained with a silver stain. Numerous spores are present.

disseminate to other organs. In the intestine it simulates idiopathic IBD or it may cause malacoplakia (318). In tissue, the fungus grows to be a large, round, oval cell measuring 5 to 15 μm in diameter. It reproduces by single or multiple budding. The distinctive feature of the fungus in tissue is an occasional large cell that, when hemisected, reveals peripheral buds protruding from a thin-walled, round mother cell that sometimes looks like a ship's wheel. The fungi are often surrounded by a granulomatous reaction combined with pyogenic inflammation (Fig. 13.117).

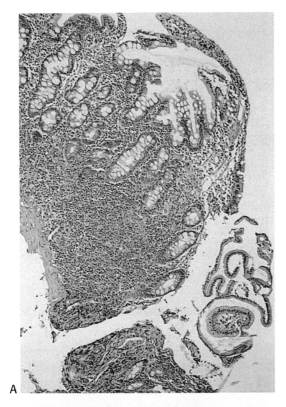

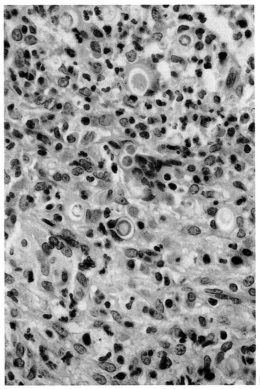

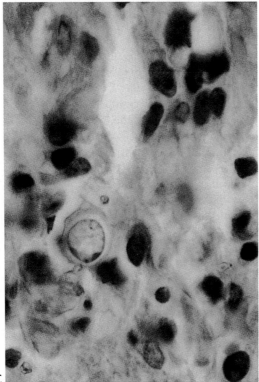

FIG. 13.117. South American blastomycosis. **A:** A portion of intestinal mucosa with regenerative features and an intense inflammatory reaction that separates the base of the glands from the muscularis mucosae. **B:** Medium magnification shows mononuclear cells surrounding spherular structures with a prominent clear space. **C:** A large spore with the typical tissue retraction surrounding the spore. (Case courtesy of Dr. Marian Trevisan, Faculdade Medicina Unicamp, Campinas, Brazil.)

Histoplasmosis

Histoplasma is a dimorphic, facultative intracellular fungus. It grows as a mycelium in the soil and as a yeast within infected cells. It thrives in areas of heavy accumulations of bird or bat excrement. It is endemic in a broad area centered around the Ohio and Mississippi River valleys in the United States, in the Caribbean, and in Central and South America. Skin testing reveals that most people living in endemic areas become infected. Gastrointestinal histoplasmosis affects both immunocompromised and immunocompetent individuals in endemic and nonendemic areas. The skin test for histoplasmosis is often negative in patients with gastrointestinal disease (319). Disseminated histoplasmosis is rare. It affects infants with immature immune systems, persons with defective cellular immunity, AIDS patients, and some patients without an identifiable immunologic defect. It is estimated that disseminated histoplasmosis develops in 55% of infected immunocompromised patients and 4% of immunocompetent patients (320,321). Immunity to histoplasmosis most closely resembles that described for tuberculosis except that the acquired immunity may not be as long-lived so that reinfection occurs more commonly. The course of the infection is mild in most immunocompetent individuals but the organism can produce progressive disseminated infections in individuals compromised by hematologic malignancies, cytotoxic therapy, or HIV infection.

Infections originate in the respiratory tract. Esophageal compression is common. Approximately one third of patients with disseminated disease have small and large bowel intestinal involvement (322). During the early phase of infection macrophages recognize, bind, and ingest the organism, providing it with access to a permissive intracellular environment for replication (323). Exceptional (usually AIDS) patients present with primary gastrointestinal histoplasmosis (324). Intestinal histoplasmosis presents as chronic diarrhea or with symptoms similar to those of IBD. Patients with untreated fatal infections exhibit large collections of organism-containing macrophages, whereas those with localized disease show discrete hyperemia, hemorrhage, mucosal nodules, ulcers that measure up to 4 cm in greatest diameter (319), and inflammation. Endoscopy in patients with disseminated disease reveals the presence of numerous, variably ulcerated, yellowish, submucosal plaques bulging into the intestinal lumen (Fig. 13.118).

A spectrum of gastrointestinal lesions can be found including diffuse lymphohistiocytic infiltration, ulcers, and lymphohistiocytic nodules that usually involve the mucosa and submucosa but that can extend into the muscularis propria, serosa, and mesentery (Figs. 13.119 and 13.120). The lesions contain numerous eosinophils, neutrophils, and plasma cells in addition to macrophages and lymphocytes. Giant cells and granulomas are rare. Well-formed granulomas are only present in 8% of patients (319). Superficial mucosal ulceration is often present over the lymphohistiocytic nodules and the ulcers and nodules frequently lie above Peyer patches. (319). The fungus-containing macrophage collections morphologically resemble those seen in various disorders. However, the *Histoplasma* within them have a distinctive appearance. *Histoplasma* spores have rigid cell walls and average approximately 3 μm in diameter. During the process of fixation, the protoplasm retracts from the wall leaving a clear space that gives the impression of an unstained capsule. The tissue may also contain viable budding fungi. Following therapy (with drugs such as amphotericin B), one sees degenerating and dead organisms. Long

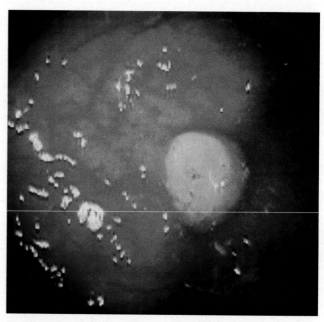

FIG. 13.118. Endoscopic features of histoplasmosis. The colon demonstrates elevated, nodular, yellowish, mucosal plaques.

after remission, one may find fungal cell wall remnants within macrophages.

Cytology preparations made from lesions that present as masses may suggest a diagnosis of a signet ring cell carcinoma due to the presence of large numbers of vacuolated cells (325).

Aspergillosis

Patients most at risk for developing *Aspergillus* infections are those undergoing prolonged periods of immunosuppression following transplantation. Risk factors for the infection include the duration of the granulocytopenia and the use of corticosteroids, cytoreductive agents, and broad-spectrum antibiotics (326). Most infections involve the esophagus, but colonic disease occurs. Colonic lesions are characterized by submucosal ulcers with confluent necrosis, which present with lower GI bleeding (327, 328). Angioinvasive aspergillosis complicating immune suppression and pancytopenia may present as neutropenic enterocolitis. The angioinvasive fungi cause intravascular thrombosis, ischemic necrosis of the cecum, and a relatively mild lymphocytic and histiocytic infiltrate.

The diagnosis of invasive aspergillosis depends on the presence of typical hyphae in the tissues. The lesion somewhat resembles mucormycosis, which also tends to penetrate blood vessels and disseminate through the vasculature. However, in contrast to *Mucor*, which has irregular branching, *Aspergillus* has a regular dichotomous branching pattern of hyphae, all apparently advancing in the same direction.

Mucormycosis

Invasive mucormycosis affects the gut, particularly in malnourished individuals or those on chemotherapy. The large

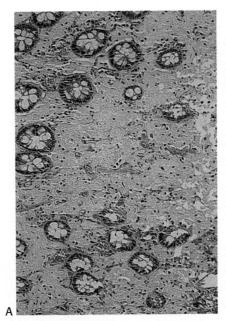
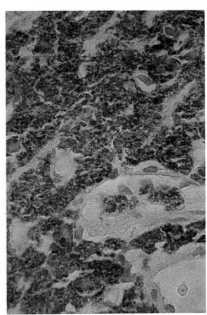

FIG. 13.119. Colonic histoplasmosis. These figures come from the lesion seen endoscopically in Figure 13.118. **A:** The lamina propria is diffusely infiltrated by foamy histiocytic cells. The epithelium appears normal. **B:** Gomori stain shows numerous fungal organisms.

bowel follows the stomach in order of frequency of involvement (329,330). Patients develop mucosal ulcers (330) that lead to bloody diarrhea (329). Characteristic pleomorphic, broad, aseptate, irregularly branched hyphae invade the tissues. The hyphae of *Mucor* measure 3 to 5 μm in diameter.

Cryptococcal Infections

Gastrointestinal cryptococcal infections are rare, occurring either as part of disseminated disease or as an isolated finding. They complicate AIDS, hematologic malignancies, and hyperimmunoglobulinemia, recurrent infection syndrome (331) or occur in patients on corticosteroid therapy (332). They usually present as pulmonary infections but rare cases exist of disease confined to the large bowel (331). The infection produces a granulomatous colitis that mimics Crohn disease.

Trichoderma Infections

Trichoderma longibrachium may cause colonic infections in the immunocompromised patient. The fungus is a branching septated organism that has angioinvasive abilities. There is a long main branch that produces shorter side branches terminating in phialides (333). It produces ulcers and ischemic colitis.

Basidiobolomycosis

Basidiobolo ranarum typically infects the skin in patients in the tropical climates of Africa and Southeast Asia (334). The organisms are irregularly branched, thin-walled, occasionally septated hyphae typically surrounded by a thick eosinophilic (Splendore-Hoeppli phenomenon). Sporelike

spherules measuring 20 to 40 μm may also be present; these contain a central nucleuslike structure (335). Prominent tissue eosinophilic infiltrates and palisading caseating granulomas surround pale fungal hyphae. The granulomas center on the muscularis propria and extend into the subserosa and attached fat and into the submucosa. The organisms cause marked mural thickening with fibrosis. Yellow nodules measuring up to 3 cm in diameter may be seen. The gross appearance of the bowel suggests Crohn disease.

Algal Infections

Prototheca species are common, unicellular, achlorophyllous saprophytes that belong to the genus of colorless, eukaryotic algae that grows slowly on conventional bacteriologic media. They occur in wet parts of the environment, such as rivers and wells. Two species, *Prototheca wickerhamii* and *Prototheca zopfii*, cause human infections. They have a characteristic morphology (336). The roughly spherical cysts vary in size from 1.3 to 16.1 μm. Smaller cysts are unicellular; the larger ones are internally divided into 2 to 20 daughter cysts (337). The rectum may become infected. Histologically, chronic inflammatory cells, including eosinophils and histiocytes, surround the organisms (Fig. 13.121). A vaguely granulomatous inflammation is present but there are no compact, well-formed granulomas.

Protozoan Infections

Amebiasis

Amebiasis has a worldwide distribution; it is more prevalent in the tropics than in temperate climates where it emerges as a sporadic disease or as epidemic outbreaks. One acquires amebiasis through the ingestion of fecally contaminated

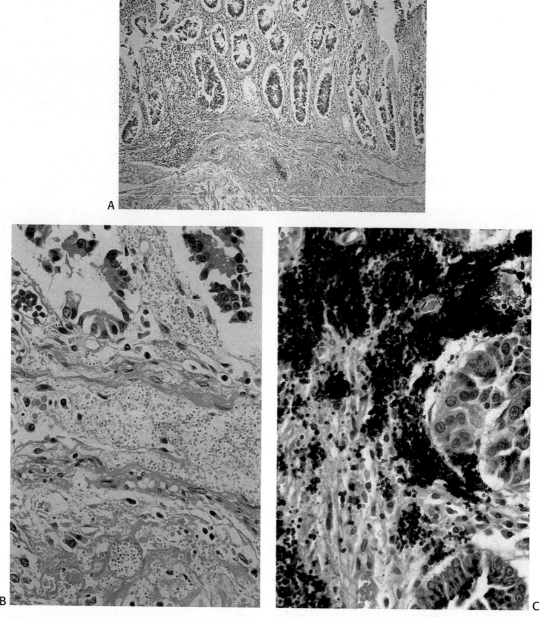

FIG. 13.120. Colonic histoplasmosis. **A:** Low-power hematoxylin and eosin–stained section shows a colonic mucosa with nonspecific inflammation. **B:** Higher magnification shows numerous grayish blue, rounded structures corresponding to the fungus in the tissues in the absence of granulomatous inflammation. **C:** Silver stains highlight the fungi.

food or water. Therefore, the risk of infection is greatest in areas with primitive or nonexistent sanitation or where human feces are used as fertilizer. The disease also spreads via colonic irrigation with infected water, as may occur in chiropractic, homeopathic, naturopathic, or nutritional therapy programs (338). The disorder may also be transmitted via anal intercourse (339). In the United States amebiasis is most commonly seen in immigrants from and travelers to developing countries. The disease is more severe in the very young and the very old (340).

Four species of the genus *Entamoeba* inhabit humans (Fig. 13.122) but only *Entamoeba histolytica* is pathogenic. *E.*

histolytica has two life forms: The invasive motile tropho-zoite, which measures 12 to 50 μm in size, and the 10- to 20-μm cyst (Fig. 13.123). Trophozoites contain a single nucleus with fine peripheral chromatin and a central karyosome. The karyosome appears as a tiny, darkly stained dot in the center of the nucleus and is often difficult to see (341). Trophozoites have a thin cell membrane and some-times exhibit fingerlike projections known as pseudopodia. The cytoplasm generally contains vacuoles.

Amoebae propagate through cysts, the resistant form in their life cycle. Cysts frequently contain highly refractile, cigar-shaped structures with rounded ends. *E. histolytica*

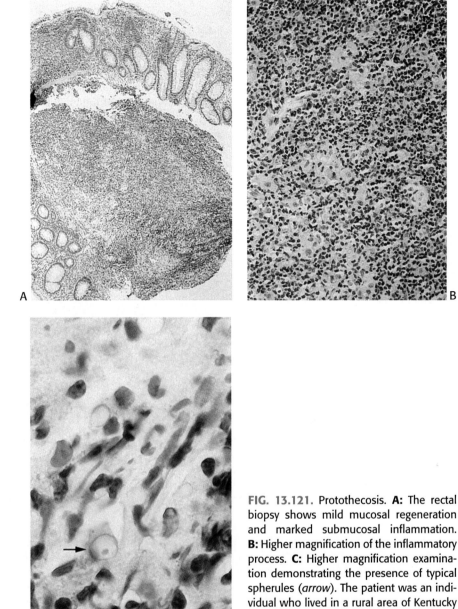

FIG. 13.121. Prototothecosis. **A:** The rectal biopsy shows mild mucosal regeneration and marked submucosal inflammation. **B:** Higher magnification of the inflammatory process. **C:** Higher magnification examination demonstrating the presence of typical spherules (*arrow*). The patient was an individual who lived in a rural area of Kentucky and bathed regularly in well water.

cysts passed in the stool are immediately infectious. They can survive outside the host for weeks to months in moist environments. Ingested cysts, unlike trophozoites, resist gastric acid, the water chlorine concentrations used in sewage systems, and storage at room temperature. Following ingestion, the organism excysts, usually in the region of the ileocecal valve. The cyst wall dissolves, liberating trophozoites. The trophozoites use the galactose and N-acetyl-D-galactosamine–specific lectin to adhere to colonic mucins and thereby colonize the large intestine (342). The trophozoites also secrete cytolytic enzymes (343), enabling them to pass through the intestinal epithelium, disrupting the tissues and liberating red blood cells that they ingest. Trophozoites digest a small cavity in the mucosal wall where they grow and divide by binary fission. Interaction of

the parasite with the intestinal epithelium causes an inflammatory response marked by activation of nuclear factor $\kappa\beta$ and the secretion of lymphokines (344). The infection may remain limited to the GI tract for years or it may extend to the liver and other organs. Specific and sensitive tests for the diagnosis *E. histolytica* in stool are now available and include antigen detection and PCR (340).

The disease affects individuals of all ages, including infants (345). The severity of the disease varies considerably. Amebiasis often remains asymptomatic or it may produce severe disease and death. Symptomatic amebiasis presents in three ways: (a) as a localized bowel infection with the typical symptoms of dysentery, including rectal bleeding; (b) as a localized granulomatous lesion that commonly affects the cecum and closely mimics a carcinoma; or (c) with hepatic

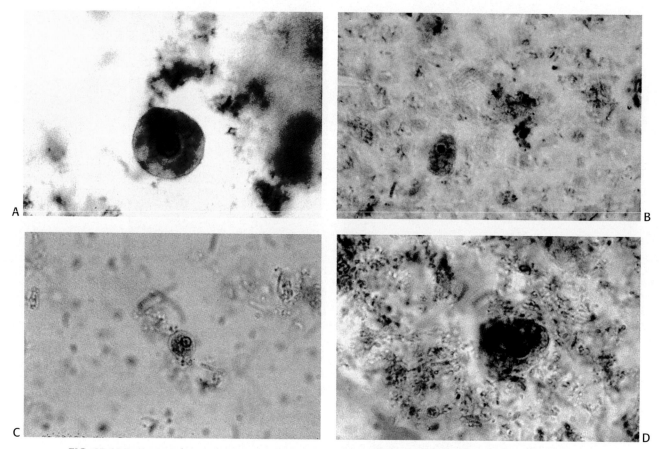

FIG. 13.122. *Entamoeba.* **A:** *Entamoeba coli* is generally considered nonpathogenic. The trophozoite seen here on stained smear is similar in size to the trophozoite of *Entamoeba histolytica* but is distinguished by its larger irregular karyosome and coarser peripheral chromatin. **B:** *Entamoeba nana* is also generally considered nonpathogenic. The trophozoite seen here is smaller than the trophozoite of *E. histolytica* and is distinguished by its prominent karyosome. **C:** On stained smears, the trophozoite of *Entamoeba hartmanni* may be confused with that of *E. histolytica* because of its usually central compact karyosome. The *E. hartmanni* trophozoite is smaller than that of *E. histolytica,* however. **D:** The *E. histolytica* trophozoite is distinguished on trichrome-stained smears by its size (usually 20 to 50 μm) and its nuclear morphology. The single nucleus has a central compact karyosome and finely granular peripheral chromatin. (A–D courtesy of Dickson Despomier, Ph.D., Department of Parasitology, Columbia University, New York, NY.)

involvement, causing amebic hepatitis or amebic liver abscesses.

The two most common symptoms of the dysenteric presentation include intermittent bloody diarrhea and lower abdominal cramps. In severe disease, the symptoms simulate ulcerative colitis and toxic megacolon, especially in geographic areas where amebiasis is not endemic. Like IBD, chronic amebic colitis may begin insidiously and exhibit cyclic remissions. Patients experience gradually increasing lower abdominal discomfort, loose stools, malodorous flatus, and recurrent bouts of diarrhea. Intermittent constipation also occurs. Over a period of 3 to 4 days, the number of stools may increase to 25 per day with weakness and prostration. Nausea, vomiting, and right-sided cramps are usual. Amebic colitis often persists for weeks, months, or years. Patients may also show a mild anemia or mildly elevated white blood count. Amebiasis also causes proctitis in children, with the disease often remaining limited to the rectum (346). Individuals particularly at high risk for developing

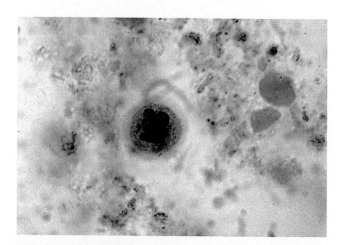

FIG. 13.123. The *Entamoeba histolytica* cyst is distinguished on trichrome stain by nuclear morphology identical to that of the trophozoite and one or more chromatoid bodies with rounded ends. (Courtesy of Dickson Despomier, Ph.D., Department of Parasitology, Columbia University, New York, NY.)

chronic proctitis without diarrhea include immigrants or travelers from endemic areas. Unusual manifestations of amebic colitis include acute necrotizing colitis, toxic megacolon, ameboma, and perianal ulceration with the potential formation of a fistula (340).

Complications of amebiasis result from the migration of the parasite through the bowel wall into adjacent structures (Fig. 13.124). The bowel wall usually becomes severely stenotic due to inflammation with abscess formation and fibrosis. Perforation and fistulae between bowel loops are rare and usually fatal (347). The most serious complication of amebiasis is venous invasion with parasitic migration through the portal system to establish amebic hepatitis or hepatic amebic abscesses, usually involving the right lobe of the liver. Hepatic involvement affects <5% of those with amebic dysentery (348). Hepatic abscesses can perforate into the subphrenic space, right pleural cavity, or right lung. Pericarditis may also occur (349). Colonic carcinoma may follow amebiasis and there is an increased frequency of polyps at the site of amebic ulceration.

Both ova and trophozoites are found in stool specimens or rectal scrapings. Stool examination also often shows the presence of Charcot-Leyden crystals. Stool examination (Figs. 13.122 and 13.123) for motile trophozoites is a simple and easy way to establish the diagnosis. Various immuno-

logic tests help make or confirm the diagnosis, including detection of amebic antigens in stool specimens or serum antibodies by fluorescent antibody techniques (350). Serologic tests may be particularly useful because they show superior sensitivity and predictive value in recognizing invasive disease than do biopsies (351).

Resected specimens often exhibit diffuse mucosal and mural involvement, sometimes producing a pattern grossly resembling IBD, especially Crohn disease (Fig. 13.125). The most extensive lesions affect the cecum, appendix, and rectosigmoid, but they may also be scattered throughout the bowel and be particularly prominent in the hepatic flexure.

The earliest amebic lesions appear as small, yellow mucoid elevations containing semifluid, necrotic material infected with the parasite. When the lesions rupture into the lumen, the organisms continue to proliferate, undermining the adjacent intact mucosa to leave discrete, oval-shaped ulcers with overhanging edges extending into the submucosa. The flat, nonindurated ulcers tend to lie on the long axis of the bowel wall, and they exhibit a characteristic hyperemic edge. A ragged, yellowish white membrane covers the ulcer floor, particularly in severe cases. The ulcers may become confluent, leaving isolated patches of intact, hyperemic mucosa among extensive areas of necrosis and extensive inflammatory polyposis.

Although invasive amebiasis is characterized by disruption and invasion of the colonic mucosa by amebic trophozoites (Fig. 13.126), histologic examination of biopsies can be nondiagnostic since often all one sees are inflammation, ulceration, and a fibrinous exudate. Biopsies should be taken from the ulcer edges, especially because this is where the organisms are most numerous. The trophozoites also sometimes lie in the overlying fibrinous exudate. For this reason, enemas should be avoided prior to biopsy, as the luminal mucus and exudate, potentially containing the trophozoites, will be removed in the process.

Few histopathologic changes are pathognomonic except for the presence of the trophozoite. Trophozoites may or may not be seen on the initial examination (Fig. 13.126). The pathologist must be able to recognize *E. histolytica* in its trophozoite form and to distinguish it from nonpathogenic amebas that may inhabit the human large intestine. Typical organisms are large, round to ovoid, varying in diameter from 6 to 40 μm. They contain a voluminous, pinkish purple cytoplasm with a distinctive foamy, vacuolated, or granular appearance. The cytoplasm is PAS positive and, unlike nonpathogenic amoebas, contains ingested red blood cells (352). Erythrophagocytosis is easily demonstrated with Heidenhain iron hematoxylin stains. The organisms must be distinguished from macrophages, which tend to be smaller and less intensely PAS positive, and contain a clearly identified nucleus. *Balantidium coli* infections produce similar histologic changes to those of amebic colitis. However, *B. coli* measure 30 × 150 × 40 μm contrasting with *Entamoeba*, which measure 30 to 40 μm in largest diameter. In tissue sections, the ameba may be surrounded by a clear space, a shrinkage

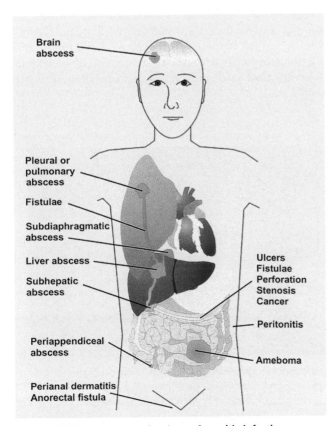

FIG. 13.124. Complications of amebic infections.

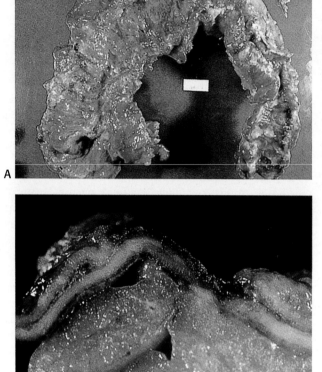

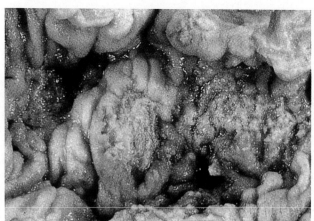

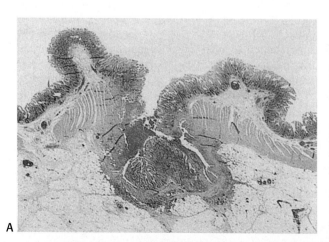

FIG. 13.125. *Entamoeba histolytica.* **A:** This colon manifests effects of severe amebiasis due to *E. histolytica.* There are multiple irregular deep ulcers. **B, C:** Having gained access through the colonic mucosa, the invasive *E. histolytica* spread laterally and deeply through the submucosa, undermining the remaining mucosa.

artifact produced by fixation (352). When one suspects the disease, one may wish to perform serologic tests to confirm the presence of the infection. Alternatively, a prophylactic trial of metronidazole may be indicated.

Patients who undergo surgical resection are typically those with severe obstructing amebic disease or transmural inflammation. The proximal colon is usually involved, although the rest of the colon, including the rectum, the anal canal, and even the distal ileum, may be affected. Early lesions show mucosal swelling and ulceration. A surface exudate composed of mucin, fibrin, and inflammatory cells develops as the superficial ulceration evolves. Amoebae are most readily detected in this exudate (352).

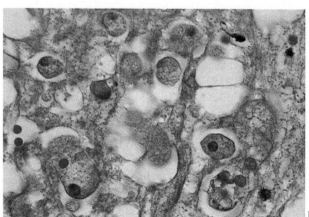

FIG. 13.126. *Entamoeba histolytica.* **A:** Typical flask-shaped ulcer of *E. histolytica.* Here much of the mucosa has been spared as the ameba has eroded through submucosa and muscularis. **B:** Trophozoites of *E. histolytica* are distinguished by their size, nuclear morphology, and phagocytosis of erythrocytes in hematoxylin and eosin–stained sections.

Developing ulcers have irregular, hyperemic mucosal outlines with markedly undermined, overhanging edges, producing a characteristic flasklike shape. The extensive undermining leads to widespread ulceration and even perforation. As the ulcers extend, the organisms may also be found in tissue spaces and small vessels. When amoebae invade tissues, they usually aggregate (Fig. 13.126) and are generally present in areas of necrosis and tissue disruption. In patients with severe disease, trophozoites may extend through the bowel wall to lie freely in the abdominal cavity or in the serosal fat. The mucosa exhibits a chronic inflammatory response characterized by minimal, moderate, or extensive lamina propria infiltrates containing lymphocytes, histiocytes, plasma cells, eosinophils, and prominent lymphoid follicles. Pronounced edema and congestion accompany these changes, along with goblet cell depletion, neutrophil emigration, and early crypt abscesses. Necrosis follows extensive edema.

Amebic ulcers develop slowly, usually allowing cellular proliferation and fibrosis to occur, often protecting against perforation. Some lesions eventually heal without significant scarring, but others progress to chronic fibrosis with persistent or recurrent focal ulceration. Prolonged inflammation leads to the production of inflammatory pseudopolyps and strictures (353). Secondary bacterial infection of the ulcers is common and, if present, complicates the histologic features.

Patients with longstanding infections and exuberant tissue reactions develop tumorous, exophytic, cicatricial, inflammatory masses known as amebomas (Fig. 13.127). Amebomas develop in the cecum, appendix, and rectosigmoid, in decreasing order of frequency. They also develop at the hepatic flexure, transverse colon, and splenic flexure (354). They usually occur in untreated or inadequately treated patients with amebiasis, years after the last recognized dysenteric attack. Amebomas are usually solitary, most commonly affecting men 20 to 60 years of age. Amebomas cause numerous symptoms including alternating diarrhea and constipation, weight loss, and low-grade fever. In endemic areas, cramping, lower abdominal pain, and a palpable mass suggest the diagnosis. In the United States, these symptoms in younger individuals suggest Crohn disease or appendiceal abscesses, whereas in older individuals colon cancer or diverticulitis is suggested.

Amebomas result from persistent ulceration and granulation tissue formation, with fibroblastic proliferation and inflammation. The lesions vary in size but may measure up to 15 cm in diameter. They present as localized, often circumferential areas of bowel wall thickening, mucosal excrescences, or large tumor masses. The inflamed mucosa often bulges into the lumen and stricture formation narrows the bowel lumen. Amebomas may extend into the adjacent mesocolon. Biopsy may be required to distinguish the lesion from a carcinoma or large adenoma.

The therapy for invasive infections differs from the therapy for noninvasive disease. Noninvasive infection may be treated with paromomycin. Nitroimidazoles, particularly metronidazole, are the mainstay of therapy for invasive disease (355).

Balantidiasis

Balantidiasis has a cosmopolitan distribution, but most infections occur in tropical and subtropical regions due to ingestion of contaminated water. The disorder may also be transmitted from person to person (356). Pigs and rats serve as reservoirs for the infection (356). *B. coli*, the largest protozoan, has both a cyst and trophozoite form. It is the only ciliated protozoan known to infect humans. Oval trophozoites, measuring $30 \times 150 \times 40\ \mu m$, contain a characteristic large, kidney-shaped macronucleus and a small or round micronucleus (Fig. 13.128); cilia cover its surface. The cytoplasm contains two contractile vacuoles and numerous food vacuoles. The anterior end is pointed and contains a funnel-shaped cytosome. The oval to spherical cysts measure 40 to 65 μm in diameter. Young cysts are covered by cilia that disappear as they age. Ingested trophozoites are liberated from the cysts in the small intestine and invade the large intestine. They continue to excyst as they descend through the large intestine.

Balantidial infections cause three clinical patterns: Acute, chronic, and fulminating (357). The most common clinical pattern is chronic disease, characterized by alternating diarrhea and constipation. Symptoms can last from days to months. In contrast, patients with acute disease exhibit nausea, vomiting, anorexia, abdominal pain, and up to 30 bloody, mucus-filled bowel movements per day. Endoscopically, shallow ulcers and pseudomembranes are present (357). The fulminant form of the infection affects emaciated or debilitated patients. The stools are bloody, often frankly hemorrhagic, and patients may exsanguinate. If perforation occurs, the infection is fatal.

B. coli invades into and ulcerates the colon (Fig. 13.128), producing severe diarrhea and hemorrhage. The right half of the colon and cecum are most commonly involved, but the rectum and sigmoid can also become infected. The histologic features mimic those of amebiasis, including the presence of

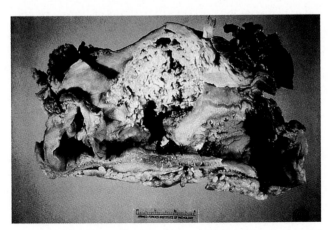

FIG. 13.127. Ameboma. The patient had chronic amebiasis and the presence of a large necrotic mass, which was resected.

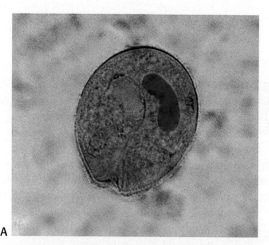
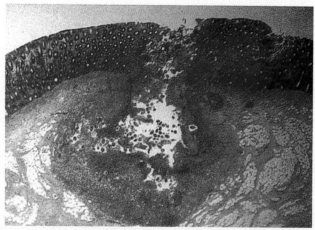

FIG. 13.128. *Balantidium coli.* **A:** The trophozoite of *B. coli* is relatively large (50 to 70 μm), ovoid shaped, and rimmed by cilia. The trophozoite has two nuclei, the larger of which is kidney bean–shaped and stains red on trichrome stain. **B:** *B. coli* invades the colon to produce ulcers similar to those seen in colonic amebiasis. The ulcers may penetrate through the entire bowel wall, as in this case. (Courtesy of Dickson Despomier, Ph.D., Department of Parasitology, Columbia University, New York, NY.)

flask-shaped ulcers containing trophozoites (358). The intervening mucosa may appear normal, edematous, or hemorrhagic. Most ulcers are superficial and multiple, but when deep ulcers develop, they perforate, particularly in fulminant disease (357). The tissues become necrotic and infiltrated with neutrophils and erythrocytes. Pseudomembranes containing neutrophils and fibrin cover the ulcers. The diagnosis rests on identifying the parasite.

Visceral Leishmaniasis

Visceral leishmaniasis (kala azar) is a parasitic disease produced by the protozoan *Leishmania donovani.* Patients present with fever, loss of appetite, occasionally diarrhea, and eosinophilia. Patients exhibit splenomegaly, hepatomegaly, anemia, and skin lesions, known as dermal leishmaniasis. The diagnosis requires microscopic identification of characteristic *Leishmania* amastigotes, culture of the organism, or serologic positivity for the protozoan (359). Microscopic diagnosis is usually carried out by bone marrow aspirate or biopsy. However, chronic visceral leishmaniasis may be first diagnosed on a rectal biopsy (359). The rectal mucosa contains well-preserved epithelium, but the intervening lamina propria is obliterated by the presence of large macrophages containing abundant cytoplasmic *Leishmania* amastigotes (Fig. 13.129). The parasitic forms are oval or round, measuring 1.5 to 3 μm in diameter, with two characteristic black dots corresponding to the nucleus and kinetoplast. The organism may also be found in the small intestine.

Blastocystis (Zierdt-Garavelli Disease)

Blastocystis hominis is a strict anaerobic protozoan that reproduces by binary division or sporulation. It is a single-celled organism found naturally in fresh water. The parasite is directly identifiable by immediate examination of feces. Infected patients present as asymptomatic carriers or with an illness consistent with an acute or chronic gastroenteritis. Organism prevalence ranges from 2% to 18% in the United States (360–362), 3% to 13% in Canada, and 3% in Great Britain.

The pathogenicity of *Blastocystis* is a topic of debate. In one study, up to 34.7% of patients who are clinically healthy harbor the organism. Symptomatic patients present with abdominal pain, watery diarrhea, constipation, anorexia, vomiting, flatulence, and weight loss. Symptoms may be present for >2 weeks. The colonic mucosa usually appears endoscopically normal, although rarely it appears erythematous and friable. The organism is usually found in the stools in patients with diarrhea, sometimes associated with signs of inflammation.

Biopsies from infected persons often appear normal. When abnormal, they may exhibit only mild nonspecific inflammation (360). Rarely, the organism causes colonic mucosal destruction but the parasite does not appear to penetrate and invade the tissues. The presence of large numbers of organisms (more than five organisms per oil immersion field), in the absence of other known bacterial, viral, or parasitic agents, should be treated. The organism may also be diagnosed in colonic cytology brushings.

Chagas Disease

Chagas disease results from infection by the parasite *Trypanosoma cruzi*, and the disease is virtually confined to South America. The entire GI tract may become involved. Patients present with achalasia, intractable constipation, megacolon, or intestinal pseudoobstruction. The infection is discussed in detail in Chapter 10.

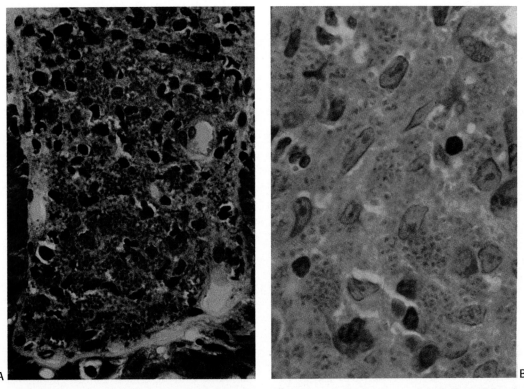

FIG. 13.129. Leishmaniasis. **A:** Gram section showing portions of the lamina propria infiltrated by the amastigote form. **B:** Methyl green–pyronine stain showing amastigote. (Pictures courtesy of Miguel Idoate, Faculty of Medicine, Universidad de Navarra, Pamplona, Spain.)

Helminthic Infections

Schistosomiasis

Schistosomiasis, also known as bilharziasis, is an infection caused by trematodes in the genus *Schistosoma*. Gastrointestinal disease results from the host's response to the schistosomal eggs and the granulomatous reaction evoked by the antigens they secrete (363). The intensity and duration of the infection determine the amount of antigen released and the severity of the chronic fibro-obstructive disease.

Schistosomiasis ranks second to malaria as a cause of serious global morbidity. Schistosomiasis infects about 200 million people worldwide (364). Three schistosomal species cause most human infections: *Schistosoma mansoni*, *Schistosoma japonicum*, and *Schistosoma haematobium*. *S. mansoni* is endemic throughout Africa and is found in many areas of Latin America and the Middle East. *S. japonicum* occurs in Asia. *S. haematobium* is endemic in Africa and in the Middle East. Rare infections with *Schistosoma intercalatum* and *Schistosoma mekongi* occur in Africa and Indochina, respectively.

Humans become infected when bathing or wading in water infected with cercaria (Fig. 13.130). The cercaria emerge from freshwater snails, penetrate the skin, enter the bloodstream, mature in the liver, and finally settle in the venous system, the intestinal wall, or the mesentery before they develop into adults. Schistosomes are the only flukes that are not hermaphroditic and in which the sexes are separate. Thus, infections by both a male and a female are required to generate ova. The female lies in the gynecophoral canal of the male. Females lay their eggs in the mesenteric veins and GI submucosal vessels. The eggs gain access to the GI lumen and the feces. If the ova reach freshwater, they hatch, releasing motile ciliated miracidia that invade snails. In the snail, the parasites undergo further development before being released again as cercaria to repeat the life cycle. The worm burden of each infected person is relatively constant because schistosomes do not multiply in the vertebrate host (365). Infection intensity increases by repeated exposures or decreases through attrition of senescent worms through the host immunity or following chemotherapy.

Infected individuals living in endemic areas often remain asymptomatic due to their acquired immunity to the organism (365). This contrasts with visitors to endemic regions who develop acute, and sometimes very severe, symptoms immediately following the first infection (366). So-called Katayama fever consists of fever, chills, eosinophilia, hepatosplenomegaly, generalized lymphadenopathy, and generalized GI symptoms (366). The syndrome develops as the females lay up to 3,500 eggs per day. Proteins in the eggs react with circulating antibodies, thereby producing a serum sickness–like syndrome (366). Other forms of schistosomiasis include hepatosplenic, pulmonary, urogenital, cerebral, and intestinal infections.

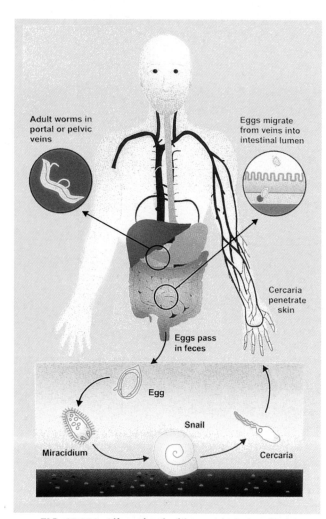

FIG. 13.130. Life cycle of schistosomiasis (see text).

The intensity of the infection varies from individual to individual. Infected persons complain of abdominal pain, diarrhea, and bloody stools. Intestinal schistosomiasis classically associates with *S. mansoni*, but *S. japonicum* and *S. haematobium* can also produce intestinal infections. Most lesions affect the rectum and left colon. Schistosomiasis also causes duodenitis in places where the parasite is endemic. It can represent a significant cause of upper GI bleeding.

Adult flukes do not cause clinical disease, probably because they incorporate host antigens as they mature. Rather, it is the numerous ova that elicit a granulomatous response (Fig. 13.131) and extensive fibrosis. Intestinal polyps and strictures develop late in the disease. Polyps detected at the time of endoscopy may represent either inflammatory polyps or adenomas. A relationship exists between schistosomiasis and colon cancer (367). Patients with heavy colonic infections do not respond well to chemotherapeutic regimens. They therefore undergo resection to treat the colonic manifestations of the disease.

Patients' tissues tend to be examined only when patients present with intussusception, mass lesions, or strictures that cause intestinal obstruction. Patients with chronic infections exhibit pronounced submucosal thickening due to fibrosis and lymphoid hyperplasia. Minute granulomas resembling tubercles are sometimes visible on the mucosal or peritoneal surfaces. Bilharzial tubercles also accumulate in the submucosa, where ova become trapped in narrow vascular channels. The granulomatous response causes single or multiple areas of focal or diffuse submucosal thickening accompanied by ulceration, hemorrhage, or stenosis, usually involving the rectum and left colon. The disease may grossly mimic CD or carcinoma. Extensive polyp formation may develop, especially in *S. japonicum* infections. Chronic schistosomiasis associated with a high parasitic burden may present as extensive (multiple) large (0.5 to 4.5 cm) serosal, distal mesenteric, and omental nodules (368), producing a lesion also referred to as the bilharzial pseudotumor or retroperitonitis (369). This condition mimics subserosal malignancy or diverticulosis. The cut surface of the lesions has a brown, crusty material reminiscent of fecaliths impacted within diverticula (369).

In the early stages of the infection one sees an acute proctitis and colitis accompanied by edema and hemorrhage as ova are discharged into the bowel lumen. Necrotic areas contain ova without a surrounding granulomatous reaction (370). Eggs in the mucosa and submucosa become surrounded by diffuse cellular infiltrates. In contrast, egg granulomas occur more frequently in the serosa and the muscularis propria (371). One may also encounter eggs in the bowel wall without any inflammation or fibrous reaction around them. Adult worms are sometimes found in mesenteric veins or venules. Morphologic features of chronic infection include localized or diffuse mucosal or serosal ulcers, strictures due to extensive granulomatous or fibrous reactions, pericolic masses, polyposis, and masses of granulation tissue.

The diagnosis rests on finding schistosomal eggs and the colitis they induce. The eggs measure 100 to 180 μm in length and about 70 μm in width. Those of *S. mansoni* are marginally longer than those of *S. japonicum* and exhibit a distinctive subterminal lateral spine. The shell has a light brown, translucent appearance and, in the case of *S. mansoni*, contains acid-fast material. This feature is diagnostically helpful if only the shell fragments are present.

Anisakiasis and Strongyloidiasis

Anisakiasis usually involves the stomach and small intestine; only rarely does it involve the colon (372). Colonic involvement is usually right sided, involving an intestinal segment measuring in length from 10 to 15 cm. The outlines of the worms can sometimes be seen, measuring approximately 0.7 mm in width and 12 to 20 mm in length. The intestinal wall surrounding the worms becomes markedly thickened (372). This parasite is discussed further in Chapters 4 and 6. *Strongyloides* infections occasionally involve the large bowel. Their clinical and pathologic features are discussed in Chapter 6.

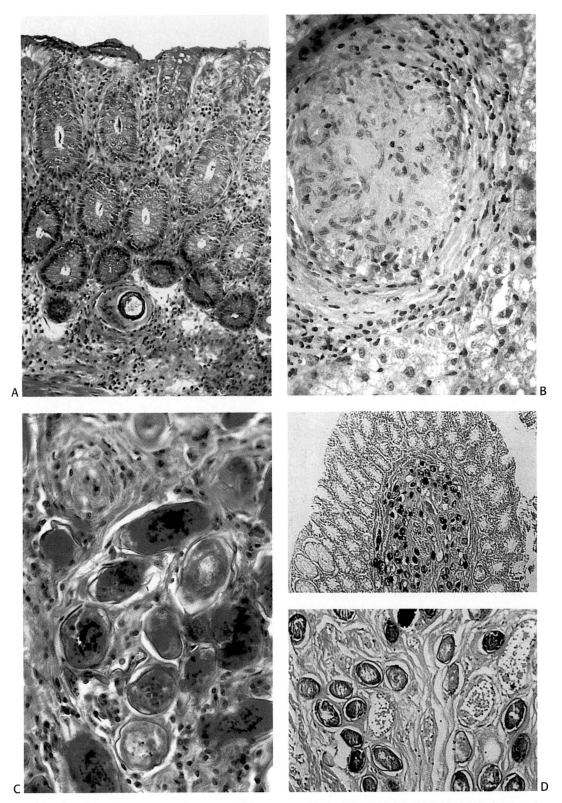

FIG. 13.131. Schistosomiasis. **A:** Colonic mucosa with schistosomes in the lamina propria. **B:** Granulomas in colonic schistosomiasis. **C:** Multiple worms and eggs in the colonic wall. **D:** The inflammatory reaction and fibrosis surround schistosomal eggs (*bottom*) deposited in the colonic submucosa and have produced a polyp (*top*).

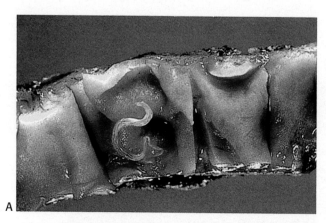
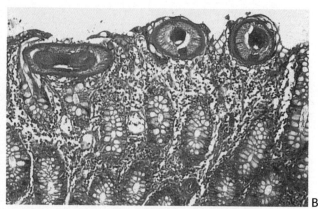

FIG. 13.132. *Trichuris trichuria.* **A:** Aborigine who had a colectomy for rectal bleeding. The *T. trichuria* is attached to the mucosa. (Courtesy of Robin Cooke, MD, Department of Pathology, Royal Brisbane Hospital, Brisbane, Australia.) **B:** The adult female *T. trichuria* threads its narrow anterior end through the superficial colonic mucosa. The broad posterior end deposits eggs into the intestinal lumen.

Trichuriasis (Whipworm)

Trichuriasis, an intestinal infection of humans caused by *Trichuris trichuria,* ranks as the third most common intestinal parasite worldwide, infecting approximately 700 million persons. The organism is most prevalent in tropical and subtropical regions. In the United States, trichuriasis is the most common intestinal helminthic infection (373). It also is the most common helminthic infection in Americans returning from tropical areas. In temperate zones, the infection most frequently affects institutionalized, mentally retarded patients (374).

Adult whipworms are found in the large intestine with their anterior ends deeply embedded in the mucosa (Fig. 13.132). They measure 30 to 50 μm in length and possess a threadlike anterior two thirds with a stouter posterior third, producing a whiplike structure. The female lays about 5,000 eggs each day. The bile-stained eggs measure 50 to 54 $\times$ 22 to 23 μm and have a bipolar barrel shape with a three-layer shell. *T. trichuria* mature inside the egg. The eggs (Fig. 13.133) must incubate for at least 3 weeks in soil before the infective larvae emerge. *Trichuris* eggs are sensitive to desiccation and a combination of heat and low humidity is detrimental to their survival. Exposure to sunlight kills them. Infection occurs when ova are ingested in fecally contaminated food and water. After ingestion, eggs hatch in the small intestine and the larvae embed themselves in the intestinal villi. They then migrate to the large intestine, where they mature into adults in about 3 months.

The severity and consequences of *Trichuris* infections vary widely. Patients with mild infections usually remain asymptomatic. The parasites have particularly severe adverse health effects in young, malnourished populations. Patients often have infections with multiple organisms. Patients present with abdominal pain, diarrhea, nausea, vomiting, constipation, and anorexia. Severe infections associate with mucous and bloody diarrhea, tenesmus, and abdominal pain. Rectal prolapse, volvulus, or intussusception compli-

cates some infections (375). The diagnosis is usually made by finding ova in the stool.

The worms typically inhabit the cecum where they burrow into the mucosa, but they can live anywhere in the colon, appendix, or lower ileum (376). Mechanical injury caused by the adult worms induces atrophy, degeneration, and intestinal necrosis (374,375). If the worms obstruct the mouths of the crypts, they become dilated, containing mucus, fibrin, and acute inflammatory cells. Moderate to severe infections associate with subepithelial hemorrhage and inflammation consisting of lymphocytes, eosinophils, and plasma cells.

NEUTROPENIC ENTEROCOLITIS (TYPHLITIS)

Neutropenic enterocolitis, also known as typhlitis, agranulocytic colitis, neutropenic enteropathy, and ileocecal syndrome,

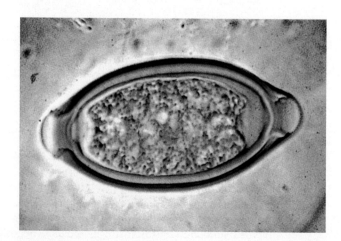

FIG. 13.133. The egg of *Trichuris trichuria* is found in the stool. It is typically bile stained and barrel shaped, with distinctive polar prominences. (Courtesy of Dickson Despomier, Ph.D., Department of Parasitology, Columbia University, New York, NY.)

traditionally affects children treated for leukemia and other conditions. It may complicate chemotherapy for solid tumors (377). However, the disorder also affects healthier, nonterminal, neutropenic children and adults with solid tumors and other conditions including AIDS. The incidence of neutropenic colitis is increasing, particularly in patients with acute myelogenous leukemia undergoing high-dose cytosine arabinoside chemotherapy. Although direct mucosal cytotoxicity from cytotoxic drugs may contribute to the disorder, it is not a prerequisite for neutropenic enterocolitis to occur.

Most patients are profoundly granulocytopenic, with their neutrophil count measuring <500 to 1,000 cells/mm^3. Patients are typically neutropenic for at least a week before symptom onset (378). Patients usually present with a dramatic onset of fever, watery or bloody diarrhea, right abdominal quadrant pain, abdominal distention, rebound tenderness, nausea, and vomiting (378). The presence of fever, rigors, and shock suggest the development of sepsis or colonic perforation. The disorder is often fatal unless aggressively treated, usually with resection of the involved bowel segment. Mortality rates range between 5% and 100% and average 40% to 50%. Death results from cecal perforation, bowel necrosis, and sepsis.

The pathogenesis of the syndrome is illustrated in Figure 13.134. The chemotherapy damages the GI mucosa by destroying the rapidly dividing epithelium. Alternatively, mucosal neoplastic infiltrates may cause breaks in the mucosal barrier. Loss of mucosal integrity coupled with the neutropenia allows bacteria to invade the bowel wall and sepsis to develop. In children, the infections usually result from *Pseudomonas* or *E. coli*, whereas in adults *C. septicum* is the most common infecting organism. Ischemia also plays a role in the genesis of the lesion. The ischemia likely results from vascular invasion by bacteria or the production of bacterial toxins followed by the development of a disseminated intravascular coagulopathy. One often sees small thrombi within the mucosal and submucosal capillaries. Other causes of ischemia include perivascular neoplastic infiltrates, episodes of hypotension following sepsis, or mucosal hemorrhage complicating severe thrombocytopenia or the presence of angioinvasive fungi. The process preferentially involves the cecum due to the luminal stasis that occurs at this site. The relatively poor vascular supply of the cecum further predisposes to ischemic injury. Rarely, other bowel segments become involved.

The gross features of neutropenic enterocolitis vary due to the influence of its multiple etiologic factors. The changes range from mucosal erythema and localized areas of hemorrhagic necrosis with moderate degrees of edema to severe transmural edema and diffuse transmural hemorrhagic necrosis (Figs. 13.135 and 13.136). Usually, the bowel appears markedly thickened, edematous, and dusky, with scattered serosal ecchymoses (Fig. 13.135). The mucosa often appears beefy red, eroded, and ulcerated. Pseudomembranes develop. The edema gives the bowel wall a boggy or myxoid appearance. The submucosal edema is so severe that fluid oozes from the cut surfaces of the specimen. When the process is transmural, perforation may occur.

A severe necrotizing colitis is present with marked transmural submucosal edema, vasculitis, stromal hemorrhage, and patchy to complete epithelial necrosis (Figs. 13.136 to 13.138). Degenerated epithelial cells detach from the basement membrane and lie within dilated glandular lumens. This process starts superficially (Fig. 13.137) and progressively involves the remainder of the crypt, frequently reaching its base (Fig. 13.138) and producing the glandular

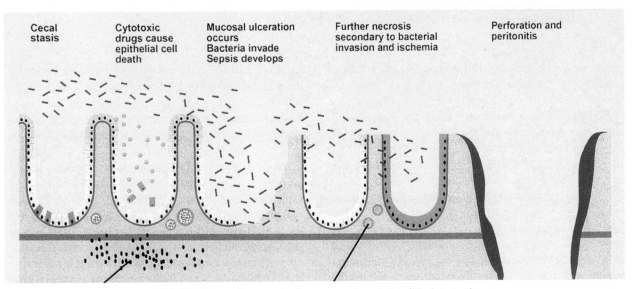

FIG. 13.134. Pathogenesis of neutropenic enterocolitis (see text).

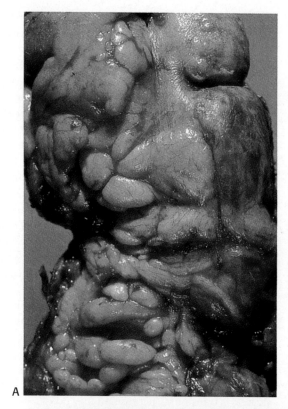

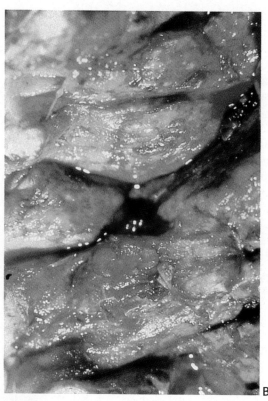

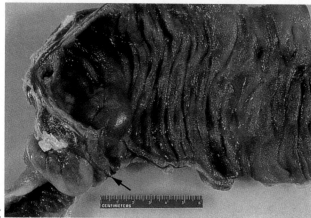

FIG. 13.135. Gross appearance of neutropenic enterocolitis. A and B are from the same specimen. **A:** A dilated bowel with an erythematous serosal surface. Early adhesions are beginning to form. **B:** Opened specimen showing a boggy mucosa without ulceration due to marked submucosal edema. **C:** Another specimen that has much more mucosal erythema. The ileocecal valve bulges into the cecal lumen. The marked submucosal edema can be seen where the bowel wall is cut in cross section (*arrow*).

dropout typical of ischemia. The mucosa becomes variably ulcerated and a pseudomembrane containing fibrin and necrotic cellular debris covers the luminal surface (Fig. 13.137). In severe cases, the bowel exhibits transmural necrosis and degeneration of the muscularis propria. Vascular damage produces subtle or profuse intramural and intraluminal hemorrhage, and fibrin thrombi are often present in the submucosal vessels. Additionally, changes characteristic of chemotherapeutic injury (Fig. 13.137), including prominent apoptosis in the crypts, focal crypt dropout, and glandular regeneration, are often present. Numerous bacteria often are present in the pseudomembrane overlying the damaged epithelium. One may also occasionally see bacteria invading the mucosa and submucosa or lying within macrophages or the interstitial spaces (Fig. 13.138). One may

also find evidence of the pre-existing neoplastic condition in the form of leukemic infiltrates within the bowel wall. There is a striking paucity of inflammation, given the degree of mucosal damage, and neutrophils are absent. *The absence of neutrophils in the face of significant cell injury allows one to make the diagnosis of neutropenic enterocolitis.* Patients may develop secondary infections that may complicate the histologic pattern. These most commonly are *Candida* or CMV infections.

The histologic features overlap with *C. difficile*–associated pseudomembranous colitis. However, *C. difficile*–associated pseudomembranous colitis has large numbers of neutrophils present in the exudate, while patients with neutropenic enterocolitis lack a neutrophilic infiltrate. The features also overlap with ischemic enterocolitis and infectious enterocolitis,

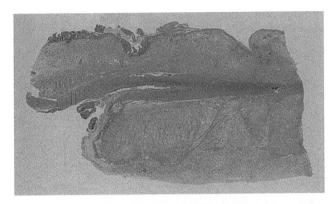

FIG. 13.136. Neutropenic enterocolitis. Whole mount section showing the marked submucosal and subserosal edema. The muscularis propria is the eosinophilic band that has somewhat of a V shape between the two lighter areas. The mucosa is variably ulcerated.

but the absolute lack of neutrophilic infiltrates only occurs in ischemia prior to reperfusion injury and neutropenic enterocolitis.

PHLEGMONOUS COLITIS

Phlegmonous colitis is a very rare disorder that presents as submucosal cellulitis. It is rarer than its gastric counterpart, discussed in Chapter 4 (379). The bowel appears thickened and congested with submucosal edema and expansion. The mucosa is intact but the folds are thickened due to the submucosal edema. An intense neutrophilic infiltrate is present in the submucosa, which variably spreads into the muscularis propria. It associates with various bacterial infections, but often an organism is not identified.

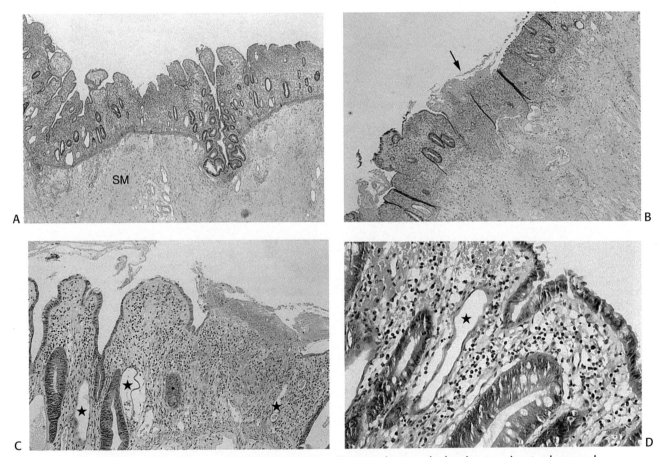

FIG. 13.137. Neutropenic enterocolitis. **A:** Low-magnification photograph showing prominent submucosal edema (*SM*). The mucosa is also edematous, but not as severely as the submucosa. There appear to be dilated vessels in the mucosa, but these in fact represent attenuated crypts. The surface is variably ulcerated. **B:** Portion of mucosa with focal ulceration and a densely adherent pseudomembrane (*arrow*). The pseudomembrane appears slightly basophilic due to the presence of numerous bacteria. The lamina propria underlying this is congested. **C:** Higher magnification showing the submucosal edema and focal erosions. The glands in the mucosa appear hyperchromatic or attenuated. Some crypts have died and are lined by flattened, atrophic cells (*stars*). Other crypts appear regenerative. **D:** Higher magnification showing an atrophic crypt (*star*) among several regenerating crypts. Note the absence of acute inflammation in all of the figures.

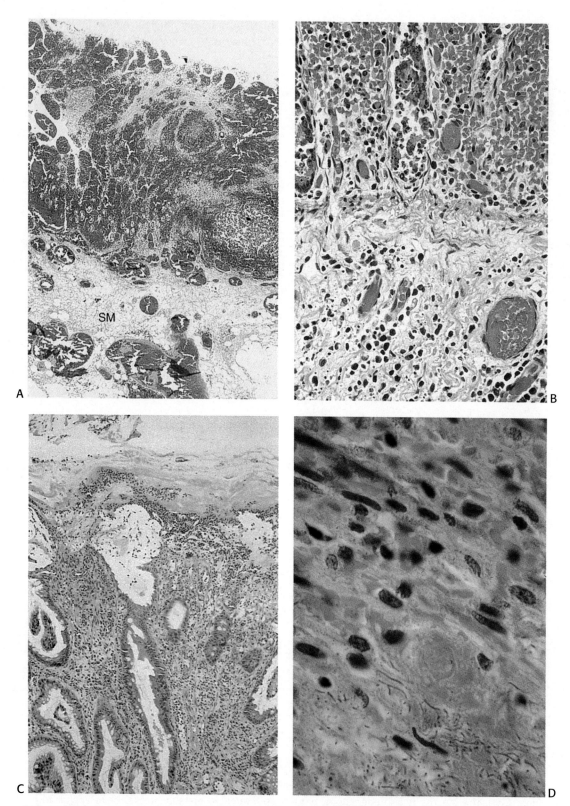

FIG. 13.138. Neutropenic enterocolitis. This case differs from that shown in Figure 13.137 by having a much more hemorrhagic mucosa. **A:** The submucosa (*SM*) is congested and the vessels are markedly dilated. **B:** Higher magnification showing marked hemorrhagic necrosis and several residual crypt bases. Vascular congestion is also present. These changes are consistent with ischemic damage that occurs in neutropenic enterocolitis. Note the absence of neutrophils. **C:** Another area of a third specimen showing early damage of the superficial portion of the crypt. The changes mimic those seen in *Clostridium difficile* colitis. **D:** Numerous bacteria are present in the tissues. They are also present in a capillary. No neutrophils are present.

MICROSCOPIC COLITIS

General Comments

Some patients with chronic idiopathic diarrhea have histologic evidence of colitis even though their colons appear normal by barium enema and by colonoscopy; such patients have the entity known as microscopic colitis (380). The term *microscopic colitis* has been used to include several distinct but probably related diseases, including collagenous colitis and lymphocytic colitis, although more accurately it is lymphocytic colitis that has been traditionally called microscopic colitis. The term microscopic colitis has also been used more broadly to include the finding of colitis in the absence of endoscopic abnormalities. As a result, the diagnosis could include IBD, especially Crohn disease and eosinophilic colitis and potentially other mild forms of colitis. This leads to confusion and we prefer to not make a diagnosis of microscopic colitis but to use more specific diagnoses of either lymphocytic colitis or collagenous colitis since these entities are well characterized.

Reports showing a progression of lymphocytic colitis to collagenous colitis have led to the suggestion that the formation of the subepithelial collagen band develops at a later stage in the disease process as a result of continued inflammation and subsequent fibrosis and that the two disorders are variations of the same disease (381).

Since patients with lymphocytic and collagenous colitis present with a history of watery, nonbloody, persistent or intermittent diarrhea, often lasting several years, it is reasonable to consider these two disorders as part of the watery diarrhea–colitis syndrome (WDCS), a distinct form of chronic colitis (382).

It is likely that similar immune abnormalities affect both groups of patients. They both have a significant increase in mean numbers of intraepithelial lymphocytes (IELs) with significantly more CD8+ than CD4+ IELs. Most IELs bear the TCR$\alpha\beta$; TCR$\gamma\delta$–bearing cells are not increased. CD4+ helper T cells predominate in the lamina propria. The colonic epithelium abnormally expresses human leukocyte antigen (HLA)-DR antigens. These findings suggest that a major histocompatibility complex (MHC)-restricted immune mechanism can be involved in the pathogenesis of both diseases (383). There is also an association with various gastrointestinal and autoimmune disorders. Two associations are particularly prominent: Degenerative osteoarticular disease and celiac disease (381,384,385). There are also reports of patients with these diseases who subsequently develop either autoimmune thyroid diseases, ulcerative colitis or Crohn disease (386), primary biliary cirrhosis, and the CREST syndrome (387). Lymphocytic colitis is more common than collagenous colitis in patients who develop Crohn disease (388). A family has been reported in which different family members had ulcerative colitis, Crohn disease, and collagenous colitis (389).

There is also a relationship between both diseases and the uses of some drugs, especially aspirin, NSAIDs, ticlopidine, lansoprazole, and flutamide. There may also be a relationship with smoking (390). Overall, the natural history of both collagenous colitis and lymphocytic colitis is benign and in some patients the disease resolves spontaneously.

Collagenous Colitis

The diagnosis *collagenous colitis* describes patients who suffer from chronic, watery diarrhea and who have subluminal deposits of a collagenous ground substance beneath the surface epithelium at the lamina propria interface (391). The female-to-male ratio is 10:1, with an age range of 23 to 86 and a mean of 54 to 66 years (385). The incidence of the disease in individuals who suffer from chronic diarrhea ranges from 0.3% to 5%. The incidence is reported to be about 16 cases per 100,000 population (384). The disorder sometimes affects children (392) and families (393).

Postulated etiologies include immune dysregulation leading to colonic inflammation, abnormalities in collagen synthesis, abnormalities in the pericryptal myofibroblasts, mast cell or eosinophil abnormalities, "plasmatic vasculosus," drugs, and bacterial toxins (394–399). Plasmacytic vasculosus is a theory that proposed leakage of plasma proteins and fibrinogen through the subepithelial capillary walls and their subsequent replacement by collagen. Surface epithelial damage appears to cause the secretory diarrhea, whereas the thickened subepithelial collagen table appears to represent a variable response to the surface damage. The injury may result from bile acid malabsorption (400), mast cell infiltrates (395), prostaglandin effects (401), or drug exposures. A significant percentage of patients with collagenous colitis have a history of using NSAIDs or antibiotics (402). *Yersinia* infections may also trigger the development of collagenous colitis (403).

The symptoms vary in duration and intensity and long periods of remission have been described. Symptoms include watery, nonbloody diarrhea with up to 20 stools per day. The diarrhea can last for months or decades. Colicky abdominal pain occurs frequently. Nausea, vomiting, flatulence, incontinence, and weight loss vary in frequency. Patients may also present with protein-losing enteropathy (404). Rarely, collagenous colitis associates with chronic constipation (405) in the absence of watery diarrhea. The disorder typically involves the colon, although the small bowel and stomach may be involved, particularly in patients with celiac disease or other autoimmune disorders. Collagenous colitis exhibits spontaneous remissions and relapses; occasionally the disease resolves spontaneously (406,407). In some patients it resolves following treatment with drugs or by diverting the fecal stream.

The histologic hallmark of collagenous colitis is mucosal colonic inflammation associated with a broad, continuous, hypocellular, eosinophilic, linear, subepithelial, fibrous band immediately subjacent to the surface epithelium (Fig. 13.139). This collagen band measures 10 to 70 μm in thickness, with a mean of 12 to 30 μm (408), and it surrounds subluminal capillaries and myofibroblasts. A thickness of at least 30 mm provides the greatest consistency in establishing the diagnosis (409). There is little if any extension of the thickened collagen

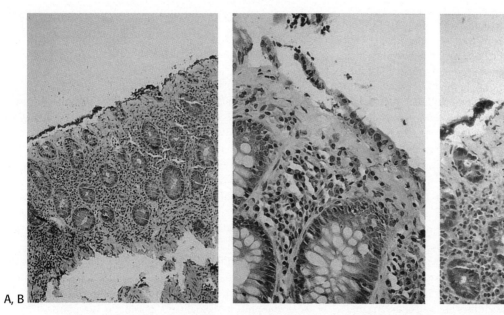

A, B   C

FIG. 13.139. Collagenous colitis. **A:** A dense, irregular, eosinophilic band lies below the luminal surface. **B:** Higher magnification showing the acellular dense band underneath an epithelium that is beginning to lift off the surface. **C:** The subepithelial band is relatively inhomogeneous and there is chronic inflammation in the lamina propria.

table around the crypts, except in cases demonstrating marked intercryptal subepithelial thickening. In addition to its thickness, the relative inhomogeneity and irregularity of the collagen layer at its lower borders helps distinguish it from the normal subepithelial basement membrane (Figs. 13.139 and 13.140). The thickened subepithelial layer stains light pink with PAS and green with Masson trichrome stains. Congo red stains are negative. The thickened collagen table predomi-

nantly contains collagen IV and tenascin (410–412). Plasma cells, mast cells, and multinucleated giant cells may be underneath, or embedded within, the thickened collagen table. The changes are most marked in the proximal colon and the distal bowel may be spared. In one study biopsies from the transverse colon were more likely to be diagnostic of the disorder than biopsies from the rectosigmoid or right colon (409). The lesion is often continuous, but it may also exhibit a patchy

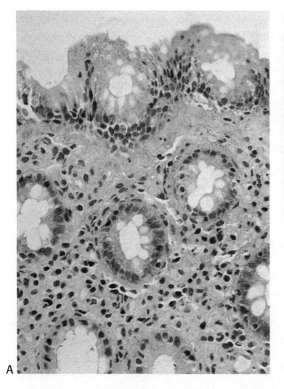

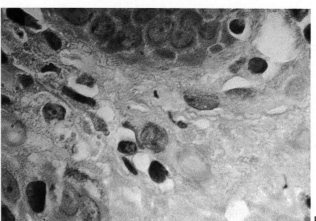

A   B

FIG. 13.140. Collagenous colitis. **A:** Medium magnification showing the band underlying the surface epithelium. **B:** High magnification demonstrating the presence of numerous cells within this thickened band (A, B: trichrome stain).

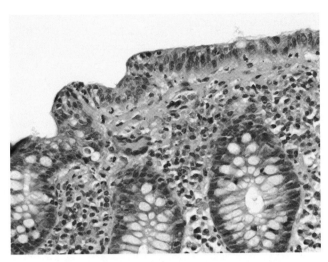

FIG. 13.141. Collagenous colitis with subluminal giant cell.

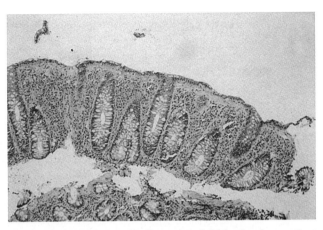

FIG. 13.142. Subluminal collagen band thickening in a patient with diverticulosis. The changes mimic those seen in collagenous colitis except for the fact that there is a branched crypt. Regenerative features should not be present in collagenous colitis.

distribution, particularly early in the disease course or as it resolves (413,414). As the disease is treated, the basement membrane thickening disappears (407).

The diagnosis of collagenous colitis not only requires a thickened collagen table, but also the presence of changes characteristic of colitis, including epithelial damage and intraepithelial lymphocytosis. Damaged epithelial cells appear flattened, mucin depleted, vacuolated, and irregularly oriented. Focally, small strips of interglandular surface epithelium lift off their basement membrane and a subepithelial cleft filled with neutrophils and eosinophils forms. Rarely, subepithelial multinucleated giant cells are present (Fig. 13.141) (415,416). Epithelial nuclei may appear slightly enlarged and minimally pseudostratified, but mitotic figures are not prominent. The glands sometimes appear slightly more basophilic than normal due to mild regeneration. Paneth cell metaplasia, which is usually a marker of IBD, may occasionally be seen and may predict the severity of the disease (385). In one study Paneth cell metaplasia was present in up to 44% of biopsies from patients with collagenous colitis (417). Pseudomembranes have also been described in collagenous colitis (402).

The intraepithelial lymphocytosis in collagenous colitis is not as dramatic as that seen in lymphocytic colitis (382). IELs are seen in the colon and may also be present in the terminal ileum (418). Focally, the superficial lamina propria contains slightly to moderately increased numbers of lymphocytes, plasma cells, and mast cells admixed with variable numbers of eosinophils and neutrophils. Eosinophils can be focally prominent and degranulating (396). The subepithelial tissues may show prominent vascularity. Neutrophilic cryptitis is often focally present (381), perhaps reflecting the exposure to NSAIDs or other drugs. The mucosal thickness remains normal and the glandular architecture is maintained without crypt elongation, atrophy, irregularity, or branching.

Patients with collagenous colitis may also have collagenous gastritis (419) and/or collagenous duodenitis or enteritis (420). We recently encountered a patient with extensive subepithelial collagen deposits throughout the gastrointestinal tract without evidence of celiac disease and NSAID or other drug use in whom there was no obvious etiology for the extensive changes that were present. The patient became extremely malnourished and eventually required total parenteral nutritional support.

Subepithelial collagen thickening occurs in various diseases, so that one must make the diagnosis of collagenous colitis in the proper clinical and histologic settings (421). Tangential sectioning of normal colon results in artifactually thickened basement membranes and such cases can be wrongly interpreted as collagenous colitis. If biopsies lack the characteristic inflammation, a thick basement membrane should be ignored. The differential diagnosis of collagenous colitis also includes lymphocytic colitis, UC, ischemic colitis, radiation colitis, amyloidosis, progressive systemic sclerosis and infectious colitis, colonic mucosal prolapse syndrome, fecal stream diversion, and diverticular disease (Fig. 13.142). Biopsies with increased subepithelial collagen deposits from patients without microscopic colitis generally come from the rectum or rectosigmoid. Features that distinguish the diseases that mimic collagenous colitis are listed in Table 13.22.

Patients may spontaneously recover from their disease or they may require treatment with antidiarrheal agents or even steroids. Mesalazine and budesonide are effective treatments for the disease and the drugs are well tolerated (422). However, there is a high risk of relapse after stopping 8 weeks of treatment (423). Patients who appear to have NSAID-related collagenous colitis or those with increased inflammation in the lamina propria tend to require steroids to treat the disease (424).

Lymphocytic Colitis

Lymphocytic colitis typically presents in elderly patients with chronic diarrhea. Patients with lymphocytic colitis exhibit a more variable age range than those with collagenous colitis; it occurs at all ages and it may be a more heterogeneous disease than collagenous colitis. The disorder affects both men and

TABLE 13.22 Distinguishing Characteristics of Diseases that May Mimic Collagenous Colitis on Biopsy

Collagenous colitis	Subluminal collagen thickening; intraepithelial lymphocytosis; inflammation in upper mucosa
Ulcerative colitis	Diffuse continuous process with numerous crypt abscesses, cryptitis, glandular destruction, and signs of chronicity; no subluminal collagen thickening
Radiation colitis	Mucosal telangiectasia, submucosal vascular changes, atypical fibroblasts, fibrosis
Infectious colitis	Diffuse lamina propria inflammation, significant neutrophils in lamina propria; usually no subluminal collagen thickening
Mucosal prolapse syndrome	Glandular distortion, mucosal ulceration, mucosal hyperplasia, mucosal fibrosis, perpendicular smooth muscle fibers in lamina propria
Ischemic colitis	Coagulative necrosis, fibrin thrombi, architectural distortion if disease chronic, mucosal fibrosis, glandular dropout
Amyloidosis	Perivascular, muscular, or lamina propria eosinophilic deposits; positivity with Congo red stains
Progressive systemic sclerosis	Fibrosis along all basement membranes, including crypts
Diverticulosis	Chronic inflammation, thickened basement membranes
Diversion colitis	Prominent nodular lymphoid hyperplasia, ulceration, acute inflammation, aphthous ulcers, cryptitis

women almost equally (390,425). In one study the incidence of lymphocytic colitis was three times higher than that of collagenous colitis (426). Patients with lymphocytic colitis present with chronic watery diarrhea that can be intermittent or continuous, ranging in duration from 2 months to 25 years. The watery diarrhea results from markedly decreased water absorption (425). Related symptoms may include mild crampy abdominal pain, moderate weight loss, and an essentially normal physical examination (382). Up to one third of patients with celiac disease have lymphocytic colitis (427). An association also exists between lymphocytic colitis and tropical sprue (428) and collagenous gastritis or enterocolic lymphocytic phlebitis (429) as well as with various autoimmune diseases. These include rheumatoid arthritis, sicca syndrome, uveitis, idiopathic pulmonary fibrosis, diabetes, pernicious anemia, autoimmune thyroid disease (430), and idiopathic thrombocytopenic purpura (384). Some patients have increased antinuclear antibodies, antiparietal cell antibodies, and antimicrosomal titers. Lymphocytic colitis patients have an increased frequency of HLA A1 and a decreased frequency of HLA A3 compared to control populations (402). There is also an association with the use of some drugs including NSAIDs, ranitidine, flutamide, Cyclo-FORT, gold salts, bentazepam and ticlopidine, carbamazepine, cimetidine, simvastin, and vinburnine (385,426,431,432). In addition, some patients develop lymphocytic colitis following infections. The lymphocytic colitis in such patients may represent either a resolving bacterial or viral infection or a persistent immune response following the infection.

The most distinctive feature of lymphocytic colitis is the presence of increased intraepithelial lymphocytes, particularly at the luminal surface (Fig. 13.143). Significantly increased numbers of intraepithelial cytotoxic T lymphocytes populate the surface epithelium (433). To be of diagnostic significance, the increased lymphocytes must number at least 15 per 100 epithelial cells (434). This threshold compares an average of 4 to 5 lymphocytes per 100 epithelial cells in the normal colon, inflammatory bowel disease, and infectious colitis (425); a mean of 8.4 in patients with celiac disease without colonic epithelial lymphocytosis; and a mean of 25 to 32.4 in patients with lymphocytic colitis without concurrent celiac disease. Sometimes the lymphocytes stack up in a vertical array between the enterocytes. Increased IELs may also be seen in the terminal ileum (418). The lamina propria contains increased numbers of lymphocytes, eosinophils, or neutrophils, although the lamina propria inflammation tends to be less than that seen in collagenous colitis and there tend to be few numbers of eosinophils. Occasionally, subepithelial multinucleated giant cells are present (415). Paneth cell metaplasia and an increased number of mast cells can also be seen. Goblet cell mucin may be reduced. Other prominent features include surface epithelial damage with cellular loss and epithelial detachment, infiltration of the surface epithelium with eosinophils and neutrophils, and minimal crypt distortion or active cryptitis (425). Increased apoptosis may be present in some patients. The increased number of eosinophils and apoptotic activity may warrant questioning the patient concerning drug use so that one can determine if the changes disappear following drug cessation. Unlike collagenous colitis, the histologic features of lymphocytic colitis are usually uniform throughout the large bowel.

Increased intraepithelial lymphocytes are common to several diseases (Table 13.23), but when diffusely present they are more likely to be associated with lymphocytic colitis. Focal lesions, sometimes taking the form of lymphoid aggregates, are more likely to be seen associated with polyps,

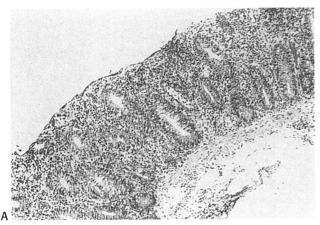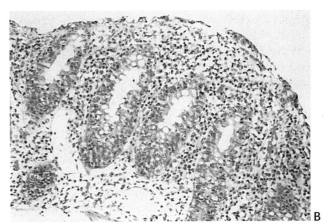

FIG. 13.143. Lymphocytic colitis. **A:** The photograph shows a hypercellular colonic biopsy. The hypercellularity is due to a lymphocytic infiltrate in the lamina propria and the epithelium. There is no architectural distortion. **B:** Higher magnification showing the intraepithelial lymphocytosis and the infiltration of the lamina propria by lymphocytes.

diverticula, or Crohn disease (433). Intraepithelial lymphocytosis may also be encountered in proximal biopsies of patients with ulcerative colitis and distally in patients with Crohn disease (91).

Atypical Lymphocytic Colitis

Lymphocytic colitis consists of the classic triad of nonbloody watery diarrhea, normal endoscopic features, and colonic epithelial lymphocytosis. Recently a group of patients has been recognized as having atypical lymphocytic colitis. These patients have the classic histologic features but they lack either the appropriate clinical or endoscopic findings (434). The patients may present with constipation rather than diarrhea, as well as hematochezia, or have macroscopic evidence of colitis at endoscopy. The histologic abnormality may also be an incidental finding. Thus, atypical lymphocytic colitis appears to be a heterogeneous group of diseases and includes patients with idiopathic constipation, coexisting lymphocytic colitis, IBD, or possibly infectious colitis (434).

Some patients who have what appears to be focal lymphocytic colitis subsequently develop Crohn disease. However, endoscopic abnormalities are present and there are moderate numbers of neutrophils in the tissue alerting one to the possibility that the disease is not lymphocytic colitis but Crohn disease (388).

TABLE 13.23 Large Intestinal Disorders Associated with Increased Intraepithelial Lymphocytes

Lymphocytic colitis
Collagenous colitis
Gluten-sensitive enteropathy
Brainerd diarrhea
Inflammatory bowel disease
Graft vs. host disease
AIDS enteropathy

Large Intestinal Changes in Celiac Disease

Patients with celiac disease may show histologic abnormalities in the rectal mucosa. These consist of increased populations of mucosal plasma cells, lymphocytes, and mast cells, especially in untreated patients or in patients rechallenged with gluten. CD3+ lymphocytes and activated CD25 lymphocytes expressing IL-2 receptors increase in the lamina propria, usually subjacent to the basal lamina. CD8+ IELs are also present. The inflammatory cells disappear (except for the mast cells) on dietary gluten restriction. The absence of neutrophils suggests that the lesion is not a conventional inflammatory-type proctitis but one induced by the gluten in the fecal stream and represents a cell-mediated form of response (435).

The changes in celiac disease may be identical to those seen in lymphocytic colitis. However, the colonic mucosa in patients with untreated celiac disease tends to lack surface epithelial abnormalities and an increased cellularity of the lamina propria, and there is lack of watery diarrhea when gluten is removed from the diet. In contrast, patients with refractory celiac disease may show colonic abnormalities indistinguishable from lymphocytic colitis. However, there may be differences in the number of CD8+ IELs in the two diseases, with more being present in lymphocytic colitis. (436).

Brainerd Diarrhea

The term *Brainerd diarrhea* is applied to the syndrome of chronic watery diarrhea characterized by abrupt onset, marked urgency to defecate, frequent fecal incontinence, abdominal cramps, weight loss, and fatigue in the absence of other systemic symptoms. The diarrhea typically lasts from 1 month to 3 years with a median duration of about 16 months (437–441). Most cases occur among patient cohorts following epidemic exposures to an unknown agent. The disease was named after Brainerd, Minnesota, where more than 100 residents developed watery diarrhea after drinking unpasteurized milk from a local dairy.

Colonic biopsies reveal surface epithelial lymphocytosis without mucosal architectural distortion, surface degenerative changes, or thickened subepithelial collagen. There is usually not an increase in the mononuclear cells of the lamina propria. The degree of surface epithelial lymphocytosis is greater than that seen in control specimens, similar to that seen in collagenous colitis, and less than that seen in lymphocytic colitis. Acute focal colitis similar to that seen in acute infectious colitis may also be seen in addition to the epithelial lymphocytosis (437). The disorder can only be diagnosed in conjunction with epidemiologic data that indicate that the patient is part of an epidemic colitis with a common point source.

LESIONS ASSOCIATED WITH INCREASED NUMBERS OF EOSINOPHILS

Occasionally one encounters biopsies in which the most striking change is a marked increase in the number of eosinophils. Their presence can suggest a drug or allergic reaction (Fig. 13.144) (442,443) or the presence of a parasitic infection. However, in the colon they also commonly associate with chronic disorders. The number of lamina propria eosinophils varies significantly, differing by a factor of 40 in different regions of the country (444). Their numbers may also differ seasonally. In children, the cecum and appendix appear to have the highest concentrations of eosinophils in comparison with the distal intestine.

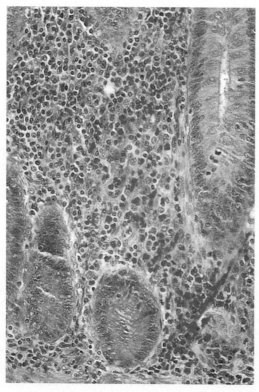

FIG. 13.144. Allergic enteritis. The lamina propria of this portion of the colon is intensely infiltrated by eosinophils.

Food Allergies

Up to 45% of the population report adverse reactions to food (445). The incidence appears to be increasing, although this may reflect increased patient and physician reporting of allergic symptoms (446). Food sensitivity occurs particularly commonly in infants and young children. Definitive diagnosis of a food allergy requires the demonstration of an unequivocal clinical reaction after a controlled food challenge and elimination of the symptom complex subsequent to removal of the offending food.

The increased susceptibility of young infants to food allergic reactions results from their general immunologic immaturity and the overall immaturity of their gastrointestinal tracts (447,448). The majority of allergic reactions to food are IgE-mediated, mast cell–dependent, immediate hypersensitivity-type reactions. The interaction of an antigen with an antibody or immunocyte triggers the allergic reaction. It is mediated by soluble factors from activated neutrophils, mast cells, and macrophages, or by direct membrane interactions between immune cells and antigens on their cell surfaces. Cytokine and inflammatory mediators are released that act directly on the epithelium, endothelium, or muscle, or indirectly through nerves and mesenchymal cells. The immediate consequences of these mediators include a local change in vascular permeability, stimulation of mucus production, increased muscle contraction, stimulation of pain fibers, recruitment of inflammatory cells, edema of mucosal epithelial villi, increased protein loss from the gut, and increased absorption of foreign antigens. Also, as a result, eosinophils, lymphocytes, and monocytes are attracted to the reaction site, where they release additional inflammatory mediators and cytokines. Repeated ingestion of an allergen stimulates mononuclear cells to secrete histamine-releasing factors, some of which interact with IgE molecules bound to basophils and mast cell surfaces (449). If significant mast cell degranulation occurs, mast cell mediators may provoke potentially fatal systemic anaphylaxis.

Cow's Milk and Soy Intolerance

A common form of allergic colitis is cow's milk and soy formula intolerance (450). It may also develop in breastfed infants, probably as the result of transfer of potentially immunogenic substances (especially cow-milk–derived β-lactoglobulin) from the maternal diet into the breast milk (451). Food allergy, whether IgE or non-IgE mediated, affects males and females equally and at any age, but occurs more often in infants and young children with a prevalence of 0.5% to 3%. Allergic proctitis commonly affects young infants who present with rectal bleeding, with or without associated diarrhea (452). Common symptoms include vomiting, pain, weight loss, an allergic history, anemia, and peripheral eosinophilia. Patients may also present with constipation (453).

The fact that food hypersensitivity reactions occur more commonly in the pediatric population and tend to decrease in incidence with increasing age suggests that immaturity of the intestinal barrier function, immaturity of the mucosal immune system, or both are important in the pathogenesis of the disorder (454,455). This is supported by the fact that as the infants age, the allergy disappears due to the development of IgG antibodies, which prevent the allergic reaction.

The degranulating eosinophils release a number of biologically active mediators, including major basic protein, eosinophil-derived neurotoxin, eosinophilic cationic protein, and eosinophilic peroxidase, all of which may be cytotoxic and lead to epithelial injury. They also produce platelet-activating factor, a substance shown to cause intestinal injury in experimental animals (456). The eosinophils have surface receptors for complement components and leukotrienes. Eosinophils also express surface receptors for IgG and a low affinity receptor for IgE and IgA (457). The fact that eosinophils can bind IgA and then degranulate is important because the gut is the major site of IgA production.

Allergic colitis involves any colonic segment, but the rectosigmoid is preferentially affected (458,459). Endoscopic features include focal erythema, a friable-appearing mucosa, and increased mucosal nodularity suggestive of lymphoid hyperplasia. Zones of entirely normal mucosa separate the abnormal areas. Severe cases may show decreased mucosal vascularity, multiple superficial aphthous erosions, or ulcers covered by a surface exudate.

Histologically, one sees increased numbers of eosinophils populating the lamina propria, epithelium, and muscularis mucosae (Fig. 13.144). A particularly characteristic feature is the presence of large numbers of eosinophils in the lamina propria (>60 eosinophils/10 high-powered field [hpf]), as well as numerous intact or degranulated eosinophils located in the base of the mucosa and interspersed among muscle fibers of the muscularis mucosae (450,458,459). The eosinophils are the major cell type in cryptitis and crypt abscesses (Fig. 13.145). Often the eosinophilic aggregates closely associate with lymphoid nodules. The intensity of the eosinophilic infiltrates varies, not only between biopsies at

different sites but within individual biopsy specimens. Although the eosinophils are thought to mediate the injury, no significant correlation exists between the number of mucosal eosinophils, patient age, illness duration, endoscopic appearance, or type of inciting formula.

The overall mucosal architecture is maintained in allergic proctocolitis without histologic features of chronicity, such as distorted, branched, or atrophic crypts; Paneth cell metaplasia; basally located lymphoid aggregates; or diffuse plasmacytosis. The eosinophilia represents an excellent marker for infantile allergic proctocolitis, but given the focal distribution of the lesion, multiple mucosal biopsy specimens must be obtained, and several levels of each should be examined (450,458,459).

Recognition of the disease is important because pediatric patients with allergic proctitis generally respond promptly to dietary changes.

Eosinophilic Gastroenteritis

Eosinophilic gastroenteritis tends to affect older children and young adults, and predominantly involves the proximal gut, especially the esophagus, stomach, and small intestine. The colon is one of the least commonly affected sites (450). Rare patients with colonic disease also have biliary tract involvement (460). Symptoms include diarrhea, rectal bleeding, abdominal pain, and fever. Barium enema and colonoscopy disclose changes indistinguishable from CD, usually confined to the right colon. Some patients also have coexisting IBD and/or cholangitis (460). Histologically, the mucosa, submucosa, or muscularis propria is infiltrated by eosinophils (Fig. 13.146). Eosinophilic gastroenteritis is discussed in detail in Chapter 6.

Pericryptal Eosinophilic Enterocolitis

Some patients who present with chronic watery diarrhea have connective tissue diseases and eosinophilic infiltrates around the intestinal crypts. The infiltrates localize to the deep mucosa,

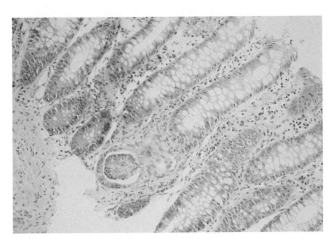

FIG. 13.145. Eosinophilic colitis. A crypt abscess is present that consists almost entirely of eosinophils. There are also increased numbers of eosinophils in the lamina propria.

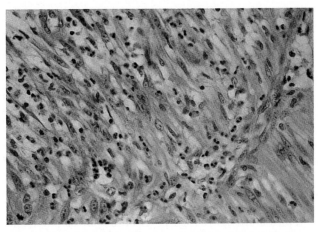

FIG. 13.146. Eosinophilic gastroenteritis. The photograph shows an intense infiltration of the muscularis propria by eosinophils.

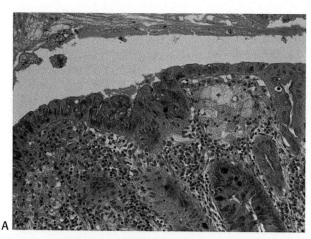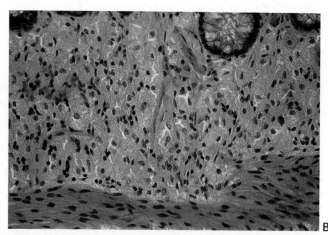

FIG. 13.147. Mucosal histiocytic infiltrates. **A:** Superficial cluster of pale histiocytic cells lies under the free surface. **B:** A group of histiocytic cells separates the base of the glands from the muscularis mucosae.

separating the crypt bases from the muscularis mucosae and penetrating into the superficial submucosa. Patients with these findings exhibit chronic diarrhea that resolves with steroid therapy (461). The patients lack gross structural abnormalities.

"Eosinophilic Colitis"

We make a diagnosis of eosinophilic colitis if we see eosinophils infiltrating the crypts or if there are focal collections of 10 or more eosinophils per hpf, in the absence of other identifiable abnormalities such as collagenous colitis, lymphocytic colitis, IBD, infection, diverticular disease, or neoplasia. We make an effort to determine if these changes occur alone or, more importantly, if there are associated increased apoptoses in the crypt bases. If these are present then we interpret the changes as most likely representing a drug reaction. In some cases, the patients will eventually be diagnosed with Crohn disease. However, in other patients the cause of the changes is never determined. It is our anecdotal experience that we make this diagnosis more often when the general public is suffering from bouts of hay fever or other seasonal allergies.

DISORDERS ASSOCIATED WITH GRANULOMAS AND MACROPHAGE COLLECTIONS

Granulomas and collections of macrophages complicate various gastrointestinal conditions, as extensively discussed in Chapter 6. Macrophage collections take the form of both compact caseating or noncaseating granulomas or they appear as diffuse infiltrates. Structures that can simulate macrophage collections or granulomas include germinal centers of the lymphoid follicles, cross sections of smooth muscle, or tangential cutting of the pericryptal myofibroblast sheath.

Small mucosal macrophage collections are common and represent a nonspecific reaction to low-grade injury. The macrophages contain foamy vacuoles or basophilic granules and they are usually scattered singly or in small clusters in

the upper or lower lamina propria (Fig. 13.147). The macrophages often stain with mucin stains (Fig. 13.148) and increase in number following mucosal injury. Small, loose collections of macrophages also lie in the lamina propria adjacent to sites of crypt rupture (*mucin granulomas*).

Occasional small granulomas can complicate almost any infection. Granulomas with central caseating necrosis constitute the histologic hallmark of tuberculosis or *Yersinia* infections (see Chapter 6). Well-formed granulomas occur in approximately 50% of cases of colonic CD (see Chapter 11) and their detection relates to the disease distribution. *Xanthogranulomas* and foreign body granulomas complicate the presence of foreign material, such as barium (Fig. 13.89), feces, talc, food, and sutures or reactions to the transmural inflammation associated with appendicitis or diverticulitis. Deep granulomatous lesions can involve the submucosa and contain foamy histiocytes and fibroblastic cells infiltrated by lymphocytes, plasma cells, and foreign material. These occur very commonly beneath invasive carcinomas (Fig. 13.149) or are associated with diverticulosis.

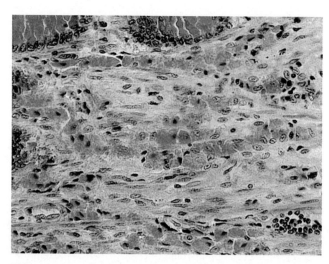

FIG. 13.148. Muciphages in the lamina propria stained with mucicarmine stain. These may be quite prominent, particularly in patients with previous mucosal injury.

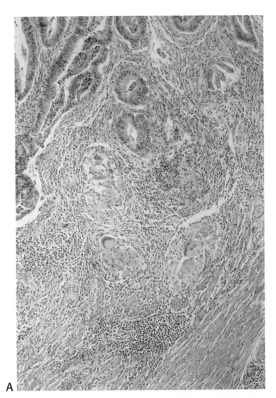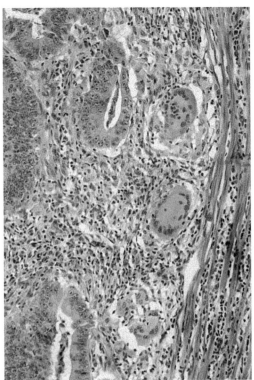

FIG. 13.149. Granulomas associated with carcinoma. **A:** A colonic carcinoma invades into the muscularis propria. Its invasive front is surrounded by an inflammatory response, which consists of granulomas and chronic inflammatory cells. **B:** Giant cells at higher magnification.

One also sees diffuse macrophage collections in *Mycobacterium avium-intracellulare* infections, Whipple disease, histoplasmosis, storage diseases, immunodeficiencies, and even algal infections. Another disorder characteristically associated with granulomatous inflammation is malakoplakia (see below).

Lamina Propria Muciphages

Muciphages, as first documented, are macrophages in the lamina propria that contain mucoproteins and are demonstrated by positive reaction with various mucin stains (462). They occur in up to 50% of rectal biopsies (462,463). These cells can be found throughout the colon in various situations and they reflect previous occult and clinically unimportant mucosal damage (463). Patients may present clinically with diarrhea, hematochezia, bowel habit change, constipation, hemorrhoids, and abdominal pain. Endoscopically, they present as nodules or polyps or they may be found incidentally (462,463). The mucosa may show regenerative or hyperplastic changes. In most cases the macrophages are located superficially (463). It may be prudent to stain for fungal or acid-fast organisms if the clinical situation warrants it.

Xanthomas

Xanthomas represent collections of PAS-positive macrophages confined to the mucosa or occupying a part of the bowel wall

(Fig. 13.150). Most commonly they are small mucosal aggregates of foamy cells lying in the upper lamina propria and resembling gastric xanthomas (see Chapter 4). However, we have seen cases in which there are extensive collections of foamy cells involving multiple areas of the colon and the mucosa and upper submucosa. The foamy cells contain lipid-like material and are mucicarmine negative. They more than likely represent a nonspecific response to a past injury.

Malakoplakia

Malakoplakia is a distinctive rare granulomatous disease that usually involves the urinary bladder. The colon is the most common site of extraurogenital involvement. Patients with colonic malakoplakia range in age from 6 weeks to 88 years and show an equal sex distribution (464,465). This disease is seldom diagnosed clinically. Rather, the diagnosis usually rests on pathologic examination of the tissues. The GI tract, particularly the large bowel, is the dominant site of involvement in children (465). Malakoplakia complicates various diseases (Table 13.24). Recently it has been found to complicate paracoccidiomycosis (318). Most patients are symptomatic. Adults present with rectal bleeding, diarrhea, and abdominal pain (465). Patients with extensive disease experience intractable diarrhea, bowel obstruction, ulcers, fistulae, and even death. Children present with fevers, failure to thrive, bloody diarrhea, and malnutrition. Endoscopically, gastrointestinal malakoplakia assumes three gross forms:

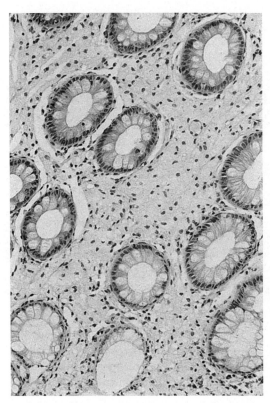

FIG. 13.150. Colonic xanthoma. The lamina propria is diffusely infiltrated with foamy histiocytes. The specimen was negative for acid-fast bacilli and fungi, and the patient had no history of a storage disease.

TABLE 13.24   **Diseases Associated with Colonic Malakoplakia**

Inflammatory bowel disease
Carcinomas
Villous adenomas
Lymphoreticular diseases
Neurofibromatosis
Immune deficiency
α-Chain disease
Miliary tuberculosis
Infection
   Tuberculosis
   Mycobacterium avium-intracellulare infection
   Klebsiella
   Escherichia coli

(a) unifocal lesions, (b) widespread mucosal multinodular lesions, and (c) large mass lesions. Surgical resection is usually curative in limited disease.

Malakoplakia results from an abnormal macrophagic response with defective bacterial degradation. This may result from an immunologic abnormality affecting cellular digestion, absence of the necessary lysosomal enzymes (466), or decreased levels of cyclic guanosine monophosphate (GMP) (467).

Grossly, colonic involvement is segmental or diffuse, with the rectosigmoid and cecum being the most commonly affected sites. Early lesions appear soft, flat, and yellowish tan (Fig. 13.151). Later, lesions become raised and tan-gray, with an irregular hyperemic margin and a central depressed area. Submucosal lesions secondarily elevate the mucosa into soft

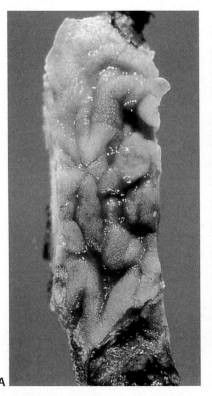

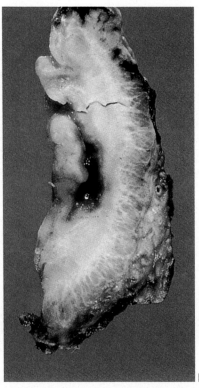

FIG. 13.151. Rectal malakoplakia. **A:** The specimen viewed en face shows a lumpy, bumpy mucosal surface. **B:** Cross section through the bowel wall shows the mucosa to the left and the serosa to the right. The process diffusely infiltrates the bowel wall.

A   B

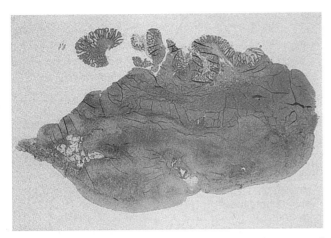

FIG. 13.152. Whole mount photograph showing the extent of the inflammation, which is primarily submucosal.

yellow-tan plaques or nodules. Often the overlying mucosa appears intact. Malakoplakia most frequently presents as one or more polypoid lesions ranging in size from 3 mm to 4 cm. Intestinal lesions extend deeply into the intestinal wall (Fig. 13.152) leading to perforation and fistula formation. The lesion may mimic tumors and/or associate with tumors.

The focal or diffuse multinodular masses consist of numerous granular cells with eosinophilic cytoplasm called von Hansemann cells, which contain giant polyphagolysosomes. These contain various forms of mineralized debris and partially digested bacteria (466). The presence of characteristic

intracellular and extracellular Michaelis-Gutmann bodies clinches the diagnosis (Fig. 13.153). Michaelis-Gutmann bodies vary in size from 2 to 10 μm and have a round, dense, or targetoid appearance due to the presence of concentric laminations. These stain blue with hematoxylin and are highlighted with the Von Kossa stain for calcium or with iron stains. They also contain lipid and are PAS and Alcian blue positive. Because malakoplakia tends to associate with both adenomas and carcinomas, the tissues should be carefully evaluated for the presence of coexisting neoplastic conditions.

Malakoplakia superficially resembles several other disorders, including storage diseases, Whipple disease, MAI, and fungal infections because of the macrophage collections, but none of these disorders contains the pathognomonic Michaelis-Gutmann bodies. Special stains serve to identify the specific infections in fungal or tuberculous lesions.

Sarcoidosis

Sarcoidosis is a chronic multisystem granulomatous disease of unknown etiology. The characteristic histologic lesions include noncaseating granulomas containing multinucleated giant cells in the absence of identifiable infectious diseases or foreign bodies. GI disease is uncommon (468). The stomach is the most frequently affected gastrointestinal organ but the colon may become involved (Fig. 13.154). Colonic sarcoidosis usually remains asymptomatic but it may cause constricting obstructive lesions resembling carcinoma on a barium

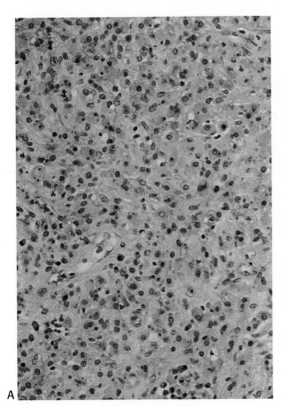
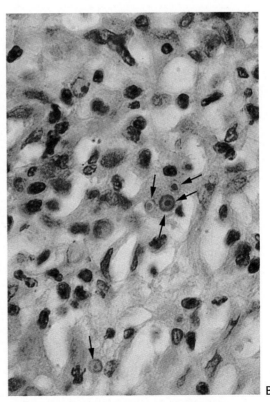

FIG. 13.153. Malakoplakia. **A:** Histiocytic cells intermingle with lymphocytes and plasma cells. **B:** Higher magnification shows typical Michaelis-Guttman bodies with their characteristic targetoid appearance (*arrows*).

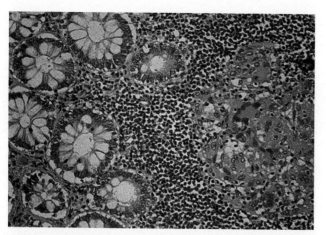

FIG. 13.154. Colonic biopsy in a patient with known sarcoid. The compact granuloma is noncaseating and surrounded by a cuff of lymphocytes.

enema. The disease also mimics CD, especially when it involves the ileocecal region (469). Not all patients with GI disease have intrathoracic involvement (470). Systemic sarcoidosis is generally extremely responsive to corticosteroid therapy, with improvement often occurring after only a few days of treatment (468).

Wegener Granulomatosis

Wegener granulomatosis is a disease of unknown etiology characterized by the presence of necrotizing granulomas of the upper and lower respiratory tract, vasculitis, and glomerulonephritis (471). Other affected organs include the intestinal tract. Wegener granulomatosis may mimic IBD when it presents as acute granulomatous colitis (471). Patients may develop nausea, vomiting, abdominal pain, and a bloody mucoid rectal discharge. The diagnosis is confirmed by the presence of characteristic palisading granulomas with a central area of necrosis that contains multinucleated giant cells surrounding small arteries and veins.

INTESTINAL CHANGES ASSOCIATED WITH IMMUNOLOGIC INJURY

HIV Infections

Epidemiology

AIDS results from infection by HIV. It associates with a number of defining abnormalities (Table 13.25). More than 30 million people are infected with HIV-1 worldwide. Epidemiologically,

---

TABLE 13.25 Definition of AIDS

Any patient with one or more of the following reliably diagnosed diseases in the absence of known cause of immunodeficiency; laboratory evidence regarding HIV infection either positive or not available:
- Candidiasis of esophagus, trachea, bronchi, or lungs
- Cryptococcosis, extrapulmonary
- Cryptosporidiosis with diarrhea persisting more than 1 month
- Cytomegalovirus disease, extranodal, in patient older than 1 month of age
- Herpes simplex virus infection with ulceration persisting more than 1 month
- Kaposi sarcoma in patient under 60 years of age
- Lymphoma, brain (primary), in patient under 60 years of age
- Lymphoid interstitial pneumonia or pulmonary lymphoid hyperplasia in child under 13 years of age
- *Mycobacterium avium-intracellular* or *Mycobacterium kansasii* disease, disseminated
- Pneumocystosis
- Progressive multifocal leukoencephalopathy

Any patient with one or more of the following reliably diagnosed diseases plus laboratory evidence of HIV infection:
- Bacterial infections, multiple or recurrent, in child under 13 years of age
- Coccidioidomycosis, disseminated
- HIV encephalopathy
- Histoplasmosis, disseminated
- Isosporiasis with diarrhea persisting more than 1 month
- Kaposi sarcoma at any age
- Lymphoma, brain (primary), at any age
- Other non-Hodgkin lymphoma of certain types
- Disseminated mycobacteriosis caused by mycobacteria other than *Mycobacterium tuberculosis*
- Tuberculosis, extrapulmonary
- *Salmonella* (nontyphoid) septicemia, recurrent
- HIV wasting syndrome

the major risk groups for developing AIDS vary depending on geographic locale. In Africa and Asia, the major risk group is sexually active heterosexuals; women are more often infected than men (472,473). In contrast, in the United States, over 70% of cases affect men having sex with men. Another 15% develop in intravenous drug users. Other high-risk groups include prostitutes, hemophiliacs, children born to HIV-positive mothers, patients transfused with infected blood or blood products, and heterosexual contacts of any of the above groups (474). HIV-infected mothers pass the virus transplacentally, at the time of delivery through the birth canal or through breast milk. AIDS especially affects Hispanics and African Americans (475). The AIDS patient population in the United States is disproportionately male, black, and poor (476). Women represented 18% of all cases in the United States in 1994. Sexual transmission is now the dominant route by which women become infected (477). Substantial declines have occurred in AIDS incidence and death in recent years (475), probably due to an increased awareness in at-risk populations and the introduction of antiretroviral therapies.

Since 1996, profound changes have taken place in the epidemiology, clinical presentation, complications, and management of HIV infections, largely due to the introduction of highly active antiretroviral treatment (HAART). As a result, gastrointestinal complications have dramatically decreased and there has been a substantial decline in the number of opportunistic infections associated with the infection (478). However, while HAART is effective in suppressing opportunistic infections, the antiretroviral medications cause GI side effects in up to 10% of cases (479). Currently, drug-induced side effects and nonopportunistic diseases are among the most common causes of GI symptoms in HIV-positive patients (478,480).

Etiology

Two HIVs exist: HIV-1 and HIV-2; both belong to the lentivirus family of nononcogenic retroviruses. HIV-1 is the predominant virus in the United States, Europe, and eastern Africa. HIV-2 infection predominates in parts of western Africa. Many fewer AIDS cases develop in HIV-2–infected than in HIV-1–infected populations. Viral transmission is similar for both viruses, except that perinatal transmission occurs less frequently in HIV-2 infections. HIV-2 also has a longer latency period before AIDS appears, the course is less aggressive, and the mortality rate is less than in HIV-1 infection. HIV-2–infected patients typically have a lower viral load and higher CD4 counts than HIV-1–infected individuals. HIV easily mutates leading to the emergence of new viral strains that can resist immune attack or drug therapy or alter the clinical or histopathologic features of the disease. The number of active replicating viruses is proportional to the number of CD4+ lymphocytes.

The virion contains two single RNA strands, structural proteins, and the enzymes required for viral replication. HIV genes encode core proteins (GAG), reverse transcriptase, protease, an endonuclease (Pol), and envelope glycoproteins (Env). At least five other genes exert regulatory

functions that may affect viral pathogenicity: vif, tat3, rev, nef, and vpr. The viruses use the enzyme reverse transcriptase to transcribe viral RNA into proviral DNA in host cells. The proviral DNA resides in the cells during viral latency. The lipid envelope surrounding the viral core derives from the host cell surface as the virions bud from the infected cell. As a result, this lipid envelope contains host membrane protein remnants as well as the viral envelope glycoprotein gp120 and the transmembrane protein gp41, two proteins involved in viral attachment and entry into host cells (481).

The CD4 protein and its coreceptor, CXCR4, and possibly CD26 on helper T-cell surfaces, serve as high-affinity receptors for the viral envelope gp120, mediating rapid, firm, cellular attachments. T-cell trophic viruses requiring CXCR4 for entry are termed X4 viruses (482).

Some HIV strains (named R5 viruses to reflect their coreceptor requirement) bind to macrophages via the β chemokine receptor CCR5 (483–485). Genetic polymorphisms in the chemokine receptor genes that mediate HIV disease progression affect disease expression (486). Cells with an absent or reduced CCR5 expression or a CCR5 mutation have a reduced sensitivity to HIV infection (487), and these cells are resistant to HIV infection even in the face of a high risk of infection (487).

Pathophysiology

The most common mode of HIV-1 infection is sexual transmission through the anogenital mucosa. Monocytes, macrophages, dendritic cells, and CD4+ T lymphocytes are the primary viral targets (481). The virus is initially acquired via one of the following: Rectal mucosal tears, M cells overlying lymphoid follicles, direct infection of the rectal epithelium, or infection of lamina propria dendritic cells (488) subjacent to the anorectal epithelium. HIV-1 viruses adhering to the luminal membranes of rectal M cells are endocytosed and delivered to intraepithelial lymphocytes, macrophages, and the mononuclear cells of the lymphoid follicles (489). The infected cells fuse with CD4+ lymphocytes and spread into deeper tissues. Within 2 days of the initial infection, viruses can be detected in draining internal iliac lymph nodes. Shortly thereafter, systemic dissemination occurs.

The gastrointestinal mucosa serves as an important reservoir for HIV, with lamina propria macrophages frequently harboring the virus (489,490). The gastrointestinal epithelium and lamina propria are also a rich source of CD4+ T cells. There are also abundant CD4+ T cells in the regional lymph nodes. The intestinal mucosa becomes profoundly and selectively depleted of CD4+ cells within days of the infection, even before similar changes occur in peripheral lymphoid tissues. In contrast, CD8+ T cells increase early in the infection and then display increased levels of activation antigens and abnormal MHC-restricted HIV-specific and -nonspecific cytotoxic abilities. A specific increase in apoptotic CD8+ T cells eventually leads to their depletion (490). A nearly complete absence of CD4+

intraepithelial lymphocytes and decreased CD11+ intraepithelial lymphocytes characterize the intestinal mucosa of severely ill AIDS patients (491).

Host factors also play a major role in the pathogenesis of HIV-related disease. A complex network of endogenous cytokines provides a delicate balance between HIV induction and suppression. The β-chemokines RANTES, MIP-1α, and MIP-1β act as suppressors of macrophage-trophic HIV strains (492) and elevated β-chemokine expression levels probably help control HIV load and replication in individuals who do not progress to AIDS (493).

Clinicopathologic Features

Acute HIV-1 infection is a transient symptomatic illness associated with high viral titers and a robust immunologic antiviral response (494). Signs and symptoms of an acute HIV-1 infection occur within days to weeks of the initial viral exposure, and include the first gastrointestinal symptoms. The most common systemic signs and symptoms include fever, fatigue, a rash, headache, lymphadenopathy, pharyngitis, myalgia, arthralgia, aseptic meningitis, retro-orbital pain, weight loss, depression, GI distress, night sweats, and oral or genital ulcers. The acute illness lasts for a few days to more than 10 weeks, but averages <14 days in length (495). Since the early signs and symptoms are nonspecific, acute HIV-1 infections are frequently confused with other viral illnesses. Initial laboratory studies may show lymphopenia and thrombocytopenia, but atypical lymphocytes are infrequent. Standard serologic tests only become positive 3 to 4 weeks after the initial infection (496). Severe and prolonged symptoms correlate with rapid disease progression (497). After the initial infection, there is a rapid viremia with widespread viral dissemination, seeding of lymphoid organs (498), and entrapment by follicular dendritic cells (499). Individuals with the highest viral loads have the highest rates of disease progression (500).

AIDS develops after a long latent period, averaging 7 to 10 years following the initial infection. During the latency period, the immune system remains relatively intact, preventing most secondary infections, but viral replication actively continues in lymphoid tissues. A CD4 count <500/mL heralds the development of clinical AIDS. A drop to <200/mL defines AIDS and indicates a high probability of developing AIDS-related infections, neoplasms, and death.

Diarrhea affects 30% to 50% of North American and European and 90% of African HIV-infected patients (472,501). AIDS patients who present with diarrhea have a greater degree of immunosuppression than those without diarrhea, predisposing the gut to the infections that contribute to morbidity and death. Diarrhea occurred in up to 90% of patients in the pre-HAART era. More recent data suggest that diarrhea is still a frequent complaint, but is more commonly attributable to drug-induced injury or non–HIV-related pathologic processes. Diarrhea in HIV infected patients results from the presence of (a) enteric

pathogenic infections, (b) complications of the drugs used to treat the infection, (c) the presence of *AIDS enteropathy* or *AIDS gastropathy,* (d) AIDS-related motility disturbances, and (e) tumor development. Often it is impossible to attribute any AIDS-associated gastrointestinal sign or symptom to a specific underlying cause, since patients usually have numerous intestinal pathologies (Table 13.26). The coccidian parasites *Cryptosporidium parvum, Isospora belli,* and *Cyclospora* and the microsporidia account for at least 50% of cases of persistent diarrhea in the industrialized and developing world with

---

TABLE 13.26   **Intestinal Lesions in AIDS**

Infections
  Bacterial
    Spirochetosis
    Salmonella typhimurium
    Shigella species
    Mycobacterium tuberculosis
    Mycobacterium avium-intracellulare
    Escherichia coli
    Campylobacter species
    Aeromonas hydrophilia
    Neisseria gonorrhoeae
    Lymphogranuloma venereum
    Syphilis
    Chlamydial species
  Viral
    Ebstein-Barr virus
    Cytomegalovirus
    Herpes simplex virus
    HIV
  Parasites
    Entamoeba histolytica
    Giardia lamblia
    Cyclospora species
    Enterobius vermicularis
    Cryptosporidium
    Toxoplasma
    Taenia saginata
    Isospora belli
    Microsporidia group
    Leishmania species
    Strongyloides
    Blastocystis hominis
  Fungi
    Candida
    Histoplasma
    Blastocystic hominis
    Pneumocystis carinii
    Aspergillus fumigatus
    Cryptococcus neoformans
HIV enteropathy
HIV ganglioneuritis
Tumors
  Kaposi sarcoma
  Lymphomas
Drug effects

major contributions from *Mycobacterium avium* complex (MAC) and other bacteria, as well as CMV infection (502). These infections are all discussed in Chapter 6.

The gastrointestinal manifestations of HIV change according to the stage of the infection. Early and intermediate gastrointestinal manifestations include diarrhea without detectable pathogens (AIDS enteropathy) and low-grade bacterial overgrowth. Well-established infections, particularly parasitic infections and viral infections, characterize late-stage disease. Severe recurrent systemic and/or gastrointestinal parasitic, viral, fungal, and protozoal infections along with the development of neoplasms and other HIV-associated pathologies often result in a fatal outcome.

Biopsies performed on AIDS patients with gastrointestinal symptoms are done to determine whether the gut is directly affected by the AIDS virus (e.g., AIDS enteropathy) or whether complications such as opportunistic infections or the development of neoplasia (e.g., Kaposi sarcoma, lymphoproliferative disorders) have developed.

HIV Enteropathy

HIV enteropathy, also know as AIDS enterocolitis or AIDS enteropathy in its broadest sense, refers to gastrointestinal damage resulting from an HIV infection. *A more specific definition of AIDS enteropathy is the presence of chronic (>1 month's duration) diarrhea, malabsorption, and wasting without evidence of an enteric infection after complete evaluation* (503).

Multiple enteric pathogenic bacteria also cause diarrhea in AIDS patients. Patients may have one or more infections, including *C. jejuni* or *Campylobacter fetus, C. difficile, Enterobacter aerogenes, Salmonella, S. flexneri, Klebsiella*, and other Gram-negative bacilli. The most common infection found in the large bowel is CMV followed by *M. avium*. Patients may also have fungal or parasitic infections (Table 13.26). The degree of inflammation seen in AIDS enteropathy correlates with mucosal levels of p24 antigen and clinical symptoms.

Proposed explanations for HIV-associated enteropathy include any or all of the following: (a) the presence of an occult enteric infection (504), (b) the direct effect of the virus on the gastrointestinal epithelium, (c) the indirect effects of a localized immunologic dysfunction, (d) an immune-mediated enterocolitis, (e) a drug-induced change, or (f) an effect of some of the coexisting nutritional deficiencies. Arguments in favor of a direct HIV-related viral cytopathic effect include the identification of the virus in epithelial cells by in situ hybridization analysis in the absence of other pathogens.

The colonoscopic mucosal pattern shows diffuse abnormalities consisting of contact bleeding, edema, superficial ulcerations, exudates, and/or loss of the normal vascular pattern. The features are nonspecific and diagnosis is by exclusion of other pathologies, especially opportunistic infections.

One often sees nonspecific intestinal inflammation in AIDS-associated enteropathy. It consists of degranulating eosinophils, activated lymphocytes, and plasma cells with increased numbers of intraepithelial and lamina propria T lymphocytes (505).

Early in the disease, the lymphocyte density is normal but lymphoid depletion develops in patients suffering from full-blown AIDS. In this latter phase, macrophage and eosinophilic infiltrates are prominent and apoptosis is common. In end-stage disease, opportunistic infections are present together with eosinophilia, neutrophilia, apoptosis, and tissue injury.

Either the mucosal T-cell alterations in AIDS or the direct viral infection of the enterocytes may alter mucosal architecture, producing an enteropathy or colopathy characterized by epithelial damage and crypt hyperplasia. The epithelial mitotic index varies with respect to disease duration and severity; they increase early and then decrease.

Colonic biopsies show a more or less normal architecture with nonspecific inflammatory changes with a mixed cell infiltrate, including intraepithelial lymphocytosis, focal crypt epithelial cell apoptosis, endothelial tubuloreticular bodies, lymphocytes, and monocytes. Colonic biopsies show changes that sometimes resemble microscopic colitis (Fig. 13.155). HIV nucleic acid is identified by in situ hybridization. The degree of inflammation correlates with mucosal levels of p24 antigen and clinical symptoms, suggesting an etiologic role for HIV (506). Other changes include atrophy of single crypts coexisting with crypts that appear regenerative (Fig. 13.156). It is unclear as to whether this results from the infection itself or from a combination of the infection and the medications that the patients receive. The crypts superficially resemble dilated lymphatics. However, lymphatics are not present in the mucosa, and closer examination discloses that the cystic spaces in the lamina propria are lined by variably flattened epithelium; often, the lumens contain apoptotic cells. Vascular calcification with intimal fibrosis, fragmentation of

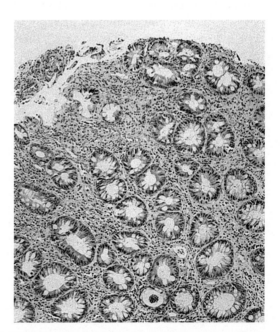

FIG. 13.155. Colonic biopsy in an AIDS patient with changes superficially resembling those found in patients with microscopic colitis. However, the epithelium appears regenerative and shows increased basophilia. Other specific changes are absent.

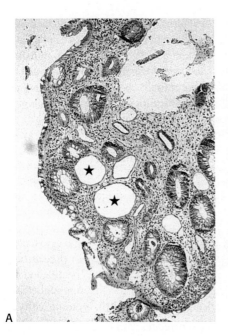

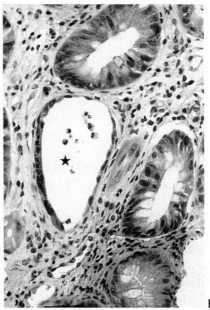

A

B

FIG. 13.156. Colonic crypt atrophy in an AIDS patient. **A:** Note the regenerative glands as well as what appear to be cystically dilated spaces (*stars*). **B:** One of these spaces seen at higher magnification (*star*). The left side of the space shows residual epithelium. On the right side of the space one sees flattened cells whose identity might be difficult to interpret in the absence of special stains or in the absence of the more cuboidal epithelium seen on the left side. The glandular lumen contains apoptotic debris.

the internal elastic lamina, and fibrosis of the media with luminal narrowing, changes designated as AIDS arteriopathy, develop in the small to medium-sized systemic arteries including those in the gastrointestinal tract and within the mesocolon. This may lead to secondary ischemic changes and mucosal ulceration. Neuromuscular alterations are common (Fig. 13.157).

One may also see small xanthomas that superficially may suggest the presence of MAC or Whipple disease, but these are negative for microorganisms. Small xanthomatous lesions are relatively common in the colon and probably represent nonspecific responses to mucosal damage resulting from many etiologies. In our experience, it is always wise to stain biopsies containing these xanthomas for the presence of mycobacteria and fungi, especially if the xanthomatous foci are prominent.

The changes of AIDS enteropathy may resemble microscopic colitis, celiac disease, or GVHD. The clinical setting, HIV testing, and antigliadin or antiendomysial antibody status serve to distinguish among these possibilities.

Treatment

A recent panel of experts recommended that immediate therapy be considered for persons with acute HIV infections (507). Early treatment restores the virus-specific cellular immune responses required to control the early viremia (508) so that they may limit the extent of viral dissemination, restrict damage to the immune system, protect antigen-presenting cells, and reduce the chance of disease progression. However, there are drawbacks to the institution of such therapy, and recent trends are leaning toward more conservative treatment

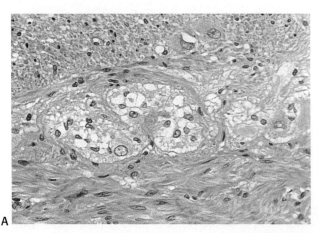

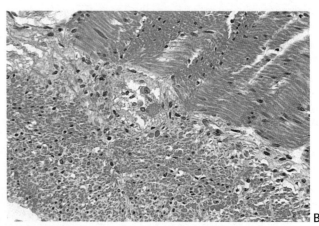

A

B

FIG. 13.157. Neuromuscular changes in AIDS. **A:** The myenteric ganglia often demonstrate mild nonspecific vacuolar degeneration. **B:** The external muscle coat often shows marked atrophy of individual myofibers. This may result either from the viral infection itself or from treatment.

with HAART. Recent recommendations are that HAART be instituted at a time when CD4 counts suggest an immediate risk of progression to AIDS, or in patients at risk of dying (509). Risks of early therapy include the adverse effects of these drugs on the quality of the patient's life as well as potential serious side effects that may result from drug toxicity. In addition, the duration of the beneficial effects of HAART is currently unknown. Previously treated patients are known to experience a poorer response to reinstitution of HAART, perhaps as a result of acquisition of some degree of drug resistance (510). Updates for treatment guidelines are available from the World Wide Web site of the HIV/AIDS Treatment Information Service (ATIS) at http://www.hivatis.org.

Graft-Versus-Host Disease

GVHD most commonly follows bone marrow or solid organ transplantation, and represents the response of immunocompetent donor cells to the histocompatibility antigens of the recipient. Less commonly, it complicates maternal–fetal cell transfer in immunodeficient children (511) or transfusion of nonirradiated cells and blood products (512,513). Although GVHD may affect any organ, intestinal GVHD is particularly important because of its frequency, severity, and impact on the general condition of the patient. The incidence of GVHD is possibly higher in African Americans than in other individuals (514).

Acute GVHD occurs in three phases: Epithelial cell injury caused by the conditioning regimen; activation of donor T cells by antigens presented by the recipient's dendritic cells; and apoptosis induced by activated T cells, cytokines, and cells of the innate immune system (520). HLA disparities between donor and recipient are the major predisposing factor. Other factors include the ages of the donor and the recipient, sex mismatch (female donor and male recipient), mismatched minor histocompatibility antigens in HLA-matched transplants, the source and dose of the transplanted hematopoietic stem cells, the intensity of the preparative regimen, and prophylaxis against GVHD or T-cell deletion of the graft (521,522).

CD8+, CD3+, and TiA1+ cytotoxic T cells mediate epithelial cell death (515,516). CD8 cells recognize class II MHC-restricted antigens producing the lymphokines that lead to the development of the enteropathy associated with GVHD (517). Apoptosis may occur through the Fas/Fas ligand pathway (518). Patients who are homozygous for a common variant in the promoter region of the interleukin-10 gene are at a low risk for GVHD after stem cell transplantation (519).

The endoscopic appearance of the mucosa in acute GVHD ranges from edema and erythema to ulcers and mucosal sloughing (523).

Mucosal biopsy provides a sensitive test for detecting GVHD. Apoptotic bodies are the sine qua non of the diagnosis. However, the biopsy should not be done during the first 3 weeks of immunosuppressive therapy because all patients will show some inflammation in the immediate posttransplant period. The lesions of acute GVHD range from necrosis of

TABLE 13.27	Histologic Grading of Graft Versus Host Disease

Grade	Features
1	Mild necrosis of individual crypts
2	Crypt abscesses and crypt cell flattening
3	Crypt dropout
4	Flat mucosa

individual crypt cells to total mucosal loss (Table 13.27). Apoptotic bodies collect at the crypt bases in the intestine, and in the neck region of the gastric glands (Fig. 13.158). The crypt bases contain vacuolated cells with karyolytic debris in cellular lacunae, producing "popcorn lesions." The cells are also sometimes called "exploding crypt cells." As a result, the base of the glands may appear dilated and contain apoptotic debris. As the lesions evolve, an entire crypt may drop out, creating single crypt loss. Acute colitis and neutrophilic infiltrates accompany the apoptosis and crypt dropout. The mucosal architecture is progressively lost with ulceration, mucosal denudation, and submucosal edema. The epithelium may appear degenerated and cuboidal. In some cases, the epithelium appears as a flattened monolayer. Ulcer healing leads to fibrosis and stricture formation. The lamina propria contains a relatively sparse mononuclear cell infiltrate.

In chronic GVHD, one sees segmental lamina propria fibrosis and submucosal fibrosis extending to the serosa. These lesions occur throughout the entire length of the gut from the esophagus to the colon.

Occasional patients pass ropy, tan material resembling strands of sloughed mucosal tissue, known as mucosal casts, per rectum. The composition of the material is rarely clear-cut. It usually contains fibrin, neutrophils, cellular debris, bacteria, or fungi, and very little identifiable tissue (524). The presence of free intestinal epithelium may be confirmed by immunostaining for cytokeratin (524). *C. difficile* infection may associate with gastrointestinal GVHD and a high mortality rate. It is postulated that the toxins produced by the bacteria increase the severity of the GVHD (525).

The changes of GVHD mimic certain infections, particularly *Salmonella* with its neutrophilic collections in the bases of the crypts (Fig. 13.158). Histologic changes resembling GVHD in the colon may develop in patients with CMV infections (526,527), malignant thymomas (Fig. 13.159) (528), severe T-cell deficiencies (529), and common variable immunodeficiency (530). Some patients have autoimmune diseases. This entity probably overlaps with autoimmune enteropathy. Histologic features similar to those of GVHD may also be due to drug injury particularly due to mycophenolate l, a drug used to reduce acute graft rejection in solid organ transplant patients (526).

The surrounding mucosa may show changes that mimic IBD. The mucosa may demonstrate mild to moderate architectural distortion (villiform surface with crypt branching and atrophy). However, the lamina propria is typically

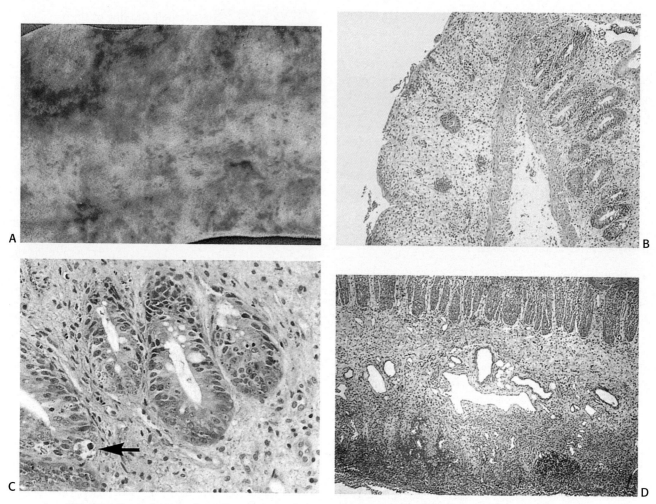

FIG. 13.158. Graft-versus-host disease (GVHD). **A:** Gross appearance of the bowel in a patient with severe GVHD demonstrates the presence of atrophy and numerous petechiae. **B:** Segmental crypt loss and necrosis are typical in marked GVHD. In the area to the right, one sees a few intact glands. **C:** Higher power magnification of the intact glands demonstrates the presence of single-cell necrosis (*arrow*). **D:** Inflammation extends through the bowel wall to involve the serosa, which is markedly thickened. (Courtesy of Drs. Meyerson, Sale, and Schulman, Fred Hutchinson Cancer Center, Seattle, WA.)

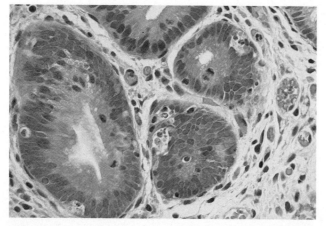

FIG. 13.159. Colonic biopsy in a patient with a malignant thymoma showing prominent "popcorn" apoptotic lesions in the crypt bases.

hypocellular with prominent small blood vessels. The lamina propria may appear to be focally fibrotic. It is unclear whether these changes are part of the GVHD or complicate the superimposed infections that may develop (531).

Omenn Syndrome

Omenn syndrome is an autosomal recessive severe combined immunodeficiency syndrome that clinically and pathologically resembles GVHD. It is characterized by an expansion of an oligoclonal T-cell population (532). Hypereosinophilia and hypogammaglobulinemia are present.

Autoimmune Colitis

Autoimmune colitis complicates autoimmune enteropathy. The colitis presents as a mild intraepithelial lymphocytosis producing a pattern resembling lymphocytic colitis, or the epithelium contains large numbers of degranulating eosinophils and mast cells superimposed on a background of mucosal atrophy (Fig. 13.160). These changes often associate with endoscopic evidence of colitis and the changes are not restricted to the large bowel. The patients lack the clinical stigmata of celiac disease. The patients often have evidence of other autoimmune diseases, such as juvenile diabetes, autoimmune hepatitis, or autoimmune thyroiditis. This disorder is discussed further in Chapter 6.

VASCULAR LESIONS

A number of vascular lesions affect the large intestine. In this chapter we will deal with nonneoplastic vascular abnormalities. Vascular tumors are covered in Chapter 19.

Portal Colopathy

Patients with portal hypertension often develop hematochezia, Hemoccult-positive stools, and anemia. Some patients develop hemorrhoids (533); most patients have esophageal varices. Seventy percent of patients have a mosaic mucosal vascular pattern or multiple vascular ectasias. The ectasias cause both acute and chronic gastrointestinal bleeding (534). Other endo-

scopic mucosal abnormalities include edema, erythema, granularity, and friability, features often seen in colitis (535). Histologically, increased numbers of small vessels with prominent branching lie in the upper and midmucosa. The dilated, tortuous mucosal capillaries may show irregular thickening and arterialization of their walls. Vascular diameters can measure 20 ± 2 micra in the ascending colon and 30 ± micra in the rectum (536). These findings associate with edema of the lamina propria and mild chronic inflammatory changes (537). The typical signs of portal hypertension are present, including dilation and tortuosity of the mesenteric veins. Neither signs of chronic liver disease nor stigmata suggestive of severe portal hypertension correlate with the endoscopic findings. The colonic lesions resemble those found in portal gastropathy, an entity discussed in Chapter 4.

Varices

Esophageal varices are well known, but it is not generally appreciated that varices can involve the rest of the GI tract (538). Adhesions or enterostomies favor the formation of intestinal varices if portal hypertension is present. Patients with pancreatitis and splenic vein thrombosis also develop colonic varices (539). Colonic varices may also occur on a familial basis in the absence of portal hypertension (540). Mean patient age is 50 and there is a slight male predominance. Sites where

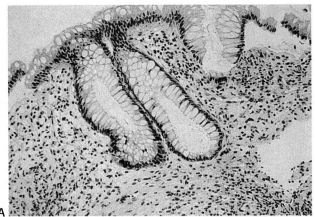

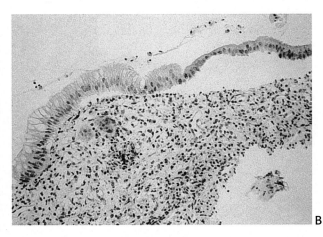

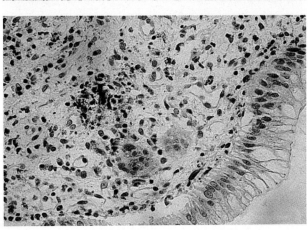

FIG. 13.160. Autoimmune colitis in a 9-month-old child. **A:** A rectal biopsy demonstrating the presence of severe glandular atrophy. **B:** This specimen is from another area and demonstrates regenerating mucosa on the upper right-hand surface. The mucosa has become simplified without glands. Several glands are being destroyed by an eosinophilic infiltrate. This is seen better at higher magnification in **C.**

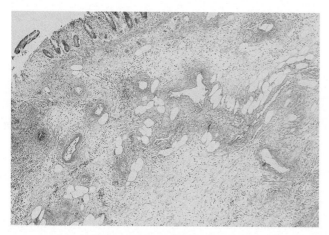

FIG. 13.161. Colonic varices.

varices form reflect the embryonic juxtaposition of visceral and systemic vascular plexuses. Portal hypertension not only causes dilation of the pre-existing natural shunts with creation of collateral vessels, but also reopens embryonic vessels, particularly the periumbilical veins, producing the caput medusae.

In patients with portal hypertension, the coronary azygous system is the primary portal–systemic channel in 50% of cases; in 25% the inferior mesenteric and internal iliac systems represent the primary portal–systemic channel. Portal–systemic communications also exist in the rectum. Prominent dilated vessels are present in the submucosa (Fig. 13.161). The histology of the varices resembles that of esophageal varices (see Chapter 2).

Dieulafoy Vascular Malformations

Dieulafoy vascular malformations, also known as caliber-persistent submucosal arteries, are rare but well-known causes of upper GI bleeding. They also affect the colon, although they rarely (541) lead to massive bleeding. A large submucosal artery lies in close contact with the mucosa, often attached to the muscularis mucosae; the vessel is oversized for the site. In the colon, the lesions arise in the ascending colon or cecum, and the preferential involvement of this site may be the result of the vascular architecture. Their histology resembles their gastric counterpart (see Chapter 4).

Angiodysplasia

The most common type of colonic vascular dysplasia is angiodysplasia, which usually involves the right colon, although it does affect other sites as well. Most regard angiodysplasia as a degenerative disease of the elderly in which malformed vessels present in the submucosa extend into the overlying mucosa. Numerous studies show an association between bleeding from angiodysplasias and the presence of aortic stenosis (542). Valve replacement causes cessation of the recurrent bleeding. This suggests that the aortic stenosis does not cause the lesion but contributes to bleeding

from it. Arteriovenous malformations (AVMs) also associate with chronic renal failure, coagulation disorders, defective platelet aggregation, and warfarin therapy for artificial heart valves and diverticular disease (61). Coagulation abnormalities contribute to episodic bleeding.

Most patients with bleeding have a deficiency of the largest multimers of von Willebrand factor induced by a latent acquired von Willebrand disease (543). Bleeding from angiodysplasia can be massive and recurrent.

The true incidence of angiodysplasia is unknown because the lesion is difficult to demonstrate surgically and pathologically. Angiodysplasias are an incidental finding in 3% to 6% of individuals undergoing colonoscopy and affect up to 25% of the elderly. They usually occur in persons older than 50 years of age, although they can affect individuals of any age. Average patient age is 70 years. The lesions are frequently multiple and primarily involve the cecum and right colon.

Selective mesenteric arteriography has been the preferred way to diagnose angiodysplasia. The hallmarks of the lesion include (a) an early filling vein that visualizes within 4 to 5 seconds after contrast material is injected; (b) a vascular tuft that represents an abnormal vascular structure, best seen in the arterial phase and usually located at the termination of a branch in the ileocolic artery; and (c) a slowly emptying, densely opacified, intramural vein that remains visualized after the other mesenteric veins have emptied. However, recent studies suggest that helical computed tomography (CT) angiography is a sensitive, specific, well-tolerated, and minimally invasive tool for diagnosing colonic angiodysplasia (544).

Most angiodysplasias are mucosal and submucosal lesions (Fig. 13.162) that are not always visible externally to the surgeon or the pathologist. A helpful way to identify the vascular abnormality is to have the surgeon cannulate the major vessels at the time of the resection, leaving the cannulas in place. When the specimen is received in the laboratory, the pathologist can inject a combination of India ink and a radiopaque dye into the specimen and then x-ray it. The specimen can then be fixed and sections taken in the area of the abnormal vasculature. The India ink will remain visible within the abnormal vessels (Fig. 13.162).

Grossly, the lesions usually consist of small (1 to 2 mm or less) or larger (>5 mm), cherry-red, fan-shaped mucosal lesions with a tense central vessel and radiating foot processes (545). Mucosal erosions may be present. The lesions are often multiple and flat. If the lesion is examined under the dissecting microscope, one sees multiple, often coalescent vascular channels with adjacent arteries and veins standing out as "coral reefs" against the normal capillary "honeycomb" pattern of the colonic mucosa. Sometimes a gross specimen is received in which the angiodysplasia has been cauterized, in which case the lesion may appear as a heaped-up ulcer.

Histologically, angiodysplasia consists of dilated, distorted vessels lined by endothelium and rarely by a small amount of smooth muscle. Enlarged arteries are also present

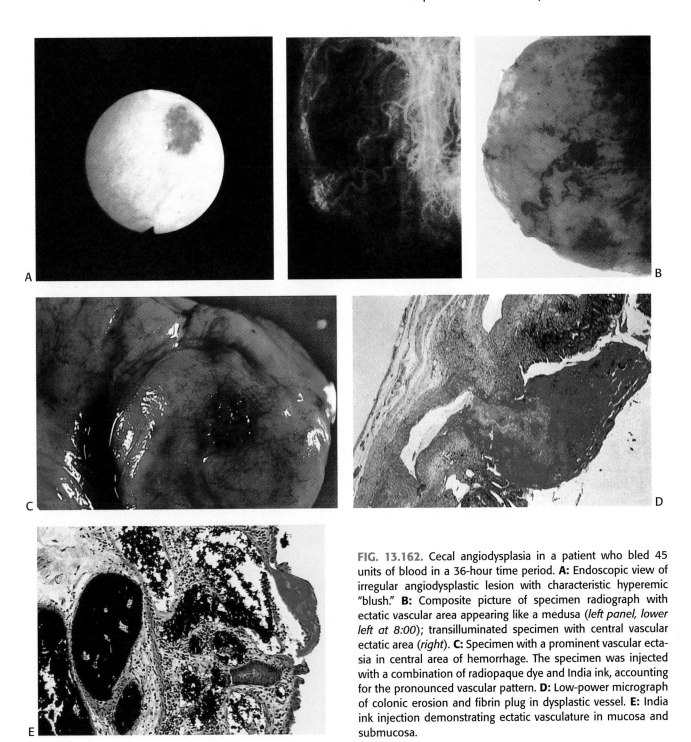

FIG. 13.162. Cecal angiodysplasia in a patient who bled 45 units of blood in a 36-hour time period. **A:** Endoscopic view of irregular angiodysplastic lesion with characteristic hyperemic "blush." **B:** Composite picture of specimen radiograph with ectatic vascular area appearing like a medusa (*left panel, lower left at 8:00*); transilluminated specimen with central vascular ectatic area (*right*). **C:** Specimen with a prominent vascular ectasia in central area of hemorrhage. The specimen was injected with a combination of radiopaque dye and India ink, accounting for the pronounced vascular pattern. **D:** Low-power micrograph of colonic erosion and fibrin plug in dysplastic vessel. **E:** India ink injection demonstrating ectatic vasculature in mucosa and submucosa.

(Fig. 13.162). The lesions are ectasias of the normal vasculature rather than true malformations. The pattern of involvement points to dilation of submucosal veins as the initial morphologic change, lending credibility to the notion that recurrent obstruction plays a role in its etiology. Repeated obstructions during the muscular contraction and distention of the colon result in dilation and tortuosity of submucosal veins and retrograde involvement of the venules of the arteriolar capillary venular units. Ultimately, the capillary rings surrounding the crypts dilate and the competency of

the precapillary sphincters is lost, producing a small arteriovenous communication.

The earliest abnormality is the presence of dilated (twice the normal diameter), thin-walled, submucosal veins that may occur in the absence of mucosal involvement. The dilated, thin-walled vessels are not sclerotic. An occasional venous tributary pierces the muscularis mucosae and joins dilated venules and capillaries of the mucosa. The architecture of the colonic crypts is not altered and the lamina propria is not significantly inflamed.

More extensive involvement leads to increased numbers of dilated and deformed mucosal and submucosal vessels, eventually distorting the mucosal architecture. Late-stage lesions show a mixture of the early lesions and dilated and tortuous mucosal capillaries and venules. As the lesions advance, the proliferating blood vessels displace the crypts. Only a layer of endothelial cells may separate the vascular channels from the intestinal lumen. Arterialization of the veins, which is recognized as hypertrophy of both the intima and smooth muscle, only occurs in advanced stages of the disease (545). Submucosal arteries are normal or moderately dilated. Occasionally, they reveal mild to moderate sclerotic changes sometimes associated with atheromatous emboli. Organized and recanalized thrombi may be present in larger submucosal veins. Some vascular ectasias extend full thickness from the serosa through the muscularis propria to the submucosa and mucosa. The presence of distorted and dysplastic vessels distinguishes this lesion from hemangiomas.

Arterial Dysplasia of the Colonic Arteries

In arterial dysplasia, the arterial vasculature varies significantly from one intestinal area to another. In some areas, the vessels appear dysplastic due to the irregularity of their walls and adventitia. They exhibit fibrous, annular thickening with medial destruction. The internal elastic layer is variably absent. The absence of the elastica allows aneurysmal dilation and subsequent rupture (546). In some segments, the vascular lumen may be completely obliterated by thrombi or variable degrees of fibrosis. Previous bleeding sites organize and are recognized by an abundance of iron-containing histiocytes and chronic inflammatory cells. In other segments, the arterial wall appears relatively normal, although mild abnormalities of the inner elastic membrane and moderate disorganization of the media and muscular layer are present.

The etiology of arterial dysplasia is unknown and many factors have been postulated, including embryologic variations, hormonal influences, autoimmune mechanisms, and trauma (546). Clinical signs and symptoms usually develop secondary to ischemic complications.

Vascular Changes in Homocystinuria

Homocystinuria causes changes in the vasculature simulating fibromuscular dysplasia. The vascular changes consist of fibroblastic intimal proliferations and narrowing of the vascular lumen, in the absence of inflammation and fibrinoid necrosis. The changes resemble those seen in atherosclerosis and may lead to intestinal ischemia.

PNEUMATOSIS COLI

Pneumatosis coli consists of gas-filled cysts within the bowel wall. Pneumatosis is asymptomatic or accompanied by constipation or diarrhea. The lesion may also be detected endo-scopically or radiographically. Most often colonic disease follows mucosal ulceration due to ischemia, necrotizing enterocolitis, infection, and other causes. In the colon it may present endoscopically as a small mucosal elevation or polyp. It may also present as an intussusception (547). The cysts are found in all bowel layers. They are lined by epithelioid macrophages, multinucleated giant cells, and a variable chronic inflammatory cell infiltrate. An exceptional example of cysts containing spirochetes in a patient with coexisting spirochetosis was recently reported.

CONNECTIVE TISSUE DISORDERS

Marfan Syndrome

Marfan syndrome is a connective tissue disorder that primarily affects the skeleton, eyes, and cardiovascular system. Diverticula develop in children and in young patients with Marfan syndrome presumably due to the defective collagen.

Ehlers-Danlos Syndrome

Ehlers-Danlos syndrome is a genetically determined, connective tissue disorder that results from mutations in the gene for type III procollagen (COL3A1) (548,549). It has multiple clinically distinct phenotypes, each showing different inheritance patterns and different biochemical abnormalities. The disease is characterized by hyperextensible skin, hypermobile joints, tissue fragility, and wide, thin scars frequently overlying bony prominences. Patient survival is shortened largely secondary to vascular rupture. The age at death ranges from 6 to 73 years with a median lifespan of 48 years (550). Ehlers-Danlos syndrome type IV is particularly lethal and characteristically presents with numerous problems, including rupture of major vessels with colorectal bleeding, prolapse, diverticulosis, diverticulitis, and spontaneous perforation (550,551). Bowel rupture usually occurs in the sigmoid colon and it accounts for approximately a quarter of major complications in young people (550). Small bowel and gastric perforation is much less common. Tissue fragility and poor wound healing contribute to surgical complications or death. Complications include wound dehiscence, evisceration, hemorrhage from abdominal vessels, fistulas, and adhesions. Some patients have recurrent perforations (550). The perforation and diverticulitis result from abnormal motility (451). Histopathologic examination of the arteries in patients with Ehlers-Danlos syndrome exhibits widespread structural abnormalities in the vessel wall in addition to aneurysms and rupture.

LYSOSOMAL STORAGE DISEASES

The lysosomal storage disorders result from various enzymatic defects, which include the absence of an enzyme activator or a protective protein, lack of a substrate activator protein, lack of a transport protein required for egress from the lysosome, defects in posttranslational processing, or synthesis of catalytically inactive proteins (552). The sites that are affected are those where the specific substrates need to be metabolized. Lysosomal storage diseases are usually classified into three categories: (a) sphingolipidoses (Gaucher disease); (b) mucopolysaccharidoses (Hurler and Hunter diseases); and (c) glycogen storage disease (Pompe disease) (Table 13.28). All three categories show variable severity and time of onset. The lysosomal disorders are usually diagnosed by enzymatic assay of white blood cells or fibroblasts or by rectal biopsies. Acid phosphatase stains highlight the intracellular inclusions present in lysosomal storage diseases. The tissues may also be examined by PAS, Luxol fast blue, and Sudan black stains, and for acid phosphatase activity, as well as examined under ultraviolet light to show accumulations of autofluorescent material (553). Most individuals advocate use of both histologic and ultrastructural examination to document the disease (553). Because the stored substances are often lipids, frozen sections are necessary to demonstrate the abnormal accumulations. Thus, when such a disease is suspected, a piece of unfixed tissue must be snap-frozen for further analysis.

Batten Disease (Neuronal Ceroid Lipofuscinosis)

Batten disease is the most common neuronal storage disease of children. It is classified into congenital, infantile, late infantile, early juvenile, and juvenile based on its pathology and age of onset. The abnormal nerves stain with Luxol fast blue (554). Patients with infantile Batten disease exhibit delayed development, including microcephaly, hyperkinesis, and neurologic problems. Neurophysiologic examinations are abnormal. In order to make the diagnosis on rectal biopsy, one needs to see neurons that can be highlighted by Sudan black or acid phosphatase staining. The patients develop seizures and dementia. Vacuolated lymphocytes are absent.

Hurler and Hunter Syndromes

The mucopolysaccharidoses include Hurler and Hunter syndromes. Patients with these syndromes have genetically determined deficiencies of the lysosomal enzymes involved in the degradation of mucopolysaccharides leading to their accumulation in the cell. Patients with Hurler syndrome accumulate heparin sulfate and dermatan sulfate, as do patients with Hunter syndrome. Hurler syndrome is inherited in an autosomal recessive manner, whereas Hunter syndrome is inherited as an X-linked recessive disorder. The patients present with involvement of many organs, including the GI tract (555). Ultrastructurally, the intracellular, membrane-bound lysosomes contain variable amounts of opaque, flocculent lamellae representing mucopolysaccharides. Fibroblasts, endothelium, and smooth muscle cells may appear vacuolated (556).

TABLE 13.28	Examples of Lysosomal Storage Diseases Affecting the Gastrointestinal Tract	
Disease	**Enzyme Deficiency**	**Major Stored Substance**
Glycogen storage disease		
Type 2–Pompe disease	α-1,4-Glucosidase (lysosomal glucosidase)	Glycogen
Sphingolipidoses		
GM1-gangliosidosis	GM1-ganglioside β-galactosidase	GM1-ganglioside, galactose-containing oligosaccharides
GM2-gangliosidosis	Hexosaminidase A	GM2-ganglioside
Tay-Sachs disease	Hexosaminidase A and B	GM2-ganglioside, globaside
Sandhoff disease	Ganglioside activator protein	GM2-ganglioside
GM2-gangliosidosis, AB variant		
Fabry disease	α-Galactosidase A	Ceramide trihexoside
Gaucher disease	Glucocerebrosidase	Glucocerebroside
Niemann-Pick disease	Sphingomyelinase	Sphingomyelin
Mucopolysaccharidoses		
Hurler syndrome	α-L-Iduronidase	Heparan sulfate
Hunter syndrome	L-Iduronosulfate sulfatase	Dermatan sulfate
		Heparan sulfate
		Dermatan sulfate
Lipid storage diseases		
Wolman disease	Acid lipase	Cholesterol esters, triglycerides

Niemann-Pick Disease

Niemann-Pick disease results from absence of sphingomyelinase, so that sphingomyelin accumulates in many organs throughout the body, including the viscera. In severe cases, extreme visceral accumulations are present along with progressive wasting, and patients often die in the first few years of life. Macrophages accumulate sphingomyelin in many tissues, including the lamina propria. They can be highlighted with the use of special stains for lipids, including Sudan black and oil red O. Ultrastructurally, macrophages contain membranous cytoplasmic bodies that resemble concentric lamellated myelin figures. Parallel palisaded lamellae impart an appearance of zebra bodies (557).

Gangliosidoses

Tay-Sachs disease is the prototype of the gangliosidoses. It results from a deficiency of the enzyme hexosaminidase A. This disease is particularly prevalent among Ashkenazi Jews. Hexosaminidase A catalyzes the degradation of GM2 ganglioside and because of the absence of the enzyme, this material accumulates within the cells, particularly of the nervous system (558). Patients also develop diarrhea and autonomic dysfunction, including motility disturbances. Adult GM1 gangliosidosis is a recently identified rare form of hereditary neuronal storage disease. It has a benign clinical course and cerebral lesions are restricted to the basal ganglia (559).

Rectal biopsies play a role in the diagnosis of gangliosidosis by demonstrating characteristic changes in the autonomic neurons (560). The biopsies need to be deep enough to include the submucosal plexus. Ultrastructurally, ganglion, Schwann, perithelial, and endothelial cells and histiocytes all contain characteristic electron-dense bodies, zebra bodies, and membranous cytoplasmic bodies (556). Patients with Tay-Sachs disease have these bodies in neural tissue. In contrast, patients with Sandhoff disease (hexosaminidase AB deficiency) exhibit similar structures in nerves as well as mesenchymal tissues, such as endothelial cells and fibroblasts (556). Membrane-bound clear vacuoles are also occasionally seen in the cytoplasm of rectal and cutaneous fibroblasts. The axons of the unmyelinated nerves appear normal (560).

Glycogen Storage Diseases

Glycogen storage disease IA and 1B result from a deficiency or defective transport of the microsomal enzyme glucose-6-phosphatase in liver, kidney, and intestinal mucosa. Impaired gluconeogenesis, fasting hypoglycemia, hepatomegaly, lactic acidosis, hyperlipidemia, hyperuricemia, impaired platelet function, and bleeding diathesis are common to both diseases. Glycogen storage disease 1B is additionally complicated by recurrent pyogenic infections caused by apparent neutropenia and neutrophil dysfunction (561). Patients with

these disorders demonstrate changes indistinguishable from Crohn disease, including ileal mucosal irregularities, colitis, granulomas, and stenosis involving the right side of the colon (562). Perianal abscesses are common. The bowel lesions may result from neutrophil deficiencies. Because a similar enteritis develops in patients with neutrophil deficiency states, treatment of the patients with colony-stimulating factors results in decreased bowel inflammation (563).

Lipid Storage Diseases

Fabry Disease

Fabry disease, an X-linked disorder of lipid metabolism, results from a deficiency of the enzyme α-galactosidase A that leads to ceramide trihexosidase accumulation. Malabsorption sometimes affects patients with small intestinal involvement. Patients with Fabry disease also present with enterovesical fistulae and lymphadenopathy. Foamy, lipid-containing, vacuolated neurons and nerve fibers of Meissner plexus, vascular endothelial cells, muscularis mucosae, and histiocytes are all strongly positive with Sudan black, Luxol fast blue, PAS, and oil red O stains on frozen sections. Ultrastructural examination shows the presence of zebralike, lamellar, lysosomal inclusions (564).

Tangier Disease

Patients with Tangier disease have abnormal apolipoprotein metabolism (565), hemolytic anemia, and lipid-containing macrophage accumulation in many tissues, including the gastrointestinal lamina propria. These accumulations most commonly affect the large intestine, but they can occur anywhere in the gut. They present as yellow to orange nodules and streaks. Histologically, these streaks and nodules contain collections of foamy, lipid-containing histiocytes.

Wolman Disease

Wolman disease (lysosomal acid esterase deficiency) is a lethal heritable disorder affecting children. It is characterized by hepatosplenomegaly, enlarged calcified adrenals, and a generalized visceral infiltration by foamy histiocytes containing neutral fats and cholesterol. Affected individuals develop persistent diarrhea and they rarely survive for more than 1 year. Fat-laden histiocytes containing cholesterol and triglycerides infiltrate the superficial lamina propria. The mucosal accumulations are most marked in the jejunum (553).

Cholesterol Ester Storage Disease

Cholesterol ester storage disease is a rare inherited disorder of lipid metabolism also due to a deficiency of lysosomal acid esterase, but it exhibits a much more benign clinical course than Wolman disease. The liver and spleen enlarge and serum cholesterol becomes elevated. Numerous foamy macrophages filled with cholesterol esters populate the muscularis mucosae and submucosa. Lipid droplets accumulate due to a block in the transport of cholesterol into lacteals. They are found in macrophages in the lamina propria of both the large and small intestine, alongside the lacteal endothelium, in the smooth muscle, and in vascular pericytes. The mucosal histiocytes containing the cholesterol esters and carotenes impart an orange tinge to the mucosal surface. The myenteric plexus appears vacuolated secondary to cholesterol ester deposits. The epithelium appears normal.

Peroxisomal Disorders

The normal intestinal epithelium contains numerous elliptical peroxisomes filled with coarsely granular material. These are absent in Zellweger syndrome (a lethal condition), and as a result, patients accumulate very-long-chain fatty acids. Other peroxisomal defects include neonatal adrenoleukodystrophy and infantile Refsum disease. The diagnosis is usually made by a combination of detecting metabolic abnormalities in very-long-chain fatty acids, bile acids, pipecolic acid, and phytanic acid, and demonstration of the absence of peroxisomes in intestinal biopsies (566,567).

CYSTIC FIBROSIS

Cystic fibrosis (CF), the most frequent lethal autosomal recessive disease in Caucasians, is caused by more than 1,000 different mutations in the *cystic fibrosis transmembrane conductance regulator (CFTR)* gene listed in the cystic fibrosis mutation database located at https://www.genet.sickkids.on.ca/cftr/. As a consequence of the wide spectrum of mutations that are present, the clinical presentation of CF varies widely from monosymptomatic disease to multiorgan involvement (568). Some CFTR mutations confer residual CFTR function in rectal epithelia, which results in a milder clinical phenotype (569).

The median survival of patients with cystic fibrosis in North America has increased to 31 years and as a result there is an increased incidence of large intestinal complications. The distal intestinal obstruction syndrome is more common in older patients, is a frequent cause of abdominal pain, and may lead to intussusception. The prevalence of Crohn disease in cystic fibrosis patients is 17 times that of the general population. Patients with CF develop various intestinal complications, including rectal prolapse, intussusception, volvulus, pneumatosis, bleeding, fecal impactions (570), and a fibrosing colonopathy from the therapy as discussed in the section on drug injury. Right-sided microscopic colitis may also develop and there may be an increased incidence of colon cancer (571). Intestinal biopsy specimens from these patients may show hyperdistended goblet cells with an abundant layer of mucus attached to the epithelial surfaces. This disorder is discussed in detail in Chapter 6.

AMYLOIDOSIS

All known types of amyloid affect the gastrointestinal tract, including amyloid A (AA), amyloid of lambda (AL), or kappa light chain origin, transthyretin amyloid (ATTR), and $\beta2$-microglobulin ($\beta2M$). They may be distinguished using a panel of immunohistochemical markers (572). A recent study showed that the most common forms of large intestinal amyloid were AL amyloid followed by AA and ATTR. There were also cases in which the classification of the amyloid type was uncertain (572). Gastrointestinal amyloidosis generally presents as a motility disorder, ulcers, areas of hemorrhage, or pseudotumors.

The colorectum also develops α_2-microglobulin deposits, the latter affecting patients on long-term dialysis (573). The development of the amyloidosis correlates with the time on dialysis (574). Patients with α_2-microglobulin deposits exhibit two patterns of amyloid deposition: A vascular pattern and a gastrointestinal pattern. The vascular pattern may be subtle and not be evident in H&E-stained sections but can be highlighted by stains for amyloid or a microglobulin immunostain (574). The amyloid deposits may associate with mild mucosal abnormalities and regeneration or there may be ischemic damage. The severity of the mucosal changes reflects the severity of the vasculopathy. In the gastrointestinal pattern the amyloid deposits in the interstitium of the mucosa, submucosa, and muscularis propria. This pattern coexists with the vascular pattern. The amyloid deposits range from barely visible amyloid without mural expansion to amyloid tumors in the muscularis propria (573–575).

Rectal biopsies are commonly obtained in patients suspected of having amyloidosis, but it is essential that the biopsies be large enough to permit inspection of the submucosal vasculature. In ordinary H&E-stained sections, amyloid appears as a pink, hyalinized thickening of the vessel walls or as a more diffuse eosinophilic infiltrate in the lamina propria, submucosa, or muscular layer (Fig. 13.163). The lesions may be inapparent in mild cases. Tumoral amyloid is often accompanied by giant cells. Special stains for the amyloid include crystal violet (Fig. 13.163), thioflavin, and Congo red coupled with polarized light to demonstrate the characteristic apple-green birefringence.

LESIONS PRESENTING AS POLYPS

Normally, the dynamic process of cell division is balanced by exfoliation from the luminal surface. If an imbalance occurs, either because of increased replication or decreased exfoliation, a polyp results. Broadly speaking, the word *polyp* simply denotes any mucosal elevation. Polyps may consist of benign or malignant epithelial proliferations, inflammatory infiltrates localized in the lamina propria, or deeper, submucosal or intramural mesenchymal proliferations, malformations, or even metastatic tumors. The three most common colorectal

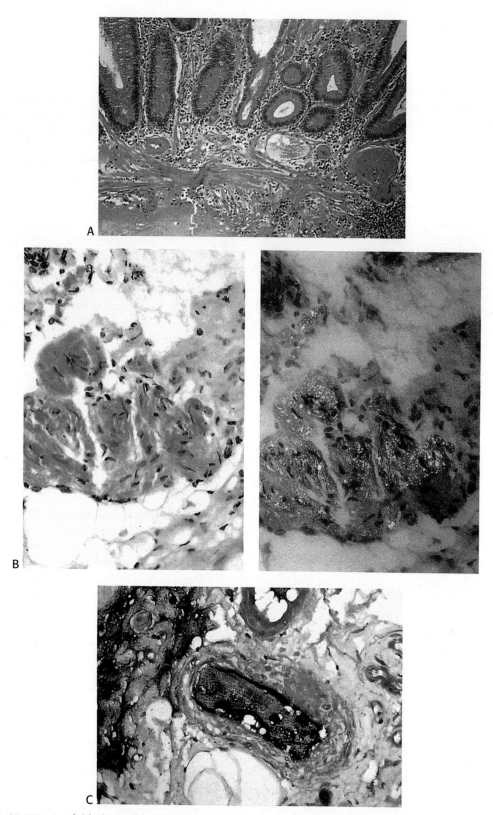

FIG. 13.163. Amyloidosis. **A:** The amyloid affects not only the small blood vessels, but also the muscularis mucosae. **B:** Congo red stain (*left*) of amyloidosis involving the smooth muscle fibers. The specimen is seen by polarized light on the right demonstrating the typical apple-green birefringence. **C:** Crystal violet stain in patient with amyloidosis in a rectal biopsy involving the submucosal vessel. An area of smudgy purplish discoloration is seen at about 2 o'clock in the blood vessel.

polyps are inflammatory, hyperplastic, and adenomatous (see Chapter 14).

Hyperplastic Polyps

Hyperplastic polyps are one of the most common polyp types seen in the adult colon. They share risk factors with adenomas and colon cancer including dietary fiber, calcium, and total fat intake; smoking; body mass index; and alcohol consumption. They often arise in a colon harboring adenomatous polyps or carcinomas (576,577). They often cluster in large numbers around colon carcinomas. Hyperplastic polyps increase in frequency with age in some populations, but not all studies confirm this (578,579). The hyperplastic polyp:adenoma ratio is highest in those parts of the world with the highest incidences of colorectal carcinoma and it falls to unity in low-risk regions (580). These lesions remain asymptomatic and are found incidentally at the time of colonoscopy or resection.

The relationship between hyperplastic polyps and the subsequent development of adenomas and carcinomas remains controversial. Hyperplastic polyps have been regarded by most observers as innocuous and nonneoplastic and unrelated to colorectal cancers, whereas others regard them as possible precursors of colorectal neoplasia (581). This issue has been clouded by the recognition of mixed hyperplastic–adenomatous polyps. Mixed polyps combine the features of both hyperplastic and adenomatous polyps without intermediate forms between them. This may be explained by the engulfment of a pre-existing hyperplastic polyp by a spreading adenoma, by stimulation of the mucosa at the advancing edge of an adenoma, or by the development of an adenoma in a hyperplastic polyp. The hyperplastic component alone does not predispose to carcinoma, but the presence of a coexisting adenomatous component does have malignant potential. It is also clouded by the inclusion of the serrated adenomas and the polyps of the hyperplastic polyposis syndrome, which are different entities that somewhat resemble hyperplastic polyps. These lesions are discussed in Chapters 12 and 14. Hyperplastic polyps are generally not regarded as having a direct relationship to colonic cancers (582,583).

The fact that the vast majority of hyperplastic polyps arise in the colons of patients with concomitant adenomas (584) has prompted speculation that hyperplastic polyps are biomarkers of colorectal neoplasia and that the associations are causally related. Some suggest that hyperplastic polyps may be a marker for an environmental factor implicated in the progression of adenomas to carcinomas (585). Alternatively, individuals may be constitutionally prone to the development of both the adenomas and hyperplastic polyps, and they may require similar environmental conditions for their development. The lesions, or at least some of the lesions, may not be as innocuous as once believed since they contain a variety of genetic abnormalities. There is evidence of dysregulated cell proliferation and apoptosis (582,586,587). The

presence of clonal genetic alterations, including *K-ras* (588–590), *BRAF* (590), and *TGFβRII* mutations; DNA microsatellite instability; and loss of the APC, p53, p16 genes and a tumor suppressor gene on chromosome 1p has led to the suggestion that hyperplastic polyps are "neoplastic" but lack malignant potential (591). There is also methylation of the DNA repair gene O^{6}methylguanine DNA methyltransferase (MGMT) in some hyperplastic polyps (592).

It appears that a subset of "hyperplastic polyps" may be a biomarker of increased risk or even represent a subtype carrying a significant malignant potential (592). These are now commonly referred to as *sessile serrated polyps* or *sessile serrated adenomas* as discussed further in Chapter 14. Identical DNA microsatellite alterations can be found in the hyperplastic and adenomatous regions of mixed hyperplastic–adenomatous polyps, suggesting that the two lesions are sequentially related (591). Features that might suggest the presence of a hyperplastic polyp with malignant potential include those listed in Table 13.29 (591).

Hyperplastic polyps are pale, sessile nodules usually developing on the crest of mucosal folds. The lesions are often multiple and appear as small mucosal elevations (Fig. 13.164), usually measuring <5 mm in diameter and rarely measuring >1 cm; most arise in the sigmoid and rectum. Their surfaces appear smooth and glistening, and the lesions are usually slightly paler than the surrounding mucosa. Hyperplastic polyps are significantly smaller and lighter in color than adenomas. Endoscopically, it is not possible to distinguish between small adenomas and hyperplastic polyps, so the lesions tend to be biopsied.

Hyperplastic polyps consist of groups of elongated hyperplastic colonic crypts. The upper half of the crypt contains characteristic intraluminal papillary infoldings. These infoldings result from an expanded replication zone and a slower rate of maturation that give the crypt a serrated or saw-toothed appearance (593). While the proliferative zone is lengthened, it is still restricted to the bottom of the crypt. Epithelium lining the crypts contains a mixture of absorptive, goblet, and endocrine cells (594). Absorptive columnar cells predominate over goblet cells. The upper part of the crypts appears crowed by a population of hypermature goblet cells, which are usually larger than normal due to intracellular mucin accumulations. The nuclei remain in a basal

---

TABLE 13.29 **Features that May Indicate "Hyperplastic Polyps" with a Malignant Potential**

- Unusual numbers (more than 20)
- Unusual size (>10 mm)
- Location in the proximal colon
- Presence of high-grade dysplasia
- Coincidental adenomas
- First-degree relatives with high-risk hyperplastic polyps
- First-degree relatives with colon cancer

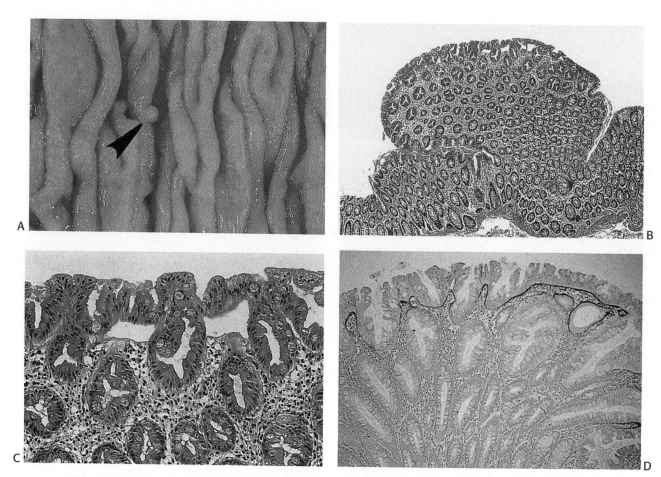

FIG. 13.164. Hyperplastic polyp. **A:** The hyperplastic polyps usually occur on mucosal folds and have the same color as the surrounding mucosa (*arrowhead*). **B:** Low-power view of a hyperplastic polyp. **C:** Higher power magnification demonstrates the stellate lumens and thickened collagen table. **D:** Higher power magnification of the thickened collagen table stained with antibodies to collagen IV.

location and are typically enlarged and vesicular with a prominent nucleolus. Atypical mitoses are rare. The bases of the crypts appear hyperchromatic and immature, resembling adenomatous epithelium. However, unlike adenomas, the epithelium matures as one progresses up the crypt toward the lumen. A large proportion of hyperplastic polyps also contain a hybrid epithelium with bidirectional differentiation toward both gastric foveolar and colonic epithelium in the same crypt (595). The replicative zone of the crypt, which contains mitotically active cells, is expanded and may comprise its lower half (Fig. 13.164). A hyperplastic pericryptal myofibroblast sheath associates with the hyperplastic epithelium. It produces an increased amount of collagen, a feature best appreciated under the free surface where there is a thickened collagen table. These lesions may become inflamed and when they do they may appear mucin depleted.

Serrated crypts, a hallmark of the hyperplastic polyp, may be seen in the regenerative mucosa in a number of settings including IBD, mucosal prolapse, and juvenile polyps. The major entity in the differential diagnosis of the hyperplastic

polyp is the serrated adenoma discussed in Chapter 14. The two lesions are compared in Table 13.30.

Inverted Hyperplastic Polyp

A variant of the hyperplastic polyp, the so-called inverted hyperplastic polyp, may simulate a carcinoma and may appear to invade the underlying submucosa. The lesions affect both sexes and patients are generally older than 50 years. The lesions tend to develop in the rectum or sigmoid and range in size from 0.2 to 1 cm with a mean size of 0.5 (596). These lesions resemble hyperplastic polyps, but instead of being solely exophytic, groups of glands lie beneath the level of the mucosa, forming one or more lobulated submucosal nodules (Fig. 13.165). There may also be a mixed pattern of lobules and distorted crypts. The overlying mucosa contains glands typical of hyperplastic polyps arranged as a sessile nodule or in a flat patch. Pedunculation is absent. The endophytic nodules show a peripheral hyperbasophilic proliferative zone and a central area of pale, more mature cells with characteristic serrated tubular profiles seen

TABLE 13.30 Hyperplastic Polyp Versus Serrated Adenoma

Feature	Hyperplastic Polyp	Serrated Adenoma
Size	Generally <0.5	Generally >0.5
Mitoses	A few at the crypt base	Abundant, the length of the crypt
Nuclear atypia	Mild at base	Mild to marked, the length of the crypt
Surface maturation	Hypermature	Immature
Crypt dilation	Surface	Base
Cytoplasmic eosinophilia	No	Yes
Surface nuclear stratification	No	Yes
Horizontal crypts	No	Yes
Collagen table	Thicker than normal	Thinner than normal

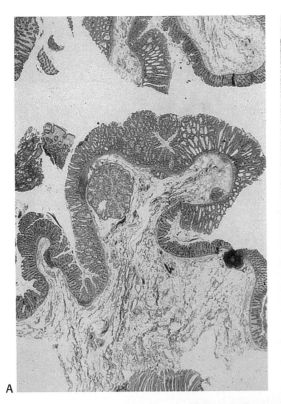

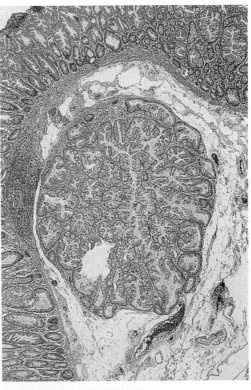

A

B

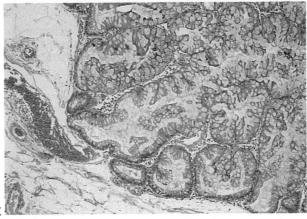

C

FIG. 13.165. Inverted hyperplastic polyp. **A:** Low magnification showing the presence of a prominent mucosal fold that contains an area of epithelium within the submucosa. This is seen better at higher magnification in **B.** The epithelium appears hyperplastic with a gradient of differentiation extending from the periphery of the lesion to its center. The crypt bases lie radially arranged at the periphery of this lesion. **C:** Higher magnification showing the edge of the lesion with the crypt bases and the serrated lumen as one approaches the center of the lesion. The absence of cytologic atypia distinguishes this from an invasive carcinoma. The presence of the glandular infoldings and prominent goblet cells distinguishes this lesion from colitis cystica profunda. Cytologically, the cells appear histologically identical to those seen in hyperplastic polyps.

in hyperplastic polyps. In contrast to the usual exophytic hyperplastic polyp, the endophytic elements exhibit a more complex growth pattern, sometimes demonstrating back-to-back glandular arrangements and intraluminal budding. The epithelial lining lacks dysplasia. Occasionally, lymphoid nodules intermingle with the lesions. Multiple endophytic lesions may be present. The muscularis mucosae appears to stretch thinly around the deep aspect of smaller lesions and is incomplete around larger nodules (596,597). When cut tangentially, one may see splaying and dissociation of the muscularis mucosae. Downward extension of hyperplastic tubules projecting into the submucosal lymphatics when sectioned obliquely simulates invasion. Fresh hemorrhage, vascular congestion, or hemosiderin may be present around the glands. The lesions arise secondary to trauma-induced protrusion of the glands through breaks in the muscularis mucosae, often near lymphoid aggregates.

Inflammatory Fibroid Polyp

Inflammatory fibroid polyps are uncommon tumorlike lesions arising in the submucosa. They are most common in the stomach and small intestine (see Chapters 2 and 4), but they occasionally develop in the rectum. Rectal lesions demonstrate the same histology as those occurring more proximally. The histology of these lesions is discussed further in Chapter 6.

Fibroblastic Polyps

Fibroblastic polyps are a recently described distinctive type of colorectal mesenchymal polyp (598,599). The lesions develop in individuals ranging in age from 37 to 84 with a mean of 60 years and with a moderate female predominance. They occur almost exclusively in the left and distal colon and generally measure <10 mm in size. They are solitary lesions that occur alone or coexist with hyperplastic polyps. They contain a mucosal proliferation of bland, plump, monomorphic spindled cells with oval nuclei arranged as bundles parallel to the surface or as haphazardly arranged sheets with focal periglandular or perivascular arrangements. Some polyps display a vague zoning arrangement with superficial bundles of spindle cells arranged parallel to the surface changing to deeper haphazardly arranged sheets of cells. There may be a thin rim of uninvolved, mildly inflamed lamina propria separating the fibroblastic cells from the superficial lining. The proliferating spindle cells can lead to a wide separation and disorganization of the crypts. The muscularis mucosae may appear slightly disorganized.

There may also be a subset of lesions that contain serrated crypts that are referred to as mixed *fibroblastic–hyperplastic polyps.* The spindle cell areas in fibroblastic polyps are positive for vimentin and negative for S100 protein, c-kit, epithelial membrane antigen, cytokeratin, CD34, CD68, COX-2, and factor XIIIa. Ultrastructurally they exhibit the features of fibroblastic cells (598,599).

Inflammatory Pseudopolyps

Inflammatory pseudopolyps are not true mucosal proliferations. Rather, they are areas of inflamed regenerating mucosa that project into the colonic lumen. As a result they may grossly resemble pedunculated or sessile adenomas (Fig. 13.166). Exceptionally, they may be very large, owing principally to an expansion of the stromal fibrous tissue. Such polyps often have an irregular surface. They have no malignant potential but their presence does not rule out other lesions in the colon. Inflammatory polyps occur most frequently in patients with colitis and sites of mucosal injury, including ulcers and anastomoses. They often appear as multiple, small sessile, sometimes ulcerated polyps.

The ulcerated mucosa is partially replaced by exuberant, edematous granulation tissue admixed with an intense inflammatory cell infiltrate. The lamina propria contains dilated crypts with both epithelial degeneration and regeneration and variable surface erosion. The crypts typically appear irregularly branched, dilated, and regenerative. Cryptitis and crypt abscesses may be prominent. Occasionally, hyperchromatic mucin-depleted regenerative epithelium simulates adenomatous epithelium. However, in contrast to adenomatous tissue, the epithelium usually shows evidence of maturation toward the surface. In patients with ulcerative colitis the changes mimic dysplasia, but the inflammatory background should alert one to being careful to not overdiagnose the lesions as dysplasia. The lesions may also contain marked atypia as described below. The lesions may also mimic juvenile polyps and the polyps of some of the rare polyposis syndromes discussed in Chapter 12. A knowledge of the clinical features (the presence of a polyposis syndrome or a colitis) helps distinguish between these possibilities.

Inflammatory Polyps with Bizarre Stromal Cells

A small group of inflammatory polyps contain bizarre stromal cells that may be mistaken for a malignancy. Most lesions occur in middle-aged or elderly patients (600,601). Large, bizarre, mesenchymal cells are present. These appear as atypical, spindled, stellate, epithelioid, or large round cells within the lamina propria or in granulation tissue. They have abundant amphophilic cytoplasm, vesicular nuclei, and large eosinophilic inclusionlike nucleoli. Because of the inclusion-like nature of the nuclei, the cells may be confused with CMV infections, but immunohistochemical stains for CMV are negative. They are usually dispersed in a zone under the ulcerated or regenerated mucosa without infiltrating the deeper stroma (Fig 13.167). Sometimes the atypical cells blend into the granulation tissue. Multinucleated and giant cell forms are also present. Rarely, atypical pale epithelioid cells form round, cohesive clusters resembling acini or vascular structures (600,601). Lack of staining with cytokeratin rules out a carcinoma. Mitotic figures are uncommon and atypical mitoses are absent. The cells do not contain mucin

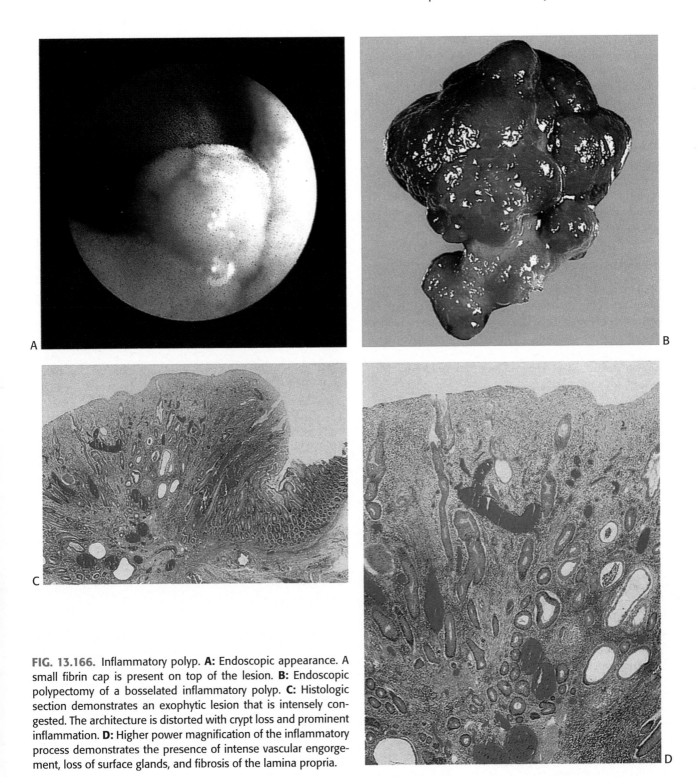

FIG. 13.166. Inflammatory polyp. **A:** Endoscopic appearance. A small fibrin cap is present on top of the lesion. **B:** Endoscopic polypectomy of a bosselated inflammatory polyp. **C:** Histologic section demonstrates an exophytic lesion that is intensely congested. The architecture is distorted with crypt loss and prominent inflammation. **D:** Higher power magnification of the inflammatory process demonstrates the presence of intense vascular engorgement, loss of surface glands, and fibrosis of the lamina propria.

or glycogen. These cells lie within the inflammatory exudate and any associated epithelial elements usually appear benign or reactive in nature. They stain strongly for vimentin and sometimes for muscle-specific actin, a phenotype that is consistent with reactive fibroblasts or myofibroblasts (601).

Misinterpretation of these reactive changes can result in unnecessary radical surgery. These lesions can be particularly confusing when encountered in small biopsies in which the entire tissue context is lost. However, immunostains should resolve their true nature, but in case of doubt the area can be rebiopsied.

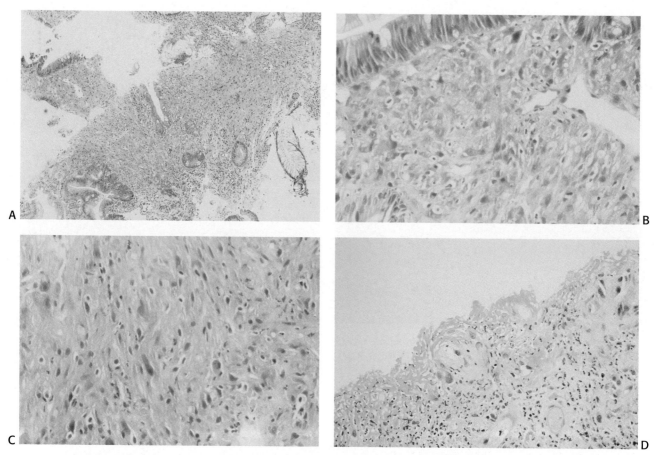

FIG. 13.167. Inflammatory polyp with stromal atypia. **A:** This low-magnification picture shows that there is significant disruption of the colonic mucosal architecture. **B:** Higher magnification shows the regenerative glands and a lamina propria filled with a proliferation of very atypical epithelioidlike spindle cells. These cells were cytokeratin, actin, S100, CD34, and CD117 negative. **C:** The usual mononuclear cells of the lamina propria are replaced by a spindle cell proliferation. **D:** Section from a different polyp with atypia that centers around the capillaries.

Inflammatory Cap Polyps

Inflammatory cap polyps develop in the setting of anorectal mucosal prolapse, affecting patients of all ages. The patients present with diarrhea, mucoid stools, gastrointestinal bleeding, and/or tenesmus. The lesions usually arise in the rectosigmoid and are often multiple, measuring in size from a few millimeters to 2 cm (602). The lesions lie on the crests of the mucosal folds separated by normal or edematous mucosa. They likely arise secondary to transitory mild ischemia that occurs when the mucosa and submucosa prolapse.

These nonneoplastic lesions consist of elongated, tortuous hyperplastic crypts. These are frequently dilated and inflamed. There is acute and chronic inflammation in the lamina propria and a characteristic cap of inflamed granulation tissue and fibrin covers the mouths of adjacent crypts (Fig. 13.168). The polyps may mimic hyperplastic polyps or adenomas, except for the distinctive covering cap. The stroma frequently contains hyperplastic frayed smooth muscle

bundles extending up from the muscularis mucosae, a feature commonly seen in anorectal mucosal prolapse.

Lymphoid Polyps and Lymphonodular Hyperplasia

Large intestinal lymphoid polyps and focal lymphoid hyperplasia most commonly arise in the rectum. They may reflect a reactive change to a prior inflammatory episode. Most patients are children, adolescents, or adults under the age of 50. Prolapse of a rectal mass, rectal bleeding, constipation, diarrhea, and discomfort may be presenting symptoms. The lesion presents as single or multiple sessile polyps or as a cobblestoned Mucosa. The "polyps" measure from 0.5 to 5 cm in diameter and have an intact mucosal surface. Some lesions appear to result from a hypersensitivity reaction to food because the patients have high IgE levels and increased intestinal permeability (603). Histologically the lesions are well circumscribed and they often have prominent germinal

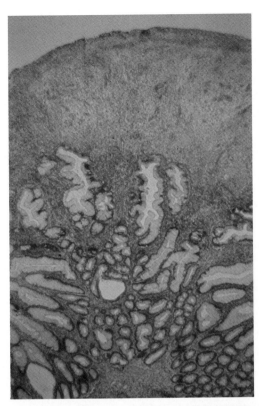

FIG. 13.168. Inflammatory cap polyp. The regenerative glands at the bases are covered by a cap of granulation tissue that spans the surface of many glands. (Photograph courtesy of Dr. Geraint Williams, University of Wales, Cardiff, Wales.)

centers. The lymphocytes are well differentiated without atypia or mitoses.

Bilharzial Polyp

An interesting inflammatory polyp that is rare in the United States but common in Egypt and other tropical countries is the bilharzial polyp. It results from schistosomal infections. Grossly, the polyps are hard and as they develop they become polypoid. They are covered by a layer of normal mucosa but their inner core consists of a mass of granulomatous tissue, ova, and, occasionally, female worms (Fig. 13.131). A true stalk gradually develops.

Juvenile Polyps

Juvenile (or retention) polyps develop most commonly in children, but they may occur in persons of any age. They present as single or multiple lesions. They invariably have a smooth, lobulated surface. The histologic features are predominantly inflammatory with a variable but usually prominent degree of cystic dilation of the glands admixed with inflammation and regeneration. These lesions are discussed further in Chapter 12.

Peutz-Jeghers Polyps

Peutz-Jeghers polyps contain a mature epithelium lining arborizing proliferations of the muscularis mucosae. They occur as part of an autosomal dominant syndrome that includes polyps in the stomach and intestines, as well as mucocutaneous pigmentation and genital tumors. The polyps tend to involve the small bowel but they may also involve the colon, either as solitary lesions or as part of PJS. This syndrome is discussed further in Chapter 12.

Isolated Colonic Hamartomas

Colonic hamartomas are localized, nonneoplastic growths usually consisting of disorganized overgrown normal mature tissues whose cellular elements are similar to those of the organ in which the lesion is found. GI hamartomas are usually thought of as belonging to patients with PJS. However, other rare hamartomas occur. Hamartomas identical to those found in PJS affect patients with tuberous sclerosis (604,605). Rare lesions consist of a mixture of mature adipose tissue lying between simple benign glands (605). Other lesions consist of a proliferation of smooth muscle cells lying between the glands (Fig. 13.169). These lack the typical arborizing pattern of Peutz-Jeghers polyps.

Inflammatory Myoglandular Polyps

Inflammatory myoglandular polyps (IMGs) are a unique subset of colorectal polyps (606). Patients range in age from 15 to 78 years, and they lack evidence of IBD or other inflammatory colitides. Endoscopic examination reveals solitary pedunculated, smooth-surfaced, red polyps. The pedunculated polyps occur in the left colon, particularly in the sigmoid, and often have a long stalk. They may be asymptomatic and found at the time of screening colonoscopy or they may cause rectal bleeding. They measure up to 2.5 cm in diameter and their cut surface reveals the presence of mucin-filled cysts. The spherical head of the polyps consists of hyperplastic glands, often with a serrated appearance or with occasional cystic dilation. The surface of the polyp appears eroded, without a fibrinous exudate. It is also covered by regenerating epithelium. Acute and chronically inflamed granulation tissue with engorged capillaries is present in the lamina propria. Many neutrophils populate the eroded areas at the periphery of the lesion. Hemosiderin deposition in the lamina propria is common.

The polyps superficially resemble juvenile polyps, inflammatory polyps, and Peutz-Jeghers polyps. However, their unique feature is the presence of radially arranged smooth muscle in the central lamina propria. Smooth muscle bundles are unusual in inflammatory and juvenile polyps. The presence of the inflammation and the cystically dilated glands are unusual for Peutz-Jeghers polyps.

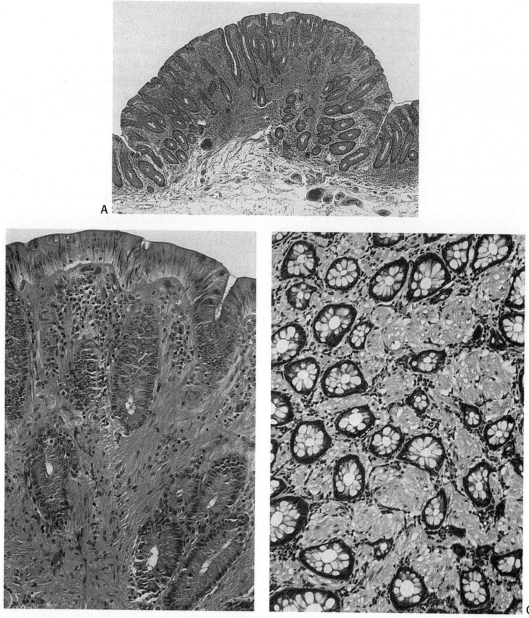

FIG. 13.169. Colonic hamartoma. **A:** Cross section through a "polyp" that demonstrates an intermingling between bands of smooth muscle and the glands. There is no clear demarcation between the smooth muscle proliferation and the muscularis mucosae. The lack of clear demarcation of the smooth muscle bundles from the intimately admixed glands distinguishes the lesion from a leiomyoma arising from the muscularis mucosae. The lesion arose in the transverse colon, distinguishing it from an area of prolapse. **B:** The lesion at higher magnification with the intermingling of smooth muscle bundles and glands. **C:** Specimen from another lesion cut in cross section showing the intermingled mixture of the smooth muscle bundles and glands.

Polyps due to Atheromatous Emboli

Rare atheromatous emboli-associated polyps have been described in the colon (607,608). The polyps are multiple, ranging from 0.3 to 1.9 cm in greatest dimension, and they usually localize to a specific colonic segment. They have an edematous submucosa and a superficially ulcerated mucosa. Microscopically, arterioles within the submucosa contain organized atheroemboli. The overlying mucosa is largely replaced by granulation tissue with focal coagulative necrosis present in the residual mucosa. The remainder of the bowel is unremarkable (608).

Granuloma Pyogenicum

The intestinal counterpart of pyogenic granuloma presents as an ulcerated, polypoid growth with either a sessile or pedunculated configuration. Histologically, it consists of lobular

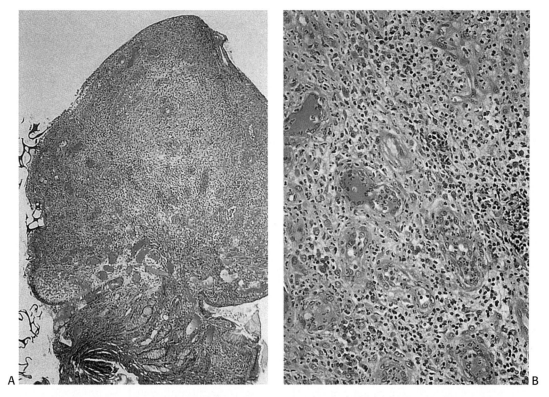

FIG. 13.170. Pyogenic granuloma. **A:** Typical configuration of the pyogenic granuloma arising from the mucosal surface. **B:** Higher power magnification showing the granulation tissue components.

proliferations of variably sized capillaries in an edematous stroma. The capillaries are lined by a single layer of flattened or rounded endothelial cells supported by sparse spindle cells and a delicate collagenous stroma. Endothelial swelling may be prominent. Capillary endothelial hyperplasia is absent. The stroma contains variable numbers of inflammatory cells and varying degrees of edema (Fig. 13.170). This angiomatous lesion has an unclear pathogenesis.

Filiform Polyposis

Filiform polyposis usually accompanies IBD. However, it occasionally is seen in the absence of known CD or UC. It presents as localized clusters of multiple fingerlike mucosal extensions, which can reach several centimeters in length (Fig. 13.171). Histologic sections demonstrate the presence of mucosal extensions supported by submucosa. The overlying

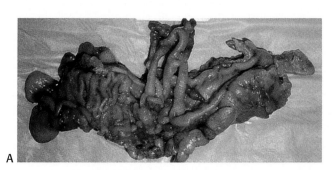
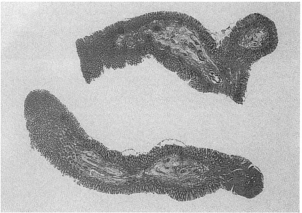

FIG. 13.171. Filiform polyposis. **A:** Gross specimen illustrating the presence of a cluster of fingerlike mucosal extensions. **B:** Biopsy from this patient showing the presence of tissue lined on both sides by colonic epithelium. It is relatively normal and supported by a submucosa containing strands of smooth muscle.

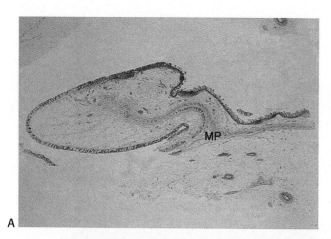
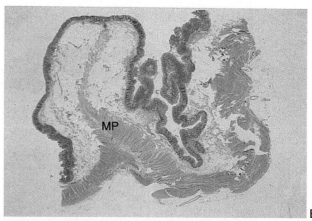

FIG. 13.172. Lipomatous hypertrophy of the ileocecal valve. **A:** Pedunculated polyp from the cecum that has a short, narrow stalk. The muscularis propria (*MP*) extends to the middle of the lesion. The majority of the lesion consists of fatty tissue. It is not well demarcated and contained within a fibrous capsule, as would be expected for a lipoma. **B:** A similar lesion that was less obviously pedunculated. The muscularis mucosae extends into the center of the lesion and nonencapsulated fatty tissue lies on either side.

mucosa generally appears relatively normal except in the case of IBD. These lesions may be received as biopsy specimens, in which case all one gets are long, fingerlike extensions of mucosa with a central submucosal core containing variable smooth muscle fibers. Often the thin structures show mucosa on both sides of the specimen.

Lipomatous Hypertrophy of the Ileocecal Valve

The ileocecal valve sometimes presents as a cecal polyp, usually as the result of lipomatous hypertrophy. This lesion is easily identified because it consists of an expansion of the submucosal fatty tissues. These do not form a well-rounded mass. Generally, the muscularis propria is thrown up into this polypoid projection and is usually seen in the center of the lesion (Fig. 13.172).

Prominent Mucosal Folds

Prominent mucosal folds may appear to the endoscopist as a polypoid lesion and may therefore be biopsied. These are usually areas of mucosal prolapse and they occur most frequently in patients with an underlying motility disorder including diverticular disease. They are discussed further in Chapter 10.

Reactive Fibromuscular Proliferations

Reactive fibromuscular proliferations consist of mucosal and submucosal proliferating mature smooth muscle cells often admixed with vessels, neural tissue, and even ganglion cells. These lesions usually complicate other disorders such as IBD. They vary in size from several millimeters to 3 or 4 cm in diameter. The mucosa generally appears regenerative with

branched crypts. Evidence of active inflammation is absent. However, there may be mild chronic inflammation both in the mucosa and in the submucosa. The underlying submucosa is variably obliterated by a proliferation of smooth muscle cells, vessels, and neural tissue. Immunostains of such lesions generally show a mixture of actin-positive cells intermingled with S100- or synaptophysin-positive cells corresponding to neural tissue. The demarcation between the muscularis mucosae and the underlying submucosa is lost. These lesions may progress on to a more mature and densely cellular stromal core that consists almost exclusively of smooth muscle tissue intermingled with other normal elements. The submucosa becomes completely obliterated. The etiology of these lesions is obscure, but they appear to represent reparative responses (Fig. 13.173).

ENDOMETRIOSIS AND ENDOSALPINGIOSIS

Colonic involvement occurs in 3% to 34% of women with endometriosis. Patients range in age from 28 to 56 years (609). Recurrent, crampy, mild abdominal pain is the most common presenting symptom. Patients may also present with nausea, vomiting, diarrhea, constipation, small-caliber stools, fever, anorexia, weight loss, hematochezia, a mass, intestinal obstruction, and infertility. Because of the predominantly serosal and subserosal location of the tissue, rectal bleeding is infrequent. An episodic and cyclic nature of the intestinal symptoms just prior to menstruation clinically suggests the diagnosis. However, symptoms coincide with menstruation in <50% of cases (610). Extensive and deep involvement of the intestinal wall (Fig. 13.174) or the inflammatory adhesions produced by resolution of recurrent episodes of bleeding may lead to intestinal obstruction,

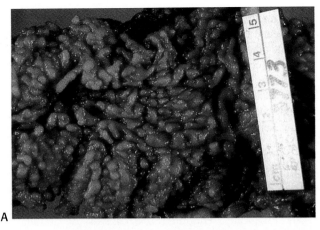

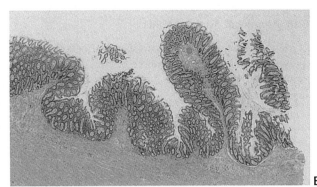

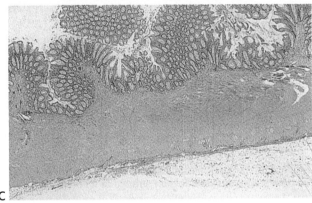

FIG. 13.173. Reactive fibromuscular proliferations. A through C are from the same specimen. **A:** Grossly innumerable short, stubby, mucosal projections are present. **B:** These consist of mucosal elevations by a proliferation of smooth muscle mixed with vessels and nerves. There is complete loss of the demarcation between the muscularis mucosae, submucosa, and muscularis propria. **C:** Higher magnification showing the obliteration of these normal landmarks.

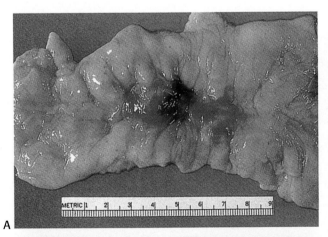

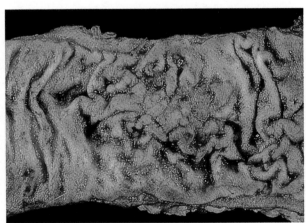

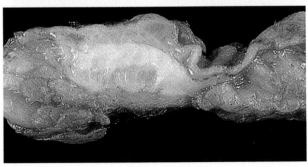

FIG. 13.174. Endometriosis. **A:** Gross appearance of the fresh specimen with prominent mucosal puckering and localized hemorrhage. **B:** Fixed specimen with submucosal endometriosis. **C:** Cross section through the bowel wall of previous specimen demonstrates prominent mucosal fibrosis.

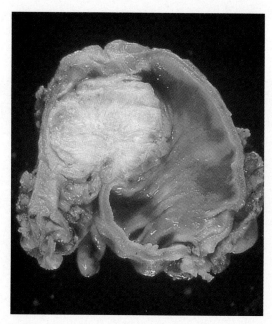

FIG. 13.175. Endometriosis presenting grossly as a cecal carcinoma.

volvulus, or intussusception. Rarely, the disorder presents as an acute abdomen. Terminal ileal disease mimics malignancy, strictures from previous radiotherapy, CD, ischemia, and infections such as *Yersinia* and tuberculosis (Fig. 13.175).

Intestinal endometriosis commonly affects those parts of the bowel that lie in proximity to genital organs. The sigmoid is the most commonly affected portion of the large bowel, followed by the rectum (611), with these two sites accounting for 70% of cases. The lesions present grossly as intramural masses of strictures or stenosis, polyps, or submucosal masses simulating a carcinoma. The serosal surface is often puckered secondary to extensive subserosal fibrosis. This may lead to secondary stricture formation. The presence of a hard annular growth that usually spares the mucosa may simulate a carcinoma. Adhesions to adjacent structures may develop. Cut sections of the bowel wall may disclose the presence of small intramural tarry or chocolate cysts.

Histologically, endometriosis consists of islands of endometrial tissue in the serosa, muscularis propria, submucosa, or rarely the mucosa of the GI tract (Fig. 13.176). Rarely, endometriosis extends into pericolonic soft tissues, invades blood vessels and their lumens, infiltrates nerves, and spreads to the pericolonic lymph nodes. Since the heterotopic endometrial tissue functions in a manner analogous to eutopic endometrial tissue, it cycles through both the proliferative and secretory phases of the menstrual cycle, and it may slough as in menstruation. As a consequence of the sloughing and bleeding, there may be regeneration of the endometrial tissues or scarring with evidence of prior hemorrhage.

The diagnosis is easily made when one identifies endometrial glands surrounded by endometrial stroma. The endometrial glands are distinguishable from colonic glands due to

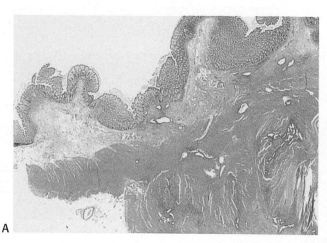

A

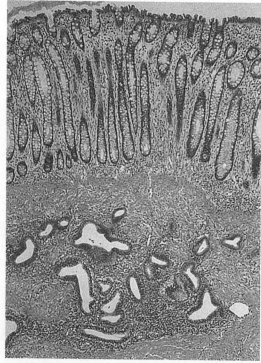

B

FIG. 13.176. Histologic sections of the lesion shown in Figure 13.175. **A:** Endometrial glands and stroma are present in the submucosa and muscularis propria. **B:** Higher magnification demonstrates the irregular arrangement of the glands surrounded by endometrial stroma.

TABLE 13.31 Comparison of Endometriosis and Colitis Cystica Profunda

Feature	Endometriosis	Colitis Cystica Profunda
Epithelium	Non–mucin-secreting endometrial glands; sometimes the glands appear dilated	Mucin-producing colorectal epithelium
Stroma	Dense and spindled	Loose lamina propria
Stromal changes, hemosiderin and fibrosis	May be present	May be present
CEA immunoreactivity	−	+

CEA, carcinoembryonic antigen.

their lack of mucin and the presence of ciliated cells. The endometrial stroma differs from normal lamina propria in that the tissue appears more compact and the stromal cells appear elongated with slightly rounded nuclei. There is often a zone of hemorrhage or fibrous tissue containing hemosiderin. In some instances the amount of endometrial stroma is disproportionate to the glandular component. In its most extreme form one may only see islands of extensive fibrosis containing hemosiderin-laden macrophages and it may be difficult to recognize the true nature of the lesion.

The surrounding mucosa may show signs of chronic injury including architectural distortion, lymphoplasmacytic infiltrates, pyloric metaplasia, ischemia, segmental acute colitis and ulceration, and rarely fissures. There may be evidence of mucosal prolapse (609). The intestinal wall may show marked concentric smooth muscle hyperplasia and hypertrophy, neuronal hypertrophy and hyperplasia, fibrosis, and serositis (609).

Endometriosis may mimic colitis cystica profunda (see Fig. 13.50), and the distinction between the two lesions can be difficult. The major difference between the two entities lies in the nature of the epithelium and its surrounding stroma (Table 13.31), particularly in the absence of the typical endometrial stroma accompanying the endometrial-lining epithelium. The lesions might also mimic ischemia or CD. This is particularly true when superficial mucosal biopsies are examined that show architectural distortion. The presence of crypt abscesses and cryptitis may further suggest the diagnosis of IBD. Rarely, areas of endometriosis may show extensive myxoid changes that may lead to an erroneous diagnosis of pseudomyxoma peritonei (612). Areas of endometriosis may also give rise to neoplasms including endometrioid adenocarcinomas, müllerian adenosarcomas, endometrial stroma sarcomas, endometrioid adenofibroma with borderline malignancy adenocarcinoma in situ, and atypical hyperplasia (613).

Endosalpingiosis is characterized by the presence of benign glands lined by ciliated tubal-type epithelium. The cells are believed to derive from the peritoneal mesothelial cells as part of the secondary müllerian system. It is one of the triad of nonneoplastic secondary müllerian lesions, the others being endometriosis and endocervicosis (614). It may

affect the colon, where it is usually found as an incidental finding. Rarely it presents as a mass simulating a neoplasm (614). The histologic features are illustrated in Chapter 8.

Inflammatory Pseudotumors

Any transmural inflammatory process, such as CD or diverticulitis, may present clinically as a mass lesion. Usually fistulae with an exuberant secondary inflammatory reaction cause the lesions. These inflammatory pseudotumors consist of variable admixtures of fat necrosis and fibrous proliferation. Radiologically, fibrous stranding is seen in the area of the lesion. Mesothelial cells may become entrapped within the inflammatory masses, leading to the development of mesothelial inclusion cysts or inducing marked mesothelial hyperplasia. If the lesion develops as a result of an abscess, one may see the residual acute and/or chronic inflammation associated with the abscess or one may see marked xanthogranulomatous inflammation. Additionally, if the mass results from fistulization from the bowel lumen, foreign material, particularly food or feces, may be present.

EFFECTS OF SURGERY AND THERAPEUTIC PROCEDURES
Endoscopic Thermal Injury

Endoscopic resection of colorectal polyps is currently a standard practice. In general, the resection margin passes through the submucosa. Less than 1% of patients perforate following the procedure (615). Perforations could result from the surgical resection of the colonic wall or from thermal injury. The postendoscopic resection sites show a range of mucosal changes including ulceration. Submucosal changes include inflammation, granulation tissue, fibrosis, and vascular proliferations. If changes are present in the muscularis propria, they may have a "skip" appearance. These consist of patchy muscular depletion or necrosis in the inner muscular layer with or without accompanying fibrosis. Ink may also be seen (615).

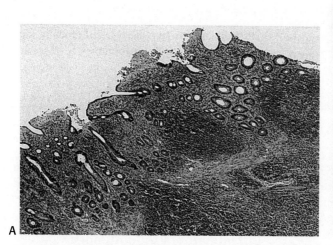
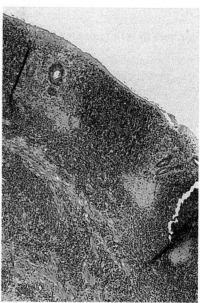

FIG. 13.177. Diversion colitis. The specimen is from a patient who had a previous resection for Crohn disease. The specimen is from the diverted segment. **A:** Marked lymphonodular hyperplasia with variable ulceration of the surface. **B:** This specimen is from an area of marked glandular atrophy. The bases of the glands are widely separated from the muscularis mucosae. The lamina propria is intensely infiltrated by lymphocytes and plasma cells.

Diversion Colitis

The term *diversion colitis* refers to the inflammation that occurs in the defunctionalized intestinal segment following diversion of the fecal stream. The changes may remain asymptomatic or give rise to rectal bleeding or discharge (616,617). Its importance lies in the inability to differentiate it from other types of proctitis, such as ulcerative colitis. The lesion completely resolves following restoration of the continuity of the fecal stream.

The pathophysiology of the changes are thought to relate to a decrease in mucosal nutrition since short-chain fatty acids that derive from the bacterial fermentation of starch and proteins are the main metabolic fuels for colonocytes, especially distally (618). A change in the bacterial flora in the defunctionalized segment may also lead to the inflammation.

Patients with diversion colitis present with continuing GI symptoms, including constipation or diarrhea with mucoid or bloody discharge and crampy abdominal pain. Endoscopically, the bowel may show erythema; petechial hemorrhages; mucosal friability; mucosal nodularity, sometimes surrounded by aphthous ulcers; nonspecific colitis; and inspissated mucus (619). Patients may also present with the underlying disorder for which the original colonic surgery and diversion were performed, such as IBD.

Inflammation develops in up to 72% of patients (Fig. 13.177). Biopsies taken from the distal diverted intestine show relatively nonspecific changes, including aphthous ulcers, focal crypt abscesses, surface exudates, surface epithelial cell degeneration, and prominent follicular hyperplasia.

It is the lymphoid hyperplasia that produces the fine mucosal nodularity. Many of the mucosal lymphoid follicles have overlying small, punctate erosions forming classic aphthous ulcers. With time, the mucosal inflammation becomes more extensive, leading to the development of ulcers and inflammatory pseudopolyps. Inflammation occurs diffusely throughout the lamina propria and is mainly chronic in nature, but it may include some neutrophils with consequent cryptitis and crypt abscess formation. Subsequently, muciphages may become prominent in the lower half of the lamina propria.

The feature that serves to distinguish diversion colitis from other forms of colitis is the consistent presence of lymphoid follicular hyperplasia (620). This lymphoid hyperplasia is particularly striking in patients with CD (Fig. 13.177), even in those who had a lack of histologic evidence in Crohn disease in the defunctionalized rectum prior to diversion. Severe cases of diversion colitis histologically resemble ulcerative colitis. However, the lack of crypt distortion and the presence of lymphoid follicular hyperplasia resembling follicular proctitis should lead to the correct diagnosis in patients without pre-existing IBD. Intramucosal granulomas sometimes form in response to ruptured crypts, possibly leading to an erroneous diagnosis of CD. However, again, the lack of diffuse mucosal inflammation, crypt distortion, and true granulomas should help avoid this diagnosis. In patients who have had pre-existing IBD, particularly CD, the diagnosis is more difficult and clinically the question is whether the inflammation is recurrence of CD or development of diversion colitis. In

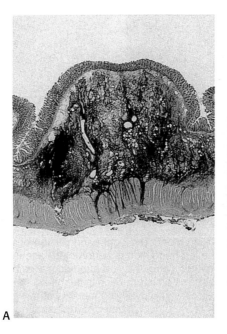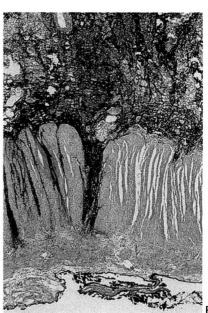

FIG. 13.178. Colonic tattoo. **A:** Low-mount photograph demonstrating the presence of a collection of India ink in the submucosa dissecting its way through the muscularis propria. **B:** Higher magnification.

some instances, it may be impossible to tell the difference and resolution of the question relies on mucosal restoration following reanastomosis.

Colostomies

Colostomies undergo various changes. If the patient has had IBD, inflammation may represent disease remission at the colostomy site. Colostomies also develop nonspecific inflammation, usually manifesting as an increase in the number of mononuclear cells infiltrating the lamina propria. The mucosa usually appears chronically damaged as evidenced by the presence of branched or irregularly shaped glands. Focal ischemia and features of mucosal prolapse are generally present.

Intestinal Effects of Endoscopic Tattooing

GI tattooing is sometimes used to mark specific features of the GI mucosa at the time of endoscopy. It is used to facilitate the location of biopsy sites or other sites of interest at the time of subsequent biopsy or surgery. Permanent tattoos are used for the long-term endoscopic follow-up of polyps or other suspicious lesions. The tattoos are produced by introduction of nondegradable pigments into the submucosa. The most commonly used substance is India ink, but others include methylene blue and indocyanine green. Submucosal injection of sterile ink produces a zone of blue-black discoloration that is grossly visible from both the mucosal and serosal surfaces. Of the various substances used to produce the tattoos, only India ink and indocyanine green persist for as long as 7 days.

Adverse effects following colonoscopic injection of India ink include focal peritonitis, abscess, fat necrosis, and inflammatory pseudotumors (621). The mechanisms by which India ink produces its effects are unknown. Adverse effects may result from the invasion of tissue by GI flora or from toxic ingredients in the preparation itself (622).

Histologically, one sees an architecturally normal mucosa with an irregular circumscribed area of black pigment deposition within the submucosa. The pigment lies within the cytoplasm of histiocytes as well as extracellularly (Fig. 13.178). Early reactions to India ink include necrosis, edema, and neutrophilic infiltrates into the submucosa and muscularis propria. Vessels are inflamed but without fibrinoid necrosis. In contrast, early reactions to methylene blue include ischemic ulceration, necrosis, and eosinophilic infiltration in the submucosa as well as fibrinoid necrosis of the vessel walls. Obliterative intimal fibrosis complicates the repair of the methylene blue injuries. These changes are absent from colons injected with India ink (623).

Because of the inflammation associated with these agents, some advocate that the injection site be completely resected at the time of definitive surgery (623). When handling such specimens, one should report whether the ink site has been completely removed and the extent of the damage associated with the ink.

Other Effects

Ureterosigmoidostomy replaced urinary diversion by ileal conduits. These procedures may be complicated by the development of polypoid lesions at the site of ureteric implantation. The lesions that develop are often multiple and include adenomatous polyps, juvenile polyps, inflammatory polyps, and carcinomas.

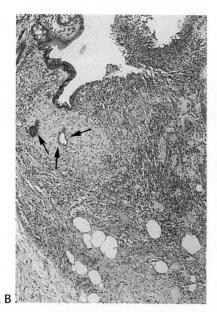
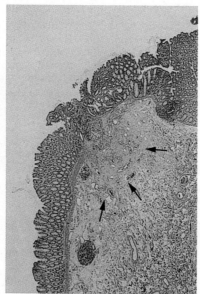
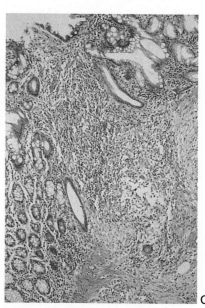

A, B   C

FIG. 13.179. Previous biopsy sites. **A:** A re-epithelializing ulcer. The right-hand portion of the ulcer is lined by granulation tissue and inflammatory cells. The left-hand side is undergoing regeneration. Underlying the regenerating epithelium are entrapped glands (*arrows*). The submucosa is intensely inflamed. **B:** An area of a polypectomy site (*arrows*) that shows an interruption in the muscularis mucosae and an area of increased fibrous density in the submucosa. The overlying mucosa shows granulation tissue and inflammatory cells. **C:** Higher magnification of the mucosal defect demonstrating the inflammatory cells and giant cells. There is significant glandular distortion to the side of the lesion and one might interpret such a focal lesion as representing Crohn disease, if one did not have the entire history.

Previous biopsy sites may cause interpretive problems, particularly due to features induced by repair. Fortunately, most such lesions are examined in a subsequent resection specimen so that the lesions can be evaluated in their complete clinical context. The area of the biopsy site will vary histologically, depending on the time interval that elapsed between the biopsy and resection or subsequent biopsy. The biopsy may cause displacement of glands into the underlying submucosa. These glands may appear reactive and may cause interpretive problems, particularly if there is a question of invasive carcinoma (Fig. 13.179).

Anastomoses are sometimes examined to exclude the presence of recurrent tumor if a mass develops in the area. If a mass is located low in the rectum, the patient may undergo a needle biopsy to determine its etiology. Many times all one finds is a dense cicatricial fibrosis with no tumor. The mucosa overlying the anastomotic site usually appears hyperplastic and regenerative. One may also encounter suture material in such a site.

MISCELLANEOUS LESIONS

Torsion of Appendices Epiploica (Epiploic Appendagitis)

The appendices epiploica lie along the entire colon from the cecum to the upper part of the rectum. Torsion or vascular thrombosis causes their infarction (Fig. 13.180), hemorrhage

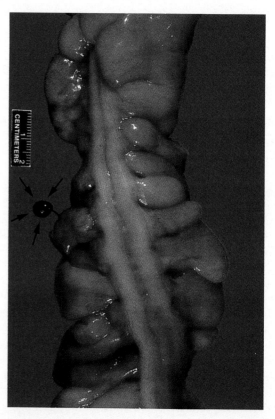

FIG. 13.180. Infarcted appendix epiploica (*arrows*). The appendix epiploica hangs by a thin strand from the pericolonic fat. It has undergone torsion and become infarcted, hence its dark color.

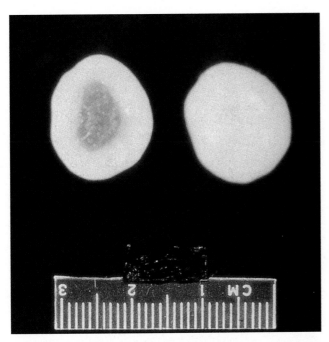

FIG. 13.181. "Peritoneal mouse." Cross section of a hard, whitish nodule containing yellowish material in its center, giving it the appearance of a cross section of a hard-boiled egg.

into the fatty tissues, abscess, or stricture formation. Appendices epiploica may also autoamputate and lie freely in the peritoneal cavity, where they may calcify and turn into "peritoneal mice" (Fig. 13.181). Histologically, they consist of fat that may appear infarcted and completely surrounded by a dense fibrous capsule or may show variable degrees of fat necrosis and calcification, again surrounded by fibrous material.

Irritable Bowel Syndrome

Irritable bowel syndrome is the most common gastrointestinal disorder encountered in general and gastroenterology practices (624,625). It is characterized by abdominal pain, altered bowel habits (diarrhea or constipation), bloating, or the passage of mucus per rectum. A number of criteria have been advanced to standardize the clinical diagnosis (626). The condition develops in women more often than men, often in those with underlying depression or anxiety. Subtle but nonspecific histopathologic changes can be found in patients with this diagnosis. These include increased numbers of mucosal lymphocytes, mast cells, endocrine cells, and nerve cells as summarized by Kirsch and Riddell (627).

Submucosal Colonic Edema (Colonic Urticaria)

Colonic urticaria causes a characteristic mucosal distortion consisting of reticular, polygonal, or mosaic radiographic patterns and broad areas of submucosal edema. The condition results from obstruction or hypersensitivity reactions

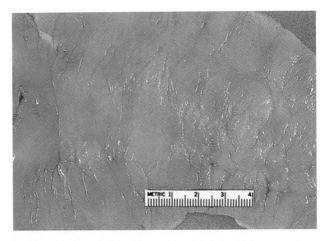

FIG. 13.182. Colonic urticaria. The bowel wall is edematous, with loss of the normal architecture.

(628). The lesion has been likened to the skin of a giraffe or a leopard (Fig. 13.182).

Pseudolipomatosis

Snover et al (629) defined the lesion known as pseudolipomatosis. These authors showed that the lesions do not contain fat cells but represent entrapped gas within the lamina propria (Figs. 13.183 and 13.184). The spaces are also not dilated lymphatics because they lack an endothelial lining. Changes of pseudolipomatosis extend from the stomach to

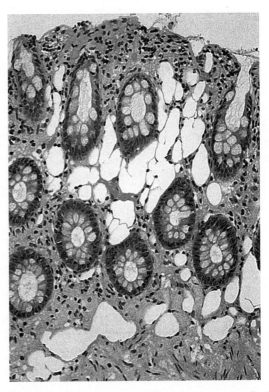

FIG. 13.183. Irregular intramucosal cystic spaces are the hallmark of pseudolipomatosis coli. Note the lack of inflammation.

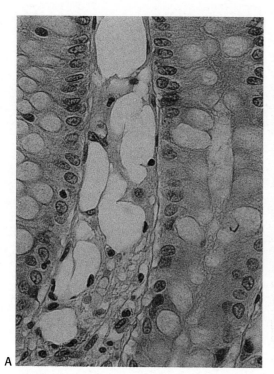
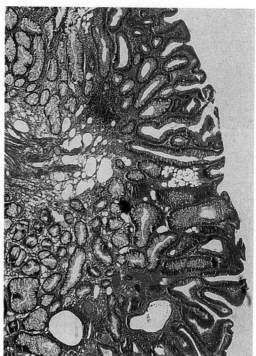

FIG. 13.184. Mucosal pseudolipomatosis. **A:** High magnification of such a lesion. Numerous air-filled cysts are present between two glands. **B:** An adenomatous polyp containing mucosal pseudolipomatosis. It is identified as collections of air-filled bubbles in the mucosa.

the rectum, and involve normal as well as abnormal tissues. It is our belief that this common finding results from the dissection of the intraluminal air that is introduced into the mucosa of the GI tract at the time of endoscopy. The lesion has no known clinical consequence.

Elastofibromatous Change

Elastofibromatous change can develop in the large intestine. The tissues demonstrate smudgy, granulofibrillar, eosinophilic deposits (Fig. 13.185). The elastofibromatous changes consist

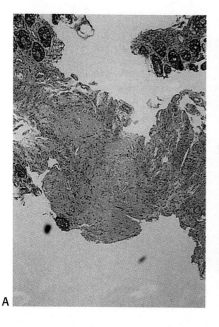
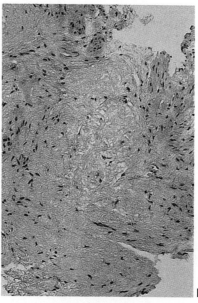

FIG. 13.185. Colonic elastosis. A and B represent a biopsy specimen. The lesion presented as a colonic nodule. **A:** The nodule consists of somewhat basophilic, granular-appearing material. **B:** This material stained positively with an elastic tissue stain.

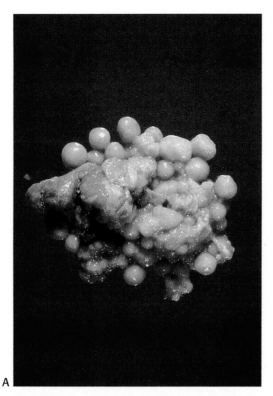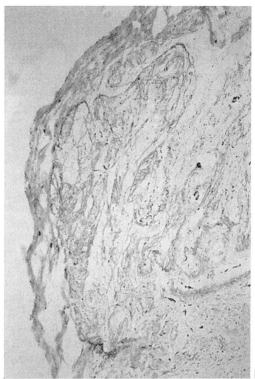

A   B

FIG. 13.186. Myxoglobulosis. **A:** Gross appearance of a "mass" found in the cecal lumen. **B:** Cross section through one of the spherules demonstrating the presence of layered, amorphous debris. The majority of the material consisted of mucin.

of eosinophilic deposits that do not stain with Congo red stains but exhibit the histochemical and ultrastructural properties of elastic fibers similar to those found in elastofibromas (630). The lesion develops following injury in genetically susceptible individuals. The pathogenesis of the lesion is unclear.

Myxoglobulosis

Myxoglobulosis is a disorder that normally affects the appendix but occasionally occurs in the cecum (Fig. 13.186). The lesion is usually identified grossly by the presence of a collection of opaque globules of variably calcified, amorphous material without an underlying architecture. This material represents concretions of mucin. In the appendix, the lesion typically associates with mucoceles, but there are no known associations in the cecum. This entity is discussed further in Chapter 8.

REFERENCES

1. Saegesser F, Loosli H, Robinson JWL, et al: Ischemic diseases of the large intestine. *Int Surg* 1981;66:103.
2. Fenoglio CM, Kaye GI, Lane N: Distribution of human colonic lymphatics in normal, hyperplastic, and adenomatous tissue. *Gastroenterology* 1973;64:51.
3. Fenoglio CM, Richart RM, Kaye GI: Comparative ultrastructural features of normal, hyperplastic, and adenomatous human colonic epithelium. *Gastroenterology* 1975;69:100.
4. Colony PC: Structural characterization of colonic cell types and correlation with specific functions. *Dig Dis Sci* 1996;41:88.
5. Kaye GI, Fenoglio CM, Pascal RR, Lane N: Comparative electron microscopic features of normal, hyperplastic, and adenomatous human colonic epithelium: variations in cellular structure relative to the process of epithelial differentiation. *Gastroenterology* 1973;64:926.
6. Cheng H, Bjerknes M, Amar J: Methods for the determination of epithelial kinetic parameters of human colonic epithelium isolated from surgical and biopsy specimens. *Gastroenterology* 1984;86:78.
7. Dobbins WO III: Diagnostic pathology of the intestine and colon. In: Trump BF, Jones RT (eds). *Diagnostic Electron Microscopy.* New York: John Wiley and Sons, 1978, pp 253–260.
8. Hull BE, Staehelin LA: The terminal web. A reevaluation of its structure and function. *J Cell Biol* 1979;81:67.
9. Goldman H, Ming SC: Mucins in normal and metaplastic gastrointestinal epithelium: histochemical distribution. *Arch Pathol* 1968; 85:580.
10. Filipe MI: Mucins in the human gastrointestinal epithelium: a review. *Invest Cell Pathol* 1979;2:195.
11. Jass JR, Roberton AM: Colorectal mucin histochemistry in health and disease: a critical review. *Pathol Int* 1994;44:487.
12. Chang S-K, Dohrman AF, Basbaum CB, et al: Localization f mucin (MUC2 and MUC3) messenger RNA and peptide expression in human normal intestine and colon cancer. *Gastroenterology* 1994;107: 28.
13. Nabeyama A, LeBlond CP: "Caveolated cells" characterized by deep surface invaginations and abundant filaments in mouse gastrointestinal epithelia. *Am J Anat* 1974;140:147.
14. Potten CS, Booth C, Prithchard DM: The intestinal epithelial stem cell; the mucosal governor. *Int J Exp Pathol* 1997;98:219.
15. Neutra MK, Padykula HA: The gastrointestinal tract. In: Weiss L (ed). *Modern Concepts of Gastrointestinal Histology.* Amsterdam: Elsevier, 1983, pp 693–700.
16. Powell DW, Mifflin RC, Valentich JD, et al: Myofibroblasts. I. Paracrine cells important in health and disease. *Am J Physiol* 1999;277:C1.

17. Neal JV, Potten CS: Circadian rhythms in the epithelial cells and the pericryptal fibroblast sheath in three different sites in the murine intestinal tract. *Cell Tissue Kinet* 1981;14:581.

18. Kaye GI, Lane N, Pascal RR: The colonic pericryptal fibroblast sheath: replication, migration and cytodifferentiation of a mesenchymal rabbit and human colon. *Gastroenterology* 1968;54:852.

19. Pascal RR, Gramlich TL, Parker KM, et al: Geographic variations in eosinophil concentration in normal colonic mucosa. *Mod Pathol* 1997;10:363.

20. Heller RS, Stoffers DA, Hussain MA, et al: Misexpression of the pancreatic homeodomain protein IDX-1 by the HOXa-4 promoter associated with agenesis of the cecum. *Gastroenterology* 1998;115:381.

21. James R, Erler T, Kazenwadel J: Homeobox gene expression in the intestinal epithelium of adult mice. *J Biol Chem* 1994;269:15229.

22. Dott NM: Anomalies of intestinal rotation: their embryology and surgical aspects: report of 5 cases. *Br J Surg* 1923;11:251.

23. Winters WD, Weinberger E, Hatch EI: Atresia of the colon in neonates: radiologic findings. *Am J Radiol* 1992;159:1273.

24. Kim PC, Superina RA, Ein S: Colonic atresia combines with Hirschsprung's disease: a diagnostic and therapeutic challenge. *J Pediatr Surg* 1995;30:1216.

25. Santulli TV, Blane WA: Congenital atresia of the intestine. Pathogenesis and treatment. *Ann Surg* 1961;154:939.

26. Carvalho F, Pereira F, Enes C: Cystic duplication of the rectum – report of two clinical cases. *Eur J Pediatr Surg* 1998;8:170.

27. Michael D, Cohen CRG, Northover JMA: Adenocarcinoma within a rectal duplication cyst: case report and literature review. *Am R Coll Surg England* 1999;81:205.

28. Williams KL: Acute solitary ulcers and acute diverticulitis of the caecum and ascending colon. *Br J Surg* 1960;47:351.

29. Wolff M: Heterotopic gastric epithelium in the rectum: a report of three new cases with a review of 87 cases of gastric heterotopia in the alimentary canal. *Am J Clin Pathol* 1971;55:604.

30. Srinivasan R, Loewenstine H, Mayle JE: Sessile polypoid gastric heterotopia of rectum. A report of 2 cases and review of the literature. *Arch Pathol Lab Med* 1999;123:222.

31. Kalani BP, Vaezzadeh MK, Sieber WK: Gastric heterotopia in rectum complicated by rectovesical fistula. *Dig Dis Sci* 1983;28:378.

32. Carlei F, Pietroletti R, Lomanta D, et al: Heterotopic gastric mucosa of the rectum: characterization of endocrine and mucin-producing cells by immunocytochemistry and lectin histochemistry. *Dis Colon Rectum* 1989;32:159.

33. Evans CS, Goldman RL: Seromucinous (salivary) ectopia of the perianal region. *Arch Dermatol* 1987;123:1277.

34. Mills SE, Walker AN, Stallings RG, et al: Retrorectal cystic hamartoma. Report of three cases, including one with a perirenal component. *Arch Pathol Lab Med* 1984;108:737.

35. Davis M, Whitley ME, Haque AK, et al: Xanthogranulomatous abscess of a müllerian duct remnant. A rare lesion of the rectum and anus. *Dis Colon Rectum* 1986;29:755.

36. Jain D, Matel M, Reyes-Mugica M, Parkash V: Heterotopic nephrogenic rests in the colon and multiple congenital anomalies: possibly related association. *Pediatr Dev Pathol* 2002;5:587.

37. Rodkey GV, Welch CE: Diverticulitis of the colon; evolution in concept and therapy. *Surg Clin North Am* 1965;45:1231.

38. Munakata A, Nakaji S, Takami H, et al: Epidemiologic evaluation of colonic diverticulosis and dietary fiber in Japan. *Tohoku J Exp Med* 1993;171:145.

39. Segal I, Solomon A, Hunt JA: Emergency of diverticular disease in the urban South African black. *Gastroenterology* 1977;72:215.

40. Levy N, Stermer E, Simon J: The changing epidemiology of diverticular disease in Israel. *Dis Colon Rectum* 1985;28:416.

41. Ryan P: Changing concepts in diverticular disease. *Dis Colon Rectum* 1983;26:12.

42. Horner JL: Natural history of diverticulosis of the colon. *Am J Dig Dis* 1958;3:343.

43. Trowell H: The development of the concept of dietary fiber in human nutrition. *Am J Clin Nutr* 1978;31:S53.

44. Painter NS, Burkitt DP: Diverticular disease of the colon: a deficiency disease of Western civilization. *BMJ* 1971;2:450.

45. Sugihara K, Muto T, Morioka Y, Asano A: Diverticular disease of the colon in Japan. A review of 615 cases. *Dis Colon Rectum* 1984;27:531.

46. Parks TG: Natural history of diverticular disease of the colon. A review of 521 cases. *BMJ* 1969;4:639.

47. Chappuis CW, Cohn I Jr: Acute colonic diverticulitis. *Surg Clin North Am* 1988;68:301.

48. Plasvic BM, Raider L, Drnobsek VH, Kogutt MS: Association of rectal diverticula and scleroderma. *Acta Radiol* 1995;36:96.

49. Almy TP, Howell DA: Diverticular disease of the colon. *N Engl J Med* 1980;302:324.

50. Schauer PR, Ramos R, Ghiatas AA, Sirinek KR: Virulent diverticular disease in young obese men. *Am J Surg* 1992;164:443.

51. Casarella WJ, Kanter IE, Seaman WB: Right-sided colonic diverticula as a cause of acute rectal hemorrhage. *N Engl J Med* 1972;286:450.

52. Lichtiger S, Kornbluth A, Salomon P, et al: Lower gastrointestinal bleeding. In: Taylor MB, Gollan JL, Peppercorn MA, et al (eds). *Gastrointestinal Emergencies*. Baltimore: Williams and Wilkins, 1992, pp 358–368.

53. Campbell K, Steele RJ: Non-steroidal anti-inflammatory drugs and complicated diverticular disease: a case-control study. *Br J Surg* 1991;78:190.

54. Tranaeus A, Heimburger O, Granqvist S: Diverticular disease of the colon: a risk factor for peritonitis in continuous peritoneal dialysis. *Nephrol Dial Transplant* 1990;5:141.

55. Galbraith P, Bagg MN, Schabel SI, et al: Diverticular complications of renal disease. *Gastrointest Radiol* 1990;15:259.

56. Farmakis N, Tudor RG, Keighley MRB: The 5-year natural history of complicated diverticular disease. *Br J Surg* 1994;81:733.

57. Muhletaler CA, Berger JL, Robinette CL Jr: Pathogenesis of giant colonic diverticula. *Gastrointest Radiol* 1981;6:217.

58. Whiteway J, Morson BC: Elastosis in diverticular disease of the sigmoid colon. *Gut* 1985;26:258.

59. Meyers MA, Alonzo DR, Gray GF, Baer JW: Pathogenesis of bleeding colonic diverticulosis. *Gastroenterology* 1976;71:577.

60. Kelly JK: Polypoid prolapsing mucosal folds in diverticular disease. *Am J Surg Pathol* 1991;15:871.

61. Mudhar HS, Balsitis M: Colonic angiodysplasia and true diverticula: is there an association? *Histopathology* 2005;46:81.

62. Makapugay LM, Dean PJ: Diverticular disease-associated chronic colitis. *Am J Surg Pathol* 1996;20:94.

63. Mellor MFA, Drake DG: Colonic volvulus in children: value of barium enema for diagnosis and treatment in 14 children. *AJR Am J Roentgenol* 1994;162:1157.

64. Ballantyne G, Brandner M, Beart R, et al: Volvulus of the colon. Incidence and mortality. *Ann Surg* 1985;202:83.

65. Frizelle FA, Wolff BG: Colonic volvulus. *Adv Surg* 1996;29:131.

66. Jain BL, Seth KK: Volvulus of intestine: a clinical study. *Ind J Surg* 1968;30:239.

67. Jordan GL Jr, Beahrs OH: Volvulus of the cecum as a postoperative complication: report of six cases. *Ann Surg* 1953;137:245.

68. Habr Gama A, Haddad J, Simonsen O, et al: Volvulus of the sigmoid colon in Brazil: a report of 230 cases. *Dis Colon Rectum* 1976;19:314.

69. Hsu H-Y, Kao C-L, Huang L-M, et al: Viral etiology of intussusception in Taiwanese childhood. *Pediatr Infect Dis J* 1998;17:893.

70. Bavikatty NR, Goldblum JR, Abdul-Karim FW, et al: Florid vascular proliferation of the colon related to intussusception and mucosal prolapse: potential diagnostic confusion with angiosarcoma. *Mod Pathol* 2001;14:1114.

71. Ihre T: Internal procidentia of the rectum: treatment and results. *Scand J Gastroenterol* 1972;7:643.

72. Stewart JR, Gladen HE: Procidentia in identical twins. Report of cases and analysis of treatment options. *Dis Colon Rectum* 1984;27:608.

73. Madigan MR, Morson BC: Solitary ulcer of the rectum. *Gut* 1969;10:871.

74. Groff DB, Nagaraj HS: Rectal prolapse in infants and children. *Am J Surg* 1990;160:531.

75. Rittmeyer C, Nakayama D, Ulshen MH: Lymphoid hyperplasias causing recurrent rectal prolapse. *J Pediatr* 1997;131:487.

76. Jan IA, Saleem N, Ali M, et al: Rectal prolapse: an unusual presentation of malacoplakia in a child. *J Coll Physicians Surg Pak* 2003;13:536.

77. Dreznik Z, Vishne TH, Kristt D, et al: Rectal prolapse: a possibly under recognized complication of anorexia nervosa amenable to surgical correction. *Int J Psychiatry Med* 2001;31:347.

78. Corman ML: Rectal prolapse in children. *Dis Colon Rectum* 1985;28:535.

79. Li S, Hamilton SR: Malignant tumors in the rectum simulating solitary rectal ulcer syndrome in endoscopic biopsy specimens. *Am J Surg Pathol* 1998;22:106.

80. Rutter KRP, Riddell RH: The solitary ulcer syndrome of the rectum. *Clin Gastroenterol* 1975;4:505.

81. Goodall HB, Sinclair ISR: Colitis cystica profunda. *J Pathol Bacteriol* 1957;73:33.

82. Zidi SH, Marteau P, Piard F, et al: Enterocolitis cystica profunda lesions in a patient with unclassified ulcerative enterocolitis. *Dig Dis Sci* 1994;39:426.

83. Magidson J, Lewin K: Diffuse colitis cystica profunda. *Am J Surg Pathol* 1981;5:4.

84. Archibald SD, Jirsch DW, Bear RA: Gastrointestinal complications of renal transplantation: 2. The colon. *Can Med Assoc J* 1978;119:1301.

85. Shah RJ, Fenoglio-Preiser C, Bleu BL, Giannella R: Usefulness of colonoscopy with biopsy in the evaluation of patients with chronic diarrhea. *Am J Gastroenterol* 2001;96:1091.

86. Calhoun BC, Gomes F, Robert ME, Jain D: Sampling error in the standard evaluation of endoscopic colonic biopsies. *Am J Surg Pathol* 2003;27:254.

87. Levine DS, Haggitt RC: Normal histology of the colon. *Am J Surg Pathol* 1989;13:966.

88. Gupta J, Shepherd NA: Colorectal mass lesions masquerading as chronic inflammatory bowel disease on biopsy. *Histopathology* 2003; 42:476.

89. Xin W, Brown PI, Greenson JK: The clinical significance of focal active colitis in pediatric patients. *Am J Surg Pathol* 2003;27:1134.

90. Volk EE, Shapiro BD, Easley KA, et al: The clinical significance of a biopsy based diagnosis of focal active colitis: a clinicopathologic study of 31 cases. *Mod Pathol* 1998;11:789.

91. Greenson JK, Robert SA, Carpenter SL, et al: The clinical significance of focal active colitis. *Hum Pathol* 1997;28:729.

92. Saunders DR, Sillery J, Rachmilewitz D, et al: Effect of bisacodyl on the structure and function of rodent and human intestine. *Gastroenterology* 1977;72:849.

93. Leriche M, Devroede G, Sanchez G, et al: Changes in the rectal mucosa induced by hypertonic enemas. *Dis Colon Rectum* 1978;21:227.

94. Meisel JL, Bergman D, Graney D, et al: Human rectal mucosa: proctoscopic and morphological changes caused by laxatives. *Gastroenterology* 1977;72:1274.

95. Pockros PJ, Foroozan P: Golytely lavage versus a standard colonoscopy preparation: effect on a normal colonic mucosal histology. *Gastroenterology* 1985;88:545.

96. Koutroubakis IE, Sfiridaki A, Theodoropoulou A, Kouromalis EA: Role of acquired and hereditary thrombotic risk factors in colon ischemia of ambulatory patients. *Gastroenterology* 2001;121:561.

97. Crummy AB, Whittaker WB, Morrissey JF, Cossman FP: Intestinal infarction secondary to retroperitoneal fibrosis. *N Engl J Med* 1971; 285:28.

98. Lucas W, Schroy PC III: Reversible ischemic colitis in a high endurance athlete. *Am J Gastroenterol* 1998;93:2231.

99. Abel ME, Russell TR: Ischemic colitis: comparison of surgical and nonoperative management. *Dis Colon Rectum* 1983;26:113.

100. Boley SJ, Brandt LJ, Veith FJ: Ischemic disorders of the intestine. *Curr Probl Surg* 1978;15:1.

101. Zelenock GB, Strodel WE, Knot JA, et al: A prospective study of clinically and endoscopically documented colonic ischemia in 100 patients undergoing aortic reconstructive surgery with aggressive colonic and direct pelvic revascularization, compared with historic controls. *Surgery* 1989;106:771.

102. Boley SJ: Colonic ischemia—25 years later. *Am J Gastroenterol* 1990; 85:931.

103. Whitehead R, Gratama S: The large intestine. In: Whitehead R (ed). *Gastrointestinal and Oesophageal Pathology*. Edinburgh: Churchill Livingstone, 1995, pp 657–682.

104. Fagin RR, Kirsner JB: Ischemic diseases of the colon. *Adv Intern Med* 1973;17:343.

105. Robinson JWL, Mirkovitch V, Winistorfer B, et al: Response of the intestinal mucosa to ischemia. *Gut* 1981;22:512.

106. Norris HT: Ischemic bowel disease: its spectrum. In: Yardley JH, Morson BC, Abell MR (eds). *The Gastrointestinal Tract* (International Academy of Pathology Monograph). Baltimore: Williams and Wilkins, 1977.

107. Griffiths JD: Surgical anatomy of the blood supply of the rectal colon. *Ann R Coll Surg Engl* 1956;19:241.

108. Dignan CR, Greenson JK: Can ischemic colitis be differentiated from *C. Difficile* colitis in biopsy specimens? *Am J Surg Pathol* 1997;21:706.

109. Markoglou C, Avgerinos A, Mitrakou M, et al: Toxic megacolon secondary to acute ischemic colitis. *Hepatogastroenterology* 1993;40:188.

110. Thomas DFM, Fernie D, Malone M, et al: Association between *Clostridium difficile* and enterocolitis in association with Hirschsprung's disease. *Lancet* 1968;1:78.

111. Kapur VK, Subramaniam R: Tropical enterocolitis in children. *Acta Paediatr Suppl* 1994;396:94.

112. Toner M, Condell D, O'Briain DS: Obstructive colitis. Ulceroinflammatory lesions occurring proximal to colonic obstruction. *Am J Surg Pathol* 1990;14:719.

113. Gratama S, Smedts F, Whitehead R: Obstructive colitis: an analysis of 50 cases and a review of the literature. *Pathology* 1995;27:324.

114. Komorowski RA, Cohen EB, Kauffman HM, et al: Gastrointestinal complications in renal transplant recipients. *Am J Clin Pathol* 1986;86:161.

115. Rivera-Nieves J, Bamias G, Alfert J, et al: Intestinal ischemia and peripheral gangrene in a patient with chronic renal failure. *Gastroenterology* 2002;122:495.

116. Robson WL, Leung AK: Henoch-Schonlein purpura. *Adv Pediatr* 1994; 41:163.

117. Schwarz DA, Stark M, Wright J: Segmental colonic gangrene: a previously unreported complication of adult hemolytic uremic syndrome. *Surgery* 1994;116:107.

118. Kaplan BS, Chesney RW, Drummond KN: Hemolytic uremic syndrome in families. *N Engl J Med* 1975;292:1090.

119. Ray CG, Tucker VL, Harris DJ, et al: Enteroviruses associated with the hemolytic uremic syndrome. *Pediatrics* 1970;46:378.

120. Koster F, Levin J, Walker L, et al: Hemolytic-uremic syndrome after shigellosis, relation to endotoxemia and circulating immune complexes. *N Engl J Med* 1978;298:927.

121. Drummond KN: Hemolytic uremic syndrome then and now. *N Engl J Med* 1985;312:116.

122. Kimura Y, Kashima K, Daa T, et al: Phlebosclerotic colitis coincident with carcinoma in an adenoma. *Pathol Int* 2003;53:721.

123. Yao T, Iwashita A, Hoashi T, et al: Phlebosclerotic colitis: value of radiography in diagnosis – report of three cases. *Radiology* 2000;214:188.

124. Abu-Alfa AK, Ayer U, West AB: Mucosal biopsy finding and venous abnormalities in idiopathic myointimal hyperplasia of the mesenteric veins. *Am J Surg Pathol* 1996;20:1271.

125. Wright CL, Cacala S: Enterocolic lymphocytic phlebitis with lymphocytic colitis, lymphocytic appendicitis and lymphocytic enteritis. *Am J Surg Pathol* 2004;28:542.

126. Lie JT: Mesenteric inflammatory veno-occlusive disease (MIVOD): an emerging and unsuspected cause of digestive tract ischemia. *Vasa* 1997;26:91.

127. Lavu K, Minocha A: Mesenteric inflammatory veno-occlusive disorder: a rare entity mimicking inflammatory bowel disorder. *Gastroenterology* 2003;125:236.

128. Flaherty MJ, Lie JT, Haggitt RC: Mesenteric inflammatory veno-occlusive disease. A seldom recognized cause of intestinal ischemia. *Am J Surg Pathol* 1994;18:779.

129. Tuppy H, Haidenthaler A, Schandalik R, Oberhuber G: Idiopathic enterocolic lymphocytic phlebitis: a rare cause of ischemic colitis. *Mod Pathol* 2000;13:897.

130. Hoffman BI, Katz WA: The gastrointestinal manifestations of systemic lupus erythematosus: a review of the literature. *Semin Arthritis Rheum* 1980;9:237.

131. Helliwell TR, Flook D, Whitworth J, Day DW: Arteritis and venulitis in systemic lupus erythematosus resulting in massive lower intestinal hemorrhage. *Histopathology* 1985;9:1103.

132. Pardi DS, Tremaine WJ, Rothenberg HJ, Batts KP: Melanosis coli in inflammatory bowel disease. *J Clin Gastroenterol* 1998;26:167.

133. Smith B: Effect of irritant purgatives on the myenteric plexus in man and the mouse. *Gut* 1968;9:139.

134. Walker NI, Bennett RE, Axelsen RA: Melanosis coli: a consequence of anthraquinone-induced apoptosis of colonic epithelial cells. *Am J Pathol* 1988;131:465.

135. Byers RJ, Marsh P, Parkinson D, Haboubi NY: Melanosis coli is associated with an increase in colonic epithelial apoptosis and not with laxative use. *Histopathology* 1997;30:160.

136. Benavides SH, Morgante PE, Monserrat AJ, et al: The pigment of melanosis coli: a lectin histochemical study. *Gastrointest Endosc* 1997; 46:131.

137. Meyer CT, Brand M, DeLuca VA, Spiro HM: Hydrogen peroxide colitis: a report of three patients. *J Clin Gastroenterol* 1981;3:31.

138. Herreiros JM, Munjoin MA, Sanchez S, Garrido M: Alcohol-induced colitis. *Endoscopy* 1983;15:121.

139. Fortson WC, Tedesco FJ: Drug-induced colitis: a review. *Am J Gastroenterol* 1984;79:878.

140. Wootton FT, Rhodes DF, Lee WM, Fitts CT: Colonic necrosis with Kayexalate sorbitol enemas after renal transplantation. *Ann Intern Med* 1989;111:947.

141. Scott TR, Graham SM, Schweitzer EJ, Bartlett ST: Colonic necrosis following sodium polystyrene sulfonate (Kayexalate)-sorbitol enema in a renal transplant patient. *Dis Colon Rectum* 1993;36:607.

142. Kaufmann HJ, Taubin HL: Nonsteroidal anti-inflammatory drugs activate quiescent inflammatory bowel disease. *Ann Intern Med* 1987;107:513.

143. Price AB: Pathology of drug-associated gastrointestinal disease. *Br J Clin Pharmacol* 2003;56:477.

144. Lee FD: Importance of apoptosis in the histopathology of drug-related lesions in the large intestine. *J Clin Pathol* 1993;46:118.

145. Fellows IW, Clarke JMF, Roberts PF: Non-steroidal anti-inflammatory drug-induced jejunal and colonic diaphragm disease: a report of two cases. *Gut* 1992;33:1424.

146. Baert F, Hart J, Blackstone MO: A case of diclofenac-induced colitis with focal granulomatous change. *Am J Gastroenterol* 1995;90:1871.

147. ReMine SG, Melrath DC: Bowel perforation in steroid treated patients. *Ann Surg* 1980;192:581.

148. Papadimitriou JC, Cangro CB, Lustberg A, et al: Histologic features of mycophenolate mofetil-related colitis: a graft-versus-host disease-like pattern. *Int J Surg Pathol* 2003;11:295.

149. Behrend M: Adverse gastrointestinal effects of mycophenolate mofetil: aetiology, incidence and management. *Drug Saf* 2001;24:645.

150. Woywodt A, Choi M, Schneider W, et al: Cytomegalovirus colitis during mycophenolate mofetil therapy for Wegener's granulomatosis. *Am J Nephrol* 2000;20:468.

151. Crane PW, Clark C, Sowter C, et al: Cyclosporine toxicity in the small intestine. *Transplant Proc* 1990;22:2432.

152. Gabe SM, Bjarnason I, Tolou-Ghamari Z, et al: The effect of tacrolimus (FK506) on intestinal barrier function and cellular energy production in humans. *Gastroenterology* 1998;115:67.

153. Schwartzentruber D, Lotze MT, Rosenberg SA: Colonic perforation. An unusual complication of therapy with high-dose interleukin-2. *Cancer* 1988;62:2350.

154. Fam AG, Paton TW, Shamess CJ, Lewis AJ: Fulminant colitis complicating gold therapy. *J Rheumatol* 1980;7:479.

155. Wong V, Wyatt J, Lewis F, Howdle P: Gold induced enterocolitis complicated by cytomegalovirus infection: a previously unrecognized association. *Gut* 1993;34:1002.

156. Wright A, Benfield GFA, Felix-Davies D: Ischemic colitis and immune complexes during gold therapy for rheumatoid arthritis. *Ann Rheum Dis* 1984;43:495.

157. Jackson CW, Haboubi NY, Whorwell PJ, Schofield PF: Gold induced enterocolitis. *Gut* 1986;27:452.

158. Miller SS, Muggia AL, Spiro HM: Colonic histologic changes induced by 5-fluorouracil. *Gastroenterology* 1962;43:391.

159. Floch MH, Hellman L: The effect of 5-fluorouracil in rectal mucosa. *Gastroenterology* 1965;48:430.

160. Beck PL, Wong JF, Swaminathan S, et al: Chemotherapy and radiotherapy–induced intestinal damage is regulated by intestinal trefoil factor. *Gastroenterology* 2004;126:796.

161. Sandmeir D, Chaubert P, Bouzourene H: Irinotecan-induced colitis. *Int J Surg Pathol* 2005;13:215.

162. Sparano JA, Dutcher JP, Kaleya R, et al: Colonic ischemia complicating immunotherapy with interleukin-2 and interferon-alpha. *Cancer* 1991;68:1538.

163. deSilva P, Deb S, Drummond RD, Rankin R: A fatal case of ischemic colitis following long-term use of neuroleptic medication. *J Intellect Disabil Res* 1992;36:371.

164. Deana DG, Dean PJ: Reversible ischemic colitis in young women: association with oral contraceptive use. *Am J Surg Pathol* 1995;19:454.

165. Tedesco FJ, Volpicelli NA, Moore FS: Estrogen- and progesterone-associated colitis: a disorder with clinical and endoscopic features mimicking Crohn's colitis. *Gastrointest Endosc* 1982;28:274.

166. Friedel D, Thomas R, Fisher RS: Ischemic colitis during treatment with alosteron. *Gastroenterology* 2001;120:557.

167. Pawel BR, de Chadarevian JP, Franco ME: The pathology of fibrosing colonopathy of cystic fibrosis: a study of 12 cases and review of the literature. *Hum Pathol* 1997;28:395.

168. Smyth RL, Ashby D, O'Hea U, et al: Fibrosing colonopathy in cystic fibrosis: results of a case-control study. *Lancet* 1995;346:1247.

169. Eckardt VF, Kanzler G, Remmele W: Anorectal ergotism: another cause of solitary rectal ulcers. *Gastroenterology* 1986;91:1123.

170. Riddell RH: The gastrointestinal tract. In: Riddell RH (ed). *Pathology of Disease Induced and Toxic Diseases.* New York: Churchill Livingstone, 1972, pp 515–540.

171. Martin P, Manley PN, Depew WT: Isotretinoin-associated proctosigmoiditis. *Gastroenterology* 1987;93:606.

172. Shpilberg O, Ehrenfeld M, Abramowich D, et al: Ergotamine induced solitary rectal ulcer. *Postgrad Med J* 1990;66:483.

173. Janower ML: Hypersensitivity reactions after barium studies of the upper and lower gastrointestinal tract. *Radiology* 1986;161:139.

174. Stringer DA, Hassall E, Ferguson AC, et al: Hypersensitivity reaction to single contrast barium studies in children. *Pediatr Radiol* 1993;23:587.

175. Lutzger LG, Factor SM: Effects of some water-soluble contrast media on the colonic mucosa. *Diagn Radiol* 1976;118:545.

176. Wallace JF: Disorders caused by venoms, bites and stings. In: Petersdorf RG, Adams RD, Braunwald E, et al (eds). *Harrison's Principles of Internal Medicine,* 10th ed. New York: McGraw-Hill, 1983, pp 1241–1261.

177. Anderson RE, Witkowski LJ, Pontius GV: Radiation stricture of the small intestine. *Surgery* 1955;38:605.

178. DeCosse JJ, Rhodes RS, Wentz WB, et al: The natural history and management of radiation induced injury of the gastrointestinal tract. *Ann Surg* 1969;170:369.

179. Novak JM, Collins JT, Donowitz M, et al: Effects of radiation on the human gastrointestinal tract. *J Clin Gastroenterol* 1979;1:9.

180. Paris F, Fuks A, Kang P, et al: Endothelial apoptosis as the primary lesion initiating intestinal radiation damage in mice. *Science* 2001;293:293.

181. Maj JG, Paris F, Haimovitz-Friedman A, et al: Microvascular function regulates intestinal crypt response to radiation. *Cancer Res* 2003;63:4338.

182. Sedgwick DM, Howard GCW, Ferguson A: Pathogenesis of acute radiation injury to the rectum: a prospective study in patients. *Int J Colorectal Dis* 1994;9:23.

183. Sandler RS, Sandler DP: Radiation-induced cancers of the colon and rectum: assessing the risk. *Gastroenterology* 1983;84:51.

184. Hauer-Jensen M, Ricter KK, Wang J, et al: Changes in transforming growth factor β1 gene expression and immunoreactivity levels during development of chronic radiation enteropathy. *Radiat Res* 1998;150:673.

185. Fajardo LF, Prionas SD, Kwan HH, et al: Transforming growth factor β1 induces angiogenesis in vivo with a threshold pattern. *Lab Invest* 1996;74:600.

186. Hauer-Jensen M: Late radiation injury of the intestine. Clinical, pathophysiological and radiobiological aspects. A review. *Acta Oncol* 1990; 92:401.

187. Gelfand MD, Teper M, Katz LA, et al: Acute irradiation proctitis in man. Development of eosinophilic abscesses. *Gastroenterology* 1968; 54:49.

188. Leupin N, Curschmann J, Kranzbühler H, et al: Acute radiation colitis in patients treated with short-term preoperative radiotherapy for rectal cancer. *Am J Surg Pathol* 2002;26:498.

189. Kang SK, Chou RH, Dodge RK, et al: Gastrointestinal toxicity of transperineal interstitial prostate brachytherapy. *Int J Radiation Oncology Phys* 2002;53:99.

190. Falcone RE, Carey LC: Colorectal trauma. *Surg Clin North Am* 1988;68:1307.

191. Cooper A, Floyd T, Barlow B, et al: Major blunt abdominal trauma due to child abuse. *J Trauma* 1988;28:1483.

192. Jeffrey RB, Federle MP, Stein SM, Crass RA: Intramural hematoma of the cecum following blunt trauma. *J Comp Assist Tomogr* 1982;6:404.

193. Westcott JL, Smith JR: Mesentery and colon injuries secondary to blunt trauma. *Radiology* 1975;114:597.

194. Altner PC: Constrictive lesions of the colon due to blunt trauma to the abdomen. A critical review of management of right colon injuries. *Surg Gynecol Obstet* 1964;118:1257.

195. Chilmindris C, Boyd DR, Carson LE, et al: A critical review of management of right colon injuries. *J Trauma* 1971;11:651.

196. Goosney DL, Knoechel DG, Finlay BB: Enteropathogenic E. coli, salmonella and shigella: masters of host cell cytoskeletal exploitation. *Emerging Infect Dis* 1999;5:216.

197. Levine MM, Levine OS: Changes in human ecology and behavior in relation to the emergence of diarrheal diseases, including cholera. *Proc Natl Acad Sci USA* 1994;91:2390.

198. Pai C, Nimet AH, Lior H, et al: Epidemiology of sporadic diarrhea due to verocytotoxin-producing *Escherichia coli*: a two-year prospective study. *J Infect Dis* 1988;157:1054.

199. Pai CH, Gordon R, Sims HV, Bryan LE: Sporadic cases of hemorrhagic colitis associated with *Escherichia coli* 0157:H7. *Ann Intern Med* 1984;101:738.

200. Horing E, Gopfert D, Schroter G, von Gaisberg U: Frequency of microorganisms isolated from biopsy specimens in chronic colitis. *Endoscopy* 1991;23:325.

201. Johnson WM, Lior H, Bezanson GS: Cytotoxic *Escherichia coli* 0157:H7 strain associated with an outbreak of hemorrhagic colitis. *Infect Immun* 1986;51:953.

202. Edelman R, Karmali MA, Fleming PA: Summary of international symposium and workshop on infections due to verocytotoxin (Shiga-like toxin) producing *Escherichia coli*. *J Infect Dis* 1988;157:1102.

203. Tarr PI, Neill MA, Clausen CR, et al: Genotypic variation in pathogenic *Escherichia coli* 0157:H7 isolated from patients in Washington, 1984-1987. *J Infect Dis* 1989;159:344.

204. Phillips AD, Navabpour D, Hicks S, et al: Enterohaemorrhagic *Escherichia coli* 0157:H7 target Peyer's patches in humans and cause attaching/effacing lesions in both human and bovine intestine. *Gut* 2000;47:377.

205. Tesh VL, O'Brien AD: The pathogenic mechanism of Shiga toxin and the Shiga-like toxins. *Mol Microbiol* 1991;5:1817.

206. Karmali MA, Petric M, Steele BT, Lim C: Sporadic cases of haemolytic-uraemic syndrome associated with faecal cytotoxin and cytotoxin-producing *Escherichia coli* in stools. *Lancet* 1983;1:619.

207. Buteau C, Proulx F, Chaibou M, et al: Leukocytosis in children with *Escherichia coli* 0157:H7 enteritis developing the hemolytic-uremic syndrome. *Pediatr Infect Dis J* 2000;19:642.

208. Dundas S, Todd WT, Stewart AI, et al: The central Scotland *Escherichia coli* 0157:H7 outbreak: risk factors for the hemolytic uremic syndrome and death among hospitalized patients. *Clin Infect Dis* 2001;33:923.

209. Ostroff SM, Kobayashi JM, Lewis JH: Infections with *Escherichia coli* 0157:H7 in Washington State. The first year of statewide disease surveillance. *JAMA* 1989;262:355.

210. Marshall W, McLimans C, Yu P, et al: Results of a 6-month survey of stool cultures for *Escherichia coli* 0157:H7. *Mayo Clin Proc* 1990;65:787.

211. Centers for Disease Control and Prevention: Outbreaks of *Escherichia coli* 0157:H7 infection and cryptosporidiosis associated with drinking unpasteurized apple cider—Connecticut and New York, October, 1996. *MMWR Morb Mortal Wkly Rep* 1997;46:4.

212. Waters JR, Sharp JCM, Dve VJ: Infection caused by *Escherichia coli* 0157:H7 in Alberta, Canada, and in Scotland: a five-year review, 1987-1991. *Clin Infect Dis* 1994;19:834.

213. Brewster DH, Brown MI, Robertson D, et al: An outbreak of *Escherichia coli* 0157 associated with a children's paddling pool. *Epidemiol Infect* 1994;112:441.

214. Swerdlow DL, Woodruff BA, Brady RC, et al: A waterborne outbreak in Missouri of *Escherichia-coli* 0157:H7 associated with bloody diarrhea and death. *Ann Intern Med* 1992;117:812.

215. Doyle MP, Schoeni JL: Isolation of *Escherichia coli* 0157:H7 from retail fresh meats and poultry. *Appl Environ Microbiol* 1987;53:2394.

216. Ryan CA, Tauxe RV, Hosek GE, et al: *Escherichia coli* 0157:H7 diarrhea in a nursing home: clinical, epidemiological and pathological findings. *J Infect Dis* 1986;154:631.

217. Easton L: *Escherichia coli* 0157: occurrence, transmission and laboratory detection. *Br J Biomed Sci* 1997;54:57.

218. Doyle MP, Schoeni JL: Survival and growth characteristics of *Escherichia coli* associated with hemorrhagic colitis. *Appl Environ Microbiol* 1984;48:855.

219. Burnens AP, Zbinden R, Kaempf L, et al: A case of laboratory acquired infection with *Escherichia coli* 0157:H7. *Zentralbi Bakteriol* 1993;279:512.

220. Griffin PM, Tauxe R: The epidemiology of infections caused by *Escherichia coli* 0157:H7, other enterohemorrhagic *E. coli* and the associated hemolytic uremic syndrome. *Epidemiol Rev* 1992;13:60.

221. Griffin PM, Olmstead LC, Petras RE: *Escherichia coli* 0157:H7–associated colitis: a clinical and histological study of 11 cases. *Gastroenterology* 1990;99:142.

222. Hunt CM, Harvey JA, Youngs ER, et al: Clinical and pathological variability of infection by enterohaemorrhagic (Vero cytotoxin producing) *Escherichia coli*. *J Clin Pathol* 1989;42:847.

223. Lamps LW, Schneider EN, Havens JM, et al: Molecular diagnosis of *Campylobacter jejuni* infection in cases of focal active colitis. *Am J Surg Pathol* 2006;30:782.

224. Cartwright KA, Evans BG: Salmon as a food-poisoning vehicle: two successive *Salmonella* outbreaks. *Epidemiol Infect* 1988;101:249.

225. Centers for Disease Control: Multistate outbreak of *Salmonella poona* infections—United States and Canada, 1991. *MMWR Morbid Mortal Wkly Rep* 1991;40:549.

226. Ingersoll B: U. S. agencies move at last to unscramble mess they've made of combating *Salmonella* in eggs. *Wall Street Journal*, January 9, 1990, p A16.

227. Rampling A: *Salmonella enteritidis* five years on. *Lancet* 1993;342:317.

228. Rodrigue DC, Tauxe RV, Rowe B: International increase in *Salmonella enteritidis*: a new pandemic? *Epidemiol Infect* 1990;105:21.

229. Christie AB: *Infectious Disease: Epidemiologic and Clinical Practice,* 4th ed., Vol. 1. New York: Churchill Livingstone, 1987, pp 101–120.

230. Bozkurt S, Celik F, Guler K: Massive lower gastrointestinal bleeding in typhoid fever. *Int Surg* 2004;89:172.

231. Takeuchi A: Electron microscope studies of experimental salmonella infection. I. Penetration into the intestinal epithelium by Salmonella typhimurium. *Am J Pathol* 1967;50:109.

232. Garcia del Porillo F, Finlay BB: Salmonella invasion of nonphagocytic cells induces formation of macropinosomes in the host cell. *Infect Immunol* 1994;62:4641.

233. Galan JE: Molecular and cellular bases of Salmonella entry into host cells. *Curr Top Microbiol Immunol* 1996;209:43.

234. Noffsinger A, Fenoglio Preiser CM, Gilinsky N, Maru D: Benign gastrointestinal diseases. Armed Forces Institute of Pathology Press, Washington, DC, in press.

235. Finlay BB, Falkow S: Salmonella as an intracellular parasite. *Mol Microbiol* 1989;3:1833.

236. Dronfield MW, Fletcher J, Langman MJS: Coincident salmonella infections and ulcerative colitis: problems of recognition and management. *Br J Med* 1974;i;99.

237. Black PH, Kunz LJ, Swartz MN: Salmonellosis – a review of some unusual aspects. *N Engl J Med* 1960;262:864.

238. Centers for Disease Control: *Shigella Surveillance: Annual Tabulation Summary, 1999.* Atlanta, GA: U.S. Department of Health and Human Services, CDC, 2000.

239. Centers for Disease Control: Shigella sonnei outbreak among men who have sex with men – San Francisco, California, 2000-2001. *MMWR Morbid Mortal Wkly Rep* 2001;50:922.

240. Lee LA, Ostroff SM, McGee HB, et al: An outbreak of shigellosis at an outdoor music festival. *Am J Epidemiol* 1991;133:608.

241. Reeve G, Martin DL, Pappas J, et al: An outbreak of shigellosis associated with the consumption of raw oysters. *N Engl J Med* 1989;321:224.

242. Morduchowicz G, Huminer D, Siegman-Igra Y: *Shigella* bacteremia in adults. A report of five cases and review of the literature. *Arch Intern Med* 1987;147:2034.

243. Keusch GT: Shigella. In: Gorbach SL (ed). *Infectious Diarrhea.* Boston: Blackwell Scientific, 1986, pp 31–50.

244. O'Brien AD, Marques LRM, Newland JW, et al: Shiga and shigalike toxins. *Microbiol Ther* 1984;14:25.

245. Upadhyay S, Neely JA: Toxic megacolon and perforation caused by *Shigella*. *Br J Surg* 1989;76:1217.

246. Islam MM, Azad AK, Bardhan PK, et al: Pathology of shigellosis and its complications. *Histopathology* 1994;24:65.

247. Caldwell GR, Reiss-Levy EA, deCarle DJ, Hunt DR: *Shigella dysenteriae* type I enterocolitis. *Aust NZ J Med* 1986;16:405.

248. Raghupathy P, Date A, Shastry JCM, et al: Haemolytic-uraemic syndrome complicating *Shigella* dysentery in south Indian children. *BMJ* 1978;1:1518.

249. Bennish ML: Potentially lethal complications of shigellosis. *Rev Infect Dis* 1991;4:S319.

250. Maurelli AT, Blackmon B, Curtiss R III: Temperature-dependent expression of virulence genes in *Shigella* species. *Infect Immunol* 1984;43:195.

251. Sansonetti PJ, Arondel J, Cantey JR, et al: Infection of rabbit Peyer's patches by Shigella flexneri: effect of adhesive or invasive bacterial phenotypes on follicle-associated epithelium. *Infect Immunol* 1996;64:2751.

252. Perdomo OJ, Cavaillon JM, Huerre M, et al: Acute inflammation causes epithelial invasion and mucosal destruction in experimental shigellosis. *J Exp Med* 1994;180:1307.

253. Adam T, Arpin M, Prevost MC, et al: Cytoskeletal rearrangements and the functional role of T-plastin during entry of Shigella flexneri into HeLa cells. *J Cell Biol* 1995;129:367.

254. Bernardini ML, Mounier J, d'Hautville H, et al: Identification of icsA, a plasmid locus of Shigella flexneri that governs bacterial intra- and intercellular spread through interaction with F-actin. *Proc Natl Acad Sci USA* 1989;86:3867.

255. Zeile WL, Purich DL, Southwick FS: Recognition of two classes of oligoproline sequences in prolifin-mediated acceleration of actin-based Shigella motility. *J Cell Biol* 1996;133:49.

256. Kadurugamuwa JL, Rhodes M, Wehland J, Timmis KN: Intercellular spread of Shigella flexneri through a monolayer mediated by membranous protrusions and associated with reorganization of the cytoskeletal protein vinculin. *Infect Immunol* 1991;59:3463.

257. Allaoui A, Mounier J, Prevost MC, et al: icsB, a Shigella flexneri virulence gene necessary for the lysis of protrusions during intracellular spread. *Mol Microbiol* 1992;6:1605.

258. Hilbi H, Zychlinsky A, Sansonnetti PJ: Macrophage apoptosis in microbial infections. *Parasitology* 1997;115:S79.

259. McDonald LC, Kilgore GE, Thompson A, et al: An epidemic toxin gene-variant of *Clostridium difficile*. *N Engl J Med* 2005;353:2433.

260. Loo VG, Poirier L, Miller MA: A predominantly clonal multi-institutional outbreak of *Clostridium difficile*-associated diarrhea with high morbidity and mortality. *N Engl J Med* 2005;353:2442.

261. Johnson S, Clabots CR, Linn FV, et al: Nosocomial *clostridium difficile* colonisation and disease. *Lancet* 1990;336:97.

262. Qualman SJ, Petrie M, Karmali A, et al: *Clostridium difficile* invasion and toxin circulation in fatal pediatric pseudomembranous colitis. *Am J Clin Pathol* 1990;94:410.

263. Reinke CM, Messick CR: Update on *clostridium difficile*-induced colitis. *Am J Hosp Pharm* 1994;51:14.

264. Collignon A, Jeantils V, Cruaud P, et al: Prevalence of *Clostridium-difficile* and toxin-A in faecal samples of HIV infected patients. *Pathol Biol* 1993;41:415.

265. Fekety R, Kim K-H, Brown D, et al: Epidemiology of antibiotic-associated colitis: isolation of *Clostridium difficile* from the hospital environment. *Am J Med* 1981;70:906.

266. Kyne L, Warny M, Qamar A, Kelly CP: Asymptomatic carriage of *Clostridium difficile* and serum levels of IgG antibody against toxin A. *N Engl J Med* 2000;242:390.

267. Kyne L, Warny M, Qamar A, Kelly CP: Association between antibody response to toxin A and protection against *Clostridium difficile* diarrhea. *Lancet* 2001;357:189.

268. Riegeler M, Sedivy R, Pothoulakis C, et al: Clostridium difficile toxin B is more potent than toxin A in damaging human colonic epithelium in vitro. *J Clin Invest* 1995;95:2004.

269. Pothoulakis C, LaMont JT: Microbes and microbial toxins: paradigms for microbial-mucosal interactions II. The integrated response of the intestine to *Clostridium difficile* toxin. *Am J Physiol* 2001;280:G178.

270. He D, Sougioultzis S, Hagen S, et al: Clostridium difficile toxin A triggers human colonocyte IL-8 release via mitochondrial oxygen radical generation. *Gastroenterology* 2002;122:1048.

271. Savidge TC, Pan W-H, Newman P, et al: *Clostridium difficile* toxin B is an inflammatory enterotoxin in human intestine. *Gastroenterology* 2003;125:413.

272. Pituch H, Van Leeuwen W, Maquelin K, et al: Toxin profiles and resistance to macrolides and new fluoroquinolones as epidemicity determinants of clinical isolates of clostridium difficile from Warsaw Poland. *J Clin Microbiol* 2007;Feb 21 (E pub).

273. Kazakova SV, Ware K, Baughman B, et al: A hospital outbreak of diarrhea due to emerging epidemic strains of *Clostridium difficile*. *Arch Int Med* 2006;166:2518.

274. Mattia AR, Doern GV, Clark J, et al: Comparison of four methods in the diagnosis of *Clostridium difficile* disease. *Eur J Clin Microbiol Infect Dis* 1993;12:882.

275. DiPersio JR, Varga FJ, Conwell DW, et al: Development of a rapid enzyme immunoassay for *Clostridium difficile* toxin A and its use in the diagnosis of *C. difficile*-associated disease. *J Clin Microbiol* 1991;29:2724.

276. Boondeekhun HS, Gurutler V, Odd ML, et al: Detection of *Clostridium-difficile* enterotoxin gene in clinical specimens by the polymerase chain reaction. *J Med Microbiol* 1993;38:384.

277. Viscidi RP, Bartlett JG: Antibiotic associated pseudomembranous colitis in children. *Pediatrics* 1981;67:381.

278. Tedesco FJ, Corless JK, Brownstein RE: Rectal sparing in antibiotic-associated pseudomembranous colitis: a prospective study. *Gastroenterology* 1982;83:1259.

279. Schnitt SJ, Antonioli DA, Goldman H: Massive mural edema in severe pseudomembranous colitis. *Arch Pathol Lab Med* 1983;107:211.

280. Wang K, Weinrach D, Lal A, et al: Signet-ring cell change versus signet-ring cell carcinoma. A comparative analysis. *Am J Surg Pathol* 2003;27:1429.

281. Schiffman R: Signet-ring cells associated with pseudomembranous colitis. *Am J Surg Pathol* 1996;20:599.

282. Bartlett JG: Antibiotic-associated diarrhea. *N Engl Med* 2002;346.

283. Sougioultziz S, Kyne L, Drudy D, et al: Clostridium difficile toxoid vaccine in recurrent C difficile-associated diarrhea. *Gastroenterology* 2005;128:764.

284. Kornbluth AA, Danzig JB, Bernstein LH: *Clostridium septicum* infection and associated malignancy: report of 2 cases and review of the literature. *Medicine* 1989;68:30.

285. Katlic MR, Derkac WM, Coleman WS: *Clostridium septicum* infection and malignancy. *Ann Surg* 1981;193:361.

286. Collier PE, Diamond DL, Young JC: Nontraumatic *Clostridium septicum* gangrenous myonecrosis. *Dis Colon Rectum* 1983;26:703.

287. Borriello SP, Welch AR, Larson HE, Barclay F: Enterotoxigenic *Clostridium perfringens:* a possible cause of antibiotic-associated diarrhoea. *Lancet* 1984;1:305.

288. Mapstone NP, Dixon MF: Vasculitis in ileocaecal tuberculosis: similarities to Crohn's disease. *Histopathology* 1992;21:477.

289. Nichol CS: Some aspects of gonorrhea in the female with special reference to infection of the rectum. *Br J Vener Dis* 1948;24:713.

290. Klausner JD, Kohn R, Kent C: Etiology of clinical proctitis among men who have sex with men. *Clin Infect Dis* 2004;38:300.

291. Gad A, Wllen R, Furugard K, et al: Intestinal spirochaetosis as a cause of long-standing diarrhoea. *Ups J Med Sci* 1977;82:47.

292. Palejwala AA, Evans R, Campbell F: Spirochaetes can colonize colorectal adenomatous epithelium. *Histopathology* 2000;37:282.

293. Uhlemann ER, Fenoglio-Preiser C: Intestinal spirochetosis. *Am J Surg Pathol* 2005;29:982.

294. Gebbers J-O, Ferguson DJ, Mason C, et al: Spirochetosis of the human rectum associated with an intraepithelial mast cell and IgE plasma cell response. *Gut* 1987;28:588.

295. Bayerdorffer E, Schwarzkopf-Steinhauser G, Ottenjann R: New unusual forms of colitis. Report of four cases with known and unknown etiology. *Hepatogastroenterology* 1986;33:187.

296. Roberts IM, Parenti DM, Albert MB: Aeromonas hydrophile-associated colitis in a male homosexual. *Arch Intern Med* 1987;147:1502.

297. Deutsch SF, Wedzina W: Aeromonas sobria-associated left-sided segmental colitis. *Am J Gastroenterol* 1997;92:2104.

298. Cowgill R, Quan SHQ: Colonic actinomycosis mimicking carcinoma. *Dis Colon Rectum* 1978;22:45.

299. Whitaker BL: Actinomycetes in biopsy material obtained from suture line granulomata following resection of the rectum. *Br J Surg* 1964;51:445.

300. Davis BT, Thiim M, Zukerberg LR: Case 2-2006: A 31 year old, HIV-positive man with rectal pain. *N Engl J Med* 2006;354:284.

301. Spaargaren J, Fennema HS, Morre SA, et al: New lymphogranuloma venereum Chlamydia trachomatis variant, Amsterdam. *Emerg Infect Dis* 2005;11:1090.

302. Nieuwenhuis RF, Ossewaarde JM, Gotz HM, et al: Resurgence of lymphogranuloma venereum in Western Europe: an outbreak of chlamydia trachomatis serovars L2 proctitis in the Netherlands among men who have sex with men. *Clin Infect Dis* 2004;39:996.

303. Schachter J, Osoba AO: Lymphogranuloma venereum. *Br Med Bull* 1983;39:151.

304. Morson BC: Anorectal venereal disease. *Proc R Soc Med* 1964;57:179.

305. Levine JS, Smith PD, Brugge WR: Chronic proctitis in male homosexuals due to lymphogranuloma venereum. *Gastroenterology* 1980;79:563.

306. Turnbull PC: Introduction: anthrax history, disease and ecology. *Curr Top Microbiol Immunol* 2002;271:1.

307. Bhat P, Mohan DN, Srinivasa H: Intestinal anthrax with bacteriological investigations. *J Infect Dis* 1985;152:1357.

308. Derizhanov SM: *Pathologic Anatomy and Pathogenesis of the Intestinal Form of Anthrax*. Smolensk Institute of Pathology Anatomy, Western Oblast Government Printing House, Moscow, Russia, 1935.

309. Huang E-S, Roche JK: Cytomegalovirus DNA and adenocarcinomas of the colon: evidence for latent viral infection. *Lancet* 1978;1:957.

310. Ho M: Epidemiology of cytomegalovirus infections. *Rev Infect Dis* 1990;12:7.

311. Kyriazis AP, Mitra SK: Multiple cytomegalovirus-related intestinal perforations in patients with acquired immunodeficiency syndrome. *Arch Pathol Lab Med* 1992;116:495.

312. Goodman ZD, Boitnott JK, Yardley JH: Perforation of the colon associated with cytomegalovirus infection. *Dig Dis Sci* 1979;24:376.

313. Foucar E, Mukai K, Foucar K, et al: Colon ulceration in lethal cytomegalovirus infection. *Am J Clin Pathol* 1981;76:788.

314. Sonsino E, Mouy R, Foucaud P, et al: Intestinal pseudoobstruction related to cytomegalovirus infection of myenteric plexus. *N Engl J Med* 1984;311:196.

315. Shintaku M, Inoue N, Sasaki M, et al: Cytomegalovirus vasculitis accompanied by and exuberant fibroblastic reaction in the intestine of an AIDS patient. *Acta Pathol Jpn* 1991;41:900.

316. Kaufman RH, Gardner HL, Rawls WE, Young RL: Clinical features of herpes genitalis. *Cancer Res* 1973;33:1446.

317. Waugh MA: Ano-rectal herpesvirus hominis infection in men. *J Am Vener Dis Assoc* 1976;3:68.

318. Rocha N, Suguiama EH, Maia D, et al: Intestinal malakoplakia associated with paracoccidiomycosis: a new association. *Histopathology* 1997;30:79.

319. Lamps LW, Molna CP, West AB, et al: The pathologic spectrum of gastrointestinal and hepatic histoplasmosis. *Am J Clin Pathol* 2000;113:64.

320. Huang CT, McGarry T, Cooper S, et al: Disseminated histoplasmosis in the acquired immune deficiency syndrome: report of five cases from a nonendemic area. *Arch Intern Med* 1987;147:1181.

321. Sathapatayavongs B, Batteiger BE, Wheat J, et al: Clinical and laboratory features of disseminated histoplasmosis during two large urban outbreaks. *Medicine* 1983;62:26.

322. Cole ACE, Ridley DS, Wolfe HRI: Bowel infection with *Histoplasma duboisii. J Trop Med Hyg* 1965;68:92.

323. Newman SL: Macrophages in host defense against Histoplasma capsulatum. *Trends Microbiol* 1999;7:67.

324. Cimponeriu D, LoPresti P, Lavelanet M, et al: Gastrointestinal histoplasmosis in HIV infection: two cases of colonic pseudocancer and review of the literature. *Am J Gastroenterol* 1994;89:129.

325. Mullick SS, Mody DR, Schwartz MR: Cytology of gastrointestinal histoplasmosis. A report of two cases with differential diagnosis and diagnostic pitfalls. *Acta Cytol* 1996;40:989.

326. Saral R: Candida and Aspergillus infections in immunocompromised patients: an overview. *Rev Infect Dis* 1991;13:487.

327. Kinder RB, Jourdan MH: Disseminated aspergillosis and bleeding colonic ulcers in renal transplant patient. *J R Soc Med* 1985;78:338.

328. Denning DW, Stevens DA: Antifungal and surgical treatment of invasive aspergillosis: review of 2,121 published cases. *Rev Infect Dis* 1990;12:1147.

329. Michalack DM, Cooney DR, Rhodes KH, et al: Gastrointestinal mucormycosis in infants and children: a cause of gangrenous intestinal cellulitis and perforation. *J Pediatr Surg* 1980;16:320.

330. Parra R, Arnau E, Julia A, et al: Survival after intestinal mucormycosis in acute myelogenous leukemia. *Cancer* 1986;58:2717.

331. Hutto JO, Bryan CS, Green FL, et al: Cryptococcosis of the colon resembling Crohn's disease in a patient with the hyperimmunoglobulinemia E-recurrent infect (Job's syndrome). *Gastroenterology* 1988;94:808.

332. Washington K, Gottfried MR, Wilson ML: Gastrointestinal cryptococcosis. *Mod Pathol* 1991;4:707.

333. Richter S, Cormican MG, Pfaller MA, et al: Fatal disseminated *Trichoderma longibrachitum* infection in an adult bone marrow transplant patient: species identification and review of the literature. *J Clin Microbiol* 1999;37:1154.

334. Binford CH, Connor DH: *Pathology of Tropical and Extraordinary Diseases.* Washington, DC: Armed Forces Institute of Pathology, 1976, pp 591–593.

335. Yousef OM, Smilack JD, Kerr DM, et al: Gastrointestinal basidiobolomycosis. Morphologic findings in a cluster of six cases. *Am J Clin Pathol* 1999;11:610.

336. Sudman MS: Prototheticosis. A critical review. *Am J Clin Pathol* 1974;61:10.

337. Cox GE, Wilson JD, Brown P: Prototheticosis: a case of disseminated algal infection. *Lancet* 1974;2:379.

338. Istre GR, Kreiss K, Hopkins RS, et al: An outbreak of amebiasis spread by colonic irrigation at a chiropractic clinic. *N Engl J Med* 1982; 307:339.

339. Allason-Jones E, Mindel A, Sargeunt P, Williams P: *Entamoeba histolytica* as a commensal intestinal parasite in homosexual men. *N Engl J Med* 1986;315:353.

340. Haque R, Huston CD, Hughes M, et al: Amebiasis. *New Engl J Med* 2003;348:1565.

341. Connor DH, Neafie RC, Meyers WM: Amebiasis. In: Binford CH, Connor DH (eds). *Pathology of Tropical and Extraordinary Diseases,* Vol. 1. Washington, DC: Armed Forces Institute of Pathology, 1976.

342. Petri WA Jr, Mann BJ, Haque R: The bittersweet interface of parasite and host: lectin-carbohydrate interactions during human invasion by the parasite *Entamoeba histolytica. Annu Rev Microbiol* 2002;56:39.

343. Reed S, Bouvier J, Pollack AS, et al: Cloning of a virulence factor of *Entamoeba histolytica. J Clin Invest* 1993;91:1532.

344. Seydel KB, Li E, Zhang Z, Stanley SL Jr: Epithelial cell iniated inflammation plays a crucial role in early tissue damage in amebic infection of human intestine. *Gastroenterology* 1998;115:1446.

345. Sotelo-Avila C, Kline MW, Silberstein MJ, Desai K: Bloody diarrhea and pneumoperitoneum in a 10-month-old girl. *J Pediatr* 1988;113:1098.

346. Merritt RJ, Coughlin E, Thomas DW, et al: Spectrum of amebiasis in children. *Am J Dis Child* 1982;136:785.

347. Turner GR, Millikan M, Carter J Jr, Hinshaw D: Surgical significance of fulminant amoebic colitis: report of perforation of the colon with peritonitis. *Am Surg* 1965;31:757.

348. Jenkinson SG, Hargrove MD: Recurrent amebic abscess of the liver. *JAMA* 1975;232:277.

349. Shookhoff HB: Amebic pericarditis. *JAMA* 1973;223:923.

350. Healy GR: Immunologic tools in the diagnosis of amebiasis: epidemiology in the United States. *Rev Infect Dis* 1986;8:239.

351. Patterson M, Healy GR, Shabot JM: Serologic testing for amoebiasis. *Gastroenterology* 1980;78:136.

352. Pittman FE, El-Hashimi WK, Pittman JC: Studies of human amebiasis. II. Light and electron-microscopic observations of colonic mucosa and exudate in acute amebic colitis. *Gastroenterology* 1973;65:588.

353. Levine SM, Stover JF, Warren JG, et al: Ameboma, the forgotten granuloma. *JAMA* 1971;215:1461.

354. Radke RA: Ameboma of the intestine: an analysis of the disease as presented in 78 collected and 41 previously unreported cases. *Ann Intern Med* 1955;43:1048.

355. Powell SJ, MacLeod I, Wilmot AL, Elsdon-Dew E: Metronidazole in amoebic dysentery and amoebic liver abscess. *Lancet* 1966;2:1329.

356. Arean VM, Echevarria R: Balantidiasis. In: Marcial-Rojas RA (ed). *Pathology of Protozoal and Helminthic Diseases.* Baltimore: Williams and Wilkins, 1971, p 234.

357. Castro J, Vazquez-Iglesias JL, Arnal-Monreal F: Dysentery caused by *Balantidium coli:* report of two cases. *Endoscopy* 1983;15:272.

358. Neafie RC: Balantidiasis. In: Binford CH, Connor DH (eds). *Pathology of Tropical and Extraordinary Diseases.* Washington, DC: Armed Forces Institute of Pathology, 1976, p 325.

359. Idoate MA, Vazquez JJ, Civeria P: Rectal biopsy as a diagnostic procedure of chronic visceral leishmaniasis. *Histopathology* 1993;22:589.

360. Sheehan DJ, Runcher BG, McKitrick JC: Association of *Blastocystis hominis* with signs and symptoms of human disease. *J Clin Microbiol* 1986;24:548.

361. Garcia LS, Bruckner DA, Claney MN: Clinical relevance of *Blastocystis hominis. Lancet* 1984;2:1233.

362. Lee MG, Rawlins SC, Didier M, DeCeulaer K: Infective arthritis due to *Blastocystis hominis. Ann Rheum Dis* 1990;49:192.

363. Boros DL, Warren KS: Delayed hypersensitivity-type granuloma formation and dermal reaction induced and elicited by a soluble factor isolated from *Schistosoma mansoni* eggs. *J Exp Med* 1970;132:488.

364. Chotsulo L, Engels D, Montresor A, Savioli L: The global status of schistosomiasis and its control. *Acta Trop* 2000;77:41.

365. Malek EA: *Snail-Transmitted Parasitic Diseases,* Vol. 1. Boca Raton: CRC Press, 1980, pp 179–185.

366. Nash TE, Cheever AW, Ottesen EA, Cook JA: Schistosome infections in humans: perspectives and recent findings. *Ann Intern Med* 1982;97:740.

367. Ming-Chai C, Jen-Chun H, P'Ei-Yu, et al: Pathogenesis of carcinoma of the colon and rectum in *Schistosoma japonica.* A study of 90 cases. *Chin Med J* 1965;84:513.

368. El-Afifi S: Intestinal bilharziasis. *Dis Colon Rectum* 1964;7:1.

369. Prosser JM, Kasznica J, Gottlieb LS, Wade G: Bilharzial pseudotumors—dramatic manifestation of schistosomiasis: report of a case. *Hum Pathol* 1994;25:98.

370. Neves J, Raso P, Pinto DD, et al: Ischemic colitis (necrotizing colitis, pseudomembranous colitis) in acute schistosomiasis mansoni: report of two cases. *Trans R Soc Trop Med Hyg* 1993;87:449.

371. Miyake M: Schistosomiasis japonicum. In: Marcial-Rojas RA (ed). *Pathology of Protozoal and Helminthic Diseases.* Baltimore: Williams and Wilkins, 1971, pp 414–421.

372. Matsumoto T, Iida M, Kimura Y, et al: Anisakiasis of the colon: radiologic and endoscopic features in six patients. *Radiology* 1992;183:97.

373. Centers for Disease Control: *Intestinal Parasite Surveillance Summary 1978.* Atlanta, GA: Centers for Disease Control, 1979.

374. Neafie RC, Connor DH: Trichuriasis. In: Binford CH, Connor DH (eds). *Pathology of Tropical and Extraordinary Diseases.* Washington, DC: Armed Forces Institute of Pathology, 1976, pp 415–420.

375. Ramirez-Weiser R: Trichuriasis. In: Marcial-Rojas RA (ed). *Pathology of Protozoal and Helminthic Diseases.* Baltimore: Williams and Wilkins, 1971, pp 658–663.

376. Sun T: Trichurasis (trichocephaliasis). In: Sun T (ed). *Pathology and Clinical Features of Parasitic Diseases.* New York: Masson, 1982, pp 151–157.

377. Kronawitter U, Kemeny NE, Blumgart L: Neutropenic enterocolitis in a patient with colorectal carcinoma. *Cancer* 1997;80:656.

378. Wade DS, Nava HR, Douglass HO: Neutropenic enterocolitis. Clinical diagnosis and treatment. *Cancer* 1992;69:17.

379. Blei ED, Abrahams C: Diffuse phlegmonous gastroenterocolitis in a patient with an infected peritoneojugular venous shunt. *Gastroenterology* 1983;84:636.

380. Flejou JR, Bogomoletz WV: Les colites microscopiques: colite collagène et colite lymphcytaire. Un concept unitaire? *Gastroenterol Clin Biol* 1993;17:T28.

381. Jesserun J, Yardley J, Lee E, et al: Microscopic and collagenous colitis: different names for the same condition? *Gastroenterology* 1986;91:1583.

382. Bogomoletz WV: Collagenous, microscopic and lymphocytic colitis. An evolving concept. *Virchows Arch A Pathol Anat* 1994;424:573.

383. Mosnier J-F, Larvol L, Barge J, et al: Lymphocytic and collagenous colitis: an immunohistochemical study. *Am J Gastroenterol* 1996;91:709.

384. Giardiello FM, Bayless TM, Jessurun J, et al: Collagenous colitis: physiologic and histopathologic studies in seven patients. *Ann Intern Med* 1987;106:46.

385. Goff JS, Barnett JL, Pelke T, Appleman HD: Collagenous colitis: histopathology and clinical course. *Am J Gastroenterol* 1997;92:57.

386. Giardiello FM, Jackson F, Lazenby A: Metachronous occurrence of collagenous colitis and ulcerative colitis. *Gut* 1991;32:447.

387. Bowling TE, Price AB, Al-Adnani M, et al: Interchange between collagenous and lymphocytic colitis in severe disease with autoimmune associations requiring a colectomy: a case report. *Gut* 1996;38:788.

388. Goldstein NS, Gyorfi T: Focal lymphocytic colitis and collagenous colitis. Patterns of Crohn's colitis? *Am J Surg Pathol* 1999;23:1075.

389. Chutkam R, Sternthal M, Janowitz HD: A family with collagenous colitis, ulcerative colitis and Crohn's disease. *Am J Gastroenterol* 2000;95:3640.

390. Baert F, Wouter K, D'Haens G, et al: Lymphocytic colitis: a distinct clinical entity? A clinicopathological confrontation of lymphocytic and collagenous colitis. *Gut* 1999;45:375.

391. Lindstrom CG: "Collagenous colitis" with watery diarrhea new entity? *Pathol Eur* 1976;11:87.

392. Gremse DA, Boudreaux CW, Manci EA: Collagenous colitis in children. *Gastroenterology* 1993;104:906.

393. Jarnerot G, Hertervig E, Granno C, et al: Familial occurrence of microscopic colitis: a report on five families. *Scand J Gastroenterol* 2001; 36:959.

394. Rams H, Rogers AI, Gandhur-Mnaymneh L: Collagenous colitis. *Ann Int Med* 1987;106:108.

395. Molas G, Flejou JR, Potet F: Microscopic colitis, collagenous colitis and mast cells. *Dig Dis Sci* 1990;35:920.

396. Levy AM, Yamazaki K, Van Keulen VP, et al: Increased eosinophil infiltration and degranulation in colonic tissue from patients with collagenous colitis. *Am J Gastroenterol* 2001;96:1522.

397. Kingham JGC, Levison DA, Morson BC, et al: Collagenous colitis. *Gut* 1996;27:570.

398. Hwang WS, Kelly JK, Shaffer EA, et al: Collagenous colitis: a disease of pericryptal fibroblast sheath? *J Clin Pathol* 1986;149:33.

399. Andersen T, Andersen JR, Tvede M, et al: Collagenous colitis: are bacterial cytotoxins responsible? *Am J Gastroenterol* 1993;88:375.

400. Rampton DS, Baithun SI: Is microscopic colitis due to bile-salt malabsorption? *Dis Colon Rectum* 1987;30:950.

401. Rask-Madsen J, Grove O, Hansen MGJ, et al: Colonic transport of water and electrolytes in a patient with secretory diarrhea due to collagenous colitis. *Dig Dis Sci* 1983;28:1141.

402. Giardiello FM, Hansen FC III, Lazenby AJ, et al: Collagenous colitis in setting of nonsteroidal antiinflammatory drugs and antibiotics. *Dig Dis Sci* 1990;35:257.

403. Bohr J, Nordfelth R, Jarnerot G, Tysk C: Yersinia species in collagenous colitis: a serologic study. *Scand J Gastroenterol* 2002;37:711.

404. Brenet P, Dumontier I, Benhaimiseni MC, et al: Collagenous colitis: a new cause of intestinal protein loss. *Gastroenterol Clin Biol* 1992; 16:182.

405. Leigh C, Elahmady A, Mitros FA, et al: Collagenous colitis associated with chronic constipation. *Am J Surg Pathol* 1993;17:81.

406. Bogomoletz WV, Adnet JJ, Birembaut P, et al: Collagenous colitis: an unrecognized entity. *Gut* 1980;21:164.

407. Debongnie JC, DeGalocsy C, Caholessur MO, Haot J: Collagenous colitis: a transient condition? *Dis Colon Rectum* 1984;27:672.

408. Saul SH: The watery diarrhea–colitis syndrome. A review of collagenous and microscopic/lymphocytic colitis. *Int J Surg Pathol* 1993; 1:65.

409. Offner FA, Jao RV, Lewin KJ, et al: Collagenous colitis: a study of the distribution of morphological abnormalities and their histological detection. *Hum Pathol* 1999;30:451.

410. Aigner T, Neureiter D, Müller S, et al: Extracellular matrix composition and gene expression in collagenous colitis. *Gastroenterology* 1997; 113:113.

411. Anagnostopoulos D, Riecken EO: Tenascin labeling in colorectal biopsies: a useful marker in the diagnosis of collagenous colitis. *Histopathology* 1999;34:425.

412. Salas A, Fernandez-Bañares F, Casalots J, et al: Subepithelial myofibroblasts and tenascin expression in microscopic colitis. *Histopathology* 2003;43:48.

413. Carpenter HA, Tremaine WJ, Batts KP, et al: Sequential histologic evaluations in collagenous colitis. *Dig Dis Sci* 1993;37:1903.

414. Tanaka M, Mazzoleni G, Riddell RH: Distribution of collagenous colitis: utility of flexible sigmoidoscopy. *Gut* 1992;33:65.

415. Libbrecht L, Croes R, Ectors N, et al: Microscopic colitis with giant cells. *Histopathology* 2002;40:335.

416. Sandmeier D, Bouzourene H: Microscopic colitis with giant cells: a rare new histopathologic subtype. *Int J Surg Pathol* 2004;12:45.

417. Ayata G, Ithamukkala S, Sapp H, et al: Prevalence and significance of inflammatory bowel disease-like morphological features in collagenous and lymphocytic colitis. *Am J Surg Pathol* 2002;6:1414.

418. Sapp H, Ithamukkala S, Brien TP, et al: The terminal ileum is affected in patients with lymphocytic or collagenous colitis. *Am J Surg Pathol* 2002;26:1484.

419. Freeman HJ: Collagenous mucosal inflammatory diseases of the gastrointestinal tract. *Gastroenterology* 2005;129:338.

420. Schreiber FS, Eidt S, Hidding M, et al: Collagenous duodenitis and collagenous colitis: a short clinical course as evidenced by sequential endoscopic and histologic findings. *Endoscopy* 2001;33:555.

421. Lazenby AJ, Yardley JH, Giardiello FM, Bayless TM: Pitfalls in the diagnosis of collagenous colitis: experience with 75 cases from a registry of collagenous colitis at The Johns Hopkins Hospital. *Hum Pathol* 1990;21:905.

422. Miehlke S, Heymer P, Bethke B, et al: Budesonide treatment for collagenous colitis: a randomized double-blind, placebo-controlled, multicenter trail. *Gastroenterology* 2002;123:978.

423. Bonderup OK, Hansen JB, Birket-Smith L, et al: Budesonide treatment of collagenous colitis: a randomized, double blind, placebo-controlled trial with morphometric analysis. *Gut* 2003;52:248.

424. Abdo A, Raboud J, Freeman HJ, et al: Clinical and histological predictors of response to medical therapy in collagenous colitis. *Am J Gastroenterol* 2002;97:1164.

425. Bo-Linn GW, Vendrell DD, Lee E, Fordtran JS: An evaluation of the significance of microscopic colitis in patients with chronic diarrhea. *J Clin Invest* 1985;75:1559.

426. Fernandez-Bañares F, Salas A, Forné M, et al: Incidence of collagenous and lymphocytic colitis: a 5-year population based study. *Am J Gastrointrol* 1999;94:4189.

427. DuBois RN, Lazenby AJ, Yardley JH, et al: Lymphocytic enterocolitis in patients with "refractory sprue." *JAMA* 1989;262:935.

428. Puri AS, Khan EM, Kumar M, et al: Association of lymphocytic (microscopic) colitis with tropical sprue. *J Gastroenterol Hepatol* 1994;9:105.

429. Groisman GM, Meyers S, Harpaz N: Collagenous gastritis associated with lymphocytic colitis. *J Clin Gastroenterol* 1996;22:134.

430. Cindoruk M, Tuncer C, Dursun A, et al: Increased colonic intraepithelial lymphocytes in patients with Hashimoto's thyroiditis. *J Clin Gastroenterol* 2002;34:237.

431. Fernandez-Bañares F, Salas A, Esteve M, et al: Collagenous and lymphocytic colitis: evaluation of clinical and histological features, response to treatment, and long term follow-up. Am J Gastroenterol 2003;98:340.

432. Berrebi D, Sautet A, Flejou J-F, et al: Ticlopidine induced colitis: a histopathological study including apoptosis. J Clin Pathol 1998;51:280.

433. Mills LR, Schuman BM, Thompson WO: Lymphocytic colitis—a definable clinical and histological diagnosis. Dig Dis Sci 1993;38:1147.

434. Wang N, Dumot JA, Achkar E, et al: Colonic epithelial lymphocytosis without a thickened subepithelial collagen table. Am J Surg Pathol 1999;23:1068.

435. Ensari A, Marsh MN, Loft DE, et al: Morphometric analysis of intestinal mucosa. V. Quantitative histological and immunocytochemical studies of rectal mucosae in gluten sensitivity. Gut 1993;34:1225.

436. Fine KD, Lee EL, Meyer RL: Colonic histopathology in untreated celiac sprue or refractory sprue: is it lymphocytic colitis or colonic lymphocytosis? Hum Pathol 1998;29:1433.

437. Bryant DA, Mintz ED, Puhr ND, et al: Colonic epithelial lymphocytosis associated with an epidemic of chronic diarrhea. Am J Surg Pathol 1996;20:1002.

438. Mintz ED, Parsonnet J, Osterholm MT: Chronic idiopathic diarrhea. N Engl J Med 1993;328:1713.

439. Osterholm MT, MacDonald KL, White KE, et al: An outbreak of a newly recognized chronic diarrhea syndrome associated with raw milk consumption. JAMA 1986;256:484.

440. Parsonnet J, Trock SC, Bopp CA, et al: Chronic diarrhea associated with drinking untreated water. Ann Intern Med 1989;10:985.

441. Martin DL, Hoberman LJ: A point source outbreak of chronic diarrhea in Texas: no known exposure to raw milk. JAMA 1986;256:469.

442. Marshak RH, Linder A, Maklansky D, Gelb A: Eosinophilic gastroenteritis. JAMA 1981;245:1677.

443. Zora JA, O'Connell EJ, Sachs MI, Hoffman AD: Eosinophilic gastroenteritis: a case report and review of the literature. Ann Allergy 1984;53:45.

444. Pascal RR, Gramlich TL: Geographic variations of eosinophil concentration in normal colonic mucosa. Mod Pathol 1993;6:51A.

445. Bender AE, Matthews DR: Adverse reactions to foods. Br J Nutr 1981;46:403.

446. Crowe SE, Perdue MH: Gastrointestinal food hypersensitivity: basic mechanisms of pathophysiology. Gastroenterology 1992;103:1075.

447. Sampson HA, Mendelson L, Rosen JP: Fatal and near-fatal anaphylactic reactions to food in children and adolescents. N Engl J Med 1992;327:380.

448. Sampson HA, Metcalfe D: Food allergies. JAMA 1992;268:2840.

449. Sampson HA, Broadbent KR, Bernhisel-Broadbent J: Spontaneous release of histamine from basophils and histamine-releasing factor in patients with atopic dermatitis and food hypersensitivity. N Engl J Med 1989;321:228.

450. Goldman H, Proujansky R: Allergic proctitis and gastroenteritis in children. Am J Surg Pathol 1986;10:75.

451. Lake AM, Whitington PF, Hamilton SR: Dietary protein-induced colitis in breast-fed infants. J Pediatr 1982;101:906.

452. Jenkins HR, Pincott JR, Soothill JF, et al: Food allergy: the major cause of infantile colitis. Arch Dis Child 1984;59:326.

453. Iacono G, Cavataio F, Montalto G, et al: Intolerance of cow's milk and chronic constipation in children. N Engl J Med 1998;339:1100.

454. Crowe SE, Perdue MH: Gastrointestinal food hypersensitivity: basic mechanisms of pathophysiology. Gastroenterology 1992;103:1075.

455. Wershil BK, Walker WA: The mucosal barrier, IgE-mediated gastrointestinal events, and eosinophilic gastroenteritis. Gastroenterol Clin North Am 1992;21:387.

456. Sun XM, Hsueh W: Platelet-activating factor produces in vivo complement activation and tissue injury in mice. J Immunol 1991;147:509.

457. Monteiro RC, Hostoffer RW, Cooper MD, et al: Definition of immunoglobulin A receptors on eosinophils and their enhanced expression in allergic individuals. J Clin Invest 1993;92:1681.

458. Odze RD, Wershil BK, Leichtner AM, Antonioli DA: Allergic colitis in infants. J Pediatr 1995;126:163.

459. Odze RD, Bines J, Leichtner AM, et al: Allergic proctocolitis in infants: a prospective clinical-pathologic biopsy study. Hum Pathol 1993;24:668.

460. Schoonbroodt D, Horsmans Y, Laka A, et al: Eosinophilic gastroenteritis presenting with colitis and cholangitis. Dig Dis Sci 1995;40:308.

461. Clouse R, Alpers D, Hockenbery D, DeSchryver-Kecskemeti K: Pericrypt eosinophilic enterocolitis and chronic diarrhea. Gastroenterology 1992;103:168.

462. Azzopardi JG, Evans DJ: Mucoprotein-containing histiocytes (muciphages) in the rectum. J Clin Pathol 1996;19:368.

463. Bejarano PA, Aranda-Michel J, Fenoglio-Preiser C: Histochemical and immunohistochemical characterization of foamy histiocytes (muciphages and xanthelasma) of the rectum. Am J. Surg Pathol 2000;24:1009.

464. Satti MB, Abu-Melha A, Taha OM, Al-Idrissi HY: Colonic malacoplakia and abdominal tuberculosis in a child. Report of a case with review of the literature. Dis Colon Rectum 1985;28:353.

465. Long JP, Althausen AF: Malakoplakia J: a 25-year experience with a review of the literature. J Urol 1989;141:1328.

466. Lewin K, Harell G, Lee A, Crowley J: An electron-microscopic study: demonstration of bacilliform organisms in malacoplakic macrophages. Gastroenterology 1974;66:28.

467. Abdou NI, NaPombejara C, Sagawa A, et al: Malacoplakia: evidence for monocyte lysosomal abnormality correctable by cholinergic agonist in vitro and in vivo. N Engl J Med 1977;297:1413.

468. Israel H, Sones M: Sarcoidosis. Clinical observation on one hundred sixty cases. Arch Intern Med 1958;102:766.

469. Bulger K, O'Riordan M, Purdy S, et al: Gastrointestinal sarcoidosis resembling Crohn's disease. Am J Gastroenterol 1988;83:1415.

470. Hilzenrat N, Spanier AL, Lamoureux E, et al: Colonic obstruction secondary to sarcoidosis: nonsurgical diagnosis and management. Gastroenterology 1995;108:1556.

471. Fauci AS, Haynes BF, Katz P, Wolff SM: Wegener's granulomatosis. Prospective clinical and therapeutic experience with 85 patients for 21 years. Ann Intern Med 1983;98:76.

472. Chin J: Current and future dimensions of the HIV/AIDS pandemic in women and children. Lancet 1990;336:221.

473. Rawandan HIV Seroprevalence Study Group: Nationwide community-based serological survey of HIV-1 and other human retrovirus infections in a central African country. Lancet 1989;1:941.

474. World Health Organization and Centers for Disease Control: Statistics from the World Health Organization and the Centers for Disease Control. AIDS 1990;4:605.

475. Centers for Disease Control: Trends in AIDS incidence, deaths, and prevalence–United States, 1996. JAMA 1997;277:874.

476. Bozette SA, Berry SH, Duan N, et al: The care of HIV-infected adults in the United States. N Engl J Med 1998;339:1897.

477. Cu-Urvin S, Flanigan TP, Rich JD, et al: Human immunodeficiency virus infection and acquired immunodeficiency syndrome among North American women. Am J Med 1996;101:316.

478. Monkemuller KE, Wilcox CM: Investigation of diarrhea in AIDS. Can J Gastroenterol 2000;14:933.

479. Bonfanti P, Valsecchi L, Parazzini F, et al: Incidence of adverse reactions in HIV patients treated with protease inhibitors: a cohort study. J Acquir Immune Defic Syndr 2000;23:236.

480. Call SA, Heudebert G, Saag M, Wilcox CM: The changing etiology of chronic diarrhea in HIV-infected patients with CD4 cell counts less than 200 cells/mm³. Am J Gastroenterol 2000;95:3142.

481. Levy JA: Infection by human immunodeficiency virus–CD4 is not enough. N Engl J Med 1996;335:1528.

482. Berger EA, Doms RW, Fenyo EM, et al: A new classification for HIV-1. Nature 1998;391:240.

483. Alkhatib G, Combadiere C, Broder CC, et al: CC CKR5: A RANTES, MIP1-alpha, MIP 1beta receptor as a fusion cofactor for macrophage-tropic HIV-1. Science 1996;272:1955.

484. Palella FJ Jr, Delaney KM, Moorman AC, et al: Declining morbidity and mortality among patients with advanced human immunodeficiency virus infection. N Engl J Med 1998;338:853.

485. Zaitseva M, Blauvelt A, Lee S, et al: Expression and function of CCR5 and CXCR4 on human Langerhans cells and macrophages: implications for HIV primary infection. Nat Med 1997;3:1369.

486. Mummidi S, Ahuja SS, Gonzalez E, et al: Genealogy of the CCR5 locus and chemokine system gene variants associated with altered rates of HIV-1 disease progression. Nat Med 1998;4:786.

487. Liu R, Paxton WA, Choe S, et al: Homozygous defect in HIV-1 coreceptor accounts for resistance for some multiply-exposed individuals to HIV-infection. Cell 1996;86:367.

488. Sneller MC, Strober W: M cells and host defense. J Infect Dis 1986;154:737.

489. Amerongen HM, Weltzin R, Farnet CM, et al: Transepithelial transport of HIV-1 by intestinal M cells: A mechanism for transmission of AIDS. J Acquir Immune Defic Syndr 1991;4:760.

490. Lewis DE, Tang DS, Adu-Oppong A, et al: Anergy and apoptosis in CD8⁺ T cells from HIV-infected persons. *J Immunol* 1994;153:412.

491. Ellakany S, Whiteside TL, Schade RR, van Thiel DH: Analysis of intestinal lymphocyte subpopulations in patients with AIDS and AIDS-related complex. *Am J Clin Pathol* 1987;87:356.

492. Cocchi F, De Vico AL, Garzino-Demo A, et al: Identification of RANTES, MIP-1α, and MIP-1β as the major HIV suppressor factors produced by CD8+ T cells. *Science* 1995;270:1811.

493. Weiss RA: HIV receptors and the pathogenesis of AIDS. *Science* 1996;272:1885.

494. Kahn JO, Walker BD: Acute human immunodeficiency virus type I infection. *N Engl J Med* 1998;339:33.

495. Schacker T, Collier AC, Hughes J, et al: Clinical and epidemiological features of primary HIV infection. *Ann Intern Med* 1996;125:257.

496. Busch MP, Lee LL, Satten GA, et al: Time course of detection of viral and serologic markers preceding human immunodeficiency virus type 1 seroconversion: implications for screening of blood and tissue donors. *Transfusion* 1995;35:91.

497. Balslev E, Thomsen KH, Weisman K: Histopathology of acute human immunodeficiency virus exanthema. *J Clin Pathol* 1990;43:201.

498. Cavert W, Notermans DW, Staskus K, et al: Kinetics of response in lymphoid tissues to antiretroviral therapy of HIV-1 infection. *Science* 1997;276:960.

499. Heath SL, Tew TG, Tew JG, et al: Follicular dendritic cells and human immunodeficiency virus infectivity. *Nature* 1995;377:740.

500. Mellors JW, Rinaldo CR Jr, Gupta P, et al: Prognosis in HIV-1 infection predicted by the quantity of virus in plasma. *Science* 1996;272:1167.

501. Janoff EN, Smith PD: Perspectives on gastrointestinal infections in AIDS. *Gastroenterol Clin North Am* 1988;17:451.

502. Farthing MJG, Kelly MP, Veitch AM: Recently recognised microbial enteropathies and HIV infection. *J Antimicrob Chemother* 1996;37:61.

503. Simon D, Brandt LJ: Diarrhea in patients with the acquired immunodeficiency syndrome. *Gastroenterology* 1993;105:1238.

504. Ullrich R, Zeitz M, Heise W, et al: Mucosal atrophy is associated with loss of activated T cells in the duodenal mucosa of human immunodeficiency virus (HIV)-infected patients. *Digestion* 1990;46:302.

505. Ferreira RC, Forsyth LE, Richman PI, et al: Changes in the rate of crypt epithelial cell proliferation and mucosal morphology induced by a T-cell-mediated response in human small intestine. *Gastroenterology* 1990;98:1255.

506. Kotler DP, Reka S, Clayton F: Intestinal mucosal inflammation associated with human immunodeficiency virus infection. *Dig Dis Sci* 1993;38:1119.

507. Carpenter CC, Fischl MA, Hammer SM, et al: Antiretroviral therapy for HIV infection in 1997: updated recommendations of the International AIDS Society–USA panel. *JAMA* 1997;277:1962.

508. Rosenberg ES, Billingsley JM, Caliendo AM, et al: Vigorous HIV-1 specific CD4+ T cell responses associated with control of viremia. *Science* 1997;278:1447.

509. Panel on Clinical Practices for Treatment of HIV Infection (2004): Guidelines form the use of antiretroviral agents in HIV-1 infected adults and adolescents. Available at: http://aidsinfo.nih.gov/guidelines/. Accessed January 1, 2007.

510. Mocraft A, Lundgren JD: Starting highly active antiretroviral therapy: why, when and response to HAART. *J Antimicrob Chemother* 2004;54:10.

511. Grogan TM, Odom RB, Burgess JH: Graft-vs-host reaction. *Arch Dermatol* 1977;113:806.

512. Anderson KC, Weinstein HJ: Transfusion-associated graft-versus-host disease. *N Engl J Med* 1990;323:315.

513. Dinsmore RE, Straus DJ, Pollack MS, et al: Fatal graft-v-host disease following blood transfusion in Hodgkin's disease documented by HLA typing. *Blood* 1980;55:831.

514. Easaw S, Lake D, Beer M, et al: Graft-versus-host disease. Possible higher risk for African American patients. *Cancer* 1996;78:1492.

515. Burdick JF, Vogelsang GB, Smith WJ, et al: Severe graft-versus-host disease in a liver-transplant recipient. *N Engl J Med* 1988;318:689.

516. Takata M: Immunohistochemical identification of perforin-positive cytotoxic lymphocytes in graft-versus-host disease. *Am J Clin Pathol* 1995;103:324.

517. Glucksburg H, Storb R, Fefar A, et al: Clinical manifestations of graft-versus-host disease in human recipients of marrow from HLA-matched sibling donors. *Transplantation* 1984;18:295.

518. Nagata S: Apoptotic by death factor. *Cell* 1997;88:355.

519. Lin MT, Storer B, Martin PJ, et al: Relation of an interleukin-10 promoter polymorphism to graft-versus-host disease and survival after hematopoietic cell transplantation. *N Engl J Med* 2003;349:2201.

520. Ferrara JLM, Yani G: Acute graft versus host disease: pathophysiology, risk factors and prevention strategies. *Clin Adv Hematol Oncol* 2005;3:415.

521. Couriel D, Caldera H, Champlin RE, Komanduri K: Acute graft-versus-host disease: pathophysiology, clinical manifestations and management. *Cancer* 2004;101:1936.

522. Socié G: Graft-versus-host disease – from the bench to the bedside? *N Engl J Med* 2005;33:1396.

523. Ponec RJ, Hackman RC, McDonald GB: Endoscopic and histologic diagnosis of intestinal graft-versus-host disease after marrow transplantation. *Gastrointest Endosc* 1999;49:612.

524. Silva MR, Henne K, Sale GE: Positive identification of enterocytes by keratin antibody staining of sloughed intestinal tissue in severe GVHD. *Bone Marrow Transplant* 1993;12:35.

525. Chakrabarti S, Lees A, Jones SC, et al: Clostridium difficile infection in allogeneic stem cell transplant recipients is associated with severe graft-versus-host disease and non-relapse mortality. *Transplant* 2000;26:871.

526. Gulbuhce HE, Brown CA, Wick M, et al: Graft-versus-host disease after solid organ transplant. *Am J Clin Pathol* 2003;119:568.

527. Snover DC: Mucosal damage simulating acute graft-versus-host reaction in cytomegalovirus colitis. *Transplantation* 1985;39:669.

528. Kornacki S, Hansen F, Lazenby A: Graft-versus-host-like colitis associated with malignant thymoma. *Am J Surg Pathol* 1995;19:224.

529. Snover DC, Filipovich AH, Ramsay NKC, et al: Graft-versus-host disease-like findings in pre-bone marrow transplantation biopsies of patients with severe T cell deficiency. *Transplantation* 1985;39:95.

530. Washington K, Stenzel TT, Buckley RH, et al: Gastrointestinal pathology in patients with common variable immunodeficiency and X-linked agammaglobulinemia. *Am J Surg Pathol* 2000;20:1240.

531. Asplund S, Gramlich TL: Chronic mucosal changes of the colon in graft-versus-host disease. *Mod Pathol* 1998;11:513.

532. Brooks EG, Filipovich AH, Padgett JW, et al: T-cell receptor analysis in Omenn's syndrome: evidence for defects in gene rearrangements and assembly. *Blood* 1999;93:242.

533. Ghoshal UC, Biswass PK, Roy G, et al: Colonic mucosal changes in portal hypertension. *Trop Gastroenterol* 2001;22:25.

534. Kozarek RA, Botoman VA, Bredfeldt JE, et al: Portal colopathy: prospective study of colonoscopy in patients with portal hypertension. *Gastroenterology* 1991;101:1192.

535. Bini EJ, Lascarides CE, Micale PL, Weinshel EH: Mucosal abnormalities of the colon in patients with portal hypertension: an endoscopic study. *Gastrointest Endosc* 2000;52:511.

536. Ponce Gonzalez JF, Dominguez Adame Lanzuna E, Martin Zurita I, Morales Mendez S: Portal hypertensive colopathy: histologic appearance of the colonic mucosa. *Hepatogastroenterology* 1998;45:40.

537. Lamps LW, Hunt CM, Green A, et al: Alterations in colonic mucosal vessel in patents with cirrhosis and noncirrhotic portal hypertension. *Hum Pathol* 1998;28:527.

538. Gudjonsson H, Zeiler D, Gamelli RL, Kaye MD: Colonic varices. Report of an unusual case diagnosed by radionuclide scanning, with review of the literature. *Gastroenterology* 1986;91:1543.

539. Burbige EJ, Tarder J, Carson S, et al: Colonic varices, a complication of pancreatitis with splenic vein thrombosis. *Am J Dig Dis* 1978;23:752.

540. Hawkey CJ, Amar SS, Daintith H, et al: Familial varices of the colon occurring without evidence of portal hypertension. *Br J Radiol* 1985;58:677.

541. Farrell DJ, Bennett MK: Dieulafoy's vascular malformation as a cause of large intestinal bleeding. *J Clin Pathol* 1992;45:363.

542. Richter JM, Christensen MR, Colditz GA, Nishioka NS: Angiodysplasia: natural history and efficacy of therapeutic interventions. *Dig Dis Sci* 1989;34:1542.

543. Veyradier A, Balian A, Wolf M, et al: Abnormal von Willebrand factor in bleeding angiodysplasias of the digestive tract. *Gastroenterology* 2001;120:346.

544. Junquera F, Quiroga S, Saperas E, et al: Accuracy of helical computed tomographic angiography for the diagnosis of colonic angiodysplasia. *Gastroenterology* 2000;119:292.

545. Mitsudo S, Boley SJ, Barndt LJ, et al: Vascular ectasias of the right colon in the elderly: a distinct pathological entity. *Hum Pathol* 1979;10:585.

546. Imahori SC: Gastrointestinal arterial fibromuscular dysplasia of childhood. *Arch Pathol Lab Med* 1989;113:9.

547. Stern MA, Chey WD: Pneumatosis coli and colonic intussusception. *N Engl J Med* 2001;345:964.

548. Black CM, Gathercole LJ, Baily AJ, et al: The Ehlers-Danlos syndrome: an analysis of the structure of the collagen fibres of the skin. *Br J Dermatol* 1980;102:85.

549. Pope FM, Jones PM, Wells RS, et al: EDS IV (acrogeria): new autosomal dominant and recessive types. *J R Soc Med* 1980;73:180.

550. Pepin M, Schwarze U, Superti-Frga A, Byers PH: Clinical and genetic features of Ehlers-Danlos syndrome type IV, the vascular type. *N Engl J Med* 2000;342:673.

551. Beighton P, De Paepe A, Steinmann B, et al: Ehlers-Danlos syndromes: revised nosology, Villefranche 1997. *Am J Med, Genet* 1998;77:31.

552. Tager JM: Inborn errors of cellular organelles: an overview. *J Inherit Metab Dis* 1987;10:3.

553. Lake BD: Storage involving the alimentary tract. In: Whitehead R (ed). *Gastrointestinal and Oesophageal Pathology.* Melbourne: Churchill Livingstone, 1995, pp 343–349.

554. Rapola J, Santavuori P, Savilahti E: Suction biopsy of rectal mucosa in the diagnosis of infantile and juvenile types of neuronal ceroid lipofuscinoses. *Hum Pathol* 1984;15:352.

555. Muenzer J: Mucopolysaccharidoses. *Adv Pediatr* 1986;33:269.

556. Taniike M, Yamano T, Shimada M, et al: Ultrastructural pathology of rectum and skin biopsies specimens in lysosomal storage diseases. *Acta Histochem Cytochem* 1990;23:81.

557. daSilva V, Vassella F, Bischoff A, et al: Niemann-Pick's disease. Clinical, biochemical and ultrastructural findings in a case of infantile form. *J Neurol* 1975;211:61.

558. Arey JB: The lipidoses: morphologic changes in the nervous system in Gaucher's disease, G_{m2}-gangliosidoses and Niemann-Pick disease. *J Clin Lab Sci* 1975;5:475.

559. Goldman JE, Katz D, Rapin DP, Suzuki K: Chronic G_{M1}-gangliosidosis presenting as dystonia: I. Clinical and pathological features. *Ann Neurol* 1981;9:465.

560. Ikeda S, Ushiyama M, Nakano T, Kikkawa T: Ultrastructural findings of rectal and skin biopsies in adult G_{m1}-gangliosidosis. *Acta Pathol Jpn* 1986;36:1823.

561. Greene HL: Glycogen storage disease. *Semin Liver Dis* 1982;2:291.

562. Roe TF, Thomas DW, Gilsanz V, et al: Inflammatory bowel disease in glycogen storage disease type Ib. *J Pediatr* 1986;109:55.

563. Couper R, Kapelushnik J, Griffiths AM: Neutrophil dysfunction in glycogen storage disease Ib: association with Crohn's like colitis. *Gastroenterology* 1991;100:549.

564. Tome FM, Fardeau M, Lenour G: Ultrastructure of muscle and sensory nerve in Fabry's disease. *Acta Neuropathol* 1977;38:187.

565. Herbert PN, Forte T, Heinen RJ, Fredrickson DS: Tangier disease. *N Engl J Med* 1978;299:519.

566. Schutgens RBH, Heymans HSA, Wanders RJA, et al: Peroxisomal disorders: a newly recognized group of genetic diseases. *Eur J Pediatr* 1986;144:430.

567. Shimozawa N, Suzuki Y, Orii T, et al: Biochemical and morphologic aspects of peroxisomes in the human rectal mucosa: diagnosis of Zellweger syndrome simplified by rectal biopsy. *Pediatr Res* 1988;24:723.

568. Tsui LC, Durie P: Genotype and phenotype in cystic fibrosis. *N Engl J Med* 1993;329:1308.

569. Hirtz S, Gonska T, Seydewitz HH, et al: CFTR Cl- channel function in native human colon correlates with the genotype and phenotype in cystic fibrosis. *Gastroenterology* 2004;127:1085.

570. Eggermont E: Gastrointestinal manifestations in cystic fibrosis. *Euro J Gastroenterol Hepatol* 1996;8:731.

571. Chaun H: Colonic disorders in adult cystic fibrosis in adult cystic fibrosis. *Can J Gastroenterol* 2001;15:586.

572. Kebbel A, Röcken C: Immunohistochemical classification of amyloid in surgical pathology revisited. *Am J Surg Pathol* 2006;30:673.

573. Araki H, Muramoto H, Oda K, et al: Severe gastrointestinal complications if dialysis-related amyloidosis in two patients on long-tern hemodialysis. *Am J Nephrol* 1996;16:149.

574. Jimenez RE, Price DA, Pinkus GS, et al: Development of gastrointestinal α2-microglobulin amyloidosis correlates with time on dialysis. *MMWR Morb Mortal Wkly Rep* 1998;22:729.

575. Borczuk A, Mannion C, Dickson D, Alt E: Intestinal pseudo-obstruction and ischemia secondary to both $β_2$-microglobulin and serum A amyloid deposition. *Mod Pathol* 1995;8:577.

576. Zauber A, Winawer SJ, Diaz B, et al: National Polyp Study: the association of colonic hyperplastic polyps and adenomas. *Am J Gastroenterol* 1988;83:1060.

577. Cappell MS, Fordo KA: Spatial clustering of multiple hyperplastic, adenomatous and malignant colonic polyps in individual patients. *Dis Colon Rectum* 1989;32:641.

578. Williams AR, Balasooriya BA, Day DW: Polyps and cancer of the large bowel: a necropsy study in Liverpool. *Gut* 1982;23:835.

579. Clark JC, Collan Y, Eide TJ, et al: Prevalence of polyps in an autopsy series from areas with varying incidence of large-bowel cancer. *Int J Cancer* 1985;36:179.

580. Jass JR, Young PJ, Robinson EM: Predictors of presence, multiplicity, size and dysplasia of colorectal adenomas. A necropsy study in New Zealand. *Gut* 1992;33:1508.

581. Blue MG, Sivak MV, Achkar E, et al: Hyperplastic polyps seen at sigmoidoscopy are markers for additional adenomas seen at colonoscopy. *Gastroenterology* 1991;100:564.

582. Fenoglio CM, Lane N: The anatomical precursor of colorectal carcinoma. *Cancer* 1974;34:819.

583. Goldman H, Ming SC, Hickock D: Nature and significance of hyperplastic polyps of the human colon. *Arch Pathol* 1970;89:349.

584. Provenzale D, Garrett J, Condon S, Sandler R: Risk for colon adenomas in patients with rectosigmoid hyperplastic polyps. *Ann Intern Med* 1990;113:760.

585. Jass JR: Relations between metaplastic polyp and carcinoma of the colorectum. *Lancet* 1983;1:28.

586. Fenoglio-Preiser CM: When is a hyperplastic polyp not a hyperplastic polyp? *Am J Surg Pathol* 1999;23:1001.

587. Carr NJ, Monihan JM, Nzeako UC, et al: Expression of proliferating cell nuclear antigen in hyperplastic polyps, adenomas and inflammatory cloacogenic polyps of the large intestine. *J Clin Pathol* 1995;48:46.

588. Giarneiri E, Nagar C, Valli S, et al: BCL2 and BAX expression in hyperplastic and dysplastic rectal polyps. *Hepatogastroenterology* 2000;47:159.

589. Otori K, Oda Y, Sugiyama K, et al: High frequency of K-ras mutations in human colorectal hyperplastic polyps. *Gut* 1997;40:660.

590. Chan TL, Zhao W, Cancer Genome Project, et al: BRAF and KRAS mutations in colorectal hyperplastic polyps and serrated adenomas. *Cancer Res* 2003;63:4878.

591. Iino H, Jass J, Simms LA, et al: DNA microsatellite instability in hyperplastic polyps, serrated adenomas and mixed polyps: a mil mutator pathway for colorectal cancer? *J Clin Pathol* 1999;52:5.

592. Jass JR: Hyperplastic polyps of the colorectum – innocent or guilty? *Colon Rectum* 2001;44:163.

593. Hayashi T, Yatani R, Apostol J, Stemmermann GN: Pathogenesis of hyperplastic polyps of the colon. A hypothesis based on ultrastructure and in vitro kinetics. *Gastroenterology* 1974;66:347.

594. Longacre TA, Fenoglio-Preiser CM: Mixed hyperplastic adenomatous polyps/serrated adenomas. A distinct form of colorectal neoplasia. *Am J Surg Pathol* 1990;14:524.

595. Koike M, Inada K, Nakanisi H, et al: Cellular differentiation status of epithelial polyps of the colorectum: the gastric foveolar cell-type in hyperplastic polyps. *Histopathology* 2003;42:357.

596. Yantiss RK, Goldman H, Odze RD: Hyperplastic polyp with epithelial misplacement (inverted hyperplastic polyp): a clinicopathologic and immunohistochemical study of 19 cases. *Mod Pathol* 2001;14:869.

597. Sobin LH: Inverted hyperplastic polyps of the colon. *Am J Surg Pathol* 1985;9:265.

598. Groisman GM, Polak-Charcon S, Appleman HD: Fibroblastic polyp of the colon: clinicopathological analysis of 10 cases with emphasis on its common association with serrated crypts. *Histopathology* 2006; 48:431.

599. Eslami-Varzaneh F, Washington K, Robert ME, et al: Benign fibroblastic polyps of the colon. A histologic, immunohistochemical and ultrastructural study. *Am J Surg Pathol* 2004;28:374.

600. Jessurun J, Paplanus SH, Nagle RB, et al: Pseudosarcomatous changes in inflammatory polyps of the colon. *Arch Pathol Lab Med* 1986;110:833.

601. Shekitka KM, Helwig EB: Deceptive bizarre stromal cells in polyps and ulcers of the gastrointestinal tract. *Cancer* 1991;67:2111.

602. Esaki M, Matsumoto M, Kobayashi H, et al: Cap polyposis of the colon and rectum: an analysis of endoscopic findings. *Endoscopy* 2001;33:262.

603. Gottrand F, Erkan T, Turck D, et al: Food induced bleeding from lymphonodular hyperplasia in the colon. *Pediatr Forum* 1993;147:821.

604. Devroede G, Lemieux B, Masse S, et al: Colonic hamartomas in tuberous sclerosis. *Gastroenterology* 1988;94:182.

605. Davis E, Chow C, Miyai K: A hamartoma of the colon with unusual features. *Endoscopy* 1991;23:349.

606. Nakamura S, Kino I, Akagi T: Inflammatory myoglandular polyps of the colon and rectum. A clinicopathological study of 32 pedunculated polyps, distinct from other types of polyps. *Am J Surg Pathol* 1992;16:772.

607. Cheville JC, Mitros FA, Vanderzalm G, Platz CE: Atheroemboli-associated polyps of the sigmoid colon. *Am J Surg Pathol* 1993;17:1054.

608. Gramlich TL, Hunter SB: Focal polypoid ischemia of the colon: atheroemboli presenting as a colonic polyp. *Arch Pathol Lab Med* 1994;118:308.

609. Yantiss RK, Clement PB, Young RH: Endometriosis of the intestinal tract. A study of 44 cases of a disease that may cause diverse challenges in clinical and pathological evaluation. *Am J Surg Pathol* 2001;25:445.

610. Badawy SZA, Freedman L, Numann P, et al: Diagnosis and management of intestinal endometriosis: a report of five cases. *J Reprod Med* 1988;33:851.

611. Weed JC, Ray JE: Endometriosis of the bowel. *Obstet Gynecol* 1987;69:727.

612. Clement PB, Granai CO, Young RH, Scully RE: Endometriosis with myxoid change: a case simulating pseudomyxoma peritonei. *Am J Surg Pathol* 1994;18:849.

613. Yantiss RK, Clement PB, Young RH: Neoplastic and pre-neoplastic changes in gastrointestinal endometriosis. A study of 17 cases. *Am J Surg Pathol* 2000;24:513.

614. McCluggage WG, Clements WDB: Endosalpingiosis of the colon and appendix. *Histopathology* 2001;39:645.

615. Matsukuma S, Goda K, Sakai Y, et al: Histopathlogic studies of colorectal postendoscopic resection sites. "Skipping electrothermal injury" associated with endoscopic resection procedures. *Am J Surg Pathol* 1999;23:459.

616. Glotzer DJ, Glick ME, Goldman H: Proctitis and colitis following diversion of the fecal stream. *Gastroenterology* 1981;80:438.

617. Ma CK, Gottlieb C, Haas PA: Diversion colitis: a clinicopathologic study of 21 cases. *Hum Pathol* 1990;21:429.

618. Mortensen PB, Clausen MR: Short chain fatty acids in the human colon: relation to gastrointestinal health and disease. *Scand J Gastroenterol* 1996;31:132.

619. Edwards CM, George B, Warren B: Diversion colitis – new light through old windows. *Histopathology* 1999;34:1.

620. Yeong ML, Bethwaite PB, Prasad J, Isbister WH: Lymphoid follicular hyperplasia—a distinctive feature of diversion colitis. *Histopathology* 1991;19:55.

621. Park SI, Genta RS, Romeio DP, Weesner RE: Colonic abscess and focal peritonitis secondary to india ink tattooing of the colon. *Gastrointest Endosc* 1991;37:68.

622. Hammond DC, Lane FR, Mackeigan JM, Passinault WJ: Endoscopic tattooing of the colon: clinical experience. *Am Surg* 1993;59:205.

623. Lane KL, Vallera R, Washington K, Gottfried MR: Endoscopic tattoo agents in the colon: tissue responses and clinical implications. *Am J Surg Pathol* 1996;20:1266.

624. Mitchell CM, Drossman DA: Survey of the AGA membership relating to patients with functional gastrointestinal disorders. *Gastroenterology* 1987;92:1282.

625. Olden KW: Diagnosis of irritable bowel syndrome. *Gastroenterology* 2002;122:1701.

626. Lembo TJ, Fink RN: Clinical assessment of irritable bowel syndrome. *J Clin Gastroenterol* 2002;35:S31.

627. Kirsch RH, Riddell R: Histopathological alterations in irritable bowel syndrome. *Mod Pathol* 2006;19:1638.

628. Seaman WB, Clements JL: Urticaria of the colon: a nonspecific pattern of submucosal edema. *AJR Am J Roentgenol* 1982;138:545.

629. Snover DC, Sandstad J, Hutton S: Mucosal pseudolipomatosis of the colon. *Am J Clin Pathol* 1985;84:575.

630. Enjoji M, Sumiyoshi K, Sueyoshi K: Elastofibromatous lesion of the stomach in a patient with elastofibroma dorsi. *Am J Surg Pathol* 1985;9:233.

Epithelial Neoplasms of the Colon

The large intestine gives rise to a host of neoplasms. In this chapter we will focus on epithelial neoplasms. Neuroendocrine tumors are covered in Chapter 17, hematologic malignancies in Chapter 18, and mesenchymal tumors in Chapter 19.

COLONIC ADENOMAS AND CARCINOMAS

Colorectal carcinoma is one of the most common neoplasms affecting individuals living in industrialized nations. Colorectal cancer is the fourth ranking cancer worldwide, accounting for approximately 9% of all cancers (1). The lifetime risk of developing colorectal carcinoma in the United States is approximately 5.5% for both men and women, with an approximately 2% chance of dying from the disease (2). Most carcinomas develop from adenomas, their precursor lesion. These adenomas occur sporadically or as part of a polyposis syndrome (see Chapter 12). Adenomas are benign by definition, although they are neoplastic and may harbor an invasive carcinoma. Carcinomas also arise in areas of dysplasia in patients with idiopathic inflammatory bowel disease (IBD) (see Chapter 11).

Considerable advances have occurred in our understanding of the molecular events associated with the progression of colorectal carcinoma since the publication of the first edition of this book. Complex interactions between inherited and acquired genomic and other biologic changes associate with both benign and malignant large bowel neoplasia. Colon cancer is highly curable if it is diagnosed in its early stages.

Incidence

Colorectal cancer exhibits at least a 25-fold variation in occurrence worldwide (1,3). It is most common in the industrialized countries of Western and Eastern Europe, North America, New Zealand, and Australia (Fig. 14.1), while its incidence is low in Africa and Asia (1,4). These large geographic differences in colorectal cancer incidence are most likely explained by different environmental and dietary exposures. Migrants from countries where colon cancer risk is low to high-risk countries show a rapid increase in their colon cancer rates (1,5). A rapid increase in colorectal cancer frequency occurring in Japan parallels its increasing prosperity and westernization (4). This phenomenon is equivalent to a migration in time rather than space and suggests that indigenous Japanese, like those who have migrated to the United States, will acquire levels of colorectal cancer risk equivalent to, or higher than, those of U.S. whites. In fact, colorectal cancer rates for Japanese individuals born in the United States are now higher than those for U.S. whites (6).

The overall and subsite frequency of colorectal cancer also shows considerable intranational ethnic variation, a phenomenon best documented in the United States and New Zealand. It is difficult to determine whether these differences have a genetic or environmental basis, given the different cultural and socioeconomic backgrounds of the ethnic groups within these countries. In the United States, the highest incidence rates in the Surveillance, Epidemiology, and End Results (SEER) registries for the years 2000 to 2003 were in Black males (72.9 of 100,000) followed by White males (61.4 of 100,000), Black females (56.1 of 100,00), Asian males (51.2 of 100,000), Hispanic males (47.3 of 100,000), White females (44.7 of 100,000), Asian females (35.7 of 100,000), and Hispanic females (32.7 of 100,000) (2).

Mortality

In 2006, an estimated 55,170 people died of colorectal cancer in the United States (2). Overall, the age-adjusted mortality rate for colorectal cancer among all ethnic groups in the United States has declined since 1975 (2). However, SEER mortality data for the years 2000 to 2003 show a significantly higher mortality for black Americans with colorectal cancer than their white compatriots (2). Mortality rates are lowest for Asian and Hispanic colorectal cancer patients in the United States.

Etiology

It is important to recognize that colon cancers and rectal cancers associate with different risk factors. This is consistent with the observation that colon cancers rise in

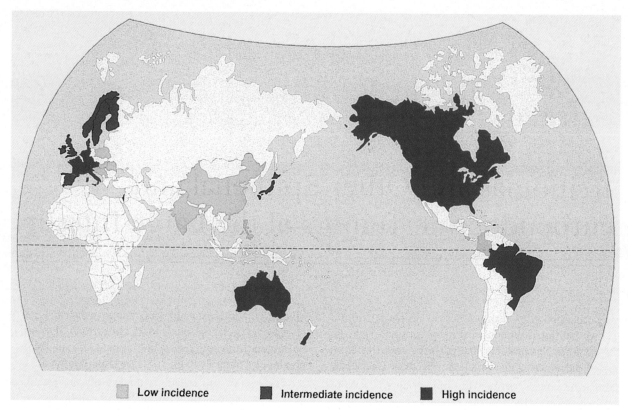

FIG. 14.1. Map showing the geographic variation in colon cancer incidence worldwide. Countries indicated in *red* represent areas of high incidence, those in *green* intermediate incidence, and those in *yellow* a low incidence of the disease.

frequency among migrants from low- to high-risk areas, while rectal cancers exhibit a fairly stable incidence (4). Moreover, the colonic subsites also show considerable variation in cancer incidence and in cancer-associated risk factors. Thus, right-sided cancers generally constitute a larger proportion of colorectal cancers in low-risk populations than in high-risk groups and show smaller postmigration increases than do left-sided cancers. That said, it should be noted that the progression of the neoplastic process from adenoma to carcinoma is similar throughout all segments of the large bowel, and that the risk factors for carcinoma and adenoma are similar (7).

Environmental and genetic influences probably play roles at different points in the neoplastic progression. Several well-characterized colon cancer syndromes indicate that inherited susceptibility plays an important role in the pathogenesis of colorectal cancer (see Chapter 12). Conversely, epidemiologic, experimental, and migrant studies clearly indicate environmental influences in the genesis of the disease. Diet may alter endogenous characteristics, such as the bowel flora, which in turn influence the conversion of ingested foods into potential carcinogens. Other environmental factors, such as physical activity, occupational exposures, or ethanol, may further influence these interactions. The interaction of environmental factors with genetic factors is complex and currently under intense scrutiny.

Genetic Factors

Familial forms of colon cancer fall into several categories: (a) patients with a polyposis syndrome, (b) patients with defined colon cancer family syndromes, and (c) patients who appear to have sporadic cancers but who have other family members with colon cancer. Genetic influences are best defined in two autosomal dominant syndromes: Familial adenomatous polyposis (FAP) and hereditary nonpolyposis colon cancer syndrome (HNPCC) (see Chapter 12). Hereditary polyposes account for approximately 1% of all colorectal carcinomas, HNPCC accounts for another approximately 5%, and perhaps 30% or more of sporadic carcinomas may be inherited (8).

Neoplasia in Asymptomatic First-degree Relatives of Persons with Colon Cancer

The presence of a colorectal cancer in a first-degree relative (sibling or parent) represents an important colon cancer risk factor. It may increase a person's lifetime risk from 1.8-fold to as high as eightfold that of the general population (9). The effect of family history is greatest for younger individuals (i.e., those younger than 45 years of age). Asymptomatic patients with one first-degree relative with colorectal cancer have nearly double the risk of developing adenomas or cancers than asymptomatic individuals without a family history; the cancer often affects younger persons (9–12). The incidence of colonic neoplasms among first-degree relatives of colorectal cancer patients ranges from 15% to 20% (13). These trends are even more pronounced in those having more than one affected relative (14,15). Familial clusters of colorectal cancer could arise on the basis of a shared gene pool, a shared environment, or a combination of both.

Relationship between Colon Cancer and Energy Balance

Reduced physical activity and obesity have emerged as consistent epidemiologic associations with colon cancer risk (7,16–23) and probably account for the association of this cancer with sedentary occupations, weight gain since age 25, body mass index, family income, and the rural/urban gradient in colon cancer frequency. Colon cancer is also associated with central adiposity independent of body mass index (22). Excess energy intake over energy expenditure may also account, at least in part, for the association of colon cancer with fat intake, since fat is a major source of energy (16). It is of interest that rectal cancer does not share these risks (7). The mechanism that accounts for the association between a positive energy balance and colon cancer has not been identified, but it has been proposed that physical activity may stimulate hormonal release, activating neural reflex mechanisms that enhance propagative peristalsis and increased colonic motility. This, in turn, leads to decreased mucosal contact with intraluminal carcinogens.

In addition, the insulin resistance that commonly affects obese individuals may also play a role (24). Type 2 diabetes associates with a threefold increase in colorectal cancer risk compared with the nondiabetic population (25). In addition, colon cancer patients exhibit greater degrees of glucose intolerance and insulin resistance than patients without colorectal cancer (26). Insulin has growth and metabolic effects that could impact the colonic epithelium predisposing to cancer development. Insulin stimulates proliferation and inhibits apoptosis in colorectal cancer cell lines, and promotes growth of colon tumors in experimental animals (27–29). The metabolic effects of insulin lead to increased concentrations of glucose and triglycerides that may additionally result in an environment in which transformed colonocytes have greater available energy sources. Insulin may also affect cell-signaling pathways by activating insulinlike growth factor, protein kinase C, and mitogen-activated protein (MAP) kinase, leading to increased mitotic activity and potential carcinogenesis (30).

Nongenetic Host Factors

Intestinal epithelium is exposed to a complex luminal environment that plays an etiologic role in colorectal tumorigenesis. Variably digested food passes into the colonic lumen from the small bowel and mixes with bile acids and other luminal constituents (Fig. 14.2). The luminal contents vary with the

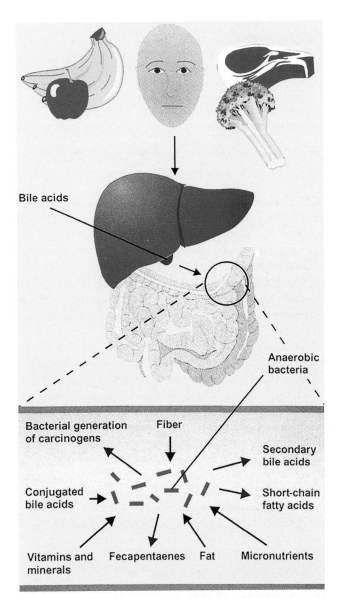

FIG. 14.2. Nongenetic factors involved in colon carcinogenesis. Dietary substances, including fruits, vegetables, and meats, influence the composition of the luminal contents of the gut. Ingested substances such as fat, fiber, vitamins, and minerals interact with bile acids and the luminal anaerobic bacterial population, producing some carcinogenic and mutagenic molecules, as well as cytoprotective substances. The level of production of each of these molecules varies depending on the composition of the luminal contents.

diet. Millions of bacteria are present in the gut lumen, and many of these generate energy by degrading and fermenting plant cell material (31). The effects of the bacterial flora are noted in Table 14.1. One byproduct, butyrate, slows cell proliferation and facilitates access of DNA repair enzymes.

Dietary Factors

The vast literature associated with the relation of diet to colorectal cancer continues to generate controversy. This is

TABLE 14.1 Effects of Colonic Bacterial Flora

Deconjugate bile acid to form secondary bile acids
Produce butyrate and other short-chain fatty acids
Activate procarcinogens
Form diacylglycerol
Ferment polysaccharides, protein, and glycoproteins
Synthesize fecapentaene
Adsorb hydrophobic molecules

due, in part, to differences in the methods employed to measure dietary variables and to the comparatively small increases in risk that can be demonstrated with even the strongest dietary associations. The three methods for dietary studies are ecologic studies that relate cancer incidence to per capita food consumption, and two analytic methods—the case control method, which assesses dietary practices of patients who have been diagnosed with cancer, and prospective cohort studies, which measure dietary exposures in healthy subjects who are followed until cancer develops. Each method has built-in flaws. Ecologic studies do not identify the dietary patterns of specific cancer patients, which may actually differ from those of the general population. Dietary data collected prospectively in cohort studies may not hold true for the future, and dietary measurements taken at the time of cancer diagnosis may reflect the influence of disease upon food preferences rather than past experience. Moreover, complex interrelationships exist between energy balance, fat and meat consumption, fiber, alcohol intake, and micronutrients, making it difficult to tease out the relative impact of any one variable upon the risk of colon cancer. The following discussion summarizes the pertinent trends in this field of study.

Fat and Animal Protein

These two items are combined because they are highly correlated in dietary intake studies. In many of the published dietary analyses, fat intake is inferred from meat consumption, so that it is not possible to assess their individual impact on colon cancer risk. The origin of the hypothesis that a high-fat diet favors the development of colon cancer dates from the early correlation studies of Burkitt (32) that showed that colon cancer and coronary heart disease (CHD), as well as their precursors adenomatous polyps and atherosclerosis, were seldom encountered in black Africans who consume very low levels of dietary fat (33). Subsequent studies in other populations showed a strong correlation between national per capita fat consumption and both colon cancer and CHD. It has been well established that a high fat intake favors CHD, and it is therefore reasonable to suggest that this also holds true for colon cancer. Furthermore, there is a strong international correlation between the mortality rates from colon cancer and CHD (34), although France (low CHD and high colon cancer rates) and Finland (high CHD

and low colon cancer rates) are exceptions. Kolonel (35) reviewed 14 correlational studies and found that six favored a fat–colon cancer connection and eight did not. In spite of these inconsistencies, he pointed out that dietary variability in fat intake in homogenous populations may not be great, and that intergroup correlational studies may be more likely to show true associations than case control or cohort studies, which show similar interstudy inconsistencies (35). The mechanisms by which a high-fat diet could associate with an increased risk of colon cancer are as follows:

1. As a source of calories. In sedentary males, even the small excess of energy intake over expenditure that is provided by a diet with 30% of calories derived from fat has resulted in quite impressive long-term weight gain, an identified risk factor for colon cancer (36).
2. As a surrogate marker for protein intake. Animal protein in the form of red meat appears to have a strong, consistent, independent association with colon cancers, while the association of fat with colon cancer disappears after controlling for red meat (7).
3. Diets high in fat and meat and poor in fiber associate with formation of hydroxyl radicals in feces, a factor that could lead to oxidative injury to DNA of colonic epithelial cells and subsequent neoplastic transformation (37).

Fibers, Fruits, and Vegetables

Many of the existing and proposed intervention studies designed to lower the frequency of colon cancer have been justified by epidemiologic studies that have shown that an inverse relationship exists between this cancer and the intake of fruits, vegetables, and selected micronutrients. This inverse association shows considerable interstudy consistency. As in the case of fat and red meat consumption, there is a strong correlation among these food items, so it is difficult to weigh the contribution of any one variable toward the decrease in large bowel cancer risk. The mechanisms by which fiber may protect against colon cancer are summarized in Table 14.2. In addition to fiber, green leafy vegetables and fruits are sources of antioxidant vitamins and substances that inhibit carcinogenesis (Table 14.3).

Micronutrients

The role of dietary vegetables in colorectal cancer prevention is more complex than just their fiber effects (Table 14.4). Vegetables contain numerous other substances, including antioxidants, folate, micronutrients such as carotenoids and ascorbate, and nonnutrients such as phenols, flavonoids, isothiocyanates, and indoles that possess potent anticarcinogenic properties (38–41). An abundant plant constituent, inositol hexaphosphate (phytic acid), is a powerful inhibitor of iron-mediated production of hydroxyl radicals, and it suppresses hydroxyl radical generation and lipid peroxidation. Consumption of vitamins D, A, C, and E and the

TABLE 14.2 Potential Benefits of Fiber in the Diet

Increases fecal mass
Decreases mucosal contact time with potential carcinogens
Increases intestinal transit time
Increases defecation frequency
Binds various reactive compounds
Dilutes intestinal contents
Has direct antitoxic effects against carcinogens and cocarcinogens
Blocks free radical formation
Substitutes for dietary fat
Reduces time for bacterial conversion of bile acids
Increases production of hydrogen, methane, and short-chain fatty acids
Adsorbs organic and inorganic substances, including bile salts
Decreases dehydroxylation of bile acids

TABLE 14.3 Dietary Influences in Colon Cancer

Normal colon bacteria convert bile acids to carcinogenic compounds, especially in individuals who consume high-fat, low-fiber diets.
Oxygen radicals and lipid peroxidation products form by diet-induced metabolic activation of procarcinogens.
Heterocyclic amines form due to cooking of meats.
Nutrient antioxidants, minerals, and trace elements in fruits and vegetables inhibit toxicity of luminal carcinogenic compounds by (a) quenching free radicals, (b) enhancing cell repair mechanisms, (c) increasing cellular immunity, and (d) regulating proliferation.

micronutrients calcium, selenium, and diallyl sulfide or almethyl trisulfide (substances found in garlic) also reduces colorectal cancer risk. Garlic is the vegetable with the strongest inverse association with colon cancer risk (40,42). The anticarcinogenic effects of garlic and other allium vegetables result from the induction of detoxifying enzymes, a reduction in tumor proliferation, or antibacterial activity (40).

Vitamin C, an antioxidant abundant in fruits and vegetables, may inhibit the formation of fecal mutagens, thus protecting against colon cancer development. Vitamin C and E supplementation decreases the number of recurrent rectal adenomas following polypectomy (43,44). Vitamin E and selenium function as antioxidants and could protect against carcinogenesis by neutralizing the toxic effects of free radicals, particularly those originating from fat metabolism.

Alterations in calcium and vitamin D metabolism may explain the geographic variation in colon cancer death rates, which tend to increase with increasing latitude and decreasing sunlight intensity, since sunlight exposure profoundly affects vitamin D metabolism. Mortality rates from colorectal cancer in the American northeast are nearly three times those found in the American south for both urban and rural populations. Colon cancer is uncommon at low latitudes and almost disappears within 10 degrees of the equator (45). An exception to this is Japan. However, the Japanese consume a diet rich in fish containing large amounts of vitamin D (46).

In some studies (45) but not others (47,48), increased dietary calcium consumption inversely correlates with colon cancer incidence and mortality. Calcium reduces colonic epithelial cell proliferation (49,50) and decreases the effects of bile acids and fatty acids on the colonic epithelium by converting them to insoluble calcium soaps. Calcium effects are modulated in part by interactions with 1,25-dihydroxy-vitamin D_3 and fatty acids (51).

An inverse relationship also exists between selenium levels and colorectal cancer risk (52). Selenium serves as a cofactor for glutathione peroxidase, which protects cells from oxidative damage. It is also probably involved in prostaglandin and antibody synthesis. A number of other micronutrients may play a role in lowering colorectal cancer incidence (Table 14.4) (53).

Alcohol Consumption

Alcohol significantly increases the risk of developing rectal cancer, whether assessed on the basis of total amount

TABLE 14.4 Beneficial Properties of Certain Micronutrients in Possible Risk Lowering in Colorectal Cancer

Micronutrient	Mechanism of Action
Calcium	Increases cellular adhesion, decreases cellular proliferation
Vitamin D	? Retards in vitro growth of human cancer cells, lowers level of ornithine decarboxylase in rats
Vitamin C	Prevents formation of N-nitro-nitrosamines, has antioxidant properties, decreases tumor development after carcinogen administration
Vitamin E	Free-radical scavengers shown both to inhibit and to promote colon tumor growth in carcinogenesis models
Selenium	Cofactor for the anticarcinogen glutathione peroxidase
Diallyl sulfide (garlic compound)	Inhibits carcinogen-induced nuclear injury
Allyl methyltrisulfide (garlic compound)	Increases activity of glutathione-S-transferase, which may inactivate carcinogens

consumed or as percent of total calories (54–58). Alcohol shows a weaker association with colon cancer, exhibiting a dose response only when assessed on the basis of presence of total calories (54). This may reflect the contribution of alcohol to a positive energy balance among heavy consumers. Additionally, substantial alcohol consumption increases the risk of adenomas and cancers due to abnormal DNA methylation (59). Cirrhosis itself may represent an independent risk factor for adenoma development; alcohol may increase the risk (60).

Smoking

Both rectal cancer and adenoma incidence is significantly elevated among users of chewing tobacco, snuff, pipes, and cigars and among current and former cigarette smokers. Cancer risk significantly increases with pack years and an earlier age of first use (61,62). It is estimated that tobacco use causes 16% of colon cancer deaths and 22% of rectal cancer deaths in a study conducted among U.S. veterans (61). The induction period for colorectal cancers is at least 35 years. Smoking may act as a tumor initiator (61). In addition, recent studies have linked smoking to microsatellite instability, CpG island methylator phenotype (CIMP), and *BRAF* mutations in colon cancers (63,64).

Occupational Factors

Rectal cancer, and to a lesser extent sigmoid cancer, associates with occupations in which dusts or fumes are inhaled, especially if the jobs are held for long time periods and when a person is young. An increased cancer risk exists among workers exposed to wood and metal dusts, plastics, fumes, organic solvents (65,66), cement, and fiberglass. Cancer risk also increases with exposure to asbestos (67). Both asbestos fibers and ferruginous bodies may be found in the tumor tissue of such patients (68). Thus, occupations associated with increased colon cancer risk include asbestos workers, pattern makers, carpet workers, steel workers, railway employees, those in the auto building or housing industry, and dry cleaners (69). Finally, individuals with sedentary jobs are more likely to develop colorectal cancer than those with active jobs.

Relationship to Atherosclerosis and Cholesterol and Lipoprotein Levels

A high fat intake over a long period of time increases serum cholesterol and β-lipoprotein levels (70). Data on the relationship between cholesterol levels and the development of colorectal adenomas and carcinomas are contradictory. Several cohort studies (71–73) have shown an inverse association between cholesterol levels and colon cancer risk. This inverse relation is strongest with right-sided cancers and attenuates with increasing time between testing and diagnosis, so that by 10 years the association is no longer apparent

(72). This suggests that the effect is a marker for undiagnosed colon cancer, since it is not observed with gastric or rectal carcinoma (71–73). Other studies have established a positive association between serum cholesterol levels and cancer risk (74). Of interest is the occasional association of Muir-Torre syndrome with familial hyperlipidemia (75). The e4 allele of apolipoprotein E may protect an individual from developing proximal colonic adenomas and carcinomas (76).

Association with Diverticulosis

There is an increased incidence of left-sided colon cancer in patients with diverticular disease, and it was Burkitt who first suggested that adenomas or cancers were likely to coexist in the same population (77). The coexistence of adenomas and diverticule (Fig. 14.3) is especially true in Western populations, but it occurs less commonly in Asian populations

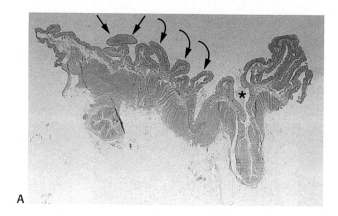

A

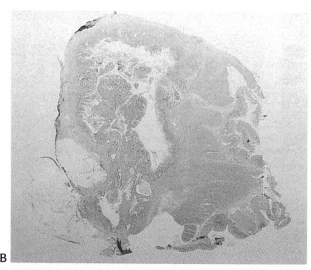

B

FIG. 14.3. Diverticulosis and adenoma. **A:** This bowel contains several polypoid mucosal structures. The *straight arrows* indicate an adenomatous polyp. The *curved arrows* highlight the prolapsing folds that create the accordion pleated mucosal pattern characteristic of diverticular disease. **B:** An adenoma arises from the epithelium lining the diverticulum and projects into the lumen. The normal colonic mucosa is seen on the right.

where the incidence of diverticulosis is lower and the diverticula tend to be right sided (78). Stemmermann and Yatani (79) showed that adenomas and diverticula both increase in migrant populations, presumably due to dietary influences. It is unlikely that the diverticula themselves predispose to neoplastic development or vice versa.

Relationship to Idiopathic Inflammatory Bowel Disease

Patients with both ulcerative colitis and Crohn disease exhibit an increased risk of developing colorectal cancer, as extensively discussed in Chapter 11.

Socioeconomic Factors and Urbanization

In most countries, colorectal cancer incidence is higher among urban residents than among rural ones (80), perhaps due to dietary influences. Some patient populations also exhibit a significant association between social standing, as measured by highest level of education, and colon cancer risk (81,82).

Hormonal Factors

Sex Hormones

Several observations suggest a role for sex hormones in colon cancer development. Women have an excess of right-sided colon cancers at all ages and a relationship may also exist with parity, which may protect against the development of colorectal cancer (83). Exogenous hormones may significantly reduce the risk of large bowel cancer, especially rectal cancers (84,85), although this is controversial (86,87). Reproductive or hormonal factors may influence bile acid metabolism, physical activity, or other variables. Up to 70% of colonic tumors are estrogen receptor (ER) positive (88). The clinical significance of ER positivity in colon cancer remains unclear.

Gastrin

Gastrin is usually made by gastric antral G cells where it stimulates gastric acid secretion, thereby facilitating protein digestion and preventing bacterial overgrowth. It also functions as a gastrointestinal growth-promoting hormone, sometimes leading to the development of colonic tumors. Total plasma gastrin levels are significantly elevated in some colon cancer patients (89). The tumors contain gastrin mRNA, progastrin, and gastrin (89–91). It remains unclear whether gastrin from the tumors acts as an autocrine growth factor and what the contribution of the serum gastrin is to colorectal carcinoma growth. However, Seitz et al (92) followed serum gastrin levels following colon cancer treatment and found that tumor recurrences associated with increasing serum gastrin levels. This led the authors to suggest autocrine secretion of gastrin by the tumor (92).

Growth Hormone

Acromegaly, a clinical syndrome characterized by growth of bones, soft tissues, and visceral organs, results from excessive growth hormone secretion. Acromegalic patients exhibit an increased adenoma and colon cancer risk (93,94). This risk is higher in males than in females. Acromegalic patients with colonic neoplasia tend to be young and display aggressive disease. The colons of such patients also exhibit increased cell proliferation (95).

Radiation

Radiation plays an etiologic role in a minority of colorectal carcinomas. Rectal tumors are most likely to develop in patients treated with radiotherapy for cervical, uterine, or prostatic carcinomas. Women irradiated for gynecologic cancers have a relative risk for subsequent colorectal cancer of 2.0 to 3.6 (96). Some tumors arise in radiation-induced strictures, sometimes associated with areas of colitis cystica profunda.

Schistosomiasis

Patients infested by *Schistosoma japonicum* have an increased incidence of colorectal neoplasms (97). Carcinomas arising in this setting occur at an earlier age and are often multicentric. The adenomas and carcinomas arise on a background of schistosomal colitis, often with preceding areas of dysplasia. The dysplasia can be either focal or diffuse and occurs in flat mucosa, in pseudopolyps, or at the edge of ulcers. The histologic appearance of the tumors resembles that occurring in noninfected individuals, except that the parasitic ova are admixed with the neoplasm (Fig. 14.4).

Relationship to Gallstones and Cholecystectomy

The role of cholecystectomy as a risk factor for colorectal cancer is controversial. Individuals who are older than 60 years of age and who have undergone cholecystectomy >10 years previously may exhibit a mildly increased risk of developing colorectal adenomas (98) and cancers, especially in the right colon (99–101). Cholecystectomy alters the proportion of secondary bile acids, including deoxycholic acid, in the bile by increasing enterohepatic cycling and allowing greater exposure to intestinal bacteria. Part of the association between colon cancer and cholelithiasis may relate to the identification of asymptomatic cholelithiasis in patients who undergo imaging of the liver as part of their clinical workup for potential metastatic colon cancer. Alternatively, common risk factors for gallstones and colon cancer may explain the apparent association (102).

Role of Ureterosigmoidostomy, Ileal Conduits, Ileostomy, and Anastomoses

A number of polypoid lesions complicate ureteral implantation into the bowel. Ureterosigmoidostomy increases colon

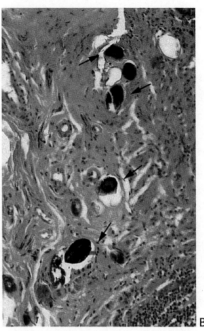

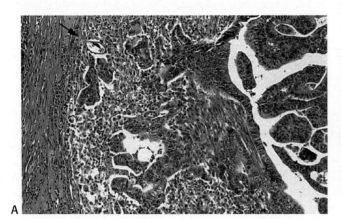

FIG. 14.4. Schistosomiasis and colon cancer. **A:** Adenomatous polyp with early invasive carcinoma arising in a patient with schistosomiasis. Clusters of *Schistosoma* ova are identifiable in the region of the muscularis mucosae on the left. **B:** Higher magnification of the calcified ova in the submucosa (*arrows*).

cancer risk by as much as 500 times in patients who have undergone the procedure (103). Adenomas develop up to 10 to 20 years following the ureterosigmoidostomy (103,104); carcinomas can arise as late as 53 years later (105,106).

Experimental data suggest that activation of fecal carcinogens by the diverted urine may increase cell proliferation and cause chronic inflammation (107). Ileal conduits are less prone to develop neoplasms (108). Colon cancer also develops at other anastomotic sites and in colostomies (109,110). Increased proliferative activity around anastomoses may explain some of the increased cancer risk (111).

Role of Gastric Surgery

Some studies suggest that patients who have undergone remote peptic ulcer surgery have an increased risk of developing colorectal cancer (112). It is postulated that increased levels of both carcinogens and unconjugated and secondary bile acids in the gastric juice after the peptic ulcer surgery increase the colon cancer risk (112), and truncal vagotomy may alter bile acid metabolism (113). However, other studies have not found an increased incidence of large bowel cancer following gastric surgery for benign disease (114).

Relationship to Skin Tags

Skin tags may constitute a marker for the presence of colonic neoplasia, since they occur more frequently in patients with colorectal cancer. It is likely that the patients have inherited a gene with pleiotropic effects involving both the skin and gut epithelium (115).

Other Factors

Tumors sometimes arise in malformations, and such tumors may exhibit unusual histologies, such as adenosquamous carcinomas (116). Patients with congenital anomalies of the urinary tract may also exhibit an increased colorectal cancer risk (117). Patients with pernicious anemia (118), diabetes mellitus (119), celiac disease (120), or AIDS (121) may have an increased risk of developing colorectal adenocarcinoma.

COLON CANCER PREVENTION

Colon cancer prevention strategies fall into three major categories: (a) identification and removal of precursor and early lesions, (b) dietary alterations, and (c) chemoprevention. Disease prevention falls into primary and secondary modalities. Primary prevention is defined as prevention of disease by some active intervention before the disease occurs. The second form of disease prevention is called secondary prevention, which involves detecting a disease before it is symptomatic and implementing an intervention to prevent the clinical manifestations of the disease, such as by removing a colonic adenoma thereby preventing its progression to adenocarcinoma.

If an improvement in colon cancer survival is to occur, increased efforts need to focus on primary prevention as well as on early detection and removal of premalignant and malignant lesions. Since epidemiologic, animal, and biochemical studies suggest that diets high in total calories and fat and low in various dietary fibers, vegetables, and micronutrients associate with an increased incidence of colorectal cancer, one

TABLE 14.5	Screening Options of Patients at Average Risk for Colorectal Cancer	
Screening Method	Interval	Consequences of a Positive Test
Fecal occult blood testing	Annual	Colonoscopy
Flexible sigmoidoscopy	Every 5 years	Polypectomy for distal polyps; possibly colonoscopy
Combined FOBT and sigmoidoscopy	FOBT annually, sigmoidoscopy every 5 years	
Colonoscopy	Every 10 years	Polypectomy; surgery for cancers or lesions that are not endoscopically resectable
Double-contrast barium enema	Every 5 years	Colonoscopy

FOBT, fecal occult blood testing.

primary means of prevention would be dietary education and diet modification. There are no data on the efficacy of this approach; therefore, most attention has focused on early detection of colonic neoplasms and chemoprevention.

Screening for Colorectal Adenomas and Carcinomas

Early Detection of Colorectal Cancer

The beneficial effects of early adenoma detection and removal were initially reported by Gilbertson in 1974 (122). Several more recent trials based on sigmoidoscopy or colonoscopy have reported a significant reduction in mortality as a result of screening (123–125). Case control studies indicate a reduction in the mortality rate from distal colorectal cancers in the magnitude of 60% to 85% (126). All studies indicate that the cancers detected have a more favorable stage when the patients are in a screening program (127). The reduction in cancer mortality results from (a) identification of early curable cancers, (b) identification and removal of premalignant polyps, and (c) the benefits of subsequent surveillance.

Screening recommendations vary depending on whether a patient falls into a high- or average-risk category. Therefore, asymptomatic individuals should have their risk evaluated to include an analysis of inherited syndromes, personal history of adenomas, or colorectal cancer and IBD (126,127).

Screening of Average-risk Populations

In 1995, an expert panel was assembled by the U.S. Agency for Health Care Policy and a consortium of gastroenterological societies to prepare clinical guidelines for colorectal cancer screening. The panel's initial report was published in 1997 (128) and later updated in 2003 (128). Screening for colorectal carcinoma is recommended for all persons aged 50 and older using one of several possible strategies: fecal occult blood testing (FOBT), flexible sigmoidoscopy, a combination of FOBT and sigmoidoscopy, colonoscopy, and double-

contrast barium enema (Table 14.5). The rationale for presenting patients with a number of screening options lies in the fact that no single test is of unequivocal superiority to the others, and giving patients a choice of methodologies may increase the likelihood that screening will occur.

Screening for High-risk Patients

Individuals with one or more relatives with colon cancer or adenomatous polyps or those with known colorectal cancer syndromes should undergo screening beginning at an earlier age and at shorter intervals than are recommended for those at average risk for colorectal cancer (Table 14.6) (128).

Chemoprevention

Cancer chemoprevention is defined as the prevention of cancer by the administration of one or more chemical entities either as individual drugs or naturally occurring dietary constituents. The three major types of chemopreventive agents are (a) inhibitors of carcinogen formation, (b) blocking agents, and (c) suppressing agents. Blocking agents inhibit tumor initiation, while suppressing agents act as inhibitors of tumor promotion and progression. An individual agent may belong to more than one class.

Significant interest lies in decreasing the incidence of both adenomas and carcinomas in patients enrolled in chemoprevention trials. Substances of current interest include antioxidants, nonsteroidal anti-inflammatory drugs (NSAIDs), and calcium, vitamin D, and other micronutrients.

Aspirin and Other Nonsteroidal Anti-inflammatory Drugs

Evidence strongly supports the notion that aspirin and other NSAIDs prevent the development and progression of gastrointestinal adenomas and carcinomas. Three separate lines of investigation indicate a correlation between NSAID use and a reduction in colorectal cancer: (a) some epidemiologic studies show a 40% to 60% decrease in the relative risk of

TABLE 14.6 Screening Recommendations for Patients at High Risk for Colorectal Cancer

Familial Risk Category	Screening Recommendation
First-degree relative with colorectal cancer or an adenoma diagnosed at an age ≥60 years, or two second-degree relatives with colorectal cancer	Same as average risk, but beginning at age 40
Two or more first-degree relatives with colon cancer, or one first-degree relative with colorectal cancer or an adenoma diagnosed at age ≤60 years	Colonoscopy every 5 years, beginning at age 40, or 10 years younger than the youngest affected relative, whichever comes first
One second- or third-degree relative with colorectal cancer	Same as average risk
Gene carrier or at risk for familial adenomatous polyposis	Sigmoidoscopy annually beginning at age 10–12
Gene carrier or at risk for attenuated familial adenomatous polyposis	Colonoscopy annually beginning in the late teens or early 20s because of the preponderance of proximal polyps in this group
Gene carrier or at risk for hereditary nonpolyposis colorectal cancer syndrome	Colonoscopy every 1–2 years, beginning at age 20–25, or 10 years younger than the youngest affected relative, whichever comes first

colorectal carcinoma and an approximately 70% risk reduction in adenoma incidence in individuals taking NSAIDs compared with those not taking them (129–136); (b) NSAIDs alter the biology of FAP, since sulindac administration results in a striking reduction in adenoma size and number (137–140); (c) experimental models show their chemopreventive effects as judged by a reduction in the frequency and number of premalignant/malignant lesions (141–143). Several recent clinical trials involving patients at high risk for colorectal cancer development have shown a significant reduction in adenoma development in those patients receiving daily aspirin (144,145).

NSAIDs exert their effects through inhibition of two enzymes involved in prostaglandin synthesis, cyclooxygenase (COX)-1 and COX-2. Both enzymes play key roles in the biosynthetic pathway by which arachidonic acid is converted into prostaglandin (PG) E_2, PGD_2, $PGF_{2\alpha}$, PGI_2, and thromboxane A_2. COX-1 is normally expressed in most tissues, while COX-2 expression is normally low. However, COX-2 is rapidly up-regulated by proinflammatory cytokines and many tumor regulators (146). In addition, COX-2, but not COX-1, is commonly overexpressed in colorectal adenomas and carcinomas (147). Evidence suggests that the COX-2–derived prostaglandin PGE_2 may play a direct role in malignant progression in colon cancer (148,149). PGE_2 appears to promote transactivation of the epidermal growth factor receptor, and may, through a complex series of steps, stabilize β-catenin within colonic epithelial cells leading to cell proliferation (150).

Calcium Supplementation

Calcium supplementation reduces intestinal proliferation (151–153) and alters the composition of intestinal bile acids, increasing the concentration of cholic acid, decreasing chenodeoxycholic acid, and increasing total fecal bile acid excretion. Calcium counteracts the effects of fatty and bile acids by binding them, making them insoluble and harmless (154). Several randomized trials have demonstrated

reduction in colorectal adenoma development in patients receiving daily calcium supplementation (155–157). Consumption of dairy products containing calcium and vitamin D also reduces colorectal cancer risk in a dose-dependent fashion (158). The beneficial effects of calcium supplementation may extend for years following cessation of calcium supplements (157).

ADENOMAS

Adenomas, the benign glandular neoplasms that precede colon cancer development, originate from the intestinal epithelium. They occur singly or multiply. When multiple, the patients may have a genetic syndrome (see Chapter 12).

Biologic Alterations in Adenomas

Despite their differing structure, all adenomas share two basic features of neoplasia, dysregulated proliferation and the failure to fully differentiate. The dysregulated proliferation is evidenced by an upward shift in the proliferative compartment (Fig. 14.5). This shift can be highlighted with the use of proliferation markers, such as with the antibody MIB-1 (Fig. 14.6) or by other labeling techniques. Mitotic figures, including abnormal ones, are present throughout the entire length of the hyperchromatic, adenomatous epithelium.

It has always been believed that adenomas form because the rate of cellular proliferation exceeds that of cellular exfoliation. However, today we know that cellular exfoliation is not the only mechanism for removing cells from the crypt. Cells also undergo apoptosis. In the normal colon, most apoptosis occurs near the luminal surface (159) consistent with a model of colorectal cell differentiation and senescence, which culminates in physiologic cell death as the cells migrate upward from the proliferative compartment in the basal crypt. This process is under the influence of the autocrine growth inhibitory apoptosis-inducing effect of transforming growth factor-β (TGF-β) (160). In contrast to the normal crypt, adenomas contain numerous apoptotic

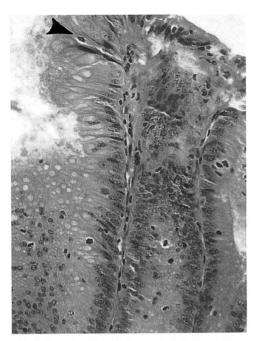

FIG. 14.5. The surface of an adenoma demonstrating the presence of increased numbers of mitoses. One mitotic figure is near the top of the mucosa (*arrowhead*).

cells (Fig. 14.7), which often lie at the adenoma base, a reversal of the normal distribution. This observation led Moss et al (161) to suggest that adenomas exhibit a reversed epithelial cell migration and an inward growth pattern directed toward the crypt base rather than toward the lumen. The shift in the location of the apoptotic figures is accompanied by a shift in TGF-β–immunoreactive cells from the adenoma surface to the base. The apoptosis-related bcl-2 family of proteins also exhibit altered expression in adenomas (162–164).

Adenomas also show abnormalities in epithelial cell differentiation. Morphologically and phenotypically, adenomatous epithelium resembles replicating cells normally present in the crypt base. Tall cells with prominent, elongated, hyperchromatic nuclei produce a characteristic "picket fence" pattern (Figs. 14.7 to 14.9) as they line the adenomatous glands. The adenomatous epithelium contains incompletely differentiated goblet cells and absorptive cells at all levels of the crypt, including the free surface (Fig. 14.9). This adenomatous pattern contrasts with the pattern of progressive differentiation seen in normal crypts. Normally, cells at the crypt base appear basophilic. As they move up the crypt toward the lumen, the cells become larger and increasingly more

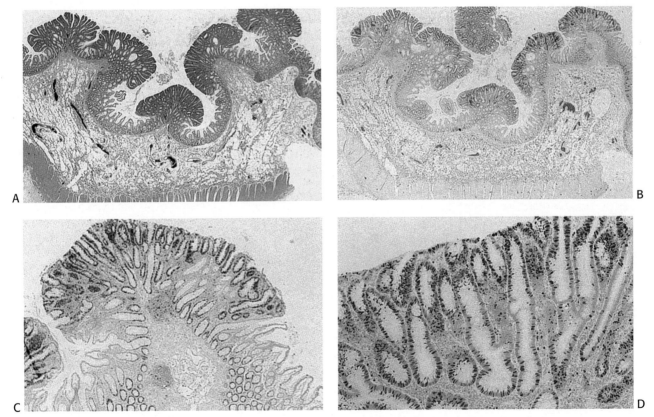

FIG. 14.6. Proliferation in adenomatous polyps. **A:** Multiple adenomas are present in the colonic mucosa from this patient with familial polyposis. **B:** Immunohistochemical staining for the proliferation marker Ki-67 using the MIB-1 antibody demonstrates a prominent band of proliferating cells at the luminal surface of the polyps. **C:** Higher magnification demonstrating the shift of the proliferation zone to the mucosal surface in an adenomatous polyp. In contrast, the adjacent nonneoplastic mucosa demonstrates the normal proliferation pattern with MIB-1–positive cells restricted to the base of the glands. **D:** Higher-power view showing numerous proliferating neoplastic cells in the superficial mucosa of the adenoma.

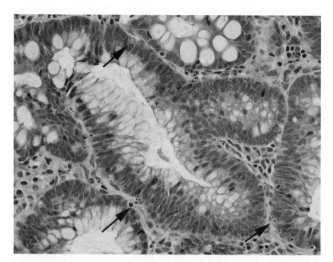

FIG. 14.7. Apoptosis in adenomatous polyps. An adenomatous gland contains scattered apoptotic cells (*arrows*). Apoptosis is commonly seen at the bases of the neoplastic glands.

eosinophilic. Mitoses disappear. A mixed cell population is present (Fig. 14.10). A gradient of differentiation appears, which is most evident histologically in the goblet cells, since goblet cells acquire increasingly larger supranuclear mucin accumulations as they mature.

Adenoma Growth

Small adenomas represent neoplastic clonal populations of colonic epithelial cells, suggesting that they arise from a single abnormal precursor stem cell. Adenomas begin in a single crypt (Fig. 14.11) and then grow by replacing normal epithelium in a centrifugal manner. Unicryptal adenomas are rare and most typically affect patients with FAP (see

Chapter 12). New adenomatous glands result from infolding of the neoplastic surface epithelium. The neoplastic cells appear to cluster at the luminal aspect of the mucosa without extending to the base of the glands (Fig. 14.12). Normal-appearing mucosa lies below the adenomatous glands (Fig. 14.12). In 86% of early tubular adenomas, the number of gland openings along the polyp surface is larger than the number of gland bases; this difference increases with polyp size (165). Additionally, gland proliferation predominates in the upper crypts and along the surface of the lesions (Fig. 14.6). Early adenomas present as small growths with a very benign tubular histology.

A small proportion of tubular adenomas increases in size and develop villous features and cytologic characteristics of high-grade dysplasia. The progression of most small adenomas is slow and occurs over several years. On average, small adenomas double their diameter in 10 years (166). In one study, small adenomas doubled during a 2-year observation period, but none of the adenomas observed over time exceeded 5 mm in size at the time of resection, nor did any show high-grade dysplasia or carcinoma (166). Another estimate of the projected increased growth relates to lesional volume. There is a 52% mean volume increase after 2 years (166).

Some adenomas ultimately progress to invasive cancers. However, it should be remembered that not all adenomas progress, and that some stay stable or may even regress and disappear while new ones form in the same colon (167).

Incidence

Incidence rates of adenomas vary considerably throughout the world. Geographic areas exhibiting a high risk for colon cancer also exhibit a high risk for adenoma development and

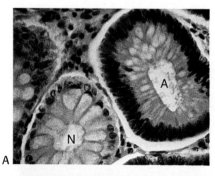

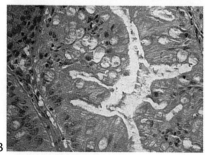

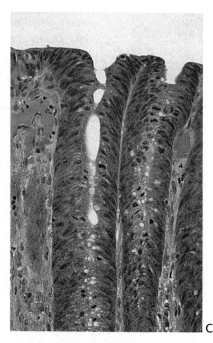

FIG. 14.8. Comparison of epithelium in normal crypts and crypts from hyperplastic and adenomatous polyps. **A:** Cross section of an adenomatous gland (*A*) and a normal gland (*N*). The adenomatous gland is lined by hyperchromatic cells, which demonstrate prominent crowding. The epithelium appears somewhat mucin depleted. In contrast, the nonneoplastic gland to the left is lined by cells with small, round, basally located nuclei without evidence of crowding. Numerous goblet cells are present. **B:** Hyperplastic polyps are lined by cells with very small, round nuclei and abundant eosinophilic cytoplasm. Note the serrated architecture of the gland. **C:** Horizontal section of an adenomatous crypt demonstrating immature cells that fail to mature as they reach the luminal surface. The nuclei are crowded and, in some areas, appear pseudostratified.

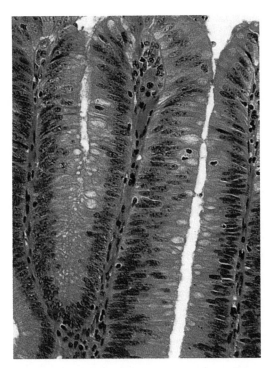

FIG. 14.9. Typical picket fence appearance of an adenomatous polyp.

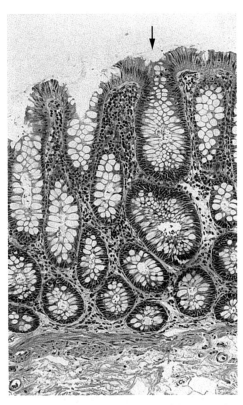

FIG. 14.11. Unicryptal adenoma. A single crypt is present, which is lined with crowded, hyperchromatic, adenomatous epithelium (*arrow*). The surrounding crypts contain nonneoplastic epithelium and demonstrate the normal pattern of differentiation. This section was taken from the colon of a patient with familial polyposis coli.

vice versa. The incidence in the general population varies from 0% to 69% depending on the country of origin (168–170) and on how the adenomas are detected (171). The incidence of adenomas depends on several other factors, including (a) whether one is examining data from an autopsy study versus an endoscopic screening study, (b) the

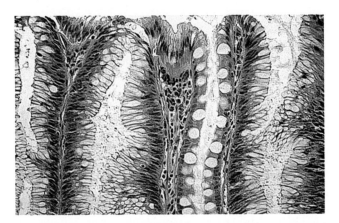

FIG. 14.10. Comparison of differentiation in adenomatous and nonneoplastic glands. The nonneoplastic gland in the center of the photograph demonstrates the normal pattern of progressive differentiation. Goblet cells and absorptive cells line the gland. The colonocyte nuclei are small, round, and basally placed. No mitotic figures are seen. In contrast, the adenomatous glands on either side show no evidence of differentiation toward the luminal surface. All of the cells appear similar and demonstrate crowded, pseudostratified, hyperchromatic nuclei.

age of the patient, and (c) whether or not the patient has a hereditary colon cancer syndrome.

Some patient populations have an extremely low adenoma incidence. For example, no adenomas were found among 14,000 autopsies performed on the South African Bantu (172), and Medillin, Colombia, which has a low incidence of colorectal cancer, also has a low incidence of adenomas (173). In Western populations, the average prevalence rate for adenomas from flexible sigmoidoscopy screening is 10%, and colonoscopic screening prevalence averages 25% (174). Adenomas accounted for 68% of all polyps removed by colonoscopy in the National Polyp Study (175). In the 50- to 59-year age group, population screening studies and autopsy studies show an adenoma prevalence rate of 41.3% to 69% (176), increasing in advancing years up to 88% in centenarians (177). Arminsky and McLean (178) documented a 7.5% increase in adenoma incidence per decade.

These data contrast with incidences of only 2.8% to 50% and a mean of 10% among autopsied patients (179,180). Low prevalence rates from autopsy series reflect geographic variations and various methodologic biases, including the fact that usually the autopsies are performed by numerous individuals with colorectal examinations ranging from a casual inspection to examinations with a hand lens. The

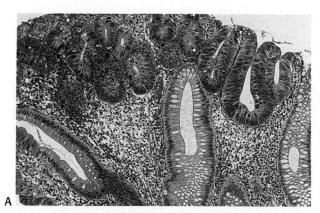
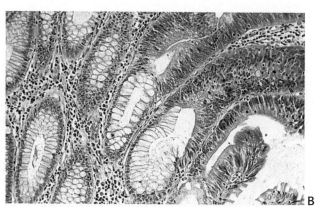

FIG. 14.12. Early adenomatous polyp. **A:** Adenomas develop from infolding of neoplastic surface epithelium. Adenomatous epithelium is seen overlying normal appearing crypts. **B:** The neoplastic cells extend into the crypts, displacing the normal epithelium in a "snowplow" fashion.

most reliable autopsy data derive from those studies performed by a single, experienced investigator. Another confounding variable is whether the data include autopsies on children as well as on adults. Autopsy series containing large numbers of children would be expected to have lower prevalence rates due to the fact that adenomas are age-related lesions. In carefully performed studies, 46.9% to 69% of cases have at least one adenoma (178,181).

Patient Age and Sex

Age and male sex correlate with adenoma development (170,175,182). Adenomas show a sharp rise in incidence in patients without hereditary adenomatous polyp syndromes at about age 40, and adenoma incidence peaks at age 60 or 70 years. In the National Polyp Study, adenomas occurred more frequently in men than women, 61.6% versus 38.4%. Patient mean age was 62 ± 11 years. Of these, 21% reported a family history of colon cancer and 12% had a family history of colonic polyps. Forty-three percent had a family history of another cancer. Thirty-nine percent had more than one adenoma (175). These authors found that the prevalence of adenomas increased 21% in the 6th to the 8th decades (53%). The prevalence of polyps in patients aged 50 to 70 years is 30% to 50%, and the likelihood of cancer developing is 6% (183).

Lesion Location

Based on endoscopic studies, most sporadic adenomas arise in the rectosigmoid (66% to 77%), where 97% are amenable to endoscopic removal (184). However, following endoscopic removal of all adenomas from the colon, adenomas have a higher incidence on the right side of the bowel in the initial follow-up period and then become more evenly distributed with time (184). Adenomas also shift from a distal to a proximal location as patients age (168–171,185). Thus, left-sided adenomas occur more commonly in younger age groups and right-sided lesions increase in frequency in

individuals older than 65 years of age. HNPCC patients have a predominance of right-sided adenomas at all ages. FAP patients have predominantly left-sided lesions and, since patients undergo prophylactic colectomy, it is unknown whether the adenoma distribution would shift toward right-sided lesions with age.

Some adenomas cluster (Fig. 14.13). This means that multiple adenomas tend to occur closer together than would be expected from the general distribution of adenomas. This phenomenon occurs in all colonic segments but is less pronounced in the rectum than in other parts of the large intestine (186).

Frequency of Multiple Polyps

Individuals with one adenoma have a 40% to 55% likelihood of having additional synchronous lesions (184,187,188). The additional adenomas are detected at the same time as the initial adenoma (synchronous adenomas) or at a different time (metachronous adenomas). The prevalence of multiple adenomas increases with age. Nine percent of individuals younger than 60 years, 17% of people between 60 and 74 years, and 28% of people older than 75 years have three or more adenomas. Multiple adenomas also arise with increased frequency at ureterosigmoidostomy sites and in patients with hereditary colon cancer syndromes and FAP. Sometimes a single sessile adenoma may appear as multiple adenomas. It may be difficult to separate a single lesion from multiple lesions if one is unaware of the gross appearance of the lesion (Fig. 14.14).

The incidence of synchronous neoplasms in patients with an index rectosigmoid adenoma measuring <5 mm in diameter, with an index rectosigmoid adenoma measuring >5 mm, or with a rectosigmoid carcinoma is 34%, 53%, and 73%, respectively (188). The synchronous neoplasm is an adenoma measuring >5 mm in diameter is 13%, 40%, and 64%, respectively (188). The incidence of large intestinal adenomas occurring synchronously with carcinomas is approximately double that of adenomas occurring alone. Metachronous adenomas, compared to index adenomas,

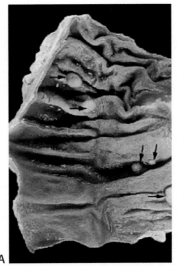
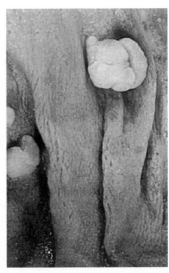

FIG. 14.13. Adenomatous polyps. **A:** This resected segment of colon contains multiple small adenomas. The polyps tend to cluster together (*arrows*). **B:** Higher magnification demonstrating the typical raspberrylike appearance of the adenomatous polyps.

tend to be smaller, tubular, only mildly dysplastic, and more uniformly distributed (189). The substantial prevalence of proximal colonic neoplasms, including advanced lesions, in asymptomatic, average-risk patients with rectosigmoid adenomas measuring <5 mm in diameter warrants colonoscopy in these patients in order to detect them (189).

A relationship exists between adenoma multiplicity and histologic findings. In patients with a single adenoma, 38.8% are villous, whereas those with multiple adenomas have a 60.1% chance of having at least one villous adenoma (190).

Patients with multiple adenomas are also more likely to harbor at least one adenoma that contains high-grade dysplasia (13.8%) versus patients with a single adenoma (7.3%).

Recurrent Adenomas

"Recurrent" adenomas result from the appearance of new adenomas, continued growth of an incompletely resected adenoma, or detection of a previously undetected but pre-existing adenoma. The overall recurrence rates for new adenomas are

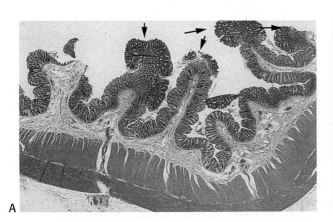

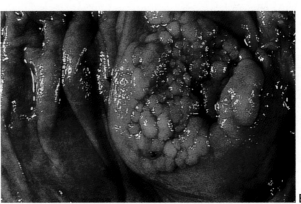

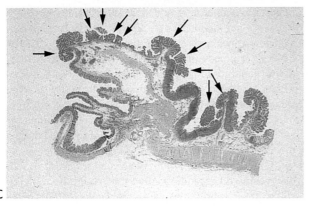

FIG. 14.14. Comparison of the appearance of multiple adenomas and a large lesion simulating multiple adenomas. **A:** Patient with familial polyposis and multiple adenomas (*arrows*). **B:** Gross specimen demonstrating a large sessile adenoma straddling the ileocecal valve and extending into the ileum. **C:** Histologic appearance of the lesion shown in B. If one had not seen the gross specimen, the multiple polypoid excrescences (*arrows*) might suggest the presence of multiple adenomas.

estimated at 20% to 60% with average follow-up times of 3 to 10 years after index polypectomy (171,183,184,191). Most recurrences occur in the first 2 years following polypectomy. The estimated time to finding new adenomas is 58 months for patients clear on the first colonoscopy and 16 months for patients who had adenomas on the first examination. In 18% of patients, the adenomas arise proximal to the splenic flexure (192,193). Villous tumors, particularly broadly sessile ones, usually have a less well-defined border than do tubular adenomas and, therefore, have a greater tendency to recur after local resection than smaller, pedunculated adenomas.

Endoscopic follow-up studies to evaluate new adenomas are hampered by the fact that as many as 25% to 27% of adenomas measuring <5 mm in diameter and up to 6% of adenomas measuring 1 cm in diameter are missed during one endoscopic examination (194,195). Right-sided adenomas are missed more often (27%) than left-sided adenomas (21%) (194). Lesions measuring up to 8 cm in diameter may be missed, and some of these may contain areas of malignancy (196).

Adenoma Incidence in Hereditary Colon Cancer Syndromes

Relatives of individuals with colorectal cancer have an adenoma prevalence rate of 39%. Patients with FAP or its variants (see Chapter 12) have an increased incidence of colonic adenomas. These are multiple and occur at a younger age than they do in the general population. FAP patients have the largest number of adenomas, although some patients have the attenuated form of the disease. Thirty percent of HNPCC patients have at least one adenoma and 20% have multiple adenomas. It is unusual to find more than five adenomas in HNPCC patients (197,198). Table 14.7 compares polyp numbers in the HNPCC and FAP hereditary syndromes.

Clinical Features and Diagnosis

Adenomas develop in diverse clinical settings. They either occur sporadically or arise in the setting of a hereditary syndrome such as a polyposis syndrome (FAP) or HNPCC. Sometimes the clinical features result from associated diseases such as diverticulosis (diverticulitis). Small adenomas, ranging up to 1.0 cm in maximum diameter, usually remain asymptomatic unless they are located in the rectosigmoid, in which case they may bleed when their surfaces become traumatized by the passage of well-formed, hardened stool. Larger lesions become symptomatic, with the symptoms depending on polyp size and location. Bleeding is the most frequent symptom, followed by a profuse, watery, or mucoid rectal discharge. Bleeding occurs more often in left-sided lesions than right-sided ones (199). At most, the patient may notice a slight reddish discoloration of the stool after defecating. The bleeding is seldom severe. Factors correlating with severe hemorrhage include adenoma size, pedunculation, and a villous growth pattern (199). The incidence of bleeding increases with increasing adenoma size and once a carcinoma develops within the adenoma. Villous tumors are more likely to bleed than tubular ones, since they tend to be larger and have a statistically higher incidence of coexisting carcinoma. The most common symptoms of villous lesions include bleeding, mucous diarrhea, constipation, and tenesmus (200). Some adenomas lead to incontinence, prolapse, and anemia. If the adenomas are large enough, they may cause changes in bowel habits or intussusception. Cecal lesions that block the appendiceal orifice may produce symptoms mimicking acute appendicitis. Ominous signs and symptoms associated with adenomas include obstruction and abdominal pain.

Other clinical features develop in individuals with distinctive polyposis syndromes in whom extraintestinal manifestations may herald the presence of intestinal lesions. These are discussed in Chapter 12.

Endoscopic Features

Small (<5 mm) colorectal polyps commonly affect individuals older than 50 years of age (201) and adenomas account for 60% to 66% of these small lesions (167,202–204). The

---

TABLE 14.7 Comparison of Hereditary Nonpolyposis Colon Cancer (HNPCC) and Familial Adenomatous Polyposis (FAP)

	HNPCC	FAP
Onset	Early	Early
Adenoma, number	<10	>100
Adenoma histology	Tubular adenomas	Tubular adenomas
Polyp distribution	Mainly right side	Left or total
Degree of dysplasia in adenoma	High grade	Low grade
Cancer distribution	Mainly right side	Random or mostly rectal
Other cancers	See Figure 20.3	See Figure 17.15
Proportion of adenomas becoming malignant	High	Low
Types of polyps	Adenomas, hyperplastic polyps, mixed hyperplastic–adenomatous polyps	Adenomas

gross endoscopic appearance may suggest the correct diagnosis. However, the endoscopic diagnosis is only correct in 82% of smaller polyps (Fig. 14.15), so histologic examination is required for confirmation (205). The current wisdom is that distal small adenomas represent biomarkers of risk for colorectal neoplasia, warranting a complete colonoscopy in the patient and lifetime surveillance for colon cancer (167). Recently, attention has focused on the development of fluorescence endoscopic imaging and high-resolution chromoendoscopy, which might provide morphologic detail of diminutive colorectal polyps that might correlate with polyp histology and eliminate the need for a biopsy and/or subsequent colonoscopy.

Gross Features

Grossly, adenomas assume one of three major growth patterns: (a) pedunculated, (b) sessile, or (c) flat or depressed (Fig. 14.16).

Pedunculated and Sessile Adenomas

Most sporadic colorectal adenomas appear as exophytic, mucosal protrusions. They range in size from invisible

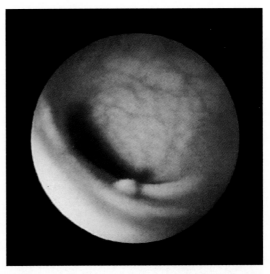

FIG. 14.15. A diminutive adenomatous polyp is present in the lower center of the photograph. The endoscopic features of such small lesions are not distinctive and require biopsy and histologic examination to confirm their neoplastic nature.

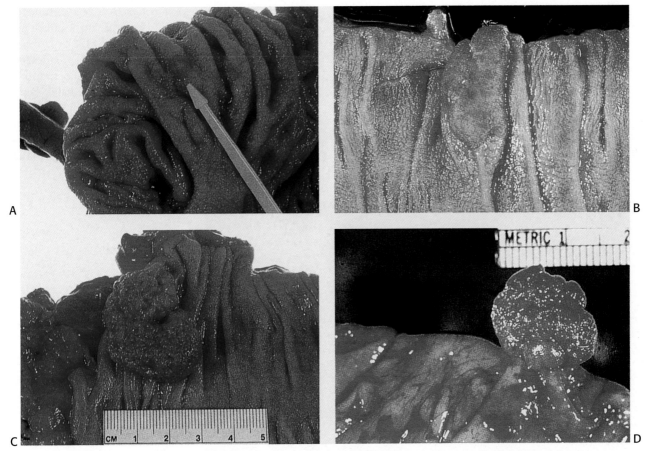

FIG. 14.16. Gross appearance of adenomatous polyps. **A:** Small adenoma on mucosal fold. **B:** Larger plaque-like lesion. **C:** Large sessile raspberrylike lesion. **D:** Pedunculated adenoma.

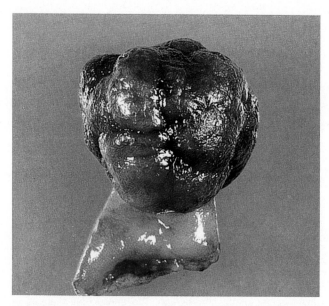

FIG. 14.17. Gross appearance of a pedunculated adenoma with the typical lobulated head and a stalk covered by normal mucosa.

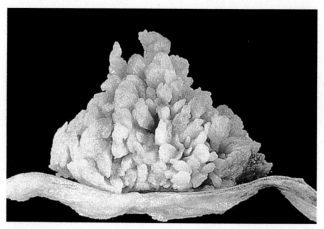

FIG. 14.19. Villous adenoma composed of long fingerlike fronds.

unicryptal lesions to large sessile adenomas sometimes measuring >20 cm in greatest dimension. Adenoma size generally correlates with gross growth pattern.

Adenomas measuring only 1 or 2 mm grossly resemble hyperplastic polyps. These minute adenomas have smooth surfaces and lack lobulations, and their color often resembles that of the normal mucosa. However, when such lesions are examined under a dissecting microscope, they exhibit characteristic pit patterns that differ from those seen in either small carcinomas or hyperplastic polyps.

Polyp architecture depends in part on whether the adenoma has a tubular, villous, or tubulovillous histologic pattern. The typical tubular adenoma presents as a small,

spherical, and variably pedunculated lesion, with its surface broken into lobules by intercommunicating clefts in larger lesions (Figs. 14.16 and 14.17). Larger lesions appear redder than the surrounding mucosa (Fig. 14.17), unless the patient has melanosis coli, in which case the lesions may appear lighter. Larger lesions exhibit a lobulated, bosselated or villous, raspberrylike, friable surface. In surgical material, approximately 90% of adenomas appear variably pedunculated and normal mucosa lines their stalks. The stalk ranges in length from several millimeters to a few centimeters. Tubulovillous adenomas tend to be larger than tubular adenomas, with a mean diameter of 19.0 mm (178).

Villous adenomas fall into three types: (a) flat, carpet-like masses; (b) lobulated, bulky, sessile masses; and (c) pedunculated lesions with short, broad pedicles. Sessile adenomas tend to be large, shaggy lesions covered by fingerlike fronds (Figs. 14.18 and 14.19). Generally, adenomas appear as grossly homogeneous, soft lesions without induration, ulceration, or fixation. Areas of pigmentation

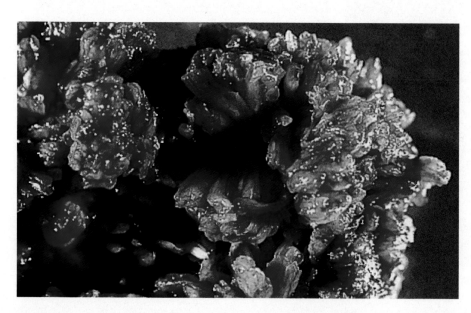

FIG. 14.18. Villous adenomas are composed of many fingerlike fronds that give them a shaggy appearance.

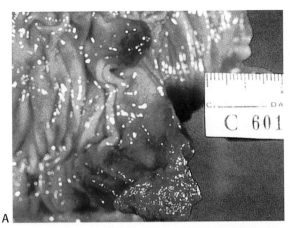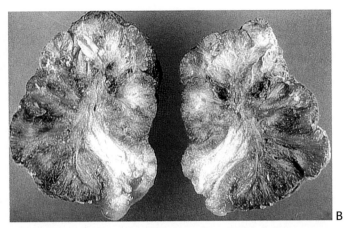

FIG. 14.20. Hemorrhage within polyps. **A:** The entire surface of these two polyps is markedly reddened due to hemorrhage. **B:** Cut surface of a polyp with hemorrhage and secondary fibrosis.

may indicate previous hemorrhage, fibrosis, pseudoinvasion, or previous fulguration (Fig. 14.20). Areas of ulceration, depression, or firmness suggest the possibility of a coexisting carcinoma (Fig. 14.21). Villous adenomas can be multiple and often associate with other adenomas, polyps, or separate carcinomas.

Villous adenomas often have ill-defined edges and attach to the mucosa by a broad base, often extending over wide mucosal areas. Because villous adenomas are less well circumscribed than tubular adenomas, with less well-defined edges than pedunculated adenomas, villous adenomas have a greater tendency to recur after local excision. Large, circumferential, carpeting, benign villous rectal adenomas are rare (Fig. 14.22) but problematic. They recur after the initial excision and may require repeated excision or diathermy to control the recurrences. Adenomas tend to be larger in males and to be largest in the rectum, followed by the ascending colon, cecum, and sigmoid colon. Adenomas also tend to be larger in individuals with multiple adenomas (206).

Adenomas Containing Carcinoma

The incidence of cancer in an adenoma increases as the size of the adenoma increases. Thirty percent of villous adenomas >5 cm contain an invasive carcinoma (207). However, even a 4-mm adenoma may contain an invasive cancer (208). Conversely, we have encountered exceptionally large sessile adenomas measuring >20 cm in greatest diameter without malignant change.

Flat (Depressed) Adenomas

Flat adenomas constitute a special subgroup of adenomas with a greater potential for malignant transformation while still small than is exhibited by exophytic adenomas

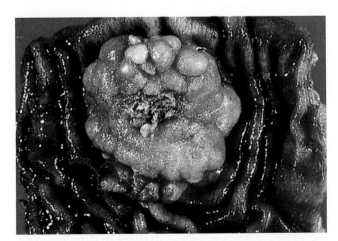

FIG. 14.21. Adenomatous polyp with a central depression representing carcinomatous transformation within the lesion. Additionally, the bowel is affected by melanosis coli but the polyp is not.

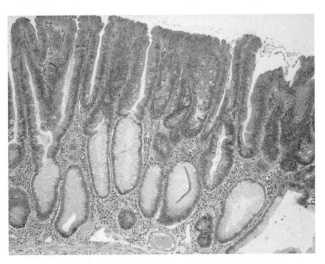

FIG. 14.22. Large, carpetlike, sessile rectal adenoma.

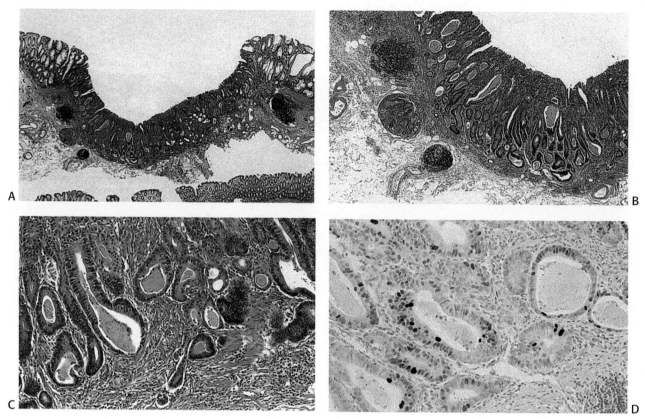

FIG. 14.23. Depressed adenoma. **A:** Low-power photomicrograph demonstrating a depressed lesion, which contains crowded glands lined by a hyperchromatic and mucin-depleted epithelium. **B:** At slightly higher power, the epithelium appears adenomatous with crowded, hyperchromatic nuclei. **C:** On higher power, there is evidence of high-grade dysplasia, and a focus of early invasion into the muscularis mucosae is seen. **D:** Immunohistochemical staining with antibodies to p53 demonstrate p53 overexpression, suggesting that the p53 gene may be mutated in this case.

Fig. 14.23). The terms *superficial, flat,* and *depressed adenoma* are all used synonymously to describe this entity. Flat adenomas can be single or multiple (209). Because flat or depressed adenomas display little or no mucosal elevation, they can be very difficult to see endoscopically and pathologically, especially in the proximal colon (210). They are often more clearly delineated endoscopically after spraying the mucosa with methylene blue or indigo carmine (211–214).

Endoscopically, flat adenomas are recognized as plaquelike lesions with vague redness or discoloration. They tend to be small, usually not exceeding 1 to 2 cm in diameter (Fig. 14.24). Flat adenomas are much more readily identified in colectomy specimens following fixation than they are at the time of endoscopy, presumably because the gross features become highlighted following formalin fixation (209). The failure to recognize these flat lesions may account for the lingering concept of de novo colorectal carcinoma (215). Depressed adenomas tend to arise more commonly in the right colon than elsewhere (215). They occur in the HNPCC syndrome, sporadically, or in patients with FAP (216). The frequency of flat adenoma is 50.7% in HNPCC patients. Flat adenomas have a high incidence of high-grade dysplasia and a high asso-

ciation with synchronous and metachronous invasive colorectal carcinomas.

Histologic Features

Histologically, adenomas fall into four categories: Tubular, tubulovillous, villous, and flat or depressed

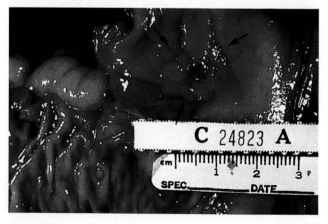

FIG. 14.24. Grossly flat adenomas appear plaquelike and slightly redder than the surrounding mucosa.

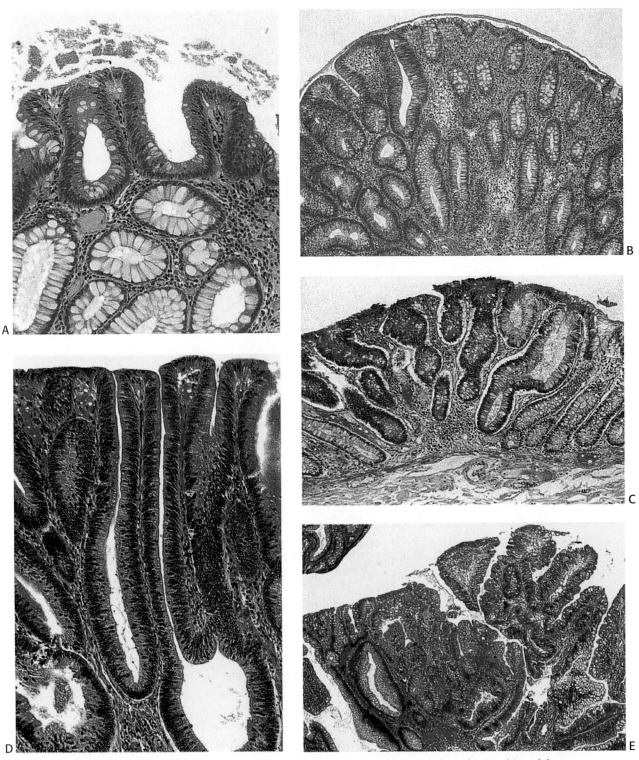

FIG. 14.25. Spectrum of pure tubular to pure villous adenomas. A through H show the transition of the pure tubular to the pure villous lesion. **A–C:** Pure tubular lesions. **D:** Early villous change is apparent by the elongation and crowding of the glands. **E:** Mixed tubular villous lesion, although it is predominantly tubular. (*continues*)

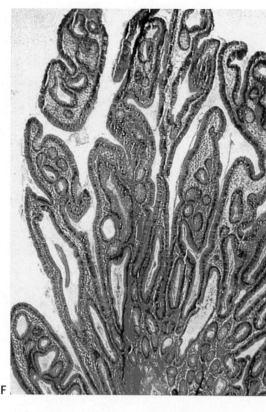

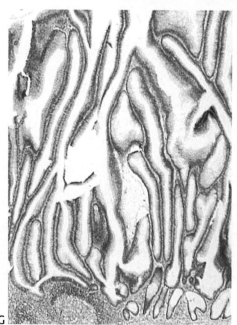

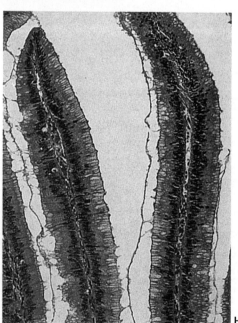

FIG. 14.25. *Continued* **F:** Tubular villous adenoma, predominantly villous, showing some tubular glands within the villous fronds. **G:** Pure villous adenoma. **H:** Delicate fronds of the pure villous adenoma.

lesions. Large or sessile adenomas are generally predominantly villous lesions, whereas smaller, pedunculated adenomas usually display a tubular or tubulovillous architecture (Fig. 14.25). Although most villous adenomas are large, small villous adenomas do exist. Some tubular adenomas may become large and sessile, and some pedunculated adenomas exhibit villous features. Many adenomas histologically show a mixture of both tubular and villous growth patterns.

Tubular Adenomas

The most common adenoma is tubular, accounting for 68% to 87.1% of adenomas in several studies (175,217,218),

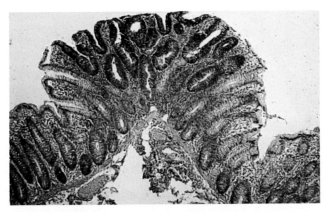

FIG. 14.26. In this small adenoma, the normal architecture of the mucosa is preserved. However, the epithelium lining the crypts has been replaced by neoplastic cells. The neoplastic glands are hyperchromatic, and the cells are crowded and pseudostratified.

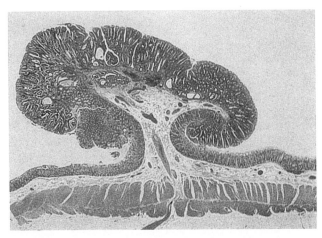

FIG. 14.28. Cross section through a pedunculated adenomatous polyp. The stalk is lined by normal colonic epithelium, while the adenomatous epithelium of the polyp head thickens the mucosa.

depending on whether or not one allows for up to a 25% villous component in tubular lesions (217). Tubular adenomas maintain their original crypt architecture, but adenomatous epithelium replaces the normal colonic epithelium in lining the crypts (Fig. 14.26). Small tubular adenomas always have dysplastic (adenomatous) surface epithelium overlying nondysplastic epithelium in the crypt base. Lamina propria separates the closely packed adenomatous crypts (Fig. 14.27). The lamina propria may contain increased numbers of lymphocytes, plasma cells, and eosinophils. When the adenomatous tubules grow, they may branch, sometimes producing an irregular architecture. In pedunculated polyps, adenomatous epithelium remains confined to the mucosa of the head of the polyp. The stalk consists of normal mucosa, including the muscularis mucosae and submucosal tissue, in continuity with the major part of the bowel wall (Fig. 14.28). Focal cystic tubular dilation (Fig. 14.29), inflammation,

hemorrhage, or erosion can all secondarily affect adenomas, especially at their surface. Small superficial tubular adenomas composed of an adenomatous epithelium that produces some mucin are occasionally overlooked. Their neoplastic nature can be confirmed using an antibody to Ki-67. The strongly immunoreactive cells will be confined to the surface, and more weakly positive cells will be at the crypt bases (Fig. 14.6).

Villous Adenomas

Approximately 20% of asymptomatic persons screened by colonoscopy have villous adenomas, a third of which contain high-grade dysplasia. Slightly <2% contain invasive carcinoma (219). Villous adenomas consist of elongated fingerlike nonbranching fronds of dysplastic epithelium extending outward from the muscularis mucosae to the colonic lumen

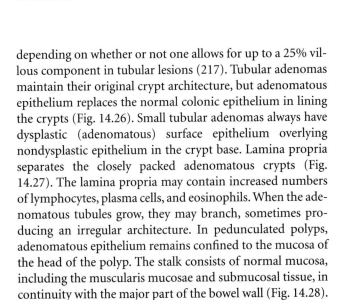

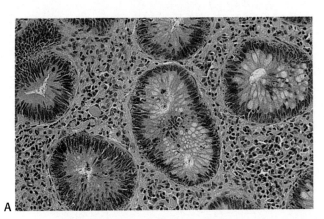

FIG. 14.27. Tubular adenoma. **A:** The lamina propria separating the adenomatous glands contains numerous lymphocytes, plasma cells, and eosinophils. **B:** The adenoma depicted in this photograph demonstrates more dysplasia than that in A. The nuclei lining the glands are stratified and have lost much of their polarity. The surrounding lamina propria contains scattered mononuclear cells and eosinophils.

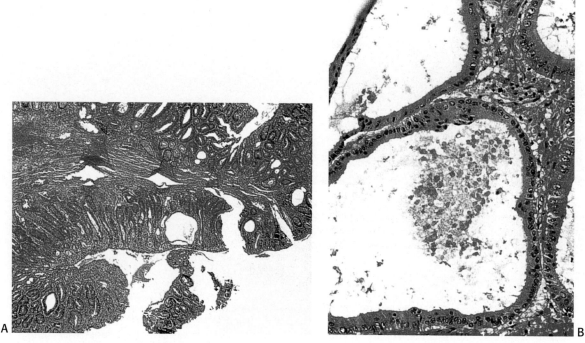

FIG. 14.29. Adenoma with cysts. **A:** Multiple small cystic spaces reside with the adenomatous epithelium. **B:** Higher-power magnification demonstrates inspissated mucus and inflammatory cells.

(Fig. 14.30). The villi contain cores of lamina propria covered by a single layer of adenomatous epithelium (220). Konishi and Morson (217) defined villous lesions as those that contain >80% of a villous component.

Tubulovillous Adenomas

Tubulovillous adenomas contain a mixture of both tubular and villous growth patterns or have broad villi containing tubular structures (Fig. 14.31). The villi may be blunt and short. Konishi and Morson (217) define tubulovillous lesions as those that contain from 20% to 79% villous components. Fung and Goldman (221) estimated that a villous component is present in 35% to 75% of all adenomas measuring >1 cm in greatest diameter.

Cell Types in Adenomas

Adenomas contain a mixture of variably differentiated absorptive cells, goblet cells, intermediate cells, endocrine cells, and Paneth cells. An abrupt transition between adenomatous and normal colonic epithelial cells is often seen, with the adenomatous cells displacing the nonneoplastic cells of the crypt creating a "snowplow" effect (Fig. 14.32). Most adenomas show some ability to partially differentiate into immature mucus-producing cells called oligomucous cells (222,223). However, the

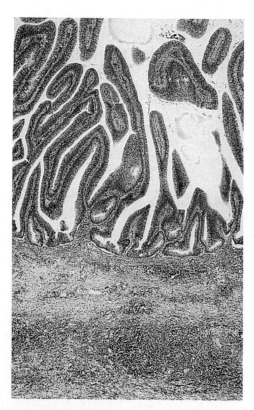

FIG. 14.30. Villous adenomas are characterized by long finger-like fronds lined by neoplastic epithelium.

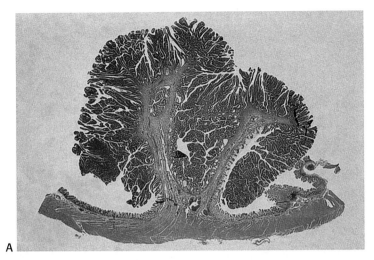

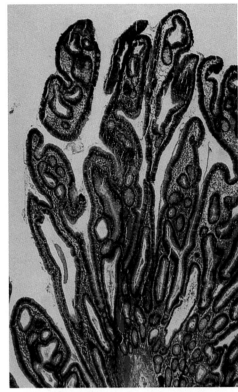

FIG. 14.31. Tubulovillous adenoma. **A:** Whole mount section of a tubulovillous adenoma demonstrating a mixture of tubular and villous architectures. **B:** On higher power, villous fronds and tubular glands are identifiable.

mucus content of the adenomatous epithelium varies (Fig. 14.33). Adenomas may demonstrate true goblet cell formation, although these cells often have an eccentric nucleus and are referred to as *dystrophic goblet cells* (Fig. 14.33). Occasionally, large numbers of mucin-producing cells are present in villous adenomas, especially those associated with potassium loss. Endocrine cells are discernible in 59% to 85% of adenomas if special stains are used to detect them (Fig. 14.34). Paneth cells are present in approximately 10% (Fig. 14.35), and squamous differentiation (Fig. 14.36) occurs in approximately 4% of lesions. Paneth cells are easily recognized in hematoxylin and eosin–stained sections due to their prominent supranuclear, eosinophilic, cytoplasmic granules. The Paneth cells are neoplastic, as evidenced by their cytologic features (Fig. 14.35). Some cells exhibit both mucinous and Paneth cell differentiation. Adenomas that contain squamous epithelium probably act as the precursor lesions for adenosquamous carcinomas, adenoacanthomas, or pure squamous cell carcinomas. Adenomas may also contain foci of osseous metaplasia, melanocytes (224), or areas of gastric mucosa (Fig. 14.37). The presence of these various cell types reflects stem cell potential to differentiate along several cell lineages (220). The presence of these various cell types in adenomas has no clinical significance.

Muscle Fibers in Adenomas

When adenomas form, the underlying muscularis mucosae frays, sending small fingerlike muscular extensions short

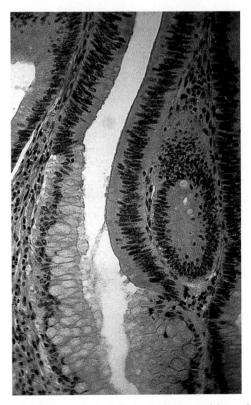

FIG. 14.32. Adenomatous cells grow downward from the surface, undermining the nonneoplastic mucosa like a snow plow. The resulting abrupt transition from neoplastic and nonneoplastic epithelium is evident in the photograph.

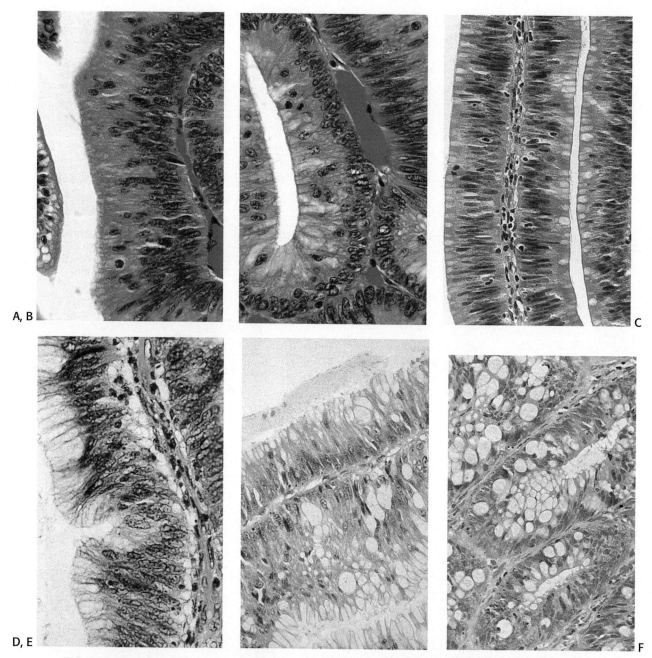

FIG. 14.33. Mucin production in adenomatous epithelium. **A:** Adenoma with almost no intracytoplasmic mucin. **B–F:** Increasing degrees of mucin content in adenomatous cells. Note the presence of dystrophic goblet cells in E and F. Dystrophic goblet cells demonstrate a loss of polarity and, as a result, are not basally located. They often contain an eccentric nucleus, giving them a signet ring cell–like appearance.

distances into the overlying interglandular stroma (Fig. 14.38). The muscular component is most evident at the junction of the head and stalk of the adenoma, where it may form a broad muscular zone. The muscularis mucosae of the stalk merges with the muscular zone of the adenoma. The deeper border of the muscular zone is not as distinct in pedunculated lesions as in sessile ones. The thick muscular zone disappears when invasive cancer develops in the adenoma (225).

Vasculature in Adenomas

The lymphatic plexus begins in the area of the muscularis mucosae, and it may accompany the distorted fibers of the muscularis into the overlying mucosa. However, lymphatics never extend higher than the bases of the crypts (Fig. 14.39).

The microvasculature of adenomas has an organization similar to that of the normal colon, but the capillaries and

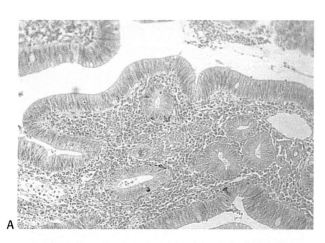

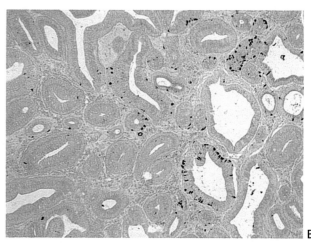

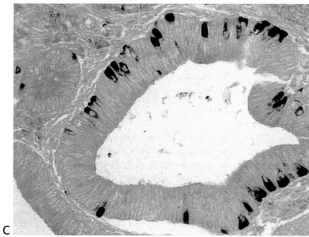

FIG. 14.34. Endocrine differentiation in adenomas. **A:** Grimelius stain demonstrating the presence of endocrine cells. **B:** Chromogranin immunoreactivity in adenoma demonstrating focal collections of endocrine cells within the adenomatous glands. **C:** Higher-power magnification of one of these glands demonstrating the large numbers of endocrine cells within the adenomatous crypt.

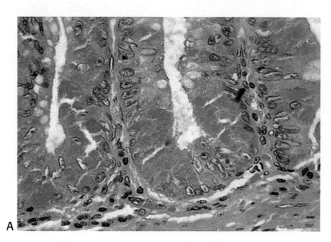

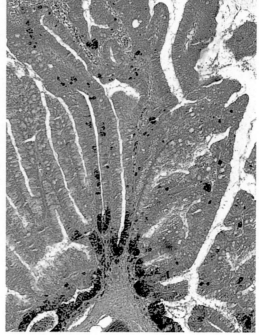

FIG. 14.35. Paneth cell differentiation in adenomas. **A:** Neoplastic Paneth cells are intermingled with other cells in the adenoma. **B:** Immunohistochemical localization of lysozyme within the Paneth cells of a villous adenoma.

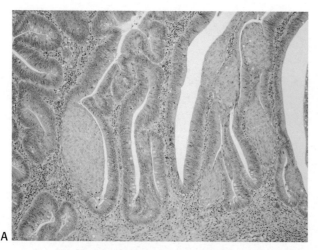
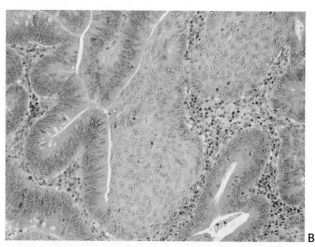

FIG. 14.36. Squamous differentiation in adenomas. **A:** Contiguous adenomatous glands and islands of squamous epithelium are seen. The junction between the squamous epithelium and adenomatous epithelium is abrupt. **B:** A squamous morule surrounds residual colonic gland.

venules appear elongated and have increased diameters compared to the vessels present in the normal lamina propria. Microvessel density increases in the spaces between the neoplastic cells. It also increases as the severity of the dysplasia increases (226).

Pseudocarcinomatous Entrapment (Pseudoinvasion)

A recognized histologic pitfall in diagnosing adenomas is the presence of pseudoinvasive foci surrounded by areas of hemosiderin deposition and fibrosis. Its significance is its

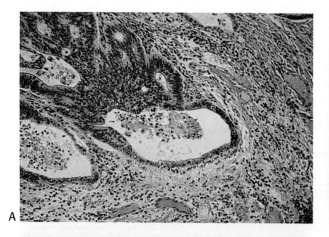
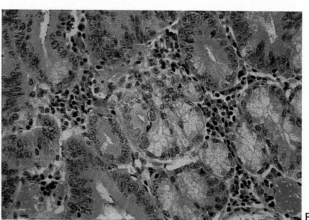
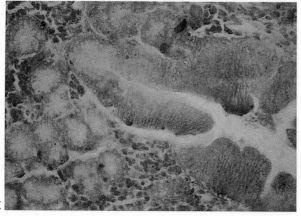

FIG. 14.37. Unusual cell types in adenomas. **A:** Melanocytes in an adenoma containing an area of carcinoma in situ. **B:** Pyloric gland differentiation in the base of an adenoma. **C:** Immunoperoxidase stain for gastrin in the polyp with pyloric epithelium.

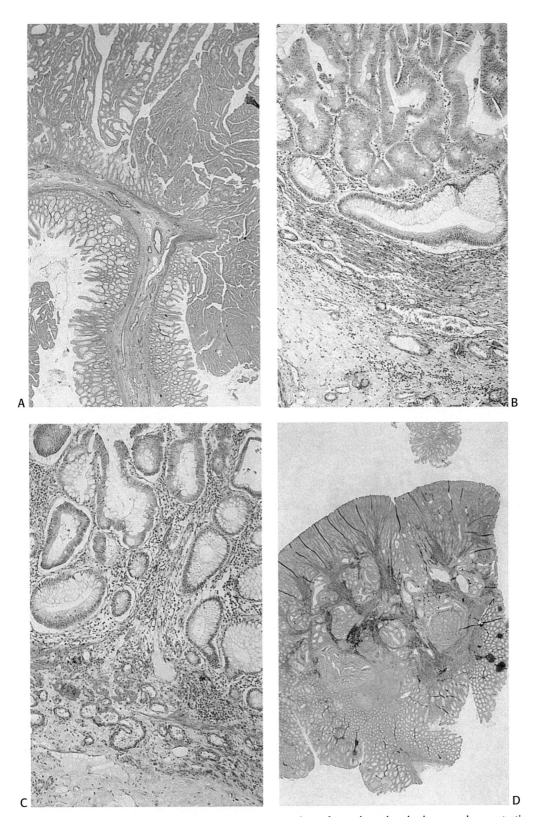

FIG. 14.38. Smooth muscle in adenomas. **A:** Low-power view of a pedunculated adenoma demonstrating abundant smooth muscle within the stalk of the polyp. The muscle is highlighted with immunohistochemical stains to actin. **B:** The muscularis mucosae of this adenomatous polyp is frayed and somewhat thickened. Thick bundles of muscle fibers surround the adenomatous epithelium. The actin stain also highlights the submucosal vessels within the stalk. **C:** Muscle fibers often extend upward from the muscularis mucosae into the lamina propria between the adenomatous glands. **D:** Adenoma with pseudocarcinomatous entrapment. Low magnification highlights the thick muscle bundles separating the lobules of adenomatous epithelium. These are not irregular and infiltrated, as could be seen in the case of an invasive carcinoma.

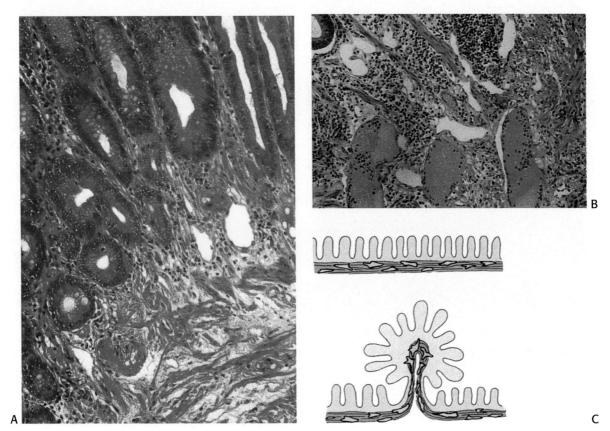

FIG. 14.39. Lymphatics in adenomas. **A:** The bases of the crypts are seen overlying a somewhat disorganized muscularis mucosae. The dilated lymphatics are present in the space between the muscularis mucosae and the base of the crypts. **B:** Higher-power magnification of this region demonstrating dilated lymphatics (*open spaces*) and congested capillaries. Fibers of the muscularis mucosae are also seen. **C:** Illustration of lymphatic distribution (*yellow*) in normal colonic mucosa (*top*) and in an adenomatous polyp (*bottom*). The lymphatics start as a plexus around the muscularis mucosae.

resemblance to invasive carcinoma and its potential to be misdiagnosed, thereby leading to needless colonic resections. Pseudocarcinomatous entrapment, variously termed *colitis cystica profunda, submucosal cysts, pseudocarcinomatous invasion,* or *epithelial misplacement,* affects a small proportion of pedunculated adenomas. Affected adenomas usually measure >1 cm in diameter, have at least a 1-cm stalk, and originate in the sigmoid colon (64% to 85%) (227).

Repeated episodes of torsion lead to hemorrhage, inflammation, and ulceration of the adenoma. As a result, the adenomatous epithelium herniates through the muscularis mucosae into the underlying submucosa. The presence of thick-walled and occasionally thrombosed submucosal blood vessels supports the concept of torsion and subsequent ischemia as the initiating event. Forceps biopsies may also cause epithelial displacement into the underlying submucosa (Figs. 14.40 and 14.41). The adenomatous tissue may be pulled further into the stalk by contraction of fibrous tissue as the biopsy site heals. The changes reflect the time elapsed from the biopsy procedure and the polyp resection. Displaced cells become embedded within capillary-rich granulation tissue during the first week following the biopsy. Subsequent submucosal fibrosis results in persistent submucosal mucin pools (228).

Histologically, one recognizes areas of pseudoinvasion by the presence of adenomatous epithelium in a submucosa without cytologic evidence of malignancy (Figs. 14.40 and 14.41). The displaced glands sometimes lie in continuity with the neoplastic tissue overlying it, and the degree of dysplasia in the displaced glands often resembles that of the glands immediately overlying it. The displaced glands may also coexist with nonneoplastic glands that were displaced along with the neoplastic ones, providing assurance that the submucosal glands are displaced rather than invasive (Fig. 14.41). Normal lamina propria surrounds displaced adenomatous glands (as opposed to a desmoplastic response surrounding an invasive carcinoma) (Figs. 14.42 and 14.43). If the epithelial displacement occurs immediately prior to the polypectomy, the glands may be surrounded by a narrow rim of granulation tissue. Fresh or old hemorrhage with hemosiderin deposits in the fibrotic stroma surrounding the displaced glands is known as *siderogenous desmoplasia* (Figs. 14.44 and 14.45). Hemosiderin also deposits in the lamina propria and in the fibrotic stroma surrounding the glands and thick-walled blood vessels. This contrasts with the lack of hemosiderin deposition in areas of true invasive carcinoma.

Rarely, areas of high-grade dysplastic mucosa become entrapped in the submucosa, a change that represents an even

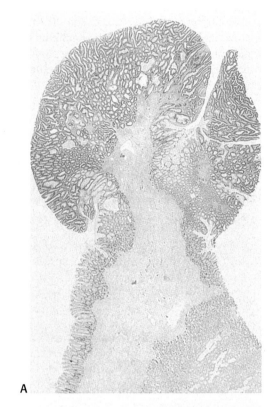

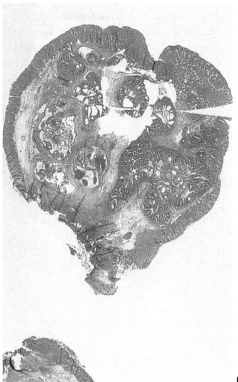

A

B

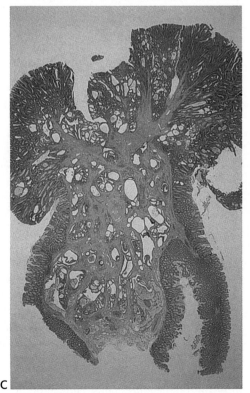

C

FIG. 14.40. Comparison of pseudocarcinomatous entrapment and invasive cancer. **A:** Pedunculated adenomatous polyp without pseudoinvasion or invasive cancer. The stalk consists of fibrous tissue, smooth muscle, vessels, and nerves. No glandular structures are present. **B:** In pseudoinvasion, glands that are cytologically benign are entrapped within the stalk. These glands are surrounded by normal lamina propria, and a desmoplastic response is absent. The glands exhibit a lobulated arrangement. **C:** In invasive carcinoma, cytologically malignant glands are present in the submucosa. These glands are surrounded by desmoplastic stroma and lack the lobulated arrangement seen in pseudoinvasion.

greater diagnostic challenge to the pathologist (Fig. 14.46). Features suggesting pseudoinvasion are listed in Table 14.8.

Occasionally, the displaced glands undergo cystic dilation with rupture and epithelial lining loss or atrophy (Fig. 14.47). Sometimes, the mucinous material within the submucosa calcifies. The distinction between a mucus-secreting invasive

adenocarcinoma and cystically dilated pseudoinvasive glands may also be difficult. Pseudoinvasive glands usually appear regular, sometimes exhibiting a lobular distribution in the submucosa. In contrast, mucinous carcinomas display an irregular distribution of angular glands or nests of atypical cells. No lamina propria surrounds the cysts or glands; instead,

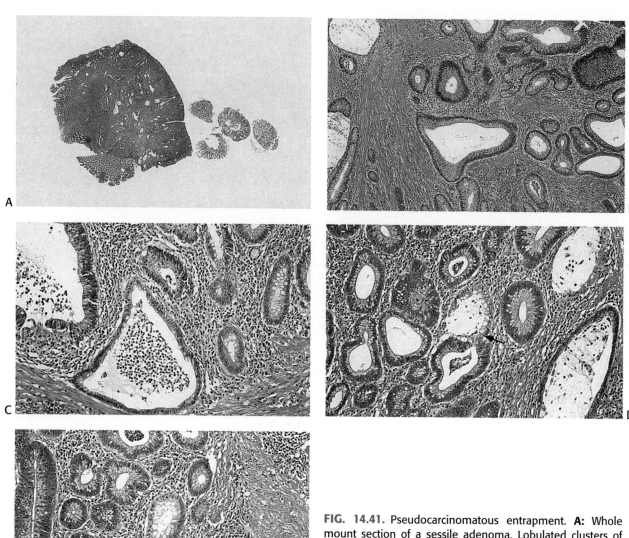

FIG. 14.41. Pseudocarcinomatous entrapment. **A:** Whole mount section of a sessile adenoma. Lobulated clusters of glands lie in the submucosa surrounded by dense muscle bands. **B:** The glands show no evidence of high-grade dysplasia and are surrounded by normal-appearing lamina propria. **C:** Higher-power view of mildly dysplastic glands surrounded by lamina propria. **D, E:** Displaced adenomatous glands are admixed with displaced nonneoplastic glands (*arrows*).

TABLE 14.8 **Features Suggesting Pseudoinvasion in Adenomas**

Direct continuity of submucosal glands with surface adenoma

Presence of lamina propria surrounding the neoplastic glands

Presence of hemosiderin

Lack of desmoplasia

Lack of cytologic features of malignancy

Presence of an admixture of adenomatous glands with normal colonic epithelium in the submucosa

Presence of an admixture of benign adenomatous glands with frankly malignant glands

Marked disorganization of the muscularis mucosae

---

a desmoplastic stroma usually lacking hemosiderin deposits is present. Focal stromal desmoplasia may be present.

Differentiating pseudocarcinomatous entrapment in adenomas from localized colitis cystica profunda or the mucosal prolapse syndromes (see Chapter 13) is also usually not difficult, since in the latter, the submucosal cysts are covered by an ulcerated, normal, or hyperplastic-appearing epithelium. The overlying epithelium is not adenomatous in prolapse or colitis cystica profunda. These lesions are compared in Table 14.9

Flat Adenomas

Flat or depressed adenomas are a variant of tubular adenoma with little or no mucosal elevation. By definition, the thickness

TABLE 14.9 Comparison of Colitis Cystica Profunda, Adenoma with Pseudoinvasion, and Invasive Cancer in Adenoma

Lesion	Surface	Sub-mucosa	Lamina Propria in the Sub-Mucosa	Desmo-Plasia	Muscular Zone	Nonneo-Plastic Glands the Sub-Mucosa	Archi-Tecture of Displaced Glands	Sidero Genous Desmo-Plasia
Colitis cystica profunda	Nonneoplastic	Displaced nonneo-plastic glands	Often	No	Thickened	Yes	Often	Lobular
Adenoma with pseudo-invasion	Adenoma with variable degrees of dysplasia	Displaced glands with variable degrees of dysplasia	Yes	No	Thickened bands	Often	Often	Lobular
Adenoma with invasive cancer	Neoplastic with variable degrees of dysplasia	Irregular malignant glands	No	Yes	Invaded by tumor	No	Not usually	Irregular infiltration

of the adenomatous mucosa does not exceed twice that of the nonadenomatous mucosa in flat adenomas (Fig. 14.48). The adenomatous changes concentrate near the luminal surface. A disproportionate number of flat adenomas contain high-grade dysplasia (41% to 42%) as determined by a

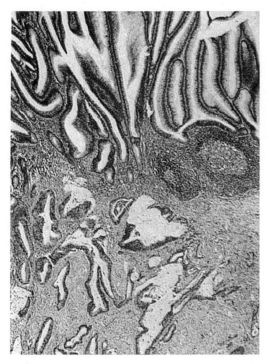

FIG. 14.42. Invasive carcinoma arising in a villous adenoma. In contrast to the lesion shown in Figure 14.41, the glands within the stroma are associated with a prominent desmoplastic response.

higher nuclear:cytoplasmic ratio and degree of cellular atypia than typically seen in polypoid adenomas (209,216). They are also more likely to harbor an invasive carcinoma than their polypoid counterparts (229).

Flat adenomas contain crowded adenomatous tubules with diameters that are smaller than those seen in the more common polypoid, tubular adenomas. This feature increases the glandular density when compared to elevated tubular adenomas. The adenomatous tubules tend to occupy the full thickness of the lamina propria at the center of the lesion with superficial growth to the periphery. Depressed adenomas measuring <1 mm in diameter show horizontal growth between the normal adjacent crypts, often leaving normal crypts entrapped as residual islands (Fig. 14.48), whereas polypoid adenomas tend to grow expansively without including remnants of the normal crypts.

The mean labeling index for proliferating cells is higher in depressed adenomas than in nondepressed adenomas, but lower than seen in intramucosal carcinomas (215). Flat lesions are also more commonly aneuploid, and demonstrate differential expression of many genes compared with normal mucosa or polypoid adenomas (209,230–232). For example, Ras gene mutations are significantly more common in flat than polypoid adenomas, and epigenetic changes occur less frequently (231).

Hypersecretory Adenomas

Secretory adenoma represents a special variant of villous adenoma, usually arising in the rectum. Patients present with profuse watery diarrhea, severe fluid and electrolyte loss, elevated blood urea nitrogen, reduced serum sodium, and hypokalemia

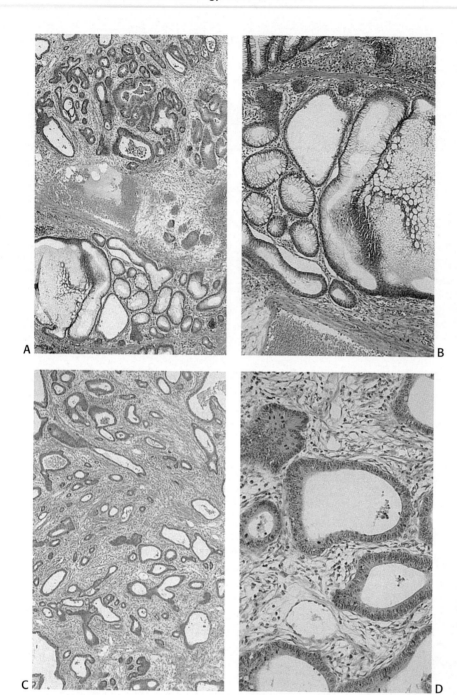

FIG. 14.43. Adenoma with pseudocarcinomatous entrapment compared with invasive carcinoma. **A:** Low-power photomicrograph demonstrating the presence of pseudoinvasion. The displaced pseudoinvasive glands appear lobulated and are surrounded by lamina propria. Thick muscle bundles surround the glands and stroma. **B:** Higher-power view of the area of pseudoinvasion. The glands demonstrate low-grade dysplasia and are surrounded by lamina propria. **C:** Invasive carcinoma. Malignant glands infiltrate the submucosa. These glands are surrounded by a desmoplastic stroma. **D:** Higher magnification of the invasive carcinoma. The irregular glands are lined by disorganized cells with hyperchromatic, irregular nuclei. A prominent desmoplastic response surrounds the malignant glands.

due to hypersecretion of fluid and an electrolyte-rich mucus. These abnormalities return to normal once the adenoma is excised. Characteristically, the mucous diarrhea is most severe in the morning after the stool has accumulated during sleeping hours. The secretion may be mediated by cyclic nucleotides (233). Histologically, pale, mucus-filled cells line the villi of hypersecretory adenomas (Fig. 14.49).

Clear Cell Adenomas

Rare adenomas contain clear cells. Usually the areas of clear cell differentiation intermingle with areas of more traditional adenoma (Fig. 14.50). The clear cells tend to exhibit minimal atypia and often contain basal nuclei. The apical cytoplasm is filled with pale, foamy-appearing cytoplasm. The nuclei are round and appear minimally pseudostratified. In another variant of clear cell adenoma, the pseudostratified nuclei exhibit clear cytoplasmic contents above and below the nuclei in a pattern somewhat reminiscent of endometrium. These areas of clear cell adenoma presumably give rise to the clear cell carcinomas that are sometimes encountered in the colon. There is no known clinical significance to the presence of the clear cells in the adenoma.

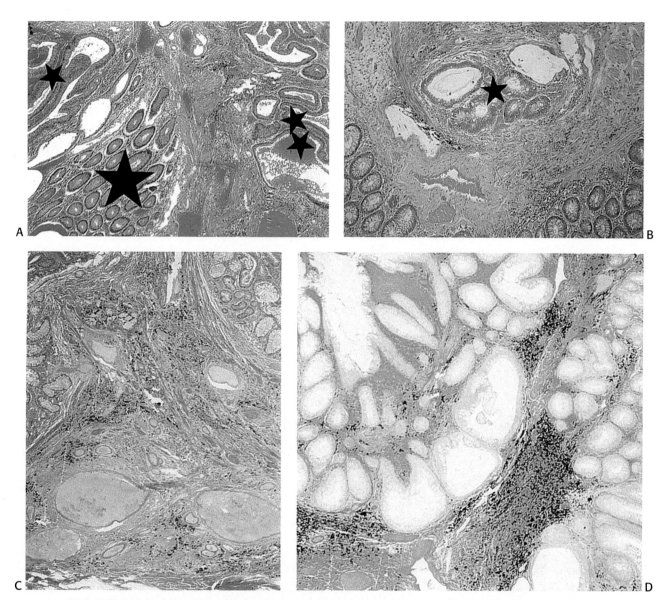

FIG. 14.44. Pseudocarcinomatous entrapment. **A:** Adenomatous epithelium has herniated into the submucosa (*double stars*), which is recognizable by the presence of large blood vessels. The herniated adenomatous glands present within the stalk of the adenoma. The normal stalk mucosa (*large star*) changes to adenomatous epithelium (*small single star*). **B:** A trapped adenomatous gland within the submucosa of the head of the polyp (*star*). **C:** Siderogenous desmoplasia within the submucosa of the head of the polyp. The brownish color comes from the presence of hemosiderin-laden macrophages. **D:** Iron stain demonstrating the presence of large amounts of iron in the submucosa.

Adenoma–Carcinoma Sequence

Adenomas constitute the obligate precursor lesion for most colorectal carcinomas (Fig. 14.51). The earliest lesions consist of pseudostratified immature, mildly dysplastic, adenomatous cells. The adenoma may be of any of the types discussed in previous sections. In some cases, one may see a continuous histologic spectrum of increasing degrees of dysplasia culminating in the development of an invasive carcinoma (Figs. 14.52 to 14.54). This neoplastic continuum can be diagrammed schematically (Fig. 14.55) and can also be

shown histologically (Fig. 14.52). Carcinomas are more likely to arise in larger adenomas than smaller ones. Observations supporting the concept that most colorectal cancers develop from adenomas are listed in Table 14.10.

Diagnosis of Adenomas

The histologic features of adenomas may be defined as low- and high-grade dysplasia, carcinoma in situ, intramucosal carcinoma, and invasive carcinoma. Low-grade dysplasia

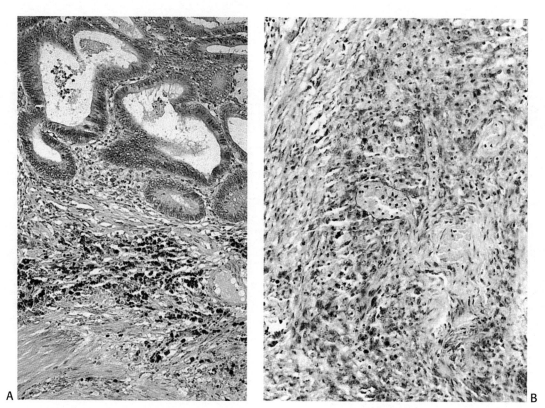

FIG. 14.45. Siderogenous desmoplasia. **A:** The stroma of this adenomatous polyp contains prominent hemosiderin deposits within the fibrous stroma surrounding entrapped glands. Hemosiderin pigment is also present in the lamina propria. **B:** Hemosiderin within the submucosa in another polyp.

and high-grade dysplasia are defined in the following section. High-grade dysplasia consists of cytologically malignant cells that remain confined within the basement membrane of the original colonic crypt. It is recognizable by the presence of marked cytologic atypia, the loss of cellular polarity, and the occasional formation of solid nests of

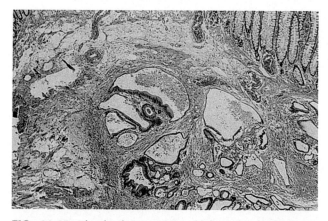

FIG. 14.46. Glands demonstrating high-grade dysplasia are present in the submucosa of this adenoma. These glands represent pseudocarcinomatous entrapment because they are surrounded by lamina propria, and there is no associated desmoplastic response.

dysplastic cells, sometimes including dystrophic goblet cells (Fig. 14.52). Extension of the neoplastic cells through the basement membrane of the crypt into the surrounding lamina propria can be designated an *intramucosal carcinoma* (Fig. 14.53) (169). Areas of intramucosal carcinoma show greater glandular irregularity and greater glandular density than carcinoma in situ. Intramucosal carcinoma may occupy the entire mucosal thickness, or it may represent a small focal area within the adenoma. Once intramucosal carcinomas reach the deep mucosa, the neoplastic cells may mingle with frayed fibers of the muscularis mucosae and may gain access to lymphatics and may theoretically metastasize (Fig. 14.56). This is extraordinarily rare. Invasion into, but not through, the muscularis mucosae is still intramucosal carcinoma.

Since neither intraepithelial neoplasia nor intramucosal carcinoma has a clinically significant potential for metastasis (if all neoplastic tissue is removed), the lesions do not require additional treatment. In fact, we rarely use the term *intramucosal carcinoma* because of the clinical misinterpretation of the significance of the lesion that can occur as a result of the word *carcinoma*. A carcinoma of the large bowel is not considered to be invasive and clinically significant until it invades through the muscularis mucosae into the underlying submucosa (Fig. 14.57). Submucosal invasion is most easily recognized by the intermingling of the malignant glands

TABLE 14.10 Adenoma–Carcinoma Sequence

Arguments Cited in Support of the Concept

1. Similar distribution of adenoma and carcinomas
2. Colorectal carcinoma frequently coexists with adenoma in the same lesion
3. Prevalence rates of adenomas and carcinomas in countries at various magnitudes of colon carcinoma risk show correlation between the two
4. A similar anatomic distribution exists for adenomas and carcinomas
5. Increased frequency of carcinoma in patients with adenomas
6. Adenomas present in patients who develop metachronous carcinomas show a significant excess of severe dysplasia compared to adenomas present in patients in whom second cancer did not develop
7. Adenomas occur with increased frequency in colons containing carcinomas
8. Increasing age of patients with increasing degrees of atypia and areas of invasive cancer (age succession adenoma–carcinoma)
9. Residual adenomas can be found in some patients with cancer
10. Production of both adenomas and carcinomas in laboratory animals
11. Endoscopic removal of adenomas reduces the expected incidence of carcinoma by 85%
12. All patients with familial adenomatous polyposis syndrome develop cancer if adenoma-bearing colon is not removed
13. Absence of carcinoma in situ outside the area of adenoma
14. Areas of direct transition are identifiable
15. Patients who have adenomas identified endoscopically refuse therapy and eventually return with an invasive carcinoma at the same site
16. De novo carcinoma extremely rare
17. Failure to demonstrate carcinoma in normal mucosa despite the countless thousands of polyp and colon sections examined histologically each year
18. Presence of an adenoma places a patient at increased lifetime risk for developing colon cancer
19. Growth of adenomatous cells in vitro results in cell populations that acquire the features of carcinoma in situ or invasive carcinoma
20. Chromosomal constitution in adenomatous and carcinomatous tissue similar
21. Antigenic relatedness between adenomas and carcinomas
22. DNA content of benign adenomas is intermediate between normal colon and cancer
23. Enzyme patterns similar in adenomas and carcinomas. Adenomas differ from hyperplastic polyps and normal mucosa
24. Similar oncogenes found in some adenomas and carcinomas

Arguments Cited Against the Concept

1. Different distribution of adenomas and carcinomas in some studies
2. Same incidence of carcinoma developing in patients with and without polyps
3. Failure to demonstrate areas of adenoma in "small" carcinomas
4. Failure to demonstrate carcinomas in adenomas

with normal submucosal structures, including medium-sized blood vessels, fat, nerves and ganglia, and larger lymphatics (Fig. 14.58). A prominent desmoplastic response often accompanies even early invasion (Fig. 14.59).

Low-grade Dysplasia

By definition, all adenomas contain at least low-grade dysplasia. Low-grade dysplasia consists of stratified dysplastic epithelium that retains its columnar shape. The nuclei are spindle or oval shaped. The stratified nuclei tend to remain in the basal epithelium extending no more than three quarters of the height of the epithelium. There is minimal nuclear hyperchromasia. Minor cytologic variations, such as varia-

tions in mucin content, nuclear pleomorphism, differences in chromatin distribution, and variations in cell size and shape, frequently occur in adenomatous epithelium, especially in larger lesions (Fig. 14.60). These findings represent features of the underlying neoplastic process and, in the absence of significant atypia or architectural alterations, have no clinical significance. Such changes are insufficient to warrant a diagnosis of high-grade dysplasia.

Occasionally, it is difficult to distinguish a small tubular adenoma from reactive epithelium present in an inflamed mucosa. One approach that we find works well is to examine the degree of differentiation of the epithelium along the length of the tubular crypt. Reactive glands appear more basophilic than normal, and the nuclei may exhibit pseudostratification.

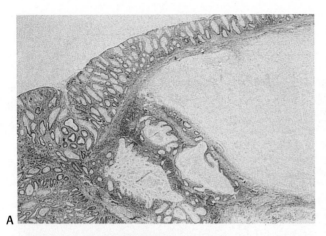

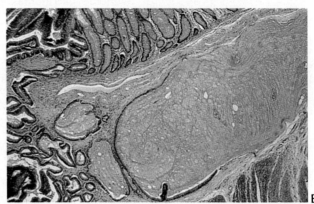

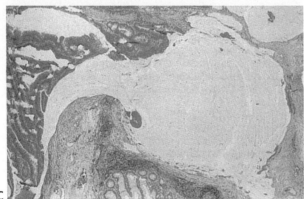

FIG. 14.47. Pseudocarcinomatous entrapment. **A:** Sometimes entrapped glands undergo cystic dilation, resulting in large mucin-filled pools within the submucosa underlying the adenoma. **B:** Higher magnification demonstrating cystically dilated mucin filled glands, which are partially lined by adenomatous epithelium. **C:** In some cases, the epithelial lining atrophies or is lost, leaving only pools of mucin within the submucosa. In such cases, careful scrutiny for irregular, atypical glands or nests of cells is warranted to rule out the presence of a mucinous carcinoma.

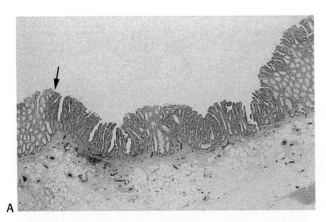

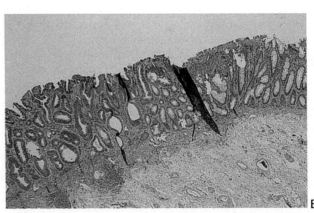

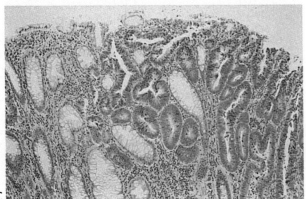

FIG. 14.48. Flat adenoma. **A:** Low-power photomicrograph of a flat adenoma. The adenoma is approximately the same thickness or thinner than the adjacent nonneoplastic colonic mucosa indicated by the *arrow.* **B:** The adenomatous epithelium is concentrated at the surface in this flat adenoma and is overgrowing some residual nonneoplastic glands seen on the right-hand side of the photograph. **C:** Higher-power magnification demonstrating adenomatous glands admixed with nonneoplastic glands at the edge of a flat adenoma. The neoplastic epithelium shows high-grade dysplasia characterized by nuclear stratification and loss of cell polarity.

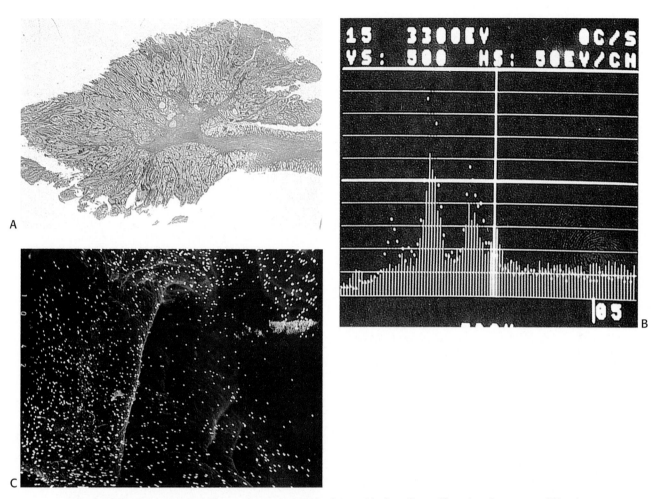

FIG. 14.49. Hypersecretory villous adenoma. **A:** Pale clear epithelium lines villous fronds. **B:** X-ray diffraction study of the lesion. *Bar lines* represent the elements found in the adenomatous tissue. *Dotted lines* represent the elements found in the surrounding normal mucosa. The *single vertical line* indicates a peak present only in the adenomatous tissue. Its energy level measures 3,300 electron-volts corresponding to the Ka show of potassium. **C:** Using the window indicated in B, the potassium was mapped to the lesion. No localization was found on the normal mucosa (not shown). However, the villous fronds showed the presence of large amounts of potassium (*white dots*).

These changes extend from the crypt base toward the luminal surface. Mitotic activity is present in the basophilic regenerating cells. If the entire gland is not replaced by basophilic epithelium, then its restriction to the bottom portion of the crypt serves to identify the epithelium as regenerative (Fig. 14.61). Conversely, in small adenomas the adenomatous glands appear more basophilic at the surface of the lesion and nonneoplastic epithelium lies below it. The mitotic activity is at the surface. Ki-67 immunostains help highlight the proliferating compartments. When the entire crypt appears immature, the epithelium may be either regenerative or adenomatous. Then one must rely on the histologic context in which the glands are found to distinguish between these two possibilities. In a setting of active inflammation, the glands are most likely to be regenerative. The one disorder in which these distinctions are particularly difficult is ulcerative colitis, as discussed in Chapter 11.

High-grade Dysplasia

High-grade dysplasia is present when the nuclei consistently come to the surface of the epithelium (Fig. 14.60). High-grade dysplasia also includes loss of the columnar shape with cellular rounding, increasing nuclear:cytoplasmic ratios, nuclear irregularity, loss of polarity, development of cellular pleomorphism, and heaping up of cells (Fig. 14.62). The cells may remain confined to the basement membrane of the original crypt, or they may extend into the surrounding lamina propria, assuming a dense cribriform pattern (Fig. 14.63) that obliterates the intervening stroma. Glandular density increases (506). It is not uncommon for the surface of adenomas to exhibit focal loss of nuclear polarity. These changes probably reflect the passage of intestinal contents over their surface stimulating reactive changes. Very reactive changes may exaggerate the cytologic features of the epithelium, causing it to

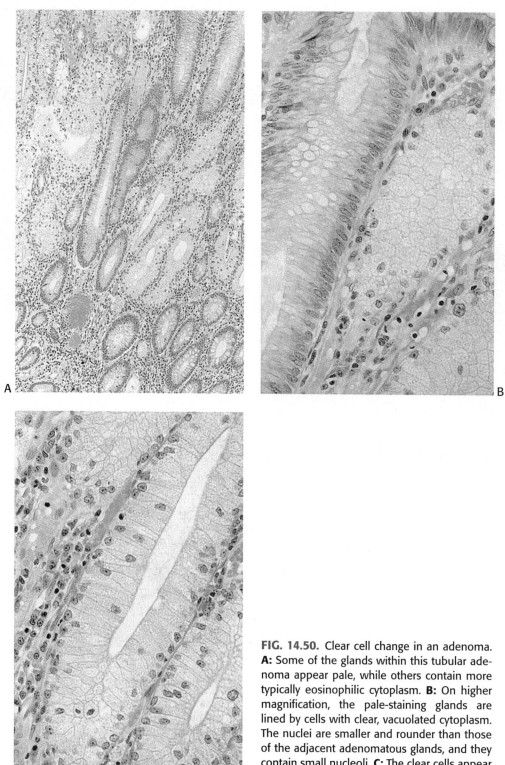

FIG. 14.50. Clear cell change in an adenoma. **A:** Some of the glands within this tubular adenoma appear pale, while others contain more typically eosinophilic cytoplasm. **B:** On higher magnification, the pale-staining glands are lined by cells with clear, vacuolated cytoplasm. The nuclei are smaller and rounder than those of the adjacent adenomatous glands, and they contain small nucleoli. **C:** The clear cells appear mildly stratified in some areas. These cells contain abundant glycogen.

resemble high-grade dysplasia, particularly if papillary tufting forms. However, the presence of associated inflammation should alert one to the possibility that the changes are reactive in nature. If the changes are minor, they should be disregarded and not used to diagnose high-grade dysplasia.

High-grade dysplasia represents the extreme end of the spectrum of abnormal histologic changes short of invasive carcinoma in the adenoma–carcinoma continuum. The presence of high-grade dysplasia strongly correlates with a contiguous invasive carcinoma. Overall, approximately 5%

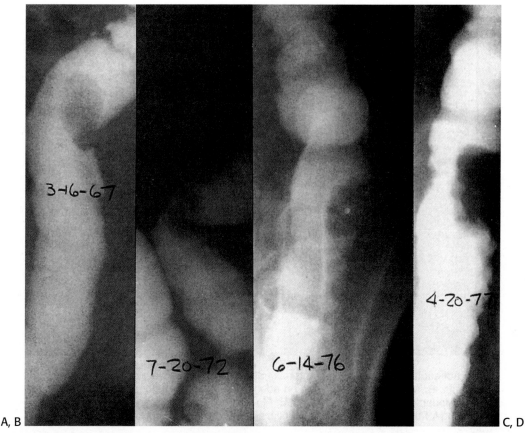

FIG. 14.51. Serial barium enema examination of descending colon shows transformation of pedunculated polyp (**A**) becoming wider at base (**B**) then sessile with malignant change (**C**) and obvious malignant tumor (**D**).

of adenomas contain high-grade dysplasia or carcinoma in situ at the time of presentation (175). Individual adenomas may contain transitions between high-grade and low-grade dysplasia. The percentage of adenomas containing high-grade dysplasia increases significantly with increasing adenoma size, villous architecture, multiplicity of adenomas, and age older than 60 years (189,234). The odds ratio for high-grade dysplasia is 20 for adenomas >1 cm and for adenomas containing a >75% villous component (189). Patients with multiple adenomas are more likely to have at least one adenoma with high-grade dysplasia (13.8%) than patients with a single adenoma (7.8%). The incidence of high-grade dysplasia in patients with a single tubular adenoma, multiple tubular adenomas, a single villous adenoma, and multiple villous adenomas is 2.8%, 4.6%, 16%, and 22%, respectively.

Adenomas Containing Cancer

The diagnosis of invasive carcinoma is made when the carcinoma extends into and through the muscularis mucosae, and one can demonstrate the tumor in the submucosa of the bowel wall or in the submucosa of the stalk of an adenoma. The stroma of both the head of the polyp and the underlying submucosa of the bowel wall appears much looser than the

lamina propria, and lacks the large population of lymphocytes and histiocytes typically seen in the lamina propria. This diagnosis is made either on a polypectomy specimen or on a biopsy of sessile lesions. Diagnosing areas of invasive carcinoma on a midsagittal section of a pedunculated adenoma is often easier than making a diagnosis of invasion on a small forceps biopsy of a larger lesion. Biopsy fragments in which the neoplastic cells mingle with the fat, medium-sized blood vessels, nerve trunks, ganglia, or large lymphatics can be diagnosed as invasive lesions. Desmoplasia often surrounds the invading glands. The glands themselves have irregular, angulated contours and show cytologic features of malignancy. Areas of invasion must be distinguished from areas of pseudoinvasion as discussed previously. Invasive cancer is present in 2.5% of adenomas at the time of presentation (175).

Carcinomas develop in the geographic centers of adenomas and spread centrifugally, replacing the pre-existing adenomatous epithelium. Several factors predispose to carcinoma development, including adenoma size, growth pattern, dysplasia grade, and patient age (169,189). Both growth pattern and dysplasia grade correlate with lesional size. Small adenomas have the lowest risk of malignant transformation, but this risk is not completely negligible. Most adenomas <1 cm in diameter usually show low-grade

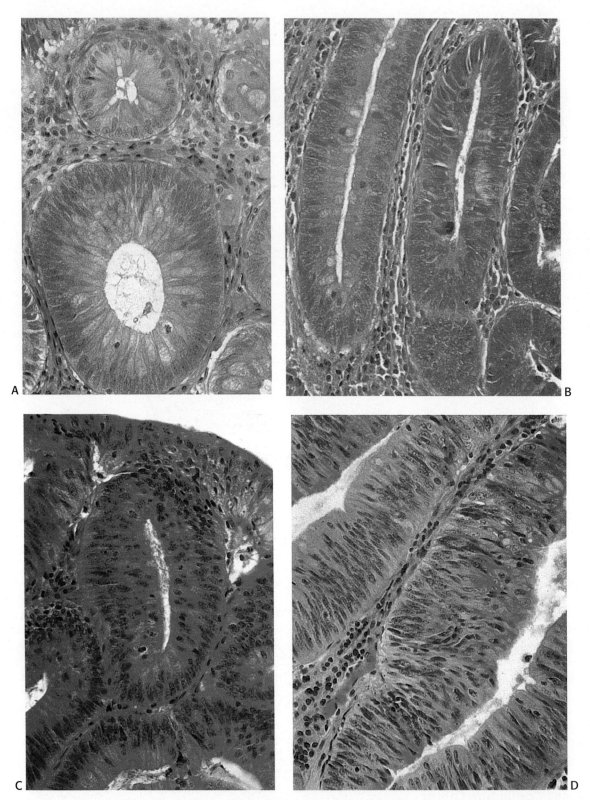

FIG. 14.52. Adenoma with progressive degrees of dysplasia. **A:** Small tubular adenomatous gland with very little atypia. **B:** Mild epithelial atypia in an adenoma. **C:** Mild to moderate epithelioid atypia in an adenoma. **D:** Moderate atypia in an adenoma. (*continues*)

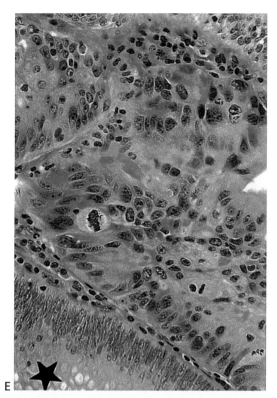

FIG. 14.52. *Continued* **E:** Moderate to severe atypia in an adenoma and severe atypia qualifying for the diagnosis of intraepithelial carcinoma or carcinoma in situ. A small fragment of residual nonatypical adenomatous epithelium is indicated by the *star*.

dysplasia and have a very low malignant potential. The risk of cancer developing in such adenomas is only 5% at 15 years. When high-grade dysplasia is present, the rate of malignancy rises to 27%. The larger the adenoma, the more likely one is to encounter a villous architecture and high-

grade dysplasia. Actuarial analysis reveals a cumulative risk of developing cancer in adenomas that are not removed at 5, 10, and 20 years of 2.5%, 8%, and 24%, respectively. Additional cancers occur at a site remote from the initial polyp, yielding a 35% risk for the development of cancer at any site over 20 years (193). It is estimated that the conversion rate of adenomas to cancer is 0.25% per year (235).

Even though adenomas clearly constitute the precursor lesion for most carcinomas, a vast gap exists in the prevalence rates of adenomas and carcinomas, indicating that some 90% to 95% of adenomas will never become malignant during a person's lifetime (168). This fact offers the challenge of developing markers for identification of those adenomas that have a high probability of progressing to an invasive carcinoma.

Prognosticators of Metastatic Risk of Cancers Present in Adenomas

Patients who have a carcinoma diagnosed following endoscopic polypectomy present a therapeutic challenge, since invasive carcinomas arising in an adenoma are at risk for developing metastases. The clinician faces the therapeutic decision as to whether or not polypectomy alone is adequate therapy or whether the patient requires a definitive surgical resection. Therefore, the metastatic risk must be determined (Table 14.11) to plan future therapy. The presence or absence of invasion into the submucosa of the bowel wall is the most critical prognostic factor (236). The metastatic risk is low if only the submucosa of the head of a pedunculated adenoma (Fig. 14.57) is invaded. In contrast, sessile and semi-sessile adenomas containing an invasive carcinoma will most likely have invasion into the submucosa of the bowel wall and, therefore, will be at higher risk for metastasis than early invasive carcinomas arising in pedunculated adenomas

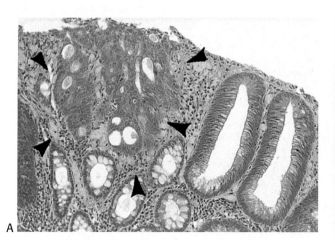

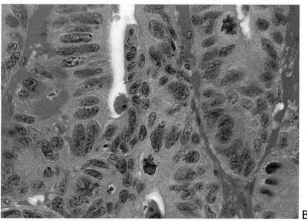

FIG. 14.53. Intramucosal carcinoma. **A:** A small tubular adenoma containing a focus of intramucosal carcinoma (*arrowheads*). These cells are atypical, and the architecture is distorted, with the glands invading the lamina propria. Several adjacent tubular adenomatous glands are seen. **B:** Higher-power magnification of the area of intramucosal carcinoma demonstrating the high mitotic activity and back-to-back gland pattern, as well as the loss of polarity.

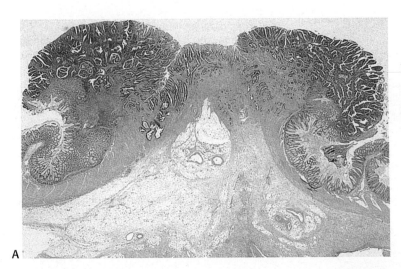
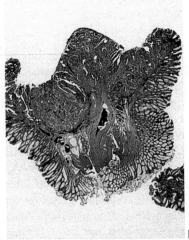

A   B

FIG. 14.54. Invasive carcinoma arising in a sessile adenoma. **A:** Whole mount section of a sessile adenoma demonstrating an area of invasive carcinoma within the central portion of the specimen. **B:** Another polyp containing infiltrating glands within the submucosa. Almost no residual adenomatous glands are present.

(Fig. 14.57). Carcinomas arising in sessile and semi-sessile adenomas with invasion into the submucosa of the bowel wall should be regarded as any other invasive colorectal carcinomas.

Carcinomas arising in pedunculated adenomas cause the biggest clinical question with regard to further management. Some of these lesions require further therapy; others do not (217,237–242). The incidence of nodal metastasis in colonic resections following polypectomies is extremely small in most series. The highest reported incidence was 25% in the series reported by Collacchio et al (241). However, many of these polyps were pathologically not early carcinomas. Most patients who develop nodal metastases are individuals with unfavorable histologic features, including adenomas that contain poorly differentiated carcinomas and exhibit lymphatic or vascular invasion and/or have positive resection margins (Table 14.11) (242,243). If these parameters are present,

35.7% of patients have lymph node metastasis (242). In contrast, adenomas containing well-differentiated or moderately differentiated cancers that are completely excised have a probability of having residual or metastatic cancer of <1% (Fig. 14.64) (236,240–242,244,245). In one large, multi-institutional study, an adverse outcome was present in 19.7% of individuals with an unfavorable histology, 8.6% with indefinite unfavorable histology, and 21% to 33% of patients with cancer at or near (within 1 mm) the cautery margin (244). The presence of cancer at or near the margin significantly associates with an adverse outcome, even in the absence of other unfavorable parameters.

Adenomas Containing Carcinoid Tumors

Adenomas containing carcinoid tumors are rare. They fall within a general category of composite tumors and arise

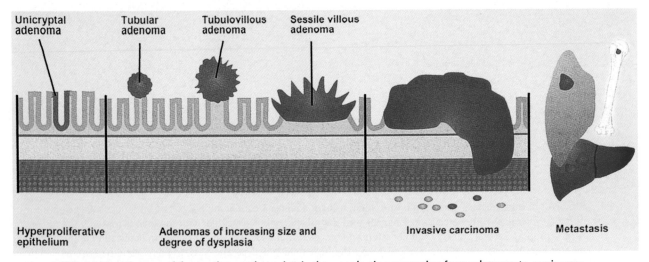

Unicryptal adenoma   Tubular adenoma   Tubulovillous adenoma   Sessile villous adenoma

Hyperproliferative epithelium   Adenomas of increasing size and degree of dysplasia   Invasive carcinoma   Metastasis

FIG. 14.55. Diagram of the continuum that exists in the neoplastic progression from adenoma to carcinoma.

TABLE 14.11	Risk Factors for Metastases from Cancer Arising in a Pedunculated Adenoma

Poorly differentiated carcinoma
Presence of lymphatic invasion
Tumor present at the resection margin
Presence of submucosal invasion of bowel wall

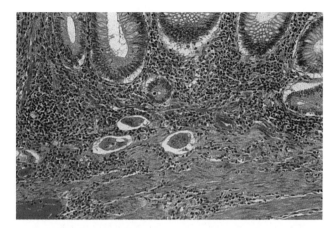

FIG. 14.56. Clusters of neoplastic cells lie within lymphatic channels in the muscularis mucosae of an adenomatous polyp. The adenoma did not contain invasive carcinoma, but did harbor an intramucosal carcinoma that abutted the muscularis mucosae.

either from a common stem cell exhibiting multidirectional differentiation or from multiple cellular events affecting several cell lineages. Adenomas often contain endocrine cells, but, despite the frequency of endocrine cells, they are seldom associated with synchronous carcinoid tumors. Carcinoid tumors in adenomas may arise via several mechanisms (246). Such lesions may arise from a common stem cell, or alternatively, the adenoma and the carcinoid tumor may arise from separate cell lineages, with their appearance in the same lesion representing collision of two separate tumors. Patients with carcinoid tumors have an increased incidence of additional malignancies, many of which arise in the gastrointestinal tract. One could postulate that substances produced by the carcinoid tumor stimulate the adjacent colonic mucosa to proliferate, ultimately leading to neoplastic transformation. Additionally, growth-regulating substances produced by carcinoid tumors could also play a role (247–249).

Pathologic Evaluation of Polyps

When one receives polyp biopsies or polypectomy specimens, it is important to record all of the pathologic features, including the number of tissue fragments received, their size, their gross morphology (i.e., pedunculated or sessile), and their locations. This is especially important in today's world of cost containment, in which one may receive multiple polyps from different sites in a single specimen container. Endoscopists should be careful to limit handling of specimens to polyps in the same colorectal subsite. The presence of unsuspected invasive tumor among one of several polyps derived from different segments of the bowel would not allow identification of the segment requiring further resection. Under this circumstance, it is important to diagnose each tissue piece, if one can determine that each represents a separate polyp. It helps to interpret the number of lesions if the endoscopist indicates the number of polypoid lesions biopsied and/or removed on the requisition. This facilitates a diagnosis of each lesion.

All lesions should be submitted for pathologic examination to (a) adequately classify the lesions histologically, (b) determine the degree of dysplasia, and (c) detect foci of invasive malignancy. Adenomas should be fixed prior to cutting.

Small specimens often contract into balls once they are removed from the endoscope due to contraction of the muscularis mucosae. Tissue fixation ensures retention of the ball

shape, making identification of the resection site difficult. This artifact can be avoided by having the endoscopist place sessile polyps on a firm matrix, such as a piece of paper or Gelfoam, before placing the specimen in the fixative.

If the lesion is pedunculated and received in a fresh state, it can be fixed in such a way that the stalk is pinned to a piece of cork and the specimen is floated upside down in the fixative so as to straighten out the stalk, thereby facilitating examination of the relationship between the head and the underlying stalk. Ideally, the endoscopist should indicate the stalk of larger adenomas by placing a needle at its base when the polyp is removed from the endoscope. In this way, the polypectomy margin can be identified later (Fig. 14.65). Realistically, this almost never happens. Occasionally, the pathologist and the endoscopist disagree as to whether a stalk is present or how long the stalk is, since the stalk often retracts into the head of the adenoma. In many lesions, it is possible to identify the excision edge of the specimen due to the presence of prominent cautery effect. However, some specimens defy accurate orientation so that the assessment of margins may be impossible. In this case, the margins are reported as not evaluable.

Once fixed, midsagittal sections should be taken to include both the head and stalk of pedunculated polyps. The landmarks of adenoma morphology are shown in Figure 14.66. The entire lesion should be examined histologically. Multiple step-sections of the adenoma may pick up a small invasive focus that might be missed on examination of a single section. Inadequate sampling of adenomas underestimates the presence of cancer. Hermanek et al (250) estimate that a single section through the center of an adenoma results in an error rate of 14% in evaluating the adequacy of the resection and that 10% of invasive carcinomas will be overlooked.

Sessile and semi-sessile adenomas should also be properly oriented. If the lesion is large (i.e., >3 cm), with an obvious

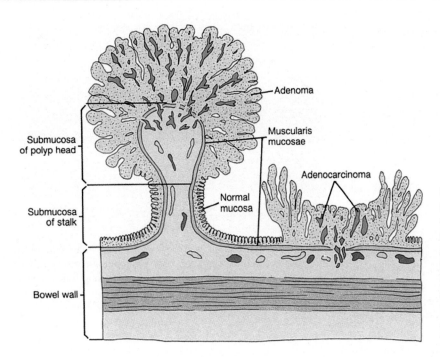

FIG. 14.57. Determination of depth of invasion is a critical pathologic assessment. Levels of invasion in a pedunculated adenoma (*left*) versus a sessile adenoma (*right*). The *green areas* are zones of carcinoma. Invasion below the muscularis mucosae in a sessile lesion places the level of invasion into the submucosa of the bowel wall, increasing the risk of metastasis. This contrasts with the invasive carcinoma in a pedunculated polyp, where the invasion is limited to the polyp head.

cancer in it, then several sections should be taken through the most deeply invasive areas and of the junction with the normal mucosa. Some lesions measure up to 18 cm or more in diameter, and it would be unrealistic to submit the entire lesion at the time of initial evaluation. In such large lesions, it is helpful to bread-loaf the entire specimen into several millimeter slices and then lay the slices out on a board to look for areas of invasive cancer. If cancer is present, one should submit the areas with deepest gross penetration into the bowel wall. If cancer is not evident grossly, preliminary sections through the center of the polyp are taken. If no invasive cancer is identified in the initial sections, the rest of the tissue should be progressively submitted until either an inva-sive cancer is identified and staged or the entire lesion has been examined histologically.

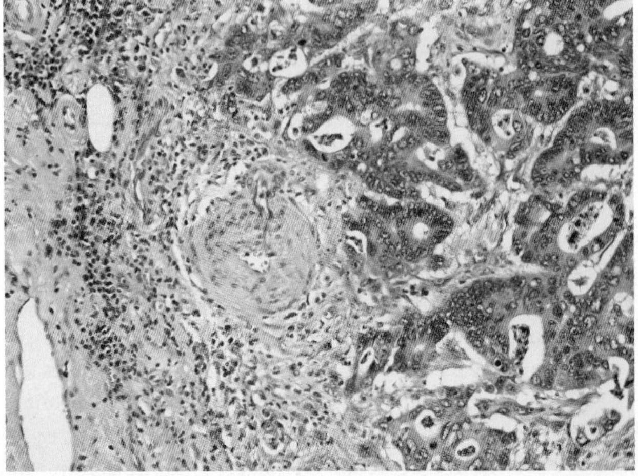

If an adenoma containing high-grade dysplasia is only biop-sied or removed in a piecemeal fashion, one may not be able to determine whether an invasive carcinoma is present or not. The histologic classification of fractional biopsies of smaller adenomas (<1.7 cm) are in 88.9% agreement with the final diagnosis in the polypectomy specimen, whereas the reliability of the biopsies in accurately diagnosing adenomas >1.7 cm is only 27.68%. Invasive carcinomas are frequently missed in biopsies taken of larger lesions (251). Reasons for the poor pre-dictability of the biopsy relate to the fact that larger adenomas tend to be villous, with invasive carcinoma developing in the center of the lesion. These centrally invasive foci tend to retract due to the tumor-associated desmoplasia. As a result, the vil-lous fronds fall into the center of the lesion, covering the inva-sive component. Also, villous fronds at the periphery of the lesion are more accessible for biopsy than the cells in the central scarred carcinoma. Cytologic evaluation of adenomas can aug-ment the diagnostic yield of malignancy (Fig. 14.67), particu-larly if the brush dislodges malignant cells from the center of the lesion where cancer is likely to be present. However, as with superficial biopsies, it is usually not possible to cytologically distinguish between invasive and noninvasive foci.

Pathology Report

The pathologist must carefully word pathology reports of colorectal adenomas to facilitate clear communication with the clinician and appropriate therapy. The pathology report should state the highest degree of dysplasia present in the adenoma, whether or not it has villous features, the com-pleteness of its removal, and the presence or absence of inva-sive tumor. If invasive cancer is present, it should be reported

FIG. 14.58. Invasive adenocarcinoma within the submucosa. The submucosa is easily identified by the presence of a large submucosal blood vessel.

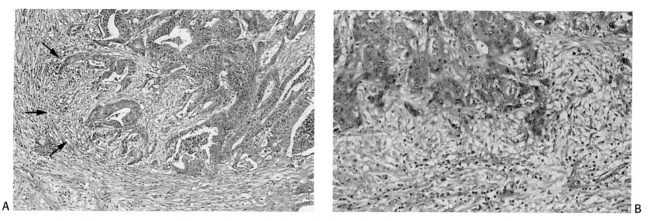

FIG. 14.59. Invasive carcinoma. **A:** Irregular glands infiltrate the submucosa creating a ragged invasive margin, especially prominent in the area marked by the *arrows*. **B:** Desmoplastic response surrounding an invasive cancer.

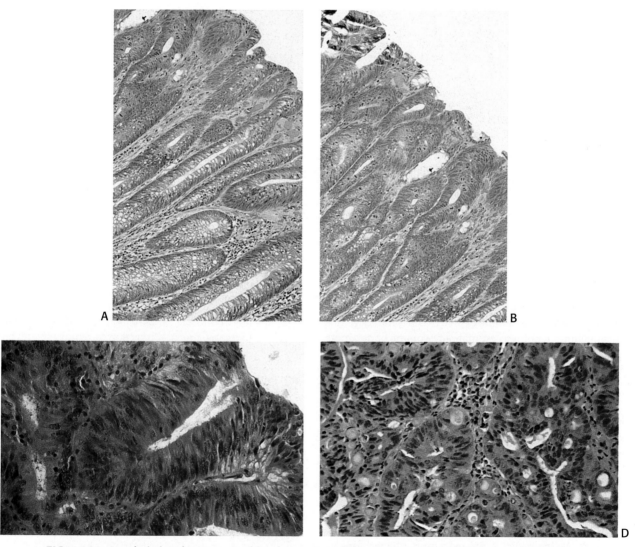

FIG. 14.60. Dysplasia in adenomas. **A:** This adenomatous polyp contains cells with little or no atypia and, therefore, represents only low-grade dysplasia. **B:** Adenomatous polyp with minor cytologic alterations including numerous mitoses and mild nuclear pleomorphism. The changes in this polyp are common in larger polyps and do not warrant a diagnosis of high-grade dysplasia. **C:** High-grade dysplasia characterized by cellular disorganization and more marked cytologic atypia. The degree of nuclear pleomorphism is sufficient in this area so that it might be called intraepithelial carcinoma. In many areas the cells are truly stratified. **D:** Stratification of cells to the luminal surface of the glands is a feature of high-grade dysplasia.

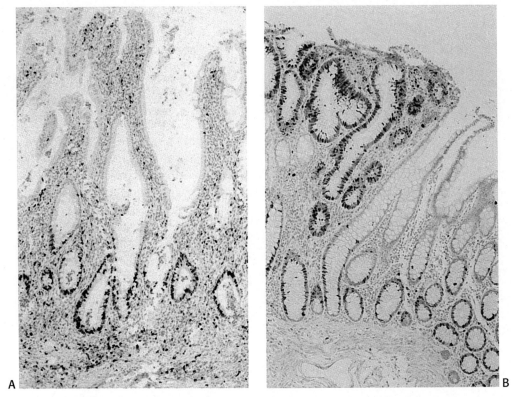

FIG. 14.61. Proliferation in normal and regenerative colonic mucosa versus adenomas. **A:** Ki-67 immuno-stain using the monoclonal antibody MIB-1. This section was taken from an area of active mucosal regeneration in a patient with inflammatory bowel disease. Large numbers of proliferating cells are identifiable in the regenerating crypts. Note the restriction of the proliferative zone to the base of the glands. **B:** In adenomas, cell proliferation is dysregulated, and the proliferating cells appear in the superficial portion of the mucosa. The normal pattern of proliferation in the basal crypts is present in the adjacent nonneoplastic mucosa (*right*). Note that fewer proliferating cells are present in this area than in A.

in terms of the depth of its invasion, involvement of the stalk or cautery margin, the presence or absence of lymphatic and vascular involvement, and the degree of differentiation. It is also sometimes helpful to estimate the volume of adenoma replaced by the carcinoma.

Treatment

Most experienced endoscopists recommend complete removal of polyps and their submission for histologic analysis (203,218). Small polyps may be either hyperplastic polyps or adenomas, and the size of a polyp does not predict its histologic features (205). It is important to note, however, that even small polyps may have advanced histologic features and, therefore, should be carefully examined histologically. Larger polyps may be removed with cautery snare, while small sessile polyps may be biopsied and ablated with hot biopsy forceps, laser ablation, or photodynamic therapy. Pedunculated polyps and sessile polyps with small mucosal attachment areas can be completely removed. However, endoscopic excision may not be possible when the lesion lies in an inaccessible site or if the polyp measures more than 2 cm in diameter and is sessile, especially if it has a broad attachment area to the

colonic wall. Large sessile lesions usually undergo multiple forceps biopsies to determine if they contain a carcinoma. Incompletely removed, wide-based, sessile polyps may require endoscopic mucosal resection to remove the remaining neoplasm. If complete endoscopic resection cannot be performed, surgical resection may be required. Following complete removal of a pedunculated adenoma containing an invasive cancer, most endoscopists perform a colonoscopy 2 to 6 months and 1 year later before reverting to a general follow-up scheme (252). The endoscopist may sometimes place a tattoo at the polypectomy site in order to identify it later (Fig. 14.68). Guidelines for clinical follow-up of patients with adenomas are summarized in Table 14.12.

ABERRANT CRYPT FOCI

Aberrant crypt foci (ACF) constitute putative preneoplastic lesions originally described in experimental animal models of colorectal cancer (253–255). ACF have been proposed as intermediate biomarkers in carcinogenesis studies (253–257). Their detection involves examining colons cleaned with Krebs-Ringers solution. The colons are cut open along their

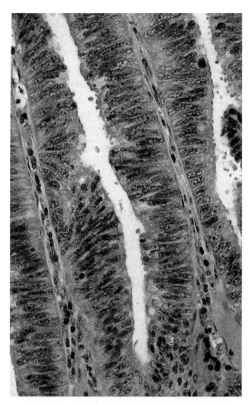

FIG. 14.62. High-grade dysplasia is characterized by increased nuclear:cytoplasmic ratios, nuclear irregularity, and true nuclear stratification.

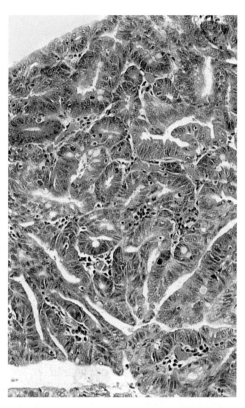

FIG. 14.63. In intramucosal carcinoma, cells extend through the basement membrane into the lamina propria. Often the glands develop a cribriform or back-to-back architecture.

longitudinal axis, fixed flat in buffered formalin, and then placed in a Krebs-Ringers solution containing 0.2% methylene blue for approximately 30 minutes. This preparation is then placed on a glass slide, mucosal side up, and examined under a light microscope at a magnification of 40× with transillumination (253). ACF consist of clusters of abnormally large, darkly staining, slightly elevated mucosal crypts (Fig. 14.69).

ACF vary from single altered glands to plaques of 412 abnormal crypts/focus (258). Aberrant crypts are three times larger in diameter than normal crypts and have oval or slit-shaped lumina rather than the usual circular lumina of the normal mucosa. They are slightly elevated above the mucosal

surface when viewed microscopically (258). They consist of histologically diverse lesions.

The mean proportion of the altered colonic mucosa and the number of foci with aberrant crypts/cm² colonic mucosa is higher in patients with colon cancer than in patients without colon cancer or predisposing conditions and is highest in patients with polyposis syndromes (256,258–260). ACF from patients with FAP appear dysplastic (256), whereas those from patients with colon cancer range from almost normal to hyperplastic to dysplastic. ACF may play a role in the early steps of human colon cancer development, particularly since dysplasia is often present.

TABLE 14.12 Guidelines for Colonoscopic Surveillance after Polypectomy

Colonoscopic and Pathologic Findings	Recommended Interval to Next Colonoscopy
Small, rectal, hyperplastic polyps	10 years
	Other interval determined by patient's colorectal cancer risk
1–2 low-risk adenomas[a]	5–10 years
3–10 low risk adenomas	3 years
Any high-risk adenoma[b]	3 years
>10 adenomas	<3 years
Inadequately removed adenomas	2–6 months

[a]Low grade dysplasia
[b]High grade dysplasia

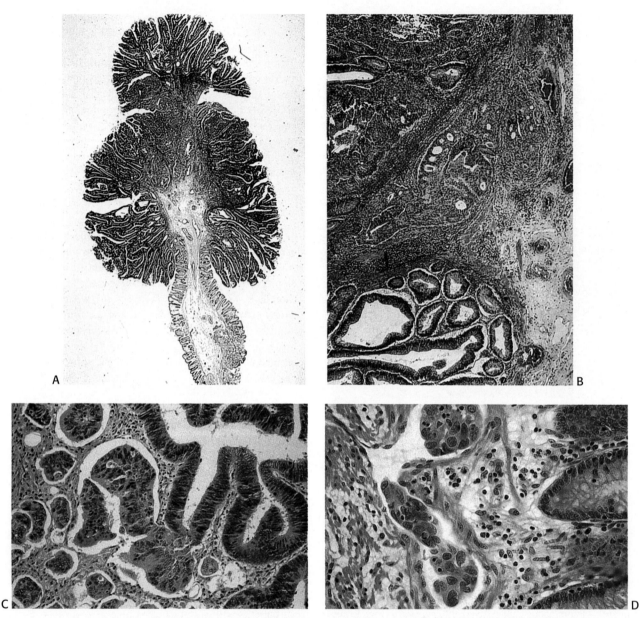

FIG. 14.64. Carcinoma arising in the head of a polyp that was later shown to have metastasized. **A:** Polypectomy specimen demonstrating the presence of an adenomatous polyp. A small area of carcinoma is present within the lesion and invades only the superficial portion of the submucosa of the head of the polyp. **B:** High-power magnification demonstrating the tumor invading the submucosa. **C:** There are well-differentiated and poorly differentiated glands. **D:** Tumor cells are present in the lymphatics of the polyp stalk.

SERRATED POLYPS

Serrated Adenomas

Serrated adenomas constitute 1% to 2% of colorectal adenomas (261,262). Patients range in age from 15 to 88 years, with a mean of 63 years. The serrated adenomas are distributed throughout the colorectum but with a predisposition of larger lesions (measuring >1 cm) to involve the right colon. They occur as single or multiple lesions. Multiple lesions may form part of a polyposis syndrome (see Chapter 12). The adenomas may be pedunculated or sessile. Serrated ade-

nomas lack any gross features that allow their distinction from ordinary adenomas.

Histologic examination at low magnification discloses a pattern of serrated glands lining the crypts, producing a pattern reminiscent of the glands in hyperplastic polyps (Fig. 14.70). However, the stratified cells lining the glands appear less mature than those found in hyperplastic polyps, and they are dysplastic (Figs. 14.70 to 14.72). Serrated adenomas are distinguished by the presence of goblet cell immaturity, upper zone and surface mitoses, and prominent nucleoli. Monotonous, mucin-depleted, often eosinophilic

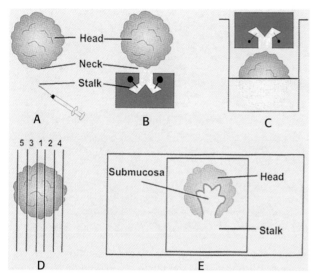

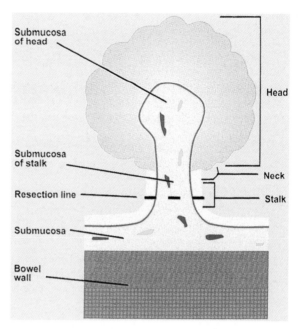

FIG. 14.65. Diagram of the handling of a polypectomy specimen in the laboratory. **A:** The base of the polyp is indicated by the endoscopist, who places a needle into the cut portion of the stalk. **B:** The polyp is pinned to a corkboard and allowed to fix while inverted in formalin **(C). D:** The fixed polyp is serially sectioned and processed for histologic evaluation **(E).**

FIG. 14.66. Landmarks of adenomas.

cells exhibiting nuclear pseudostratification and occasional loss of the polarity line the glands (Fig. 14.71). However, some serrated adenomas contain significant amounts of mucin. Nuclear:cytoplasmic ratios are greater in serrated adenomas than in hyperplastic polyps but slightly less than those seen in traditional adenomas. As the cells become increasingly atypical, they lose their stratification and the nuclei become rounder, more pleomorphic, and large. Additionally, glandular crowding and luminal budding begin to appear (Fig. 14.72). The surfaces of serrated adenomas, particularly those that are sessile, may show papillary tufting. The collagen table underlying the free surface is not as thickened as in hyperplastic polyps and is thinner than that seen

in the normal mucosa, resembling more the collagen table of adenomas (234).

Serrated adenomas often contain foci of high-grade dysplasia, and in one study, 11% contained areas of intramucosal carcinoma (261). Carcinomas can also develop within serrated adenomas (169,261) (Fig 14.73).

Sessile Serrated Polyps

Torlakovic and Snover recognized in 1996 that the "hyperplastic polyps" seen in association with hyperplastic polyposis differed morphologically from traditional hyperplastic polyps (263). In addition, Goldstein et al (264) found similar

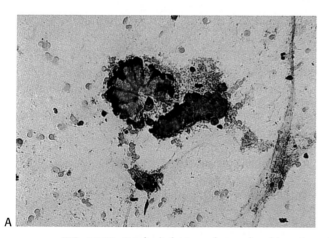

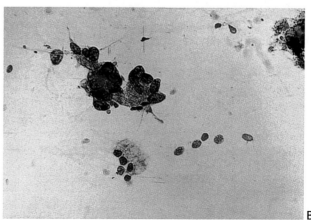

FIG. 14.67. Cytologic features from a brushing of a colonic polyp. **A:** Normal colonic cells are present along with atypical (adenomatous) cells. **B:** Malignant cells retrieved from a brushing specimen of the polyp.

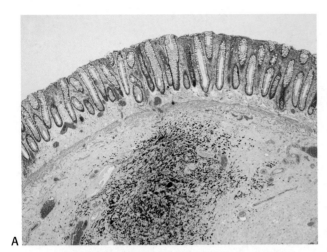

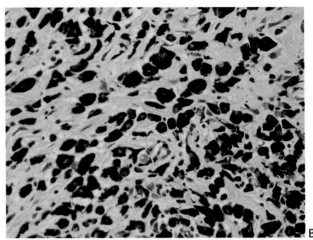

FIG. 14.68. Submucosal tattoo. **A:** Endoscopic mucosal resection of a previous polypectomy site. A submucosal collection of histiocytes containing black pigment is present. This represents the tattoo site placed by the endoscopist at the time of the initial polypectomy. **B:** Higher-power view showing histiocytes containing granular black India ink pigment.

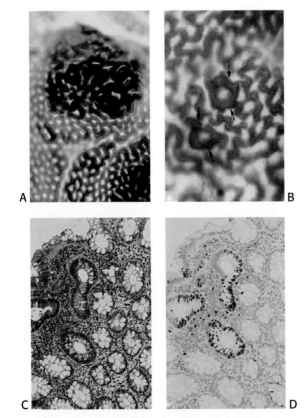

FIG. 14.69. Aberrant crypt foci. **A:** Methylene blue staining of the colonic mucosa from a patient with familial polyposis reveals foci of dark staining representing aberrant crypt foci. **B:** Smaller aberrant crypt focus (*arrows*) consisting of two or three abnormally staining glands. **C:** Histologic section of an aberrant crypt focus identified by methylene blue staining. The glands in this case appear adenomatous. **D:** Ki-67 immunostaining of the section shown in C demonstrates abnormal proliferation in the aberrant crypts.

features among serrated polyps that preceded the development of microsatellite instability (MSI)-positive colon cancers. The morphologic criteria for these so-called sessile serrated polyps are summarized in Table 14.13.

These sessile serrated polyps make up approximately 2% of all polyps removed colonoscopically, and may account for as much as 8% of polyps that would have previously been characterized as hyperplastic polyps (262). Sessile serrated polyps have a tendency to be right sided, large (>1 cm), sessile, and endoscopically poorly circumscribed, sometimes mimicking enlarged folds (262–264). It is important to note, however, that similar polyps may be found on the left side of the colon, and should be still be diagnosed as sessile serrated polyps. We prefer the term *sessile serrated polyp* over the

TABLE 14.13 Major Histologic Features of Sessile Serrated Polyps

Abnormal proliferation/dysmaturation
    Nuclear atypia in middle/upper crypts
    Oval nuclei in middle crypts
    Prominent nucleoli in middle/superficial crypts
    Dystrophic goblet cells
    Irregular distribution of goblet cells
    Mitoses in middle/upper crypts
Architectural abnormalities
    Basal crypt dilation
    Horizontal orientation of deep crypts
    Prominent serrations
    Serration to base of crypt
    Inverted crypts
Other features
    Lack of thickened basement membrane
    Focal loss of hMLH1 positivity

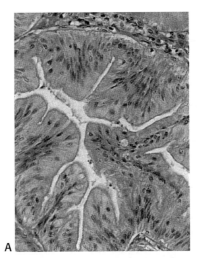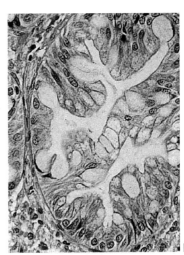

FIG. 14.70. Hyperplastic polyp versus serrated adenoma. Although the glandular architectures of hyperplastic polyps and serrated adenomas are similar, there are distinct cytologic differences between the two. **A:** Serrated adenomas are composed of less mature cells with elongated, hyperchromatic nuclei resembling those found in adenomas. **B:** The cells of hyperplastic polyps are mature, with small, round, basally arranged nuclei.

other terms commonly used in the literature (*sessile serrated adenoma, giant hyperplastic polyp*) because it reflects the fact that these lesions lack the traditional-type dysplasia seen in other adenomas of the colon, including serrated adenoma.

Histologically, sessile serrated polyps differ from hyperplastic polyps in that they demonstrate exaggerated serration of the crypts, with the serrated epithelium extending all the way into the crypt base. This deep serration is often accompanied by gland dilation and a peculiar form of crypt branching that imparts a bootlike appearance to the colonic gland (Fig. 14.74). In contrast, in hyperplastic polyps, crypt serration is usually confined to the superficial one half of the gland, and the basal crypt is straight and tubular, like that seen in normal colon. Sessile serrated polyps also demonstrate an abnormal pattern of proliferation with extension of mitotic figures into the mid- and upper crypts (Fig. 14.75). These polyps also show more cytologic atypia than is usually seen in hyperplastic polyps, especially in the upper regions of the crypts. In sessile serrated polyps, the nuclei present in the upper crypt are mildly enlarged and vesicular and may contain prominent nucleoli (Fig. 14.76). In contrast, nuclei in the upper crypts of hyperplastic polyps appear "hypermature" with small, basally located nuclei and inconspicuous nucleoli (Fig. 14.77).

Some polyps contain coexisting serrated and adenomatous epithelium. Such lesions likely represent pre-existing sessile serrated polyps in which superimposed adenomatous changes have developed. Histologically, mixed serrated–adenomatous polyps consist of discrete areas of traditional adenomatous epithelium that may be tubular, tubulovillous, or villous, although most commonly it is tubulovillous, lying adjacent to, or intermingled with, areas of serrated polyp. These lesions differ from true serrated adenomas in that the adenomatous areas have the traditional appearance with straight or tubular lumens, contrasting with the serrated lumens seen in serrated adenomas. Additionally, the adenomatous epithelium appears more basophilic than many of the epithelial cells lining serrated adenomas. Occasionally, however, these polyps may contain an admixture of sessile serrated polyp, serrated adenoma, and traditional adenoma (Fig 14.78).

Molecular Evidence for the "Serrated Pathway" of Colorectal Cancer

Triggered by morphologic observations, molecular studies now provide convincing evidence that a pathway from serrated polyps (sessile serrated polyp and serrated adenoma) to colorectal carcinoma exists. Studies examining molecular alterations in serrated adenomas demonstrated different genetic alterations than those traditionally seen in the adenoma–carcinoma sequence (265–268). For example, *APC, KRAS,* and *TP53* mutation and loss of heterozygosity are uncommon, chromosomal instability is absent, and immunostaining for the Wnt pathway transcriptional activator β-catenin shows a normal membranous distribution consistent with the presence of wild-type *APC* and *CTNNB1* genes. Eventually, studies began to demonstrate a set of changes in serrated adenomas that were also present in sessile serrated polyps and a subset of colorectal cancers. These changes include mutations of *BRAF* (269–271), microsatellite instability (272–274) mutation of *TGF-β RII* (273), loss of expression of the DNA repair genes *MGMT* (O-6-methylguanine-DNA methyltransferase) (267,275) and *MLH1*, and widespread DNA methylation abnormalities (271,273). The reasons for the variations in genetic signatures are that serrated adenomas are not homogeneous lesions, pathologists have different diagnostic thresholds for serrated adenoma/sessile serrated polyp, and types of serrated adenoma may differ according to anatomic region in the colon or the population under study.

Natural History of Serrated Polyps and Clinical Implications

Knowledge of the true frequency of hyperplastic polyps, serrated adenomas, and sessile serrated polyps is important because it will allow estimation of the true rate of malignant conversion of these lesions. In one study, residual serrated polyp was observed adjacent to 5.8% of colorectal carcinomas (276). This is probably an underestimate of the true incidence

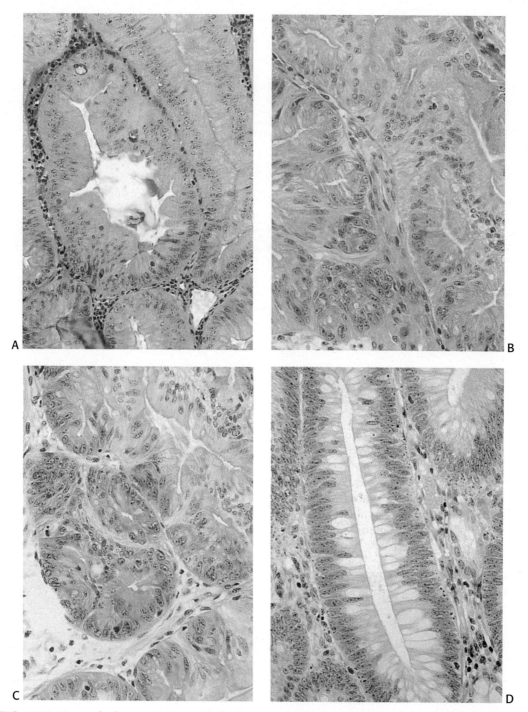

FIG. 14.71. Serrated adenoma. **A:** Serrated adenomas are lined by eosinophilic, mucin-depleted cells. There is minimal nuclear stratification. **B:** The cells have a higher nuclear:cytoplasmic ratio and demonstrate more nuclear atypia and loss of polarity than seen in hyperplastic polyps. **C:** Another serrated adenoma demonstrating loss of nuclear polarity and mild atypia. **D:** Tubular adenomas demonstrate a greater degree of nuclear crowding than occurs in serrated adenomas. In addition, the nuclei are larger and more elongated.

of colorectal cancer originating in serrated polyps because most tumors outgrow and destroy the precursor lesion, or because superimposed adenomatous changes obscure the original serrated nature of the polyp. Some studies suggest that as many as 20% of colorectal cancers demonstrate wide-

spread defects in DNA methylation (so-called CIMP positive), and that many (if not all) of these may arise within serrated polyps (277). Combining the various types of serrated polyp with malignant potential, it is likely that the rate of conversion to malignancy would be at least as great as for adenomas.

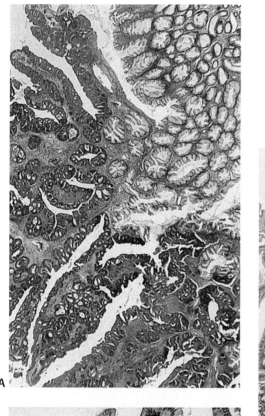

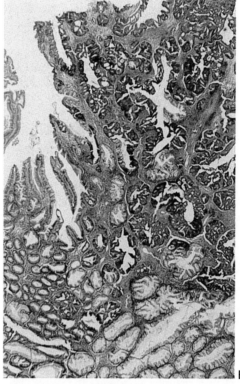

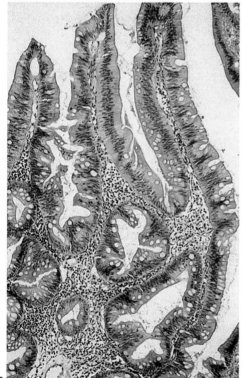

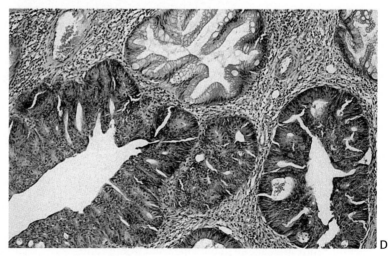

FIG. 14.72. Serrated adenoma containing high-grade dysplasia. **A:** At low power, a sharp line of demarcation is identifiable between the typical serrated adenoma (*upper right*) and the serrated adenoma with high-grade dysplasia (*lower left*). **B:** The glands containing high-grade dysplasia appear hyperchromatic compared to those without dysplasia. **C:** Higher-power view of the serrated adenoma in an area lacking high-grade dysplasia. The cells demonstrate eosinophilic cytoplasm and slightly crowded nuclei. There is little stratification of the cells. **D:** Higher magnification in an area with high-grade dysplasia. The dysplastic glands demonstrate prominent nuclear stratification and a greater degree of crowding than is seen in the nondysplastic gland in the upper portion of the photograph. The nuclear:cytoplasmic ratio is high, and glandular budding is seen.

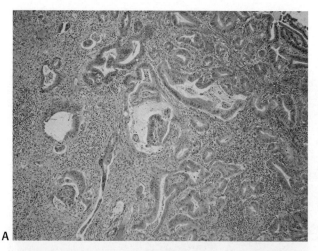

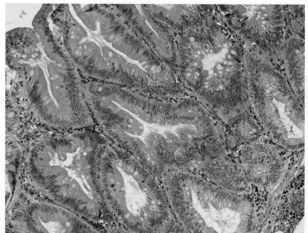

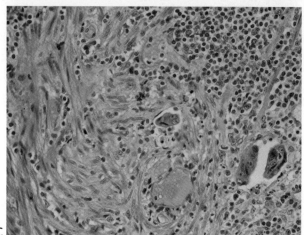

FIG. 14.73. Carcinoma arising in a serrated adenoma. **A:** Invasive adenocarcinoma extends into the submucosa of this polyp. The glands are angulated, and are focally surrounded by a desmoplastic stroma. **B:** The overlying epithelium shows features of a serrated adenoma. **C:** A focus of lymphatic invasion is present.

Any serrated lesion 1 cm or more in greatest dimension should probably be followed in a manner analogous to that for traditional adenomas. Such lesions require follow-up to ensure that they were completely excised at the time of colonoscopy. The interval for follow-up of these lesions is unknown at the present time, but repeat colonoscopy every 2 to 5 years is probably reasonable (278).

ADENOCARCINOMA

Incidence and Death Rates

The highest incidence rates for colon cancer occur in North America, Australia, and New Zealand, as discussed previously in this chapter. The risk for colorectal cancer rises significantly after age 40 in both men and women and doubles in each succeeding decade until age 75 (279). From 2000 to 2004, the median age at diagnosis for cancer of the colon and rectum was 71 years of age (2).

Approximately 1% were diagnosed between 20 and 34 years of age, 3.6% between 35 and 44, 11.1% between 45 and 54, 17.8% between 55 and 64, 25.7% between 65 and

74, 28.6% between 75 and 84, and 12.2% after 85 years of age. The incidence of a second primary colorectal malignancy increases in patients with one or more colorectal cancers (280). An increased colorectal cancer risk exists in the conditions listed in Table 14.14.

TABLE 14.14   Individuals at High Risk of Developing Colorectal Carcinoma

Patients with present or past colorectal adenoma
Patients with previous colorectal carcinomas
Patients in families with hereditary nonpolyposis colon cancer
Patients with a family history of colon cancer
Patients with familial adenomatous polyposis syndromes:
    Familial polyposis coli
    Gardner syndrome
    Oldfield syndrome
    Turcot syndrome
    Zanca syndrome
    Peutz-Jeghers syndrome
    Juvenile polyposis
Patients with ulcerative colitis
Patients with Crohn disease
Patients with some forms of infectious colitis

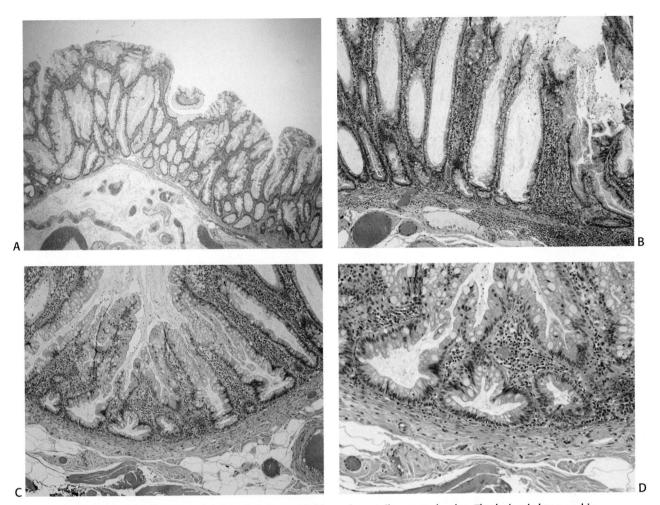

FIG. 14.74. Sessile serrated polyp. **A:** Low-power view of a sessile serrated polyp. The lesion is large and is composed of crypts with exaggerated serration and dilation. **B:** Another sessile serrated polyp with prominent crypt dilation. **C:** The bases of many of the crypts are branched, or bend at right angles in an orientation parallel to the muscularis mucosae. **D:** Higher power showing the configuration of the bases of the crypts.

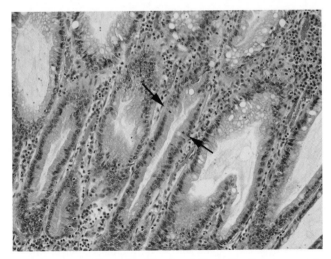

FIG. 14.75. Sessile serrated polyp. Mitotic figures are seen in the mid- to upper portion of the crypts (*arrows*). In the normal colonic glands mitotic figures are confined to the lower third of the crypt.

Family history is important in assessing colorectal cancer risk, especially in patients younger than 50 years of age. Genetic factors play a significant role in at least 20% of patients with colorectal cancer. Approximately 1% of the total cancer burden is contributed by FAP, 5% is associated with HNPCC, and 15% is contributed by other forms of familial cancer. HNPCC patients have an excess of proximal colonic cancers, while patients with FAP have predominantly left-sided cancers. FAP and HNPCC are discussed more extensively in Chapter 12.

Differences in the death rates from colorectal cancer relate to differences in socioeconomic factors, diet, population longevity, genetic factors, and the quality of available medical care (169). In the United States, death from colorectal carcinoma is uncommon before age 30 in the general population, but rises significantly after age 50. The overall 5-year relative survival rate for 1996–2003 from 17 SEER geographic areas was 64%. Five-year relative survival rates by race and sex were 64.9% for white

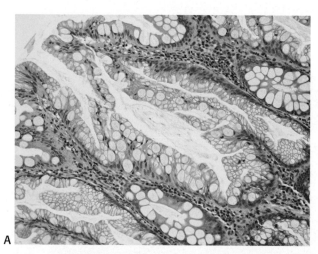

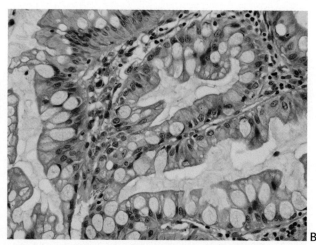

FIG. 14.76. Sessile serrated polyp. A: The upper portions of the crypts are lined by cells with enlarged nuclei compared with the normal epithelium. Dystrophic goblet cells are also present. **B:** Higher-power view showing the enlarged but uniform nuclei.

men, 64.9% for white women, 55.2% for black men, and 54.7% for black women (2). Colorectal cancer is declining in incidence and it is being detected at earlier stages of disease, leading to increased survival and decreased mortality rates.

Sexual Differences

In North America and Australia (areas with high rates of colorectal cancer) and in Japan and Italy (countries with rapidly rising rates), the age-adjusted incidence of colorectal cancer

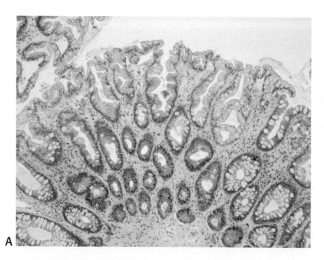

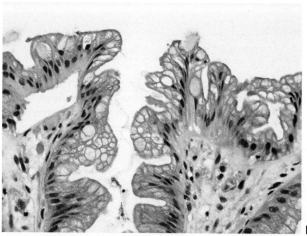

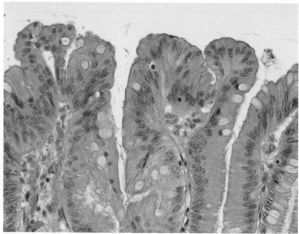

FIG. 14.77. Hyperplastic polyp. A: Low-power view of a hyperplastic polyp. The superficial portion of the crypts appears serrated, but the bases are straight and tubular. No dilation of the glands is present. **B:** Higher magnification of the superficial crypt epithelium of a hyperplastic polyp. The nuclei are small and hyperchromatic. **C:** Superficial crypt in a sessile serrated polyp taken at the same magnification as B. The nuclei are larger than those of the hyperplastic polyp, and the chromatin is less dense.

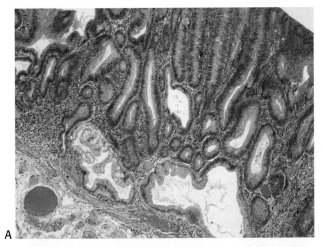

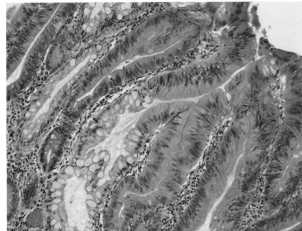

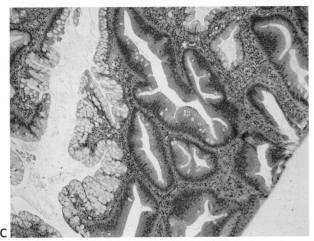

FIG. 14.78. Sessile serrated polyp with superimposed adenomatous change. **A:** The residual dilated and serrated crypts of a sessile serrated polyp are seen in the deep mucosa. The superficial portions of the colonic crypts have been replaced by adenomatous epithelium. **B:** Cells resembling those of a serrated adenoma are seen displacing the epithelium of a typical sessile serrated polyp. **C:** Sessile serrated polyp and serrated adenoma admixed in the same polyp.

for men exceeds that for women. Women have higher rates of right-sided neoplasms and develop their cancers at an earlier age than men (281,282). Men exhibit a decline in the proportion of sigmoid cancers with an increase in transverse and descending colon cancer as they age. In some regions of the world, such as Southern Asia, rectal cancers occur more commonly in males, whereas colonic carcinomas affect both sexes equally (283).

Racial Differences

In the United States, the highest colon cancer risk affects blacks, followed by whites. Intermediate levels exist in persons of Asian or Pacific Island descent. The lowest colorectal cancer risk is observed in Hispanics and Native Americans (2). A statistically significant percentage of black patients have proximally located lesions (284). Sixty percent of whites with colon cancers develop sigmoid cancer compared to 36.6% of blacks. Of all colonic cancers in blacks, 35% develop in the right colon, versus 24% in whites (284–286). The implication of this finding is that screening sigmoidoscopy may miss a significant proportion of colonic adenomas or carcinomas in black populations.

Location

Colon cancer risk varies by subsite within the colon (279). The location of colorectal carcinomas reflects screening practices, environmental and genetic factors, sexual and racial differences, and patient age. In low-risk countries, carcinomas of the cecum and ascending colon occur more frequently than carcinomas of the left colon, whereas in high-risk countries, colorectal carcinomas more commonly arise in the rectosigmoid region (169), a distribution similar to that seen in the United States (287). Right-sided colon carcinomas increase in incidence as patients age, particularly in women, with a progressive decline in the incidence of sigmoid and rectal lesions (285,288,289).

Colorectal carcinomas may also develop rarely in J-pouch reservoirs following low anterior resections (290) or in intestinal tissue transplanted into other sites, such as in neovaginas (291) or into the bladder as a bladder extender.

Multiple Tumors

Patients with colorectal cancer have a predisposition for developing more than one colorectal neoplasm, including both adenomas and carcinomas. In fact, the large bowel is the organ most frequently involved by multiple primary malignant tumors (291–296). Patients with multiple tumors also have a greater chance of developing carcinoma in other organs of the body (293). Not surprisingly, such patients often have one of the hereditary forms of colon cancer. Multiple tumors occur commonly in patients with polyposis syndromes, HNPCC (see Chapter 12), and chronic IBD (see Chapter 11).

Multiple neoplasms may be synchronous (Fig. 14.79) or metachronous. Synchronous cancers are twice as frequent as metachronous ones (293,295). Synchronous neoplasms affect 35.9% of patients; 25.7% of the lesions are adenomas (294). The incidence rates of synchronous colorectal cancers range from 1.5% to 12% (292–296). Synchronous cancers often remain confined to the same region of the bowel, probably having arisen from clustered adenomas. However, since synchronous carcinomas can also be widely separated, a complete colonoscopy must be performed in every patient with colon cancer to search for additional tumors in other intestinal segments.

Metachronous tumors occur in 1.6% of patients with colorectal cancer (297). Patients with metachronous tumors tend to be somewhat younger when they originally present than patients with only single colon cancers; patients with synchronous lesions tend to be somewhat older (298). The incidence of metachronous tumors increases as the follow-up increases. Several large series, with prolonged follow-up, have reported intervals of 8.5 to 11 years between the development of the initial tumor and the subsequent development of a metachronous lesion (292,299,300). Up to 64% of patients have their second tumor discovered within 5 years of the first tumor, 45% within 3 years, and 20% within 1 year. The cumulative risk of a colon cancer survivor developing a metachronous growth increases from 3.5% after the resection of one cancer to 8% after the removal of two (299).

Clinical Features

Since colorectal carcinoma develops over a long period of time, it is not surprising that symptoms may be absent or are so slowly progressive that the patient fails to notice them. Thus, the patient may present with relatively minimal symptoms when diagnosed. From 5% to 12.5% of patients may remain asymptomatic (301,302). The clinical presentation depends on whether the tumors develop in the right or left colon and whether they are early or advanced (Fig. 14.80). Initial symptoms of colon carcinoma are usually vague and nonspecific. The symptoms and signs may relate directly to the gastrointestinal tract, or they may be constitutional in nature. Weight loss and malaise commonly occur, but these symptoms are often disregarded by the patient due to their nonspecificity. Cancers of the cecum and ascending colon are often flat or polypoid, and the stool is soft in this location. As a result, right-sided lesions often remain clinically "silent" because they fail to cause obstruction or visible melena. Weakness, malaise, fatigue, and weight loss in such patients may occur secondary to iron deficiency anemia. Cardiac failure or angina pectoris may be presenting symptoms in anemic patients.

Changes in bowel habits affect 22% to 58% of patients with colorectal carcinoma (302,303) and occur most frequently when the neoplasm arises in the left colon. The changes are often minimal, but progressive, and include diarrhea and a sensation of incomplete rectal emptying or incontinence. As the tumor grows and progressively encircles the bowel wall, the stool caliber decreases and constipation, obstipation, and other signs of bowel obstruction appear.

Rectal bleeding is the initial complaint in approximately 50% of patients (303). This nonspecific symptom can present as subtle degrees of bleeding, which may not be visible and are only manifested by the presence of an iron deficiency anemia. Frank hematochezia sometimes

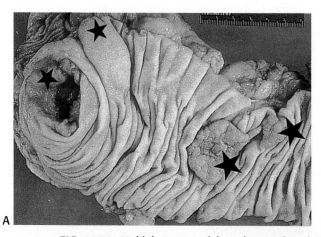
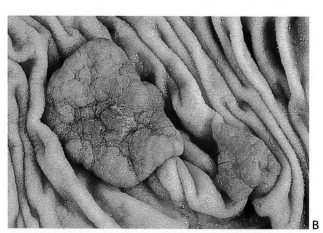

FIG. 14.79. Multiple tumors of the colon. A: Three lesions are present and two are indicated by *stars*. In the smallest lesion, the star is placed to the side of the lesion so as not to obliterate it. One of the lesions completely surrounds the ileocecal valve. **B:** Two of the lesions are seen at higher power. The larger one contains invasive carcinoma.

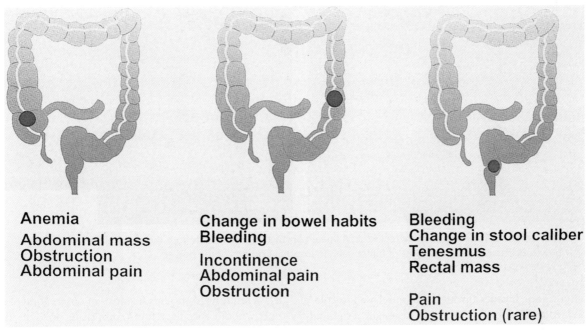

Anemia
Abdominal mass
Obstruction
Abdominal pain

Change in bowel habits
Bleeding

Incontinence
Abdominal pain
Obstruction

Bleeding
Change in stool caliber
Tenesmus
Rectal mass

Pain
Obstruction (rare)

FIG. 14.80. The clinical symptoms that develop in patients with colon cancer depend on location of the tumor. Early symptoms are shown in *black*, and late symptoms are shown in *blue*.

develops. Rectal bleeding develops in about 70% of left-sided lesions, but often goes unnoticed by the patient. Fewer than 25% of patients with right-sided tumors notice any blood in the stools, probably because the blood becomes admixed with the feces. In a prospective study of patients presenting to general practitioners with a complaint of rectal bleeding, 10.3% of these patients had a colon cancer (304).

The issue of rectal bleeding is complicated these days by the use of NSAIDs, either to treat arthritic conditions or as prophylaxis for cardiovascular disease. These drugs are well known to cause intestinal bleeding. Rectal bleeding should never be attributed to NSAIDs, hemorrhoids, or rectal fissures, especially in older individuals, unless a malignancy has been ruled out. Some low-lying lesions are easily felt by a rectal examination (Fig. 14.81).

Abdominal pain is the presenting complaint in approximately 50% of patients with colon cancer. It is more likely to occur in patients with colon cancer rather than in those with rectal tumors (303). Pain often occurs in advanced colorectal cancer when the tumor invades the serosa (Fig. 14.82) or adjacent tissues. Occasionally, an obstructing, but not deeply penetrating, tumor may cause rupture of a diverticulum proximal to it. Lower abdominal pain is occasionally a symptom of cecal or ascending colonic lesions. Pain from left colonic lesions may result from varying degrees of bowel obstruction proximal to a constricting carcinoma (Fig. 14.83). Carcinomas at the ileocecal valve may mimic Crohn disease or cause appendicitis by obstructing the appendiceal lumen.

Approximately 20% of patients who present with colonic ischemia (so-called obstructive colitis) have a coexisting car-

cinoma causing the ischemia. Usually, the ischemic area develops proximal to the tumor and is separated from the tumor by a segment of normal-appearing colon. The tumor may also lie within the ischemic area (Fig. 14.84).

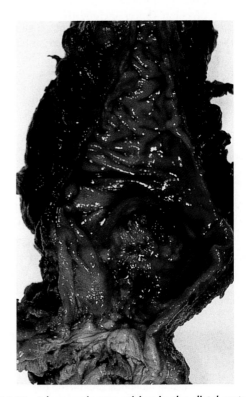

FIG. 14.81. Adenocarcinoma arising in the distal rectum just above the anal canal. This polypoid lesion was palpable on rectal examination.

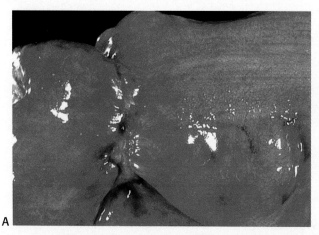
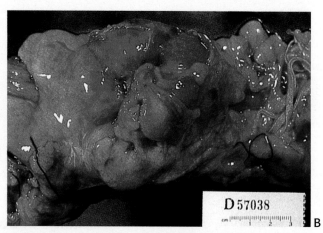

FIG. 14.82. Serosal aspect of the colon. **A:** A linear constricting lesion seen from the external surface of the bowel. **B:** There are large masses of tumor seen in external portions of the bowel.

When a tumor invades through the bowel wall, a colo-colo fistula may develop (Fig. 14.85). Occasionally, a sigmoid carcinoma presents as an acute bowel obstruction or acute perforation with peritonitis. Peritonitis results from perforation of the bowel by a deeply invasive tumor or tumor extension into a diverticulum. Patients may also present with small bowel obstruction, particularly when the small bowel becomes adherent to, or invaded by, a colonic cancer.

Uncommonly, an otherwise clinically silent advanced carcinoma, most often involving the cecum, presents as an abdominal mass or hepatomegaly due to metastases. Unusual presentations of colon cancer include the development of gluteal abscesses or colocutaneous fistulae, fevers of unknown origin, or pyogenic arthritis.

Delays in the diagnosis of symptomatic patients fall into three major categories: (a) delays in scheduling initial or subsequent office visits or laboratory tests resulting in an average delay of 3 weeks (31% of delays), (b) physician-related delays resulting from a misdiagnosis or observation of symptoms without specific action (comprising 46% of all diagnostic delays and resulting in an average delay of 18 weeks), and (c) patient-related delays resulting in an average delay of 12 weeks (305). Children with colon cancers are especially likely to undergo a delay in diagnosis due to the failure to recognize the possibility of this disorder, especially if a family history for colorectal cancer does not exist.

Colorectal Cancers Arising in Polyposis Syndromes

Cancers developing in the polyposis syndromes are discussed in Chapter 12.

Colorectal Cancers Arising in Inflammatory Bowel Disease

Carcinomas developing in the setting of IBD are discussed in Chapter 11.

Colon Cancer in Young Patients

Colon cancer develops in <1% of individuals in the first 2 decades of life (306,307). Colon cancer has been found in a fetus, but the youngest living patient was 9 months old at the time of diagnosis (308). Young patients with colon cancer are likely to have FAP, HNPCC, another hereditary cancer syndrome (see Chapter 12), or IBD (see Chapter 11). However, occasionally colorectal cancer also develops in young patients without any predisposing known cause (306).

Symptom duration ranges from days to months. Tumors arising in the cecum usually have a shorter period of symptom duration (306). The nonspecific signs and symptoms resemble ordinary childhood abdominal diseases, including acute appendicitis (309,310). Abdominal pain and vomiting are usually present, but distension and the presence of a mass and a change in bowel habits are rare. Weight loss occurs late

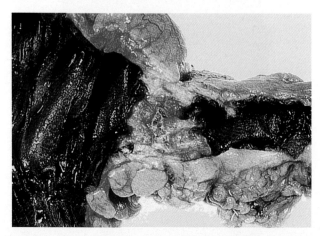

FIG. 14.83. Constricting adenocarcinoma of the colon. The proximal portion of the bowel is markedly dilated as a result of the obstruction produced by the tumor. In addition, the patient has melanosis coli.

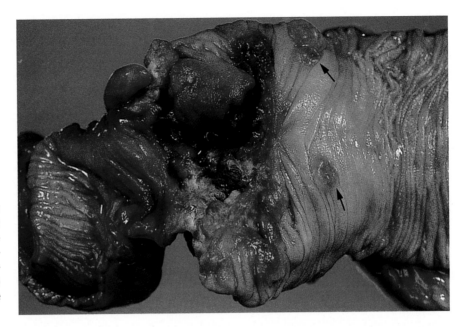

FIG. 14.84. Annular carcinoma with ischemia. The ischemic areas lie within and immediately adjacent to the carcinoma, and are identified by the presence of a greenish tan pseudomembrane. Several satellite lesions (*arrows*) stud the mucosal surface adjacent to the carcinoma.

in the disease. Anemia and visible evidence of bleeding almost exclusively associate with left-sided and rectal tumors (311).

It is common for young patients to experience a marked delay in their diagnosis due to their age. Therefore, they often have high-stage tumors at the time of diagnosis (306–308,312). The average delay between symptom onset and treatment is 6.5 months (313). Eighty-six percent of young patients have metastases at the time of diagnosis (314). Primary tumors arise throughout the large bowel. In one study, 25% of tumors involved the right colon, 24% the left colon, and 11% the rectum; 60% occurred in females (314). The predominant histologic type in children and adolescents is a poorly differentiated, mucin-producing carcinoma, contrasting with an incidence in adults of only 5% to 15% (309–312,315–318). A positive family history for colon cancer is present in 38% of patients.

Young patients appear to have a worse prognosis than their older counterparts, with 5-year survivals of 10% or less

(309,315,319). The median overall survival is 4 to 8 months in those diagnosed late in the disease, compared with 24 months in patients who are diagnosed earlier (306). The most significant factor associated with survival is stage at presentation (307,313,314,318). Survival is also affected by the histologic type of tumor, tumor resectability, extent of bowel wall invasion, and presence of lymph node capsular invasion (314), which is an especially sensitive marker for short-term survival (307,314). Common sites of recurrence involve the ovaries and the omentum (307).

Colorectal Cancer Arising During Pregnancy

Colorectal carcinomas developing during pregnancy are extremely rare, estimated to affect <0.002% of pregnant women (320). Most carcinomas arise in the rectum and rectosigmoid (321). Predisposing factors, including FAP or IBD, are often present in this younger age group. Common complaints include abdominal pain and distension, nausea, vomiting, constipation, and bleeding (321). A delay in diagnosis is a significant problem, since the symptoms are often attributed both by the patient and the physician to the pregnancy itself. Complications include intestinal obstruction, bowel perforation, cancer perforation, and obstruction to the descent of the fetus by the tumor. Extensive metastatic lesions are often present at the time of surgery. No patient with colorectal carcinoma diagnosed during pregnancy reported in the literature has survived for more than 5 years. Choice of therapy depends on the operability of the tumor and the age of the fetus at the time of diagnosis.

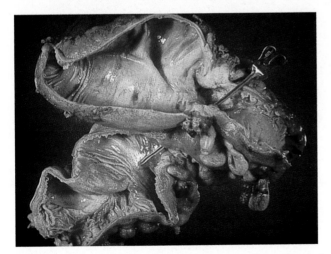

FIG. 14.85. Adenocarcinoma invading into an adjacent loop of large intestine and creating a colo-colo fistula.

Gross Features

Small carcinomas measuring 1 to 2 cm in diameter are usually red, granular, buttonlike lesions that are variably elevated

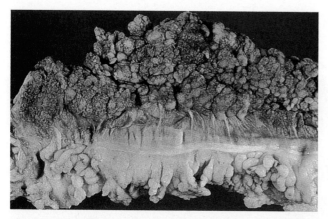

FIG. 14.86. Polypoid adenocarcinoma. A large exophytic tumor mass extends into the colonic lumen. The surface is lobular or papillary and demonstrates no evidence of ulceration.

above the tan mucosal surface. They are often sharply circumscribed, and grossly resemble adenomas (Fig. 14.79). Some are elevated only a few millimeters, whereas others are almost hemispherical in shape. Their consistency at this stage varies depending on the relative proportions of carcinoma, pre-existing adenoma, and the amount of coexisting stromal desmoplasia. As carcinoma replaces the adenoma, the tumor becomes firmer and paler (Fig. 14.79).

The gross appearance of colorectal carcinomas may be polypoid, fungating (exophytic), ulcerating, stenosing, or diffusely infiltrating. The polypoid type of carcinoma forms an exophytic intraluminal mass that has little in the way of surface ulceration (Fig. 14.86). It generally appears nodular,

lobular, or papillary, and often contains residual adenoma. Approximately two thirds of all tumors are ulcerating; one third appear fungating. Bulky, fungating cancers often arise in the cecum and ascending colon (Fig. 14.87). Fungating lesions are basically papillary lesions with more ulceration. The ulceration destroys the underlying papillary architecture, leaving residual exophytic components. This type of tumor often has a raised or rolled border, and residual adenoma may be present. It tends to grow into the lumen and to extend along one wall, especially in the spacious cecum. Although it may occupy a large proportion of the colonic lumen, it rarely causes obstruction. The central part of these lesions typically feels firm, corresponding to the area of carcinoma. If soft areas are present, particularly at the edges of the lesion, this usually represents residual adenoma. This type of tumor often remains asymptomatic until blood loss results in anemia. The intraluminal tumor mass often exceeds the intramural tumor in volume (Fig. 14.88).

Ulcerating carcinomas (Fig. 14.89) deeply invade into the colonic wall. The edge of an infiltrating carcinoma is only slightly elevated above the surrounding normal mucosa, or it may be completely flat. The diffusely infiltrative type of carcinoma infiltrates a segment of the intestinal wall, often in a circumferential fashion, without forming a nodular mass.

Adenocarcinomas arising in the transverse and descending colon usually become infiltrative and ulcerating, producing annular, constricting tumors (Fig. 14.90). They appear irregularly round, with raised, pale pink or white edges and central excavations (Fig. 14.83). They probably begin as locally infiltrative carcinomas that progressively encircle the bowel wall. These tumors obstruct the lumen and exhibit a

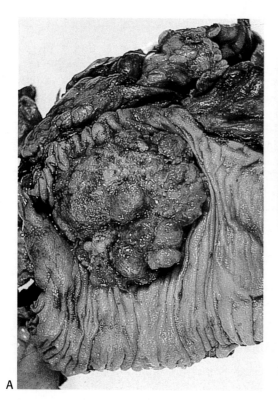

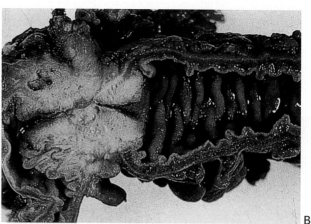

FIG. 14.87. Bulky carcinomas involving the cecum. **A:** A large exophytic lesion is present. **B:** The lesion almost completely blocks the cecum.

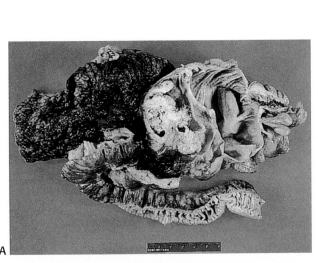

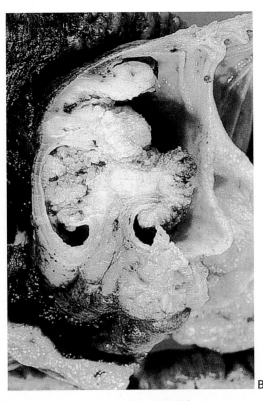

FIG. 14.88. Perforated adenocarcinoma of the colon. **A:** The entire colectomy specimen. **B:** Higher-power magnification showing the tumor itself.

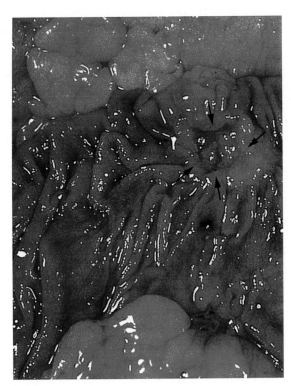

characteristic "apple core" or "napkin ring" appearance on barium contrast radiographs (Fig. 14.91). Except for their circumferential growth, their appearance resembles that of infiltrative carcinomas. Lateral intramural extension beyond the macroscopic border is unusual. The bowel usually dilates proximal to the tumor, with attenuation of the mucosal folds (Fig. 14.83). These tumors thicken the bowel wall and

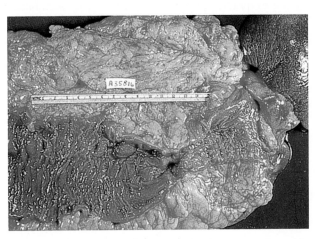

FIG. 14.89. Small ulcerative adenocarcinoma indicated by the *arrows.*

FIG. 14.90. Transverse colectomy and splenectomy. A napkin-ring lesion is present in the colon.

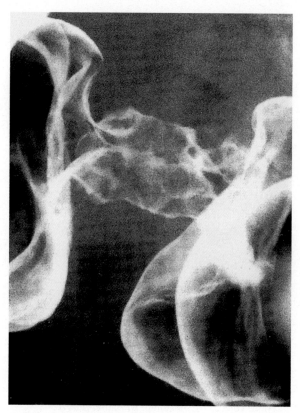

FIG. 14.91. Double-contrast enema demonstrates characteristic appearance of annular infiltrating adenocarcinoma.

obliterate the muscularis propria, a feature best seen on the cut surface (Figs. 14.92 and 14.93). The tumors are firm due to the desmoplastic stromal reaction they induce. The intramural tumor volume may be at least as great as the luminal portion. When the tumors extend completely through the bowel wall, they may involve contiguous structures such as the small intestine, another part of the colon, or the stomach. Central necrosis and ulceration of a transmural tumor may cause perforation and peritonitis (Fig. 14.88). Combined or atypical growth patterns are not unusual; part of a tumor may be exophytic and the rest relatively flat (Fig. 14.92). Multilobed tumors suggest that close synchronous carcinomas coalesced (Fig. 14.94).

Diffuse infiltrating colorectal carcinomas are uncommon, but when they are present, they convert the colon into a rigid tube. This pattern of involvement resembles gastric linitis plastica. A fourth pattern of growth is the recently recognized flat or superficial carcinoma, which arises from flat adenomas. These carcinomas often appear as a flat plaque on the mucosal surface with extensive intramural invasion.

Histologic Features

General Comments

Ninety to ninety-five percent of all large bowel tumors are ordinary adenocarcinomas (322). They are usually easily rec-

ognizable as moderately to well-differentiated, gland-forming adenocarcinomas (Fig. 14.95). Twenty-five percent are well differentiated, 60% are moderately differentiated, and 15% are poorly differentiated (322). Tall, malignant, columnar cells with a high mitotic rate line large, irregular glands (Fig. 14.95). Well-differentiated carcinomas may demonstrate intraglandular papillary infoldings. The cells show cytologic anaplasia, although one may encounter malignant tumors that are so well differentiated that it is impossible to render a diagnosis of malignancy, except for the presence of glands infiltrating the bowel wall (Fig. 14.96). Even early invasive cancers usually induce a strong desmoplastic response. This aids in the diagnosis of minimally invasive carcinomas (Figs. 14.59 and 14.97). However, there are some colorectal carcinomas that invade the bowel wall without inducing much of a desmoplastic response. Such tumors may cause a diagnostic problem, particularly if the patient has associated diverticulosis. In such cases, it may be impossible to tell whether the lesion is invasive or not. In many cases, there is no histologic difference between the superficial portion of the tumor and deeply invasive or metastatic tumor. In other cancers, the deeper tumor may differ histologically from the surface. Mucin production ranges from virtually none to tumors producing so much mucin that they are designated as mucinous carcinomas. Many exophytic carcinomas exhibit a papillary structure composed of histologically malignant cells. However, the infiltrating intramural component is usually less obviously papillary, exhibiting moderately to well-differentiated glandular structures (Fig. 14.95). Rare tumors have a prominent papillary component even in their invasive parts (Fig. 14.96).

Residual adenomatous mucosa may be present at the edge of a malignancy, especially in smaller tumors. The majority of small carcinomas associated with residual adenomas are well differentiated. Some small polypoid carcinomas lack residual adenoma. These are only superficially invasive and are designated as polypoid carcinomas (Fig. 14.98).

One may also see hyperplastic glands adjacent to neoplasms. The mucosa appears taller and more tortuous than normal, with an increase in the number of goblet cells. This is probably a reactive change that occurs in response to mucosal abnormalities and is termed *transitional mucosa*. This mucosa differs histochemically from the surrounding normal mucosa (323).

Occasional colorectal adenocarcinomas mimic urinary bladder villous adenomas. Distinguishing a primary bladder adenocarcinoma from spread of a colonic carcinoma to the bladder may be impossible without consideration of factors other than the histology (324). Asbestos workers who develop colonic carcinomas may show the presence of asbestos bodies within the colonic tissue as well as in the mesentery (68).

Colonic adenocarcinomas invade through the wall, either in an expanding or an infiltrative growth pattern. Approximately 75% of tumors have relatively well-circumscribed, advancing margins, but 25% are more diffusely infiltrative. The expanding pattern consists of

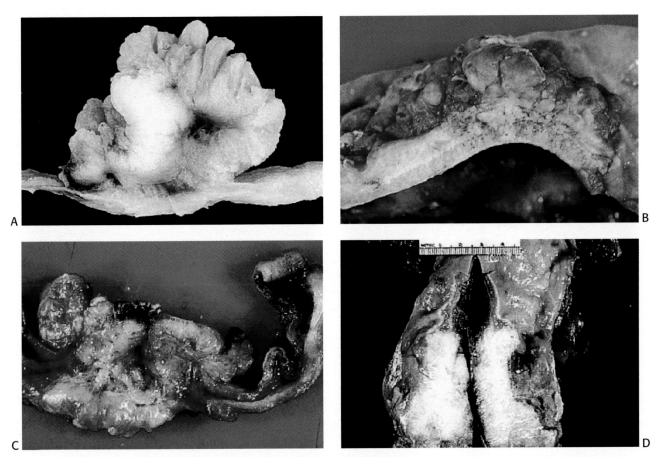

FIG. 14.92. Adenocarcinoma. **A:** Cut surface of the bowel demonstrating the presence of an invasive carcinoma that is arising in a villous adenoma. The carcinoma is recognizable by the presence of the dense white tissue. Residual villous fronds are also seen. **B:** Cross sections through a flat lesion demonstrating carcinoma penetrating the bowel wall. **C:** Invasive carcinoma extending into the omental fat. **D:** Fixed specimen. Tumor extends into the pericolic fat.

nodular aggregates of neoplastic glands. Infiltrative tumors consist of individual cells or small glands infiltrating through the wall. Infiltrative tumors generally lack an inflammatory response, whereas this reaction is present in the expanding lesions. Expanding carcinomas usually exhibit a polyploid or fungating growth pattern, whereas infiltrative carcinomas are usually ulcerative or diffusely infiltrative.

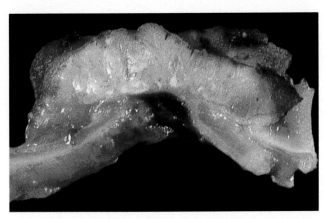

FIG. 14.93. Cut section through a colonic adenocarcinoma. The tumor obliterates the muscularis propria and invades to the serosal surface.

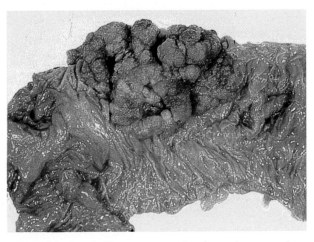

FIG. 14.94. Large bulky mass suggesting the coalescence of several lesions.

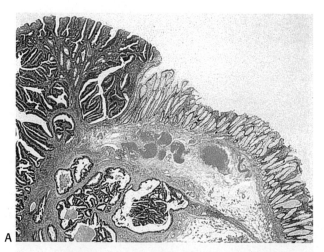
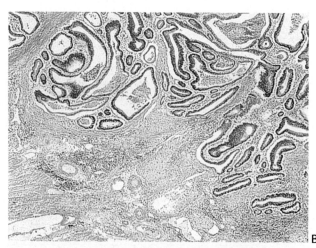

FIG. 14.95. Well-differentiated adenocarcinoma. **A:** A villous adenoma is seen at the surface. A well-differentiated adenocarcinoma invades the submucosa and extends under the normal mucosa. **B:** Higher-power magnification showing the well-differentiated glands and the invasive portion of the tumor.

Histologic Grading

Histologic grading is a routine practice in the pathologic reporting of large bowel cancer and is used as a prognostic indicator. Histologic grading is mainly gauged on a tumor's architectural features. Well-formed glands are present in >75% of the tumors that are well differentiated, in 25% to 75% of moderately differentiated tumors, and in <25% of poorly differentiated carcinomas. In well-differentiated carcinomas, well-formed glands are lined by cells that maintain their nuclear polarity (Fig. 14.95). The glands resemble those present in adenomas. Poorly differentiated tumors predominantly consist of solid tumors composed of cells showing a loss of nuclear polarity and considerable nuclear pleomorphism (Fig. 14.99). Moderately differentiated tumors fall in between these two extremes (Fig. 14.100). Occasionally, one portion of a tumor appears well differentiated while another

area is poorly differentiated (Fig. 14.101). The histologic grade is assigned according to the least differentiated area found, even though this may appear to be quantitatively insignificant. Tumor giant cells are sometimes present (Fig. 14.102). The cells in the solid areas may be completely anaplastic, or they may exhibit a signet ring morphology (Fig. 14.102).

Occasionally, one observes totally undifferentiated carcinomas that consist of large sheets of malignant cells. They contain abundant cytoplasm and minimal mucinous differentiation and, therefore, require further analysis to determine their epithelial nature. This can be confirmed by the use of immunostains for cytokeratin.

The agreement between the grade of a biopsy and corresponding resected tumor varies from 52% to 69%. Only 52% of poorly differentiated tumors are diagnosed as such in a preoperative biopsy. The poor predictive value is not improved by taking multiple biopsies (325). Thus, the grade

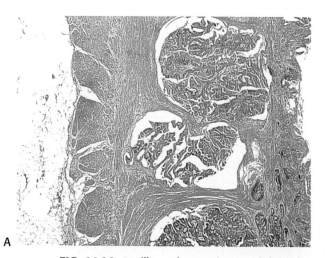
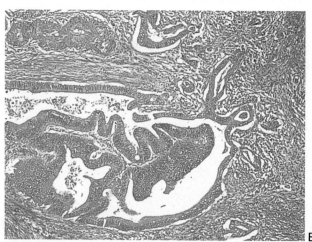

FIG. 14.96. Papillary adenocarcinoma of the colon. **A:** Low-power magnification demonstrating the presence of tumor extending into the muscularis propria. **B:** Higher-power magnification demonstrates the well-formed papillary structures.

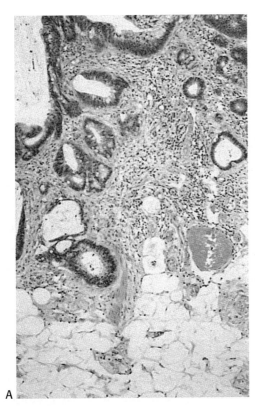
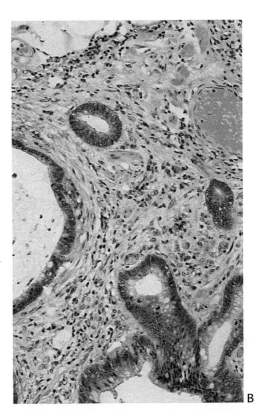

FIG. 14.97. Minimally invasive adenocarcinoma. **A:** Low-power photomicrograph demonstrating the presence of neoplastic glands in the superficial submucosa. **B:** On higher magnification, one can appreciate the desmoplastic stroma, which surrounds the invasive glands.

of colorectal carcinoma cannot be accurately assessed on a preoperative biopsy.

Cell Types in Carcinomas

A number of cell types are present in colorectal adenocarcinomas. These include variably differentiated enterocytes, goblet cells, Paneth cells, endocrine cells (Fig. 14.103), squamous cells, melanocytes, and trophoblastic cells. Multipotential

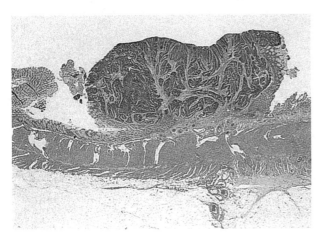

FIG. 14.98. Polypoid carcinoma. An exophytic tumor without residual adenoma of the epithelium is seen.

crypt stem cells can differentiate into these, and perhaps other cell types, thereby producing colorectal carcinomas that exhibit a number of distinctive histologic patterns. Some tumors are rich in Paneth cells, especially papillary carcinomas and mucinous tumors (326–328). The round, supranuclear granules of both normal and neoplastic Paneth cells stain red with hematoxylin and eosin stains. The Paneth cells lie interspersed singly or in small groups among the goblet cells. The Paneth cells are not mitotically active, but they do show obvious signs of neoplasia, including loss of polarity, cellular anaplasia, and an increased nuclear:cytoplasmic ratio. There is also marked variation in the number, shape, and electron density of Paneth cell granules. The presence of these cells has no impact on the biology of the tumor.

Neuroendocrine cells are present in 8% to 51% of colorectal carcinomas (329–332). The endocrine cells usually appear at the edges of glands and may have clear or granular eosinophilic cytoplasm, allowing their histologic recognition. Their presence can also be confirmed using special stains or immunostains. Some authors indicate that there is no prognostic significance of neuroendocrine differentiation in colorectal adenocarcinomas (327,328), but others do not share this view (332–336).

Stromal Components

The stroma of colorectal carcinomas has largely been ignored, but the recent introduction of peritumoral lymphocytic

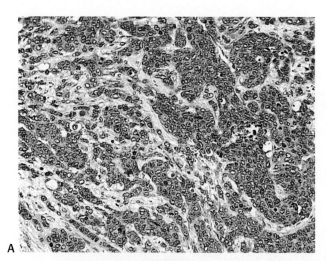
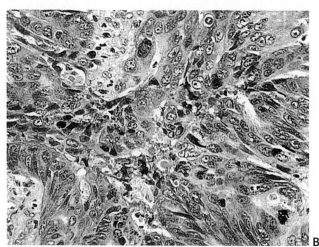

FIG. 14.99. Poorly differentiated adenocarcinoma. **A:** Irregular nests of tumor cells without obvious glandular differentiation. **B:** The cells are large and highly anaplastic.

infiltration into the Jass (337) staging system calls attention to the need to evaluate this feature. The stromal component of colonic carcinomas varies from little or no stroma (see Fig. 14.108) to frankly scirrhous tumors (Fig. 14.104). Stromal fibroblasts actively proliferate. The activated fibroblasts produce collagen and other connective tissue proteins that induce the desmoplastic reaction. Prominent stromal elastosis surrounds some invasive carcinomas; a conspicuous proliferation of elastic fibers is also present in the vascular media of blood vessels lying in proximity to tumor cells (338).

Colorectal carcinomas may also exhibit a peritumoral lymphocytic infiltrate, which can be judged as conspicuous or inconspicuous using the Jass criteria (337,339). These infiltrates consist of mast cells, eosinophils, macrophages, lymphocytes, plasma cells, and S100 protein–positive dendritic cells. Cytotoxic T lymphocytes constitute the majority of the infiltrating cells. The costimulatory molecules B7.1 (CD80) and B7.2 (CD86) by macrophages along the invasive margin of colon cancers is in accordance with the clinicopathologic studies that suggest that peritumoral lymphocytic infiltrates have a favorable prognostic factor. The presence of these cellular infiltrates suggests that there is an ongoing immune response potentially directed against the tumor cells.

Another type of reaction developing around tumors is a Crohn-like reaction (Fig. 14.105). It is characterized by the presence of discrete lymphoid aggregates, often with germinal centers ringing the periphery of invasive carcinoma. It is typically found at the interface of the muscularis propria and pericolic fibroadipose tissue. The magnitude of the Crohn-like reaction correlates with patient survival (340).

Tumor Vessels

Neovascularization of colorectal carcinomas results in a disorganized vascular pattern of nodular capillary clusters and capillary sheets of frequently interanastomosing vessels. They may also almost completely pack the interstitial spaces, making the overall vascular volume of carcinomas greater than that of adenomas or the normal colon. These changes

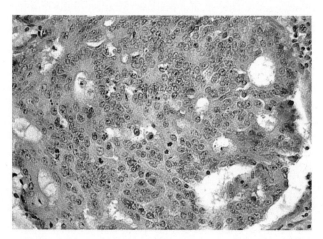

FIG. 14.100. Moderately differentiated adenocarcinoma.

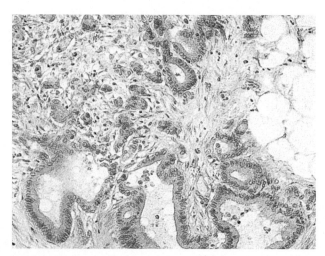

FIG. 14.101. An invasive component of this carcinoma is both well differentiated and poorly differentiated.

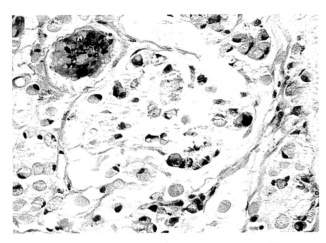

FIG. 14.102. A signet ring cell tumor is present with a large tumor giant cell.

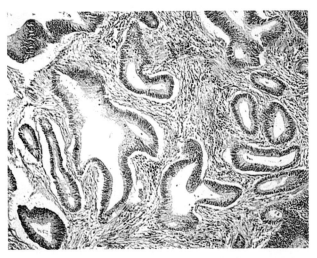

FIG. 14.104. Marked desmoplastic responses seen surrounding the invasive malignant glands.

are focal and occur even in intramucosal carcinoma. Most capillaries have a long tortuous course and numerous capillary sprouts. Tumor microvessel diameters are greater than normal (341).

The intratumoral blood vessels display various structural abnormalities, including endothelial cell proliferation, endothelial fenestrations, multilayered basement membranes, and thickened perivascular tissues. These features may result from repeated damage or may represent the effects of vascular remodeling (341). Red blood cells within the vessels also appear morphologically abnormal (341), perhaps explaining the propensity of colon cancers to form thrombi and produce the ischemia sometimes associated with them. The abnormal vessels may also facilitate intravascular invasion by the neoplasm.

Cancer Arising in Diverticula

Because colon cancer and diverticulosis often coexist in a specimen, the carcinomas may extend down into the diverticula

(Fig. 14.106). When the orifice of a diverticulum is blocked by the tumor, diverticulitis may develop. Carcinomas may also develop within the diverticulum itself. Staging of such lesions poses problems. Because of the increased penetration of the wall inherent in the diverticular location, a conservative approach would mandate that one stage such lesions at the maximum level of extension in the bowel wall, even if it is in the diverticulum. The reason for making this statement is that virtually nothing is known about the subsequent biology of these lesions, and as a result, one should probably be conservative in the approach to this problem.

Pathologic Characteristics of Sporadic Colorectal Cancers with Microsatellite Instability

Microsatellite unstable (MSI) sporadic colon cancers differ phenotypically from microsatellite stable (MSS) tumors. In addition, the prognosis of MSI sporadic cancers may differ

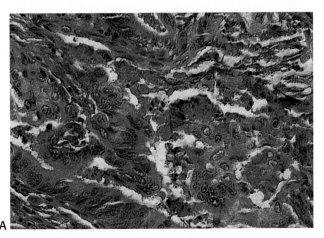

A

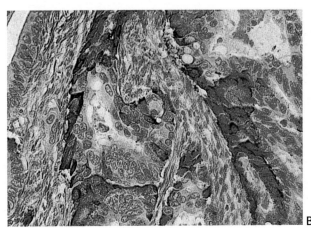

B

FIG. 14.103. Endocrine differentiation. **A:** A typical adenocarcinoma containing large numbers of endocrine cells. **B:** Grimelius stain demonstrates the presence of numerous endocrine cells.

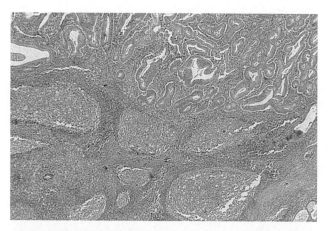

FIG. 14.105. Colonic adenocarcinoma with a marked Crohn-like tissue reaction. Well-formed lymphoid aggregates with prominent germinal centers lie at the margins of the tumor.

from that of MSS neoplasms (342–347), making their recognition of potential importance in patient management. Patients with sporadic MSI cancers tend to be somewhat younger than other patients (60 ± 5 years, range 22 to 83, vs. 66 ± 1, range 27 to 90). MSI tumors have a marked tendency to develop proximal to the splenic flexure (94% vs. 34%). In comparison to MSS proximal tumors, MSI tumors have more frequent exophytic growth and large size, poor differentiation, extracellular mucin, a Crohn-like lymphoid reaction, and a trend toward less frequent p53 product overexpression by immunohistochemistry (348,349).

Mucinous differentiation (>30% of the tumor) occurs in 39% to 75% of adenocarcinomas with an MSI phenotype and only 19% of MSS adenocarcinomas (348–350). Also, the plexiform pattern of the growth of the carcinoma significantly associates with the MSI phenotype (349). The plexiform pattern of growth is characterized by richly anastomosing and branching glandular spaces or cords in well- and poorly differentiated cancers, respectively (349). The plexiform pattern (irregular tubular differentiation) represents an

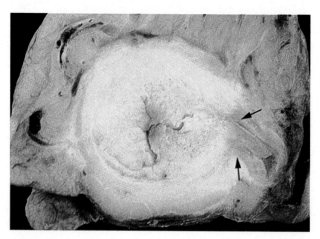

FIG. 14.106. Multiple diverticula with carcinoma extending into one (*arrows*).

early step of mucinous differentiation and should not be considered independent of it.

Flat Carcinomas

Flat carcinomas consist of slightly elevated, flat, or depressed lesions. This lesion is not rare in Japan, where it was first described, although it is rare in Europe and North America. Flat adenomas and adenocarcinomas resemble one another endoscopically and grossly. Softness of the intestinal wall and flabbiness of the tumor during endoscopy are clues to diagnosing adenoma endoscopically, whereas an endoscopic feature that suggests a cancer is stiffness of the tumor (212). Early cancers of the superficial type may appear nonpolypoid, flat, or depressed (Fig. 14.107). The height of the lesion does not exceed 50% of the tumor diameter (212,351). The mean size of small, flat colorectal cancers ranges from 1 to 20 mm with a mean of 6.7 mm, and is significantly smaller than polypoid lesions. When compared to polypoid lesions, flat colorectal cancers are more often proximally located, are less frequently well differentiated, and have fewer adenomatous remnants.

Controversy continues to surround superficial lesions, since disagreement exists concerning whether they represent true invasive carcinomas or areas of flat intramucosal carcinoma. Nonetheless, small carcinomas with clear-cut submucosal invasion do exist (Fig. 14.108). By the time they are detected, superficial adenocarcinomas may overgrow their associated adenomatous tissue (352), causing the tumor to resemble de novo carcinoma (351,353). Residual adenoma is present in only 8.1% of lesions. Only 40% of flat adenomas with a diameter <10 mm remain confined to the mucosa (212). The invasive tumors tend to be well or moderately differentiated.

Carcinomas that arise in flat adenomas develop from the base of lesions and may appear solid and/or cystic (Figs. 14.108 and 14.109). Epithelial cells in the basal parts of the crypts immediately adjacent to lymphocytic aggregates frequently show decreased amounts of mucus and cytoplasmic basophilia as well as increased nuclear:cytoplasmic ratios and mitotic figures suggesting active cellular proliferation (352). Even though superficial cancers invade only into the submucosa, they still may metastasize to the regional lymph nodes. Cancers invading the submucosa frequently develop lymphatic and/or vascular permeation. Lymphatic and vascular permeation occurs even when the lesions are small and may be more prevalent away from the rectosigmoid.

One rare form of flat carcinoma presents as an inverted, transmural, solid, and cystic lesion covered by a flat adenoma. The tumor may appear well differentiated, extending into the serosa and demonstrating a lobulated topography in the absence of a desmoplastic inflammatory stromal reaction. This pattern has been termed *endophytic malignant transformation* (354). Such transformation must be distinguished from the misplaced glandular epithelium as seen in localized colitis cystica profunda (354). Follicular lymphocytic aggregates frequently are observed in superficial-type adenocarcinomas but rarely in superficial adenomas (352).

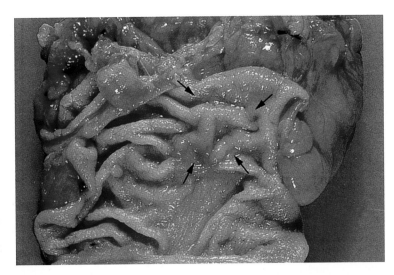

FIG. 14.107. Flat carcinoma with a plaquelike appearance (*arrows*). It is distinguishable from a flat adenoma because of its firm consistency, not its gross appearance. A small polypoid hyperplastic polyp is present nearby.

Carcinomas Associated with Schistosomiasis

Carcinomas arising in the setting of schistosomiasis (*S. japonicum*) often arise on a background of granulomatous colitis with mild to severe dysplasia. The dysplasia is either focal or diffuse in its distribution and occurs in flat mucosa, pseudopolyps, or regenerating epithelium at the edges of ulcers. These dysplastic changes represent the pathologic basis for the future malignant development of schistosomal colitis and resemble the changes found in longstanding chronic ulcerative colitis (355). Some tumors are multicentric (355). The patients have colitis for 2 to 20 years (355).

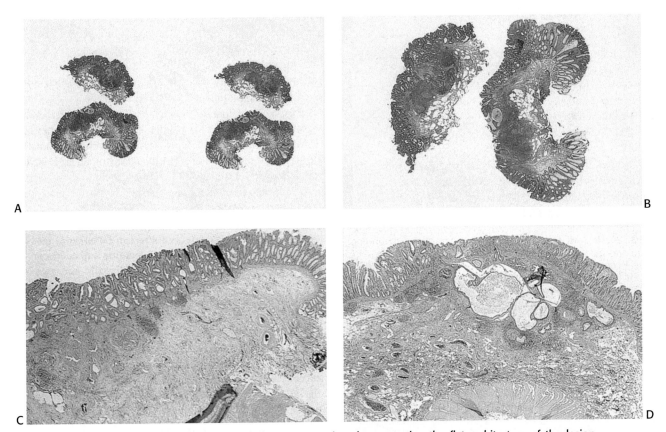

FIG. 14.108. Flat carcinoma. **A:** Whole mount section demonstrating the flat architecture of the lesion. **B:** Slightly higher magnification showing a flat lesion that invades into the submucosa. The lesion is surrounded by a prominent lymphoid reaction. **C:** Low-power photomicrograph of another flat carcinoma. Invasive carcinoma is present extending into the submucosa on the left side of the photograph. This cancer is arising in a flat adenoma. **D:** Flat carcinoma with cystic dilation of the invading glands. The tumor invades into the submucosa and is associated with a lymphocytic response.

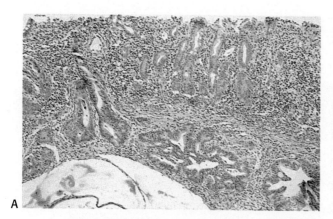

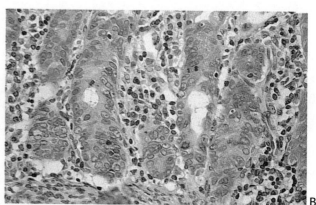

A

B

FIG. 14.109. Flat carcinoma. **A:** Flat carcinoma invading into the submucosa. The invasive glands are lined by cells with clearly malignant cytologic features. Some glands are cystically dilated and filled with mucin. The epithelial lining of such glands may be absent or atrophic. **B:** Higher-power magnification demonstrating nuclear pleomorphism, loss of polarity, and numerous mitotic figures in the malignant glands.

Schistosomal ova are abundant throughout the bowel wall associated with fibrous proliferations (Fig. 14.4).

Special Histologic Types of Colorectal Carcinoma

Mucinous Carcinomas

Many ordinary adenocarcinomas contain a mucinous component (Figs. 14.110 and 14.111), but when >50% of the tumor is mucinous, the tumor is classified as a mucinous adenocarcinoma (314,356,357). Mucinous tumors account for 10% to 15% of colorectal carcinomas (358,359) and 33% of rectal cancers (358). There are two subtypes of mucinous carcinoma: Colloid carcinoma and signet ring cell carcinoma. In colloid carcinomas, the mucin is extracellular, whereas in signet ring carcinomas, the mucin is intracellular in location. In both types, the material secreted is an acid mucopolysaccharide that stains with periodic acid–Schiff (PAS), mucicarmine, and acidic aniline blue stains. Like ordinary adenocarcinomas, both

signet ring carcinomas (Fig. 14.112) and colloid carcinomas arise in adenomas, particularly villous adenomas (358,360). Residual adenoma may be present in up to 31% of mucinous carcinomas (358,360). Mucinous carcinomas sometimes metastasize within the intestinal mucosa, creating many new polypoid lesions in the remaining mucosa. One extraordinary example of this was a patient who had >100 "polyps" (361).

Mucinous carcinomas differ clinically and pathologically from ordinary carcinomas. These tumors often affect young patients (314) and those with HNPCC. Seventy-nine to eighty-three percent of colorectal cancers in patients in the first 3 decades of life are predominantly mucinous, approximately equally divided between the signet ring and the colloid types (307,314). The delay in diagnosis in young people accounts for the very poor prognosis of mucinous carcinomas, especially in young patients (314,358). Mucinous carcinomas are more likely to invade adjacent viscera (29% vs. 10%) and show more extensive lymph node involvement beyond the pericolonic region (50% vs. 26%) than nonmucinous carcinomas (362). Disease recurrences occur more frequently in patients with colloid (51.7%) or signet ring carcinoma (100%) as compared

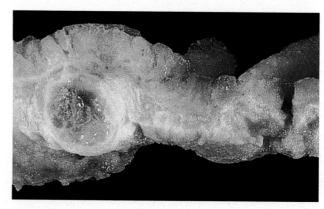

FIG. 14.110. The colon contains a large fungating mucinous tumor. Grossly, the mucinous areas may be appreciated on cut section, where they appear soft and gelatinous (not shown).

FIG. 14.111. Cross section of the bowel wall in a patient with a colloid carcinoma.

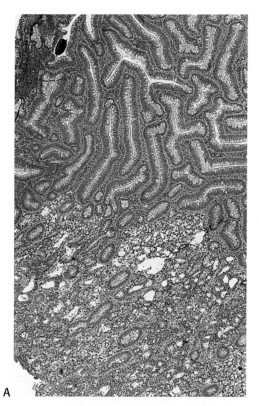 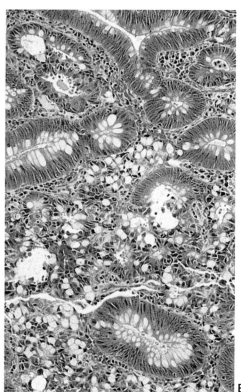

FIG. 14.112. Signet ring cell carcinoma arising in an adenomatous polyp. **A:** Low-power photomicrograph demonstrating the advancing margin of the early signet ring cell carcinoma (*bottom*). The adenomatous glands are separated by individually infiltrating cells with pale, vacuolated cytoplasm. **B:** On higher power, the signet ring cells are clearly seen. They contain abundant cytoplasmic mucin that pushes the nucleus to the periphery of the cell, giving it a signet ring appearance.

with ordinary adenocarcinomas. This justifies a more aggressive surgical approach, including extensive nodal dissection and resection of adjacent organs that seem to be macroscopically affected (362). Some patients with mucinous carcinomas develop pseudomyxoma peritonei or Trousseau syndrome (venous thrombophlebitis in patients with carcinoma). The latter may lead to cerebrovascular accidents (363).

Overall, mucinous carcinomas have a significantly worse prognosis, with a 5-year survival rate of 17% to 18% and a median survival of 33 months (364). The prognosis is worst in rectal mucinous tumors (358,359,365,366). In one study, the prognosis was found to be worse with tumors of high mucin content (>80%) than in those with a moderate mucinous content (60% to 80%) (366). The poor prognosis results in part from the tendency of mucinous tumors to dissect through the bowel wall in an infiltrative pattern.

Finding a significant mucinous component in the preoperative biopsy correlates well with similar findings in the resection specimen. In one study, 83% of mucinous carcinoma–positive biopsy specimens exhibited >25% mucinous carcinoma in the corresponding resection specimen, whereas only 10% of biopsies negative for mucinous carcinoma contained >25% mucinous carcinoma in the surgical specimen. Similarly, 83% of mucinous carcinoma–positive biopsy speci-

mens revealed carcinoma at the B2 or higher stage upon resection compared with 63% of mucinous carcinoma–negative biopsy specimens (356).

Colloid Carcinomas

Colloid carcinomas represent 10% to 15% of all carcinomas of the large bowel (358,359). Colloid carcinomas often arise in villous adenomas (367,379), in areas of villous dysplasia in ulcerative colitis (358), or in an anorectal fistula (368). The tumors may appear as very large, bulky, gelatinous neoplasms lacking fibrosis or scarring but containing large mucinous areas. The mucinous pools allow the tumor to dissect easily along tissue planes. The presence of the mucin makes surgical extirpation difficult (357).

Colloid carcinomas are diagnosable when one sees (a) malignant-appearing glands disrupted by the presence of abundant, extruded, intraluminal mucin; (b) mucin pools in the connective stroma; and (c) superficial pools of mucin containing free-lying ribbons or clusters of malignant cells. Columnar cells may line the large mucinous pools (Figs. 14.113 and 14.114). The epithelium may appear extremely well differentiated. Other tumors consist of irregular glands, trabecular groups of cells, or clumps of cells lying free in

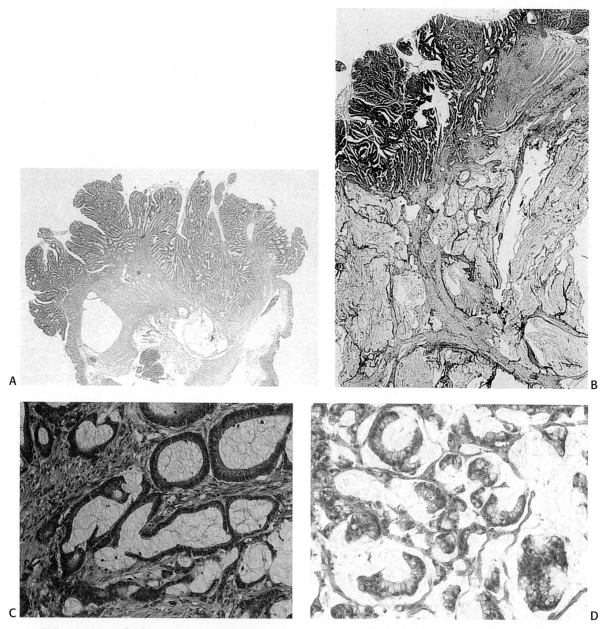

FIG. 14.113. Colloid carcinoma. **A:** Whole mount section of a colloid carcinoma arising in an adenoma. Isolated small mucinous pools are present. **B:** A more extensive colloid carcinoma underlies the villous adenoma. Large mucinous cysts are present. **C:** Histologic pattern of moderately cellular tumor with small mucinous lakes lined by well-differentiated epithelial cells. **D:** Highly differentiated colloid carcinoma demonstrating the presence of malignant mucin-filled epithelial cells floating free in mucinous pools. There is an attempt at gland formation. (*continues*)

mucinous lakes. Colloid carcinomas may demonstrate extensive lymphatic involvement or extensive submucosal spread, appearing to track along the submucosa and undermining the mucosa (369). Colloid carcinomas exhibit a propensity for lymph node metastases, reduced tubule differentiation, less lymphocytic infiltration, and more proximal distribution compared with nonmucinous tumors (367,370). A tendency for proximal distribution probably associates with the finding that HNPCC patients tend to have proximal lesions that exhibit a mucinous histology.

Signet Ring Cell Carcinomas

The second type of mucinous tumor is the "intracellular" type or signet ring cell carcinoma. The signet ring variety of mucinous carcinoma, although uncommon, tends to affect younger individuals. Patients present with changes in bowel habits, weight loss, and blood and mucus in the stools. Signet ring cell carcinomas account for approximately 1.1% of all colorectal carcinomas (364). Patients range in age from 18 to 29 years (360). Patients with signet ring carcinoma tend to

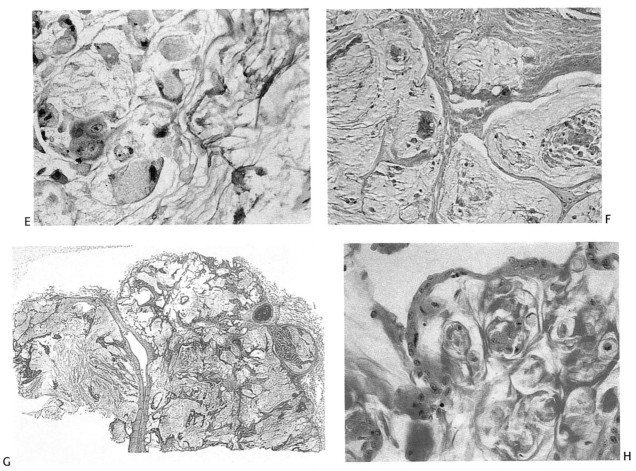

FIG. 14.113. *Continued* **E:** Mucin-filled anaplastic cells are seen. **F:** Large mucinous pools with malignant cells isolated within the mucin. **G:** Cross section through the bowel wall demonstrating massive replacement by mucinous carcinoma. **H:** Mucinous carcinoma with signet ring features.

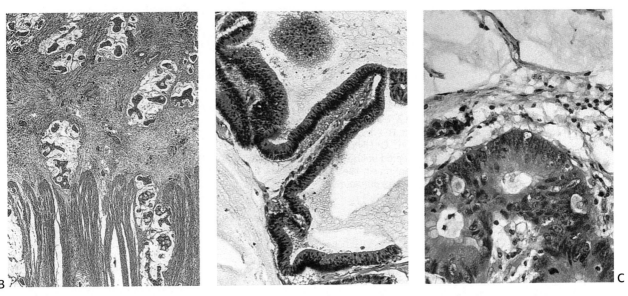

FIG. 14.114. Colloid carcinoma. **A:** Low-power view of a colloid carcinoma infiltrating through the submucosa into the muscularis propria. **B:** Pools of mucin are present, which contain ribbons of neoplastic cells. The tumor cells are well differentiated, demonstrating crowded, hyperchromatic nuclei reminiscent of adenomatous epithelium. **C:** In other areas, clusters of cells are present within a desmoplastic stroma. Some of these cells form glands. They appear more atypical than the cells depicted in B. A pool of mucin lies above the cell cluster.

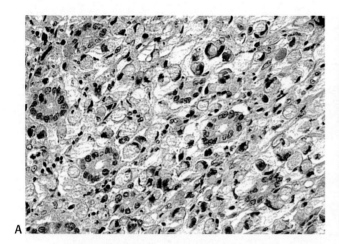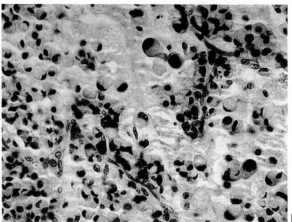

FIG. 14.115. Signet ring carcinoma. **A:** Many neoplastic signet rings are seen infiltrating around more differentiated tubular structures. **B:** A more poorly differentiated signet ring tumor without evidence of glandular differentiation.

have more extensive disease at the time of diagnosis than do those with ordinary adenocarcinoma (371). This has been attributed to delay in diagnosis, because many of the patients are young and the disease clinically resembles IBD. As many as 30% of patients with signet ring carcinoma have ulcerative colitis, further complicating recognition of the cancer (372). Furthermore, the tumor tends to spread intramurally with relative sparing of the mucosa, making it difficult to see radiographically, endoscopically, or grossly. There are few symptoms early in its course. The diffuse intramural infiltration by neoplastic cells may, at first, suggest an inflammatory process. Diffuse and circumferential bowel wall infiltration produces a thick, rigid, intestinal segment creating colonic linitis plastica (372). Advanced lesions present with constriction of the intestinal wall, widespread lymph node metastases, and spread to the peritoneal surfaces.

The histologic diagnosis of signet ring carcinoma depends on finding a preponderance (>50%) of poorly differentiated tumor cells with copious intracytoplasmic mucin pushing the nuclei to the cell periphery (Figs. 14.115 and 14.116). Some tumor cells may appear extremely anaplastic. However, not all signet ring cell carcinomas display a classic signet ring morphology. Rather, they contain cells with a fine, foamy cytoplasm and a central nucleus (Fig. 14.117).

The differential diagnosis of signet ring cell carcinomas involves a primary glandular neoplasm, a metastasis from another site such as the stomach or breast (Fig. 14.118), and adenocarcinoid tumors. Since linitis plastica with signet ring carcinoma has its greatest frequency in the stomach, secondary involvement of the colon by a gastric cancer must be considered when colonic linitis plastica is encountered. If residual adenoma is present, one can be reasonably confident that the lesion is primary, although we have seen rare cancers metastatic to an adenomatous polyp (373). Patient history and immunostains are extremely important in ruling out a metastatic tumor. Adenocarcinoid tumors tend to grow in a more organoid fashion than signet ring cell carcinomas, and

the cells appear more cohesive than the widely separated, more discohesive cells typical of colonic signet ring cell tumors.

Overall, signet ring cell carcinomas behave aggressively (371,374), with most patients presenting at stage III or IV. The overall 5-year survival in one series was 9.4% (374). Seventy-five percent of patients with T2 disease survived 5 years, compared with 5.1% and 0% of patients with T3 and T4 tumors, respectively.

Linitis Plastica

The term *linitis plastica* (Greek for linen cloth or net) was first described by Lietaud in 1779, but credit for the first case is given to Andrau, who, in 1829, described the condition. Primary linitis plastica of the colon was first described by Laufman and Saphir (375). Since the term *linitis plastica* is a gross term, several different histologic forms of cancer may produce the changes.

Linitis plastica is characterized by diffuse infiltration of neoplastic cells into a hollow viscus with significant desmoplastic response, imparting a rigid, fibrotic, thickened appearance to the wall of the organ (375). Both primary and secondary carcinomas can cause a colonic linitis plastica. Some cases of linitis plastica occur secondary to involvement by a gastric carcinoma (376). Grossly, the intestine appears diffusely thickened, particularly in the area of the submucosa. Eighty percent of primary lesions develop distal to the splenic flexure. In contrast, linitis plastica resulting from a metastatic gastric carcinoma usually affects the transverse colon, since metastases occur hematogenously via the gastrocolic ligament (377).

Linitis plastica affects individuals from age 20 to 60 years, with an average age of 51 to 56 years (377,378). The clinical features are usually limited to lower gastrointestinal symptoms, most often including altered bowel habits and abdominal or rectal pain, or melena. The average symptom duration prior to diagnosis is 3 months (377). Some patients have pre-existing ulcerative colitis (377).

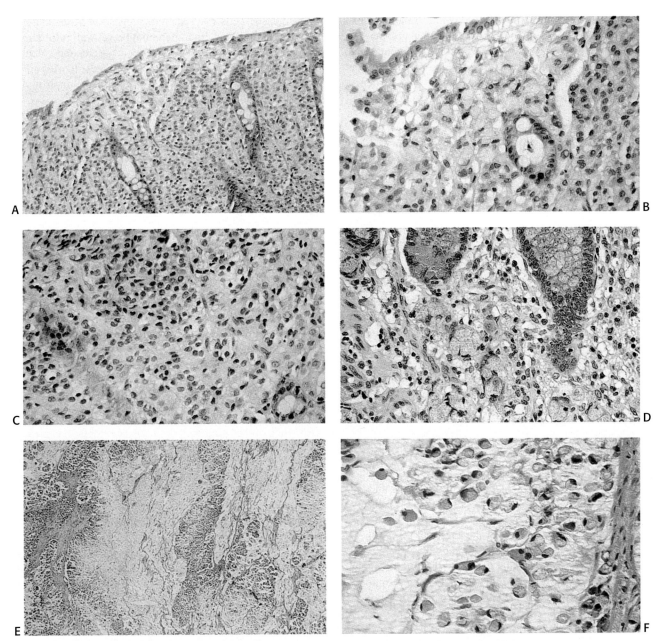

FIG. 14.116. Signet ring cell carcinoma. **A:** The lamina propria of the colon has been expanded by a population of infiltrating tumor cells. **B:** On higher power, the infiltrating cells are discohesive and contain abundant intracytoplasmic mucin, which displaces the nucleus to the periphery of the cell. A residual nonneoplastic gland is present in the central portion of the photograph. Often, the cells lack the indented nuclei more typical of signet ring cells. As a result, the tumor superficially resembles a xanthoma. **C:** Signet ring cells infiltrate the deep mucosa and superficial submucosa. **D:** Signet ring cell carcinoma in the area of the ileocecal valve. The tumor cells infiltrate individually and in small clusters. The nuclei are eccentric, and many appear atypical. **E:** In some signet ring cell tumors, mucinous lakes form as in colloid carcinomas. **F:** Typical signet ring cells are present floating in these mucin pools.

Radiologically, the disease simulates primary inflammatory disorders, such as Crohn disease, diverticulitis, and others. The mucosa may be relatively spared by the tumor, with the majority of the lesion infiltrating the submucosa (375). Radiologically, linitis plastica lacks an intraluminal mass or areas of ulceration. Rather, the bowel wall appears diffusely thickened. These changes may be seen more easily on computed tomography (CT) or magnetic resonance imaging (MRI) than on a barium enema.

Because there is frequently a lack of an apparent mucosal lesion, endoscopically directed biopsies should be deep enough to include the submucosa in order to provide a more accurate diagnosis. Grossly, the margins of the lesion are tapered and appear poorly delineated. The mucosa usually

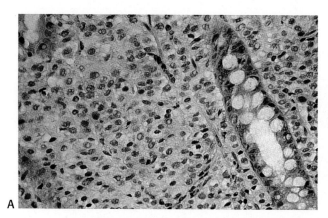

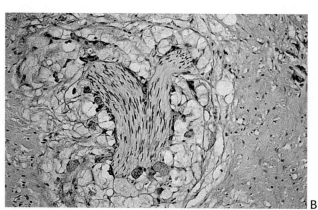

FIG. 14.117. Signet ring cell carcinoma. **A:** Not all signet ring cells show the classic morphology. In this case, the signet ring cells resemble histiocytes with central nuclei with vesicular chromatin and inconspicuous nucleoli. **B:** More classic signet ring cell carcinoma demonstrating perineural invasion.

appears intact, although it may be ulcerated. Histologically, linitis plastica consists of diffusely infiltrating, darkly stained, small, atypical cells that may have a signet ring appearance (Fig. 14.119). Abortive gland formation may also be present.

The tumors spread early, via lymphatic dissemination and/or by local extension (Fig. 14.120). Both peritoneal seeding and regional lymph node metastases are often present at the time of initial surgery. Seventy-five percent of patients have lymph

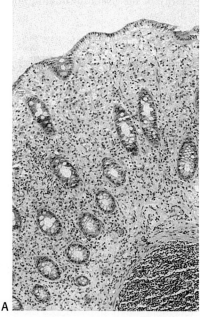

FIG. 14.118. Metastatic breast cancer in colon. **A:** Low-power photomicrograph demonstrating a population of cells expanding the lamina propria. **B:** Higher-power view of the infiltrating cells. They contain abundant eosinophilic cytoplasm and round central nuclei. Some classic signet ring cells are also present. **C:** Immunohistochemical staining with antibodies to gross cystic disease protein confirm that these cells represent metastatic breast carcinoma.

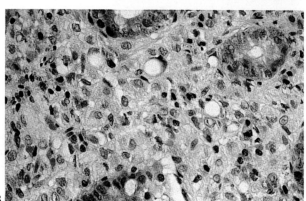

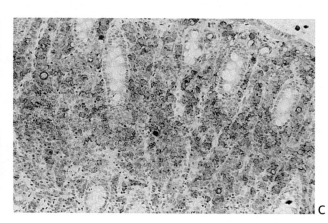

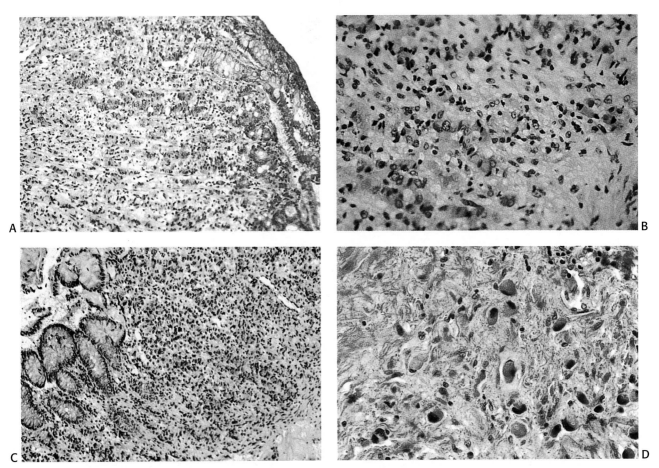

FIG. 14.119. Linitis plastica. **A:** Low-power magnification of tumor replacing the mucosa. **B:** The neoplastic cells subtly infiltrate the tissues. **C:** Most of the malignant cells are mucicarmine positive. **D:** The number of neoplastic cells may be quite small, as illustrated here.

nodal metastases, and 38% have peritoneal metastases. Females often have metastases to the uterus, ovaries, and fallopian tubes. Diffuse carcinomatosis of the abdomen or pelvis frequently occurs (378). Liver metastases are present in a low percentage of patients. Spread to bone and lung is rare (377). The prognosis is poor, with a mean duration of survival of only 8.3 months after diagnosis (377).

Squamous Cell–containing Carcinomas

The incidence of squamous and adenosquamous carcinoma ranges between 0.1 and 0.5 cases per 1,000 colonic malignancies (379,380). The tumors show an increased incidence in patients with chronic ulcerative colitis (379). Squamous cell carcinomas may also develop in patients with Crohn disease and longstanding rectal fistulae. The tumors that arise in the setting of IBD may result from hyperstimulation of intestinal stem cells due to an ongoing chronic inflammatory response. This could lead to stem cell hyperplasia and a broad spectrum of tumor types, including those containing squamous differentiation. A simple proliferation of basal cells may replace the damaged epithelium. Further demands for cell replacement lead to basal cell anaplasia and the

inability to differentiate normally, resulting in tumors that become glandular, become squamous, or show mixed cell populations. In this setting, the carcinoma need not develop in a pre-existing adenoma. Other adenosquamous and squamous carcinomas arise in adenomas, perhaps from those containing squamous morules (Fig. 14.36). Pure squamous cell carcinomas occur less commonly than adenoacanthomas or adenosquamous cancers.

Both sexes are equally affected (380). Hypercalcemia complicates the clinical picture in some patients due to production of parathormone by the tumor (381–383). Humoral calcemia of malignancy is diagnosed on the basis of an elevated parathormone level and positive tumor immunoreactivity to parathormone hormone (381). Colonic tumors containing areas of squamous differentiation are treated in the same fashion as ordinary adenocarcinomas.

Adenosquamous Carcinomas and Adenoacanthomas

No gross features distinguish adenosquamous carcinomas or adenoacanthomas from ordinary adenocarcinomas. Adenosquamous carcinomas usually occur in young patients who

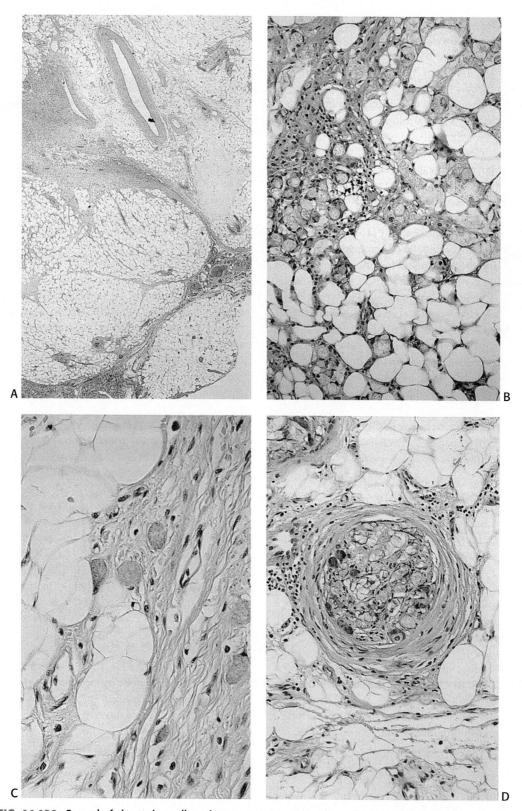

FIG. 14.120. Spread of signet ring cell carcinoma. **A:** Low-power view of the mesenteric fat from a patient with signet ring cell carcinoma. Clusters of hyperchromatic cells are present, which appear to be puckering the serosal surface. **B:** On higher power, clusters of signet ring cells are present within the mesenteric fat. **C:** Individual signet ring cells infiltrate the fat and fibrous tissue of the subserosa. **D:** Vascular invasion is also present.

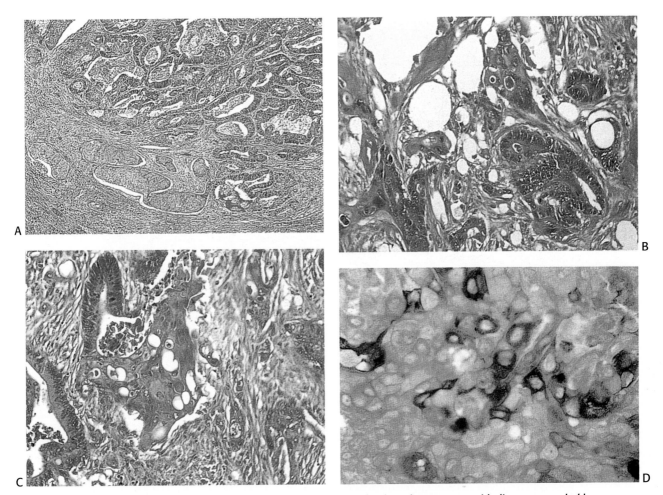

FIG. 14.121. Adenosquamous carcinoma. **A–C:** Neoplastic glands and squamous epithelium surrounded by desmoplastic tissue response. These are shown better in B and C. **D:** Cytokeratin staining in an adenosquamous carcinoma.

tend to present with advanced disease. They follow a highly aggressive course when compared with classic colorectal adenocarcinomas (380,384), with an overall 5-year survival of approximately 30% (384). Distant metastases occur early.

Histologically, adenosquamous carcinomas consist of an admixture of malignant glands and malignant squamous cells with variable keratinization (Fig. 14.121). Rarely, the tumors combine a mucinous and/or signet ring cell adenocarcinoma with a squamous cell component (385). The tumors often show extensive lymphatic invasion. When the tumors metastasize, the metastases may contain both glandular and squamous cell components or either component by itself. Rare tumors combine adenosquamous elements with areas of carcinoid differentiation. In this situation, the three elements intimately intermingle with one another. Such lesions exhibit the biologic behavior of the underlying adenosquamous carcinoma and not the carcinoid tumor.

Adenoacanthomas refer to those adenocarcinomas that contain a benign squamous cell component. These lesions are not grossly distinctive. Adenoacanthomas account for <0.2% of all colonic malignancies (386).

Squamous Carcinomas

The following criteria are required to diagnose a primary intestinal squamous cell carcinoma (387): (a) no evidence of primary squamous carcinoma exists in any other site that could provide a source of metastasis or direct extension to the bowel, (b) the affected bowel segment is not a squamous-lined fistula, (c) no continuity exists between the tumor and the anal squamous epithelium, and (d) no glandular differentiation is present. When these strict diagnostic criteria are met, squamous carcinomas of the colorectum are exceedingly rare. A recent estimate from SEER data in United States demonstrated that squamous cell carcinoma comprised 0.3% of all colorectal carcinomas (388). Squamous cell carcinomas develop in patients who have had previous radiation therapy (389), ulcerative colitis (389–391), schistosomiasis (389,392), congenital malformations (393), and chronic sinuses. These associations suggest that chronic inflammation stimulates reserve cells in the crypt to become squamous and neoplastic. Some patients have metachronous colonic carcinomas (394).

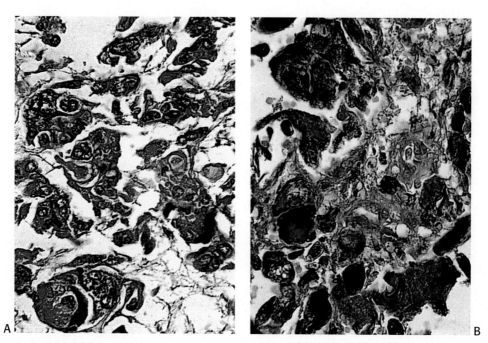

FIG. 14.122. Colon cancer. **A**: Carcinoma with choriocarcinomatous differentiation. **B** is stained with antibody to human chorionic gonadotropin.

No gross features identify a colon cancer as a squamous carcinoma. Most squamous carcinomas are large, ulcerated lesions. They may be confined to a small polyp (395). Most tumors arise in the rectum, but they may also arise in other colonic sites (388). The tumors range in differentiation from well to poorly differentiated. Histologically, well-differentiated intestinal squamous cell carcinomas show prominent areas of keratinization, intercellular bridges, keratin pearls, lack of gland formation, and no stainable mucin. Keratin formation may be inconspicuous in poorly differentiated tumors. The tumors metastasize to the regional lymph nodes and to the liver (389). The overall 5-year survival for colorectal squamous cell carcinomas is 49% (388).

Basaloid (Cloacogenic) Carcinomas

The extremely rare colonic basaloid carcinomas resemble basaloid tumors of the anal canal, but they arise far from the pectinate line in the sigmoid colon. The tumors are exophytic or ulcerating masses with clinical features similar to adenocarcinoma. Basaloid tumors may produce parathyroid hormone or adrenocorticotropic hormone (396). They are aggressive lesions capable of metastasis. Histologically, the tumors resemble their anal counterparts. They consist of islands of small, poorly differentiated cells separated by connective tissue. Small foci of keratinized cells are present. Peripheral palisading is often present. Basaloid carcinomas probably arise from the undifferentiated crypt cell. Alternatively, these could be considered to represent poorly differentiated squamous cell carcinomas.

Carcinosarcomas

Colonic carcinosarcomas deeply invade the bowel wall, metastasize widely, resist multiagent chemotherapy, and cause early patient death. The tumors consist of a carcinoma or adenosquamous carcinoma admixed with a sarcoma showing osseous, cartilaginous, and nonspecific spindle cell differentiation. Both the sarcomatous and carcinomatous areas are cytokeratin immunoreactive (397). Although called a carcinosarcoma of the colon, this lesion is probably more analogous to the so-called spindle cell carcinomas that arise more commonly in the esophagus (see Chapter 3).

Carcinoma with Germ Cell Elements

Primary intestinal adenocarcinomas may contain various germ cell elements.

Choriocarcinoma

Buckley and Fox (398) showed that 43% of morphologically typical adenocarcinomas of the large bowel contain human chorionic gonadotropin (hCG)-positive cells. However, the development of intestinal carcinoma that contains cells that morphologically resemble syncytiotrophoblasts or cytotrophoblasts is rare (399–402). Occasional intestinal carcinomas contain a mixture of adenocarcinoma and choriocarcinoma. Nearly all of the cases that have been described are typical adenocarcinomas with markedly elevated serum hCG levels. Rare pure colonic choriocarcinomas also exist (403). Women are affected three times more often than men (399,404). Patients range in age from 28 to 84 years, with a mean of 54 years. The mean age is 79 years for men and

46 years for women. The prognosis of patients with choriocarcinoma is poor; survival is <5 months.

The tumors arise anywhere in the colon and rectum, although there is a tendency for them to involve the left side of the colon (398–400,405). Histologically, the tumors typically consist of variably differentiated adenocarcinomas containing cells that appear less well differentiated, often with great variations in the size and shape of the tumor cells. Cytotrophoblastic areas consist of solid sheets of large, clear or pale, mononuclear cells with defined cell membranes and variable numbers of cytoplasmic PAS-positive granules. Scattered mononucleated or multinucleated giant cells with features of syncytiotrophoblasts (Fig. 14.122) are also present. These bizarre cells have abundant eosinophilic cytoplasm. The tumors often exhibit marked hemorrhagic necrosis. Such tumors may represent metaplastic derivatives of the proliferating neoplastic cells (398). hCG immunostains stain not only the large syncytiotrophoblasticlike cells, but also the adenocarcinomatous cells (401). There is a tendency for the positive cells to be located at the periphery of the tumor (405). This pattern recapitulates the peripheral distribution in normal trophoblastic tissue in relationship to the growing embryo, a distribution that helps find and invade host blood vessels. This may account for the increased aggressiveness of these tumors.

These tumors metastasize widely to the liver, lymph nodes, lungs, and spleen (399–402). In some cases, when these neoplasms metastasize, the metastasis is a choriocarcinoma, whereas the primary lesion does not contain obvious areas of choriocarcinoma. However, staining the primaries with an antibody to hCG usually discloses a small fraction of atypical epithelial elements that are hCG positive (401). Syncytiotrophoblastic differentiation may also gradually increase with advancing distance from the primary lesion in the metastases (401).

hCG-containing cells are found in 80% of mucinous and 92% of poorly differentiated carcinomas, even in the absence of trophoblastic differentiation (406). hCG is detected more frequently in carcinomas invading the entire bowel wall (67%) than in those confined to the submucosa or muscularis (30%). Seventy-nine percent of cases have lymph node and/or hepatic metastases in the setting of hCG positivity in the primary tumor and only 32% without metastases show hCG immunoreactivity. The immunohistologic detection of hCG in colorectal carcinomas may be a biologic marker of prognostic significance (406).

Mixed Choriocarcinoma–Endodermal Sinus Tumors

Rare colorectal adenocarcinomas contain areas of endodermal sinus tumor admixed with choriocarcinoma (407). Patients with these tumors develop elevated serum α-fetoprotein (AFP) and hCG levels. The various histologic components merge imperceptibly with one another. The tumors metastasize to regional lymph nodes. The immunophenotype of the tumor varies depending on the area in which it is examined.

Adenocarcinomatous areas show strong carcinoembryonic antigen (CEA) immunoreactivity and weak AFP activity. Areas of primary choriocarcinoma are strongly positive with antibodies to hCG and negative for AFP and CEA, and areas of nodal metastases resembling yolk sac tumor are weakly positive for hCG and CEA and strongly positive for AFP.

Teratomas

Teratomas have been described in the colon (408–410). An unusual patient was reported who had a polypoid lesion that histologically contained evidence of a teratoma with differentiation along all three germ layers. In the patient reported by Mauer et al (408), the surface of the polyp consisted of pigmented skin with hair extending from the surface. Tumors arise in the cecum, descending colon, sigmoid, and rectum and present with variable symptoms, including pain, rectal bleeding, abdominal mass, intestinal intussusception, and perforation. Coexistent conditions include schistosomiasis (410), adenocarcinoma (411), and ulcerative colitis (409). Most colorectal teratomas arise within the intestinal wall in the muscularis or submucosa. It is distinctly unusual for tumors to arise in the mucosa, such as in the case presented by Mauer et al (408). The presence of surface hair represents a pathognomonic feature of this lesion.

Endodermal Sinus Tumors

A rare example of a pure endodermal sinus tumor arising in the colon of a 3-year-old boy has been reported (412). Its histologic features were identical to the same tumor arising in the ovary or testis.

Extrauterine Müllerian Tumors

Tumors considered to be of müllerian origin occur in extrauterine sites but are rare. Such lesions may arise via transformation either of areas of endometriosis (413) or of multipotential peritoneal cells lining the serosal surface (414). By far the more common route appears to be transformation of areas of endometriosis (413). Primary malignant mixed müllerian tumors may also arise primarily in the colon or rectum (414). Histologically, the tumors exhibit a full range of histologies simulating those that originate in the endometrial cavity (Figs. 14.123 and 14.124). They contain mixtures of neoplastic epithelial and mesenchymal elements. The mesenchymal components can be either heterologous or homologous in nature in a manner resembling primary endometrial tumors.

Adenocarcinoma with Osseous Metaplasia

Foci of osseous metaplasia occasionally occur in colorectal carcinomas (Fig. 14.125), particularly mucin-secreting neoplasms (415). Necrosis, inflammation, pre-existing calcification, increased stromal vascularity, and extracellular mucin

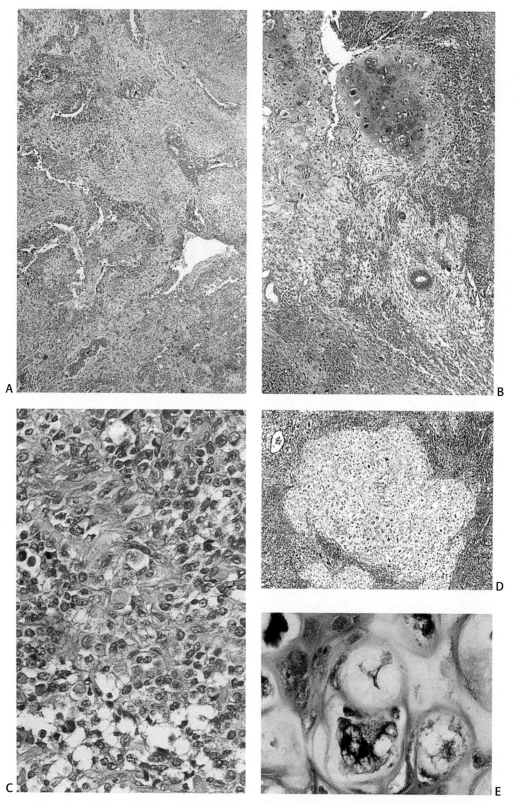

FIG. 14.123. Extrauterine malignant mixed müllerian tumor. **A:** Low-power photomicrograph demonstrating a malignant glandular proliferation surrounded by stroma containing numerous bizarre cells. **B:** Higher-power view demonstrating a mixture of malignant glandular and stromal elements. A focus of cartilaginous differentiation is present in the upper portion of the photograph. **C:** Malignant mesenchymal component resembling rhabdomyosarcoma. **D:** Chondrosarcomatous component. **E:** Higher-power view demonstrating bizarre giant cells within the chondrosarcomatous component of the tumor.

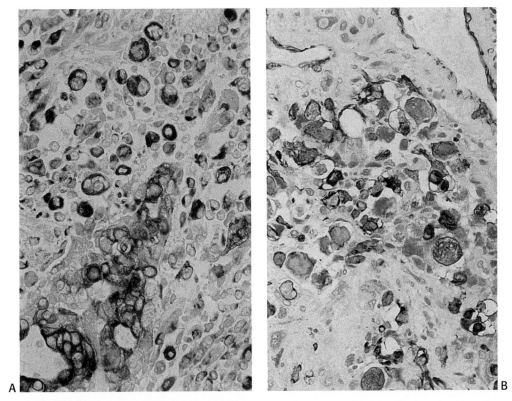

FIG. 14.124. Extrauterine malignant mixed müllerian tumor. **A:** Immunohistochemical staining for cytokeratin is positive in the epithelial component of the neoplasm (*dark blue*), and rhabdomyoblasts stain with an antibody to desmin (*red*). **B:** Actin stains also highlight mesenchymal cells with rhabdomyosarcomatous features.

deposition all associate with heterotopic bone formation in tumors. Clinically, the presence of the metaplastic bone probably has no significance. The tumor cells may secrete an unknown substance that stimulates the bone formation (416). Inflammation may also play a role in the osseous metaplasia (415). The heterotopic ossification occurs in either the primary lesion or the metastasis. Usually no predisposing cause can be identified for the ossification.

The metaplastic bone appears histologically benign and its production is stimulated by the stroma, probably in response to reparative processes. The bone formation is characterized by the appearance of osteoblastlike cells at the surfaces of the mineral deposit. These osteoblastic cells may develop from pre-existing mesenchymal cells within the stroma surrounding tumors. These osteoblastic cells may form a matrix, which then calcifies through the action of

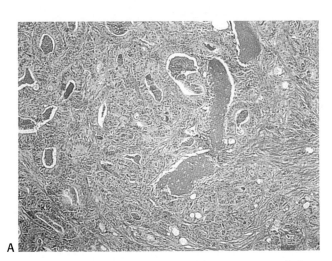
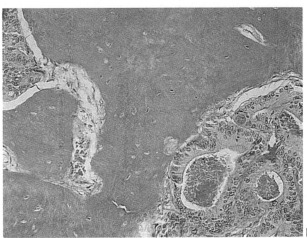

FIG. 14.125. Carcinoma with osseous metaplasia. **A:** This moderately well-differentiated carcinoma is associated with the presence of several islands of metaplastic bone. **B:** These are seen with high-power magnification.

enzymes, such as alkaline phosphatase and carbonic anhydrase (416).

Stem Cell Carcinomas

Some forms of highly malignant colonic carcinomas consist of mixtures of undifferentiated cells focally intermingling with neuroendocrine, exocrine, and squamous cells, sometimes arranged in an organoid manner (417,418). The predominant histologic pattern in such tumors is that of a small cell undifferentiated carcinoma, but adenocarcinoma, colloid, and squamous differentiation are also found. Histochemical and immunohistochemical findings of such tumors reflect the individual components. The glandular portions tend to be PAS, Alcian blue, and mucicarmine positive. CEA immunoreactivity occurs in the glandular and squamous components. The neuroendocrine components may stain with antibodies to synaptophysin, neuron-specific enolase (NSE), Leu-7, and sometimes chromogranin. Cytokeratin immunostains may stain all the components, but the pattern of staining differs. Well-differentiated glandular or squamous areas tend to be the most strongly positive. The neuroendocrine areas stain like small cell carcinomas. Such tumors usually fail to make any known hormonal product. The tumors arise anywhere in the colon, and all that have been reported in the literature metastasized and had very short survival periods, presumably reflecting the presence of the small cell component, which places them in a poor prognostic group. Liver metastases are frequent.

Pleomorphic (Giant Cell) Carcinoma

Pleomorphic, or giant cell, carcinomas may arise in the large bowel. Prognosis is poor due to early tumor spread, with only a few months of postoperative survival. Histologically, the tumors consist of solid sheets of poorly cohesive cells broken into clusters by delicate stromal strands. The tumor growth is predominantly intramural, with most of the luminal surface being covered by an intact mucosa. Central ulceration can be seen. Adenomatous changes are generally not seen in the adjacent epithelium. The tumors consist of a mixture of giant cells, small polygonal cells, and spindle cells. The giant cells are identical to those seen in giant cell carcinomas of the lung. Nuclei are pleomorphic, with distinct nuclear membranes, a vesicular chromatin pattern with irregular clumping, and one or more prominent nucleoli. The nuclei are pushed to the edge of the cells, often resulting in a bent or reniform eccentric nucleus. The cellular size varies, with the larger cells having two or more nuclei. Typical and atypical mitoses are frequently present. Lymphocyte tumor cell emperipolesis is frequently seen. The spindle cells and smaller polygonal cells have a smaller amount of cytoplasm, and the nuclei do not appear as pleomorphic but otherwise show similar characteristics. The proportion of the different cell types present varies among tumors. Because these pleomorphic carcinomas exhibit some differentiation characteristics of carcinoid tumors, some regard them as poorly differentiated variants of neuroendocrine carcinomas. Ultrastructurally, one may see evidence of glandular as well as endocrine differentiation. Intracytoplasmic perinuclear whorls of intermediate filaments and dense core secretory granules are present. The tumors immunohistochemically contain keratin-, vimentin-, epithelial membrane antigen (EMA)-, NSE-, and chromogranin-immunoreactive cells. These tumors are negative for mucin.

Other Carcinoma Types

Rare colon cancers form psammoma bodies (Fig. 14.126) or display a clear cell morphology (Fig. 14.127). Clear cell carcinomas consist of uniform cells with clear cytoplasm due to the presence of intracytoplasmic glycogen. These lesions should not be confused with metastatic renal cell carcinoma or other metastatic clear cell cancers. A carcinoma has also been described with rhabdoid features (419). It is important to recognize that such patterns can represent primary colon tumors and do not necessarily imply the presence of a metastasis.

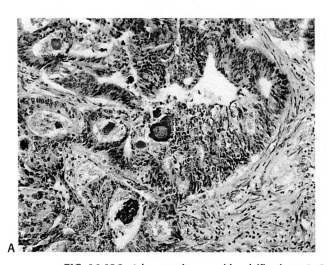
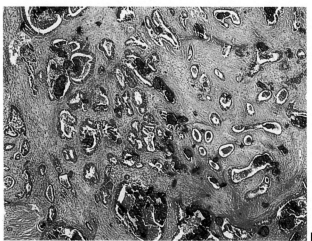

FIG. 14.126. Adenocarcinoma with calcifications. **A:** Carcinoma with psammoma body–like structures within lumens. **B:** Scirrhous carcinoma with microcalcifications.

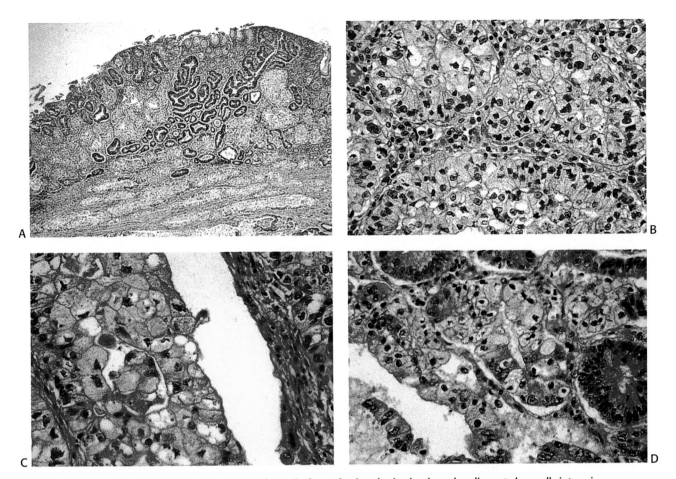

FIG. 14.127. Clear cell carcinoma. **A:** The typical neoplastic colonic glands and malignant clear cells intermingle. **B:** Clear cell carcinoma component at higher power resembles renal cell carcinoma. **C:** Periodic acid–Schiff stain of clear cell carcinoma is focally positive. **D:** Mucicarmine stain of clear cell carcinoma is negative.

Chumas and Lorelle (420) described an anorectal adenocarcinoma that grossly was deeply pigmented and resembled a melanoma. Histologically and ultrastructurally, the tumor was a moderately differentiated adenocarcinoma whose neoplastic epithelium contained both compound melanosomes and epithelial cells containing mucin droplets. Intermediate stages of melanosome formation were absent, suggesting that the carcinoma cells had phagocytosed melanin produced by adjacent normal anal melanocytes.

Finally, small cell carcinomas (SCCs) arise in the large intestine. These are discussed with the other neuroendocrine lesions in Chapter 17.

Biopsy Interpretation of Colorectal Neoplasia

Biopsies are taken to confirm the clinical suspicion of a carcinoma, ascertain its histologic type, and grade the neoplasm. The diagnosis of carcinoma in a biopsy specimen should never be made unless there is unequivocal evidence of invasion. In some cases, one receives fragments of malignant glands that, if they were found within the submucosa, would be easily diagnosable as an invasive cancer. However, because only tissue fragments are present in the absence of

submucosal structures, one cannot make the diagnosis of invasive carcinoma. Such a lesion may be only intramucosal carcinoma. Even the presence of desmoplasia surrounding malignant glands does not necessarily confirm the diagnosis of invasion unless one clearly sees submucosal structures. Submucosal invasion can be most easily confirmed if one sees the presence of large blood vessels, nerves, or ganglia adjacent to the malignant cells.

Some masses that clinically appear to be adenocarcinomas turn out to be other lesions that may not require surgery, such as lymphomas. The masses may also represent metastases from other sites, such as from a melanoma or breast cancer, and the biopsy is performed merely to document the presence of the metastasis.

Judging the degree of dysplasia of a neoplasm on a biopsy is difficult, since biopsies often underestimate the histologic grade. Biopsies are particularly helpful if one is able to demonstrate forms of tumor that are particularly aggressive, such as mucinous or signet ring cell, undifferentiated, or small cell carcinomas.

A positive biopsy should always be obtained before either irradiation or radical surgery is contemplated. In order to be representative, it is prudent to perform several

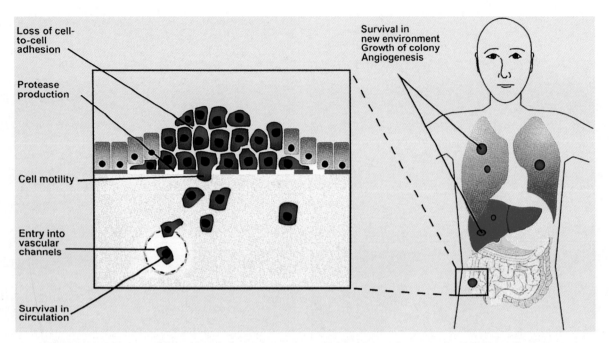

FIG. 14.128. Diagram demonstrating the steps necessary for invasion and metastasis of cancer cells (*green*). The initial step for tumor spread involves loss of cell-to-cell and cell-to-basement membrane adhesion. This occurs through loss of cadherins, catenins, and integrins. Next, the cells must break through the basement membrane, a process that is facilitated by production of proteolytic enzymes such as collagenases, cathepsins, and hyaluronidase, as well as loss of inhibitors of metalloproteinases. Cells may then enter the submucosa, where they access vascular and lymphatic channels through secondary invasion. At the metastatic site, the cells must arrest, adhere to the endothelium, and then migrate out of the vascular system. In order to survive in their new environment, tumor cells must produce angiogenic factors to promote the ingrowth of a new vascular supply. Tumor cells must also evade host immunologic defenses, a process that may occur through production of altered human leukocyte antigen and other tumor-specific antigens.

biopsies from different areas of larger lesions. Biopsies from the edges of lesions may show only adenoma or areas of transitional mucosa, whereas central biopsies may show fibrinous exudate or granulation tissue from an ulcerating lesion.

Tumor Spread

While it is not the intention of this text to provide an in-depth treatise with respect to the general mechanisms of tumor spread, it is important that the process be understood in a general way, both to understand the biology of the process and because pathologists are often involved in the delineation of the factors involved in tumor invasion and metastasis. When tumors spread, they do so by escaping from normal cellular growth controls. This process occurs both locally and distantly and involves interactions between the neoplastic cells and their surrounding environment. Multiple steps are required for invasion and metastasis to occur. Many of the steps are well defined. Some involve the generation of new blood vessels within the tumor (angiogenesis). This increased vascularization increases the probability that tumor cells can reach the bloodstream and colonize secondary sites. During invasion and metastasis, individual tumor cells attach to

other cells and/or to matrix proteins. Adhesion molecules play a critical role in these cellular attachments. The neoplastic cells translocate across extracellular matrix barriers (invade). In order for this to happen, specific proteinases lyse the matrix proteins. Many factors, including matrix components, stimulate tumor cell migration. Once the metastatic cells finally reach a secondary site and colonize it, they must grow in that site. Growth factors stimulate metastatic cells to proliferate at these secondary sites. Figure 14.128 illustrates these processes.

Colorectal adenocarcinomas spread intramurally or intraluminally, by perineural, lymphatic, and/or venous invasion; by direct extension to contiguous structures; by seeding the peritoneal cavity or serosal membranes; or by implantation in surgical wounds and anastomotic sites.

Intramural Growth

Once a tumor develops, it may grow in several directions. In some cases, it first protrudes into the lumen, whereas in others it invades deeper into the colonic wall. The tumors extend through the bowel wall, either progressing in an orderly fashion through the various intestinal wall layers or extending through the area of the penetrating vessels (Fig. 14.129).

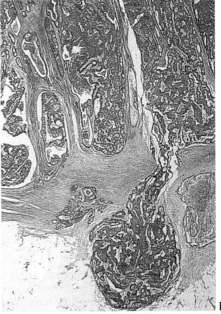

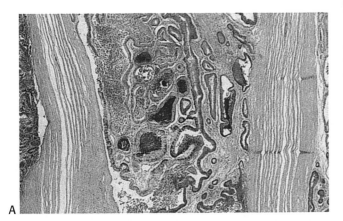

FIG. 14.129. Intramural growth of colon carcinoma. **A:** Infiltrating glands are present within the muscularis propria. **B:** Penetration through the full thickness of the bowel wall may occur as a result of tumor extension along the penetrating vessels.

Mural penetration results in direct involvement of adjacent organs or tissues, peritoneal seeding, or both.

The extent of the longitudinal spread is important at the time of surgical resection, since it impacts the length of the resection margin. Longitudinal or superficial spread, both proximal and distal to the origin of tumor, is often minimal, usually being <1 to 2 cm (421,422). In one study of rectal cancers, 74% of the tumors demonstrated the same degree of lateral extension in the deeper portions of the bowel wall as was seen grossly. In 21% of cases, the tumor spread beyond the gross margin by <5 mm, and in 5% of cases the tumor histologically extended for 5 to 15 mm beyond the gross margin (423). Tumors with distal spread of >1 cm are usually advanced Dukes C tumors (422,424).

Distal margins of 2 cm are generally considered to be safe for all patients. However, Kameda et al (425) noted that intramural spread can exceed 2.1 cm in infiltrative tumors, leading them to recommend that resection margins be 2 cm for localized carcinomas and 3 cm for infiltrative carcinomas. Colloid and signet ring cell tumors are an exception to the rule and should probably be resected with wider margins due to their tendency to infiltrate and dissect through the bowel wall (422).

Superficial Spread

Rare tumors spread superficially along the mucosa. Cecal carcinomas can extend into the appendix and the terminal ileum, replacing the native appendiceal and ileal mucosa and invading the underlying muscularis propria (426).

Extension to Adjacent Organs

Direct extension to adjacent organs occurs in approximately 10% of colorectal carcinomas, mainly in large advanced cancers with nodal and distant metastases. Colorectal cancers may penetrate adjacent segments of the small or large intestine and cause obstruction, peritonitis, or fistulae. Carcinomas of the hepatic flexure, transverse colon, or splenic flexure may extend directly into the liver, pancreas, spleen, gallbladder, and stomach. Carcinomas of the ascending and descending colon may involve the retroperitoneum. Vesicocolic and vesicorectal fistulae result from tumor extension to the bladder. Rectovaginal or colovaginal fistulae result when cancers invade into the vagina. Cecal carcinomas may extend into the lateral abdominal gutter and into the abdominal wall.

Direct Extension of Rectal Carcinomas into the Prostate or Bladder

Such patients often present with genitourinary symptoms; gastrointestinal manifestations are less common. Histologically, some lesions involving the bladder mimic primary villous adenomas of the bladder. Distinguishing a primary bladder carcinoma from a colonic carcinoma may not be possible based on histopathologic grounds alone. The bladder may give rise to adenocarcinomas, including the enteric mucin- or colloid-producing lesions and signet ring cell morphologies (427), morphologies identical to those of colorectal neoplasms. Other features, such as the presence of dirty necrosis within the tumor, may serve as a clue to a colonic origin. Urinary bladder adenocarcinomas resemble their intestinal counterparts not only morphologically but also histochemically, immunohisto-chemically, and ultrastructurally so that it may not be possible to use special stains to distinguish the two lesions.

Peritoneal Spread

Tumor spread within the peritoneal cavity occurs most commonly in poorly differentiated carcinomas, particularly mucinous tumors. Approximately 10% of patients undergoing resection for colorectal adenocarcinoma can be expected to develop peritoneal tumor foci. Peritoneal involvement by carcinoma is usually verifiable by cytologic examination of the ascites fluid that is usually present (169).

Better differentiated carcinomas may produce only a few peritoneal nodules, whereas signet ring cell carcinomas often produce diffuse intra-abdominal seeding (Fig. 14.120). Colloid carcinomas produce pseudomyxoma peritonei.

Lymphatic and Lymph Node Spread

Colon cancers frequently metastasize to the regional lymph nodes. The incidence of lymphatic invasion ranges from 8% to 73% and increases with tumor stage and grade (428,429). Lymphatic invasion is also more common in tumors of the colon than in rectosigmoid or rectal lesions (15% vs. 10%) (430). Tumors with intramural and extramural blood vessel invasion have the highest incidence of lymphatic invasion compared with blood vessel invasion–negative tumors (52% vs. 5%).

Intestinal carcinoma first enters the lymphatics in the bowel wall when it penetrates the muscularis mucosae (Fig. 14.130). The first lymph nodes to become involved are those closest to the tumor in the bowel wall. Metastases usually progress from one lymph node to the next in a fairly orderly fashion, following normal lymph flow. Normal lymphatic flow is through the lymphatic channels along the major arteries, with several echelons of lymph nodal involvement: Pericolic, intermediate, and principal or the so-called high-point nodes. The latter become involved only after more proximal ones contain metastases. Rarely, one sees discontinuous or skip metastases. If tumors lie between two major vascular pedicles, the lymphatic flow may drain in either or both directions.

Blockage of normal lymph flow in advanced carcinomas sometimes produces atypical routes of tumor spread, including what has been called *retrograde lymphatic spread*. In such cases, intramural lymphatics lying at some distance from the primary tumor become filled with malignant cells.

Rectal carcinomas first metastasize to the perirectal lymph nodes at the level of the primary tumor or immediately above it and then spread to the next group of lymph nodes. In patients with late-stage rectal carcinomas, hemorrhoidal lymphatics become blocked and the tumor spreads laterally or in a downward direction. Pericolonic lymph nodes along the mesenteric border of the pelvis may become involved at this stage.

Low rectal carcinomas involving the pectinate line may metastasize to both inguinal and mesenteric lymph nodes. Morson and Dawson (431) reported a 2% incidence of inguinal node involvement in rectal adenocarcinomas and a 7% incidence among carcinomas of the distal rectum. Lymph node metastases are unilateral in most patients, but they can be bilateral in as many as a third of cases.

The histologic features of the tumor within the lymph nodes vary considerably. Often, the lymph node is totally replaced by obvious tumor (Figs. 14.131 and 14.132). In other situations, dense sclerosis largely replaces the lymph node in such a way that it may be difficult to recognize the presence of metastatic tumor. In still other situations, one may only see mucinous pools representing areas of metastasis from colloid carcinomas without any obvious cellular components. Generally speaking, an extracolonic tumor focus in which no residual nodal tissue is identifiable can be considered to represent nodal metastasis when the lesion has a rounded smooth contour reminiscent of a lymph node. Nodules with an irregular contour are not considered nodal metastases, but are thought to represent extracolonic venous invasion.

Since the number of lymph nodes involved by metastatic tumor affects the prognosis (432–435), the lymph nodes should be carefully identified when the resection specimen is examined grossly. However, despite the strong prognostic significance of nodal metastases, meticulous lymph node dissection is often overlooked. Wide variation exists in both the number of lymph nodes identified in a resection specimen and the number of nodal metastases identified.

Controversy exists with regard to the number of lymph nodes that must be examined to yield a reliable assessment of nodal status in patients with colorectal cancer. In 1990, the Working Party Report to the World Congresses of Gastroenterology proposed that at least 12 lymph nodes be sampled to adequately stage a patient (436). However, more recent reports suggest that this number may not be adequate. Goldstein et al (437) found that the number of node-positive patients continued to increase until 17 to 20 lymph nodes had been examined, and suggested that at least 17 nodes be sampled for adequate staging. Similarly, a study by Wong et al found that at least 14 lymph nodes needed to be assessed before a node positivity rate similar to that of the National Cancer Data Bank could be achieved (438). Other studies suggest that at least 20 lymph nodes should be examined (433). These studies do clearly indicate that to accurately stage a colorectal cancer patient, as many nodes as possible should be evaluated, and that nodal counts of less than 12 to 14 should be considered inadequate for staging and should prompt the pathologist to go back to the specimen in an attempt to recover additional lymph nodes.

Venous Spread

Colon cancer also spreads by venous permeation (Fig. 14.133), a feature present in 17% to 61% of cases. Venous invasion

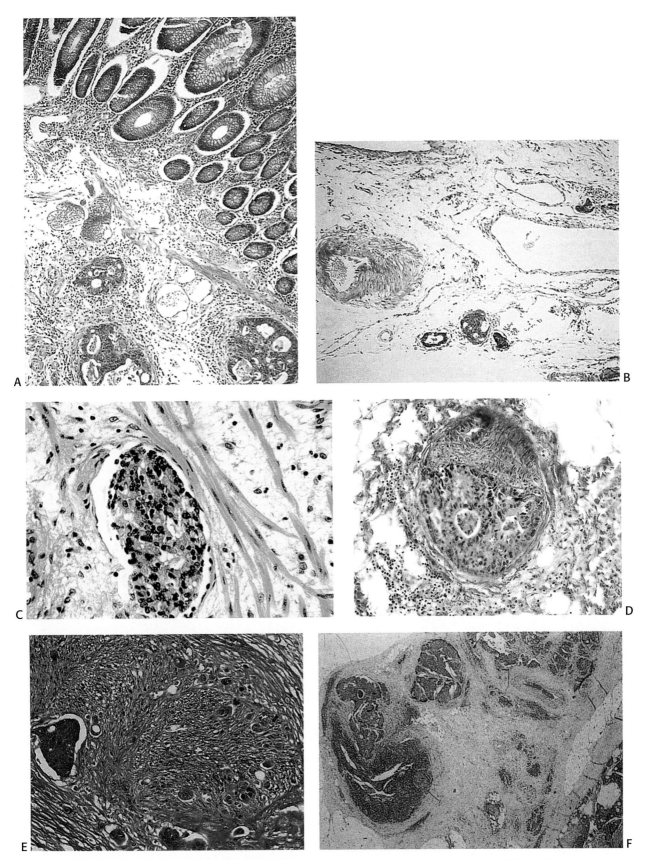

FIG. 14.130. Lymphatic involvement of tumor. **A:** Submucosal lymphatics are completely filled with tumor cells that underlie the normal mucosa adjacent to the tumor. **B:** Tumor in serosal lymphatics. **C:** Tumor cells in lymphatic at higher power. **D:** Perineural invasion. **E:** Perineural invasion. The nerve is stained brown with an antibody to neuron-specific enolase. **F:** Direct lymph node extension by carcinoma.

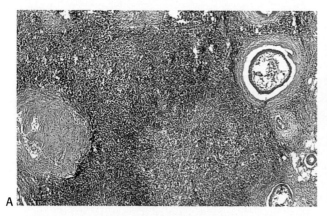

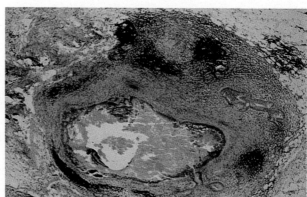

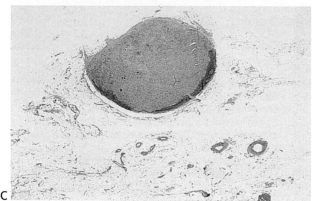

FIG. 14.131. Lymph node metastases. **A:** Isolated well-formed glands are present within the lymph node parenchyma. **B:** This lymph node contains pools of mucin partially lined by malignant cells. Much of the node has been replaced. **C:** Near-complete replacement of a lymph node by a poorly differentiated adeno-carcinoma.

increases with tumor stage and grade (439,440). Among 700 resected specimens examined by Morson and Dawson (431), 50% had tumor extension into intramural veins and 35% had permeation of extramural veins. Talbot et al (439) reported intramural blood vessel invasion in 31% of cases, with 69% of these being extramural. Minsky et al (441) showed that 61% of cases had intramural vascular invasion and 23% had extramural invasion. If elastic tissue or immunostains for actin are not used, blood vessel invasion will be correctly identified in only 16% to 41% of cases (441–443).

Venous involvement correlates with regional lymph node involvement and poor differentiation, and usually results in liver metastases. Venous invasion is present in 89.5% of patients with synchronous colorectal carcinoma and hepatic metastases and in 75% of individuals with metachronous hepatic metastases as compared to 15.4% of patients with Dukes C tumors who survive for 5 years without recurrence (444).

The distal rectum has a dual venous drainage. The regional vascular drainage of a growth in the upper third of the rectum occurs centrally along the course of the inferior mesenteric artery. In the lower rectum, there is an additional route along the middle rectal vessels. The middle and inferior hemorrhoidal veins pass through the pelvis and drain directly into the inferior vena cava. Therefore, distal rectal tumors are more likely to produce isolated pulmonary metastases than hepatic metastases (445). Bony metastases

involving the sacrum and vertebral bodies occur via the vertebral venous plexus of Batson (446).

The histologic features of venous invasion fall into three types: (a) tumor cells distinct from the vein walls (the floating type); (b) tumor cells filling the venous lumen, with or without a recanalized space in the center of the vein (i.e., the filling type); and (c) tumors growing in the lumen associated with a vascular thickening and an inflammatory reaction with its walls and the surrounding tissue (i.e., the occlusive type) (Fig. 14.134). The occlusive type of venous invasion may protect against subsequent recurrent disease, since inflammatory damage to the venous walls around the intravenous tumor appears to reduce the likelihood of distant metastases (444).

Perineural or Intraneural Spread

Another way a tumor spreads is via perineural or intraneural extension. Carcinomas may extend along perineural spaces for distances as great as 10 cm from the primary tumor (440). The incidence of perineural invasion varies from 14% to 32% (440,447) and increases with both tumor stage and grade.

Tumor Implantation

Implantation refers to the release of tumor cells from the primary tumor and their deposition on another surface. This

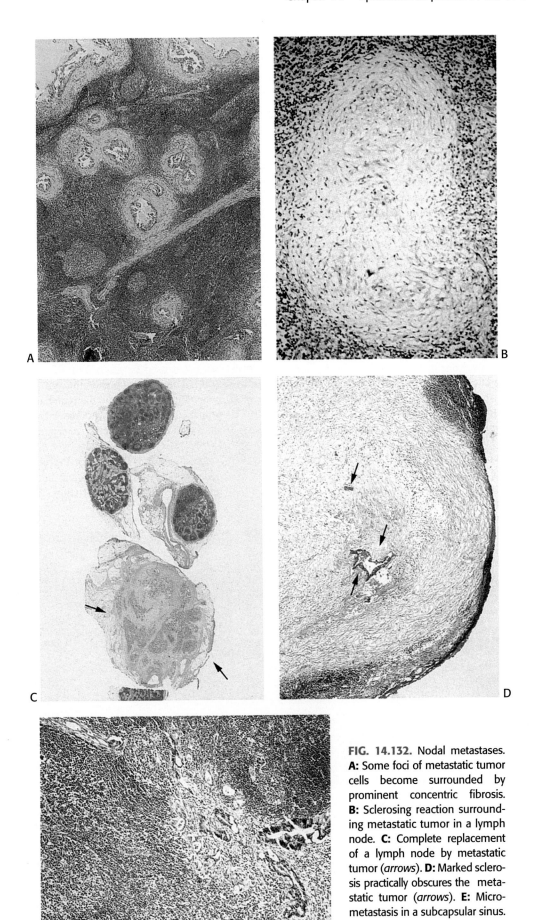

FIG. 14.132. Nodal metastases. **A:** Some foci of metastatic tumor cells become surrounded by prominent concentric fibrosis. **B:** Sclerosing reaction surrounding metastatic tumor in a lymph node. **C:** Complete replacement of a lymph node by metastatic tumor (*arrows*). **D:** Marked sclerosis practically obscures the metastatic tumor (*arrows*). **E:** Micrometastasis in a subcapsular sinus.

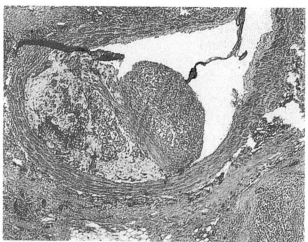

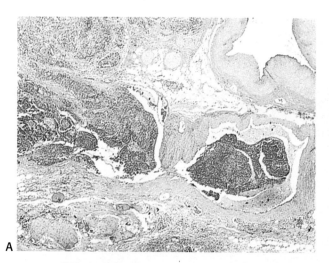

FIG. 14.133. Venous invasion. **A:** Venous invasion by carcinoma. **B:** A tumor thrombus is seen and attached to vessel wall.

occurs when exfoliated tumor cells are shed intraluminally or from the serosal surface into the peritoneum. Tumor implantation also results from surgical manipulations, when tumor cells deposit on wound surfaces (Fig. 14.135).

Experimentally, surgical trauma enhances tumor growth (448). Maximum enhancement occurs when the healing process has progressed between 2 and 8 days, with a peak between 5 and 7 days. A lesser growth enhancement occurs if

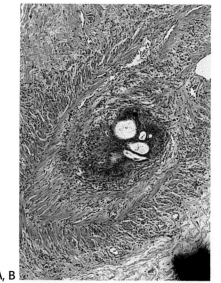

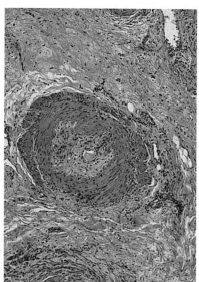

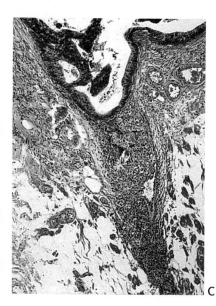

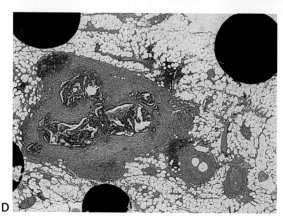

FIG. 14.134. Venous invasion. **A:** A tumor embolus is present in a medium-sized vein. The tumor cells fill the lumen of the vessel, and there is an associated inflammatory response extending into the vessel wall. **B:** Venous invasion with fibrosis and recanalization. The tumor cells are difficult to identify. **C:** Vascular invasion with associated inflammation. **D:** Adenocarcinoma with somewhat papillary architecture fills the vein lumen.

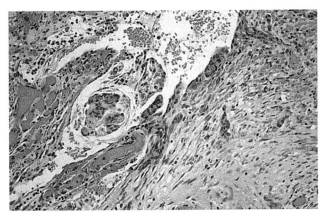

FIG. 14.135. Malignant cells within reactive tissue on the serosal surface of the colon following surgical resection.

TABLE 14.15	Incidence of Metastases in Colonic Versus Rectal Tumors	
Metastatic Sites	Colon Carcinoma	Rectal Carcinoma
Liver	75.5%	61.9%
Lung	47.7%	64.2%
Lymph nodes	77%	70.4%
Peritoneum	49.4%	25.4%
Adrenals	13.8%	18.7%
Ovary	17.3%	3.6%
Bone	11.7%	19.4%
Pleura	11.3%	12.7%
Brain	6.3%	8.2%
Kidney	5.0%	4.5%
Skin	5.0%	3.0%
Spleen	6.7%	2.2%

cells reach the anastomosis within 2 hours of its formation (448). The clinical implication is that enhanced tumor growth occurs in colonic anastomoses in the first few hours following surgery when tumor cells encounter healing tissues.

Suture line recurrences usually result from viable tumor cells in the bowel lumen that implant in fibrin present at the anastomotic site or via direct implantation by sutures. To prevent this, the surgeon will often ligate the area of bowel to be resected and irrigate it with tumoricidal agents. Retrograde lymphatic spread accounts for a few suture line recurrences. Anastomotic recurrences affect 0% to 36% of patients, with the variation resulting from differences in patient selection, operating techniques, and methods of follow-up evaluation (449–452).

Tumor implants may occur in abdominal or peritoneal wounds or at the anastomotic site. Tumor implants in abdominal wounds and colostomy sites usually result from contamination by a perforated tumor or from instruments and hands that have contacted the tumor.

Extranodal Metastases

Patients with colorectal carcinoma develop distant metastases. The liver is the primary site of hematogenous metastases, followed by the lung. Liver metastases are present at the time of diagnosis in 15% to 25% of patients and will develop in 60% of patients with progressive disease. Involvement of other sites, in the absence of liver or lung metastases, is rare. The incidence of metastases varies with tumor size and location (Table 14.15) and involvement of the regional lymph nodes. Overall, 75% to 77% of distant metastases involve the liver (Fig. 14.136) (431,453,454), 5% to 50% involve the lung (Fig. 14.137), and 5% to 8% involve the brain (431,455). Patients with liver metastases may show secondary metastases to lymph nodes draining the liver.

The incidence of bone metastases ranges from 0.96% to 11% (431,456). Rectal carcinomas metastasize to bones more frequently than colonic carcinomas (456) due to their venous drainage, since rectal tumors lie adjacent to the paravertebral

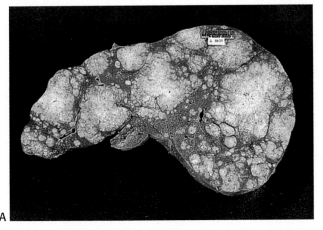
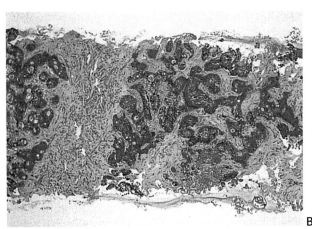

A   B

FIG. 14.136. Metastatic disease in the liver. **A:** Numerous large metastatic tumor nodules in liver. **B:** Needle biopsy of the liver containing metastatic colon cancer.

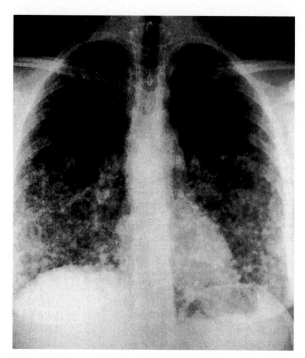

FIG. 14.137. Chest film demonstrates numerous metastases to both lungs from colonic adenocarcinoma.

venous plexus (Batson plexus). The distribution of bone metastasis is mainly to the vertebrae, followed by the pelvis. Patients with occult tumors may initially present with osseous metastases (457).

The most common secondary ovarian neoplasm to mimic an ovarian primary tumor is metastatic large intestinal adenocarcinoma. Approximately 40% of metastatic adenocarcinomas in the ovary originate from the colon. Ovarian metastases occur by hematogenous or peritoneal spread, or through seeding of contiguous structures and draining lymph nodes. Ovarian metastases affect 23% of women with colon cancer (458,459). Patients range in age from 47 to 80 years, with an average age of 60 years. Most patients have abdominal pain and a pelvic mass. One rare metastatic tumor stimulated estrogen production, which manifested as postmenopausal uterine bleeding (460).

The ovarian tumors and the large bowel carcinomas are discovered synchronously in 56% of cases; in 44% they are metachronous. Adenocarcinoma metastatic to ovaries has a very poor prognosis. Seventy percent of patients die within 1 to 19 months of detection (459). Tumors initially classified as Dukes B lesions and later found to have ovarian metastases have a worse prognosis than Dukes B lesions without ovarian metastases. Dukes A tumors do not metastasize to the ovary (461,462).

When colorectal tumors metastasize to the ovary, they frequently form large cystic or solid masses with smooth outer contours and the metastases are often unilateral, thus resembling primary endometrioid or mucinous ovarian adenocarcinomas (462). Most metastatic tumors show hemor-

rhage and necrosis. Both ovaries are involved in up to 50% of the cases.

The most characteristic microscopic features of ovarian metastases are garland and cribriform growth patterns, intraluminal necrosis, segmental destruction of glands, and absence of squamous metaplasia.

Less common metastatic sites include the spleen (463), biliary tract (464), pancreas, peripancreatic lymph nodes (465), adrenals (466), breast, testis (467), skin (468), umbilicus (469), oral cavity (470), vagina (471), epididymis (472), tracheobronchial tree (473), skeletal muscle (474), kidney, thyroid, ureter (475), left supraclavicular lymph nodes (476), heart (477), pericardium (478), gingiva (479), stomach, meninges (480), choroid (481), thumb (482), penis (483,484), and nail beds (485).

Intestinal Metastases

Autometastasis of colon cancers can occur, particularly among mucinous tumors (361). The metastases appear as mucosal polyps. In the patient reported by Buckmaster et al (361), the mucosa was studded by >100 uniform polyps measuring 0.5 to 1 cm. The mucosa between the polyps appeared normal. Histologically, the polyps contained metastatic signet ring cell carcinoma.

Colorectal Carcinoma Staging

All cancer staging systems seek to identify clinical and pathologic features that predict clinical outcome (prognosis) or, in some cases, guide therapy. Numerous schemes have been developed to stage colorectal carcinoma. The theme common to all staging systems is the depth of invasion into the bowel wall and the presence or absence of lymph node involvement. For decades, the Dukes classification scheme was the standard.

In 1932, Dukes (486) refined the Lockhart and Mummery classification devised in 1926 and established the staging system that bears his name. In that system, Dukes stage A tumors remained confined to the bowel wall (submucosa or muscularis propria) with no serosal invasion (486,487). Dukes stage B tumors extended through the muscularis propria to the serosa and beyond. Dukes stage C tumors exhibited metastases in regional lymph nodes. The Dukes original 3-year survival rates were 80%, 73%, and 7%, respectively, for A, B, and C lesions (486). In 1954, Denoix (488) proposed the TNM cancer classification system based on disease extent. Beahrs and Myers (489) adapted the TNM system. The TNM staging system has now been adopted by the Union International Contre Cancer (UICC) and the American Joint Commission on Cancer (AJCC).

Although no staging system is absolutely perfect, most today advocate the use of the AJCC/UICC TNM staging classification of colorectal cancer, and it is the system shown here in order to help promote its use on an international basis (Table 14.16). The TNM classification for carcinomas of the colon and rectum is compatible with the Dukes classification,

TABLE 14.16 **Staging for Colorectal Carcinoma—American Joint Committee on Cancer**

Primary Tumor (T)

TX	Primary tumor cannot be assessed
T0	No evidence of primary tumor
Tis	Carcinoma is situ (intraepithelial or invasion of lamina propria)[a]
T1	Tumor invades submucosa
T2	Tumor invades muscularis propria
T3	Tumor invades through the muscularis propria into the subserosa, or into nonperitonealized pericolic or perirectal tissues
T4	Tumor directly invades other organs or structures or perforates the visceral peritoneum[b,c]

Regional Lymph Nodes (N)

NX	Regional lymph nodes cannot be assessed
N0	No regional lymph node metastasis
N1	Metastasis in one to three regional lymph nodes
N2	Metastasis in four or more regional lymph nodes

Distant Metastasis (M)

MX	Presence of distant metastasis cannot be assessed
M0	No distant metastasis
M1	Distant metastasis

Stage Grouping

Stage	T	N	M	Dukes[d]
Stage 0	Tis	N0	M0	—
Stage I	T1	N0	M0	A
	T2	N0	M0	A
Stage IIA	T3	N0	M0	B
Stage IIB	T4	N0	M0	B
Stage IIIA	T1–2	N1	M0	C
Stage IIIB	T3–4	N1	M0	C
Stage IIIC	Any T	N2	M0	C
Stage IV	Any T	Any N	M1	D

Histopathologic Type

This staging classification applies to carcinomas that arise in the colon, rectum, or appendix. The classification does not apply to sarcomas, lymphomas, or carcinoid tumors of the large intestine or appendix. The histologic types include adenocarcinoma, mucinous carcinoma (colloid type) (>50% mucinous carcinoma), signet ring cell carcinoma (>50% signet ring cell), squamous cell carcinoma, adenosquamous carcinoma, small cell carcinoma, undifferentiated carcinoma, and carcinoma NOS.

[a] Tis includes cancer cells confined within the glandular basement membrane (intraepithelial) or lamina propria (intramucosal) with no extension through the muscularis mucosae into the submucosa.
[b] Direct invasion in T4 includes invasion of other segments of the colorectum by way of the serosa, for example, invasion of the sigmoid colon by carcinoma of the cecum.
[c] Tumor that is adherent to other organs or structures, macroscopically, is classified as T4. However, if no tumor is present in the adhesion, microscopically, the classification should be T3.
[d] Comparison with Dukes classification.

but it adds greater precision in the identification of some of the prognostic subgroups. Like the Dukes classification, the TNM classification is based on the depth of tumor invasion into the wall of the intestine, extension to adjacent structures, and the number of regional lymph nodes involved, as well as on the presence or absence of distant metastases. The TNM classification applies to both clinical and pathologic staging. However, most colorectal carcinomas are staged after pathologic examination of the resected specimen and surgical exploration of the abdomen (490).

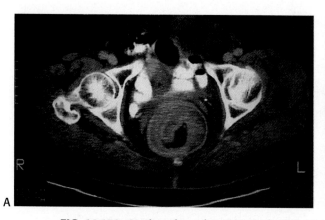 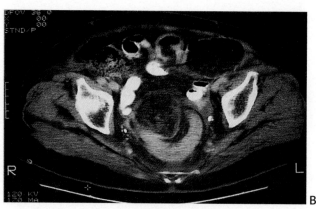

FIG. 14.138. Staging of rectal carcinoma. **A:** Computed tomographic scan demonstrates a rectal carcinoma that has produced an intussusception. **B:** At another level, a mass is present, which infiltrates into the perirectal soft tissue.

Once colorectal cancer has been confirmed by imaging studies and biopsy, it is important that one accurately stage the tumor. Preoperative staging aims to accurately assess tumor extent prior to treatment so that more precise treatment can be planned. This is usually done utilizing MRI, CT, and endosonography. Early reports suggested that CT was an excellent preoperative staging method because of its cross-sectional anatomic capabilities and its ability to detect metastases (491) (Fig. 14.138). Early studies reported accuracy rates of 85% to 90% (492,493); these were later revised to 50% to 75% (494–496). In general, sensitivity, specificity, and accuracy are higher in more advanced stages of the disease than in early cases. This is due to the inability of CT to accurately diagnose tumor microinvasion into the pericolonic fat or to determine the presence of metastatic tumor in normal-sized lymph nodes.

Because of their fixed position in the pelvis, the rectum and sigmoid are particularly well suited to CT evaluation. Tumors in the ascending and descending colon are also readily evaluated because of their usually fixed position. Tumors of the flexures, transverse colon, and sigmoid are less easily examined by CT because of the interference from colonic peristalsis and diaphragmatic excursions. MRI suffers from some of the same limitations as CT (495,497).

Rectal cancers are often staged utilizing endoscopic ultrasound (EUS) (Fig. 14.139). Indications for EUS in the management of rectal lesions are as follows: (a) to determine the suitability of large polyps or small rectal cancers for endoscopic mucosal resection or transanal excision, (b) to determine whether preoperative chemotherapy and radiation are needed for larger rectal lesions, and (c) for surveillance after surgery for rectal cancer (498). EUS is more accurate than pelvic CT or MRI in defining the depth of tumor invasion (498–501). EUS detects tumor penetration beyond the muscularis propria (T3 disease), with an accuracy of 70% to 90%

in most series (502–505), but may overstage T2 lesions as a result of inflammatory and desmoplastic reactions or retraction of the muscularis propria in earlier stage lesions (506). EUS is also not as sensitive in detecting local lymph node involvement as it is in assessing depth of tumor invasion. The accuracy is 70% to 75%, still greater than that for CT or MRI (507). EUS-guided fine needle aspiration of suspicious-appearing nodes may improve the accuracy of lymph node staging (508). Previous radiotherapy may alter the endosonographic staging of rectal cancer and hamper radiographic interpretations (509).

Intraoperative laparoscopic ultrasonography may be used to aid in the detection of liver metastases in patients with colorectal cancer and, therefore, may increase the accuracy of intraoperative staging.

Detection of Recurrent Cancer

After therapy, patients may undergo special imaging studies to identify local tumor recurrence or secondary tumor growth elsewhere, especially in patients with rising CEA levels (510,511). CT, positron emission tomography (PET)-CT, and MRI are useful in detecting recurrent colorectal carcinomas, especially following abdominal peritoneal resection. These techniques can detect recurrent tumor at a time when the patient is still asymptomatic and CEA levels are still normal (512). The limitations of CT in detecting recurrent tumor resemble those seen in preoperative staging (i.e., the inability to detect microscopic invasion of pericolonic or perirectal fat and the inability to detect tumor in normal-sized lymph nodes).

Prognosis

Many factors influence the prognosis of patients with colorectal cancer, including the presence of pre-existing diseases such as familial polyposis, ulcerative colitis, or HNPCC, as

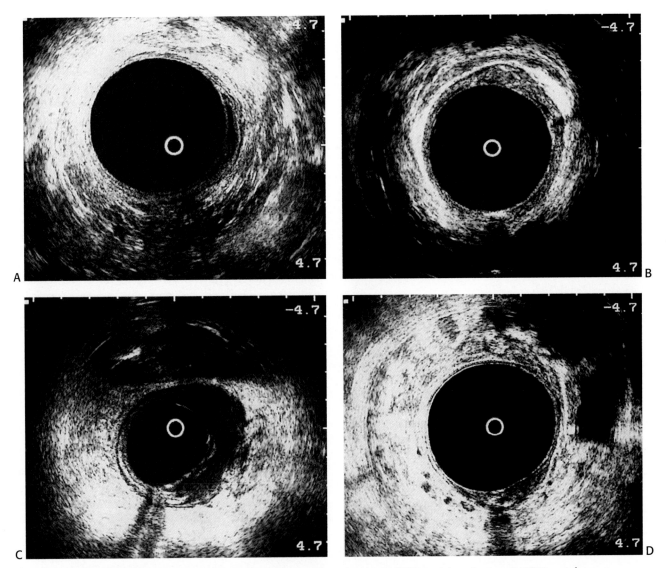

FIG. 14.139. Transrectal ultrasound. **A:** T1N0 rectal carcinoma. **B:** T2N0 rectal carcinoma. **C:** T3N0 rectal carcinoma. **D:** T3N1 rectal carcinoma. (Photographs courtesy of Dr. Janice Rafferty, Department of Surgery, University of Cincinnati, Cincinnati, OH.)

well as tumor growth characteristics, including the presence of vascular or lymphatic invasion, tumor size and grade, and, to some extent, the method and extent of treatment. Patient sex, tumor site within the colon, and the presence of perforation or obstruction also affect prognosis (428,450,513–519). Prognostic factors are listed in Table 14.17.

Prognostic variables fall into several categories: Those that are proven, those that are probable, and those that are not yet established. Prognostic factors considered to be proven include tumor stage and grade, the presence of vascular invasion, and the status of the radial margins. Probable prognostic factors include tumor site, tumor perforation or obstruction, lymphatic and perineural invasion, histologic patterns of lateral tumor margins, and peritumoral lymphoid cells or lymphoid aggregates. The most important prognostic factor is the pathologic extent of disease (tumor stage).

Tumor Stage

The most significant prognostic feature is the degree of bowel wall penetration by a tumor (Figs. 14.140 and 14.141), the presence or absence of lymph node metastases, and the presence or absence of distant metastases. The former is most accurately assessed by histologic examination of full-thickness sections of the tumor obtained from the deepest area of tumor penetration into the bowel wall. The overall 5-year survival rate among patients with localized disease, regional disease, and distant metastasis is 91.8%, 65.8%, and 8.8%, respectively (371).

By Cox multivariate analysis, the number of positive lymph nodes remains the best discriminant of survival. The cutoff of the number of nodes that need to be positive before a prognostic difference is seen differs from three to six

TABLE 14.17	Prognostic Factors for Colorectal Carcinoma

Pathologic Factors

Tumor stage
Extent of local invasion of carcinoma
Lymph node metastasis
Number of lymph nodes with metastasis
Distant metastasis
Type of carcinoma
Growth pattern of carcinoma
Margin from tumor
Radial margins
Nature of invasive margin
Grade of differentiation of carcinoma
Vascular permeation by carcinoma
Perineural invasion by carcinoma
Serosal involvement by carcinoma
Intraperitoneal spread
Inflammatory reaction to carcinoma
Lymph node reaction
Tumor location
Fibrosis in carcinoma
Location of carcinoma
Size and shape of carcinoma
Proliferation status
DNA ploidy of carcinoma
Extent of treatment

Clinical Factors

Age of patient
Sex of patient
Symptoms and their duration
Presence of perforation or obstruction
Serum carcinoembryonic antigen level

(450,514,520). In one study, survival fell to 60% when one to four lymph nodes were involved and to 20% when more than five were involved (431). The ratio of the number of involved nodes to the number of nodes examined may be an even better predictor of prognosis (432,435).

The concept of tumor staging is likely to change sometime in the future, by incorporating either the concept of minimal residual disease (i.e., the detection of micrometastases) or the potential of "molecular upstaging." "Molecular upstaging" might occur if a specific prognostic factor identifies patients in a lower stage whose tumors are likely to behave in a manner analogous to higher stage lesions. Both the "molecular upstaging" and the detection of minimal residual disease may allow patients to be selected for systemic therapy at an earlier stage when the metastatic burden is low and presumably the disease more treatable and may lead to new staging systems.

Histologic Grade and Type

Tumor differentiation (histologic grade) is next in importance prognostically (521) since, regardless of the depth of tumor invasion, poorly differentiated adenocarcinomas

associate with lymph node metastases in >50% of cases. In contrast, moderately differentiated and well-differentiated tumors have fewer lymph node metastases (522). Grade also correlates with the likelihood of venous and local spread, as well as lymphatic and bowel wall penetration (487,450).

Tumor type also influences prognosis. Among the various histologic subtypes of colon cancer, mucinous carcinomas, small cell carcinomas, and signet ring cell carcinomas demonstrate a much worse prognosis than ordinary adenocarcinomas (358,523).

Tumor Location

Disparate findings exist concerning the influence of tumor location and patient prognosis. This probably results from the impact of various genetic syndromes that predispose patients to develop carcinomas in either the left or right side of the colon. Generally, it is said that the 5-year survival is lower for patients with colon cancers at or below the peritoneal reflection compared to those arising above the reflection (429,524). The majority of late recurrences are also found in tumors arising in the descending colon, sigmoid colon, and rectum. In one large study, carcinomas of the left colon had the most favorable prognosis, whereas those situated in the sigmoid and rectum had a worse outcome (525).

Gross Growth Pattern

Ulcerated as opposed to polypoid or sessile, exophytic cancers have a poorer prognosis and are more likely to spread locally and distantly (83% vs. 45% vs. 38%, respectively) (450,521,536). These statistics result from the fact that exophytic tumors have a lower frequency of mural penetration when compared with ulcerating tumors (24% vs. 39% to 46%) (450). There are also fewer hematogenous metastases (23% vs. 31%) in exophytic tumors. In contrast, flat carcinomas are more frequently deeply invasive when compared with polypoid cancers (67% vs. 23%) and exhibit lymphatic invasion more often (41% vs. 16%) (527,528).

Tumor Multiplicity

The prognosis in patients with multiple carcinomas depends on factors found in individual tumors. Tumor multiplicity by itself does not impact survival. Survival relates to the most adverse factors found in any one tumor.

Tumor Margins

Because some tumors spread laterally in the bowel wall, surgeons must be careful to resect the lesions in a way that does not leave residual tumor in the proximal and distal margins of resection. Were tumor to remain, the patient would be likely to develop a local recurrence at the anastomotic site. Rectal tumors, resected with a short distal margin of grossly normal tissue (low anterior resection), are especially prone to local recurrence due to the presence of intramural extension.

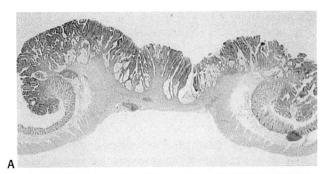

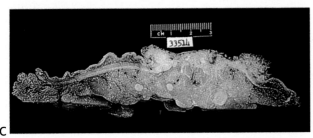

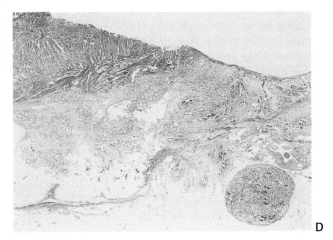

FIG. 14.140. Cross section through the bowel wall demonstrating the presence of invasive tumor. **A:** A well-differentiated carcinoma arising in an adenoma is seen. It extends to the muscularis propria but does not invade through it. **B:** Tumor invading the muscularis propria. **C:** Cross section through the bowel demonstrating the presence of an invasive tumor and tumor metastatic to the lymph nodes (*white spots* in adipose tissue). **D:** Whole mount section of the Dukes C lesion.

The nature of the tumor margins affects recurrence rate, and the nature of an adequate resection margin for colorectal carcinoma has been debated for years. Devereux and Deckers (529) followed 214 patients for a minimum of 2 years and found that a surgical margin of >5 cm associated with a 9% anastomotic recurrence rate in Dukes stage B lesions. Those with tumor margins measuring <5 cm had a 43% recurrence rate. Among Dukes stage C lesions, there was a 17% anastomotic recurrence rate whether the margins were shorter or longer than 5 cm (529). The only exception to this

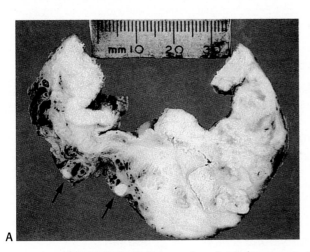

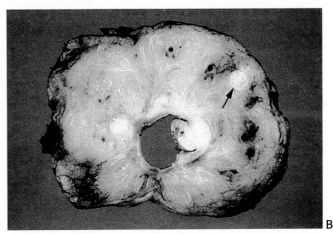

FIG. 14.141. Radial margins of rectal cancer. **A:** The tumor has completely destroyed the bowel wall and extends into the pericolic adipose tissue. A lymph node is present, which contains metastatic tumor. Tumor extends to the radial margin, which is inked. **B:** Strands of tumor infiltrate the pericolic fat in this section. Tumor is not present in the radial margin, but a pericolonic lymph node is positive and lies close to the radial margin. (Photographs courtesy of Dr. Geraint Williams, Department of Pathology, Coleg Meddygaeth Prifysgol Cymru, University of Wales College of Medicine, Health Park, Cardiff CF4 4XN, UK.)

is when satellite lesions develop and are grossly visible on the mucosal surface. Thus, it appears that 5 cm constitutes an adequate resection margin in Dukes stage B and C colorectal cancers. However, in the rectum, one may not have the luxury of such distances, and then one might wish to take advantage of the fact that most tumors do not extend further than 2 cm, unless they are already advanced lesions (422,424).

Radial Margins

In rectal cancer, local spread beyond the bowel wall is a proven prognostic determinant (487,530). Any involvement of the mesorectal (deep radial or circumferential) margin strongly predicts subsequent local recurrence (531–534). In fact, these margins may be more important than the lateral margins in determining prognosis. Local failure is more likely to occur in patients with positive radial margins compared with those with negative radial margins (85% vs. 3%). Twenty to thirty-three percent of patients with rectal cancer who have negative proximal and distal longitudinal margins have positive radial margins (530–534). Five-year survival is significantly greater in patients with <4 mm of mesorectal spread than in those with >4 mm of mesorectal spread (55% vs. 25%). Mesorectal spread is a prognostic factor that is independent of the presence of lymph node metastases (530). There are also significant differences in survival in patients with either Dukes B or C tumors with slight and extensive mesorectal spread (66% vs. 37% and 30% vs. 18%, respectively).

Lymphatic Permeation

An increasing degree of lymphatic invasion associates with a lower survival (430,535,536), and the degree of lymphatic invasion increases with tumor stage and grade (428,429, 484,486). However, by proportional hazards analysis, Minsky et al (430) demonstrated that the presence of lymphatic invasion is an independent prognostic factor for survival. The presence of lymphatic invasion also correlates with local recurrence rate (429).

Venous Invasion

The literature contains inconsistent results with respect to the impact of venous invasion on the presence of visceral metastasis, survival, and tumor recurrence. This is due, in part, to inconsistent ways of identifying venous spread. The presence of extramural invasion and thick-walled veins portends a worse prognosis than intramural invasion (169,439). A strong correlation exists between the presence of tumor in extramural veins and death due to metastatic disease. The incidence of blood vessel invasion increases with tumor grade and stage. Patients whose tumors have vascular invasion show a significant decrease in survival (74% in blood vessel–positive tumors vs. 85% in blood vessel–negative

tumors) (441,537). Actuarial survival significantly further decreases in patients with extramural vascular invasion from 72% to 35% (441). Blood vessel invasion is an independent prognostic factor for survival in some studies (442,447, 538,539) but not in others (441,540).

Aneurysmal distension; inflammatory damage of the walls of invaded veins, a thrombus cap, or endothelial cell mantle covering intravenous tumor; and a clearly defined stroma in the intravenous growth all appear to exert a protective effect on patient survival, whereas permeation of capillaries in the venous walls, the presence of loose clumps of tumor cells in the veins, and direct contact between the tumor cells and venous blood appear to adversely impact survival (439).

Perineural Invasion

The incidence of perineural invasion significantly increases in stage III tumors, and a significant difference exists in local recurrence rates and 8-year survival rates between patients with stage III lesions with perineural invasion and patients with stage III lesions without perineural invasion (540). Patients with perineural invasion also have more local recurrences in anastomotic sites than those without it. The 5-year actuarial survival is also lower in patients with perineural invasion than in those without it (7% vs. 35%) (447,541).

Obstruction and Perforation

Obstruction and perforation may reduce patient survival (526,542–544). Patients with large bowel carcinomas that present with complete obstruction have a decreased 5-year survival, even within the same stage (526,543). When the perforation results from extensive tumor invasion of the bowel wall, the patients exhibit very poor prognosis (526). When tumors perforate freely into the peritoneal cavity, virtually no patient survives (542).

Nature of the Invasive Margin

Patients who have tumors with pushing, rather than infiltrating, margins have a better prognosis (86% vs. 14%) (544). Those tumors that diffusely infiltrate the neighboring tissue exhibit a worsened prognosis (545). The presence of a poorly defined tumor border, the lack of an inflammatory reaction, and the presence of pronounced fibrosis (desmoplasia) associate with an unfavorable stage distribution.

Peritumoral Lymphocytic Infiltration

Patients whose tumors show a prominent peritumoral lymphocytic infiltrate, the cuff of mononuclear cells that borders the leading edge of invasive colorectal carcinomas, have an improved survival (544,546,547).

Crohn-like Lymphoid Reaction

The presence of lymphoid aggregates within the muscularis propria or pericolic fibrous adipose tissue in patients with invasive carcinomas has been termed a *Crohn-like lymphoid reaction* and it correlates with an improved survival (340,546).

Reactive Lymph Nodes

A number of investigators have shown that an apparent immunologic response in the draining lymph nodes correlates with improved survival in patients with colorectal cancer (452,548,549). An even greater increase in survival is present when sinus histiocytosis coexists with a local inflammatory reaction to the tumor in its primary location (548). Paracortical lymphoid hyperplasia also appears to correlate with an improved prognosis (452), whereas reactive germinal centers do not (548).

Presence of Residual Disease

Survival estimates in patients who have gross residual disease following surgical resection is 8% at 3 years and 0% at 5 years. Statistically significant factors relative to survival include the amount of residual tumor (microscopic vs. gross), treatment method, intraoperative electron beam irradiation (IORT) versus no IORT, and the type of resection (550).

Peritoneal and Serosal Involvement

Local peritoneal involvement is a strong predictor of intraperitoneal recurrence or persistent and pelvic recurrence, and it may predict local recurrence after surgery for upper and middle rectal carcinomas (532). It significantly associates with palliative surgery, extent of local spread, and mucinous subtype. The prognostic significance of local spread beyond the bowel wall, particularly to serosal surfaces, is less well studied. Several staging systems, including the TNM classification, include serosal involvement as a prognostic stage (518,519). Patients with free-lying tumor cells are more likely to have intraperitoneal recurrences and/or persistence than those with local peritoneal involvement.

DNA Content

Increasing proliferation and DNA abnormalities accompany the progression of colorectal carcinomas from adenomas (551). Aneuploidy is a consistent finding in colorectal carcinomas (Fig. 14.142) (551–553), ranging in incidence from 46% to 93% (554–558). The frequency of aneuploidy increases with tumor stage.

Populations of aneuploid cells also exist in the histologically normal mucosa adjacent to colorectal cancers. In one study, 62% of colorectal cancers were aneuploid and 48% were associated with an adjacent aneuploid, nonneoplastic mucosa. Mucosa adjacent to diploid cancers only had diploid characteristics. These changes were observed for distances as

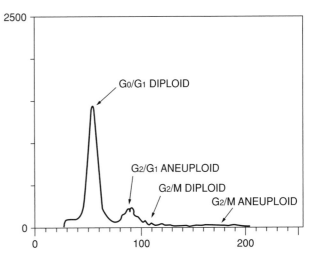

FIG. 14.142. Flow cytometric evaluation of ploidy in colon cancer. A large population of diploid cells is present, probably representing a combination of normal mucosa, stroma, and inflammatory cells. A smaller aneuploid peak represents that at least a proportion of the tumor cells is present.

large as 10 cm from the primary tumor. Histologically, the mucosa generally displays diffuse, generally mild, and reactive mucosal abnormalities. These findings suggest the presence of a field effect (556).

Some studies have demonstrated that DNA aneuploidy associates with decreased survival following surgery (559–565), although in multivariate analysis, only two recent studies have demonstrated ploidy to represent an independent prognostic variable. Other studies have shown no impact of ploidy on prognosis (566–572). As a result, the recent American Society of Clinical Oncology (ASCO) does not recommend that ploidy analysis be performed in the workup of patients with colorectal cancer (573).

Molecular Alterations

Among the various molecular alterations that exist in colorectal carcinoma, none has been unequivocally shown to be of clinical utility in determining prognosis or guiding therapy. As a result, current ASCO guidelines do not recommend the use of microsatellite instability, *ras* mutation, *p53* mutation, or chromosome 18q loss of heterozygosity analysis for assessing prognosis or guiding therapy in colorectal cancer (573).

Patient Variables

Patient Age

Data with respect to patient age and prognosis are conflicting, especially in young people. Very elderly patients often present emergently and therefore undergo emergency surgeries, which have a higher mortality rate than elective surgeries (574). Young individuals, particularly children, also are believed to have a very poor prognosis. Explanations for this include a large number of mucinous adenocarcinomas (309,315,575) and a delay in the diagnosis of the disease, resulting in late-stage disease. Fifty-three percent of young patients have high-grade tumors compared with only 20% of older patients (575). However, when stage-adjusted survival is analyzed, other reports suggest that there is no difference in relative prognosis for younger age patients (306,316,576,577). Some even suggest that colorectal cancer patients younger than 40 years of age have an even better prognosis than older patients, if all tumors are considered irrespective of their histopathologic diagnosis (578). The discrepancy in outcome may result from the inclusion of young individuals with HNPCC (see Chapter 12).

Gender

In some studies, women tend to have a more favorable prognosis than men (443,579,580), but other studies do not confirm this (581).

Race

Colorectal cancer staging shows that African American and non-Hispanic white low-income patients have higher stages of both colon and rectal cancers (285). In 1974 to 1976, the black–white difference in 5-year survival rates for all stages combined was 5% (45% in blacks and 50% in whites). In 1986 to 1991, it widened to a statistically significant 10% difference (52% in blacks and 62% in whites) (582). Currently, the difference in mortality from colorectal cancer in African Americans versus Caucasian Americans remains at approximately 10% (2). Some factors related to the higher stage of disease relate to decreased access to health care. However, even when patients are compared stage for stage, 5-year survival rates still differ. This may be related, in part, to the fact that blacks are less likely to have an associated lymphoid reaction compared with whites (582). Other pathologic findings, such as differences in blood vessel, lymphatic invasion, necrosis, and mucinous type of histology, did not account for the difference in another study (582).

Presence of Symptoms

Patients in whom colorectal cancer is detected by screening techniques tend to be treated at an earlier age and, therefore, have an improved chance of cure. This, in fact, has resulted in a decline in colon cancer–associated deaths. Symptomatic patients tend to have a poorer survival than asymptomatic patients. Hemorrhage and/or rectal bleeding associate with an improved prognosis, perhaps due to mucosal erosions that manifest early and lead to early interventions (526). However, these findings are controversial (523,526).

Treatment

While it is not the intent of this book to provide extensive discussions of therapy, it is important for pathologists to have an understanding of the therapeutic options as well as the therapeutic procedures so that they can be more knowledgeable in their evaluation of biopsies and/or resection specimens. The treatment of malignant tumors depends on sev-

eral factors. The first is the presence or absence of disseminated disease, and the second is the probability of local recurrence. These are determined by pathologic factors that relate to the clinical stage of the tumor.

Colonic Resection

The standard therapy for colorectal carcinomas is surgical resection. The type of surgery performed depends on the site and extent of the tumor, and on the anatomy and the lymphatic drainage patterns (Fig. 14.143). Extensive resections may cure patients who would die if only less radical surgery were performed (583). Carcinomas of the ascending colon and cecum are treated by ileocolectomy. Tumors located beneath the peritoneal reflection are treated by an abdominal perineal resection. Carcinomas arising in other portions of the large bowel are treated by anterior resection.

The surgical treatment requires excision of an adequate amount of normal colon proximal and distal to the tumor and adequate lateral margins if the tumor is adherent to a contiguous structure. It also requires adequate removal of the regional lymph nodes. Lymphadenectomy not only is necessary for staging, but it also serves as a therapeutic procedure. Removal of intermediate and more central (principal) lymph nodes requires ligation and division of multiple main vascular trunks.

Extended resections may also be done in individuals who have cancers that extend into adjacent organs, such as the duodenum or the pancreatic head. En bloc resection, with the achievement of tumor-free margins, can afford long-term survival advantages to such patients (584). Small segmental resections with the removal of only the paracolic lymph nodes are usually reserved for patients who are medically poor risks or individuals who already have evidence of liver metastasis or peritoneal seeding. For patients with obstructing carcinomas, staged procedures are generally accepted.

Preoperative colonoscopy is essential for optimal surgical management of patients with colorectal cancer because it detects synchronous neoplasms that can be removed at the time of surgery. The planned surgical approach is tailored to the colonoscopic findings. Subtotal colectomy is the procedure of choice in the management of patients with polyposis syndromes, HNPCC, and synchronous colon cancers, and it is generally thought to be the primary procedure when cancer of the colon is associated with synchronous adenomatous polyps in areas other than those normally included within the scope of the regional operation. Other possible indications for subtotal colectomy include previous transverse colostomy for obstruction, associated severe diverticular disease, and age younger than 50 years with a positive family history.

Resection of Rectal Lesions

The surgical strategy differs in the three parts of the rectum and depends on the endosonographic or CT-determined tumor stage (Table 14.18) and tumor differentiation (585).

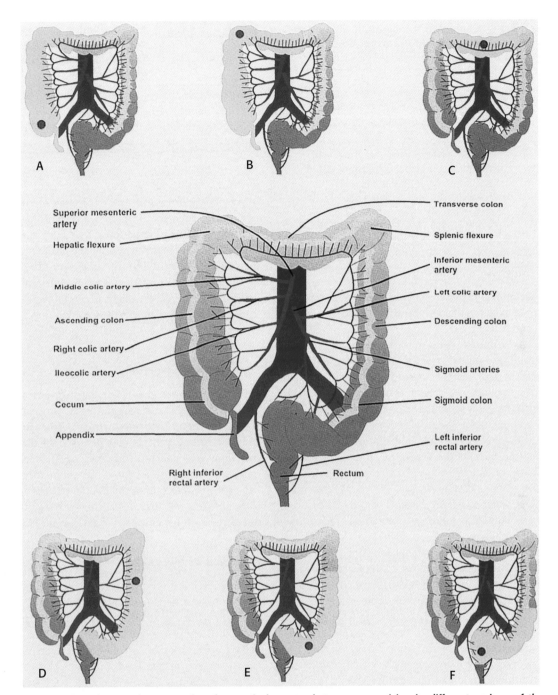

FIG. 14.143. Diagram demonstrating the surgical approach to cancers arising in different regions of the colon. The cancers are represented in *green* and the extent of the resections in *yellow*.

The treatment options for those tumors that lie below the peritoneal reflection (the extraperitoneal rectum) differ from those that lie above the peritoneal reflection (intraperitoneal rectum). Patients with tumors arising in the intra-abdominal rectum are treated in a manner similar to those with a more proximal colonic tumor.

The rectum is typically divided into thirds:

1. Upper third—Tumors arising in the upper third have their lower edge 11 to 12 cm from the anal verge. These lesions are usually removed by anterior or low anterior resection followed by restoration of bowel continuity via an end-to-end or side-to-end anastomosis.
2. Middle third—Cancers arising in the middle third of the rectum arise 6 to 11 cm from the anal verge. These patients may undergo abdominal perineal resection with permanent colostomy, but this does not yield superior results to those achieved with sphincter-saving surgical treatments for the same types of tumors (586). Thus, every effort is usually made to restore intestinal continuity for patients with cancers. The success of this procedure depends on the expertise of the surgeon and patient

TABLE 14.18   **Computed Tomographic Staging of Primary and Recurrent Colonic Tumors**

Stage I	Intraluminal mass without thickening of colon wall
Stage II	Thickened colon wall (>5 mm) or pelvic mass without invasion of adjacent structures or extension to pelvic sidewalls
Stage IIIA	Thickened colon wall or pelvic mass with invasion of adjacent structures but not to pelvic sidewalls or abdominal wall
Stage IIIB	Thickened colon wall or pelvic mass extending to pelvic sidewalls and/or abdominal wall without distant metastases
Stage IV	Metastatic disease with or without local abnormality

TABLE 14.19   **Adverse Pathologic Features Requiring Potential Additional Therapy Following Local Excision of Rectal Tumors**

Tumor budding—moderate to poor differentiation
Poorly demarcated in base of front
Tumor extension—to the middle or deep submucosa
Lymphatic invasion

factors, including the presence of associated disorders, the presence of collateral blood flow, prostatic size, body habitus, and pelvic width.

3. Lower third—Tumors arising in the lower 5 cm of the rectum require abdominal perineal resection. Abdominal sacral resection or stapled low anterior resections are sometimes feasible, and restorative proctectomy with coloanal anastomosis is used in selected patients (587).

Patients with early lesions may undergo local procedures, including full-thickness local excision, fulguration, endocavitary irradiation, or brachytherapy. Local excision alone can be performed endoscopically, transanally, transsphincterally, transsacrally, or transcoccygeally. Patients who have advanced rectal cancers may also undergo nonradical therapeutic approaches, including local excision, fulguration, cryosurgery, or endocavitary radiation. These patients usually have advanced local disease that would necessitate resection of a nearby adjacent vital structure or are medically high-risk patients (588).

One of the most important features concerning limited treatment is appropriate case selection, since smaller, lower grade tumors that are T1 or early T2 have the best results. Pretreatment staging plays an important role in selecting the patients for conservative management. Key factors to determine are (a) tumor differentiation, (b) tumor depth (T classification), and (c) lymph node status (N classification). Biopsy, endorectal ultrasound, and pelvic CT, as well as MRI, are used to aid in this assessment. The tumors should be small, superficial, and well differentiated (589,590). Well-differentiated T1 and T2 rectal lesions, particularly those measuring <3 cm in diameter, may be managed by local excision. In contrast, moderately or poorly differentiated T1 and T2 tumors, regardless of their size, are managed best by radical techniques (591). When adverse pathologic features are found in a local excision specimen (Table 14.19), the disease-free survival is improved by immediate surgical salvage as opposed to salvage resection at the time of a clinical recurrence (94% vs. 56%) (592). The implication of these localized therapeutic approaches is that the pathologist is likely to be called upon

to provide careful assessment of biopsies of low rectal lesions in order to identify the presence of lymphatic or vascular invasion or histologic patterns that may associate with an adverse outcome. Similarly, once the limited resection specimen has been received in the laboratory, the pathologist will be called upon to provide an accurate determination of the presence of factors that might necessitate additional surgery. These include involvement of deep margins, the presence of lymphatic or vascular invasion, and poor differentiation.

Laparoscopic Colectomy

Laparoscopic approaches have gained acceptance due to a possible reduction in the major stresses associated with major abdominal surgery and to initiatives designed to hasten patient convalescence. Recent studies have shown that laparoscopic colectomy is as safe and efficacious as open colectomy in the treatment of many patients with colon cancer (593–595). Laparoscopic resection of small rectal cancers may also be feasible, but data are currently lacking with regard to use of this technique for more advanced rectal lesions (593,595).

Resection of Metastatic Lesions

Hepatic resection for colorectal carcinoma metastases is the most common hepatic operation performed in the United States, and the operation is likely to become more prevalent (596,597). However, only 8% to 27% of all patients with hepatic metastases from colorectal cancers are suitable for hepatic resection. Selection of patients likely to benefit from surgery remains controversial and subjective. Survival is affected by patient age, size of the largest metastasis, CEA levels, stage of the primary tumor, disease-free interval, number of liver nodules, and status of the resection margins (598,599). Patients should have clear resection margins of >1 cm (600).

In the absence of nodal disease or direct invasion, patients with unilobar solitary tumors of any size or unilobar multiple tumors (less than four) of <2 cm (stages I and II) have the highest survival rates. Survival estimates of 95%, 65%, and 49% at 1, 3, and 5 years, respectively, following hepatic resections have been observed in patients when all gross metastatic tumor was removed (600,601). Patients with bilobar involvement (multiple tumors of any size or a large single metastasis [stage IVa]) have survival rates of 88%, 28%,

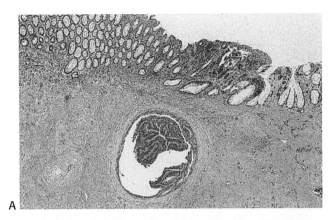

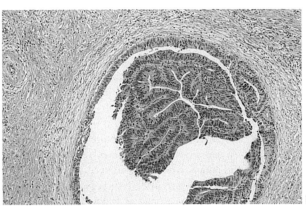

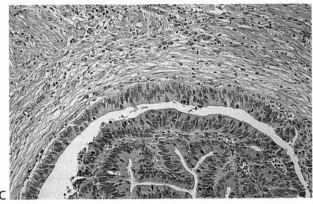

FIG. 14.144. Effects of preoperative radiation. **A:** Low-power view demonstrating a small focus of residual well-differentiated adenocarcinoma. The surrounding stroma is fibrotic, and the overlying colonic mucosa shows radiation damage. **B:** Higher-power view of the adenocarcinoma. The tumor is surrounded by desmoplastic, reactive stroma. **C:** Higher-power view of the carcinoma.

and 20% at 1, 3, and 5 years, respectively. Patients with nodal involvement or extrahepatic disease (stage IVb) experience the poorest outcome, with 1-, 3-, and 5-year survival rates of 80%, 12%, and 0%, respectively (600,602).

Chemotherapy

An important advance in cancer treatment was made when it was found that adjuvant therapy significantly improves the survival of patients with colorectal cancer. In the 1980s, adjuvant 5-fluorouracil (5-FU) was shown to decrease the risk of colorectal cancer recurrence, and since that time 5-FU with leucovorin became the mainstay in the postoperative treatment of patients with stage III colorectal cancer (603–610). More recently, the addition of oxaliplatin to 5-FU/leucovorin has been shown to improve disease-free survival among stage III colon cancer patients (611,612). The benefit of adjuvant treatment for stage II patients is still debated, and most reserve chemotherapy for stage II patients at high risk for recurrent disease (613,614).

Hepatic Arterial Infusion

Unlike portal vein infusion of chemotherapeutic agents, hepatic arterial infusion is designed to treat metastatic disease in the liver. Hepatic metastases derive their blood supply from the hepatic artery. In contrast, hepatocytes are nourished by the portal circulation. Hepatic arterial infusion

chemotherapy maximizes tumor exposure to the drug, thereby minimizing systemic toxicity. A number of trials have demonstrated significantly higher response rates (40% to 60% for intra-arterial therapy compared with 10% to 20% for systemic drug administration), but none has revealed substantial survival benefits (615–619).

Radiotherapy

Radiotherapy plays a role in the management of some colorectal cancers (620), and its role is especially well established in rectal cancers. Radiotherapy may be used preoperatively, postoperatively, or to treat recurrent disease.

Preoperative Chemoradiation

Preoperative radiation combined with 5-FU administration followed by either local excision or radical resection allows sphincter preservation in many patients with locally advanced rectal tumors (621,622). In addition, this treatment improved rates of local tumor recurrence and decreased acute and long-term toxicity of adjuvant chemotherapy (622). As a result, pathologists often receive resection specimens from patients who have been treated preoperatively. In such specimens, residual tumor may be difficult to detect grossly, and lymph nodes may be small and hard to find. If tumor is present, it may show radiation effects (Fig. 14.144) as may the surrounding tissues (Fig. 14.145).

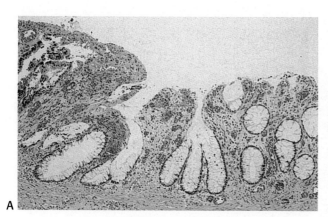
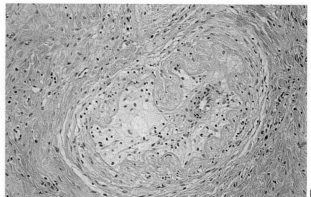

FIG. 14.145. Radiation effects. **A:** Colonic mucosa overlying a rectal cancer treated with preoperative radiation. The mucosa shows architectural distortion and changes closely resembling ischemia. **B:** Submucosal vessel with intimal thickening secondary to radiation damage. The vessel contains the foamy histiocytes typical of radiation injury.

Adjuvant Radiotherapy

Adjuvant pelvic radiation reduces local recurrence after conventional resection, particularly when it is used in combination with 5-FU–based chemotherapy after resection of transmural (T3 and T4) and node-positive (N1, N2, and N3) tumors (621). Older patients may tolerate radiation less well than younger ones and may be at increased risk for radiation-related small bowel damage, so the radiation therapist should pay attention to techniques that limit the amount of small bowel in the irradiated field (623).

Local Recurrence

Recurrences correlate with tumor stage, the number of lymph nodes affected by metastases, tumor spread in the mesorectum, mucinous histology, vascular and lymphatic invasion, and the distance of the distal margin of resection from the tumor. Rectal carcinomas associate with a higher local recurrence rate than seen in colonic tumors. Overall, recurrence rates range from 10% to 25% (533). Approximately 8% of Dukes A lesions, 25% to 31% of patients with stage B2 cancers, and approximately 50% of those with stage C tumors will develop pelvic recurrence after surgical resection (587,624). Several clinicopathologic features predict local recurrences of rectal cancer. Extension of tumor through the bowel wall and nodal involvement are most important.

Patients with advanced rectal cancer may undergo palliative resection since it provides good relief of local symptoms, but the procedure does not prolong survival. If palliative excision is impossible, endoscopic transanal resection may be used to remove obstructing lesions lying below the peritoneal reflection; alternatively, frail patients may undergo laser ablation (625).

Tumor Markers of Colorectal Carcinomas

A number of tumor markers are associated with colorectal carcinomas. Some of these represent gains in the expression of a protein, whereas others represent loss of expression. Some of these play a role in monitoring the clinical course of patients with colorectal carcinoma, whereas others may aid in determining the prognosis of a given patient.

Tumor markers associated with colorectal cancers are listed in Table 14.20. Monoclonal antibodies to many of these antigens have become widely available. These antibodies can be radiolabeled and used to delineate areas of occult

TABLE 14.20 Tumor Markers Associated with Colorectal Carcinoma

Carcinoembryonic antigen (CEA)
Carcinoma antigen 19.9 (CA19.9)
Carcinoma antigen 50 (CA50)
Carcinoma antigen 242 (CA242)
Alkaline phosphatase
α_1-Antitrypsin
Sucrase-isomaltase
TAG72391
TAG171A
Blood group antigens
Sialyl Lex
Sialosyl-Tn
T antigen
Mucoproteins
Muc-1
Colon-ovarian tumor antigen (COTA)
Growth factors and receptors
p glycoprotein
E-cadherin

recurrent colorectal carcinoma in patients with rising serum levels (626–631). Antibodies may also be used to detect micrometastases intraoperatively by utilizing a handheld gamma-detecting probe to assess the extent of colorectal cancer in patients previously injected with radiolabeled antibodies (632). However, each antigen has the potential to shed into the circulation, either spontaneously or upon tumor lysis. Thus, antigens such as CEA, TAG72, and 171A can be detected in histologically normal lymph nodes adjacent to sites of colorectal carcinoma (633), since the antigen is taken up by antigen-presenting cells in lymph nodes. In the lymph nodes, the antigens are processed and antigenic fragments interact with circulating antibody, creating a false-positive uptake of radiolabeled antibody in histologically normal lymph nodes. This effect varies among different antigens and among different antibodies against the same antigen. There is no evidence that any single antigen acts as an ideal tumor marker (633).

Carcinoembryonic Antigen

CEA, the first colorectal cancer antigen (634), is the prototype of an oncofetal antigen. It is expressed in both fetal and adult cells, particularly in tumors. Most colorectal carcinomas make CEA (Fig. 14.146). Only about 3% of tumors are CEA negative. CEA is expressed at the apical border and intracytoplasmically in mucus-secreting cells. It is also expressed in adenomas and in IBD.

CEA levels, once thought to be potentially useful for screening patients for the presence of colorectal carcinoma, are much more important as indicators of carcinoma relapse (634–636). Serum levels rise in patients with recurrent disease before clinical evidence of tumor growth. Current ASCO guidelines recommend that CEA levels be evaluated every 3 months in patients with stage II or III colorectal cancer, and that testing be continued for at least 3 years following surgery or systemic therapy (573). Elevations in the CEA level should prompt a

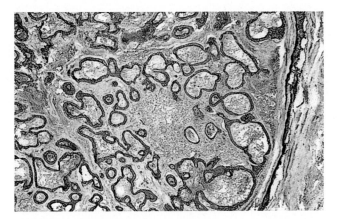

FIG. 14.146. Lymph node metastasis from a colon cancer demonstrating strong immunoreactivity for carcinoembryonic antigen.

search for metastatic or recurrent disease. Increases in CEA levels occurring within 1 or 2 weeks following chemotherapy, however, should be interpreted with caution since tumor lysis may result in CEA release into the blood (637).

Keratins

Immunocytochemically, colorectal carcinomas are invariably positive for keratin. Not all keratins are expressed by colon cancers, however. The differential expression of certain keratin molecules, but not others, helps identify colorectal carcinomas and distinguishes them from other carcinomas. Most commonly, colon cancers are positive for cytokeratin-20 and negative for cytokeratin-7. This expression pattern may be diagnostically useful in distinguishing between colorectal and pulmonary adenocarcinomas (638). Immunostains for keratins are also useful in detecting evidence of micrometastases or minimal residual disease.

CA-19

CA-19, a carbohydrate cell surface antigen newly synthesized by cancer cells (639), is related to the blood group antigen Lea (640) and is present in approximately 80% of colonic carcinomas as well as in benign lesions and in dysplasias. Elevated serum levels are found in approximately 50% of cancer patients. Current data, however, do not support its clinical use for monitoring colorectal cancer patients (573).

Growth Factors and Their Receptors

TGF-α is sometimes increased in colorectal carcinomas. The level does not correlate with histologic stage or grade (641). Epidermal growth factor receptor (EGFR) expression increases in lymph node–positive patients when compared with node-negative colorectal cancers (642). The extent of EGFR expression may also influence patient survival. Patients in whom >50% of their tumor cells stain with an antibody to EGFR have a poorer prognosis than those in whom <50% of the cells are positive.

Hepatocyte growth factor (HGF) promotes tumor invasion and metastasis and is overexpressed in colon cancers. HGF binds to the receptor, encoded by the C-met gene, and increases signal transduction.

Adhesion Molecules

E-cadherin is expressed in the normal colon and is downregulated in colon cancer (643). Patients surviving >5 years exhibit significantly higher levels of E-cadherin mRNA than those surviving <5 years (644).

Molecular Changes in Colorectal Cancer

Many investigations into the genetic basis of colorectal cancer development took advantage of the existence of hereditary syndromes that increase patient susceptibility to colon carcinoma. The histologic progression of the disease involves alterations in key genes and their protein products, including oncogenes, tumor suppressor genes, and DNA mismatch repair (MMR) genes, as well as epigenetic changes in the promoters of many genes.

Specific genes tend to be mutated at specific times during neoplastic progression to colon cancer, but it is the accumulation of a critical number of genetic alterations, rather than their specific order, that governs the appearance of neoplasia. There are essentially three pathways that exist in the development of colorectal cancers: A chromosomal instability pathway similar to that affecting patients with FAP, a microsatellite instability pathway similar to that seen in association with HNPCC, and an epigenetic or methylator pathway. Each of these pathways will be discussed below. It is important to note, however, that considerable overlap exists in these pathways and, therefore, an individual tumor may show alterations common to more than a single pathway.

Chromosomal Instability Pathway

Colorectal cancers arising via the chromosomal instability pathway demonstrate hyperploidy; allelic losses involving chromosomes 17p, 18q, 18p, and 22q; ras oncogene mutations; and frequent mutations in the tumor suppressor genes APC and p53. These tumors are those that arise via the now familiar multistep progression in the adenoma–carcinoma sequence initially described by Vogelstein et al in 1990 (645) (Fig. 14.147).

APC Gene

FAP is an autosomal dominant disorder characterized by the onset of multiple colorectal polyps and a predisposition to

colorectal carcinoma (see Chapter 12). FAP patients have inactivating germ line mutations in the *adenomatous polyposis coli (APC)* gene located on chromosome 5. *APC* gene somatic mutations are also present in sporadic colorectal adenomas and carcinomas (646–652). Likewise, mice carrying *APC* germ line mutations (MIN mice) are predisposed to develop intestinal tumors (653).

Alterations in the APC locus occur early in the neoplastic progression, occurring in small adenomas (654). *APC* mutations are homogeneously present throughout small adenomas, but are absent from the normal epithelium of the adenoma stalks (655). Sixty percent of colorectal cancers and 63% of adenomas have at least one somatic mutation in the *APC* gene. The mutations found in the adenomas resemble those found in the cancers (654). A second event promotes the transition from abnormally proliferating epithelium to adenoma formation (645,656–661). Inactivation of the second *APC* allele, through allelic loss or mutation alone, affects 35% to 70% of adenomas and 35% to 45% of cancers (645,647,648,654,658,661–664), raising the possibility that this is a frequent, but nonobligatory, step in colon cancer progression.

Most mutations result in truncation of the carboxy terminus of the *APC*-encoded protein (647,652,665–669), suggesting that this part of the protein is important in mediating its growth-suppressing effects (660,669). *APC* is a negative regulator of colonic epithelial proliferation (670) and functions as a part of the Wnt signaling pathway. Under normal circumstances, *APC* directs ubiquitin-mediated degradation of cytoplasmic β-catenin, preventing it from reaching the nucleus of the cell, where it interacts with transcription factors, ultimately resulting in cell proliferation. Adenomas lacking *APC* mutations frequently show mutations in β-catenin, which result in activation of the same Wnt signaling

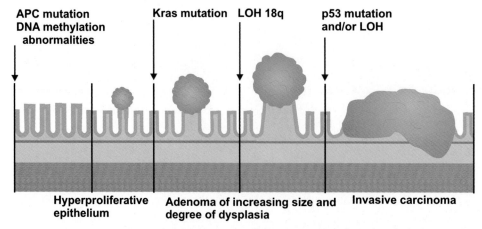

FIG. 14.147. Diagram depicting the chromosomal instability pathway for the development of colorectal carcinoma. The earliest changes that occur involve alterations in DNA methylation and mutations in the APC gene. These changes may precede the development of histologically recognizable abnormalities. Mutations in the k-ras gene occur in small adenomas, with loss of tumor suppressor genes on chromosome 18q occurring later. p53 mutations are late occurrences that probably play a role in the transformation of large, dysplastic adenomas to frankly invasive carcinomas.

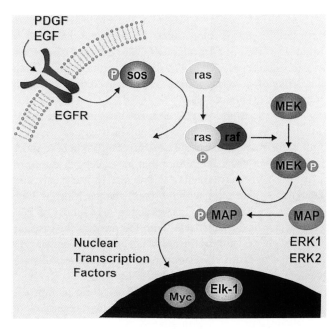

FIG. 14.148. Diagram of the role of ras in the cell.

pathway (671,672). APC function is discussed in detail in Chapter 12.

ras Genes

ras protooncogenes function in normal cell growth and differentiation (673) via their role as G proteins, participating in signal transduction from growth factor receptors on the cell membrane (Fig. 14.148) (674). Various growth signals lead to p21 ras activation, a step required for transmission of the signal (675). *ras* guanosine triphosphate (GTP) activates various cellular targets, stimulating enzymatic cascades that lead to cell cycle progression, changes in cytoskeletal organization, cell adhesion, and cell proliferation. Mutations in codons 12, 13, or 61 convert *ras* protooncogenes to oncogenes and result in autonomous cell growth and proliferation (673,674).

Most mutations in colorectal neoplasms affect codon 12 of the *K-ras* gene. Rare mutations involve the *N-ras* gene (645,676–680). ras mutations occur during the intermediate stages of adenoma growth (645,681) rather than early in the neoplastic continuum or as a later change associated with carcinoma development. *ras* mutations generally follow *APC* mutations. They are infrequent in small adenomas, occurring more commonly in larger adenomas with high-grade dysplasia (645,682). Similar timing of *K-ras* mutations occurs in tumors from patients with FAP and with sporadic adenomas, although *K-ras* mutations occur more frequently in sporadic adenomas than in FAP-associated adenomas (683,684–686). The incidence of *K-ras* mutations in adenomas and primary colorectal carcinomas ranges from 12% to 75% and 21% to 65%, respectively (645,674,677,682,687–693). *K-ras* mutations remain stable throughout the natural history of human colorectal cancers (694), resulting in identical *ras*

mutations both in the primary tumor and its metastases. ras mutations occur in both the diploid and aneuploid cells of adenomas and carcinomas (677), but they are more common in aneuploid tumors (677,693). This suggests that *K-ras* mutations occur before aneuploidy develops (677).

Although *ras* mutations occur relatively early during colorectal tumor development, they do not play a major role in the genesis of flat adenomas and carcinomas (695–697). They occur in only 16% to 23% of flat adenomas and 17% to 23% of flat carcinomas (695–698) compared with 67% of polypoid adenomas and 76% of cancers. Even mildly dysplastic adenomas or small (<5 mm) adenomas exhibit a higher mutation incidence when they are polypoid (62% and 57%, respectively) compared to their flat counterparts (23% and 19%, respectively). These data suggest that *K-ras* mutations correlate with adenoma morphology or clinical features, and that flat cancers may associate with different molecular alterations than those seen in the usual adenoma–carcinoma sequence (699).

p53 Gene

The *p53* gene, located on the short arm of chromosome 17, is the most frequently mutated gene identified to date in human cancers and is now widely recognized as a tumor suppressor gene. *p53* deletions and/or mutations are oncogenic. The *p53* gene encodes a short-lived phosphoprotein (700); its oligomers bind DNA and it acts as a transcription factor (701). It contains several separate functional domains that contribute to its regulation (702–708).

The p53 protein plays numerous roles within the cell. It is implicated in the control of cell proliferation, differentiation, DNA repair and synthesis, and programmed cell death (709–712). p53 causes G1 cell cycle arrest in response to DNA damage, hypoxia, and other stresses (Fig. 14.149) (713–715), allowing the injured cell time to repair the alterations in its DNA before entering the S phase of the cell cycle. G1 arrest results from transcriptional activation of p21$^{WAF1/CIP1}$A (716,717). p21$^{WAF1/CIP1}$A has a p53 binding site located near its promoter (716,718–720), and it acts as a universal inhibitor of the cyclin-CDC2 or cyclin-CDK complexes, which drive the main events of the cell cycle (718–720). p53 also regulates the G2/M-cell cycle transition (721). Loss of this cell cycle checkpoint control results in potential replication of damaged DNA and its passage to daughter cells. p53 also directs cells into a pathway of programmed cell death in cases in which the DNA damage is too severe to be repaired (709,711,712).

Cells that lack the wild-type *p53* lack cell cycle checkpoint activity, and these cells undergo gene amplification at high frequencies (722). Loss of the normal growth regulatory activity of the wild-type protein provides cells with a selective growth advantage, promotes genetic instability, diminishes the probability of apoptosis, and contributes to unregulated cell growth (708,722–724). It is important to note, however, that p53 mutations alone are insufficient to initiate a cancer;

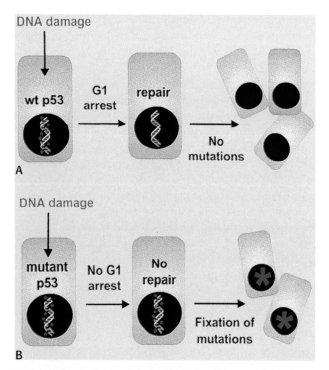

FIG. 14.149. Role of p53. **A:** Cells that sustain DNA damage but contain wild-type p53 arrest in the G1 phase of the cell cycle. DNA repair occurs and cell replication proceeds, producing daughter cells without DNA abnormalities. **B:** If a cell containing mutant p53 sustains DNA damage, arrest does not occur in G1, and the damaged DNA is replicated and passed down to daughter cells.

mutations at additional tumor suppressor or oncogene loci are necessary for complete malignant transformation (710).

Missense point mutations resulting in faulty *p53* proteins are the most prevalent type of *p53* alterations seen in human tumors (710). Other alterations range from complete deletion of the gene to the generation of stop codons, both resulting in protein absence.

Although the wild-type *p53* acts as a tumor suppressor, mutant *p53* may sometimes exert a dominant negative effect (705,725,726). The polypeptides of mutated *p53* have a longer half-life than the wild-type protein. As a result, they accumulate in cancer cells and form oligomeric protein complexes with wild-type p53 subunits, thereby functionally inactivating them (705–728). Therefore, *p53* mutations may result in complete or near complete loss of normal p53 function, although the normal allele has not been lost. Small mutations in the *p53* coding sequence weaken the ability of p53 to bind to DNA binding sites (729). Eventually, though, the second allele is also inactivated in most tumors and p53 function is lost entirely (730). Most colorectal cancers are hemizygous for p53 (731,732), retaining an allele that is almost always mutated (703,731,733–735). Patients with colorectal carcinomas demonstrate mutations in all regions of exons 5 through 8 of the *p53* gene. Only one third of mutations occur at the hotspot codons 175, 248, 273, and 282 (734,735).

Loss of heterozygosity (LOH) of the *p53* locus associates with later stages of colon cancer development. *p53* LOH is found in <10% of adenomas (645,736) and in 31% to 78% of carcinomas (645,736–738). *p53* mutations occur in both flat and polypoid adenomas, but usually only those with high-grade dysplasia (739).

The association of *p53* abnormalities with the most advanced stages of colorectal neoplasia suggests that *p53* mutations mark those neoplasms that tend to behave more aggressively (740). Carcinomas that have allelic deletions of 17p have a greater tendency to give rise to metastatic and fatal disease than those without such a change. Most of these tumors have total loss of p53 function (731). Loss of heterozygosity on 17p correlates with the presence of vascular and lymphatic vascular invasion (741). Allelic loss of p53 shows a significant association with the presence of distant metastases and shortened survival (742,743).

p53 immunoreactivity (Fig. 14.150) is found in approximately 47% to 50% of colorectal carcinomas, regardless of the allelic status. p53 immunoreactivity tends to increase with tumor stage. Patients with p53-positive tumors show a more advanced stage with a higher incidence of lymph node and liver metastases. p53 nuclear overexpression may represent an independent predictor of survival in lymph node–positive colorectal cancer patients (744).

Loss of Heterozygosity on Chromosome 18q

Since allelic loss of the long arm of chromosome 18 occurs commonly in colorectal carcinomas, it was expected that a tumor suppressor gene resided in this area (645,745). This region contains at least two putative tumor suppressor genes, *DCC* (deleted in colon cancer) and *DPC4* (deleted in pancreatic cancer, locus 4) or Smad4. Although originally thought to be lost in a significant proportion of colorectal cancers, the DCC gene seems not to be involved in colorectal carcinogenesis (746). Homozygous deletions and/or mutations in Smad4, however, occur in xenografts and cell lines derived from colorectal cancer, as well as in 10% to 35% of primary colorectal cancers (747–750).

Smad4 was first identified as a tumor suppressor gene in pancreatic cancers and was initially designated as *DPC4* (751). The human Smad4 gene contains 11 exons with a predicted 552 amino acid coding sequence, and encodes a protein important in the TGF-β superfamily of signaling proteins. TGF-β signals are transduced by two kinds of receptors, receptor I (RI) and II (RII), which have serine/threonine kinase activity. Upon the binding of TGF-β to TGF-βRII, this receptor activates TGF-βRI by phosphorylation. TGF-βRI, in turn, phosphorylates the intracellular target Smad2 or Smad3. Phosphorylated Smad2 or Smad3 bind Smad4 and the resulting Smad complex translocates to the nucleus. This protein complex interacts with DNA directly or indirectly, regulating transcription of target genes and leading to the regulation of cellular proliferation.

The frequency of Smad4 mutation increases with the progression from adenoma to carcinoma. In one study, mutations

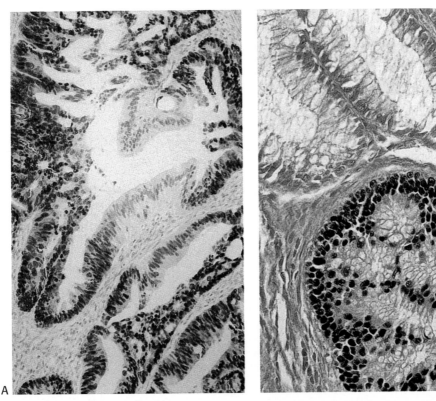

FIG. 14.150. p53 immunohistochemistry. **A:** Moderately differentiated colon cancer demonstrating strong p53 immunoreactivity. Such strong staining often indicates the presence of p53 mutation. **B:** p53 immunoreactivity is present in the neoplastic tissue at the bottom right, but the adjacent nonneoplastic colonic mucosa is p53 negative.

were found in 0 of 40 adenomas, 10% of intramucosal carcinomas, 7% of invasive carcinomas without distant metastasis, and 35% of primary invasive carcinomas with distant metastasis (752). These *Smad4* gene mutations included frameshift, nonsense, and missense mutations. Loss of the wild-type allele was also detected in 95% of invasive and metastatic carcinomas. In another study (753), Smad4 expression was detected by immunohistochemistry in all adenomas or stage I adenocarcinomas, but was observed in only 8% of stage II, 6% of stage III, and 22% of stage IV cancers. These data again suggest that inactivation of Smad4 is a late event in colorectal carcinogenesis.

The status of chromosome 18q abnormalities also may have prognostic value in patients with stage II colorectal cancer (754,755), since the survival in patients with stage II cancer and chromosome 18 allelic loss resembles that seen in patients with stage III disease. In contrast, patients with stage II disease who do not have chromosome 18 allelic losses in their tumors show a survival rate similar to that of patients with stage I disease and may not require additional therapy (755).

Microsatellite Instability Pathway

Mismatch Repair Genes

A new category of genes found to be important in human cancers was discovered through investigation of HNPCC families. These are known as the mismatch repair (MMR) genes. MMR genes act in concert with other genes to remove mismatches, stabilize the DNA strand, and resynthesize a new DNA strand. This process, known as mismatch repair, plays an essential role in stabilizing the genome (756,757). Inherited abnormalities in mismatch repair also occur in two other rare colorectal cancer syndromes, Muir-Torre and Turcot syndromes.

At least six different human mismatch repair genes exist including MLH1, MSH2, MSH3, MSH6, PMS1, and PMS2. These genes are the human counterparts of *Escherichia coli* and yeast mismatch repair genes, and their products selectively bind DNA base to base mispairs and insertion–deletion loop mismatches, initiating the repair process (Fig. 14.151). When the mismatch repair pathway is inactivated, affected cells demonstrate a 100- to 1,000-fold increased mutation rate (758,759). Repetitive sequences are especially sensitive to mutation and are mutated at the highest rate. Replication errors probably result from somatic slippage of DNA polymerase during DNA replication and accumulate in the absence of correct repair mechanisms. As a result, tumors arising in patients with such mismatch repair defects are characterized by instability in the length of microsatellite sequences.

Germline mutations occur in *MLH1* in 33%, *MSH2* in 31% to 40%, and *PMS2* in 4% of HNPCC kindreds (760).

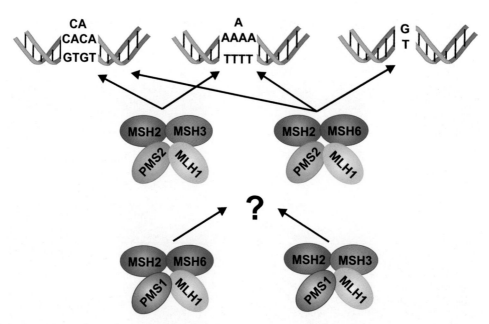

FIG. 14.151. DNA mismatch repair. The mismatch repair proteins form a variety of complexes that repair different types of errors. MLH1, MSH2, MSH3, and PMS2 form a complex that is responsible for correcting loop mismatches; MLH1, MSH2, MSH6, and PMS2 perform a similar function, but also correct mispaired bases. The function of some combinations of proteins is not yet understood.

Patients with Muir-Torre syndrome develop their susceptibility due to the inheritance of a frame shift mutation in the *MSH2* gene in one family and a nonsense mutation in the *MSH2* gene in another family (761). Microsatellite instability and somatic inactivation of MMR genes also occurs in approximately 15% of sporadic colorectal carcinomas (762–765). Unlike HNPCC-associated tumors, mutation is not the mechanism by which the MMR genes are silenced. Instead, sporadic colorectal cancers show epigenetic silencing, most commonly of the *MLH1* promoter, by means of promoter methylation (766,767). Like their HNPCC counterparts, sporadic lesions with MMR defects tend to occur on the right side of the colon and tend to be mucinous, poorly differentiated, and DNA diploid. Patients with sporadic MSI-positive tumors also have increased survival compared to those without MSI (768). The MSI phenotype also occurs in neoplastic lesions in patients with ulcerative colitis (769,770).

Microsatellite alterations in neoplastic tissues are traditionally separated into three categories: MSS, low-level MSI (MSI-L), and high-level MSI (MSI-H). MSI-L occurs when <30% of tested microsatellite loci demonstrate instability, while MSI-H is defined as instability at >30% of loci. A National Cancer Institute workshop recommended the use of five specific microsatellite markers to distinguish between MSI-L and MSI-L neoplasms (771). Making the distinction between MSI-L and MSI-H phenotypes is of significance since the underlying genetic alterations differ.

Defective DNA mismatch repair of the type seen in patients with HNPCC usually is associated with alterations in the *MLH1* or *MSH2* mismatch repair genes (772–775).

Tumors in these patients are MSI-H and demonstrate an increased frequency of mutation in both repetitive microsatellite poly(G) and poly(A) sequences. When such mutations occur in repetitive elements within genes known to regulate cellular proliferation, growth, or differentiation, they may directly contribute to neoplastic transformation. The most commonly targeted gene in MSI-H colon cancers is the *TGF-βRII*. Other genes containing repetitive sequences may also be altered (776–788) (Table 14.21).

The relationship between microsatellite instability and other genetic alterations commonly found in colorectal cancers is not well understood. Alterations in the Wnt signaling pathway occur in colonic neoplasms regardless of their MSI status (789). Mutations in *APC* are found in 21% of MSI-H colon cancers (790, 791). In addition, 22% to 31% of MSI-H tumors contain ras mutations (792). Mutations in *p53* are less common in MSI-H than MSS colon cancers, but do occur (790,792,793).

Epigenetic Pathway

Methylation Abnormalities

The finding of aberrant MLH1 promoter methylation in sporadic MSI-H colon cancers dramatically illustrated the role epigenetic changes play in inactivating critical genes for the development of cancer (766,767,794). Since this observation, aberrant methylation has been well described at multiple genetic loci in a variety of human cancers (795,796). Hypermethylation of CpG islands occurs normally with aging at some loci, but cancer-associated methylation abnormalities involve different genes (Table 14.22). For example,

| TABLE 14.21 | Target Genes of Frameshift Mutations in MSI-H Colon Carcinomas |

Gene	Function	Repeat Type	Consequence
TGF-βRII	Tumor suppressor	$(A)_{10}$	Loss of tumor suppressor activity
IGFIIR	Tumor suppressor	$(G)_9$	Loss of tumor suppressor activity
Bax	Apoptosis promoter	$(G)_8$	Loss of apoptotic signaling
MSH3	Mismatch repair gene	$(A)_8$	Loss of MMR function with increase in mutation rate
MSH6	Mismatch repair gene	$(C)_8$	Loss of MMR function with increase in mutation rate
TCF4	Transcription factor	$(A)_9$	Increased transcriptional activity
MBD4	Methyl-CpG binding thymine glycosylase	$(A)_{10}$	Possible increase in MMR deficiency
PTEN	Tumor suppressor	$(A)_6$ exon 7, $(A)_6$ exon 8	Loss of tumor suppressor activity
RIZ	Tumor suppressor	$(A)_8$ exon 8 $(A)_9$ exon 8	Loss of tumor suppressor activity
AXIN2	Wnt signaling pathway	4 repeats in exon 7	TCF-dependent transcriptional activation
Activin RII	Serine threonine kinase in TGF-β pathway	$(A)_8$ exon 10, $(A)_8$ exon 3	Loss of tumor suppressor activity

MMR, mismatch repair; RII, receptor II; TGF, transforming growth factor.

| TABLE 14.22 | Genes Inactivated by Promoter Methylation in Colon and Colon Cancer |

Gene	Location	Age-related Methylation	Methylation in Colon Cancer (%)
ER	6q25.1	Yes	>90
MYOD1	11p15.4	Yes	>90
N33	8p22	Yes	80
RARβ1	3p24	Yes	80
IGF2	11p15.5	Yes	70
PAX6	11p13	Yes	70
CSPG2	5q12-14	Yes	70
HPP1/TPEF	2q33	Yes	60–80
RASSF1	3p21.3	Yes	50
THBS2	6q27	Yes	50
CALCA	11p15	No	50
HIC1	17p13.3	No	50
HLTF	3q25-26	No	50
WT1	11p13	No	50
P16	9p21	No	40
MGMT	10q26	No	30
TIMP3	22q12-13	No	27
MDR1	7q21.1	No	20–30
RARβ2	3p24	Yes	10–30
COX-2	1p25.2-3	Yes	10–20
MLH1	3p21.3	No	10–20
P14/ARF	9p21	No	10–20
APC	5q21	No	10–20
CACNA1G	17q22	No	10–20
RIZ1	1p36	No	10–20
THBS1	15q15	No	10–20
LKB1/STK11	19p13.3	No	5–10
EGFR	7p12	Yes	0

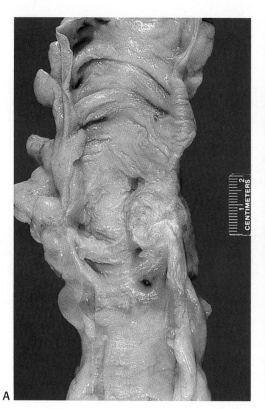
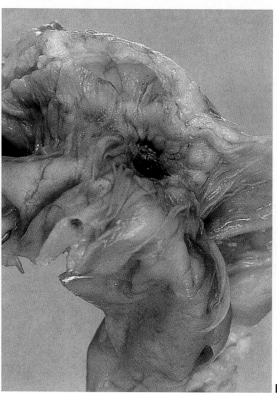

A   B

FIG. 14.152. Metastatic carcinoma. **A:** The rectal mucosa appears irregular, the bowel wall is thickened, and the lumen is narrowed secondary to involvement by contiguous spread of prostate carcinoma. **B:** An ulcerated lesion is present in the colon, which represents a focus of metastatic pancreatic cancer.

mutation of *p16* has not been described in colon cancer, but methylation of the *p16* promoter is detected in 40% of colon cancers (797) and has been found in colon adenomas. This observation suggests that aberrant promoter methylation occurs early in the adenoma–carcinoma sequence, a finding confirmed in other studies as well (798,799). In fact, observations that some colorectal cancer patients tend to show widespread methylation abnormalities involving multiple loci has led to the concept of the CIMP (800–802). The causes underlying CIMP are not yet understood.

CIMP-positive colorectal cancers appear to represent a distinct phenotype and, therefore, may represent a distinct pathway to colorectal cancer development. CIMP-positive colon cancers tend to be poorly differentiated, and arise more commonly in the right colon in older patients (803–806). The CIMP is also strongly associated with sessile serrated polyps and serrated adenomas (807,808). CIMP-positive tumors can be divided into two groups, those that are MSI positive and those that are MSS with a high frequency of *K-ras* mutations (275,803). The MSI-H tumors occurring in association with CIMP develop as a result of methylation of the *MLH1* promoter (797). *Ras* gene mutations that are seen in the MSS group of CIMP-positive tumors may result from methylation of the *MGMT* promoter, an alteration that increases the frequency of G to A mutations (809).

SECONDARY TUMORS

The large bowel may be the site of metastasis or extension from a number of tumors. It may also be involved by direct invasion or extension, intraperitoneal seeding, hematogenous dissemination, lymphatic metastasis, or intraluminal or intramural dissemination. The most common mode of secondary colonic involvement is peritoneal seeding; therefore, it is most common to see metastatic nodules deriving from either ovarian cancers (810,811) or mucinous colonic or appendiceal neoplasms. The anterior wall of the rectum at the Douglas pouch is probably the most common site for the discovery of peritoneal seeding (812). Other common locations include the sigmoid colon, transverse colon, and along both paracolic gutters (813). The rectum may also be affected by direct extension of tumor from the prostate or cervix (Fig. 14.152) (811). When prostate cancers invade the rectum, patients may present with signs and symptoms of rectal disease and an absence of genitourinary symptoms. Secondary involvement by extension along mesenteric reflections occurs in the transverse colon, where neoplasms of either the stomach or pancreas extend into the colon (Fig. 14.152) (814). Anal tumors, particularly melanomas, can extend into the rectum. Malignant mesotheliomas may metastasize and present as colonic polyps (815). The lesions may closely resemble primary adenocarcinomas.

Metastases from ovarian, breast, or lung carcinomas (816,817) are the most common in females, whereas gastrointestinal tract and lung tumors are the most common source of metastatic lesions in males. Other causes of secondary colorectal cancer include bladder, kidney, pancreas, prostate, and cervical cancer. Metastases from malignant melanoma to the gastrointestinal tract are fairly common, particularly in the small bowel (818,819), but in the colon they are infrequent and usually remain asymptomatic. We have also seen an unusual case of diffuse intraperitoneal spread of melanoma.

Tumor implants produce slight puckering of the bowel, with development of perpendicular transverse folds or stripes (811). Occasionally, they may produce a polypoid lesion that may induce an intussusception (820). They may also cause obstruction, bleeding, or perforation (816,817). At times, they become large enough to cause intussusception (819,820). Metastases infiltrate the colonic wall, producing annular lesions mimicking primary colonic carcinomas or diffusely simulating a linitis plastica (821). A metastatic lesion is often suggested by the presence of a neoplastic mass that primarily occupies the submucosa, muscularis propria, or serosa, and leaves the overlying mucosa intact. Carcinomas can also metastasize to adenomas (373,822).

DISTINGUISHING COLONIC NEOPLASMS FROM NEOPLASMS FROM OTHER SITES

There are two types of problems one encounters with respect to metastatic carcinomas of the colon. The first is determining if a tumor in the intestine is primary or secondary, and the second reflects the need to distinguish a colorectal carcinoma metastatic to other sites from a primary tumor in that site.

When colon cancers metastasize, particularly in individuals with multiple primary cancers, distinguishing a metastatic colonic tumor from either a primary lung tumor or a metastasis from another site may be histologically difficult. One histologic feature helpful in suggesting the presence of a colonic primary lesion is the presence of "dirty necrosis" (324,823). This feature is particularly helpful when present in biopsy specimens. It is less helpful in cytology specimens, since intact tissues are usually not obtained. More often, however, one relies on the use of a panel of antibodies to distinguish between a variety of possible primary sites of origin. A battery of immunostains may help resolve this clinical conundrum. Antibodies to specific cytokeratins may help delineate the site of the primary lesion. Colon carcinomas are usually negative for cytokeratin-7 but positive for cytokeratin-20 (824,825). Used alone, neither cytokeratin immunostaining nor cytokeratin-20 immunostaining reliably separates the tumors. For example, the immunophenotype of cytokeratin-7+ cytokeratin-20– occurs in 86% of pulmonary adenocarcinomas and 0% of colonic carcinomas. Conversely, the cytokeratin-7– cytokeratin-20+ immunophenotype occurs in 77% of colon cancers and 0% of pulmonary

tumors (638). TTF-1 immunoreactivity may also aid in distinguishing primary lung from metastatic colon cancers.

Cytokeratin-7 immunostaining also helps distinguish metastatic colon cancers from ovarian primaries (Fig. 14.153). In one study, all but one of the primary metastatic colonic carcinomas were negative for cytokeratin-7, whereas all the primary and metastatic ovarian carcinomas were positive for cytokeratin-7. The tumors metastatic to the ovary were all positive for cytokeratin-20 and CEA. Among the primary ovarian carcinomas, none of six serous, three of seven endometrioid, and 3 of 11 mucinous tumors were positive for cytokeratin-20. Ten of the primary ovarian tumors were negative for CEA using both monoclonal and polyclonal antibodies.

EVALUATION OF RESECTION SPECIMENS
General Comments

The unopened bowel should be carefully examined upon receipt from the operating room, then opened and pinned to a corkboard for fixation in 10% buffered formalin. Those specimens that are received partially opened or, worse yet, received in formalin unopened and allowed to fix over a weekend tend to become fixed in distorted positions, making it extremely difficult to establish normal anatomic relationships as well as the various pathologic features that are present. In the worst case, one may have extreme difficulty determining the exact anatomic location of a tumor and in obtaining accurate measurements to the nearest resection margins.

Inspection of the unopened bowel provides important information. Dilation is indicative of obstruction, and it informs the examiner that the dilated portion is the proximal part of the specimen. Retraction of the serosal surface in the region of a palpable mass indicates serosal invasion (Fig. 14.82). Palpation of the serosal surface discloses the circumferential extent of the tumor so that one can avoid transecting the tumor when opening the bowel, unless it is completely annular. The mesentery and pericolonic fat should be carefully examined for lymph nodes and evidence of gross vascular invasion. Those extensively involved by metastases are enlarged, hard, and white on cut surface. Grossly, venous invasion may be evident.

The surgical specimen should be opened along the antimesenteric border, unless palpation of the specimen indicates that a tumor lies in this area, in which case the bowel should be opened taking care to avoid sectioning through the middle of the tumor. The resection specimen should be described, particularly with respect to the distance to the nearest margins, if these are close to the tumor. After having been opened, cleaned, and described, the specimen is pinned to a corkboard and immersed floating upside down in formalin for a number of hours to obtain adequate fixation. The specimen should be photographed. This can be done when it is received fresh or following fixation. Some details become more obvious after the fixation.

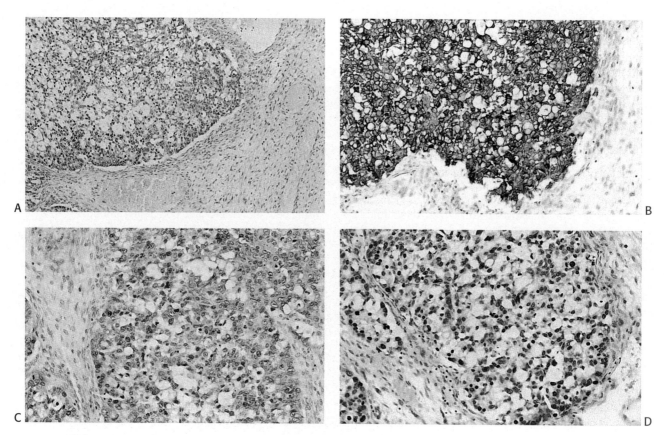

FIG. 14.153. Colon carcinoma metastatic to ovary. **A:** The ovary contains a poorly differentiated mucinous adenocarcinoma. **B:** Cytokeratin-20 immunostains are strongly positive. **C:** Immunohistochemical staining for cytokeratin-7 is negative. **D:** Negative HAM56 staining.

Evaluation of Tumor Margins

One could question whether there is any justification for the routine histologic examination of bowel resection margins in colorectal carcinoma resection specimens, particularly large colectomy specimens in which the extent of the surgical resection is determined by the vascular supply. Most tumors rarely extend >1.5 cm laterally in the bowel wall unless the tumor has a mucinous histology. Certainly any tumor that is >5 cm from the nearest margin, is not poorly differentiated, and does not have a mucinous or signet ring histology is not likely to involve the tumor margins. What is more important is the examination of the degree of intramural spread of the tumor. This is particularly true for rectal cancers that lie below the peritoneal reflection. The deep radial margins represent an important prognostic indicator and should be evaluated carefully. In order to adequately assess the radial margins, the specimen should be inked at the time it is received.

Lymph Node Examination

Tumor stage is the single most important prognosticator for patients with colorectal carcinoma; therefore, an attempt to identify nodal metastases is very important in handling the resection specimen. The nodes most likely to become involved are those closest to the tumor. Pericolic lymph nodes may be obtained in one of several ways. The fat adjacent to the colon (the mesocolic fat) can be meticulously dissected off the muscularis propria and then searched by a variety of techniques (see below), or a rim of immediately adjacent fatty tissue may be left on the specimen with the sections taken in such a way as to include this fatty tissue. Since the nodal metastases occur progressively from those closest to the tumor to those most distant from it, these are the most likely to be positive. As noted in the TNM staging system (Table 14.16), the number of positive lymph nodes distinguishes the N status.

There are several ways to search for minute lymph nodes in resection specimens for adenocarcinoma. Lymph nodes can be removed from the fresh or fixed specimen, or the fatty tissues can be placed in a clearing solution. Using a clearing technique, metastases are found in 45% to 78% of small lymph nodes measuring <5 mm in diameter (535,826,827). Detection of these small lymph nodes containing metastases is important in accurately staging rectal carcinomas (827). Several groups identified a significantly greater number of nodes and a greater number of lymph nodes with metastases in the cleared specimens compared with noncleared specimens (828–830). Traditional dissection showed metastases in 43.7% of patients, but after fat clearance a further 4.8%

were found to be lymph node positive (828). Unfortunately, clearing techniques increase the turnaround time for the resection signout. However, in contrast, Jass et al (831) found no significant difference in the number of lymph nodes harvested when traditional dissection and fat clearance methods were compared. The difference in the number of lymph nodes found by traditional dissection versus those found during clearing depends, of course, on the meticulousness with which the initial dissection is done.

Identification of Extramural Venous Invasion

A debate exists concerning the optimum method for demonstrating venous invasion (440). Attempts to document this have included venous radiography, primary macroscopic preparation, injection of silver solutions, and histochemical techniques. Extramural venous invasion is found in 11% to 54.1% of colorectal carcinomas (439). Dirschmid et al (832) compared tangential sectioning of the fat beneath the tumor with perpendicular sectioning of the same tissue for detecting extramural venous invasion. Sections taken tangentially proved a more accurate estimation of venous involvement: 54.1% compared with 16.6% of colonic tumor (441,832) and 75% versus 36% of rectal cancers (439,832).

When venous invasion is identified, a note should be made in the report as to whether it was grossly identifiable (V2) or microscopic (V1) and whether it is intramural, extramural, or both.

Sections To Be Taken

At least three histologic sections should be taken from each tumor present in the specimen. These sections should be taken through the full thickness of the bowel wall, so that the depth of invasion can be assessed. One or two sections should be taken of the subserosal connective tissue and fat in a plane parallel to the long axis of the colon, so that extramural venous or perineural extension of the tumor can be detected. Other sections should include the proximal and distal margins, any other mucosal lesions that are present, one or two sections of the uninvolved colonic mucosa, and a section of the appendix if it is included in the resection. Lymph nodes should be carefully identified and submitted by location (i.e., adjacent to tumor, proximal and distal).

Reporting of Resected Large Intestinal Carcinomas

The Association of Directors of Anatomic and Surgical Pathology (ADASP) has formulated a series of recommendations for the reporting of resected large intestinal carcinomas. The recommendations are divided into four major areas: (a) items that provide an informative gross description; (b) additional diagnostic features that are recom-

mended to be included in the report, if possible; (c) optional features that may be included in the final report; and (d) a checklist. These recommendations are listed below (833).

A. Gross description
  1. How the specimen was received—fresh, in formalin, opened, unopened, etc.
  2. How the specimen was identified—labeled with (name and number) and designated as (e.g., right colon)
  3. Part(s) of intestine received, length of each segment, other structures received—terminal ileum, appendix, anal canal, attached/adherent organs, and identified vessels
  4. Tumor description
     • Site in intestine
     • Proximity to nearest margin
     • Gross subtype (e.g., polypoid, annular, constricting, ulcerating, infiltrative, plaque, or linitis plastica)
     • Dimensions (three if possible)
     • Macroscopic depth of penetration
     • Appearance of serosa adjacent to tumor (e.g., retracted)
  5. Presence of features of obstruction (proximal dilation)
  6. Presence of perforation
  7. Status of residual bowel—polyps, IBD, diverticula, ulcers, and strictures
  8. Lymph nodes identified
  9. Tissue submitted for special investigation (e.g., flow cytometry) should be specified
B. Diagnostic information
  1. Site of tumor and part of bowel resected
  2. Histologic type
     • Adenocarcinoma; not otherwise specified
     • Mucinous (colloid) carcinoma (>50% mucinous)
     • Signet ring cell carcinoma (>50% signet ring cells)
     • Adenosquamous carcinoma
     • Small cell undifferentiated (oat cell) carcinoma
     • Undifferentiated carcinoma
     • Other (specify)
  3. Histologic grade—a modification of the World Health Organization (WHO) classification is recommended for adenocarcinoma not otherwise specified (NOS) only
     • Well differentiated—complex or simple tubules, easily discerned nuclear polarity, and uniform-sized nuclei
     • Moderately differentiated—complex, simple, or slightly irregular tubules, nuclear polarity just discerned or lost
     • Poorly differentiated—highly irregular glands or an absence of glandular differentiation with loss of nuclear polarity

4. Depth of infiltration—the authors' recommendations are based on those in the TNM classification
   • Into the submucosa but not into the muscularis propria (T1)
   • Into but not through the muscularis propria (T2)
   • Through the muscularis propria and into the subserosal fat or pericolonic or perirectal adipose tissue (T3)
   • Reaching the serosa or peritoneal surface (T4)
   • Into adjacent organs (T4)
   • With perforation if present
5. Lymph node metastases—stated as number of involved nodes and total number of nodes
6. Presence of mesenteric deposits (since these are included in the TNM classification)
7. Other sites biopsied for metastatic disease—peritoneum, adjacent organs, liver, and ovary
8. Adequacy of local excision—radial/proximal/distal resection margins. Assessment of proximal and distal margins is routine in the bowel as in other organs. In the rectum the deep margin (radial [lateral] margin) should be assessed. The radial margin is defined as the point at which the tumor reaches the closest to a deep (lateral, circumferential) resected margin and is usually the deepest point of invasion in the rectum. For the large intestine outside of the rectum, the "lateral" surgical resection margin is the mesenteric border of resection and is usually widely free of tumor unless dissection has deliberately been carried out close to the bowel wall. The antimesenteric serosal surface of the nonrectal large intestine is not a radial resection margin.
9. Other significant disease (e.g., IBD, other tumors, polyps, FAP, diverticular disease and its complications, ulcers, and strictures)
10. If information required for prognosis or therapy is not available (e.g., no nodes found or radial margin not assessable), this should be stated specifically in the report.

Other features that may be evaluated because they probably have prognostic significance are listed in Table 14.23.

TABLE 14.23 **Other Features That May Be Described**

1. Nature of the advancing edge—regular or irregular/infiltrative
2. Inflammatory infiltrate—e.g., Crohn-like, lymphocytic, or eosinophilic
3. Lymph vessel infiltration
4. Perineural infiltration
5. Venous infiltration (extramural veins only)

REFERENCES

1. Parkin DM, Bray F, Ferlay J, Pisani P: Global cancer statistics, 2002. *CA Cancer J Clin* 2005;55:74.
2. SEER Stat Fact Sheets: Cancer of the Colon and Rectum. Available at: http://seer.cancer.gov/statfacts/html/colorect. Accessed December 30, 2006.
3. Shibuya K, Mathers CD, Boschi-Pinto C, et al: Global and regional estimates of cancer mortality and incidence by site: II. Results for the global burden of disease 2000. *BMC Cancer* 2002;2:37.
4. Parkin DM: International variation. *Oncogene* 2004;23:6329.
5. McMichael AJ, McCall MG, Hartshorne JM, et al: Patterns of gastrointestinal change in European migrants to Australia. The role of dietary change. *Int J Cancer* 1980;25:431.
6. Parkin DM, Bray F, Devesa S: Cancer burden in the year 2000: the global picture. *Eur J Cancer* 2001;37:S4.
7. Potter JD: Nutrition and colorectal cancer. *Cancer Causes Control* 1996;7:127.
8. Leppert M, Burt R, Hughes JP, et al: Genetic analysis of an inherited predisposition to colon cancer in a family with a variable number of adenomatous polyps. *N Engl J Med* 1990;322:904.
9. Fuchs CS, Giovannucci EL, Colditz GA, et al: A prospective study of family history and the risk of colorectal cancer. *N Engl J Med* 1994;331:1669.
10. Ponz de Leon M, Sassatelli R, Sacchette C, et al: Familial aggregation of tumors in the three-year experience of a population-based colorectal cancer registry. *Cancer Res* 1989;49:4344.
11. Bishop D, Hall N: The genetics of colorectal cancer. *Eur J Cancer* 1994;30:1946.
12. St. John DJ, McDermott FT, Hopper JL, et al: Cancer risk in relatives of patients with common colorectal cancer. *Ann Intern Med* 1993;118:785.
13. Ponz de Leon M: Prevalence of hereditary nonpolyposis colorectal carcinoma (HNPCC). *Ann Med* 1994;26:209.
14. Rozen P, Fireman Z, Figer A, et al: Family history of colorectal cancer as a marker of potential malignancy within a screening program. *Cancer* 1987;60:248.
15. Bazzoli F, Fossi S, Sottili S, et al: The risk of adenomatous polyps in asymptomatic first-degree relatives of persons with colon cancer. *Gastroenterology* 1995;109:783.
16. Lyon JL, Mahoney AW, West DW, et al: Energy intake: Its relationship to colon cancer risk. *J Natl Cancer Inst* 1987;78:853.
17. Little J, Logan RFA, Hawtin PG, et al: Colorectal adenomas and energy intake, body size and physical activity—a case-control study of subjects participating in the Nottingham faecal occult blood screening programme. *Br J Cancer* 1993;67:172.
18. Gorham ED, Garland CF, Garland FC: Physical activity and colon cancer risk. *Int J Epidemiol* 1989;18:728.
19. Le Marchand L, Wilkens LR, Kolonel LN, et al: Associations of sedentary lifestyle, obesity, smoking, alcohol use and diabetes with the risk of colorectal cancer. *Cancer Res* 1997;57:4787.
20. Caan BJ, Coates AO, Slattery ML, et al: Body size and the risk of colon cancer in a large case-control study. *Int J Obes Relat Metab Disord* 1998;22:178.
21. Russo A, Franceschi S, La Vecchia C, et al: Body size and colorectal-cancer risk. *Int J Cancer* 1998;78:161.
22. Dietz AT, Newcomb PA, Marcus PM, Storer BE: The association of body size and large bowel cancer risk in Wisconsin women. *Cancer Causes Control* 1995;6:30.
23. MacInnis RJ, English DR, Hopper JL, et al: Body size and composition and colon cancer risk in men. *Cancer Epidemiol Biomarkers Prev* 2004;13:533.
24. Gunter MJ, Leitzmann MF: Obesity and colorectal cancer: epidemiology, mechanisms and candidate genes. *J Nutr Biochem* 2006;17:145.
25. Khaw KT, Wareham N, Bingham S, et al: Preliminary communication: glycated hemoglobin, diabetes, and incident colorectal cancer in men and women: a prospective analysis from the European prospective investigation into cancer—Norfolk study. *Cancer Epidemiol Biomarkers Prev* 2004;13:915.
26. Yam D, Fink A, Mashiah A, Ben-Hur E: Hyperinsulinemia in colon, stomach and breast cancer patients. *Cancer Lett* 1996;104:129.
27. Wu X, Fan Z, Masui H, et al: Apoptosis induced by an anti-epidermal growth factor receptor monoclonal antibody in a human colorectal carcinoma cell line and its delay by insulin. *J Clin Invest* 1995;95:1897.
28. Tran TT, Medline A, Bruce WR: Insulin promotion of colon tumors in rats. *Cancer Epidemiol Biomarkers Prev* 1996;5:1013.

29. Corpet DE, Jacquinet C, Peiffer G, Tache S: Insulin injections promote growth of aberrant crypt foci in the colon of rats. *Nutr Cancer* 1997;27:316.

30. Prentki M: New insights into the pancreatic beta-cell metabolic signaling in insulin secretion. *Eur J Endocrinol* 1996;134:272.

31. McGarr SE, Ridlon JM, Hylemon PB: Diet, anaerobic bacterial metabolism, and colon cancer: a review of the literature. *J Clin Gastroenterol* 2004;39:98.

32. Burkitt DP: Relationship as a clue to causation. *Lancet* 1970;2:1237.

33. Trowell H, Burkitt D: *Western Diseases: Their Emergence and Prevention* (Preface). London: Arnold, 1981.

34. Segi M, Kurihara M, Tsukahara Y: *Mortality for Selected Causes in 30 Countries (1950–61)*. Tokyo: Kosai, 1966, p 188.

35. Kolonel L: Fat and colon cancer: how firm is the epidemiologic evidence? *Am J Clin Nutr* 1987;45(1 suppl):336.

36. Nomura AM, Heilbrun LK, Stemmermann GN: Body mass index as a predictor of cancer in men. *J Natl Cancer Inst* 1985;74:319.

37. Erhardt JG, Lim SS, Bode JC, Bode C: A diet rich in fat and poor in dietary fiber increases the in vitro formation of reactive oxygen species in human feces. *J Nutr* 1997;127:706.

38. Wattenberg LW: Inhibition of carcinogenic effects of polycyclic hydrocarbons by benzyl isothiocyanate and related compounds. *J Natl Cancer Inst* 1977;58:195.

39. Deluca HF, Ostrem V: The relationship between the vitamin D system and cancer. *Adv Exp Med Biol* 1987;206:413.

40. Steinmetz KA, Potter JD: Vegetables, fruits and cancer. II. Mechanisms. *Cancer Causes Control* 1991;2:427.

41. Steinmetz KA, Kushi LH, Bostick RM, et al: Vegetables, fruit, and colon cancer in the Iowa Women's Study. *Am J Epidemiol* 1994;139:1.

42. Giovannucci E, Willett WC: Dietary factors and risk of colon cancer. *Ann Med* 1994;26:443.

43. Dion PW, Bright-See EB, Smith CC: The effect of dietary ascorbic acid and alpha-tocopherol in fecal mutagenicity. *Mutat Res* 1988;102:27.

44. Bussey HJ, DeCosse JJ, Deschner EE, et al: A randomized trial of ascorbic acid in polyposis coli. *Cancer* 1982;50:1434.

45. Sorenson AW, Slattery ML, Ford MH: Calcium and colon cancer: a review. *Nutr Cancer* 1988;11:135.

46. Kono S, Imanishi K, Shinchi K, Yanai F: Relationship of diet to small and large adenomas of the sigmoid colon. *Jpn J Cancer Res* 1993;84:13.

47. Alder RJ, McKeown-Eyssen G: Calcium intake and risk of colorectal cancer. *Front Gastrointest Res* 1988;14:177.

48. Heilbrun LK, Hankin JH, Nomura AM, Stemmermann GN: Colon cancer and dietary fat, phosphorus, and calcium in Hawaiian and Japanese men. *Am J Clin Nutr* 1986;43:306.

49. Newmark H, Lipkin M: Calcium, vitamin D, and colon cancer. *Cancer Res* 1992;52(7 suppl):2067s.

50. Pence B: Role of calcium in colon cancer prevention: experimental and clinical studies. *Mutat Res* 1993;290:87.

51. Lointier P, Wargovich MJ, Saez S, Levin B: The role of vitamin D3 in the proliferation of human colon cancer in vitro. *Anticancer Res* 1987;7:817.

52. Nelson RL: Dietary minerals and colon carcinogenesis. *Anticancer Res* 1987;7:259.

53. Milsom JW: Pathogenesis of colorectal cancer. *Surg Clin N Am* 1993;73:1.

54. Stemmermann GN, Nomura AMY, Chyou PH, Yoshizawa C: Prospective study of alcohol and large bowel cancer. *Dig Dis Sci* 1990;35:1414.

55. Cope GF, Wyatt JL, Pinder IF, et al: Alcohol consumption in patients with colorectal adenomatous polyps. *Gut* 1991;32:70.

56. Riboli E, Cornee J, Macquart-Moulin G, et al: Cancer and polyps of the colorectum and lifetime consumption of beer and other alcoholic beverages. *Am J Epidemiol* 1991;134:157.

57. Akhter M, Kuriyama S, Nakaya N, et al: Alcohol consumption is associated with an increased risk of distal colon and rectal cancer in Japanese men: the Miyagi Cohort Study. *Eur J Cancer* 2007;43:383.

58. Moskal A, Norat T, Ferrari P, Riboli E: Alcohol intake and colorectal cancer risk: a dose-response meta-analysis of published cohort studies. *Int J Cancer* 2007;120:664.

59. Sandler RS, Lyles CM, Peipins LA, et al: Diet and risk of colorectal adenomas—macronutrients, cholesterol and fiber. *J Natl Cancer Inst* 1993;85:884.

60. Naveau S, Chaput JC, Bedossa P, et al: Cirrhosis as an independent risk factor for colonic adenomas. *Gut* 1992;33:535.

61. Heineman EF, Zahm SH, McLaughlin JK, Vaught JB: Increased risk of colorectal cancer among smokers: results of a 26-year follow-up of US veterans and a review. *Int J Cancer* 1994;59:728.

62. Giovannucci E, Colditz GA, Stampfer MJ, et al: A prospective study of cigarette smoking and risk of colorectal adenoma and colorectal cancer in United States women. *J Natl Cancer Inst* 1994;86:192.

63. Samowitz WS, Albertson H, Sweeney C, et al: Association of smoking, CpG island methylator phenotype, and V600E BRAF mutations in colon cancer. *J Natl Cancer Inst* 2006;98:1731.

64. Slattery ML, Curtin K, Anderson K, et al: Associations between cigarette smoking, lifestyle factors, and microsatellite instability in colon tumors. *J Natl Cancer Inst* 2000;92:1831.

65. Schottenfeld D, Warshauer ME, Zauber AG, et al: Study of cancer mortality and incidence in wood shop workers of the General Motors Corporation. Report prepared for the Occupational Health Advisory Board of United Auto Workers, April 18, 1980.

66. Swanson GM, Belle SH, Burrows RW: Colon cancer incidence among model makers and pattern makers in the automobile manufacturing industry: a continuing dilemma. *J Occup Med* 1985;27:567.

67. Weiss W: Asbestos and colorectal cancer. *Gastroenterology* 1990;99:876.

68. Ehrlich A, Gordon RE, Dikman SH: Carcinoma of the colon in asbestos-exposed workers: analysis of asbestos content in colon tissue. *Am J Ind Med* 1991;19:629.

69. Fredriksson M, Bengtsson N, Hardell L, Axelson O: Colon cancer, physical activity, and occupational exposures. *Cancer* 1989;63:1838.

70. Booth S, Lacey RW: Effect of recent food on estimation of high-density lipoprotein and total cholesterol in normal subjects. *Ann Clin Biochem* 1982;19:176.

71. Sherwin RW, Wentworth DN, Cutler JA, et al: Serum cholesterol levels and cancer mortality in 361,662 men screened for the Multiple Risk Factor Intervention Trial. *JAMA* 1987;257:943.

72. Stemmermann GN, Chyou PH, Kagan A, et al: Serum cholesterol and cancer mortality in Japanese-American men: The Honolulu Heart Program. *Ann Intern Med* 1991;151:969.

73. Sorlie PD, Feinleib M: The serum cholesterol-cancer relationship: an analysis of trends in the Framingham study. *J Natl Cancer Inst* 1982;69:989.

74. Mannes GA, Maier A, Thieme C, et al: Relationship between the frequency of colorectal adenoma and the serum cholesterol level. *N Engl J Med* 1986;315:1634.

75. Rodenas JM, Herranz MT, Tercedor J, et al: Muir-Torre syndrome associated with a family history of hyperlipidemia. *J Am Acad Dermatol* 1993;28:285.

76. Kervinen K, Södervik H, Mäkelä J, et al: Is the development of adenoma and carcinoma in proximal colon related to apolipoprotein E phenotype? *Gastroenterology* 1996;110:1785.

77. Burkitt DP: Related disease related cause? *Lancet* 1969;2:1229.

78. Code PE, Chan KW, Chan YT: Polyps and diverticula of the large intestine: a necropsy survey in Hong Kong. *Gut* 1985;26:1045.

79. Stemmermann GN, Yatani R: Diverticulosis and polyps of the large intestine. A necropsy study of Hawaii Japanese. *Cancer* 1973;31:1260.

80. Baquet CR, Horm JW, Gibbs T, et al: Socioeconomic factors and cancer incidence among blacks and whites. *J Natl Cancer Inst* 1991;83:551.

81. Van Loon AJ, van den Brandt PA, Golbohm RA: Socioeconomic status and colon cancer incidence: a prospective cohort study. *Br J Cancer* 1995;71:882.

82. Weiderpass E, Pukkala E: Time trends in socioeconomic differences in incidence rates of cancer of gastro-intestinal tract in Finland. *BMC Gastroenterol* 2006;6:41.

83. Davis FG, Furner SE, Persky V, Koch M: The influence of parity and exogenous female hormones on the risk of colorectal cancer. *Int J Cancer* 1989;43:587.

84. Chute CG, Willett WC, Colditz GA, et al: A prospective study of reproductive history and exogenous estrogens on the risk of colorectal cancer in women. *Epidemiology* 1991;2:201.

85. Calle EE, Miracle-McMahill HL, Thun MJ, et al: Estrogen replacement therapy and risk of fatal colon cancer in a prospective cohort of postmenopausal women. *J Natl Cancer Inst* 1995;87:517.

86. Marcus PM, Newcomb PA, Young T, et al: The association of reproductive and menstrual characteristics and colon and rectal cancer risk in Wisconsin women. *Ann Epidemiol* 1995;5:303.

87. Wu-Williams AH, Lee M, Whittemore AS: Reproductive factors and colorectal cancer risk among Chinese females. *Cancer Res* 1991;51:2307.

88. Takeda H, Yamakawa M, Takahashi T, et al: An immunohistochemical study with an estrogen receptor-related protein (ER-D5) in human colorectal cancer. *Cancer* 1992;69:907.

89. Ciccotosto G, McLeish A, Hardy K, Shulkes A: Expression, processing, and secretion of gastrin in patients with colorectal carcinoma. *Gastroenterology* 1995;109:1142.

90. Baldwin GS, Zhang QX: Measurement of gastrin and transforming growth factor a messenger RNA levels in colonic carcinoma cell lines by quantitative polymerase chain reaction. *Cancer Res* 1992;52:2261.

91. Finley GG, Koski RA, Melhem MF, et al: Expression of the gastrin gene in the normal human colon and colorectal adenocarcinoma. *Cancer Res* 1993;53:2919.

92. Seitz JF, Giovannini M, Monges G, et al: Serum gastrin levels in colorectal cancers—evolution after treatment. *Gastroenterol Clin Biol* 1992;16:385.

93. Brunner JE, Johnson CC, Zafar S, et al: Colon cancer and polyps in acromegaly: increased risk associated with family history of colon cancer. *Clin Endocrinol* 1990;32:65.

94. Vasen HFA, Van Erpecum KJ, Roelfsema F, et al: Increased prevalence of colonic adenomas in patients with acromegaly. *Eur J Endocrinol* 1994;131:235.

95. Cats A, Dullaart RP, Kleibeuker JH, et al: Increased epithelial cell proliferation in the colon of patients with acromegaly. *Cancer Res* 1996;56:523.

96. Sandler RS, Sandler DP: Radiation-induced cancers of the colon and rectum: assessing the risk. *Gastroenterology* 1983;84:51.

97. Guo W, Zheng W, Li JY, et al: Correlations of colon cancer mortality with dietary factors, serum markers and schistosomiasis in China. *Nutr Cancer* 1993;20:13.

98. Mannes AG, Weinzierl M, Stellaard F, et al: Adenomas of the large intestine after cholecystectomy. *Gut* 1984;25:863.

99. Turunen MJ, Kivilaakso EO: Increased risk of colorectal cancer after cholecystectomy. *Ann Surg* 1981;194:639.

100. Weiss NS, Daling JR, Chow WH: Cholecystectomy and the incidence of cancer of the large bowel. *Cancer* 1982;49:1713.

101. Schottenfeld D, Winawer SJ: Cholecystectomy and colorectal cancer. *Gastroenterology* 1983;85:966.

102. Narisawa T, Yamazaki Y, Kusaka H, et al: Clinical observation on the association of gallstones and colorectal cancer. *Cancer* 1991;67:1696.

103. Rivard JY, Bedard A, Dionne L: Colonic neoplasms following uterosigmoidostomy. *J Urol* 1975;113:781.

104. Sheldon CA, McKinley CR, Hartig PR, Gonzalez R: Carcinoma at the site of ureterosigmoidostomy. *Dis Colon Rectum* 1983;26:55.

105. Harford FJ, Fazio VW, Epstein LM, Hewitt CB: Rectosigmoid carcinoma occurring after ureterosigmoidostomy. *Dis Colon Rectum* 1984;27:321.

106. Cuesta MA, Donner R: Adenocarcinoma arising at an ileostomy site: report of a case. *Cancer* 1976;37:949.

107. Crissey MM, Steele GD, Gittes RF: Rat model for carcinogenesis in ureterosigmoidostomy. *Science* 1980;207:1079.

108. Tomera KM, Unni KK, Utz DC: Adenomatous polyp in ileal conduit. *J Urol* 1982;128:1025.

109. Takami M, Hanada M, Kimura M, et al: Adenocarcinoma arising at a colostomy site. Report of a case. *Dis Colon Rectum* 1983;26:50.

110. Weshler Z, Sulkes A, Rizel S: Carcinoma of the colon following ureterocolostomy. *Dis Colon Rectum* 1979;22:434.

111. Roe R, Fermor B, Williamson RCN: Proliferative instability and experimental carcinogenesis at colonic anastomoses. *Gut* 1987;28:808.

112. Offerhaus GJ, Tersmette AC, Tersmette KW, et al: Gastric, pancreatic, and colorectal carcinogenesis following remote peptic ulcer surgery. Review of the literature with emphasis on risk assessment and underlying mechanism. *Mod Pathol* 1988;1:352.

113. Mullan FJ, Wilson HK, Majury CW, et al: Bile acids and the increased risk of colorectal tumours. *Br J Surg* 1990;77:1085.

114. Fisher SG, Davis F, Nelson R, et al: Large bowel cancer following gastric surgery for benign disease: a cohort study. *Am J Epidemiol* 1994;139:684.

115. Dunlop MG: Inheritance of colorectal cancer susceptibility. *Br J Surg* 1990;77:245.

116. Hickey WF, Corson J: Squamous cell carcinoma arising in a duplication of the colon: case report and literature review of squamous cell carcinoma of the colon and of malignancy complicating colonic duplication. *Cancer* 1981;47:602.

117. Atwell JD, Taylor I, Cruddas M: Increased risk of colorectal cancer associated with congenital anomalies of the urinary tract. *Br J Surg* 1993;80:785.

118. Talley NJ, Chute CG, Larson DE, et al: Risk for colorectal adenocarcinoma in pernicious anemia: a population-based cohort study. *Ann Intern Med* 1989;111:738.

119. Williams J, Walsh D, Jackson J: Colon carcinoma and diabetes mellitus. *Cancer* 1984;54:3070.

120. Swinson CM, Slavin G, Coles EC, Booth CC: Coeliac disease and malignancy. *Lancet* 1983;1:111.

121. Danzig JB, Brandt LJ, Reinus JF, Klein RS: Gastrointestinal malignancy in patients with AIDS. *Am J Gastroenterol* 1991;86:715.

122. Gilbertsen VA: Proctosigmoidoscopy and polypectomy in reducing the incidence of rectal cancer. *Cancer* 1974;34:936.

123. Citarda F, Tomaselli G, Capocaccia R, et al: Efficacy in standard clinical practice of colonoscopic polypectomy in reducing colorectal cancer incidence. *Gut* 2001;48:812.

124. Thiis-Evensen E, Hoff GS, Sauar J, et al: Population-based surveillance by colonoscopy: effect on the incidence of colorectal cancer. Telemark Polyp Study I. *Scand J Gastroenterol* 1999;34:414.

125. Newcomb PA, Storer BE, Morimoto LM, et al: Long-term efficacy of sigmoidoscopy in the reduction of colorectal cancer incidence. *J Natl Cancer Inst* 2003;105:82.

126. Selby JV, Friedman GD, Quesenberry CP Jr, Weiss NS: A case-control study of screening sigmoidoscopy and mortality from colorectal cancer. *N Engl J Med* 1992;326:653.

127. Levin B, Bond J: Colorectal cancer screening: recommendations of the U.S. preventive services task force. *Gastroenterology* 1996;111:1381.

128. Winawer S, Fletcher R, Rex D, et al: Colorectal cancer screening and surveillance: clinical guidelines and rationale-update based on new evidence. *Gastroenterology* 2003;124:544.

129. Muscat JE, Stellman SD, Wynder EL: Nonsteroidal antiinflammatory drugs and colorectal cancer. *Cancer* 1994;74:1847.

130. Thun M, Namboodiri M, Heath CW Jr: Aspirin use and reduced risk of fatal colon cancer. *N Engl J Med* 1991;325:1593.

131. Peleg I, Maibach H, Brown S, Wilcox M: Aspirin and nonsteroidal anti-inflammatory drug use and the risk of subsequent colorectal cancer. *Arch Intern Med* 1994;154:394.

132. Rosenberg L, Palmer JR, Zauber AG, et al: A hypothesis; nonsteroidal anti-inflammatory drugs reduce the incidence of large-bowel cancer. *J Natl Cancer Inst* 1991;83:355.

133. Suh O, Mettlin C, Petrelli NJ: Aspirin use, cancer, and polyps of the large bowel. *Cancer* 1993;72:1171.

134. Marnett LJ: Aspirin and the potential role of prostaglandins in colon cancer. *Cancer Res* 1992;52:5575.

135. Logan RF, Little J, Hawtin PG, Hardcastle JD: Effect of aspirin and non-steroidal anti-inflammatory drugs on colorectal adenomas: case-control study of subjects participating in the Nottingham faecal occult blood screening programme. *Br Med J* 1993;307:285.

136. Gann PH, Manson JE, Glynn RJ, et al: Low-dose aspirin and incidence of colorectal tumors in a randomized trial. *J Natl Cancer Inst* 1993;85:1220.

137. Giardiello FM, Hamilton SR, Krush AJ, et al: Treatment of colonic and rectal adenomas with sulindac in familial adenomatous polyposis. *N Engl J Med* 1993;328:1313.

138. Labayle D, Fischer D, Vielh P, et al: Sulindac causes regression of rectal polyps in familial adenomatous polyposis. *Gastroenterology* 1991;101:635.

139. Nugent KP, Farmer KC, Spigelman AD, et al: Randomized controlled trial of the effect of sulindac on duodenal and rectal polyposis and cell proliferation in patients with familial adenomatous polyposis. *Br J Surg* 1993;80:1618.

140. Spagnesi MT, Tonelli F, Dolara P, et al: Rectal proliferation and polyp occurrence in patients with familial adenomatous polyposis after sulindac treatment. *Gastroenterology* 1994;106:362.

141. Rao CV, Tokumo K, Rigotty J, et al: Chemoprevention of colon carcinogenesis by dietary administration of piroxicam, alpha-difluoromethylornithine, 16 alpha-fluoro-5-androsten-17-one, and ellagic acid individually and in combination. *Cancer Res* 1991;51:4528.

142. Reddy BS, Nayini J, Tokumo K, et al: Chemoprevention of colon carcinogenesis by concurrent administration of piroxicam, a nonsteroidal antiinflammatory drug with D,L-alpha-difluoromethylornithine, an ornithine decarboxylase inhibitor, in diet. *Cancer Res* 1990;50:2562.

143. Reddy BS, Rao CV, Rivenson A, Kelloff G: Inhibitory effect of aspirin on azoxymethane-induced colon carcinogenesis in F344 rats. *Carcinogenesis* 1993;14:1493.

144. Baron JA, Cole BF, Sandler RS, et al: A randomized trial of aspirin to prevent colorectal adenomas. *N Engl J Med* 2003;348:891.

145. Sandler RS, Halabi S, Baron JA, et al: A randomized trial of aspirin to prevent colorectal adenomas in patients with previous colorectal cancer. *N Engl J Med* 2003;348:883.

146. Subbaramaiah K, Dannenberg AJ: Cyclooxygenase 2: a molecular target for cancer prevention and treatment. *Trends Pharmacol Sci* 2003;24:96.

147. Eberhardt CE, Coffey RJ, Radhika A, et al: Up-regulation of cyclooxygenase 2 gene expression in human colorectal adenomas and adenocarcinomas. *Gastroenterology* 1994;107:1183.

148. Hull MA, Ko SC, Hawcroft G: Prostaglandin EP receptors: targets for treatment and prevention of colorectal cancer? *Mol Cancer Ther* 2004;3:1031.

149. Kawamori T, Uchiya N, Sugimura T, Wakabayashi K: Enhancement of colon carcinogenesis by prostaglandin E_2 administration. *Carcinogenesis* 2003;24:985.

150. Castellone MD, Teramoto H, Gutkind JS: Cyclooxygenase-2 and colorectal cancer chemoprevention: the b-catenin connection. *Cancer Res* 2006;66:11085.

151. Wargovich M, Isbell G, Shabot M, et al: Calcium supplementation decreases rectal epithelial cell proliferation in subjects with sporadic adenoma. *Gastroenterology* 1992;103:92.

152. Barsoum GH, Hendrickse C, Winslet MC, et al: Reduction of mucosal crypt cell proliferation in patients with colorectal adenomatous polyps by dietary calcium supplementation. *Br J Surg* 1992;79:581.

153. Reshef R, Rozen P, Fireman Z, et al: Effect of a calcium-enriched diet on the colonic epithelial hyperproliferation induced by N-methyl-N-nitro-N-nitrosoguanidine in rats on a low calcium and fat diet. *Cancer Res* 1990;50:1764.

154. Newmark HL, Wargovich MJ, Bruce WR: Colon cancer and dietary fat, phosphate, and calcium: a hypothesis. *J Natl Cancer Inst* 1984;72:1323.

155. Wallace K, Baron JA, Cole BF, et al: Effect of calcium supplementation on the risk of large bowel polyps. *J Natl Cancer Inst* 2004;921.

156. Bonithon-Kopp C, Kronborg O, Giacosa A, et al: Calcium and fibre supplementation in prevention of colorectal adenoma recurrence: a randomised intervention trial. European Cancer Prevention Organisation Study Group. *Lancet* 2000;356:1300.

157. Grau MV, Baron JA, Sandler RS, et al: Prolonged effect of calcium supplementation on risk of colorectal adenomas in a randomized trial. *J Natl Cancer Inst* 2007;99:129.

158. Cho E, Smith-Warner SA, Spiegelman D, et al: Dairy foods, calcium and colorectal cancer: a pooled analysis of 10 cohort studies. *J Natl Cancer Inst* 2004;96:1015.

159. Gavrieli Y, Sherman Y, Ben-Sasson SA: Identification of programmed cell death via specific labeling of nuclear DNA fragmentation. *J Cell Biol* 1992;119:493.

160. Wang CY, Eshleman JR, Wilson JK, Markowitz S: Both transforming growth factor-β and substrate release are inducers of apoptosis in a human colon adenoma cell line. *Cancer Res* 1995;55:5101.

161. Moss SF, Liu TC, Petrotos A, et al: Inward growth of colonic adenomatous polyps. *Gastroenterology* 1996;111:1425.

162. Hague A, Moorghen M, Hicks D, et al: Bcl-2 expression in human colorectal adenomas and carcinomas. *Oncogene* 1994;9:3367.

163. Krajewska M, Moss SF, Krajewski S, et al: Elevated expression of Bcl-X and reduced Bax in primary colorectal adenocarcinomas. *Cancer Res* 1996;56:2422.

164. Sinicrope FA, Ruan SB, Cleary KR, et al: Bcl-2 and p53 oncoprotein expression during colorectal tumorigenesis. *Cancer Res* 1995;55:237.

165. Cole JW, McKalen A: Studies on the morphogenesis of adenomatous polyps in the human colon. *Cancer* 1963;16:998.

166. Hoff G: Colorectal polyps. Clinical implications: screening and cancer prevention. *Scand J Gastroenterol* 1987;22:769.

167. O'Brien M, O'Keane J, Zauber A, et al: Precursors of colorectal carcinoma. *Cancer* 1992;70:1317.

168. Johannsen G, Momsen O, Jacobsen NO: Polyps of large intestine in Aarhus, Denmark. *Scand J Gastroenterol* 1989;24:799.

169. Fenoglio-Preiser CM, Perzin K, Pascal RR: *Tumors of the Large and Small Intestine.* AFIP Fascicle, 2nd Series. Washington, DC: AFIP, 1990.

170. Clark JC, Collan Y, Eide TJ, et al: Prevalence of polyps in an autopsy series from areas with varying incidence of large-bowel cancer. *Int J Cancer* 1985;36:179.

171. Neugut AI, Jacobson JS, Ahsan H, et al: Incidence and recurrence rates of colorectal adenomas: a prospective study. *Gastroenterology* 1995;108:402.

172. Bremner CG, Ackerman L: Polyps and carcinoma of the large bowel in the South African Bantu. *Br J Cancer* 1970;26:991.

173. Restrepo C, Correa P, Duque E, Cuello C: Polyps in a low-risk colonic cancer population in Colombia, South America. *Dis Colon Rectum* 1981;24:29.

174. Giacosa A, Frascio F, Munizzi F: Epidemiology of colorectal polyps. *Tech Coloproctol* 2004;8:S243.

175. Winawer SJ, Zauber A, Diaz B, et al: The National Polyp Study: overview of program and preliminary report of patient and polyp characteristics. In: Steele G, (ed): *Basic and Clinical Perspectives of Colorectal Polyps and Cancer.* New York: Alan R. Liss, 1988, p 35.

176. Vatn MH, Stalsberg H: Polyps of the large intestine in Oslo: a prospective autopsy study. *Cancer* 1982;49:819.

177. Chapman I: Adenomatous polypi of large intestine: incidence and distribution. *Ann Surg* 1963;157:223.

178. Arminski TC, McLean DW: Incidence and distribution of adenomatous polyps of the colon and rectum based on 1,000 autopsy examinations. *Dis Colon Rectum* 1964;7:249.

179. Ekelund G: *On Colorectal Polyps and Carcinoma with Special Reference to Their Interrelationship.* Sweden: Malmo General Hospital, University of Lund, 1974.

180. Hoff G, Foerster A, Vatn MH, Gjone E: Epidemiology of polyps in the rectum and sigmoid colon. Histological examination of resected polyps. *Scand J Gastroenterol* 1985;20:677.

181. Rickert R, Auerbach O, Garfinkel L, et al: Adenomatous lesions of the large bowel. An autopsy survey. *Cancer* 1979;43:1847.

182. Neugut AI, Jacobson JS, DeVivo I: Epidemiology of colorectal adenomatous polyps. *Cancer Epidemiol Biomarkers Prev* 1993;2:159.

183. Atkin WS, Morson BC, Cuzick J: Long-term risk of colorectal cancer after excision of rectosigmoid adenomas. *N Engl J Med* 1992;326:658.

184. Winawer SJ, O'Brien MJ, Wayne JD, et al: Risk and surveillance of individuals with colorectal polyps. *Bull WHO* 1990;68:789.

185. Bernstein M, Feczko P, Halpert R, et al: Distribution of colonic polyps: increased incidence of proximal lesions in older patients. *Radiology* 1985;155:35.

186. Eide TJ, Stalsberg H: Polyps of the large intestine in Northern Norway. *Cancer* 1978;42:2839.

187. Winawer SJ, St. John J, Bond J, et al: Screening of average-risk individuals for colorectal cancer. *Bull WHO* 1990;68:505.

188. Tripp MR, Morgan TR, Sampliner RE, et al: Synchronous neoplasms in patients with diminutive colorectal adenomas. *Cancer* 1987;60:1599.

189. O'Brien MJ, Winawer SJ, Zauber AG, et al: The National Polyp Study: patient and polyp characteristics associated with high grade dysplasia in adenomas. *Gastroenterology* 1990;98:371.

190. Winawer SJ, Schottenfeld D, Flehinger BJ: Colorectal cancer screening. *J Natl Cancer Inst* 1991;83:243.

191. Neugut AI, Lauthenbach I, Abi-Rached B, Forde KA: Incidence of adenomas after curative resection for colorectal cancer. *Am J Gastroenterol* 1996;91:2096.

192. Neugut AI, Johnsen CM, Forde KA, Treat MR: Recurrence rates for colorectal polyps. *Cancer* 1985;55:1586.

193. Stryker SJ, Wolff BG, Culp CE, et al: Natural history of untreated colonic polyps. *Gastroenterology* 1987;93:1009.

194. Rex D, Cutler C, Lemmel G, et al: Colonoscopic miss rates of adenomas determined by back-to-back colonoscopies. *Gastroenterology* 1997;112:24.

195. Rex CK, Lehman GA, Ulbright TM, et al: The yield of a second screening flexible sigmoidoscopy in average-risk persons after one negative examination. *Gastroenterology* 1994;106:593.

196. Glick S, Teplick S, Balfe D, et al: Large colonic neoplasms missed by endoscopy. *AJR Am J Roentgenol* 1989;152:513.

197. Jass JR: Colorectal adenomas in surgical specimens from subjects with hereditary non-polyposis colorectal cancer. *Histopathology* 1995;27:263.

198. Lanspa SJ, Jenkins JX, Watson P, et al: Adenoma follow-up in at-risk Lynch syndrome family members. *Anticancer Res* 1993;13:1793.

199. Sobin LH: The histopathology of bleeding from polyps and carcinomas of the large intestine. *Cancer* 1985;55:577.

200. Stulc JP, Petrelli NJ, Herrera L, Mittelman A: Colorectal villous and tubulovillous adenomas equal to or greater than four centimeters. *Ann Surg* 1988;207:65.

201. Rex DK, Lehman LA, Hawes RH, et al: Screening colonoscopy in asymptomatic average risk persons with negative fecal occult blood tests. *Gastroenterology* 1991;100:64.

202. Gottlieb LS, Winawer SJ, Sternberg S, et al: National polyp study (NPS): the diminutive polyp. *Gastrointest Endosc* 1984;30:143.

203. Tedesco FJ, Hendrix JC, Pickens CA, et al: Diminutive polyps: histopathology, spatial distribution, and clinical significance. *Gastrointest Endosc* 1982;28:1.

204. Waye JD, Frankel A, Braunfeld SF: The histopathology of small colon polyps. *Gastrointest Endosc* 1980;26:80.

205. Chapuis PH, Dent OF, Goulston KJ: Clinical accuracy in the diagnosis of small polyps using the flexible fiberoptic sigmoidoscope. *Dis Colon Rectum* 1982;25:669.

206. Jass JR, Stewart SM, Schroeder D, Lane MR: Screening for hereditary non-polyposis colorectal cancer in New Zealand. *Eur J Gastroenterol Hepatol* 1992;4:523.

207. Lescher TC, Dockerty MB, Jackman RJ, Beahrs OH: Histopathology of the larger colonic polyp. *Dis Colon Rectum* 1967;10:118.

208. Urbanski S, Haber G, Kortan P, Marcon N: Small colonic adenomas with adenocarcinoma. *Dis Colon Rectum* 1983;31:58.

209. Wolber RA, Owen DA: Flat adenomas of the colon. *Hum Pathol* 1991;22:70.

210. Riddell RH: Flat adenomas and carcinomas: seeking the invisible? *Gastrointest Endosc* 1992;38:721.

211. Kuramoto S, Ihara I, Sakai S, et al: Depressed adenoma in the large intestine. Endoscopic features. *Dis Colon Rectum* 1990;33:108.

212. Kuramoto S, Oohara T: Flat early cancers of the large intestine. *Cancer* 1989;64:950.

213. Hunt DR, Cherian M: Endoscopic diagnosis of small flat carcinoma of the colon. Report of three cases. *Dis Colon Rectum* 1990;33:143.

214. Iishi H, Tatsuta M, Tsutsui S, et al: Early depressed adenocarcinomas of the large intestine. *Cancer* 1992;69:2406.

215. Hamilton SR: Flat adenomas: what you can't see can hurt you. *Radiology* 1993;187:309.

216. Kubota O, Kino I, Nakamura S: A morphometrical analysis of minute depressed adenomas in familial polyposis coli. *Pathol Int* 1994;44:200.

217. Konishi F, Morson BC: Pathology of colorectal adenomas: a colonoscopic survey. *J Clin Pathol* 1982;35:830.

218. Konishi F, Muto T, Kamiya J, et al: Histopathologic comparison of colorectal adenomas in English and Japanese patients. *Dis Colon Rectum* 1984;27:515.

219. DiSario JA, Foutch PG, Mai HD, et al: Prevalence of malignant potential of colorectal polyps in asymptomatic, average-risk men. *Am J Gastroenterol* 1991;86:941.

220. Fenoglio-Preiser C: Colonic polyp histology. *Semin Colon Rectal Surg* 1991;2:234.

221. Fung CH, Goldman H: The incidence and significance of villous change in adenomatous polyps. *Am J Clin Pathol* 1970;53:21.

222. Balazs M: Electron-microscopic study of the villous adenoma of the colon. *Virchows Arch A Pathol Anat* 1980;387:193.

223. Ioachim N, Delaney W, Madrazo A: Villous adenoma of the colon and rectum: an ultrastructural study. *Cancer* 1974;34:586.

224. Bansal M, Fenoglio CM, Robboy SJ, King DW: Are metaplasias in colorectal adenomas truly metaplasias? *Am J Pathol* 1984;115:253.

225. Fulcheri E, Baracchini P, Lapertosa G, Bussolati G: Distribution and significance of the smooth muscle component in polyps of the large intestine. *Hum Pathol* 1988;19:922.

226. Skinner SA, Frydman GM, O'Brien PE: Microvascular structure of benign and malignant tumors of the colon in humans. *Dig Dis Sci* 1995;40:373.

227. Cheung DK, Attiyeh FF: Pseudo-carcinomatous invasion of colonic polyps. *Dis Colon Rectum* 1981;24:399.

228. Dirschmid K, Kiesler J, Mathis G, et al: Epithelial misplacement after biopsy of colorectal adenomas. *Am J Surg Pathol* 1993;17:1262.

229. Richter H, Slezak P, Walch A, et al: Distinct chromosomal imbalances in nonpolypoid and polypoid colorectal adenomas indicate different genetic pathways in the development of colorectal neoplasms. *Am J Pathol* 2003;163:287.

230. Kita H, Hikichi Y, Hikami K, et al: Differential gene expression between flat adenoma and normal mucosa in the colon in a microarray analysis. *J Gastroenterol* 2006;41:1053.

231. Takahashi T, Nosho K, Yamamoto H, et al: Flat-type colorectal advanced adenomas (laterally spreading tumors) have different genetic and epigenetic alterations from protruded-type advanced adenomas. *Mod Pathol* 2007;20:139.

232. Postma C, Hermsen M, Coffa J, et al: Chromosomal instability in flat adenomas and carcinomas of the colon. *J Pathol* 2005;205:514.

233. Jacob H, Schlondorff D, St. Onge G, Bernstein L: Villous adenoma depletion syndrome. Evidence for a cyclic nucleotide-mediated diarrhea. *Dig Dis Sci* 1985;30:637.

234. Jorgensen OD, Kronborg O, Fenger C: The Funen adenoma follow-up study—characteristics of patients and initial adenomas in relation to severe dysplasia. *Scand J Gastroenterol* 1993;28:239.

235. Eide TJ: The age-, sex-, and site-specific occurrence of adenomas and carcinomas of the large intestine within a defined population. *Scand J Gastroenterol* 1986;21:1083.

236. Haggitt RC, Glotzbach RE, Soffer EE, et al: Prognostic factors in colorectal carcinomas arising in adenomas: implications for lesions removed by endoscopic polypectomy. *Gastroenterology* 1985;89:328.

237. Waye JD, Lewis BS, Frankel A, Geller SA: Small colon polyps. *Am J Gastroenterol* 1988;83:120.

238. Lipper S, Kahn LB, Ackerman LV: The significance of microscopic invasive cancer in endoscopically removed polyps of the large bowel. *Cancer* 1983;52:1691.

239. Cranley JP, Petras RE, Carey WD, et al: When is endoscopic polypectomy adequate therapy for colonic polyps containing invasive carcinoma. *Gastroenterology* 1986;91:419.

240. Wilcox GM, Beck JR: Early invasive cancer in adenomatous colonic polyps (malignant polyps). Evaluation of the therapeutic options by decision analysis. *Gastroenterology* 1987;92:1159.

241. Collacchio TA, Forde KA, Scantlebury VP: Endoscopic polypectomy: inadequate treatment for invasive colorectal carcinoma. *Ann Surg* 1981;194:704.

242. Coverlizza S, Risio M, Ferrari A, et al: Colorectal adenomas containing invasive carcinoma. Pathologic assessment of lymph node metastatic potential. *Cancer* 1989;64:1937.

243. Nicholls RJ, Zinicola R, Binda GA: Indications for colorectal resection for adenoma before and after polypectomy. *Tech Coloproctol* 2004;8:S291.

244. Cooper HS, Deppisch LM, Gourley WK, et al: Endoscopically removed malignant colorectal polyps: clinicopathologic correlations. *Gastroenterology* 1995;108:1657.

245. Winawer SJ, Witt TR: Cancer in a colonic polyp, or malignant colonic adenomas; is polypectomy sufficient? *Gastroenterology* 1981;81:625.

246. Lyda MH, Fenoglio-Preiser CM: Composite adenoma-carcinoid tumors of the colon. *Arch Pathol* 1998;122:262.

247. Ahlman H, Wangberg B, Nilsson O: Growth regulation in carcinoid tumors. *Endocrinol Metab Clin North Am* 1993;22:889.

248. Nilsson O, Wangberg B, McRae A, et al: Growth factors and carcinoid tumours. *Acta Oncol* 1993;32:115.

249. Nilsson O, Wangberg B, Kolby L, et al: Expression of transforming growth factor and its receptors in human neuroendocrine tumors. *Int J Cancer* 1995;60:645.

250. Hermanek P, Sobin LH, Fleming ID: What do we need beyond TNM? *Cancer* 1996;77:815.

251. Pugliese V, Gatteschi B, Aste H, et al: Value of multiple forceps biopsies in assessing the malignant potential of colonic polyps. *Tumori* 1981;67:57.

252. Levine JS, Ahnen DJ: Adenomatous polyps of the colon. *N Engl J Med* 2006;355:2551.

253. Bird RP: Observation and quantification of aberrant crypts in the murine colon treated with a colon carcinogen: preliminary findings. *Cancer Lett* 1987;37:147.

254. Bird RP, McLellan EA, Bruce WR: Aberrant crypts, putative precancerous lesions, in the study of the role of diet in the aetiology of colon cancer. *Cancer Surv* 1989;8:189.

255. Caderni G, Bianchini F, Mancina A, et al: Effect of dietary carbohydrates on the growth of dysplastic crypt foci in the colon of rats treated with 1,2-dimethylhydrazine. *Cancer Res* 1991;51:3721.

256. Pretlow TP, Barrow BJ, Ashton WS, et al: Aberrant crypts: putative preneoplastic foci in human colonic mucosa. *Cancer Res* 1991;51:1564.

257. Gregorio C, Losi L, Fante R, et al: Histology of aberrant crypt foci in the human colon. *Histopathology* 1997;30:328.

258. Otori K, Sugiyama K, Hasebe T, et al: Emergence of adenomatous aberrant crypt foci (ACF) from hyperplastic ACF with concomitant increase in cell proliferation. *Cancer Res* 1995;55:4743.

259. Roncucci L, Medline A, Bruce W: Classification of aberrant crypt foci and microadenomas in human colon. *Cancer Epidemiol Biomarkers Prev* 1991;1:57.

260. Roncucci L, Stamp D, Medline A, et al: Identification and quantification of aberrant crypt foci and microadenomas in the human colon. *Hum Pathol* 1991;22:287.

261. Longacre TA, Fenoglio-Preiser CM: Mixed hyperplastic adenomatous polyps/serrated adenomas: a distinct form of colorectal neoplasia. *Am J Surg Pathol* 1990;14:524.

262. Higuchi T, Sugihara K, Jass JR: Demographic and pathological characteristics of serrated polyps of the colorectum. *Histopathology* 2005;47:32.
263. Torlakovic E, Snover DC: Serrated adenomatous polyposis in humans. *Gastroenterology* 1996;110:748.
264. Goldstein NS, Bhanot P, Odish E, Hunter S: Hyperplastic-like colon polyps that preceded microsatellite-unstable adenocarcinomas. *Am J Clin Pathol* 2003;119: 778.
265. Ajioka Y, Watanabe H, Jass JR, et al: Infrequent K-ras codon 12 mutation in serrated adenomas of human colorectum. *Gut* 1998;42:680.
266. Uchida H, Ando H, Maruyama K, et al: Genetic alterations of mixed hyperplastic adenomatous polyps in the colon and rectum. *Jpn J Cancer Res* 1998;89:299.
267. Sawyer EJ, Cerar A, Hanby AM, et al: Molecular characteristics of serrated adenomas. *Gut* 2002;51:200.
268. Yamamoto T, Konishi K, Yamochi T, et al: No major tumorigenic role for beta-catenin in serrated as opposed to conventional colorectal adenomas. *Br J Cancer* 2003;89:152.
269. Chan TL, Zhao W, Leung SY, et al: *BRAF* and *KRAS* mutations in colorectal hyperplastic polyps and serrated adenomas. *Cancer Res* 2003; 63:4878.
270. Kambara T, Simms LA, Whitehall VL, et al: *BRAF* mutation and CpG island methylation: an alternative pathway to colorectal cancer. *Gut* 2004;53:1137.
271. Yang S, Jarraye FA, Mack C, et al: BRAF and KRAS mutations in hyperplastic polyps and serrated adenomas of the colorectum: relationship to histology and CpG island methylation status. *Am J Surg Pathol* 2004;28:1452.
272. Iino H, Jass JR, Simms LA, et al: DNA microsatellite instability in hyperplastic polyps, serrated adenomas, and mixed polyps: a mild mutator pathway for colorectal cancer? *J Clin Pathol* 1999;52:5.
273. Park SJ, Rashid A, Lee JH, et al: Frequent CpG island methylation in serrated adenomas of the colorectum. *Am J Pathol* 2003;162:815.
274. Konishi K, Yamochi T, Makino R, et al: Molecular differences between serrated and conventional colorectal adenomas. *Clin Cancer Res* 2004;10:3082.
275. Whitehall VL, Walsh MD, Young J, et al: Methylation of O-6-methylguanine-DNA methyltransferase characterizes a subset of colorectal cancer with low level DNA microsatellite instability. *Cancer Res* 2001;61:827.
276. Makinen MJ, George SM, Jernvall P, et al: Colorectal carcinoma associated with serrated adenoma—prevalence, histological features, and prognosis. *J Pathol* 2001;193:286.
277. Hawkins N, Norrie M, Cheong K, et al: CpG island methylation in sporadic colorectal cancer and its relationship to microsatellite instability. *Gastroenterology* 2002;122:1376.
278. Cunningham KS, Riddell RH: Serrated mucosal lesions of the colorectum. *Curr Opin Gastroenterol* 2006;22:48.
279. Parkin DM, Muir CS, Whelan SL, et al: *Cancer Incidence in Five Continents.* Vol 6, IARC Scientific Publication No. 120. Lyon, France: International Agency for Research on Cancer, 1992.
280. Enblad P, Adami HO, Glimelius B, et al: The risk of subsequent primary malignant disease after cancer of the colon and rectum. A nationwide cohort study. *Cancer* 1990;65:2091.
281. McMichael AJ, Potter JD: Do intrinsic sex differences in lower alimentary tract physiology influence the sex-specific risks of bowel cancer and other biliary and intestinal diseases? *Am J Epidemiol* 1983;118:620.
282. Vobecky J, Leduc C, Devroede G: Sex differences in the changing anatomic distribution of colorectal carcinoma. *Cancer* 1984;54:3065.
283. Singh JP, Maini VK, Bhatnagar MS: Large-bowel malignancy. Epidemiology and gut motility studies in South Asia. *Dis Colon Rectum* 1984;27:10.
284. Thomas CR, Jarosz R, Evans N: Racial differences in the anatomical distribution of colon cancer. *Arch Surg* 1992;127:1241.
285. Steele GD: The national cancer data base report on colorectal cancer. *Cancer* 1994;74:1979.
286. Johnson H, Carstens R: Anatomical distribution of colonic carcinomas: interracial differences in a community hospital population. *Cancer* 1986;58:997.
287. Ziegler RC, Devesa SS, Fraumeni JF, et al: Epidemiologic patterns of colorectal cancer. In: DeVita VT Jr, Hellman S, Rosenberg SA (eds): *Important Advances in Oncology.* Philadelphia: JB Lippincott, 1986, p 209.
288. Lieberman DA, Weiss DG, Bond JH, et al: Use of colonoscopy to screen asymptomatic adults for colorectal cancer. Veterans Affairs Cooperative Study Group 380. *N Engl J Med* 2000;343:162.
289. Slattery M, Friedman G, Potter J, et al: A description of age, sex, and site distributions of colon carcinoma in three geographic areas. *Cancer* 1996;78:1666.
290. Stebbing JF, Mortensen NJM: Carcinoma in a colon J pouch reservoir after low anterior resection for villous adenoma. *Br J Surg* 1995;82:172.
291. Andryjowicz E, Qizilbash AH, DePetrillo A, et al: Adenocarcinoma in a cecal neovagina—complication of irradiation: report of a case and review of literature. *Gynecol Oncol* 1985;21:235.
292. Lee T-K, Barringer M, Myers RT, Sterchi JM: Multiple primary carcinomas of the colon and associated extracolonic primary malignant tumors. *Ann Surg* 1982;195:501.
293. Lasser A: Synchronous primary adenocarcinomas of the colon and rectum. *Dis Colon Rectum* 1978;21:20.
294. Slater G, Aufses A, Szporn A: Synchronous carcinoma of the colon and rectum. *Surgery* 1990;171:283.
295. Parkash O: Multiple primary malignancies: a statistical study based on autopsy data from 1943–1972. *Virchows Arch* 1977;375:281.
296. Langevin JM, Nivatvongs S: The true incidence of synchronous cancer of the large bowel. A prospective study. *Am J Surg* 1984;147:330.
297. Kiefer PJ, Thorson AG, Christensen MA: Metachronous colorectal cancer. *Dis Colon Rectum* 1986;29:378.
298. Welch JP: Multiple colorectal tumors. An appraisal of natural history and therapeutic options. *Am J Surg* 1981;142:274.
299. Heald RJ, Bussey HJ: Clinical experiences at St. Marks' Hospital with multiple synchronous cancers of the colon and rectum. *Dis Colon Rectum* 1975;18:6.
300. Bussey HJR, Wallace MH, Morson BC: Metachronous carcinoma of the large intestine and intestinal polyps. *Proc R Soc Med* 1967;60:208.
301. De Leon ML, Schoetz DJ Jr, Coller JA, Veidenheimer MC: Colorectal cancer: Lahey Clinic Experience, 1972-76; an analysis of prognostic indicators. *Dis Colon Rectum* 1987;30:237.
302. Speights MO, Johnson MW, Stoltenberg PH, et al: Colorectal cancer: current trends in initial clinical manifestations. *South Med J* 1991;84:575.
303. Barillari P, de Angelis R, Valabrega S, et al: Relationship of symptom duration and survival in patients with colorectal carcinoma. *Eur J Surg Oncol* 1989;15:441.
304. Goulston KJ, Cook I, Dent OF: How important is rectal bleeding in the diagnosis of bowel cancer and polyps. *Lancet* 1986;2:261.
305. Funch D: Diagnostic delay in symptomatic colorectal cancer. *Cancer* 1985;56:2120.
306. Odone V, Chang L, Caces J, et al: The natural history of colorectal carcinoma in adolescents. *Cancer* 1982;49:1716.
307. Rao BN, Pratt CB, Fleming ID, et al: Colon carcinoma in children and adolescents. A review of 30 cases. *Cancer* 1985;55:1322.
308. Kern WH, White WC: Adenocarcinoma of colon in a 9-month old infant. *Cancer* 1958;11:855.
309. Radhakrishnan CN, Bruce J: Colorectal cancers in children without any predisposing factors. A report of eight cases and review of the literature. *Eur J Pediatr Surg* 2003;13:66.
310. Andersson A, Bergdahl L: Carcinoma of the colon in children: a report of six new cases and review of the literature. *J Pediatr Surg* 1976;11:967.
311. Goldthron J, Canizaro P: Gastrointestinal malignancies in infancy, childhood, and adolescence. *Surg Clin North Am* 1986;66:845.
312. Steinberg J, Tuggle D, Postier R: Adenocarcinoma of the colon in adolescents. *Am J Surg* 1988;156:460.
313. Adloff M, Arnaud J, Schloegel M, et al: Colorectal cancer in patients under 40 years of age. *Dis Colon Rectum* 1986;29:322.
314. Mills SE, Allen MS Jr: Colorectal carcinoma in the first three decades of life. *Am J Surg Pathol* 1979;3:443.
315. Kravarusic D, Feigin E, Dlugy E, et al: Colorectal carcinoma in childhood: a retrospective multicenter study. *J Pediatr Gastroenterol Nutr* 2007;44:209.
316. Umpleby HC, Williamson RCN: Carcinoma of the large bowel in the first four decades. *Br J Surg* 1984;71:272.
317. Petrek JA, Sandberg WA, Bean PK: The role of gender and other factors in the prognosis of young patients with colorectal cancer. *Cancer* 1985;56:952.
318. Domergue J, Ismail M, Astre C, et al: Colorectal carcinoma in patients younger than 40 years of age. *Cancer* 1988;61:835.
319. Chantada GL, Perelli VB, Lombardi MG, et al: Colorectal carcinoma in children, adolescents and young adults. *J Pediatr Hematol Oncol* 2005;27:39.
320. McLean DW, Arminski TC, Bradley GT: Management of primary carcinoma of the rectum diagnosed during pregnancy. *Am J Surg* 1955;90:816.

321. Minter A, Malik R, Ledbetter L, et al: Colon cancer in pregnancy. *Cancer Control* 2005;12:196.

322. Qizilbash AH: Pathologic studies in colorectal cancer: a guide to the surgical pathology examination of colorectal specimens and review of features of prognostic significance. *Pathol Annu* 1982;17:1.

323. Robey-Cafferty SS, Ro JY, Ordonez NG, Cleary KR: Transitional mucosa of colon. A morphological, histochemical, and immunohisto-chemical study. *Arch Pathol Lab Med* 1990;114:72.

324. Silver SA, Epstein JI: Adenocarcinoma of the colon simulating primary urinary bladder neoplasia—a report of nine cases. *Am J Surg Pathol* 1993;17:171.

325. Thomas GDH, Dixon MF, Smeeton NC, Williams NS: Observer varia-tion in the histological grading of rectal carcinoma. *J Clin Pathol* 1983; 36:385.

326. Shousha S: Paneth cell-rich papillary adenocarcinoma and a mucoid adenocarcinoma occurring synchronously in colon: a light and elec-tron microscopic study. *Histopathology* 1979;3:489.

327. Gibbs NM: Incidence and significance of argentaffin and Paneth cells in some tumours of the large intestine. *J Clin Pathol* 1967;20:826.

328. Shousha S: Signet-ring cell adenocarcinoma of rectum: a histological, his-tochemical and electron microscopic study. *Histopathology* 1982;6:341.

329. Smith DM, Haggitt RC: The prevalence and prognostic significance of argyrophil cells in colorectal carcinomas. *Am J Surg Pathol* 1984; 8:123.

330. Pagani A, Papotti M, Abbona C, Bussolati G: Chromogranin gene expressions in colorectal adenocarcinomas. *Mod Pathol* 1995;8:626.

331. Park JG, Choe GY, Helman LJ, et al: Chromogranin—A expression in gastric and colon cancer tissues. *Int J Cancer* 1992;51:189.

332. Ho SB, Toribara NW, Bresalier RS, Kim YS: Biochemical and other markers of colon cancer. *Gastroenterol Clin North Am* 1988;17:811.

333. Arends JW, Wiggers T, Verstijnen K, Bosman FT: The occurrence and clinicopathological significance of serotonin immunoreactive cells in large bowel carcinoma. *J Pathol* 1986;149:97.

334. De Bruine AP, Wiggers T, Beek C, et al: Endocrine cells in colorectal adenocarcinomas: incidence, hormone profile and prognostic rele-vance. *Int J Cancer* 1993;54:765.

335. Hamada Y, Oishi A, Shoji T, et al: Endocrine cells and prognosis in patients with colorectal carcinoma. *Cancer* 1992;69:2641.

336. Jansson D, Gould VE, Gooch GT, et al: Immunohistochemical analysis of colon carcinomas applying exocrine and neuroendocrine markers. *Acta Pathol Microbiol Immunol Scand* 1988;96:1129.

337. Jass JR: Lymphocytic infiltration and survival in rectal cancer. *J Clin Pathol* 1986;39:585.

338. Martinez-Hernandez A, Catalano E: Stromal reaction to neoplasia: colonic carcinomas. *Ultrastruct Pathol* 1980;1:403.

339. Jass JR, Atkin WS, Cuzick I, et al: The grading of rectal cancer: histo-logical perspectives and a multivaritate analysis of 447 cases. *Histopathology* 1986;10:437.

340. Graham DM, Appelman HD: Crohn's-like lymphoid reaction and col-orectal carcinoma: a potential histologic prognosticator. *Mod Pathol* 1990;3:332.

341. Djaldetti M, Fishman P, Chaimoff C, et al: Severe alterations of red blood cells from the vessels of colorectal tumors. *Arch Pathol Lab Med* 1985;109:62.

342. Sinicrope FA, Rego RL, Halling KC, et al: Prognostic impact of microsatellite instability and DNA ploidy in human colon carcinoma patients. *Gastroenterology* 2006;131:729.

343. Thibodeau SN, Bren G, Schaid D: Microsatellite instability in cancer of the proximal colon. *Science* 1993;260:816.

344. Lothe RA, Peltomaki P, Meling GI, et al: Genomic instability in col-orectal cancer: relationship to clinicopathological variables and family history. *Cancer Res* 1993;53:5849.

345. Halling KC, French AJ, McDonnell DK, et al: Microsatellite instability and 8p allelic imbalance in stage B2 and C colorectal cancers. *J Natl Cancer Inst* 1999;91:1295.

346. Gryfe R, Kim H, Hsieh ET, et al: Tumor microsatellite instability and clinical outcome in young patients with colorectal cancer. *N Engl J Med* 2000;342:69.

347. Kakar S, Aksoy S, Burgart LJ, Smyrk TC: Mucinous carcinoma of the colon: correlation with loss of mismatch repair enzymes with clinico-pathologic features and survival. *Mod Pathol* 2004;17:696.

348. Kim H, Jen J, Vogelstein B, Hamilton SR: Clinical and pathological characteristics of sporadic colorectal carcinomas with DNA replica-tion errors in microsatellites. *Am J Pathol* 1993;145:148.

349. Risio M, Reato G, di Celle P, et al: Microsatellite instability is associated with the histological features of the tumor in nonfamilial colorectal cancer. *Cancer Res* 1996;56:5470.

350. Mecklin JP, Svendsen LB, Peltomaki P, Vasen HF: Hereditary nonpoly-posis colorectal cancer. *Scand J Gastroenterol* 1994;29:673.

351. Kuramoto S, Oohara T: Minute cancers arising de novo in the human large intestine. *Cancer* 1988;61:829.

352. Minamoto T, Sawaguchi K, Ohta T, Itoh T: Superficial-type adenomas and adenocarcinomas of the colon and rectum: a comparative mor-phological study. *Gastroenterology* 1994;106:1436.

353. Wada R, Matsukuma S, Abe H, et al: Histopathological studies of superficial-type early colorectal carcinoma. *Cancer* 1996;77:44.

354. Begin LR, Gordon PH, Alpert LC: Endophytic malignant transforma-tion within flat adenoma of the colon: a potential diagnostic pitfall. *Virchows Arch A* 1993;422:415.

355. Ming-Chai C, Chi-Yuan C, Pei-Yu C, Jen-Chun H: Evolution of col-orectal cancer in schistosomiasis. Transitional mucosal changes adja-cent to large intestinal carcinoma in colectomy specimens. *Cancer* 1980;46:1661.

356. Younes M, Katikaneni PR, Lechago J: The value of the preoperative mucosal biopsy in the diagnosis of colorectal mucinous adenocarci-noma. *Cancer* 1993;72:3588.

357. Connelly JH, Robey-Cafferty SS, Cleary KR: Mucinous carcinoma of the colon and rectum: an analysis of 62 stage B and C lesions. *Arch Pathol Lab Med* 1991;115:1022.

358. Symonds DA, Vickery AL: Mucinous carcinoma of the colon and rec-tum. *Cancer* 1976;37:1891.

359. Sundblad AS, Paz RA: Mucinous carcinoma and their relation to polyps. *Cancer* 1982;50:2504.

360. Liu IO, Kung IT, Lee JM, Boey JH: Primary colorectal signet-ring cell carcinoma in young patients: report of 3 cases. *Pathology* 1985;17:31.

361. Buckmaster MJ, Sloan DA, Ellis JL, Schwartz RW: Mucinous adenocar-cinoma of the colon metastatic to the intestinal mucosa. *Surgery* 1994;115:767.

362. Yamamoto S, Mochizuki H, Hase K, et al: Assessment of clinicopatho-logic features of colorectal mucinous adenocarcinoma. *Am J Surg* 1993;166:257.

363. Amico L, Caplan L, Thomas C: Cerebrovascular complications of mucinous cancers. *Neurology* 1989;39:522.

364. Secco GB, Fardelli R, Campora E, et al: Primary mucinous adenocarci-nomas and signet-ring cell carcinomas of colon and rectum. *Oncology* 1994;51:30.

365. Green JB, Timmcke AE, Mitchell WT, et al: Mucinous carcinoma: just another colon cancer? *Dis Colon Rectum* 1993;36:49.

366. Umpleby HC, Ranson DL, Williamson RC: Peculiarities of mucinous colorectal carcinoma. *Br J Surg* 1985;72:715.

367. Sasaki O, Atkin WS, Jass JR: Mucinous carcinoma of the rectum. *Histopathology* 1987;11:259.

368. Jones EA, Morson BC: Mucinous adenocarcinoma in anorectal fistu-lae. *Histopathology* 1984;8:279.

369. Horton KM, Jones B, Bayless TM, et al: Mucinous adenocarcinoma at the ileocecal valve mimicking Crohn's disease. *Dig Dis Sci* 1994;39:2276.

370. Halvorsen TB, Seim E: Influence of mucinous components on survival in colorectal adenocarcinomas: a multivariate analysis. *J Clin Pathol* 1988;41:1068.

371. Kang H, O'Connell JB, Maggard MA, et al: A 10-year outcomes evalu-ation of mucinous and signet ring cell carcinoma of the colon and rec-tum. *Dis Colon Rectum* 2005;48:161.

372. Ojeda VJ, Mitchell KM, Walters MN, Gibson MJ: Primary colorectal linitis plastica type of carcinoma: report of two cases and review of the literature. *Pathology* 1982;14:181.

373. Wiltz O, O'Toole K, Fenoglio CM: Breast carcinoma metastatic to a solitary adenomatous polyp in the colon. *Arch Pathol Lab Med* 1984;108:318.

374. Makino T, Tsujinaka T, Mishima H, et al: Primary signet-ring cell car-cinoma of the colon and rectum: report of eight cases and review of 154 Japanese cases. *Hepatogastroenterology* 2006;53:845.

375. Laufman H, Saphir O: Primary linitis plastica type of carcinoma of the colon. *Arch Surg* 1951;62:79.

376. Coe FO: Linitis plastica. *South Med J* 1931;24:477.

377. Amorn Y, Knight WA: Primary linitis plastica of the colon: report of two cases and review of the literature. *Cancer* 1978;41:2420.

378. Stevens WR, Ruiz P: Primary linitis plastica carcinoma of the colon and rectum. *Mod Pathol* 1989;2:265.

379. Crissman JD: Adenosquamous and squamous cell carcinoma of the colon. *Am J Surg Pathol* 1978;2:47.

380. Chevinsky AH, Berelowitz M, Hoover HC: Adenosquamous carcinoma of the colon presenting with hypercalcemia. *Cancer* 1987;60:1111.

381. Links M, Ho H, Clingan P, Diamond T: Hypercalcaemia in a patient with fatal adenosquamous carcinoma of the colon. *Med J Aust* 1994;160:286.

382. Thompson JT, Paschold EH, Levine EA: Paraneoplastic hypercalcemia in a patient with adenosquamous cancer of the colon. *Am Surg* 2001;67:585.

383. Fujita T, Fukuda K, Nishi H, et al: Paraneoplastic hypercalcemia with adenosquamous carcinoma of the colon. *Int J Clin Oncol* 2005;10:144.

384. Cagir B, Nagy MW, Topham A, et al: Adenosquamous carcinoma of the colon, rectum and anus: epidemiology, distribution, and survival characteristics. *Dis Colon Rectum* 1999;42:258.

385. Boscaino A, Orabona P, Donofrio V, et al: Adenosquamous carcinoma of the colon—case report of an unusual type. *Tumori* 1993;79:288.

386. Erasmus LJ, van Heerden JA, Dahlin DC: Adenoacanthoma of the colon. *Dis Colon Rectum* 1978;21:196.

387. Cooper HS: Carcinoma of the colon and rectum. In: Norris HT (ed). *Pathology of the Colon, Small Intestine and Anus.* New York: Churchill Livingstone, 1983, p 201.

388. Kang H, O'Connell JB, Leonardi MJ: Rare tumors of the colon and rectum: a national review. *Int J Colorectal Dis* 2007;22:183.

389. Williams GT, Blackshaw WAJ, Morson BC: Squamous carcinoma of the colorectum and its genesis. *J Pathol* 1979;129:139.

390. Comer TP, Beahrs OH, Dockerty MB: Primary squamous cell carcinoma and adenoacanthoma of the colon. *Cancer* 1971;28:1111.

391. Hohm WH, Jackman RJ: Squamous cell carcinoma of the rectum complicating ulcerative colitis: report of two cases. *Proc Staff Meetings Mayo Clin* 1964;39:249.

392. Wiener MT, Polayes SH, Yidi R: Squamous cell carcinoma with schistosomiasis of the colon. *Am J Gastroenterol* 1962;37:48.

393. Adair HM, Trowell JE: Squamous cell carcinoma arising in a duplication of the small bowel. *J Pathol* 1981;133:25.

394. Lyttle JA: Primary squamous carcinoma of the proximal large bowel. Report of a case and review of the literature. *Dis Colon Rectum* 1983; 26:279.

395. Dixon CF, Dockerty MB, Powelson MH: Squamous cell carcinoma of the mid-rectum: report of a case. *Proc Staff Meetings Mayo Clin* 1954; 29:420.

396. Strate RW, Richardson JD, Bannayan GA: Basosquamous (transitional cloacogenic) carcinoma of the sigmoid colon. *Cancer* 1977;40:1234.

397. Weidner N, Zekan P: Carcinosarcoma of the colon. Report of a unique case with light and immunohistochemical studies. *Cancer* 1986;58:1126.

398. Buckley CH, Fox H: An immunohistochemical study of the significance of HCG secretion by large bowel adenocarcinomata. *J Clin Pathol* 1979;32:368.

399. Park CH, Reid JD: Adenocarcinoma of the colon with choriocarcinoma in its metastases. *Cancer* 1980;46:570.

400. Ordonez NG, Luna MA: Choriocarcinoma of the colon. *Am J Gastroenterol* 1984;79:39.

401. Metz KA, Richter HJ, Leder LD: Adenocarcinoma of the colon with syncytiotrophoblastic differentiation: differential diagnosis and implications. *Pathol Res Pract* 1985;179:419.

402. Nguyen GK: Adenocarcinoma of the sigmoid colon with focal choriocarcinoma metaplasia: a case report. *Dis Colon Rectum* 1982;25:230.

403. Le DT, Austin RC, Payne SN, et al: Choriocarcinoma of the colon: report of a case and review of the literature. *Dis Colon Rectum* 2003;46:264.

404. Rodilla IG, Val-Bernal JF, Cabrera E, Fernandez FA: Primary choriocarcinoma of the rectum in a man. *Int J Surg Pathol* 1995;3:131.

405. Shousha S, Chappell R, Matthews J, Cooke T: Human chorionic gonadotrophin expression in colorectal adenocarcinoma. *Dis Colon Rectum* 1986;29:558.

406. Campo E, Palacin A, Benasco C, et al: Human chorionic gonadotropin in colorectal carcinoma. *Cancer* 1987;59:1611.

407. Ostor AG, McNaughton WM, Fortune DW, et al: Rectal adenocarcinoma with germ cell elements treated with chemotherapy. *Pathology* 1993;25:243.

408. Mauer K, Waye J, Lewis B, Szporn A: The hairy polyp: a benign teratoma of the colon. *Endoscopy* 1989;21:148.

409. Zalatnai A, Dubecz S, Harka I, Banhidy F Jr: Malignant teratoma of the left colon associated with chronic ulcerative colitis. *Virchows Arch A* 1987;411:61.

410. El-Khatib Y: Pedunculated teratoma of rectum infected with bilharziasis. *Br J Surg* 1972;59:655.

411. Russell P: Carcinoma complicating a benign teratoma of the rectum. *Dis Colon Rectum* 1974;17:550.

412. Cho KJ, Myong NH, Jang JJ: Effusion cytology of endodermal sinus tumor of the colon. *Acta Cytol* 1991;35:207.

413. Lott JV, Rubin RJ, Salvati EP, Salazar GH: Endometrioid carcinoma of the rectum arising in endometriosis: report of a case. *Dis Colon Rectum* 1978;21:56.

414. Mira JL, Fenoglio-Preiser CM, Husseinzadeh N: Malignant mixed mullerian tumor of the extraovarian secondary mullerian system. Report of two cases and review of the English literature. *Arch Pathol Lab Med* 1995;119:1044.

415. Haque S, Eisen R, West B: Heterotopic bone formation in the gastrointestinal tract. *Arch Pathol Lab Med* 1996;120:666.

416. Kumasa S, Mori H, Mori M, et al: Heterotopic bone formation in tumor stromal tissue: Immunohistochemical considerations. *Acta Histochem Cytochem* 1990;23:427.

417. Damjanov I, Amenta PS, Bosman FT: Undifferentiated carcinoma of the colon containing exocrine, neuroendocrine and squamous cells. *Virchows Arch A* 1983;401:57.

418. Novello P, Duvillard P, Grandjouan S, et al: Carcinomas of the colon with multidirectional differentiation. Report of two cases and review of the literature. *Dig Dis Sci* 1995;40:100.

419. Chetty R, Bhathal PS: Caecal adenocarcinoma with rhabdoid phenotype. An immunohistochemical and ultrastructural analysis. *Virchows Arch* 1993;422:179.

420. Chumas JC, Lorelle CA: Melanotic adenocarcinoma of the anorectum. *Am J Surg Pathol* 1981;5:711.

421. Williams NS, Dixon MF, Johnston D: Reappraisal of the 4 centimetre rule of distal excision for carcinoma of the rectum: a study of distal intramural spread and of patients survival. *Br J Surg* 1983;70:150.

422. Madsen P, Christiansen J: Distal intramural spread of rectal carcinomas. *Dis Colon Rectum* 1986;29:279.

423. Lazorthes F, Voigt JJ, Roques J, et al: Distal intramural spread of carcinoma of the rectum correlated with lymph nodal involvement. *Surg Gynecol Obstet* 1990;170:45.

424. Sidoni A, Bufalari A, Alberti PF: Distal intramural spread in colorectal cancer: a reappraisal of the extent of distal clearance in fifty cases. *Tumori* 1991;77:514.

425. Kameda K, Furusawa M, Mori M, Sugimachi K: Proposed distal margin for resection of rectal cancer. *Jpn J Cancer Res* 1990;81:100.

426. Lin JI, Cogbill CL, Athota PJ, et al: Superficial spreading adenocarcinoma of appendix, cecum, and terminal ileum. *Dis Colon Rectum* 1980;23:587.

427. Braun EV, Ali M, Fayemi AO, Beaugard E: Primary signet-ring cell carcinoma of the urinary bladder; review of the literature and report of a case. *Cancer* 1981;47:1430.

428. Michelassi F, Block GE, Vannucci L, et al: A 5- to 21-year follow-up and analysis of 250 patients with rectal adenocarcinoma. *Ann Surg* 1988; 208:379.

429. Michelassi F, Vannucci L, Ayala JJ, et al: Local recurrence after curative resection of colorectal adenocarcinoma. *Surgery* 1990;108:787.

430. Minsky BD, Mies C, Rich TA: Lymphatic vessel invasion is an independent prognostic factor for survival in colorectal cancer. *Int J Rad Oncol Biol Phys* 1989;17:311.

431. Morson BC, Dawson IMP: *Gastrointestinal Pathology.* 2nd Ed. Oxford: Blackwell Scientific, 1979, p 648.

432. Chang GJ, Rodriguez-Bigas MA, Skibber JM, Moyer VA: Lymph node evaluation and survival after curative resection of colon cancer: systematic review. *J Natl Cancer Inst* 2007;99:433.

433. Le Voyer TE, Sigurdson ER, Hanlon AL, et al: Colon cancer survival is associated with increasing number of lymph nodes analyzed: a secondary survey of intergroup trial INT-0089. *J Clin Oncol* 2003; 21:2912.

434. Berger AC, Sigurdson ER, Le Voyer T, et al: Colon cancer survival is associated with decreasing ratio of metastatic to examined lymph nodes. *J Clin Oncol* 2005;23:8706.

435. Lee HY, Choi HJ, Park KJ, et al: Prognostic significance of metastatic lymph node ratio in node-positive colon cancer. *Ann Surg Oncol* 2007;14:1712.

436. Fielding LP, Arsenault PA, Chapuis PH, et al: Working report to the World Congresses of Gastroenterology, Sydney 1990. *J Gastroenterol Hepatol* 1991;6:325.

437. Goldstein NS, Weldons S, Coffey M, et al: Lymph node recovery from colorectal resection specimens removed for adenocarcinoma: trends

over time and a recommendation for a minimum number of lymph nodes to be removed. *Am J Clin Pathol* 1996;106:209.

438. Wong JH, Severino R, Honnebier MB, et al: Number of nodes examined and staging accuracy in colorectal carcinoma. *J Clin Oncol* 1999;17:2896.

439. Talbot IC, Ritchie S, Leighton M, et al: Invasion of veins by carcinoma of rectum: method of detection, histological features and significance. *Histopathology* 1981;5:141.

440. Seefeld P, Bargen JA: The spread of carcinoma of the rectum: invasion of lymphatics, veins and nerves. *Ann Surg* 1943;118:76.

441. Minsky BD, Mies C, Recht A, et al: Resectable adenocarcinoma of the rectosigmoid and rectum. 2. The influence of blood vessel invasion. *Cancer* 1988;61:1417.

442. Griffin MR, Bergstralh EJ, Coffey RJ, et al: Predictors of survival after curative resection of carcinoma of the colon and rectum. *Cancer* 1987;60:2318.

443. Lapertosa G, Baracchini P, Fulcheri E, Tanzi R: Prognostic value of the immunocytochemical detection of extramural venous invasion in Dukes' C colorectal adenocarcinomas. *Am J Pathol* 1989;135:939.

444. Ouchi K, Sugawara T, Ono H, et al: Histologic features and clinical significance of venous invasion in colorectal carcinoma with hepatic metastasis. *Cancer* 1996;78:2313.

445. Berge T, Ekelund G, Mellner C, et al: Carcinoma of the colon and rectum in a defined population: an epidemiological, clinical and postmortem investigation of colorectal carcinoma and coexisting benign polyps in Malmo, Sweden. *Acta Chir Scand* 1973;438:1.

446. Batson OV: The vertebral system of veins as a means of cancer dissemination. *Prog Clin Cancer* 1967;3:1.

447. Krasna MJ, Flancbaum L, Cody RP, et al: Vascular and neural invasion in colorectal carcinoma: incidence and prognostic significance. *Cancer* 1988;61:1018.

448. Skipper D, Cooper AJ, Marston JE, Taylor I: Exfoliated cells and in vitro growth in colorectal cancer. *Br J Surg* 1987;74:1049.

449. Cirocco WC, Schwartzman A, Golub RW: Abdominal wall recurrence after laparoscopic colectomy for colon cancer. *Surgery* 1994;116:842.

450. Cohen AM, Wood WC, Gunderson LL, Shinnar M: Pathological studies in rectal cancer. *Cancer* 1980;45:2965.

451. Manson PN, Corman ML, Coller JA, Veidenheimer MC: Anastomotic recurrence after anterior resection for carcinoma; Lahey clinic experience. *Dis Colon Rectum* 1976;19:219.

452. Pihl E, Hughes ESR, McDermott FT, et al: I. Carcinoma of the rectum and rectosigmoid: cancer specific long-term survival. A series of 1061 cases treated by one surgeon. *Cancer* 1980;45:2902.

453. Russell AH, Tong D, Dawson LE, Wisbeck W: Adenocarcinoma of the proximal colon. Sites of initial dissemination and patterns of recurrence following surgery alone. *Cancer* 1984;53:360.

454. Weiss L, Grundmann E, Torhorst J, et al: Haematogenous metastatic patterns in colonic carcinoma: an analysis of 1541 necropsies. *J Pathol* 1986;150:195.

455. Takahura K, Sano K, Hoho S: *Metastatic Tumors of the CNS.* Tokyo: Igaku-Shoin, 1982.

456. Besbeas S, Stearns M Jr: Osseous metastases from carcinoma of the colon and rectum. *Dis Colon Rectum* 1978;24:266.

457. Hoehn JL, Ousley JL, Avecilla CS: Occult carcinoma of the colon and rectum manifesting as osseous metastasis. *Dis Colon Rectum* 1979;22:129.

458. Pitluk H, Poticha S: Carcinoma of the colon and rectum in patients less than 40 years of age. *Surgery* 1983;157:335.

459. Daya D, Nazerali L, Frank G: Metastatic ovarian carcinoma of large intestinal origin simulating primary ovarian carcinoma. A clinicopathologic study of 25 cases. *Am J Clin Pathol* 1992;97:751.

460. Brennecke SP, McEvoy MI, Seymour AE, et al: Caecal adenocarcinoma metastatic to ovary inducing increased oestrogen production and postmenopausal bleeding. *Aust NZ J Obstet Gynaecol* 1986;26:158.

461. Herrera LO, Ledesma EJ, Natarajan N, et al: Metachronous ovarian metastases from adenocarcinoma of the colon and rectum. *Surg Gynecol Obstet* 1982;154:531.

462. Lash RH, Hart WR: Intestinal adenocarcinomas metastatic to the ovaries: a clinicopathologic evaluation of 22 cases. *Am J Surg Pathol* 1987;11:114.

463. Inaba S, Tanaka T, Yamagishi H, et al: A case of colon cancer metastasizing to the spleen. *Jpn J Clin Oncol* 1984;14:425.

464. Dyess DL, Ferrara JJ, Webb WA: Metastatic colon carcinoma to the biliary tract mimicking choledocholithiasis. *Am Surg* 1989;55:71.

465. Charnsangavej C, Whitley NO: Metastases to the pancreas and peripancreatic lymph nodes from carcinoma of the right side of the colon—CT findings in 12 patients. *AJR Am J Roentgenol* 1993;160:49.

466. Cedermark BJ, Blumenson LE, Pickren JW, et al: The significance of metastases to the adrenal glands in adenocarcinoma of the colon and rectum. *Surg Gynecol Obstet* 1977;144:537.

467. Moore J, Law D, Moore E, Dean C: Testicular mass: an initial sign of colon carcinoma. *Cancer* 1982;49:411.

468. Reingold IM: Cutaneous metastases from internal carcinoma. *Cancer* 1966;19:162.

469. Zeligman I, Schwilm A: Umbilical metastasis from carcinoma of the colon. *Arch Dermatol* 1974;110:911.

470. Rusthoven JJ, Fine S, Thomas G: Adenocarcinoma of the rectum metastatic to the oral cavity. Two cases and a review of the literature. *Cancer* 1984;54:1110.

471. Raider L: Remote vaginal metastases from carcinoma of the colon. *AJR Am J Roentgenol* 1966;97:944.

472. Burger R, Guthrie TH: Metastatic colonic carcinoma to epididymis. *Urology* 1973;2:566.

473. Carlin BW, Harrell JH, Olson LK, Moser KM: Endobronchial metastases due to colorectal carcinoma. *Chest* 1989;96:1110.

474. Araki K, Kobayashi M, Ogata T, Takuma K: Colorectal carcinoma metastatic to skeletal muscle. *Hepatogastroenterology* 1994;41:405.

475. Gattoni F, Baldini U, Avogadro A, et al: Un raro caso di metastasi ureterale da neoplasia del colon. *Radiol Med* 1986;72:595.

476. Cervin J, Silverman J, Loggie B, Geisinger K: Virchow's node revisited. Analysis with clinicopathologic correlation of 152 fine-needle aspiration biopsies of supraclavicular lymph nodes. *Arch Pathol Lab Med* 1995;119:727.

477. Nishida H, Grooters RK, Coster D, et al: Metastatic right atrial tumor in colon cancer with superior vena cava syndrome and tricuspid obstruction. *Heart Vessels* 1991;6:125.

478. Kacenelenbogen R, Devriendt J, De Reuck M, et al: Cardiac tamponade as first manifestation of colonic cancer. *Arch Intern Med* 1984;144:622.

479. Rentschler RE, Thrasher TV: Gingival and mandibular metastases from rectal adenocarcinoma: case report and 20 year review of the English literature. *Laryngoscope* 1982;92:795.

480. Arora YR: Colonic carcinoma presenting with meningeal metastases. *J R Coll Surg Edinb* 1973;18:376.

481. Schneider PA, Bosshard C: Aderhautmetastasen bei Kolonkarzinom. *Klin Monatsbl Augenheilkd* 1978;172:513.

482. Guttmann G, Stein I: Metastatic tumor of the thumb from adenocarcinoma of the colon. *Int Surg* 1968;49:217.

483. Banerjee CK, Lim KP, Cohen NP: Penile metastasis: an unusual presentation of metastatic colonic cancer. *J R Coll Surg Edinb* 2002;47:763.

484. Perdomo JA, Hizuta A, Iwagaki H, et al: Penile metastasis secondary to cecum carcinoma: a case report. *Hepatogastroenterology* 1998;45:1589.

485. Drury BJ: Adenocarcinoma of the rectum with metastasis to the nailbed of the finger. *Calif Med* 1959;91:35.

486. Dukes CE: Cancer of the rectum: an analysis of 1000 cases. *J Pathol Bacteriol* 1940;50:527.

487. Dukes CE, Bussey HJ: The spread of rectal cancer and its effect on prognosis. *Br J Cancer* 1958;12:309.

488. Denoix PF: French Ministry of Public Health National Institute of Hygiene Monograph No. 4. Paris, 1954.

489. Beahrs OH, Myers MH: *Manual for Staging of Cancer.* 2nd ed. American Joint Committee on Cancer. Philadelphia: JB Lippincott, 1983.

490. Greene FL, Page DL, Fleming ID, et al (eds): *AJCC Cancer Staging Manual.* 6th ed. New York: Springer, 2002.

491. Thompson W, Trenkner S: Staging colorectal carcinoma. *Radiol Clin North Am* 1994;32:25.

492. Dixon AK, Fry IK, Morson BC, et al: Preoperative computed tomography of carcinoma of the rectum. *Br J Radiol* 1981;54:655.

493. Thoeni RF, Moss AA, Schnyder P, Margulis AR: Detection and staging of primary rectal and rectosigmoid cancer by computed tomography. *Radiology* 1981;141:135.

494. Thoeni RF: CT evaluation of carcinomas of the colon and rectum. *Radiol Clin North Am* 1989;27:731.

495. Hodgman CG, MacCarty RL, Wolff BG, et al: Preoperative staging of rectal carcinoma by computed tomography and 0.15 T magnetic resonance imaging: preliminary report. *Dis Colon Rectum* 1986;29:446.

496. Angelelli G, Macarini L, Lupo L, et al: Rectal carcinoma: CT staging with water as contrast medium. *Radiology* 1990;177:511.

497. Butch RJ, Stark DD, Wittenberg J: Staging rectal cancer by MR and CT. *AJR Am J Roentgenol* 1986;146:1155.
498. Savides TJ, Master SS: EUS in rectal cancer. *Gastrointest Endosc* 2002;56(4 suppl):S12.
499. Kwok H, Bissett IP, Hill GL: Preoperative staging of rectal cancer. *Int J Colorectal Dis* 2000;15:9.
500. Meyenberger C, Huch Boni RA, Bertschinger P, et al: Endoscopic ultrasound and endorectal magnetic resonance imaging: a prospective, comparative study for preoperative staging and follow-up of rectal cancer. *Endoscopy* 1995;217:469.
501. Thaler W, Watzka S, Martin F, et al: Preoperative staging of rectal cancer by endoluminal ultrasound vs. magnetic resonance imaging. *Dis Colon Rectum* 1994;37:1189.
502. Durdey P, Williams NS: Pre-operative evaluation of patients with low rectal carcinomas. *World J Surg* 1992;16:430.
503. Beynon J, Roe AM, Foy DM, et al: Preoperative staging of local invasion in rectal cancer using intraluminal ultrasound. *J R Soc Med* 1987;80:23.
504. Anderson BO, Hann LE, Enker WE, et al: Transrectal ultrasonography and operative selection for early carcinoma of the rectum. *J Am Coll Surg* 1994;179:513.
505. Solomon MJ, McLeod RS: Endoluminal transrectal ultrasonography: accuracy, reliability, and validity. *Dis Colon Rectum* 1993;36:200.
506. Hawes RH: New staging techniques. Endoscopic ultrasound. *Cancer* 1993;71(12 suppl):4207.
507. Harewood GC: Assessment of publication bias in the reporting of EUS performance in staging rectal cancer. *Am J Gastroenterol* 2005;100:808.
508. Bhutani MS: Recent developments in the role of endoscopic ultrasonography in diseases of the colon and rectum. *Curr Opin Gastroenterol* 2007;23:67.
509. Muller-Schimpfle M, Brix G, Schlag P, et al: Recurrent rectal cancer: diagnosis with dynamic MR imaging. *Radiology* 1993;189:881.
510. Collier BD, Foley WD: Current imaging strategies for colorectal cancer. *J Nucl Med* 1993;34:537.
511. Collier BD, Abdel-Nabi H, Doerr RJ, et al: Immunoscintigraphy performed with In-111-labeled CYT-103 in the management of colorectal cancer: comparison with CT. *Radiology* 1992;185:179.
512. McCarthy SM, Barnes D, Deveney K, et al: Detection of recurrent rectosigmoid carcinoma: prospective evaluation of CT and clinical factors. *AJR Am J Roentgenol* 1985;144:577.
513. Coburn MC, Pricolo VE, Soderberg CH: Factors affecting prognosis and management of carcinoma of the colon and rectum in patients more than eighty years of age. *J Am Coll Surg* 1994;179:65.
514. Cohen AM, Tremiterra S, Candela F, et al: Prognosis of node-positive colon cancer. *Cancer* 1991;67:1859.
515. Heys SD, Sherif A, Bagley JS, et al: Prognostic factors and survival of patients aged less than 45 years with colorectal cancer. *Br J Surg* 1994;81:685.
516. Harrison JC, Dean PJ, El-Zeky F, Vander Zwaag R: Impact of the Crohn's-like lymphoid reaction on staging of right-sided colon cancer: results of multivariate analysis. *Hum Pathol* 1995;26:31.
517. Galandiuk S, Wieand HS, Moertel CG, et al: Patterns of recurrence after curative resection of carcinoma of the colon and rectum. *Surg Gynecol Obstet* 1992;174:27.
518. Newland RC, Dent OF, Lyttle MN, et al: Pathologic determinants of survival associated with colorectal cancer with lymph node metastases—a multivariate analysis of 579 patients. *Cancer* 1994;73:2076.
519. Newland RC, Dent OF, Chapuis PH, Bokey L: Survival after curative resection of lymph node negative colorectal carcinoma. A prospective study of 910 patients. *Cancer* 1995;76:564.
520. Malassagne B, Valleur P, Serra J, et al: Relationship of apical lymph node involvement to survival in resected colon carcinoma. *Dis Colon Rectum* 1993;36:645.
521. Bjerkeset T, Morild I, Mork S, Soreide O: Tumor characteristics in colorectal cancer and their relationship to treatment and prognosis. *Dis Colon Rectum* 1987;30:934.
522. Brodsky JT, Richard GK, Cohen AM, Minsky BD: Variables correlated with the risk of lymph node metastasis in early rectal cancer. *Cancer* 1992;69:322.
523. Minsky BD, Mies C, Rich TA, et al: Colloid carcinoma of the colon and rectum. *Cancer* 1987;60:3103.
524. Michelassi F, Ewing C, Montag A, et al: Prognostic significance of ploidy determination in rectal cancer. *Hepatogastroenterology* 1992;39:222.
525. Wolmark N, Wieand HS, Rockette HE, et al: The prognostic significance of tumor and location and bowel obstruction in Dukes B and C colorectal cancer: findings from the NSABP clinical trials. *Ann Surg* 1983;198:743.
526. Steinberg SM, Barkin JS, Kaplan RS, Stablein DM: Prognostic indicators of colon tumors: the Gastrointestinal Tumor Group experience. *Cancer* 1986;57:1866.
527. Tada S, Yao T, Iida M, et al: A clinicopathologic study of small flat colorectal carcinomas. *Cancer* 1994;74:2430.
528. Moreira LF, Iwagaki H, Hizuta A, et al: Outcome in patients with early colorectal carcinoma. *Br J Surg* 1992;79:436.
529. Devereux DF, Deckers PJ: Contributions of pathologic margins and Dukes' stage to local recurrence in colorectal carcinoma. *Am J Surg* 1985;149:323.
530. Cawthorn SJ, Parums DV, Gibbs NM, et al: Extent of mesorectal spread and involvement of lateral resection margin as prognostic factors after surgery for rectal cancer. *Lancet* 1990;335:1055.
531. Adam IJ, Mohamdee MO, Martin IG, et al: Role of circumferential margin involvement in the local recurrence of rectal cancer. *Lancet* 1994;344:707.
532. Shepherd NA, Baxter KJ, Love SB: Influence of local peritoneal involvement on local recurrence and prognosis in rectal cancer. *J Clin Pathol* 1995;48:849.
533. Abulafi AM, Williams NS: Local recurrence of colorectal cancer: the problem, mechanisms, management and adjuvant therapy. *Br J Surg* 1994;81:7.
534. Ng IO, Luk IS, Yuen ST, et al: Surgical lateral clearance in resection of rectal carcinomas: a multivariate analysis of clearance in resected rectal carcinomas. *Cancer* 1993;71:1972.
535. Kotanagi H, Fukuoka T, Shibata Y, et al: The size of regional lymph nodes does not correlate with the presence or absence of metastasis in lymph nodes in rectal cancer. *J Surg Oncol* 1993;54:252.
536. Shirouzu K, Isomoto H, Morodomi T, Kakegawa T: Carcinomatous lymphatic permeation: prognostic significance in patients with rectal carcinoma—a long term prospective study. *Cancer* 1995;75:4.
537. Willett CG, Lewandrowski K, Donnelly S, et al: Are there patients with stage I rectal carcinoma at risk for failure after abdominoperineal resection? *Cancer* 1992;69:1651.
538. Horn A, Dahl O, Morild I: Venous and neural invasion as predictors of recurrence in rectal adenocarcinoma. *Dis Colon Rectum* 1991;34:798.
539. Wiggers T, Arends JW, Volovics A: Regression analysis of prognostic factors in colorectal cancer after curative resections. *Dis Colon Rectum* 1988;31:33.
540. Shirouzu K, Isomoto H, Kakegawa T: Prognostic evaluation of perineural invasion in rectal cancer. *Am J Surg* 1993;165:233.
541. Bognel C, Rekacewicz C, Mankarios H, et al: Prognostic value of neural invasion in rectal carcinoma: a multivariate analysis on 339 patients with curative resection. *Eur J Cancer* 1995;31A:894.
542. Welch JP, Donaldson GA: Management of severe obstruction of the large bowel due to malignant disease. *Am J Surg* 1974;127:492.
543. Kelley WE, Brown PW, Lawrence W, et al: Penetrating, obstructing and perforating carcinomas of the colon and rectum. *Arch Surg* 1981;116:381.
544. Thynne GS, Weiland LH, Moertel C, Silvers A: Correlation of histopathologic characteristics of primary tumor and uninvolved regional lymph nodes in Dukes' Class C colonic carcinoma with prognosis. *Mayo Clin Proc* 1980;55:243.
545. Nacopoulou L, Azaris P, Papacharalampous N, Davaris P: Prognostic significance of histologic host response in cancer of the large bowel. *Cancer* 1981;47:930.
546. Harrison JC, Dean PJ, El-Zeky F, Vander Zwaag R: From Dukes through Jass: pathological prognostic indicators in rectal cancer. *Hum Pathol* 1994;25:498.
547. Ohtani H, Naito Y, Saito K, Nagura H: Expression of costimulatory molecules B7-1 and B7-2 by macrophages along invasive margin of colon cancer: a possible antitumor immunity? *Lab Invest* 1997;77:231.
548. Patt DJ, Brynes RK, Vardiman JW, Coppleson LW: Mesocolic lymph node histology is an important prognostic indicator for patients with carcinoma of the sigmoid colon: an immunomorphologic study. *Cancer* 1975;35:1388.
549. Tsakraklides V, Wanebo HJ, Sternberg SS, et al: Prognostic evaluation of regional lymph node morphology in colorectal cancer. *Am J Surg* 1975;129:174.
550. Suzuki K, Gunderson LL, Devine RM, et al: Intraoperative irradiation after palliative surgery for locally recurrent rectal cancer. *Cancer* 1995;75:939.

551. Armitage NC, Robins RA, Evans DF, et al: The influence of tumor cell DNA abnormalities on survival in colorectal cancer. *Br J Surg* 1985; 72:828.

552. Bauer KD, Bagwell CB, Giaretti W, et al: Consensus review of the clinical utility of DNA flow of cytometry in colorectal cancer. *Cytometry* 1993;14:486.

553. Bauer KD, Lincoln ST, Vera-Roman JM, et al: Prognostic implications of proliferative activity and DNA aneuploidy in colonic adenocarcinoma. *Lab Invest* 1987;57:329.

554. Fischbach W, Zidianakis Z, Luke G, et al: DNA mapping of colorectal neoplasms: a flow cytometry study of DNA abnormalities and proliferation. *Gastroenterology* 1993;105:1126.

555. Grigolato P, Berenzi A, Benetti A, et al: Cytometric ploidy and proliferative activity in colorectal carcinoma. *Eur J Histochem* 1994;38:163.

556. Ngoi SS, Staiano-Coico L, Godwin TA, et al: Abnormal DNA ploidy and proliferative patterns in superficial colonic epithelium adjacent to colorectal cancer. *Cancer* 1990;66:953.

557. Silvestrini R, D'Agnano I, Faranda A, et al: Flow cytometric analysis of ploidy in colorectal cancer: a multicentric experience. *Br J Cancer* 1993;67:1042.

558. Steinbeck RG, Heselmeyer KM, Neugebauer WF, et al: DNA ploidy in human colorectal adenocarcinomas. *Anal Quant Cytol Histol* 1993; 15:187.

559. Barratt PL, Seymour MT, Stenning SP, et al: DNA markers predicting benefit from adjuvant fluorouracil in patients with colon cancer: a molecular study. *Lancet* 2002;360:1381.

560. Bazan V, Migliavacca M, Zanna I, et al: DNA ploidy and S-phase fraction, but not p53 or NM23-H1 expression, predict outcome in colorectal cancer patients: result of a 5-year prospective study. *J Cancer Res Clin Oncol* 2002;128:650.

561. Berczi C, Bocsi J, Bartha I, et al: Prognostic value of DNA ploidy status in patients with rectal cancer. *Anticancer Res* 2002;22:3737.

562. Chen HS, Sheen-Chen SM, Lu CC: DNA index and S-phase fraction in curative resection of colorectal adenocarcinoma: analysis of prognosis and current trends. *World J Surg* 2002;26:626.

563. Geido E, Sciutto A, Rubagotti A, et al: Combined DNA flow cytometry and sorting with k-ras2 mutation spectrum analysis and the prognosis of human sporadic colorectal cancer. *Cytometry* 2002;50:216.

564. Purdie CA, Piris J: Histopathological grade, mucinous differentiation and DNA ploidy in relation to prognosis in colorectal carcinoma. *Histopathology* 2000;36:121.

565. Salud A, Porcel JM, Raikundalia B, et al: Prognostic significance of DNA ploidy, S-phase fraction, and P-glycoprotein expression in colorectal cancer. *J Surg Oncol* 1999;72:167.

566. Buglioni S, D'Agnano I, Vasselli S, et al: p53 nuclear accumulation and multiploidy are adverse prognostic factors in surgically resected stage II colorectal cancers independent of fluorouracil-based adjuvant therapy. *Am J Clin Pathol* 2001;116:360.

567. Ko JM, Cheung MH, Kwan MW, et al: Genomic instability and alterations in APC, MCC and DCC in Hong Kong patients with colorectal carcinoma. *Int J Cancer* 1999;84:404.

568. Flyger HL, Larsen JK, Nielsen HJ, Christensen IJ: DNA ploidy in colorectal cancer, heterogeneity within and between tumors and relation to survival. *Cytometry* 1999;38:293.

569. Lammering G, Taher MM, Gruenagel HH, et al: Alteration of DNA ploidy status and cell proliferation induced by preoperative radiotherapy is a prognostic factor in rectal cancer. *Clin Cancer Res* 2000;6:3215.

570. Russo A, Migliavacca M, Zanna I, et al: p53 mutations in L3-loop zinc-binding domain, DNA-ploidy, and S phase fraction are independent prognostic indicators in colorectal cancer: a prospective study with a five-year follow-up. *Cancer Epidemiol Biomarkers Prev* 2002;11:1322.

571. Sampedro A, Salas-Bustamante A, Lopez-Artimez M, et al: Cell cycle flow cytometric analysis in the diagnosis and management of colorectal carcinoma. *Anal Quant Cytol Histol* 1999;21:347.

572. Sinicrope FA, Hart J, Hsu HA, et al: Apoptotic and mitotic indices predict survival rates in lymph node-negative colon carcinomas. *Clin Cancer Res* 1999;5:1793.

573. Locker GY, Hamilton S, Harris J, et al: ASCO 2006 update of recommendations for the use of tumor markers in gastrointestinal cancer. *J Clin Oncol* 2006;24:5313.

574. Mulcahy H, Patchett S, Daly L, O'Donoghue D: Prognosis of elderly patients with large bowel cancer. *Br J Surg* 1994;81:736.

575. Recio P, Bussey HJ: The pathology and prognosis of carcinoma of the rectum in the young. *Proc R Soc Lond* 1965;58:789.

576. Safford KL, Spebar MJ, Rosenthal D: Review of colorectal cancer in patients under age 40 years. *Am J Surg* 1981;142:767.

577. Simstein NL, Kovalcik PJ, Cross GH: Colorectal carcinoma in patients less than 40 years old. *Dis Colon Rectum* 1978;2:169.

578. Enblad G, Enblad P, Adami HO, et al: Relationship between age and survival in cancer of the colon and rectum with special reference to less than 40 years of age. *Br J Surg* 1990;77:611.

579. de Mello J, Struthers L, Turner R, et al: Multivariate analysis as aides to diagnosis and assessment of prognosis in gastrointestinal cancer. *Br J Cancer* 1983;48:341.

580. McDermott FT, Hughes ES, Pihl E, et al: Comparative results of surgical management of single carcinomas of the colon and rectum: a series of 1939 patients managed by one surgeon. *Br J Surg* 1981; 68:850.

581. Fielding LP, Phillips RK, Fry JS, Hittinger R: Prediction of outcome after curative resection for large bowel cancer. *Lancet* 1986;2:904.

582. Chen VW, Fenoglio-Preiser CM, Wu XC, et al: Aggressiveness of colon cancer in Blacks and Whites. *Cancer Epidemiol Biomarkers Prevent* 1997;6:1087.

583. Abcarian H: Operative treatment of colorectal cancer. *Cancer* 1992; 70:1350.

584. Curley SA, Evans DB, Ames FC: Resection for cure of carcinoma of the colon directly invading the duodenum or pancreatic head. *J Am Coll Surg* 1994;179:587.

585. Hildebrandt U, Schuder G, Feifel G: Preoperative staging of rectal and colonic cancer. *Endoscopy* 1994;26:810.

586. Williams NS: The rationale of preservation of the anal sphincter in patients with low rectal cancer. *Br J Surg* 1984;71:575.

587. Paty PB, Enker WE, Cohen AM: Treatment of rectal cancer by low anterior resection with coloanal anastomosis. *Ann Surg* 1994;219:365.

588. Ottery FD, Bruskewitz RC, Weese JL: Endoscopic transrectal resection of rectal tumors. *Cancer* 1986;57:563.

589. Grem JL: Current treatment approaches in colorectal cancer. *Semin Oncol* 1991;18:17.

590. Karita M, Tada M, Okita K, Kodama T: Endoscopic therapy for early colon cancer: the strip biopsy resection technique. *Gastrointest Endosc* 1991;37:128.

591. Willett CG, Compton CC, Shellito PC, Efird JT: Selection factors for local excision or abdominoperineal resection of early stage rectal cancer. *Cancer* 1994;73:2716.

592. Baron PL, Zakowski MF: Immediate vs. salvage resection after local treatment for early rectal cancer. *Dis Colon Rectum* 1995;38:177.

593. Bruch HP, Esnaashari H, Schwander O: Current status of laparoscopic therapy of colorectal cancer. *Dig Dis* 2005;23(2):127.

594. Stocchi L, Nelson H: Laparoscopic colon resection for cancer. *Adv Surg* 2006;40:59.

595. Kienle P, Weitz J, Koch M, Buchler MW: Laparoscopic surgery for colorectal cancer. *Colorectal Dis* 2006;8(suppl 3):33.

596. Silen W: Hepatic resection for metastases from colorectal carcinoma is of dubious value. *Arch Surg* 1989;124:1021.

597. Steele G Jr, Ravikumar TS: Resection of hepatic metastases from colorectal cancer. Biologic perspective. *Ann Surg* 1989;210:127.

598. Cady B, Stone MD: The role of surgical resection of liver metastases in colorectal carcinomas. *Semin Oncol* 1991;18:399.

599. Nordlinger B, Guiguet M, Vaillant JC, et al: Surgical resection of colorectal carcinoma metastases to the liver. *Cancer* 1996;77:1254.

600. Fortner JG: Recurrence of colorectal cancer after hepatic resection. *Am J Surg* 1988;155:378.

601. Wagner JS, Adson MA, van Heerden JA, et al: The natural history of hepatic metastases from colorectal cancer. A comparison with resective treatment. *Ann Surg* 1984;199:502.

602. Gayowski TJ, Iwatsuki S, Madariaga JR, et al: Experience in hepatic resection for metastatic colorectal cancer: analysis of clinical and pathologic risk factors. *Surgery* 1994;116:703.

603. Wolmark N, Fisher B, Rockette H, et al: Postoperative adjuvant chemotherapy or BCG for colon cancer: results from NSABP protocol C-01. *J Natl Cancer Inst* 1988;80:30.

604. Laurie JA, Moertel CG, Fleming TR, et al: Surgical adjuvant therapy of large-bowel carcinoma: an evaluation of levamisole and the combination of levamisole and fluorouracil. The North Central Cancer Treatment Group and the Mayo Clinic. *J Clin Oncol* 1989;7:1447.

605. Windle R, Bell PR, Shaw G: Five year results of a randomized trial of adjuvant 5-fluorouracil and levamisole in colorectal cancer. *Br J Surg* 1987;74:569.

606. Moertel CG, Fleming TR, Macdonald JS, et al: Levamisole and fluorouracil for adjuvant therapy of resected colon carcinoma. *N Engl J Med* 1990;322:352.

607. Moertel CG, Fleming TR, Macdonald JS, et al: Fluorouracil plus levamisole as effective adjuvant therapy after resection of stage III colon carcinoma: a final report. *Ann Intern Med* 1995;122:321.

608. Francini G, Petrioli R, Lorenzini L, et al: Folinic acid and 5-fluorouracil as adjuvant chemotherapy in colon cancer. *Gastroenterology* 1994;106:899.

609. O'Connell MJ, Mailliard JA, Kahn MJ, et al: Controlled trial of fluorouracil and low-dose leucovorin given for 6 months as postoperative adjuvant therapy for colon cancer. *J Clin Oncol* 1997;15:246.

610. Taal BG, Van Tinteren H, Zoetmulder FA: Adjuvant 5FU plus levamisole in colonic or rectal cancer: improved survival in stage II and III. *Br J Cancer* 2001;85:1437.

611. Andre T, Boni C, Mounedji-Boudiaf L, et al: Oxaliplatin, fluorouracil, and leucovorin as adjuvant treatment for colon cancer. *N Engl J Med* 2004;350:2343.

612. De Gramont A, Boni C, Navarro M, et al: Oxaliplatin/5-FU/LV in the adjuvant treatment of stage II and III colon cancer: efficacy results with a median follow-up of 4 years. *J Clin Oncol* 2005;23:246S.

613. Samantas E, Dervenis C, Rigatos SK: Adjuvant chemotherapy for colon cancer: evidence on improvement in survival. *Dig Dis* 2007; 25:67.

614. Wolpin BM, Meyerhardt JA, Mamon HJ, Mayer RJ: Adjuvant treatment of colorectal cancer. *CA Cancer J Clin* 2007;57:168.

615. Hohn DC, Stagg RJ, Friedman MA, et al: A randomized trial of continuous intravenous versus hepatic intraarterial floxuridine in patients with colorectal cancer metastatic to the liver: the Northern California oncology group trial. *J Clin Oncol* 1989;7:1646.

616. Kemeny N, Daly J, Reichman B, et al: Intrahepatic or systemic infusion of fluorodeoxyuridine in patients with liver metastases from colorectal carcinoma: a randomized trial. *Ann Intern Med* 1987;107:459.

617. Kemeny N: Management of liver metastases from colorectal cancer. *Oncology* 2006;20:1161.

618. Martin JK, O'Connell MJ, Wieand HS, et al: Intra-arterial floxuridine versus systemic fluorouracil for hepatic metastases from colorectal cancer. *Arch Surg* 1990;125:1022.

619. Rougier P, Hay JM, Oliver JM, et al: A controlled multicentric trial of intrahepatic artery chemotherapy versus standard palliative treatment for colorectal liver metastases. *Proc Am Soc Clin Oncol* 1990;9:104.

620. Sischy B, Gunderson L: The evolving role of radiation therapy in management of colorectal cancer. *CA Cancer J Clin* 1986;36:351.

621. Ng A, Recht A, Busse P: Sphincter preservation therapy for distal rectal carcinoma. *Cancer* 1997;79:671.

622. Sauer R, Becker H, Hohenberger W, et al: Preoperative versus postoperative chemoradiotherapy for rectal cancer. *N Engl J Med* 2004;351:1731.

623. Farniok KE, Levitt SH: Role of radiation therapy in the treatment of colorectal cancer—implications for the older patient. *Cancer* 1994; 74(7 suppl):2154.

624. Biggers OR, Beart RW, Ilstrup DM: Local excision of rectal cancer. *Dis Colon Rectum* 1986;29:374.

625. Baigrie RJ, Berry AR: Management of advanced rectal cancer. *Br J Surg* 1994;81:343.

626. Siccardi AG, Buraggi GL, Colella AC, et al: Immunoscintigraphy of adenocarcinomas by means of radiolabeled F(ab')2 fragments of an anti-carcinoembryonic antigen monoclonal antibody: a multicenter study. *Cancer Res* 1989;49:3095.

627. Patt YZ, Podoloff DA, Curley S, et al: Technetium 99m labeled IMMU-4, a monoclonal antibody against carcinoembryonic antigen, for imaging of occult recurrent colorectal cancer in patients with rising serum carcinoembryonic antigen levels. *J Clin Oncol* 1994;12:489.

628. La Valle GJ, Chevinsky A, Martin EW: Impact of radioimmunoguided surgery. *Semin Surg Oncol* 1991;7:167.

629. Kuhn JA, Corbisiero RM, Buras RR, et al: Intraoperative gamma detection probe with presurgical antibody imaging in colon cancer. *Arch Surg* 1991;126:1398.

630. Corbisiero RM, Yamauchi DM, Williams LE, et al: Comparison of immunoscintigraphy and computerized tomography in identifying colorectal cancer: individual lesion analysis. *Cancer Res* 1991;51:5704.

631. Doerr RJ, Abdel-Nabi H, Merchant B: Indium 111 ZCE-025 immunoscintigraphy in occult recurrent colorectal cancer with elevated carcinoembryonic antigen level. *Arch Surg* 1990;125:226.

632. Cote R, Houchens D, Hitchcock C, et al: Intraoperative detection of occult colon cancer micrometastases using 125I-radiolabeled monoclonal antibody CC49. *Cancer* 1996;77:613.

633. Mariani-Costantini R, Muraro R, Ficari F, et al: Immunohistochemical evidence of immune responses to tumor associated antigens in lymph nodes of colon carcinoma patients. *Cancer* 1991;67:2880.

634. Gold P, Freeman SO: Specific carcinoembryonic antigens of the human digestive system. *J Exp Med* 1965;122:467.

635. Arnaud JP, Koehl C, Adloff M: Carcinoembryonic antigen (CEA) in diagnosis and prognosis of colorectal carcinoma. *Dis Colon Rectum* 1980;23:141.

636. Midiri G, Amanti C, Benedetti M, et al: Correlation between serial CEA levels and surgery in patients with colorectal carcinoma. *J Surg Oncol* 1981;17:341.

637. Sorbye H, Dahl O: Carcinoembryonic antigen surge in metastatic colorectal cancer patients responding to oxaliplatin combination chemotherapy: implications for tumor marker monitoring and guidelines. *J Clin Oncol* 2003;21:4466.

638. Loy TS, Calaluce RD: Utility of cytokeratin immunostaining in separating pulmonary adenocarcinomas from colonic adenocarcinomas. *Am J Clin Pathol* 1994;102:764.

639. Luk GD, Desai TK, Conteas CN, et al: Biochemical markers in colorectal cancer: diagnostic and therapeutic implications. *Gastroenterol Clin North Am* 1988;17:931.

640. Magnani JL, Nilsson B, Brockhaus M, et al: A monoclonal antibody-defined antigen associated with gastrointestinal cancer is a ganglioside containing sialated lacto-N-fucopentose. *J Biol Chem* 1982;257:14365.

641. Liu C, Woo A, Tsao MS: Expression of transforming growth factor-alpha in primary human colon and lung carcinomas. *Br J Cancer* 1990; 62:425.

642. Steele RJ, Kelly P, Ellul B, Eremin O: Epidermal growth factor receptor expression in colorectal cancer. *Br J Surg* 1990;77:1352.

643. Shapiro M, Fannon AM, Kwong PD, et al: Structural basis of cell-cell adhesion by cadherins. *Nature* 1995;374:327.

644. Dorudi S, Sheffield JP, Poulsom R, et al: E-cadherin expression in colorectal cancer: an immunohistochemical and in situ hybridization study. *Am J Pathol* 1993;142:981.

645. Vogelstein B, Fearon ER, Hamilton SR, et al: Genetic alterations during colorectal-tumor development. *N Engl J Med* 1988;319:525.

646. Groden J, Thliveris W, Samowitz W, et al: Identification and characterization of the familial adenomatous polyposis coli gene. *Cell* 1991;66:589.

647. Joslyn G, Carlson M, Thliveris A, et al: Identification of deletion mutations and three new genes at the familial polyposis locus. *Cell* 1991;66:601.

648. Miyoshi Y, Nagase H, Ando H, et al: Somatic mutations of the APC gene in colorectal tumor: mutation cluster region in the APC gene. *Hum Mol Genet* 1992;1:229.

649. Nagase H, Nakamura Y: Mutations of the APC (adenomatous polyposis coli) gene. *Hum Mutat* 1993;2:425.

650. Nagase H, Miyoshi Y, Horii A, et al: Correlation between the location of germ-line mutations in the APC gene and the number of colorectal polyps in familial adenomatous polyposis patients. *Cancer Res* 1992;52:4055.

651. Nishisho I, Nakamura Y, Miyoshi Y, et al: Mutations of chromosome 5q21 genes in FAP and colorectal cancer patients. *Science* 1991;253:665.

652. Powell SM, Zilz N, Beazer-Barclay Y, et al: APC mutations occur early during colorectal tumorigenesis. *Nature* 1992;359:235.

653. Moser AR, Pitot HC, Dove WF: A dominant mutation that predisposes to multiple intestinal neoplasia in the mouse. *Science* 1990;247:322.

654. Powell SM, Zilz N, Beazer-Barclay Y, et al: APC mutations occur early during colorectal tumorigenesis. *Nature* 1992;359:235.

655. Tsao J, Shibata D: Further evidence that one of the earliest alterations in colorectal carcinogenesis involves APC. *Am J Pathol* 1994;145:531.

656. Bodmer WF, Bailey CJ, Bodmer J, et al: Localization of the gene for familial adenomatous polyposis on chromosome 5. *Nature* 1987; 328:614.

657. Leppert M, Dobbs M, Scambler P, et al: The gene for familial polyposis coli maps to the long arm of chromosome 5. *Science* 1987;238:1411.

658. Rees M, Leigh SE, Delhanty JD, Jass JR: Chromosome 5 allele loss in familial and sporadic colorectal adenomas. *Cancer* 1989;59:361.

659. Okamoto M, Sasaki M, Sugio K, et al: Loss of constitutional heterozygosity in colon carcinoma from patients with familial polyposis coli. *Nature* 1988;331:273.

660. Smith KJ, Levy DB, Maupin P, et al: Wild-type but not mutant APC associates with the microtubule cytoskeleton. *Cancer Res* 1994;54:3672.

661. Solomon E, Voss R, Hall V, et al: Chromosome 5 allele loss in human colorectal carcinomas. *Nature* 1987;328:616.

662. Ashton-Rickardt PG, Dunlop MG, Nakamura Y, et al: High frequency of APC loss in sporadic colorectal carcinoma due to breaks clustered in 5q21-22. *Oncogene* 1989;4:1169.

663. Law DJ, Olschwang S, Monpezat JP, et al: Concerted nonsyntenic allelic loss in human colorectal carcinoma. *Science* 1989;241:961.

664. Miyoshi Y, Ando H, Nagase H, et al: Germ-line mutations of the APC gene in 53 familial adenomatous polyposis patients. *Proc Natl Acad Sci USA* 1992;89:4452.

665. Nakatsuru S, Yanagisawa A, Ichii S, et al: Somatic mutation of the APC gene in gastric cancer: frequent mutations in very well differentiated adenocarcinoma and signet-ring cell carcinoma. *Hum Mol Genet* 1992;1:559.

666. Aceto G, Cristina-Curia M, Veschi S, et al: Mutations of APC and MYH in unrelated Italian patients with adenomatous polyposis coli. *Hum Mutat* 2005;26:394.

667. Miyaki M, Konishi M, Kikuchi-Yanoshita R, et al: Characteristics of somatic mutation of the adenomatous polyposis coli gene in colorectal tumors. *Cancer Res* 1994;54:3011.

668. Su LK, Johnson KA, Smith KJ, et al: Association between wildtype and mutant APC products. *Cancer Res* 1993;53:2728.

669. Munemitsu S, Souza B, Muller O, et al: The APC gene product associates with microtubules in vivo and promotes their assembly in vitro. *Cancer Res* 1994;54:3676.

670. Baeg GH, Matsumine A, Kuroda T, et al: The tumour suppressor gene product APC blocks cell cycle progression from G0/G1 to S phase. *EMBO J* 1995;14:5618.

671. Van de Wetering M, Sancho E, Verweij C, et al: The β-catenin/Tcf-4 complex imposes a crypt progenitor phenotype on colorectal cancer cells. *Cell* 2002;111:241.

672. Uthoff SM, Eichenberger MR, McAuliffe TL, et al: Wingless-type frizzled protein receptor signaling and its putative role in human colon cancer. *Mol Carcinog* 2001;31:56.

673. Barbacid M: Ras genes. *Annu Rev Biochem* 1987;56:779.

674. Bos JL: Ras oncogenes in human cancer: a review. *Cancer Res* 1989;49:4682.

675. Medema RH, Bos JL: The role of p21 ras in receptor tyrosine kinase signaling. *Crit Rev Oncog* 1993;4:615.

676. Bell SM, Kelly SA, Hoyle JA, et al: c-Ki-ras gene mutations in dysplasia and carcinomas complicating ulcerative colitis. *Br J Cancer* 1991;64:174.

677. Burmer GC, Loeb LA: Mutations in the KRAS2 oncogene during progressive stages of human colon carcinoma. *Proc Natl Acad Sci USA* 1989;86:2403.

678. Finkelstein SD, Sayegh R, Christensen S, Swalsky PA: Genotypic classification of colorectal adenocarcinoma—biologic behavior correlates with K-ras-2 mutation type. *Cancer* 1993;71:3827.

679. Finkelstein S, Sayegh R, Bakker A, Swalsky P: Determination of tumor aggressiveness in colorectal cancer by K-ras-2 analysis. *Arch Surg* 1993;128:526.

680. Nagata Y, Abe M, Kobayashi K, et al: Glycine to aspartic acid mutations at codon 13 of the c-Ki-ras gene in human gastrointestinal cancers. *Cancer Res* 1990;50:480.

681. Shibata D, Schaeffer J, Li ZH, et al: Genetic heterogeneity of the c-K-ras locus in colorectal adenomas but not in adenocarcinomas. *J Natl Cancer Inst* 1993;85:1058.

682. Ranaldi R, Gioacchini A, Manzin A, et al: Adenoma-carcinoma sequence of colorectum. Prevalence of K-ras gene mutation in adenomas with increasing degree of dysplasia and aneuploidy. *Diagn Mol Pathol* 1995;4:198.

683. Miyaki M, Seki M, Okamoto M, et al: Genetic changes and histopathological types in colorectal tumor from patients with familial adenomatous polyposis. *Cancer Res* 1990;50:7166.

684. Ando M, Takemura K, Maruyama M, et al: Mutations in c-K-ras 2 gene codon 12 during colorectal tumorigenesis in familial adenomatous polyposis. *Gastroenterology* 1992;103:1725.

685. McLellan EA, Owen RA, Stepniewska KA, et al: High frequency of K-ras mutations in sporadic colorectal adenomas. *Gut* 1993;34:392.

686. Sasaki M, Sugio K, Sasazuki T: K-ras activation in colorectal tumors from patients with familial polyposis coli. *Cancer* 1990;65:2576.

687. Breivik J, Meling GI, Spurkland A, et al: K-ras mutation in colorectal cancer: relations to patient age, sex and tumor location. *Cancer* 1994;69:367.

688. Halter SA, Webb L, Rose J: Lack of ras mutations and prediction of long-term survival in carcinoma of the colon. *Mod Pathol* 1992;5:131.

689. Forrester K, Almoguera C, Han K, et al: Detection of high incidence of K-ras oncogenes during human colon tumorigenesis. *Nature* 1987;327:298.

690. Ohmura M, Hattori T: A possible multiclonal development in human colonic carcinomas. *J Cancer Res Clin Oncol* 1995;121:321.

691. Ronai Z: Ras oncogene detection in pre-neoplastic lesions: possible applications for diagnosis and prevention. *Oncol Res* 1992;4:45.

692. Rochlitz C, Heide I, Kant E, et al: Position specificity of Ki-ras oncogene mutations during the progression of colorectal carcinoma. *Oncology* 1993;50:70.

693. Suchy B, Zietz C, Rabes HM: K-ras point mutations in human colorectal carcinomas: relation to aneuploidy and metastasis. *Int J Cancer* 1992;53:30.

694. Losi L, Benhatter J, Costa J: Stability of K-ras mutations throughout the natural history of human colorectal cancer. *Eur J Cancer* 1992;28A:1115.

695. Minamoto T, Sawaguchi K, Mai M, et al: Infrequent K-ras activation in superficial-type (flat) colorectal adenomas and adenocarcinomas. *Cancer Res* 1994;54:2841.

696. Yamagata S, Muto T, Uchida Y, et al: Lower incidence of K-ras codon 12 mutation in flat colorectal adenomas than in polypoid adenomas. *Jpn J Cancer Res* 1994;85:147.

697. Yamagata S, Muto T, Masaki T, et al: Polypoid growth and K-ras codon 12 mutation in colorectal cancer. *Cancer* 1995;75:953.

698. Fujimori T, Satonaka K, Yamamura-Idei Y, et al: Non-involvement of ras mutations in flat colorectal adenomas and carcinomas. *Int J Cancer* 1994;57:51.

699. Hasegawa H, Ueda M, Watanabe M, et al: K-ras gene mutations in early colorectal cancer. Flat elevated vs polyp-forming cancer. *Oncogene* 1995;10:1413.

700. Reich NC, Levine AJ: Growth regulation of a cellular tumor antigen, p53, in non-transformed cells. *Nature* 1984;308:199.

701. Lin J, Chen J, Elenbaas B, Levine AJ: Several hydrophobic amino acids in the p53 aminoterminal domain are required for transcriptional activation, binding to mdm-2 and the adenovirus 5 E1B 55kd protein. *Genes Dev* 1994;8:1235.

702. Cho Y, Gorina S, Jeffrey P, et al: Crystal structure of a p53 tumor suppressor-DNA complex: a framework for understanding how mutations inactivate p53. *Science* 1994;265:346.

703. Nigro JM, Baker SJ, Preisinger AC, et al: Mutations in the p53 gene occur in diverse human tumour types. *Nature* 1988;342:705.

704. Pietenpol JA, Tokino T, Thiagalingam S, et al: Sequence-specific transcriptional activation is essential for growth suppression by p53. *Proc Natl Acad Sci USA* 1994;91:1998.

705. Srivastava S, Wang S, Tong YA, et al: Dominant negative effect of a germ-line mutant p53: a step fostering tumorigenesis. *Cancer Res* 1993;53:4452.

706. Tarunina M, Jenkins JR: Human p53 binds DNA as a protein homodimer but monomeric variants retain full transcription transactivation activity. *Oncogene* 1993;8:3165.

707. Vogelstein B, Kinzler KW: p53 function and dysfunction. *Cell* 1992;70:523.

708. Srinivasan R, Roth JA, Maxwell SA: Sequence-specific interaction of a conformational domain of p53 with DNA. *Cancer Res* 1993;53:5361.

709. Clarke AR, Purdie CA, Harrison DJ, et al: Thymocyte apoptosis induced by p53 dependent and independent pathways. *Nature* 1993;362:849.

710. Levine AJ, Momand J, Finlay CA: The p53 tumour suppressor gene. *Nature* 1991;315:453.

711. Lowe SW, Schmitt EM, Smith SW, et al: p53 is required for radiation-induced apoptosis in mouse thymocytes. *Nature* 1993;362:847.

712. Shaw P, Bovey R, Tardy S, et al: Induction of apoptosis by wild type p53 in a human colon tumor-derived cell line. *Proc Natl Acad Sci USA* 1992;89:4495.

713. Graeber TG, Osmanian C, Jacks T, et al: Hypoxia-mediated selection of cells with diminished apoptotic potential in solid tumors. *Nature* 1996;379:88.

714. Lane DP: p53, guardian of the genome. *Nature* 1992;358:15.

715. Tlsty TD, Margolin BH, Lum K: Differences in the rates of gene amplification in non-tumorigenic and tumorigenic cell lines as measured by Luria-Delbrück fluctuation analysis. *Proc Natl Acad Sci USA* 1989;86:9441.

716. El-Deiry W, Tokino T, Velculescu VE, et al: WAF1, a potential mediator of p53 tumor suppression. *Cell* 1993;75:817.

717. Waldman T, Lengauer C, Kinzler KW, Vogelstein B: Uncoupling of S phase and mitosis induced by anticancer agents in cells lacking p21. *Nature* 1996;381:713.

718. Harper JW, Adami GR, Wei N, et al: The p21 Cdk-interacting protein Cip1 is a potent inhibitor of G1 cyclin-dependent kinases. *Cell* 1993;75:805.

719. Noda A, Ning Y, Venable SF, et al: Cloning of senescent cell-derived inhibitors of DNA synthesis using an expression screen. *Exp Cell Res* 1994;211:90.

720. Xiong Y, Hannon GJ, Zhang H, et al: p21 is a universal inhibitor of cyclin kinases. *Nature* 1993;366:701.

721. Cross SM, Sanchez CA, Morgan CA, et al: A p53-dependent mouse spindle check point. *Science* 1995;267:1353.

722. Livingstone LR, White A, Sprouse J, et al: Altered cell cycle arrest and gene amplification potential accompany loss of wild type p53. *Cell* 1992;70:923.

723. Hartwell L: Defects in a cell cycle checkpoint may be responsible for the genomic instability of cancer cells. *Cell* 1992;71:543.

724. Yin Y, Tainsky MA, Bischoff FZ, et al: Wild type p53 restores cell cycle control and inhibits gene amplification cells with mutant p53 alleles. *Cell* 1992;70:937.

725. Milner J: A conformation hypothesis for the suppressor and promoter function of p53 in cell growth control and cancer. *Proc R Soc Lond Ser B Biol Sci* 1991;245:139.

726. Milner J, Medcalf EA: Cotranslation of activated mutant p53 with wild type drives the wild-type p53 protein into the mutant conformation. *Cell* 1991;65:765.

727. Kern S, Pietenpol JA, Thiagalingam S, et al: Oncogenic forms of p53 inhibit p53-regulated gene expression. *Science* 1992;256:827.

728. Farmer G, Bargonetti J, Zhu H, et al: Wild-type p53 activates transcription in vitro. *Nature* 1992;358:83.

729. Kern SE, Kinzler KW, Bruskin A, et al: Identification of p53 as a sequence-specific DNA-binding protein. *Science* 1991;252:1708.

730. Baker SJ, Fearon ER, Vogelstein B: Suppression of human colorectal carcinoma cell growth by wild-type p53. *Science* 1990;249:912.

731. Baker SJ, Fearon ER, Nigro JM, et al: Chromosome 17 deletions and p53 gene mutations in colorectal carcinomas. *Science* 1989;244:217.

732. Baker SJ, Preisinger AC, Jessup JM, et al: p53 gene mutations occur in combination with 17p allelic deletions as late events in colorectal tumorigenesis. *Cancer Res* 1990;50:7717.

733. Shaw P, Tardy S, Benito E, et al: Occurrence of Ki-ras and p53 mutations in primary colorectal tumors. *Oncogene* 1991;6:2121.

734. Van den Broek MH, Renault B, Fodde R, et al: Sites and types of p53 mutations in an unselected series of colorectal cancers in the Netherlands. *Anticancer Res* 1993;13:587.

735. Van den Broek MH, Jhanwar SC, Fodde R, et al: P53 mutations in colorectal cancers in the patients of metropolitan New York. *Anticancer Res* 1993;13:1769.

736. Ohue M, Tomita N, Monden T, et al: A frequent alteration of p53 gene in carcinoma in adenoma of colon. *Cancer Res* 1994;54:4798.

737. Khine K, Smith DR, Goh HS: High frequency of allelic deletion on chromosome 17p in advanced colorectal cancer. *Cancer* 1994;73:28.

738. Cunningham J, Lust JA, Schaid DJ, et al: Expression of p53 and 17p allelic loss in colorectal carcinoma. *Cancer Res* 1992;52:1974.

739. Aoki T, Takeda S, Yanagisawa A, et al: APC and p53 mutations in de novo colorectal adenocarcinomas. *Hum Mutat* 1994;3:342.

740. Kern SE, Fearon ER, Tersmette KW: Clinical and pathological associations with allelic loss in colorectal carcinoma. *JAMA* 1989;261:3099.

741. Takanishi DM Jr, Angriman I, Yaremko ML: Chromosome 17p allelic loss in colorectal cancer. *Arch Surg* 1995;130:585.

742. Hamelin R, Laurent-Puig P, Olschwang S, et al: Association of p53 mutations with short survival in colorectal cancer. *Gastroenterology* 1994;106:42.

743. Dix BR, Robbins P, Soong R, et al: The common molecular genetic alterations in Dukes' B and C colorectal carcinomas are not short-term prognostic indicators of survival. *Int J Cancer* 1994;59:747.

744. Zeng ZS, Sarkis AS, Zhang ZF, et al: p53 nuclear overexpression: an independent predictor of survival in lymph node—positive colorectal cancer patients. *J Clin Oncol* 1994;12:2043.

745. Vogelstein B, Fearon ER, Kern SE, et al: Allelotype of colorectal carcinomas. *Science* 1989;244:207.

746. Fazeli A, Dickinson SL, Hermiston ML, et al: Phenotype of mice lacking functional deleted in colorectal cancer (DCC) gene. *Nature* 1997;386:796.

747. Thiagalingam S, Lengauer C, Leach FS, et al: Evaluation of candidate tumour suppresser genes on chromosome 18 in colorectal cancers. *Nat Genet* 1996;13:343.

748. MacGrogan D, Pegram M, Slamon D, Bookstein R: Comparative mutational analysis of DPC4 (Smad4) in prostatic and colorectal carcinomas. *Oncogene* 1997;15:1111.

749. Takagi Y, Kohmura H, Futamura M, et al: Somatic alterations of the DPC4 gene in human colorectal cancers in vivo. *Gastroenterology* 1996;111:1369.

750. Koyama M, Ito M, Nagai H, et al: Inactivation of both alleles of the DPC4/SMAD4 gene in advanced colorectal cancers: identification of seven novel somatic mutations in tumors from Japanese patients. *Mutat Res* 1999;406:71.

751. Harn SA, Schutte M, Hoque AT, et al: DPC4, a candidate tumor suppresser gene at human chromosome 18q21.1. *Science* 1996;271:350.

752. Miyaki M, Iijima T, Konishi M, et al: Higher frequency of Smad4 gene mutation in human colorectal cancer with distant metastasis. *Oncogene* 1999;18:3098.

753. Maitra A, Molberg K, Albores-Saavedra J, Lindberg G: Loss of Dpc4 expression in colonic adenocarcinomas correlates with the presence of metastatic disease. *Am J Pathol* 2000;157:1105.

754. Shibata D, Reale M, Lavin P, et al: The DCC protein and prognosis in colorectal cancer. *N Engl J Med* 1996;335:1727.

755. Jen J, Kim H, Piantadosi S, et al: Allelic loss of chromosome 18q and prognosis in colorectal cancer. *N Engl J Med* 1994;331:213.

756. Modrich P: Methyl-directed DNA mismatch correction. *J Biol Chem* 1989;264:6597.

757. Modrich P: Mechanisms and biological effects of mismatch repair. *Annu Rev Genet* 1991;25:229.

758. Parsons R, Li GM, Longley MJ, et al: Hypermutability and mismatch repair deficiency in RER+ tumor cells. *Cell* 1993;75:1227.

759. Bhattacharyya NP, Skandalis A, Ganesh A, et al: Mutator phenotypes in human colorectal carcinoma cell lines. *Proc Natl Acad Sci USA* 1994;91:6319.

760. Papadopoulos N, Nicolaides NC, Wei Y-S, et al: Mutation of a MutL homolog in hereditary colon cancer. *Science* 1994;263:1625.

761. Kolodner R, Hall N, Lipford J, et al: Structure of the human MSH2 locus and analysis of two Muir-Torre kindreds for msh2 mutations. *Genomics* 1994;24:516.

762. Aaltonen LA, Peltomaki P, Mecklin JP, et al: Replication errors in benign and malignant tumours from hereditary nonpolyposis colorectal cancer patients. *Cancer Res* 1994;54:1645.

763. Ionov Y, Peinado MA, Malkhosyan S, et al: Ubiquitous somatic mutations in simple repeated sequences reveal a new mechanism for colonic carcinogenesis. *Nature* 1993;363:558.

764. Thibodeau SN, Bren G, Schaid D: Microsatellite instability in cancer of the proximal colon. *Science* 1993;260:816.

765. Liu B, Nicolaides NC, Markowitz S, et al: Mismatch repair gene defects in sporadic colorectal cancers with microsatellite instability. *Nature Genet* 1995;9:48.

766. Kane M, Loda M, Gaida G, et al: Methylation of the *hMLH1* promoter correlates with lack of expression of hMLH1 in sporadic colon tumors and mismatch repair-defective human tumor cell lines. *Cancer Res* 1997;57:808.

767. Veigl M, Kasturi L, Olechnowicz J, et al: Biallelic inactivation of *hMLH1* by epigenetic gene silencing, a novel mechanism causing human MSI cancers. *Proc Natl Acad Sci USA* 1998;95:8698.

768. Lothe RA, Peltomaki P, Meling GI, et al: Genomic instability in colorectal cancer: relationship to clinicopathologic variables and family history. *Cancer Res* 1993;53:5849.

769. Heinen CD, Noffsinger AE, Belli J, et al: Regenerative lesions in ulcerative colitis are characterized by microsatellite mutation. *Genes Chrom Cancer* 1997;19:170.

770. Suzuki H, Harpaz N, Tarmin L, et al: Microsatellite instability in ulcerative colitis-associated colorectal dysplasias and cancers. *Cancer Res* 1994;54:4841.

771. Boland CR, Thibodeau SN, Hamilton SR, et al: A National Cancer Institute work-shop on microsatellite instability for cancer detection and familial predisposition: development of international criteria for

the determination of microsatellite instability in colorectal cancer. *Cancer Res* 1998;58:5248.

772. Fishel R, Lescoe MK, Rao MRS, et al: The human mutator gene homolog *MSH2* and its association with hereditary nonpolyposis colon cancer. *Cell* 1993;75:1027.

773. Bronner CE, Baker SM, Morrison PT, et al: Mutation in the DNA mismatch repair gene homologue hMLH1 is associated with hereditary non-polyposis colon cancer. *Nature* 1994;368:258.

774. Leach FS, Nicolaides NC, Papadopoulos N, et al: Mutations of a mutS homolog in hereditary nonpolyposis colorectal cancer. *Cell* 1993; 75:1215.

775. Papadopoulos N, Nicolaides NC, Wei YF, et al: Mutation of the mutL homolog in hereditary colon cancer. *Science* 1994;263:1625.

776. Rampino N, Yamamoto H, Ionov Y, et al: Somatic frameshift mutations in the BAX gene in colon cancers of the microsatellite mutator phenotype. *Science* 1997;275:967.

777. Myeroff LL, Parsons R, Kim S-J, et al: A transforming growth factor beta receptor type II gene mutation common in colon and gastric but rare in endometrial cancer with microsatellite instability. *Cancer Res* 1995;55:5545.

778. Markowitz S, Wang J, Myeroff L, et al: Inactivation of the type II TGFβ receptor in colon cancer cells with microsatellite instability. *Science* 1995;268:1336.

779. Parsons R, Myeroff L, Liu B, et al: Microsatellite instability and mutations of the transforming growth factor b type II receptor gene in colorectal cancer. *Cancer Res* 1995;55:5548.

780. Souza RF, Lei J, Yin J, et al: A transforming growth factor β1 receptor type II mutation in ulcerative colitis-associated neoplasms. *Gastroenterology* 1997;112:40.

781. Liu W, Dong X, Mai M, et al: Mutations in AXIN2 cause colorectal cancer with defective mismatch repair by activating β-catenin/TCF signaling. *Nat Genet* 2000;26:146.

782. Riccio A, Aaltonen LA, Godwin AK, et al: The DNA repair gene MBD4 (MED1) is mutated in human carcinomas with microsatellite instability. *Nat Genet* 1999;23:266.

783. Malkohosyan S, Rampino N, Yamamoto H, Perucho M: Frameshift mutator mutations. *Nature* 1996;382:499.

784. Duval A, Iacopetta B, Ranzani GN, et al: Variable mutation frequencies in coding repeats of TCF-4 and other target genes in colon, gastric and endometrial carcinoma showing microsatellite instability. *Oncogene* 1999;18:6806.

785. Bader S, Walker M, Hendrich B, et al: Somatic frameshift mutations in the MBD4 gene of sporadic colon cancers with mismatch repair deficiency. *Oncogene* 1999;18:8044.

786. Guanti G, Resta N, Simone C, et al: Involvement of PTEN mutations in the genetic pathways of colorectal cancerogenesis. *Hum Mol Genet* 2000;9:283.

787. Chadwick RB, Jiang GL, Bennington GA, et al: Candidate tumor suppressor *RIZ* is frequently involved in colorectal carcinogenesis. *Proc Natl Acad Sci USA* 2000;97:2662.

788. Piao Z, Fang W, Malkhosyan S, et al: Frequent frameshift mutations in RIZ in sporadic gastrointestinal and endometrial carcinomas with microsatellite instability. *Cancer Res* 2000;60:4701.

789. Huang J, Papadopoulos N, McKinley A, et al: APC mutations in colorectal tumors with mismatch repair deficiency. *Proc Natl Acad Sci USA* 1996;93:9049.

790. Konishi M, Kikuchi-Yanoshita R, Tanaka K, et al: Molecular nature of colon tumors in hereditary nonpolyposis colon cancer, familial polyposis, and sporadic colon cancer. *Gastroenterology* 1996;111:307.

791. Miyaki M, Iijima T, Kimura J, et al: Frequent mutation of betacatenin and APC genes in primary colorectal tumors from patients with hereditary nonpolyposis colorectal cancer. *Cancer Res* 1999; 59:4506.

792. Fujiwara T, Stolker JM, Watanabe T, et al: Accumulated clonal genetic alterations in familial and sporadic colorectal carcinomas with widespread instability in microsatellite sequences. *Am J Pathol* 1998;153: 1063.

793. Eshleman J, Casey G, Kochera M, et al: Chromosome number and structure both are markedly stable in RER colorectal cancers and are not destabilized by mutation of p53. *Oncogene* 1998;17:719.

794. Herman J, Umar A, Polyak K, et al: Incidence and functional consequences of *hMLH1* promoter hypermethylation in colorectal carcinoma. *Proc Natl Acad Sci USA* 1998;95:6870.

795. Baylin SB, Herman JG: DNA hypermethylation in tumorigenesis: epigenetics joins genetics. *Trends Genet* 2000;16:168.

796. Jones P, Laird P: Cancer epigenetics comes of age. *Nat Genet* 1999; 21:163.

797. Toyota M, Ho C, Ahuja N, et al: Identification of differentially methylated sequences in colorectal cancer by methylated CpG island amplification. *Cancer Res* 1999;59:2307.

798. Chan AO, Broaddus RR, Houlihan PS, et al: CpG island methylation in aberrant crypt foci of the colorectum. *Am J Pathol* 2002;160:1823.

799. Rashid A, Shen L, Morris JS, et al: CpG island methylation in colorectal adenomas. *Am J Pathol* 2001;159:1129.

800. Whitehall VL, Wynter CV, Walsh MD, et al: Morphological and molecular heterogeneity within nonmicrosatellite instability-high colorectal cancer. *Cancer Res* 2002;62:6011.

801. van Rijnsoever M, Grieu F, Elsaleh H, et al: Characterisation of colorectal cancers showing hypermethylation at multiple CpG islands. *Gut* 2002;51:797.

802. Toyota M, Ahuja N, Ohe-Toyota M, et al: CpG island methylator phenotype in colorectal cancer. *Proc Natl Acad Sci USA* 1999;96:8681.

803. Toyota M, Ohe-Toyota M, Ahuja N, Issa JP: Distinct genetic profiles in colorectal tumors with or without the CpG island methylator phenotype. *Proc Natl Acad Sci USA* 2000;97:710.

804. Malkohosyan SR, Yamamoto H, Piao Z, Perucho M: Late onset and high incidence of colon cancer of the mutator phenotype with hypermethylated hMLH1 gene in women. *Gastroenterology* 2000;119:598.

805. Shannon BA, Iacopetta BJ: Methylation of the hMLH1, p16 and MDR1 genes in colorectal carcinoma: associations with clinicopathologic features. *Cancer Lett* 2001;167:91.

806. Burri N, Shaw P, Bouzourene H, et al: Methylation silencing and mutations of the p14ARF and p16INK4a genes in colon cancer. *Lab Invest* 2001;8:217.

807. Chan AO, Issa JP, Morris JS, et al: Concordant CpG island methylation in hyperplastic polyposis. *Am J Pathol* 2002;160:529.

808. Jass JR, Biden KG, Cummings M, et al: Characterisation of a subtype of colorectal cancer combining features of the suppressor and mild mutator pathways. *J Clin Pathol* 1999;52:455.

809. Esteller M, Toyota M, Sanchez-Cespedes M, et al: Inactivation of the DNA repair gene O6-methylguanine-DNA methyltransferase by promoter hypermethylation is associated with G to A mutations in K-ras in colorectal tumorigenesis. *Cancer Res* 2000;60:2368.

810. Ginaldi S, Lindell MM Jr, Zornoza J: The striped colon: a new radiographic observation in metastatic serosal implants. *AJR Am J Roentgenol* 1980;134:453.

811. Rubesin SE, Levine MS, Bezzi M, et al: Rectal involvement by prostatic carcinoma: barium enema findings. *AJR Am J Roentgenol* 1989;152:53.

812. Gedgaudas RK, Kelvin FM, Thompson WM, et al: The value of the preoperative barium-enema examination in the assessment of pelvic masses. *Radiology* 1983;146:609.

813. Feczko PJ, Collins DD, Mezwa DG: Metastatic disease involving the gastrointestinal tract. *Radiol Clin North Am* 1993;31:1359.

814. Meyers MA: Intraperitoneal spread of malignancies and its effect on the bowel. *Clin Radiol* 1981;32:129.

815. Masangkay A, Susin M, Baker R, et al: Metastatic malignant mesothelioma presenting as colonic polyps. *Hum Pathol* 1997;28:993.

816. Wegener M, Borsch G, Reitemeyer E, Schafer K: Metastasis to the colon from primary bronchogenic carcinoma presenting as occult gastrointestinal bleeding: report of a case. *Z Gastroenterol* 1988;26:358.

817. Pang JA, King WK: Bowel hemorrhage and perforation from metastatic lung cancer: report of three cases and a review of the literature. *Aust NZ J Surg* 1987;57:779.

818. Geboes K, De Jaeger E, Rutgeerts P, et al: Symptomatic gastrointestinal metastases from malignant melanoma. A clinical study. *J Clin Gastroenterol* 1988;10:64.

819. Silverman JM, Hamlin JA: Large melanoma metastases to the gastrointestinal tract. *Gut* 1989;30:1783.

820. Fawaz F, Hill GJ: Adult intussusception due to metastatic tumors. *South Med J* 1983;75:522.

821. Libshitz HI, Lindell MM, Dodd GD: Metastases to the hollow viscera. *Radiol Clin North Am* 1982;20:487.

822. Tiszlavicz L: Stomach cancer metastasizing into a solitary adenomatous colonic polyp. *Orv Hetil* 1990;131:1259.

823. Flint A, Lloyd R: Colon carcinoma metastatic to the lung. Cytologic manifestations and distinction from primary pulmonary adenocarcinoma. *Colon Carcinoma* 1992;36:230.

824. Berezowski K, Stastny J, Kornstein M, et al: Cytokeratins 7 and 20 and carcinoembryonic antigen in ovarian and colonic carcinoma. *Mod Pathol* 1995;9:426.

825. Mobus VJ, Moll R, Gerharz CD, et al: Establishment of new ovarian and colon carcinoma cell lines—differentiation is only possible by cytokeratin analysis. *Br J Cancer* 1994;69:422.

826. Herrera L, Villarreal JR: Incidence of metastases from rectal adenocarcinoma in small lymph nodes detected by a clearing technique. *Dis Colon Rectum* 1992;35:783.

827. Andreola S, Leo E, Belli F, et al: Manual dissection of adenocarcinoma of the lower third of the rectum specimens for detection of lymph node mestastases smaller than 5 mm. *Cancer* 1996;77:607.

828. Scott K, Grace R: Detection of lymph node metastases in colorectal carcinoma before and after fat clearance. *Br J Surg* 1989;76:1165.

829. Hida J, Mori N, Kubo R, et al: Metastases from carcinoma of the colon and rectum detected in small lymph nodes by the clearing method. *J Am Coll Surg* 1994;178:223.

830. Cawthorn SJ, Gibbs NM, Marks CG: Clearance technique for the detection of lymph nodes in colorectal cancer. *Br J Surg* 1986;73:58.

831. Jass JR, Miller K, Northover JM: Fat clearance method versus manual dissection of lymph nodes in specimens of rectal cancer. *Int J Colon Dis* 1986;1:155.

832. Dirschmid K, Lang A, Mathis G, et al: Incidence of extramural venous invasion in colorectal carcinoma. *Hum Pathol* 1996;27:1227.

833. Association of Directors of Anatomic and Surgical Pathology: Recommendations for the reporting of resected large intestinal carcinomas. *Hum Pathol* 1996;27:5.

CHAPTER 15

The Nonneoplastic Anus

EMBRYOLOGY

The anal canal develops from the distal hindgut. Early in development, the hindgut, allantois, and urogenital tracts end in a common cloaca. Later, the urogenital septum divides the hindgut into the anterior urogenital and posterior gastrointestinal compartments. Distally, the cloacal membrane, composed of an ectodermal and endodermal layer, separates the endodermally derived hindgut from the ectoderm. It ruptures at approximately the seventh week of gestation, at which time the urogenital septum is almost completely formed and normal anatomic relationships are established. Cloacal membrane remnants are converted to the urogenital and anal membranes. These membranes eventually dehisce, allowing orifices to be established for the urogenital and anal structures. Mesoderm later invades the perianal region, forming the external sphincter. The dentate line and anal papillae are remnants of the anal membrane.

If the cloacal membrane persists for longer than normal, the inferior abdominal muscles and the pubic bones develop in a lateral unfused position. If the cloacal membrane ruptures before the urogenital septum separates the bladder from the hindgut, cloacal exstrophy occurs (1). Incomplete separation of the cloaca results in an abnormal connection between the rectum and bladder, urethra, or vagina and imperforate anus (1). Figure 15.1 shows the embryology of the anus with the progressive development of the cloaca and formation of the primitive urogenital sinus with eventual separation of the urogenital sinus into the urinary bladder and the anorectal canal.

DEFINITIONS

In the most commonly accepted definition, the *anal canal* extends from the perineal skin to the lower end of the rectum at the upper border of the internal sphincter at the anorectal ring. It ranges in length from 3 to 4 cm (2,3). The *anal verge* marks the junction of the anal canal and the perineal skin. It is identified microscopically by the appearance of cutaneous adnexa. The *dentate* or *pectinate line* marks the junction between the anal canal and the rectum (Fig. 15.2) and it lies in the center of the anal canal.

Sixteen mucosal longitudinal folds, known as the *anal columns of Morgagni,* and homologous structures in the lower rectum, known as the *rectal columns of Morgagni,* cover the underlying blood vessels. These are separated by the anal sinuses or the *sinuses of Morgagni*. The anal columns connect to one another at the dentate line by anal or semilunar valves. *Anal papillae* are toothlike, raised projections located on the top of the anal columns that represent ridges of squamous mucosa directly joining the rectal mucosa. Both anal crypts and papillae show marked individual variations and they are often absent. Under the valves, the mucosa joins the hairless skin of the transitional zone in the irregular pectinate line (Fig. 15.3). The external anal sphincter consists of voluntary skeletal muscle arranged as a tube surrounding the internal sphincter. The internal anal sphincter represents the terminal end of the circular smooth layer of the muscularis propria and contains fascicles of involuntary smooth muscle fibers ensheathed in connective tissue. The conjoined longitudinal coat represents the most caudal extension of the longitudinal coat joined by a few striated muscle fibers from the levator ani. It traverses the anal canal between the internal and external sphincters. The internal anal sphincter plays an important role in anal continence and maintenance of resting anal canal pressure.

The dual origin of the vascular supply of the anal canal reflects its dual embryology. Most of the anal canal is supplied by the rectal arteries, a continuation of the inferior mesenteric artery. The inferior anal canal is supplied by the inferior rectal arteries, branches of the internal pudendal arteries. The mucocutaneous junction forms a watershed zone between these two vascular supplies. Terminal vascular branches form tiny arteriovenous anastomoses with the submucosal plexus (Fig. 15.4). Above the dentate line, the vessels form a series of hollow communicating spaces surrounded by connective tissue in a structure that resembles a glomerulus. This system is known as the *corpus cavernosum recti.*

Venous drainage of the superior anal canal is via the superior rectal veins, tributaries of the inferior mesenteric vein. Above the mucocutaneous level, veins drain into the portal venous system. Below this, veins drain into the pudendal veins. The lymphatic drainage of the proximal

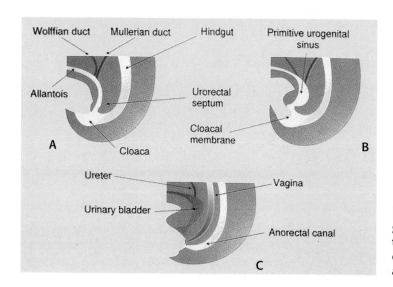

FIG. 15.1. Embryology of the anus. **A–C** show the progressive development of the cloaca and formation of the primitive urogenital sinus with eventual separation of the urogenital sinus into the urinary bladder and the anorectal canal. See text for further details.

two thirds of the anal canal is into the inferior mesenteric lymph nodes. Distal rectal lymphatics drain laterally along the course of the inferior or medial hemorrhoidal vessels into the para-aortic lymph nodes ending in the hypogastric, obturator, and internal iliac nodes. Alternatively, they follow the superior rectal artery to drain into nodes in the sigmoid mesocolon near the origin of the inferior mesentery artery (Fig. 15.4). Distally, the lymphatics have a more complex arrangement. Some anal canal lymphatics connect with rectal lymphatics (4); others cross the anal verge and pass along the genital femoral sulcus on either side, terminating in the inferomedial superficial inguinal lymph nodes (Fig. 15.4) (5). The lymphatics of the lower anal canal drain to the inguinal lymph nodes. Occasionally, connections exist with the common iliac, middle, and lateral sacral, lower gluteal, external iliac, and deep inguinal nodes (6). This organization is reflected in the metastatic spread of anal tumors (Fig. 15.4).

HISTOLOGIC FEATURES

The anal canal mucosa contains four distinctive zones: (a) the *colorectal zone* immediately distal to the rectum (Fig. 15.5); (b) the *transitional zone*, roughly corresponding to the area of the anal columns with its distal border approximately at the level of the anal valves and sinuses; (c) the *smooth*

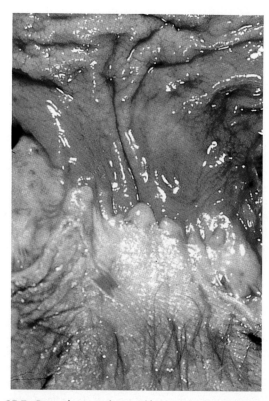

FIG. 15.3. Resection specimen of lower rectum and anal canal. At the bottom there is a rim of wrinkled perianal skin. Above this is the squamous zone. The anal transitional zone is the pale pink region separating the tan-brown rectal mucosa from the white squamous zone.

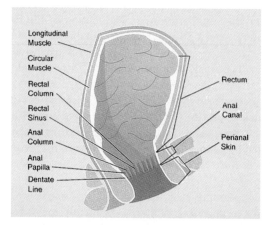

FIG. 15.2. Anal canal. The figure shows the relationship of the anal musculature to the rectum, anal columns, and anal papillae as well as the perianal skin.

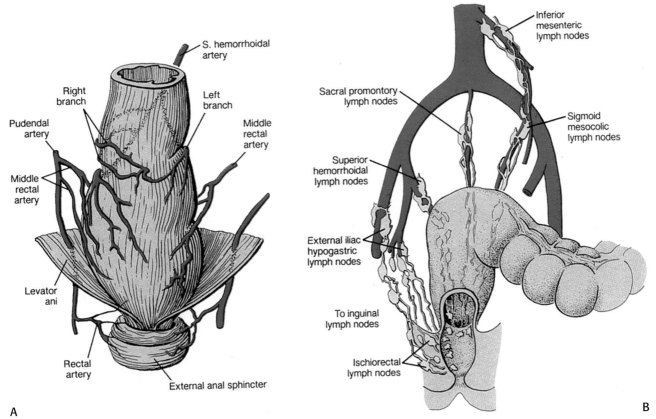

FIG. 15.4. Normal anatomy. **A:** Arterial blood supply of rectum. (Adapted from Grant JCB. *Grant's Atlas of Anatomy.* Baltimore: Williams and Wilkins, 1962.) **B:** Lymph node drainage of the anus.

zone below the anal columns covered by uninterrupted nonkeratinizing squamous epithelium devoid of skin appendages (Fig. 15.6); and (d) the *distal zone*, composed of keratinizing squamous epithelium. The lower anal canal ends at the anal verge, where the squamous mucosa merges with perianal skin. The squamous mucosa of the anal canal lacks the hair and skin appendages seen in the perianal skin.

The mucosa of the *colorectal zone* resembles rectal mucosa except that the crypts may appear shorter and more irregular (Fig. 15.5). The *transitional zone* has irregular outlines and varying locations and extents (7). The cells form four to nine layers and contain transitional, intermediate, or cloacogenic epithelium (Fig. 15.7). The basal layer contains the proliferative compartment. Basal cells are small with

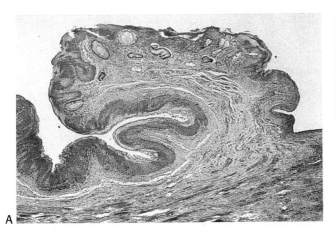
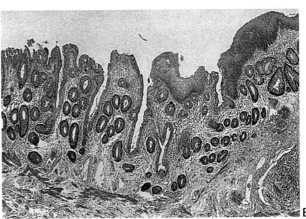

FIG. 15.5. Normal anal canal. **A:** Section through the area of the anal valves demonstrating the transitions of different forms of epithelium in the area. Transitional, rectal, and squamous mucosa is visible. **B:** Nonkeratinizing squamous mucosa covers colorectal glands. In other areas, transitional epithelium covers the glandular epithelium.

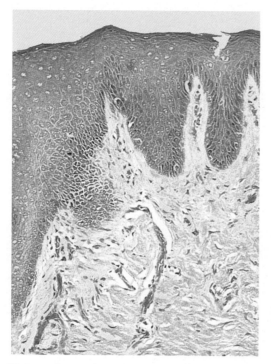

FIG. 15.6. Anal zone showing the presence of nonkeratinizing squamous epithelium. The underlying submucosa is densely fibrotic.

nuclei arranged perpendicularly to the basement membrane. The junction with the underlying tissues is sharp and abrupt. The shape of intermediate cells is usually between that of basal cells and surface cells. Surface cells have a polygonal, columnar, cuboidal, or flattened shape (Fig. 15.7) and resemble bladder or immature metaplastic squamous epithelium, especially when they contain sparse mucus.

They sometimes resemble immature goblet cells (8). Mature goblet cells may also be present. The cells in this zone express cytokeratins (CKs) 7 and 19, but not cytokeratin 20 (9). Mitoses are rare unless there has been mucosal injury. Squamous epithelium often covers the anal columns. Melanocytes may be present in this zone, although these are more prominent in the anal squamous epithelium (10). Endocrine cells lie above the dentate line in the colorectal mucosa, in the transitional mucosa, in anal ducts and glands, in crypts, and in perianal sweat glands (11).

Anal glands discharge into the anal crypts through four to eight long tubular *anal ducts* (Fig. 15.8) that follow a tortuous course through the lamina propria before penetrating the internal sphincter musculature. Occasionally, anal ducts extend upward above the level of the anal valves, explaining the origin of certain unusual submucosal neoplasms in the proximal anal canal (see Chapter 16). The epithelial lining of the ducts varies, often appearing squamous at the gland opening, transitional with or without cylindric glands in the middle, and simple columnar in its deepest part. Transitional epithelium contains four to six cell layers at the duct origin and two to three cell layers when the ducts penetrate the muscle. Goblet cells are present in large numbers, particularly in their terminal portions before they enter the anal crypts. Anal glands are strongly positive for CK7, but negative for CK20. A characteristic feature of the anal glands is the presence of intraepithelial microcysts.

The nonkeratinizing epithelium of the anal canal changes into keratinizing stratified squamous epithelium with numerous melanocytes at the anal verge (Fig. 15.9). Dendritic pigmented cells may also be quite prominent, extending into the suprabasal region (Fig. 15.10). The skin immediately around the anus forms the "zona cutanea." Sweat glands are

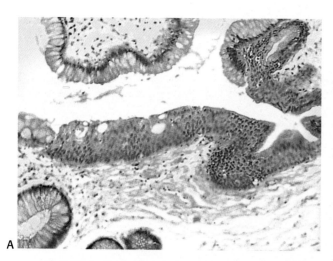

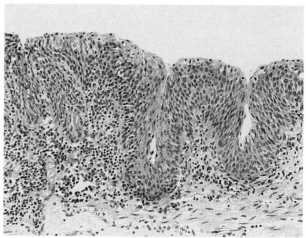

FIG. 15.7. Anal transitional zone. **A:** The surface is covered by columnar epithelium and cuboidal to polygonal cells resembling immature squamous epithelium. Microcysts are present in the epithelium. Rectal-type glands are present in the underlying lamina propria. **B:** Higher magnification of the cells in the transitional zone demonstrating the presence of immature squamous epithelium arising from a prominent basal cell layer. The superficial cells show sparse mucin production. The lamina propria contains lymphocytes. Scattered smooth muscle fibers are also present.

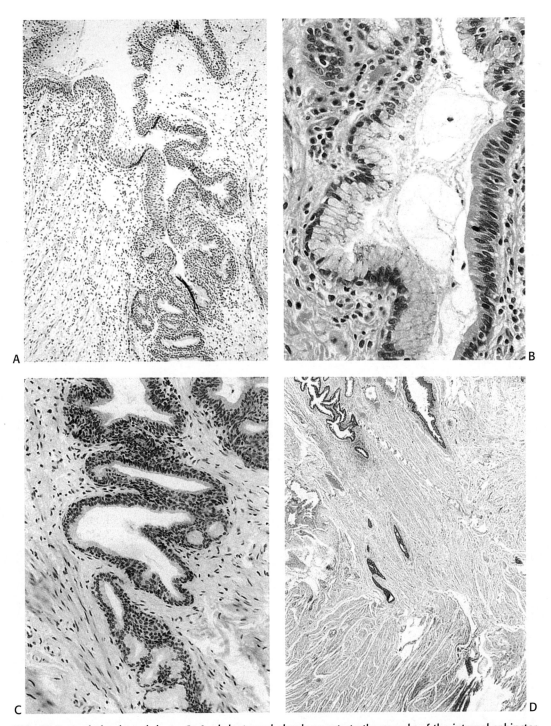

FIG. 15.8. Anal glands and ducts. **A:** Anal ducts and glands penetrate the muscle of the internal sphincter. The epithelium is similar to that seen in the anal transitional zone epithelium. **B:** A portion of anal gland lined by mucin-secreting columnar epithelium and by nonmucinous columnar epithelium. **C:** Higher magnification of the glands in the area of transitional epithelium. In the superficial parts mucin-secreting cells are seen overlying the more immature underlying cells. **D:** Higher magnification of the deepest portions of the glands demonstrating the deep penetration of the anal ducts and glands into the underlying musculature.

absent from the area immediately bordering the anus, but an elliptical zone measuring 1.5 cm in width lying at a distance of 1 to 1.5 cm from the anus contains simple tubular glands called circumanal glands (Fig. 15.11). Anogenital sweat glands have a long excretory duct opening at the skin surface and a wide coiled secretory part with multiple lateral extensions that form diverticula and branches. The ducts are lined by a two-layered pseudostratified epithelium and myoepithelium and by a luminal layer of tall columnar cells with conspicuous snouts (12).

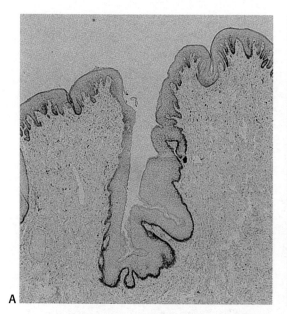
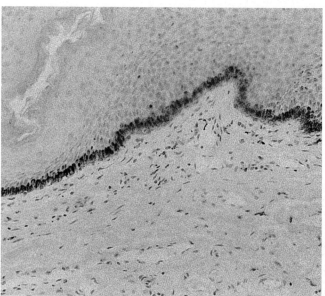

FIG. 15.9. A: Pigmented epithelium from the nonkeratinizing portion of the anus. The tissue comes from a black individual and demonstrates prominent deeply pigmented melanocytes in the basal layer of the epithelium. **B:** Higher magnification of A.

The submucosal connective tissue of the upper anal canal is loose, but in the pecten, denser fibroelastic tissue anchors the epithelium to the superficial portion of the internal sphincter, creating a submucosal barrier at the dentate line. The internal venous plexus in the proximal two thirds of the anal canal may give the mucosa a plum-colored or purplish appearance. This plexus is modified into three specialized vascular anal cushions in the left lateral, right anterior, and right posterior zones of the anal canal. These consist of submucosal anastomosing networks of arterioles and venules with arterial venous communications that have a resemblance to erectile tissue (13).

CONGENITAL ANOMALIES

Anorectal malformations are among the most common gastrointestinal (GI) congenital abnormalities, affecting 1 in every 2,000 to 5,000 live-born infants (14,15). They vary from minor, narrowing defects to serious, complex defects. Anal atresia occurs in many different syndromes (Table 15.1), and 22% to 72% of patients have associated anomalies affecting the vertebrae, gastrointestinal tract, and urologic and genital systems (14,16). The most common defects are the *VATER-* or *VACTERL*-associated anomalies (see Chapter 2). The VATER association includes vertebral defects, anal atresia, tracheoesophageal fistula, esophageal atresia, and radial and renal abnormalities (16). Cardiac defects, a single umbilical artery, and prenatal growth deficiency may also be present. In the

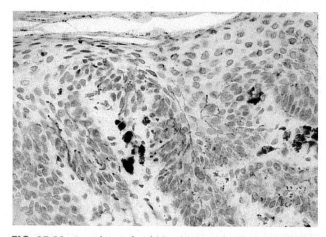

FIG. 15.10. Prominent dendritic pigmented cells lie within the basal layer of the epithelium. They send long processes into the overlying epithelium. The underlying lamina propria contains melanophages. Some of the squamous cells in the upper portions of the mucosa have acquired melanin pigment.

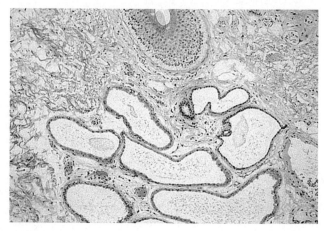

FIG. 15.11. Perianal zone demonstrating the simple tubular circumanal glands.

TABLE 15.1	Selected Abnormalities Associated with Anal Atresia

Townes-Brocks syndrome
Cloacal exstrophy and the OEIS complex
VATER syndrome
VATERL syndrome
CHARGE syndrome
Fraser-Jacquier-Chen syndrome
Pallister-Hall syndrome
Smith-Lemli-Opitz II syndrome
McKusick-Kaufman syndrome
Opitz-Frias syndrome
Caudal regression syndrome
Sacral agenesis syndrome

TABLE 15.2	Classification of Anorectal Malformations

Males

High malformations
  Anorectal agenesis
    Rectoprostatic urethral fistula[a]
    Without fistulas
  Rectal atresia
Intermediate malformations
  Rectobulbar urethral fistula
  Anal agenesis without fistula
Low malformations
  Anocutaneous fistula
  Anal stenosis

Females

High malformations
  Anorectal agenesis
    Rectovaginal fistula
    Without fistula
  Rectal atresia
Intermediate malformations
  Rectovestibular fistula
  Rectovaginal fistula
  Anal agenesis without fistula
Low malformations
  Anovestibular fistula
  Anocutaneous fistula[a]
  Anal stenosis
Cloacal malformations

[a]Includes vaginal or vulvar fistulae.

Townes-Brocks syndrome, an autosomal dominant condition, patients have two or more of the following manifestations: (a) anorectal malformation (imperforate anus, anteriorly placed anus, or anal stenosis); (b) hand malformations (preaxial polydactyly, broad bifid thumb, or triphalangeal thumb); and (c) external ear malformations (microtia, i.e., "satyr" or "lop" ear; preauricular tags or pits) with sensorineural hearing loss. Additionally, urinary tract malformations, mental retardation, and a pericentric inversion of chromosome 16 have been described (17,18). It is unclear whether syndromes with similar abnormalities, such as the VATER, caudal regression, or sacral agenesis syndromes, are distinct and different syndromes or variations of the same one. The *Currarino triad* combines with congenital anorectal stenosis, a scimitar-shaped sacral defect, and a presacral mass. The disorder is familial in approximately 50% of cases (19). Most frequently, the presacral mass is either an anterior sacral meningocele or benign teratoma.

Anorectal anomalies result from arrested development of the caudal region of the gut during fetal life. When the urorectal septum fuses abnormally with the cloacal membrane or when the anal and genital tubercles develop abnormally, the rectum opens in abnormal spots in the perineum or female external genitalia. Thus, many anal anomalies involve stenosis, occlusive membranes, or agenesis with or without fistulas to the perineal skin, urethra, bladder, vulva, or vagina. Their classification relies on the relationship of the terminal bowel to the levator muscles that form the pelvic diaphragm (Table 15.2) (20). These anomalies are high or supralevator deformities when the bowel ends above the pelvic floor and low or translevator deformities when the bowel ends below the pelvic floor. High anorectal malformations are less common than the low type, but the high type more frequently associates with other anomalies (21).

The etiology of these defects remains uncertain. Vascular accidents are postulated to cause localized defects (22). Mesodermal abnormalities may explain patterns of multiple malformations. Diabetes and drug ingestion (thalidomide, phenytoin, and Tridione) are more common in mothers of infants with anorectal malformations (21–23), while occupa-

tional exposures to potential teratogens are more common in fathers of children with anorectal malformations. Other potential etiologic associations include maternal AIDS, exposures to x-rays, severe trauma, a retained intrauterine device, gestational age <38 weeks, and Down syndrome (24).

Animal models that disrupt the SONIC hedgehog signal transduction pathway lead to a spectrum of developmental anomalies that strongly resemble those present in the VACTERL syndrome, suggesting that they play a role in the development of the VACTERL complex in humans (25,26). (Sonic hedgehog is an endoderm-derived signaling molecule that induces hindgut mesodermal gene expression.) Cases of Townes-Brocks syndrome (TBS) are often sporadic, but mutations in the gene encoding the SALL-1 zinc finger transcription factor (27) may explain the familial form of the disease. Further, the diagnosis can be confirmed by finding the mutation (28). Recently, a gene responsible for the Currarino triad has been mapped to 7q36, near the locus of the gene for holoprosencephaly (29).

Imperforate Anus

Imperforate anus results from failure of the cloacal membrane to perforate. Consequently, the anus does not open

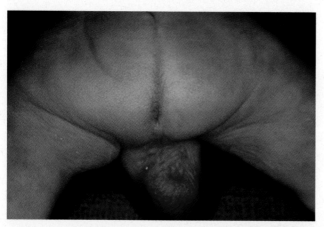

FIG. 15.12. Picture of a male infant with anal atresia. Note the absence of an opening from the anal canal onto the perineum.

normally into the perineum (Fig. 15.12). Imperforate anus more commonly affects males than females, and can be divided into four major groups: (a) stenosis alone (11%), (b) imperforate anus with only a thin membrane separating the anus and rectum (4%), (c) imperforate anus with a widely separated anus and rectum (76%), and (d) normal anus with the rectum ending some distance above it (9%) (14,30). Fistulae often form between the rectum and the urogenital system. In males, the fistulae tend to be urinary (urethra, 25%; bladder, 33%; perineum, 42%), and in females, rectourinary and rectogenital (vaginal, 84%; perineum, 14.5%; bladder, 1.5%). Rarely, the rectum opens to the scrotum, the undersurface of the penile shaft, or the prepuce (31). Patients with imperforate anus may also have an associated hyperreflexic or atonic urinary bladder (32).

Imperforate anus also occurs in the urorectal septum malformation sequence, a rare congenital malformation affecting females that is characterized by ambiguous external genitalia, disordered/malformed internal genitalia, and imperforate anus, vagina, and urethra. Other abnormalities include renal agenesis or dysplasia, pulmonary hypoplasia, congenital heart defects, and vertebral anomalies (33). The thymic-renal-anal-lung dysplasia syndrome is an autosomal recessive abnormality characterized by a unilobed or absent thymus, renal and ureter agenesis/dysgenesis, intrauterine growth retardation, and imperforate anus (34). Renal, anal, and lung dysplasia is shared with three syndromes: Fraser-Jacquier-Chen (35), Pallister-Hall (PH) (36), and Smith-Lemli-Opitz II (37). Imperforate anus may also complicate prune belly syndrome (38), Eagle-Barrette syndrome (39), or the OEIS complex (omphalocele-exstrophy-imperforate anus-spinal defect syndrome).

Low Abnormalities

Low abnormalities are common (40% of abnormalities) and include ectopic (perineal, vestibular, vulvar) anus. Fistulas may or may not be present; associated abnormalities are rare. The anus opens anterior to its normal position, sometimes in

the vulva. The ectopic anorectum lies below the puborectalis muscle. In contrast, congenital rectovestibular or rectovaginal fistula opens into the vagina or the vulva but above the puborectalis muscle (40). In a related anomaly, the covered anus, a bar of skin derived from the lateral genital folds, covers the anal canal. An anocutaneous fistula passes anteriorly from the anal canal to the exterior at the perineal raphe. A misplaced external sphincter with conjoined fibers inserted behind the elongated, ventrally angulated terminal canal can functionally obstruct fecal passage even in patients with an adequate anal canal and anal orifice. These anomalies can generally be treated with relatively localized surgery with a good outcome.

Intermediate Abnormalities

Intermediate abnormalities are rare (15%) and include proximal anal canal stenoses. The terminal bowel appears dilated and thickened (41), and a shortened anal canal lies within the levator diaphragm. Other changes depend on the sex of the individual. In males, there is a clear separation between fibers running toward the pubis and others running toward the perineal body and bulbocavernosus muscle ventrally. Striated muscle fibers of the pubococcygeus muscle associate with the bowel wall. Fibers of the puborectalis may be present dorsally and laterally (42). Girls with a rectovestibular fistula lack the perineal body (central tendon) that normally lies between the rectum and vagina. Fascicles of the pubococcygeus and the external sphincter become displaced laterally.

High (Supralevator) Abnormalities

Supralevator anomalies account for 40% of anal abnormalities and include anorectal agenesis. Anorectal agenesis is a relatively primitive defect reflecting a cloaca that has not divided into separate urinary and alimentary canals. For this reason, the defect is also referred to as *primitive cloaca, cloacal persistence,* or *rectocloacal fistula.* The rectum reaches the upper surface of the pelvic floor, but the entire anal canal and pelvic floor musculature are absent. The rectum opens into a posterior urethra or bladder in males and into a posterior vaginal fornix in females. Failure of the müllerian systems to fuse normally creates two uteri that open into the globular cloacal cavity. Trisomy 4 is found in some patients (43). These abnormalities have a severe prognosis and more complicated surgical repair because of the obstruction and the common association with other congenital anomalies involving the vertebrae and urinary tract as well as defective innervation of the pelvic musculature. The musculature when it is examined may show hypoplasia of the muscularis propria, and there may be evidence of oligoneuronal hypoganglionosis or neuronal dysplasia.

Cloacal Exstrophy and the OEIS Complex

The OEIS syndrome is the most severe spectrum of birth defects involving the GI tract (and other sites). It affects 1 in

200,000 to 400,000 pregnancies and has an unknown cause. The male-to-female incidence is 3:1. The disease is usually sporadic in nature. However, it can affect siblings from separate pregnancies, suggesting that some cases may have a genetic basis (44). Some patients have trisomy 18; others may have prenatal exposures to methamphetamines or other recreational drugs or maternal heparin use (45).

There is usually exstrophy of the urinary bladder and small or large intestines, anal atresia, colonic hypoplasia, omphalocele, and external genitalia anomalies (46). Other less frequent abnormalities include meningocele, spina bifida, unilateral hypoplasia of the kidney, single umbilical artery, Meckel diverticulum, and colonic duplication (47). The exstrophy–epispadias sequence includes, in increasing order of severity, phallic separation with epispadias, pubic diastasis, cloacal exstrophy, and the OEIS complex. Cloacal exstrophy is also a complex spectrum of malformations that is often fatal. In addition to an imperforate anus, the babies have an omphalocele, two exstrophic bladders between which there is an open cecum, and a blindly ending colon hanging down in the pelvis from the cecum (48).

Caudal Dysplasia (Caudal Regression Syndrome)

The caudal dysplasia syndrome associates with sacral vertebral anomalies, abnormalities in the pelvis and lower limbs, anal and genital defects, absent fibula, short femoral bones, and meningomyelocele (49). Heart anomalies and tracheoesophageal fistula may also be present. In its severest form, sirenomelia is present (50). The anal malformations include a complete covered anus with or without fistula formation and rectal atresia. Caudal regression syndrome associates with maternal diabetes or prediabetes (50). Other syndromes that closely resemble caudal dysplasia include the Aschcraft syndrome of familial hemisacrum (51) and the Cohn-Bay-Nielsen syndrome of familial hemisacrum (52).

Anorectal Cysts (Hindgut Cysts, Tailgut Cysts)

Some developmental cysts represent sequestered duplications; others represent a form of teratoma; still others are thought to arise from embryonic remnants of the tailgut or the neuroenteric canal (53,54) (Fig. 15.13). Early in development, the embryo possesses a true tail, which reaches its largest diameter at 35 days of gestation (8 mm). The anus develops above the tail on day 56 of gestation (35 mm), by which time the tail completely regresses (55,56). The neuroenteric canal, the connection between the amnion and the yolk sac, forms around day 16 and obliterates once the notochord forms. Remnants of this canal can give rise to presacral cysts (55).

Developmental cysts lie anterior to the coccyx or lower sacrum. Most cases are asymptomatic and found incidentally. They present as retrorectal or posterior anal masses in children and young adults, more commonly affect females

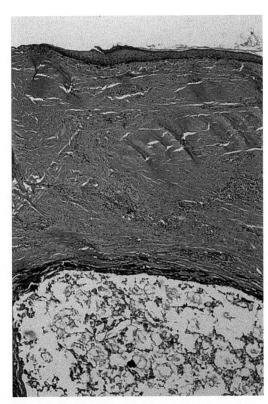

FIG. 15.13. Anal cyst. The unilocular cyst in the bottom of the photograph contains amorphous debris without a lining. This probably represents a tailgut cyst. Smooth muscle fibers do not surround the entirety of the lesion, ruling out a duplication cyst.

than males, and often coexist with other congenital abnormalities, including spina bifida and stenosis. Although these lesions are congenital anomalies, they most commonly present in patients with an average age of 36 (55). Complications include infection, bleeding, or malignant degeneration.

The lesions usually appear multicystic and may measure many centimeters in diameter. Rarely, a unilocular cyst is present. The cysts do not communicate with one another, but are separated by a dense fibrous connective tissue stroma. Squamous, transitional, simple, mucinous, columnar, and/or ciliated columnar epithelia line the cystic spaces. The lumen may be filled with mucin or gelatinous material. The lesions also contain disorganized smooth muscle bundles. Anal developmental cysts differ from duplication cysts in that the musculature of duplication cysts appears much more orderly than the haphazard muscular orientation seen in anorectal developmental cysts. There is no evidence of dysplasia and no teratomatous elements are present. Benign retrorectal cystic teratomas should only be diagnosed when there is evidence of differentiation into all three germ cell layers (54).

In contrast to the cysts derived from tailgut remnants that are usually small and multilocular with satellite cysts, *hindgut cysts* resemble duplication cysts. They are larger, unilocular, and surrounded by a variably thick muscle layer

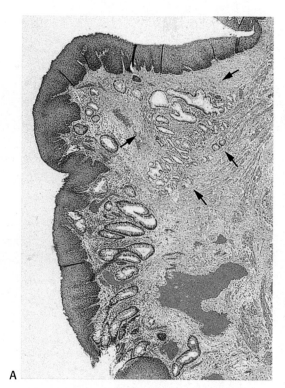
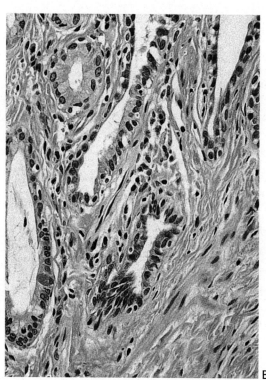

FIG. 15.14. Ectopic gastric mucosa in the anal canal. **A:** Low-power magnification showing gastric glands in the submucosa (*arrows*). **B:** Higher magnification showing that the gastric epithelium has some characteristics of gastric antral glands.

(57). They often contain heterotopic tissue such as pancreatic or gastric tissue. The cysts grow slowly and frequently remain asymptomatic unless they grow large enough to cause pressure, fullness, constipation, urinary and/or fecal incontinence, perineal pain, and/or numbness. Infected cysts may lead to retrorectal abscesses and fistula formation (52). Duplication cysts resemble duplication cysts described in Chapters 6 and 13. When they contain ectopic gastric mucosa, peptic ulcers may develop. The differential diagnosis includes anal duct cyst, hindgut cyst, and tailgut cyst.

Ectopic Tissues

Ectopic prostatic tissue in the anal submucosa (58,59) presents as a presacral mass or abnormal bowel movements, although this is rare (59). Grossly, the lesion may appear as a multiloculated cyst containing thick, milky tan-yellow fluid. Hyperplastic smooth muscle fibers and dilated prostatic glands arranged in a dense fibromuscular stroma are present. The epithelium demonstrates a range of morphologic appearances. Typical cuboidal prostatic glandular epithelium lines the majority of the glands. In many glands, the cells pile up into small papillae containing thin, fibrovascular cores. Glandular hyperplasia may be present. Focally, features of low-grade prostatic intraepithelial neoplasia may be present (59). The epithelium is positive for prostate-specific antigen.

Mucinous tissues of the *salivary gland type* have been reported in the rectal submucosa. Even more rarely, they occur in the perianal region (60). Anorectal *müllerian duct remnants* often associate with other müllerian abnormalities. These lesions become detectable when secondary changes develop in them, such as abscesses (61).

Gastric and/or *pancreatic heterotopias* occur in the anorectal region either alone or complicating a duplication or hindgut cyst (62). They present as hemorrhoids, a polyp, or fistulae, but histologic examination of the tissue demonstrates the presence of heterotopic epithelium with the presence of pyloric glands (Fig. 15.14) and/or pancreatic tissue. When parietal cells are present in the heterotopic tissue, peptic ulceration may ensue. We have also seen neoplasia develop in the heterotopic tissues.

ANAL DUCT CYSTS

Anal gland cysts develop along the entire course of the anal glands in the anal transitional zone, especially in the space between the internal and external sphincters. They may present as presacrococcygeal masses closely related to the anorectal junction. They are usually lined by the epithelium of the anal transitional zone and anal glands. Variable numbers of mucin-secreting cells are present at the surface. The lesions result from mucus retention due to inflammation or trauma.

ANORECTAL PROLAPSE (PROCIDENTIA)

Anorectal prolapse affects both adults and children. Histologically, the anal mucosa may appear acanthotic, hyperkeratotic, congested, and chronically inflamed (Fig. 15.15). Inflammatory cloacogenic polyps may form (see Chapter 13). Other major features of prolapse are discussed in Chapter 13.

ANAL FISSURES

Anal fissures are longitudinal mucosal lacerations in the distal anal canal that disrupt the skin at their distal ends. They start at the anal verge and can extend to the dentate line. Most are located in the posterior midline, with 10% to 15% occurring anteriorly. "Off the midline" fissures suggest that a predisposing disorder, such as Crohn disease, HIV/AIDS, tuberculosis, syphilis, sexual abuse, or anal carcinoma, may be present. Not infrequently, the anal skin at the lower margin of the fissure becomes inflamed, producing an edematous sentinel pile at the lower edge of the fissure. Chronic anal fissures frequently present with the triad of fissures, sentinel tags, and hypertrophied anal papillae (Fig. 15.16).

This is a disorder of young adults, affecting both sexes equally. Fissures are often caused by local trauma such as the passage of hard stool or explosive diarrhea. The perianal sphincter muscle often goes into spasm, pulling the edges of the fissure apart, impairing defecation and leading to further mucosal tearing with subsequent bowel movements. Persistent hypertonia and spasm of the internal anal sphincter

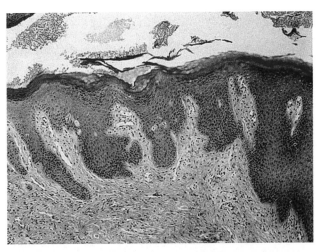

FIG. 15.15. Anal mucosa in prolapse. Widened acanthotic rete pegs extend deep into the underlying submucosa. The surface shows marked hyperkeratosis and parakeratosis. Little acute or chronic inflammation is present.

leads to a secondary reduction in the blood flow and localized ischemic ulceration (63). The clinical hallmark of an anal fissure is pain during, and especially after, defecation. The pain is often severe enough for patients to avoid bowel movements altogether. Bright red blood may be seen on the toilet tissue.

The microscopic features are nonspecific and consist of acute or chronic inflammation, depending on the stage of the disease. Acute inflammation and granulation tissue line the center of the fistulous tract and chronic inflammation

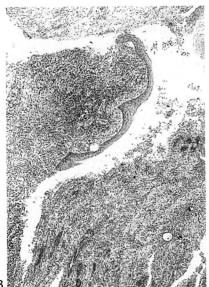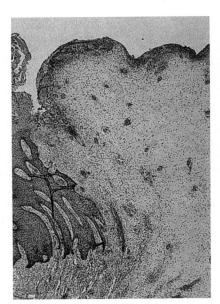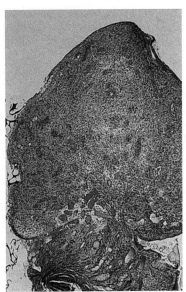

A, B   C

FIG. 15.16. Anal fissures. **A:** Low magnification showing an anal fissure. Residual squamous epithelium is present in one portion of the field. The underlying tissues are intensely inflamed. Acute inflammation, edema, granulation tissue, and mucosal erosion are evident. **B:** As fissures heal, the epithelium becomes more hyperplastic and acanthotic as seen on the left-hand side of the picture. **C:** Sometimes the edges of the lesion develop granuloma pyogenicum.

lies deeper in the lesion. Prominent dilated capillaries, fibrosis, edema, and regenerating squamous epithelium are often present. Pyogenic granulomas may develop at the healing edge. With the passage of time, chronic fissures develop thickened skin margins, and fibers of the internal anal sphincter become visible at the fissure's base.

The differential diagnosis usually includes some form of infection and Crohn disease. For this reason, the tissue should be examined carefully for the presence of organisms and granulomas.

The majority of fissures are superficial and heal quickly. Treatment of both acute and chronic fissures includes dietary modification, increased fluid intake, and sitz baths. Chronic fissures may be treated with sphincterotomy, topical glyceryl trinitrate ointment, and injection of botulinum toxin into the anal sphincter (64).

ANORECTAL AND PERIANAL ABSCESSES AND FISTULAE

Anorectal abscesses and fistulae share similar pathogenetic mechanisms and often coexist. Microbiologic data demonstrate two major groups of lesions. One consists of the anal equivalent of cutaneous abscesses usually resulting from Gram-positive cocci. These almost never develop into fistulae and are treated by simple drainage. The second group causes more morbidity and often associates with fistula formation. Various enteric or dermal organisms may be cultured from the abscess cavities (65–67). Some of these infections are invasive and necrotizing (67). These infections often start in the anal glands, resulting in an abscess. If the abscess drains into the anal lumen, the infection usually subsides. Extension to other sites results in fistula in ano or an abscess often in an intersphincteric location. Abscesses also complicate other conditions (Table 15.3). Males and females are affected about equally, and patients range in age from

teenagers to the elderly. Perianal abscesses that develop in infants often result from infected diaper rash most commonly caused by *Staphylococcus* or enteric bacteria. Perianal abscesses in older children complicate inflammatory bowel disease, immunodeficiency, or leukemia. Patients present with pain, drainage, and fever.

As with any abscess, histologic examination shows the presence of a localized collection of acute and chronic inflammatory cells. The center of the abscess may become cavitary secondary to the presence of liquefaction necrosis (Fig. 15.17). The differential diagnosis includes presacral epidermal inclusion cysts, infected sebaceous cysts, hidradenitis suppurativa, Crohn disease, Bartholin gland abscesses, pilonidal sinus, and carcinoma.

The term *fistula* implies the presence of an inflammatory tract between two epithelial-lined surfaces, whereas *sinus* refers to a tract with only one open end. *Fistula in ano* is the tunnel that connects an internal opening, usually an anal crypt at the base of the column of Morgagni at the dentate line, with an external opening, usually on the perianal skin. Most anal fistulae represent a complication of infection of the anal glands, as noted above. The diagnosis is made by seeing blood, pus, and sometimes stool draining from an external opening. Long tracts may have secondary openings along their course. If the tract is chronic, it may be palpated as a subcutaneous cord. The average patient age is 38 years. Fistulas may also associate with Crohn disease, postoperative and perirectal/anal trauma, radiation, infections, and neoplasms. Anal fistulae may also develop in patients with heterotopic gastric mucosa due to the presence of oxyntic mucosa and secondary peptic ulceration (62), or they may complicate cow's milk protein allergy in children (68). Anal fistulas are often complex lesions involving different tissues and causing varying degrees of sphincter involvement and destruction. Fistulas are classified into four main types based on the site to which they extend (Table 15.4) (69). The opening of an anal fistula is usually within 5 cm of the anus.

Fistulae may be difficult to identify in a gross specimen. Uncomplicated chronic fistulae are often identified by the presence of a cordlike thickening that may be better appreciated by palpation than by visual inspection of the specimen. One may also probe the fistulous tract in order to identify it. Injection of methylene blue or some other dye helps delineate the fistula course. The histologic features reflect the duration of the process, with more acute lesions containing numerous acute inflammatory cells and granulation tissue along the length of the fistula. Eventually, the fistulous tract becomes fibrotic and may be lined by hyperplastic squamous epithelium, which can produce a secondary epidermoid cyst (Fig. 15.18). Remnants of anal gland epithelium may also be seen. If intestinal contents gain access to the fistula or if the patients are treated with oil-based medications, giant cell reactions or granulomas may develop.

The differential diagnosis of fistula in ano is shown in Table 15.5. Of these entities, Crohn disease is the lesion most likely to be confused with a simple fistula, especially since

TABLE 15.3	Diseases Complicated by Anorectal Abscesses

Hidradenitis suppurativa
Crohn disease
Infections
   Tuberculosis
   Chlamydial infections
   Actinomycosis
   Staphylococcal
   Gram-negative bacteria
Infected cysts
Deep fissures
Foreign bodies
Malignancies
Trauma
Previous surgery

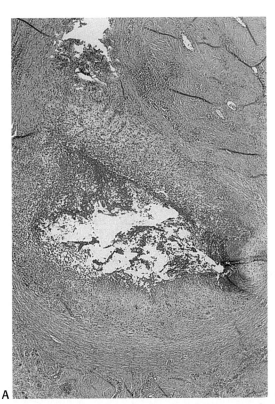
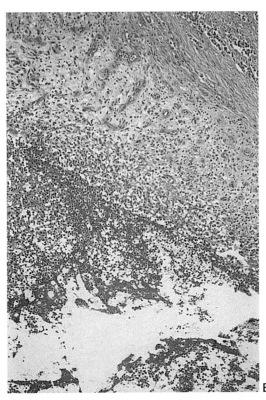

FIG. 15.17. Perianal abscess. A: An abscess is present deep in the anal wall. Its center has undergone lique-faction necrosis. **B:** Higher magnification showing the liquefaction necrosis surrounded by organizing granulation tissue and older fibrosing reparative tissue.

TABLE 15.4 **Classification of Anal Fistulae**

A. Intersphincteric: The tract runs between the internal and external sphincteric muscle. It is low if it runs low into the skin and high if it runs under the rectum.
  1. Simple low tract
  2. High blind tract
  3. High tract with rectal opening
  4. Rectal opening without a perineal opening
  5. Retrorectal extension
  6. Secondary to pelvic disease
B. Transsphincteric: In this variety, the tract runs through the external sphincteric and through the ischiorectal fossa to the perianal gland.
  1. Uncomplicated
  2. High blind tract
C. Suprasphincteric: The tract runs between and above the intersphincteric space above the external sphincteric space and back into the ischiorectal fossa to the perianal gland.
  1. Uncomplicated
  2. Blind tract
D. Extrasphincteric: This is secondary to pelvic sepsis rather than anal gland infarction and discharges through the ischiorectal fossa to the skin.
  1. Secondary to anal fistula
  2. Secondary to trauma
  3. Secondary to anal rectal disease
  4. Secondary to pelvic inflammation

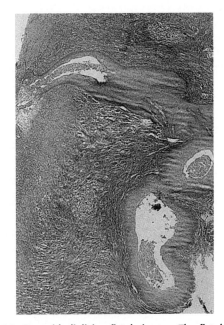

FIG. 15.18. Re-epithelializing fistula in ano. The fistulous tracts are lined by squamous epithelium. The surrounding soft tissue is fibrotic and inflamed.

TABLE 15.5 Differential Diagnosis of Fistula in Ano

Inflammatory bowel disease
   Crohn disease
   Ulcerative colitis
Sigmoid diverticulitis
Infections
   Tuberculosis
   Actinomycosis
   Lymphogranuloma venereum
   Syphilis
   Chlamydial infections
Hidradenitis suppurativa
Pilonidal sinus with perianal extension
Behçet syndrome
Infected perianal sebaceous cysts
Anal duct carcinoma
Trauma
Buschke-Lowenstein tumors

only about 50% of fistulae developing in the setting of Crohn disease contain sarcoidlike granulomas suggesting the diagnosis (see Chapter 11). Hidradenitis suppurativa is differentiated by the presence of multiple perianal skin openings and the fact that the opening in the anal canal lies distal to the dentate line. Pilonidal sinus with perianal extension and infected perianal sebaceous cysts are also in the differential diagnosis. Lastly, carcinomas, mostly low grade, may develop in longstanding fistulae after many decades. Anal duct carcinomas may also present clinically as chronic fistulous tracts.

HEMORRHOIDS

Hemorrhoids are enlarged hemorrhoidal cushions (70). The hemorrhoidal cushions lie in the submucosa and consist of a connective tissue cushion surrounding arteriovenous communications between terminal branches of the superior rectal arteries and the superior, inferior, and middle rectal arteries (70). Most people have three of these cushions lying at 4, 7, and 11 o'clock when they are in the lithotomy position. The anal cushions are believed to play a role in anal continence since they become engorged with blood and project into the lumen during defecation. With advancing age, the connective tissue and muscle fibers that anchor the vascular cushions to the underlying sphincter mechanism may become attenuated and deteriorate, allowing the hemorrhoids to slide into the anal canal and become congested, bleed, and prolapse (71). Hereditary and environmental factors, as well as individual habits, may account for variations in hemorrhoid size, presentation, or symptoms. Factors that predispose to hemorrhoid formation include increasing age, chronic diarrhea, prolonged sitting, chronic straining, pregnancy, low-fiber diets, anal sphincter spasm, and tumors (71). Hemorrhoids are classified based on their location with respect to the dentate line. *Internal hemorrhoids* lie above the dentate line and are covered by rectal mucosa. *External hemorrhoids* develop below the dentate line covered by the squamous mucosa of pecten or the perianal skin. Terms used to describe hemorrhoids are listed in Table 15.6.

The exact incidence of hemorrhoidal disease is unknown, but it is thought that 4.4% to 25% of adults have them (72). The peak incidence is between ages 45 and 65. Hemorrhoids rarely develop in individuals under the age of 30, except in

TABLE 15.6 Terminology and Classification of Lesions Associated with Hemorrhoids

External skin tag	Redundant fibrotic skin at the anal verge usually resulting from previous thrombosed external hemorrhoids or previous anal surgery
External hemorrhoids	Dilated venules at the inferior hemorrhoidal plexus located below the dentate line
Internal hemorrhoids	The anal cushions located above the dentate line that prolapse
First-degree hemorrhoids	Anal cushions that slide down beyond the dentate line upon straining and that bleed in defecation
Second-degree hemorrhoids	Anal cushions that prolapse through the anus on straining but reduce spontaneously
Third-degree hemorrhoids	Anal cushions that prolapse through the anus upon straining or exertion and that require manual replacement into the anal canal
Fourth-degree hemorrhoids	Prolapsed hemorrhoid that stays out all the time and cannot be reduced
Strangulated hemorrhoids	When a sphincter spasm occurs in the presence of irreducible prolapsed hemorrhoids, both the external and internal hemorrhoids become engorged, the blood supply is compromised, and the hemorrhoids become strangulated

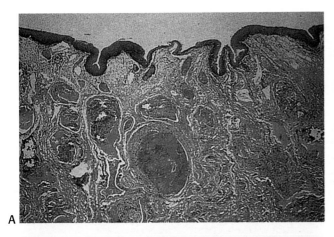

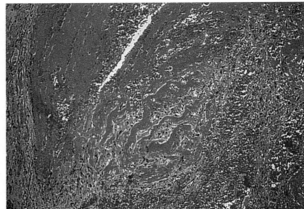

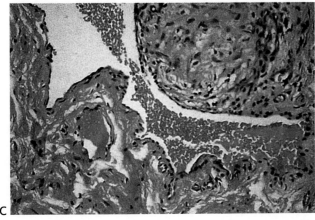

FIG. 15.19. Hemorrhoids. **A:** Prominent dilated hemorrhoidal plexus within the anal transitional zone. The central large vessel is partially thrombosed. **B:** High magnification of the thrombosed vessel shown in A. Prominent lines of Zahn are seen. **C:** Further organization of a thrombosis within a hemorrhoid.

pregnant women. Both sexes are affected equally. Generally external hemorrhoids remain asymptomatic unless they become thrombosed, in which case they present as an acutely painful perianal lump. Resolution of the thrombosis leads to persistent skin tags. Patients complain of bright red blood on toilet tissue or coating the stool and a vague feeling of rectal discomfort. Painless bleeding is the most common sign of hemorrhoids. Anorectal discomfort increases when the hemorrhoids enlarge or prolapse through the anus, an event often accompanied by edema and sphincteric spasm. Complications include superficial ulceration, necrosis, inflammation, fissure formation, and infarction.

External hemorrhoids are visible on the anal verge and perianal skin. They are actually skin tags that represent residual redundant skin that can easily be seen when the buttocks are parted. They do not bleed because they are covered by squamous epithelium. These are usually seen in young and middle-aged patients and cause few symptoms unless they become thrombosed, when they can become quite painful. The changes resolve spontaneously with eventual fibrosis; some lesions require surgical removal.

It is necessary to histologically examine hemorrhoids because other diseases present clinically as hemorrhoids, including carcinoid tumors and malignant melanoma (73). Excised hemorrhoids often contain dilated, thick-walled

submucosal vessels and smaller vascular spaces that are frequently hemorrhagic and thrombosed (Fig. 15.19). Variable degrees of ulceration and fibrosis are present. As the lesions resolve, intravascular papillary endothelial hyperplasia and recanalization commonly occur (Fig 15.20). The intravascular endothelial cell proliferations can appear quite cellular and the endothelial lining might show mild pleomorphism and rare mitoses. A single layer of endothelial cells characteristically covers these papillae. The key to differentiating the lesion from an angiosarcoma is the confinement of the changes to the pre-existing vascular spaces. One can identify the pre-existing venous walls with the use of elastic tissue stains. Furthermore, the vascular spaces fail to interanastomose with one another.

Hemorrhoids may be treated nonoperatively with sclerotherapy, cryotherapy, rubber-band ligation, bipolar diathermy, electrotherapy, or infrared photocoagulation, or they may be treated surgically.

ANAL PAPILLAE, SKIN TAGS, AND FIBROEPITHELIAL POLYPS

Anal tags (fibroepithelial polyps) are present in 45% of patients who undergo proctoscopic examination. They are

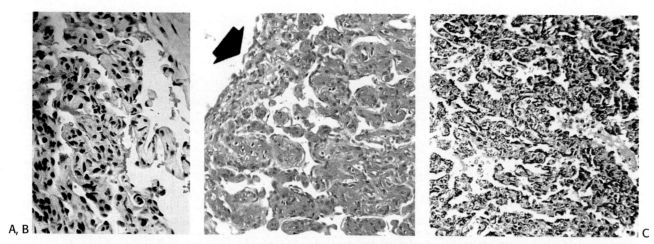

A, B   C

FIG. 15.20. Thrombosed hemorrhoids **A:** High magnification of the intravascular proliferation. The venous edge is in the upper right-hand corner. The lumen contains a proliferation of endothelial cells and fibrous tissue representing an organizing blood clot. **B:** A similar lesion in a later stage of evolution. The lesion is confined within the area of the venous wall (*arrow*). **C:** In contrast to the lesion shown in A and B, the vascular channels of this angiosarcoma freely interanastomose with one another and they are lined by atypical endothelial cells. Such lesions are not confined with vascular lumina but freely invade into adjacent tissues.

believed to be acquired lesions. They represent hyperplastic projections of the anal mucosa and submucosa (Fig. 15.21) in the region of the anal columns that enlarge and protrude into the anal lumen in response to irritation, infections, or injury. The surface epithelium is always squamous in nature and it overlies loose fibroconnective tissue. These anal tags clinically resemble hemorrhoids, but unlike hemorrhoids, they do not contain the thick-walled vessels with evidence of recent remote organizing thrombi. They may resemble fibroepithelial polyps or skin tags arising on cutaneous sites. Not uncommonly, reactive atypical stromal cells with large, multiple, peripherally located, vesicular nuclei are present (Fig. 15.22). These appear round to oval and uniform, arranged in a linear, rosette, or grapelike fashion. Their nuclei may also be crowed

or overlapping. They lack pleomorphism, hyperchromasia, and mitotic figures. Many atypical stromal cells are round to elongated; others have irregular or stellate contours. The cytoplasm appears deep reddish blue and finely vacuolated, with indistinct borders. The stromal cells are randomly scattered in the subepithelial connective tissue of the anal mucosa, beneath the squamous epithelium. In most cases, they are diffusely arranged, but occasionally, focal aggregates of atypical cells are seen. Mast cells are often a prominent accompaniment to these cells (74–76). The giant cells are negative with antibodies to cytokeratin, actin, desmin, S100, and factor VIII and are strongly positive for vimentin, CD34, and a_1-antichymotrypsin (76). The relative acellularity of the lesion, its lack of mitotic activity, and its overall reactive appearance distinguish the lesion from a neoplasm.

ANORECTAL VARICES

Anorectal varices are dilated submucosal veins that connect the middle and inferior hemorrhoidal veins in patients with portal hypertension. They differ from hemorrhoids (77), but the two entities may coexist and both can bleed. Anorectal varices are small, usually <5 mm in diameter, but may be >5 mm. The risk of bleeding correlates with their size. Their histology resembles that of esophageal varices.

DIEULAFOY LESION

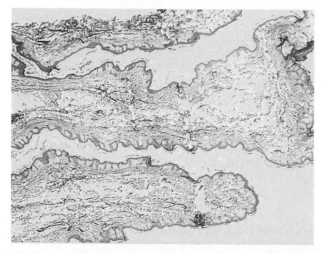

FIG. 15.21. Anal skin tags. They consist of fibrovascular tissue and are covered by mature squamous epithelium. In their early stages of formation they contain prominent inflammation. As these mature, anal inflammation goes away.

Dieulafoy lesions are an unusual source of massive bleeding and were first described in the stomach. They have since been discovered in other sites exceeding the anus, although this is the rarest site of occurrence (78). The histology of this lesion is described in detail Chapter 4.

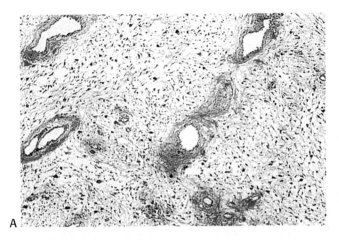

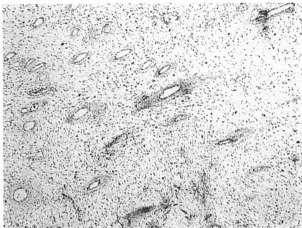

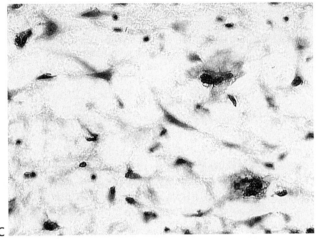

FIG. 15.22. Anal papillae. A: Pseudosarcomatous appearance with the presence of an edematous stroma containing prominent hyalinized blood vessels. The blood vessels are arranged perpendicularly to the surface. **B:** Atypical stromal cells are present in the edematous stroma. **C:** Immature stellate cells and bubbly multinucleated cells that may mimic a liposarcoma.

INFECTIONS

Syphilis

Virtually all anal syphilitic infections result from sexual activity. Syphilis affects 5% of male homosexuals with anorectal symptoms (79). Anorectal syphilitic infections in children suggest the presence of sexual abuse. Anorectal syphilis may go undiagnosed, especially when it remains asymptomatic, because clinicians routinely fail to examine the anorectal area for the presence of chancres and apparently trivial lesions frequently resemble other nonvenereal inflammatory diseases. Symptomatic lesions are misdiagnosed as idiopathic anal ulcers, fissures, nonspecific proctitis, or polyps (80).

Spirochetes penetrating the epithelium incite a focal inflammatory reaction with the formation of a chancre (81). The chancre begins as a papule, but it then ulcerates and acquires raised borders that appear as a punched-out, eroded, or ulcerated painless papule with a raw indurated base and serous exudate. Anal chancres may cause pain on defecation and rectal bleeding. Chancres persist for days to a month but usually disappear within 2 weeks. Other lesions associated with syphilitic infections include polyps and smooth, lobulated masses that may resemble neoplasms

(79). The secondary stage of syphilis begins 6 to 8 weeks after the onset of the disease. The symptoms resemble a flu-like illness, with generalized lymphadenopathy and generalized or localized skin and mucosal eruptions (81). The lesions appear as macules, papules, tubercles, or pustules. At this stage, single or multiple condyloma lata form. Coexisting sexually transmitted infections such as herpesvirus, *Neisseria gonorrhoeae,* or *Chlamydia trachomatis* may be present.

The histologic features of the lesion are nonspecific, with superficial ulceration associated with an underlying dense inflammatory cell infiltrate that is usually rich in plasma cells. Thick-walled blood vessels with prominent endothelial cells or an obliterative endarteritis containing a mixed inflammatory infiltrate and numerous plasma cells (Fig. 15.23) may be seen. Crypt abscesses and granulomas may also be present. The organisms spread from the chancre via lymphatics to the regional lymph nodes, which become enlarged and hard. The diagnosis is clinched by the demonstration of spirochetes in fixed tissue by the appropriate immunostains or silver stains. One can also demonstrate the spirochete in fluids and tissues using dark field microscopy, immunofluorescent staining, or silver stains (Fig. 15.23). The diagnosis should always be confirmed serologically.

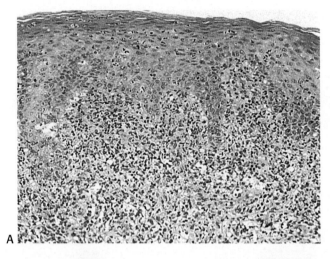

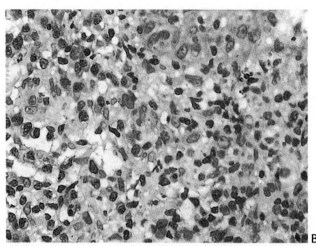

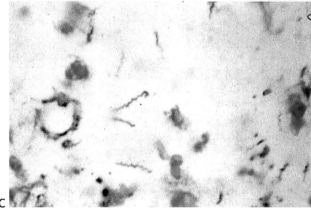

FIG. 15.23. Syphilitic proctitis. **A:** The mucosa is inflamed. **B:** Large numbers of chronic inflammatory cells including plasma cells are present. **C:** Warthin-Starry stain of an anal smear demonstrating the spirochetes. (A and B courtesy of Dr. T. Merlin, Albuquerque, NM.)

Gonorrhea

Anorectal gonorrhea results from anal intercourse or it represents secondary genital–anal spread in patients with gonococcal cervicitis or urethritis. The prevalence of gonococcal infections is increased in homosexual males, prostitutes, and sexually abused children. A recent increase in cases has been linked to the perception that HIV/AIDS is a less serious disease than previously believed because of the availability of highly active antiretroviral therapies and thus the practice of safe sex is declining (82). Infected patients generally remain asymptomatic, but they might also present with mild anal burning, pain, discharge, or bleeding. Endoscopy reveals a hyperemic edematous anorectal mucosa with a purulent discharge in the anal crypts (83) or perianal abscesses (84). The anorectum may also appear normal. The diagnosis is confirmed by finding the organism (*Neisseria gonorrhoeae*) in stained smears of the discharge (Fig. 15.24) and/or by culturing it on Thayer-Martin medium.

Histologically, an acute or subacute proctitis develops, including the area of the anal crypts and ducts. IgA-secreting plasma cells, lymphocytes, and neutrophils may be present in the infiltrate. Ulcers may be present, although this is uncommon (85). Since the features are nonspecific, culture or Gram stain on the tissues is required in order to identify the organism.

Tuberculosis

Anorectal tuberculosis is rare except in those countries where pulmonary and intestinal tuberculosis are common. GI infections tend to affect those areas of the gut that contain prominent lymphoid tissue, including the anorectum. Anorectal tuberculosis presents as a mass, an ulceration, fissures, fistulae,

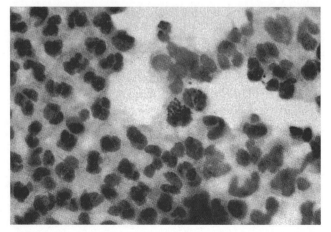

FIG. 15.24. Anal smear showing gonococcal organisms within cells. (Courtesy of Dr. T. Merlin, Albuquerque, NM.)

or abscesses. The fistulae tend to be complex and associated with the lower rectal sphincter. Secondary tracts are common (86). Verrucous, warty anal masses also develop. The diagnosis requires organism identification by culture or in tissue sections. Caseating granulomas containing multinucleated giant cells are present. Organisms are identifiable using Ziehl-Neelsen stains. In chronic tuberculosis or in anal fistulae, organisms are sparse or absent. In such cases, it may be difficult to differentiate anorectal tuberculosis from Crohn disease.

Donovanosis

Donovanosis, a highly contagious, venereally transmitted, chronically progressive, autoinoculable ulcerating disease, involves the skin, mucosa, and lymphatics of the perianal and genital area (87). It is endemic in the tropics (88) and rare in the United States. The ratio of affected males to females is 10:1. The incubation period ranges from 8 days to 1 year, but most lesions appear within a month after sexual exposure (89). The disease results from intracellular microorganisms identifiable morphologically as the Donovan body seen in tissue smears using a rapid Giemsa test (90). Microbial cultures (91) and a polymerase chain reaction (PCR) test are diagnostic (92). The causative bacteria are *Calymmatobacterium granulomatous,* Gram-negative pleomorphic bacteria that are antigenically related to *Klebsiella* species. Other venereal diseases, particularly syphilis, frequently coexist with donovanosis.

The infection starts as a firm papule or subcutaneous nodule that progressively ulcerates. Classically, there are four types of lesions: (a) ulcerogranulomatous, the most common type, which consists of beefy red, nontender ulcers that bleed easily and may become extensive if left untreated; (b) hypertrophic or verrucous inflammatory dry nodules that usually have an irregular edge; (c) necrotic, foul-smelling deep ulcers causing tissue destruction; and (d) dry, sclerotic, or cicatricial lesions with fibrosis and scar formation (90). The infection consists of inflammatory nodules, fissures, fistulae, and extensive fibrosis. The scarring fibrosis leads to deformity and strictures.

Marked acanthosis and pseudoepitheliomatous hyperplasia are present. The inflamed lamina propria contains a heavy infiltrate of plasma cells, neutrophils, and a few lymphocytes. Capillaries and blood vessels appear prominent. Donovan bodies are present in enlarged histiocytes. They are best seen in air-dried smears made by crushing biopsy tissue between them and then fixing the slides in methanol and staining them with a Wright-Giemsa stain or Warthin-Starry stain. Donovan bodies appear as rounded coccobacilli lying within cystic cytoplasmic spaces in the mononuclear cells. They resemble bluish black safety pins due to bipolar chromatin condensations (90). As the disease progresses, the infection produces a destructive lymphadenopathy. Complications of the disease include deep ulcers, chronic scarring, lymphedema, and exuberant epithelial proliferations grossly resembling carcinoma. Perianal donovanosis also resembles condylomata lata of secondary syphilis. Locally destructive lesions and secondary infections may lead to severe morbidity or even death. Squamous cell carcinomas may complicate longstanding disease.

Chancroid

Chancroid results from infection by *Haemophilus ducreyi*. It is in the differential diagnosis of anogenital herpes, syphilis, and lymphogranuloma venereum. Chancroid is a common cause of genital ulcer disease in many developing countries (93) and has recently been established as a significant sexually transmitted disease in the United States (94). The organism produces single or multiple painful anal ulcers at the inoculation site and abscesses in the draining lymph nodes. When multiple ulcers are present, they often differ in their stage of development (Fig. 15.25). The ulcer begins as a macule that rapidly becomes pustular and ruptures, leaving a shallow saucer-shaped ulcer surrounded by a narrow erythematous margin. The ulcers have ragged edges and a base

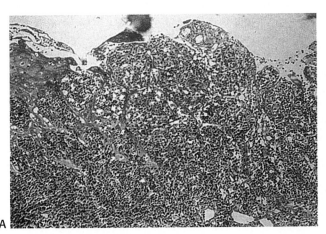
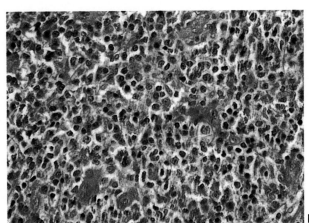

FIG. 15.25. Chancroid. A: Anal ulcer in a patient with chancroid proven by culture. **B:** Higher-power magnification shows the presence of acute and chronic inflammation.

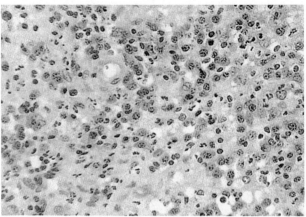

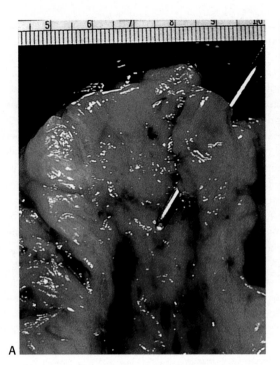

FIG. 15.26. Lymphogranuloma venereum (LGV). **A:** Gross specimen in a patient with LGV proctitis. The anorectum is thickened and fibrotic. A probe is inserted through a fistulous tract. Numerous areas of ulceration and hemorrhage are present. **B:** The lesion demonstrates a prominent acute and chronic inflammatory infiltrate. Because of the marked acute inflammation in this lesion, granulomas are not present.

covered by a grayish necrotic exudate. Gram stains made from the ulcer exudates are unreliable (95), and bacterial isolation is difficult because the organisms are difficult to grow. Recently developed monoclonal antibodies allow rapid detection of the organism (96).

Histologic sections of well-developed chancroid ulcers reveal three distinct layers: The superficial layer consists of red blood cells, polymorphonuclear leukocytes, histiocytes, fibrin, necrotic debris, and intra- and extracellular Gram-negative coccobacilli (*H. ducreyi*) at the base of the ulcer. Vascular proliferations and edema characterize the middle layer. Thrombosis with subsequent tissue necrosis and ulceration may result from endothelial swelling. The deep layer contains a dense infiltrate of plasma cells, lymphocytes, and polymorphonuclear leukocytes (97).

Lymphogranuloma Venereum

Lymphogranuloma venereum (LGV) is a tropical and subtropical chronic scarring sexually transmitted disease, caused by *C. trachomatis* serovars L1, L2, and L3. It is rare in the Western world. Infections caused by LGV strains of *C. trachomatis* affect travelers from endemic areas or patients with sexual contacts from endemically infected populations. The disease also develops in HIV-infected patients (98). In women, anorectal infections also result from spread of infected secretions along the perineum or by spread via the pelvic lymphatics. Some patients may have other diseases, including genital herpes or syphilis (99).

Patients usually present with anorectal pain; proctitis; a mucous, purulent, bloody rectal discharge; diarrhea; inguinal adenopathy; or spontaneously draining fistulae.

Patients also have nonspecific systemic symptoms including fever and leukocytosis. Sigmoidoscopy reveals a friable ulcerative process with the disease limited to the anorectum. Late (years later) complications include the formation of anorectal fissures, fistulae, strictures, and carcinomas (Fig. 15.26).

The anorectal lesions consist of hemorrhagic inflammation and regional lymphadenitis. The primary lesion is usually a small and painless papule or ulcer that may escape detection. HIV-infected patients tend to present with deeper, larger, and multiple ulcers (100). The papule ulcerates and develops into a painless elevated area of beefy red granulation tissue. In chronic cases, the ulcers are large and irregularly shaped with serpiginous extensions (100). Anorectal fissures and fistulae develop (101). Other patients develop granulomatous masses. Since LGV is an obligate intracellular pathogen, it replicates within epithelial cells and histiocytes at the primary site of infection. The histologic findings include granulomas with giant cells, crypt abscesses, extensive inflammation, neuromatous hyperplasia, and extensive fibrosis (Fig. 15.26). As a result, the disease is an exact mimic of Crohn disease. As the disease becomes more chronic, the overlying epithelium becomes acanthotic. The inflammatory infiltrate loses its neutrophils and becomes more mononuclear in nature with the presence of large numbers of lymphocytes and plasma cells (Fig. 15.27). Spontaneous healing occurs after several months, leaving inguinal scars.

Organisms spread via lymphatics to the regional lymph nodes, where they produce inguinal or femoral lymphadenitis. High anal infections produce hypogastric and deep iliac lymphadenitis. Initially, the nodes remain discrete, but as

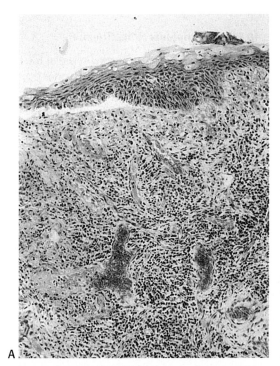
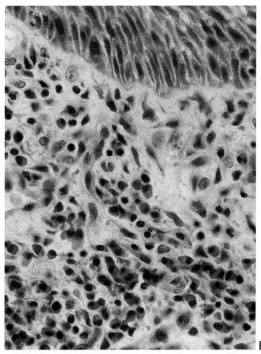

FIG. 15.27. Chronic lymphogranuloma venereum. **A:** A thinned squamous epithelium shows superficial ballooning degeneration. The underlying tissues appear congested and inflamed. **B:** Large numbers of lymphocytes and plasma cells are present. At this stage in the disease neutrophils are absent.

progressive periadenitis develops, they become matted, fluctuant, and suppurative. The overlying skin becomes fixed, inflamed, and thinned. Patients finally develop multiple draining fistulae. Histologic involvement of the nodes initially shows characteristic small stellate abscesses surrounded by histiocytes. These abscesses coalesce to produce large necrotic suppurative foci.

Complications of untreated anorectal infections include perirectal abscesses; fistula in ano; rectovaginal, rectovesical, and ischiorectal fistulae; anorectal strictures; and squamous cell carcinoma. Secondary bacterial infection contributes to the complications. The differential diagnosis of the inflamed anorectal mucosa includes ulcerative colitis, Crohn disease, amebiasis, syphilis, gonorrhea, carcinoma, and infection with herpes simplex virus, *Yersinia* species, *Campylobacter* species, and *Clostridium difficile*.

Nonlymphogranuloma Venereum Chlamydial Infections

C. trachomatis is one of the most common sexually transmitted diseases in the United States, striking 4 million Americans each year (102). The infection rate among men having sex with men ranges from 4% to 7.2% (103). Patients present with nonspecific lower genital tract infections in women and a nonspecific urethritis in men. Common symptoms include pruritus and anal and perianal pain. The infection induces a nonspecific inflammatory response rather than the granulomatous inflammation more typical of LGV. Endoscopically, a nonspecific

proctitis with friable granular and edematous mucosa is present. Currently a PCR assay exists to detect this organism (104).

Fungal Infections

Fungal infections are rare in the anorectal mucosa. Candidiasis primarily affecting debilitated individuals may cause anal abscesses, fissures, and fistulae. *Candida* species that infect this area include *Candida albicans, Candida guilliermondi,* and *Candida parapsilosis* (105,106). Rare *Histoplasma* infections affect the anus in patients with disseminated disease (107). *Paracoccidioidomycosis* may present in the anal and perianal region in patients with disseminated disease (108). It starts as a small, painless, erythematous plaque with well-defined edges, but with growth, the central areas become eroded and granulomatous. The lesions eventually develop into abscesses, which drain spontaneously, creating painful ulcerated lesions (108). *Nocardia brasiliensis* (85%) and *Actinomadura madurae* (10%) may cause perianal infections, particularly among agricultural workers (109). The differential diagnosis includes anal sinuses, hidradenitis, and cutaneous tuberculosis.

Viral Infections

Anogenital herpetic infections result from *herpes simplex virus* (HSV) II (110) as the result of direct inoculation during anal intercourse. Strong independent associations for the presence of HSV II antibodies are found in patients

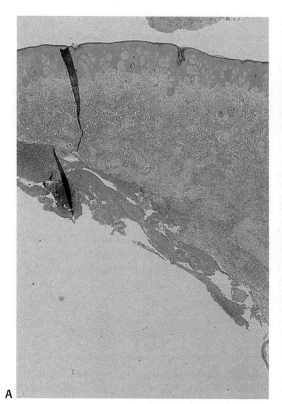
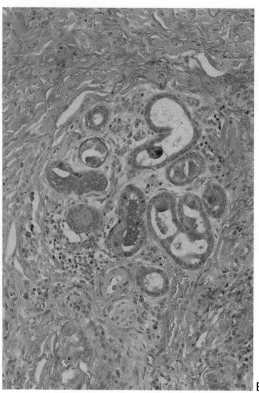

FIG. 15.28. Cytomegalovirus (CMV) infection. **A:** The tissue was removed from this HIV-positive person because of persistent fissures and fistulae. The epithelium overlying the fistula is acanthotic with prominent hyperkeratosis. **B:** Numerous CMV inclusions are present in the epithelium of the skin adnexal structures. They are also present in other areas in the endothelial cells and macrophages in the soft tissues.

with a homosexual orientation, increasing number of years of sexual activity, increasing number of lifetime partners, number of past gonococcal infections, and having receptive anal and/or vaginal contact (110). The clinical presentation usually begins with itching and perianal soreness. Severe anorectal pain follows. Patients also present with fever, inguinal adenopathy, tenesmus, constipation, anorectal discharge, and bleeding. Neurologic symptoms develop in the distribution of the sacral roots in some patients. HSV also produces severe proctitis and chronic perianal ulcers.

Grossly, herpetic lesions appear as erythematous nodules with small clustered vesicles that rupture, giving rise to larger ulcerations. The perianal skin and anal canal are most frequently involved, but the distal rectal mucosa might also become infected. The disease often resolves within a couple of weeks, but recurrences are common. One confirms the diagnosis by viral culture of the vesicular fluid, serologic studies, or histologic examination. Histologically, herpetic infections resemble those occurring in other cutaneous and mucosal surfaces. The histologic characteristics of HSV proctitis include the presence of multinucleated cells, intranuclear inclusions, and lymphocytic infiltration around the submucosal vessels. The inclusions typically affect the epithelial cells.

Characteristic giant cells containing prominent intranuclear inclusions (Cowdry bodies) are generally identified in early lesions. Immunoperoxidase stains may confirm the diagnosis.

Cytomegalovirus (CMV) can produce anal ulcerations and histologic features resembling those found in the esophagus (see Chapter 2). Nuclear inclusions are identified in endothelial cells, macrophages, and the epithelium of the adnexal structures of the perianal skin (Fig. 15.28). Infections with *human papillomavirus* (HPV) produce koilocytosis, condylomata, and cancers in the perianal skin and lower anal canal. For a more detailed description of these relationships, see Chapter 16.

Enterobiasis

Enterobiasis (pinworm, or oxyuriasis), an intestinal infection of humans, results from infection by *Enterobius vermicularis*. The worm infects approximately 200 million people worldwide. The female averages 10 mm in length and the male averages 3 mm. The organisms live with their heads attached to the mucosa of the cecum, appendix (see Chapter 8), and adjacent intestine. The gravid female migrates through the anal canal at night, deposits approximately 10,000 eggs on the perianal skin, and dies. Each egg contains an embryo

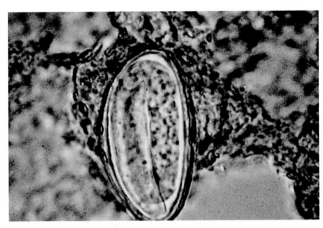

FIG. 15.29. Enterobius vermicularis egg in stool. A larval form is present in the center of the ovum.

(Fig. 15.29), which develops into an infective larva within a few hours. After the egg is ingested, the larva emerges in the small intestine and migrates distally to the cecum. In less than a month's time, newly developed gravid females discharge ova in the perianal region.

In humans, infections occur by direct transfer of ova from the anus to the mouth by way of contaminated fingers. The most common symptom, pruritus ani, is most troublesome at night, a feature related to the nocturnal migration of the gravid females. Examination for ova of material obtained from the perianal skin by means of Scotch tape preparation represents the preferred detection method. Occasionally, the organism causes anal abscesses or perianal sepsis. Perianal tissues may show the presence of an intense and acute eosinophilic inflammatory exudate with histiocytes. Scattered eosinophilic microabscesses may contain the parasitic ova.

GRANULOMATOUS ANORECTAL DISORDERS DUE TO FOREIGN MATERIAL

Anorectal granulomas may have numerous etiologies. The most common include infections (tuberculosis, LGV, syphilis), Crohn disease, and foreign material. Infectious etiologies have already been discussed. In this section, noninfectious causes of anorectal granulomas will be covered.

Oleogranuloma

Oleomas, oleogranulomas, or paraffinomas are foreign body reactions to unabsorbable oily substances. Previously these materials were used to treat hemorrhoids; they are seldom used today. The most severe reactions occur against mineral oils. The oleogranulomas may develop rapidly after the oil enters tissues or they may appear months to years later. The lesions localize to the anal canal just above the dentate line or they can extend into the rectum or even into the perirectal

fat. The granulomatous response produces a firm, yellowish gray submucosal mass or ulcer that may become fixed to other structures (111).

The histologic features reflect the stage of development. In early phases, an acute inflammatory response is present, which may also contain numerous eosinophils. Increasing fibrosis and zones of mononuclear cells, epithelioid cells, giant cells, and a peripheral proliferating fibrous connective tissue gradually replace the acute inflammation (Fig. 15.30). The fat is not easily identified in tissues that undergo routine processing but can be easily seen in frozen sections using fat stains. However, this is generally not necessary because the morphology is so distinctive. The differential diagnosis of the lesion includes pneumatosis intestinalis, lymphangioma, mucosal lipomatosis, or some forms of liposarcoma. However, unlike liposarcomas, which contain intracellular fat vacuoles and show cellular atypia, oleogranulomas are characterized by the presence of extracellular lipid collections and they lack atypical cells. The spaces are far more irregular than those seen in lymphangiomas. The open spaces are also far more irregular than typically seen in pneumatosis intestinalis.

Barium Granulomas

Barium sulfate, used as a contrast medium to GI radiologic procedures, is not an irritant, but when it extravasates into tissues, it accumulates within macrophages and giant cells, producing tumorous masses, fibrosis, and strictures. Barium granulomas result either from mechanical trauma during radiologic procedures or from barium entering mucosal defects due to inflammation, fistulae, or diverticula. Histologically, a typical foreign body reaction develops with histiocytes surrounding greenish gray barium sulfate crystals as described in greater detail in Chapter 13.

Ivalon Tumor

Ivalon, a polyvinyl sponge, is sometimes inserted into the anorectal region to treat rectal prolapse. It may elicit a fibroblastic and granulomatous response, producing a localized hard anorectal mass. Numerous multinucleated giant cells surround the Ivalon pieces lining up along their edges. Because the Ivalon superficially resembles pieces of bone surrounded by osteoblasts, care must be taken not to misinterpret the lesion as a bone tumor. Histologic examination shows that the irregular eosinophilic structures contain no cells (112).

Foreign Body Granulomas

One may also see granulomatous reactions around material inserted into fissures or fistulae in an effort to treat them. This may include portions of gauze or other packing

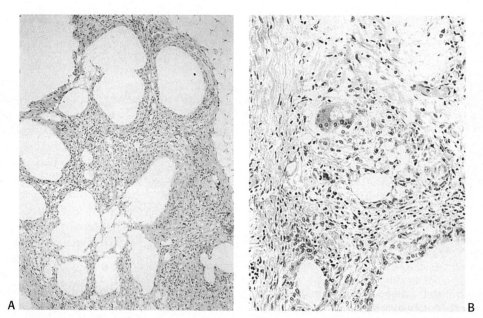

FIG. 15.30. Oleoma. A: Numerous irregularly shaped and sized cystic spaces are present in the tissues. These spaces are far more irregular than typically seen in pneumatosis intestinalis. **B:** Higher magnification showing giant cells admixed with acute and chronic inflammatory cells in fibrous tissue. The fat is not evident in this lesion due to extraction during tissue processing.

materials. Occasionally, remnants of suture material with a surrounding suture granuloma may also be present.

INFLAMMATORY CLOACOGENIC POLYP

Inflammatory cloacogenic polyp (ICP) is a nonneoplastic polyp that results from transitional zone prolapse. It presents as a small sessile polyp at the anorectal junction in patients in their 5th to 7th decades. Histologic features of ICPs show some overlap with the prolapse-associated changes seen in the rectum (see Chapter 13). They contain anal transitional zone epithelium and may exhibit a complex tubulovillous growth pattern. Simple columnar colonic or transitional epithelium containing goblet cells and compressed absorptive cells line the villous projections. Hyperplastic smooth muscle fibers from the muscularis mucosae extend perpendicularly into a normal or inflamed lamina propria (Figs. 15.31 and 15.32). The surfaces of the lesions may be eroded and there may be fibromuscular effacement of the lamina propria. Displaced epithelium and cysts containing variable amounts of mucin and inflammatory cells may lie in the submucosa. The surface epithelium is frequently hyperplastic. The importance of recognizing an ICP lies in distinguishing it from an adenoma, which it may closely resemble. However, the overall benign reactive appearance of the glandular epithelium and the fibromuscular hyperplasia of the muscularis mucosae and lamina propria in ICPs should make this distinction possible. The lesion also differs from Peutz-Jeghers polyps, which only very rarely involve the anal canal

and characteristically contain thick arborizing muscle bundles. Rarely, these lesions may contain areas of anal intraepithelial neoplasia (113).

RADIATION-INDUCED CHANGES

Radiation-induced changes often affect the anus because the common therapy for advanced cervical, prostatic, or rectal cancers frequently includes radiotherapy. The changes may be acute or chronic, depending on the time the tissues are examined in relation to the time when the radiation was administered. Acute changes present as areas of ulceration with fibrinoid necrosis of the vasculature (Fig. 15.33). Chronic changes are typically identified when anal tissues are examined for other reasons, most commonly hemorrhoids. At this time one sees fibrosis and atypical radiation fibroblasts. There may also be damage to the myenteric plexus, with fibrosis and neural hyperplasia. Vascular changes similar to those described elsewhere in this book are also present.

DISORDERS PRIMARILY INVOLVING THE PERIANAL SKIN

Itching of the perianal skin or *pruritus ani* is more common in males and has an extensive etiology. Leakage of stool onto the perianal skin is a common factor. It may also

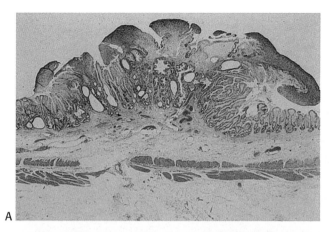
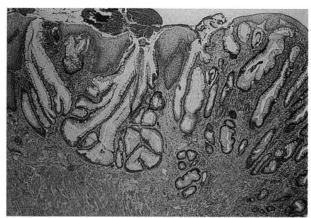
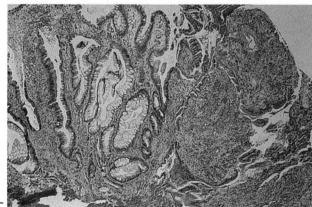

FIG. 15.31. Inflammatory cloacogenic polyp. The histologic features of cloacogenic polyps differ depending on whether they arise in the transitional mucosa **(A, B)** or in the rectal mucosa **(C)**. In the transitional mucosa, the lesion consists of both squamous epithelium and glandular epithelium with regenerative features (A,B). Those that originate in the rectal mucosa do not contain squamous epithelium but demonstrate a villiform architecture and regenerative features (C). The lesion may distort the muscularis mucosae, obliterating the usual landmarks between the lamina propria, muscularis mucosae, and underlying submucosa, as seen best in B. Note that the glands demonstrate a somewhat lobular architecture with branching (B). Although they are hyperplastic, no cytologic features of malignancy are present within them. In C, the villiform architecture is evident, as is the regenerative nature of the mucosa. On the right-hand side of the lesion, one sees prominent granulation tissue.

be a manifestation of various dermatologic diseases, infections, and poor hygiene, as well as being idiopathic in nature. The perianal areas either appear normal or reddened and excoriated due to patients' tendency to scratch. The skin may also appear smooth and atrophic with superficial abrasions. When the disease becomes chronic, the affected surfaces appear thickened with multiple irregular radial folds. Epidermal hyperplasia, variable degrees of hyperkeratosis, hydrops of the prickle cells, dermal edema, and dermal inflammation characterize pruritus ani (Fig. 15.34). If the patient has been scratching the area, the inflammation may appear acute in nature. Otherwise, it usually consists of lymphocytic and mononuclear cell infiltrates.

Epidermal inclusion cysts develop in the perianal skin and they are identical to their cutaneous counterparts. Rare

epidermoid cysts develop at the end of an anal fistula when epithelial ingrowth has occurred. These lack all the germ cell layers characteristic of retrorectal dermoid cysts (benign teratomas).

Perianal bacterial dermatitis is a common dermatologic condition in infants and children and can be caused by various conditions, including candidiasis, diaper dermatitis, seborrheic dermatitis, and eczema. Group A β-hemolytic streptococci, *Streptococcus pyogenes,* and *Staphylococcus aureus* also rarely cause this condition (114). These lesions are characterized by perianal erythematous patches with clearly defined borders, sometimes associated with a functional disturbance. The histologic features are that of an acute or chronic dermatitis.

Molluscum contagiosum, a contagious viral disease, is characterized by the appearance of multiple small waxy

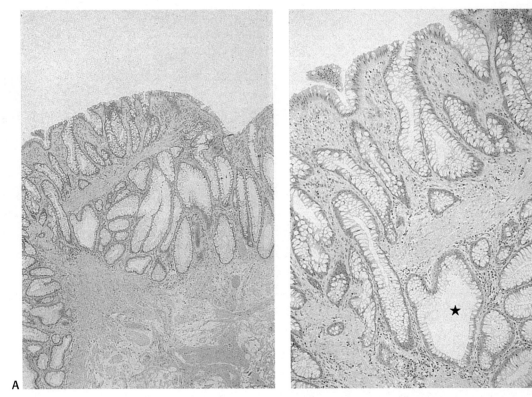

FIG. 15.32. Inflammatory cloacogenic polyp. **A:** The muscularis mucosae appears hypertrophic and extends in broad bands into the overlying mucosa. The glands are hyperplastic and branched. **B:** The intersecting bands of smooth muscle tissue separate the regenerative glands from one another (*star*).

papules that have characteristic umbilicated centers. The most common sites of involvement include the abdominal skin as well as the skin of the perineum, thigh, penis, scrotum, and vulva. In addition, the buttock and perianal regions are sometimes affected. Histologically, the lesions consist of a

lobular epidermal proliferation that extends to the dermis (Fig. 15.35). The most characteristic portion of the lesion is the presence of prominent inclusion bodies.

An infective *necrotizing fascitis* known as *Fournier gangrene* was originally described in the scrotum, but it can

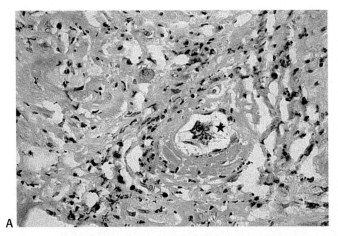
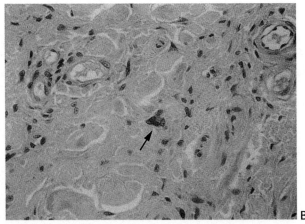

FIG. 15.33. Anorectal region radiation changes in a patient who had received radiotherapy for a gynecologic malignancy 3 months previously. **A:** Acute changes. Note the fibrinoid necrosis surrounding the vessels (*star*), acute and chronic inflammation, and presence of atypical stromal cells. **B:** Soft tissues from the anal region of a patient who had received radiotherapy for cervical cancer 25 years prior to the resection of this tissue. Note the presence of an atypical multinucleated stromal cell (*arrow*).

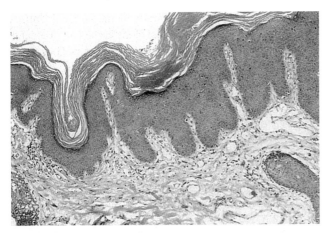

FIG. 15.34. Pruritus ani. Mild nonspecific reactive changes are present with mild superficial submucosal inflammation and capillary ectasia. The hyperplastic squamous epithelium is hyperkeratotic with a prominent granular cell layer.

also develop in the perianal area in both men and women. Males are afflicted more commonly than females (115). Diabetes is an important predisposing factor. There may also be a relationship with alcoholism, the presence of malignancies, and poor socioeconomic status (115). The common denominator of all of the risk factors (diabetes, alcoholism, leukemia, and HIV) is impaired host resistance due to reduced cellular immunity. The major sources of sepsis are the local skin, anus, and rectum. Intestinal lesions are the most common foci of sepsis and include ruptured appendicitis, colonic carcinoma, and diverticulitis (115). Many types of organisms, singly or in combination, are encountered in this disorder (116). Organisms that have been identified include *Clostridium, Klebsiella, Streptococcus, Staphylococcus, Bacteroides,* and *Corynebacterium* species and coliforms. Their synergistic activities inflict devastat-

ing necrotizing fasciitis on the patient. The suppurative bacterial infection leads to thrombosis of small subcutaneous vessels, secondary ischemia, and gangrene of the overlying skin.

Hidradenitis suppurativa is both an acute and a chronic inflammatory process involving the skin and subcutaneous tissues in areas where apocrine glands exist. The initiating event is occlusion of the apocrine duct by a keratinous plug due to ductal dilation and stasis. Secondary bacterial infection ensues. The infection can then rupture extending into the surrounding tissues. The chronic cyclic nature of the disease leads to fibrosis and hypertrophic scarring of the skin. Subcutaneous sinus tracts, abscesses, ulcers, and scars develop. The sinus tracts lie superficial to the sphincteric muscle and often involve the lower part of the anal canal, distal to the dentate line.

Patients present with tender, painful, subcutaneous nodules that rupture after about a week. Subcutaneous tunneling of infection occurs, often resulting in fibrosis. Grossly, the skin appears blotchy with areas of red and white discoloration. Pus drains from multiple sinus tract openings. These lesions may appear localized or may involve a large perianal area, each extending to the buttocks. Secondary anal fistulae may develop. The lesion may be confused with fistula in ano or anorectal Crohn disease. Although the sinus tracts in hidradenitis suppurativa may enter the anal canal, they are shallow and lie superficial to the internal sphincter and have no relationship with the dentate line (117). Histologically, the inflammation consists of plasma cells, lymphocytes, and giant cells. The squamous epithelium shows downward ingrowth. Treatment consists of antibiotics. In rare cases, extensive excision of the involved area cures the problem. Rarely, carcinoma complicates this disorder. Nevi may develop in the perianal skin. These resemble the junctional, intradermal, or compound nevi seen on other cutaneous surfaces.

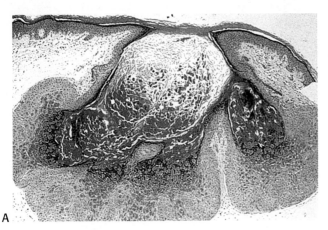

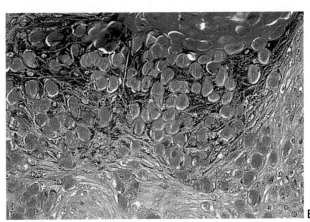

FIG. 15.35. Molluscum contagiosum. **A:** Molluscum contagiosum present in the perianal skin. **B:** Characteristic eosinophilic viral inclusions are present deep in the core of the lesion.

REFERENCES

1. Jones KL: *Smith's Recognizable Patterns of Human Malformation,* 5th ed. Philadelphia: WB Saunders, 1997.
2. Nivatvongs S, Stern HS, Fryd DS: The length of the anal canal. *Dis Colon Rectum* 1981;24:600.
3. Rociu E, Stoker J, Eijkemans MJ, Lameris JS: Normal anal sphincter anatomy and age- and sex-related variations at high-spatial-resolution endoanal MR imaging. *Radiology* 2000;217:395.
4. Blair JB, Holyoke EA, Best RR: A note on the lymphatics of the middle and lower rectum and anus. *Anat Rec* 1950;108:635.
5. Slanetz CA, Herter FP: The large intestine. In: Hagensen CD, Feind CR, Herter FP, et al (eds). *The Lymphatics in Cancer.* Philadelphia: WB Saunders, 1972, p 489.
6. Caplan I: The lymphatic vessels of the anal region—a study and investigation about 50 cases. *Folia Angiol* 1976;24:260.
7. Fenger C: The anal transitional zone. Location and extent. *Acta Pathol Microbiol Scand A* 1979;87:379.
8. Fenger C, Knoth M: The anal transitional zone: a scanning and transmission electron microscopic investigation of the surface epithelium. *Ultrastruct Pathol* 1981;2:163.
9. Williams GR, Talbot IC, Northover JM, Leigh IM: Keratin expression in the normal anal canal. *Histopathology* 1995;26:39.
10. Clemmensen OJ, Fenger C: Melanocytes in the anal canal epithelium. *Histopathology* 1991;18:237.
11. Fetissof F, Dubois MP, Assan R, et al: Endocrine cells in the anal canal. *Virchows Arch A Pathol Anat* 1984;404:39.
12. Van der Putte SC: Ultrastructure of the human anogenital sweat gland. *Anat Rec* 1993;235:583.
13. Thomson WH: The nature of haemorrhoids. *Br J Surg* 1975;62:542.
14. Kiesewetter WB, Turner CR, Sieber WK: Imperforate anus. *Am J Surg* 1964;107:412.
15. Shaul DB, Harrison EA: Classification of anorectal malformations—initial approach, diagnostic tests, and colostomy. *Semin Pediatr Surg* 1997;6:187.
16. Smith DW: Recognizable patterns of human malformation. In: *Major Problems in Clinical Pediatrics,* 3rd ed. Philadelphia: WB Saunders, 1982.
17. Ferraz FG, Nunes L, Ferraz ME, et al: Townes-Brocks syndrome: report of a case and review of the literature. *Ann Genet* 1989;32:120.
18. Friedman PA, Rao DW, Aylsworth AS: Six patients with the Townes-Brocks syndrome including five familial cases and an association with a pericentric inversion of chromosome 16. *Am Soc Hum Genet* 1987;41(3 suppl):A60.
19. Currarino G, Coln D, Votteler T: Triad of anorectal, sacral and presacral anomalies. *Am J Roentgenol* 1981;137:395.
20. Santulli TV, Kiesewetter WB, Bill AH Jr: Anorectal anomalies. A suggested international classification. *J Pediatr Surg* 1970;5:281.
21. Boocock GR, Donnai D: Anorectal malformation: familial aspects and associated anomalies. *Arch Dis Child* 1987;62:576.
22. Hoyme HE, Jones KL, Dixon SD, et al: Prenatal cocaine exposure and fetal vascular disruption. *Pediatrics* 1990;85:743.
23. Ives EJ: Thalidomide and anal anomalies. *Can Med Assoc J* 1962;87:670.
24. Torres R, Levitt MA, Tovila JM, et al: Anorectal malformations and Down's syndrome. *J Pediatr Surg* 1998;33:194.
25. Mo R, Kim JH, Zhang J, et al: Anorectal malformations caused by defects in sonic hedgehog signaling. *Am J Pathol* 2001;159:765.
26. Kim J, Kim P, Hui CC: The VACTERL association: lessons from the sonic hedgehog pathway. *Clin Genet* 2001;59:306.
27. Kohlhase J, Liebers M, Backe J, et al: High incidence of R276X SALL1 mutation in sporadic but not familial Townes-Brocks syndrome and report of the first familial case. *J Med Genet* 2003;40:e127.
28. Kohlhase J: SALL1 mutations in Townes-Brocks syndrome and related disorders. *Hum Mutat* 2000;37:30.
29. Lynch SA, Bond PM, Copp AJ, et al: A gene for autosomal dominant sacral agenesis maps to the holoprosencephaly region at 7q36. *Nat Genet* 1995;11:93.
30. Ashcraft KW, Holder TM: Congenital anal stenosis with presacral teratoma. *Ann Surg* 1965;162:1091.
31. Keith A: Malformation of the hind end of the body. *BMJ* 1908;ii:1736.
32. Ralph DJ, Woodhouse CRJ, Ransley PG: The management of the neuropathic bladder in adolescents with imperforate anus. *J Urol* 1992;148:366.
33. Escobar LF, Weaver DD, Bixler D, et al: Urorectal septum malformation sequence. Report of six cases and embryological analysis. *Am J Dis Child* 1987;141:1021.
34. Rudd NL, Curry C, Chen KTH, et al: Thymic-renal-anal-lung dysplasia in sibs: a new autosomal recessive error of early morphogenesis. *Am J Med Genet* 1990;37:401.
35. Fraser FC, Jequier S, Chen MF: Chondrodysplasia, situs inversus totalis, cleft epiglottis and larynx hexadactyly of hand and feet, pancreatic cystic dysplasia, renal dysplasia/absence, micropenis and ambiguous genitalia, imperforate anus. *Am J Med Genet* 1989;34:401.
36. Hall JG, Pallister PD, Clarren SK, et al: Congenital hypothalamic hamartoblastoma, hypopituitarism, imperforate anus and postaxial polydactyly—a new syndrome? Part I: clinical, causal and pathogenetic considerations. *Am J Med Genet* 1980;7:47.
37. Curry CJR, Carey JC, Holland JS, et al: Smith-Lemli-Opitz syndrome type II: multiple congenital anomalies with male pseudohermaphroditism and frequent early lethality. *Am J Med Genet* 1987;26:45.
38. Salihu HM, Tchuniguem G, Aliyu MH, Kouam L: Prune belly syndrome and associated malformations. A 13 year experience from developing country. *West Indian Med J* 203;52:281.
39. Aliyu MH, Salihu HM, Kouam L: Eagle-Barrett syndrome: occurrence and outcomes. *East Afr Med J* 2003;80:595.
40. Ruiz-Moreno F, Gerdo-Ceballo A, Lozano-Saldivar G: Vaginal anus. *Dis Colon Rectum* 1980;23:306.
41. Brent L, Stephens FD: Primary rectal ectasia: a quantitative study of smooth muscle cells in normal and hypertrophied human bowel. *Prog Pediatr Surg* 1976;9:41.
42. deVries PA, Cox KL: Surgery of anorectal anomalies. *Surg Clin North Am* 1985;65:1139.
43. Van Allen MI, Ritchie S, Toi A, et al: Trisomy 4 in a fetus with cyclopia and other anomalies. *Am J Med Genet* 1993;6:1947.
44. Smith NM, Chambers HM, Furness ME, Haan EA: The OEIS complex (omphalocele-exstrophy-imperforate anus-spinal defects): recurrence in sibs. *J Med Genet* 1992;29:730.
45. Keppler-Noreuil KM: OEIS complex (omphalocoele-exstrophy-imperforate anus-spinal defects): a review of 14 cases. *Am J Med Genet* 2002;107:271.
46. Carey JC, Greenbaum B, Hall BD: The OEIS complex (omphalocele, exstrophy, imperforate anus, spinal defects). *Birth Defects* 1978;14:253.
47. Von Geldern CE: The etiology of cloacal exstrophy and allied malformations. *J Urol* 1959;82:134.
48. Hendren WH: Cloaca, the most severe degree of imperforate anus. *Ann Surg* 1998;228:331.
49. Passarge E, Lenz W: Syndrome of caudal regression in infants of diabetic mothers: observations of further cases. *Pediatrics* 1966;37:672.
50. Stewart JM, Stoll S: Familial caudal regression anomalad and maternal diabetes. *Lancet* 1964;2:1124.
51. Ashcraft KW, Holder TM, Harris DJ: Familial presacral teratomas. *Birth Defects* 1975;11:143.
52. Cohn J, Bay-Nielsen E: Hereditary defect of the sacrum and coccyx with anterior sacral meningocele. *Acta Pediatr Scand* 1969;58:268.
53. Louw JH, Cywes S, Cremin BJ: Anorectal malformations: classification and clinical features. *S Afr J Surg* 1971;9:11.
54. Mills SE, Walker AN, Stallings RG, et al: Retrorectal cystic hamartoma. Report of three cases, including one with a perirenal component. *Arch Pathol Lab Med* 1984;108:737.
55. Hjermstad BM, Helwig EB: Tailgut cysts. Report of 53 cases. *Am J Clin Pathol* 1988;89:139.
56. Levert LM, Van Rooyen W, Van den Bergen HA: Cysts of the tailgut. *Eur J Surg* 1996;162:149.
57. Bale PM: Sacrococcygeal developmental abnormalities and tumours in children. *Persp Pediatr Pathol* 1984;8:9.
58. Tekin K, Sungurtekin U, Aytekin FO, et al: Ectopic prostatic tissue of the anal canal presenting as rectal bleeding. *Dis Colon Rectum* 2002;45:979.
59. Fulton RS, Rouse RV, Ranheim EA: Ectopic prostate: case report of a presacral mass presenting with obstructive symptoms. *Arch Pathol Lab Med* 2001;125:286.
60. Shindo K, Bacon HE, Holmes EJ: Ectopic gastric mucosa and glandular tissue of a salivary type in the anal canal. *Dis Colon Rectum* 1972;15:57.
61. Davis M, Whitley ME, Haque AK, et al: Xanthogranulomatous abscess of a müllerian duct remnant. A rare lesion of the rectum and anus. *Dis Colon Rectum* 1986;29:755.

62. Parkash S, Veliath AJ, Chandrasekaran V: Ectopic gastric mucosa in duplication of the rectum presenting as a perianal fistula. *Dis Colon Rectum* 1982;25:225.

63. Schouten WR, Briel JW, Auwerda JJ, De Graaf EJ: Ischaemic nature of anal fissure. *Br J Surg* 1996;83:63.

64. American Gastroenterological Association: AGA technical review on the diagnosis and care of patients with anal fissure. *Gastroenterology* 2003;124:235.

65. Grace RH, Harper IA, Thompson RG: Anorectal sepsis: microbiology in relation to fistula-in-ano. *Br J Surg* 1982;69:401.

66. Fry GA, Martin WJ, Dearing WH, et al: Primary actinomycosis of the rectum with multiple perianal and perineal fistulae. *Mayo Clin Proc* 1965;40:296.

67. Bode WE, Ramos R, Page CP: Invasive necrotizing infection secondary to anorectal abscess. *Dis Colon Rectum* 1982;25:416.

68. Iacono G, Cavataio F, Montalto G, Carrocci A: Cows milk protein allergy as a cause of anal fistula and fissure. *J Allergy Clin Immunol* 1998;101:125.

69. Parks AG, Morson BC: The pathogenesis of fistula-in-ano. *Proc R Soc Med* 1962;55:751.

70. Thompson WHF: The nature of hemorrhoids. *Br J Surg* 1975;62:542.

71. Haas PA, Fox TA, Haas GP: The pathogenesis of hemorrhoids. *Dis Colon Rectum* 1984;27:442.

72. Nelson RL, Abcarian H, Davis FG, Persky V: Prevalence of benign anorectal disease in a randomly selected population. *Dis Colon Rectum* 1995;38:341.

73. Fenoglio CM: Routine pathological examination of hemorrhoids. *JAMA* 1984;252:2067.

74. Groisman GM, Amar M, Polak-Charcon S: Multinucleated stromal cells of the anal mucosa: a common finding. *Histopathology* 2000;36:224.

75. Groisman GM, Polak-Charcon S: Fibroepithelial polyps of the anus: a histologic, immunohistochemical, and ultrastructural study, including comparison with the normal anal subepithelial layer. *Am J Surg Pathol* 1998;22:70.

76. Sakai Y, Matsukuma S: CD34+ stromal cells and hyalinized vascular changes in the anal fibroepithelial polyps. *Histopathology* 2002;41:230.

77. Hosking SW, Smart HL, Johnson AG, Triger DR: Anorectal varices, haemorrhoids and portal hypertension. *Lancet* 1989;8634:349.

78. Azimuddin K, Stasik JJ, Rosen L, et al: Dieulafoy's lesion of the anal canal: a new clinical entity. Report of two cases. *Dis Colon Rectum* 2000;43:423.

79. Quinn TC, Stam WE, Godell SE, et al: The polymicrobial origin of intestinal infections in homosexual men. *N Engl J Med* 1983;309:576.

80. Smith D: Infectious syphilis of the anal canal. *Dis Colon Rectum* 1963;6:7.

81. Catterall RD: Sexually transmitted diseases of the anus and rectum. *Clin Gastroenterol* 1975;4:659.

82. Rietmeijer CA, Paatanik JL, Judson FN, Douglas JM: Increases in gonorrhea and sexual risk behaviors among men who have sex with men: a 12 year trend analysis at the Denver Metro Health Clinic. *Sex Transm Dis* 2003;30:562.

83. Rice RJ, Thompson SE: Treatment of uncomplicated infections due to Neisseria gonorrhoeae. A review of clinical efficacy and in vitro susceptibility studies from 1982 through 1985. *JAMA* 1986;255:1739.

84. El-Dhuwaib Y, Ammori BJ: Perianal abscess due to Neisseria gonorrhoeae. *Eur J Clin Microbiol Infect Dis* 2003;22:422.

85. McMillan A, Lee FD: Sigmoidoscopic and microscopic appearance of the rectal mucosa in homosexual men. *Gut* 1981;22:1035.

86. Kraemer M, Gill SS, Seow-Choen F: Tuberculous anal sepsis: report of clinical features in 20 cases. *Dis Colon Rectum* 2000;43:1589.

87. Remigio PA: Granuloma inguinale. In: Sun T (ed). *Sexually Related Infectious Diseases: Clinical and Laboratory Aspects.* Philadelphia: Field and Wood, 1986, p 15.

88. Hudson BJ, vanderMeijden WI: A survey of sexually transmitted diseases in five STD clinics in Papua New Guinea. *PNG Med J* 1999;37:152.

89. Sehgal VN, Sharma HK: Donovanosis. *J Dermatol* 1992;19:932.

90. O'Farrell N: Donvanosis. *Sex Transm Infect* 2002;78:452.

91. Kharsany AB, Hoosen AA, Kiepiela P, et al: Growth and cultural characteristics of Calymmatobacterium granulomatous—the etiological agent of granuloma inguinale (sonovanosis). *J Med Microbiol* 1997;46:579.

92. Carter J, Bowden FJ, Sriprakash KS, et al: Diagnostic polymerase chain reaction for donovanosis. *Clin Infect Dis* 1996;23:1168.

93. Nasanze H, Fast MV, D'Costa LJ, et al: Genital ulcers in Kenya: Clinical and laboratory study. *Br J Vener Dis* 1981;57:378.

94. Schmid GP, Sanders LL, Blount JH, Alexander ER: Chancroid in the United States. Reestablishment of an old disease. *JAMA* 1987;258:3265.

95. Deacon RB, Albritton DC, Olansky S, Kaplan WA: Simplified procedure for the isolation and identification of Haemophilus ducreyi. *J Invest Dermatol* 1956;26:399.

96. Karim QN, Finn GY, Easmon CSF, et al: Rapid detection of Haemophilus ducreyi in clinical and experimental infections using monoclonal antibody: a preliminary evaluation. *Genitourin Med* 1989;65:361.

97. Fung JC: Chancroid (Haemophilus ducreyi). In: Sun T (ed). *Sexually Related Infectious Diseases: Clinical and Laboratory Aspects.* Philadelphia: Field and Wood, 1986, p 15.

98. Nieuwenhuis RF, Ossewaarde JM, van der Meijden WI, Neumann HA: Unusual presentation of early lymphogranuloma venereum in an HIV-1 infected patient: effective treatment with 1 g erythromycin. *Sex Transm Infect* 2003;79:453.

99. Scieux C, Barnes R, Bianchi A, et al: Lymphogranuloma venereum: 27 cases in Paris. *J Infect Dis* 1989;60:662.

100. Rothenberg RB: Lymphogranuloma venereum. In: Freedberg IM, (ed). *Fitzpatrick's Dermatology in General Medicine.* New York: McGraw Hill, 1999, pp 2591–2594.

101. Mabey D, Peeling RW: Lymphogranuloma venereum. *Sex Transm Infect* 2002;78:90.

102. Washington AE, Johnson RE, Sanders KK Jr: Chlamydia trachomatis infections in the United States. What are they costing us? *JAMA* 1987;257:2070.

103. Manavi K, McMillan A, Young H: The prevalence of rectal chlamydial infection amongst men who have sex with men attending the genitourinary medicine clinic in Edinburgh. *Int J STD AIDS* 2004;15:162.

104. Lister NA, Tabrizi SN, Fairley CK, Garland S: Validation of Roche COBAS Amplicor assay for the detection of Chlamydia trachomatis in rectal and pharyngeal specimens by omp1 PCR assay. *J Clin Microbiol* 2004;43:239.

105. Gagneur A, Sizun J, Vernotte E, et al: Low rate of Candida parapsilosis-related colonization and infection in hospitalized preterm infants: a one-year prospective study. *J Hosp Infect* 2001;48:193.

106. Jarvis WR: Epidemiology of nosocomial fungal infections, with emphasis on Candida species. *Clin Infect Dis* 1995;20:1526.

107. Earle JHO, Highman JH, Lockey E: A case of disseminated histoplasmosis. *BMJ* 1984;i:607.

108. Costa Vieira RA, Lopes A, Oliveira HV, et al: Anal paracoccidioidomycosis: an unusual presentation of disseminated disease. *Rev Soc Bras Med Trop* 2001;34:583.

109. Chavez G, Estrada R, Bonifaz A: Perianal actinomycetoma experience of 20 cases. *Int J Dermatol* 2002;41:491.

110. van de Laar MJ, Termorshuizen F, Slomka MJ, et al: Prevalence and correlates of herpes simplex virus type 2 infection: evaluation of behavioral risk factors. *Int J Epidemiol* 1998;27:127.

111. Hernandez V, Hernandez IA, Bethrong M: Oleogranuloma simulating carcinoma of the rectum. *Dis Colon Rectum* 1967;10:205.

112. Hulman G, Kirkham JS: Ivalon sponge presenting as an extrarectal mass. *Histopathology* 1990;16:502.

113. Hanson IM, Armstrong GR: Anal intraepithelial neoplasia in an inflammatory cloacogenic polyp. *J Clin Pathol* 1999;52:393.

114. Herbst RA: Perineal streptococcal dermatitis/disease. *Am J Clin Dermatol* 2003;4:555.

115. Eke N: Fournier's gangrene: a review of 1726 cases. *Br J Surg* 2000;87:718.

116. Salvino C, Harford FJ, Dobrin PB: Necrotizing infections of the perineum. *South Med J* 1993;86:908.

117. Culp CE: Chronic hidradenitis suppurativa of the anal canal. *Dis Colon Rectum* 1983;26:669.

Neoplastic Lesions of the Anus

GENERAL COMMENTS

Anal tumors are predominantly squamous in nature, and while they are rare, they have shown an increase in recent years due to the high prevalence of human papilloma virus (HPV) and HIV infections. Tumors arise in both the anal canal and the perianal areas. These include condylomata, intraepithelial neoplasias, invasive carcinomas, neuroendocrine tumors (see Chapter 17), malignant melanomas, mesenchymal tumors (see Chapter 19), hematologic malignancies (see Chapter 18), and secondary tumors.

CONDYLOMATA

Condylomata are benign squamous papillomas caused by HPV infections that exhibit characteristic viral features. They are also commonly referred to as *anogenital warts*. Of note, while they develop in the anal canal, these tumors are not included in the latest World Health Organization (WHO) classification of anal canal tumors (Table 16.1) (1). Anorectal and perianal condylomata frequently develop in individuals who engage in anal intercourse (2). Their incidence has increased by 50% in recent decades (3), a fact attributed to changes in sexual practices. HIV-infected persons have a high prevalence of anal HPV infections and the neoplasms that develop as a result of the infection. Most patients are male, many of whom admit to having sex with other men. Patients with anal condylomata frequently have coexisting penile, perineal, perianal, anorectal junction, or vulvar lesions. Many patients have recurrent lesions.

Anogenital warts also affect children as the result of increased early sexual activity; sexual abuse; and acquisition of the virus from the tissues of the birth canal at the time of delivery. The anatomic distribution of anal condylomata in children differs from that seen in adults. Seventy-seven percent of boys have perianal disease compared with 8% of adults. Affected children range in age from birth to 17 years, with an average of 5.5 years (4).

Condylomata result from infection by HPV types 1, 2, 6, 7, 10, 11, 16, and 18. HPV 6 and 11 represent the most common HPV types found in genital warts (Fig 16.1) (5). Marked atypia or the presence of carcinoma suggests a coexisting HPV 16 or 18 infection.

Condylomata develop in the anal transitional zone or on the perianal skin (Figs. 16.2 and 16.3). The gross features vary widely, with the spectrum of lesions ranging from single to multiple growths and from small benign "bumps" to extensive papillary, warty, cauliflowerlike superficial tumors covering large mucosal areas. Tumors that develop in the anal canal tend to have an acuminate or flat gross appearance. Those arising in the perianal areas tend to be more papillary in nature. Fifty percent of patients with perianal warts have condylomata in the anal canal (6). Nonkeratinized condylomata have a characteristic soft pinkish purple appearance, whereas keratinized lesions appear gray-white. Occasional tumors are pigmented. Smaller lesions are smooth, translucent, and almost vesiclelike. Smaller lesions may coalesce into larger ones, especially in immunosuppressed individuals and diabetics.

Condylomata consist of benign, acanthotic, papillomatous, squamous growths with variable thickening of the stratum corneum, superficial parakeratosis, and dyskeratosis (Fig. 16.4). The rete ridges appear elongated, broadened, and blunted, mimicking the pattern of pseudoepitheliomatous hyperplasia. A normally oriented basal cell layer measuring one to three cells in thickness lies at the base of the neoplastic proliferation. The cells above the basal layer show an orderly progression of squamous cell maturation, a pattern contrasting with the disorderly cellular maturation seen in Bowen disease or squamous cell carcinoma. A well-defined border separates the proliferating squamous epithelium from its underlying supporting stroma. The superficial cells appear large and contain clear cytoplasm with a central hyperchromatic nucleus and perinuclear halo, features known as koilocytosis (Fig. 16.5). Koilocytosis along with anisokaryosis, nuclear hyperchromasia, and the presence of binucleate cells correlate with the presence of HPV. Sometimes koilocytes are absent, perhaps secondary to resolution of the viral infection. Scattered mitotic figures, some of which may appear bizarre, may be present in the acanthotic epithelium. The stroma contains chronic inflammation, and the tissue may appear edematous with vascular dilation.

Some condylomata grow in a flat pattern (Fig. 16.2) similar to that seen in the cervix. Such lesions, sometimes referred to as *condyloma planum*, show koilocytosis (Fig. 16.5) and

TABLE 16.1	World Health Organization Classification of Anal Carcinomas

Carcinomas of the anal canal

Squamous cell carcinoma
  Large cell keratinizing
  Small cell nonkeratinizing (transitional)
  Basaloid
Adenocarcinoma
  Rectal type
  Anal gland
  Carcinomas arising in fistulas
Small cell carcinoma
Undifferentiated

Carcinomas of the anal margin

Keratinizing or nonkeratinizing squamous cell carcinoma
Verrucous carcinoma (giant condyloma)
Bowen disease
Bowenoid papulosis
Basal cell carcinoma
Paget disease
Sweat gland tumors

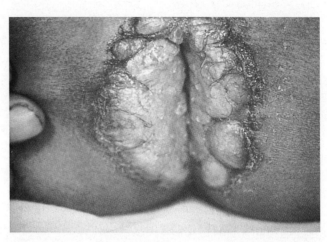

FIG. 16.2. Flat condyloma diffusely involving the perianal region.

other cytologic features of condylomata but lack the prominent acanthotic growth pattern typical of the more common condyloma acuminatum.

Condylomata may contain areas of intraepithelial neoplasia or invasive carcinomas (Fig. 16.6). The gross appearance cannot be used to distinguish between condylomata with and without areas of high-grade dysplasia or early invasive carcinoma. These diagnoses can only be made following histologic examination of biopsies or resected lesions. Subtle and/or abrupt transitions occur from benign condylomatous areas to the more malignant areas. Areas of typical condyloma, carcinoma in situ, and invasive carcinoma often coexist. With the development of dysplasia, the cells become disorganized, mitoses appear above the basal layer, and the number of dyskeratotic cells increases. Invasive cancers usually develop in the centers of the lesions. The diagnosis of invasive carcinoma is made once the neoplastic cells pass through the basement membrane. Malignant foci are characterized by marked loss of cellular maturation, severe nuclear pleomorphism, an increased nuclear:cytoplasmic ratio, and stromal desmoplasia surrounding invasive cell nests. The histology of the malignant cell populations is discussed further below. There does not appear to be any difference in the biology of condylomata with and without areas of dysplasia in terms of the likelihood of recurrence.

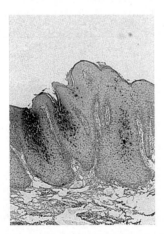

FIG. 16.1. Condyloma. In situ hybridization for human papillomavirus.

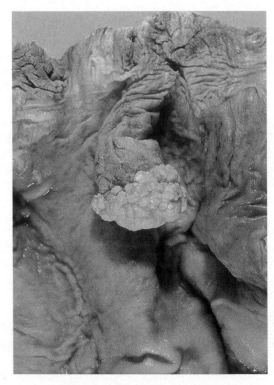

FIG. 16.3. Pedunculated condyloma.

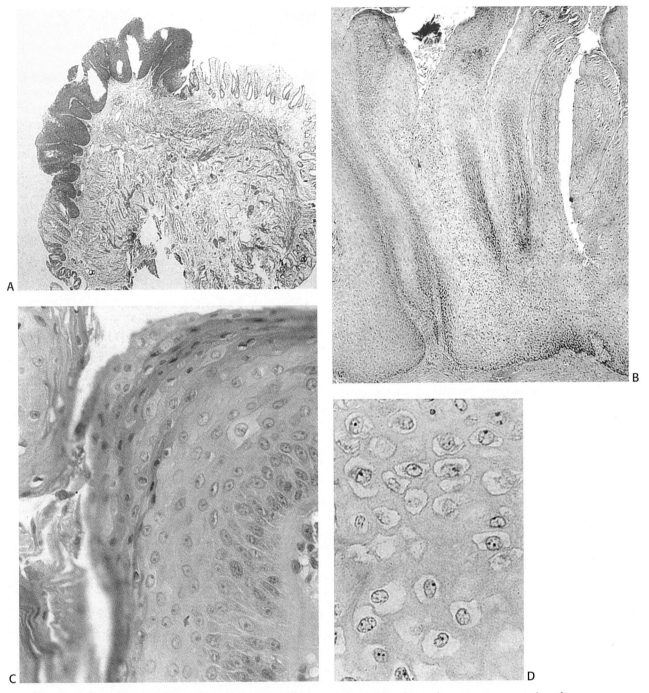

FIG. 16.4. Condyloma acuminatum. **A:** A condyloma extends from the anal squamous mucosa into the anal canal abutting on the rectal mucosa. **B:** High-power magnification demonstrates the acanthotic squamous proliferation. **C:** High magnification demonstrating the parakeratosis. **D:** Koilocytosis.

Because of their location, condylomata often become secondarily inflamed, and reactive changes can be mistaken for areas of dysplasia. Inflamed condylomata are characterized by the presence of interstitial inflammation and edema, superficial vacuolization independent of koilocytosis, and variable degrees of basal cell hyperplasia and hypertrophy. In

contrast to dysplasia, the basal nuclei do not appear irregular, and they exhibit a more or less orderly pattern of maturation. The nuclei are nonoverlapping, contrasting with areas of intraepithelial neoplasias.

Anal and perianal warts may be treated with podophyllotoxin and/or imiquimod at home or by various surgical or

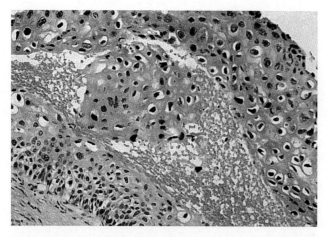

FIG. 16.5. Flat condyloma demonstrating prominent koilocytosis and a disorderly cellular arrangement.

cryotherapy procedures in the office (7). Venereal warts treated with podophyllin may appear histologically alarming and mimic dysplasia.

LESIONS OF THE ANAL CANAL

Intraepithelial Neoplasia

The terminology of anal canal intraepithelial neoplasia has changed over the last few decades. These lesions were originally referred to as squamous dysplasia and carcinoma in situ. In the last edition of this book we termed these lesions anal canal intraepithelial neoplasias. Currently the terminology is evolving to a designation of *anal squamous intraepithelial lesions (ASILs)* in a manner analogous to the terminology used in the classification of cervical neoplasias. Like cervical

squamous intraepithelial lesions (SILs), ASILs are divided into low-grade (LSILs) and high-grade (HSILs) lesions. Indeed, as will be seen, cervical SILs and ASILs share common histologies and etiologies. In all of these lesions the neoplastic cells are confined to the area above the basement membrane.

ASILs originate in both the transitional and squamous zones of the anal canal, often at the squamocolumnar junction, a feature shared with cervical neoplasia. Furthermore, the transitional zone often contains immature squamous epithelium, a cell type that may be particularly vulnerable to infection by high-risk HPV types. HPV infections play a critical role in the development of ASILs and anal carcinoma (8), and an HSIL is considered to be the immediate precursor lesion for invasive squamous cell carcinoma. SILs have been noted in the mucosa adjacent to invasive tumors in 70% to 84% of patients (9,10).

Risk factors for anal HPV infection include HIV positivity (in both men and women), high-risk lifestyles, a history of smoking (11), and organ transplantation. The frequency of HPV in HSILs and LSILs is high among men who have sex with men, especially in those with HIV infections. Approximately 95% of HIV-infected gay men and 65% of HIV-negative gay men develop HPV infections of the anal canal or the perianal skin (12). The prevalence is also high among HIV-positive drug users, and in these patients there may not be a history of anal intercourse (13). The high risk for HPV infections in HIV-infected persons relates in part to the low CD4 cell counts present in these patients. Patients with CD4+ cell counts $<500 \times 10^6$ cells/L are especially at risk. The benefits of high activity antiretroviral therapy (HAART) in restoring immune function and reducing opportunistic infections means that many patients are living longer than prior to HAART (14). As a result, the incidence of HPV infections and ASILs has increased in HAART-treated patients (15). HPV genotypes 6 and 11 associate with LSILs,

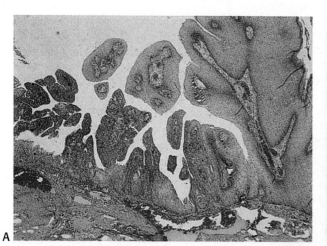

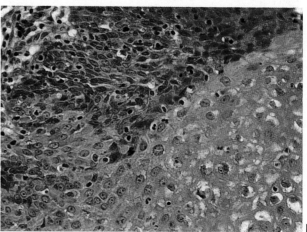

FIG. 16.6. Carcinoma in situ arising in an anal condyloma. **A:** The area of malignant transformation is shown in the left-hand part of the figure. At the right is residual benign condyloma. **B:** Higher magnification showing the junction of the area of carcinoma in situ (*upper left*) with the more benign koilocytotic cells in the lower right.

whereas HPV genotypes 16 and 18 associate with HSILs (16). The progression of LSILs to HSILs occurs over a short period of time (2 to 4 years) in HIV-infected homosexual men (12,17). The average age of patients with SILs is younger than that of patients with invasive carcinomas. The relationship of HPV to anal neoplasia is discussed further in the next section.

The prevalence of ASILs is significantly higher in men with evidence of anal HPV infections, including the presence of anal warts or the presence of flat, white epithelium. In such patients, dysplasia is present in up to 36% of cases by cytologic evaluation and in 92% of patients by biopsy. As many as a third of the patients have HSILs (18). Of women with anal HPV infections, 35.7% have cervical intraepithelial neoplasia (CIN); some also have ASILs. Additionally, vaginal or vulvar intraepithelial neoplasia may extend to the anus. ASILs are also demonstrable in 0.2% to 2.3% of minor surgical specimens, such as hemorrhoids. ASILs are seen with increased frequency in incidental surgical specimens from homosexual men (19).

Patients may present with bleeding or pruritus, or they may remain completely asymptomatic. ASILs may present as eczematoid or papillomatous areas, papules, or macules. Anoscopy facilitates the detection of ASILs and the delineation of their extent. Indigo carmine dye spraying of the mucosa may help define the limits of the lesions (20). Examination of biopsies and cytologic preparations is required to detect or confirm the presence of LSILs and HSILs. Unfortunately, the agreement among pathologists or cytologists for the diagnosis of ASIL is only moderate (21,22).

The histologic features of ASILs resemble those of CIN. ASILs consist of a thickened proliferating epithelium (Fig. 16.7) containing undifferentiated cells with a high

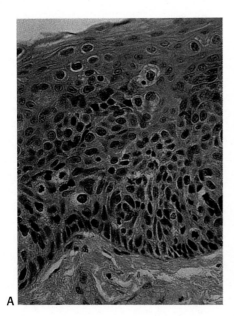

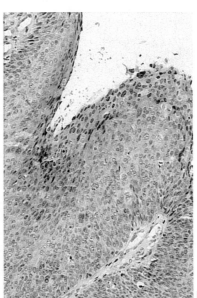

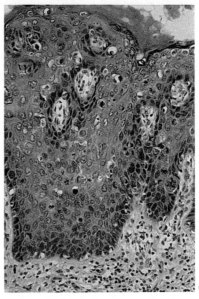

FIG. 16.7. Anal canal intraepithelial neoplasia (ACIN). **A:** Note the proliferation of atypical cells with numerous and sometimes abnormal mitotic figures. The process does not extend all the way to the surface. **B:** Cells appear smaller and more hyperchromatic with extension of abnormal-appearing nuclei all the way to the free surface. Some koilocytotic changes are also evident. **C:** Even when the mucosa is tangentially cut, as evidenced by cross sections of numerous stromal cores, it is possible to diagnose ACIN by virtue of the disorderly appearance of the epithelium and the presence of increased and abnormal mitoses.

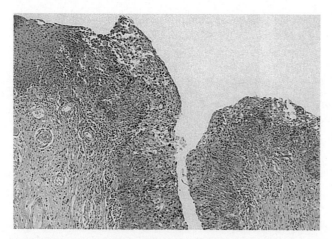

FIG. 16.8. Sometimes anal intraepithelial neoplasias become markedly infiltrated with lymphocytes as shown in this illustration.

nuclear:cytoplasmic ratio extending from the basal layer toward the mucosal surface (5). There is often an abrupt transition between the normal and the dysplastic epithelium. Varying degrees of nuclear pleomorphism and mitotic activity are present. The lesions may or may not show superficial hyperkeratosis or parakeratosis, contrasting with perianal lesions. The cytologically malignant cells lose their normal polarity, overlapping with one another throughout the neoplastic disorderly epithelium. The basal cells appear hyperplastic. The lesions grow in a flat fashion or they form neoplastic acanthotic fingers. Variable thicknesses of the mucosa may be replaced by the neoplastic cells. When the neoplastic proliferation occupies two thirds or more of the mucosal thickness, the lesion is classified as an HSIL. Neoplastic proliferations occupying less than two thirds of the mucosa are classified as an LSIL. Pigmented dendritic cells often lie among the neoplastic cells. A prominent lymphocytic infiltrate may underlie the neoplastic proliferation (Fig. 16.8).

The neoplastic cells may extend into underlying anal glands. Alternatively, one may see entrapped, normal-appearing anal transitional zone epithelium, not yet replaced by the neoplastic process. The neoplastic cells may also extend into skin appendages. These extensions may reach a median depth of 1.14 mm for involved hair follicles and 1.44 mm for the involved sweat glands with a range up to 2.2 mm. This means that to completely eradicate the disease, tissue destruction or removal must reach a depth of at least 2.2 mm below the adjacent basement membrane (23).

Because of the effectiveness of cervical screening programs in reducing the incidence of cervical neoplasia, the use of anal-rectal cytology (ARC) is increasing in evaluating anal HPV-related diseases in high-risk individuals (men who have sex with men and HIV-infected persons). ARC is an accurate, noninvasive, and cost-effective screening method for ASILs (24). Its sensitivity for detecting biopsy-proven ASILs was 69% in HIV-positive men and 47% in HIV-negative men at the first visit in one study. Repeat cytology increased the sensitivity to 81% and 50%, respectively, in these two groups of men (25). ARC is also used to examine HIV-infected adolescents or those with high-risk sexual behavior (26).

ARC does not require anoscopy or special patient preparation before the examination other than refraining from receptive anal intercourse before the examination. The areas to be sampled should include the anal canal and the area of the anorectal junction, but not the perianal skin. They are collected using a tap water-moistened swab. If the sample is to be examined in a liquid-based cytology preparation, the swab is placed in the preservative vial and agitated to release the harvested cells. Alternatively, the swab can be smeared on a glass slide in a manner analogous to the conventional cervical Pap smear. The cytologic specimens can also be used for oncogenic HPV testing.

ARCs are interpreted according to the Bethesda 2001 guidelines modified for this site. Thus, the cytologic features are divided into atypical squamous cell lesions, LSILs, and HSILs (27). The second edition of the *Bethesda System Atlas* provides guidelines for specimen interpretation and evaluation of the adequacy of ARC (27). If the specimen contains metaplastic cells and rectal cells, one can be certain that the transitional zone has been sampled. LSILs are characterized by the presence of koilocytes and superficial and high intermediate cells with an increased nuclear:cytoplasmic ratio. Binucleate cells are common. The nuclear membrane is often irregular and angular. Chromatin clumping and hyperchromasia may also be present. Atypical parakeratotic cells may be present, especially in men with increasing degrees of immunodeficiency (28). HSILs consist of intermediate cells or immature squamous metaplastic cells. They have high nuclear:cytoplasmic ratios with nuclear enlargement. Coarse chromatin is present in the nuclei along with irregular wrinkled nuclear membranes. Nucleoli are inconspicuous. These cells may be dispersed singly or arranged in clusters. Parakeratosis is common. Of note, the features of HSILs and invasive carcinoma overlap somewhat since the typical tumor diathesis background picture of invasive cancer is often absent from the invasive anal canal lesions.

HSILs are treated to prevent the development of invasive carcinomas using excisional or ablative techniques (29); some clinicians require complete excision of the lesion with histologically negative margins. However, the lesions may be difficult to remove completely so that recurrences are common. LSILs tend to be followed and some cases spontaneously regress over time.

Anal Canal Carcinomas: General Comments

The terminology for anal carcinomas has been confusing for decades due to the fact that the histology of the anal canal is relatively complex, as discussed in Chapter 15, and the histologies of the tumors can be quite variable. Thus, terms such as *cloacogenic, keratinizing or nonkeratinizing squamous, basaloid, transitional, mucoepidermoid,* and *adenoid cystic carcinomas* have been applied to tumors arising in this site. The reproducibility of these diagnoses was also problematic in part because some of the terms were used interchangeably. A recent study showed that the subdivision of the squamous cell variants that arise in this site has a low level of intra- and interpathologist reproducibility (30). Others have shown that there is little or no prognostic significance in separating these tumors into their variant histologic patterns (31–34). Furthermore, all of these patterns show an etiologic association with HPV infections. Because of these concerns, the current WHO classification eliminated many of these terms. The current simplified WHO classification of anal tumors is more practical and reproducible (Table 16.1) (1).

Squamous Cell Carcinomas

The vast majority of anal canal carcinomas are squamous cell carcinomas (SCCs). These are far more common in the anal canal than in the anal margin (35), and in some ways they are more similar to genital malignancies than they are to other gastrointestinal cancers.

Epidemiology and Patient Demographics

Anal carcinomas are rare tumors, accounting for only 1.5% of gastrointestinal tumors. Studies based on data from the Surveillance, Epidemiology, and End Results (SEER) program show that anal canal cancer incidence has increased in the United States, especially in cities such as San Francisco, where the incidence has doubled. The incidence of anal cancer in the United States is 0.5 per 100,000 population for men and 0.8 per 100,000 for women (36). The recent increase among men having sex with men suggests that homosexual men belong to an increased–risk group. HPV can be found in 88% to 98% of men having sex with men (37–39). The incidence rate for anal cancer for single males is 6.1 times that of married males. This excess is limited to squamous variants (40). There is also an increased incidence among HIV-positive men, despite the introduction of HAART (41). HAART-treated HIV-infected persons are living longer so that it is likely that the natural history of anal HPV infections and anal cancer will change and likely increase. Further, there is evidence that because of the availability of better therapies, individuals are practicing much less safe sex.

Anal canal tumors develop in all adult age groups, but women tend to present in their 5th and 7th decades (31,36). Men between the ages of 20 and 49 have a higher incidence of squamous cell carcinomas than women (36). The age of patients with HPV-related anal tumors is significantly less than that of patients with HPV-negative tumors (42).

Etiology and Predisposing Factors

The etiology of anal SCCs is multifactorial and represents an interaction between both genetic and environmental factors. Decades ago, anal cancer was thought to develop in areas that were chronically inflamed as the result of benign conditions such as fissures, fistulae, hemorrhoids, or Crohn disease (43–46). Today these factors are not believed to play a major role in the pathogenesis of anal cancer. Numerous epidemiologic studies have shown that the strongest risk factors for anal carcinoma include HPV infection (11,16,47,48), lifetime number of sexual partners (39,49), cigarette smoking (particularly in women) (48), genital warts (a manifestation of HPV infection) (49,50), receptive anal intercourse (11,39,49), and HIV infection (11,51–53). The risk of invasive carcinoma in HPV-infected individuals increases in the setting of HIV, perhaps related to the decrease in anal mucosal Langerhans cells (54). Females who engage in anal intercourse show a strong association with the disease (55), as do those with HIV infections (48), previous infection with herpesvirus or *Chlamydia trachomatis,* or a positive or questionable cervical Pap smear. Squamous cell carcinoma involving the anal canal is more often positive for high-risk HPV (92%) than perianal SCC (64%) (56).

HPV DNA is present in 81% of anal SCCs in both males and females. HPV types 16, 18, and 33 play important etiologic roles in the genesis of the tumors (5). HPV 31, 35, and 51 are also present in some tumors. It is not uncommon to find a mixture of the "benign" HPV 6 or 11 coexisting with the "malignant" HPV 16 and 18 in the same lesion. HPV 16 or 18 infections predispose individuals to increased cancer risk through the accumulation of mutational events that eventually lead to chromosomal instability and the conversion of premalignant to invasive growths. High-risk HPVs encode three oncogenes: E5, E6, and E7. The E6 and E7 viral proteins bind and inactivate the tumor suppressor proteins p53 and Rb, respectively, leading to subsequent uncontrolled cell proliferation (57). E5 is thought to transform cells by modulating growth factor receptors, and the epidermal growth factor receptor (EGFR) is required for the hyperplastic properties of E5 (58). HPV is more likely to be present in tumors with the following features: Basaloid histology, adjacent SIL, poor or absent keratinization, and a predominance of small or medium-sized tumor cells (51).

Host immune defenses also play an important role in the genesis of anal cancer because anal cancers occur more commonly in immunosuppressed individuals such as HIV-infected and transplant patients. These patients show a strong association with HPV infections, which occur at a younger age; are multifocal, persistent, and recurrent; and progress rapidly (59).

Clinical Features

The signs and symptoms of anal SCCs are often nonspecific, so that 76% of cancers are initially diagnosed as benign lesions. The clinical manifestations relate to tumor size and the extent of mural invasion. Patients with anal cancer present with rectal bleeding, pruritus, pain, discharge, swelling, and perianal ulceration. As the tumors grow, patients develop worsening pain, changes in bowel habits, incontinence, the

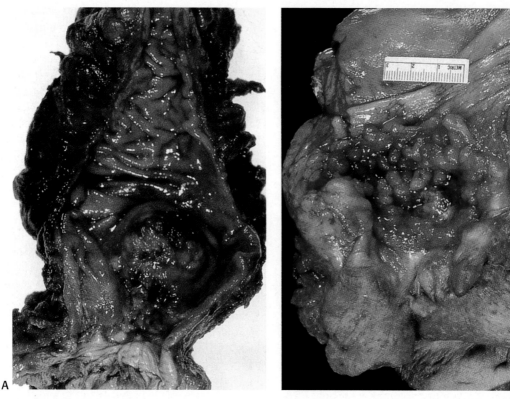

FIG. 16.9. Anal canal carcinomas. **A:** Obstructing carcinoma in the anal canal. **B:** Ulcerating and exophytic squamous cell carcinoma.

sensation of a rectal mass, tenesmus, weight loss, diarrhea, ulceration, incontinence, and fistulae (60). Symptom duration may range up to 4 years, with most patients being symptomatic for more than 6 months (61). Many patients have enlarged inguinal lymph nodes at the time of presentation. Squamous cell carcinomas appear to behave more virulently in men than in women (62).

Pathologic Features

Most anal canal SCCs arise at or above the dentate line in the area of the transitional epithelial zone (Fig. 16.9). Larger tumors in the middle or lower canal may grow into the anal orifice, but most anal canal tumors are not visible at this site. Tumors arising in condylomata may appear as indurated polypoid masses or as mucosal or submucosal plaques. They may also appear as an ulcer or fissure with slightly raised indurated margins. The color of the tumor may differ from that of the surrounding mucosa. The tumors range in size from 0.5 cm to up to 15 cm in diameter (63). Larger tumors appear as areas of ulceration or as fungating masses that may become fixed to the underlying structures.

The tumors consist of invasive elongated and angulated tumor nests that contain large pale eosinophilic squamous cells (Fig. 16.10) with or without areas of keratinization. The tumor cells have prominent cytoplasmic borders, but intercellular

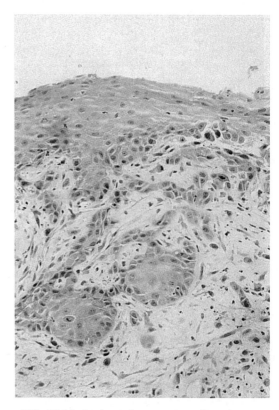

FIG. 16.10. Anal canal squamous cell carcinoma.

junctions are often absent. The cells may contain a clear or granular cytoplasm. Better differentiated tumors may demonstrate peripheral palisading, a pattern that disappears as the tumors become less differentiated. Central necrosis may be present. The hyperchromatic nuclei appear round, ovoid, and vesicular, containing numerous mitotic figures. Rarely, keratinizing large cell SCC components are present (Fig. 16.11). Basaloid areas may be present. These consist of small to intermediate-sized basaloid cells with minimal keratinization, peripheral palisading, comedolike necrosis in the center of the lobular tumor islands (Fig 16.12), and the possible deposition of basement membrane–like material (which imparts an adenoid cystic–like pattern) (64). Tumor areas resembling adenoid cystic carcinoma may show prominent perineural invasion (Fig. 16.13). The basaloid areas are compared to perianal basal cell carcinomas in Table 16.2. The cells of what was previously termed *transitional cell carcinoma* consist of larger elongated cells containing plentiful clear (Fig. 16.14) or slightly eosinophilic cytoplasm arranged in anastomosing cords and islands that are sharply demarcated from the surrounding stroma. The cells at the epithelial stromal junction may show an attempt at palisading. Tumors that contain foci of mucin secretion or small mucin lakes were previously termed *mucoepidermoid carcinomas* (Fig. 16.15); they are currently termed *squamous cell carcinomas*

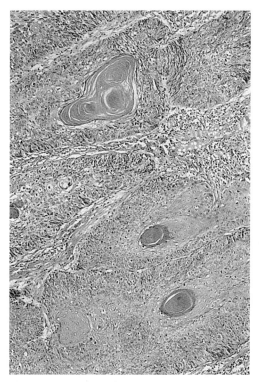

FIG. 16.11. Squamous cell anal canal carcinoma. Note the prominent central keratinization. The surrounding stroma is desmoplastic.

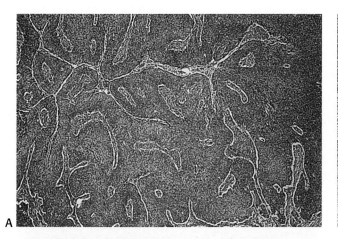

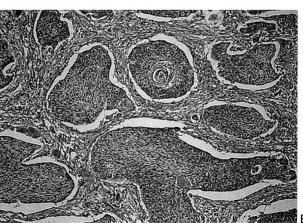

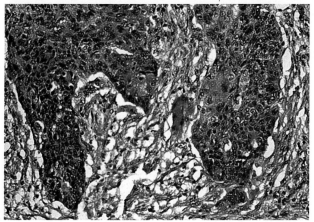

FIG. 16.12. Anal canal carcinoma. **A:** Low-power magnification of one of the squamous variants demonstrating a somewhat basaloid appearance. **B:** Higher-power magnification of the lesion shown in A. **C:** Small neoplastic cells are present. Focal squamous differentiation is seen.

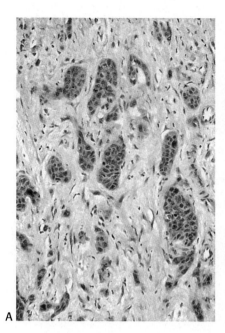

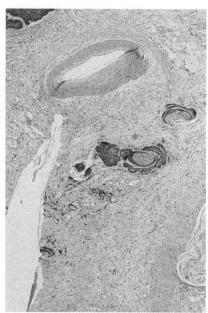

FIG. 16.13. Squamous cell carcinoma. **A:** Infiltrating nests of large, well-demarcated cells without obvious squamous differentiation. **B:** Prominent perineural invasion is present mimicking an adenoid cystic pattern.

with mucinous microcysts (1). Sarcomatoid carcinomas (65) and *anal clear cell variants* also occur (66).

SCCs often show a progression of squamous cell lesions that may include condylomata, SILs, and invasive carcinoma. In other instances, the tumor appears to "drop off" an overlying more or less normal-appearing squamous epithelium (Fig. 16.16). The tumors are often positive for EGFR (Fig 16.17) and p53 protein.

In earlier classifications of anal canal tumors, a grading system was proposed based on two criteria: The presence or absence of squamous cell elements and the degree of differentiation of the transitional cell component (67). However, the current classification advises against grading these tumors since generally the only tissue that is available is a small biopsy, which may not be representative of the entire tumor (1).

Spread of Anal Canal Cancer

Anal canal SCCs spread locally to the lower rectum, to the anal sphincter, and into the ischiorectal fossa. The submu-

cosal layer is very narrow in the anal canal and hence, the mucosa lies very close to the anal sphincter, explaining why anal canal carcinomas often infiltrate this structure. Local perineal invasion with involvement of the posterior vaginal septum, prostate, or bladder affects 15% to 20% of patients. Lateral growth into the ischiorectal fossa may present as an abscess, a fistula, or eventual annular stenosis.

Lesions of the middle and proximal anal canal spread to the mesorectal, superior hemorrhoidal, and inferior mesenteric lymph nodes. Mesorectal node involvement occurs in up to 56% of tumors measuring >4 cm. Metastasis to inguinal lymph nodes occurs in 10% to 25% of tumors and approximately 25% have bilateral lymph node involvement (68). Lower rectal lesions preferentially spread toward the hemorrhoidal lymph nodes and, later, to the superficial inguinal lymph nodes. Up to 44% of lymph node metastases affect lymph nodes measuring <5 mm in diameter, with most positive lymph nodes lying above the peritoneal reflection. Because of the small size of the perianal and perirectal

TABLE 16.2   Comparison of the Basaloid Variant of Squamous Cell Carcinoma and Basal Cell Carcinoma

Characteristic	Basaloid Variant	Basal Cell Carcinoma
Tumor location	Usually anal canal	Usually anal margin
Peripheral palisading	Often inconspicuous	Prominent
Cell characteristics	Highly pleomorphic	Minimal pleomorphism
Invasiveness	Highly invasive	Locally invasive
Metastatic potential	High	Low
CEA	Positive	Negative
EMA	Positive	Negative
Ber-EP4	Negative	Positive
CK 19, 22, AE1	Positive	Negative

CEA, carcinoembryonic antigen; EMA, epithelial membrane antigen.

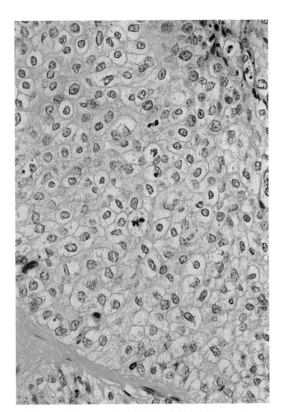

FIG. 16.14. Squamous cell carcinoma with the so-called transitional cell pattern and prominent clear cell features.

lymph nodes, many anal canal SCCs are understaged due to failure to find the lymph nodes (69).

Vascular invasion develops less frequently than lymphatic spread, affecting 10% of patients. Hematogenous spread causes distant metastases in the liver, lung, skin, brain, perineum, or spinal cord. Distant metastases affect up to 10% of patients at the time of diagnosis (62); another 10% to 15% of patients develop metastases during the course of their disease. The American Joint Committee on Cancer (AJCC) staging scheme for anal canal carcinomas is presented in Table 16.3.

Prognosis

The prognosis of anal carcinomas depends on the site of origin, tumor size, depth of invasion, extent of local spread, and nodal status (31,62,70,71). Tumor size inversely correlates with prognosis and strongly associates with tumor stage. Lesions that only invade into the submucosa have an excellent prognosis (31). Tumor size is one of the most important prognostic factors, with most tumors measuring <2 cm in diameter being amenable to cure (71). Tumors measuring >8 cm demonstrate a 5-year survival rate of 31% to 47.3%, contrasting with those measuring <8 cm, which have a 75% 5-year survival rate (62). Tumor stage is also important and in part relates to tumor size. Five-year survival rates for early-stage disease are 65% to 71.3% for stage I compared with 23.1% to 33% for stage IV disease (72,73). Patients with distant metastases have a 5-year survival rate of 11%. Patients whose tumors show a squamous histology have a 5-year survival rate of 57.5% compared with 41.3% for adenocarcinoma (73). Patients with inguinal lymph node metastases have a poor prognosis, with a 5-year survival rate of <20% (74).

Tumor location is also important. Squamous cell carcinomas arising at the anal margin have a better prognosis than those arising in the anal canal, likely due to the fact that those at the anal margin present as smaller tumors that are more easily cured by local excision (see below). DNA ploidy analysis does not consistently reach independent prognostic significance relative to histologic grade or tumor stage when examined in multivariate analysis (75). However, p53 overexpression may associate with an inferior outcome for patients with anal canal tumors treated with chemoradiation (76).

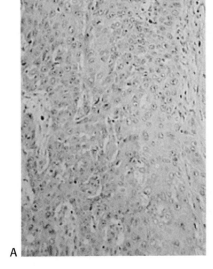
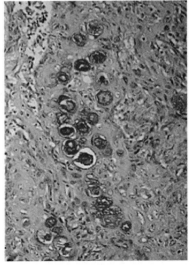

FIG. 16.15. Squamous cell carcinoma with mucinous microcysts. **A:** Hematoxylin and eosin–stained section showing what appears to be a predominantly squamous cell carcinoma. **B:** Mucin stain demonstrating prominent mucin accumulations in the squamous proliferation.

A   B

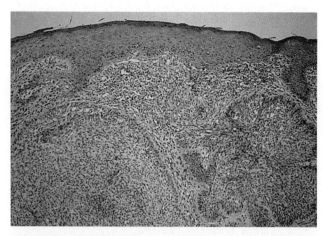

FIG. 16.16. Basaloid variant of squamous cell carcinoma. Note the prominent peripheral palisading of the malignant cells in the underlying stroma. The overlying epithelium appears normal.

Treatment

Currently the most effective therapy is the early detection of the tumors and their precursors. In recent years, surgery alone has been replaced by the organ-sparing combination of radiotherapy and chemotherapy as the primary treatment in patients with anal squamous cell cancers (71,77). Because the tumors may spread to the rectal mesenteric, hypogastric, and inguinal lymph nodes, these sites should be included in the initial radiation management of the tumors (78). Surgery is usually reserved for residual or recurrent disease. In contrast, most patients with adenocarcinomas undergo aggressive surgery with radiation and chemotherapy for control of local disease and treatment of metastatic disease (73,79). The overall 5-year survival rate for patients with anal canal tumors is 60% to 80% for patients undergoing combined radiation therapy and chemotherapy and around 60% for

those undergoing abdominoperineal resection (74). Virtually all anal canal carcinomas strongly express EGFR (Fig. 16.17) and EGFR expression correlates with the proliferative rate of the tumors (80), suggesting that the tumors may be effectively treated with EGFR-targeted therapies. The role of HPV vaccines as a way to prevent the tumors is still to be determined.

Adenocarcinomas: General Comments

Anal adenocarcinomas account for 8% to 19% of anal carcinomas (74,81) and fall into several groups, including those that arise from the colorectal mucosa in the upper anal canal, the anal glands, and their draining ducts and those arising in

TABLE 16.3 TNM Staging of Carcinomas of the Anal Canal

Primary tumor

TX	Primary tumor cannot be assessed
T0	No primary tumor
Tis	Carcinoma in situ
T1	<2 cm in greatest dimension
T2	2–5 cm in greatest dimension
T3	>5 cm in greatest dimension
T4	Invasion of adjacent organ

Regional lymph nodes

NX	Lymph nodes cannot be assessed
N0	No lymph node metastases
N1	Perirectal lymph nodes involved
N2	Unilateral internal iliac and/or inguinal lymph nodes involved
N3	Bilateral internal iliac and/or inguinal lymph nodes involved or perirectal and inguinal lymph nodes involved

Distant metastases

MX	Cannot be assessed
M0	Absent
M1	Present

Stage grouping

Stage 0	Tis	N0	M0
Stage I	T1	N0	M0
Stage II	T2	N0	M0
	T3	N0	M0
Stage IIIA	T1	N1	M0
	T2	N1	M0
	T3	N1	M0
	T4	N0	M0
Stage IIIB	T4	N1	M0
	Any T	N2	M0
	Any T	N3	M0
Stage IV	Any T	Any N	M1

Adapted from the American Joint Committee on Cancer (AJCC). *Cancer Staging Manual,* 6th ed. Springer-Verlag, New York, NY, 2001.

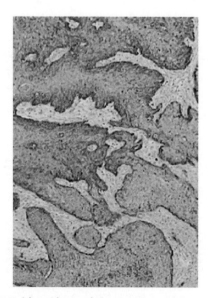

FIG. 16.17. Epidermal growth factor receptor immunoreactivity.

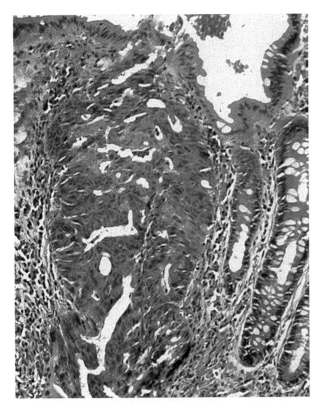

FIG. 16.18. Rectal-type anal canal adenocarcinoma.

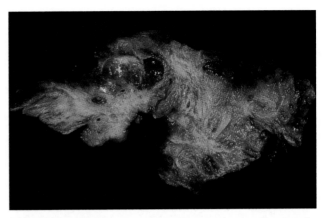

FIG. 16.19. Gross features of anal duct carcinoma showing the presence of prominent deep cystic spaces.

fistulae. All of these tumors are graded in the same way as rectal adenocarcinomas (1).

Adenocarcinomas of the Rectal Type

Adenocarcinomas arise in the upper part of the anal canal from the rectal-type epithelium present at this site, or they represent extensions of primary rectal adenocarcinomas with the majority representing extensions of rectal carcinomas. These tumors show no relationship to HPV infections. They present clinically in the same way as anal canal SCCs. Grossly and histologically, primary anal adenocarcinomas resemble their rectal counterparts (Fig. 16.18) (see Chapter 14). Like their rectal counterparts, the tumors may contain variable numbers of endocrine cells. These range from isolated endocrine cells to tumors showing combined features of adenocarcinoma and carcinoid (82).

Anal Gland Carcinoma

Anal gland carcinoma is a rare and controversial entity. Their rarity and confusion with adenocarcinomas arising in fistulae make statements concerning their demographics difficult. The latest WHO classification stresses an origin from the anal glands or the ducts that drain them in order to classify these tumors as anal gland neoplasms (1). However, a complicating feature is the fact that some anal fistulae may result from infections in the anal glands. Anal gland carcinomas

primarily affect older men (83). The etiology of these tumors is unknown.

The tumors lie within the submucosa of the anal canal (Fig. 16.19), sometimes producing a submucosal mass. The overlying mucosa usually appears normal unless the tumor has extended to the mucosa, in which case a small erosion may be present. A tumor that arises near the orifice of the anal duct may appear as a small polypoid, rough, ulcerated area in the anal crypt at the dentate line.

The current WHO classification stresses the fact that the tumor acini be lined by cuboidal cells with little or no mucin production (1). However, we have seen mucinous adenocarcinomas developing in this region that coexisted with intraepithelial neoplasia in the anal ducts so that the WHO criteria appear to be overly restrictive to us. Others have also described mucinous carcinomas arising from the anal glands (84,85). We believe that anal duct carcinomas may show two different histologic patterns. One pattern that corresponds to the strict definition of the WHO classification consists of collections of very well-differentiated glands lined by mildly atypical columnar cells with hyperchromatic nuclei and scattered, scant mucin droplets in the cytoplasm; cellular stratification (Fig. 16.20); and papillary formations. Occasionally, one appreciates coexisting intraepithelial malignancy in early lesions (Fig. 16.21). The other pattern, the *colloid variant*, consists of prominent acellular to paucicellular mucinous pools. These mucinous pools (Fig. 16.22) separate the layers of the anorectal wall and adjacent soft tissues as the tumors penetrate the deeper tissue. Epithelial cells may be quite sparse, requiring a diligent search for their presence. Once found, they may manifest little cellular atypia. Malignant glands extending into the anal canal at the pectinate line become surrounded by fibrous tissue containing acute and chronic inflammatory cells and mucinous pools. Signet ring cells may lie in the pools of mucin. The overlying mucosa generally appears intact. Tumors arising from the anal glands express a CK7+/CK20− phenotype (83), a feature shared with benign intramuscular anal glands (86,87).

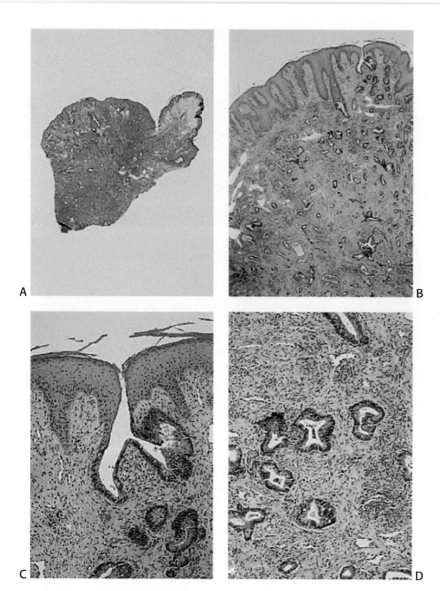

FIG. 16.20. Well-differentiated anal duct carcinoma. **A:** Low-power photograph showing a polypoid mass in the anal canal. **B:** Higher magnification shows the presence of a well-differentiated adenocarcinoma diffusely infiltrating the underlying tissues. Two residual anal ducts can be seen lined by neoplastic epithelium. The acanthotic squamous epithelium also has evidence of pagetoid spread of the anal duct carcinoma. This is illustrated at higher power in Figure 16.23. **C:** Higher magnification of one of the anal ducts demonstrating the neoplastic epithelium. **D:** Higher magnification of some of the infiltrating ducts. (Case courtesy of Dr. G. Boren, St. Francis-St. George Hospital, Cincinnati, OH.)

Generally, anal duct carcinomas spread in an annular extraluminal manner around the anal canal. Recurrences are common. Metastases occur early, perhaps because the tumors arise in normal ducts that already lie deep in the anal wall. Metastatic spread primarily affects pelvic and periaortic lymph nodes; hematogenous metastases occur late. The tumor may also spread in a pagetoid fashion (Fig. 16.23). The tumors are treated surgically. Advanced lesions may receive chemoradiation.

Adenocarcinomas Arising in Anal Fistulae

Well-differentiated adenocarcinomas may develop within an anorectal fistula. These fistulae may be congenital or acquired in nature and some may result from infections in the anal glands and their ducts. These anal fistulae may be lined by anal duct epithelium (88). Because of the relative prevalence of fistula in ano and perirectal abscesses, these initially insidious, slowly growing tumors often remain clinically unsuspected for long periods of time (84,89). Clinical features that suggest their presence include a long history of painful buttock masses associated with discomfort on defecation and occasionally clear mucous discharge. Approximately 15% of patients remain asymptomatic. While the tumors grow slowly, they can be locally aggressive lesions.

Grossly, the tumor presents as a submucosal mass. The tumor typically penetrates the anal sphincter. Cross sections of the anus typically reveal the presence of innocuous-appearing cysts deeper in the anal wall. These tumors tend to be small (89) and may exhibit a yellowish tan color (89). The tumors are typically colloid-type adenocarcinomas. Treatment of this aggressive tumor represents a surgical challenge due to its infiltrative growth pattern, often into the perirectal tissues. Such lesions require wide excisions to remove the entire tumor. Some also advocate the use of radiation therapy or chemoradiation to treat the lesion (90).

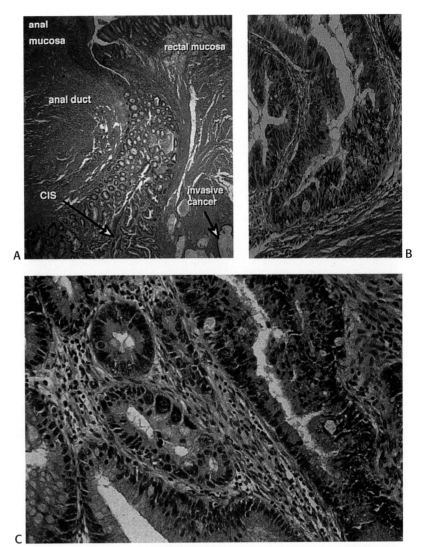

FIG. 16.21. Anal duct carcinoma. **A:** An anal duct extends from the overlying mucosa. The epithelium becomes neoplastic in the deeper part (*long arrow*). An area of invasion is illustrated as well (*short arrow*). **B:** Higher magnification showing the in situ transformation of the anal duct epithelium. **C:** Varying degrees of neoplasia of the pre-existing anal duct.

Other Tumors

Some tumors that develop in the anal canal are undifferentiated. They lack sufficient differentiation to be classified as either squamous or glandular in nature (Fig. 16.24). These tumors are relatively rare and when they develop, they tend to be characterized by a high mitotic activity and an aggressive clinical course. The most anaplastic and most lethal of the anal canal tumors are *small cell carcinomas*. These are discussed further in Chapter 17.

ANAL MARGIN LESIONS

Bowenoid Papulosis

Bowenoid papulosis is an AIDS-defining illness in adults with HIV infections. It consists of one or more pigmented anogenital macules (91). The lesions present as reddish brown to violaceous papules and plaques, sometimes with a verrucous appearance. They remain confined to the perianal area or diffusely involve the anogenital region. Bowenoid papulosis may spread into the anal canal. Pruritus and irritation may develop, although usually the lesions remain asymptomatic. The clinical differential diagnosis includes condylomata, verruca vulgaris, and nevus. The disease is linked to HPV types 16, 18, 31, 32, 34, 39, 42, 51, 52, and 53, with the overwhelming majority of cases linked to HPV 16 (92–94). Bowenoid papulosis, unlike typical squamous cell carcinoma in situ, affects young patients, peaking in incidence during the 3rd decade. The duration of the lesions ranges from a few weeks to several years. The disease is chronic and slowly progressive.

Most lesions measure only a few millimeters in diameter (91). Histologically, bowenoid papulosis appears sharply demarcated from the surrounding normal epithelium. Elongated epidermal rete ridges (irregular acanthosis), occasional significant papillomatosis, varying degrees of hyperkeratosis, focal hypergranulosis, and frequent parakeratosis histologically characterize the lesion (Fig. 16.25). The squamous epithelium matures in an orderly fashion but

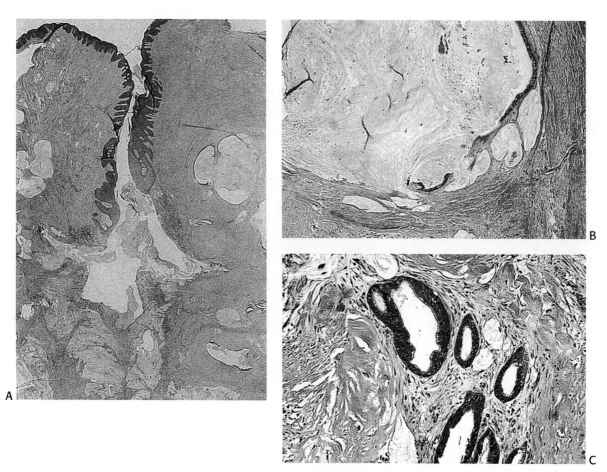

FIG. 16.22. Anal duct carcinoma. **A:** Large mucinous pools that contain scant numbers of malignant cells are present. The central structure represents either a pre-existing fistula or a perianal duct that has become lined by squamous epithelial cells. **B:** High-power magnification of the neoplastic areas in one of the more acellular ones demonstrating large mucinous pools and sparse cells. **C:** Part of the deeper invasive portion of the lesion that is more cellular and demonstrates the presence of neoplastic glands. (Case courtesy of Dr. A. Chang, U.S. Naval Hospital, Norfolk, VA.)

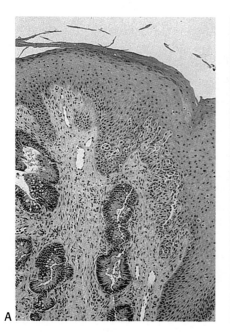

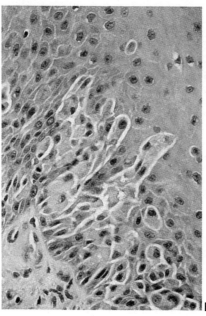

FIG. 16.23. Pagetoid spread of well-differentiated anal duct carcinoma. **A:** Low magnification showing the presence of the infiltrating anal duct carcinoma in the underlying submucosa. Prominent pagetoid spread is seen in the overlying epidermis. **B:** Higher magnification of the pagetoid spread. (Case courtesy of Dr. G. Boren, St. Francis-St. George Hospital, Cincinnati, OH.)

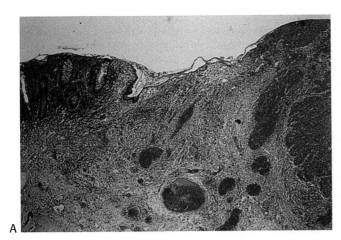

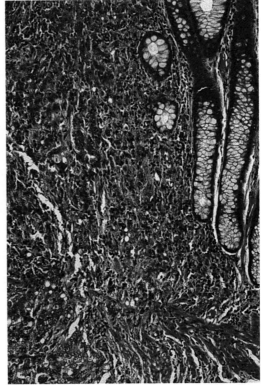

FIG. 16.24. Poorly differentiated anal canal carcinoma. **A:** The tumor arises in the rectal zone of the anal canal and is present at the extreme right-hand portion of the photograph surrounded by a prominent lymphocytic infiltrate. **B:** Higher magnification of the neoplasm shows the presence of infiltrating poorly differentiated cells without obvious glandular or squamous differentiation.

hyperchromatic nuclei and dyskeratotic cells lie at all levels of the epithelium. Frequent and atypical mitoses and atypical keratinocytes with pleomorphic nuclei can be seen. Nuclear viral inclusions are present in the granular and parakeratotic areas (Fig. 16.26) (94). These basophilic bodies, sometimes with a halo, represent a consistent diagnostic feature of Bowenoid papulosis that distinguishes it from ASIL. The tumor spreads intraepidermally and the underlying basement membrane remains intact without invasion through it. The dermal papillae may contain dilated tortuous vessels and a superficial lymphohistiocytic infiltrate.

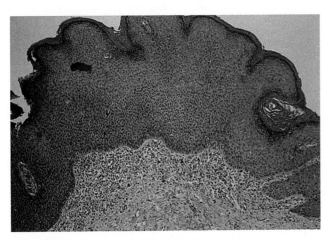

FIG. 16.25. Bowenoid papulosis. Notice the broad hyperkeratotic proliferation of relatively uniform cells.

Bowen Disease

Bowen disease, a form of intraepithelial squamous cell carcinoma, may involve the perianal skin diffusely or in a multicentric fashion (94). The disease mainly affects the elderly. Most lesions are detected in individuals not clinically suspected of having the disease (95). An association with HPV 58 is reported in one case (96). The most common presenting symptoms include itching, burning, pain, or bleeding. Anal Bowen disease acts as a chronic, slow-growing tumor that usually spreads intraepidermally. At least 5% of tumors become invasive and 27% of these metastasize (97).

Grossly, Bowen disease presents as a slightly raised, firm, irregular, erythematous, or reddish brown plaque with a scaly, eczematoid appearance. Ulceration and fissuring may occur. The characteristic microscopic features include a plaquelike epidermal lesion characterized by acanthosis, hyperkeratosis, and/or parakeratosis with a disorderly proliferation of dysplastic dyskeratotic squamous cells throughout the full thickness of the epithelium. The variably sized cells appear disorganized and contain pleomorphic hyperchromatic nuclei (Fig. 16.27). Multinucleated giant cells, vacuolated cells, and mitotic figures appear at all levels in the epidermis. The presence of a pyknotic nucleus encircled by a clear halo suggests the presence of an HPV infection. In the perianal region, accessory skin structures, including hair follicles and sweat glands, become involved by intraepithelial disease extension. A mononuclear inflammatory infiltrate invades the upper dermis. The lesion differs from bowenoid papulosis by virtue of the orderly maturation and absence of

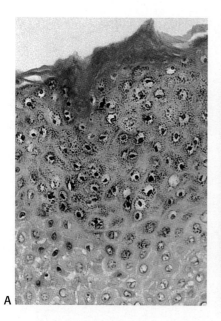
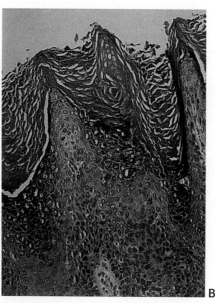

FIG. 16.26. Bowenoid papulosis. **A:** Superficial portion of the mucosa demonstrating marked prominence of the granular cell layer. **B:** Note the presence of atypical cells in the lower portions of the epithelium and the prominent granular cell layer. Marked hyperkeratosis covers the lesion.

pilosebaceous epithelial involvement of the latter lesion, as compared to the disorderly pattern of epithelial cells and involvement of the pilosebaceous units as seen in Bowen disease. Additionally, bowenoid papulosis appears more sharply confined than Bowen disease.

Bowen disease is usually included in the differential diagnosis of perianal intraepithelial neoplasias along with Paget disease and malignant melanoma because of the presence of large, pale vacuolated cells with prominent perinuclear halos in the basal area. Immunohistochemical stains help distinguish these lesions from one another (Table 16.4). The disorder is treated with wide local excision (98).

Basal Cell Carcinoma

Basal cell carcinomas normally develop in sun-exposed regions, but they may develop in the anal margin and perianal skin. The tumors present as indurated, sometimes ulcer-

ated areas. They histologically resemble the various patterns seen in the more common cutaneous basal cell carcinomas. Numerous, often bizarre mitoses may be present. These indolent lesions should be differentiated from the more aggressive basaloid carcinomas, which metastasize early, often causing patient death. As with elsewhere in the body, basal cell carcinomas respond to local excision. The two lesions are compared in Table 16.2 (99).

Squamous Cell Carcinoma

Anal margin carcinomas are defined as tumors arising below the dentate line but still having a considerable portion of the tumor located in the anal canal. They account for 25% of all SCCs. A slight male predominance exists for anal margin tumors. Anal margin SCC presents in various forms, often following a long history of perianal problems such as bleeding, pain, the sensation of a mass, and pruritus. SCCs present

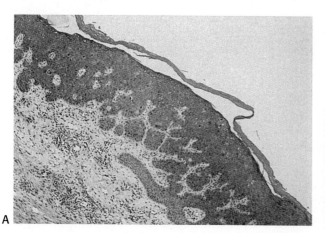
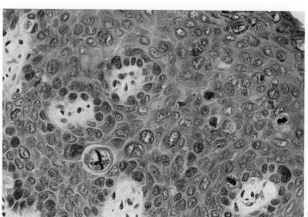

FIG. 16.27. Bowen disease. **A:** Note the presence of prominent acanthotic epithelium containing neoplastic cells. **B:** Higher magnification shows the cytologic atypia and the presence of abnormal mitotic figures.

TABLE 16.4   Special Stains in Intraepithelial Neoplasms

	Paget Disease (Primary)	Paget Disease (Secondary)	Bowen Disease	Melanomas
Special stains				
Mucicarmine	+	+	−	−
PAS	+	+	−	−
Alcian blue	+	+	−	−
Fontana Masson	−	−	−	+
Immunostains				
CEA	+	+	−	+[a]
Gross cystic disease fluid protein	+	−	−	−
CK8 + 18	+	+	−	−
CK7/20	+/−	+/+	−	−
CK5 + 14	−	−	+	−
S100	−	−	−	+
HMB45	−	−	−	+
MELAN-A	−	−	−	+
Vimentin	−	−	−	+
NSE	−	+/−	−	+/−

[a] May be positive when polyclonal antibodies are used. They are negative with monoclonal antibodies.
PAS, periodic acid–Schiff; CEA, carcinoembryonic antigen; NSE, neuron-specific enolase.

as slowly growing, hard, small nodules that often become ulcerated. The lesions appear exophytic, resembling the condylomata from which many arise. Anal margin tumors tend to grow circumferentially around the anus. The differential diagnosis of anal margin tumors includes leukoplakia, malignant melanoma, intraepithelial adenocarcinoma, extramammary Paget disease, basal cell carcinoma, condyloma acuminata, and certain skin disorders such as lichen sclerosus et atrophicus.

Anal margin SCCs are usually well-differentiated (Fig. 16.28) or moderately differentiated (Fig. 16.28) keratinizing squamous carcinomas that behave like skin cancers. Areas of intraepithelial neoplasia may be present. The invasive tumors contain large cells, often with prominent cell borders and areas of keratinization (Fig. 16.28). The irregularly arranged cells may show peripheral palisading and they contain numerous mitoses. Tumor size relates to the extent of microscopic infiltration. Tumors measuring >2 cm are more likely to infiltrate deeply. Carcinomas of the anal margin tend to express CK5/6 and CK13, but unlike anal canal tumors, CK7, CK18, and CK19 are rarely expressed. Anal margin tumors express cadherin; this antigen is lost in anal canal lesions (100).

The prognosis is better than that of SCCs arising in the anal canal. The most important prognostic factor is the status of the regional lymph nodes. T1 and T2 lesions receive radiation to the tumor but not the inguinal lymph nodes (101,102). T3 and T4 tumors are treated with radiation to the tumor and the inguinal lymph nodes and chemotherapy to avoid sphincter-damaging surgical procedures. Because of the differences in the sites to be irradiated, some advocate the use of sentinel node biopsy to accurately assess the nodal status in an effort to better guide the radiation therapy (103).

Verrucous Carcinoma (Giant Condylomata)

Verrucous carcinomas arise on many mucosal surfaces, including the anorectum (104), and some cases associate with HPV 6, 11, 16, and 18 infections (105,106). Different viral genotypes often coexist in different areas of the tumors (107). The lesions are rare despite the increased incidence of anal condylomata and anal carcinomas. Although the distinction between verrucous carcinoma and giant condyloma is difficult, practically speaking the distinction between the two lesions is probably unnecessary because adequate local excision is the treatment of choice for both. In fact, the latest WHO classification regards giant condylomata (Buschke-Lowenstein tumors) as the same entity (1).

Verrucous carcinomas have a male:female incidence of 2.7:1 and the mean age at presentation is 43.9 years (108). The most common presenting symptoms include perianal mass, pain, abscess or fistula, and bleeding. No correlations exist between clinical presentation, tumor size, symptom duration, and tumor behavior. These large cauliflowerlike masses may ulcerate, spread superficially, and burrow through soft tissues to form sinus tracts and fistulae involving large areas of the perineum, pelvis, genital tract, and buttocks. These fistulae and abscesses predispose the patient to chronic sepsis (105,109). Clinically, the tumors can be misinterpreted as fistulae, hidradenitis suppurativa, condyloma acuminatum, benign squamous papilloma, pseudoepitheliomatous hyperplasia, or epidermodysplasia verruciformis. Underdiagnosis results from failure to biopsy a lesion not thought to be clinically significant or examination of nonrepresentative superficial biopsies.

Grossly, verrucous carcinomas present as pale, exophytic, cauliflowerlike masses with a papillomatous surface arising

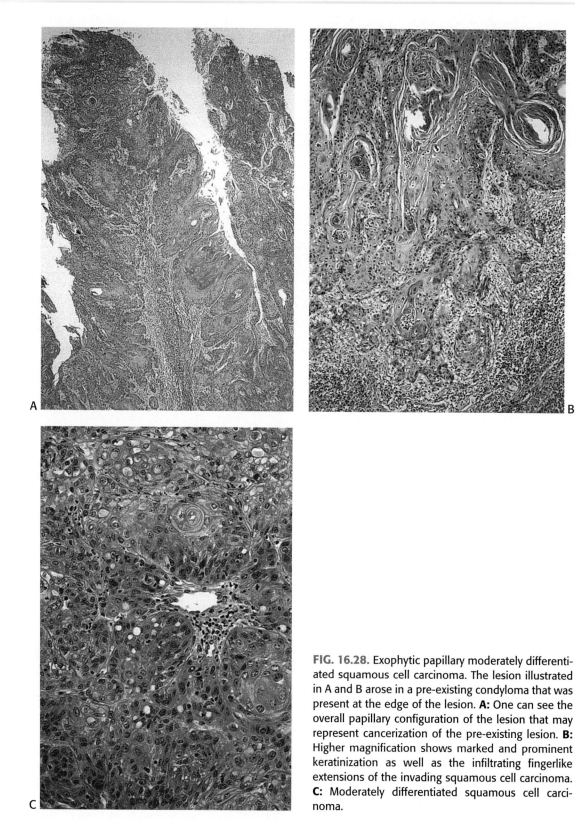

FIG. 16.28. Exophytic papillary moderately differentiated squamous cell carcinoma. The lesion illustrated in A and B arose in a pre-existing condyloma that was present at the edge of the lesion. **A:** One can see the overall papillary configuration of the lesion that may represent cancerization of the pre-existing lesion. **B:** Higher magnification shows marked and prominent keratinization as well as the infiltrating fingerlike extensions of the invading squamous cell carcinoma. **C:** Moderately differentiated squamous cell carcinoma.

in the perianal skin, anal canal, or distal rectal mucosa. Histologically, they consist of locally expansile papillary proliferations supported by vascularized connective tissue stromal cords. The lesions exhibit accentuated acanthosis, papillomatosis, and thickened, elongated rete ridges when compared to condylomata (Fig. 16.29). Prominent mitotic activity and koilocytosis are usually present. Broad, bulbous, acanthotic fingers of squamous epithelium push into the underlying stroma in verrucous carcinoma rather than invading it in the irregular fashion commonly seen in

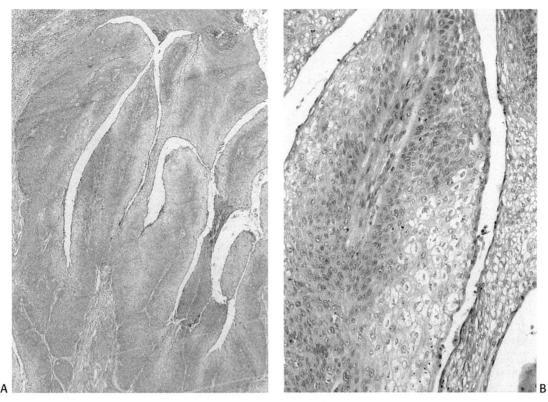

FIG. 16.29. Verrucous carcinoma. **A:** Lesion showing prominent papillary spiked epithelium and broad acanthotic bulging into the underlying stroma. **B:** Higher magnification showing the prominent koilocytotic atypia on the somewhat disorderly epithelium at the stromal epidermal junction.

ordinary invasive SCC. The epithelium characteristically appears well differentiated and the plane of the basement membrane appears intact. The individual cells evidence more atypia and a less orderly maturation than do the cells comprising giant condylomata. The deep, broadly infiltrative margins also distinguish the lesion from the more common condyloma acuminatum.

Verrucous carcinomas grow slowly with local tissue destruction and invasion. Recurrences are common. Local metastases rarely develop, in contrast to ordinary SCC. Distant metastases do not occur. Treatment consists of wide local excision to ensure that the deep margins are histologically free of tumor. Verrucous carcinomas that invade the rectal sphincter or extend beneath the muscle require an abdominal–perineal resection. Radical surgery may cure up to 61% of patients (110). Inadequately excised tumors recur in a wreathlike pattern. Chemotherapy may only cure approximately 25% of patients (110). Chemotherapy and focused radiation therapy may be used in certain cases of recurrent or extensive disease with unpredictable responses (108).

Paget Disease

Malignant mucous-producing cells infiltrating the perianal epidermis characterize Paget disease Perianal Paget disease often presents as a pruritic, painful, bleeding, indurated, or oozing eczematous lesion that grossly appears flaky and white. The lesion may also appear as a well-circumscribed, reddish brown, and plaquelike, velvety, moist, and/or eroded lesion. Clinically, Paget disease mimics Bowen disease, malignant melanoma, leukoplakia, and other dermatoses. The disease usually affects elderly Caucasians. Mean patient age is 61 years, with a range of 35 to 82 years (111); males and females are about equally affected (112). Occasionally, the disease is familial in nature (113).

Extramammary Paget disease falls into two groups: Primary Paget disease of cutaneous origin and Paget disease secondary to an underlying internal malignancy. The tumor cells of cutaneous extramammary Paget disease may originate from the intraepidermal cells of apocrine gland ducts, from adnexal stem cells, or from pluripotential keratinocyte stem cells (114,115). Secondary anal Paget disease complicates anal canal carcinomas (111,116,117), anal duct cancers, rectal tumors (118), and neuroendocrine carcinomas (119). Other associated internal cancers include carcinomas of the stomach and colon, as well as cancers of the pelvic region (111). The Paget cells may or may not be contiguous with the underlying adenocarcinoma. Abundant, large, pale, clear or basophilic cells arranged singly or in clusters infiltrate all levels of the squamous epithelium (Fig. 16.30). Hyperchromatic nuclei, multiple nuclei, and mitoses can be seen. Occasionally, glandular structures are present. Often, cell clusters accumulate in the lower portion of the rete pegs,

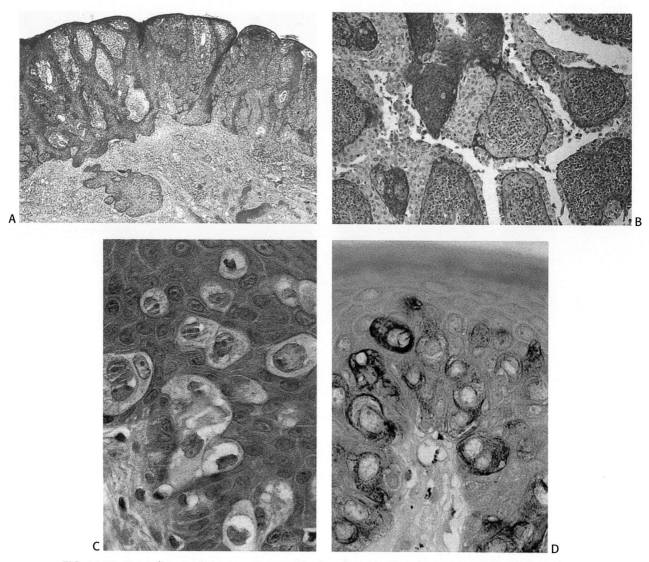

FIG. 16.30. Paget disease. **A:** Low-power magnification demonstrating the presence of isolated malignant Paget cells. **B:** Higher-power magnification of a different lesion showing numerous pagetoid cells surrounding the fibrovascular cores. **C:** Higher-power magnification of the pagetoid cells and **(D)** carcinoembryonic antigen stain.

widening them and compressing the basal cells. Paget cells also extend to the epithelial outer root sheaths of the pilary complex and apocrine sweat ducts. Other microscopic features include hyperkeratosis, parakeratosis, acanthosis, and epithelial hyperplasia. The hyperplasia may be extensive enough to be reminiscent of fibroepithelioma of Pinkus (120,121) or papillomatous hyperplasia (121). If the number of Paget cells is small, the papillomatous lesion may resemble a condyloma acuminatum (121). An inflammatory infiltrate containing lymphocytes, plasma cells, histiocytes, polymorphonuclear leukocytes, eosinophils, and mast cells lies beneath the affected epidermis. The involved epithelium usually remains intact, but ulcers do occur when large accumulations of Paget cells are present. This slow-growing malignancy may remain localized for years. Eventually it becomes invasive, sometimes culminating in metastatic adenocarcinoma. An invasive component is present in up to 44% of patients (112).

One of the difficulties in evaluating patients with perianal Paget disease is the fact that individual malignant cells are often present at a large distance from the grossly visible margin of the lesion, and may form multicentric or satellite lesions without obvious continuity with other Paget cells or with a primary neoplasm (122). The mean size of the lesion is 3.0 cm in diameter, with a range of 0.4 to 12 cm. When the tumor cells lie at a distance from the main lesion, isolated Paget cells may be extremely difficult to identify histologically and may resemble melanocytes present in the normal basal layer or even Langerhans cells. For this reason, we typically stain the margins of resections for Paget disease with special stains in cases in which clear cells are present to rule out the presence of Paget cells.

The cells comprising both primary and secondary Paget disease stain with mucin stains (periodic acid–Schiff [PAS], mucicarmine, and Alcian blue) and carcinoembryonic antigen (CEA). However, the lesions show a variable immunophenotype depending on whether the disease is primary or secondary to an internal malignancy. Primary forms of the disease stain positively with antibodies to CEA, CK7, and gross cystic disease fluid protein (GCDFP) (123,124). The tumor cells express gastric surface-type mucin MUC1, which is a mammary-type mucin (125), as well as HER2/neu (126). The *HER2/neu* gene is amplified, potentially making this disease one that can be treated with HER2-targeted therapy. Androgen receptors are also frequently expressed (127). Paget disease complicating a rectal malignancy will demonstrate a Muc2/CK7+/CK20+/GCDFP–phenotype (128–130). Paget disease complicating other tumor types will show the immunophenotype of the underlying cancer. The differential diagnosis includes lentiginous melanoma or Bowen disease and can be distinguished by the use of special stains (see Table 16.4).

Extramammary Paget disease should be completely excised. The type of operation performed depends on whether or not an underlying cancer can be identified, the type and site of the cancer, and the extent and location of the Paget disease. When carcinoma of the rectum is present, abdominoperineal resection is usually performed. Paget disease associated with carcinoma of perianal or cutaneous sweat glands can be treated with wide excision. However, Paget disease almost always extends beyond its clinically visible involved margin, making one-stage resection difficult. Some physicians perform tissue mapping with multiple tissue biopsies before definitive surgery is undertaken to define the limits of the lesion. More recently, photodynamic diagnosis is being used as a less invasive and less expensive way to map the lesional limits (131). Mohs microscopic surgery also has the potential to avoid radical excision in some patients.

Intraoperative frozen sections are also sometimes used to define the surgical margins and reduce the need for further operations (116). Nonetheless, frequent recurrences characterize the disease; recurrence rates may reach 61%. The average time to recurrence is over 2.5 years (116). Overall and disease-free survival at 5 years is 59% and 64%, respectively, and at 10 years is 33% and 39%, respectively. Some patients die of metastatic disease.

Photodynamic therapy may be used to treat patients with residual disease (132). Adjuvant chemotherapy may be used in patients with aggressive disease (112). The role of radiotherapy in this disease is controversial (133).

Adnexal Tumors

Sweat gland tumors rarely develop in the anogenital region, almost always affecting middle-aged white women (134). Patients generally complain of a lump that has been present for less than a year, swelling, itching, pain, or ulceration. *Hidradenoma papilliferum* primarily affects women between the ages of 30 and 50. The tumors present as spherical, circumscribed lesions usually measuring <1 cm in diameter. An unusual example of a 2-cm ulcerated perianal lesion was reported recently (135). The tumors display both glandular and papillary areas (Fig. 16.31). The glandular areas are lined by a double layer of tall columnar epithelial cells that show active decapitation secretion and one or two layers of cuboidal flattened myoepithelial cells resting on a well-defined thin basement membrane. The slender papillary structures contain scanty connective tissue cores. The epithelial cells contain mucinophilic, PAS-positive, diastase-resistant granules. Occasionally, cysts with focal epithelial proliferations are seen.

Perianal *apocrine carcinoma* arising in a benign apocrine adenoma was recently reported (136). Characteristic two–cell layers with both apocrine epithelial cells and myoepithelial

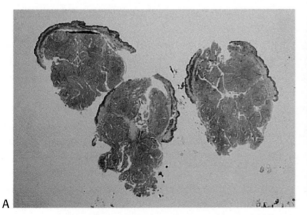 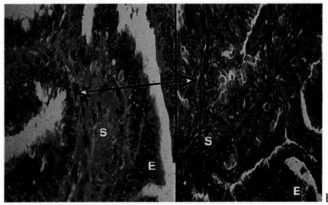

FIG. 16.31. Perianal hidradenoma. **A:** Note the presence of a polypoid mass that appears lobulated at low power. **B:** Higher magnification shows the presence of a prominent stromal component covered by two cell layers, one next to the stroma, which is spindled and flat and illustrated by the *arrow,* and the more cuboidal epithelium (*E*). The myoepithelial cells, which represent the flattened cells overlying the stroma (*S*), are highlighted by staining with smooth muscle actin.

cells were present in the benign portions. There was loss of the myoepithelial layer in the malignant component and the glands became more irregular and angular.

Sclerosing sweat duct carcinomas also arise in this location (137). The tumors are locally aggressive as they are highly infiltrative and perineural invasion is common. There is minimal cytologic atypia and few mitotic figures (137).

Trichoepitheliomas are uncommon benign tumors that develop from the follicular-sebaceous-apocrine unit. Two clinical forms are described: Multiple trichoepithelioma, which has a family history and starts to appear during puberty, mainly affecting the face; and giant solitary trichoepithelioma, which has no family history and generally appears during adulthood and has a predilection for involving the perianal area (138,139). The tumors contain nests of basaloid cells with follicular differentiation. The cells are frequently heavily glycogenated. Horny cysts are also present. Areas of transformation to basal cell carcinoma may be present in the giant perianal tumors (140).

MALIGNANT MELANOMA

Anal melanomas account for 0.1% to 1.07% of all anal tumors and approximately 1% of all primary melanomas (141). The annual incidence of primary anal melanoma is 0.016 per 100,000 population (142). Although melanomas are uncommon, the anal canal is the most common site for a primary gastrointestinal tumor (142) and anorectal melanomas account for 24% of all mucosal melanomas (143). Anal melanoma, a disease of adult Caucasians, has a mean age at diagnosis of 58 to 64 years and a range of 22 to 96 years (144). There is a female preponderance of cases (145). HIV infection has been implicated as a risk factor in young, mostly male patients (145).

The most common presenting symptoms are nonspecific and include rectal bleeding followed by pain, the sensation of a mass, constipation, diarrhea, abdominal pain, weight loss, and tenesmus (141). Some lesions present as hemorrhoids. Since the initial clinical diagnosis is incorrect in as many as 80% of cases (67), symptoms are often present for several months before the diagnosis is made. As a result, the tumors may attain a large size before being correctly diagnosed. Rarely, a metastasis to the inguinal lymph nodes leads to the discovery of an advanced occult primary tumor. Advanced disease may also present with neurologic complications, including sciatica. Metastases are present at the time of diagnosis in more than half of patients. The etiology of anorectal melanoma remains unknown. While sun exposure represents a major cause of the cutaneous forms of the disease (146), the inverse association of melanoma incidence with latitude is a striking contrast to the situation that exists with cutaneous and ocular melanomas (146).

Although melanomas develop throughout the anus, two thirds arise in the proximal portion of the pecten and transitional zone around the dentate line (Fig. 16.32). They range

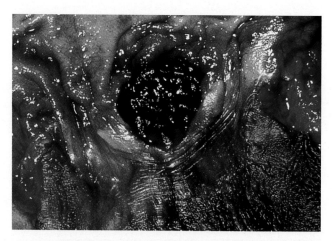

FIG. 16.32. Ulcerated malignant melanoma.

in size from a few millimeters to >10 cm, with a mean diameter of 4.1 cm (144). Smaller lesions appear sessile, but as they become bulky they form protuberant, polypoid masses, which prolapse through the anal orifice, becoming secondarily ulcerated (144). Polypoid lesions tend to invade the submucosa, whereas more sessile lesions invade deeper into the underlying muscle layers. Small, warty projections may surround a larger lesion. The degree of tumor pigmentation varies. Twenty to fifty percent of tumors are pigmented; others are amelanotic in nature (142).

When melanomas are detected, they are usually deeply invasive lesions. However sometimes *melanoma in situ* is seen. This lesion consists of proliferations of neoplastic, variably pigmented neoplastic cells that remain confined to the mucosa. Tumors range in thickness from 0.5 mm to >20 mm. Only a minority of patients have lesions that measure <2 mm, but these patients have excellent survival rates. One can use an optical micrometer to measure tumor thickness in invasive lesions. One measures from the mucosal surface or from the surface of an area of ulceration to the point of deepest penetration of the lesion.

Invasive melanomas display histologic and immunohistochemical similarities with cutaneous melanomas. They exhibit considerable variability in tumor cell size and shape, both from tumor to tumor and within a given lesion. The cells are often large with an epithelioid appearance and finely distributed pigment giving the cytoplasm a dusty-tan appearance. The large hyperchromatic nuclei (Fig. 16.33) usually measure about 1.5 to 2 times the diameter of the nuclei of the surrounding keratinocytes. The nuclei of most neoplastic cells appear elongated with well-dispersed chromatin. Multinucleated and polymorphic giant cells are common in melanoma and exceptional in adenocarcinoma and squamous cell carcinomas. Some tumors (small round cell melanomas) contain atypical round cells resembling lymphocytes (Fig. 16.34). Others have spindle cells arranged in interlacing fascicles resembling a sarcoma. Polygonal cells predominate in the more cellular areas. A nesting or trabecular pattern can be seen, especially superficially. Deeper

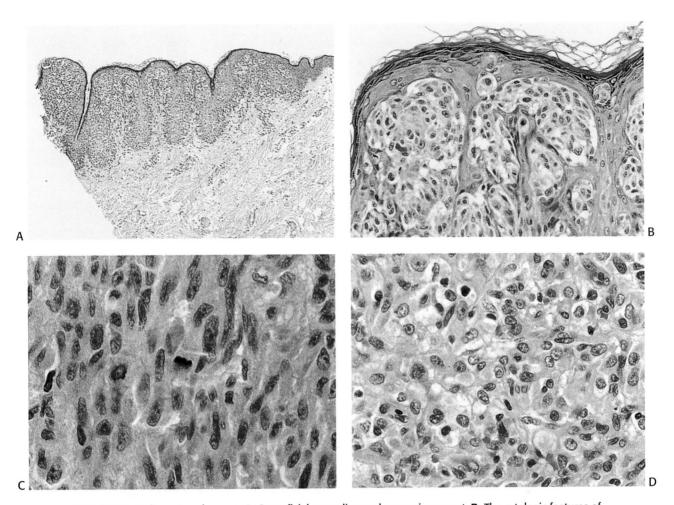

FIG. 16.33. Malignant melanoma. **A:** Superficial spreading melanoma is present. **B:** The cytologic features of the lesion are clearer here. **C:** The presence of numerous mitoses is evident. **D:** Another malignant melanoma that had metastasized to the inguinal lymph nodes from the anal region.

invasive portions of the tumor tend to grow in solid sheets. The cells may also form alveolar patterns and/or aggregates resembling carcinoid tumors. The intercellular material consists of collagen fibers and a basophilic matrix. Mitotic activity varies and occasionally can be extremely difficult to detect. Other anorectal melanomas appear very cellular and frequently anaplastic with large numbers of mitoses. *Desmoplastic melanomas* also can arise in the anus (147). They resemble their cutaneous counterparts.

Prominent *junctional melanocytic atypia* extends laterally from 0.7 to 1.7 cm from the neoplasm (146) in 20% to 75% of patients (144), especially in those tumors arising in the anorectal zone (67). These junctional changes are most likely to be seen with smaller tumors. The junctional component may be above or lateral to the invasive component, and many microscopic sections may be needed to demonstrate its presence. Junctional melanocytes concentrate in the basal and suprabasal layers and vary in shape from a spindle cell morphology to epithelioid cells, sometimes focally arranged in groups (in thèques). The presence of junctional changes (Fig. 16.35) identifies that the lesion is a primary anal melanoma.

Intraepithelial extensions of malignant melanoma may be confused with Paget disease. However, the use of special stains (Table 16.4) eliminates this dilemma (148). Antibodies to S100 protein can be used but they are less specific than HMB45. However, we have encountered anal melanomas, especially of the small cell type, that are negative with HMB45 but are S100 positive. Because both markers are positive independent of melanin synthesis, they are particularly helpful in establishing the diagnosis in amelanotic lesions. Melanomas metastatic to the anorectal area may be CEA positive when polyclonal antibodies are used to detect CEA. This immunoreactivity is not seen with monoclonal antibodies for CEA.

Analysis of the tumors for the presence and nature of *BRAF* and *ras* mutations may help distinguish between cutaneous melanomas and anal melanomas. The latter lack the *BRAF* V599E exon 15 mutation and *ras* mutations characteristic of cutaneous melanomas (149,150). However, rare anal melanomas may contain novel *BRAF* mutations in exon 15 and exon 11 (150). Allelic loss of the *NF1* gene has also been reported in a patient with neurofibromatosis and anal melanoma (151).

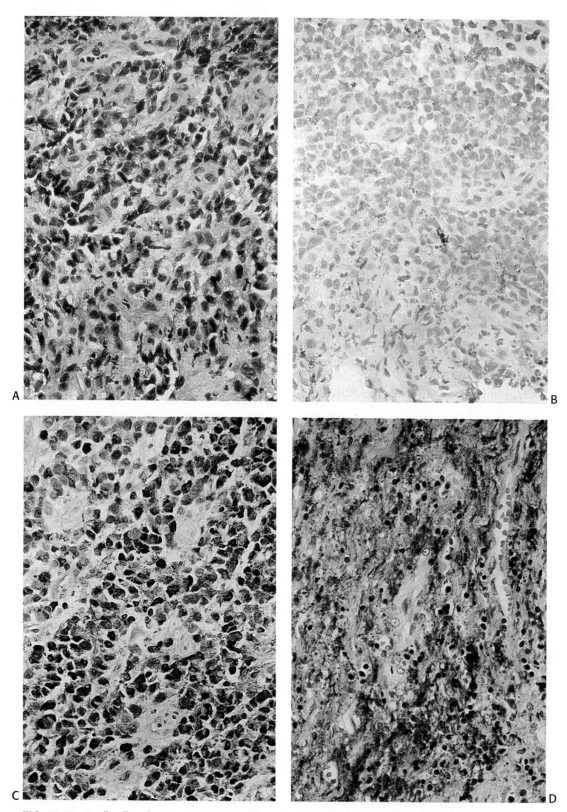

FIG. 16.34. Small cell melanoma. **A:** Hematoxylin and eosin appearance of the small cells with features not typical of the usual melanoma. One sees fine brownish pigment scattered among the cells. **B:** HMB45 immunostain showing the lack of immunoreactivity. The brown pigmentation, however, is seen more easily in this preparation. **C:** S100 immunostain showing strong immunoreactivity. **D:** This patient underwent radiotherapy for treatment of the disease and then resection. D comes from the resection specimen in which no residual tumor cells were identified but instead prominent pigmentation was present. This pigment represented extravasated melanin granules diffusely distributed throughout the stroma.

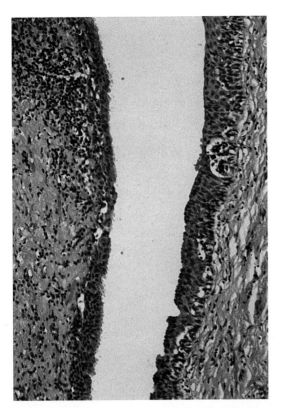

FIG. 16.35. Junctional activity in the transitional epithelium adjacent to an invasive melanoma. Note the prominent intraepithelial collections of melanocytic cells.

Although anal canal melanomas may appear deceptively benign, they behave in a highly malignant fashion and invade the lower rectum early in the course of the disease. They invade deeply and extend into the perianorectal tissues. Rarely, they directly invade the bladder, prostate, vagina, or sacrum. They may also spread laterally in the submucosa, producing variably polypoid, discontinuous satellite lesions. Anorectal melanomas also disseminate via lymphatic and hematogenous routes to lymph nodes, lungs, liver, brain, bone, and skin (67). They also spread through the lymphatic system along the superior hemorrhoidal vessels laterally to the iliac and obturator nodes and via the perianal lymphatics to the medial superficial inguinal lymph nodes (144).

Anal melanoma has a very poor prognosis. The overall 5-year survival is approximately 10% to 33%. Average patient survival is 9 months to 2.8 years. The survival rate (and prognosis) of primary anorectal melanomas is directly related to tumor size and thickness (81,146,152,153). Patients with lesions measuring between 2 and 3 mm in thickness survive 50 months. The mean survival of patients with 3- to 5-mm lesions is 8 months, and those patients with lesions measuring 5.7 to 9 mm have a mean survival of 14 months (141). Patients with stage I disease develop local or regional pelvic recurrences. Mean survival for patients with stage I disease is 29 months, compared with 11 months for patients with stage II disease or 9 months for patients with stage III disease. In the absence of distant metastases at the time of surgery, overall survival increases to 20% to 30% (153). Tumor proliferative rate may also have prognostic significance, with tumors with a Ki-67 labeling index of >40% having a worse prognosis than those with a lower labeling index (154).

Radical excision may cure patients with lesions measuring <3 mm in depth. Some patients with metastatic anorectal melanomas may have major responses or partial responses to chemotherapy (155). In large lesions, not curable by radical surgery, more conservative local approaches using excision or cryotherapy may achieve local palliation, as may treatment with intratumoral injections of interferon-β along with systemic chemotherapy (156).

TUMORS DEVELOPING IN CONGENITAL ANOMALIES

Neoplasms may develop in various congenital abnormalities involving the anorectal region. We have seen neoplastic transformation involving heterotopic gastric mucosa. Tumors also develop in tailgut cysts including carcinoid tumors (157), adenocarcinomas (158), adenosquamous carcinomas (159), and carcinomas with prominent meningothelial proliferations (160). The histologic features of the tailgut cysts are described in Chapter 15.

LESIONS DEVELOPING IN THE ANOGENITAL MAMMARYLIKE GLANDS

Apocrine fibroadenomas histologically resembling mammary intracanalicular fibroadenomas arise in the perianal skin. The ducts are lined by a double layer of epithelial cells, a low cuboidal cell at the base with an eosinophilic columnar cell at the luminal side. Occasional papillary proliferations are present (161). The irregularly sized nuclei contain a fine chromatin pattern. Occasional mitoses can be seen. Occasionally, elongated and compressed spindle-shaped cells lie between the basal portion of the epithelium and the underlying basement membrane. Both exocrine and apocrine glandular epithelium can be present. Sebaceous differentiation or areas of *pseudoangiomatous stromal hyperplasia* (162) may also be seen. Myoepithelial cells are easily recognizable. They can be highlighted utilizing antibodies to smooth muscle actin. These tumors all behave in a benign fashion.

Adenosis tumors may develop that histologically resemble their mammary counterparts. Areas of regular as well as sclerosing adenosis are present, along with variably sized microcysts and cysts. Short papillary projections may be present along with the characteristic myoepithelial cells. Decapitation secretions are prominent (163).

TABLE 16.5 Tumors Arising in the Retrorectal Space

Liposarcoma
Hemangioepithelial sarcoma
Extra-abdominal desmoid
Lymphangioma
Osteogenic sarcoma
Osteoma
Neurofibroma
Schwannoma
Ganglioneuroma
Ependymoma
Adrenal rest tumor

RETRORECTAL TUMORS

The retrorectal region is the potential space defined by the rectum anteriorly, the sacrum posteriorly, the peritoneal reflection superiorly, and the levator ani and coccygeal muscles inferiorly. The iliac vessels and ureters define its lateral margins. Retrorectal lesions can be classified as congenital, inflammatory, neoplastic, and miscellaneous in nature. Neoplasms developing in this area are listed in Table 16.5. The most common presentation is an asymptomatic mass discovered on routine rectal examination (164). The largest percentage are chordomas (38%). Other tumors include neurogenic tumors (15%), chondrosarcomas (8%), adenocarcinomas (8%), and others. The tumors range in size from 3 to 20 cm with a median diameter of 8 cm. These tumors affect patients of all ages, with peaks in the 1st and 6th decades. Patients present with pain and constipation, as well as bowel obstruction and urinary incontinence.

Retrorectal cystic hamartomas are uncommon lesions of controversial pathogenesis that arise in the presacrococcygeal space. They develop in anatomic regions where tailgut vestiges presumably reside and appear as multicystic lesions lined by stratified squamous, transitional, seromucinous, and/or intestinal epithelium (166,167). Retrorectal cystic hamartomas contain tissues from multiple germ cell layers but they lack the dermal appendages, neural elements, or other mesenchymal derivatives, such as cartilage and bone, that are frequently seen in mature teratomas. Immature elements are never found in retrorectal cystic hamartomas. One also sees poorly organized collections of smooth muscle in the surrounding connective tissue, but well-formed smooth muscle coats characteristic of a duplication cyst are absent.

OTHER ANAL AND PERIANAL TUMORS

Various neuroendocrine tumors may develop in the anus as discussed in Chapter 17. Merkel cell tumors may arise here as well (168). Rarely, the anal canal gives rise to mesenchymal tumors including leiomyomas and leiomyosarcomas, rhabdomyosarcomas, granular cell tumors, hemangiomas, lipomas, neurilemomas, Kaposi sarcoma, leukemia, and lymphomas. These tumors resemble those discussed in Chapters 18 and 19.

Secondary tumors include metastases from various sites. Retrorectal tumors may also extend into the anus.

SPECIMEN EXAMINATION

A protocol for examining specimens from patients with carcinomas of the anus and the anal canal is presented in reference 169.

REFERENCES

1. Fenger C, Frisch M, Marti MC, Parc R: Tumors of the anal canal. In: Hamilton SR, Aaltonen LA (eds). *World Health Organization Classification of Tumors. Pathology and Genetics of Tumors of the Digestive System.* Lyons, France: IARC Press, 2000, pp 147–155.
2. Peters RK, Mack TM: Patterns of anal carcinoma by gender and marital status in Los Angeles County. *Br J Cancer* 1983;48:629.
3. Frazer IH, Medley G, Crapper RM, et al: Association between anorectal dysplasia, human papillomavirus and human immunodeficiency virus infection in homosexual men. *Lancet* 1986;2:657.
4. Patel R, Groff DB: Condylomata acuminata in childhood. *Pediatrics* 1972;50:153.
5. Noffsinger A, Witte D, Fenoglio-Preiser CM: The relationship of human papillomaviruses to anorectal neoplasia. *Cancer* 1992;70:1276.
6. Kuypers JM, Kiviat NB: Anal papillomas virus infections. In: Surawicz C, Owen R (eds). *Gastrointestinal and Hepatic Infections.* Philadelphia: WB Saunders Company, 1995, pp 279–285.
7. Von Krogh G, Lacey CJN, Gross G, et al: European guideline for the management of anogenital warts. *Int J STD AIDS* 2001;12:40.
8. Croxson T, Chabon AB, Rorat E, et al: Intraepithelial carcinoma of the anus in homosexual men. *Dis Colon Rectum* 1984;27:325.
9. Fenger C, Nielsen VT: Precancerous changes in the anal canal epithelium in resection specimens. *Acta Pathol Microbiol Immunol Scand A* 1986;94:63.
10. Beckmann AM, Daling JR, Sherman KJ, et al: Human papillomavirus infection and anal cancer. *Int J Cancer* 1989;43:1042.
11. Holly EA, Ralston ML, Darragh TM, Greenblatt RM: Prevalence and risk factors for anal squamous intraepithelial lesions in women. *J Nat Cancer Inst* 2001;93:843.
12. Palefsky JM, Holly EA, Ralston ML, et al: Prevalence and risk factors for human papillomavirus infection of the anal canal in human immunodeficiency virus (HIV)-positive and HIV-negative homosexual men. *J Infect Dis* 1998;177:361.
13. Piketty C, Darragh TM, Da Costa M, et al: High prevalence of anal human papillomavirus infection and anal cancer precursors among HIV-infected persons in the absence of anal intercourse. *Ann Int Med* 2003;183:453.
14. Martin F, Bower M: Anal intraepithelial neoplasia in HIV positive people. *Sex Transm Inf* 2001;77:327.
15. Horster S, Thoma-Greber E, Siebeck M, Bogner JR: Is anal carcinoma a HAART-related problem? *Eur J Med Res* 2003;30:142.
16. Palefsky JM, Holly EA, Gonzales J, et al: Detection of human papillomavirus DNA in anal intraepithelial neoplasia and anal cancer. *Cancer Res* 1991;51:1014.
17. Critchlow CW, Surawicz CM, Holmes KK, et al: Prospective study of high grade anal squamous intraepithelial neoplasia in a cohort of homosexual men: influence of HIV infection, immunosuppression and human papillomavirus infection. *AIDS* 1995;9:1255.
18. Medley G: Anal smear test to diagnose occult anorectal infection with human papillomavirus in men. *Br J Vener Dis* 1984;60:205.
19. Nash G, Allen W, Nash S: Atypical lesions of the anal canal mucosa in homosexual men. *JAMA* 1986;256:873.

20. Yamaguchi T, Moriya Y, Fujii T, et al: Anal canal squamous cell carcinoma in situ, clearly demonstrated by indigo carmine dye spraying: report of a case. *Dis Colon Rectum* 2000;43:1161.

21. Colquhoun P, Nogueras JJ, Dipasquale B, et al: Interobserver and intraobserver bias exists in the interpretation of anal dysplasia. *Dis Colon Rectum* 2003;46:1332.

22. Lytwyn A, Salit IE, Raboud J, et al: Interobserver agreement in the interpretation of anal intraepithelial neoplasia. *Cancer* 2005;103:1447.

23. Skinner PP, Ogunbiyi OA, Scholefield JH, et al: Skin appendage involvement in anal intraepithelial neoplasia. *Br J Surg* 1997;84:675.

24. Goldie SJ, Kuntz KM, Weinstein MC, et al: Cost-effectiveness of screening for anal squamous intraepithelial lesions and anal cancer in human immunodeficiency virus-negative homosexual and bisexual men. *Am J Med* 2000;108:634.

25. Palefsky JM, Holly EA, Hogeboom CJ, et al: Anal cytology as a screening tool for anal squamous intraepithelial lesions. *J Acquir Immune Defic Syndr Hum Retrovirol* 1997;14:415.

26. Moscicki A-B, Durako SJ, Houser J, et al: Human papillomavirus infection and abnormal cytology of the anus in HIV-infected and uninfected adolescents. *AIDS* 2003;17:311.

27. Darragh T, Birdsong G, Luff R, Davey D: In: Solomon D, Nayar R (eds). *The Bethesda System for Reporting Cervical Cytology: Definitions, Criteria and Explanatory Notes,* 2nd ed. New York: Springer-Verlag, 2004.

28. Sayers SJ, McMillan A, McGoogan E: Anal cytological abnormalities in HIV-infected homosexual men. *Int J STD AIDS* 1998;9:37.

29. Chin-Hong PV, Palefsky JM: Natural history and clinical management of anal human papillomavirus disease in men and women infected with human immunodeficiency virus. *Clin Infect Dis* 2002;35;1127.

30. Fenger C, Frisch M, Jass JJ, et al: Anal cancer subtype reproducibility study. *Virchows Arch* 2000;436:229.

31. Dougherty BG, Evans HL: Carcinoma of the anal canal. A study of 79 cases. *J Clin Pathol* 1985;83:159.

32. Shepherd NA, Scholefield JH, Love SB, et al: Prognostic factors in anal squamous carcinoma: a multivariate analysis of clinical, pathological and flow cytometric parameters in 235 cases. *Histopathology* 1990;16:545.

33. Boman BM, Moertel CG, O'Connell MJ, et al: Carcinoma of the anal canal: a clinical and pathologic study of 188 cases. *Cancer* 1984;54:114.

34. Licitra L, Spinazze S, Docci R, et al: Cancer of the anal region. *Crit Rev Oncol Hematol* 2002;43:77.

35. Jass JR, Sobin LH, Morson BC: *Histological Typing of Intestinal Tumors.* Berlin: Springer Verlag, 1989.

36. Johnson LG, Madeleine MM, Newcomer LM, et al: Anal cancer incidence and survival: the surveillance, epidemiology and end results experience, 1973-2000. *Cancer* 2004;101:281.

37. Melbye M, Cote TR, Kessler L, et al: High incidence of anal cancer among AIDS patients. *Lancet* 1994;343:636.

38. Daling JR, Madeline MM, Johnson LG, et al: Human papillomavirus, smoking and sexual practices in the etiology of anal cancer. *Cancer* 2004;101:270.

39. Frisch M, Glimelius B, van den Brule AJC: Sexually transmitted infection as cause of anal cancer. *N Engl J Med* 1997;337;1350.

40. Peters RK, Mack TM, Bernstein L: Parallels in the epidemiology of selected anogenital carcinomas. *J Nat Cancer Inst* 1984;72:609.

41. Palefsky JM: Anal squamous intraepithelial lesions in human immunodeficiency virus-positive men and women. *Semin Oncol* 2000;27:471.

42. Heino P, Goldman S, Lagerstedt U, Dillner J: Molecular and serological studies of human papillomavirus among patients with anal epidermoid carcinoma. *Int J Cancer* 1993;53:377.

43. Slater G, Greenstein A, Aufses AH Jr: Anal carcinoma in patients with Crohn's disease. *Ann Surg* 1984;199:348.

44. Daly JJ, Madrazo A: Anal Crohn's disease with carcinoma in situ. *Dig Dis Sci* 1989;25:464.

45. Buckwalter JA, Jurayj MN: Relationship of chronic anorectal disease to carcinoma. *Arch Surg* 1957;75:352.

46. Kline RJ, Spencer RJ, Harrison EG Jr: Carcinoma associated with fistula-in-ano. *Arch Surg* 1964;89:989.

47. Bjorge T, Engeland A, Luostarinen T, et al: Human papillomavirus infection as a risk factor for anal and perianal skin cancer in a prospective study. *Br J Cancer* 2002;87:61.

48. Durante AJ, Williams AB, Da Cossta M, et al: Incidence of anal cytological abnormalities in a cohort of human immunodeficiency virus-infected women. *Cancer Epid Bomarkers Prevent* 2003;12:638.

49. Daling JR, Weiss NS, Hislop TG, et al: Sexual practices, sexually transmitted diseases and the incidence of anal cancer. *N Engl J Med* 1987; 317:973.

50. Sobhani I, Vaugnat A, Walker F, et al: Prevalence of high grade dysplasia and cancer in the anal canal in human papillomavirus infected individuals. *Gastroenterology* 2001;120:857.

51. Frisch M, Smith E, Grulich A, Johansen C: Cancer in a population-based cohort of men and women in registered homosexual partnerships. *Am J Epidemiol* 2003;157:966.

52. Palefsky JM, Holly EA, Ralston ML, et al: High incidence of high grade squamous intra-epithelial lesions among HIV-positive and HIV-negative homosexual and bisexual men. *AIDS* 1998;12:495.

53. Grulich AE, Li Y, McDonald A, et al: Rates of non-AIDS-defining cancers in people with HIV infection before and after AIDS diagnosis. *AIDS* 2002;16:1155.

54. Sobhani I, Walker F, Roudot-Thoraval F, et al: Anal carcinoma: incidence and effect of cumulative infections. *AIDS* 2004;18:1561.

55. Moscicki A-B, Hills NK, Shiboski S, et al: Risk factors for abnormal anal cytology in young heterosexual women. *Cancer Epidemiol Biomarkers Prevent* 1999;8:173.

56. Frisch M, Fenger C, van den Brule AJC, et al: Variants of squamous cell carcinoma of the anal canal and perianal skin and their relation to human papillomaviruses. *Cancer Res* 1999;59;753.

57. Kubbutat M, Stites DP, Farhat S, et al: Role of E6 and E7 oncoproteins in HPV-induced anogenital malignancies. *Semin Virol* 1996;7:295.

58. Williams SMG, Disbrow GL, Schlegel R, et al: Requirement of epidermal growth factor receptor for hyperplasia induced by E5, a high risk human papillomavirus oncogene. *Cancer Res* 2005;6:6534.

59. Penn I: Cancers of the anogenital region in renal transplant recipients. Analysis of 65 cases. *Cancer* 1986;68:611.

60. Klotz RG, Pamukcoglu T, Souilliard DH: Transitional cloacogenic carcinoma of the anal canal. Clinicopathologic study of 373 cases. *Cancer* 1967;20:1727.

61. Sawyers JL: Squamous cell cancer of the perianus and anus. *Surg Clin North Am* 1972;52:935.

62. Papillon J, Montbarbon MD: Epidermoid carcinoma of the anal canal. *Dis Colon Rectum* 1987;30:324.

63. Wong CS, Tsao MS, Sharma V, et al: Prognostic role of p53 expression in epidermoid carcinoma of the anal canal. *Int J Radiation Oncol Biol Phys* 1999;45:9.

64. Chetty R, Serra S, Hsieh E: Basaloid squamous carcinoma of the anal canal with an adenoid cystic pattern. *Am J Surg Pathol* 2005;29:1668.

65. Kuwano H, Iwashita A, Enjoji M: Pseudosarcomatous carcinoma of the anal canal. *Dis Colon Rectum* 1983;26:123.

66. Watson PH: Clear-cell carcinoma of the anal canal: a variant of anal transitional zone carcinoma. *Hum Pathol* 1990;21:350.

67. Morson BC, Sobin LH: Histological typing of intestinal tumours. In: *International Histological Classification of Tumours,* No. 15. Geneva: World Health Organization, 1976, p 67.

68. Clark J, Petrelli N, Herrera L, et al: Epidermoid carcinoma of the anal canal. *Cancer* 1986;57:400.

69. Wade DS, Herrera L, Castillo NB, Petrelli NJ: Metastases to the lymph nodes in epidermoid carcinoma of the anal canal studies by a clearing technique. *Surg Gynecol Obstet* 1989;169:238.

70. Schraut WH, Wang C-H, Dawson PJ, et al: Depth of invasion, location, and size of cancer of the anus dictate operative treatment. *Cancer* 1983;51:1291.

71. Ryan DP, Compton CC, Mayer RJ: Carcinoma of the anal canal. *N Engl J Med* 2000;342:792.

72. Pintor MP, Northover JM, Nicholls RJ: Squamous carcinoma of the anus at one hospital from 1948 to 1984. *Br J Surg* 1989;76:806.

73. Myerson RJ, Karnell LH, Menck HR: The National Cancer Data Base report on carcinoma of the anus. *Cancer* 1997;80:805.

74. Deans GT, McAleer JJ, Spence RA: Malignant anal tumors. *Br J Surg* 1994;81:500.

75. Scott NA, Beart RW Jr, Weiland LH, et al: Carcinoma of the anal canal and flow cytometric DNA analysis. *Br J Cancer* 1989;60:56.

76. Bonin SR, Pajak TF, Russell AH, et al: Overexpression of p53 protein and outcome of patients treated with chemoradiation for carcinoma of the anal canal. *Cancer* 1999;85:1226.

77. Hung A, Crane C, Delcos M, et al: Cisplatin-based combined modality therapy for anal carcinoma. *Cancer* 2003;97:1195.

78. Cohen AM, Wong WD: Anal squamous cell cancer nodal metastases: prognostic significance and therapeutic considerations. *Surg Oncol Clin N Am* 1996;5:203.

79. Rousseau DL, Petrelli NJ, Kahlenberg MS: Overview of anal cancer for the surgeon. *Surg Oncol Clin N Am* 2004;13:249.

80. Hui YZ, Noffsinger AE, Miller MA, et al: Strong epidermal growth factor receptor expression but not Her2/neu expression correlates with cell proliferation in anal canal carcinomas. *Int J Surg Pathol* 1999;7:193.

81. Klas JV, Rothenberger DA, Wong WD, Madoff RD: Malignant tumors of the anal canal: the spectrum of disease, treatment and outcomes. *Cancer* 1999:85:1686.

82. Anagnostopoulos GK, Arvanitidis D, Sakorafas G, et al: Combined carcinoid-adenocarcinoma tumor of the anal canal. *Scand J Gastroenterol* 2004;39:198.

83. Hobbs CM, Lowry MA, Owen D, Sobin LH: Anal gland carcinoma. *Cancer* 2001;92:2045.

84. Winkelman J, Grosfeld J, Bigelow B: Colloid carcinoma of anal gland origin. Report of a case and review of the literature. *Am J Clin Pathol* 1964;42:395.

85. Wong AY, Rahilly MA, Adams W, Lee CS: Mucinous anal gland carcinoma with perianal pagetoid spread. *Pathology* 1998;30:1.

86. Li SC, Waters BL, Simmons-Arnold L, Beatty BG: Cytokeratin 7 and 20 expression in rectal adenomas, rectal adenocarcinomas, anal glands and junctional rectal mucosa. *Mod Pathol* 2001;14:90A.

87. Williams GR, Talbot IC, Northover JMA, Leigh IM: Keratin expression in the normal anal canal. *Histopathology* 1995;26:39.

88. Thomas RM, Sobin LH: Gastrointestinal cancer: incidence and prognosis by histological type. SEER population based data: 1973-1987. *Cancer* 1995;75:154.

89. Close AS, Schwab RL: A history of the anal ducts and anal duct carcinoma. *Cancer* 1955;8:979.

90. Nishimura T, Nozue M, Suzuki K, et al: Perianal mucinous carcinoma successfully treated with a combination of external beam radiotherapy and high dose rate interstitial brachytherapy. *Br J Radiol* 2000;73:661.

91. Fenoglio-Preiser CM, Perzin K, Pascal RR: *Tumors of the Large and Small Intestine.* AFIP Fascicle, 2nd Series. Washington, DC: AFIP, 1990.

92. Degner AM, Laino L, Accappaticcio G, et al: Human papillomavirus-32-positive extragenital Bowenoid papulosis (BP) in a HIV patient with typical genital BP localization. *Sex Transm Dis* 2004;31:619.

93. Schwartz RA, Janniger CK: Bowenoid papulosis. *J Am Acad Dermatol* 1991;24:261.

94. Ikenberg H, Gissmann L, Gross G, et al: Human papillovirus-type-16-DNA in genital Bowen's disease and in Bowenoid papulosis. *Int J Cancer* 1983;32:563.

95. Strauss RJ, Fazio VW: Bowen's disease of the anal and perianal area. A report and analysis of twelve cases. *Am J Surg* 1979;137:231.

96. Grodsky L: Unsuspected anal cancer discovered after minor anorectal surgery. *Dis Colon Rectum* 1967;10:471.

97. Graham JH, Helwig EB: Bowen's disease and its relationship to systemic cancer. *Arch Dermatol* 1961;83:738.

98. Cleary RK, Schaldenbrand JD, Fowler JJ, et al: Treatment options for perianal Bowen's disease. Survey of American Society of Colon and Rectal Surgeons members. *Am Surg* 2000;66:866.

99. Alvarez-Canas MC, Fernandez FA, Rodilla IG, Val-Bernal JF: Perianal basal cell carcinoma: a comparative histologic, immunohistochemical, and flow cytometric study with basaloid carcinoma of the anus. *Am J Dermatopathol* 1996;18:371.

100. Behrendt G, Hansmann M: Carcinomas of the anal canal and anal margin differ in their expression of cadherin, cytokeratins and p53. *Virch Arch* 2001;439:782.

101. Charnley N, Choudhury A, Chesser P, et al: Effective treatment of anal cancer in the elderly with low dose chemoradiation. *Br J Cancer* 2005;92:1221.

102. Newlin HE, Zlotecki RA, Morris CC, et al: Squamous cell carcinoma of the anal margin. *J Surg Oncol* 2004;86:55.

103. Perera D, Pathma-Nathan N, Rabbit P, et al: Sentinel node biopsy for squamous cell carcinoma of the anus and anal margin. *Dis Colon Rectum* 2003;46:1027.

104. Gingrass PJ, Bubrick MP, Hitchcock CR: Anorectal verrucous squamous carcinoma. Report of two cases. *Dis Colon Rectum* 1978;21:120.

105. Gissmann L, DeVilliers EM, zur Hausen H: Analysis of human genital warts (condylomata acuminata) and other genital tumors for human papillomavirus type 6 DNA. *Int J Cancer* 1981;29:5124.

106. Wells M, Robertson S, Lewis F, Dixon MF: Squamous carcinoma arising in a giant perianal condyloma associated with human papillomavirus types 6 and 11. *Histopathology* 1988;12:319.

107. Soler C, Chardonnet Y, Allibert P, et al: Detection of multiple types of human papillomavirus in a giant condyloma from a grafted patient. Analysis by immunohistochemistry, in situ hybridisation, Southern blot and polymerase chain reaction. *Virus Res* 1992;23:193.

108. Trombetta LJ, Place RJ: Giant condyloma acuminatum of the anorectum: trends in epidemiology and management: report of a case and review of the literature. *Dis Colon Rectum* 2001;44:1878.

109. Knoblich R, Failing JF Jr: Giant condyloma acuminatum (Buschke-Lowenstein tumor) of the rectum. *Am J Clin Pathol* 1967;48:389.

110. Chu QD, Vereidis MP, Libbey NP, Wanebo HJ: Giant condyloma acuminatum (Buschke-Lowenstein tumor) of the anorectal and perianal regions. Analysis of 42 cases. *Dis Colon Rectum* 1994;36:950.

111. Helwig EB, Graham JH: Anogenital (extramammary) Paget's disease. A clinicopathological study. *Cancer* 1963;16:387.

112. McCarter MD, Quan SHQ, Busam K, et al: Long term outcome of perianal Paget's disease. *Dis Colon Rectum* 2003;46:612.

113. Kuehn PG, Tennant R, Brenneman AR: Familial occurrence of extramammary Paget's disease. *Cancer* 1973;31:145.

114. Lloyd J, Flanagan AM: Mammary and extramammary Paget's disease. *J Clin Pathol* 2000;53:742.

115. Regauer S: Extramammary Paget's disease—a proliferation of adnexal origin? *Histopathology* 2006;48:723.

116. Stacy D, Burrell MO, Franklin EW: Extramammary Paget's disease of the vulva and anus: use of intraoperative frozen-section margins. *Am J Obstet Gynecol* 1986;155:519.

117. Giltman LI, Osborne PT, Coleman SA, Uthman EO: Paget's disease of the anal mucosa in association with carcinoma demonstrating mucoepidermoid features. *J Surg Oncol* 1985;28:277.

118. Arminski TC, Pollard RJ: Paget's disease of the anus secondary to a malignant papillary adenoma of the rectum. *Dis Colon Rectum* 1973; 16:46.

119. Guo L, Kuroda N, Miyazaki E, et al: Anal canal neuroendocrine carcinoma with Pagetoid extension. *Pathol Int* 2004;54:630.

120. Yamamoto O, Yasuda H: Extramammary Paget's disease with superimposed herpes simplex infection: immunohistochemical comparison with cases of the two respective diseases. *Br J Dermatol* 2003;48:1258.

121. Brainard JA, Hart WR: Proliferative lesions associated with anogenital Paget's disease. *Am J Surg Pathol* 2000;24:543.

122. Belcher RW: Extramammary Paget's disease: enzyme histochemistry and electron microscopic study. *Arch Pathol Lab Med* 1972;94:59.

123. Mazoujian G, Pinkus GS, Haagenssen DE: Extramammary Paget's disease—evidence for origin. *Am J Surg Pathol* 1984;8:43.

124. Onishi T, Watanabe S: The use of cytokeratins 7 and 20 in the diagnosis of primary and secondary extramammary Paget's disease. *Br J Dermatol* 2001;142:243.

125. Kondo Y, Kashima K, Daa T, et al: The ectopic expression of gastric mucin in extramammary and mammary Paget's disease. *Am J Surg Pathol* 2002;26:617.

126. Tanskanen M, Jahkola T, Asko-Seljavaara S, et al: Her 2 oncogene amplification in extramammary Paget's disease. *Histopathology* 2003;42:575.

127. Liegl B, Horn L-C, Moinfar F: Androgen receptors are frequently expressed in mammary and extramammary Paget's disease. *Mod Pathol* 2005;18:1283.

128. Kuan SF, Montag AG, Hart J, et al: Differential expression of mucin genes in mammary and extramammary Paget's disease. *Am J Surg Pathol* 2001;25:1469.

129. Goldblum JR, Hart WR: Perianal Paget's disease. A histologic and immunohistochemical study of 11 cases with and without associated rectal adenocarcinoma. *Am J Surg Pathol* 1998;22:170.

130. Nowak MA, Guerriere-Kovach P, Pathan A, et al: Perianal Paget's disease. Distinguishing primary and secondary lesions using immunohistochemical studies including gross cystic disease fluid protein-15 and cytokeratin 20 expression. *Arch Pathol Lab Med* 1998;122:1077.

131. Arki Y, Noake T, Hata H, et al: Perianal Paget's disease treated with a wide excision and gluteal fold flap reconstruction guided by photodynamic diagnosis. *Dis Colon Rectum* 2003;46:1563.

132. Runfola MA, Weber TK, Rodriguez-Bigas MA, et al: Photodynamic therapy for residual neoplasms of the perianal skin. *Dis Colon Rectum* 2000;43:499.

133. Brown RSD, Lankester KJ, McCormack MM, et al: Radiotherapy for perianal Paget's disease. *Clin Oncol* 2002;14:272.

134. Meeker JH, Neubecker RD, Helwig EB: Hidradenoma papilliferum. *Am J Clin Pathol* 1962;37:182.

135. Handa Y, Yamanaka N, Inagaki H, Tomita Y: Large ulcerated perianal hidradenoma papilliferum in a young female. *Dermatol Surg* 2003;29:790.

136. MacNeill KN, Riddell RH, Ghazarian D: Perianal apocrine adenocarcinoma arising in a benign apocrine adenoma; first case report and review of the literature. *J Clin Pathol* 2005;58:17.

137. Murata S, Fujita S, Sugihara K, et al: Sclerosing sweat duct carcinoma in the perianal skin: a case report. *Jpn J Clin Oncol* 1997;27:197.

138. Tatnall FM, Jones EW: Giant solitary trichoepitheliomas located in the perianal area: report of three cases. *Br J Dermatol* 1986;115:91.

139. Clark J, Ioffreda M, Helm KF: Multiple familial trichoepitheliomas: a folliculosebaceous-apocrine genodermatosis. *Am J Dermatopathol* 2002;24:402.

140. Martinez CA, Priolli DG, Piovesan HP, Waisberg J: Nonsolitary giant perianal trichoepithelioma with malignant transformation into basal cell carcinoma: report of a case and review of the literature. *Dis Colon Rectum* 2004;47:773.

141. Wanebo HJ, Woodruff JM, Farr GH: Anorectal melanoma. *Cancer* 1981;47:1891.

142. Morson BC, Volkstadt H: Malignant melanoma of the anal canal. *J Clin Pathol* 1963;16:126.

143. Chang AE, Karnell LH, Menck HR: The national cancer data base report on cutaneous and noncutanaeous melanoma. *Cancer* 1998;1664.

144. Cooper PH, Mills SE, Allen S: Malignant melanoma of the anus: report of 12 patients and analysis of 255 additional cases. *Dis Colon Rectum* 1982;25:693.

145. Cagir B, Whiteford MH, Topham A, et al: Changing epidemiology of anorectal melanoma. *Dis Colon Rectum* 1999;42:1203.

146. Pack GT, Oropeza R: A comparative study of melanoma and epidermoid carcinoma of the anal canal: a review of twenty melanomas and twenty-nine epidermoid carcinomas. *Dis Colon Rectum* 1967;10:161.

147. Ackermann DM, Polk HC Jr, Schrodt GR: Desmoplastic melanoma of the anus. *Hum Pathol* 1985;16:1277.

148. Fitzgibbons P, Chaurushiya P, Nichols P, et al: Primary mucosal malignant melanoma: an immunohistochemical study of 12 cases with comparison to cutaneous and metastatic melanomas. *Hum Pathol* 1989;20:269.

149. Gorden A, Osman I, Gai W, et al: Analysis of BRAF and NRAS mutations in metastatic melanoma tissues. *Cancer Res* 2003;63:3955.

150. Helmke BM, Mollenhauer J, Herold-Mende C, et al: BRAF mutations distinguish anorectal from cutaneous melanoma at the molecular level. *Gastroenterology* 2004;127:1815.

151. Ishii S, Shiiba K, Mizoi T, et al: Allelic loss of the NF1 gene in anal malignant melanoma in a patient with neurofibromatosis type I. *Int J Clin Oncol* 2001;6:2001.

152. Das G, Gupta S, Shukla PJ, Jagannath P: Anorectal melanoma: a large clinicopathological study from India. *Int Surg* 2003;8:21.

153. Ross M, Pezzi C, Pezzi T, Meurer D, et al: Patterns of failure in anorectal melanoma. A guide to surgical therapy. *Arch Surg* 1990;125:313.

154. Ben-Izhak O, Bar-Chana M, Sussman L, et al: Ki67 antigen and PCNA proliferation markers predict survival in anorectal malignant melanoma. *Histopathology* 2002;41:519.

155. Kim KB, Sanguino AM, Hodges C, et al: Biochemotherapy in patients with metastatic anorectal mucosal melanoma. *Cancer* 2004;100:1478.

156. Ulmer A, Metzger S, Fierlbeck G: Successful palliation of stenosing anorectal melanoma by intratumoral injections with natural interferon-beta. *Melanoma Res* 2002;12:395.

157. Mathieu A, Chamlou R, Le Moine F, et al: Tailgut cyst associated with carcinoid tumor: case report and review of the literature. *Histol Histopathol* 2005;20:1065.

158. Maruyama A, Murabayashi K, Hayashi M, et al: Adenocarcinoma arising in a tailgut cyst: report of a case. *Jpn J Surg* 1998;28:1319.

159. Krivokapic Z, Dimitrijevic I, Barisic G, et al: Adenosquamous carcinoma arising within a retrorectal tailgut cyst: case report. *World J Gastroenterol* 2005;11:6225.

160. Andea AA, Klimstra DS: Adenocarcinoma arising in a tailgut cyst with prominent meningothelial proliferation and thyroid tissue: case report and review of the literature. *Virch Arch* 2005;446:316.

161. Assor D, Davis JB: Multiple apocrine fibroadenomas of the anal skin: case reports. *Am J Clin Pathol* 1977;68:397.

162. Kazakov DV, Bisceglia M, Mukensnabl P, Michal M: Pseudoangiomatous stromal hyperplasia in lesions involving anogenital mammary-like glands. *Am J Surg Pathol* 2005;29:1243.

163. Kazakov DV, Bisceglia M, Sima R, Michal M: Adenosis tumor of anogenital mammary-like glands: a case report and demonstration of clonality by HUMARA assay. *J Cutan Pathol* 2006;33:43.

164. Hobson KG, Ghaemmaghami V, Roe JP, et al: Tumors of the retrorectal space. *Dis Colon Rectum* 2005;48:1964.

165. Cody HS, Marcove RC, Quan SH: Malignant retrorectal tumors: 28 years experience at Memorial Sloan-Kettering Cancer Center. *Dis Colon Rectum* 1981;24:501.

166. Caropreso PE, Wengert PA Jr, Milford HE: Tailgut cyst: a rare retrorectal tumor. Report of a case and review. *Dis Colon Rectum* 1975;18:597.

167. Gius JA, Stout AP: Perianal cysts of vestigial origin. *Arch Surg* 1938;37:268.

168. Patterson C, Musselman L, Chorneyko K, et al: Merkel cell (neuroendocrine) carcinoma of the anal canal. *Dis Colon Rectum* 2003;46:676.

169. Rickert RR, Compton CC: Protocol for the examination of specimens from patients with carcinomas of the anus and anal canal. *Arch Pathol Lab Med* 2000;124:21.

Gastrointestinal Neuroendocrine Lesions

GENERAL ORGANIZATION OF THE GASTROINTESTINAL SYSTEM

The gastrointestinal neuroendocrine system (GNES) is the largest and most complex endocrine organ in the body (1). The gut contains numerous neuroendocrine (NE) cells that produce many peptide hormones. Since NE cells exhibit endocrine, paracrine, and neurotransmitter functions (Fig. 17.1), they are best termed *NE cells* rather than *endocrine cells*. They constitute a complex system that regulates many gastrointestinal (GI) functions. Some NE secretions act as true peptide hormones. Gastrin, secretin, and cholecystokinin (CCK) are secreted into the blood to reach their target organs (stomach, pancreas, and gallbladder); soon thereafter they are metabolized and eliminated. Other peptides, such as somatostatin, are released into the local subepithelial connective tissue or directly onto other cell types via long basal cytoplasmic processes in a paracrine fashion. Neurons interact with gastrointestinal endocrine cells, endocrine cells interact with other endocrine cells, and endocrine cells may influence neurons (1,2). In addition, many GI hormones interact with the hypothalamic-pituitary axis to orchestrate the secretory activity and motility necessary for effective digestion (1), including acid, bicarbonate, and enzyme secretion and local blood flow. The GNES also interacts with the immune system (1). Immune responses alter neural and endocrine function, and in turn, neural and endocrine activity modifies immunologic functions. Finally, some GI hormones enhance metabolic levels and promote GI growth.

NE cells are widely distributed throughout the epithelia of the stomach, intestines, distal esophagus, and anus. Their overall density, contents, and structure differ in various parts of the gut. Most NE cells lie within the epithelium, but some are also present in the lamina propria of the stomach and the appendix. Endocrine cells are sensitive to chemical and mechanical stimuli, to which they respond by releasing extracellular mediators. At least 14 types of NE cells populate the GI mucosa (Table 17.1) (2). Some peptides are produced solely in the upper GI tract and are stimulated only for a short time following meals; others are scattered throughout the gut and are exposed to prolonged stimulation. Gastrin is primarily a gastric antral hormone; CCK, secretin, gastric

inhibitory polypeptide, and motilin are mainly upper small intestinal hormones; and enteroglucagon and neurotensin are lower intestinal peptides. In contrast, vasoactive intestinal polypeptide (VIP), substance P, enkephalins, bombesin, somatostatin, and other substances are produced more diffusely throughout the gut.

NE cells may be open or closed, depending on whether or not they reach the gastrointestinal lumen (Fig. 17.2). Closed endocrine cells fail to reach the lumen, suggesting that they do not react to luminal stimuli. Instead, they probably react to other stimulants, such as distension, temperature, and neural or hormonal factors. "Open" cells extend from the basal lamina to the lumen. Most open endocrine cells reach the lumen in a narrow specialized area containing tufts of microvilli and a centriole that acts as a sensor of the luminal contents.

Identification of Neuroendocrine Cells

NE cells can sometimes be recognized in routinely stained sections by the presence of pyramidally shaped eosinophilic or clear cells lying along the basement membrane. Eosinophilic granules, which generally are smaller than those seen in Paneth cells, may be visible and lie diffusely distributed throughout the cell or in a subnuclear location (Fig. 17.3). Since not all NE cells are immediately recognizable in hematoxylin and eosin (H&E)-stained sections, numerous techniques have been devised to detect their presence. The earliest techniques involved reactions with various heavy metals, especially silver (Table 17.2), and ultrastructural evaluation. In this country, these techniques have largely been abandoned due to their expense, the difficulty in performing them well, and the more recent development of a number of immunostains that reliably detect endocrine cells. Immunologic markers of neuroendocrine differentiation include antibodies to neuron-specific enolase (NSE), protein gene product (PGP) 9.5, synaptophysin, and chromogranin (CgA). Of these, NSE is the least specific. CgA is a secretory granule that is located alongside specific hormones in large dense-core vesicles of neuronal and NE cells (3). It is secreted in tumors; the amount present in the blood correlates with the tumor burden. NE cells containing amines (histamine and serotonin) regularly exhibit CgA immunoreactivity.

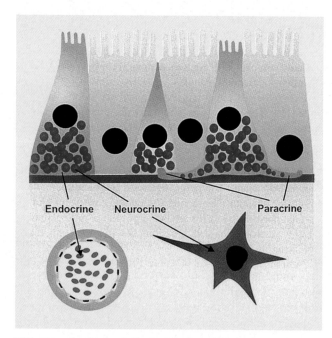

FIG. 17.1. Endocrine cells have endocrine functions whereby the contents of their secretory granules are released into the circulation to have an effect at a location distant from the site of production. They also have neurocrine effects influencing neuronal functions. Long basal extensions of endocrine cells that touch other endocrine cells or nearby epithelial cells mediate paracrine effects.

Other peptide-containing endocrine cells are heterogeneous in their CgA immunoreactivity. We prefer synaptophysin immunostains since they reliably detect a wide variety of gastrointestinal NE cells. These antibodies and the silver-based techniques allow the identification of endocrine cells but do not provide information with respect to their hormonal products. Specific cell types can be identified immunohistochemically using antibodies directed against the specific hormone that the cells are known to produce.

In this chapter, we will first discuss normal gastrointestinal NE cell populations. This will be followed by a discussion of gastrointestinal NE cell proliferations. These include hyperplastic lesions as well as NE tumors.

NORMAL GASTROINTESTINAL NEUROENDOCRINE CELL POPULATIONS

Esophagus

NE cells lie scattered among the basal cells in approximately 25% of normal individuals (4). They are also present in the mucous glands (5).

Stomach

There are at least eight distinct gastric endocrine cell types, including enterochromaffin (EC), enterochromaffinlike (ECL),

TABLE 17.1 **Gastrointestinal Endocrine Cells**

Cell Name	Location	Main Product
D	Stomach Small intestine Appendix Large intestine	Somatostatin
D1	Stomach Small intestine Appendix Large intestine	Unknown
EC	Stomach Intestines Appendix Submucosal glands	Serotonin
ECL	Stomach Intestines Appendix Submucosal glands	Histamine
G	Pylorus Duodenum	Gastrin
I	Small intestine	Cholecystokinin
K	Small intestine	Gastrin-releasing peptide

L	Intestine	Enteroglucagon,
		  pancreatic
		  polypeptidelike
		  peptide

M	Small intestine	Motilin
N	Small intestine Appendix	Neurotensin
P	Stomach Small intestine	? Gastrin-releasing peptide
PP	Small intestine	Pancreatic polypeptide
S	Small intestine	Secretin
X	Gastric antrum	Unknown

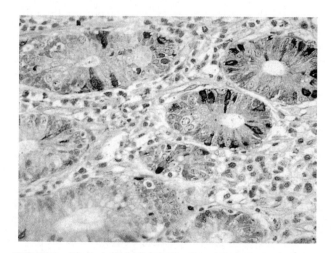

FIG. 17.2. Open and closed endocrine cells in normal colonic mucosa stained with an antibody to chromogranin.

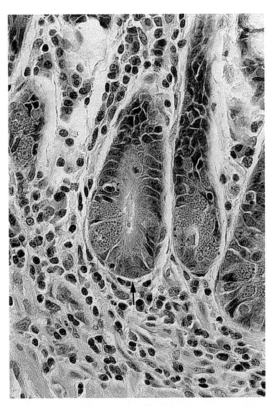

FIG. 17.3. Cross section of several crypt bases showing a mixture of cell types. The endocrine cell highlighted by the *arrow* lies beneath other cell types.

TABLE 17.2	Special Stains Used to Detect Neuroendocrine Cells
Argentaffin cells	Cells with granules that precipitate silver from ammoniacal silver nitrate solutions
Enterochromaffin cells	Cells that react with potassium dichromate
Argyrophilic cells	Cells that precipitate silver only if an external reducing agent is present

D, D1, P, G, X, and ghrelin-producing cells (Table 17.1) (6). Three cell types (ECL, G, and D) account for >75% of the gastric NE cell mass. NE cells appear as cuboidal or short columnar cells scattered among the gastric epithelia, usually in the glands (Fig. 17.4). Less commonly they occur in the glandular neck. NE cells rarely reach the foveolae; they are absent from the surface. Their composition and distribution differ in the oxyntic and antral mucosa. Approximately 50% of antral NE cells are G cells (gastrin producing), 30% are serotonin-producing EC cells, and 15% are somatostatin-producing D cells. The remaining 5% consist of other cell types. The predominant NE cell in the fundus is the histamine-producing ECL cell. There are also a few X cells with an unknown secretory product, ghrelin-producing cells, and EC cells. Most gastric NE cells are closed. They lie along the basement membrane and are covered by nonendocrine epithelium that prevents their contact with the glandular lumen.

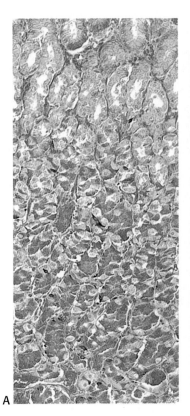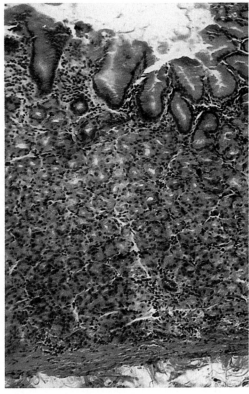

FIG. 17.4. Argyrophilic endocrine cells in the normal fundus stain with Grimelius stain **(A).** Corresponding hematoxylin and eosin stain **(B).**

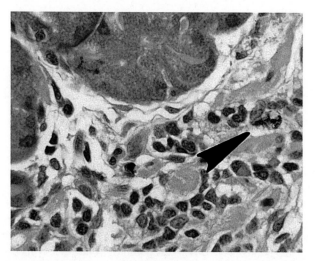

FIG. 17.5. Widely scattered endocrine cells (*arrow*) within the lamina propria. Chromogranin immunostain.

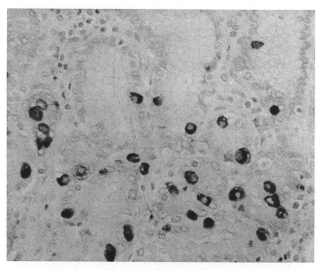

FIG. 17.6. Antral G cells stained with gastrin immunostain.

They contain numerous basally located hormone-containing granules. The NE cells secrete their hormones into the intercellular space, where they diffuse into capillaries. Scattered endocrine cells are occasionally found in the lamina propria near the base of glands apparently unattached to epithelium. They exist singly (Fig. 17.5) or in clusters and are seen in the antrum or antrocorpus junction. Lamina propria endocrine cells occur predominantly in the stomach of patients with gastritis, but they can also be found in the normal stomach.

G Cells

G cells are large, round or oval cells (7) that produce gastrin. They mainly lie in the neck region of the antral glands trailing off toward the gland base. G cells normally have an irreg-

ular and random spatial distribution that ranges between one and three to four cells per gland. They contain variably dense cytoplasmic granules measuring 150 to 200 in μm diameter. Argyrophilic and argentaffinic stains fail to detect most G cells (7), but they are easily identified by CgA or synaptophysin stains. They are also identifiable using gastrin-specific immunohistochemical stains (Fig. 17.6).

The number of antral G cells varies, depending on the acid content of the stomach, the presence of proliferative stimuli, and gastric location. G cells are most numerous on the greater curvature. Gastrin promotes acid and pepsinogen secretion (Fig 17.7), gastric motility, and gastric oxyntic mucosal proliferation. In sustained hypergastrinemia, parietal cells, ECL cells, and surface mucosal cells increase in number. The trophic effect of gastrin is most marked on ECL cells (8). Parietal cell mass and G-cell density are interrelated.

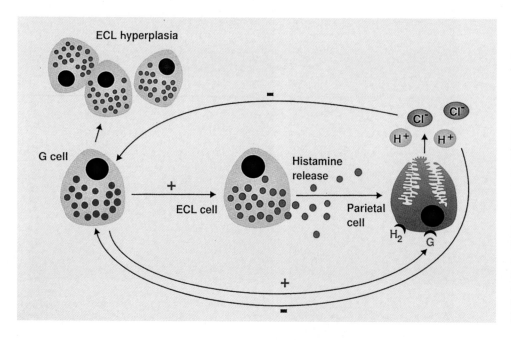

FIG. 17.7. Gastrin effects on enterochromaffinlike (ECL) cells. Gastrin release stimulates ECL hyperplasia by binding to gastrin receptors on ECL cells. This results in hyperplasia of ECL cells as well as histamine release. The histamine released from the ECL cells binds to histamine receptors on G cells leading to acid secretion. Gastrin also acts directly on parietal cells by binding to gastrin receptors present on these cells, again causing acid secretion. Acid produced by the parietal cell negatively regulates gastrin secretion through a feedback loop.

Hypochlorhydria causes G-cell proliferation and increased gastrin transcription.

Enterochromaffin Cells

EC cells are the most numerous NE cell populations in the gut and they are widely found in many sites including the stomach. They are sparse in the mucous neck portion but are quite numerous in the lower half of the gland. Their overall distribution is patchy; areas with numerous EC cells alternate with areas containing few or none. They are especially numerous in areas of intestinal metaplasia (9). These cells are described further below.

D Cells

D cells secrete somatostatin and are uniformly distributed throughout the antral and oxyntic mucosa (Fig. 17.8). Approximately 20% of gastric D cells have basal axonal-like cytoplasmic processes with terminal expansions that allow D cells to function in a paracrine fashion (10). Most antral D cells are open cells that act as receptors, interacting with luminal contents. A feedback mechanism exists in which intraluminal acid stimulates somatostatin secretion. In the fundus, D cells are closed. Somatostatin secretion from D cells inhibits gastric acid, gastrin and intrinsic factor secretion, and acetylcholine release.

Enterochromaffinlike Cells

ECL cells are confined to the oxyntic mucosa, where they represent the dominant NE cell type, constituting 40% to 45% of oxyntic NE cells (6). ECL cells express CCK-2 (gastrin) receptors, which mediate histamine secretion and ECL cell growth (11,12). ECL cells decrease in number after antrectomy due to reduced gastrin levels. The pyramidally shaped ECL cells are closed with a broad base that directly abuts the basement membrane of oxyntic glands. They are randomly scattered throughout the lower and middle thirds of the glands (11). Their lateral processes extend to, and terminate on, parietal cell surfaces, allowing them to act in a paracrine fashion. They also act in an endocrine fashion. ECL cells can be identified by silver stains, or more specifically, by antibodies against histamine, histidine decarboxylase, and vesicular monoamine transporter 1 and 2 (VMAT 1 and 2) (13). ECL cells are a self-renewing population.

Ghrelin-producing Cells

Ghrelin is a recently discovered peptide that is produced by about 20% of endocrine cells in the oxyntic mucosa. These cells appear to differ from the ECL, EC, D, and probably X cells also present in this area (14). Ghrelin stimulates release of growth hormone (15), stimulates food intake, and modulates sleep (16). It also has an antiproliferative effect in neoplastic tissues (17) and stimulates gastric contractility (18). The hormone localizes to polygonal or flask-shaped endocrine cells in the oxyntic mucosa. These cells appear larger than the adjacent cells (19).

Small Intestine

While NE cells constitute <1% of all intestinal epithelial cells, numerous subpopulations of NE cells are present in this site (20). NE cells lie interspersed among absorptive cells and goblet cells in the crypts (Fig 17.9) and on the villi (Fig. 17.10), and some are found within Brunner glands. They share a common origin from the crypt epithelial stem cell (21). Each subpopulation has a distinct distribution along the cranial–caudal axis and along the crypt–villus axis, thereby producing an integrated response to various stimuli and facilitating normal secretory, absorptive, and motor functions.

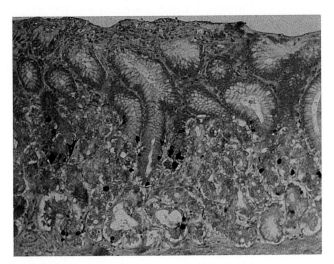

FIG. 17.8. Somatostatin-containing cells are quite numerous in the antrum.

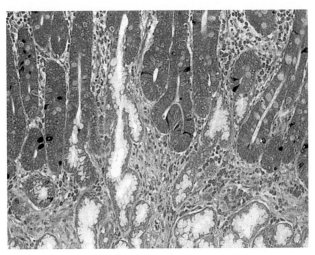

FIG. 17.9. Small intestinal enterochromaffin (EC) cells stained with an antibody to serotonin.

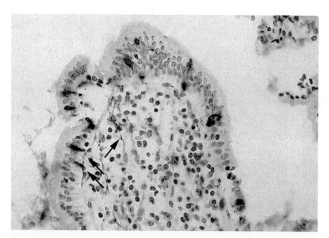

FIG. 17.10. Synaptophysin immunostain demonstrating endocrine cells along the surface of the villi, as well as numerous intramucosal nerves (*arrows*).

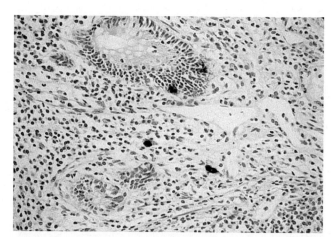

FIG. 17.11. Endocrine cells in the epithelium of the appendix. Chromogranin stain demonstrates endocrine cells in the crypt epithelium as well as in the lamina propria.

EC cells have an almost exclusively intraepithelial location resting on the basement membrane and projecting into the lumen with their apical portions. They are evenly distributed between crypts and villi. They are recognizable by their bright red granules. Others appear clear. Their cytoplasm is occupied by a large number of secretory granules. The major secretory product is serotonin, but subsets of EC cells also produce minor amounts of tachykinins, enkephalins, and motilin (7). Serotonin is synthesized from the amino acid tryptophan by hydroxylation and decarboxylation in the EC cell cytoplasm and subsequently transported into secretory granules by an active transport mechanism. Upon specific membrane simulation, granules are translocated to the cell membrane and released by exocytosis. Serotonin may influence adjacent cells by paracrine mechanisms or reach distant cells via the circulation. Release of serotonin in response to an acid pH, hypertonic glucose, amino acids, and noxious stimuli affects nerve endings that evoke mucosal hyperemia, secretion, and peristalsis (22).

The duodenum and jejunum harbor a large number of different NE cell types; the spectrum gradually narrows as one proceeds distally (23). The duodenum contains EC cells, D cells, and cells immunoreactive for CCK and gastrin. *Gastric inhibitory polypeptide–containing cells* occur in the midzone of the duodenal glands and to a lesser extent in the jejunum (24). *Motilin-immunoreactive cells* populate the duodenum and upper jejunum. *Substance P cells* in the proximal small intestine occur mainly in the crypts and lower villi, whereas *secretin-containing cells* are found nearly exclusively on villi. Brunner glands also contain NE cells producing and storing somatostatin, gastrin, CCK, and peptide YY (25).

Appendix

The appendix contains two populations of EC cells: Those in the crypts and those in the lamina propria (Fig. 17.11). They occur singly or in small clusters, and are more common in adults than in children. Lamina propria NE cells lie scattered near the base of the crypts, apparently unattached to crypt epithelium. They are invariably part of a structure termed the enterochromaffin cell–nerve fiber complex (26) that contains a mixture of endocrine cells, neurons, Schwann cells, and unmyelinated nerve processes all surrounded by an external lamina that is continuous with that of adjacent peptidergic nerve fibers. The EC cell–nerve fiber complex facilitates integration between intestinal endocrine cells and the enteric nervous system. Crypt endocrine cells tend to lie near the base of the crypts. Both crypt and lamina propria endocrine cells contain serotonin, somatostatin, enteroglucagon vasoactive intestinal polypeptide, and substance P. More endocrine cells populate the distal appendix than the proximal appendix. ECL cells, D cells, L cells, and N cells are also present.

Large Intestine, Rectum, and Anus

The colon has the least number of NE cells of any region of the GI tract, except the esophagus. The endocrine cell population in this region is heterogeneous in nature (Table 17.1). NE cells appear as small round or pyramidal cells lying on the basement membrane and scattered among the nonendocrine epithelial cells. They are most numerous in the base of the crypts and appear clear or they contain prominent eosinophilic basal granules. The latter are released by pinocytosis from the basal and lateral surfaces of the cells. Secretory products of these cells exert a paracrine modulating effect on neighboring exocrine and endocrine cells. When these products cross the basal membrane, they enter the bloodstream reaching target organs, where they exert endocrine effects. The neural effects of these cells are exerted as the hormones diffuse to synapses.

Anal endocrine cells lie above the dentate line in the colorectal mucosa, in the transitional mucosa, in anal ducts and glands, in crypts, and in perianal sweat glands. Like endocrine cells elsewhere, they lie close to the basement membrane. Endocrine cells are absent in the pectineal folds and perianal skin.

MOLECULAR FEATURES OF GASTROINTESTINAL ENDOCRINE TUMORS

Neuroendocrine tumors (NETs) exhibit a series of genetic aberrations, including point mutations, gene deletions, DNA methylation, chromosomal losses, and chromosomal gains involving both oncogenes and tumor suppressor genes. Several genetic syndromes with mutations in tumor suppressor genes, including multiple endocrine neoplasia type 1 (MEN-1) and neurofibromatosis type I (NF1), associate with the development of gastrointestinal NE tumors. MEN-1, an autosomal dominant disorder, associates with mutations in the *MEN1* gene on chromosome 11q13. *MEN1* encodes the protein menin, which binds Jun1, inhibiting Jun1-activated transcription (27,28). Mutations and/or loss of heterozygosity (LOH) at the *MEN1* locus occur in 40% to 75% of gastrointestinal NE tumors (27,29). The frequency of this event differs depending on tumor site and whether the tumors are sporadic or arise as part of the MEN-1 syndrome. For example, foregut and some midgut NETs have frequent deletions and mutations in the *MEN1* gene (30). *MEN1* LOH is present in 33% of midgut carcinoid tumors (31). Type II gastric carcinoids show LOH at the *MEN1* locus in 75% of tumors as compared to 16% of type I gastric carcinoids (32). LOH at the *MEN1* locus appears to be an important prerequisite to switch hypergastrinemia-induced ECL proliferations from a hyperplastic to a neoplastic state (31). Further, the presence of 11q13 LOH in gastric carcinoid tumors of patients without hypergastrinemia suggests that inactivation of the *MEN1* gene alone can cause ECL cell tumors (33). *Reg-a* gene alterations may be important in gastric ECL carcinoids (34). Mutation of the *Reg-a* gene could contribute to the development of ECL cell carcinoid tumors by allowing unrestrained stimulating effects of gastrin (34). Alterations in the *MEN1* gene also occur in 25% to 40% of sporadic gastrinomas (35).

LOH at locations distal to 11q13 at the location of the *succinate ubiquinone oxidoreductase subunit D* (SDHD) tumor suppressor gene is also implicated in the development of midgut (rather than foregut) carcinoids (36). Twenty-two percent of duodenal and ileal carcinoids show alterations at the *SDHD* locus (36). A number of other chromosomal gains and losses develop in NETs, but losses at 18qter, 11q22-24, and 16q are the most common genetic defects in midgut carcinoids (37,38). LOH at chromosome 18q is seen in 67% of midgut tumors (37). Fifteen percent of midgut tumors show abnormalities of the X chromosome (39). Inactivation of the $p16^{INK\alpha}$/*CDKN2A tumor* suppressor gene on chromosome 9p21 is also common in NE tumors. $p16^{INK\alpha4}$ inactivation occurs by either gene deletion or methylation of CpG islands (40) and is observed in 50% to 52% of sporadic gastrinomas (35). Other abnormalities found in gastrinomas include

aneuploidy, mismatch repair defects, amplification of the HER2/neu protooncogene (41), and other genetic changes.

Almost 80% of gastrointestinal NETs demonstrate nuclear and cytoplasmic β-catenin expression and 37.5% contain an exon 3 mutation (42). Another gene that may be important in the development of NETs is the *PDCD4* (*programmed cell death protein 4*) gene (43). *PDCD4* is a newly described tumor suppressor gene that suppresses cell proliferation and lies close to the *MEN1* gene on chromosome 11q13. Sporadic endocrine tumors arising in several sites frequently show loss of its expression.

NF1 is an autosomal dominant disorder resulting from mutations in the *NF1* gene located at 17q11. These mutations lead to premature truncation of neurofibromin, the tumor suppressor gene product. Some NF1 patients develop duodenal somatostatinomas (44) or gangliocytic paragangliomas. Several genes are frequently methylated in GI NETs including *p14, p16, MGMT, THBS1, RARβ, ER,* and *COX2* (37,45). p16 methylation is more frequent in older patients and associates with metastasis (45). The *Ras-association domain family 1, isoform A (RASSF1A)* gene is also frequently methylated in these neoplasms and associates with lymph node metastasis (45). Allelic losses of chromosomes 11q, 16q, and 1q may be important in the pathogenesis of goblet cell carcinoids and ileal carcinoids (46).

Immunohistochemical studies describe overexpression of the antiapoptotic bcl2 protein in gastric endocrine cell hyperplasia (47) and loss of E-cadherin expression in two thirds of malignant rectal carcinoid tumors (48). p53 expression is rare in small intestinal NETs (49) but occurs in up to 16% of carcinoid tumors (50). *p53* mutations are found in up to 25% of appendiceal goblet cell carcinoids as well as in some conventional appendiceal carcinoids (51). Ki-67 staining and p53 staining may serve as prognostic factors in some tumors (52,53).

Transforming growth factor-α (TGF-α) is expressed in 72% of gastrointestinal carcinoid tumors and most tumors also express its receptor, epidermal growth factor receptor (EGFR) (37). Gastrin-releasing peptide (GRP) is expressed in a proportion of NETs and gastrin-releasing peptide receptor (GRPR) is expressed in the majority of such tumors. Both GRP and GRPR are coexpressed in some gastrointestinal NETs, although GRP is not expressed by normal gastrointestinal neuroendocrine cells (54). Other proteins that are frequently expressed include c-myc, c-erbB2, and c-jun (55). These tumors also frequently express the somatostatin receptor subtype 2, a factor that may help select patients suitable for somatostatin analog treatment (56).

NEUROENDOCRINE CELL HYPERPLASIA

The term *NE cell hyperplasia* signifies a nonneoplastic, nonautonomous proliferation (more than two times normal) of NE cells leading to increased numbers of NE cells per unit area and increases in their total cell mass (57). It develops in

TABLE 17.3 Proliferative Endocrine Cell Lesion	
Histologic Pattern	Definition
Simple hyperplasia	Increase in single cells in glands
Linear hyperplasia	Forms of chains of five or more endocrine cells and equals two chains per millimeter
Micronodular hyperplasia	Nodules of endocrine cells with more than five endocrine cells in glands or crypts that do not exceed the diameter of the gastric glands
Adenomatoid hyperplasia	The presence of five or more coalescing nodules
Dysplasia	Enlargement and fusion of enterochromaffinlike nodules measuring <0.5 mm in diameter. These contain relatively atypical cells and may have microinvasion or newly formed stroma
Intramucosal or invasive carcinoids	Endocrine cell growths measuring >0.5 mm or invading the submucosa

various chronic inflammatory conditions, including chronic atrophic gastritis (CAG), *Helicobacter pylori* gastritis, celiac disease, and inflammatory bowel disease (IBD). It also complicates the use of gastric acid–suppressing therapies, which leads to chronic hypergastrinemia in most patients (58).

NE cell hyperplasia results from a combination of a prolonged cell half-life, augmented replication of mature cells, and/or differentiation of a larger fraction of uncommitted stem cells into specific NE cell types. Each of these mechanisms may be triggered by loss of normal inhibitory influences on NE cell proliferation, a lack of normal negative feedback mechanisms, or the trophic action of stimulating substances. Additionally, autocrine mechanisms may stimulate a cell's own proliferation. The local tissue microenvironment may also play a significant role in inducing the hyperplasia.

The stages in the progression of hyperplastic neuroendocrine lesions are shown in Table 17.3. *Simple or diffuse hyperplasia*, the earliest hyperplastic stage, is characterized by a diffuse increase in NE cells scattered singly or in clusters of up to three cells per gland. The cells may appear enlarged, especially in the lower third of the mucosa. *Linear hyperplasia* is diagnosed when linear, semi-linear, or daisy-chain–like ECL cell configurations are present. The next stage, *micronodular hyperplasia,* consists of solid micronodular NE cell nests measuring 100 to 150 μm in size (the average diameter of a gastric gland) (57,59,60). These may be bounded by an intact basement membrane continuous with that of the rest of the gland or lie in the basal glandular portion of the mucosa dissociated from the glands lying free in the lamina propria abutting the muscular mucosae. *Adenomatoid hyperplasia* consists of a close aggregation of five or more interglandular micronodular lesions, each with an intact basement membrane. As each micronodule enlarges, it breaks down its basement membrane and the cells develop cytologic atypia with an increased nuclear:cytoplasmic ratio, thereby qualifying for a diagnosis of a dysplasia. This dysplastic stage marks the borderline between the hyperplastic stages preceding it and the neoplastic stage of a fully developed carcinoid tumor

following it. It is the earliest "point of no return" in the hyperplasia–neoplasia sequence of ECL proliferation (57). These lesions include enlarging micronodules, fusing micronodules, microinvasive lesions, and nodules with newly formed stroma. The *carcinoid* stage is characterized by nodular infiltrating growths measuring >0.5 mm in diameter. These steps may be seen in proliferative NE cell lesions involving many cell types including G, ECL, EC, D, and L cells.

Often, gastrointestinal NE cell hyperplasia is unsuspected (61), since most lesions do not release enough hormones or other secretory products to produce significant biochemical abnormalities or to give rise to specific clinical syndromes. Furthermore, even though hyperplasia may be present, the lesions may not be visible endoscopically or grossly. Additionally, NE cell hyperplasias often remain unrecognized even when standard H&E-stained sections are examined due to their rarity and the difficulty in recognizing increased numbers of endocrine cells among the other epithelial cells present in the glands. Sometimes, it is only when suspicions of the gastroenterologist and/or pathologist cause the specimen to be stained a neuroendocrine marker that the increased number of endocrine cells becomes apparent.

Neuroendocrine Cell Hyperplasia in the Esophagus

NE cell hyperplasia in the esophagus usually develops in the setting of Barrett esophagus (BE). It is a common event affecting up to 90% of cases of BE. The majority of the cells are EC cells (62).

Neuroendocrine Cell Hyperplasia in the Stomach

G-cell Hyperplasia

G cells become hyperplastic in any condition that lowers gastric acid concentrations, including extensive multifocal gastritis,

TABLE 17.4	Conditions Associated with Hypergastrinemia and G-cell Hyperplasia

Chronic atrophic gastritis
Pernicious anemia
Primary G-cell hyperplasia and hyperfunction
Gastric ulcer
Gastric carcinoma
Retained excluded antrum
Helicobacter pylori infections
Multiple endocrine neoplasia type 1
Acromegaly
Gastric outlet obstruction
Gastric distention
Prior vagotomy
Chronic renal failure with uremia
Zollinger-Ellison syndrome
Chronic hypercalcinosis
Long-term therapy with H_2 receptor blockers
Long-term therapy with protein pump inhibitors

pernicious anemia, vagotomy, and prolonged treatment with proton pump inhibitors (Table 17.4; Figs. 17.12 to 17.14). G-cell hyperplasia following *vagotomy* results from a combination of chronic antral distention, decreased acid secretion, and release from vagally mediated inhibitors of G-cell proliferation. G-cell hyperplasia in *acromegaly* results either from the patients also having the MEN-1 syndrome or from unidentified trophic factors secreted by the pituitary.

Primary antral G-cell hyperplasia and hyperfunction is a rare pediatric disorder in which G-cell hyperplasia, hyperfunction, or both occur without a clear cause (63). This entity, also known as *pseudo-Zollinger-Ellison syndrome*, causes clinical and biochemical features resembling those seen in Zollinger-Ellison syndrome (ZES) but the patients lack a gastrin-producing tumor. The hypergastrinemia reverts to normal following antrectomy. Most familial cases result from a genetic defect in normal regulation of G-cell function or proliferation. Patients with nonfamilial forms of the disease have increased antral G-cell sensitivity to intragastric food stimulation (64).

The distribution of hyperplastic G-cell populations in primary and secondary antral G-cell hyperplasia is similar with increased G-cell numbers in the lower and middle thirds of the antral glands. Occasionally, longstanding diffuse antral G-cell hyperplasia progresses to multiple small micronodular G-cell clusters (Fig. 17.14) that eventually give rise to G-cell tumors (gastrinomas). Gastrin also stimulates oxyntic mucosal growth and increases the progenitor cell labeling index in this area.

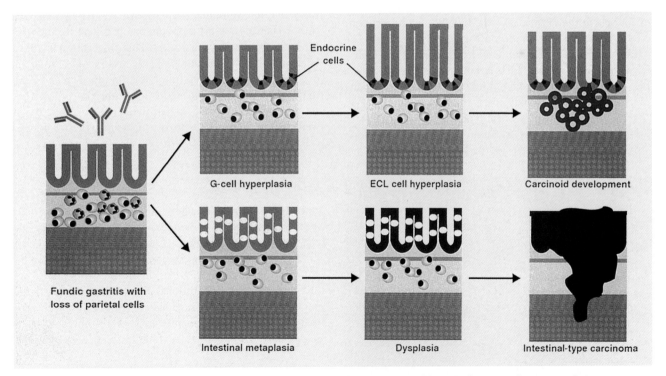

FIG. 17.12. Progression of autoimmune gastritis to carcinoid tumors and intestinal-type carcinomas. Patients with autoimmune gastritis develop G-cell hyperplasia in response to an antibody-mediated attack on the parietal cells that subsequently leads to decreased acid production. The hyperplastic G cells produce increased amounts of gastrin, leading to both foveolar hyperplasia as well as ECL cell hyperplasia. The ECL cell hyperplasia progresses further to the development of ECL micronests and eventually carcinoid tumors. At the same time, the gastric epithelium may become intestinalized in response to epithelial loss from the immunologic attack. This intestinal epithelium becomes dysplastic and can progress to intestinal-type carcinomas.

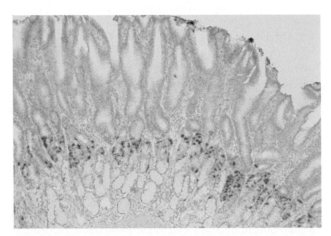

FIG. 17.13. Linear G-cell hyperplasia highlighted by gastrin immunostain.

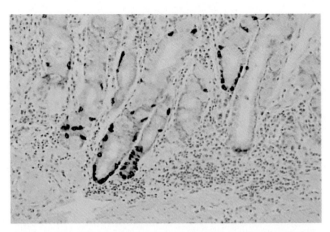

FIG. 17.15. Chromogranin immunostain showing linear hyperplasia.

Enterochromaffinlike Cell Hyperplasia

ECL cells are extremely sensitive to the stimulatory effects of gastrin, undergoing secondary hyperplasia in chronic hypergastrinemic states (65). Hypergastrinemia results in increased proliferation of both pluripotential stem cells and mature ECL cells (66). Gastrin also stimulates ECL function, as reflected by an increase in histamine decarboxylase activity and histamine release (67). The ECL hyperplasia is reversible if the hypergastrinemia is removed. ECL lesions develop exclusively in the oxyntic mucosa. In CAG, the hyperplastic cells are present only in the atrophic fundic glands and pyloric metaplastic glands but not in the intestinal metaplastic glands. Hyperplastic ECL lesions range from a diffuse ECL cell hyperplasia through linear and nodular aggregates to intramucosal and frankly invasive carcinoid tumors (Figs. 17.15 and 17.16). Patients with hypergastrinemia due to *H. pylori* infections or the chronic use of proton pump inhibitors (68) develop ECL cell hyperplasia, but carcinoid tumors are rare.

The most frequent histologic change in ECL cells in ZES patients is a diffuse hyperplasia, affecting more than half of ZES patients. Linear hyperplasia affects approximately 18% of patients, whereas micronodular hyperplasia is infrequent (59). Dysplastic ECL lesions can also develop. The topographic distribution of linear hyperplasia often localizes to the greater curvature and does not correspond to that of the ECL cell micronodular hyperplasia, dysplasia, and ECL tumor, changes that are more uniformly distributed between the lesser and greater curvatures. This observation led Bordi to suggest that the linear hyperplasia occurring in the setting of ZES may not be a step in the micronodular hyperplasia–dysplasia–NET (carcinoid) sequence. Rather, linear hyperplasia may represent a self-limited lesion (59). Antrectomy as well as some pharmacologic treatments may reverse the ECL cell hyperplasia.

D-cell Hyperplasia

Antral D-cell hyperplasia develops in patients with duodenal ulcer disease (69). Extensive gastric D-cell hyperplasia was reported in a 37-year-old woman with dwarfism, obesity, dryness of the mouth, and goiter. The D-cell density in this patient was increased 39-fold in the gastric fundus and 25-fold in the antrum. Antral G cells were increased 2.3-fold and they showed pronounced hypertrophy (69). The hypersomatostatinemia may have interfered with pituitary hormone release at an early age, thereby resulting in the dwarfism.

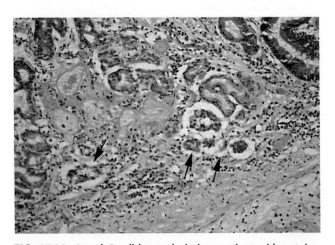

FIG. 17.14. Antral G-cell hyperplasia in a patient with autoimmune gastritis. Note the clusters of endocrine cells in the lamina propria (*arrows*). The lesion is visible even without a gastrin or neuroendocrine immunostain. The hyperplastic focus corresponds to an area of micronodular hyperplasia.

Hyperplasia of Ghrelin-producing Cells

Pericarcinoidal oxyntic mucosal ghrelin cell hyperplasia consistently occurs in patients with CAG. The ghrelin-producing cells are larger than their normal counterparts and appear polygonal or flask shaped. Diffuse, linear, and nodular forms of hyperplasia occur (19).

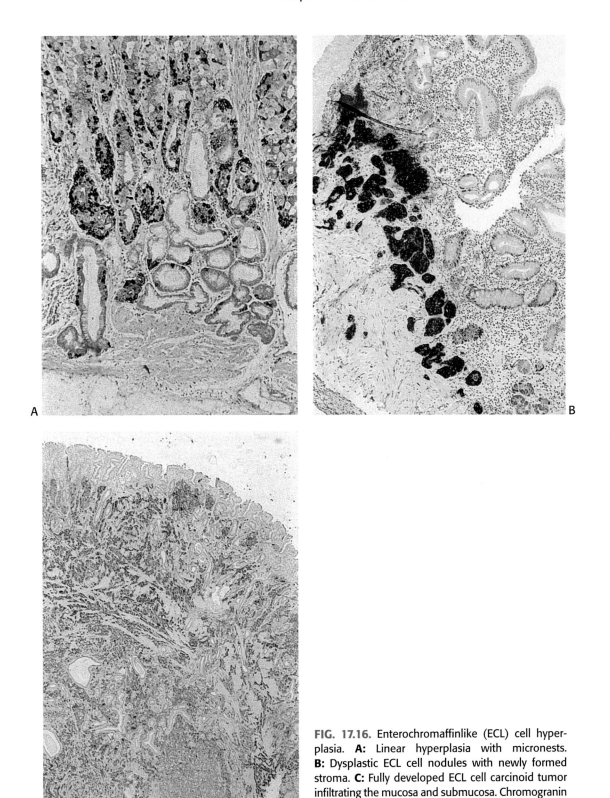

FIG. 17.16. Enterochromaffinlike (ECL) cell hyperplasia. **A:** Linear hyperplasia with micronests. **B:** Dysplastic ECL cell nodules with newly formed stroma. **C:** Fully developed ECL cell carcinoid tumor infiltrating the mucosa and submucosa. Chromogranin immunostain.

Neuroendocrine Cell Hyperplasia in the Intestines

EC cell hyperplasia occurs in the intestines in three major settings: Celiac disease, inflammatory bowel disease, and adjacent to carcinoid tumors. D-cell hyperplasia may be pre-

sent in patients with somatostatinomas and MEN-1. In the setting of celiac disease, hyperplastic NE cells are irregularly distributed within the crypts, often associated with increased numbers of Paneth cells. Goblet cells are normal or occasionally increased in number. The subepithelial basement

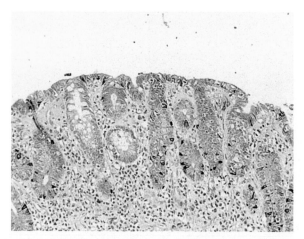

FIG. 17.17. Endocrine cell hyperplasia in the completely flattened small intestinal mucosa of a patient with celiac disease. Chromogranin immunostain.

TABLE 17.5	World Health Organization Classification of Endocrine Tumors

Well-differentiated endocrine tumors (carcinoid tumors)—benign or low-grade malignancy
Well-differentiated endocrine carcinomas (malignant carcinoids)
Poorly differentiated endocrine carcinomas (small cell carcinoma)
Mixed endocrine–exocrine tumors (such as adenocarcinoids)
Rare neuroendocrinelike lesions

membrane may appear normal or thickened (Fig. 17.17) (70). These changes progress with increased mucosal flattening and expansion of the crypt cells. Pyloric metaplasia may develop. The abnormalities are most marked on the crests of mucosal folds.

Endocrine cell hyperplasia affects as many as 40% of IBD patients (71). Paneth cell metaplasia distal to the hepatic flexure, pyloric metaplasia, and endocrine cell hyperplasia often indicate a long history of colitis (72). IBD patients may also develop very small NE tumors, called microcarcinoids. They are not grossly evident and are typically detected in biopsy specimens performed for other reasons or in resection specimens. When present, these lesions lie in the muscularis mucosae and upper submucosa (73). The cells are arranged in a trabecular fashion and consist of multiple small islands of large, pale, eosinophilic cells.

Endocrine cell micronests (ECMs) occur in the minor and major duodenal papillae and are usually immunoreactive for somatostatin and pancreatic polypeptide (74). Some of the lesions break off the ductules of the pancreatic duct or represent atrophic or degenerating islets. Some patients exhibit rectal endocrine cell hyperplasia or focal NE micronests, often surrounding rectal carcinoid tumors (Fig. 17.18) (75). Microcarcinoids may develop in areas of diversion colitis (76).

TERMINOLOGY OF NEUROENDOCRINE TUMORS

NE tumors range from classic carcinoid tumors to small cell carcinomas. They may be classified according to their location, the normal cell counterpart toward which differentiation is occurring, and whether they are benign, of borderline malignancy, of low-grade malignancy, or of high-grade malignancy (77,78). Tumors of mixed endocrine and glandular lineage are classified separately. Carcinoid tumors are classically defined as low-grade, potentially malignant, epithelial neoplasms showing NE differentiation. They most frequently develop in the gastrointestinal system. The term *carcinoid tumor*, as commonly used by pathologists, encompasses a wide spectrum of neoplasms that originate from various NE cells. However, it has become clear that not all gastrointestinal carcinoid tumors are the same. Rather, they reflect the products they secrete and the cells from which they arise. Thus, gastric carcinoids differ substantially from ileal carcinoids, which differ significantly from appendiceal lesions. Current estimates indicate that the various gastrointestinal carcinoid tumors produce as many as 40 different secretory products (79). These tumors may be referred to by the name of the cell population from which they arise (such as ECL tumors), by the hormones they produce (such as gastrinoma), or by their location in the gut (such as midgut carcinoid). It has recently been suggested that these tumors be called *well-differentiated neuroendocrine tumors* (78), terminology adopted by the latest World Health Organization (WHO) classification (Table 17.5) (77). However, to avoid confusion, the term *carcinoid* was not entirely abandoned in the revised classification.

WELL-DIFFERENTIATED NEUROENDOCRINE TUMORS (CARCINOID TUMORS)

Fifty-four to eighty-five percent of all carcinoid tumors arise in the GI tract (80). They develop anywhere, from the esophagus to the anus, but they are decidedly unusual in the esophagus and anus. The widespread use of endoscopy, ultrasonography, computerized tomography, magnetic resonance imaging, and other imaging techniques have significantly enhanced the detection of previously undetectable lesions. For this reason, there appears to have been an increase in the incidence of gastrointestinal carcinoid tumors as well as a shift in the relative proportions of tumors arising in various sites (81). In a recent population-based cancer registry study, the gastrointestinal tract accounted for 54% of NETs. Within the gut, the small intestine was the most common site (44.7%), followed by the rectum (19.6%), appendix (16.7%), colon (10.6%), and stomach (7.2%) (81).

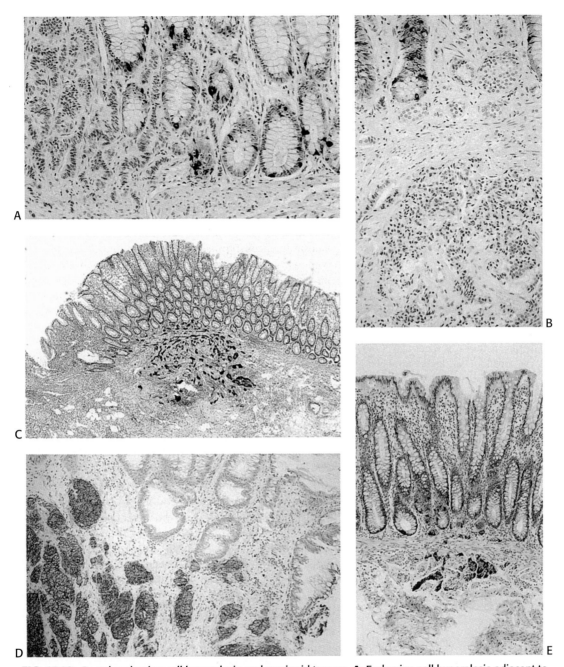

FIG. 17.18. Rectal endocrine cell hyperplasia and carcinoid tumors. **A:** Endocrine cell hyperplasia adjacent to a carcinoid tumor (chromogranin immunostain). Note that the carcinoid tumor (*left*) is chromogranin negative. **B:** A carcinoid tumor lies in the superficial submucosa. The overlying rectal mucosa shows endocrine cell hyperplasia. **C:** Small rectal carcinoid found incidentally at the time of histologic examination. **D:** Synaptophysin-stained adenocarcinoid tumor. **E:** Microcarcinoid straddling the muscularis mucosae. This was one of multiple small carcinoid tumors present in the rectum of this patient. There is overlying endocrine hyperplasia in the colonic mucosa.

Some NETs develop in unusual locations, such as in Meckel diverticula (Fig. 17.19) (82), cystic duplications (83), and the mesentery (84). These neoplasms often arise on a background of NE cell hyperplasia.

Foregut NETs include esophageal, gastric, and proximal duodenal tumors. Midgut lesions include distal duodenal, small intestinal, ascending colon, and proximal transverse colon tumors. Hindgut NETs include distal transverse colon, descending colon, and rectal tumors. While this concept is probably outdated today, it has historical value since tumors derived from these embryologic origins differ clinically, histochemically, and immunohistochemically. Foregut and hindgut tumors are typically argentaffin negative in contrast with midgut tumors, which are argentaffinic.

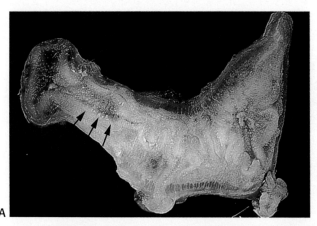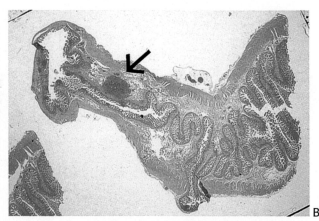

A   B

FIG. 17.19. Incidental carcinoid arising in Meckel diverticulum. **A:** The lesion is not readily visible in the gross specimen unless one looks carefully for it (*arrows*). **B:** The tumor (*arrow*) is well demarcated but unencapsulated.

NETs are usually easily diagnosed because of their distinctive histologic appearance. They exhibit five histologic patterns (Table 17.6) (85). The tumors contain cytoplasmic secretory granules identifiable by the techniques previously discussed. A tumor should only be diagnosed as a carcinoid tumor if it displays the classic histologic architecture of trabecular, insular, or ribbonlike cell clusters with little or no cellular pleomorphism and sparse mitoses. The presence of focal endocrine differentiation in a tumor lacking classic histologic features should not be diagnosed as a NET.

The clinical behavior of this group of tumors is often unpredictable and the traditional morphologic criteria of malignancy have limited applicability to NETs. Tumor biology is influenced by tumor size, location, stage, evidence of metastasis, and histologic features (78). Thus, tumors arising in the appendix are often found incidentally and are usually small and seldom metastasize (86). In contrast, ileal and jejunal tumors are frequently already metastatic to the regional lymph nodes and liver when they are first diagnosed (87). Patient prognosis may also be influenced by the clinical setting in which the tumors arise, the presence or absence of the carcinoid syndrome, and the underlying molecular abnormalities. These features are discussed further in the context of the site-specific NETs.

Some NETs may present early when there is an overt syndrome such as that related to a gastrinoma, but other tumors present at a late stage with liver metastases and the carcinoid syndrome and metastatic tumor in the liver. The measurement of tumor markers in the circulation of patients with NETs may be useful and is of threefold importance. It often establishes the diagnosis, it is useful in monitoring disease progression and response to treatment, and it may serve as a prognostic marker. For example, circulating CgA is elevated in approximately 90% of malignant gastrointestinal NETs (88). In addition, many neoplastic NE cell proliferations express somatostatin receptors (SSTRs), allowing new diagnostic and therapeutic strategies to be developed. Somatostatin analogs reduce secretion via inhibitory G proteins and therefore may lead to marked symptom relief. By using radiolabeled somatostatin analogs, tumors can be localized scintigraphically or during surgery with the aid of scintillation detection (radioguided surgery). Residual tumors may be treated with radionuclide therapy since radionuclides are internalized into tumor cells after SSTR binding (89).

One problem that arises in the diagnosis of NETs is distinguishing a gastrointestinal carcinoid tumor from a pulmonary carcinoid tumor. The panel of cytokeratin (CK)-20/CK-7 and thyroid transcription factor (TTF)-1 antibodies may distinguish among these lesions, since pulmonary tumors do not express CK-20 and GI tumors usually do not express TTF-1 or CK-7 (90).

Esophageal Carcinoid Tumors

Esophageal NETs are very rare, accounting for 0.05% of all gastrointestinal carcinoids and 0.02% of all esophageal carcinomas. The majority of patients are males with an age range of 30 to 82 and a mean age of 56 to 63 years (91,92). The tumors usually develop in the lower esophagus, are typically solitary lesions, and may arise in association with adenocarcinoma in the setting of Barrett esophagus (92). Patients present with dysphagia. The development of the carcinoid syndrome is extremely rare (93). The tumors tend to be large, measuring up to 12 cm in diameter, and they

TABLE 17.6	**Histologic Patterns of Carcinoid Tumors**
Type I	Solid, nodular, and insular cords
Type II	Trabeculae or ribbons with frequent anastomosing patterns
Type III	Tubules and glands or rosettelike patterns
Type IV	Poor differentiation or atypical patterns
Type V	Mixed tumors

TABLE 17.7   Types of Gastric Carcinoid Tumors

Type I	ECL cell tumors associated with type A (autoimmune) chronic atrophic gastritis[a]
Type II	ECL cell tumors associated with combined MEN-1 and Zollinger-Ellison syndrome[a]
Type III	Sporadic ECL tumors
Type IV	Non-ECL tumors (gastrin-, serotonin-, and ACTH- secreting tumors)
Type V	ECL cell tumors associated with achlorhydria and parietal cell hyperplasia[a]

[a]Hypergastrinemic states.
ACTH, adrenocorticotropic hormone; ECL, enterochromaffinlike; MEN-1, multiple endocrine neoplasia type 1.

may be restricted to the lamina propria or deeply infiltrate the esophageal wall (92,94,95). Some tumors appear polypoid. Metastases are present in approximately 50% of cases (95). Histologically, foregut NETs contain anastomosing ribbons, solid nests, trabeculae, acini, or rosettes. The cells are usually round or polygonal but they may appear oval or cylindrical and may have a high mitotic rate (4 mitoses/10 high-powered field [hpf]) (94,95). Carcinoid tumors that arise in the setting of BE-associated adenocarcinoma exhibit endocrine cell hyperplasia in the associated adenocarcinoma. The tumors are reported to have a poor prognosis even in the absence of metastases (95), but this issue may be confused by the inclusion of atypical carcinoids or even small cell carcinomas in some reports of these lesions (92). Long-term survivors are reported (96) even with nodal metastases.

Gastric Carcinoid Tumors

Gastric NETs arise from endocrine cells of the gastric mucosa, usually the ECL cells. They develop in five settings, four of which associate with ECL cell hyperplasia (Table 17.7). ECL-type tumors are frequently classified according to the Rindi classification that recognizes the first three types of tumors listed in Table 17.7 (97). Table 17.8 shows the latest WHO classification of gastric endocrine cell tumors (78). Tumors arising in the various settings differ significantly in their biologic behavior (98,99). In a large series of ECL carcinoids, 79% were associated with CAG, 10% of patients had ZES, and 11% of tumors were sporadic (97).

In the past, gastric NETs accounted for about 4% of the total number of gastrointestinal carcinoids (100) and 0.3% of gastric neoplasms (141). However, these lesions have become more common, related to improved diagnostic methods including endoscopy and immunohistochemistry and heightened awareness of their existence. They are now estimated to account for 11% to 30% of GI NETs (101). In Japan, a country with extensive use of gastric endoscopy, the stomach is the second most common site of NETs. The increased use of acid-suppressing therapies may also account for an increasing incidence of ECL cell proliferative lesions. Up to 100% of patients on high-dose acid suppressive therapies develop hypergastrinemia (58) and the possibility of developing NETs.

ECL cell proliferations (diffuse, linear, and/or micronodular hyperplasias) and their more advanced equivalents (ECL cell dysplasia and ECL carcinoid tumors) all associate with chronic hypergastrinemia (102). However, hypergastrinemia alone appears to be insufficient to induce carcinoid

TABLE 17.8   Classification of Neuroendocrine Tumors of the Stomach

Well-Differentiated Neuroendocrine Tumor (Carcinoid)

Benign: Nonfunctioning, confined to mucosa–submucosa, nonangioinvasive, <1 cm in size
• ECL tumor of corpus–fundus (usually multiple) associated with chronic atrophic gastritis or MEN-1
• Serotonin-producing or (very rare) gastrin-producing tumor

Benign or low-grade malignant (uncertain malignant potential): Nonfunctioning, confined to mucosa–submucosa with or without angioinvasion, 1–2 cm in size
• ECL tumor with chronic atrophic gastritis or MEN-1 or sporadic
• Serotonin-producing or (very rare) gastrin-producing tumor

Well-Differentiated Neuroendocrine Carcinoma (Malignant Carcinoid)

Low-grade malignant: Invasion of the muscularis propria and beyond of metastases, >2 cm in size
• Nonfunctioning, usually sporadic ECL cell carcinoma, rarely in chronic atrophic gastritis or MEN-1 or serotonin or gastrin producing
• Functioning with serotonin-producing carcinoma (atypical carcinoid syndrome) or gastrin-producing carcinoma (gastrinoma)

Poorly Differentiated Neuroendocrine Carcinoma

High-grade malignant

ECL, enterochromaffinlike; MEN-1, multiple endocrine neoplasia type 1.

development as evidenced by the fact that ZES patients without the MEN-1 syndrome rarely develop gastric carcinoids despite prolonged serum gastrin levels more than 10-fold normal (99). In contrast, patients with familial MEN-1 who develop ZES, develop type II carcinoids 30 times more frequently than the normal population. These carcinoid tumors affect 13% to 30% of all MEN ZES cases (103). Therefore, both endocrine and genetic factors are implicated in the pathogenesis of type I and type II gastric carcinoids.

Genetic traits, as in patients with MEN-1; other genetic alterations, as discussed earlier; overexpression of the gastrin receptor gene or growth factors such as EGF or TGF-α; and alterations in the local microenvironment may all play a role in the subsequent development of the carcinoid tumors. Other substances may also play a role in tumor development. Recently it has been shown that pituitary adenylate cyclase–activating polypeptide and vasoactive intestinal polypeptide are even more potent modulators of ECL hyperplasia than gastrin (102). The reg-protein may also control ECL cell numbers by restraining the stimulatory effect of gastrin.

Neuroendocrine Tumors Arising in the Setting of Chronic Atrophic Gastritis (Type I Tumors)

Type I carcinoids account for approximately 74% to 79% of all gastric NETs. Five to ten percent of patients with CAG and hypergastrinemia develop ECL carcinoids (98,102). The demographics of the lesion mimic those of autoimmune gastritis. More than 70% of cases develop in older women with a mean age of 63 years (98,99). Type I carcinoids develop in part from the hypergastrinemia that results from loss of parietal cell mass and decreased acid output as a consequence of the autoimmune gastritis (98,99). Tumors developing in this setting arise on a background of ECL cell hyperplasia and dysplasia (Fig. 17.20). In more than half of the cases, the tumors are multifocal.

Type I carcinoids are the most "benign" of the gastric carcinoid tumors (104). They present as small, tan submucosal nodules or polyps in the corpus usually measuring <1 cm. Most measure only 1 to 3 mm in diameter; 97% are <1.5 cm in diameter. The tumors tend to be limited to the mucosa and submucosa, with only 7% invading the muscularis propria. They infrequently cause liver metastases (2% to 5% of cases) (98).

Most tumors are characterized by small microlobular aggregates formed by regularly distributed cells that may create a mosaiclike pattern. They consist of solid nests, trabeculae, ribbons, tubular structures, or a combination of these patterns. The cytoplasm appears slightly eosinophilic, slightly basophilic, or amphophilic. Cytoplasmic granules may or may not be seen on routine preparations. The cells contain centrally located, round or oval, monomorphic nuclei, with generally inapparent nucleoli and little or no nuclear pleomorphism or mitotic activity. Angioinvasion is rare. The background mucosa shows the typical features of CAG, often with intestinal metaplasia.

The tumor cells are argyrophilic but not argentaffinic. They are consistently immunoreactive for NE markers including CgA, synaptophysin, and NSE. The tumor cells, as well as the surrounding hyperplastic endocrine cells, are positive for the newly discovered hormone ghrelin (19). VMAT-2 is a specific marker for ECL tumors. The cells variably produce mucin (105). A small population of tumor cells

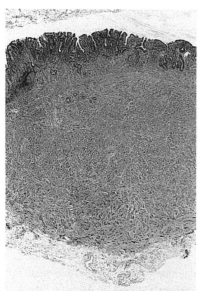 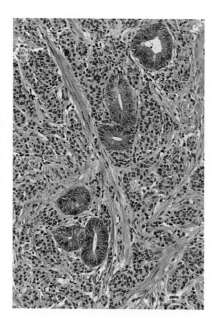 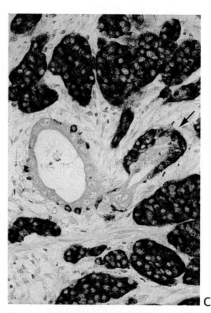

A, B   C

FIG. 17.20. Carcinoid tumor. **A:** Low-power view demonstrates a proliferation of small, uniform cells within the deep mucosa and submucosa. **B:** The cells are arranged in nests and rosettelike structures. There is no nuclear pleomorphism and mitotic figures are not seen. Residual gastric glands lie among the tumor cells. **C:** The endocrine differentiation of this lesion is highlighted by the chromogranin stain. A focus of linear endocrine hyperplasia is present in a residual gastric gland (*arrow*).

may be positive for serotonin, gastrin, somatostatin, pancreatic polypeptide, or α-human chorionic gonadotropin (α-hCG). A few ECL cell tumors produce histamine and 5-hydroxytryptophan (5-HT); when these lesions metastasize they may produce an atypical carcinoid syndrome (97).

Type I carcinoid tumors may regress after gastrin levels decrease, usually by antrectomy (106) or treatment with somatostatin analogs (107). These treatments result in resolution, regression, or stabilization of many ECL tumors (108). At some stage, however, ECL cell proliferations may become irreversible, making it difficult to estimate the degree of tumor regression following treatment. It is hard to predict which of multiple ECL tumors have progressed beyond the point of gastrin dependence and are autonomous in their growth. The octreotide suppression test may predict a beneficial outcome from antrectomy (109). The tumors may also be removed surgically or endoscopically depending on their size and number (110). Biopsy and observation are other possible therapeutic options. Gastrectomy is reserved for patients with extensive tumor involvement of the gastric wall, to control bleeding, or in patients in whom the tumors progress (110).

When the tumors metastasize, it is usually to the regional lymph nodes; distant metastases are rare. They almost never cause the death of the patient (98). The generally better prognosis of this type of gastric NET relates in part to earlier diagnosis because the patients are commonly seen for symptoms related to the underlying CAG. Alternatively, the better prognosis may relate to the intrinsically benign nature of tumors arising in this setting.

Neuroendocrine Tumors Arising in the Setting of Multiple Endocrine Neoplasia Type 1–Zollinger-Ellison Syndrome (Type II Carcinoid Tumors)

Type II carcinoids represent 6% to 10% of all gastric NETs. The tumors do not show any gender predilection and occur at an earlier age than type I tumors with a median age at development of 50 years (98). Gastric carcinoids arising in the setting of ZES usually associate with MEN-1 (98). The ECL cell NETs develop in the oxyntic mucosa and are frequently multiple (136). They are the consequence of hypergastrinemia resulting from a gastrin-secreting NE cell neoplasm (often a pancreatic islet cell tumor). Rare sporadic ZES-associated gastric carcinoids also occur, although generally these patients only have simple linear hyperplasia (57).

ECL NETs arise on a background of parietal cell hypertrophy and hyperplasia and ECL cell hyperplasia and dysplasia. Since the patients present with a hypertrophic gastropathy characteristic of ZES, the gastric folds appear thickened. In addition, there are usually multiple, small tumor nodules. ECL tumors occurring in this setting are more likely to measure >1.5 cm and to produce local lymph node metastases (30%) and liver metastases (10%) than type I tumors (98). The histologic features of the tumors resemble type I gastric carcinoids described above.

Octreotide can control the hypergastrinemia, leading to regression of related ECL cell hyperplasia and NETs (111). Removal of all gastrinomas in patients with type II ECL carcinoids results in carcinoid tumor regression (112).

Neuroendocrine Tumors Arising in the Setting of Achlorhydria and Parietal Cell Hyperplasia

Recently two patients were reported with multiple gastric carcinoids arising in the setting of marked hypergastrinemia, associated with achlorhydria and hypertrophic parietal cells. The parietal cell hyperplasia caused mucosal thickening. Focal intestinal metaplasia was present. There were also areas of ciliated metaplasia. Multiple intramucosal and invasive carcinoid tumors involving the gastric body and fundus arose on a background of marked ECL cell hyperplasia. The largest tumor nodule measured 1.3 cm in diameter. A micrometastasis was present in a regional lymph node. The oxyntic mucosa showed marked parietal cell hyperplasia and hypertrophy. Some of the parietal cells appeared vacuolated and many displayed protrusions of their apical cytoplasm into dilated oxyntic glands filled with inspissated eosinophilic material. (113,114). This presentation appears to represent a rare form of gastric carcinoids associated with an intrinsic acid secretion abnormality as supported by the ultrastructural demonstration of the lack of the parietal cell canalicular system (114) and the failure of the parietal cells to stain with an antibody directed at the α and β subunits of the H^+/K^+-ATPase proton pump (113).

Sporadic Gastric Neuroendocrine Tumors (Type III Carcinoids) (Well-differentiated Neuroendocrine Carcinomas)

Sporadic NETs are most common in men (74%), with a mean age of 55 years (98). They are unassociated with CAG and hypergastrinemia and represent a proliferation of various cell types including ECL, EC, and X cells. They are usually single lesions that do not arise on a background of NE cell hyperplasia. The incidence of multiple type III carcinoids is only 1% (98). The tumors occur anywhere in the stomach. Unlike type I and type II tumors, type III tumors are aggressive and larger than other gastric NETs. They generally present as a mass lesion mimicking the clinical presentation of adenocarcinomas with bleeding, obstruction, or metastasis as presenting findings. Patients may present with an atypical carcinoid syndrome with cutaneous flushing in the absence of diarrhea. Tumors producing these clinical symptoms usually produce histamine and 5-HT (115).

Grossly, type III tumors often appear as smooth, round, yellow, submucosal nodules measuring >2 cm in diameter (Fig. 17.21). They are usually covered by an intact mucosa, although larger lesions may develop an irregularly shaped, reddened depression or surface ulceration. Histologically, type III NETs exhibit various growth patterns, including trabecular, gyriform, medullary or solid, glandular, or rosette, or a mixture of all of these (Fig. 17.22). Often they show a

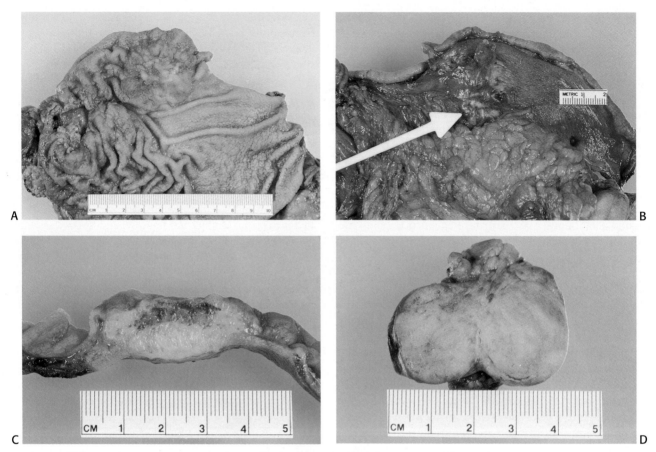

FIG. 17.21. Gross appearance of sporadic gastric carcinoid tumor. **A:** Opened stomach showing the tumor. **B:** The tumor extends to the serosal surface (*arrow*). **C:** Cut surface of the tumor showing that it extends through the gastric wall. **D:** Metastatic tumor in a perigastric lymph node.

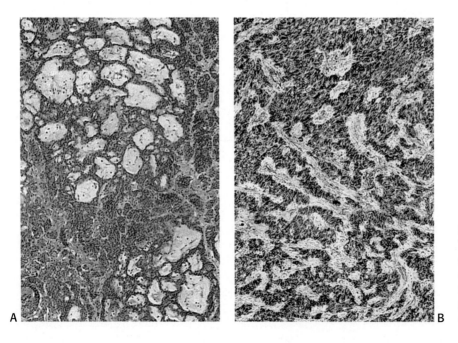

FIG. 17.22. Gastric carcinoid tumor. **A:** The tumor is composed of solid nests, ribbons, and glandlike structures. The cells are uniform and mucin has accumulated in many areas. **B:** Chromogranin stain highlights the cords of cells.

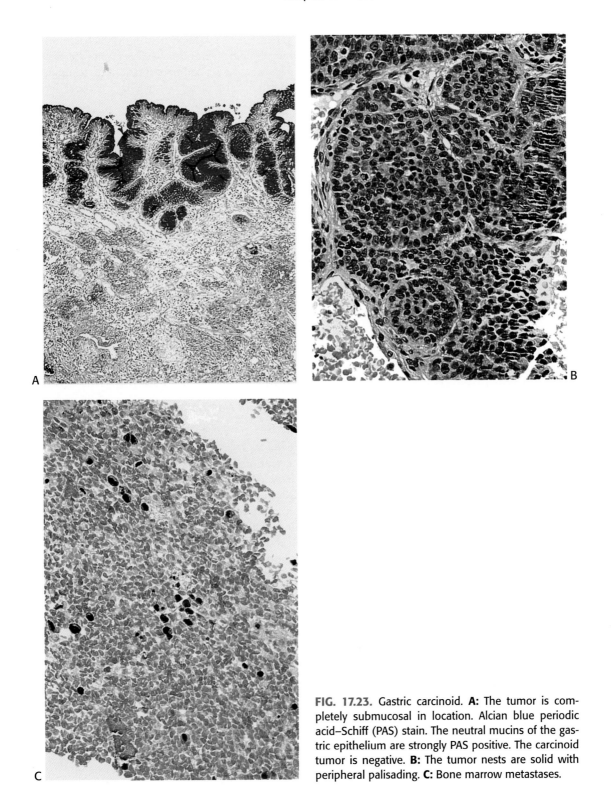

FIG. 17.23. Gastric carcinoid. **A:** The tumor is completely submucosal in location. Alcian blue periodic acid–Schiff (PAS) stain. The neutral mucins of the gastric epithelium are strongly PAS positive. The carcinoid tumor is negative. **B:** The tumor nests are solid with peripheral palisading. **C:** Bone marrow metastases.

prevalence of solid cellular aggregates (Fig 17.23) and large trabeculae with cellular crowding. The round, spindle-shaped, and polyhedral cells are irregularly distributed and have fairly large vesicular nuclei and prominent small, eosinophilic nucleoli. The cells may also contain smaller hyperchromatic nuclei with irregular chromatin clumping and increased mitoses. Sparse areas of necrosis may be pre-

sent. Larger tumors may invade deeply and promote a prominent fibroblastic stromal response. These lesions extend intramurally and invade vascular or lymphatic channels to produce nodal and distant metastases (116). Factors that predict aggressive behavior include cellular atypia, two or more mitoses per hpf, angioinvasion, and transmural invasion (98,117). Although tumor size correlates with a

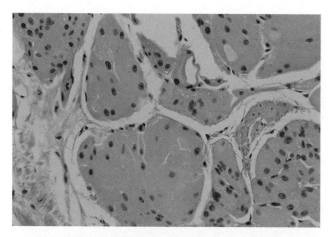

FIG. 17.24. Gastric carcinoid with oncocytic features.

tendency to metastasize, minute tumors are known to spread beyond the stomach (118). Thus, while the latest WHO criteria suggest that NETs tumors ≤1 cm are benign lesions, this criterion does not appear to be applicable to all of these tumors. Regional lymph node metastasis may be seen in tumors as small as 0.3 cm in diameter (119).

These tumors frequently express p53 and have a high KI-67 labeling rate. Rare tumors show widespread ossification or have an oncocytic appearance (Fig. 17.24). These tumors are also positive for markers of bone formation and differentiation including bone morphogenetic protein, osteopontin, and osteonectin (120). Type III carcinoid tumors often display an aggressive local behavior and metastasize. Seventy-six percent of tumors invade the muscularis propria and/or subserosa and lymph node, and distant metastases are present in 2% to 71% and 22% to 75% of cases, respectively (98). The 5-year survival in patients with sporadic carcinoids is <50%, reflecting the high rate of metastasis. The 5-year survival rate is significantly higher for localized disease (64.3%) and for those with regional metastases (29.9%) than for lesions with distant metastases (10%) (91). As noted above, patients with type I carcinoid tumors benefit from antrectomy, but this treatment has no value in sporadic carcinoid tumors (121). Therefore, it is important to distinguish between these two groups of patients. This is usually accomplished based on clinical and morphologic features, as well as on the presence or absence of adjacent ECL cell hyperplasia. The features of sporadic and hypergastrinemia-associated carcinoids are compared in Table 17.9.

Non–enterochromaffinlike Neuroendocrine Tumors

These tumors arise anywhere in the stomach and are usually single large lesions that are often highly malignant. Affected patients may present with ZES due to gastrin production by the tumor or with Cushing syndrome due to secretion of adrenocorticotropic hormone (ACTH). Serotonin-producing NETs are rare in the stomach (98). They resemble midgut carcinoids, consisting of rounded nests of tightly packed small tumor cells often showing peripheral palisading. Gastrin-producing tumors exhibit a characteristic thin trabecular pattern and the cells are strongly positive for NE markers and for gastrin. These tumors may metastasize and also cause ZES.

Small Intestinal Neuroendocrine Tumors

Duodenal Neuroendocrine Tumors

It used to be believed that duodenal NETs only accounted for 1.8% to 2.9% of gastrointestinal NETs (100), but with the advent of improved imaging and the increased use of upper endoscopy, they are currently estimated to account for up to 22% of all gut endocrine tumors (80). Gastrin cell tumors account for the largest group (62% to 65%) of tumors arising in the upper intestine, followed by somatostatin cell tumors (15% to 21%), gangliocytic paragangliomas (9%), undifferentiated tumors, and pancreatic polypeptide (PP) cell tumors (122). The WHO classification of these tumors is shown in Table 17.10. In one study, 72% of patients with duodenal NETs were male. Patient median age was 53 to 59 years with a range of 18 to 90 years (123). These tumors associate with MEN-1, ZES, and NF1. The majority of duodenal carcinoids exhibit a mixture of cribriform, insular, glandular, and solid and trabecular growth patterns. They produce various hormones as discussed below. In addition, xenin is said

TABLE 17.9   Comparison of Sporadic and Hypergastrinemia-associated Carcinoid Tumors

	Sporadic Lesions	Hypergastrinemia-associated Lesions
Chronic atrophic gastritis	Absent	Present
Endocrine cell hyperplasia	Absent	Present
Genetic associations	None	Multiple endocrine neoplasia syndrome
Size	Variable	Small
Multifocality	Usually single	Multiple
Behavior and treatment	Aggressive, do not regress following antrectomy	Benign, regress following antrectomy

TABLE 17.10 Classification of Neuroendocrine Tumors of the Duodenum and Upper Jejunum

Well-Differentiated Neuroendocrine Tumor (Carcinoid)

Benign: Nonfunctioning, confined to mucosa–submucosa, nonangioinvasive, <1 cm in size
- Gastrin-producing tumor (upper part of duodenum)
- Serotonin-producing tumor
- Gangliocytic paraganglioma (any size and extension, periampullary)

Benign or low-grade malignant (uncertain malignant potential): Nonfunctioning, confined to mucosa–submucosa with or without angioinvasion, 1 cm in size
- Functioning gastrin-producing tumor (gastrinoma), sporadic or MEN-1 associated
- Nonfunctioning somatostatin-producing tumor (ampullary region) with or without NF1
- Nonfunctioning serotonin-producing tumor

Well-Differentiated Neuroendocrine Carcinoma (Malignant Carcinoid)

Low-grade malignant: Invasion of the muscularis propria and beyond or metastases
- Functioning with gastrin-producing carcinoma (gastrinoma), sporadic or MEN-1 associated
- Nonfunctioning somatostatin-producing carcinoma (ampullary region), with or without NF1
- Nonfunctioning or functioning carcinoma (with carcinoid syndrome)
- Malignant gangliocytic paraganglioma

Poorly Differentiated Neuroendocrine Carcinoma

High-grade malignant: Functioning or nonfunctioning, poorly differentiated intermediate or small cell carcinoma

MEN-1, multiple endocrine neoplasia type 1; NF1, neurofibromatosis type 1.

to be a marker of duodenal NETs because it is exclusively expressed in these tumors, regardless of their hormonal content and functional activity (124).

G-cell Tumors (Gastrinomas)

Seventy-five percent of patients have sporadic tumors; 25% associate with MEN-1 (125). These are the most common malignant functional NET. Tumors associated with overt ZES differ from their nonfunctioning counterparts by arising earlier in life in a nonbulbar location and having a higher incidence of metastases.

Ninety percent of gastrinomas arise within the so-called "gastrinoma triangle." Its superior margin crosses the cystic and common bile ducts, its inferior margin is formed by the junction of the second and third portion of the duodenum, and the medial margin is delineated by the junction of the neck and the body of the pancreas. Approximately 15% of gastrinomas arise in extrapancreatic sites; 13% originate in the second portion of the duodenum. The remainder arise in the stomach, upper jejunum, biliary tree, and lymph nodes within the gastrinoma triangle (126). It has been suggested that precursor cells of gastrin-producing tumors become dispersed during the dorsal rotation of the ventral pancreas during embryonic development and are incorporated into lymphatic tissues (127), thereby providing the anatomic basis for primary nodal gastrinomas. There are also reports of isolated gastrin- or synaptophysin-staining cells in 15% of normal lymph nodes from the gastrinoma triangle (128,129).

Duodenal gastrinomas arising in the setting of MEN-1 are multiple, in contrast to sporadic gastrinomas, which are typically single lesions (130). The multiple tumors seen in MEN-1 patients are thought to be multiple primary lesions based on clonality studies (32). Sixteen percent of duodenal gastrinomas are incidental findings in surgical resection specimens, usually removed for peptic ulcer disease. However, some tumors are large enough to cause clinical symptoms from mass effects, including bile duct obstruction. Approximately one third of patients with gastrinomas have diarrhea. Some patients present with the ZES.

The main features of duodenal gastrinomas include their small size and submucosal location. Most develop in the first and second portions of the duodenum. The tumors may appear slightly polypoid and are often endoscopically misinterpreted as heterotopic pancreas or gastric mucosa or as an inflammatory process. The tumors range in size from 0.2 to 20 cm in diameter (131). However, they measure ≤1 cm in diameter in 62% to 80% of patients. Very small tumors are easily missed during exploratory laparotomy or during gross examination of surgical specimens. Despite their small size, these tumors commonly metastasize and nearly half demonstrate nodal metastases (126,132). Such metastases are often larger than the primary tumors, probably leading to an overdiagnosis of primary nodal gastrinomas.

Gastrinomas display a trabecular/pseudoglandular and/or solid growth pattern. The tumors appear uniform with scanty cytoplasm arranged in solid clusters and ribbons (Figs. 17.25 and 17.26). Some contain a perinuclear collection of whorled microfilaments. Angioinvasion may be present. Gastrinomas

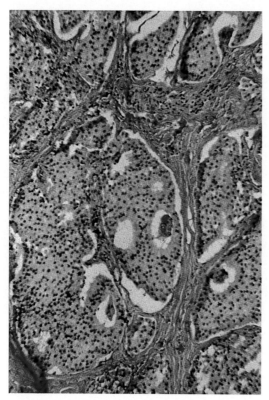

FIG. 17.25. Duodenal gastrinoma found incidentally at the time of resection for a duodenal ulcer. The tumor measured <0.4 mm in diameter.

cannot be differentiated from other functional and nonfunctional NETs based solely on their histologic appearance. Gastrin immunoreactivity in the majority of cells establishes the diagnosis. In addition, gastrinomas may produce other polypeptides including glucagon, somatostatin, serotonin, insulin, pancreatic polypeptide, ACTH, enkephalins (133), and hCG.

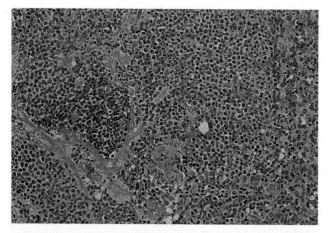

FIG. 17.26. Duodenal gastrinoma resected from the duodenum. Unlike the lesion illustrated in Figure 17.25, this tumor consisted of solid nests of cells with a very monomorphic appearance and not a prominent insular pattern.

In MEN-1, G-cell hyperplasia involving the intestinal crypts and/or Brunner glands surrounds duodenal gastrinomas. These hyperplastic foci are not seen in patients with sporadic non–MEN-1–associated gastrinomas (134). The hyperplasia may be linear, micronodular, and/or microinvasive (134). Invasive lesions are recognizable by the fact that they are in the lamina propria and surrounded by thickened collagen and may demonstrate angioinvasion. Multifocal gastrinomas originate from the diffuse proliferative changes. The histology of the microgastrinomas that accompany larger neoplasms resembles that of the larger gastrinomas. The hyperplastic lesions show increased KI-67 expression and reduced gastrin staining, suggesting that the G cells are hyperactive and release increased amounts of gastrin. hCG expression is not present in the precursor lesions, but is seen in microgastrinomas and in fully developed gastrinomas (134). This is of interest since in the stomach, hCG expression has been associated with dysplastic and neoplastic transformation (135).

Gastrinomas are generally slow-growing tumors (125,126). Markers that may predict aggressive behavior and metastases include tumor size, invasion beyond the submucosa, aneuploidy and a high S-phase fraction (136), *Her2/neu* amplification and overexpression (137), LOH of chromosome 1q9 (138), the type of gastrin produced by the tumor (139), and overexpression of EGFR and hepatocyte growth factor (HGF) (140). Prognosis also relates to the number of peptides produced. Patients with gastrinomas that produce only gastrin have 5-year survivals of 87%, contrasting with a 22% 5-year survival in patients with tumors that produce multiple circulating hormones (88). Patients with overt ZES have an increased incidence of metastases. However, survival is primarily determined by the presence of liver metastases. The frequency of liver metastases depends on the size and location of the primary tumor and the presence of MEN-1 at initial presentation (80). Among patients with sporadic gastrinomas, 34% are free of disease at 10 years as compared with none of the patients with MEN-1. However, overall, the survival appears to be better in patients with gastrinomas in the setting of MEN than for those with sporadic gastrinomas (141). Their overall 10-year survival rate is 94% (126). Patients with sporadic gastrinomas should be offered surgical exploration for possible cure of their disease (126). In addition, debulking of metastatic tumor may improve symptoms and the length of survival when cure cannot be achieved. In patients with ZES, the advent of effective acid-reducing pharmacologic agents has changed the primary morbidity of the disease from that of acid hypersecretion to one of tumor growth and spread. Thus, symptoms can be temporized using histamine receptor antagonists, proton pump inhibitors, or somatostatin analogs.

D-cell Tumors (Somatostatinomas)

Somatostatinomas account for <1% of all NETs (142). Patients range in age from 29 to 83. Fifty percent of somatostatinomas associate with NF1 (123). Somatostatinomas sometimes develop in patients with neurofibromatosis and pheochromocytoma, suggesting that this triad may constitute a new multiple endocrine neoplasia syndrome (MEN-3) (143). Somatostatinomas may also arise on a background of D-cell hyperplasia in the setting of celiac disease, suggesting a relationship between D-cell growth and chronic inflammation (144).

The somatostatinoma syndrome (diabetes mellitus, diarrhea, steatorrhea, hypo- or achlorhydria, weight loss, anemia, and gallstones) usually affects patients with pancreatic somatostatin-producing NETs; the full-blown syndrome does not usually complicate duodenal somatostatin cell tumors. However, because duodenal somatostatinomas often develop in the ampulla of Vater, they cause jaundice and intestinal obstruction early in their development, resulting in resection before the full syndrome develops.

Somatostatinomas arise in the deep portion of the mucosa or possibly in Brunner glands and have a tendency to be invasive. These are usually single, but multiple (up to 30) tumors have been described in the absence of an underlying genetic syndrome (145). The histologic patterns of somatostatinomas resemble those seen in other NETs with the exception that they display a prominent glandular pattern and contain intraglandular psammoma bodies (Fig. 17.27) (146). These result from secretion of somatostatin by the tumor cells. The Grimelius stain is positive in only about one third of cases (144). Immunohistochemical techniques show a preponderance of somatostatin-positive cells (Fig. 17.27). Other substances produced by these tumors include gastrin (147), calcitonin (148), insulin, VIP, prostaglandin E_2, substance P, serotonin, and carcinoembryonic antigen (CEA) (142,149). Somatostatinomas associated with NF1 are often pure so-matostatinomas, whereas similar tumors unassociated with NF1 are frequently multihormonal (149,150).

The combination of a striking glandular pattern with psammoma bodies and a negative Grimelius stain may lead to a misdiagnosis of adenocarcinoma. However, in contrast to most carcinomas, somatostatinomas consist of uniform cells with few mitoses, although rarely some metastatic carcinomas can appear histologically bland. Somatostatinomas frequently metastasize (143). Prognosis is better in patients in whom the tumor is detected early. Features of malignancy include extension to the muscularis propria, the sphincter of Oddi, or the pancreas; a maximum diameter of >2 cm; and the presence of mitotic figures. The liver is most commonly involved followed by regional lymph nodes and bones.

Other Hormone-producing Neuroendocrine Tumors

EC cell, serotonin-producing tumors, the classic argentaffinic midgut tumors, may develop in the duodenum (Fig. 17.28), but are rare in this site. They have the characteristic features described below for distal jejunal/ileal tumors. One percent of *insulinomas* arise in the duodenal mucosa (151), the splenic hilum, or the gastrocolic ligament. The presence of multiple

tumors suggests the diagnosis of MEN-1. Insulinomas secrete insulin autonomously; excessive insulin levels result in profound hypoglycemia with trembling, irritability, weakness, diaphoresis, tachycardia, hunger, headaches, blurred vision, personality changes, mental confusion, bizarre behavior, amnesia, obtundation, convulsions, and coma (152). Elevated plasma insulin levels and the low plasma glucose during prolonged fasting establish the diagnosis (153). The tumors histologically resemble other intestinal NETs. Insulinomas, unlike other endocrine tumors, are rarely malignant. They can be diagnosed by staining the tumors with antibodies to insulin.

Most *glucagonomas* arise in the pancreas, but primary duodenal lesions have been described (154,155). Glucagonomas secrete glucagon autonomously and patients with functional tumors present with a syndrome characterized by waxing and waning skin lesions known as neurolytic migratory erythema, abnormal glucose tolerance tests with or without clinical diabetes mellitus, hypoaminoacidemia, weight loss, normochromic-normocytic anemia, and, occasionally, glossitis, stomatitis, cheilitis, diarrhea, abdominal pain, nausea and vomiting, a tendency to venous thrombosis, and mental status changes. Histologically, glucagonomas resemble other carcinoid tumors and show no distinctive features except for the presence of glucagon-positive cells in the tumors. Even though most glucagonomas are malignant, mitotic figures and nuclear atypia are rare. The tumors are immunohistochemically positive for glucagon.

GRFomas are NETs that produce growth hormone–releasing factor resulting in acromegaly. These are rare tumors and about 30% associate with MEN-1. Ten percent develop in the small intestines, where they are often multiple, large, and metastatic. Their presence should be suspected in patients with a NET and acromegaly (156).

Nonfunctional Duodenal Neuroendocrine Tumors

Nonfunctioning duodenal NETs usually consist of serotonin-producing EC cells or calcitonin-producing cells. They do not behave aggressively unless they extend beyond the submucosa (80). These tumors may occasionally have an amyloid stroma.

Jejunal and Ileal Neuroendocrine Tumors

NETs developing in this region of the gut are typically EC cell serotonin-producing carcinoid tumors, but L-cell, glucagonlike peptide, and PP/polypeptide YY (PYY)-producing tumors also arise in this location. These tumors have an incidence of 0.28 to 0.89 per 100,000 population per year (100,157,158). They account for 23% to 28% of all GI endocrine tumors (100). Jejunal and ileal carcinoids usually develop in individuals ranging in age from the 3rd to the 10th decades of life, with a peak incidence in the 6th and 7th decades. However, the tumors may develop in children, in which case they behave aggressively. Men and women are

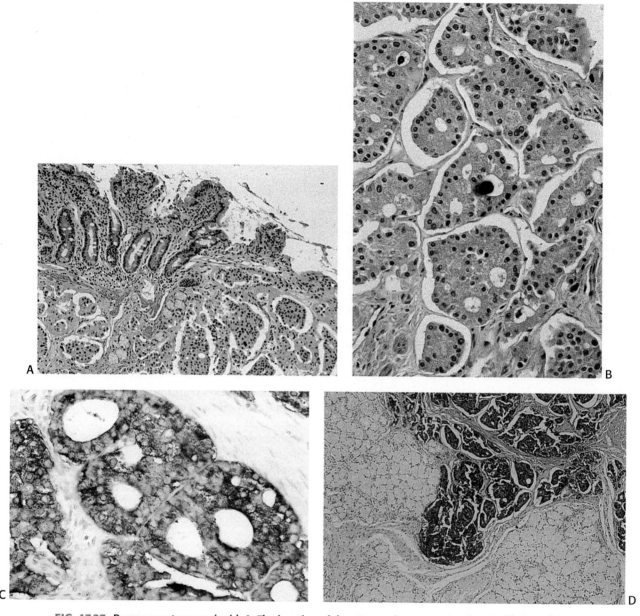

FIG. 17.27. Psammomatous carcinoid. A: The junction of the more or less normal mucosa with the adjacent tumor. **B:** Higher magnification of the tumor showing the presence of well-defined tubular cell nests without atypia. A psammoma body is seen in the center of the photograph. **C:** Synaptophysin immunostain. **D:** Somatostatin immunostain.

equally affected. Blacks are affected more than whites (100). Ileal carcinoid tumors may also complicate Crohn disease (159). The duration of the Crohn disease varies from months to years (160).

Asymptomatic small intestinal NETs may be discovered incidentally at the time of autopsy or surgery. Symptomatic lesions result from tumor mass effects, the effects of tumor-engendered fibrosis, or the presence of the carcinoid syndrome. Many symptomatic patients have a long history of intermittent crampy abdominal pain suggestive of episodic intestinal obstruction (161). The symptoms worsen with progressive intestinal obstruction; abdominal distension and

vomiting develop. Other patients present with infarction, bleeding, weight loss, diarrhea, or lymphadenopathy.

Because patient survival has increased due to somatostatin receptor 2–targeted therapy and an increasing number of other therapeutic and diagnostic options, the clinical manifestations of the fibrosis are emerging as a major issue in the morbidity and mortality of the disease (80). Contraction of the desmoplastic (fibrotic) tissue associated with the tumor causes angulation, kinking, or distortion of the bowel wall and secondary intestinal obstruction. Serosal fibrosis-producing adhesions lead to volvulus, luminal constriction of the bowel lumen, or matting together of bowel

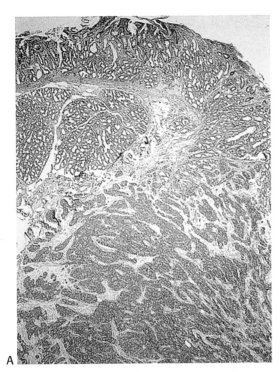
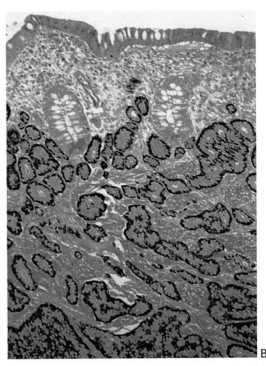

FIG. 17.28. Duodenal carcinoid tumor. **A:** The tumor consists of uniform cells arranged in solid nests and cords. **B:** Chromogranin immunostain.

loops. Fibrosis around mesenteric metastases causes fixation of the ileal mesentery to the retroperitoneum with fibrous bands obstructing the small intestine and transverse colon (162). Blood vessels caught in the mesenteric fibrosis may be secondarily compressed, leading to ischemic necrosis of the involved bowel segment. Bowel infarctions and gangrene (Fig. 17.29) (161) may also develop secondary to concentric vascular thickening (see below). Retroperitoneal fibrosis may also lead to hydronephrosis and renal failure (163).

Symptomatic tumors have usually spread beyond the site or origin. Ninety-three percent of symptomatic patients with small intestinal NETs have metastases, compared to 9% of patients whose tumors are found incidentally (161).

The carcinoid syndrome affects 10% to 18% of patients with NETs, particularly those with ileal lesions (162). The syndrome usually, but not necessarily, requires the presence of hepatic metastases so that sufficient amounts of the substances produced by the tumor can reach the systemic

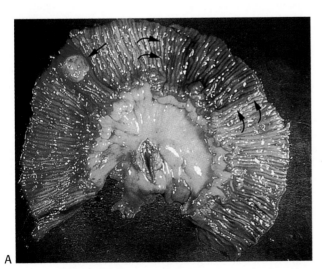
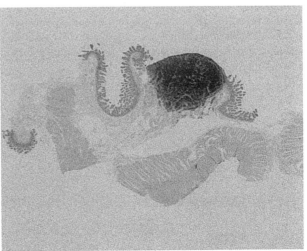

FIG. 17.29. Ileal carcinoid. **A:** The small tan-yellow circumscribed mucosal nodule is the carcinoid tumor (*arrow*). Note the associated discontinuous areas of ischemia, which appear as an area of localized erythema (*curved arrows*). **B:** Low-power micrograph showing the tumor highlighted by a chromogranin immunostain.

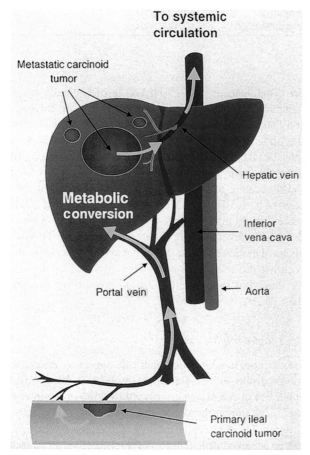

FIG. 17.30. Pathophysiology of the carcinoid syndrome (see text).

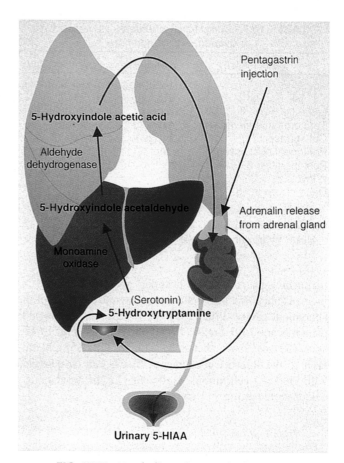

FIG. 17.31. Metabolism of serotonin (see text).

circulation without undergoing metabolic degradation. The aggregate mass of metastatic tumor in the liver often exceeds that in the primary site, allowing the metastases to produce enormous amounts of secretory products. Furthermore, the blood supply of the metastases drains directly into the systemic circulation via efferent hepatic veins, thereby sequestering the hormones from hepatic metabolism (Fig. 17.30).

Serotonin forms from the essential dietary amino acid tryptophan by hydroxylation and decarboxylation. Serotonin is broken down in the liver and lung by monoamine oxidase and reduced to 5-hydroxyindoleacetic acid (5-HIAA), a biologically inactive metabolite excreted in the urine (Fig. 17.31) (164). Provocative tests using pentagastrin (PG) elicit the release of both 5-HT and tachykinins (165). Elevated levels of >30 mg of 5-HIAA in 24 hours diagnose the syndrome.

The classic carcinoid syndrome consists of vasomotor, cardiopulmonary, and GI symptoms. The syndrome is often precipitated by alcohol or food intake, emotional stress, exercise, or straining at stool. The major clinical manifestations include paroxysms of sweating, flushing, facial and anterior chest cyanosis, wheezing or asthmalike attacks, abdominal colic, and right-sided heart failure. Mild or explosive diarrhea is the second most common symptom. Minor features include abdominal pain, edema, malabsorption with pella-

gralike or sclerodermalike skin lesions, peptic ulcers, myopathies, arthralgias, and retroperitoneal fibrosis (166).

Carcinoid heart disease affects 50% to 66% of patients with classic carcinoid syndrome (167). Endocardial or subendocardial lesions involve the right side of the heart, causing tricuspid and pulmonary valve dysfunction and repeated episodes of ventricular failure (167). Patients with extensive endocardial involvement may present with a restrictive cardiomyopathy (168). Plaquelike thickenings develop on the affected endocardium in the right atrium, papillary muscles of the tricuspid valve, valvular leaflets, and cardiac chambers. The majority of the lesion consists of an acid mucopolysaccharide-rich stromal tissue, reticulin fibers, and collagen. The cells in the plaques are smooth muscle cells, fibroblasts, and myofibroblasts (169). Pulmonary fibrosis may also occur, usually in the setting of advanced metastatic disease.

Many peptides are produced by carcinoid tumors (170–173) and these may mediate the carcinoid syndrome symptoms. Neuropeptide K (NPK), the most abundant tachykinin in the plasma of carcinoid patients and in tumor tissue extracts, may mediate the carcinoid flush. Substance P also causes flushing, hypertension, tachycardia, and increased intestinal motility (174). GI hypermotility and diarrhea probably result from 5-HT, VIP, glucagon, prostaglandins, substance P, secretin, motilin, and/or neurotensin production

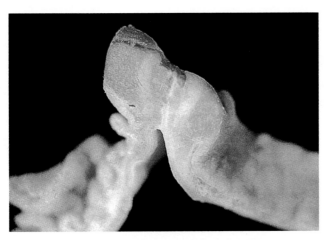

FIG. 17.32. Small intestinal carcinoid. The carcinoid tumor (*yellow area*) kinks the bowel wall because of the associated desmoplasia.

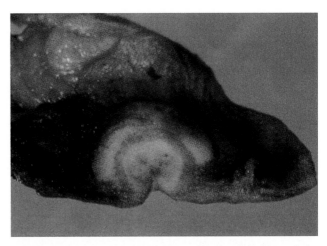

FIG. 17.34. Ileal carcinoid showing the focal kinking of the bowel wall secondary to tumor growth through the muscularis propria and secondary fibrosis with serosal adhesions.

(175). Some of the secreted substances are also implicated in the fibrosing disorders. These include serotonin, TGF-β family members, connective tissue growth factor, bone morphogenic protein, nerve growth factor-2, and platelet-derived growth factor (176,177).

Approximately 80% of small bowel carcinoid tumors develop in the ileum. Multiple tumors develop in 25% to 30% of patients (161). In some cases, dozens of tumors are present. The practical implication of this multifocality is that the entire small intestine should be carefully palpated when a small bowel carcinoid has been identified to find additional tumors. Clonality studies show that multiple tumors appear to be clonally identical, raising the possibility that these "multiple" tumors are actually metastases from a single lesion (178). Twenty-nine percent of patients also have other noncarcinoid neoplasms, possibly secondary to the production of growth factors that might induce secondary neoplasms.

NETs develop deep in the mucosa, growing slowly and extending into the underlying submucosa as well as into the overlying mucosa. They form small, firm tan, yellow, or gray-brown intramural nodules bulging slightly into the intestinal lumen (Figs. 17.32 to 17.34). They range from barely palpable thickenings to nodules measuring up to 3.5 cm in diameter (179). It is rare for primary tumors to be larger than this. Carcinoid tumors developing in the setting of Crohn disease tend to be small lesions measuring <1 cm (160). Small NETs are not encapsulated and usually demonstrate minimal invasion at their borders. Tumors that reach the lumen may ulcerate. As the tumors increase in size, they infiltrate beyond the submucosa into the muscularis propria, eventually reaching the serosa and mesentery. As the tumor becomes more deeply invasive, the bowel appears constricted or fibrotic (Fig. 17.35).

Midgut NETs demonstrate a characteristic insular (type I) growth pattern, which consists of solid nests or cords of cells

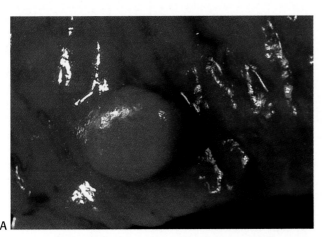
A

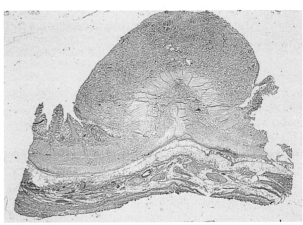
B

FIG. 17.33. Ileal carcinoid. **A:** Gross appearance of polypoid carcinoid. The mucosal surface is smooth and not ulcerated. **B:** The margins are well defined and there is no extension into muscularis propria.

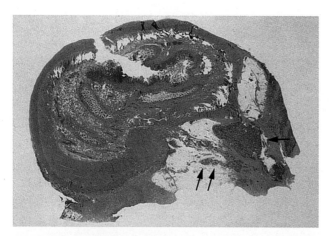

FIG. 17.35. Small bowel kinking from carcinoid tumor that grows into the serosal fat (*arrows*). Concomitant fibrosis has caused adhesions of multiple bowel loops.

with clearly defined boundaries, although the other growth patterns (Table 17.6) can also be seen. The cells lie in closely packed, round, regular, and monomorphous cell masses, buds, and islands (Figs. 17.36 and 17.37). The cells often palisade at the edges of the nests. Some tumors contain a mixture of both insular cords and tubules and rosettes. Individual cells as well as the tubular lumens may contain mucin (Fig. 17.38). Prominent capillaries represent a common feature. Rare tumors contain a dense eosinophilic stroma. NET cells usually contain a moderate amount of slightly acidophilic, slightly basophilic, or amphophilic cytoplasm. Eosinophilic cytoplasmic granules may be identified, especially at the periphery of the cellular nests (Fig. 17.38). Typical NETs demonstrate little or no cellular pleomorphism, indistinct cell borders, small nucleoli, nuclear hyperchromasia, and little mitotic activity. The relatively small, round to oval central nuclei have well-defined, regular nuclear membranes. When NETs invade the muscularis propria, they appear to insinuate themselves between the muscle fibers, spreading the fibers apart rather than destroying them (Fig. 17.39). When the tumor cells infiltrate intramural nerves, the latter become hypertrophic (Fig. 17.40). NE cell hyperplasia and small proliferating endocrine cell aggregates within the crypts may associate with small intestinal carcinoids, suggesting that such lesions originate from intraepithelial endocrine cells and subsequently infiltrate into the lamina propria (180). Up to 110 grossly visible tumors have been observed along with numerous grossly invisible EC cell microproliferations in the lamina propria. These show no apparent connections to the intracryptal endocrine cells, which do not appear to be increased (181). There are also circumstances where multiple tumors associate with increased intracryptal endocrine cells (53). These intraepithelial endocrine cells form linear proliferations or intracryptal aggregates and lamina propria endocrine cell micronodules appear to bud off them. Thus, there appeared to be an EC cell hyperplasia–carcinoid sequence similar to

the ECL cell hyperplastic continuum that occurs in the stomach.

The classic carcinoid tumor contains granules that are both argentaffinic and argyrophilic. In most tumors, argentaffin cells (Fig. 17.41) constitute the major cell population (182). The outermost cells tend to be the most argentaffinic (Fig. 17.42). The tumors stain strongly with the usual neuroendocrine immunostains. Most midgut carcinoids are multihormonal, with the most frequently encountered hormones being serotonin (Fig. 17.43), somatostatin, and gastrin. They may also produce enteroglucagon, PP, or PYY (171,182–187). Some of the substances are released into the circulation and their serum levels may serve as useful tumor makers. The two most helpful are CgA and neurokinin A (88).

Two thirds of these tumors produce CEA, 20% express prostate-specific antigen, and 7% contain S100-positive cells (80). Cytokeratin immunoreactivity is present in 68% of midgut carcinoid tumors (187). These tumors also display strong immunostaining for vascular endothelial growth factor, perhaps accounting for the rich vascularity commonly seen in these tumors. Ki-67 expression is low in these tumors, even in those that metastasize.

Concentric elastic vascular sclerosis often affects the large mesenteric vessels (Fig. 17.44), sometimes obliterating the vascular lumens, leading to ischemia (188). The elastosis and fibrosis are not confined to the vessels. It may also surround nests of tumor cells, resulting in extensive matting of involved tissues and lymph nodes, sometimes producing fibrous adhesions.

It is estimated that 1% to 35% of all small intestinal NETs metastasize (161,189). Metastases first involve the regional lymph nodes and then the liver (Figs. 17.45 and 17.46). Lymph nodes with metastases can measure up to 5 to 6 cm in diameter or they may be matted together, secondary to the tumor-associated desmoplasia. The cut surface of the nodes often has the yellow or tan color characteristic of NETs. The primary neoplasm may remain relatively small (<3.5 cm), even when extensive metastatic disease involves the lymph nodes or liver. The right lobe of the liver, which receives most of the blood supply from the ileum, is involved more often than the left. NETs may also metastasize to the ovaries (190), peritoneum (191), and spleen (192). Ovarian carcinoid tumors may present a diagnostic dilemma because the lesions may be primary in the ovary or represent a metastasis of an intestinal lesion. Features that distinguish primary from secondary ovarian carcinoid tumors are listed in Table 17.11 (190). Tumors rarely metastasize outside of the abdominal cavity (0.5% of cases). When they do, metastatic sites include the pleura, heart (193), breast (194), bone marrow (Fig. 17.46), skin (195), and eye (196). Metastases to the skin or subcutaneous tissues can be confused with Merkel cell tumors, particularly in the absence of a demonstrable primary elsewhere.

Identifying tumors that will behave aggressively can be difficult. The distinction between a benign and malignant

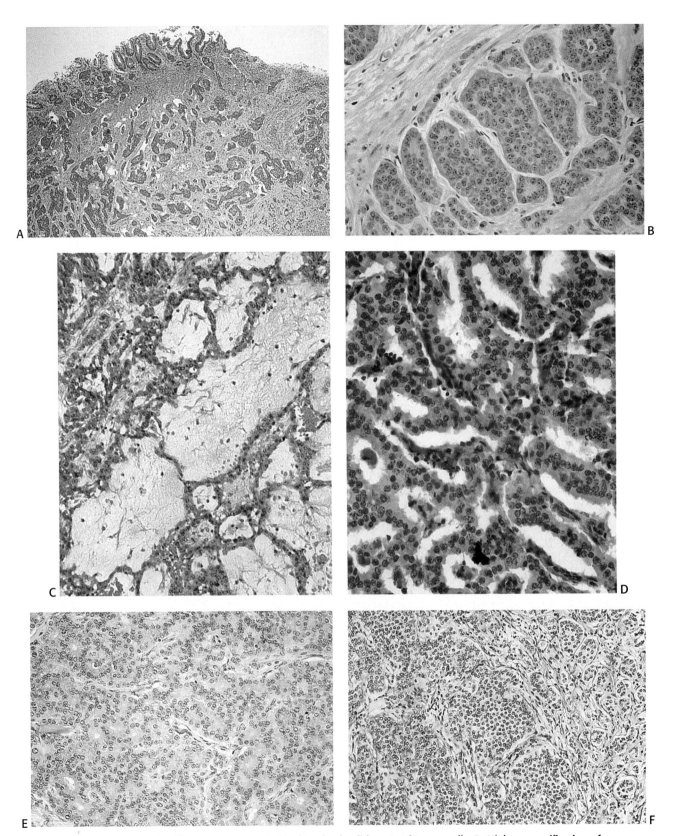

FIG. 17.36. Carcinoid tumor patterns. **A:** Varying-sized solid nests of tumor cells. **B:** Higher magnification of the lesion shown in A demonstrating solid nests and also marked tissue retraction artifact. **C:** Trabecular pattern. **D:** Higher magnification of the interanastomosing ribbons of tumor cells. **E:** Carcinoid composed of acinarlike structures. **F:** Tumor demonstrating solid nests as well as glandular structures. Some of these nests are less well differentiated than others.

TABLE 17.11	Comparison of Primary Vs. Secondary Ovarian Carcinoid Tumors	
Feature	Primary	Secondary
Age	31–79 (mean 60)	21–82 (mean 51)
Laterally	Unilateral	Bilateral
Teratomatous elements	Present	Absent
Cut surface	Homogeneous	Nodular
Peritoneal abscesses	Absent	Often present
Postoperative 5-HIAA levels	Negative	Often positive
Dead of carcinoid		
1 year	0%	38%
4 years	0%	77%

HIAA, hydroxyindoleacetic acid.

tumor traditionally relies on the presence or absence of metastases because histologic features alone do not usually allow one to predict malignancy. Factors determining their relatively malignant nature include tumor size, extent of local spread, presence of metastases at the time of diagnosis, mitotic rate, multiplicity, female gender, depth of invasion and presence of the carcinoid syndrome, increasing patient age, histologic pattern, presence of another malignancy, proliferative rate, and ploidy status (87,161,197). Approximately 2% of tumors measuring <1 cm, 50% of tumors measuring from 1 to 2 cm, and 80% of tumors measuring >2 cm metastasize (161). An increased median survival (4 years) is seen in patients with tumors displaying a mixed insular/glandular pattern (198). Patients with a pure insular and trabecular pattern have a median survival of 2.9 and 2.5 years, respectively. NETs discovered incidentally have an excellent prognosis compared to tumors in symptomatic patients. In one series of 28 patients with

operable tumors, including 11 without metastases and 17 with operable metastases, 68% survived 5 years; only 2 of the 28 patients died of metastatic carcinoid tumor within 5 years of surgical resection. In contrast, only 27% of inoperable cases survived 5 years (161). In another series, the overall 5-year survival for patients with small bowel carcinoids was 59%; the 10-year survival was 43%. The 5- and 10-year survival rates were 72% and 60% and 35% and 15%, respectively, for patients without and with hepatic metastases.

Patients with resectable jejunal and ileal NETs should undergo wide excision of the involved intestinal segment, including a mesenteric node dissection, regardless of the size of the primary tumor (199). Tumors that are nonfunctioning, measure <1 cm, are confined to the mucosa/submucosa, and are not angioinvasive are generally cured by local excision. However, even if the tumor cannot be totally excised, the surgeon should attempt to resect as much grossly visible tumor as

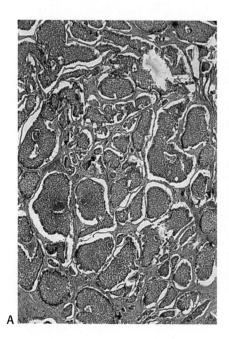 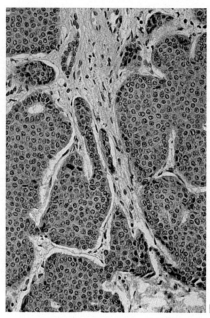

A   B

FIG. 17.37. Ileal carcinoid. **A:** The tumor islands are relatively closely packed together and a marked tissue retraction artifact is present. **B:** Higher magnification showing monomorphous cell masses. Some cells have large nuclei and small nucleoli as well as inconspicuous cytoplasm and fine chromatin. Other rare cells demonstrate gigantic nuclei. Mitoses are rare and there is less tissue retraction than seen in A.

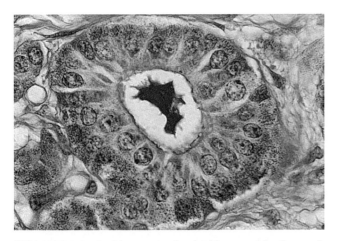

FIG. 17.38. Carcinoid tumor stained with a combination periodic acid–Schiff and chromogranin stain demonstrating luminal secretions and basal cytoplasmic neuroendocrine granules.

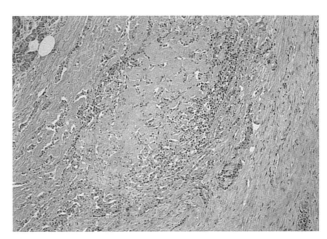

FIG. 17.39. Small separate nests of carcinoid tumor infiltrate the smooth muscle fibers of the muscularis propria without causing destruction of the native tissues.

possible, for palliation (161) and to avoid later complications such as bleeding, intestinal obstruction, or perforation. Some patients suffer more from disabling hormonal syndromes than from the tumor itself. Such patients may warrant aggressive therapy to reduce the tumor burden to achieve a comfortable life. Hepatic arterial occlusion may result in significant relief of hormonal symptoms. The 5-year survival rate of patients with hepatic metastases is 18% to 32% (100,200).

Today there is a tendency to treat patients with metastatic disease aggressively with surgery, somatostatin analogs, interferon, and possibly radiation and/or chemotherapy (80).

Neuroendocrine Tumors in Meckel Diverticulum

Carcinoid tumors developing in Meckel diverticulum have a propensity to develop in males. Patients range in age from

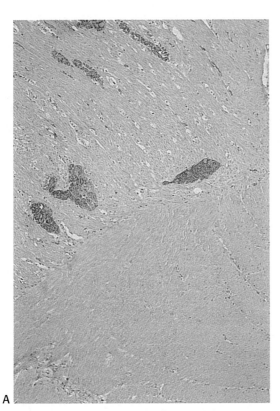

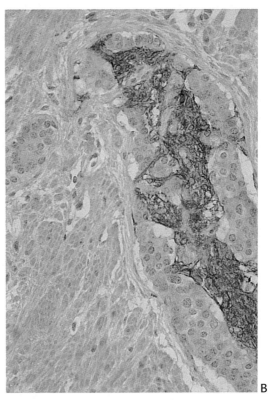

FIG. 17.40. Neural cell adhesion molecule immunostain of the wall of the small bowel demonstrating the presence of marked neural hypertrophy. **A:** Higher magnification demonstrating the hypertrophic nerves. **B:** Nerve infiltrated by tumor cells.

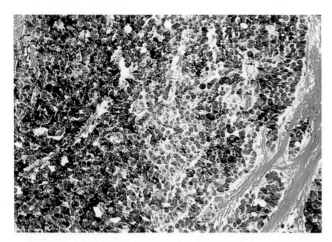

FIG. 17.41. Argentaffin-positive carcinoid tumor (Fontana-Masson stain).

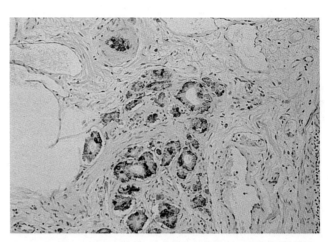

FIG. 17.43. Serotonin immunostaining of midgut carcinoid.

14 months to 82 years. Seventy-seven percent of symptomatic patients have metastases (201). It is likely that these neoplasms are more analogous to gastric ECL tumors than to small intestinal carcinoids since they likely arise in areas of heterotopic gastric mucosa.

Appendiceal Neuroendocrine Tumors

NETs account for between 50% and 85% of all of surgically diagnosed appendiceal tumors and approximately 20% of all GI carcinoid tumors (91). This number reflects a decreasing incidence from previous studies, perhaps reflecting a decline in the practice of incidental appendectomies. They affect approximately 0.02% to 1.5% of all surgically removed appendices, and 4.4% are multifocal with evidence of carcinoid tumors elsewhere (202). Appendiceal NETs affect patients ranging in age from 6 to 80 years (91,202,203), with a mean age of 49.3 years (80), some 20 years earlier than that seen for carcinoids involving other parts of the gut. Tubular

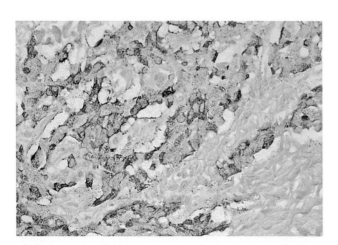

FIG. 17.42. Argyrophilic-positive carcinoid tumor. Note the prominent granular staining of the tumor nests (Grimelius stain).

carcinoids occur at a significantly younger age than goblet cell carcinoids (average 29 vs. 53 years) (123). Patients with IBD sometimes develop appendiceal NETs (160). Fourteen percent of patients also have a histologically confirmed second primary malignant tumor of some other type, with the colon, cervix, and endometrium being among the most common sites of origin (202,204). A preponderance of women exists in older age groups, whereas men predominate in younger ages. In nongynecologic patients, the most common reason for the appendectomy is acute appendicitis caused by tumor obstruction of the lumen. The carcinoid syndrome rarely occurs in association with appendiceal lesions. It generally develops in patients with widespread metastases, and appendiceal carcinoid tumors rarely give rise to distant metastases.

Unlike other gastrointestinal NETs, the cell of origin of appendiceal carcinoids is the subepithelial Kultschitzky cell, which has both endocrine and neural features (205). These subepithelial cells are more numerous toward the appendiceal tip, consistent with the observation that 70% to 80% of appendiceal carcinoid tumors occur at the tip, 5% to 22% arise in the body, and only 7% to 8% arise in the base of the appendix (202,204).

The gross appearance of the tumors varies from a subtle deformity and kinking of the appendiceal wall to a mass protruding into the lumen obliterating it or diffusely infiltrating the appendiceal wall (Fig. 17.47). It may also appear as an area of firm, gray-yellow tissue simulating distal fibrous occlusion. In some cases, the tumor produces circumferential narrowing; in other cases the lumen appears eccentrically narrowed. Ninety-five percent of tumors measure <1 cm in diameter. Carcinoid tumors usually spread by extending into the serosa (Fig. 17.48) or by permeating serosal lymphatics and veins. However, metastases are rare. Only 1% to 9% of appendiceal NETs metastasize, usually to regional lymph nodes. Distant metastases are rare (202,204).

Appendiceal NETs display several distinct histologic patterns: The typical EC cell, serotonin-producing carcinoid; the L-cell, glucagonlike peptide- and PP/PYY-producing carcinoid;

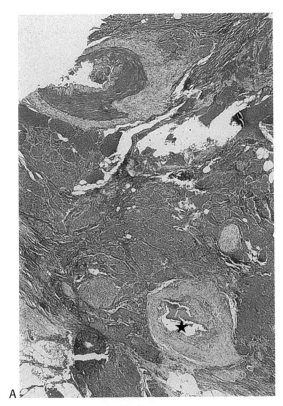
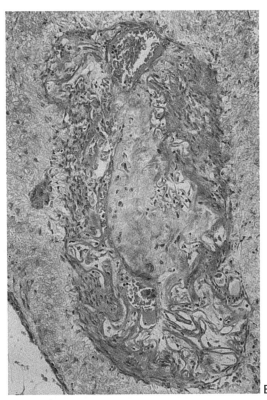

FIG. 17.44. Vascular sclerosis. **A:** Vessels on the serosal surface demonstrate varying degrees of vascular sclerosis. The vessel with the *star* is shown at higher power in B. **B:** Marked intimal medial and adventitial fibrosis. The elastin is reduplicated and the vessel is recanalized. Trichrome stain.

the tubular carcinoid; the goblet cell carcinoid; and mixed carcinoid–adenocarcinoma. The last two entities are discussed in the section on mixed endocrine–exocrine neoplasms.

EC Cell Tumors

EC cell tumors are indistinguishable from ileal carcinoids. They produce serotonin and substance P and exhibit a typical

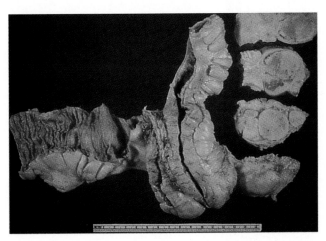

FIG. 17.45. Metastatic carcinoid involving the regional lymph nodes. Multiple tumor masses are seen on the cross section of the specimen.

insular pattern of solid nests with little nuclear pleomorphism and peripheral palisading (Soga type A pattern) (Fig 17.48). A minority of tumors exhibit glandular formations (type C patterns) or a mixture of the two (types A and C). If an acinar component is present, the cells differentiate into solid rosettes containing small amounts of inspissated mucin. If this variant is present, some of the cells may appear clear. This pattern has been termed the clear cell or balloon cell carcinoid (206). The NE granules lie scattered evenly throughout the cytoplasm or concentrate at the periphery of the tumor cell clumps, imparting a prominent eosinophilic border to the cells. Occasional cells may appear vacuolated, perhaps related to degeneration (207). These tumors are argentaffinic, argyrophilic, and positive with the usual NE cell markers and serotonin. Occasional cells stain for somatostatin, glucagon, calcitonin, CCK, gastrin, ACTH, neurotensin, motilin, and PP (208), but CEA is usually negative or only weakly positive. The majority of the tumor involves deeper layers of the appendiceal wall, often accompanied by fibrosis and hypertrophy of the muscularis propria. The tumors may show perineural or lymphatic invasion. Approximately two thirds of the tumors extend to the peritoneal surface. In the infiltrative portions of the tumor, the typical insular pattern is replaced by narrow cords and ribbons. Retraction artifacts mimic angioinvasion, but since angioinvasion is not used in the classification of appendiceal neoplasms (Table 17.12), it is not a major concern in

TABLE 17.12 Classification of Neuroendocrine Tumors of the Appendix

Well-Differentiated Neuroendocrine Tumor (Carcinoid)

Benign: Nonfunctioning, confined to appendiceal wall, nonangioinvasive, ≤2 cm in size
• Serotonin-producing tumor
• Enteroglucagon-producing tumor

Benign or low-grade malignant (uncertain malignant potential): Nonfunctioning, invading the mesoappendix, angioinvasive, >2 cm in size

Well-Differentiated Neuroendocrine Carcinoma (Malignant Carcinoid)

Low-grade malignant: Infiltrating deep in the mesoappendix, >2.5 cm in size or metastases
• Nonfunctioning or functioning serotonin-producing carcinoma (with carcinoid syndrome)

High-grade malignant: Poorly differentiated intermediate or small cell carcinoma

Mixed Exocrine–Neuroendocrine Carcinoma

Low-grade malignant
• Goblet cell carcinoid

evaluating these tumors. More aggressive tumors display nuclear pleomorphism and a higher mitotic rate than their less aggressive counterparts (179). Metastases to the peritoneum, regional lymph nodes, and liver rarely develop (204). Conventional appendiceal carcinoids tend not to express cytokeratin (209), and this factor, along with the presence of S100-positive sustentacular cells (Fig. 17.49), may make these tumors more similar to paragangliomas than to ileal NETs.

L-cell Tumors

Nonargentaffinic L-cell carcinoids are much less common than EC cell carcinoids. They produce glucagonlike peptides and PP/PYY. These tumors are usually small, measuring only 2 to 3 mm in size, and they are easily overlooked lesions on gross examination of the appendix. They consist of tubular or trabecular patterns (Soga type B) resembling rectal carcinoid tumors. The round, solid cellular nests typical of argentaffinic carcinoids are absent. The regular, neoplastic endocrine cells show little mitotic activity. Although they are nonargentaffinic, the cytoplasmic granules are frequently argyrophilic with the Grimelius technique (210), contain various peptide hormones, and react with antibodies to CgA and/or synaptophysin. The tumors also produce mucin and are cytokeratin immunoreactive (209). L-cell tumors with a dominant glandular pattern correspond to tubular carcinoids (203,211,212). L-cell tumors behave in the same way as EC tumors.

Appendiceal carcinoids have the best prognosis of all the carcinoids, probably reflecting the fact that the lesions are often detected early as well as the inherent biology of the tumor. In Godwin's (100) review of patients with appendiceal carcinoid tumors, the 5-year survival was 99%! Prognosis directly relates to tumor size, the presence of vascular or perineural invasion, and mesoappendiceal extension. Moertel found no recurrence among 108 patients with tumors measuring <1 cm, followed for 5 years. Tumors measuring 2 cm in greatest diameter may present with widespread metastases at the time of initial detection (202,204). Seventy-one percent of the patients who undergo resection survive 5 years, with a median time to subsequent recurrence of 8 years (204). These data are based on measurement of the tumor in the fresh state, and it should be kept in mind that formalin

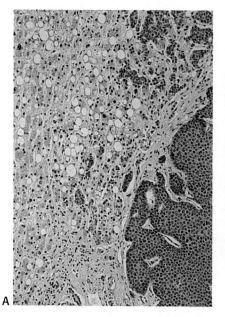
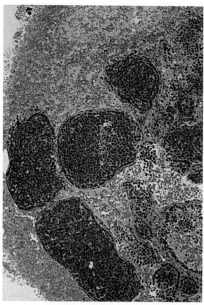

A   B

FIG. 17.46. Metastatic carcinoid. **A:** Liver metastasis. **B:** Bone marrow metastases.

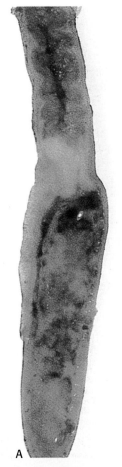

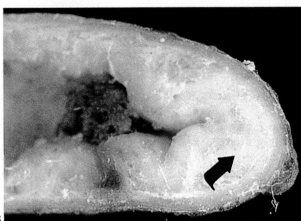

FIG. 17.47. Appendiceal carcinoid. **A:** Stricture of the appendix secondary to the presence of a carcinoid tumor. The surrounding mucosa appears inflamed due to the presence of coexisting appendicitis. The distal appendicitis results from the obstruction by the carcinoid tumor present in the middle of the appendix. **B:** Small carcinoid (*arrow*) in the distal end of the appendix. The yellow-gray area could easily be missed on gross examination. The lesion diffusely infiltrated the bowel wall and extended to the serosa.

fixation causes carcinoid tumors to shrink by almost one third of their original volume (213). Tumors measuring <2 cm in diameter with mesoappendiceal invasion may metastasize or spreading transcelomically.

TABLE 17.13	Indications for Hemicolectomy in Patients with Carcinoid Tumors

Tumor arises at appendix base
Tumor present in resection margin
Tumor extension to mesoappendix
Tumor in extra-appendiceal lymphatics
Tumor measures ≥2 cm
Evidence of metastases
High mitotic activity
Lymphatic invasion
Mucinous histology

Simple appendectomy represents adequate treatment for most tumors, but an ileocolectomy should be performed if the tumor meets one of the criteria listed in Table 17.13 (202,204). Simple appendectomy is recommended for tumors measuring <2 cm if no gross evidence of metastatic disease is found at laparotomy (204).

D-cell Tumors

These are extremely rare in the appendix. A case of a psammomatous somatostatinoma was reported in a patient with NF1. It was histologically identical to the same tumor arising in the duodenum (214).

Colonic Neuroendocrine Tumors (Carcinoids)

Large intestinal carcinoid tumors account for approximately 6% of all GI NETs (100). Patients range in age from 9 to 83 years and average 64 to 66 years of age (100). The age-adjusted incidence is 0.07 to 0.31 cases per 100,000 population per year. The tumors exhibit an equal gender distribution. Whites are more frequently affected than blacks (91). Colorectal carcinoid tumors may complicate longstanding chronic inflammatory diseases such as ulcerative colitis (215). Additionally, the incidence of NETs may be higher in Japan and Southern Asia than in Western countries (100). As with other GI carcinoid tumors, colorectal NETs associate with tumors in other sites, particularly in the GI tract. The overall incidence of secondary tumors ranges from 3% to 15% (216,217). These tumors include both adenocarcinomas as well as other carcinoid tumors.

Forty-eight percent of the NETs arise in the cecum, 16% in the ascending colon, 6% in the transverse colon, 11% in the descending colon, and 13% in the sigmoid colon; in the remainder it is difficult to tell the exact site of origin. The clinical presentation varies depending on the size and site of the tumor. The symptoms associated with these neoplasms include pain, rectal bleeding, and diarrhea. These usually result from mechanical trauma associated with the passage of solid feces over the tumor surface. Some colonic NETs cause profound and unexplained weight loss; most lack humoral manifestations. The carcinoid syndrome is uncommon, even in the presence of liver metastases. Early lesions

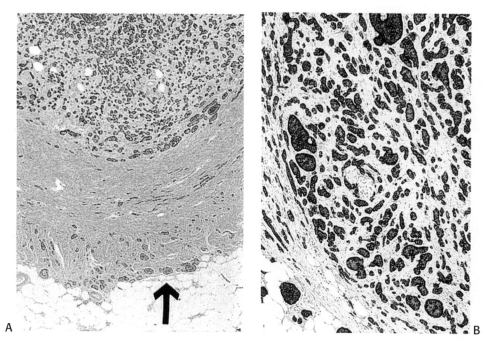

FIG. 17.48. A: Brownish stain (antibody to chromogranin) represents presence of neurosecretory granules. The tumor is present within the central fibrous occluded portion of the appendix, as well as extending all the way out to the serosa (*arrow*). **B:** Cross section through a different lesion showing central fibrous occlusion of the appendix and peripheral carcinoid tumor (brown cells) reaching the serosa.

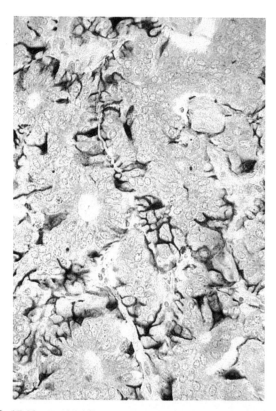

FIG. 17.49. Carcinoid tumor. S100-immunostained preparation showing the presence of prominent peripheral S100-positive sustentacular cells. Many are spider shaped.

are polypoid and tend to have an excellent prognosis following resection. More advanced tumors appear ulcerated and aggressive. Some NETs present as large bulky masses, sometimes measuring up to 16 cm in greatest diameter (216). These deeply invade the bowel wall and involve regional lymph nodes by the time they are detected.

The histology of large intestinal EC cell tumors resembles carcinoid tumors arising in the small intestine or appendix. The WHO classification of colonic NETs is shown in Table 17.14. Solid clumps or islands of uniform pale cells with peripheral cords and trabeculae are present. The cells at the periphery may appear hyperchromatic and contain bright eosinophilic granular cytoplasm. Other patterns include the formation of tubules containing luminal periodic acid–Schiff (PAS)-positive material. However, they generally exhibit a more undifferentiated pattern with clinically more aggressive features, whereas well-differentiated features such as insular, trabecular, and glandular patterns are less common (217). A significant number of hindgut NETs exhibit moderate atypia and a high mitotic rate, and these lesions tend to behave more aggressively than the average midgut carcinoid tumor. Silver stains are generally negative, although populations of argyrophilic cells and even argentaffinic cells do occur in some cases (218). CgA immunostains may be negative (219). However, synaptophysin is usually positive (219).

Colonic carcinoids exhibit the worse prognosis of all GI carcinoid tumors with an overall 5-year survival of 33% to

TABLE 17.14 **Classification of Neuroendocrine Tumors of the Ileum, Colon, and Rectum**

Well-Differentiated Neuroendocrine Tumor (Carcinoid)

Benign: Nonfunctioning, confined to mucosa–submucosa, nonangioinvasive, <1 cm in size (ileum) or ≤2cm colon and rectum
- Serotonin-producing tumor
- Enteroglucagon-producing tumor

Benign or low-grade malignant (uncertain malignant potential): Nonfunctioning, confined to mucosa–submucosa, angioinvasive, or <1 cm in size (ileum) or ≤ 2cm colon and rectum
- Serotonin-producing tumor
- Enteroglucagon-producing tumor

Well-Differentiated Neuroendocrine Carcinoma (Malignant Carcinoid)

Low-grade malignant: Invasion of the muscularis propria and beyond or metastases
- Nonfunctioning or functioning serotonin-producing carcinoma (with carcinoid syndrome)
- Nonfunctioning enteroglucagon-producing carcinoma

Poorly Differentiated Neuroendocrine Carcinoma

High-grade malignant

42% (100,200). Although tumor size and microinvasion are major prognostic features in other GI NETs, these features tend to be less useful in assessing the prognosis of colonic NETs because most of these lesions exceed 2 cm in size and involve the muscularis propria at the time of presentation (217). Mitotic rate, overall tumor grade, and the histologic pattern all influence survival (217,220).

Colonic NETs can be treated by local excision if they are found at an early stage (≤2 cm) (219). Larger tumors should be treated aggressively with a standard colonic resection and lymph node dissection. Only 16.6% of lesions <2 cm metastasize, whereas 74% of lesions >2 cm metastasize. These tumors metastasize to the lymph nodes, liver, mesentery, peritoneum, pancreas, ureters, ovaries, omentum, and, rarely, heart, diaphragm, kidney, uterus, adnexa, and colon (216).

Rectal Neuroendocrine Tumors

Rectal NETs constitute 0.7% to 1.3% of all rectal tumors (100,216,221) and 10% to 20% of all gastrointestinal NETs (100). The autopsy incidence is <0.04% (223), but this is probably an underestimate, since the rectum is rarely carefully examined at the time of autopsy. Rectal carcinoids equally affect males and females (222). The tumors develop most frequently in the 5th to 7th decades, with an age range of 1 to 93 years (222,223). Patients with IBD have an increased tumor incidence. Multiple carcinoids occur in 2% to 4.5% of rectal cases (100,223).

Overall, patients with rectal carcinoids fit into two groups: Small solitary lesions measuring <1 cm and larger lesions with the possibility of metastases. Many rectal carcinoids present as asymptomatic firm, yellowish submucosal nodules usually measuring <0.5 cm in diameter and are detected at the time of endoscopy or digital rectal examina-tion. Others appear as nodular mucosal or submucosal plaquelike thickenings, while a few appear polypoid or sessile (Fig. 17.50). These rounded neoplasms usually lack surface ulceration.

When symptoms referable to NETs are present, they usually manifest as anorectal discomfort or constipation. Patients rarely exhibit the carcinoid syndrome. Patients with the syndrome usually have extensive hepatic metastases. Less than 0.5% of patients with extensive nodal metastases but without hepatic involvement exhibit the syndrome. Rare patients with benign tumors may also exhibit the carcinoid syndrome (223). Uncommonly, the tumors present as larger, ulcerated growths (>2 cm), which may metastasize (221). Larger tumors have a capacity to invade directly into the urinary bladder.

Three histologic patterns are encountered in rectal carcinoids that are typically L-cell tumors: Ribbon, acinar, and mixed (Fig. 17.51). The ribbon pattern is the most common,

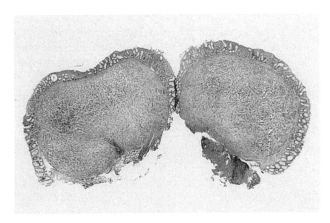

FIG. 17.50. Whole mount section of a polypoid rectal carcinoid tumor.

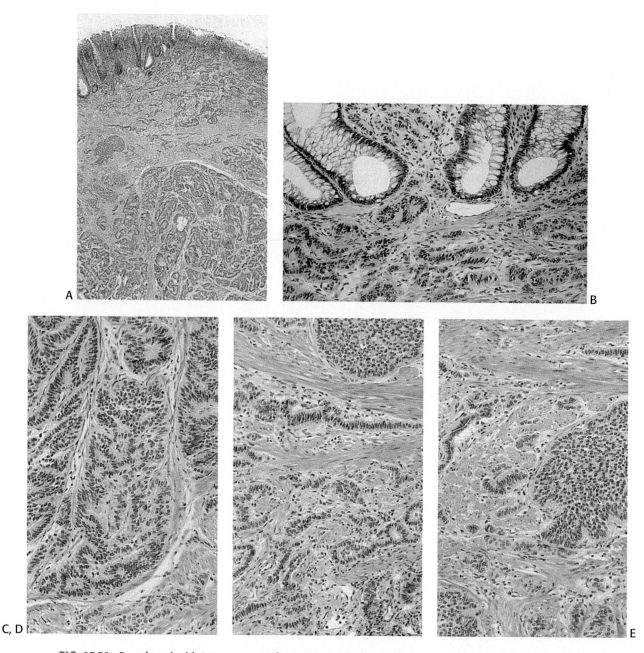

FIG. 17.51. Rectal carcinoid. **A:** Low-power photomicrograph demonstrating a carcinoid tumor, which is present in both the mucosa and submucosa of the rectum. The tumor shows solid, ribbonlike, and acinar growth patterns. **B:** The tumor infiltrates the muscularis mucosae and extends upward into the mucosa. **C:** Acinar pattern of growth. The cells have round, uniform nuclei. **D:** Ribbons of cells infiltrate the submucosa. **E:** Solid nests of uniform cells are identifiable in some areas.

followed by the mixed and acinar patterns, respectively (224). The ribbons consist of two or more cell layers arranged along a delicate vascularized connective tissue core. The ribbons may be straight, convoluted, or interlacing. In the tubular or acinar pattern, the neoplastic cells lie within a delicate fibrovascular stroma. These NETs are rarely argentaffinic, but many are argyrophilic (219). Chromogranin immunostains are often negative. However, antibodies to synaptophysin delineate the true nature of the lesion (219). Most rectal carcinoids produce multiple hor-

mones including any of the following: serotonin, glucagon, insulin, glicentin, somatostatin, pancreatic polypeptide, substance P, serotonin, endorphins, enkephalins, α-hCG, and PYY (224–229). Prostate-specific acid phosphatase is found in 80% to 100% of rectal carcinoids (230). Unlike other gastrointestinal NETs, trabecular hindgut carcinoid tumors may express vimentin. Rectal carcinoid tumors are also CEA immunoreactive (231).

NE cell hyperplasia surrounds some rectal NETs (220). Multiple rectal carcinoid tumors and numerous extraglandular exocrine cell proliferations and microcarcinoids may be present. There are also circumstances where multiple tumors associate with increased intracryptal endocrine cells (75). A rare example of a psammomatous rectal carcinoid was recently reported. However, no data were presented as to whether it produced somatostatin as is seen in duodenal psammomatous carcinoids (232).

Because most rectal carcinoids are small, the metastatic potential is low. The tumors generally have a favorable prognosis with an overall survival rate of 88.3% (220). Features of rectal endocrine tumors that suggest malignancy include presenting symptoms (221), a ribbon histologic pattern, histologic microinvasion, tumor size, spread into and beyond the muscularis propria, a diffusely infiltrating and invasive margin, ulceration, and features of atypical carcinoids (221,222,226). Tumor size is the most useful prognostic factor. Tumors <1 cm in diameter rarely (0% to 3%) metastasize (233). In contrast, tumors measuring ≥2 cm in greatest diameter exhibit regional lymph node metastases or liver metastases in 60% to 100% of cases (221,233). Tumors measuring from 1 to 1.9 cm have a 10% to 15% incidence of metastases (216,231). Metastatic sites include the lung, liver, lymph nodes (222), bone, cranium (234), and endocrine organs. Ki-67 or p53 staining does not appear to add additional information above standard histologic examination (235), and the value of ploidy assessments is controversial (236,237).

Rectal NETs are treated with surgery. Lesions measuring <1 cm in size that are purely submucosal are usually managed by a minor procedure (endoscopic removal or a transanal resection) (238). For tumors measuring 1 to 2 cm without evidence of nodal metastases, a wide excision with meticulous evaluation to exclude muscular invasion is recommended (239). Radical surgery is required for tumors >2 cm in diameter, with muscular invasion or with nodal metastases. If the tumors display atypical histologic patterns, then radical operation should be considered even if the tumor measures <2 cm. While the WHO criteria suggest that tumors ≤1 cm are benign lesions, this does not appear to be true of some rectal lesions (240). Metastases have been reported from lesions measuring 5 mm or less.

Tubular Carcinoid Tumors

Tubular carcinoids are rare tumors that most commonly develop in the appendix in younger patients, but they also develop elsewhere in the gastrointestinal tract. They tend to develop in the tip of the appendix and show little contact with the overlying mucosa. They cause an ill-defined thickening of the appendiceal wall.

The tumors have a distinctive appearance with small discrete tubules (Fig. 17.52) or linear structures in an abundant stoma. Comma-shaped structures may also be present, but solid nests are generally absent. The tumor cells have round or oval nuclei; nucleoli may be prominent in some cells. The cells contain variable amounts of eosinophilic cytoplasm.

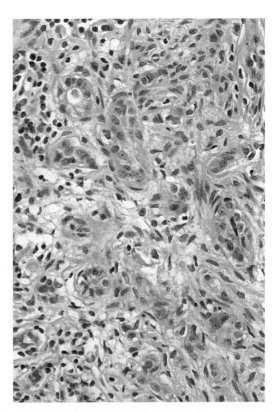

FIG. 17.52. Tubular carcinoid tumor of the appendix. The tubular structures intermingle with a proliferation of fibrous tissue. The lesion was associated with neural hyperplasia.

Occasionally, mucin is present in the lumens of the tubules. Argentaffin and argyrophilic cells are present in a majority of tumor cells (241). The tumors are positive for CgA, synaptophysin, serotonin, and IgA. S100-positive cells are absent (242).

Features that are helpful in diagnosing these tumors include an origin from the base of the crypts, an orderly growth pattern, integrity of the overlying mucosa, and absence of mitoses or cytologic atypia. Tubular carcinoids, but not other types of carcinoids, produce proglucagon mRNA (243), and they are frequently immunoreactive for glucagon, an unusual feature in other types of carcinoids. It is important to distinguish this lesion from goblet cell carcinoids that have a worse prognosis and require more aggressive treatment (241). Tubular carcinoids have a better prognosis, behaving more like classic carcinoids.

GANGLIOCYTIC PARAGANGLIOMAS

Rare neoplasms known as gangliocytic paragangliomas combine elements of three different cell lineages: Epithelioid cells resembling paraganglioma or carcinoid tumor cells; spindle cells reminiscent of Schwann cells; and ganglion cells. Most patients present in the 5th to 6th decades, with ages ranging from 17 to 80 years and a male-to-female incidence of 1.8:1 (244). NF1 patients have an increased propensity to develop gangliocytic paragangliomas.

Patients present with GI bleeding, nausea, vomiting (245), or hemorrhage (246). The extent of the bleeding may vary in both severity and chronicity, with some patients presenting with mild bleeding over several years' duration or others presenting in hypothalamic shock requiring transfusion. Obstructive jaundice develops in periampullary lesions (247).

Most gangliocytic paragangliomas arise in the medial aspect of the second part of the duodenum, especially at the ampulla of Vater. Some also originate in the jejunum (244–250), stomach, or appendix. Gangliocytic paragangliomas present as small polypoid submucosal lesions, frequently with an ulcerated mucosal surface and an average diameter of 2 cm. The lesions are usually not encapsulated and have an infiltrative pattern.

Histologically, the tumors contain a mixture of several distinct histologic patterns including (a) typical neurofibroma, with proliferating neurites and Schwann cells; (b) ganglion cells mixed with Schwann cells; and (c) proliferations of clear epithelioid cells arranged in clusters or radial patterns resembling carcinoid tumors (Fig. 17.53). The feature that distinguishes these lesions from ganglioneuromas is the presence of the carcinoidlike epithelial islands. The tumors insinuate themselves into the overlying lamina propria, often involving the underlying tissues and extending into the submucosa or the serosa.

The epithelioid cells stain positively with a variety of antibodies including chromogranin, synaptophysin, pancreatic polypeptide, neuron-specific enolase, serotonin, somatostatin, Leuenkephalin, insulin, glucagon, and vasoactive intestinal peptide. The spindle cells almost always are strongly positive for S100 protein, but may also stain with NSE, neurofilament protein, and vimentin. The ganglion cells frequently stain positively with NSE and neurofilament protein.

Gangliocytic paragangliomas usually follow a benign clinical course. With complete excision, surgical therapy is usually curative. Recurrences are possible in lesions that are incompletely excised. Rarely, gangliocytic paragangliomas metastasize (249,250). The metastases are to the regional lymph nodes; distant metastases do not occur.

NEUROENDOCRINE CARCINOMA

Most neuroendocrine carcinomas are either atypical carcinoids (well-differentiated NE carcinomas) or poorly differentiated NE carcinomas (Tables 17.5, 17.8, 17.10, 17.12, and 17.14). The tumors may be either pure or mixed with adenocarcinomatous and/or squamous cell carcinomatous components. Foci of necrosis and high mitotic indices are commonly observed in these neoplasms. CgA immunoreactivity in these lesions is generally poor, and synaptophysin represents a better marker of NE differentiation. Neuroendocrine carcinomas result from multidirectional differentiation of malignant epithelial cells.

Well-differentiated Neuroendocrine Carcinomas (Atypical [Malignant] Carcinoid Tumors)

Well-differentiated NE carcinomas have histologic features and a biologic behavior between that of typical carcinoid tumors and poorly differentiated NE carcinomas (small cell carcinomas) described below. They develop sporadically and in the setting of IBD. These lesions develop in the stomach, often in its proximal third (251); in the rectum; and in the esophagus (252). These are aggressive lesions and represent poorly differentiated forms of carcinoid tumors with increased mitotic activity and absent or limited extent of necrosis.

The cells range in appearance from uniform, large, polygonal, or fusiform types with abundant eosinophilic granular cytoplasm and round to oval nuclei similar to the cells seen in typical carcinoid tumors to pleomorphic cells with scanty cytoplasm and hyperchromatic variably sized and shaped nuclei. The pleomorphic epithelioid cells are two to three times the size of small cells with abundant eosinophilic to amphophilic cytoplasm. Mitoses range from 1 to 10/10 hpf. The tumors exhibit prominent fibroblastic host responses and obvious lymphatic invasion. There may be peripheral palisading. Neoplastic cells are arranged in sheets, trabeculae, ribbons, and nests, with necrotic foci and neuroepithelial-like rosettes (Fig. 17.54). However, sometimes definite cellular nests or trabeculae may be hard to find and often require an extensive examination of the tumor to identify them. Focal areas may resemble classic small cell carcinoma (SCC). The lesions show transmural involvement with limited mucosal involvement. The tumors are nonargentaffinic but strongly argyrophilic and they stain with the usual immunohistochemical markers of NE cell differentiation. The tumors may show vascular or lymphatic invasion; extensive local invasion, including invasion of the muscularis propria; an anaplastic appearance; cellular pleomorphism; mucin production; and necrosis. When these features are present, 50% of the tumors metastasize (250).

High-grade Neuroendocrine Carcinomas

High-grade NE cell carcinomas are typically divided into small cell carcinomas and large cell (also called intermediate cell) NE carcinomas.

Poorly Differentiated Endocrine Cell Carcinoma/Small Cell Carcinoma

SCCs are malignant epithelial tumors that are similar in morphology, immunophenotype, and behavior to pulmonary SCC (253–256). They are clinically aggressive and have an extremely poor prognosis, even when discovered at

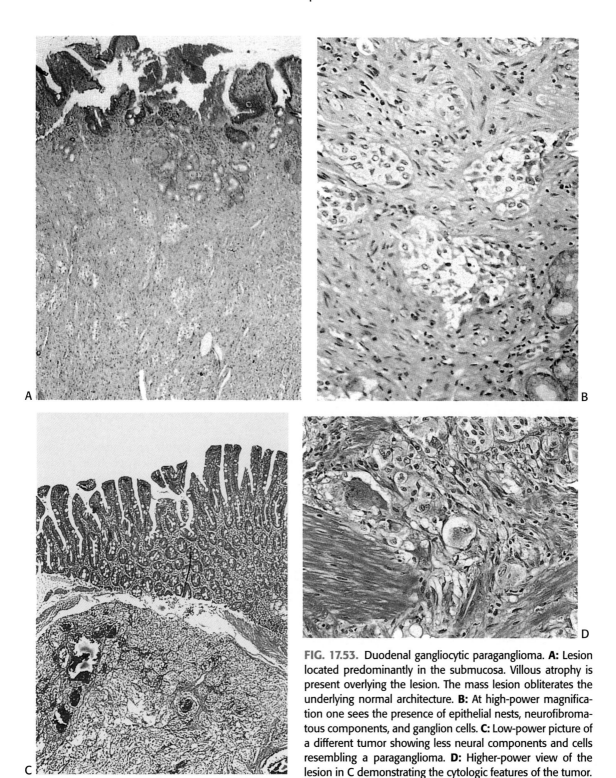

FIG. 17.53. Duodenal gangliocytic paraganglioma. **A:** Lesion located predominantly in the submucosa. Villous atrophy is present overlying the lesion. The mass lesion obliterates the underlying normal architecture. **B:** At high-power magnification one sees the presence of epithelial nests, neurofibromatous components, and ganglion cells. **C:** Low-power picture of a different tumor showing less neural components and cells resembling a paraganglioma. **D:** Higher-power view of the lesion in C demonstrating the cytologic features of the tumor.

an early stage. SCCs represent 0.1% to 1% of all GI malignancies, with the esophagus being the most common primary GI site of origin (256). Most patients present with overt distant metastases. Systemic symptoms are common. Ectopic hormone secretion may occur.

These small blue cell tumors consist of densely packed, small, and oval-, spindle-, or fusiform-shaped anaplastic cells with dark, round or oval, hyperchromatic nuclei containing coarse chromatin (Fig. 17.55). A small but discernible amount of eosinophilic to amphophilic cytoplasm without discrete cell borders surrounds the nuclei. The nuclei are approximately twice the diameter of mature lymphocytes. The small cells and intermediate cells form solid sheets, nests, and rosettes as well as ribbonlike cellular

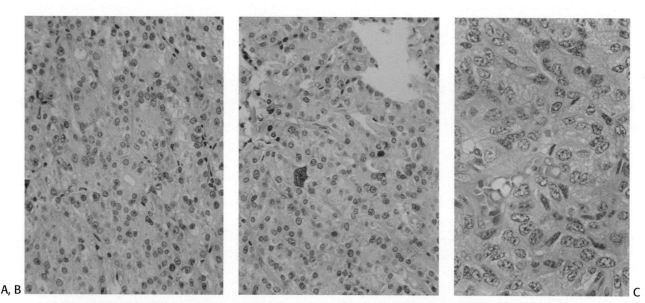

FIG. 17.54. Well-differentiated neuroendocrine carcinoma (malignant carcinoid). **A:** The tumor consists of large eosinophilic cells, vaguely arranged in closely packed cell nests. **B:** Isolated large cells may be present. **C:** Another tumor that has a histologic pattern that begins to approach large cell undifferentiated neuroendocrine carcinoma. The cells are large and the nuclei have marked chromatin clumping.

strands. Nucleoli are usually not prominent and may be completely absent. Significant nuclear molding may be present. Intermediate-sized cells and rare giant cells may intermingle with the small cells. The tumors may contain mono- and multinucleated tumor cells with large, angulated or fusiform, intensely hyperchromatic nuclei (Fig. 17.56). Crush artifacts (Azzopardi effect) are often present. Mitoses range in number from 10 to 125/10 hpf. Necrosis occurs in the central areas of the tumors (Fig. 17.57). Focal necrosis and vascular invasion are present in all cases.

The stroma varies from scanty reticulin fibers surrounding closely apposed nests of tumor to zones of marked desmoplasia. Typically, little or no inflammation associates

with the tumor. Mucin stains are negative in the tumor cells. Argyrophil reactions vary, but a few argyrophilic granules are usually present. Cytokeratin stains may show punctate perinuclear cytoplasmic reactivity. Immunostaining with antibodies to CgA are often disappointing, but antibodies to synaptophysin are strongly positive, making the latter the most reliable stain for detecting this tumor (Fig. 17.58). The tumors may also stain with NSE, Leu7, and neurofilament protein (Fig. 17.59). The tumors have a high proliferative rate and often display p53 immunoreactivity (Fig. 17.60). Recently it has been suggested that expression of human achaete-scute homolog gene-1 protein may be a more sensitive and specific marker of these highly aggressive tumors (257). The cytology of small cell carcinoma resembles that of

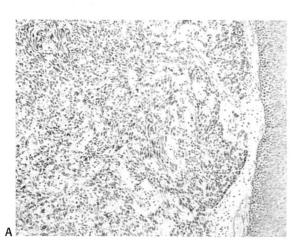

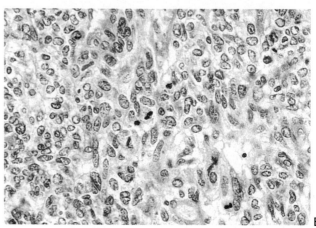

FIG. 17.55. Small cell carcinoma. **A:** Subepithelial small cell carcinoma. **B:** This highly cellular neoplasm consists of small cells with overlapping nuclei.

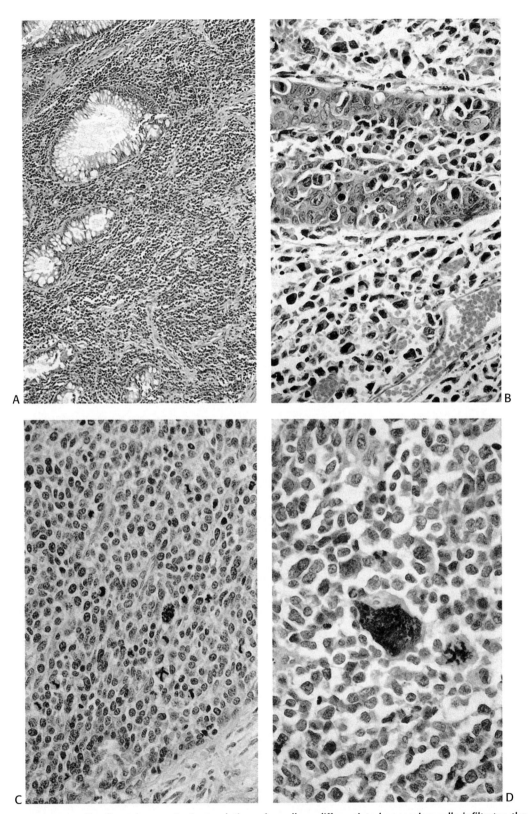

FIG. 17.56. Small cell carcinoma. **A:** A population of small, undifferentiated-appearing cells infiltrates the lamina propria. Several residual colonic crypts are present. **B:** The tumor is composed of sheets and nests of cells with hyperchromatic nuclei and scant cytoplasm. **C:** Sheets of neoplastic cells are present. A tumor giant cell is located in the center of the photograph. Note also the presence of numerous mitotic figures, some of which are very atypical. **D:** Higher-power view of a multinucleated tumor giant cell.

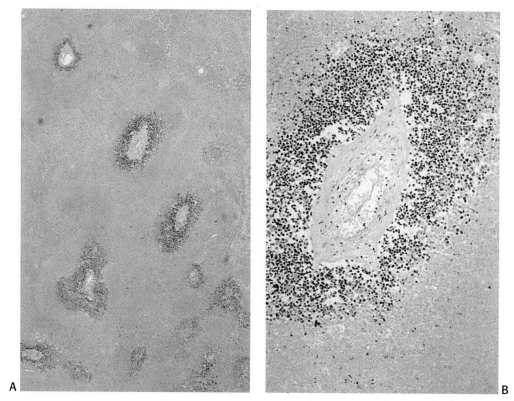

FIG. 17.57. Small cell carcinoma. **A:** This tumor demonstrates extensive necrosis. Viable tumor cells are present only surrounding vascular structures. **B:** Higher magnification demonstrating the perivascular clusters of viable tumor cells.

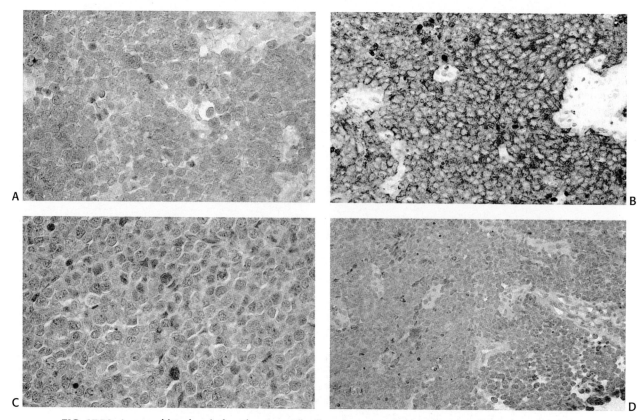

FIG. 17.58. Immunohistochemical markers in small cell carcinoma. **A:** Weak neuron-specific enolase immunoreactivity. **B:** Synaptophysin stains are almost always strongly positive in small cell carcinoma. **C:** Chromogranin immunoreactivity is often negative. **D:** Cytokeratin stain shows focal punctate cytoplasmic staining.

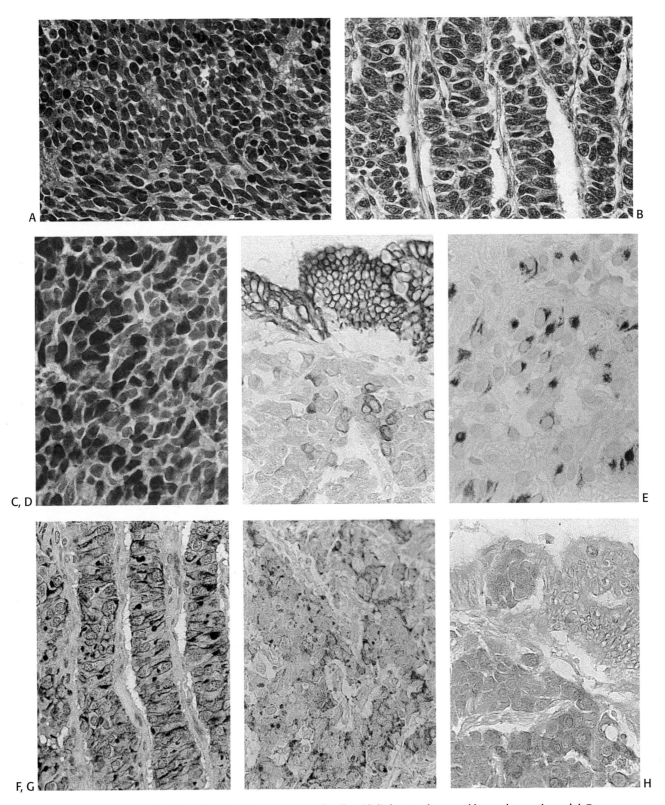

FIG. 17.59. Duodenal small cell carcinoma. **A:** Small cells with little cytoplasm and hyperchromatic nuclei. **B:** Trabecular pattern with prominent mitotic activity. **C:** Ki-67 immunoreactivity demonstrates that approximately 70% of the cells are proliferating. **D:** Focal cytokeratin immunoreactivity in small cells. The overlying ductal epithelium is strongly positive. **E:** Neurofilament positivity in the small cells. **F:** Cytokeratin positivity in the trabecular region showing strong membrane staining and strong dotlike cytoplasmic reactivity. **G:** Chromogranin immunostains decorate more than half of the tumor cells. **H:** Weak neuron-specific enolase positivity of the tumor cells. (Pictures courtesy of Dr. G. Zamboni, University of Verona, Italy.)

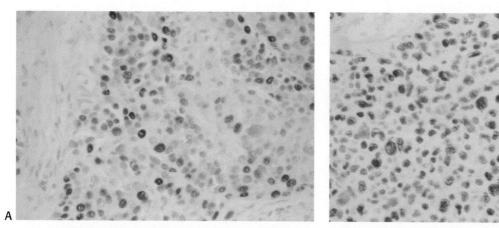

FIG 17.60. Small cell carcinoma. **A:** Ki-67 immunostain shows that these tumors have a high proliferative rate. **B:** The tumors are frequently p53 positive.

the corresponding lung tumor (Fig. 17.61). Small blue cells that are argyrophilic display the typical small cell immunophenotype. SCCs can resemble lymphomas, but the use of immunohistochemical and special stains usually resolves this differential diagnosis (Table 17.15).

Esophageal Small Cell Carcinomas

The esophagus is the most common site of extrapulmonary SCCs. Its incidence ranges from 0.5% to 7.6% of all esophageal tumors, depending on the country of origin of the patient (258,259). The tumor is more common in Japan than elsewhere in the world (260). Median patient age is 67 years, with a range of 45 to 89 years (260,261). Patients with SCC are often males in their 5th to 8th decades of life (260,261), and they often have a history of heavy smoking (260,261). There is also an association with longstanding achalasia (262). Presenting symptoms include dysphagia, weight loss, and chest pain. Most develop in the lower and middle thirds of the esophagus (261), and they may be single or multiple. The tumors range in size from 1 to 14 cm. The gross features of esophageal SCC are nonspecific, except perhaps for a tan, fleshy appearance. The tumors appear polypoid, fungating, or ulcerating. Invasion into the tracheobronchial tree causes a transesophageal fistula. In this setting it may be difficult to determine whether the tumor arises primarily in the lungs or in the esophagus.

SCCs may invade the submucosa and deeper layers of the esophageal wall. Lymphatic and blood vessel involvement is common. The overlying squamous epithelium often remains intact. Most small cell tumors demonstrate a pure small cell morphology (261), but they may also contain foci of squamous carcinoma in situ (260), invasive squamous carcinoma (261), adenocarcinoma, carcinoid tumor, or mucoepidermoid carcinoma (259), suggesting that the tumors arise from pluripotential basal cells present in the squamous epithelium or in the ducts of the submucosal glands (260). The tumors may also arise in areas of Barrett esophagus (263).

TABLE 17.15 Comparison of Small Cell Carcinoma Vs. Lymphoma

Stain	Small Cell Carcinoma	Lymphoma
H&E	Small blue cell tumor with variable history	Small blue cell tumor with variable history
Cytokeratin	±	−[a]
Vimentin	Often positive	Usually negative
Epithelial membrane antigen	±	±
Leukocyte common antigen	−	+
CD45	−	+
Chromogranin	+	−
Leu7	+	±
Neuron-specific enolase	+	−
Synaptophysin	+	−
Neurofilament protein	+	−

± indicates cases that may be positive or negative.
[a] May be positive in anaplastic large cell lymphoma and lymphocyte-depleted Hodgkin disease, myeloma, histiocytic lymphoma, and rare T- and B-cell lymphomas.
H&E, hematoxylin and eosin.

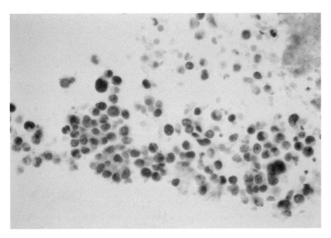

FIG 17.61. Characteristic cytologic features of small cell carcinoma are seen in this brushing from an esophageal tumor.

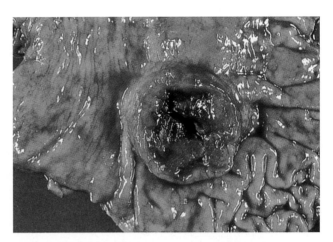

FIG. 17.62. Poorly differentiated gastric neuroendocrine carcinoma. The tumor is polypoid and demonstrates surface ulceration, necrosis, and hemorrhage. (Photograph courtesy of Dr. Onja Kim, ANSA Medical Center, Seoul, Korea.)

The tumors may produce ACTH (264), calcitonin (264), vasoactive intestinal polypeptide, gastrin, secretin parathormone, colony-stimulating factor (264), and antidiuretic hormone, causing various syndromes, including hypercalcemia, Cushing syndrome, watery diarrhea, and hypokalemia–achlorhydria (265). Microsatellite instability may be more frequent in esophageal SCC than in squamous cell carcinomas (259,266). The tumors express p53 in 50% to 100% of cases (266-268), lose Rb expression, and overexpress bcl-2 (267). Proliferating cell nuclear antigen (PCNA) labeling rates range from 64% to 91% (268).

Esophageal SCCs show more aggressive lymphatic spread than squamous cell carcinomas at an equivalent stage. As a result, the tumors tend to disseminate rapidly. Most patients have disseminated disease when first seen. Metastases of esophageal SCCs are to the abdominal and cervical lymph nodes. Median survival is 3.1 months. Survival is in the range of several weeks for untreated patients to 6 to 12 months for those receiving therapy. Some patients benefit from aggressive combination chemotherapy. In local regional disease, treatment may be initiated using chemoradiation and then if metastatic disease is excluded, surgical resection may be considered and may produce long-term remission and possibly long-term survival (269). In patients with limited stage disease, surgery with curative intent may also be considered as part of the multimodality therapy (259).

Gastric Small Cell Carcinomas

Gastric SCCs account for 6% of gastric NE tumors and are more common in men than women. The mean age of presentation is 63 years (98). SCCs are more common in the body and fundus (Fig. 17.62), although there are examples of antral tumors. The tumors exhibit the typical SCC morphology described above. They may also contain areas of adenocarcinoma and squamous cell carcinoma. Molecular analyses of these mixed tumors show identical *p53* and *ras* mutations

in all components, suggesting a monoclonal origin (270). When the tumors extend to the peritoneum, they may be diagnosed on cytologic examination of peritoneal washings. The malignant-appearing small cells are present on a necrotic background with naked hyperchromatic nuclei. Some tumor cells may contain paranuclear blue inclusions (271). Most patients with gastric small cell carcinoma die within 1 year of diagnosis (272).

Intestinal Small Cell Carcinomas

Large and small intestinal SCCs are rare tumors. They are more prevalent in Japan than in the United States. Most SCCs develop in males. It is a tumor of older adults, with ages ranging from 20 to 74 years, and a mean of 64 to 66 years (273). The majority of duodenal SCCs arise at the ampulla of Vater. Extra-ampullary duodenal SCCs are very rare (255). These ampullary tumors are grossly small (2 to 3 cm) tumors that are focally ulcerated or protuberant lesions (Fig. 17.63). Small intestinal SCCs may appear as ulcerated neoplasms.

SCCs arise anywhere within the large bowel, but are most common in the right colon (274). Colonic tumors range from localized bulky, polypoid lesions to neoplasms projecting into the bowel lumen (Fig. 17.64) or perforating the bowel wall. Annular or linitis plastica–like tumors or partly obstructing tumors may also be present. SCCs may also present as tiny foci in adenomatous polyps (256). The tumors may also develop in the setting of ulcerative colitis (274), where they may be multifocal (275). They may also arise on a background of endocrine cell hyperplasia (275). Virtually all of these undifferentiated neoplasms remain clinically silent. However, when symptoms develop, they include crampy abdominal pain, malaise, weight loss, fever, diarrhea, and rectal bleeding. In most reported cases, symptom duration is only a few weeks.

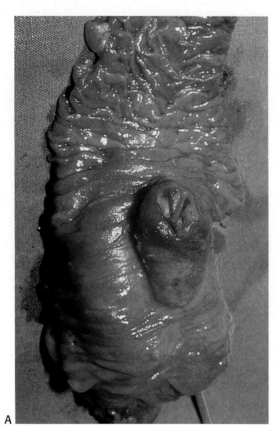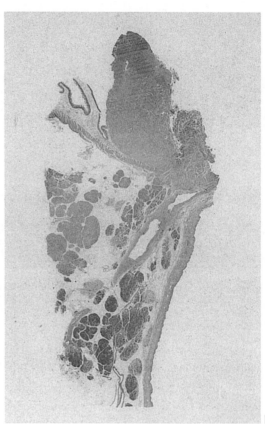

A   B

FIG. 17.63. Small cell carcinoma. A: Gross appearance of a tumor that arises at the ampulla of Vater. **B:** Whole mount of the lesion illustrated in A. The exophytic ampullary tumor has strictured the pancreatic duct. (Pictures courtesy of Dr. G. Zamboni, University of Verona, Italy.)

The tumors arising in the small bowel may show focal squamous differentiation. They often show direct invasion into the duodenum, pancreas, and/or bile duct. These aggressive tumors have a propensity for invasion and early metastasis. At the time of surgery almost all patients have metastases in the regional lymph nodes and the liver. Metastases also affect the peritoneum and lungs.

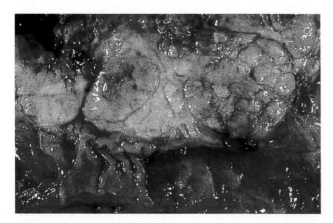

FIG. 17.64. Small cell carcinoma. A polyploid tumor mass projects into the colonic lumen.

The histologic features are typical of SCC. Overlying villous or tubulovillous adenomas are present in 45% of cases. When associated with adenomas, the interface of the adenoma with the SCC is abrupt, without evidence of transitional forms. Because of their association with adenomas and the demonstration of glandular, endocrine, squamous, and Paneth cell differentiation, most believe that SCCs arise from uncommitted "stem cells" in colorectal adenomas (274,276). The lesions may infiltrate transmurally, with limited involvement of the lamina propria, or they may be predominantly intramucosal, with only focal submucosal invasion.

The prognosis for SCCs is worse than for adenocarcinomas of comparable stage. They are able to widely disseminate from only superficially invasive foci (274). Nodal metastases are frequently present at the time the tumors are detected. Seventy-one percent of tumors metastasize to the liver. Even after aggressive treatment, patients die between 3 and 12 months following diagnosis, with 64% of patients dying within 5 months of diagnosis. However, some patients may exhibit a dramatic remission in response to a combined radiation and multidrug regimen designed to treat pulmonary SCC. However, even these remissions are usually followed by widespread metastases and death. The residual tumor may be of pure small cell histology or may have evidence of squamous cell carcinoma and/or adenocarcinoma, either along or in combination with the small cell carcinoma.

Anal Small Cell Carcinomas

The most anaplastic and most lethal of the anal canal tumors are the rare SCCs. The tumors arise in the upper part of the anal canal (276), grow rapidly, and metastasize early. The patients have an invariably fatal outcome. The differential diagnosis of these lesions includes basaloid squamous carcinomas. The latter are positive for high molecular cytokeratins, whereas SCCs are positive for neuroendocrine markers. Most patients present with advanced disease.

LARGE CELL NEUROENDOCRINE CARCINOMA

Large cell NE carcinomas (LCNECs) are rare, poorly differentiated endocrine carcinomas. They comprise <1% of colorectal cancers. Average patient age is 57 years, with a range of 29 to 86 years. The tumors develop in the colon, rectum, and anal canal (277). They have a histology intermediate between a conventional carcinoid tumor and a SCC. These malignant neoplasms are composed of large cells arranged in organoid, nested, trabecular, rosettelike, and palisading patterns that suggest NE differentiation (Fig. 17.65). In contrast to SCC, the cytoplasm is more abundant, nuclei are more vesicular, and nucleoli are prominent. Large multinucleated tumor cells may be present. The cells may appear discohesive, and there is less nuclear overlapping than is seen in typical SCC. Mitoses are easy to find, as is lymphovascular invasion. Focal necrosis is often present. As with SCCs, the tumors may exist alone or associate with adjacent adenoma or conventional adenocarcinoma. These tumors express cytokeratins mimicking the poorly differentiated adenocarcinomas that they resemble. However, in contrast to poorly differentiated adenocarcinomas, LCNECs express NE markers and lose retroblastoma (RB) expression (278).

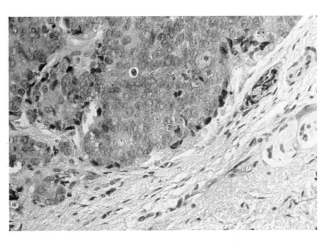

FIG. 17.65. Large cell neuroendocrine cell carcinoma.

The biologic behavior of these tumors resembles that of SCC. Most patients have metastases at the time of detection (277).

MIXED ENDOCRINE–GLANDULAR NEOPLASMS

Definitions and General Comments

Mixed endocrine–exocrine tumors constitute a heterogeneous group of rare neoplasms that includes different histopathologies and prognostic classes. The presence of occasional NE cells is common in many gastrointestinal adenocarcinomas. The degree of NE cell differentiation varies between tumors; when it is extensive the tumors may contain areas that resemble conventional carcinoids. More typically, the endocrine cells are inconspicuous and the quantity present is not obvious until the tumors are stained with NE cell markers. Carcinoid tumors or SCCs may coexist with adenomas or adenocarcinomas as composite tumors. The possible spectrum is shown in Table 17.16. The Lewin classification for these mixed neoplasms is shown in Table 17.17. These

---

TABLE 17.16 Possible Spectrum of Composite Tumors[a]

Nonendocrine Component	Endocrine Component
Adenoma	Carcinoid tumor (well-differentiated neuroendocrine tumor)
Adenocarcinoma	Malignant carcinoid (well-differentiated neuroendocrine carcinoma)
Well–poorly differentiated	Poorly differentiated neuroendocrine carcinoma
Signet ring cell	Small cell carcinoma
Diffuse gastric cancer	Intermediate cell carcinoma
Adenocarcinoma with squamous components	Pleomorphic giant cell tumor
Squamous carcinoma	Increased numbers of normal-appearing neuroendocrine cells
Pancreatic acinar differentiation	

[a]One or more elements from each of the columns can be combined with each other.

TABLE 17.17 Lewin Classification of Composite Tumors

- Carcinomas with interspersed endocrine cells
- Mixed tumors with admixed glandular and endocrine elements, each element comprising at least one third of the tumor
- Amphicrine tumors with glandular and endocrine differentiation in the same cell
- Collision tumors with juxtaposition of two elements without admixing of the two cell types

elements may intermingle with each other, as in goblet cell carcinoid tumors, or be distinctly separated from each other, as in collision tumors. The relative proportion and degree of differentiation of the glandular and endocrine components in these tumors are highly variable. The prognosis of these lesions depends on the histologic features and degree of differentiation of each of the components.

Mixed endocrine–glandular tumors may represent either the simultaneous proliferation of different cell lineages or the proliferation of multipotential stem cells capable of differentiating along multiple cell lineages. In tumors, amphicrine cells are present that contain both endocrine granules and mucin droplets. The presence of such cells supports the idea of a common precursor stem cell giving rise to two lines of differentiation within an individual cell (21).

Mutational studies support a monoclonal origin for tumors with mixed histologies when identical genetic mutations are present in each of the components as occurs in some tumors. In contrast, in collision tumors, where separate tumors may arise in close proximity to one another, there is evidence of a polyclonal origin as shown by immunohistochemical staining and genetic studies. Allelotyping studies also suggest that many mixed tumors are monoclonal in origin, whereas collision tumors have a polyclonal origin.

Goblet Cell Carcinoid

Goblet cell carcinoids have been described by a number of terms including *mucinous carcinoid, adenocarcinoid, crypt cell carcinoma,* and *microglandular carcinoma.* They exhibit features of both adenocarcinoma and carcinoid tumor. Goblet cell carcinoids may develop in the esophagus, duodenum (123,279), colon, and rectum (280,281); they are most common in the appendix. Sometimes they develop in patients with IBD (282). Goblet cell carcinoids may present with acute appendicitis or as an abdominal or pelvic mass (283).

Goblet cell carcinoids arise in any part of the appendix. They display a primarily submucosal growth pattern and appear as areas of firm whitish, sometimes mucoid discoloration. They range in size from 0.5 to 2.5 cm (209), although their exact size may be difficult to determine because of their diffusely infiltrative nature. A well-defined tumor mass may not be appreciated in lesions that grow circumferentially.

The tumors consist of uniform nests of mature-looking goblet cells arranged in small smooth-bordered cell nests (Figs. 17.66 to 17.68), small tight cellular clumps, cellular rosettes, and signet ring cells (241,283). Most cells contain abundant intracytoplasmic mucin; smaller numbers of endocrine cells with finely granular eosinophilic cytoplasm are also normally present, as are Paneth cells (283). In addition, there may be amphicrine cells present. Foci resembling Brunner glands that are lysozyme positive may also be seen (283). None of the cell types demonstrates conspicuous nuclear pleomorphism or mitotic activity.

The EC cell component varies markedly within the lesions. In a minority of lesions, the EC component represents the predominant feature; in such lesions, small parts of the tumor may be indistinguishable from a conventional carcinoid tumor. Other tumors resemble a signet ring cell carcinoma because an inconspicuous NE component is only detectable after the use of stains for NE differentiation. For this reason, we advocate that all appendiceal lesions that look like signet ring cell carcinomas be stained with NE markers to exclude the presence of the biologically less aggressive goblet cell carcinoid. Some tumors produce enough mucin to create pools of extravasated, extracellular mucus within the appendiceal wall.

The tumors arise deep in the mucosa and infiltrate the lamina propria without lymphatic or venous invasion. The mucosa is typically spared, except where the tumor touches the bases of the crypts. These tumors tend to infiltrate all layers of the bowel wall extending to the serosa in a manner resembling traditional carcinoid tumors. They often elicit a considerable desmoplastic response. Mucin stains are intensely positive in the signet ring cells and in the extracellular mucinous pools. Argentaffinic and argyrophilic cells are often present and the cells are immunoreactive with antibodies to CEA and NE markers (Fig. 17.67). Duodenal goblet cell carcinoids may produce somatostatin. Cytology preparations of peritoneal washings show small round carcinoid cells with stippled chromatin and occasional signet ring cells.

The differential diagnosis of these tumors includes tubular carcinoids, which have a better prognosis (241). In the latter tumor, all of the tumor cells are positive with NE markers, the glandular lumens contain mucin but there is no intracytoplasmic mucin, and Paneth cells are generally absent. Goblet cell carcinoids should also be differentiated from clear cell carcinoids that are considered to be variants of classic carcinoids (208). The finding of preinvasive neoplasia (adenoma or dysplasia) in the mucosa suggests that one is dealing with a carcinoma rather than an adenocarcinoid.

Goblet cell carcinoids are thought to represent a line of differentiation that is intermediate between a classic carcinoid tumor and an adenocarcinoma. Their clinical behavior supports this concept. These tumors are more aggressive than carcinoid tumors, typically behaving as a low-grade

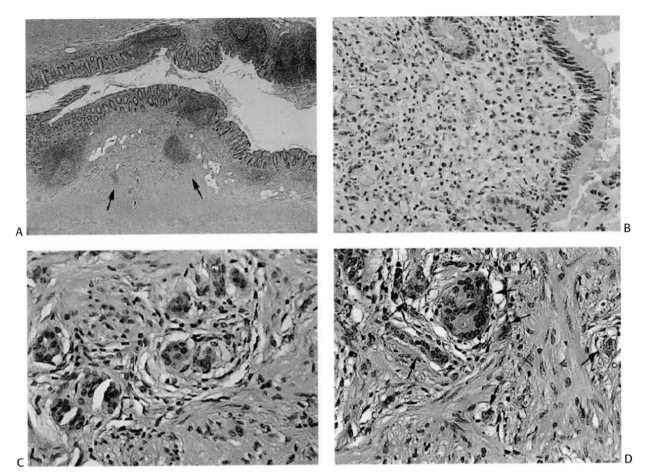

FIG. 17.66. Appendiceal goblet cell carcinoid. **A:** Longitudinal cross section of the appendix. The tumor is subtle in this low-power photomicrograph. Small tumor nests diffusely infiltrate the muscular wall (*arrows*). **B:** The tumor cells form clusters of mucin-secreting cells without lumen formation. Here they subtly infiltrate the lamina propria. **C:** Tumor cells present in the muscularis propria. Well-defined tumor cell nests are surrounded by a looser myxoid stroma. A prominent desmoplastic response as might be seen in an infiltrating adenocarcinoma is absent. **D:** Both glands (*arrows*) as well as linear arrangements (*arrow*) of the tumor are present.

carcinoma and spreading less quickly than conventional adenocarcinomas (241). Unlike adenocarcinomas, goblet cell carcinoids have a propensity for transperitoneal spread and frequent ovarian involvement. In some patients, regional lymph nodes and the liver become involved as a result of direct lymphatic or vascular dissemination. Metastases may appear as a pure carcinoid tumor or goblet cell carcinoid.

The 5-year actuarial survival of patients with goblet cell adenocarcinoids is 73% to 84% (241), and the 10- and 15-year actuarial survival estimate is 66% (241). Patients with abdominal or pelvic metastasis have a more ominous prognosis, with most patients experiencing tumor recurrence within 5 years, despite treatment. Some patients with extensive regional disease die of their cancer within a year of diagnosis (241). Thirty percent of patients with Krukenberg tumors from the appendiceal adenocarcinoids die within 5 years of their initial diagnosis.

Some authors conclude that simple appendectomy represents adequate treatment for appendiceal goblet cell carci-

noids localized to the appendix with less than mitoses per 10 hpf and no foci of cytologic atypia (241,284). Others suggest routine hemicolectomy in patients with localized disease (285) and aggressive surgical resection for patients with ovarian or other intra-abdominal or pelvic tumor or diffuse appendiceal involvement (286). These tumors may strongly express the p53 protein in the majority of the tumor cells (287).

Mixed Goblet Cell Carcinoid–Adenocarcinoma

Mixed goblet cell carcinoids–adenocarcinomas are lesions in which adenocarcinomas appear to arise from a pre-existing goblet cell carcinoid. They are most common in the appendix, the most common site of goblet cell carcinoids, but they also develop in the colon and duodenum (279,288). The tumors contain areas that show typical features of goblet cell carcinoid as well as areas that appear to be less differentiated and exhibit a more carcinomatous growth pattern with solid

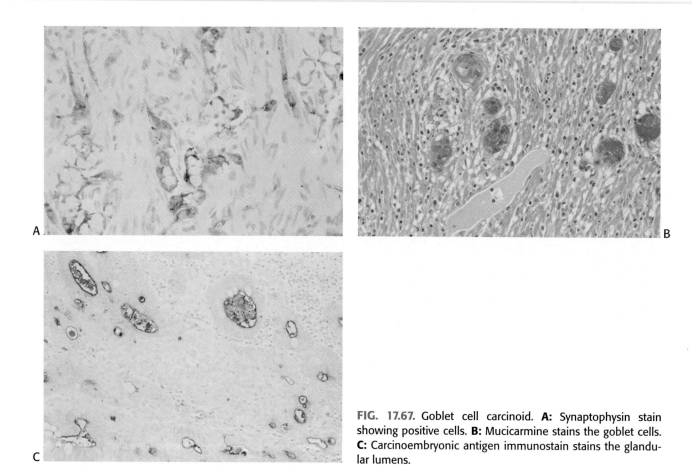

FIG. 17.67. Goblet cell carcinoid. **A:** Synaptophysin stain showing positive cells. **B:** Mucicarmine stains the goblet cells. **C:** Carcinoembryonic antigen immunostain stains the glandular lumens.

FIG. 17.68. Adenocarcinoid. **A:** Low-power photomicrograph demonstrating nests of palestaining cells within the mucosa and submucosa. **B:** The tumor is composed of clusters of cells containing abundant cytoplasmic mucin. Some of the cells resemble signet ring cells, but they lack the cytologic and architectural atypia characteristic of signet ring cell carcinomas. **C:** Synaptophysin immunostains are strongly positive.

sheets of cells, cribriform glands, or infiltrating signet ring cells in a single-file pattern. The tumors may also contain attenuated glandular cords lined by mucin-depleted cuboidal cells or mucin-containing columnar cells resembling more typical intestinal adenocarcinomas. They occur in the apparent absence of neoplastic change in the overlying mucosal epithelium (123). The lesions differ from signet ring cell carcinomas, which show much more architectural and cytologic atypia and frequently produce pools of extracellular mucin. These tumors have a propensity for transcoelomic spread, especially to the ovaries and less frequently to peritoneal surfaces (123,241,281). The tumors may also spread to lymph nodes or the liver as the result of lymphatic or vascular invasion. Aggressive tumors may be recognized by the following: the presence of lymphovascular invasion, 20 or more mitoses/10 hpf, a carcinomatous growth pattern in >50% of the tumor (presence of fused or cribriform glands, single-file pattern, densely infiltrating signet ring cells, solid sheets of cells), and spread beyond the appendix (123,241,281). Tumors with these features should be treated aggressively with radical hemicolectomy.

Pleomorphic (Giant Cell) Neuroendocrine Carcinoma

Both the large bowel and the small bowel give rise to rare NE neoplasms containing highly pleomorphic multinucleated cells. Histologically, the tumors consist of solid sheets of poorly cohesive cells broken into clusters by delicate stromal strands. They contain a mixture of eosinophilic giant cells, small polygonal cells, and spindle cells (Fig. 17.69). The giant cells are identical to those seen in giant cell carcinomas of the lung. Large pleomorphic nuclei, with distinct nuclear membranes, a vesicular chromatin pattern with irregular clumping, and one or more prominent nucleoli, are present. The nuclei may be pushed to the edge of the cells, often resulting in a bent or reniform eccentric appearance. Cell size varies, with larger cells having two or more nuclei. Numerous typical and atypical mitoses are frequently present. Lymphocyte tumor cell emperipolesis is frequently

seen. The spindle cells and smaller polygonal cells have a smaller amount of cytoplasm, and the nuclei do not appear as pleomorphic but otherwise show similar characteristics. Because these pleomorphic carcinomas contain evidence of NE differentiation, some regard them as poorly differentiated variants of neuroendocrine carcinomas. Ultrastructurally, the cells show glandular as well as endocrine differentiation. Intracytoplasmic perinuclear whorls of intermediate filaments and dense core secretory granules are present. The tumors are positive for cytokeratin, vimentin, epithelial membrane antigen (EMA), NSE, and chromogranin. They are also immunoreactive for various hormones. These tumors are mucin negative.

The differential diagnosis of the lesion includes pleomorphic carcinoma, sarcoma, and amelanotic malignant melanoma. It may closely resemble the latter. The use of special stains serves to establish the diagnosis (Table 17.18). The few tumors that the authors have seen have behaved aggressively with prominent lymphatic involvement and metastases present at the time of diagnosis. Prognosis is poor due to early tumor spread with only a few months of postoperative survival.

Composite Adenoma–Carcinoid Tumors

Adenomas containing carcinoid tumors are rare. Adenomas often contain endocrine cells but, despite the frequency of endocrine cells, they seldom give rise to a carcinoid tumor in or near the adenoma. These lesions fall within the general category of composite tumors and arise either from a common stem cell exhibiting multidirectional differentiation or from multiple cellular events affecting several cell lineages. In the colon there are two distinct patterns of adenoma–carcinoid tumors (289). In one, the carcinoid cells intimately intermingle with the adenomatous glands (Fig. 17.70); in the other, the two tumors appear to arise as separate lesions juxtaposed to one another (Fig. 17.71). The first lesion probably arose from a common stem cell. The second probably arose as a separate event, with the adenoma and the carcinoid tumor arising from separate cell lineages.

TABLE 17.18 Differential Diagnosis of Pleomorphic Neuroendocrine Carcinoma

Component	Pleomorphic Neuroendocrine Carcinoma	Sarcoma	Malignant Melanoma
Reticulin pattern	Epithelial	Mesenchymal	Intermediate
Mucin or PAS stains	Some focally positive cells	Negative	Negative
Cytokeratin	Positive	Negative	Negative
Vimentin	Often negative but some can be positive	Positive	Positive
HMB45	Negative	Negative	Positive
S100	Negative	May be positive	Positive
Synaptophysin	Positive	Negative, except in neural tumors	Usually negative
Chromogranin	May be positive	Negative, except in neural tumors	Negative
Actin	Negative	Some positive	Negative
CD117	Usually negative	GISTs positive	Negative
Myosin	Negative	Some positive	Negative

GISTs, gastrointestinal stromal tumors; PAS, periodic acid–Schiff.

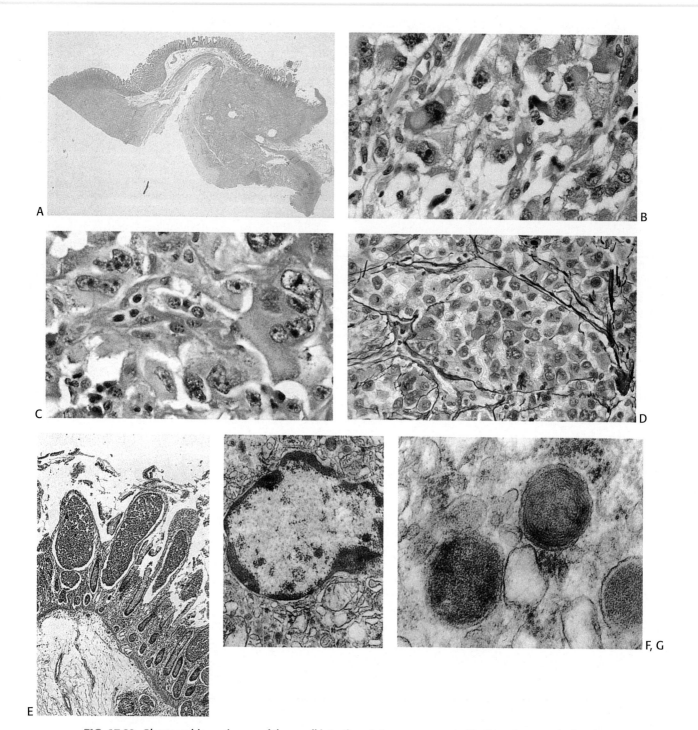

FIG. 17.69. Pleomorphic carcinoma of the small intestine. **A:** Low-power magnification photograph showing the presence of a large small intestinal tumor that diffusely invades the bowel wall. **B:** High-power magnification of individual tumor cells showing the cytologic features. Signet ring–like cells, as well as other noncohesive carcinoma cells, are present. **C:** Many of the cells have the appearance of multinucleated neoplastic giant cells. **D:** Reticulin demonstrating the carcinomatous nature of the proliferation. **E:** Marked lymphangitic spread is evidenced by the presence of submucosal lymphatic involvement, as well as dilation of the central lacteals. **F:** Paucity of neurosecretory granules; electron micrograph of one of the rare cells that contained evidence of neurosecretory granules. **G:** Higher-power magnification of the neurosecretory granules showing the typical dense core morphology.

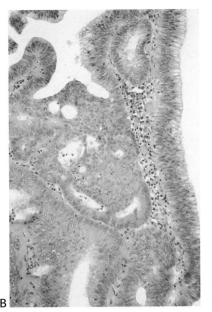
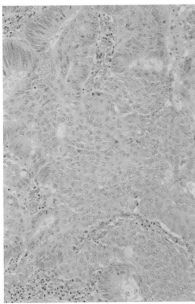
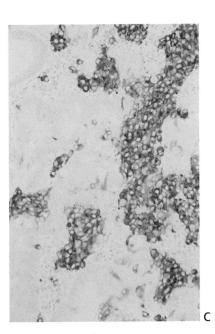

A, B   C

FIG 17.70. Carcinoid tumor intermingling with a tubular adenoma. **A:** Areas where the adenomatous epithelium is more evident. The solid areas are the carcinoid tumor. The neuroendocrine (NE) cell proliferations resemble either an area of high-grade dysplasia or a squamous morule. **B:** Another area of the same polyp with a more solid proliferation of NE cells. **C:** Synaptophysin immunostain highlights the NE cell proliferations.

One could postulate that substances produced by the carcinoid tumor stimulated the immediately adjacent mucosa to undergo increased proliferation and neoplastic transformation (290,291). The carcinoid component in both lesions was small, and we have not seen any examples of metastases from the carcinoid component. However, an ileal lesion was reported in which the carcinoid component had metastasized to the liver, peritoneum, and lymph nodes at the time of diagnosis (291). It arose in the terminal ileum producing a cecal protrusion. The lesion contained two components, an adenoma with low-grade dysplasia and a carcinoid tumor. The adenomatous component stained positively for EMA and CEA and negatively for NSE. The carcinoid component stained positively for NSE and negatively for EMA (292).

A rare example of a composite gastric adenocarcinoma and adenocarcinoid has also been reported (293).

Adenoendocrine Carcinoma

Adenoendocrine carcinomas are rare. They develop throughout the gastrointestinal tract from the esophagus to the anus (280,294). They develop sporadically as well as in sites of chronic inflammations such as in association with Barrett esophagus or in patients with IBD (186). Lewin (281) restricts the term to those tumors in which the endocrine cells comprise 30% to 50% of an adenocarcinoma. They contain a carcinomatous component that is glandular in origin; squamous cell carcinoma may also be present. In most, the glandular component resembles a high-grade adenocarcinoma (intestinal or signet ring cell type) and the endocrine component consists of either a carcinoid tumor or SCC. Some forms of highly malignant carcinomas consist of mixtures of undifferentiated cells focally intermingling with neuroendocrine, exocrine, and squamous cells, sometimes arranged in an organoid manner (Fig. 17.72). An interesting patient was recently reported who had a gastric carcinosarcoma with prominent SCC components (295). In some tumors, the cell populations are demarcated fairly well from one another, whereas in others they intermingle. The histochemical and immunohistochemical findings reflect the individual components. The glandular parts tend to be PAS, Alcian blue, and mucicarmine positive. CEA immunoreactivity occurs in the

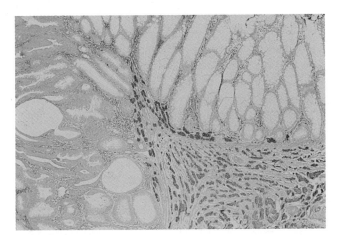

FIG 17.71. Carcinoid tumor developing beneath a tubulovillous adenoma. The neuroendocrine cell proliferation is highlighted in brown by the synaptophysin immunostain.

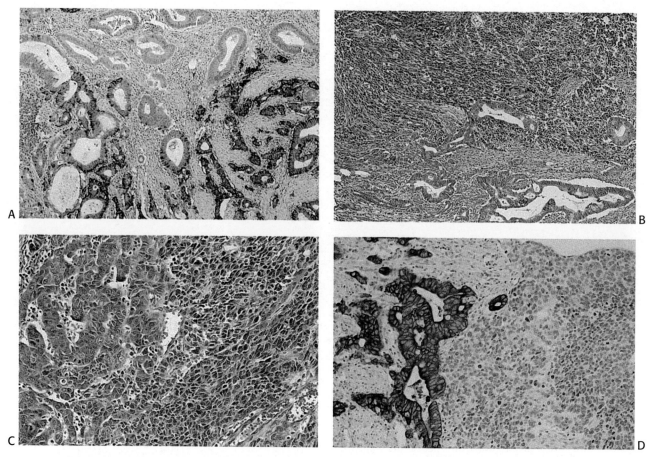

FIG. 17.72. Composite neuroendocrine tumor with adenocarcinoma. **A:** Chromogranin staining confirms the neuroendocrine differentiation in a proportion of the cells. **B:** Another area of the same tumor demonstrating adenocarcinoma adjacent to a poorly differentiated, small cell carcinoma. **C:** Higher-power view demonstrating the close apposition of the adenocarcinoma and the poorly differentiated endocrine component of the lesion. The neuroendocrine cells in this area are hyperchromatic, and the nuclear:cytoplasmic ratio is high. **D:** Chromogranin stain in another area of the tumor demonstrating positivity in the well-differentiated neuroendocrine portion of the tumor but negative staining in the small cell component.

glandular and squamous components. Argentaffin reactions are often negative. Argyrophilic reactions may be positive in the NE areas. The NE components may stain with the usual NE immunohistochemical markers. Cytokeratin immunostains may stain all the components, but the pattern of staining differs in the different areas. Well-differentiated glandular or squamous areas tend to be the most strongly positive. The NE areas stain like SCCs. When the tumors are those in which there are merely increases in the number of NE cells, the biology of the tumors resembles that of the usual adenocarcinoma of a comparable stage and grade. However, these tumors tend to be aggressive when the endocrine component is a SCC. The latter places them in a poor prognostic group and liver metastases are frequent. When reporting these tumors, one can make the diagnosis of a composite tumor, but each of the tumor types should be specified in the diagnosis along with the relevant degree of differentiation of each of the components so that the clinicians may be able to estimate the patient prognosis and treat the component types.

Composite Tumors with Pancreatic Acinar Differentiation

An unusual variant of composite tumors are tumors that show areas of glandular, endocrine, and pancreatic acinar differentiation. These may develop in the stomach (296) or the ampulla of Vater (297). The tumors are predominantly submucosal in location with focal involvement of the overlying mucosa. They infiltrate into the muscularis propria or beyond. The surrounding mucosa is normal. The cut surfaces of the tumors are smooth and gray-white to tan. The predominant histologic pattern consists of circumscribed cellular islands composed of solid nests of polygonal NE cells surrounded by numerous vessels. Small acinar lumina punctuate the nests. Another glandular component consists of well-differentiated adenocarcinoma. The cells lining the neoplastic glands may resemble foveolar cells. Interspersed goblet cells may be present. CK-7, CEA, and Muc are positive in the glandular areas. Markers of pancreatic acinar differentiation are positive in the solid areas and overlap with the

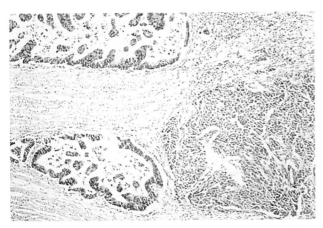

FIG. 17.73. Collision tumor with adenocarcinoma (*left*) and carcinoid tumor (*right*).

endocrine cell markers. When the tumors metastasize, all of these components are present in the metastatic lesions (296,297). Tumors such as this could result from neoplasia developing in heterotopic pancreatic or from pluripotential stem cells.

COLLISION TUMORS

Collision tumors of the gut are exceedingly rare. They consist of tumors with NE differentiation abutting an adenocarcinoma or adenoma or squamous cell carcinoma into another. The endocrine areas must be in intimate juxtaposition to a neoplastic glandular and/or squamous cell lesion, but they should not intermingle with one another (Fig. 17.73). Collision tumors occur when two tumors that have arisen at independent topographic sites meet and eventually intermingle with one another. One makes the diagnosis of a collision tumor most easily when clear-cut evidence suggests that the tumor originated in two separate epithelia with clear separation of the two components. Often, if both tumor types metastasize, the two types of growth also remain clearly separated in the metastasis. Collisions occur between SCCs and/or adenocarcinomas, and with sarcomas, lymphomas, melanomas, or metastases (155,156).

Probably the most common setting for collision tumors to occur is in the setting of CAG, where the hypergastrinemia causes the formation of ECL cell hyperplasia and multiple ECL cell carcinoids. The hypergastrinemia is also trophic for the growth of the glandular cells and varying degrees of glandular dysplasia, and neoplasia may coexist with the carcinoid tumors.

INCREASED ENDOCRINE CELLS IN TREATED ADENOCARCINOMAS

The presence of focal endocrine cells in colorectal adenocarcinomas is a frequent finding. However, NE cells may account for up to 20% of the cell population in tumors that have been treated with chemoradiation. The NE cells may form nests and cords appear deeply eosinophilic. They usually have round and uniform, but sometimes pleomorphic, nuclei. The proportion of endocrine cells significantly associates with the extent of the treatment response. Tumors treated with chemoradiation are more likely to contain abundant endocrine cells than those treated with radiotherapy alone. These cells also frequently express the p53 protein (298).

REFERENCES

1. Ahlman H, Nilsson O: The gut as the largest endocrine organ in the body. *Ann Oncol* 2001;12:S63.
2. Sundler F, Bottcher G, Ekbland E, Hakanson R: The neuroendocrine system of the gut. *Acta Oncol* 1989;28:282.
3. Winkler H, Fischer-Colbrie R: The chromogranins A and B: the first 25 years and future perspectives. *Neuroscience* 1992;49:497.
4. Solcia E, Polak JM, Larsson L-I, et al: Update on Lausanne classification of endocrine cells. In: Bloom SR, Polak JM (eds). *Gut Hormones.* 2nd ed. London: Churchill Livingstone, 1981, pp 98–100.
5. Kaduk B, Barth H: The localization of endocrine cells in the distal esophagus. *Virchows Arch A Pathol Anat Histol* 1978;377:311.
6. Solcia E, Capella C, Fiocca R, et al: The gastroenteropancreatic endocrine system and related tumors. *Gastroenterol Clin North Am* 1989;18:671.
7. Pearse AGE, Coulling I, Weavers B, Friesen S: The endocrine polypeptide cells of the human stomach, duodenum, and jejunum. *Gut* 1970;11:649.
8. Tielemans Y, Hakanson R, Sundler F, Willems G: Proliferation of enterochromaffin-like cells in omeprazole-treated hypergastrinemic rats. *Gastroenterology* 1989;96:723.
9. Inokuchi H, Kawai K, Takeuchi Y, Sano Y: Immunohistochemical study on the morphology of enterochromaffin cells in the human fundic mucosa. *Cell Tissue Res* 1984;235:703.
10. Larsson L-I: Evidence for anterograde transport of secretory granules in processes of gastric paracrine (somatostatin) cells. *Histochemistry* 1984;80:323.
11. Bordi C, D'Adda T, Azzoni C, et al: Hypergastrinemia and gastric enterochromaffin-like cells. *Am J Surg Pathol* 1995;19:8.
12. Bakke I, Qvigstad G, Sandvik AK, et al: The CCK-2 receptor is located on the ECL cell, but not on the parietal cell. *Scand J Gastroenterol* 2001;36:1128.
13. Nilsson O, Levin Jakobsen AM, Kölby L, et al: Importance of vesicle proteins in the diagnosis and treatment of neuroendocrine tumors. *Ann NY Acad Sci* 2004;1014:280.
14. Date Y, Kojima M, Hosoda H, et al: Ghrelin, a novel growth-hormone-releasing acylated peptide, is synthesized in a distinct endocrine cell type in the gastrointestinal tracts of rats and humans. *Endocrinology* 2000;141:4255.
15. Takaya K, Ariyasu H, Kanamoto N, et al: Ghrelin strongly stimulates growth hormone release in humans. *J Clin Endocrinol Metab* 2000;85:4908.
16. Asakawa A, Inui A, Kaga T, et al: Ghrelin is an appetite-stimulatory signal from stomach with structural resemblance to motilin. *Gastroenterology* 2001;120:337.
17. Cassoni P, Papotti M, Ghe' C, et al: Identification, characterization and biological activity of specific receptors for natural (ghrelin) and synthetic growth hormone secretagogues in human breast carcinomas and cell lines. *J Clin Endocrinol Metab* 2001;86:1738.
18. Masuda Y, Tanaka T, Inomata N, et al: Ghrelin stimulates gastric acid secretion and motility in rats. *Biomchem Biophys Res Commun* 2000;276:905.
19. Papotti M, Cassoni P, Volante M, et al: Ghrelin-producing endocrine tumors of the stomach and intestine. *J Endocrinol Metab* 2001;86:5052.
20. Sjolund K, Sanden G, Hakanson R, Sundler F: Endocrine cells in human intestine: an immunocytochemical study. *Gastroenterology* 1983;85:1120.
21. Cheng H, Leblond CP: Origin, differentiation and renewal of the four main epithelial cell types in the mouse small intestine. V. Unitarian

theory of the original of the four epithelial cell types. *Am J Anat* 1974;141:537.

22. Dayal Y: Neuroendocrine cells of the gastrointestinal tract: introduction and historical perspective. In: Dayal Y (ed). *Endocrine Pathology of the Gut and Pancreas.* Boca Raton, FL: CRC Press, 1991, pp 1–31.

23. Carlei F, Barsotti P, Crescenzi A, et al: Neuroendocrine epithelial cells of the main pancreatic ducts and ampulla. *Ital J Gastroenterol* 1993;25: 171.

24. Grossman MI: General concepts. In: Bloom SR, Polak JM (eds). *Gut Hormones.* Edinburgh: Churchill Livingstone, 1981, pp 17–22.

25. Bosshard A, Chery-Croze S, Cuber JC, et al: Immunocytochemical study of peptidergic structures in Brunner's glands. *Gastroenterology* 1989;97:1382.

26. Aubock L, Ratzenhofer M: Extra-epithelial enterochromaffin cell–nerve fibre complexes in the normal human appendix and in neurogenic appendicopathy. *J Pathol* 1982;136:217.

27. Chandrasekharappa SC, Guru SC, Manickam P, et al: Positional cloning of the gene for multiple endocrine neoplasia type 1. *Science* 1997;276:404.

28. Agarwal SK, Guru SC, Heppner C, et al: Menin interacts with the AP1 transcription factor JunD and represses JunD-activated transcription. *Cell* 1999;96:143.

29. Jensen RT: Carcinoid and pancreatic endocrine tumors: recent advances in molecular pathogenesis, localization, and treatment. *Curr Opin Oncol* 2000;12:368.

30. Görtz B, Roth J, Krähenmann A, et al: Mutations and allelic deletions of the *MEN1* Gene are associated with a subset of sporadic endocrine pancreatic and neuroendocrine tumors and not restricted to foregut neoplasms. *Am J Pathol* 1999;154:429.

31. D'Adda T, Keller G, Bordi C, et al: Loss of heterozygosity in 11q-13-14 regions in gastric neuroendocrine tumors not associated with multiple endocrine neoplasia type I syndrome. *Lab Invest* 1999;79:671.

32. Debelenko LV, Zhuang Z, Emmert-Buck MR, et al: Allelic deletions on chromosome 11q13 in multiple endocrine neoplasia type 1-associated and sporadic gastrinomas and pancreatic endocrine tumors. *Cancer Res* 1997;57:2238.

33. Bordi C, Falchetti A, Azzoni C, et al: Aggressive forms of gastric neuroendocrine tumors in multiple endocrine neoplasia type I. *Am J Surg Pathol* 1997;21:1075.

34. Chiba T: Is Reg gene mutation involved in development of enterochromaffin cell carcinoid tumors? *Gastroenterology* 1999;116:1489.

35. Corleto VD, Delle Fave G, Jensen RT: Molecular insights into gastrointestinal neuroendocrine tumours: importance and recent advances. *Dig Liver Dis* 2002;34:668.

36. Kytola S, Nord B, Elder EE, et al: Alterations of the SDHD gene locus in midgut carcinoids. Merkel cell carcinomas, pheochromocytomas, and abdominal paragangliomas. *Genes Chromosomes Cancer* 2002;34:325.

37. Leotlela PD, Jauch A, Holtgreve-Grez H, et al: Genetics of neuroendocrine and carcinoid tumors. *Endocr Relat Cancer* 2003;10:437.

38. Wang GC, Yao JC, Worah S, et al: Comparison of genetic alterations in neuroendocrine tumors: frequent loss of chromosome 18 in ileal carcinoid tumors. *Mod Pathol* 2005;18:1079.

39. Pizzie S, D'Adda T, Azzoni C, et al: Malignancy associated allelic losses on the X chromosome in foregut but not in midgut endocrine tumours. *J Pathol* 2002;196:401.

40. Lubomierski N, Kersting M, Bert T, et al: Tumor suppressor genes in the 9p21 gene cluster are selective targets of inactivation in neuroendocrine gastroenteropancreatic tumors. *Cancer Res* 2001;61:5905.

41. Goebel SU, Iwamoto M, Raffeld M, et al: HER-2/*neu* expression and gene amplification in gastrinomas: correlations with tumor biology, growth and aggressiveness. *Cancer Res* 2002;62:3702.

42. Fujimori M, Ikeda S, Shimizu Y, et al: Accumulation of ß-catenin protein and mutations in exon 3 of ß-*catenin* gene in gastrointestinal carcinoid tumors. *Cancer Res* 2001;61:6656.

43. Göke R, Gregel C, Göke A, et al: Programmed cell death protein 4 (PDCD4) acts as a tumor suppressor in neuroendocrine tumor cells. *Ann NY Acad Sci* 2004;1014:220.

44. Cappelli C, Agosti B, Braga M, et al: Von Recklinghausen's neurofibromatosis associated with duodenal somatostatinoma. A case report and review of the literature. *Minerva Endocrinol* 2004;29:19.

45. Liu L, Broaddus RR, Yao JC, et al: Epigenetic alterations in neuroendocrine tumors: methylation of RAS-association domain family 1, isoform A and p16 genes are associated with metastasis. *Modern Pathol* 2005;18:1632.

46. Stancu M, Wu TT, Wallace C, et al: Genetic alterations in goblet cell carcinoids of the vermiform appendix and comparison with gastrointestinal carcinoid tumors. *Mod Pathol* 2003;16:1189.

47. Azzoni C, Doglioini C, Viale G, et al: Involvement of BCL-2 oncoprotein in the development of enterochromaffin-like cell gastric carcinoids. *Am J Pathol* 1996;20:433.

48. Kawahara M, Kammori M, Kanauchi H, et al: Immunohistochemical prognostic indicators of gastrointestinal carcinoid tumours. *Eur J Surg Oncol* 2002;28:140.

49. O'Dowd G, Gosney JR: Absence of overexpression of p53 protein by intestinal carcinoid tumours. *J Pathol* 1995;175:403.

50. Cheng J, Sheu L, Meng C, et al: Expression of p53 protein in colorectal carcinoids. *Arch Surg* 1996;131:67.

51. Rammani DM, Wistuba II, Behrens C, et al: K-ras and p53 mutations in the pathogenesis of classical and goblet cell carcinoids of the appendix. *Cancer* 1999;86:14.

52. Li CC, Hirowaka M, Quian ZR, et al: Expression of E-cadherin, b-catenin, and K-67 in goblet cell carcinoids of the appendix: an immunohistochemical study with clinical correlation. *Endocr Pathol* 2002;13:47.

53. Moyana TN, Satkunam N: A comparative immunohistochemical study of jejunoileal and appendiceal carcinoids. Implications for histogenesis and pathogenesis. *Cancer* 1992;70:1081.

54. Scott N, Millward E, Cartwright EJ, et al: Gastrin releasing peptide and gastrin releasing peptide receptor expression in gastrointestinal carcinoid tumors. *J Clin Pathol* 2004;57:189.

55. Wang D-G, Johnston CF, Buchanan KD: Oncogene expression in gastroenteropancreatic neuroendocrine tumors. *Cancer* 1997;80:668.

56. Janson ET, Stridsberg M, Gobl A, et al: Determination of somatostatin receptor subtype 2 in carcinoid tumors by immunohistochemical investigation with somatostatin receptor subtype 2 antibodies. *Cancer Res* 1998;58:2375.

57. Solcia E, Bordi C, Creutzfeldt W, et al: Histopathological classification of non-antral endocrine growths in man. *Digestion* 1988;41:185.

58. Lamberts R, Creutzfeldt W, Struber HG, et al: Long-term omeprazole therapy in peptic ulcer disease: gastrin, endocrine cell growth, and gastritis. *Gastroenterology* 1993;104:1356.

59. Bordi C, Azzoni C, Ferraro G, et al: Sampling strategies for analysis of enterochromaffin-like cell changes in Zollinger-Ellison syndrome. *Am J Clin Pathol* 2000;114:419.

60. Solcia E, Fiocca R, Villani L, et al: Morphology and pathogeneses of endocrine hyperplasia, precarcinoid lesions, and carcinoids arising in chronic atrophic gastritis. *Scand J Gastroenterol* 1991;26(Suppl 180):146.

61. Dayal Y: Hyperplastic proliferations of enteroendocrine cells. *Endocr Pathol* 1994;5:4.

62. Griffin M, Sweeney EC: The relationship of endocrine cells, dysplasia and carcinoembryonic antigen in Barrett's mucosa to adenocarcinoma of the oesophagus. *Histopathology* 1987;11:53.

63. Bhagavan BS, Hofkins GA, Woel GM, Koss L: Zollinger-Ellison syndrome. Ultrastructure and histochemical observation in a child with endocrine tumorlets of gastric antrum. *Arch Pathol* 1974;98:217.

64. Cooper RG, Dockray GJU, Calam J, Walker R: Acid and gastrin responses during intragastric titration in normal subjects and duodenal ulcer patients with G cell hyperfunction. *Gut* 1985;26:232.

65. Dayal Y: Hyperplastic proliferations of the ECL cells. *Yale J Biol Med* 1992;65:805.

66. Arnold R, Frank M, Simon B, et al: Adaptation and renewal of the endocrine stomach. *Scand J Gastroenterol* 1992;27(Suppl 193):20.

67. Sandvik AK, Waldum HL, Kleveland PM, et al: Gastrin produces an immediate and dose-dependent histamine release preceding acid secretion in the totally isolated, vascularly perfused rat stomach. *Scand J Gastroenterol* 1987;22:803.

68. Lambers R, Creutzfeldt W, Stockman F, et al: Long term omeprazole treatment in man: effects on gastric endocrine cell populations. *Digestion* 1988;39:126.

69. Holle GE, Spann W, Eisenmenger W, et al: Diffuse somatostatin-immunoreactive D-cell hyperplasia in the stomach and duodenum. *Gastroenterology* 1986;91:733.

70. Sjolund K, Aluments J, Berg N-O, et al: Enteropathy of coeliac disease in adults: increased number of enterochromaffin cells in the duodenal mucosa. *Gut* 1982;23:42.

71. Gledhill A, Enticott ME, Howe S: Variation in the argyrophil cell population of the rectum in ulcerative colitis and adenocarcinoma. *J Pathol* 1986;149:287.

72. Morson BC: Pathology of ulcerative colitis. In: Kirsner JB, Shorter RG (eds). *Inflammatory Bowel Disease.* 2nd ed. Philadelphia: Lea and Febiger, 1980, p 281.

73. Matsumoto T, Jo Y, Mibu R, et al: Multiple microcarcinoids in a patient with long standing ulcerative colitis. *J Clin Pathol* 2003;56:963.

74. Noda Y, Watanabe H, Iwafuchi M, et al: Carcinoids and endocrine cell micronests of the minor and major duodenal papillae: their incidence and characteristics. *Cancer* 1992;70:1825.

75. Moyana TN, Satkunam N: Crypt cell proliferative micronests in rectal carcinoids—an immunohistochemical study. *Am J Surg Pathol* 1993; 17:350.

76. Griffiths AP, Dixon MF: Microcarcinoids and diversion colitis in a colon defunctioned for 18 years: report of a case. *Dis Colon Rectum* 1992;35:685.

77. Cappella C, Heitz PU, Höffler H, et al: Revised classification of neuroendocrine tumours of the lung, pancreas and gut. *Virchows Arch* 1995;425:547.

78. Klöppel G, Perren A, Heitz PU: The gastroenteropancreatic neuroendocrine cell system and its tumors: the WHO classification. *Ann NY Acad Sci* 2004;1014:13.

79. Delcore R, Friesen SR: Gastrointestinal neuroendocrine tumors. *J Am Coll Surg* 1994;178:187.

80. Modlin IM, Kidd M, Latich I, et al: Current status of gastrointestinal carcinoids. *Gastroenterology* 2005;128:1717.

81. Maggard, MA, O'Connell JB, Ko CY: Updated population-based review of carcinoid tumors. *Ann Surg* 2004;240:117.

82. Moyana TN: Carcinoid tumors arising from Meckel's diverticulum: a clinical, morphologic, and immunohistochemical study. *Am J Clin Pathol* 1989;91:52.

83. Smith JH, Hope PG: Carcinoid tumor arising in a cystic duplication of small bowel. *Arch Pathol Lab Med* 1985;109:95.

84. Barnardo DE, Stavrou M, Bourne R, et al: Primary carcinoid tumor of the mesentery. *Hum Pathol* 1984;15:796.

85. Soga J, Tazawa K: Pathologic analysis of carcinoids. Histologic re-evaluation of 62 cases. *Cancer* 1971;28:990.

86. Anderson JR, Wilson BG: Carcinoid tumours of the appendix. *Br J Surg* 1985;72:545.

87. Burke AP, Thomas RM, Elsayed AM, et al: Carcinoids of the jejunum and ileum. An immunohistochemical and clinicopathologic study of 167 cases. *Cancer* 1997;79:1086.

88. Ardill JES, Erikkson B: The importance of the measurement of circulating markers in patients with neuroendocrine tumors of the pancreas and gut. *Endocr Relat Cancer* 2003;10:459.

89. Wängberg B, Nilsson O, Johanson V, et al: Somatostatin receptors in the diagnosis and therapy of neuroendocrine tumors. *Oncologist* 1997;2:50.

90. Cai, Y-C, Banner B, Glickman J, et al: Cytokeratin 7 and 20 and thyroid transcription factor 1 can help distinguish pulmonary from gastrointestinal carcinoid and pancreatic endocrine tumors. *Human Pathol* 2001;32:1087.

91. Modlin IM, Sandor A: An analysis of 8305 cases of carcinoid tumors. *Cancer* 1997;79:813.

92. Hoang MP, Hobbs CM, Sobin LH, et al: Carcinoid tumor of the esophagus: a clinicopathologic study of four cases. *Am J Surg Pathol* 2002;26:517.

93. Broicher K, Hienz HA: Karzinoid-Syndrom bei im Osophagus lokalisiertem Primartumor. *Z Gastroenterol* 1974;12:377.

94. Nawroz IM: Malignant carcinoid tumour of oesophagus. *Histopathology* 1987;11:879.

95. Ready AR, Soul JO, Matthews HR: Malignant carcinoid tumor of the oesophagus. *Thorax* 1989;44:594.

96. Partensky C, Chayvialle JA, Berger F, et al: Five-year survival after transhiatal resection of esophageal carcinoid tumor with a lymph node metastasis. *Cancer* 1993;72:2320.

97. Rindi G, Luinetti O, Cornaggia M, et al: Three subtypes of gastric argyrophil carcinoid and the gastric neuroendocrine carcinoma: a clinicopathologic study. *Gastroenterology* 1993;104:994.

98. Rindi G, Bordi C, Rappel S, et al: Gastric carcinoids and neuroendocrine carcinomas: pathogenesis, pathology, and behavior. *World J Surg* 1996;20:168.

99. Borch K, Ahren B, Ahlman H, et al: Gastric carcinoids: biologic behavior and prognosis after differentiated treatment in relation to type. *Ann Surg* 2005;242:64.

100. Godwin JD II: Carcinoid tumors: an analysis of 2837 cases. *Cancer* 1975;36:560.

101. Sjoblom SM: Clinical presentation and prognosis of gastrointestinal carcinoid tumors. *Scand J Gastroenterol* 1988;23:779.

102. Solcia E, Rindi G, Larosa S, et al: Morphological, molecular, and prognostic aspects of gastric endocrine tumors. *Microsc Res Tech* 2000;48: 339.

103. Jensen RT: Gastrinoma as a model for prolonged hypergastrinemia in man. In: Walsh JH (ed). *Gastrin.* New York: Raven, 1993, pp 373–393.

104. Thomas RM, Baybick JH, Elsayed AM, Sobin LH: Gastric carcinoids: an immunohistochemical and clinicopathologic study of 104 patients. *Cancer* 1994;73:2053.

105. Mendelsohn G, de la Monte S, Dunn JL, et al: Gastric carcinoid tumors, endocrine cell hyperplasia, and associated intestinal metaplasia. Histologic, histochemical, and immunohistochemical findings. *Cancer* 1987;60:1022.

106. Jordan Jr PH, Barroso A, Sweeney J: Gastric carcinoids in patients with hypergastrinemia. *J Am Coll Surg* 2004;199:552.

107. Tomassetti P, Migliori M, Caletti GC, et al: Treatment of type II gastric carcinoid tumors with somatostatin analogues. *N Engl J Med* 2000;343: 551.

108. Hirschowitz BI, Griffith J, Pellegrin D, et al: Rapid regression of enterochromaffin-like cell gastric carcinoids in pernicious anemia after antrectomy. *Gastroenterology* 1992;102:1409.

109. Higham AD, Dimaline R, Varro A, et al: Octreotide suppression test predicts beneficial outcome from antrectomy in patients with gastric carcinoid tumor. *Gastroenterology* 1999;114:817.

110. Gilligan CJ, Lawton GP, Tang LH, et al: Gastric carcinoid tumor; the biology and therapy of an enigmatic and controversial lesion. *Am J Gastroenterol* 1995;90:338.

111. Caplin ME, Hodgson HJ, Dhillon AP, et al: Multimodality treatment for gastric carcinoid tumor with liver metastases. *Am J Gastroenterol* 1998;93:1945.

112. Richards AT, Hinder RA, Harrison AC: Gastric carcinoid tumors associated with hypergastrinemia and pernicious anemia: regression of tumors by antrectomy. *South Med J* 1987;72:51.

113. Abraham SC, Carney JA, Ooi A, et al: Achlorhydria, parietal cell hyperplasia, and multiple gastric carcinoids. A new disorder. *Am J Surg Pathol* 2005;29:969.

114. Ooi A, Ota M, Katsuda S, et al: An unusual case of multiple gastric carcinoids associated with diffuse endocrine cell hyperplasia and parietal cell hypertrophy. *Endocr Pathol* 1995;6:229.

115. Roberts LJ, Bloomgarden ZT, Marvey SR Jr, et al: Histamine from the gastric carcinoid provocation by pentagastrin and inhibition by somatostatin. *Gastroenterology* 1983;84:272.

116. Lewin KJ, Appelman HD: *Tumors of the Esophagus and Stomach.* Washington, DC: Armed Forces Institute of Pathology, 1996.

117. Moesta KT, Schlag P: Proposal for a new carcinoid tumor staging system based on tumor tissue infiltration and primary metastasis: a prospective multicentre carcinoid tumor evaluation study. (West German Surgical Oncologists' Group.) *Eur J Surg Oncol* 1990;16:280.

118. Kumashiro R, Naitoh H, Teshima K, et al: Minute gastric carcinoid tumor with regional lymph node metastasis. *Int Surg* 1989;74:198.

119. Xie S-D, Wang L-B, Song X-Y, et al: Minute gastric carcinoid tumor with regional lymph node metastasis: a case report and review of literature. *World J Gastroenterol* 2004;10:2461.

120. Yamagishi SI, Suzuki T, Ohkuro H, et al: Ossifying gastric carcinoid tumor containing bone morphogenetic protein, osteopontin and osteonectin. *J Endocrinol Invest* 2004;27:870.

121. Hirschowitz BI, Griffith J, Pellegrin D, et al: Rapid regression of enterochromaffin like cell gastric carcinoids in pernicious anemia after antrectomy. *Gastroenterology* 1992;102:1409.

122. Bordi C, D'Adda T, Azzoni C, et al: Gastrointestinal endocrine tumors; recent developments. *Endocr Pathol* 1998;9:99.

123. Burke AP, Sobin LH, Federspiel BH, et al: Carcinoid tumors of the duodenum. A clinicopathologic study of 99 cases. *Arch Pathol Lab Med* 1990;114:700.

124. Feurle GE, Anlauf M, Hamscher G, et al: Xenin-immunoreactive cells and extractable xenin in neuroendocrine tumors of duodenal origin. *Gastroenterology* 2002;123:1616.

125. Ellison EH, Wilson SD: The Zollinger-Ellison syndrome: re-appraisal and evaluation of 260 registered cases. *Ann Surg* 1964;160:512.

126. Norton JA, Fraker DL, Alexander HR, et al: Surgery to cure the Zollinger-Ellison syndrome. *N Engl J Med* 1999;341:635.

127. Passaro E Jr, Howard TJ, Sawicki MP, et al: The origin of sporadic gastrinomas within the gastrinoma triangle: a theory. *Arch Surg* 1998;133:13.

128. Herrmann ME, Ciesla MC, Chejfec S, et al: Primary nodal gastrinomas—immunohistochemical study in support of a theory. *Arch Pathol Lab Med* 2000;124:832.

129. Perrier ND, Batts KP, Thompson GB, et al: An immunohistochemical survey for neuroendocrine cells in regional pancreatic lymph nodes: a plausible explanation for primary nodal gastrinomas? Mayo Clinic Pancreatic Surgery Group. *Surgery* 1995;118:957.

130. Pipeleers-Marichal M, Somers G, Willems G, et al: Gastrinomas in the duodenums of patients with multiple endocrine neoplasia type 1 and the Zollinger-Ellison syndrome. *N Engl J Med* 1990;322:723.

131. Zogakis TG, Gibril F, Libutti SK, et al: Management and outcome of patients with sporadic gastrinoma arising in the duodenum. *Ann Surg* 2003;238:42.

132. Gibril F, Venzon DJ, Ojeaburu JV, et al: Prospective study of the natural history of gastrinoma in patients with MEN1: definition of an aggressive and a nonaggressive form. *J Clin Endocrinol Metab* 2001;86:5282.

133. Norheim I, Theodorsson-Norheim E, Brodin E, Öberg K: Tachykinins in carcinoid tumours. Their use as a tumour marker and possible role in the carcinoid flush. *J Clin Endocr Metab* 1986;63:605.

134. Anlauf M, Perren A, Meyer CL, et al: Precursor lesions in patients with multiple endocrine neoplasia type 1-associated duodenal gastrinomas. *Gastroenterology* 2005;128:1187.

135. Peghini PL, Annibale B, Azzoni C, et al: Effect of chronic hypergastrinemia on human enterochromaffin-like cells: insights from patients with sporadic gastrinomas. *Gastroenterology* 2002;123:68.

136. Metz DC, Kuchnio M, Fraker DL, et al: Flow cytometry and Zollinger-Ellison syndrome: relationship to clinical course. *Gastroenterology* 1993;105:799.

137. Goebel SU, Vortmeyer AO, Zhuang Z, et al: Identical clonality of sporadic gastrinomas at multiple sites. *Cancer Res* 2000;60:60.

138. Chen YJ, Vortmeyer A, Zhuang Z, et al: X-chromosome loss of heterozygosity frequently occurs in gastrinomas and is correlated with aggressive tumor growth. *Cancer* 2004;100:1379.

139. Fabri PJ, Johnson JA, Ellison EC: Prediction of progressive disease on Zollinger-Ellison syndrome: comparison of available preoperative tests. *J Surg Res* 1981;31:93.

140. Peghini PL, Iwamoto M, Raffeld M, et al: Overexpression of epidermal growth factor and hepatocyte growth factor receptors in a proportion of gastrinomas correlates with aggressive growth and lower curability. *Clin Cancer Res* 2002;8:2273.

141. Melvin WS, Johnson JA, Sparks J, et al: Long-term prognosis of Zollinger-Ellison syndrome in multiple endocrine neoplasia. *Surgery* 1993;114:1183.

142. Vinik AI, Strodel WE, Eckhauser FE, et al: Somatostatinomas, ppomas, neurotensinomas. *Semin Oncol* 1987;14:263.

143. Dayal Y, Tallberg KA, Nunnemacher G, et al: Duodenal carcinoids in patients with and without neurofibromatosis. *Am J Surg Pathol* 1986;10:348.

144. Capella C, Riva C, Rindi G, et al: Histopathology, hormone products and clinicopathologic profile of endocrine tumors of the upper small intestine. A study of 44 cases. *Endocr Pathol* 1991;2:92.

145. Takagi H, Miyairi J, Hata M, et al: Multiple somatostatin- and gastrin-containing carcinoids of the duodenum: report of a case treated by pancreas-sparing duodenectomy. *Hepatogastroenterology* 2003;50:711.

146. Taccagni GL, Carlucci M, Siuroni M, et al: Duodenal somatostatinoma with psammoma bodies: an immunohistochemical and ultrastructural study. *Am J Gastroenterol* 1986;81:33.

147. Alumets J, Ekelund G, Hakanson R, et al: Jejunal endocrine tumor composed of somatostatin and gastrin cells and associated with duodenal ulcer disease. *Virchows Arch A Path Anat* 1978;378:17.

148. Galmiche JP, Chayvialle JA, Dubois PM, et al: Calcitonin-producing pancreatic somatostatinoma. *Gastroenterology* 1980;78:1577.

149. Soga J, Suzuki T, Yoshikawa K, et al: Carcinoid somatostatinoma of the duodenum. *Eur J Cancer* 1990;26:1107.

150. Hough DR, Chan A, Davidson H: von Recklinghausen's disease associated with gastrointestinal carcinoid tumors. *Cancer* 1983;51:2206.

151. Miyazaki K, Funakoshi A, Nishihara S, et al: Aberrant insulinoma in the duodenum. *Gastroenterology* 1986;90:1280.

152. Glickman MH, Hart MJ, White TT: Insulinoma in Seattle: 39 cases in 30 years. *Am J Surg* 1980;140:119.

153. Pelletier G, Cortot A, Launay JM, et al: Serotonin-secreting and insulin-secreting ileal carcinoid tumor and the use of in vitro culture of tumoral cells. *Cancer* 1984;54:319.

154. Friesen SR, Hermreck AS, Mantz FA: Glucagon, gastrin and carcinoid tumors of the duodenum, pancreas and stomach. Polypeptide "apudomas" of the foregut. *Am J Surg* 1974;127:90.

155. Bordi C, De Vita O, Pilanto FP, et al: Multiple islet cell tumors with predominance of glucagon-producing cells and ulcer disease. *Am J Clin Pathol* 1987;88:153.

156. Doherty GM, Skogseid BM: *Surgical Endocrinology*. Philadelphia: Lippincott Williams and Wilkins, 2001.

157. Surveillance Epidemiology and End Results (SEER) Program: Division of cancer prevention and control. *Nat Cancer Inst* 1987.

158. Teitelbaum SL: The carcinoid. A collective review. *Am J Surg* 1972;123:3564.

159. Wood WJ, Archer R, Schaeffer JW, et al: Coexistence of regional enteritis and carcinoid tumor. *Gastroenterology* 1970;59:265.

160. Sigel JE, Goldblum JR: Neuroendocrine neoplasms arising in inflammatory bowel disease: A report of 14 cases. *Mod Pathol* 1998;11:537.

161. Moertel CG, Sauer WG, Dockerty MB, Baggenstoss AH: Life history of the carcinoid tumor of the small intestine. *Cancer* 1961;14:901.

162. Marshall J, Bodnarchuk G: Carcinoid tumors of the gut: our experience over three decades and review of the literature. *J Clin Gastroenterol* 1993;16:123.

163. Sakai D, Murakami M, Kawazoe K, et al: Ileal carcinoid tumor complicating carcinoid heart disease and secondary retroperitoneal fibrosis. *Pathol Int* 2000;50:404.

164. Feldman JM, Lee EM, Castleberry CA: Catecholamine and serotonin content of foods: effect on urinary excretion on homovanillic and 5-hydroxyindoleacetic acid. *J Am Diet Assoc* 1987;87:1031.

165. Ahlman H, Dahlstrom A, Gronstad K, et al: The pentagastrin test in the diagnosis of the carcinoid syndrome. Blockade of gastrointestinal symptoms by Ketanserin. *Ann Surg* 1985;201:81.

166. Beaton H, Homan W, Dineen P: Gastrointestinal carcinoids and the malignant carcinoid syndrome. *Surg Gynecol Obstet* 1981;152:268.

167. Yun D, Heywood JT: Metastatic carcinoid disease presenting solely as high-output heart failure. *Ann Intern Med* 1994;3120:45.

168. MacDonald RA, Robbins SL: Pathology of the heart in the carcinoid syndrome. A comparative study. *Arch Pathol* 1957;363:103.

169. Robiolio PA, Rigolin VH, Harrison JK, et al: Predictors of outcome of tricuspid valve replacement in carcinoid heart disease. *Am J Cardiol* 1995;75:485.

170. Nilsson O, Gronstad KO, Goldstein M, et al: Adrenergic control of serotonin release from a midgut carcinoid tumor. *Int J Cancer* 1985;36:307.

171. Wilander E, El-Salhy M: Immunocytochemical staining of midgut carcinoid tumors with sequence-specific gastrin antisera. *Acta Pathol Microbiol Scand* 1981;89:247.

172. Conlon JM, Deacon CF, Richter G, et al: Circulating tachykinins (substance P, neurokinin A, neuropeptide K) and the carcinoid flush. *Scand J Gastroenterol* 1987;22:97.

173. Tatemoto K, Lundberg JM, Jornvall, Mutt V: Neuropeptide K: isolation, structure and biological activities of a novel brain tachykinin. *Biochem Biophys Res Commun* 1985;128:947.

174. Okumura K, Yasue H, Ishizaka H, et al: Endothelium-dependent dilator response to substance P in patients with coronary spastic angina. *J Am Coll Cardiol* 1992;20:838.

175. Jaffe BM, Condon S: Prostaglandins E and F in endocrine diarrheagenic syndromes. *Ann Surg* 1976;184:516.

176. Waltenberger J, Lundin L, Oberg K, et al: Involvement of transforming growth factor-ß in the formation of fibrotic lesions in carcinoid heart disease. *Am J Pathol* 1993;142:71.

177. Zhang PJ, Furth EE, Cai X, et al: The role of beta-catenin, TGF beta 3, NGF2, FGF2, IGFR2, and BMP4 in the pathogenesis of mesenteric sclerosis and angiopathy in midgut carcinoids. *Hum Pathol* 2004;35:670.

178. Sherman SP, Li CY, Carney JA: Microproliferation of enterochromaffin cells and the origin of carcinoid tumors of the ileum: a light microscopic and immunocytochemical study. *Arch Pathol Lab Med* 1979;103:639.

179. Lundqvist M, Wilander E: Majority and minority cell populations in small intestinal carcinoids. *Acta Pathol Microbiol Scand A* 1982;90:317.

180. Wilander E, El-Salhy M: Immunocytochemical staining of midgut carcinoid tumors with sequence-specific gastrin antisera. *Acta Pathol Microbiol Scand* 1981;89:247.

181. Lundqvist M, Wilander E: Somatostatin-like immunoreactivity in midgut carcinoids. *Acta Pathol Microbiol Scand A* 1981;89:335.

182. Yang K, Ulich T, Chang L, et al: The neuroendocrine products of intestinal carcinoids. An immunoperoxidase study of 35 carcinoid tumors stained for serotonin and 8 polypeptide hormones. *Cancer* 1983;51:1918.

183. Wilander E, Portela-Gomes G, Grimelius L, et al: Enteroglucagon and substance P-like immunoreactivity in argentaffin and argyrophil rectal carcinoids. *Virch Arch B Cell Pathol* 1977;25:117.

184. McGrath-Linden SJ, Johnston CF, O'Connor, DT, et al: Pancreastatin-like immunoreactivity in human carcinoid disease. *Regul Pept* 1991; 33:55.

185. Theodorsson-Norheim E, Oberg K, Rosell S, et al: Neurotensin-like immunoreactivity in plasma and tumor tissue from patients with endocrine tumors of the pancreas and gut. *Gastroenterology* 1983;85:881.

186. D'Herbomez M, Gouze V: Chromogranin: a marker of neuroendocrine tumours. *Ann Biol Clin* 2002;60:641.

187. Nash SV, Said JW: Gastroenteropancreatic neuroendocrine tumors: a histochemical and immunohistochemical study of epithelial (keratin proteins, carcinoembryonic antigen) and neuroendocrine (neuron-specific enolase, bombesin and chromogranin) markers in foregut, midgut, and hindgut tumors. *Am J Clin Pathol* 1986;86:415.

188. Qizilbash AH: Carcinoid tumors, vascular elastosis, and ischemic disease of the small intestine. *Dis Colon Rectum* 1977;20:554.

189. MacDonald RA: A study of 356 carcinoids of the gastrointestinal tract. *Am J Med* 1956;21:867.

190. Robboy SJ, Scully RE, Norris HJ: Carcinoid metastatic to the ovary. A clinicopathologic analysis of 35 cases. *Cancer* 1974;33:798.

191. Robb JA, Kuster GGR, Bordin GM, et al: Polypoid peritoneal metastases from carcinoid neoplasms. *Hum Pathol* 1984;15:1002.

192. Falk S, Stutte HJ: Splenic metastasis in an ileal carcinoid tumor. *Pathol Res Pract* 1989;185:238.

193. Fine SN, Gaynor ML, Isom OW, Dannenberg AJ: Carcinoid tumor metastatic to the heart. *Am J Med* 1990;89:690.

194. Chodofe RJ: Solitary breast metastasis from carcinoid of the ileum. *Am J Surg* 1965;109:814.

195. Normal JL, Cunningham PJ, Cleveland BR: Skin and subcutaneous metastases from gastrointestinal carcinoid tumors. *Arch Surg* 1971; 103:767.

196. Harbour JW, Depotter P, Shields CL, Shields JA: Uveal metastasis from carcinoid tumor—clinical observations in nine cases. *Ophthalmology* 1994;101:1084.

197. Greenberg RS, Baumgarten DA, Clark WS, et al: Prognostic factors for gastrointestinal and bronchopulmonary carcinoid tumors. *Cancer* 1987;60:2476.

198. Johnson LA, Lavin P, Moertel CG, et al: Carcinoids: the association of histologic growth pattern and survival. *Cancer* 1983;51:882.

199. Rothmund M, Kisker O: Surgical treatment of carcinoid tumors of the small bowel, appendix, colon and rectum. *Digestion* 1994;55:86.

200. Strodel WE, Talpos G, Eckhauser F, et al: Surgical therapy for small-bowel carcinoid tumors. *Arch Surg* 1983;118:391.

201. Nies C, Zielke A, Hasse C, et al: Carcinoid tumors of Meckel's diverticula. Report on two cases and review of the literature. *Dis Colon Rectum* 1992;35:589.

202. Moertel CG, Dockerty MB, Judd ES: Carcinoid tumours of the vermiform appendix. *Cancer* 1968;21:270.

203. Parkes SE, Muir KR, al Sheyyab M, et al: Carcinoid tumours of the appendix in children 1957–1986: incidence, treatment and outcome. *Br J Surg* 1993;80:502.

204. Moertel CG, Weiland LH, Nagorney DM, Dockerty MB: Carcinoid tumor of the appendix: treatment and prognosis. *N Engl J Med* 1987;317:1699.

205. Masson P: Carcinoid tumors (argentaffin tumors) and nerve hyperplasia of the appendicular mucosa. *Am J Pathol* 1928;4:181.

206. Edmonds P, Merino MJ, Livolsi VA, et al: Adenocarcinoid (mucinous carcinoid) of the appendix. *Gastroenterology* 1984;86:302.

207. Dische FE: Argentaffin and non-argentaffin tumors of the appendix. *J Clin Pathol* 1968;21:60.

208. Burke AP, Sobin LH, Federspiel BH, et al: Appendiceal carcinoids: correlation of histology and immunohistochemistry. *Mod Pathol* 1989;2:630.

209. Wilander E, Scheibenpflug L: Cytokeratin expression in small intestinal and appendiceal carcinoids. *Acta Oncol* 1993;32:131.

210. Wilander E, Portela-Gomes G, Frimelius L, et al: Argentaffin and argyrophil reactions of human gastrointestinal carcinoids. *Gastroenterology* 1977;73:733.

211. Burke AP, Sobin LH, Federspiel BH, et al: Goblet cell carcinoids and related tumors of the vermiform appendix. *Am J Clin Pathol* 1990;94: 27.

212. Carr NJ, Sobin LH: Unusual tumors of the appendix and pseudomyxoma peritonei. *Semin Diagn Pathol* 1996;13:314.

213. Glasser CM, Bhagavan BS: Carcinoid tumors of the appendix. *Arch Pathol Lab Med* 1980;104:272.

214. MacGillivray DC, Heaton RB, Ruchin JM, Cruess DF: Distant metastasis from a carcinoid tumor of the appendix less than one centimeter in size. *Surgery* 1992;111:466.

215. Gledhill A, Hall PA, Cruse JP, Pollock DJ: Enteroendocrine cell hyperplasia, carcinoid tumours and adenocarcinoma in long-standing ulcerative colitis. *Histopathology* 1986;10:501.

216. Ballantyne GH, Savoca PE, Flannery JT, et al: Incidence and mortality of carcinoids of the colon. Data from the Connecticut Tumor Registry. *Cancer* 1992;69:2400.

217. Berardi RS: Carcinoid tumors of the colon (exclusive of the rectum). *Dis Colon Rectum* 1972;15:383.

218. Smith DM, Haggitt RC: A comparative study of generic stains for carcinoid secretory granules. *Am J Surg Pathol* 1983;7:61.

219. Al Kafaji B, Noffsinger AE, Stemmermann GN, et al: Immunohistologic analysis of carcinoid tumors. Diagnostic and prognostic significance. *Hum Pathol* 1998;29:992.

220. Modlin IM, Lye KD, Kidd M: A five-decade analysis of 13,715 carcinoid tumors. *Cancer* 2003;97:934.

221. Burke M, Shepherd N, Mann CV: Carcinoid tumors of the rectum and anus. *Br J Surg* 1987;74:358.

222. Orloff MJ: Carcinoid tumors of the rectum. *Cancer* 1971;28:175.

223. Soga J, Tazawa K: Pathologic analysis of carcinoids: histologic reevaluations of 62 cases. *Cancer* 1971;28:990.

224. O'Briain DS, Dayal Y, DeLellis RA, et al: Rectal carcinoids as tumors of the hindgut endocrine cells: a morphological and immunohistochemical analysis. *Am J Surg Pathol* 1982;6:131.

225. Fukayama M, Hayashi Y, Koike M: Human chorionic gonadotropin in the rectosigmoid colon. Immunohistochemical study on unbalanced distribution of subunits. *Am J Pathol* 1987;127:83.

226. Alumets J, Alm P, Falkmer S, et al: Immunohistochemical evidence of peptide hormones in endocrine tumors of the rectum. *Cancer* 1981;48:240915.

227. Fiocca R, Capella C, Buffa R, et al: Glucagon-, glicentin-, and pancreatic polypeptide-like immunoreactivities in rectal carcinoids and related colorectal cells. *Am J Pathol* 1980;100:81.

228. Wilander E, El-Salhy M, Lundqvist M, et al: Polypeptide YY (PYY) and pancreatic polypeptide (PP) in rectal carcinoids. An immunocytochemical study. *Virchows Arch* 1983;401:67.

229. Wilander E, Portela-Gomes G, Grimelius L, et al: Enteroglucagon and substance P-like immunoreactivity in argentaffin and argyrophil rectal carcinoids. *Virchows Arch B Cell Pathol* 1977;25:117.

230. Sobin LH, Hjermstad BM, Sesterhenn IA, Helwig EB: Prostatic acid phosphatase activity in carcinoid tumors. *Cancer* 1986;58:136.

231. Federspiel BH, Burke AP, Sobin LH, Shekitka KM: Rectal and colonic carcinoids. A clinicopathologic study of 84 cases. *Cancer* 1990;65: 135.

232. Pai SA, Kini D, Shetty K, et al: Psammomatous carcinoid of the rectum. *J Clin Pathol* 2003;56:978.

233. Caldarola VT, Jackman RJ, Moertel CG, Dockerty MB: Carcinoid tumors of the rectum. *Am J Surg* 1964;107:844.

234. Bouldin TW, Killebrew R, Bone SC, Gay RM: Metastases of rectal carcinoid to the posterior fossa. *Neurosurgery* 1979;5:496.

235. Kanter M, Lechago J: Multiple malignant rectal carcinoid tumors with immunocytochemical demonstration of multiple hormonal substances. *Cancer* 1987;60:1782.

236. Cheng JY, Lin JC, Yu DS, et al: Flow cytometric DNA analysis of colorectal carcinoids. *Am J Surg* 1994;168:29.

237. Cohn G, Erhardt K, Cedermark B, et al: DNA distribution pattern in intestinal carcinoid tumors. *World J Surg* 1986;10:548.

238. Okamoto Y, Fuji M, Tateiwa S, et al: Treatment of multiple rectal carcinoids by endoscopic mucosal resection using a device for esophageal variceal ligation. *Endoscopy* 2004;36:469.

239. Loftus JP, van Heerden JA: Surgical management of gastrointestinal carcinoids. *Adv Surg* 1995;28:317.

240. Soga J: Early-stage carcinoids of the gastrointestinal tract: an analysis of 1914 reported cases. *Cancer* 2005;103:1587.

241. Warkel RL, Cooper PH, Helwig EB: Adenocarcinoid, a mucin-producing carcinoid tumor of the appendix. *Cancer* 1978;42:2781.

242. Goddard MJ, Lonsdale RN: The histogenesis of appendiceal carcinoid tumours. *Histopathology* 1992;20:345.

243. Shaw PA, Pringle JH: The demonstration of a subset of carcinoid tumours of the appendix by in situ hybridization using synthetic probes to proglucagon mRNA. *J Pathol* 1992;167:375.

244. Kepes JJ, Zacharias DDL: Gangliocytic paragangliomas of the duodenum. A report of two cases with light and electron microscopic examination. *Cancer* 1971;27:61.

245. Scheithauer BW, Nora FE, Lechago J, et al: Duodenal gangliocytic paraganglioma. Clinicopathologic and immunocytochemical study of 11 cases. *Am J Clin Pathol* 1986;86:559.

246. Aung W, Gallagher HJ, Joyce WP, et al: Gastrointestinal haemorrhage from a jejunal gangliocytic paraganglioma. *J Clin Pathol* 1995;48:84.

247. Perrone T: Duodenal gangliocytic paraganglioma and carcinoid. *Am J Surg Pathol* 1986;10:147.

248. Hashimoto S, Kawasaki S, Matsuzawa K, et al: Gangliocytic paraganglioma of the papilla of Vater with regional lymph node metastasis. *Am J Gastroenterol* 1992;87:1216.

249. Sundararajan V, Robinson-Smith TM, Lowy AM: Duodenal gangliocytic paraganglioma with lymph node metastasis: a case report and review of the literature. *Arch Pathol Lab Med* 2003;127:139.

250. Sweeney EC, McDonnell L: Atypical gastric carcinoids. *Histopathology* 1980;4:215.

251. Xiaogang Z, Xingtao J, Huasheng W, et al: Atypical carcinoid of the esophagus: report of a case. *Ann Thorac Cardiovasc Surg* 2002;8:302.

252. Lindberg GM, Molbert KH, Vuitch MF, et al: Atypical carcinoid of the esophagus: a case report and review of the literature. *Cancer* 1997;79:1476.

253. Swanson PE, Dykoski D, Wick MR, Snover DC: Primary duodenal small cell neuroendocrine carcinoma with production of vasoactive intestinal polypeptide. *Arch Pathol Lab Med* 1986;110:317.

254. Lee CS, Machet D, Rode J: Small cell carcinoma of the ampulla of Vater. *Cancer* 1992;70:1502.

255. Zamboni G, Franzin G, Bonetti F, et al: Small-cell neuroendocrine carcinoma of the ampullary region: a clinicopathologic, immunohistochemical, and ultrastructural study of three cases. *Am J Surg Pathol* 1990;14:703.

256. Brenner B, Tang LH, Klimstra DS, et al: Small-cell carcinomas of the gastrointestinal tract: a review. *J Clin Oncol* 2004;22:2730.

257. Shida T, Furuya M, Nikaido T, et al: Aberrant expression of human achaete-scute homologue gene 1 in the gastrointestinal neuroendocrine carcinomas. *Clin Cancer Res* 2005;11:450.

258. Takubo K, Nakamura K, Sawabe M, et al: Primary undifferentiated small cell carcinoma of the esophagus. *Hum Pathol* 1999;30:216.

259. Medgyesy CD, Wolff RA, Putnam JB Jr, et al: Small cell carcinoma of the esophagus: the University of Texas M. D. Anderson Cancer Center experience and literature review. *Cancer* 2000;88:262.

260. Wu Z, Ma J-Y, Yang J-J, et al: Primary small cell carcinoma of esophagus: report of 9 cases and review of literature. *World J Gastroenterol* 2004;10:3680.

261. Casas F, Ferrer F, Farrus B, et al: Primary small cell carcinoma of the esophagus. A review of the literature with emphasis on therapy and prognosis. *Cancer* 1997;80:1366.

262. Doherty MA, McIntyre M, Arnott SJ: Oat cell carcinoma of esophagus: a report of six British patients with a review of the literature. *Int J Radiat Oncol Biol Phys* 1984;10:147.

263. Saint Martin MC, Cheifec G: Barrett esophagus-associated small cell carcinoma. *Arch Pathol Lab Med* 1999;123:1123.

264. Nagashima R, Mabe K, Takahashi T: Esophageal small cell carcinoma with ectopic production of parathyroid hormone-related protein (PHTrp), secretin, and granulocyte colony-stimulating factor (G-CSF). *Dig Dis Sci* 1999;44:1312.

265. Watson KJ, Shulkes A, Smallwood RA, et al: Watery diarrhea-hypokalemia-achlorhydria syndrome and carcinoma of the esophagus. *Gastroenterology* 1985;88:798.

266. Gonzalez LM, Sanz-Esponera J, Saez C, et al: Case report: esophageal collision tumor (oat cell carcinoma and adenocarcinoma) in Barrett's esophagus: immunohistochemical, electron microscopy and LOH analysis. *Histol Histopathol* 2003;18:1.

267. Okudela K, Ito T, Kameda Y, et al: Immunohistochemical analysis for cell proliferation-related protein expression in small cell carcinoma of the esophagus; a comparative study with small cell carcinoma of the lung and squamous cell carcinoma of the esophagus. *Histol Histopathol* 1999;14:479.

268. Kimura H, Konishi K, Inoue T, et al: Primary small cell carcinoma of the esophagus: flow cytometric analysis and immunohistochemical staining for the p53 protein and proliferating cell nuclear antigen. *J Surg Oncol* 1998;68:246.

269. Tobari S, Ikeda Y, Kurihara H, et al: Effective treatment with chemotherapy and surgery for advanced small cell carcinoma of the esophagus. *Hepatogastroenterology* 2004;51:1027.

270. Han B, Mori I, Nakamura M, et al: Combined small-cell carcinoma of the stomach: p53 and K-ras gene mutational analysis supports a monoclonal origin of three histological components. *Int J Exp Pathol* 2005;86:213.

271. Yamaguchi T, Imamura Y, Nakayama K, et al: Paranuclear blue inclusions of small cell carcinoma of the stomach: report of a case with cytologic presentation in peritoneal washings. *Acta Cytol* 2005;49:207.

272. Kusayanagi S, Konishi K, Miyasaka N, et al: Primary small cell carcinoma of the stomach. *J Gastroenterol Hepatol* 2003;18:743.

273. Burke AB, Shekitka KM, Sobin LH: Small cell carcinomas of the large intestine. *Am J Clin Pathol* 1991;95:315.

274. Mills SE, Allen MS Jr, Cohen AR: Small cell undifferentiated carcinoma of the colon. A clinicopathological study of five cases and their association with colonic adenomas. *Am J Surg Pathol* 1983;7:643.

275. Rubin A, Pandya PP: Small cell neuroendocrine carcinoma of the rectum associated with chronic ulcerative colitis. *Histopathology* 1988;13:95.

276. Gaffey M, Mills S, Lack E: Neuroendocrine carcinoma of the colon and rectum. *Am J Surg Pathol* 1990;14:101023.

277. Bernick PE, Klimstra DS, Shia J, et al: Neuroendocrine carcinomas of the colon and rectum. *Dis Colon Rectum* 2004;47:163.

278. Nassar H, Albores-Saavedra J, Klimstra DS: High-grade neuroendocrine carcinoma of the ampulla of Vater: a clinicopathologic and immunohistochemical analysis of 14 cases. *Am J Surg Pathol* 2005;29:588.

279. Jones MA, Griffith LA, West AB: Adenocarcinoid tumor of the peri-ampullary region: a novel duodenal neoplasm presenting as biliary tract obstruction. *Hum Pathol* 1989;20:198.

280. Levendoglu H, Cox CA, Nadimpalli V: Composite (adenocarcinoid) tumors of the gastrointestinal tract. *Dig Dis Sci* 1990;35:519.

281. Lewin K: Carcinoid tumors and the mixed (composite) glandular-endocrine cell carcinomas. *Am J Surg Pathol* 1987;11:71.

282. Auber F, Gambiez L, Desreumaux P, et al: Mixed adenocarcinoid tumor and Crohn's disease. *J Clin Gastroenterol* 1998;26:353.

283. Isaacson P: Crypt cell carcinoma of the appendix (so-called adenocarcinoid tumor). *Am J Surg Pathol* 1981;5:213.

284. Anderson NH, Somerville JE, Johnston CF, et al: Appendiceal goblet cell carcinoids: a clinicopathological and immunohistochemical study. *Histopathology* 1991;18:61.

285. Park K, Blessing K, Kerr K, et al: Goblet cell carcinoid of the appendix. *Gut* 1990;31:322.

286. Butler JA, Houshiar A, Lin F, Wilson SE: Goblet cell carcinoid of the appendix. *Am J Surg* 1994;168:685.

287. Horiuchi S, Endo T, Shimoji H, et al: Goblet cell carcinoid of the appendix endoscopically diagnosed and examined with *P53* immunostaining. *J Gastroenterol* 1998;33:582.

288. Shah IA, Schlageter MO, Boehm N: Composite carcinoid-adenocarcinoma of ampulla of Vater. *Hum Pathol* 1990;21:1188.

289. Lyda MH, Fenoglio-Preiser CM: Composite adenoma-carcinoid tumors of the colon. *Arch Pathol* 1998;122:262.

290. Nilsson O, Wangberg B, McRae A, et al: Growth factors and carcinoid tumours. *Acta Oncol* 1993;32:115.

291. Nilsson O, Wangberg B, Kolby L, et al: Expression of transforming growth factor alpha and its receptors in human neuroendocrine tumors. *Int J Cancer* 1995;60:645.

292. Varghese NM, Zaitoun AM, Thomas SM, et al: Composite glandular-carcinoid tumour of the terminal ileum. *J Clin Pathol* 1994;47:427.

293. Yang GCH, Rotterdam H: Mixed (composite) glandular-endocrine cell carcinoma of the stomach. *Am J Surg Pathol* 1991;15:592.

294. Fujiyoshi Y, Kuhara H, Eimoto T: Composite glandular-endocrine cell carcinoma of the stomach. Report of two cases with goblet cell carcinoid component. *Pathol Res Pract* 2005;201:823.

295. Yamazaki K: A gastric carcinosarcoma with neuroendocrine cell differentiation and undifferentiated spindle-shaped sarcoma component possibly progressing from the conventional tubular adenocarcinoma; an immunohistochemical and ultrastructural study. *Virchows Arch* 2003;442:77.

296. Jain D, Eslami-Varzaneh F, Takano AM, et al: Composite glandular and endocrine tumors of the stomach with pancreatic acinar differentiation. *Am J Surg Pathol* 2005;29:1524.

297. Moncur JT, Lacy BE, Longnecker DS: Mixed acinar-endocrine carcinoma arising in the ampulla of Vater. *Hum Pathol* 2002;33:449.

298. Shia J, Tickoo SK, Guillem JG, et al: Increased endocrine cells in treated rectal adenocarcinomas. A possible reflection of endocrine differentiation in tumor cells induced by chemotherapy and radiotherapy. *Am J Surg Pathol* 2002;26:863.

Lymphoproliferative Disorders of the Gastrointestinal Tract

In this discussion of gastrointestinal lymphoproliferative disorders the emphasis will be on neoplastic diseases. The lymphoid hyperplasias will be considered only in the context of their differential diagnosis from lymphomas. Being the most common site of primary extranodal lymphoma, the gastrointestinal tract accounts for between 30% and 50% of all cases (1,2). These lymphomas are almost exclusively of non-Hodgkin type; primary gastrointestinal Hodgkin lymphoma, although well documented, is vanishingly rare. In the West, gastrointestinal lymphoma comprises between 4% and 18% of all non-Hodgkin lymphomas, but there is some evidence that the incidence is rising (3,4). There is considerable geographic variation in the incidence of primary gastrointestinal lymphoma best illustrated by the high incidence in the Middle East. Exact figures are difficult to obtain but in the Middle East, excluding skin tumors, lymphoma as a whole is the most common malignancy, and 25% of these lymphomas arise primarily in the gastrointestinal tract (5). Considerable differences in incidence also exist between Western countries; there is, for example, a 13-fold higher incidence of primary gastric lymphoma in northeastern Italy compared to Britain (6).

DEFINITION

Nodal lymphoma frequently involves the gastrointestinal tract as a secondary phenomenon; this frequency has almost certainly been underestimated as shown by the study of Fischbach et al (7), who performed gastroscopies on newly diagnosed nodal lymphomas and found gastric involvement in over 25%, including cases of low and high histologic grade lymphoma. Strict criteria for a diagnosis of primary gastrointestinal lymphoma are, therefore, necessary if its incidence is not to be overestimated. The criteria laid down by Dawson et al in 1961 (8), which require that the lymphoma be limited to the gastrointestinal tract and its contiguous lymph nodes, are still applicable, although they do not take account of modern staging procedures, which can detect small foci of disease in the liver and bone marrow, the presence of which does not necessarily exclude a primary gastrointestinal tumor. An operational definition of primary gastrointestinal lymphoma is that lymphoma presents with the main bulk of disease in the gastrointestinal tract necessitating the direction of treatment primarily to that site. Inevitably, this definition is blurred at its edges, and some widely disseminated gastrointestinal lymphomas will not be included while occasional cases of selectively disseminated nodal lymphomas might be wrongly assigned.

SITES OF ORIGIN

The stomach is by far the most common site of primary gastrointestinal lymphoma in the West and Far East (9,10), followed by the small intestine. The opposite is true in the Middle East (5), where most arise in the small intestine and the stomach is next in frequency. In all regions, colonic, rectal, and esophageal lymphomas account for a very small minority of cases. The distribution of gastrointestinal tract lymphomas is paradoxic since the normal gastric mucosa is almost devoid of lymphoid tissue and many primary intestinal lymphomas arise proximal to the terminal ileum, where there is the greatest concentration of mucosa (gut)-associated lymphoid tissue (MALT) in the form of Peyer patches.

STAGING

The Musshoff modification of the Ann Arbor staging system for extranodal lymphoma (11) is most commonly used for staging gastrointestinal lymphomas. In stage I_E (where E signifies an extranodal site), the lymphoma is confined to the wall of the stomach or intestine. In stage II_{1E}, there is involvement of regional lymph nodes that are contiguous with the primary site, while in stage II_{2E}, there is involvement of a regional but noncontiguous lymph node group. Stage III refers to involvement of lymph nodes on both sides of the diaphragm, the spleen (stage III_S), or both (stage III_{E+S}). In stage IV, there is dissemination to the bone marrow or other nonlymphoid organs.

CLASSIFICATION OF PRIMARY GASTROINTESTINAL LYMPHOMA

With the few exceptions of other "organ-specific" lymphomas such as certain cutaneous T-cell lymphomas, splenic

TABLE 18.1 Primary Gastrointestinal Non-Hodgkin Lymphoma

B Cell

Mucosa-associated lymphoid tissue (MALT) lymphoma
  Immunoproliferative small intestinal disease
Diffuse large B-cell lymphoma
  With a MALT lymphoma component
  Without a MALT lymphoma component
Mantle cell lymphoma
Follicular lymphoma
Burkitt lymphoma
Lymphomas and lymphoproliferations associated with
  immunodeficiency
Other types of lymphoma corresponding to lymph node
  equivalents

T and NK Cell

Enteropathy associated T-cell lymphoma
Other types unassociated with enteropathy
Nasal-type NK-cell lymphoma

Rare Types

Includes conditions that may simulate lymphoma

---

marginal zone lymphoma, and some other rare entities, most lymphomas listed in the World Health Organization (WHO) lymphoma classification (12) can arise in the gastrointestinal tract. In terms of frequency, however, the types of lymphomas occurring in lymph nodes and the gastrointestinal tract are quite different, and there are also certain gastrointestinal lymphomas that do not occur in peripheral lymph nodes. A classification of primary gastrointestinal lymphomas is given in Table 18.1.

B-cell Lymphomas

Amongst B-cell lymphomas, MALT lymphoma, of which gastric MALT lymphoma is the prototype and most intensively studied, is the most interesting, if not the most common gastrointestinal lymphoma. Immunoproliferative small intestinal disease (IPSID) is a specific subtype of MALT lymphoma distinguished by its epidemiology and association with the synthesis of an abnormal α heavy chain (13,14). MALT lymphoma, including IPSID, may undergo transformation into diffuse large B-cell lymphoma (DLBCL) with loss of the characteristic histologic hallmarks of the original disease, but in at least a proportion of gastrointestinal DLBCL, careful examination will reveal residual foci of MALT lymphoma (15). However, most gastrointestinal DLBCLs, which comprise the majority of gastrointestinal lymphomas, appear to have arisen de novo without any evidence for transformation from a MALT lymphoma, and some of these express antigens such as CD10, which clearly indicates that they are not related to MALT lymphoma. Other B-cell tumors that arise in the gastrointestinal tract

include mantle cell lymphoma, which often results in the condition called lymphomatous polyposis (16); a variant of follicular lymphoma; and Burkitt lymphoma, the latter being particularly common in the Middle East (17). Immunodeficiency-associated lymphoproliferative disorders and lymphomas also tend to arise primarily in the gastrointestinal tract. Finally, any type of B-cell lymphoma other than those listed above may present primarily in the gastrointestinal tract although not necessarily arising there.

T-cell and NK-cell Lymphomas

Primary gastrointestinal T-cell lymphomas are much less common than B-cell tumors. Enteropathy associated T-cell lymphoma (EATL) (18,19), which occurs as a complication of celiac disease, is the only distinctive T-cell tumor of the intestine and, in some ways, is the equivalent of B-cell MALT lymphoma in that it appears to arise from a gut-committed T-cell. Other T-cell lymphomas less commonly arise in the gastrointestinal tract.

NK-cell lymphomas of nasal type, although, as their name suggests, are more common in the upper respiratory tract, not infrequently present as primary intestinal tumors (20).

A number of other tumors of hematopoietic tissue, including histiocytic neoplasms (21) and granulocytic sarcoma (22), may also occur as primary gastrointestinal tumors. Although these are, strictly speaking, not lymphomas, they are easily mistaken for lymphoid tumors and are included in the WHO lymphoma classification.

MALT LYMPHOMA

In formulating classifications of non-Hodgkin lymphomas, considerable attention has been paid to architectural, cytologic, and functional similarities between the various lymphomas and normal lymphoid tissue as exemplified by the peripheral lymph node. However, studies of extranodal lymphomas, particularly gastrointestinal lymphomas, have suggested that their clinicopathologic features are not related to lymph nodes but instead to the structure and function of MALT (23,24).

The anatomic distribution and structure of lymph nodes are adapted to deal with antigens carried to the node in afferent lymphatics, which drain sites at various distances from the node. Permeable mucosal sites, such as the gastrointestinal tract, however, are particularly vulnerable to pathogens and antigens since they are in direct contact with the external environment, and specialized lymphoid tissue has evolved to protect them. This MALT includes gut-associated lymphoid tissue, nasopharyngeal lymphoid tissue (the tonsils), and other less well-characterized aggregates of lymphoid tissue related to other mucosae. Gut-associated lymphoid tissue serves as the paradigm for MALT.

Histology and Immunology of MALT

MALT in the gastrointestinal tract consists of four lymphoid compartments that include organized collections of lymphoid tissue, which, when concentrated in the terminal ileum, form Peyer patches; the lamina propria lymphocytes; plasma cells and accessory cells; intraepithelial lymphocytes; and the mesenteric lymph nodes. MALT lymphomas essentially recapitulate the features of Peyer patches.

Peyer Patches

Organized lymphoid nodules are distributed throughout the small intestine, the appendix, and the colorectum. These nodules concentrate in the terminal ileum, where they collectively form the Peyer patches, the generic term applied to this compartment of MALT. Peyer patches are unencapsulated aggregates of lymphoid cells that bear a certain resemblance to lymph nodes (Fig. 18.1). Each Peyer patch nodule consists of B- and T-cell areas and associated accessory cells. The B-cell area is composed of a germinal center surrounded by a mantle zone of small B lymphocytes, which is broadest at the mucosal aspect of the follicle. Surrounding the mantle zone is a broad marginal zone in which most of the cells are small to intermediate-sized B lymphocytes with moderately abundant, pale-staining cytoplasm and nuclei with a slightly irregular outline leading to a resemblance to centrocytes. The

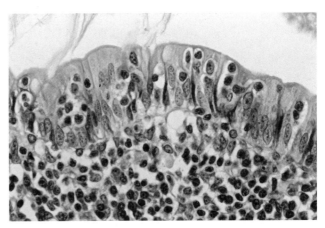

FIG. 18.2. Detail of the dome epithelium showing intraepithelial B lymphocytes constituting the lymphoepithelium that defines mucosa-associated lymphoid tissue.

marginal zone extends toward the mucosal surface and some marginal zone B cells enter the overlying dome epithelium, where they form the lymphoepithelium, which is a defining feature of MALT (Fig. 18.2). Immunohistochemical studies of Peyer patches (25–27) have shown that the B-cell follicles are identical to those of lymph nodes. In contrast to the IgM- and IgD-positive mantle zone, the peripheral marginal zone cells are IgM positive but IgD negative. Lateral to the deep aspect of the B-cell follicle, there is a T-cell zone in which high endothelial venules are prominent, equivalent to the paracortical T zone of the lymph node.

Definition of MALT Lymphoma

MALT lymphoma is listed in the WHO classification (12) under the designation "extranodal marginal zone lymphoma of mucosa associated lymphoid tissue" (MALT lymphoma) and defined as a lymphoma that recapitulates the histology of MALT (Peyer patches); the normal cell counterpart is the marginal zone B cell. MALT lymphomas arise in MALT acquired following chronic inflammation (acquired MALT) and consequently their clinical and pathologic features merge with those of the preceding chronic inflammatory disorder. MALT lymphomas consist of morphologically heterogeneous small B cells including marginal zone (centrocytelike) cells, cells resembling monocytoid cells, small lymphocytes, and scattered immunoblast and centroblastlike cells. There is plasma cell differentiation in a proportion of the cases. The infiltrate appears to arise in the marginal zone of reactive B-cell follicles, which, although reactive, are an integral part of MALT lymphomas and extends into the interfollicular region. In epithelial tissues the neoplastic cells typically infiltrate the epithelium, forming lymphoepithelial lesions (12).

Epidemiology

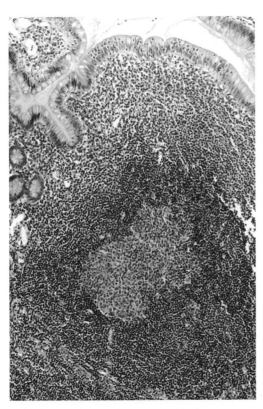

FIG. 18.1. Normal Peyer patch. A B-cell follicle with a subepithelial marginal zone covered by the dome epithelium.

MALT lymphoma comprises 7% to 8% of all B-cell lymphomas and at least 50% of primary gastric lymphomas

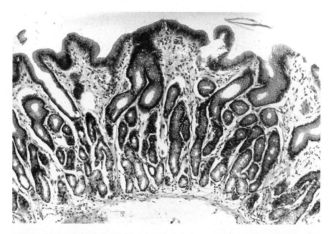

FIG. 18.3. Normal gastric antral mucosa. There is no organized lymphoid tissue.

(28,29). Most cases occur in adults with a median age of 61 years and a slight female predominance. There is a higher incidence of gastric MALT lymphoma in northeastern Italy, probably related to a high prevalence of *Helicobacter pylori*–associated gastritis in that region (6). Histologically, identical intestinal (30,31) and esophageal lymphomas also occur, but they are distinctly infrequent in comparison. A special subtype of small intestinal MALT lymphomas known as immunoproliferative small intestinal disease occurs in the Middle East, parts of the Indian subcontinent, and the Cape region of South Africa (14).

Etiology

MALT lymphomas only rarely arise from native MALT; they more usually arise from MALT that has been acquired as a result of a chronic inflammatory disorder at sites normally devoid of MALT, including the stomach (Fig. 18.3). Here MALT is commonly acquired almost always as a result of the reaction to infection with *H. pylori,* which precedes development of most cases of gastric MALT lymphoma (Fig. 18.4) (32). A similar relationship has been proposed between intestinal infection with *Campylobacter jejuni* and IPSID (33). The functional characteristics of acquired MALT and the degree to which it resembles normal MALT have not been investigated. Likewise, the factors that, in a small number of cases, result in transformation of this reactive MALT into a lymphoma that recapitulates many of its normal morphologic and functional properties remain speculative.

Helicobacter pylori *and Gastric MALT Lymphoma*

Several lines of evidence suggest that gastric MALT lymphoma arises from MALT acquired as a consequence of *H. pylori* infection. *H. pylori* can be demonstrated in the gastric mucosa of the majority of cases of gastric MALT lymphoma (Fig. 18.5) (34). The first study in which this association was

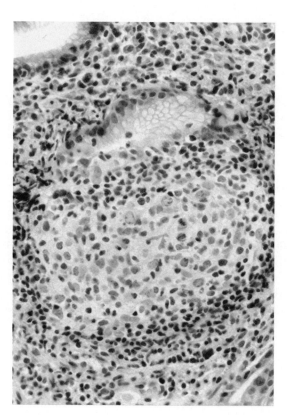

FIG. 18.4. Gastric biopsy showing *Helicobacter pylori*–associated chronic gastritis resulting in acquisition of mucosa-associated lymphoid tissue by gastric antral mucosa.

examined showed that the organism was present in over 90% of cases. Subsequent studies have shown a lower incidence (35) but also that the density and detectability of *H. pylori* decreases as lymphoma evolves from chronic gastritis (36). A subsequent case control study showed an association between previous *H. pylori* infection and the development of primary gastric lymphoma (37). More compelling evidence confirming a role for *H. pylori* in the pathogenesis of gastric lymphoma has been obtained from studies that detected the lymphoma B-cell clone in the chronic gastritis that preceded the lymphoma (36) and from a series of in vitro studies showing that lymphoma growth could be stimulated in culture by *H. pylori* strain–specific T cells when crude lymphoma cultures were exposed to the organism (38). Finally, following the initial study by Wotherspoon et al (39), several groups have confirmed that eradication of *H. pylori* with antibiotics results in regression of gastric MALT lymphoma in 75% of cases (40) (see below).

Campylobacter jejuni *and Immunoproliferative Small Intestinal Disease*

Unlike gastric MALT lymphomas, relatively few cases of IPSID, which is in any case rare, have definitively been shown to respond to broad-spectrum antibiotics. Moreover, the presumptive organism linked to IPSID has remained

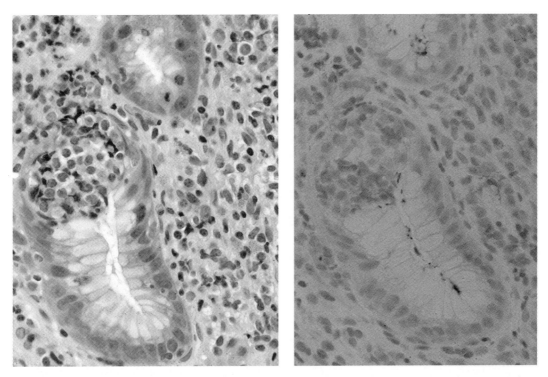

FIG. 18.5. Biopsy from a gastric mucosa-associated lymphoid tissue lymphoma showing a characteristic lymphoepithelial lesion (*left*) containing *Helicobacter pylori* (*right*).

unknown. In 2004, Lecuit et al (33), based on a single case report, suggested that *C. jejuni* may play the same role in IPSID as *H. pylori* does in gastric MALT lymphoma. Isaacson et al (unpublished) in a polymerase chain reaction (PCR) study confirmed an association between *C. jejuni* and IPSID but also detected the organism in other small intestinal lymphomas. To date, no laboratory study on the effects of *C. jejuni* on IPSID cells has been reported, and further studies on the effects of *C. jejuni* eradication are awaited.

Histology of Acquired Mucosa-associated Lymphoid Tissue

Tissues in which MALT lymphomas occur seem to mount a stereotyped response to certain known and unknown agents with accumulation of lymphoid tissue that forms Peyer patch–like structures (Fig. 18.4).

Because of its unique ability to withstand a low pH, *H. pylori* is the one organism, apart from some other, rare *Helicobacter* strains, that can survive in the human gastric mucosa. The prevalence of *H. pylori* gastritis in any given population varies from 20% to 100% depending on the locality and the age cohort (see Chapter 4). With some exceptions, the prevalence of gastric MALT lymphoma is related to that of *H. pylori* gastritis. Typically, infection results in active chronic inflammation with B-cell follicles and the formation of a lymphoepithelium by B-cell infiltration of glands immediately adjacent to the follicles (41) (Fig. 18.4)—features of acquired MALT. Between the follicles, the

gastric mucosal lamina propria is infiltrated by T lymphocytes, plasma cells, macrophages, and occasional collections of neutrophils. The lymphoid infiltrate may be extremely florid and at times difficult to distinguish from MALT lymphoma, especially when there are expanded sheets of mantle zone cells in biopsy fragments.

Immunohistochemistry is useful in delineating the B-cell follicles and distinguishing the IgM- and IgD-positive mantle zone cells from IgM-positive, IgD-negative MALT lymphoma cells. Staining for immunoglobulin light chains can be useful in detecting monoclonal B cells and plasma cells in some cases of MALT lymphoma; however, the presence of polyclonal plasma cells does not exclude the diagnosis. PCR analysis normally reveals a polyclonal B-cell population in gastritis, but there are reports of spurious monoclonality detected in gastric biopsies from patients with *H. pylori* gastritis (42). When the test is properly performed and interpreted this is extremely uncommon (43), but it is noteworthy that in patients with gastritis who have later developed MALT lymphoma, the identical monoclonal B-cell population has been detected in both lesions (36).

Clinical Presentation

Patients with gastric lymphoma usually present with nonspecific dyspepsia; severe abdominal pain and the presence of an abdominal mass are rare. The findings at endoscopy are usually those of nonspecific gastritis and/or a peptic ulcer, the presence of a mass again being unusual. Most gastric

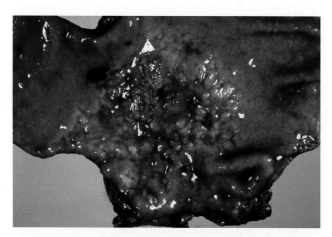

FIG. 18.6. Gastric mucosa-associated lymphoid tissue lymphoma resulting in a "cobblestone" appearance of the gastric mucosa.

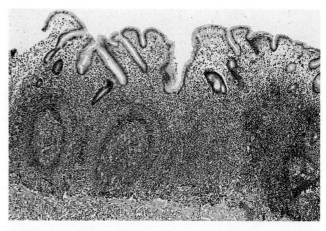

FIG. 18.7. Gastric mucosa-associated lymphoid tissue lymphoma. The infiltrate accentuates the marginal zone around B-cell follicles.

MALT lymphomas are at stage I_E at the time of diagnosis. Gastric lymph node involvement (stage I_{1E}) is present in 5% to 10% and bone marrow involvement (stage IV_E) may be found in up to 10% of cases (44).

Pathology of MALT Lymphoma

Gross Features

Macroscopically, MALT lymphomas, although sometimes forming obviously tumorous masses, frequently are indistinguishable from the inflammatory lesion that underlies the acquisition of MALT from which the lymphoma arises. Gastric MALT lymphoma, for example, may form a single dominant mass but often results in only slightly raised congested mucosa with superficial erosions easily confused at endoscopy with chronic gastritis (Fig. 18.6). MALT lymphomas are typically multifocal with small, even microscopic foci of lymphoma scattered throughout the organ involved. Each of these foci is clonally identical (45).

Histopathology

Although there are some differences determined by the site of origin, the histology of MALT lymphoma is essentially stereotyped in that, like acquired MALT, the lymphomas, especially in their early stages, recapitulate the histology of Peyer patches (46). The neoplastic B lymphocytes infiltrate around reactive B-cell follicles, external to a preserved follicular mantle, in a marginal zone distribution and spread out to form larger confluent areas, which eventually overrun some or most of the follicles (Fig. 18.7). Like marginal zone B cells, the neoplastic cells have pale cytoplasm with small to medium-sized, slightly irregularly shaped nuclei containing moderately dispersed chromatin and inconspicuous nucleoli. These cells have been called centrocyte-like because of their resemblance to germinal center centrocytes. The accumulation of more abundant pale-staining cytoplasm may

lead to a monocytoid appearance of the lymphoma cells, while in some cases the cells more closely resemble small lymphocytes (Fig. 18.8). Scattered large cells resembling centroblasts or immunoblasts are usually present, but are in the minority and do not form confluent clusters or sheets (Fig. 18.9). Plasma cell differentiation is present in up to a third of cases (Fig. 18.10) and, in gastric lymphomas, tends to be maximal beneath the surface gastric epithelium. In a subset of cases there is extreme plasma cell differentiation characterized by a subepithelial band of confluent large eosinophilic plasma cells often accompanied by lakes of extruded immunoglobulin (Fig. 18.11). Small clusters of neoplastic marginal zone cells are present often invading individual gastric glands to form lymphoepithelial lesions (Fig. 18.12). In these lesions, glandular epithelium is invaded and destroyed by discrete aggregates of lymphoma cells (Fig. 18.13). Lymphoepithelial lesions are defined as aggregates of three or more neoplastic marginal zone lymphocytes within glandular epithelium preferably associated with distortion or necrosis of the epithelium. In gastric MALT lymphoma the lesions are often accompanied by eosinophilic degeneration of the epithelium (Fig. 18.13). Lymphoepithelial lesions, although highly characteristic of MALT lymphoma, especially gastric lymphoma, are not pathognomonic. In some MALT lymphomas, such as those of the small and large intestine, they are difficult to find.

The MALT lymphoma cells sometimes specifically colonize germinal centers of the reactive follicles (47). Usually this imparts a vaguely nodular or follicular pattern to the lymphoma (Fig. 18.14). In some cases the lymphoma cells specifically target germinal centers, where they may undergo blast transformation (Fig. 18.15) or plasma cell differentiation (Fig. 18.16). The presence of transformed blasts confined to pre-existing germinal centers is not considered to be evidence of transformation to a large B-cell lymphoma.

Like other low-grade B-cell lymphomas, MALT lymphoma may undergo transformation to a diffuse large B-cell lymphoma (15). Transformed centroblast or immunoblastlike

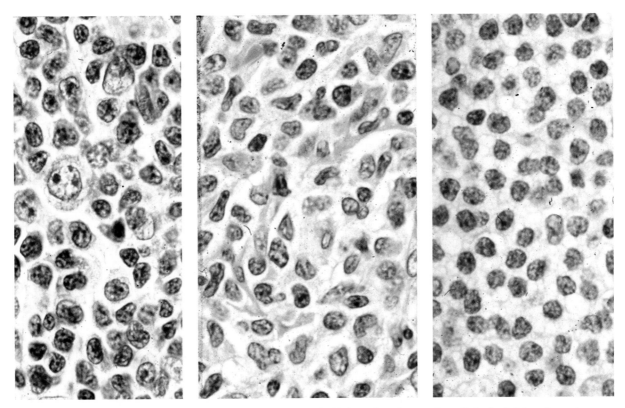

FIG. 18.8. Cytology of gastric mucosa-associated lymphoid tissue lymphoma. The cells in the left-hand panel resemble small lymphocytes and include scattered transformed blasts. Typical "centrocytelike" cells are seen in the middle panel, while the cells in the right-hand panel resemble monocytes.

cells are present in variable numbers in MALT lymphoma (Fig. 18.9) and there is some evidence that grading of MALT lymphoma according to the number of transformed cells has subtle clinical relevance (48). However, only when solid or sheetlike proliferations of transformed cells are present should the lymphoma be considered to have transformed to diffuse large B-cell lymphoma (Fig. 18.17). This transformation may or may not result in complete overgrowth of the preceding MALT lymphoma. The current recommendation is that such cases are best designated as diffuse large B-cell lymphoma; the presence or absence of concurrent MALT lymphoma and the relative proportions of both should be documented (49).

Biopsy Appearances

In small endoscopic biopsies the classic features of MALT lymphoma are not as easily observed as they are in resection

FIG. 18.9. Prominent transformed blasts in a gastric mucosa-associated lymphoid tissue lymphoma.

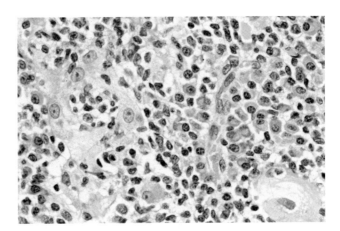

FIG. 18.10. Plasma cell differentiation in a gastric mucosa-associated lymphoid tissue lymphoma.

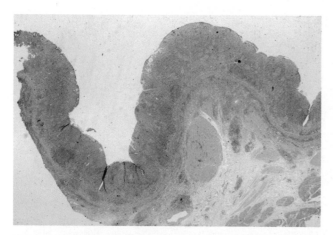

FIG. 18.11. Extreme plasma cell differentiation in gastric mucosa-associated lymphoid tissue lymphoma resulting in a subepithelial eosinophilic band.

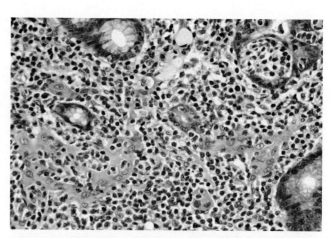

FIG. 18.13. Lymphoepithelial lesions in a case of gastric mucosa-associated lymphoid tissue lymphoma distorting glands and associated with eosinophilic change of gastric epithelium.

specimens. Reactive follicles are not as easy to define and are particularly affected by crush artefact. Equally, the cytologic appearances of marginal zone cells may not be as clear. A diffuse, dense lymphoid infiltrate in a gastric biopsy (Fig. 18.18A) should always raise suspicion, particularly if it occupies the entire biopsy fragment. Careful evaluation of the cytology of the cells is indicated (Fig. 18.18B) and identification of lymphoepithelial lesions (Fig. 18.18B) is very helpful in establishing the diagnosis.

Morphology of Gastric Mucosa-associated Lymphoid Tissue Lymphoma Following Eradication of Helicobacter pylori

Approximately 75% of gastric MALT lymphomas will respond to eradication of *H. pylori* with regression of the tumor over a period of up to 18 months (Fig. 18.19) (39). Repeated endoscopy with biopsy is necessary to determine whether or not the lymphoma is responding. The endo-

scopic appearances may revert within 6 months of the eradication of *H. pylori* but may take as long as 2 years. There is often a noticeable change in the histologic appearance of the biopsy within a few weeks with gradual clearance of the lymphoma in following months. Initially, there is disappearance of the inflammatory infiltrate accompanying the lymphoma with an empty-appearing eosinophilic lamina propria that may contain lymphoid aggregates (Fig. 18.20). These aggregates contain small B lymphocytes without transformed blasts and gradually become smaller with time. Immunohistochemistry shows that they contain few accompanying T cells and have a markedly reduced proliferation fraction compared to the original lymphoma. Such aggregates may not disappear altogether and may persist for long periods at the base of the mucosa or in the submucosa. In up to 60% of cases, B-cell monoclonality can still be demonstrated using PCR (50), suggesting that bacterial eradication represses but does not eliminate the lymphoma clone, which

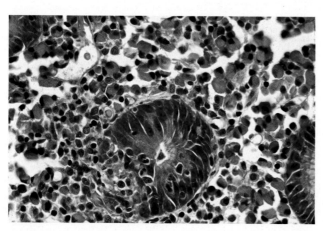

FIG. 18.12. Higher magnification of extreme plasma cell differentiation. A single lymphoepithelial lesion is present in the center.

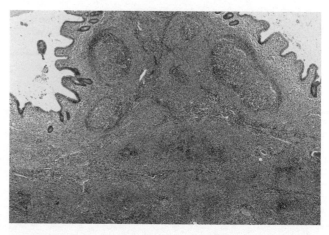

FIG. 18.14. Follicular colonization. Lymphoma cells in the marginal zone surround the follicles (*above*) and replace them (*below*), resulting in a follicular growth pattern.

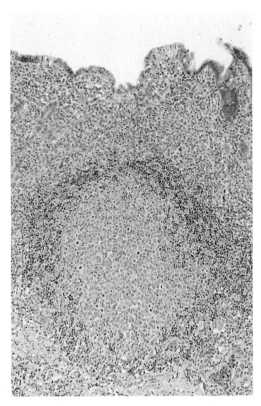

FIG. 18.15. The germinal center of a B-cell follicle has been infiltrated by transformed mucosa-associated lymphoid tissue lymphoma cells.

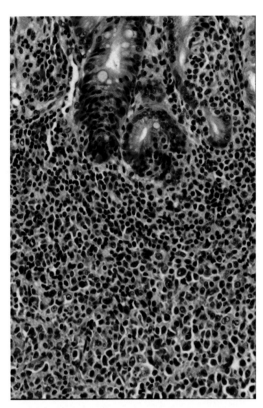

FIG. 18.17. High-grade transformation (*below*) of a gastric mucosa-associated lymphoid tissue lymphoma (*above*).

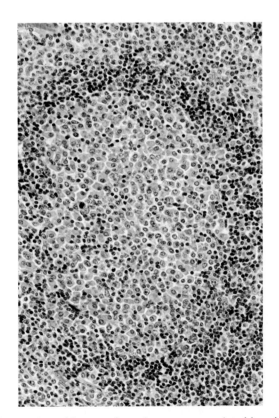

FIG. 18.16. In this case of gastric mucosa-associated lymphoid tissue lymphoma the germinal center is infiltrated by plasma cells.

is still presented in the lymphoid aggregates. The fate of these small aggregates is not completely known but it is assumed that they eventually disappear. PCR analysis may reveal persistence of the neoplastic clone after disappearance of morphologic evidence of lymphoma; however, the clinical significance of this finding is not clear. It is important not to make a diagnosis of persisting lymphoma on the basis of molecular analysis alone in the absence of good histologic evidence.

Multifocality of Gastric Mucosa-associated Lymphoid Tissue Lymphoma

Gastric MALT lymphoma typically disseminates within the stomach to form a multifocal lesion. Indirect evidence for this comes from the observation of recurrent MALT lymphomas in the gastric stump after partial gastrectomy in patients in whom clear resection margins were documented by histologic examination (51). Wotherspoon et al (52) systematically examined gastrectomy specimens of five MALT lymphomas using a "Swiss roll" technique. They showed that numerous small tumor foci with identical immunoglobulin light chain restriction to the main tumor mass were distributed throughout the gastric mucosa, including macroscopically normal regions (Figs. 18.21 and 18.22). A subsequent investigation by sequence analysis of the rearranged immunoglobulin heavy chain genes confirmed the clonal identity of these multiple tumor foci (53). Further studies by

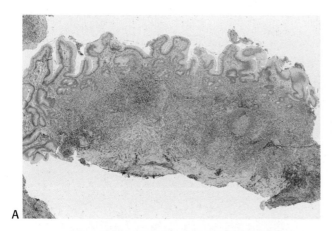

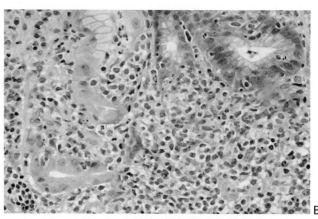

A   B

FIG. 18.18. A: Gastric biopsy showing diffuse lymphocytic infiltration of the lamina propria with residual B-cell follicles. **B:** Higher magnification shows that the infiltrating cells are "centrocyte-like" and invade individual glands to form lymphoepithelial lesions.

microdissection and clone-specific PCR demonstrated that tumor cells were frequently present in reactive lymphoid tissue that showed no histologic evidence of lymphoma (54–56).

Dissemination

Most gastric MALT lymphomas are at stage I when they present; between 4% and 17% have disseminated to regional lymph nodes, and approximately 10% have already disseminated to the bone marrow at the time of diagnosis (44,57). Gastric MALT lymphomas have a tendency to disseminate to other sites where MALT lymphomas occur, including the small intestine, salivary gland, and lung.

When MALT lymphomas disseminate to lymphoid tissue, including lymph nodes and spleen, they specifically invade the marginal zone (Fig. 18.23). This can lead to a deceptively benign or reactive appearance, especially in mesenteric lymph nodes, in which a marginal zone is normally present. Immunohistochemistry for immunoglobulin light chains can be very helpful in discriminating a normal marginal zone from disseminated MALT lymphoma (Fig. 18.24).

Subsequently, the lymphoma in the marginal zones expands to form more obvious sheets of interfollicular lymphoma. Occasionally, follicular colonization in involved lymph nodes can lead to an appearance that simulates follicular lymphoma (Fig. 18.25).

Immunohistochemistry

The immunophenotype of MALT lymphoma essentially recapitulates that of marginal zone cells (Table 18.2). The B cells are CD20, CD79a, CD21, and CD35 positive and CD5, CD23, and CD10 negative. CD43, indicative of a neoplastic phenotype, is expressed in approximately 50% of cases. The tumor cells typically express IgM and less often IgA or IgG, are IgD negative, and show immunoglobulin light chain restriction (Fig. 18.26). A significant intratumoral population of CD3-positive, predominantly CD4-positive T cells is characteristic. Expanded meshworks of follicular dendritic cells are typically detected with antibodies CD21 and CD23, corresponding to follicles that have been overrun or specifically colonized by lymphoma cells. Variable numbers of CD10- and Bcl6-positive germinal center cells may be seen in

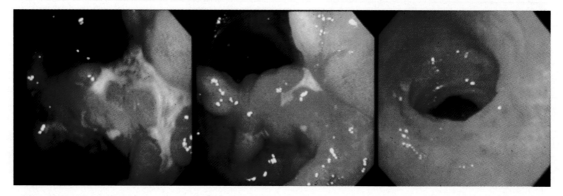

FIG. 18.19. Endoscopic appearance of a gastric mucosa-associated lymphoid tissue lymphoma at diagnosis (*left*), 10 days after eradication of *Helicobacter pylori* (*center*), and 10 months after eradication (*right*).

TABLE 18.2	Immunophenotype of Marginal Zone B Cells and Cells of MALT Lymphoma		
Antigen	Splenic MZ	Peyer Patch MZ	MALT Lymphoma
CD20	+	+	+
IgM[a]	+	+	+
IgD	−/+	−/+	−
CD5	−	−	−
CD10	−	−	−
CD21[b]	+/−	+	+
CD35[b]	+	+	+

MALT, mucosa-associated lymphoid tissue; MZ, marginal zone.

[a]Occasional case expresses IgA or IgG.

[b]In cryostat sections.

these areas, but the neoplastic MALT lymphoma cells are negative for these antigens.

Molecular Genetic Features of Mucosa-associated Lymphoid Tissue Lymphoma

Antigen Receptor Genes

In the B cells of MALT lymphoma, immunoglobulin heavy and light chain genes are rearranged and show somatic mutation of their variable regions, consistent with a postgerminal center memory B-cell derivation (53,58). Ongoing mutations are thought to occur in most cases (58). Because of the difficulty in distinguishing between acquired MALT and MALT lymphoma, particularly in small biopsies (see below), there has been a tendency to rely on molecular evidence of monoclonality detected by PCR for the diagnosis of lymphoma. This technique may fail to detect monoclonality in up to 15% of cases of overt lymphoma and thus produce false-negative results (54). There are also reports of apparently

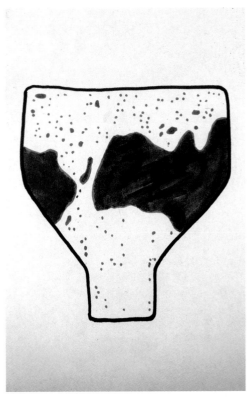

FIG. 18.21. Map of gastric lymphoma showing main tumor and multiple additional sites of involvement.

spurious monoclonality in biopsies of acquired MALT, for example, gastric biopsies showing only chronic gastritis (42,55,56), where there is no histologic evidence of malignancy. The frequency of this spurious monoclonality varies between laboratories, which suggests that technique may be a factor. These findings serve to emphasize that MALT lymphoma should not be diagnosed in the absence of clear histologic evidence. This point is underlined by the frequent finding of persistent monoclonality in small residual, clinically insignificant lymphoid aggregates that persist following eradication of *H. pylori* for the treatment of MALT lymphoma (50).

Molecular Genetic Abnormalities

A number of molecular abnormalities have been described in gastric MALT lymphoma including trisomies 3, 12, and 18 and the specific chromosomal translocations t(11;18)(q21;q21), t(1;14)(p22;q32), and t(14;18)(q32;q21). T(11;18) involves the *API2* and *MALT1* genes and generates a functional *API2–MALT1* fusion product (59–61). T(1;14) and t(14;18) juxtapose the *BCL10* and *MALT1* genes, respectively, to the immunoglobulin gene locus in 14q32 leading to deregulated expression of the oncogene (62–65). The oncogenic activities of the three chromosome translocations are linked by the physiologic role of BCL10 and MALT1 in antigen receptor-mediated nuclear factor (NF) κB activation

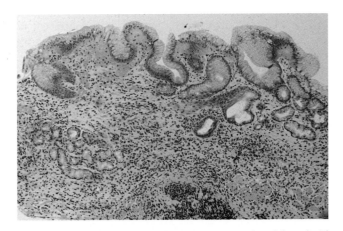

FIG. 18.20. Gastric biopsy of a mucosa-associated lymphoid tissue lymphoma after eradication of *Helicobacter pylori*. The lamina propria has an "empty" appearance and an occasional lymphoid nodule persists.

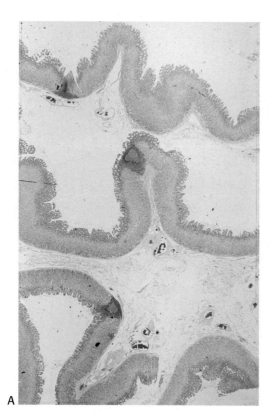
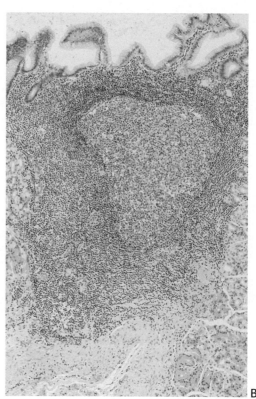

FIG. 18.22. A: Histology of a "Swiss roll" preparation showing microscopic foci of lymphoma. **B:** Higher magnification of a "microlymphoma." The lymphoma occupies the marginal zone around a reactive B-cell follicle.

(66). The three chromosome translocations occur at markedly variable incidences in MALT lymphoma of different sites but are always mutually exclusive (66). Among the three chromosome translocations, t(11;18) is the most frequent, occurring in 25% to 30% of gastric MALT lymphomas (67).

There is growing evidence suggesting that t(11;18)-positive cases are distinct from other MALT lymphomas, including those with t(1;14) or t(14;18). T(11;18)-positive MALT lymphomas rarely undergo high-grade transformation

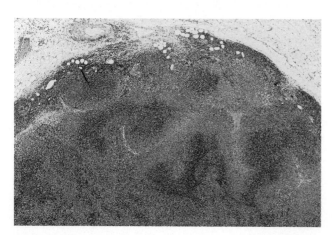

FIG. 18.23. Lymph node involvement by gastric mucosa-associated lymphoid tissue lymphoma. The tumor is distributed in the marginal zones.

(68,69), despite the fact that the translocation is significantly associated with cases at advanced stages and that these cases typically do not respond to *H. pylori* eradication (70,71). Cytogenetically, t(11;18)-positive tumors usually do not show other chromosomal aberrations, such as trisomies 3 and 18, frequently seen in t(11;18)-negative tumors, including those positive for t(1;14) and t(14;18) (72). Furthermore, t(11;18) MALT lymphomas show markedly fewer chromosomal gains and losses than translocation-negative tumors (71).

T(11;18) can be detected in paraffin-embedded tissue by reverse transcription PCR (RT-PCR), while fluorescent in situ hybridization (FISH) is useful for demonstrating all three characteristic translocations. In cases positive for t(11:18) as well as 20% of translocation-negative cases, BCL10 protein is up-regulated in the nucleus where it stains weakly (Fig. 18.27). In the much rarer t(1:14) cases, nuclear BCL10 is expressed intensely both in the nucleus and cytoplasm (Fig. 18.28). The significance of these findings remains unknown at present.

Postulated Normal Cell Counterpart of Mucosa-associated Lymphoid Tissue Lymphoma

The architectural features of MALT lymphoma, particularly in early cases, show quite clearly that the neoplastic cells are infiltrating the marginal zone around B-cell follicles (Figs. 18.7 and 18.29). In non-neoplastic lymphoid tissue a prominent marginal zone is present only in the spleen, Peyer patches,

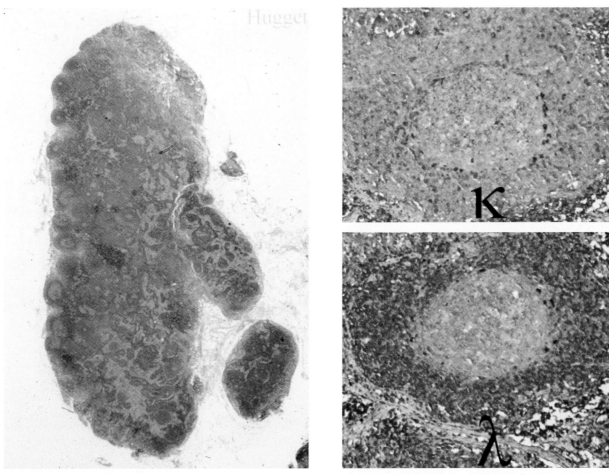

FIG. 18.24. Gastric lymph node from a case of gastric mucosa-associated lymphoid tissue lymphoma appears normal (*left*), but immunohistochemistry (*right*) shows marginal zone involvement by lymphoma showing λ immunoglobulin light chain restriction.

and mesenteric lymph nodes. This allows a comparison of the cytology and immunophenotype of normal marginal zone cells with those of MALT lymphoma. Cytologically, MALT lymphoma cells bear a close resemblance to marginal zone cells. Both are slightly larger than small lymphocytes,

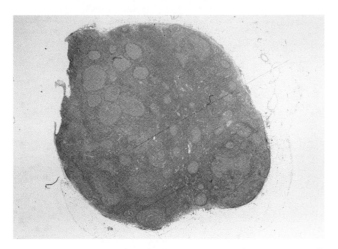

FIG. 18.25. Gastric lymph node from a case of mucosa-associated lymphoid tissue lymphoma with follicular colonization leading to a resemblance to follicular lymphoma.

have a slightly irregular nuclear outline, and moderate amounts of pale-staining cytoplasm. Interestingly, in Peyer patches collections of marginal zone cells are found within the dome epithelium. The immunophenotype of cells of the marginal zone and MALT lymphoma is virtually identical, both expressing CD20 and other pan B-cell antigens, CD21, CD35, and IgM, but not IgD.

Prognosis

MALT lymphomas are among the most indolent of all lymphomas and have a good prognosis overall regardless of stage. Five- and 10-year overall survival rates of over 80% are the rule, although progression-free survival may be somewhat lower (73). Cases in which transformation to diffuse large B-cell lymphoma has occurred have a significantly lower survival of approximately 50% at 5 years (48).

The treatment of gastric MALT lymphoma has attracted considerable attention since the initial publication showing that the lymphoma may regress following eradication of *H. pylori* with antibiotics. The follow-up of MALT lymphoma patients following eradication of *H. pylori* is rather complex, requiring repeated gastroscopy with biopsy (see above), and

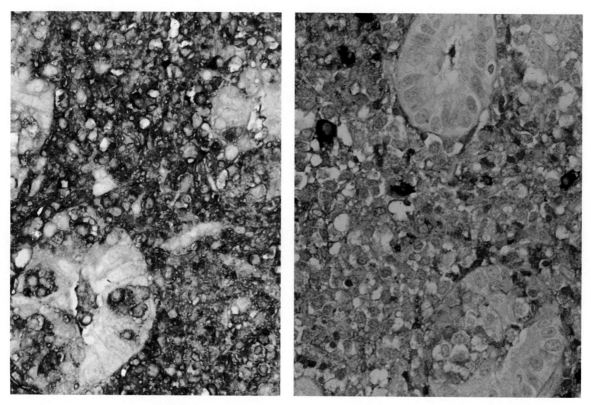

FIG. 18.26. Gastric mucosa-associated lymphoid tissue lymphoma immunostained for κ (*left*) and λ (*right*) immunoglobulin light chains. There is κ light chain restriction.

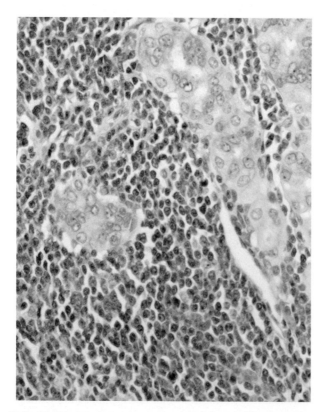

FIG. 18.27. Gastric mucosa-associated lymphoid tissue lymphoma, t(11;18) positive, immunostained for BCL10. Tumor cells are weakly positive.

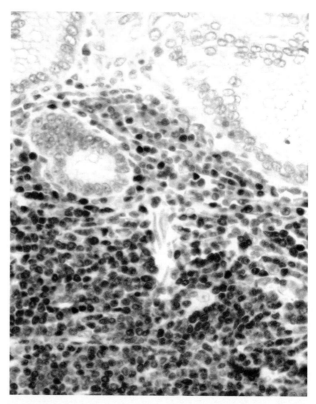

FIG. 18.28. Gastric mucosa-associated lymphoid tissue lymphoma, t(1;14) positive, immunostained for BCL10. Tumor cell nuclei are strongly positive.

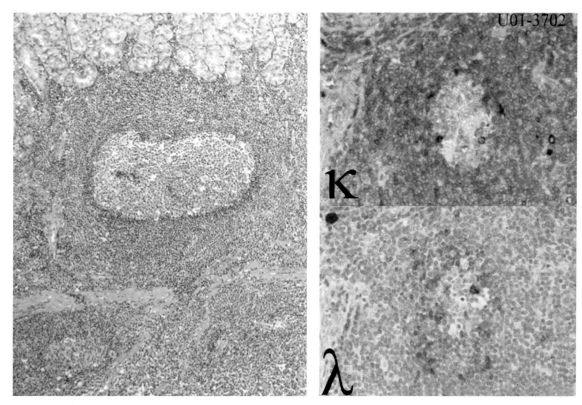

FIG. 18.29. A focus of gastric mucosa-associated lymphoid tissue lymphoma occupying the marginal zone around a reactive B-cell follicle (*left*). The tumor cells show κ immunoglobulin light chain restriction (*right*).

it would be extremely useful to be able to identify the approximately 25% of cases of gastric MALT lymphoma that do not respond to eradication of *H. pylori*. Studies using endoscopic ultrasound have suggested that if the tumor has invaded beyond the submucosa, it is less likely to respond (74,75). Equally, cases that have transformed to large B-cell lymphoma are unlikely to respond, although there are reports of complete regression in such cases (76,77). Following the cloning of t(1;14) and t(11;18) breakpoints, these translocations have been shown to have a bearing on the response to *H. pylori* eradication. T(11;18)(q21;q21), present in up to 25% of cases, is strongly associated with failure to respond to eradication of *H. pylori* (78). Interestingly, both t(1;14) and t(11;18) are associated with nuclear expression of BCL10 protein that is particularly intense in t(1;14)-positive cases. Moreover, the frequency of both t(11;18)(q21;q21) and nuclear BCL10 expression is significantly higher in tumors that have invaded or disseminated beyond the stomach (78% and 93%, respectively) than those confined to the stomach (10% and 38%, respectively) (79). These findings in part explain the results based on the use of endoscopic ultrasound and suggest that both t(11;18)(q21;q21) and BCL10 nuclear expression are associated with failure to respond to *H. pylori* eradication and with more advanced stage MALT lymphoma. Therefore, before embarking on *H. pylori* eradication as definitive therapy, the pertinent genotypic and/or immunohistochemical investigations should be carried out.

Differential Diagnosis

Reactive Versus Neoplastic Mucosa-associated Lymphoid Tissue

The distinction between acquired MALT, the precursor of MALT lymphoma, and MALT lymphoma in the early stages of evolution is often diagnostically difficult. Gastric MALT acquired as a consequence of *H. pylori* infection comprises reactive B-cell follicles without an identifiable marginal zone (Fig. 18.30). The lamina propria around the follicles is infiltrated by a mixture of inflammatory cells, including plasma cells and T lymphocytes. A lymphoepithelium can be seen adjacent to the follicles and can mimic the lymphoepithelial lesion characteristic of MALT lymphoma (Fig. 18.30B). In the presence of these intraepithelial B cells immediately adjacent to follicles, the absence of a diffuse infiltrate of IgM-positive IgD negative B lymphocytes external to the IgD- and IgM-positive mantle zone cells is very helpful in distinguishing such cases from MALT lymphoma (Table 18.2).

In the distinction between acquired MALT and MALT lymphoma, inference of monoclonality, either by the demonstration of immunoglobulin light chain restriction using immunohistochemistry or flow cytometry, is necessary. Coexpression of CD43 by B cells is a useful hint that the B-cell population is neoplastic. The use of PCR of immunoglobulin heavy chain genes to discriminate polyclonal-reactive lymphoid infiltrates from monoclonal MALT

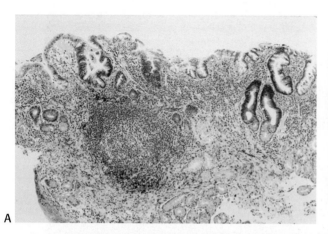
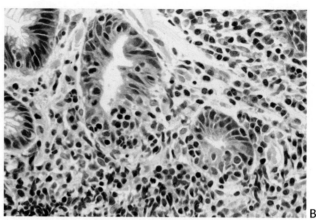

FIG. 18.30. **A:** Gastric biopsy showing *Helicobacter pylori*–associated chronic gastritis. There is a prominent B-cell follicle. **B:** High magnification of gastric glands close to the follicle showing infiltration by lymphocytes resembling a lymphoepithelial lesion. Wotherspoon score, 3 (see Table 18.3).

lymphoma is controversial but there is no doubt that, properly performed, a positive PCR result is strong evidence in favor of lymphoma. Wotherspoon et al (39) have proposed a scoring system to assist in the differential diagnosis of MALT lymphoma from chronic gastritis in biopsy specimens (Table 18.3).

Mucosa-associated Lymphoid Tissue Versus Other Small B-cell Lymphomas

Because of differences in clinical behavior and management, it is important to differentiate MALT lymphoma from the other small B-cell lymphomas that may present or involve extranodal sites (Table 18.1). These are discussed in greater detail in the section that follows on intestinal lymphomas. They include mantle cell lymphoma, lymphocytic lymphoma (chronic lymphocytic leukemia), and follicular lymphoma. The cytologic features of mantle cell lymphoma can closely simulate those of MALT lymphoma and occasional lymphoepithelial lesions may be present. However, absence of transformed blasts, together with expression of CD5 and IgD and, importantly, intranuclear expression of cyclin D1, a consequence of t(11;14), serves to distinguish mantle cell lymphoma. Small lymphocytic lymphoma (chronic lymphocytic leukemia) is characterized by small round lymphocytes, usually together with peripheral blood lymphocytosis and often with pseudofollicles, although these may be difficult to

appreciate in extranodal sites. Expression of CD5, CD23, and IgD without nuclear cyclin D1 provides further distinction from MALT lymphoma. Finally, follicular lymphoma, which may arise extranodally, can be difficult to distinguish from MALT lymphoma with follicular colonization. The transformed MALT lymphoma cells within follicles may closely resemble centroblasts but typically are CD10 and BCL6 (nuclear) negative, in contrast to the cells of follicular lymphoma, which usually express both antigens both within and between follicles. Assessment of these antigens, together with stains for follicular dendritic cells (FDCs) such as CD21 or CD23, is useful. Cytogenetic and molecular genetic analyses to detect t(11;18) and t(14;18) are also helpful. MALT lymphoma with plasmacytic differentiation can be difficult to distinguish from lymphoplasmacytic lymphoma. Occurrence in an extranodal site like the stomach (as opposed to lymph node or spleen), the characteristic Peyer patch–like architecture, and the presence of cytologically characteristic marginal zone B cells and lymphoepithelial lesions all favor a diagnosis of MALT lymphoma.

Mucosa-associated Lymphoid Tissue Lymphoma and Adenocarcinoma

There are numerous reports of synchronous gastric MALT lymphoma and adenocarcinoma (80,81). In the series of 237

TABLE 18.3	Scoring System for Distinguishing MALT Lymphoma from Chronic Gastritis	
Score	Interpretation	Histology
0	Normal	Occasional plasma cells
1	Chronic active gastritis	Lymphocyte clusters, no follicles
2	Follicular gastritis	Prominent follicles, no lymphoepithelial lesions
3	Suspicious, probably reactive	Follicles, occasional adjacent lymphoepithelial lesion, no diffuse infiltrate
4	Suspicious, probably lymphoma	Follicles, diffuse marginal zone cell infiltrate, no lymphoepithelial lesions
5	MALT lymphoma	Follicles, diffuse marginal zone cell infiltrate, lymphoepithelial lesions present

MALT, mucosa-associated lymphoid tissue.

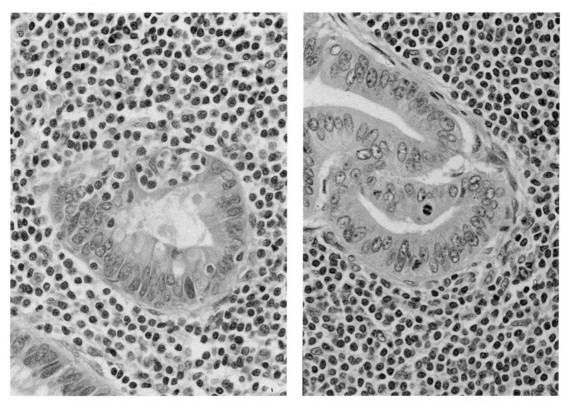

FIG. 18.31. Gastric mucosa-associated lymphoid tissue lymphoma (*left*) with synchronous adenocarcinoma (*right*). The lymphoma cells do not form lymphoepithelial lesions with the neoplastic gastric glands.

cases of gastric lymphoma reported by Nakamura et al (82), 10% of lymphomas were complicated by adenocarcinoma. Interestingly, the MALT lymphoma cells do not form lymphoepithelial lesions with neoplastic gastric epithelium (Fig. 18.31). The role of *H. pylori* in the pathogenesis of both conditions may be relevant (83).

DIFFUSE LARGE B-CELL LYMPHOMA OF THE STOMACH

DLBCL of the stomach is at least as common if not more common than MALT lymphoma. Foci of DLBCL may be seen in MALT lymphoma, suggesting that there has been transformation from one to the other as occurs in other small B-cell lymphomas (Fig. 18.17). The extent of this secondary high-grade component varies; in some cases there is a minor large cell component composed of small cohesive sheets of transformed blasts within the MALT lymphoma, while others are characterized by a predominance of large cell lymphoma with only small residual foci of MALT lymphoma, which can be difficult to find. Some cases of DLBCL of the stomach in which a MALT lymphoma component cannot be detected are transformed MALT lymphomas that have been completely overgrown by DLBCL, but others are true primary DLBCL. Those cases that are CD10 positive are unlikely to be transformed MALT lymphomas. However,

there is no difference in the clinical behavior between transformed MALT lymphoma and primary DLBCL (84).

Histopathology

The histologic features of gastric DLBCL of the stomach are no different from those found in nodal disease. The large cells may resemble centroblasts or immunoblasts but tend to have more cytoplasm than classic centroblasts, which imparts a plasmablastic appearance. Bizarre, often multinucleated cells are not uncommon and these sometimes resemble Reed-Sternberg cells (Fig. 18.32). The large cells infiltrate

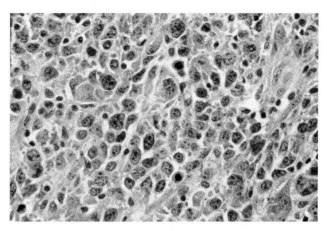

FIG. 18.32. Diffuse large B-cell gastric lymphoma.

in sheets between glands, and invasion of individual glands with formation of lymphoepithelial lesions, although it occurs, is rare. There is often an accompanying population of small lymphocytes, which can be shown with immunohistochemistry to be T cells.

Immunohistochemistry

Transformed MALT lymphomas are characteristically BCL2 and CD10 negative (85) but, in contrast to MALT lymphoma, usually express BCL6 (86). Primary gastric DLBCL, on the other hand, may be CD10 positive and a proportion are BCL2 positive. Immunostaining with CD21 may reveal numerous residual FDC meshworks that represent reactive follicles that have been overrun or colonized by the lymphoma, a finding that may suggest that the DLBCL originated as a MALT lymphoma that has transformed. Immunophenotypic characteristics do not, however, reliably distinguish transformed MALT lymphoma from primary DLBCL, which may also be CD10 negative.

Molecular Genetics

Rearrangement and/or mutations of BCL6 have been reported in a proportion of cases (87,88) and mutation with loss of heterozygosity of p53 has been described in 29% of cases of transformed MALT lymphoma (89). Cases of MALT lymphoma with t(11;18) seldom transform to DLBCL (90). Some reports have suggested that transformed MALT lymphomas differ from primary DLBCL in showing *c-myc* rearrangement in a high proportion of cases (91), but in general there is no reliable genetic property that distinguishes transformed MALT lymphoma from de novo DLBCL.

Prognosis

It is generally agreed that gastric DLBCL shows less favorable behavior than MALT lymphoma. Cogliatti et al (84) found that the 5-year survival of gastric DLBCL was significantly worse than that of MALT lymphoma (75% vs. 91%) and that there was no difference between DLBCL and transformed MALT lymphoma. Chemotherapy is the treatment of choice for gastric DLBCL but, interestingly, there are several reports of cases of gastric DLBCL that have responded to eradication of *H. pylori* (92,93).

INTESTINAL MUCOSA-ASSOCIATED LYMPHOID TISSUE LYMPHOMA

Most intestinal MALT lymphomas arise in the small intestine, colorectal lymphomas being distinctly rare. There does not appear to be any difference in behavior between the two sites, and they will therefore be considered together. IPSID is a distinctive subtype of MALT lymphoma that is associated with the synthesis of α immunoglobulin heavy chain and is

restricted in its incidence to certain geographic areas, particularly the Middle East. Immunoproliferative small intestinal disease will be described as a separate entity following discussion of the more usual intestinal MALT lymphoma that has no special epidemiologic or immunologic features. To date, there are only a few studies of intestinal lymphoma in which the cases have been analyzed taking the MALT concept into account (22,94,95).

Clinical Presentation

Most cases of small intestinal lymphoma occur in elderly patients and present with intestinal obstruction, while rectal bleeding is a more common presenting sign in colonic lymphoma. A significant number of colonic lymphomas arise in the setting of inflammatory bowel disease, but this is not a recognized risk factor for small intestinal lymphoma (96). Any segment of the intestine may be involved and most tumors occur as single lesions, although cases presenting as multiple polyposis have been recorded (97,98). The mesenteric lymph nodes are usually involved (stage II$_E$), but spread outside the abdomen including bone marrow involvement is unusual at presentation. In some cases a cryptic simultaneous gastric MALT lymphoma is present and most of these cases are thought to be examples of secondary intestinal MALT lymphoma (99).

Histopathology

The histology of MALT lymphoma of the intestine is identical to that of gastric MALT lymphoma. Reactive B-cell follicles are prominent and these are surrounded by neoplastic marginal zone cells, which often show plasma cell differentiation (Fig. 18.33). Lymphoepithelial lesions (Fig. 18.34) are not as numerous in comparison to gastric lymphoma but can almost always be found. However, care must be taken not to overinterpret their presence, especially in the terminal ileum, since intraepithelial B cells occur normally in the

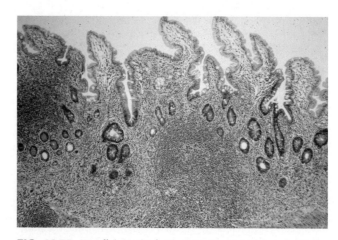

FIG. 18.33. Small intestinal mucosa-associated lymphoid tissue lymphoma.

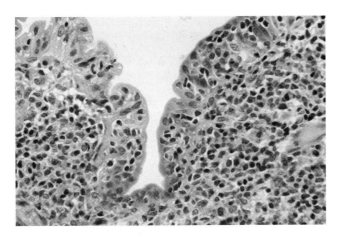

FIG. 18.34. Lymphoepithelial lesion in a small intestinal mucosa-associated lymphoid tissue lymphoma.

dome epithelium of Peyer patches and may increase in lymphoid hyperplasia. Follicular colonization may also be seen.

Differential Diagnosis

Focal Lymphoid Hyperplasia

This condition occurs in the terminal ileum and can be subdivided into a more common form seen in children and young adults and a rarer form seen in older individuals (100). In the case of young patients, the condition is known by several names including *enteritis follicularis, cobblestone ileum, nonsclerosing ileitis, pseudopolyposis lymphatica,* and *terminal lymphoid ileitis.* It occurs more frequently in males and may present as ileocecal intussusception, as an appendicitislike illness, or with bleeding. Since the diagnosis is usually made clinically, there are few histologic descriptions of this condition, but published reports describe marked hyperplasia of Peyer patches with sharply defined follicles and submucosal edema. There is no disorganization of lymphoid tissue or infiltration of the muscularis and little resemblance to lymphoma. In the adult form (101), the clinical presentation is one of weeks to years of abdominal pain, which may be associated with a mass in the right iliac fossa. The histologic features include follicular hyperplasia (Fig. 18.35) of the mucosa, which is frequently associated with ulceration, and a diffuse lymphoplasmacytic infiltrate extending deeply into the wall of the ileum, often involving the serosa. Eosinophils may be a prominent component of the infiltrate. The normal marginal zone cell component of Peyer patches participates in the hyperplastic process, leading to exaggeration of the normal association of these cells with dome epithelium. Structures resembling lymphoepithelial lesions may be seen in tangentially cut sections. The result is a picture that may closely simulate MALT lymphoma from which it can be distinguished once again by its polyclonal nature.

Diffuse Nodular Lymphoid Hyperplasia of the Intestine

Diffuse nodular lymphoid hyperplasia may occur in the small intestine, colon, or both. It is an extremely rare condition that

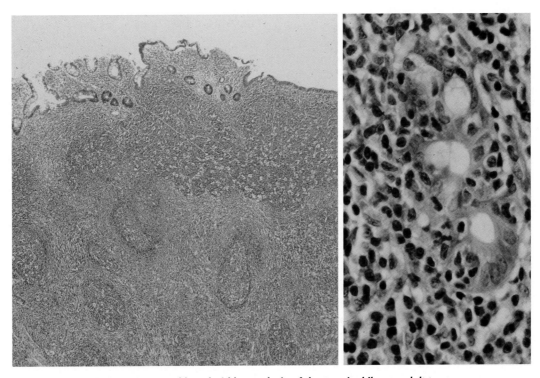

FIG. 18.35. Focal lymphoid hyperplasia of the terminal ileum, adult type.

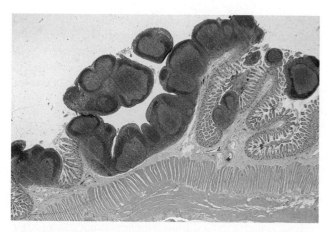

FIG. 18.36. Diffuse nodular hyperplasia of the small intestine.

involves long segments of bowel and occurs in two forms. The most well recognized of these is that associated with congenital or acquired hypogammaglobulinemia, which is only rarely associated with lymphoma (102). Histologically, there is enlargement of the mucosal B-cell follicles caused by hyperplasia of follicle centers (Fig. 18.36). These hyperplastic follicles are confined to the mucosa and surrounded by a normal-appearing mantle zone. The marginal zone is inconspicuous and there is no associated interfollicular infiltrate. In the second form of this condition (103), in which immunoglobulin deficiency is not present, there is a well-documented association with malignant lymphoma. The lymphoma is of MALT type and shows an interrelationship with the hyperplastic follicles as described above.

Prognosis

The clinical behavior of intestinal B-cell lymphoma is not as favorable as that of gastric lymphoma. Histologic grade, stage of disease, and resectability have prognostic significance. A 5-year survival of 44% to 75% is reported for intestinal MALT lymphoma and 25% to 37% for DLBCL (94,95,104). Importantly, the behavior of intestinal DLBCL is not affected by the presence or absence of a MALT component (95).

IMMUNOPROLIFERATIVE SMALL INTESTINAL DISEASE

This condition, first described by Ramot in 1965 (105), is a variant of MALT lymphoma characterized by a diffuse lymphoplasmacytic (predominantly plasmacytic) infiltrate in the upper small intestine. The disease has been most frequently reported in the Middle East but appears markedly to have declined in incidence there. Significant numbers of cases have also been reported from the Cape region of South Africa (14) and sporadic cases from elsewhere. An important distinguishing feature of IPSID is the synthesis of α heavy chain, without light chain, by the plasma cells; this can be

detected in the serum or duodenal juice in approximately two thirds of cases, hence the term α-chain disease. In the remaining one third of cases the α-chain protein is still synthesized but not secreted (106).

Clinical Presentation

Immunoproliferative small intestinal disease is a disease predominantly of young adults and usually presents with profound malabsorption. There are numerous reports describing remissions or even cure of IPSID in its early stages following the use of broad-spectrum antibiotics (107–109). There seems little doubt that the removal of either specific or nonspecific immune stimulants from the gut lumen can have a profound effect on some cases of IPSID in the early stages, but given the natural history of the disease, prolonged follow-up is needed before the term *cure* can be used with confidence. The fact that this type of MALT lymphoma is to a degree antigen responsive may be significant when considering the biology of the entire group of MALT lymphomas.

Gross Features

The macroscopic appearances of IPSID depend on the stage. In most cases there is diffuse, even thickening of the upper jejunum together with enlarged mesenteric lymph nodes. Circumscribed lymphomatous masses may be present and these may be multiple, sometimes producing multiple small intestinal polyps. The stomach is sometimes involved, but spread to other abdominal organs is rare.

Histologic Features

The histology of IPSID exemplifies all the features of MALT lymphoma with marked plasma cell differentiation. Three stages of IPSID are recognized (110). In stage A, the lymphoplasmacytic infiltrate is confined to the mucosa and mesenteric lymph nodes. In stage B, nodular mucosal lymphoid infiltrates are present and the infiltrate extends below the muscularis mucosa. Stage C is characterized by the presence of lymphomatous masses and transformation to DLBCL. The plasma cell infiltrate in the mucosa causes broadening, but not shortening, of the villi (Figs. 18.37 and 18.38). These cells are not invasive and show no evidence of mitotic division. Already present in stage A IPSID, and increasing in prominence in stage B, are aggregates of neoplastic marginal zone B cells, which cluster around epithelial crypts and form lymphoepithelial lesions (Fig. 18.39). Reactive follicles vary in number, and it is colonization of these by marginal zone cells that results in the lymphoid nodules of stage B IPSID (10) (Fig. 18.39) and the so-called follicular lymphoma variant (14,111). Transformation to DLBCL occurs in the same way as in gastric lymphoma, and the large cells frequently show bizarre cytologic features (Fig. 18.40).

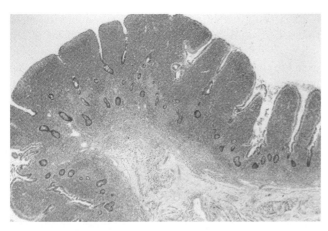

FIG. 18.37. Immunoproliferative small intestinal disease. There is diffuse mucosal plasma cell infiltration with pericryptal pale areas corresponding to aggregates of marginal zone B cells.

Lymph Node Involvement

The mesenteric lymph nodes are involved early in the course of IPSID. Initially, there is filling of the sinusoids by mature plasma cells, but later the characteristic marginal zone infiltrate of the neoplastic cells is seen (Fig. 18.41). Follicular colonization may occur in the lymph nodes usually characterized by the presence of α chain–positive plasma cells within germinal centers.

Immunohistochemistry and Molecular Genetics

Immunohistochemical studies of IPSID (13,14) confirm the synthesis of α heavy chain, without light chain, by the plasma cells, marginal zone cells, and transformed blasts (Fig. 18.42). The IgA is always of subclass IgA1 but occasional cases have been described in which both IgA1 and IgA2 have been synthesized (13). In a minority of cases immunoglobulin light chain is synthesized and when this occurs, there is light chain restriction (112). The neoplastic marginal zone cells show

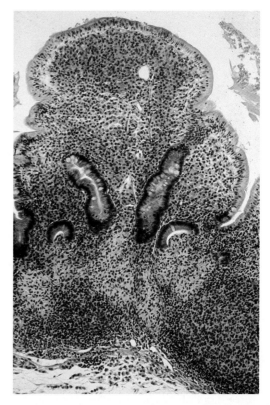

FIG. 18.39. A case of immunoproliferative small intestinal disease showing B-cell follicles and surrounding marginal zone cells that form lymphoepithelial lesions with intestinal crypts. The overlying lamina propria is heavily infiltrated by plasma cells.

the same immunophenotype as in other MALT lymphomas. In cases in which the infiltrate appears to consist only of plasma cells, staining with CD20 antibodies will often reveal clusters of B cells concentrated around small intestinal crypts and forming lymphoepithelial lesions.

Gene rearrangement studies in early (stage A and B) IPSID have shown monoclonal heavy and light chain gene rearrangement (113); t(11;18) is not found in IPSID (114).

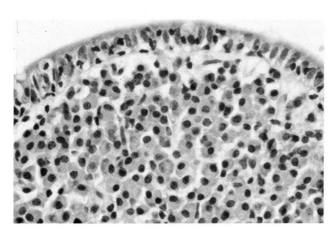

FIG. 18.38. High magnification of lamina propria plasma cells in immunoproliferative small intestinal disease.

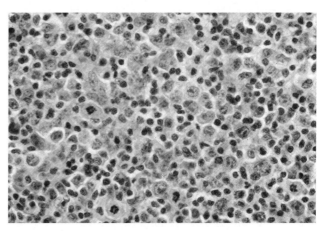

FIG. 18.40. Transformation of immunoproliferative small intestinal disease to diffuse large B-cell lymphoma.

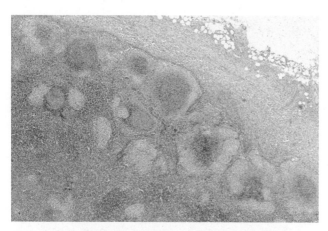

FIG. 18.41. Mesenteric lymph node from a case of immuno-proliferative small intestinal disease showing infiltration of marginal zones by pale-staining tumor B cells (compare with Figure 18.23).

Prognosis

IPSID runs a prolonged course, often over many years, and rarely spreads out of the abdomen until the terminal stages when high-grade transformation has occurred. Partial or even complete responses to broad-spectrum antibiotics have been reported (107–109).

Pathophysiology

Immunoproliferative small intestinal disease is in many ways the prototype of MALT lymphomas, exemplifying the prolonged natural history and the tendency of the lymphoma to remain localized in the abdomen with only few documented cases of spread to the periphery. Histologically, too, the marginal zonelike morphology of the lymphoid cells, the formation of lymphoepithelial lesions, plasma cell differentiation, and follicular colonization place IPSID firmly in the MALT category. The clinical indolence and response of some cases of stage A IPSID to broad-spectrum antibiotics has led to the common view that at this stage IPSID is a hyperplastic, non-neoplastic but prelymphomatous condition. However, observations on three cases of stage A IPSID in which light chain was being synthesized (112) (an uncommon event in IPSID) showed light chain restriction, and studies on a further three cases have shown clonal heavy and light chain immunoglobulin gene rearrangement (113). It is most likely, therefore, that IPSID is neoplastic de novo. How, then, can the response of some cases of stage A IPSID to antibiotics be explained? The extreme plasma cell differentiation that characterizes IPSID and that is maximal beneath the surface epithelium suggests that, although neoplastic, the lymphoid cells are not altogether autonomous and are exhibiting a degree of sensitivity to either a specific antigen or a nonspecific immune stimulant such as endotoxin. By removing the luminal source of immune stimulation, antibiotics could result in resolution of the plasma cell component of the mucosal infiltrate and even inhibit growth of the lymphoid element. In other words, the relationship between an immunologic, probably infectious agent and the lymphoma is identical to that between *H. pylori* and gastric MALT lymphoma.

MANTLE CELL LYMPHOMA (LYMPHOMATOUS POLYPOSIS)

Lymphomatous polyposis (also called multiple lymphomatous polyposis) is an uncommon but well-described disease (16,115). Most patients are over 50 years of age and there is no established sex preponderance. Presenting symptoms are those of abdominal pain, sometimes accompanied by melena, and barium studies or endoscopy reveals multiple polyps, which prove to be lymphomatous. Any part of the gastrointestinal tract may be involved, but in many of the cases the largest tumors are in the ileocecal region. The frequency of cases genuinely restricted to the gastrointestinal tract is very low, most patients having evidence of mantle cell lymphoma elsewhere.

Macroscopically, the intestinal mucosa is peppered with multiple white fleshy polyps ranging in size from 0.5 to 2 cm; much larger tumors may be present especially in the ileocecal region (Fig. 18.43). The mesenteric lymph nodes are usually obviously involved.

Histopathology

The smallest lesions consist of a single mucosal lymphoid nodule, which is diffusely replaced by lymphoma, sometimes with preservation of the reactive germinal center. The larger polyps may show either a diffuse or nodular lymphoid infiltrate that may, in some cases, be so nodular as to resemble follicular lymphoma (Fig. 18.44). Characteristically reactive "naked" germinal centers are trapped in the lymphomatous infiltrate, which appears selectively to replace their mantle zones. The nodular pattern appears to be a consequence of selective replacement of pre-existing nonneoplastic follicles by the tumor cells (16). Intestinal glands are displaced and obliterated and very occasional "lymphoepithelial lesions" (without the characteristic epithelial changes) can be seen. Typically, scattered, usually single epithelioid histiocytes and small sclerotic blood vessels are present. Cytologically, the infiltrate of mantle cell lymphoma consists of a uniform population of small to medium-sized lymphocytes with irregular nuclear contours, which resemble centrocytes (Fig. 18.45). Transformed blasts are conspicuously absent. The immunophenotype (see below) is in keeping with derivation from a subpopulation of mantle zone B cells (116). Several variants of mantle cell lymphoma are described but are beyond the scope of this book.

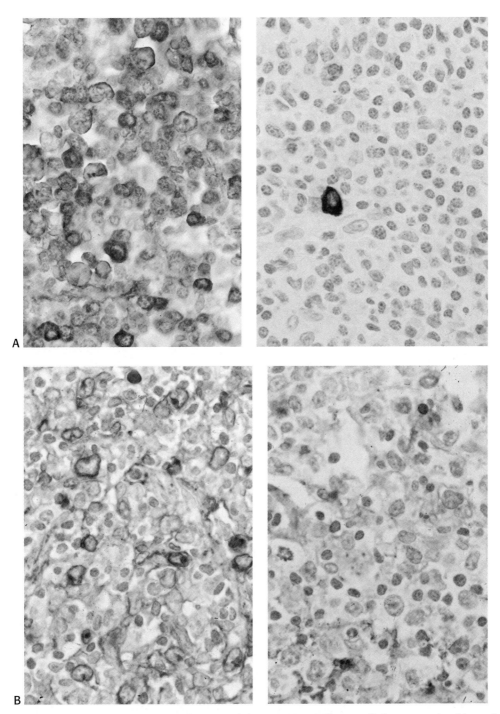

FIG. 18.42. A: Immunoproliferative small intestinal disease (IPSID) plasma cells immunostained for α chain (*left*) and κ and λ immunoglobulin light chains (*right*). **B:** Transformed IPSID immunostained for α chain (*left*) and κ and λ immunoglobulin light chains (*right*).

Immunohistochemistry and Molecular Genetics

Characteristically, the cells express pan B-cell antigens together with IgM, IgD, CD5, CD43, and, importantly, nuclear cyclin D1 (116). Other distinctive features of this type of lymphoma include negative immunostaining for CD10 and CD23 and the presence of rather loose nodular CD21-positive FDC meshworks (16).

Like its nodal counterpart, intestinal mantle cell lymphoma is characterized by t(11;14)(q13;q32) that results in *bcl-1* gene rearrangement with overexpression of nuclear cyclin D1 in almost 100% of cases (116).

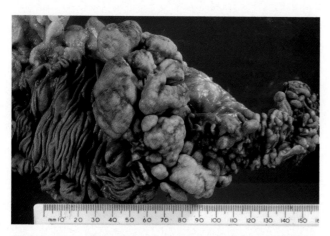

FIG. 18.43. A case of mantle cell lymphoma of the terminal ileum and cecum showing multiple polyps (lymphomatous polyposis) and cecal masses.

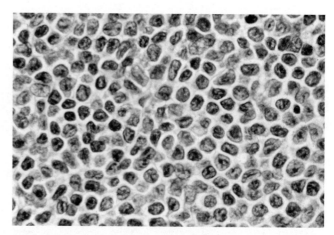

FIG. 18.45. Typical cytologic appearance of mantle cell lymphoma.

Differential Diagnosis

MALT lymphoma, follicular lymphoma, and lymphocytic lymphoma (chronic lymphocytic leukemia) can all give rise to multiple lymphomatous polyps in the intestine and, conversely, intestinal mantle cell lymphoma does not necessarily present with intestinal polyps. Moreover, all four lymphomas may be cytologically similar. Distinguishing between them is particularly difficult in small biopsies. The differential diagnosis of these small B-cell lymphomas of the intestine is summarized in Table 18.4. Monotony of the infiltrate and absence of transformed blasts favor a diagnosis of mantle cell lymphoma, but immunohistochemistry to show expression of CD5 and nuclear cyclin D1 is essential to distinguish it from the other small B-cell lymphomas.

Clinical Behavior

Like nodal mantle cell lymphoma, those presenting in the intestine have usually disseminated widely at the time of

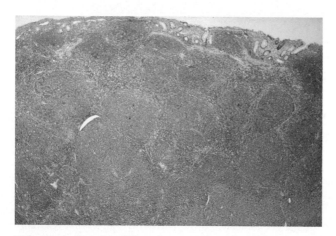

FIG. 18.44. Mantle cell lymphoma of the colon. The tumor has a follicular growth pattern.

diagnosis. Involvement of liver, spleen, bone marrow, and peripheral lymph nodes soon follows identification of the polyps. This aggressive clinical behavior is quite different from the indolent behavior of MALT lymphoma, and distinction between the two conditions is therefore important.

FOLLICULAR LYMPHOMA

Follicular lymphoma may occur as a primary tumor in the small intestine, especially in the ileocecal region and duodenum (117). From examination of the gastrointestinal tract alone it is not possible to tell whether the tumor is primary or secondary, and careful staging is necessary to determine between the two.

Histologic Features

Follicular lymphoma consists of typical neoplastic follicles composed principally of centrocytes with fewer centroblasts and usually involves the full thickness of the intestinal wall with lateral extension into the mucosa. An interfollicular diffuse infiltrate is frequently present and is usually composed of smaller lymphocytes with somewhat irregularly shaped nuclei (Fig. 18.46). This component may form rare lymphoepithelial lesions, which can cause confusion with MALT lymphoma, especially in endoscopic biopsies and if follicular colonization is a prominent feature.

A particular type of follicular lymphoma occurs in the duodenum, often in the region of the ampulla of Vater (118–120). It is often discovered incidentally at endoscopy, when the lesions appear as small mucosal nodules; these lymphomas comprise only one or two follicles restricted to the mucosa. On close inspection these follicles exhibit the characteristics of follicular lymphoma in that they lack polarity, consist principally of centrocytes, and are devoid of tingible body macrophages. Diagnosis of these tiny lesions as

TABLE 18.4	Differential Diagnosis of MALT Lymphoma			
	MALT	Mantle Cell	Follicular	Lymphocytic
Follicles	+	+	+	−(+)
Lymphoepithelial Lesions	+	−(+)	−(+)	−(+)
Cytology	CCL*	CCL	GCC**	L***
Immunoglobulin	M+,D−	M+,D+	M−/+, D−/+	M+,D+
CD20	+	+	+	+
CD5	−	+	−	+
CD10	−	−	+	−
CYCLIN D1	−	+	−	−

CCL, centrocytelike; GCC, germinal center cell; L, lymphocytic, occasionally centrocytelike; MALT, mucosa-associated lymphoid tissue.

follicular lymphoma often depends on immunohistochemical and/or molecular evidence (see below).

Immunohistochemistry and Molecular Genetics

The follicles of follicular lymphoma usually express CD10 and BCL2 and show light chain restriction (Fig. 18.47). However, 20% of cases are CD10 negative and some fail to express BCL2. CD10 is often down-regulated in the interfollicular diffuse component. One study has reported that the cells of intestinal follicular lymphomas show a tendency to express surface IgA, the preferential immunoglobulin of the mucosa immune system and rarely expressed by nodal follicular lymphomas (121). Moreover, these cells also express the α4-β7 mucosal homing receptor.

Molecular evidence of monoclonal immunoglobulin gene rearrangement is often an important consideration in distinguishing follicular lymphoma from reactive hyperplasia. In the single study quoted above, the immunoglobulin heavy chain genes of intestinal follicular lymphoma were extensively mutated consistent with antigen-based selection. BCL2 rearrangement is also present in most cases (117).

Differential Diagnosis

The morphologic and phenotypic features that are useful in distinguishing follicular lymphoma are listed in Table 18.4. In those cases where the interfollicular cells form lymphoepithelial lesions, the differential diagnosis from MALT lymphoma becomes problematic. Expression of CD10 by cells outside germinal centers is diagnostic of follicular lymphoma, as is the finding of coexpression of bcl2 and CD10 in cells within germinal centers.

DIFFUSE LARGE B-CELL LYMPHOMA OF THE INTESTINE

Diffuse large B-cell lymphomas account for 45% of small intestinal lymphomas, and a residual focus of MALT lymphoma can be identified in half of these (95). Histologically,

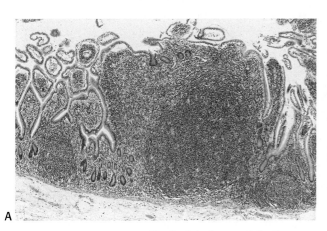
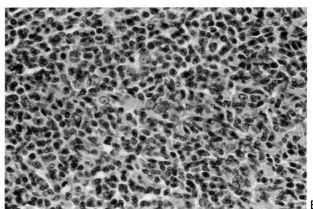

FIG. 18.46. A: Follicular lymphoma of the ileum. **B:** Higher magnification of tumor cells showing characteristic nuclear irregularity.

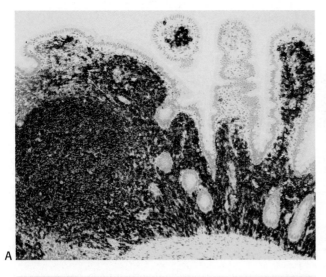

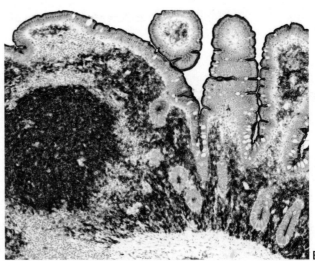

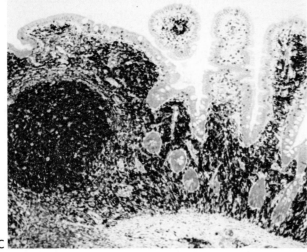

FIG. 18.47. Follicular lymphoma of the ileum. **A:** CD20. **B:** CD10. **C:** BCL2 CD10-positive cells are seen outside the B-cell follicle and this, together with BCL2 expression by germinal center B cells, is diagnostic.

the DLBCLs resemble their gastric counterparts and they exhibit the same immunohistochemical and molecular genetic features.

BURKITT LYMPHOMA

In the Middle East, primary gastrointestinal Burkitt lymphoma is a relatively common disease of children. It has been comprehensively studied in Algeria (17,122), where Burkitt lymphoma accounts for 46.5% of all childhood non-Hodgkin lymphomas and 60% of these cases arise primarily in the intestine. The disease is more common in boys and shows a peak incidence between 4 and 5 years of age. There is a predilection for the terminal ileum, but any part of the small intestine may be involved. Cases frequently present with intussusception. The cytogenetic alterations in this form of Burkitt lymphoma are similar, but possibly not identical, to those seen in the classic African form, as is the association with the Epstein-Barr virus. In Western countries, childhood gastrointestinal lymphoma is the most common

manifestation of so-called sporadic Burkitt lymphoma. This tumor, which also occurs in young adults, closely resembles endemic Burkitt lymphoma (described above).

Macroscopically, the lesions vary from localized obstructing tumors to huge masses involving long intestinal segments. Mesenteric and retroperitoneal lymph node involvement is common.

Histopathology

The histologic appearances are characteristic of classic African Burkitt lymphoma with mucosal effacement by sheets of medium-sized monomorphic blasts interspersed with phagocytic histiocytes. The blasts are characterized by a narrow rim of cytoplasm around nuclei with multiple small basophilic nucleoli and clumped chromatin (Fig. 18.48).

In Western countries, cases of so-called sporadic Burkitt lymphoma most often involve the ileocecal region and the histologic appearances may be identical. More commonly, however, there is greater cytologic variability and, unlike classic Burkitt lymphoma, immunohistochemistry may

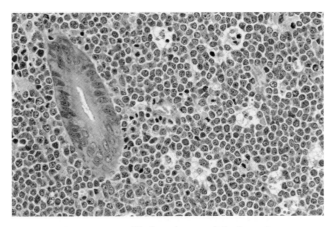

FIG. 18.48. Burkitt lymphoma of the intestine.

TABLE 18.5	Lymphoproliferative Lesions and Lymphomas Associated with Iatrogenic Immunosuppression for Organ Transplantation

Early lesions
    Reactive plasmacytic hyperplasia
    Infectious mononucleosis-like
Polymorphic posttransplant lymphoproliferative disease
Monomorphic posttransplant lymphoproliferative disease
    B-cell lymphomas
        Diffuse large B-cell lymphoma
        Burkitt lymphoma
        Plasma cell neoplasms
    T-cell lymphomas
        Peripheral T-cell lymphoma unspecified
Hodgkin lymphoma

show synthesis of cytoplasmic as well as surface immunoglobulin. The cytogenetic characteristics of these rare tumors have not been well characterized and they do not show the same consistent association with Epstein-Barr virus infection.

OTHER TYPES OF PRIMARY B-CELL LYMPHOMA CORRESPONDING TO PERIPHERAL LYMPH NODE EQUIVALENTS

There is no reason why any type of lymphoma cannot arise from mucosa-associated lymphoid tissue, but in practice, entities common in peripheral lymph nodes only infrequently arise in the gastrointestinal tract. Likewise, the rarer nodal lymphomas such as lymphocytic lymphoma and lymphoplasmacytic lymphoma hardly ever occur as primary gastrointestinal tumors. The reasons for this are obscure.

IMMUNODEFICIENCY-ASSOCIATED B-CELL LYMPHOPROLIFERATIVE CONDITIONS AND LYMPHOMA

The gastrointestinal tract is a favorite site for the occurrence of immunodeficiency-associated lymphoproliferative disorders (LPDs) and lymphomas (Table 18.5). The broad causes of the immunodeficiency include (a) primary immune disorders and immunodeficiency syndromes, (b) HIV infection, (c) iatrogenic immunosuppression for solid organ or bone marrow allografts, and (d) iatrogenic immunosuppression associated with methotrexate treatment for autoimmune disease.

There are certain histologic features that are common to lymphomas associated with all these causes of immunodeficiency; these include a predominance of a B-cell phenotype, high-grade histology, and Epstein-Barr virus (EBV) positivity. The exception is MALT lymphoma, a low-grade lesion, unassociated with EBV that has occasionally been reported in association with immunodeficiency (123,124). The LPDs

and lymphomas associated with specific causes of immunodeficiency will be discussed separately.

Primary immune disorders and immunodeficiency syndromes include conditions that result in ineffective immune surveillance such as the X-linked lymphoproliferative disorder, ataxia telangiectasia, Wiskott-Aldrich syndrome, common variable immunodeficiency, severe combined immunodeficiency, autoimmune lymphoproliferative syndrome, Nijmegan breakage syndrome, and hyper-IgM syndrome. The nature of the immune defect is highly variable between these different conditions and the LPDs and lymphomas associated with them are equally heterogeneous, although EBV is involved in most of them. The intestinal tract is a common site of involvement, where the defect in immunity may manifest as polymorphic lymphoproliferation similar to that associated with iatrogenic immunosuppression (see below) or, more commonly, as a diffuse large B-cell lymphoma. T-cell lymphomas may occur, especially in the setting of ataxia telangiectasia. Hodgkin lymphoma also occurs, but small lymphocytic lymphomas, with the exception of rare MALT lymphomas, are not seen.

HIV Infection

The gastrointestinal tract is a favored site for HIV-associated lymphomas that may include Burkitt lymphoma and its plasmacytic variant, diffuse large B-cell lymphoma, peripheral T-cell lymphoma, and unspecified and Hodgkin lymphoma. EBV is commonly found in the B-cell and Hodgkin lymphomas. MALT lymphoma has also been associated with HIV disease, where it is not associated with EBV.

Iatrogenic Immunosuppression for Solid Organ or Bone Marrow Allografts

Lymphomas that complicate iatrogenic immunosuppression, collectively known as posttransplant lymphoproliferative disorders (PTLDs), are, not surprisingly, very similar to

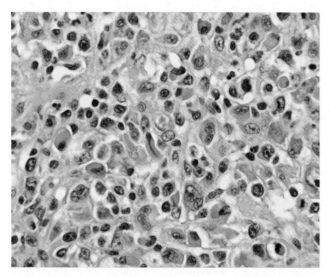

FIG. 18.49. Polymorphic posttransplant lymphoproliferative disorder. This case expressed polytypic immunoglobulin light chains and was Epstein-Barr virus negative.

those occurring in association with other forms of immunodeficiency. They are becoming increasingly common and, together with HIV-associated lymphomas, comprise the most important of the group of immunodeficiency-associated LPDs and lymphomas. Once more, the gastrointestinal tract is a common site. The spectrum of PTLDs is summarized in Table 18.5. Most PTLDs appear to be caused by EBV-induced poly- or monoclonal B-cell proliferations (125), and EBV can be demonstrated in the proliferating cells using in situ hybridization to demonstrate EBV-encoded RNA (EBER). However, approximately 20% are EBV negative and in these the underling factor driving the proliferation of the lymphoid cells is unknown. PTLDs can occur at any time after transplantation depending on the type of allograft and the agent(s) used for immunosuppression.

Early Lesions

In reactive plasmacytic hyperplasia, the intestinal lamina propria is heavily infiltrated by mature plasma cells with occasional transformed blasts forming single or multiple localized lesions but without evidence of tissue destruction. The plasma cells can be shown to synthesise both κ and λ immunoglobulin light chains. In infectious mononucleosis-like PTLD, the lesion is composed of a polymorphic proliferation of transformed B and T cells with scattered, large, sometimes multinucleated cells that resemble Hodgkin and Reed-Sternberg cells. Immunoglobulin light chain expression is again polytypic.

Polymorphic Posttransplant Lymphoproliferative Disorder

Polymorphic PTLD lesions infiltrate and destroy intestinal tissues with consequent ulceration. The lesions are com-

posed of a mixture of cell types from small lymphocytes and plasma cells to large transformed blasts (Fig. 18.49); there may be areas of necrosis and evidence of florid proliferation. The cells may or may not show evidence of EBV infection. Once more, the B cells in these lesions can be shown to synthesize polytypic light chains and PCR shows no evidence of monoclonal proliferation. Reduction in immunosuppression may lead to lesional regression in some cases (126–128), but others may resist treatment and progress to monomorphic PTLD or lymphoma.

Monomorphic Posttransplant Lymphoproliferative Disorder

Monomorphic PTLD may manifest as any type of diffuse large B-cell lymphoma, Burkitt lymphoma with or without plasmacytoid features (129) (Fig. 18.50), or plasmacytoma (130). Most are EBV positive and can be shown to be monotypic by immunohistochemistry and/or monoclonal by molecular techniques. They rarely regress following withdrawal of immunosuppressive drugs. T-cell monomorphic PTLDs occur but are distinctly rare (131).

Hodgkin Lymphoma

PTLD with the characteristics of Hodgkin lymphoma (HL) must be discriminated from polymorphic PTLD by applying the strictest criteria for the diagnosis of HL. This can be a difficult exercise compounded by the fact that HL PTLD is always EBV positive.

Methotrexate-associated Lymphoproliferative Disorders

These infrequent LPDs have been reported in patients treated with methotrexate for a variety of autoimmune diseases, especially rheumatoid arthritis (132). The intestine is the most common site of origin, and these LPDs cover the same histologic spectrum as PTLD. A few cases of follicular lymphoma have also been recorded.

ENTEROPATHY ASSOCIATED T-CELL LYMPHOMA

An association between malabsorption and intestinal lymphoma was first reported in 1937 (133), at which time it was thought that the lymphoma was in some way responsible for malabsorption. It subsequently became clear that the reverse is true (134) and that intestinal lymphoma was a complication of celiac disease or gluten-sensitive enteropathy. In 1978 Isaacson and Wright characterized celiac-associated lymphoma as a single entity, namely a variant of malignant histiocytosis (135). Later, Isaacson et al showed that both the phenotype and genotype of this disease were those of T cells rather than histiocytes (136). This type of lymphoma is now

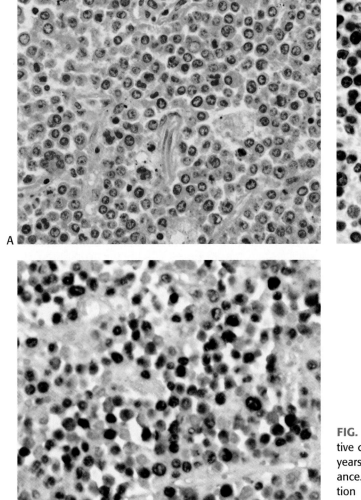

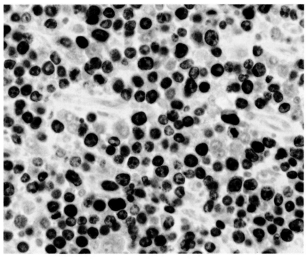

FIG. 18.50. A: Monomorphic posttransplant lymphoproliferative disorder in a patient who had received a renal transplant 8 years previously. The tumor cells have a plasmacytoid appearance. **B:** Immunostaining with Ki-67 shows a proliferation fraction of 100%. **C:** Epstein-Barr virus–encoded RNA in situ hybridization is positive.

included in the WHO classification of lymphoma as "enteropathy associated T-cell lymphoma" (EATL).

Definition

Enteropathy associated T-cell lymphoma is a tumor of intraepithelial lymphocytes showing varying degrees of transformation but usually presenting as a tumor of large lymphoid cells (5).

Epidemiology

Enteropathy associated T-cell lymphoma characteristically occurs in the 6th and 7th decades, although there are sporadic reports of cases in younger individuals. Males and females are affected equally. Most, if not all, patients with EATL have the celiac disease–associated human leukocyte antigen (HLA) DQA1 and DQB1 genotype (137). Enteropathy associated T-cell lymphoma is most common in those regions with the highest prevalence of celiac disease such as Northern Europe and very rare in regions such as the Far East, where celiac disease does not occur.

Etiology

There is strong evidence that EATL complicates celiac disease (gluten-sensitive enteropathy), discussed further in Chapter 6 (138,139). The lymphoma may complicate established celiac disease, sometimes only manifested by celiac-associated conditions such as dermatitis herpetiformis, of long standing but more usually follows a short history of adult-onset celiac disease and/or dermatitis herpetiformis. The assumption in these cases is that the patients have indeed had lifelong, albeit cryptic, gluten sensitivity. In keeping with this, in a proportion of cases there is no history of malabsorption but jejunal villous atrophy and crypt hyperplasia are found in the small intestinal mucosa when the tumor is resected. The only manifestation of celiac disease in some cases is an increase of intraepithelial T cells, while in a minority the jejunum appears normal or near normal. Studies showing that the jejunal mucosa can appear completely normal in celiac disease, so-called latency (140), provide an explanation for this finding, which was previously thought to argue against a strict association of EATL with celiac disease.

Further evidence for this association includes the identical HLA types of celiac patients and those with EATL (137), demonstration of gluten sensitivity in EATL patients, and the observation that in patients with celiac disease a gluten-free diet may protect against the development of lymphoma (141). There is controversy over the actual magnitude of the risk of lymphoma in celiac disease patients. In a recent study (142) the risk was increased sixfold, but this figure referred to lymphoma in general. Had specific risk of EATL been calculated, it would have been many times this figure.

Clinical Presentation

The most common presentation is the reappearance of malabsorption accompanied by abdominal pain in a patient with a history of adult or childhood celiac disease who has previously responded to a gluten-free diet. This may be accompanied by an ichthyotic skin rash and finger clubbing. Other presentations include the sudden onset of severe, usually gluten-insensitive malabsorption in a previously well individual or an acute abdominal emergency due to small intestinal perforation or hemorrhage. In most cases the lymphoma involves multiple segments of small intestine and has already disseminated at the time of diagnosis. Common sites of dissemination include mesenteric lymph nodes, liver, spleen, bone marrow, lung, and skin. Rarely, the lymphoma presents at one of these sites and intestinal involvement becomes apparent only later.

Gross Features

EATL may involve any part of the small intestine and occasionally other parts of the gastrointestinal tract including the colon and stomach, but in most cases arise in the jejunum. The tumor is usually, but not always, multifocal and forms ulcerating nodules, plaques, strictures, or, less commonly, large masses, which may be accompanied by benign-appearing ulcers and strictures (Fig. 18.51). The mesentery is often

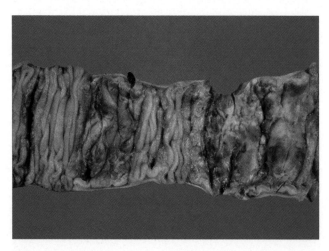

FIG. 18.51. Gross appearance of enteropathy associated T-cell lymphoma (ETL) showing multiple ulcerating lesions of the small intestine.

infiltrated and mesenteric lymph nodes are commonly involved. There is sometimes remarkably little macroscopic evidence of disease in the intestine as opposed to the mesenteric lymph nodes.

Histologic Features

The histologic features of EATL show great variation both between cases and within any single case (Fig. 18.52). The most characteristic appearance is that of a pleomorphic tumor of large lymphoid cells (Fig. 18.52A). Other cases may be composed of strikingly bizarre, often multinucleated giant cells (Fig. 18.52B) or more monomorphic cells with prominent central nucleoli leading to an immunoblastic appearance (Fig. 18.52C). In a substantial number of cases the number of inflammatory cells, particularly eosinophils, may be so great as to almost obscure the neoplastic T cells, especially in the presence of the extensive necrosis that often occurs in this variant (Fig. 18.52D). There is a subgroup of cases (143) (see below) in which the neoplastic T cells characteristically express CD56 and are only slightly larger than normal small lymphocytes. They often form monomorphic sheetlike infiltrates in the submucosa and muscularis propria (Fig. 18.53). In all variants intraepithelial tumor cells are usually prominent (Fig. 18.54). Granulomas may be present and cause confusion with Crohn disease.

The histology of the small intestinal mucosa remote from the site of the tumor is an important consideration in the diagnosis of EATL. In most cases the changes are identical to those of celiac disease. Thus, there are villous atrophy with crypt hyperplasia, plasmacytosis of the lamina propria, and increased numbers of intraepithelial lymphocytes (Fig. 18.55). Like uncomplicated celiac disease, the mucosal changes are maximal proximally and improve distally so that the lower jejunum and ileum may be normal. This must be borne in mind when the lymphoma arises in the more distal small intestine. In some cases of celiac disease the changes in the mucosa are much less severe. The villous architecture may be normal and the only hint of celiac disease is an increase in intraepithelial lymphocytes best seen in immunostained preparations. The degree of intraepithelial lymphocytosis may be spectacular and so extreme as to virtually obscure the epithelial cells. The lymphocytes are small, without neoplastic features, and in these extreme cases spill into the lamina propria, where they may merge with the lymphomatous infiltrate (Fig. 18.56).

Numerous shallow ulcers extending into the submucosa are frequently present in the mucosa remote from the lymphoma (Fig. 18.57). The bases of these ulcers contain an inflammatory infiltrate of small lymphocytes and plasma cells with an overlying acute inflammatory exudate. Episodes of ulceration followed by healing lead to scarring with stricture formation and distortion of mucosal architecture accentuated by destruction of the muscularis mucosae and the emergence of glands lined by cells of the ulceration-associated cell lineage (144), previously called pseudopyloric metaplasia.

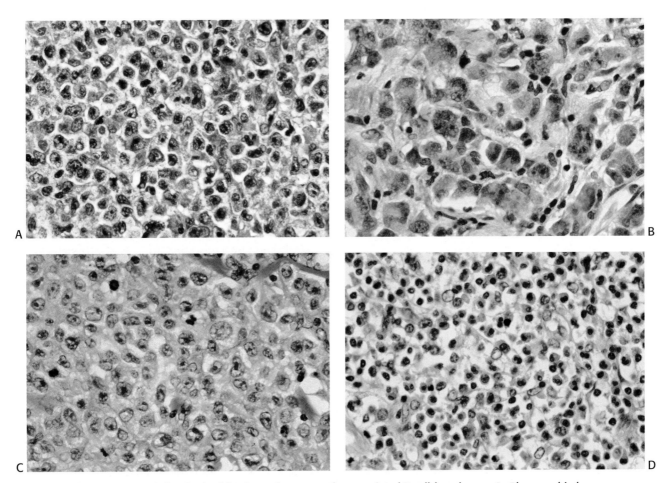

FIG. 18.52. Variation in the histology of enteropathy associated T-cell lymphoma. **A:** Pleomorphic large cell variant. **B:** Bizarre multinucleated giant cell variant. **C:** Monomorphic immunoblastic variant. **D:** Inflammatory variant.

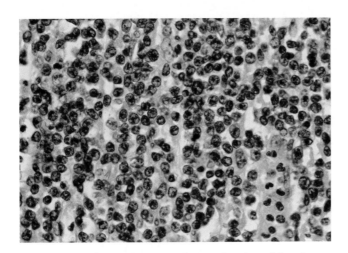

FIG. 18.53. Subtype of enteropathy associated T-cell lymphoma composed of monomorphic small cells.

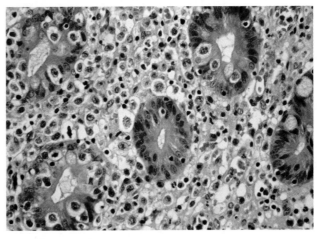

FIG. 18.54. Mucosa in enteropathy associated T-cell lymphoma showing intraepithelial invasion by tumor cells.

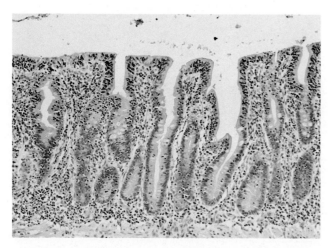

FIG. 18.55. The uninvolved mucosa in enteropathy associated T-cell lymphoma shows villous atrophy with crypt hyperplasia.

Lymph Node Involvement

The pattern of mesenteric lymph node involvement may be predominantly intrasinusoidal, paracortical, or both (Fig. 18.58). Selective necrosis of lymph nodes, often involving entire nodes, remote from the main lesion is a feature of some cases (145) (Fig. 18.59). The cause of this necrosis is obscure.

Immunohistochemistry and Molecular Genetics

In most cases of EATL the tumor cells express CD3, CD7, CD103, and granzyme B. They are usually CD4 and CD8 nega-

tive and express either the α/β or the γ/δ T-cell receptor. This immunophenotype is not consistent, however, and in some cases the cells fail to express CD3 or, more often, express CD8. Those cases of EATL composed of large anaplastic cells are usually CD30 positive. In the subset of EATL cases composed of monomorphic sheets of small lymphoid cells, the immunophenotype is distinctive in that the tumor cells express CD3, CD8, CD56, and granzyme B. The immunophenotype of the intraepithelial T cells in the uninvolved small intestinal mucosa may be normal, but more often, in common with the accompanying lymphoma, they fail to express CD8 (Fig. 18.60).

Genotypic studies of EATL have shown clonal rearrangement of the T-cell receptor (TCR) β- and γ- chain genes (146). PCR amplification of the T-cell receptor γ-chain gene has shown that the tumor cell clone can be amplified from the uninvolved mucosa in a significant number of cases. Chromosomal gains at 9q have been reported in a series of ETL cases, while a further study has shown loss of heterozygosity at chromosome 9p (147,148). Baumgartner et al showed that there was a high frequency of chromosomal alterations in EATL (149), and later the same group showed that these involved amplification of *NOTCH1* and *ABL1* genes (150). In common with some other T-cell lymphomas, EBV DNA in monoclonal form and latent membrane protein 1 have been demonstrated in EATL, particularly in cases reported from central America (151).

Postulated Normal Cell Counterpart

The immunophenotypic features of EATL approximate those of intraepithelial T lymphocytes (IELs), which are thought to

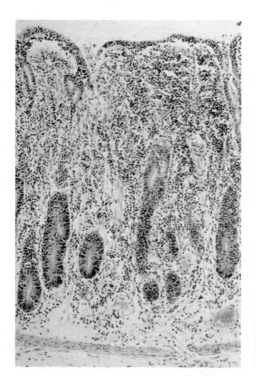

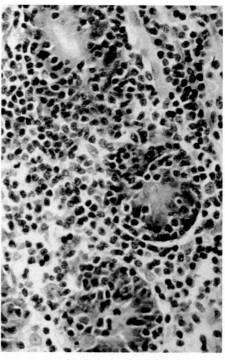

FIG. 18.56. Florid intraepithelial lymphocytosis with spillage of small intraepithelial lymphocytes into the lamina propria (*right*).

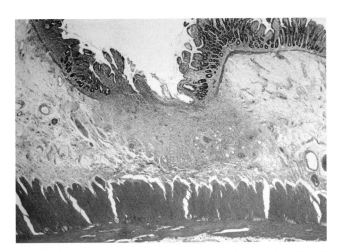

FIG. 18.57. Uninvolved mucosa in enteropathy associated T-cell lymphoma showing inflammatory ulceration.

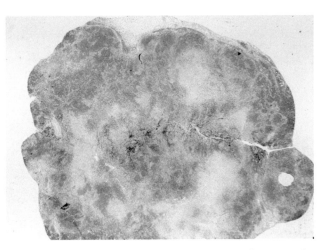

FIG. 18.59. Mesenteric lymph node from a case of enteropathy associated T-cell lymphoma showing large areas of necrosis. There was no evidence of lymphoma.

be the normal cell counterpart of this lymphoma (152). Intraepithelial lymphocytes are, however, phenotypically heterogeneous (153–155). Most are cytotoxic T cells that express CD3 and CD8 and have rearranged TCR γ-chain genes. There is a minority population of CD4- and CD8-negative IELs with rearranged γ/δ- but not α/β-chain genes. These γ/δ positive T cells comprise 10% to 15% of IELs in normal mucosa and may increase in concentration in patients with celiac disease up to a level of 30%. Finally, there is a third population of CD56-positive cells that accounts for a very small fraction of IELs that is virtually undetectable in immunostained paraffin sections (unpublished observations).

Prognosis

The clinical course of ETL is very unfavorable except in a minority of cases in which resection of a localized tumor has been followed by long remission. In most cases the

lymphoma involves multiple segments of intestine, rendering resection impossible, or has already disseminated beyond the mesenteric lymph nodes or out of the abdomen. Chemotherapy, sometimes with added bone marrow transplantation, may result in temporary remission of the disease.

REFRACTORY CELIAC DISEASE

Some cases of celiac disease become unresponsive to a gluten-free diet or may be unresponsive de novo. The term *refractory celiac disease* or, more commonly, *refractory sprue* has been used for these cases (156). While the onset of refractory celiac disease may more or less immediately precede

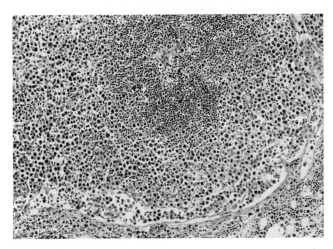

FIG. 18.58. Mesenteric lymph node showing infiltration by enteropathy associated T-cell lymphoma.

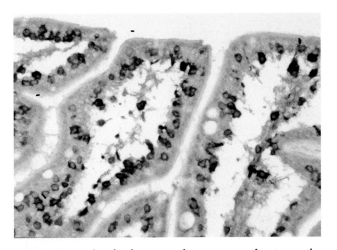

FIG. 18.60. Uninvolved mucosa from a case of enteropathy associated T-cell lymphoma double-stained for CD8 (*brown*) and CD3 (*blue*) showing increased numbers of phenotypically aberrant CD8-negative intraepithelial T cells. The main tumor was also CD3 positive, CD8 negative.

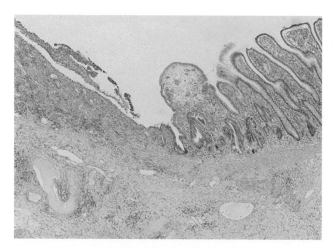

FIG. 18.61. A case of refractory celiac disease showing nonspecific inflammatory ulceration (ulcerative jejunitis).

EATL, other cases persist as refractory celiac disease for many years without the emergence of overt lymphoma. Nonspecific inflammatory ulcers of the small intestinal mucosa, identical to those that occur in EATL, are often present in refractory celiac disease, when it has been termed *ulcerative jejunitis* (Fig. 18.61) (157). Studies of TCR genes in both ETL and refractory celiac disease have now elucidated the relationship between the two conditions.

Using PCR followed by sequence analysis of TCR γ genes, Murray et al (146) showed that there was a T-cell population in the "uninvolved" enteropathic small intestinal mucosa adjacent to EATL that shared the same monoclonal TCR γ rearrangement as the lymphoma. Ashton-Key et al confirmed this finding and further showed TCR γ monoclonality in the nonspecific "inflammatory" ulcers that accompanied EATL as well as in the ulcers and intervening mucosa of refractory sprue (158). In cases where lymphoma subsequently developed, the same clone could be detected in the malignant cells by PCR and sequence analysis. Cellier et al (159) investigated cases of refractory sprue and showed that in this condition, monoclonal populations of T cells are present in the small intestinal mucosa. They showed that this monoclonal population is constituted by phenotypically abnormal CD3-positive/-negative, CD4-negative, and CD8-negative intraepithelial lymphocytes (Fig. 18.62). Cellier et al later drew together the clinical and laboratory features of refractory sprue (160). Importantly, they definitively clarified the relationship between celiac disease and refractory sprue by showing the presence of celiac disease–specific antiendomysial or antigliadin antibodies, in most cases together with other characteristics of celiac disease including a previous response to gluten withdrawal or the characteristic HLA DQA1*0501 and DQB1*0201 phenotype (137). Additionally, they showed that in all truly refractory cases, the intraepithelial lymphocytes

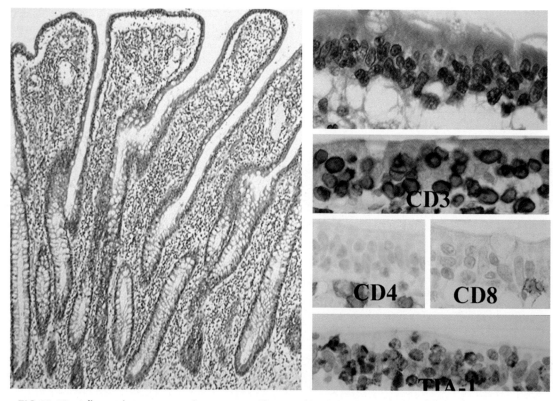

FIG 18.62. Adjacent intact mucosa in same case illustrated in Figure 18.61. Increased CD3-positive intraepithelial T cells are CD4 negative but positive for cytotoxic granules (TIA-1) (*bottom right*).

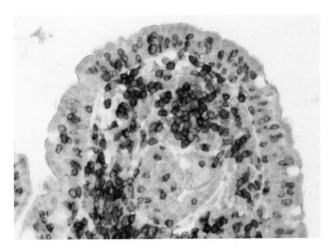

FIG 18.63. Mucosa from a case of refractory celiac disease double-stained for CD8 (*brown*) and CD3 (*blue*). There are increased numbers of CD3-positive intraepithelial T cells with an aberrant CD8-negative phenotype.

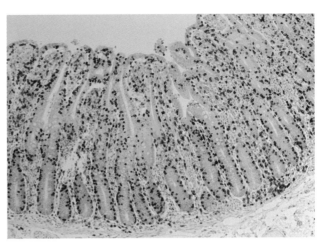

FIG. 18.64. Uninvolved mucosa from a case of CD56-positive enteropathy associated T-cell lymphoma showing large numbers of CD56-positive intraepithelial T cells.

were either monoclonal, expressed an abnormal immunophenotype, or both.

The studies summarized above raise several questions regarding the significance of the detection of a monoclonal T-cell population in the small intestine. Firstly, where exactly do these cells reside and what is their phenotype? Secondly, what is the link, if any, between these different complications of celiac disease that are characterized by monoclonal populations of T cells in enteropathic mucosa? Thirdly, is clonality synonymous with neoplasia or even malignancy? Finally, what are the implications of detecting such a population for patient management?

Bagdi et al (161) showed that in double-stained (CD8/CD3) preparations of sections of small intestine from refractory celiac disease patients with a monoclonal T-cell population in their small intestinal mucosa, there was a marked decrease in the proportion of CD8-positive intraepithelial lymphocytes (Fig. 18.63). Moreover, in cases of EATL, the cytologically bland intraepithelial lymphocytes in the intervening mucosa shared the immunophenotype and genotype of the lymphoma. Specifically, in monomorphic CD56-positive cases, these lymphocytes also expressed CD56 (Fig. 18.64). Interestingly, these clonal and immunophenotypically aberrant intraepithelial lymphocytes were often present in the crypt epithelium, in contrast to uncomplicated celiac disease, where they are confined to the surface epithelium. Moreover, these cells were widely distributed throughout the gastrointestinal tract from stomach to anus.

It would seem safe to conclude, therefore, that the monoclonal intraepithelial lymphocytes in patients with refractory sprue are neoplastic, although they are not cytologically abnormal and they do not form tumor masses. The accumulation of phenotypically aberrant, monoclonal intraepithelial lymphocytes appears to be the first step in the genesis of EATL. Patients with refractory celiac disease and/or ulcerative jejunitis are therefore suffering from a neoplastic T-cell disorder, possibly involving most of the gastrointestinal tract. Treatment of this group of patients, most of whom have severe unremitting malabsorption, is difficult. It is uncertain whether chemotherapeutic regimens appropriate for lymphoma have anything to offer in this respect or whether new strategies will need to be devised. Further, cell and molecular biologic investigations are indicated, particularly to establish the precise relationship between the neoplastic intraepithelial lymphocytes and the cells of fully developed EATL.

OTHER TYPES OF T-CELL LYMPHOMA UNASSOCIATED WITH ENTEROPATHY

Carbonnel et al described a distinctive intestinal *T-cell lymphoma composed of small CD4-positive lymphocytes* widely distributed throughout the lamina propria of the intestinal mucosa (162). In common with ETL, this suggests a specific association with native gut lymphoid tissue, in this case the lamina propria rather than the intraepithelial T-cells. These cases are characterized by a slow relentless course and prolonged survival, an unusual feature for T-cell lymphomas.

Cases of *CD56-positive T/NK-cell lymphoma of nasal type*, although typically occurring in the upper respiratory tract, not only frequently spreads to the gastrointestinal tract, but may arise there as a primary tumor (20). The lymphoma involves multiple sites, forming tumor masses. Typically, it also infiltrates long segments of intestinal mucosa, where it is associated with villous atrophy, but unlike EATL, this is seen only in mucosa infiltrated by lymphoma; the villous architecture of uninvolved mucosa is normal.

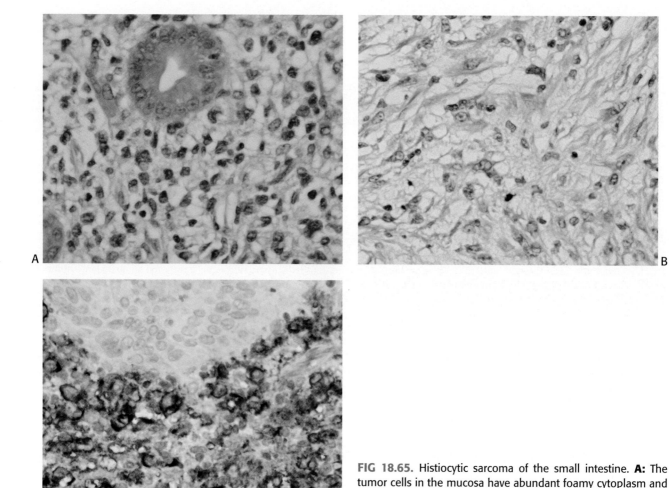

FIG 18.65. Histiocytic sarcoma of the small intestine. **A:** The tumor cells in the mucosa have abundant foamy cytoplasm and hyperchromatic, polymorphic nuclei. **B:** The tumor cells invading the serosa are spindle shaped. **C:** The tumor cells express histiocytic antigens such as CD163.

There are numerous isolated case reports of a wide variety of T-cell lymphomas arising in the gastrointestinal tract, but they do not comprise recognized clinicopathologic entities.

HISTIOCYTIC SARCOMA

True histiocytic neoplasms of the intestine are well documented (163–166). All the tumors arose in the small intestine, where they produced ulcerating masses. The tumor cells typically have abundant cytoplasm that is sometimes foamy (Fig. 18.65A). They may be bizarre, are often multinucleated, and in some case are focally arranged in a spindle cell sarcomalike pattern (Fig. 18.65B). Lymph nodes have been involved in all of the cases. The immunophenotype is that of histiocytes (macrophages), CD11c, CD163 (Fig. 18.65C), lysozyme, and CD68 positive. Cells with dendritic cell properties manifested by tortuous nuclei and focal S100 positivity are also often present. These tumors have a high mortality.

LANGERHANS CELL HISTIOCYTOSIS

Langerhans histiocytosis occasionally involves the digestive tract, where it presents as isolated foci of histiocytes with abundant eosinophilic cytoplasm and grooved or "coffee bean–like" nuclei (Fig. 18.66). The cells are typically CD1a and S100 positive (Fig.18.66B,C).

GRANULOCYTIC SARCOMA

Rarely, acute myeloid leukemia presents as an isolated gastrointestinal tumor that can easily be confused with a lymphoma (167). The characteristic, finely granular nucleus lacking nucleoli (Fig. 18.67) and the presence of eosinophil metamyelocytes should lead to the correct diagnosis. This can be confirmed by appropriate immunohistochemical staining for myeloperoxidase, CD56, CD34 (Fig. 18.67), and lysozyme. Acute leukemia usually manifests soon after the diagnosis, but intervals as long as 15 years have been reported.

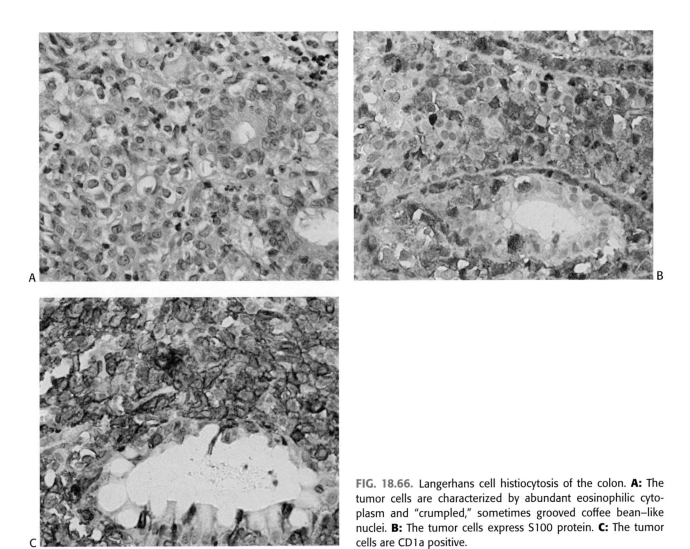

FIG. 18.66. Langerhans cell histiocytosis of the colon. **A:** The tumor cells are characterized by abundant eosinophilic cytoplasm and "crumpled," sometimes grooved coffee bean–like nuclei. **B:** The tumor cells express S100 protein. **C:** The tumor cells are CD1a positive.

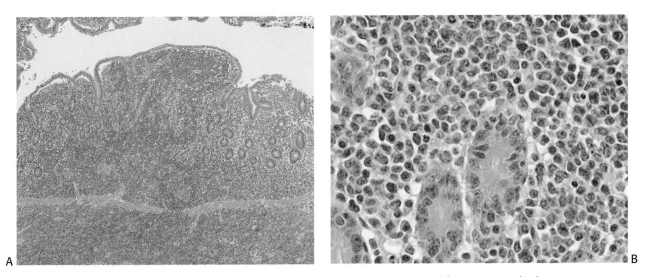

FIG. 18.67. Granulocytic sarcoma of the small intestine. **A:** There is invasion of the mucosa and submucosa. **B:** Higher magnification shows large cells with granular nuclear chromatin, lacking nucleoli. (*continues*)

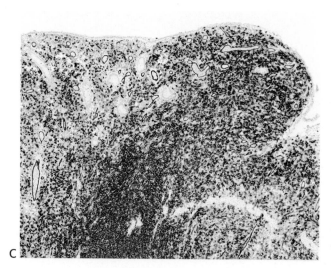

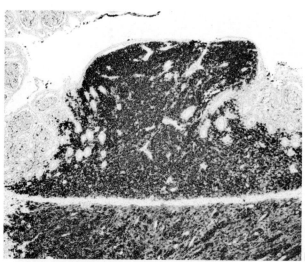

FIG. 18.67. (*Continued*) **C:** The tumor cells are CD56 positive. **D:** The tumor cells express CD34.

REFERENCES

1. Freeman C, Berg JW, Cutler SJ: Occurrence and prognosis of extranodal lymphomas. *Cancer* 1972;29:252.
2. Otter R, Bieger R, Kluin PM, et al: Primary gastrointestinal non-Hodgkin's lymphoma in a population-based registry. *Br J Cancer* 1989;60:745.
3. Azab MB, Henry-Amar M, Rougier P, et al: Prognostic factors in primary gastrointestinal non-Hodgkin's lymphoma: a multivariate analysis, report of 106 cases, and review of the literature. *Cancer* 1989;64:1208.
4. Hayes J, Dunn E: Has the incidence of primary gastric lymphoma increased? *Cancer* 1989;63:2073.
5. Salem P, Anaissie E, Allam C, et al: Non-Hodgkin's lymphomas in the Middle East. A study of 417 patients with emphasis on special features. *Cancer* 1986;58:1162.
6. Doglioni C, Wotherspoon AC, Moschini A, et al: High incidence of primary gastric lymphoma in northeastern Italy. *Lancet* 1992;339:834.
7. Fischbach W, Kestel W, Kirchner T, et al: Malignant lymphomas of the upper gastrointestinal tract. Results of a prospective study in 103 patients. *Cancer* 1992;70:1075.
8. Dawson IMP, Cornes JS, Morson BC: Primary malignant lymphoid tumours of the intestinal tract. Report of 37 cases with a study of factors influencing prognosis. *Br J Surg* 1961;49:80.
9. Mihaljevic B, Nedeljkov-Jancic R, Vujicic V, et al: Primary extranodal lymphomas of gastrointestinal localizations: a single institution 5-yr experience. *Med Oncol* 2006;23:225.
10. Nakamura S, Matsumoto T, Iida M, et al: Primary gastrointestinal lymphoma in Japan: a clinicopathologic analysis of 455 patients with special reference to its time trends. *Cancer* 2003;97:2462.
11. Musshoff K: Klinische Stadieneinteilung der Nicht-Hodgkin-Lymphome. *Strahlentherapie* 1977;153:218.
12. Jaffe E, Harris NL, Stein H, Vardiman JW (eds): *World Health Organization Classification of Tumours. Pathology and Genetics of Tumours of Haematopoietic and Lymphoid Tissues.* Lyon, France: IARC Press, 2001.
13. Isaacson PG, Dogan A, Price SK, et al: Immunoproliferative small-intestinal disease: an immunohistochemical study. *Am J Surg Pathol* 1989;13:1023.
14. Price SK: Immunoproliferative small intestinal disease: a study of 13 cases with alpha heavy-chain disease. *Histopathology* 1990;17:7.
15. Chan JKC, Ng CS, Isaacson PG: Relationship between high-grade lymphoma and low-grade B-cell mucosa-associated lymphoid tissue lymphoma (MALToma) of the stomach. *Am J Pathol* 1990;136:1153.
16. Isaacson PG, MacLennan KA, Subbuswamy SG: Multiple lymphomatous polyposis of the gastrointestinal tract. *Histopathology* 1984;8:641.
17. Ladjadj Y, Philip T, Lenoir GM, et al: Abdominal Burkitt-type lymphomas in Algeria. *Br J Cancer* 1984;49:503.
18. Isaacson P, Wright DH: Malignant histiocytosis of the intestine. Its relationship to malabsorption and ulcerative jejunitis. *Hum Pathol* 1978;9:661.
19. Isaacson PG, O'Connor NTJ, Spencer J, et al: Malignant histiocytosis of the intestine: a T-cell lymphoma. *Lancet* 1985;ii:688.
20. Lu D, Lin CN, Chuang SS, et al: T-cell and NK/T-cell lymphomas in southern Taiwan: a study of 72 cases in a single institute. *Leuk Lymphoma* 2004;45:823.
21. Brugo EA, Marshall RB, Riberi AM, et al: Preleukemic granulocytic sarcomas of the gastrointestinal tract. Report of two cases. *Am J Clin Pathol* 1977;68:616.
22. Radaszkiewicz T, Dragosics B, Bauer P: Gastrointestinal malignant lymphomas of the mucosa-associated lymphoid tissue: factors relevant to prognosis. *Gastroenterology* 1992;02:1628.
23. Isaccson P, Wright DH: Malignant lymphoma of mucosa-associated lymphoid tissue. A distinctive type of B-cell lymphoma. *Cancer* 1983;52:1410.
24. Isaacson P, Wright DH: Extranodal malignant lymphoma arising from mucosa-associated lymphoid tissue. *Cancer* 1984;53:2515.
25. Spencer J, Finn T, Isaacson PG: Human Peyer's patches: an immunohistochemical study. *Gut* 1986;27:405.
26. Spencer J, Finn T, Isaacson PG: Gut associated lymphoid tissue: a morphological and immunocytochemical study of the human appendix. *Gut* 1985;26:672.
27. Spencer J, Finn T, Pulford KAF, et al: The human gut contains a novel population of B lymphocytes which resemble marginal zone cells. *Clin Exp Immunol* 1985;62:607.
28. Ranaldi R, Goteri G, Baccarini MG, et al: A clinicopathological study of 152 surgically treated primary gastric lymphomas with survival analysis of 109 high grade tumours. *J Clin Pathol* 2002;55:346.
29. Lymphoma Classification Project: A clinical evaluation of the International Lymphoma Study Group classification of non-Hodgkin's lymphoma. *Blood* 1997;89:3909.
30. Saito T, Tamaru J, Kishi H, et al: Extranodal marginal zone B-cell lymphoma of mucosa-associated lymphoid tissue (MALT lymphoma) arising in the small intestine with monoclonal cryoglobulinemia. *Pathol Int* 2004;54:712.
31. Miyazaki T, Kato H, Masuda N, et al: Mucosa-associated lymphoid tissue lymphoma of the esophagus: case report and review of the literature. *Hepatogastroenterology* 2004;51:750.
32. Wyatt JL, Rathbone BJ: Immune response of the gastric mucosa to Campylobacter pylori. *Scand J Gastroenterol* 1988;suppl 142:44.
33. Lecuit M, Aberchin E, Martin A, et al: Immunoproliferative small intestinal disease associated with Campylobacter jejuni. *N Engl J Med* 2004;350:239.
34. Wotherspoon AC, Ortiz-Hidalgo C, Falzon MR, et al: Helicobacter pylori-associated gastritis and primary B-cell gastric lymphoma. *Lancet* 1991;338:1175.

35. Nakamura S, Yao T, Aoyagi K, et al: Helicobacter pylori and primary gastric lymphoma. A histopathologic and immunohistochemical analysis of 237 patients. *Cancer* 1997;79:3.

36. Nakamura S, Aoyagi K, Fruruse M, et al: B-cell monoclonality precedes the development of gastric MALT lymphoma in *Helicobacter pylori*-associated chronic gastritis. *Am J Pathol* 1998;152:1271.

37. Parsonnet J, Hansen S, Rodriguez L, et al: *Helicobacter pylori* infection and gastric lymphoma. *N Engl J Med* 1994;330:1267.

38. Hussell T, Isaacson PG, Crabtree JE, et al: The response of cells from low-grade B-cell gastric lymphomas of mucosa-associated lymphoid tissue to *Helicobacter pylori*. *Lancet* 1993;342:571.

39. Wotherspoon AC, Doglioni D, Diss TC, et al: Regression of primary low-grade B-cell gastric lymphoma of mucosa-associated lymphoid tissue type after eradication of Helicobacter pylori. *Lancet* 1993;342: 575.

40. Stolte M, Bayerdorffer E, Morgner A: Helicobacter and gastric MALT lymphoma. *Gut* 2002;50:III19.

41. Isaacson PG: Gastrointestinal lymphoma and lymphoid hyperplasias. In: Knowles DM (ed). *Neoplastic Hematopathology*, 2nd ed. Philadelphia: Lippincott Williams and Wilkins, 2001.

42. His ED, Greenson JK, Singleton TP, et al: Detection of immunoglobulin heavy chain gene rearrangement by polymerase chain reaction in chronic active gastritis associated with Helicobacter pylori. *Hum Pathol* 1996;27:290.

43. De Mascarel A, Dubus P, Belleanne G, et al: Low prevalence of monoclonal B-cells in Helicobacter pylori gastritis patients with duodenal ulcer. *Hum Pathol* 1998;29:784.

44. Raderer M, Wohrer S, Streubel B, et al: Assessment of disease dissemination in gastric compared with extragastric mucosa-associated lymphoid tissue lymphoma using extensive staging: a single-center experience. *J Clin Oncol* 2006;24:3136.

45. Du MQ, Diss TC, Dogan A, et al: Clone-specific PCR reveals wide dissemination of gastric MALT lymphoma to the gastric mucosa. *J Pathol* 2000;192:488.

46. Isaacson PG, Spencer J: Malignant lymphoma of mucosa-associated lymphoid tissue. *Histopathology* 1989;11:445.

47. Isaacson PG, Wotherspoon AC, Diss T, et al: Follicular colonization in B-cell lymphoma of mucosa-associated lymphoid tissue. *Am J Surg Pathol* 1991;15:819.

48. DeJong D, Boot H, Van Heerde P, et al: Histological grading in gastric lymphoma: pre-treatment criteria and clinical relevance. *Gastroenterology* 1997;112:1466.

49. Harris NL, Jaffe ES, Diebold J, et al: The World Health Organization classification of neoplasms of the hematopoietic and lymphoid tissues: report of the Clinical Advisory Committee meeting – Airlie House, Virginia, November, 1997. *Hematol J* 2000;1:53.

50. Thiede C, Wundisch T, Alpen B, et al: Long-term persistence of monoclonal B cells after cure of Helicobacter pylori infection and complete histologic remission in gastric mucosa-associated lymphoid tissue B-cell lymphoma. *J Clin Oncol* 2001;19:1600.

51. Thieblemont C, Berger F, Dumontet C, et al: Mucosa-associated lymphoid tissue lymphoma is a disseminated disease in one third of 158 patients analyzed. *Blood* 2000;95:802.

52. Wotherspoon AC, Doglioni C, Isaacson PG: Low-grade gastric B-cell lymphoma of mucosa-associated lymphoid tissue (MALT): a multifocal disease. *Histopathology* 1992;20:29.

53. Du M, Diss TC, Xu C, et al: Ongoing mutation in MALT lymphoma immunoglobulin gene suggests that antigen stimulation plays a role in the clonal expansion. *Leukemia* 1996;10:1190.

54. Diss TC, Pan L: Polymerase chain reaction in the assessment of lymphomas. *Cancer Surv* 1997;30:21.

55. Sorrentino D, Ferraccili G, DeVita S, et al: B-cell clonality and infection with Helicobacter pylori: Implications for development of gastric lymphoma. *Gut* 1996;38:837.

56. Soni M, Shabbab I, Fitzgerald M, et al: Detection of clonality in B-cell proliferation in Helicobacter pylori induced chronic gastritis in pediatric patients. *Mod Pathol* 1997;10:65A.

57. Montalbaan C, Castrillo JM, Abraira V, et al: Gastric B-cell mucosa-associated lymphoid tissue (MALT) lymphoma. Clinicopathological study and evaluation of the prognostic factors in 143 patients. *Ann Oncol* 1995;6:355.

58. Qin Y, Greiner A, Trunk MJF, et al: Somatic hypermutation in low-grade mucosa-associated lymphoid tissue-type B-cell lymphoma. *Blood* 1995;86:3528.

59. Akagi T, Motegi M, Tamura A, et al: A novel gene, MALT1 at 18q21, is involved in t(11;18) (q21;q21) found in low-grade B-cell lymphoma of mucosa-associated lymphoid tissue. *Oncogene* 1999;18:5785.

60. Dierlamm J, Baens M, Wlodarska I, et al: The apoptosis inhibitor gene *API2* and a novel 18q gene, *MLT*, are recurrently rearranged in the t(11;18)(q21;q21) associated with mucosa-associated lymphoid tissue lymphomas. *Blood* 1999;93:3601.

61. Morgan JA, Borowsky AD, Kuo F, et al: Breakpoints of the t(11;18) (q21;q21) in mucosa-associated lymphoid tissue (MALT) lymphoma lie within or near the previously undescribed gene *MALT1* in chromosome 18. *Cancer Res* 1999;59:6205.

62. Willis TG: Bcl10 is involved in t(1;14)(p22;q32) of MALT B cell lymphoma and mutated in multiple tumor types. *Cell* 1999;96:35.

63. Zhang Q, Siebert R, Yan M, et al: Inactivating mutations and overexpression of *BCL10*, a caspase recruitment domain-containing gene, in MALT lymphoma with t(1;14)(p22;q32). *Nature Genet* 1999;22:63.

64. Sanchez-Izquierdo D, Buchonnet G, Siebert R, et al: *MALT1* is deregulated by both chromosomal translocation and amplification in B-cell non-Hodgkin lymphoma. *Blood* 2003;101:4539.

65. Streubel B, Lamprecht A, Dierlamm J, et al: T(14;18)(q32;q21) involving IGH and MALT1 is a frequent chromosomal aberration in MALT lymphoma. *Blood* 2003;101:2335.

66. Isaacson PG, Du MQ: MALT lymphoma: from morphology to molecules. *Nat Rev Cancer* 2004;4:644.

67. Streubel B, Simonitsch-Klupp I, Mullauer L, et al: Variable frequencies of MALT lymphoma-associated genetic aberrations in MALT lymphomas of different sites. *Leukemia* 2004;18:1722.

68. Remstein ED, Kurtin PJ, James CD, et al: Mucosa-associated lymphoid tissue lymphomas with t(11;18)(q21;q21) and mucosa-associated lymphoid tissue lymphomas with aneuploidy develop along different pathogenetic pathways. *Am J Pathol* 2002;161:63.

69. Chuang SS, Lee C, Hamoudi RA, et al: High frequency of t(11;18) in gastric mucosa-associated lymphoid tissue lymphomas in Taiwan, including one patient with high-grade transformation. *Br J Haematol* 2003;120:97.

70. Liu H, Ruskon-Formestraux A, Lavergne-Slove A, et al: Resistance of t(11;18) positive gastric mucosa-associated lymphoid tissue lymphoma to *Helicobacter pylori* eradication therapy. *Lancet* 2000;357:39.

71. Ott G, Katzenberger T, Greiner A, et al: The t(11;18)(q21;q21) chromosome translocation is a frequent and specific aberration in low-grade but not high-grade malignant non-Hodgkin's lymphomas of the mucosa-associated lymphoid tissue (MALT-) type. *Cancer Res* 1997; 57:944.

72. Zhou Y, Ye H, Martin-Subero JI, et al: Distinct comparative genomic hybridisation profiles in gastric mucosa-associated lymphoid tissue lymphomas with and without t(11;18)(q21;q21). *Br J Haematol* 2006;133:35.

73. Cogliatti SB, Schmid U, Schumacher U, et al: Primary B-cell gastric lymphoma: a clinicopathological study of 145 patients. *Gastroenterology* 1991;101:1159.

74. Sackman M, Morgner A, Rudolph B, et al: Regression of gastric MALT lymphoma after eradication of Helicobacter pylori is predicted by endosonographic staging. MALT Lymphoma Study Group. *Gastroenterology* 1997;113:1087.

75. Nakamura S, Matsumoto T, Suekane H, et al: Predictive value of endoscopic ultrasonography for regression of gastric low grade and high grade MALT lymphomas after eradication of Helicobacter pylori. *Gut* 2001;48:454.

76. Chen LT, Lin JT, Shyu RY, et al: Prospective study of Helicobacter pylori eradication therapy in stage I(E) high-grade mucosa-associated lymphoid tissue lymphoma of the stomach. *J Clin Oncol* 2001;19:4245.

77. Alpen B, Robbecke J, Wundisch T, et al: Helicobacter pylori eradication therapy in gastric high grade non-Hodgkin's lymphoma (NHL). *Ann Haematol* 2001;80:B106.

78. Liu H, Ye H, Ruskone-Fourmestraux A, et al: T(11;18) is a marker for all stage gastric MALT lymphomas that will not respond to H. pylori eradication. *Gastroenterology* 2002;122:1286.

79. Liu H, Ye H, Dogan A, et al: T(11;18)(q21;q21) is associated with advanced MALT lymphoma that expresses nuclear BCL10. *Blood* 2001;98:1182.

80. Baron BW, Bitter MA, Baron JM, Bostwick DG: Gastric adenocarcinoma after gastric lymphoma. *Cancer* 1987;60:1876.

81. Shani A, Schutt AJ, Weiland LH: Primary gastric malignant lymphoma followed by gastric adenocarcinoma: report of 4 cases and review of the literature. *Cancer* 1978;42:2039.

82. Nakamura S, Yao T, Aoyagi K, et al: Helicobacter pylori and primary gastric lymphoma. A histopathologic and immunohistochemical analysis of 237 patients. *Cancer* 1997;79:3.

83. Parsonnet J, Friedman GD, Vandersteen DP, et al: Helicobacter pylori infection and the risk of gastric carcinoma. *N Engl J Med* 1991; 325:1127.

84. Cogliatti SB, Schmid U, Schumacher U, et al: Primary B-cell gastric lymphoma: a clinicopathological study of 145 patients. *Gastroenterology* 1991;101:1159.

85. Villuendas R, Piris MA, Orradre JL, et al: Different bcl-2 protein expression in high-grade B-cell lymphomas derived from lymph node or mucosa-associated lymphoid tissue. *Am J Pathol* 1991;139:989.

86. Omonishi K, Yoshino T, Sakuma I, et al: Bcl-6 protein is identified in high-grade but not low-grade mucosa-associated lymphoid tissue lymphomas of the stomach. *Mod Pathol* 1998;11:181.

87. Liang R, Chan WP, Kwong, YL, et al: High incidence of BCL-6 gene rearrangement in diffuse large B-cell lymphoma of primary gastric origin. *Cancer Genet Ctyogenet* 1997;97:114.

88. Liang R, Chan WP, Kwong YL, et al: Bcl-6 gene hypermutations in diffuse large B-cell lymphoma of primary gastric origin. *Br J Haematol* 1997;99:668.

89. Du M, Peng H, Singh N, et al: The accumulation of p53 abnormalities is associated with progression of mucosa-associated lymphoid tissue lymphoma. *Blood* 1995;86:4587.

90. Ott G, Katzenberger T, Greiner A, et al: The t(11;18)(q21;q21) chromosome translocation is a frequent and specific aberration in low-grade but not high-grade malignant non-Hodgkin's lymphomas of the mucosa-associated lymphoid tissue (MALT) type. *Cancer Res* 1977; 57:3944.

91. Raghoebier S, Kramer MHH, van Krieken JHJM, et al: Essential differences in oncogene involvement between primary nodal and extranodal large cell lymphoma. *Blood* 1991;78:2680.

92. Chen LT, Lin JT, Shyu, RY, et al: Prospective study of Helicobacter pylori eradication therapy in stage I(E) high-grade mucosa-associated lymphoid tissue lymphoma of the stomach. *J Clin Oncol* 2001;19:4245.

93. Alpen B, Robbecke J, Wundisch T, et al: Helicobacter pylori eradication therapy in gastric high grade non-Hodgkin's lymphoma (NHL). *Ann Haematol* 2001;80:B106.

94. Nakamura S, Matsumoto T, Takeshita M, et al: A clinicopathologic study of primary small intestine lymphoma: prognostic significance of mucosa-associated lymphoid tissue-derived lymphoma. *Cancer* 2000;88:286.

95. Domizio P, Owen RA, Shepherd NA, et al: Primary lymphoma of the small intestine: a clinicopathological study of 119 cases. *Am J Surg Pathol* 1993;17:429.

96. Greenstein AJ, Mullin GE, Strauchen JA, et al: Lymphoma in inflammatory bowel disease. *Cancer* 1992;69:1119.

97. Breslin NP, Urbanski SJ, Shaffer EA: Mucosa-associated lymphoid tissue (MALT) lymphoma manifesting as multiple lymphomatosis polyposis of the gastrointestinal tract. *Am J Gastroenterol* 1999;94:2540.

98. Yatabe Y, Nakamura S, Nakamura T, et al: Multiple polypoid lesions of primary mucosa-associated lymphoid-tissue lymphoma of colon. *Histopathology* 1998;32:116.

99. Spencer J, Diss TC, Isaacson PG: A study of the properties of a low-grade mucosal B-cell lymphoma using a monoclonal antibody specific for the tumour immunoglobulin. *J Pathol* 1990;160:231.

100. Fieber SS, Schaefer HJ: Lymphoid hyperplasia of the terminal ileum—a clinical entity? *Gastroenterology* 1966;50:83.

101. Rubin A, Isaacson PG: Florid reactive lymphoid hyperplasia of the terminal ileum in adults: a condition bearing a close resemblance to low-grade malignant lymphoma. *Histopathology* 1990;17:19.

102. Hermans PE, Huizenga KA, Hoffman HN, et al: Dysgammaglobulinemia associated with nodular lymphoid hyperplasia of the small intestine. *Am J Med* 1966;40:78.

103. Matuchansky C, Touchard G, Lemaire M, et al: Malignant lymphoma of the small bowel associated with diffuse nodular lymphoid hyperplasia. *N Engl J Med* 1985;313:166.

104. Shepherd NA, Hall PA, Coates PJ, et al: Primary malignant lymphoma of the colon and rectum. A histopathological and immunohistochemical analysis of 45 cases with clinicopathological correlations. *Histopathology* 1988;12:235.

105. Ramot B, Shahin N, Bubis JJ: Malabsorption syndrome in lymphoma of small intestine. A study of 13 cases. *Isr J Med Sci* 1965;1:221.

106. Rambaud JC, Modigliani R, Phuoc BK, et al: Non-secretory alpha-chain disease in intestinal lymphoma. *N Engl J Med* 1980;303:53.

107. Ben-Ayed F, Halphen M, Najjar T, et al: Treatment of alpha chain disease. Results of a prospective study in 21 Tunisian patients by the Tunisian-French Intestinal Lymphoma Study Group. *Cancer* 1989;63: 1251.

108. Zamir A, Parasher G, Moukarzal AA, et al: Immunoproliferative small intestinal disease in a 16-year-old boy presenting as severe malabsorption with excellent response to tetracycline treatment. *J Clin Gastroenterol* 1998;27:85.

109. Matsumoto S, Kinoshita Y, Fakuda H, et al: "Mediterranean lymphoma" treated with antibiotics. *Intern Med* 1996;35:961.

110. Galian A, Lecestre MJ, Scotto J, et al: Pathological study of alpha-chain disease, with special emphasis on evolution. *Cancer* 1977;39:2081.

111. Nemes Z, Thomázy V, Szeifert G: Follicular centre cell lymphoma with alpha heavy chain disease. A histopathological and immunohistochemical study. *Virchows Arch A Pathol Anat* 1981;394:119.

112. Isaacson PG, Price SK: Light chains in Mediterranean lymphoma. *J Clin Pathol* 1985;38:601.

113. Smith W, Price SK, Isaacson PG: Immunoglobulin gene rearrangement in immunoproliferative small intestinal disease (IPSID). *J Clin Pathol* 1987;40:1291.

114. Ye H, Liv H, Attygalle A, et al: Variable frequencies of t(11;18) in MALT lymphomas of different sites: significant association with Cag A strains of *H. Pylori* in gastric MALT lymphoma Blood 2003;102:1012.

115. O'Briain DS, Kennedy MJ, Daly PA, et al: Multiple lymphomatous polyposis of the gastrointestinal tract. A clinicopathologically distinctive form of non-Hodgkin's lymphoma of B-cell centrocytic type. *Am J Surg Pathol* 1989;13:691.

116. Banks PM, Chan J, Cleary ML, et al: Mantle cell lymphoma. A proposal for unification of morphologic, immunologic, and molecular data. *Am J Surg Pathol* 1992;16:637.

117. LeBrun DP, Kamel OW, Cleary ML, et al: Follicular lymphomas of the gastrointestinal tract. Pathologic features in 31 cases and bcl-2 oncogenic protein expression. *Am J Pathol* 1992;140:1327.

118. Misdraji J, Fernandez del Castillo C, Ferry JA: Follicle center lymphoma of the ampulla of Vater presenting with jaundice: report of a case. *Am J Surg Pathol* 1997;21:484.

119. Yoshino T, Miyake K, Ichimura K, et al: Increased incidence of follicular lymphoma in the duodenum. *Am J Surg Pathol* 2000;24:688.

120. Nadal E, Martinez A, Jimenez M, et al: Primary follicular lymphoma arising in the ampulla of Vater. *Ann Hematol* 2002;81:228.

121. Bende RJ, Smit LA, Bossenbroek JG, et al: Primary follicular lymphoma of the small intestine. a4b7 expression and immunoglobulin configuration suggest and origin from local antigen-experienced B cells. *Am J Pathol* 2003;162:105.

122. Anaissie E, Geha S, Allam C, et al: Burkitt's lymphoma in the Middle East: a study of 34 cases. *Cancer* 1985;56:2539.

123. Wotherspoon AC, Diss TC, Pan L, et al: Low grade gastric B-cell lymphoma of mucosa-associated lymphoid tissue in immunocompromised patients. *Histopathology* 1996;28:129.

124. Desar IM, Keuter M, Raemaekers JM, et al: Extranodal marginal zone (MALT) lymphoma in common variable immunodeficiency. *Net J Med* 2006;64:136.

125. Purtilo DT, Strobach RS, Okarno M, et al: Epstein-Barr virus-associated lymphoproliferative disorders. *Lab Invest* 1992;67:5.

126. Nalesnik MA, Jaffe R, Starzl TE, et al: The pathology of posttransplant lymphoproliferative disorders occurring in the setting of cyclosporine A-prednisolone immunosuppression. *Am J Pathol* 1988;133:173.

127. Knowles DM, Cesarman E, Chadburn A, et al: Correlative morphologic and molecular genetic analysis demonstrates three distinct categories of posttransplantation lymphoproliferative disorders. *Blood* 1995;85:552.

128. Starzl TE, Nalesnik MA, Porter KA, et al: Reversibility of lymphomas and lymphoproliferative lesions developing under cyclosporin-steroid therapy. *Lancet* 1984;1:583.

129. Dalton WS, Grogan TM, Meltzer PS, et al: Drug-resistance in multiple myeloma and non-Hodgkin's lymphoma: detection of P-glycoprotein and potential circumvention by addition of verapamil to chemotherapy. *J Clin Oncol* 1989;7:415.

130. Cleary ML, Warnke R, Sklar J: Monoclonality of lymphoproliferative lesions in cardiac-transplant recipients. Clonal analysis based on immunoglobulin-gene rearrangements. *N Engl J Med* 1984; 310:477.

131. Nelson BP, Nalesnik MA, Bahler DW, et al: Epstein-Barr virus-negative post-transplant lymphoproliferative disorders: a distinct entity? *Am J Surg Pathol* 2000;24:375.

132. Menke DM, Griesser H, Moder KG, et al: Lymphomas in patients with connective tissue disease. Comparison of p53 protein expression and latent EBV infection in patients immunosuppressed and not immunosuppressed with methotrexate. *Am J Clin Pathol* 2000; 113:212.

133. Fairlie NH, Mackie FP: The clinical and biochemical syndrome of lymphadenoma and allied disease involving the mesenteric lymph nodes. *BMJ* 1937;i:3792.

134. Gough KR, Read AE, Naish JM: Intestinal reticulosis as a complication of idiopathic steatorrhoea. *Gut* 1962;3:232.

135. Isaacson PG, Wright DH: Intestinal lymphoma associated with malabsorption. *Lancet* 1978;i:67.

136. Isaacson PG, O'Connor NTG, Spencer J, et al: Malignant histiocytosis of the intestine: a T-cell lymphoma. *Lancet* 1985;2:688.

137. Howell WM, Leung ST, Jones DB, et al: HLA-DRB, DQA, and −DQB polymorphism in celiac disease and enteropathy-associated T-cell lymphoma. Common features and additional risk factors for malignancy. *Hum Immunol* 1995;43:29.

138. O'Farrelly C, Feighery C, O'Briain DS, et al: Humoral response to wheat protein in patients with coeliac disease and enteropathy associated T-cell lymphoma. *BMJ* 1986;293:908.

139. Swinson CM, Slavin G, Coles EC, et al: Coeliac disease and malignancy. *Lancet* 1983;i:111.

140. O'Mahony S, Vestey JP, Ferguson A: Similarities in intestinal humoral immunity in dermatitis herpetiformis without enteropathy and in coeliac disease. *Lancet* 1990;335:1487.

141. Holmes GKT, Prior P, Lane MR, et al: Malignancy in coeliac disease—effect of a gluten free diet. *Gut* 1989;30:333.

142. Asking J, Linet M, Gridley G, et al: Cancer incidence in a population-based cohort of individuals hospitalised with celiac disease or dermatitis herpetiformis. *Gastroenterology* 2002;123:1438.

143. Chott A, Haedicke W, Mosberger I, et al: Most CD56+ intestinal lymphomas are CD8+ CD5- T-cell lymphomas of monomorphic small to medium size histology. *Am J Pathol* 1998;153:1483.

144. Wright NA, Pike C, Elia G: Induction of a novel epidermal growth factor-secreting cell lineage by mucosal ulceration in human gastrointestinal stem cells. *Nature* 1990;343:82.

145. Howat AJ, McPhie JL, Smith DA, et al: Cavitation of mesenteric lymph nodes: a rare complication of coeliac disease, associated with a poor outcome. *Histopathology* 1995;27:349.

146. Murray A, Cuevas D, Jones B, et al: Study of the immunohistochemistry and T-cell clonality of enteropathy associated T-cell lymphoma. *Am J Pathol* 1995;146:509.

147. Zettl A, Ott G, Makulik A, et al: Chromosomal gains at 9q characterize enteropathy-type T-cell lymphoma. *Am J Pathol* 2002;161:1635.

148. Obermann EC, Diss TC, Hamoudi RA, et al: Loss of heterozygosity on chromosome 9p21 is a frequent finding in enteropathy-type T-cell lymphoma. *J Pathol* 2004;202:252.

149. Baumgärtner AK, Zettl A, Chott A, et al: High frequency of genetic aberrations in enteropathy-type T-cell lymphoma. *Lab Invest* 2003; 83:1509.

150. Cejkove P, Zettl A, Baumgärtner AK, et al: Amplification of NOTCH1 and ABL1 gene loci is a frequent aberration in enteropathy-type T-cell lymphoma. *Virchows Arch* 2005;446:416.

151. Quintalla-Martinez L, Lome-Maldonado C, Ott G, et al: Primary intestinal non-Hodgkin's lymphoma and Epstein-Barr virus: high frequency of EBV-infection in T-cell lymphomas of Mexican origin. *Leuk Lymphoma* 1998;30:111.

152. Spencer J, Cerf-Bensussan N, Jarry A, et al: Enteropathy associated T-cell lymphoma (malignant histiocytosis of the intestine) is recognised by a monoclonal antibody (HML1) that defines a membrane molecular on human mucosal lymphocytes. *Am J Pathol* 1988;132:1.

153. Russell GJ, Winter HS, Fox VL, et al: Lymphocytes bearing the γδT-cell receptor in normal human intestine and celiac disease. *Hum Pathol* 1991;22:690.

154. Lundqvist C, Vladimir B, Hammarstrom S, et al: Intraepithelial lymphocytes. Evidence for regional specialization and extrathymic T-cell maturation in the human gut epithelium. *Int Immunol* 1995;7:1473.

155. Spencer J, Isaacson PG, Diss TC, et al: Expression of disulfide-linked and non-disulfide-linked forms of the T-cell receptor γ/δ heterodimer in human intestinal intraepithelial lymphocytes. *Eur J Immunol* 1989; 19:1335.

156. Trier JS: Celiac sprue. *N Engl J Med* 1991;325:1709.

157. Jewell DP: Ulcerative enteritis. *BMJ* 1983;287:1740.

158. Ashton-Key M, Diss TC, Pan LX, et al: Molecular analysis of T-cell clonality in ulcerative jejunitis and enteropathy associated T-cell lymphoma. *Am J Pathol* 1997;151:493.

159. Cellier C, Patey N, Mauvieux L, et al: Abnormal intestinal intraepithelial lymphocytes in refractory sprue. *Gastroenterology* 1998;114:471.

160. Cellier C, Delabesse E, Helmer C, et al: Refractory sprue (or cryptic enteropathy-associated T-cell lymphoma): the missing link between coeliac disease and enteropathy-associated T-cell lymphoma? Clinical, pathological, phenotypic and molecular evidence in a national cooperative study. *Lancet* 2000;356:203.

161. Bagdi E, Diss TC, Munson P, et al: Mucosal intraepithelial lymphocytes in enteropathy associated T-cell lymphoma, ulcerative jejunitis and refractory celiac disease constitute a neoplastic population. *Blood* 1999;94:260.

162. Carbonnel F, d'Almagne H, Lavergne A, et al: The clinicopathological features of extensive small intestinal CD4 T cell infiltration. *Gut* 1999;45:662.

163. Copie Bergman C, Wotherspoon AC, Norton AJ, et al: True histiocytic lymphoma: a morphologic, immunohistochemical and molecular genetic study of 13 cases. *Am J Surg Pathol* 1998;22:1386.

164. Miettinen M, Fletcher CD, Lasota J: True histiocytic lymphoma of small intestine. Analysis of tx S-100 protein-positive cases with features of interdigitating reticulum cell sarcoma. *Am J Clin Pathol* 1993;100:285.

165. Kamel OW, Gocke CD, Kell DL, et al: True histiocytic lymphoma: a study of 12 cases based on current definition. *Leuk Lymphoma* 1995;18:81.

166. Pileri SA, Grogan TM, Harris NL, et al: Tumours of histiocytes and accessory dendritic cells: an immunohistochemical approach to classification from the International Lymphoma Study Group based on 61 cases. *Histopathology* 2002;41:1.

167. Brugo EA, Marshall RP, Riberi AM, et al: Preleukemic granulocytic sarcomas of the gastrointestinal tract. Report of two cases. *Am J Clin Pathol* 1977;68:616.

CHAPTER 19

Mesenchymal Tumors

GENERAL COMMENTS

Gastrointestinal (GI) spindle cell tumors caused diagnostic confusion for decades. Previously, most were diagnosed as either smooth muscle or neural tumors. However, following decades of ultrastructural and immunohistochemical studies, and more recently genetic investigations, it is now evident that most GI mesenchymal tumors arise from interstitial cells of Cajal (ICCs), the gastrointestinal pacemaker cells. For this reason, the term *gastrointestinal pacemaker cell tumor* (GIPACT) has been suggested (1). However, the more general term *gastrointestinal stromal tumors* (GISTs) has long been in vogue and has taken hold. While GISTs are the most common GI mesenchymal tumors, an array of other mesenchymal tumor types also develop in the GI tract.

GASTROINTESTINAL STROMAL TUMORS

Demography

An estimated 5,000 to 6,000 new cases of GIST are diagnosed annually, with 10% to 30% of them being malignant (2). Most tumors are sporadic in nature, affecting individuals in their 5th or 6th decades of life. However, GISTs may arise in very young patients (3), and rare congenital tumors also exist (4). There is a slight male predominance. However, GISTs developing in the setting of the Carney triad (gastric GISTs, pulmonary chondromas, and extraadrenal paragangliomas) generally affect women under the age of 20 (5). GISTs developing in this setting are often multifocal, are purely epithelioid, and have a low risk of metastasis. GISTs arising in association with paragangliomas but without pulmonary chondromas may represent a variant of the Carney syndrome (5).

Familial GISTS develop in patients with germline-activating *KIT* (6) or *platelet-derived growth factor receptor-α* (*PDGFRA*) mutations (see below). Hyperpigmentation, mast cell tumors, and dysphagia are common to some kindreds (6). GISTS also develop in young patients with neurofibromatosis type 1 (NF1). The tumors are often multiple, usually developing in the small intestine (7). GISTs also complicate tuberous sclerosis (8) or following radiation therapy.

Cell of Origin

Most GISTs arise from CD117+ ICCs present in and around the myenteric plexus. ICCs show both myogenic and neural differentiation (1), explaining the immunohistochemical heterogeneity of the tumors that derive from them. Some GISTs originate from a CD34+ subset of ICC (9) or from primitive stem cells that can differentiate into ICC or smooth muscle cells (10).

Molecular Genetic Features

Constitutive activating *KIT* mutations occur in approximately 85% of GISTs. The *KIT* gene encodes a transmembrane tyrosine kinase receptor for stem cell factor (SCF). SCF receptor binding causes receptor dimerization and phosphorylation, inducing proliferation and inhibiting apoptosis (Fig. 19.1) (11). Activating mutations occur in exons 11 (21% to 71%), 9 (3% to 21%), 13, and 17 (Fig. 19.1) in a decreasing order of frequency (11–14). The type of *KIT* mutation is partially site and morphologically dependent (15–17). Spindle cell GISTs are most likely to contain exon 11 mutations, and exon 9 mutations most commonly affect intestinal GISTs (17). Novel germline mutations resulting in exon 8 deletions occur in familial GISTs and mastocytosis (18). *KIT* mutations range from single base pair substitutions to complex deletions/insertions. Internal tandem duplications may also be found (19). Generally, only one type of *KIT* mutation occurs in any given tumor. However, rare tumors contain two different somatic mutations. Recurrent tumors may show a different molecular phenotype than the primary tumor. So, for example, the primary tumor may show a mutation in exon 11 and the recurrence may contain both the exon 11 mutation as well as a new mutation in exon 13 (20).

Approximately 4% to 18% of GISTs harbor *PDGFRA*-activating mutations (17,21). The *PDGFRA* gene lies adjacent to the *KIT* locus and its structure and organization suggest that both genes derive from a common ancestral gene. *PDGFRA* mutations occur in exons 18, 12, and 14, with most involving exon 18 (16). Approximately 12% of GISTs lack *KIT* or *PDGFRA* mutations (16), indicating that there may be other rare, but yet unidentified genetic abnormalities that

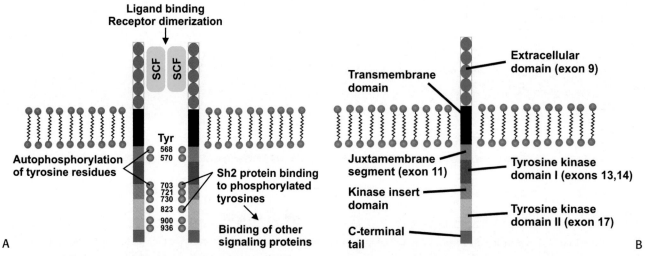

FIG. 19.1. Diagram of the kit receptor. **A:** Binding of stem cell factor to the receptor causes its dimerization, causing phosphorylation of tyrosine residues, which in turn activates downstream signals. **B:** The most common sites of mutation are illustrated.

contribute to GIST tumorigenesis. GISTs with *KIT* and *PDGFRA* mutations exhibit unique expression profiles and the genes identified by this technology may contribute to distinct clinicopathologic phenotypes. These gene products may also serve as highly selective therapeutic targets in GISTs containing *KIT* or *PDGFRA* mutations.

Familial GISTs associate with exon 8, 11, 13, and 17 *KIT* mutations (6,18) or mutations in the *PDGFRA* gene. In contrast, GISTs arising in the setting of NF1 tend to lack *KIT* or *PDGFRA* mutations (22). However, a novel *NF1* mutation has been found in this setting (23). Nonfamilial GISTs associated with paragangliomas lack germline *KIT* mutations or mutations in the *SDHA, SDHB, SDHC,* and *SDHD* genes, genes typically associated with familial paraganglioma (24).

General Clinical Features

The clinical manifestations of GISTs vary depending on the site of origin, tumor size, and layer of the gut wall from which they arise. Many benign tumors remain asymptomatic, only to be found incidentally. However, they can become symptomatic, especially when large. Symptoms include dysphagia, abdominal pain, gastrointestinal bleeding, or obstruction. GI bleeding may present as chronic anemia or, occasionally, as massive hemorrhage. Some tumors may be palpated externally or during rectal examination.

General Gross Features

GISTs most commonly arise in the stomach (60% to 70%) followed by the small intestine (20% to 30%) (particularly the duodenum) (2), the colorectum (5%), and the esophagus (<5%). NF1 patients develop intestinal GISTs; gastric tumors are less common. Patients with NF1, familial GISTs, and the Carney triad often develop multiple GISTs.

GISTs usually center around the submucosa or muscularis propria. Most are well-circumscribed lesions surrounded by a thin pseudocapsule of compressed normal tissues. GISTs appear as single nodules, plaques, or multinodular lesions. Broad-based, intraluminal polypoid lesions may also be present. The tumors grow in an endocentric (Fig. 19.2) or exocentric fashion (Fig. 19.3). Tumors with both exocentric and endocentric growth patterns have a dumbbell shape (Fig. 19.4). The overlying mucosa can be intact or ulcerated. On cut section, GISTs lack the bulging, whorled cut surface characteristic of smooth muscle tumors. Instead, the cut surface appears pink and granular with patchy areas of hemorrhage, necrosis, or cystic degeneration (Fig. 19.5). Tumors vary in size from 0.5 to 45 cm, with a median size of 6 cm.

Interstitial Cells of Cajal Hyperplasia

Patients with familial GISTs or with NF1 often show a focal or diffuse ICC hyperplasia, particularly in the area of the myenteric plexus (Fig. 19.6). This change involves many regions of the gastrointestinal tract. The hyperplastic ICCs are polyclonal in nature (25) and are CD117+ and sometimes CD34+.

Common Histologic Features

Many GISTs are identified at the time of resection, when the diagnosis is established and a determination is made as to whether the tumor is benign or malignant. GISTs may also be diagnosed on biopsy (Fig. 19.7) or cytology specimens (Fig. 19.8). However, it is not realistic to attempt to distinguish a benign from a malignant GIST on biopsy or cytologic material unless the tumor is overtly malignant, since the features of malignancy are judged by many criteria in addition to the histologic features of the tumor (see below).

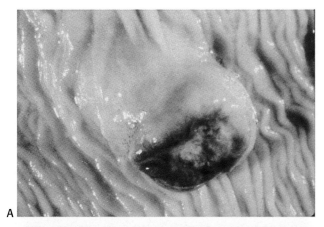

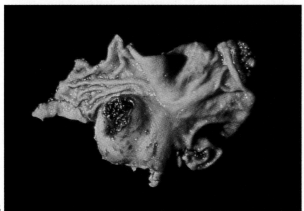

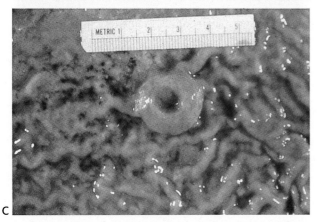

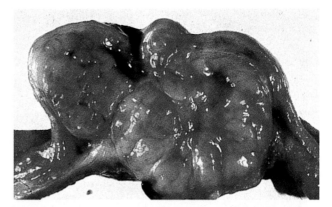

FIG. 19.3. Cut surface of a small intestinal gastrointestinal stromal tumor with a multilobulated irregular architecture.

pattern. The nuclei typically have blunt ends and are bullet or cigar shaped, but they can also be long and pointed. Some tumor cells have abundant cytoplasm; there may be areas of hyalinization and skenoid fibers. Epithelioid tumors consist of closely packed, polygonal cells. Some tumors also contain nests of small cells with an alveolar pattern. A small proportion of stromal tumors contain focal highly pleomorphic cells. These tumors usually have high mitotic rates measuring in excess of 10 mitoses/10 high-powered field (hpf).

There is a wide clinical and pathologic spectrum ranging from indolent diminutive tumors to rapidly progressing sarcomas. Therefore, they have been extensively studied to better predict their biology, often with conflicting conclusions. As a result, a group of soft tissue pathologists met and developed consensus recommendations for assessing GIST biology (26) (Table 19.1). These generally work well, but they do not take into account tumor location, so one can add some refinements to these general recommendations based on tumor location, as discussed below.

The histologic features of the more common forms of GISTs are discussed by location. There are also rare histologic variants that occur anywhere in the gut. *Gastrointestinal*

FIG. 19.2. Gastrointestinal stromal tumor (GIST) gross features. **A:** Small GIST with superficial ulceration and necrosis. The central ulcer is surrounded by a hyperemic surface consisting of granulation tissue. **B:** Large gastric leiomyoma with irregular superficial ulceration and a densely adherent clot on the surface. **C:** Small gastric GIST projecting into the lumen and producing a polypoid structure grossly resembling the nipplelike projections seen in some examples of heterotopic pancreas. At the time the stomach was removed for gross examination, it was filled with blood.

GISTs can be divided into spindle cell, epithelioid, mixed, and pleomorphic lesions. Seventy percent of tumors are predominantly spindle cell in nature (2). The spindle cell components may exhibit a storiform, palisading, or herringbone

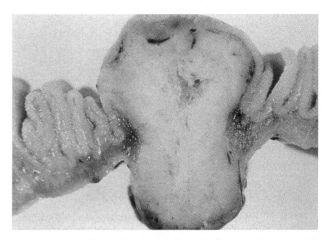

FIG. 19.4. Small intestinal gastrointestinal stromal tumor with dumbbell-shaped (exophytic and endophytic) growth pattern.

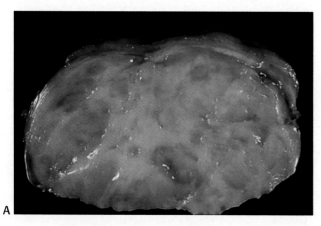

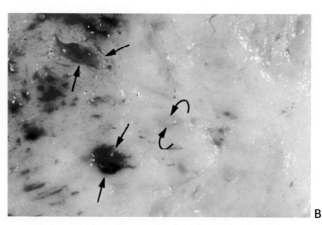

FIG. 19.5. Gastric gastrointestinal stromal tumor. **A:** Cut surface of the lesion. **B:** Higher magnification of the cut surface showing hemorrhagic cysts (*arrows*) and tan discolored areas (*curved arrows*) interspersed among tan-white solid areas.

autonomic nerve tumors (GANTs) are now known to represent a GIST variant. This variant is relatively more common in the small intestine and stomach and is relatively uncommon in the colon (27) and esophagus. The tumor contains small to intermediate-sized cells with a spindle or epithelioid appearance and a solid growth pattern. The cells exhibit long axonal processes containing cholinergic and adrenergic fibers and enveloping adjacent cells. Mitoses range from 1 to 23 mitoses/hpf (27,28).

Another histologic GIST variant contains cells with *signet ring cell features*. These tumors frequently affect women and present as small (<2.5 cm), well-circumscribed, gastric, small intestinal, or rectal serosal nodules. Histologically, the lesions are characterized by a proliferation of large, round to oval cells containing abundant clear cytoplasm with nuclear displacement toward the cellular periphery (Fig. 19.9). These signet-appearing cells merge with more typical spindled cells. The tumor cells associate with a prominent myxoid matrix. Immunohistochemistry shows a heterogeneous staining pattern with strong positivity for vimentin and variable staining for CD34, S100, and actin. In the study initially

describing these lesions (29), CD117 staining was not carried out since it predated the recognition that CD117 as a GIST marker.

The *mesotheliomalike GIST variant* typically contains epithelioid cordlike areas with pseudoglandular patterns distributed in a myxoid stroma (Fig. 19.10). GISTs with a *rhabdoid phenotype* (Fig. 19.11) contain paranuclear whorls of vimentin filaments (30). *Oncocytic variants* contain large numbers of mitochondria. *Small cell variants* contain cells with angulated nuclei that appear crowded together. Sometimes the tumor cells lie in tight perivascular whorls or balls of small spindle-shaped cells resembling paragangliomas. The *cytotoxic T-lymphocyte–rich GIST* (Fig. 19.12) arises in the stomach, esophagus, or mesentery, and resembles classic GISTs or GANTs with the exception that they are infiltrated by cytotoxic T cells (31). *NF1-associated GISTs* resemble non-NF1 spindle cell GISTs. Most contain skeinoid fibers and the tumors are typically surrounded by ICC hyperplasia. NF1-associated GISTs show dual differentiation with CD117+ ICCs and S100+ Schwann cells.

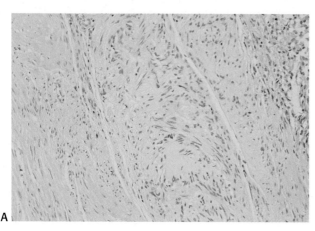

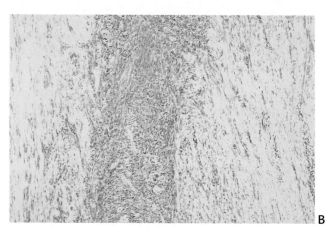

FIG. 19.6. Interstitial cells of Cajal hyperplasia. **A:** Histologically, this lesion appears as a neural hyperplasia in the area of the myenteric plexus. **B:** c-kit immunostain discloses the true nature of the lesion.

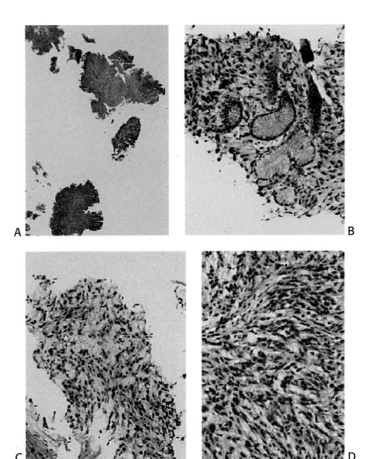

FIG. 19.7. Gastric gastrointestinal stromal tumor. **A:** This patient with known chronic active gastritis developed a mass lesion. Biopsy fragments of the most recent biopsy. The fragments differ in their appearance. The lower and middle biopsy fragments show evidence of chronic active gastritis. In the upper fragment, the gastric architecture is destroyed by the presence of an infiltrating mass. **B:** Higher magnification of an area of the upper biopsy fragment showing the replacement of the gastric mucosa by a cellular population with a high nuclear:cytoplasmic ratio that invades the lamina propria. This lesion can be diagnosed as malignant since there is mucosal invasion. **C:** Another area of the biopsy demonstrates a cellular neoplasm with a prominent myxoid stroma. **D:** This fragment is composed exclusively of spindle cells.

Esophageal Gastrointestinal Stromal Tumors

Esophageal GISTs are rare and most are malignant. They present as intramural tumors or as polyps (32). They exhibit a cellular spindle cell pattern, or show areas of epithelioid differentiation. The histologic pattern varies, ranging from sheets of cells to areas with nuclear palisading and myxoid change. Some tumors demonstrate neural differentiation. These lesions are consistently CD34+ and c-kit positive with occasional actin immunoreactivity (32).

Gastric Gastrointestinal Stromal Tumors

The stomach is the most common site of GISTs, where they are generally benign, but this is influenced by the features listed in Table 19.1 and by gastric location. There is a high frequency of malignancy in fundic and gastroesophageal GISTs, as compared with antral GISTs. Gastric GISTs show

TABLE 19.1 Consensus Recommendations for Defining Risk of Aggressive Behavior in Gastrointestinal Stromal Tumors

	Size	Mitotic Count
Very low risk	<2 cm	<5/50 hpf
Low risk	2–5 cm	<5/50 hpf
Intermediate risk	<5 cm	6–10/50 hpf
	5–10 cm	<5/50 hpf
High risk	>5 cm	>5/50 hpf
	>10 cm	Any mitotic rate
	Any size	>10/50 hpf

hpf, high-powered field.
Modified from Hirota S, Nishida T, Isozaki K, et al: Familial gastrointestinal stromal tumors associated with dysphagia and novel type germline mutation of KIT gene. *Gastroenterology* 2002;122:1493.

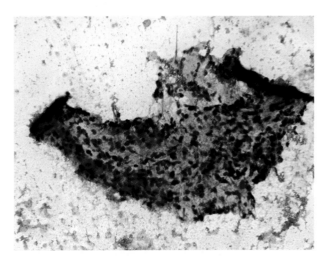

FIG. 19.8. Fine needle aspirate of a gastric gastrointestinal stromal tumor. A highly cellular tissue fragment is present that consists predominantly of spindle cells. There are no mitoses.

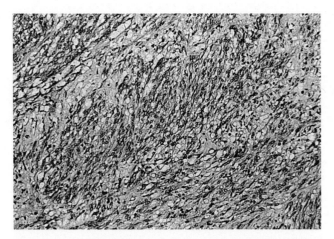

FIG. 19.9. Gastrointestinal stromal tumor with signet ring features.

two morphologic phenotypes that are relatively specific. One is a *cellular spindle cell stromal tumor* characterized by fascicles of spindle cells, often with pronounced palisades, monotonous and uniform nuclei, and perinuclear vacuoles, which indent the nucleus. Occasional large nuclei may occur.

Hyalinization and myxoid degeneration are common. Mitotic activity is low. *Epithelioid GISTs* constitute most of the remaining GISTs. The tumors contain round epithelioid cells with prominent clear cytoplasm and cytoplasmic perinuclear vacuolization. The tumor cells lie in sheets or packets rather than in fascicles; they tend to be oriented in a perivascular pattern. In the stomach, most epithelioid GISTs are benign, provided mitotic counts do not exceed five mitoses per 50 hpf (33).

There is no consensus on the appropriate classification of gastric GISTs. One can follow the consensus recommendations discussed earlier or report gastric GISTs, noting the maximum mitotic rate and maximum tumor diameter and making a comment about the adequacy of the resection margin, tumor cellularity, and the presence or absence of mucosal invasion. Alternatively, one can use one of the two classifications described below.

Trupiano et al divided gastric GISTs into benign and malignant spindle cell GISTs, benign and malignant epithelioid GISTs, and benign and malignant mixed lesions (34). The predominant cell type is determined by the presence of >75% of the tumor being represented by either spindle cells

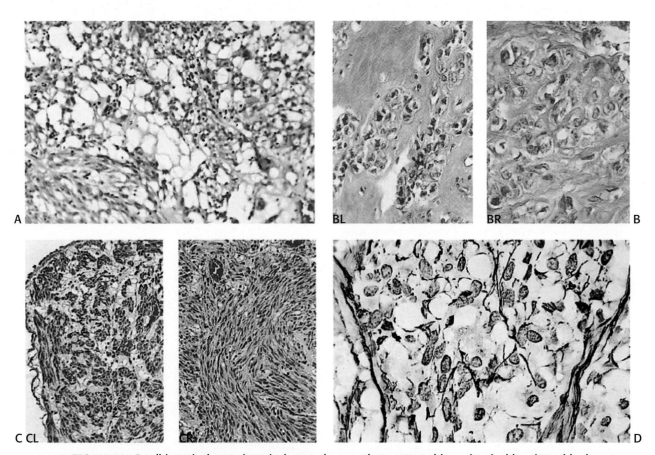

FIG. 19.10. Small intestinal gastrointestinal stromal tumor that presented in an inguinal hernia and had a pattern reminiscent of a mesothelioma. The photos are from the primary lesion in the ileum. **A:** Note the mixture of spindle cells and epithelioid areas. **B:** Ileal serosal surface showing epithelioid nests (*left*). Higher magnification (*right*). **C:** Other areas of the primary tumor. Epithelioid cells are seen on the left and spindle cells on the right. **D:** Reticulin stain demonstrating absence of reticulin.

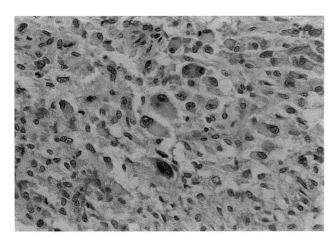

FIG. 19.11. Gastric gastrointestinal stromal tumor with a rhabdoid phenotype.

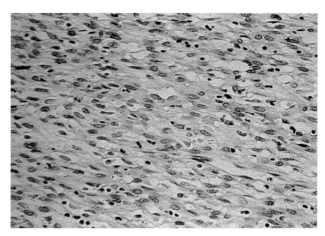

FIG. 19.12. Gastrointestinal stromal tumor with scattered cytotoxic T cells.

or epithelioid cells. Tumors that do not meet these criteria are classified as mixed tumors. Nuclear grade is considered to be high if the nuclei are large with irregular nuclear membranes and vesicular chromatin. Tumors without these features were classified as low grade (34).

According to this classification, *benign cellular spindle cell GISTs* are highly cellular tumors, with uniform spindle cells with an abundant pale to eosinophilic cytoplasm. The compact cells exhibit a patternless, fascicular, whorled, storiform, or palisading architecture. The uniform pale nuclei contain evenly distributed chromatin, inconspicuous nucleoli, and regular nuclear borders (Fig. 19.13). Mitotic activity is typically less than or equal to two figures per 50 hpf. Perinuclear vacuoles may be present. The tumor cells are often separated by a hyalinized or calcified stroma. There may be areas of liquefactive necrosis with pools of acellular material separating perivascular tumor islands (34).

Benign epithelioid GISTS, the most common gastric GISTs, consist predominantly, or exclusively, of epithelioid cells, often with well-defined borders, arranged in nests or sheets (Fig. 19.14). The cells have abundant cytoplasm that may be eosinophilic, amphophilic, or clear. There is often a condensed rim of eosinophilic cytoplasm adjacent to the nucleus with peripheral cytoplasmic clearing that is only appreciated on hematoxylin and eosin (H&E) examination, due to the fact that this is a fixation-induced artifact (Fig. 19.15). The nuclei are usually round with small nucleoli, but scattered multinucleated giant cells or cells with bizarre nuclei can be present. Mitotic figures are rare (usually two or less per 50 hpf). Stromal alterations include hyalinization and calcification (34). A rich vascular supply can cause a neuroendocrine or glomus appearance.

In contrast to benign cellular GISTs, *malignant spindle cell GISTs* are larger, more cellular tumors containing cells with a high nuclear:cytoplasmic ratio (Fig. 19.16). The cytoplasm may appear eosinophilic, basophilic, or amphophilic. The nuclei vary in size and often appear vesicular. The perinuclear vacuoles typical of benign lesions are often absent; areas of tumor necrosis are common. Individual tumor cells may be arranged in storiform or fascicular patterns. Some tumors

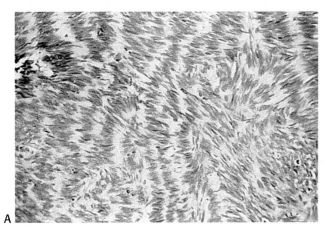

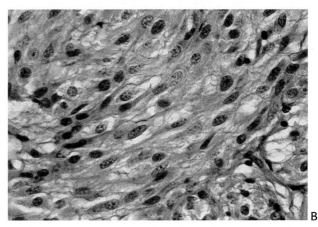

FIG. 19.13. Gastric gastrointestinal stromal tumor. **A:** Foci of spindled cell palisades • **B:** Higher magnification of the spindle cells.

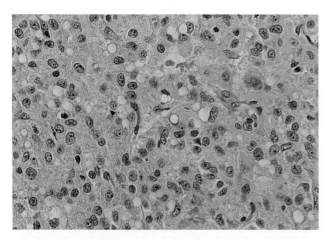

FIG. 19.14. Epithelioid gastrointestinal stromal tumor. The tumor consists of large polygonal cells.

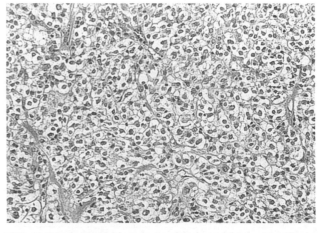

FIG. 19.15. Epithelioid gastrointestinal stromal tumor with so-called "fried egg" appearance.

show prominent nuclear palisading. Mitoses often number >10 mitoses/50 hpf. Mucosal invasion, as defined by infiltration of tumor cells across the muscularis mucosae between the glands at the base of the mucosa, may be seen (Fig. 19.7).

Malignant epithelioid GISTs consist of densely packed cells with less cytoplasm than the spindle cell variant. They are more cellular than their benign counterparts. The cells may be arranged in small acinarlike clusters or large sheets. A prominent myxoid stroma is often present. The nuclei are

frequently hyperchromatic and monotonous in appearance. Some cells are pleomorphic. However, scattered bizarre cells are more common in benign epithelioid GISTs. Since the mitotic activity overlaps with that seen in benign epithelioid tumors (unless the mitoses are numerous), mitoses cannot be used to separate benign from malignant lesions. Furthermore, because benign-appearing areas are often present in malignant epithelial GISTs, extensive sampling is required to identify the malignant component (34).

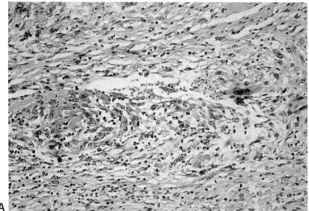

A

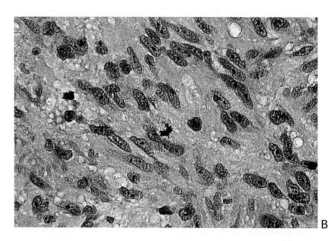

B

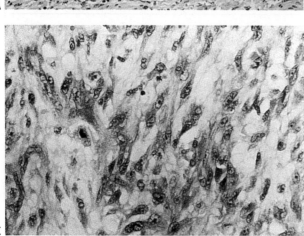

C

FIG. 19.16. Malignant spindle cell gastrointestinal stromal tumor. **A:** Low-power view showing atypical cells and focal necrosis. **B:** Medium-power view showing moderate cellular atypia and increased mitotic activity. **C:** Immature spindled and stellate cells with increased mitotic activity are present in a myxoid stroma.

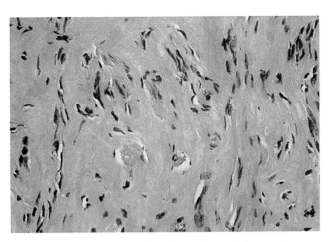

FIG. 19.17. Sclerosing spindle cell gastrointestinal stromal tumor.

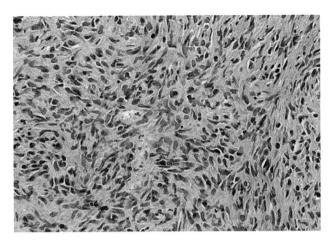

FIG. 19.18. Sclerosing epithelioid gastrointestinal stromal tumor. The figure demonstrates the presence of a densely cellular lesion with crowded nuclei. No mitotic activity is present. This area was surrounded by more typical spindle-shaped cells.

A recent large study of gastric GISTs (765 cases with long-term follow-up) delineated eight histologic subtypes of gastric GISTs, an admixture of the subtypes, and a group of tumors that were unclassified (8). The eight types are as follows:

1. *Sclerosing spindle cell GISTs* are paucicellular tumors that show extensive extracellular collagen (Fig. 19.17) spindle cells, no nuclear atypia, low mitotic activity, and common calcification. They are usually small, although 13% were >10 cm.
2. *Palisading and vacuolated spindle cell GISTs* (Fig. 19.13) consist of cellular, plump, uniform spindle cells with nuclear palisading, perinuclear vacuolization, and limited atypia; mitotic activity rarely exceeded 10 mitoses/50 hpf.
3. *Hypercellular spindle cell GISTs* contain uniformly densely packed cells with diffuse sheets of spindle cells exhibiting limited atypia, nuclear palisading, and perinuclear vacuolization. The mitotic activity rarely exceeded 15 mitoses/50 hpf.
4. *Sarcomatous spindle cell GISTs* (Fig. 19.16) contain spindle or oval cells with diffuse atypia, and the tumor cells were often in bundles separated by a myxoid stroma. The mitotic activity is >20 mitoses/50 hpf; nearly all tumors are >5 cm in diameter.
5. *Sclerosing epithelioid GISTs* (Fig. 19.18) exhibit a syncytial pattern and consist of cohesive uniform polygonal cells with indistinct cell borders and diffuse collagenous matrix. Multinucleation and low mitotic rate are characteristic.
6. *Epithelioid GISTs with discohesive patterns* (Fig. 19.19) consist of large polygonal cells with abundant cytoplasm, distinct cellular borders, discohesive growth patterns, scant interstitial matrix, multinucleation, possible focal atypia, and low mitotic rates.
7. *Hypercellular epithelioid GISTs* (Fig. 19.20) contain back-to-back epithelioid cells with well-defined borders, nuclear atypia, and a higher nuclear:cytoplasmic ratio than the epithelioid GISTs with discohesive patterns. Mitotic activity rarely was >10 mitoses/50 hpf.
8. *Sarcomatous epithelioid GISTs* contain epithelioid to rounded cells with well-defined borders, high nuclear:cytoplasmic ratios, uniform nuclei, prominent nucleoli, and conspicuous mitotic activity (>20 mitoses/50 hpf).

The tumors are also divided into eight groups, based on maximum tumor diameter and mitotic activity (Table 19.2)

TABLE 19.2 Suggested Guidelines for Assessing the Malignant Potential of Gastric Gastrointestinal Stromal Tumors of Different Sizes and Mitotic Activity

Benign (no tumor-related mortality detected)
Group 1 (≤2 cm, ≤5 mitoses/50 hpf)
Probably benign (very low malignant potential, <3% PD)
Group 2 (>2 and ≤5 cm, ≤5 mitoses/50 hpf)
Group 3a (>5 and ≤10 cm, ≤5 mitoses/50 hpf)
Uncertain or low malignant potential (no PDs but too few cases to reliably determine prognosis)
Group 4 (≤2 cm, >5 mitoses/50 hpf)
Low to moderate malignant potential (12%–15% tumor-related mortality)
Group 3b (>10 cm, ≤5 mitoses/50 hpf)
Group 5 (>2 and ≤5 cm, >5 mitoses/50 hpf)
High malignant potential (49%–86% tumor-related mortality)
Group 6a (>5 and ≤10 cm, >5 mitoses/50 hpf)
Group 6b (>10 cm, >5 mitoses/50 hpf)

hpf, high-powered field; PD, progressive disease.
Modified from Miettinen M, Sobin LH, Lasota J: Gastrointestinal stromal tumors of the stomach: a clinicopathologic, immunohistochemical, and molecular genetic study of 1765 cases with long-term follow-up. *Am J Surg Pathol* 2005;29:52.

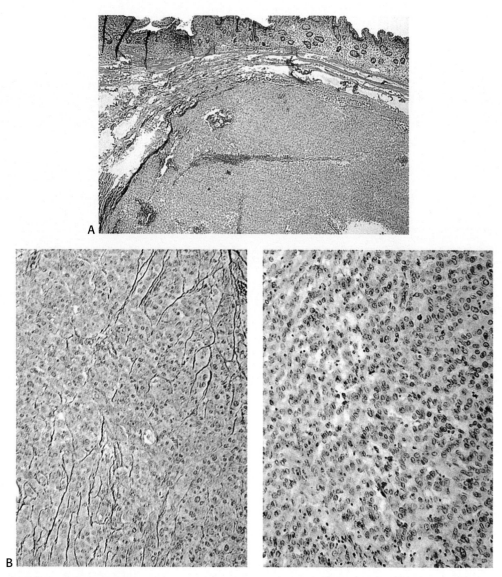

FIG. 19.19. Gastrointestinal stromal tumor (GIST) with discohesive cells. **A:** GIST arising in submucosa with a pushing margin extending to the muscularis mucosae. **B:** Composite picture of characteristic epithelioid to oval cells (*right*) and reticulin stain (*left*) circumscribing individual cells and groups of cells.

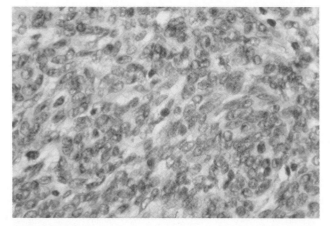

FIG. 19.20. Hypercellular epithelioid gastrointestinal stromal tumor. The mitotic activity in this cellular lesion with overlapping nuclear borders was three mitoses per 50 hpf.

(8). The spectrum from the sclerosing, palisading–vacuolated, hypercellular, to sarcomatous among spindle cell GISTs reflected increasing frequency of adverse outcome. The sarcomatous type differed significantly from the others in terms of tumor-specific survival. The epithelioid sarcomatous tumors had a slightly better prognosis than analogous spindle cell tumors. Myxoid changes may be seen in both spindle cell and epithelioid cell lesions (Fig. 19.21).

Features that appear to correlate with an aggressive clinical behavior of gastric GISTs include tumor mitotic activity, maximum tumor diameter, high nuclear grade, high cellularity, mixed cell type, mucosal invasion, tumor cell necrosis, and stromal alterations such as extensive myxoid change and absence of hyalinization (34).

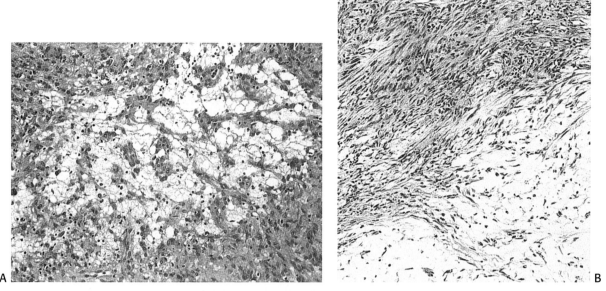

FIG. 19.21. Myxoid changes in gastrointestinal stromal tumor (GISTs). A: Focal area of myxoid degeneration showing abundant pale, amphophilic mucoid stroma. B: Another lesion demonstrating the presence of typical spindled cells of the GIST and adjacent myxoid areas.

Small Intestinal Gastrointestinal Stromal Tumors

As a group, a larger percentage of small bowel GISTs are malignant when compared to gastric GISTs. The classic benign small intestinal GIST is a small lesion (measuring <5 cm) that consists of a uniform population of cytologically bland spindle cells with abundant eosinophilic cytoplasm and overall low tumor cellularity. The cells are usually distributed in nests separated by fine fibrovascular septae producing an organoid growth pattern reminiscent of paragangliomas. Eosinophilic collagen globules (skeinoid fibers) are characteristic and are often numerous, especially in duodenal lesions (Fig. 19.22). These fibers are most common in smaller, mitotically less active tumors. Focal calcification may be present. Nuclear palisading suggestive of neural tumors occurs in many tumors. The tumors may also contain distinctive hemangiomalike, sometimes glomerularlike vascular proliferations lying between the sheets of tumor cells. Perivascular

FIG. 19.22. Small intestinal gastrointestinal stromal tumor with skeinoid fibers. A: Hematoxylin and eosin section demonstrating the presence of amorphous aggregates of eosinophilic material typical of skeinoid fibers within the tumor. The tumor cells themselves are round and epithelioid-like in appearance or more elongated. B: Periodic acid–Schiff (PAS) stain demonstrating the PAS positivity of the material.

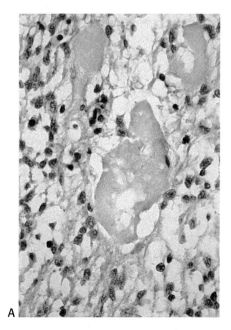
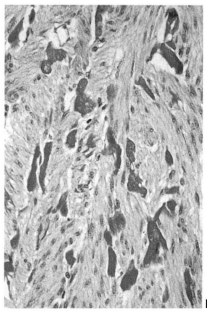

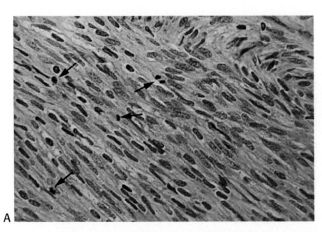
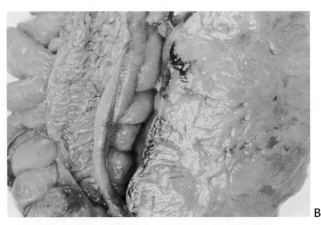

A   B

FIG. 19.23. Malignant small intestinal gastrointestinal stromal tumor. **A:** Low-power photograph showing the presence of a cellular spindle cell lesion with numerous mitoses (*arrows*). **B:** Gross features of the lesion shown in A. A mass surrounds the bowel.

hyalinization is also common (33). Mitoses are low (less than five per 50 hpf). Benign tumors lack tumor cell necrosis and mucosal invasion (35).

Most malignant small intestinal GISTs consist of highly cellular spindle cell proliferations (Fig. 19.23) with more cytologic atypia than occurs in benign tumors. The nuclei are larger with more coarsely clumped chromatin; mitoses are easily identified (greater than five per 50 hpf). The cells are typically arranged in long fascicles, as opposed to the organoid pattern seen in benign tumors. Skeinoid fibers are few in number or absent, and many, but not all, malignant small intestinal GISTs have tumor cell necrosis and/or mucosal invasion. Tumors with a conspicuous epithelioid component comprising more than 25% of the tumor are virtually always malignant (24,36,37). Since many malignant small intestinal GISTs contain benign areas, as well as malignant areas, these tumors should be well sampled to detect the malignant areas.

In one study, small intestinal GISTs were divided into the six categories shown in Table 19.3. Significant prognostic features included tumor size (>5 cm), mitoses (greater than five per 50 hpf), the presence of coagulation necrosis, an epithelioid histology, the absence of hyalinized vessels and

skeinoid fibers, and the presence of mucosal invasion (33,38).

Appendiceal and Large Intestinal Gastrointestinal Stromal Tumors

Appendiceal GISTs are spindle cell tumors that may contain skeinoid fibers. They lack atypia and mitotic activity (39). *Colorectal GISTs* are almost always spindle cell tumors, of which 50% are malignant, often with a highly aggressive clinical course. An infiltrative border, greater than 5 mitoses per 50 hpf (40), and mucosal invasion (Fig. 19.24) correlate with metastasis or death. The prognostic impact of tumor size is more controversial than in tumors arising in other locations (40). Colonic GISTs that contain skeinoid fibers have a better prognosis than those without them. Occasionally, malignant large intestinal GISTs contain osteoclastlike giant cells (40).

Anorectal GISTs are rare; most arise within the muscularis propria (41). They are generally a homogeneous group of cellular tumors composed predominantly of spindle cells; skeinoid fibers are absent. Small submucosal lesions without mitoses and pleomorphism behave in a benign fashion;

TABLE 19.3	Miettinen Classification of Small Intestinal Gastrointestinal Stromal Tumors		
Group	Size	Mitoses	Prognosis
1	≤2 cm	≤5 mitoses/50 hpf	Generally behave in benign fashion
2	>2–5 cm	≤5 mitoses/50 hpf	6% develop metastases and die of their disease
3	>5 cm	≤5 mitoses/50 hpf	31% develop metastases; median survival 18 months
4	≤2 cm	>5 mitoses/50 hpf	There were no tumors in this group
5	2–5 cm	>5 mitoses/50 hpf	50% risk intra-abdominal spread, metastasis, or death
6	7.5 cm	>5 mitoses/50 hpf	86% intra-abdominal spread or metastasis

hpf, high power field.
Modified from Miettinen M, Makhlouf H, Sobin LH, Lasota J: Gastrointestinal stromal tumors of the jejunum and ileum. A clinicopathologic, immuno-histochemical and molecular genetic study of 906 cases before Imatinib with long-term follow-up. *Am J Surg Pathol* 2006;30:477.

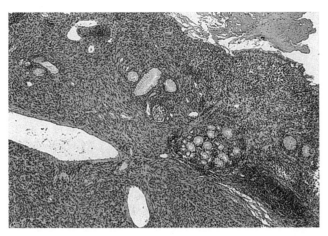

FIG. 19.24. Intestinal malignant gastrointestinal stromal tumor. The tumor diffusely invades the mucosa. Residual trapped intestinal glands are evident. A band of chronic inflammation is associated with some of the residual glands.

malignant tumors often have an infiltrative growth pattern and mitotic rates of five or more mitoses per 50 hpf. The impact of nuclear pleomorphism, necrosis, mitotic count, and intramuscular location is currently unclear (42). These tumors require long-term follow-up to determine their behavior. Deep intramuscular, cellular tumors should be considered to be malignant if they are >5 cm in diameter, infiltrate the muscularis propria, have one or more mitotic figure per 50 hpf, or contain coagulative necrosis or pleomorphism (42).

Histologic Features of Gastrointestinal Stromal Tumors Following Treatment

Treated tumors may change their histology following treatment. Spindle cell tumors may develop an epithelioid or pseudopapillary epithelioid growth pattern characterized by rounded cells with an eosinophilic cytoplasm and uniform round to ovoid nuclei. There is a dramatic decrease in tumor cell density with the formation of a myxohyaline stroma, extensive hemorrhage, necrosis, and cystic trans-

formation. There is usually a marked decrease in its proliferative rate (43). The tumor may lose its CD117 positivity with only a few residual positive cells (44). Some tumors also become CD34 negative. Some tumors become desmin positive (45).

Immunohistochemical Features of Gastrointestinal Stromal Tumors

The definitive marker for a GIST (benign and malignant) is c-kit protein (CD117) expression (26,46). However, c-kit immunoreactivity can be seen in other tumors (Table 19.4) and not all GISTs are positive. The interpretation of the staining patterns is complicated by the fact that there are several commercially available antibodies and variable staining methodologies may result in false-positive and false-negative results. Additionally, CD117 positivity may be lost in treated tumors. Efforts are currently under way to validate c-kit staining. Further, CD117 immunohistochemistry tissue microarrays are available that facilitate interlaboratory comparisons of staining results, quality assurance programs, and educational purposes (47).

The predominant CD117 staining pattern is a diffuse cytoplasmic positivity (Fig. 19.25). Membrane staining or dotlike positivity may also occur. Rarely, CD117 positivity is present in only a portion of cells. PDGFRA immunostaining can be helpful in discriminating between c-kit–negative GISTs and other mesenchymal lesions. Other mesenchymal tumors are PDGFRA negative except for a subset of desmoid tumors (48).

Approximately 70% of GISTs express CD34 (Fig. 19.26) (48). CD34 immunoreactivity varies from 47% in small intestinal GISTs to 96% to 100% in rectal and esophageal tumors. Absence of CD34 expression in benign GISTs may indicate that they arise from more mature ICCs, whereas malignant GISTs may contain dedifferentiated ICCs that also express CD34 (49).

GISTs are variably positive with both smooth muscle (Fig. 19.27) and neural markers. Smooth muscle actin expression is most common in small intestinal GISTs (47%) and most rare in rectal and esophageal GISTs (10% to 13%). When

TABLE 19.4 c-kit–expressing Tumors

Adenoid cystic salivary gland carcinoma	Fibrosarcoma	Neuroblastomas
Angiomyolipomas	GISTs	Nevi
Angiosarcoma	Kaposi sarcomas	Osteosarcomas
Chronic myelogenous leukemia	Lipomas	Rhabdomyosarcoma
Clear cell sarcomas	Malignant glioma	Seminomas
Endometrial cancer	Mast cell tumors	Small cell lung cancer
Ewing sarcomas/PNET	Melanocytic schwannomas	Synovial sarcomas
Extraskeletal chondrosarcoma	Melanomas	Thyroid tumors
Fibromatosis	Merkel cell carcinoma	Wilms tumor

GISTs, gastrointestinal stromal tumors; PNET, primitive neuroectodermal tumor.

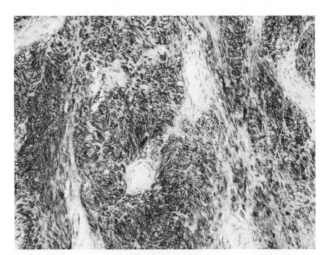

FIG. 19.25. c-kit immunostaining of a gastrointestinal stromal tumor. This tumor is strongly positive for the kit protein.

actin is expressed, it is generally focal, indicating that smooth muscle differentiation is incomplete. Heavy caldesmon, an actin-binding cytoskeleton-associated protein, is also expressed in some GISTs. Desmin staining is less common and is typically limited to scattered tumor cells, with more prominent staining in epithelioid tumors. S100 protein expression occurs in 10% to 15% of GISTs, usually in small intestinal GISTs, in a focal staining pattern. Scattered tumor cells may be cytokeratin positive. Eighty percent of GISTs stain with BCL2.

GISTs also express the intermediate filament nestin, a protein that is not expressed in other mesenchymal tumors, unless there is neural differentiation (50). Almost 100% of GISTs strongly express the *dog1* (discovered in GISTs) gene. The cell surface protein expression is highly specific for GISTs (51). PKCθ is positive in up to 96% of GISTs (52). The GANT variant of GIST may show patchy immunostaining

for neuron-specific enolase (NSE), S100, synaptophysin, vasoactive intestinal polypeptide, substance P, chromogranin, and neurofilament protein. Muscle cell markers are variably positive.

Differential Diagnosis

Because the morphologic spectrum of GISTs is wide, the differential diagnosis is also wide. It includes smooth muscle tumors, schwannomas, malignant peripheral nerve sheath tumors, solitary fibrous tumors, inflammatory fibroid tumors, synovial sarcomas, mesotheliomas, neuroendocrine tumors, glomus tumors, sarcomatoid carcinomas, malignant melanomas, and angiosarcomas. Immunohistochemical analysis is required to distinguish among the entities within this differential diagnosis (Table 19.5). CD117 expression confirms the diagnosis in most tumors. Rarely, epithelioid GISTs express CD34 in the absence of CD117. Since some epithelioid GISTs show cytokeratin immunoreactivity, coexpression of either CD34 or CD117 becomes critical to avoid misdiagnosing these cases as carcinomas. Inflammatory GISTs raise the differential diagnosis of follicular dendritic cell sarcoma, inflammatory myofibroblastic tumor, inflammatory leiomyosarcoma, inflammatory malignant fibrocytic sarcoma, and inflammatory fibroid polyps.

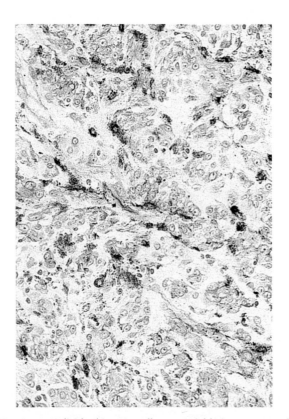

FIG. 19.27. Individual tumor cells are variably immunoreactive for actin in this gastrointestinal stromal tumor.

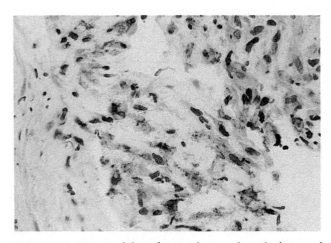

FIG. 19.26. CD34 staining of a gastric gastrointestinal stromal tumor.

TABLE 19.5 Differential Diagnosis of Gastrointestinal Stromal Tumors (GISTs)

	CD117	CD138	CD34	CR	CK	S100	Melan A	HMB45	SYN	VIM	Desmin	SM actin	HHC35	CD99
Epithelioid GISTs														
GIST	95%+	79%+	+	–	rare+	rare+	–	–	rare	+	rare	30%	50%	–
Mesothelioma	17%	+	rare	+	+	rare	–	–	–	+	rare	+	+	50%
Melanoma	>50%	20%	–	–	rare	+	+	+	rare	+	rare	50%	–	rare
Carcinoma	some types+	some types+	some types+	some types+	+	some types+	–	–	SCC & NE	some types	sarco-matoid	spindle cell	spindle cell	some types
Paraganglioma	<10%	?	–	–	–	+	–	–	–	+	–	–	–	–
Carcinoid tumor	–	+	–	–	+	ap+	–	–	–	–	–	–	rare	–
Lymphoma	50%	40%	–	rare	–	some	–	–	–	+	+	+	+	some
Leiomyoma/sarcoma	rare	60%	+	25%–	–	–	–	rare	–	+	+	+	+	30%
Spindle Cell GISTs														
GIST	+	+	+	–	rare+	rare	–	–	rare	+	rare	30%	50%	+
Schwannoma	rare	?	+	–	–	+	–	mela-notic	rare	+	–	–	–	+
Leiomyoma/sarcoma	rare	50%	+	25%	–	–	–	–	–	+	+	+	+	30%
Fibromatosis	50%	?	–	–	–	–	–	–	–	+	–	+	+	–
Mesothelioma	rare	rare	rare	+	+	rare	–	–	–	+	rare	+	+	50%
Liposarcoma	rare	?	50%	rare	some	+	–	–	–	+	5%	some	–	–
MPNST	–	–	+	–	–	+	–	–	rare	+	rare	–	rare	–
Solitary fibrous tumor	rare	–	+	–	rare	rare	–	–	–	+	–	–	–	+
Neurofibroma	–	–	+	–	–	+	40%	30%	–	+	–	15%	–	–

AP, appendix; CK, cytokeratin; CR, calretinin; MPNST, malignant peripheral nerve sheath tumors; NE, neuroendocrine lesion; SCC, small cell carcinoma; SM, smooth muscle; SYN, synaptophysin; VIM, vimentin.

TABLE 19.6   Gastrointestinal Stromal Tumors: Prognostic Factors

Tumor location
Tumor size
Presence of metastasis
Mucosal invasion
Patient age
Mitotic index (proliferation index)
Necrosis
Cytologic atypia, cellularity, nuclear pleomorphism
Atypical mitoses
Cytomorphology (epithelial vs. spindle cell)
Nature of the stroma
Kit or platelet-derived growth factor receptor-α (PDGFRA) mutational status
Loss of heterozygosity at 1p36

Prognosis

Predicting the clinical behavior of GISTs requires an evaluation of the gross, microscopic, and, possibly, immunohistochemical and molecular features of the tumors (Table 19.6). Tumor size, mitotic rate, patient age, and tumor location have been most commonly cited as the best predictors of clinical behavior at any site (26). However, some believe that tumor size and mitotic index are insufficient to provide an accurate long-term prediction of prognosis (53). Table 19.1 shows the consensus recommendations for defining risk of aggressive behavior (26), and we have previously discussed factors that appear to be important in specific anatomic locations.

Tumor size alone cannot be used to reliably separate benign from malignant gastric stromal tumors (34), since significant overlap exists between individual cases. Tumors ≥7 cm are significantly more likely to metastasize than smaller tumors. However, up to 35% of patients with an adverse outcome have tumors measuring <7 cm. Likewise, 33% of patients with a good outcome have tumors measuring ≥7 cm. Metastasis occurs in 20% of tumors <6 cm compared to 85% of those that are 6 cm or larger (44). In another study, 15% of GISTs <2.5 cm, 29% of tumors measuring 2.5 to 5 cm, 65% of tumors between 5 and 10 cm, and virtually all tumors >10 cm metastasized (54). Small intestinal tumors use a size cutoff of 5 cm (see above).

Larger tumors tend to have an especially poor prognosis, partly because surgical extirpation is difficult in such lesions and larger lesions tend to invade adjacent structures. Small size in the absence of mitotic activity does not preclude malignant behavior, however. Invasion into adjacent organs also correlates with an aggressive clinical course, as does the presence of metastases.

The impact of *proliferative index* is highly site dependent, being most unpredictable in the small bowel. It should be noted that there is often significant intratumoral variability in the mitotic activity. Mitotic counts should be performed in the most mitotically active areas of the tumor. Generally, mitotic counts are highest in the most cellular areas of the neoplasm. High-grade lesions (>10 mitoses/10 hpf) have the most dismal outcome, with 0% 10-year survival (55). One can measure proliferation in ways other than by mitotic counts, including immunostaining for proliferating cell nuclear antigen (PCNA) and Ki-67 as well by studying silver staining nucleolar organizing regions (AGNORs). All studies using these methods show a relationship between cell proliferation and prognosis, but they do not add anything to standard mitosis counting.

Tumor location helps predict outcome. Patients with esophageal tumors have the best survival, whereas the prognosis is worst for those with small intestinal GISTs (53). In stark contrast to gastric tumors, intestinal tumors >10 cm with mitotic activity of five or fewer mitoses per 50 hpf and those ≤5 cm with mitoses of greater than five mitoses per 50 hpf have a high metastatic rate (38). Benign GISTs outnumber malignant GISTs in the stomach, whereas malignant GISTs are more common in the intestine (38).

Tumor cell necrosis is more common in malignant than in benign GISTs, but benign tumors may contain necrotic areas, particularly if there has been torsion of pedunculated lesions. *Mucosal invasion* is a highly specific marker of malignancy. However, it is not a sensitive marker, since many GISTs do not infiltrate the overlying mucosa. Additionally, surface ulceration may make evaluation of this feature difficult.

Tumors in young people tend to have a better prognosis than those developing in older individuals, even when metastases are present, especially in the setting of the Carney triad. Of note, radiographic evidence of pulmonary lesions should not be taken as clinical evidence of lung metastases, especially in young women, because the pulmonary lesion may represent a benign pulmonary hamartoma in patients with the Carney triad.

The *prognostic value of KIT mutations* is controversial. Some have found that *KIT* mutations preferentially occur in malignant GISTs (56) and that the mutations have independent prognostic significance (57). Others suggest that *KIT* mutation is obligatory for GIST development, and therefore not related to tumor prognosis (58). Rather, the type or location of mutation may determine a patient's prognosis and treatment response. Mutations in exon 11 associate with a poor outcome (59). Deletions in codons 557/558 of exon 11 significantly correlate with disease recurrence and shortened survival (57). Gastric GISTs with *KIT* exon 11 deletions have a higher rate of aggressive disease than tumors with exon 11 point mutations (11).

PDGFRA mutations significantly associate with a higher frequency of epithelioid or mixed morphology; multinucleated giant cells; a low proliferation rate; a gastric, omental, or peritoneal location; and a favorable prognosis, although this is not statistically significant (8,17,60).

Treatment

Surgery is the initial treatment, with the aim to perform a complete en bloc resection of the tumor, which may include removal of adjacent organs if required. However, even after complete surgical resection, many malignant GISTs recur. When patients fail surgical treatment, they typically fail at the original tumor site, or in the peritoneum, omentum, or liver (61). These lesions may also metastasize to the ovary (62). GISTs rarely metastasize outside the abdominal cavity. Recurrences occur within the first 2 years, although low-grade tumors may not recur for decades.

Until recently, no other therapies (chemotherapy or radiation) have been effective. However, the use of targeted therapies designed to inactivate the tyrosine kinase activity of both the c-kit and PDGFRA receptors has improved patient prognosis. Imatinib, a selective adenosine triphosphate (ATP) competitive inhibitor of the tyrosine kinase activity of c-kit, decreases proliferation and induces apoptosis (63). It is very effective in treating metastatic or recurrent GISTs (64). More than 60% of patients with metastatic GISTs treated with imatinib have a major durable response, with a reduction of 70% to 90% of the tumor volume (64).

The efficacy of imatinib and the duration of the disease control may correlate with the type or location of *KIT* mutation. Eighty percent of tumors with exon 11 mutations are sensitive to imatinib treatment (65). Tumors with a novel point mutation in exon 14 in the kit ATP pocket also demonstrate imatinib sensitivity (66). In contrast, the *KIT*-D816V mutation affects the kinase catalytic domain, interfering with the imatinib-binding site, rendering the drug ineffective (67). Only 50% of tumors with exon 9 mutations respond and 20% of tumors with no mutations have a partial response. Missense mutations in the kinase domain 1 correlate with imatinib resistance (68). Cells carrying *KIT*-Del557-558/T670I or *KIT*-Ins502-503/V654A mutations are resistant to imatinib.

The location of the mutation in the *PDGFRA* gene also affects sensitivity to imatinib. Most isoforms with a substitution involving codon D842 in exon 18 (D842V, RD841-842KI, and D1842-8431M) are resistant to the drug, with the exception of D842Y. Other mutations in exon 18 (D846Y, N84K, Y849K, and HDSN845-848P) are imatinib sensitive (16). Corless et al recently proposed a molecular classification of GISTs (16) (Table 19.7).

It has now become clear that some patients with GISTs develop resistance to imatinib during chronic therapy. The resistance may be of two forms: Either primary resistance or acquired resistance after an initial benefit from the drug. Secondary mutations are found in 46% of tumors in patients with acquired resistance, most of whom had had a primary mutation in kit exon 11 (68). Most secondary mutations are located in exon 17; others occur in exons 13 and 14 (68,69).

Progressive tumors may also show an acquired PDGFRA-D842V mutation.

The next major challenge will be the treatment of tumors that become resistant to imatinib, which will presumably occur through the selection of pre-existing drug-resistant clones that carry unresponsive mutant forms of either the kit or PDGFRA receptor. It is conceivable that a combination that uses imatinib with other agents or surgery may prove the way to prevent the development of drug-resistant tumors. New drugs that are currently being developed target the ATP binding sites of various tyrosine kinases, including c-kit, to address the insensitivity of some tumors to imatinib (70). For example, a new kinase inhibitor, SU11248, has a broader spectrum of activity, inhibiting both kit and PDGFRA as well as the vascular endothelial growth factor receptor, so that it is also a powerful antiangiogenic agent. The drug is currently in clinical trials (70).

SMOOTH MUSCLE TUMORS

Leiomyomas

True gastrointestinal smooth muscle tumors exist, but they are uncommon. Leiomyomas are most common in the esophagus, anorectum, and colon. Leiomyomas constitute approximately 0.4% of all esophageal neoplasms; they are the most common benign mesenchymal esophageal tumor, followed by granular cell tumors. Esophageal leiomyomas typically affect adults; males are more commonly affected than females. Autopsy studies show very small leiomyomas (micro- or seedling leiomyomas) in approximately 8% of individuals (71). Esophageal leiomyomas develop at a younger age than GISTs, with a median age of 30 to 35 years. Esophageal leiomyomas may afflict patients with Alport syndrome or with multiple endocrine neoplasia type 1 (MEN-1) (72). We are also seeing localized leiomyomas in many of our patients undergoing resection of distal esophageal adenocarcinomas after preoperative chemoradiation. Colonic leiomyomas show a male predominance and a median age of 62.

Esophageal leiomyomas may become symptomatic or be found incidentally. Polypoid esophageal leiomyomas project into the lumen, producing retrosternal, epigastric, or noncardiac chest pain; pyrosis; and dysphagia. Esophageal tumors also cause obstruction or bleeding. Antral leiomyomas produce gastric outlet obstruction. Intestinal tumors may lead to intussusception, volvulus, and torsion. Appendiceal neoplasms remain clinically silent or produce acute appendicitis. Colonic lesions tend to remain asymptomatic, only to be discovered incidentally during the workup of the patient for occult bleeding or during colonoscopy for other reasons. Smaller colonic lesions present as polyps, especially when they originate in the muscularis mucosae (Fig. 19.28). Anorectal leiomyomas present with rectal pain, tenesmus, or constipation.

TABLE 19.7 Molecular Classification of Gastrointestinal Stromal Tumors (GISTs)

GIST Type	Comments
Sporadic GIST	
KIT mutation	
Exon 11	Best response to imatinib
Exon 9	Intermediate response to imatinib
Exon 13	Sensitive to imatinib in vitro; clinical responses observed
Exon 17	Sensitive to imatinib in vitro; clinical responses observed
PDGFRA mutation	
Exon 12	Sensitive to imatinib in vitro; clinical responses observed
Exon 18	D842V has poor response to imatinib; other mutations are sensitive
Wild type	Poor response to imatinib
Familial GIST	
KIT exon 11 (V559A, delV559, W557R)	Skin pigmentation, urticaria pigmentosa, mastocytosis
KIT exon 13 (K642E)	No skin pigmentation or mastocytosis
KIT exon 17 (D820Y)	No skin pigmentation or mastocytosis; abnormalities in esophageal peristalsis
GIST with paraganglioma	Autosomal dominant; endocrine symptoms common
Pediatric GIST	
Sporadic	KIT mutations much less frequent than in adults
Carney triad	Gastric GIST with pulmonary chondroma and/or paraganglioma; female:male ratio = 7:1; no KIT mutations identified
NF1-Related GIST	**No KIT Mutations Identified**

NF1, neurofibromatosis type 1; PDGFRA, platelet-derived growth factor receptor-α.
Modified from Corless CL, Fletcher JA, Heinrich MC: Biology of gastrointestinal stromal tumors. *J Clin Oncol* 2004;22:3813.

Leiomyomas arise from either the muscularis mucosae or muscularis propria, where they form well-demarcated nodular muscular expansions or well-demarcated intramural tumors. They may also present as small polyps projecting into the lumen. The mucosa and serosa stretch over the surface of small lesions. Leiomyomas are typically pale, firm or rubbery, occasionally lobulated, usually round or oval pinkish-white lesions with a whorled appearance resembling their uterine counterparts. Unusual tumors measure >10 cm.

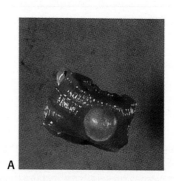
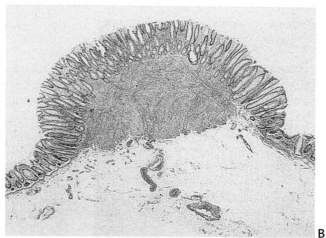

FIG. 19.28. Colonic leiomyomas. **A:** This colonic leiomyoma arises from the muscularis propria. **B:** Histologic features of a leiomyoma of the colon showing a downward proliferation of the muscularis mucosae, which elevates the mucosa. This lesion presented as a sessile polyp.

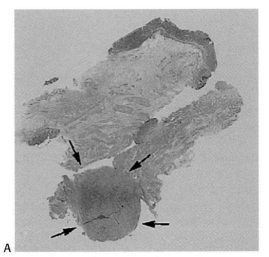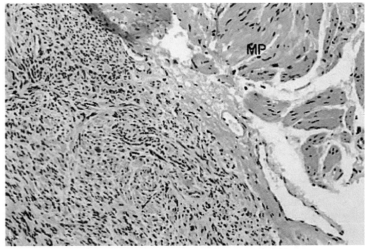

A   B

FIG. 19.29. Microleiomyoma of the stomach. **A:** Whole mount section of the stomach showing the presence of a gastric leiomyoma (*arrows*). **B:** Higher magnification showing the junction of the leiomyoma (*lower left*) and the muscularis propria (*MP*).

Esophageal and gastric leiomyomas are generally small, sessile, submucosal lesions that occasionally become pedunculated. They rarely ulcerate. Most arise in the distal esophagus, with a decreasing frequency proximally. Esophageal and gastric microleiomyomas are small (<1 cm), incidentally found microscopic lesions. They appear as tiny, whitish nodules typically involving the gastroesophageal junction, where they arise from the inner oblique muscle (Fig. 19.29). However, they can be seen anywhere in the esophagus or stomach. Many colorectal leiomyomas originate from smooth muscle cells in the muscularis mucosae (Fig. 19.28). They typically measure several millimeters in diameter, although lesions up to 2.2 cm have been described (32).

Leiomyomas are low to moderately cellular tumors containing interlacing fascicles of bland spindle-shaped, smooth muscle cells. The cells are more haphazardly arranged than in the normal muscular layers; peripherally, they may merge into the adjoining muscular layer. The cells appear hypertrophic and contain an abundant eosinophilic fibrillar cytoplasm. They often display prominent nuclear palisading. Epithelioid differentiation and hyalinization may be present. The nuclei generally appear elongated and cigar shaped, usually without significant pleomorphism. Mitotic activity is minimal or absent. Perinuclear halos are often present. Vascularity varies from tumor to tumor. Duodenal leiomyomas may contain considerable nuclear atypia, but the mitotic rates are usually less than one mitosis per 50 hpf.

Colorectal tumors may contain multiple eosinophilic globules that are positive for α-smooth muscle actin, muscle-specific actin, and desmin (73). These globules differ from the skeinoid fibers seen in GISTs. The tumor cells are positive for smooth muscle actin, are variably positive for desmin, and usually fail to express c-kit and CD34. *KIT* mutations are absent. Small leiomyomas can be safely removed by polypectomy or local enucleation. Larger lesions may require resection.

Epstein-Barr Virus–Associated Smooth Muscle Tumors

Epstein-Barr virus (EBV)-associated smooth muscle tumors are rare lesions that develop in immunocompromised individuals, particularly pediatric AIDS patients and organ transplant recipients. The lesions typically develop in children and adults under the age of 50 (74). In transplant patients, the tumors usually develop 3 or more years following the transplant surgery. The tumors differ from conventional leiomyomas in that the tumors are frequently multiple and in many small lesions the tumors appear to arise in vascular walls.

Most gastrointestinal lesions develop in the small bowel. The tumors range in size, with many tumors being only several millimeters in diameter. The tumors are relatively well differentiated with only modest nuclear atypia. Mitotic activity ranges from virtually none to levels as high as 18/10 hpf, with an average of less than three mitoses per 10 hpf (74). Focal areas of myxoid degeneration or necrosis are present in a minority of cases. The tumors contain intratumoral T lymphocytes and foci of primitive rounded cells that arise gradually or abruptly from a background of differentiated smooth muscle cells. The presence of these primitive cells has no impact on prognosis (74). Given the multiplicity of the tumors, the question arises as to whether they represent multiple independent primary tumors (i.e., independent infection events) or metastases from a single primary tumor. Most data support multiple infection events (74). Despite the fact that the histologic features of these tumors meet the criteria for leiomyosarcomas based on the Billings criteria (75), patients have an excellent prognosis, with few patients dying of their disease (74).

Leiomyomatosis

Leiomyomatosis is the term used to describe multifocal, ill-defined, smooth muscle proliferations that resemble clusters of leiomyomas or form linear constricting masses. The disorder affects males twice as frequently as females (76). Gastrointestinal leiomyomatosis may represent an isolated disorder or it can develop in patients with several syndromes, including Alport syndrome (AS), gastroesophageal-vulvar leiomyomatosis (GVL), MEN-1 (77), tuberous sclerosis (78), tracheobronchial leiomyomatosis, and pyloric stenosis (76). GVL is a rare, indolent, multifocal smooth muscle proliferation, primarily involving the gastroesophagus and vulva; it can affect other areas as well (79). Many patients also have Alport syndrome. The multiple tumors arising in the setting of MEN-1 are independent clones, although they develop through *MEN1* alterations. A hereditary defect of basement membrane is present in some patients (80).

The molecular changes of leiomyomatosis vary, depending on the background on which the tumors develop. A deletion of the *COL4A5/CLL4A6* locus located on the X chromosome (81) is present in some tumors. Patients with tuberous sclerosis show mutations in either the *TSC1* (chromosome 9q34) or *TSC2* (chromosome 16p13) tumor suppressor gene (82).

Esophageal leiomyomatosis may cause regurgitation, vomiting, failure to thrive, cough, and stridor secondary to tracheobronchial compression. The disease progresses slowly with symptoms often being present for years before the disease is correctly diagnosed. Infiltration of the esophageal myenteric plexus by hyperplastic smooth muscle cells causes manometric features resembling achalasia. Patients with GVL may present with esophageal symptoms or intestinal pseudo-obstruction (83). Clitoral hypertrophy and vulvar and periurethral leiomyomas may also be present. One patient with tuberous sclerosis presented with multiple areas of leiomyomatosis throughout the colon and prolonged constipation (84). The intestine and bowel appeared dilated proximally and the dilation decreased distally. This patient was also mentally retarded.

Esophageal leiomyomatosis usually extends from the midesophagus to the proximal stomach. Although most of the esophagus is involved, one may see dominant masses involving only a segment of the esophagus. The muscle proliferations arise from any of the muscle layers, most often the muscularis propria. Leiomyomatosis also affects extra-esophageal sites, including the tracheobronchial tree, the female genital tract, the small intestine, or the mesentery. The walls of the rectum and anal canal may be markedly thickened, and the rectum may be severely dilated.

The neoplastic proliferations present as many ill-defined, pale, sausagelike or U-shaped masses that vary in diameter.

They may grow in a semi-constricting manner, sometimes affecting long gastrointestinal segments measuring up to 35 cm in length. They may also be as small as 0.5 cm in diameter. The proliferations may extend to the serosa, and may invade adjacent normal tissues. Some nodules protrude into the colonic lumen, producing sessile polyps (84).

Histologically, leiomyomatosis consists of multiple confluent or nonconfluent well-differentiated smooth muscle proliferations and nodules arising from both the muscularis mucosae and muscularis propria. The lesions extend in a pushing manner through the muscularis mucosae into the lamina propria, but do not reach the lumen. The smooth muscle proliferations often infiltrate the myenteric plexus. The cells lose their usually parallel orientation and form fascicles, interlacing bundles, and whorls. The cells contain oval, slightly enlarged hyperchromatic nuclei. Nuclear atypia and mitoses are difficult to find. Variable amounts of collagen are present. Hyperplastic neural changes sometimes accompany the smooth muscle proliferation (77). The smooth muscle cells are positive with antibodies to actin and vimentin and are variably desmin positive. They are negative with a host of other antibodies including CD34, CD117, neurofilament, glial fibrillary acidic protein, CD34, S100, synaptophysin, CK/AE1-3, NSE, chromogranin, vasoactive intestinal polypeptide, CD31, estrogen receptor, and progesterone receptor.

Leiomyomatosis differs from multiple leiomyomas in that multiple leiomyomas are multiple circumscribed tumors with distinct pushing margins rather than poorly delineated smooth muscle proliferations. Leiomyomatosis also differs from idiopathic muscular hypertrophy, which is a rare condition in which the entire muscularis propria becomes uniformly thickened without nodule formation. GVL behaves in an indolent manner and is unlikely to be malignant. Patients with extensive leiomyomatosis may benefit from surgical resection and esophageal replacement.

Disseminated Peritoneal Leiomyomatosis (Leiomyomatosis Peritonealis Disseminata)

Disseminated peritoneal leiomyomatosis (DPL) primarily affects women in the reproductive age group, many of whom are pregnant, postpartum, or taking oral contraceptives (85). Symptoms (pelvic pain and abnormal uterine bleeding) usually result from coexisting uterine leiomyomata and not from the GI lesions. Innumerable small (several millimeters in size) smooth muscle proliferations ranging from 0.1 to 2 cm stud the serosal and peritoneal surfaces and the omentum (Fig. 19.30). There may also be larger leiomyomatous masses. These nodules consist of interwoven fascicles of smooth muscle cells that exist alone or coexist with areas of endometrial or endocervical differentiation (85,86). The proliferating cells interdigitate with one another and with proliferating fibroblasts and myofibroblasts. The lesions may show mild to moderate hypercellularity, but without coagulative necrosis, pleomorphism, or cytologic or nuclear

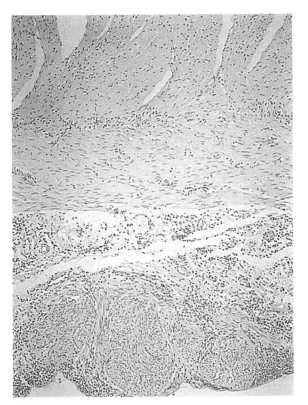

FIG. 19.30. Leiomyomatosis peritonealis disseminata. Spindle-shaped proliferating smooth muscle cells are situated between the muscularis propria and the serosa.

atypia. Mitotic figures are rare (less than two mitoses per 100 hpf). Atypical mitoses are absent. The histogenesis of DPL remains controversial, but most accept that it represents a hormonally driven metaplasia of the subcelomic mesenchyme (85). Increased levels of estrogen and progesterone receptors are seen in the smooth muscle cells (85). Most DPL cases behave in a clinically benign fashion and, in some cases, the lesions may partially or completely regress (85). Occasionally, however, DPL may progress, recur, or undergo malignant transformation (87).

Smooth Muscle Hamartomas

Smooth muscle hamartomas develop spontaneously or in the setting of tuberous sclerosis or Cowden syndrome. They present as single or multiple nodular, sessile, or, more rarely, pedunculated intestinal polyps. The hamartomas consist of proliferating, mature, spindle-shaped smooth muscle cells arranged in interlacing bundles that replace the lamina propria and entrap the epithelium (Fig. 19.31). There may also be fibrous tissue proliferation.

Smooth muscle hamartomas differ from Peutz-Jeghers–associated hamartomas in that the latter contain prominent arborizing smooth muscle proliferations that divide the epithelium and its surrounding normal-appearing lamina propria into segments. In contrast, smooth muscle hamartomas show proliferating smooth muscle cells obliterating

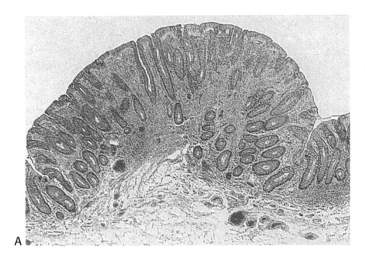

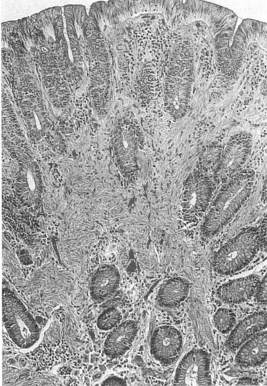

FIG. 19.31. Colonic smooth muscle hamartoma. **A:** Hamartomatous smooth muscle proliferation involving colonic lamina propria. **B:** Higher-power view demonstrating admixed muscular and fibrous tissue displacing the colonic glands. Note the lack of cellular atypia.

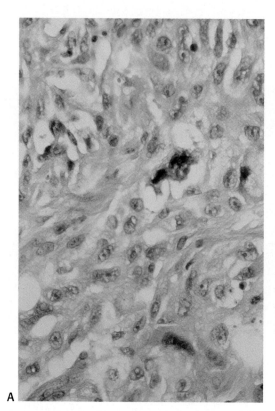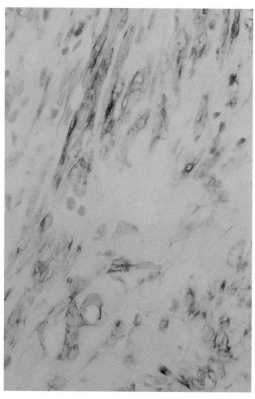

FIG. 19.32. Small intestinal leiomyosarcoma. **A:** These spindle cell lesions typically show much more pleomorphism and atypical mitoses than malignant gastrointestinal stromal tumors. **B:** Actin immunostain of the same lesion. The tumor was kit negative.

the lamina propria lying between the crypts without the prominent smooth muscle arborizations. Hamartomas also differ from leiomyomas in that leiomyomas are generally solitary and well circumscribed.

Leiomyosarcomas

True leiomyosarcomas do develop in the luminal gut, the omentum, and the mesentery, but they are not nearly as common as GISTs. Leiomyosarcomas, particularly vascular ones, affect older individuals. Leiomyosarcomas generally present in the same way as malignant GISTs, often as luminal, sometimes ulcerated, polypoid tumors (40). Grossly, the lesions appear lobular, gray-beige with pinkish tan areas and greenish areas of necrosis (50). The tumors range in size from 10 to 23 cm and may be multiple.

Gastrointestinal, omental, and mesenteric leiomyosarcomas contain well-differentiated smooth muscle cells with elongated or oval, often blunt-ended (cigar-shaped) atypical nuclei and eosinophilic cytoplasm. The tumors resemble soft tissue leiomyosarcomas. All of the tumors exhibit nuclear pleomorphism, which, unlike GISTs, can be extensive (Fig. 19.32). Coagulative necrosis is usually present; skeinoid fibers are absent. Mitotic activity is often high (sometimes >50 mitoses/50 hpf) (88). The differential diagnosis includes the entities listed in Table 19.5. Leiomyosarcomas are globally positive for α-smooth muscle actin and variably

positive for desmin. They may be focally positive for cytokeratin-18, but negative for cytokeratin-19. The tumors are negative for CD34, CD117, S110, glial fibrillary acidic protein (GFAP), and other neural markers. Leiomyosarcomas lack *KIT* mutations.

Leiomyosarcomas are treated with surgical resection. Lesions that are completely excised may be cured. However, tumors with positive tumor margins tend to recur locally as well as metastasize to the liver, causing patient death (88).

NEURAL TUMORS

Primary gastrointestinal neurogenic tumors are rare. They fall into two major groups: Those of peripheral nerve sheath origin (schwannomas, neurofibromas, ganglioneuromas, neuromas, and perineuromas) and those arising from the sympathetic or chromaffin system (neuroblastomas, ganglioneuromas, and paragangliomas).

Schwann Cell Tumors

Isolated gastrointestinal schwannomas constitute only 2% to 6% of all GI mesenchymal tumors and 0.2% of all gastric tumors. Patients range in age from 10 to 81 years with an average age of 52.6 (89). Women are slightly more commonly affected than men. Gastrointestinal Schwann cell

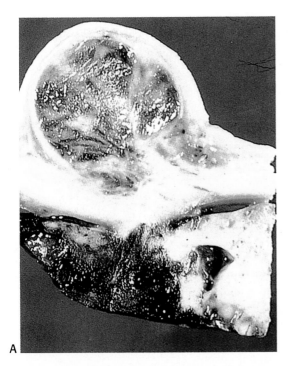

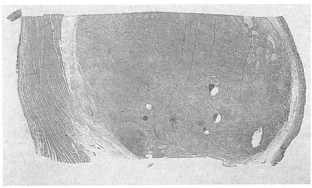

FIG. 19.33. Gastric schwannoma. **A:** Cut section of a pigmented gastric schwannoma. The overlying mucosal surface is not ulcerated. **B:** Whole mount of the lesion shown in A. Note pushing margins and lack of necrosis or hemorrhage.

tumors are particularly common in NF1 patients (90). Some patients have associated lesions (conditions), including colonic adenomas or Gorlin syndrome (90). The clinical features vary depending on lesional size and location. They present in the same ways as GISTs. Schwannomas preferentially affect the stomach (91) followed by the colon and rectum (92). Less commonly, they arise in the small intestine and esophagus. A subset of schwannomas, the benign mucosal epithelioid nerve sheath tumors, preferentially affects the colon (93), although this may reflect the large number of colonic biopsies that are examined annually.

Schwannomas average 6.4 cm in diameter with a range of 0.5 to 14 cm. Grossly and endoscopically, they resemble other mesenchymal neoplasms (Fig. 19.33). They arise in the submucosa and muscularis propria and are usually covered by an intact mucosa. Larger tumors ulcerate. These spherical or ovoid tumors may protrude into the bowel lumen in a polypoid fashion, or they may lie primarily in an intramural location or present as a subserosal mass projecting from the antimesenteric bowel surface (Fig. 19.34). Schwann cell tumors may grossly appear to be well encapsulated, but histologically they interdigitate with the surrounding stroma. Schwannomas are generally glistening, rubbery to firm, yellow, white-tan tumors, often with speckled cut surfaces resembling soft tissue schwannomas. Myxoid areas may be present. An exceptional schwannoma diffusely involved the entire large bowel (94).

Most schwannomas arise from the myenteric plexus (Fig. 19.35). Benign schwannomas consist almost entirely of Schwann cells without neurites (Fig. 19.36). They contain woven nests of compact bundles of slender, wavy S100-positive spindle cells admixed with a loose myxoid stroma. The tumor cells may also form compact fascicles, occasionally

aligning in rows or vague palisades (Verocay bodies). Some exhibit classic Antoni A and B areas, although these are commonly absent (95). Individual cells have a distinct eosinophilic cytoplasm. The dark fusiform nuclei vary in shape and size. Pleomorphism is generally mild, although some tumors focally may show significant nuclear atypia. However, even in these areas the nuclei have a uniform chromatin distribution. Mitotic activity is minimal to scanty and never exceeds five mitoses per 50 hpf. When the tumor bundles are cut transversely, the cells appear round and epithelioid. The cells are often intimately admixed with collagenous fibers highlighted by trichrome stains. Schwannomas often contain a sprinkling of lymphocytes and mast cells. Features unique to GI schwannomas include peripheral lymphoid cuffs and an uncommon microtrabecular pattern (95). The peripheral lymphoid foci sometimes contain germinal centers. GI schwannomas also differ from their soft tissue counterparts in that they often lack hyalinized blood vessels, a fibrous capsule, or degenerative changes (95).

Mucosal benign epithelioid nerve sheath tumors, a subset of GI schwannomas, show an infiltrative growth pattern and consist of spindled to predominantly epithelioid cells arranged in nests and whorls. The lesions center in the lamina propria and extend toward the mucosal surface and superficial submucosa. The proliferating cells contain uniform round to oval nuclei with frequent intranuclear pseudoinclusions and an eosinophilic fibrillary cytoplasm. The lesion may be surrounded by eosinophils (93).

The vast majority of schwannomas are benign. Histologic criteria for the diagnosis of malignancy are based on the number of mitotic figures, cellularity, nuclear atypia, and tumor necrosis. A rare esophageal malignant schwannoma measuring 8.2 cm in diameter contained a proliferation of

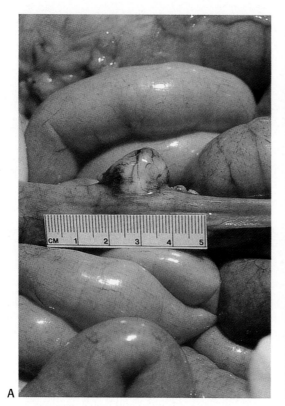
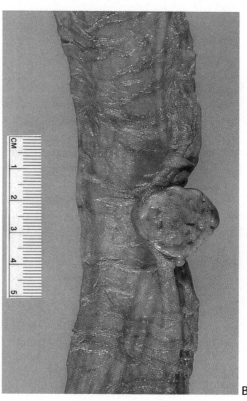

FIG. 19.34. Neurilemoma of the small bowel. **A:** Photograph of the intestines in place. A mass is present projecting from the serosal surface of the jejunum. **B:** Opened bowel demonstrating the presence of a nodular mass projecting into the serosal surface.

spindle-shaped cells with variably sized, chromatin-rich nuclei and a palisading structure. The nuclei showed marked atypia with high cellularity without necrosis and minimal mitotic activity. Nonetheless, metastases were present in the regional lymph nodes (96).

Schwannomas may show melanocytic differentiation (Fig. 19.37) and other mesenchymal elements. Tumors containing skeletal muscle cells are called Triton tumors (Fig. 19.38). Schwannomas are diffusely S100 (nuclear and cytoplasmic) and vimentin positive. Schwannomas are also immunoreactive for Leu7, laminin, GFAP, and PGP 9.5. Most tumors are also positive for nestin, a marker also commonly expressed in GISTs (50). Epithelial membrane antigen staining is limited to a few residual perineural cells. The tumors are also variably focally CD34+ (95). They are CD117, smooth muscle actin, and desmin negative unless they contain heterologous elements (Fig. 19.38).

Tumors without cytologic atypia or significant mitotic activity generally follow a benign clinical course. Malignant tumors require resection.

Perineuromas

Perineuromas are rare benign peripheral nerve sheath tumors. They generally arise in soft tissues and only a handful of cases have been reported in the stomach and intestine (77). There is a marked female predominance. The age of

diagnosis ranges from 35 to 72, with a median age of 51. Most lesions present as small sessile polyps often found during routine screening for colorectal cancers. Rare tumors present with abdominal pain or GI bleeding. One unusual case presented with intermittent abdominal pain, nausea, and vomiting, culminating as small bowel obstruction and necessitating partial resection (97).

Incidentally detected colorectal tumors range in size from 0.2 to 0.6 cm. The tumors arise in the mucosa or submucosa and measure 3 to 5 cm in size. The cut surfaces of these well-circumscribed tumors appear myxoid without necrosis. Histologically, perineuromas contain a proliferation of cytologically bland spindle cells with ovoid to tapered nuclei. The eosinophilic cells have pale, indistinct, elongated, bipolar cytoplasmic processes. The lesions may show a focally whorled growth pattern. Intramucosal lesions interdigitate with the adjacent lamina propria, sometimes entrapping hyperplastic glands; they may also infiltrate between the smooth muscle bundles of the muscularis propria. The cells lack cytologic atypia, mitotic activity, or pleomorphism. A fine collagenous stroma lies among the tumor cells.

The tumors are epithelial membrane antigen (EMA), vimentin, and neural cell adhesion molecule (NCAM) positive. EMA positivity ranges from very strong in some areas to very weak in others. This is due to the delicate nature of the cell cytoplasmic processes. Fifty percent of cases are positive for the tight junction–associated protein claudin-1 (97). All

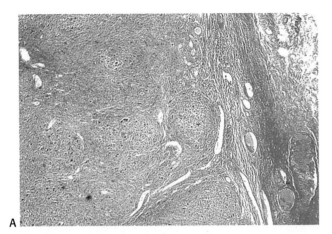

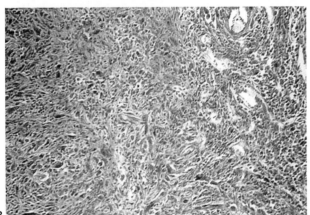

FIG. 19.35. Malignant schwannoma arising in the jejunum. **A:** The wall of the small bowel is extensively replaced by tumor cells. **B:** Area with spindle cell proliferation and giant cells.

tumors are negative for S100 protein, GFAP, neurofilament protein, smooth muscle actin, desmin, caldesmon, CD117, and keratin. The differential diagnosis includes ganglioneuromas, neurofibromas, and leiomyomas (Table 19.8).

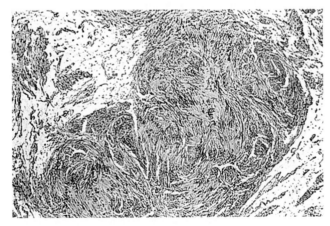

FIG. 19.36. Microscopic appearance of benign schwannoma with swirling bundles of Schwann cells. The tumor contains both Antoni A and Antoni B areas.

Neurofibromas and Neurofibromatosis

Gastrointestinal neurofibromas develop either as sporadic isolated lesions or as a more diffuse GI involvement in NF1 patients. NF1, an autosomal dominant disorder, affects at least 1 in every 3,000 people, making it one of the most common inherited human diseases. Approximately 25% of all NF1 patients develop gastrointestinal manifestations, including neurofibromas as well as other tumor types (Table 19.9).

The *NF1* gene localizes to chromosome 17q11.2. *NF1* alterations include translocations, deletions, insertions, and point mutations, all of which interrupt the coding sequence. The *NF1* gene product neurofibromin reduces signal transduction by accelerating inactivation of the ras protooncogene (98). *NF1* is a tumor suppressor gene that regulates a number of cellular processes including the extracellular signal-related kinase (ERK) mitogen-activated protein (MAP) cascade, adenyl cyclase, and cytoskeletal assembly. *NF1* mutations generally lead to an increased risk of both benign and malignant tumors, especially malignant peripheral nerve sheath tumors (MPNSTs). The development of MPNSTs is a multistage process involving many altered cell cycle regulators in addition to the biallelic inactivation of the *NF1* gene. Other altered genes include *p53* and *p16* (99,100). Neurofibromas also aberrantly express the epidermal growth factor receptor.

Recent data suggest a possible relationship between NF1 and hereditary nonpolyposis colorectal cancer syndrome. Children who are homozygous carriers of *MLH1* mutations exhibit clinical features of NF1 and early onset of extracolonic cancers including hematologic and central nervous system malignancies (101). Most of these patients do not develop gastrointestinal neoplasms, but one report of two patients with homozygous *MLH1* mutations did show

TABLE 19.8 **Intramural Perineuromas: Differential Diagnosis**

	Cell Types	IHC
GISTs	Epithelioid spindle mixed cell types	Most c-kit + Some PDGFRα + 50% caldesmon + EMA −
Schwannomas	Schwann cells	S100 ±, GFAP + EMA −
Perineuromas	Perineural cells	EMA + S100 −, NF −, GFAP − Caldesmon − Actin −
Leiomyomas	Smooth muscle cells	Actin + Caldesmon + EMA −

EMA, epithelial membrane antigen; GFAP, glial fibrillary acidic protein; GISTs, gastrointestinal stromal tumors; IHC, immunohistochemistry; NF, neurofibromatosis; PDGFRA, platelet-derived growth factor receptor-α.

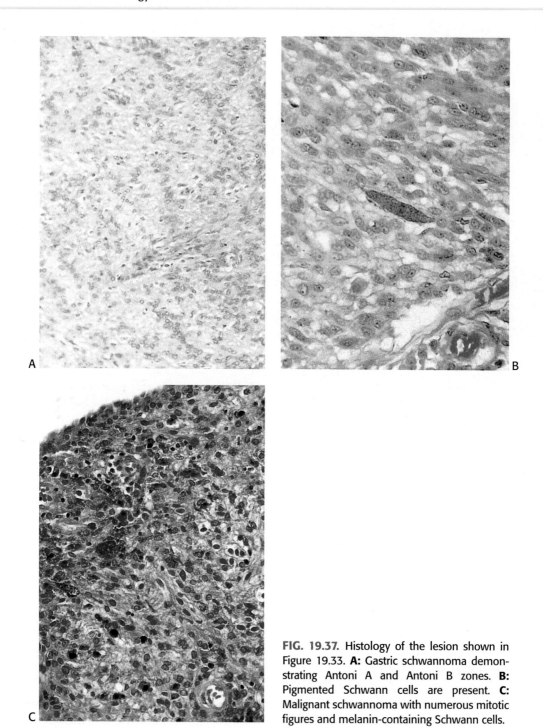

FIG. 19.37. Histology of the lesion shown in Figure 19.33. **A:** Gastric schwannoma demonstrating Antoni A and Antoni B zones. **B:** Pigmented Schwann cells are present. **C:** Malignant schwannoma with numerous mitotic figures and melanin-containing Schwann cells.

colonic and small intestinal neoplasms in addition to NF1-like features (102).

Seven important components characterize NF1 patients; two must be present to establish the diagnosis (103) (Table 19.10). In addition to the dysplastic lesions and benign and malignant tumors, NF1 patients also tend to have a smaller than normal stature, and up to 60% of patients suffer from a learning disability.

Neurofibromas, present in small numbers during childhood, becoming more numerous with growth, puberty, pregnancy, and advancing age. GI neurofibromas cause

bleeding, melena, obstruction, pain, and other problems. Megacolon and pseudo-obstruction affect 10% of patients due to neural plexus abnormalities (Fig. 19.39) (103). Neurofibromas most commonly develop in the jejunum, followed by the stomach, ileum, duodenum, colon (103), and mesentery. Rare lesions arise in the esophagus and appendix (103). The tumors are usually solitary unless the patient has NF1, in which case multiple serosal and mucosal polypoid nodules develop (Fig. 19.40) (104). Most neurofibromas arise from the myenteric plexus and project from the antimesenteric surface of the bowel. Rarely, they present as polyps.

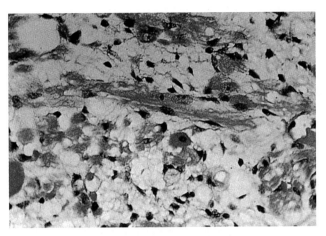

FIG. 19.38. Focus of skeletal muscle differentiation in a schwannoma. This tumor can be designated as a triton tumor.

TABLE 19.9	Gastrointestinal Lesions Seen with Increased Frequency in Neurofibromatosis Type 1 Patients

Neurofibromas
Schwannomas
Duodenal carcinoid tumors
Somatostatinomas
Gastrointestinal stromal tumors
Paragangliomas
Gangliocytic paragangliomas
Ganglioneuromas
Esophageal hyperplastic polyps
Ganglion cell abnormalities
Hyperplasia of the enteric nervous system
Gastrointestinal adenocarcinomas
Adenomas
Intestinal malignant mixed tumors

Neurofibromas appear as encapsulated or nonencapsulated spherical or cylindrical tumors.

The tumors consist of a mixture of spindle cells with wavy dark nuclei, strands of collagen, and varying amounts of a myxoid matrix. The cells include Schwann cells, perineurial cells, fibroblasts, endothelial cells, mast cells, and occasional axons, along with scattered neurites and, rarely, melanocytes (Figs. 19.41). Definitive characteristics exist for each of the five major cell types present in these lesions (Table 19.11). A storiform pattern may be seen, but this is uncommon. Neurofibromas contain large numbers of mast cells.

In NF1 patients, proliferations of nerve fibers involve the lamina propria, submucosa, and/or serosa (Fig. 19.41). Submucosal lesions that extend through the muscularis mucosae may separate the overlying crypts, causing the lesion to resemble a juvenile polyp or a perineurioma. Nerve plexuses often appear abnormal with a pronounced decrease in the number of argyrophilic neurons and a marked increase in nerve fibers, particularly in the descending and sigmoid colon. Because of the neural abnormalities, the circular and longitudinal muscle layers become both atrophic and hypertrophic. The neurofibromas are frequently plexiform in the setting of NF1.

Neurofibromas are not usually removed in the setting of NF1 due to their large number and the lack of symptoms in

small lesions. Symptomatic larger lesions or those that cause secondary problems such as volvulus or intussusception are resected. Currently, clinical trials in NF1 patients are evaluating the efficacy of epidermal growth factor receptor (EGFR) inhibitors in the treatment of these tumors.

Neuromas

Spontaneous neuromas develop almost exclusively in the appendix unless there is pre-existing trauma, in which case traumatic neuromas develop. Appendiceal neuromas are discussed in Chapter 8. *Traumatic neuromas* consist of proliferating endoneural and perineural connective tissue, Schwann cells, and regenerating neurons. When a nerve is damaged, the axon of the central stump of the distal end of the normal segment proximal to the site of injury begins to sprout by budding and then grows in a zigzag fashion. Traumatic neuromas develop near anastomotic sites or following other bowel injuries.

Malignant Peripheral Nerve Sheath Tumors

MPNSTs often affect NF1 patients and usually exhibit Schwann cell differentiation. However, since not all tumors in the group are clearly schwannian in origin, most prefer the

TABLE 19.10	Features of Neurofibromatosis

1. Six or more café-au-lait spots (macules), the greatest diameter of which measures >3 mm in prepubertal patients and >15 mm in postpubertal patients
2. Two or more neurofibromas of any type or one plexiform neurofibroma
3. Freckling in the axillary or inguinal region
4. Optic gliomas
5. Two or more Lisch nodules
6. A distinctive osseous lesion known as sphenoid dysplasia or pseudoarthrosis
7. A first-degree relative with the diagnosis of neurofibromatosis type 1 defined by the preceding criteria

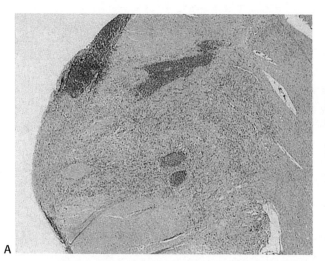
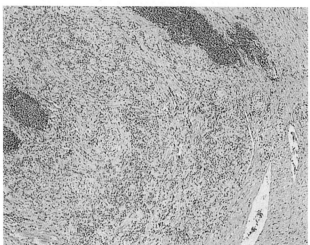

FIG. 19.39. Patient with neurofibromatosis and intestinal pseudo-obstruction. **A:** Neurofibroma arising in the myenteric plexus. **B:** Higher-power view of the same lesion demonstrating proliferation of neural cells and Schwann cells.

diagnosis of MPNST for this group of neoplasms. These tumors often associate with small or large nerves; however, similar tumors may develop in the absence of an identifiable nerve. Many MPNSTs initially appear as highly cellular fibrosarcomalike tumors. Features that suggest the diagnosis of MPNST include the presence of alternating hypocellular and hypercellular regions; the appearance of thin, comet-shaped or bullet-shaped nuclei, particularly in the hypocellular areas; nervelike whorls; tactoid bodies resembling Meissner corpuscles; nuclear palisading (a feature that may also be present in other spindle cell tumors such as leiomyosarcomas); the presence of prominent thick-walled vessels; and heterologous elements. Several histologic subtypes of MPNSTs exist. Some resemble fibrosarcomas (the most common pattern) with dense populations of spindle cells arranged in fascicles intersecting at acute angles and producing a herringbone pattern. Hypocellular areas are also present. The presence of these alternating hypercellular and hypocellular areas suggests nerve sheath origin and is reminiscent of benign Schwann cell tumors.

Other tumors resemble neurofibromas and mitotic activity is important in identifying these lesions as malignant. Other features suggestive of malignancy include the presence of focal, densely cellular lesions or necrosis. Occasional cases display extreme nuclear pleomorphism with a malignant fibrous histocytoma (MFH)-like appearance. Any tumor containing more than one mitotic figure per 20 hpf should be construed as evidence of potential malignant behavior.

Lesions that can be especially difficult to diagnose are those that are purely epithelioid in nature. These tumors typically

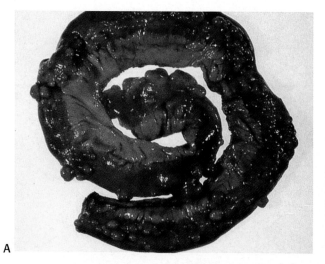
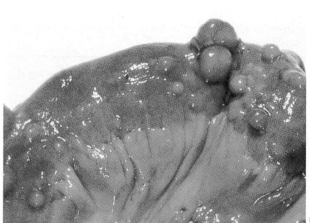

FIG. 19.40. Neurofibromatosis coli. **A:** Partial small intestinal resection demonstrating numerous small, pedunculated serosal and subserosal polypoid lesions. **B:** Higher-power view of small intestinal neurofibromatosis. (Courtesy of Dr. G. Atkinson, Department of Pathology, Presbyterian Hospital, Albuquerque, NM.)

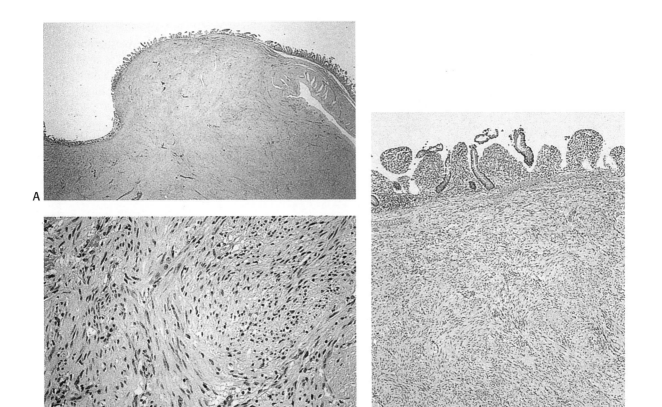

FIG. 19.41. Neurofibromatosis coli. **A:** Focal neurofibromatous proliferation elevating overlying mucosa and producing a "polyp." **B:** Interlacing bundles of neurons, Schwann cells, and fibroblasts. **C:** Area of proliferating neurons, Schwann cells, and fibroblasts arising from nerve. (Courtesy of Dr. G. Atkinson, Department of Pathology, Presbyterian Hospital, Albuquerque, NM.)

TABLE 19.11	Immunoreactivity of Cells in Neurofibromas

Schwann cells
Neuromas
  PGP 9.5
  S100
  Type IV collagen
Perineural cells
  Type IV collagen
Fibroblasts
  Type I collagen
  Type II collagen
  Fibronectin
Endothelial cells
  Factor VIII–related antigen
  Type IV collagen
Mast cells
  Factor VIII–related antigen
  Histamine
Axons
  Neurofilament protein
  PGP 9.5

grow in a nodular pattern, usually associated with necrosis, and they may be confused with either a melanoma or carcinoma since the epithelioid cells are closely packed and grow in sheets. The cytoplasm of the epithelioid cells is pale and the nuclei are usually rounded with evenly dispersed chromatin or prominent nucleoli. S100 positivity is seen in 50% to 75% of all MPNSTs. The staining is never diffuse and its positivity is as strong as in cellular schwannomas. Some MPNSTs show perineural differentiation that is recognized by significant EMA reactivity.

Ganglioneuromas

Gastrointestinal ganglioneuromas (GNs) fall into three groups: Isolated (solitary) polypoid ganglioneuromas (the most common group), ganglioneuromatous polyposis, and diffuse ganglioneuromatosis (106). All three forms predominantly affect the colon and rectum, unlike neurofibromas, which more commonly involve the small intestine and stomach. The transmural form of diffuse ganglioneuromatosis is most frequently seen in MEN-2b patients. In contrast, NF1 patients have mucosal ganglioneuromas.

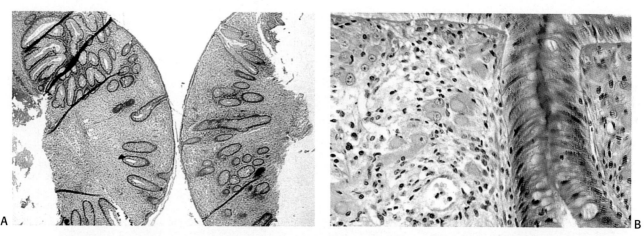

FIG. 19.42. Isolated ganglioneuroma in a patient who presented with a colonic polyp. **A:** Whole mount of polypectomy specimen. **B:** Characteristic proliferation of ganglion cells in stroma displacing the glands.

Isolated Ganglioneuromas

Isolated GNs develop in the absence of the various syndromes associated with polypoid or diffuse ganglioneuromatosis. The tumors develop equally in men and women. Isolated polypoid GNs occur at any age, but most patients are young, usually younger than 20 years of age. Most lesions are detected incidentally. Symptomatic patients present with rectal bleeding, pain, weight loss, and irritable bowel. Lesions involving the ileocecal valve may present as acute appendicitis. GNs develop in the appendix, terminal ileum, duodenum, stomach, intestines, and anus (107), presenting as small, single, sessile or pedunculated polyps that range in size from 0.1 to 2 cm in diameter.

These lesions typically develop in the mucosa or submucosa, often with a low-power pattern resembling a juvenile polyp because of the disturbed crypt architecture, cystic glands, expanded lamina propria, and smooth surface epithelium (Fig. 19.42). Closer inspection demonstrates a hypercellular and expanded lamina propria composed of S100-positive spindle cells lying in a fibrillar matrix with isolated ganglion cells (or irregular groups and nests of ganglion cells) dispersed among the spindle cells. The spindle cells merge imperceptibly with the surrounding lamina propria. In cases where one is uncertain if the large cells present in these proliferations are ganglion cells, they can be stained with antibodies to synaptophysin, NSE, or RET protein.

In another pattern, GNs appear as nodular mucosal proliferations with clustered ganglion cells admixed in varying amounts without causing significant disarray of the mucosal architecture. Another pattern of GN consists of nodular mucosal and submucosal ganglion and spindle cell proliferations suggestive of a neurofibroma. This pattern shows continuity between the mucosal and submucosal components with a microscopic plexiformlike arrangement of the neural elements sometimes involving the submucosal plexus. Patients with NF1 may show ganglioneuromas admixed with areas of plexiform neurofibroma and carcinoid tumor (Fig. 19.43).

The bulk of ganglioneuromas consist of nonmyelinated nerve fibers coursing in all fibers and accompanied by Schwann cells. A thin collagenous connective tissue capsule may surround the tumor, separating it from the overlying muscularis mucosae or other portions of the gastrointestinal wall. The number of ganglion cells varies greatly from place to place; most are arranged in clusters. Ganglion cells may also separate strands of a splayed muscularis mucosae; occasional ganglion cells are present in the mucosa proper. Most ganglion cells appear multipolar and are not pigmented. The ganglion cells are not surrounded by capsular or satellite cells. Ectopic ganglion cells in the lamina propria can occur in response to mucosal injury, but the ectopic ganglion cells associated with reparative lesions lie within a normal-appearing lamina propria without the characteristic S100-positive spindle cell proliferation seen in GNs.

The removal of isolated ganglioneuromas is curative. These lesions are benign, are not associated with systemic manifestations, and do not require long-term follow-up.

Ganglioneuromatous Polyposis

Ganglioneuromatous polyposis affects patients with familial adenomatous polyposis (108), multiple cutaneous lipomas and skin tags (106), Cowden disease (109), tuberous sclerosis (110), MEN-2b, (111), neurofibromatosis (105), colorectal carcinoma (112), and juvenile polyposis (Fig. 19.44) (113). MEN-2 patients with intestinal GNs often exhibit germline mutations in the *ret* oncogene (114). There is a slight male predominance and patients range in age from 19 to 61 years with a mean of 39 years. Diffuse gastrointestinal ganglioneuromatosis, lipomatosis, bilateral adrenal myolipomas, pancreatic telangiectasias, and a multinodular goiter may affect patients with a history of insulin-dependent diabetes, hypertension, peptic ulcer, and remote cerebral infarction (115). This may represent a rare variant of the MEN complex or a separate, previously unrecognized syndrome.

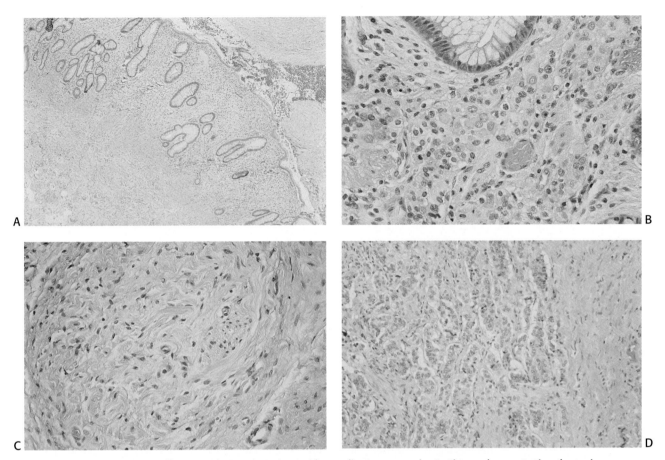

FIG. 19.43. Neurofibromatosis type 1 patient with ganglioneuromatosis. **A:** Picture demonstrating the typical low-power appearance of a ganglioneuroma. The lamina propria is infiltrated by a spindle cell proliferation that separates the glands without destroying them. **B:** Higher magnification of the lamina propria showing the spindle cells and ganglion cells. **C:** Area of neurofibromatous proliferation. **D:** The lesion had carcinoid cells intermingled with it. (Case courtesy of Dr. George Mutema, Good Samaritan Hospital, Cincinnati, OH.)

Ganglioneuromatous polyposis is distinguished by the presence of 20 to 40 innumerable sessile or pedunculated mucosal and/or submucosal tumors ranging in size from 1 mm to 2.2 cm. The lesions tend to concentrate in the colon and terminal small bowel, but they occur elsewhere, including the stomach and appendix (106). The polyps histologically resemble polypoid GNs, but they show greater variability in their neural supportive and ganglion cell content when compared to polypoid GNs. The overlying surface may ulcerate. A diffuse hyperplastic overgrowth of the various plexuses often occurs and may associate with pseudo-obstruction. Other lesions demonstrate unusual filiform mucosal projections containing clusters of ganglion cells with little or no apparent neural components.

Diffuse Ganglioneuromatosis

Diffuse ganglioneuromatosis occurs in association with congenital defects, mental retardation, NF1, MEN-2b (111), juvenile polyposis, adenomatous polyps, Cowden disease (116), carcinomas (108), or MPNSTs. The prevalence of ganglioneuromas in MEN-2b approaches 100% (11). Patients

with diffuse ganglioneuromatosis tend to be males ranging in age from 6 to 59 years with a mean age of 35. Patients with MEN-2b and diffuse ganglioneuromatosis typically present at a young age and exhibit gastroesophageal and small intestinal motility disorders (117), mimicking Hirschsprung disease. Severe constipation is usually the first and main gastrointestinal symptom, although diarrhea and diverticular disease can also be present. Patients may have extraintestinal neurofibromas, and various skeletal abnormalities are present in 81% of these patients.

Diffuse ganglioneuromatosis can extend from the lips to the rectum. The lesions vary in size from a few millimeters to 1 to 17 cm, producing stricturelike thickening of bowel segments or large irregular, nodular lesions. When the lesions are large, they may cause napkin-ring constrictions that grossly resemble carcinomas. Irregular mucosal nodular lesions can also be seen. Discrete tumor masses are usually absent. The lesions may involve the mucosa, submucosa, and subserosal plexuses. They tend to grow intramurally and to ulcerate when large. Unlike their more polypoid variants, the lesions of diffuse ganglioneuromatosis tend to be less well circumscribed. Also unlike solitary ganglioneuromas and

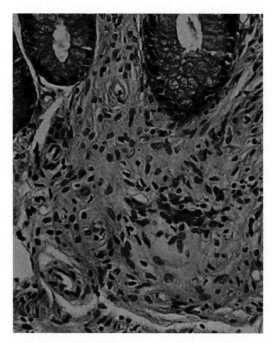

FIG. 19.44. Patient with juvenile polyposis coli and ganglioneuromatosis. Low-power magnification of the mucosa demonstrating the replacement of the muscularis mucosae with proliferation of neurofibromatouslike elements as well as isolated ganglion cells.

gangliomatous polyposis, the epicenter of diffuse ganglioneuromas lies within the muscularis propria, causing the mural thickening described previously.

Diffuse ganglioneuromatosis consists of exuberant, usually transmural proliferations of nerve fibers, ganglion cells, and supporting cells of the enteric nervous system. The growth pattern varies from fusiform hyperplastic expansions of the myenteric plexus to confluent irregular transmural ganglioneuromatous proliferations that distort the myenteric plexus and infiltrate the adjacent bowel wall. The morphologic changes are highlighted by antibodies directed at S100, GFAP, vimentin, NSE, and synaptophysin. These lesions represent a complex hyperplasia of peptidergic, cholinergic, and probably adrenergic nerve fibers instead of a selective overgrowth of any one type of nerve fiber (112). Transmural ganglioneuromas exhibit increased immunoreactivity for vasoactive intestinal polypeptide, nerve growth factor, opioid peptides, leu-enkephalin, and substance P (118). In patients with the transmural form of the disease, there may be associated intestinal neuronal dysplasia (119) and myenteric plexus hyperplasia.

PARAGANGLIOMAS

Rare gastrointestinal paragangliomas affect the esophagus, stomach, and small bowel, especially the duodenum (Fig. 19.45) (120–122). Abdominal paragangliomas are usually sporadic lesions, although familial forms have been reported

(123). These familial forms associate with germline mutations in the *SDHD, SDHC,* and *SDHB* genes (124–126). Some patients have NF1 (122), MEN-2 (127), von Hippel-Lindau disease (128), the Carney triad (5), or a variant GIST paraganglioma syndrome (5,24). In the latter setting the paragangliomas are frequently multicentric and extra-adrenal (jejunal) in location (24).

Paragangliomas may be large, measuring up to 10 cm in diameter. Unlike gangliocytic paragangliomas, they do not primarily affect the submucosa but enter the bowel from its external surface. The tumors appear grayish white with multiple cysts and hemorrhagic foci histologically resembling paragangliomas arising elsewhere. They contain spindle cells (Schwann cells) and round or polygonal epithelioid cells arranged in *Zellballen* (Fig. 19.45). The epithelioid cells are argyrophilic and surrounded by a capillary network. The tumors lack the neurofibromatous and carcinoidal components found in gangliocytic paragangliomas. Malignant tumors contain significant pleomorphism and numerous mitoses. Cellular pleomorphism alone is an unreliable criterion of malignancy, contrasting with mitotic activity and vascular invasion. There is diffuse cytoplasmic positivity for GFAP and NSE in most cells. Chromogranin A and synaptophysin immunoreactivity is more heterogeneous. The tumor cells can be focally positive for neurofilament protein. Cytokeratin stains demonstrate strong reactivity in scattered tumor cells. The tumor may also produce ectopic substances such as adrenocorticotropic hormone (ACTH) and vasoactive intestinal peptide. S100 immunostains highlight the sustentacular cells. An unusual patient with the Carney triad exhibited dual CD117 expression in both a stromal tumor and a paraganglioma (129).

GRANULAR CELL TUMORS

Gastrointestinal granular cell tumors, once thought to be rare, are now more commonly encountered due to the increased use of upper endoscopy. The tumors develop in individuals from ages 20 to 70, equally affecting men and women and often affecting blacks. Some tumors develop following radiation therapy (130). Granular cell tumors may coexist with other tumors, including GISTs, adenocarcinomas (131), other granular cell tumors, esophageal squamous cell carcinoma (132), and esophageal leiomyomatosis (133).

Granular cell tumors are often discovered incidentally at the time of endoscopy, surgery, or autopsy. Larger lesions are likely to be symptomatic. Symptoms depend on tumor location. Esophageal tumors present with dysphagia. Intestinal lesions present with intussusception, volvulus, bleeding, or a mass. Anal lesions may cause perianal discomfort and bleeding.

Granular cell tumors arise throughout the gastrointestinal tract, but are most common in the esophagus (Figs. 19.46 and 19.47) and large intestine (134). Up to 20% of lesions are multiple within a given organ. Sometimes granular cell tumors develop at several GI sites (135). Most esophageal

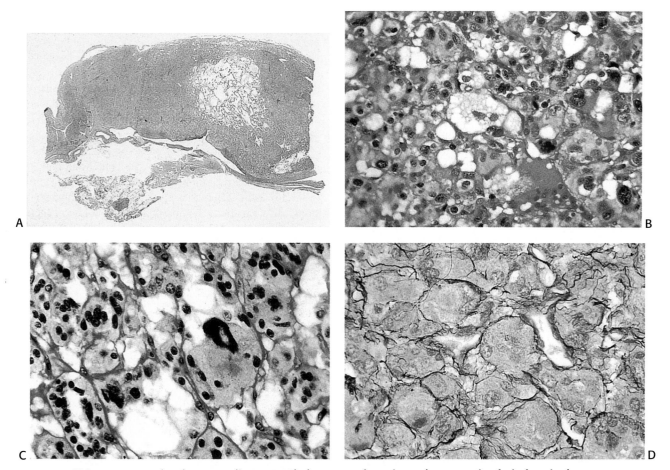

FIG. 19.45. Duodenal paraganglioma. **A:** Whole mount of specimen demonstrating foci of cystic change. **B:** Histologic features of a typical paraganglioma are present. **C:** Periodic acid–Schiff stain delineating the presence of prominent basement membranes surrounding the "Zellballen." **D:** Reticulin stain demonstrating a pattern similar to that seen in C.

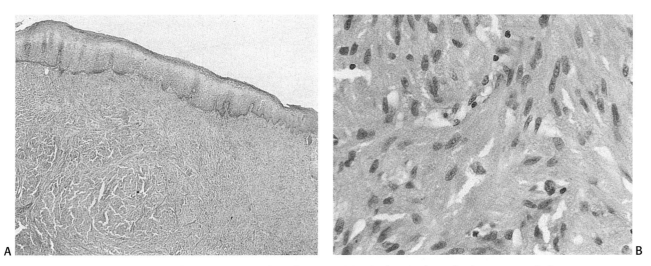

FIG. 19.46. Granular cell tumor. **A:** Granular cell tumor arising in the esophageal submucosa, replacing normal structures. **B:** Higher-power view of tumor cells, demonstrating characteristic eosinophilic granular cytoplasm.

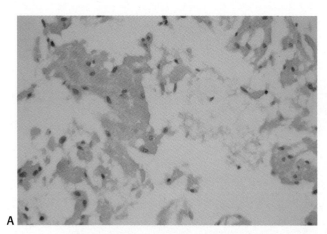

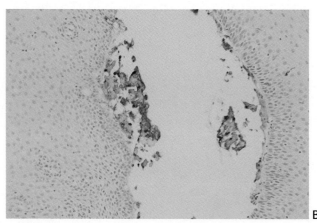

FIG. 19.47. Biopsy of esophageal granular cell tumor. **A:** The biopsy contained detached fragments of large eosinophilic cells and strips of squamous epithelium (not shown). **B:** The squamous epithelium is present and clinging to its bases is an S100-positive cell population.

granular cell tumors arise distally. Gastric granular cell tumors tend to affect the antrum. The tumors usually appear as smooth, sessile, localized, yellow–grayish white lesions measuring 1 to 4 cm in diameter. They arise in the submucosa or muscularis propria and are covered by an intact mucosa. Larger lesions are often malignant (136).

Gastrointestinal granular cell tumors resemble granular cell tumors arising elsewhere. They contain nests and cords of rounded, polygonal, occasionally elongated, infiltrating, bland cells with small dark nuclei and an abundant granular eosinophilic cytoplasm (Fig. 19.46). Variably sized coarse, red granules are periodic acid–Schiff (PAS) positive after diastase digestion. Pseudoepitheliomatous hyperplasia of the overlying squamous epithelium occurs in esophageal and anal squamous epithelium, especially in small esophageal biopsies (Fig. 19.47). Some tumors are confined to the muscularis propria or even to the adventitia (134); these deeper lesions will be missed on esophageal biopsies. Occasionally, an extensively infiltrating pattern is present in benign lesions (135).

Gastric granular cell tumors are randomly distributed between the submucosa and muscularis propria. Submucosal lesions may infiltrate or obliterate the muscularis mucosae and extend into the base of the mucosa, between individual glands. The tumor cells are neural in origin and are strongly S100 positive.

Granular cell tumors can be benign or malignant. Malignant lesions are rare (136). The following criteria suggest malignancy: Large size (>5 cm), increased cellularity, tumor cell necrosis, tumor cell spindling, increased nuclear size, large nucleoli, mitotic activity (greater than two mitoses per 10 hpf), and nuclear pleomorphism (136). Unfortunately, several studies of granular cell tumors that have metastasized found no reliable pathologic variables that allow one to distinguish benign from malignant tumors other than the presence of metastases or vascular invasion.

Granular cell tumors may resemble malignant melanomas or metastatic carcinomas. However, the bland cytologic fea-

tures should suggest that the lesion is benign. Immunohistochemical stains help elucidate the nature of the tumor. Granular cell tumors are consistently positive with antibodies to S100, vimentin, α_1-antitrypsin, α_1-antichymotrypsin, Leu7, myelin basic protein, CD68, GFAP, NSE (137), and nestin (138) and variably positive for cytokeratin (139). They may be weakly positive for CD117.

Areas of epithelial hyperplasia and the clinical impression of a mass may cause granular tumors to be misinterpreted as squamous carcinomas, particularly if only a small superficial mucosal biopsy is examined that contains hyperproliferative immature squamous cells with numerous mitoses and pseudoinvasive squamous cell tongues. The epithelial cells of pseudoepitheliomatous hyperplasia generally lack cytologic atypia and the connective tissue interface is far more complicated in invasive squamous cell carcinoma than in pseudoepitheliomatous hyperplasia.

Most esophageal granular cell tumors are small, benign tumors that can safely be left alone. They may also be removed by polypectomy or incisional biopsy. Large, symptomatic, or malignant lesions should be excised.

LIPOMAS, LIPOSARCOMAS, AND RELATED LESIONS

Gastrointestinal adipose tissue proliferations include lipomas, angiolipomas, liposarcomas, lipomatosis polyposis, and lipomatous hyperplasia of the ileocecal valve. All of these lesions are neoplastic except the last entity, which is discussed in Chapter 14.

Lipomas

Lipomas predominantly arise in the large bowel (51% to 70%), decreasing in incidence in the small bowel, stomach, and esophagus. In the stomach, the antrum is preferentially affected; in the colon, the right side is preferentially affected.

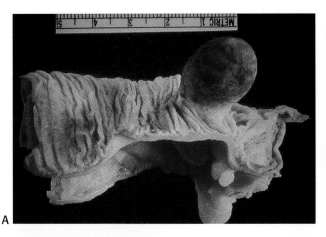
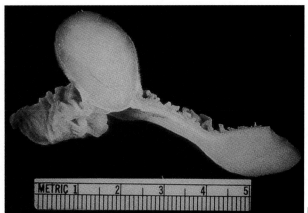
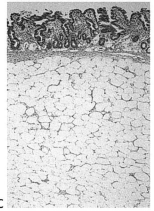

FIG. 19.48. Small intestinal lipoma. **A:** Pedunculated lesion demonstrating surface erythema. **B:** Cross section shows that the central portion of this well-encapsulated lesion consists of greasy, yellow material. **C:** Histologic features showing the presence of a submucosal lipoma that is replacing the normal submucosal structures. The lesion is well demarcated and consists of mature fat.

Large intestinal lipomas range in incidence from 0.035% to 4.4% of all intestinal neoplasms. They affect men and women equally and are less frequent in blacks than in whites. They occur in adults as well as children. Most patients with symptomatic lesions are 50 to 60 years old. Gastrointestinal lipomas are usually solitary, although some patients develop multiple lesions. Small lipomas are usually asymptomatic. Larger lesions may cause abdominal pain, intestinal obstruction, intussusception, and bleeding with iron deficiency anemia. Gastric lipomas >3 cm tend to ulcerate, causing peptic ulcer–like symptoms. Anorectal lipomas may present with rectal prolapse (140).

Most lipomas are compressible, submucosal lesions covered by an intact mucosa (Fig. 19.48). Rare lesions develop in the serosa. Small lipomas appear as a thickened fold or small polyp. Others may be large, lobulated, and pedunculated. Large lesions can twist and infarct or act as lead points of an intussusception. On cut surface, lipomas appear bright yellow, round, greasy, and encapsulated unless they have become infarcted (Fig. 19.49).

Lipomas consist of sharply circumscribed submucosal masses of mature adipose tissue with an overlying intact or eroded mucosa. Usually, a thick fibrous capsule surrounds the tumor. Secondary changes including nuclear hypertrophy, hyperchromasia, fat necrosis, fatty cysts, and foamy macrophages may be present. If extensive, these changes may mimic a liposarcoma. However, lipoblasts are absent. As the areas of fat necrosis resolve, spindle cells or atypical cellular areas remain. Such lesions are sometimes termed *atypical lipomas* (Fig. 19.50) (141). The atypical features consist of areas of cellular fibrosis, atypical hyperchromatic nuclei, and increased mitoses with the occasional atypical mitoses.

Mucosal pseudolipomatosis (air within the mucosa) may superficially resemble lipomas. Unlike true lipomas, mucosal pseudolipomatosis consists of irregularly shaped air spaces and the lesions are not encapsulated.

Angiolipomas

Angiolipomas arise in the stomach, duodenum, and colon, but they are rare (142–144). They grossly resemble lipomas. Larger lesions become hemorrhagic. These lesions are histologically identical to their extraintestinal counterparts and consist of a mixture of proliferating adipose tissue and blood vessels (Fig. 19.51). The latter consist of capillaries (complex and branching), often with a concomitant pericytic proliferation.

Lipomatosis

Diffuse lipomatous polyposis of the colon is rare, affecting both children and adults with a male predominance (145). Patients present with "polyposis," weight loss, intestinal bleeding, malabsorption, and intestinal obstruction.

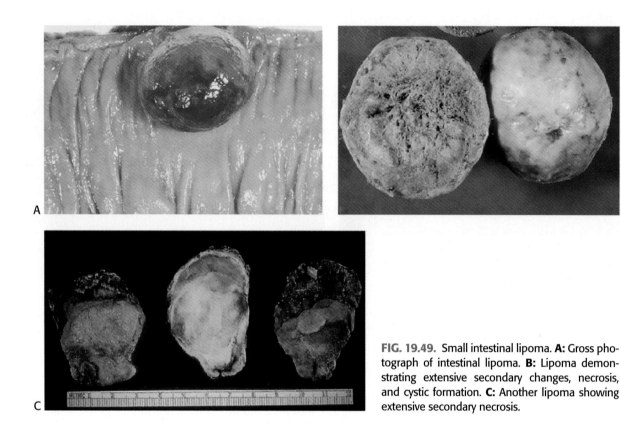

FIG. 19.49. Small intestinal lipoma. **A:** Gross photograph of intestinal lipoma. **B:** Lipoma demonstrating extensive secondary changes, necrosis, and cystic formation. **C:** Another lipoma showing extensive secondary necrosis.

Grossly, one sees dozens to hundreds of submucosal, sessile, and occasionally pedunculated lipomas accompanied by a marked but patchy increase in submucosal fat. The lipomas range in size from 0.2 to 5 cm. Larger lesions become hemorrhagic and ulcerated. The lesions may be distributed throughout the colon, or they may have a higher density in the descending and sigmoid colon (146). An exceptional patient was reported in whom there were between 700 and 1,000 polyps. The vast majority were lipomas, but multiple adenomas and hyperplastic polyps were also present (146). The lesions consist of mature fat, but unlike true lipomas,

they are not well encapsulated. The fat generally represents an extension of the submucosal into the mucosa, regularly replacing the lamina propria and sometimes displacing the glands.

Liposarcomas

Liposarcomas originate in the GI tract; more commonly, the GI tract becomes secondarily involved by the ingrowth of a retroperitoneal or mesenteric tumor. Primary gastrointestinal liposarcomas develop in adults. A rare example of a

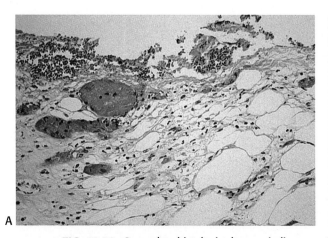
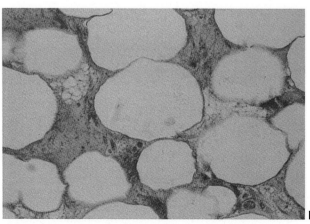

FIG. 19.50. Secondary histologic changes in lipomas. **A:** The surface of this lipoma has become eroded and shows acute inflammation and beginning fat necrosis. **B:** This infarcted lipoma has undergone coagulation necrosis and lacks nuclei.

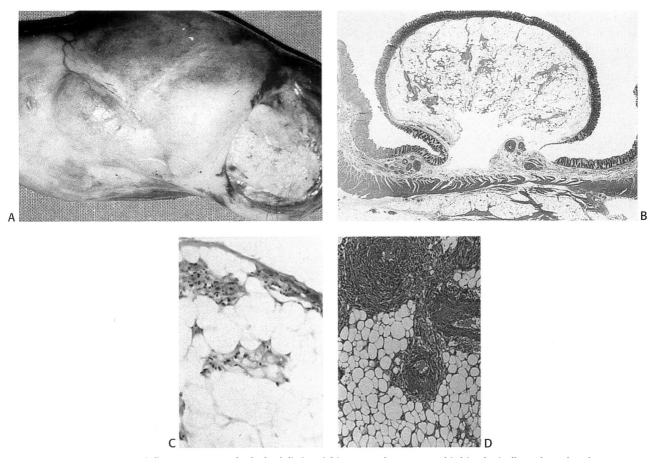

FIG. 19.51. Angiolipoma. **A:** Note the lack of distinguishing gross features. **B:** This histologically pedunculated lesion consists of a proliferation of fat and blood vessels within the submucosa, elevating an intact mucosal surface. **C:** Higher magnification of one of the less cellular areas, demonstrating the presence of mature fat and small vessels. **D:** Sometimes the vascular proliferations are more extensive than shown in this figure.

liposarcoma arising in the sigmoid mesocolon in conjunction with lipomatosis of the rectosigmoid has also been described (147). Myxoid and round cell liposarcomas associate with *TLS-CHOP* or *EWS-CHOP* fusion genes (148).

Patients present with abdominal discomfort, vomiting, or intestinal obstruction. The tumors vary in appearance from lobular, yellow, greasy masses that partially obstruct the intestinal lumen (Fig. 19.52) to soft, myxoid, almost gelatinous lesions to more solid, white, firm nodules that are sharply demarcated from surrounding mature-looking adipose tissue. Hemorrhage and necrosis are common. The tumors are generally large (2.5 to 60 cm) at the time of presentation (149). The mucosa overlying the tumor often becomes ulcerated. Primary liposarcomas grow out from the intestinal wall and spread into the mesentery. In large tumors with extensive involvement of the abdominal cavity, one may be unable to determine whether the tumor arose in the bowel or extended into it from an extragastrointestinal site.

The histologic features of gastrointestinal liposarcomas resemble liposarcomas arising in soft tissues. Well-differentiated liposarcomas show variations in adipocyte size and a scattering of mono- and multivacuolated lipoblasts with irregularly shaped, hyperchromatic nuclei that are often situated on

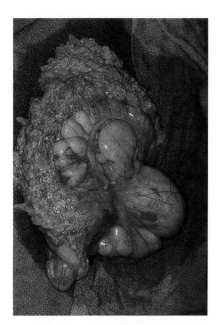

FIG. 19.52. Liposarcoma. Portion of colonic wall demonstrating the presence of a large liposarcoma that encircles the bowel. The large, irregular lobules of the tumor are distinguished from the normal-appearing mesocolon.

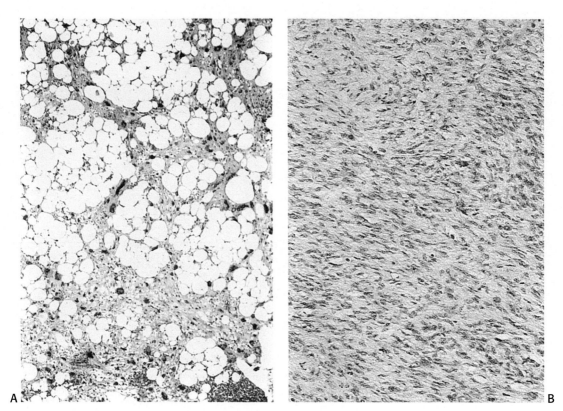

FIG. 19.53. Histologic features of liposarcoma. **A:** The tumor demonstrates atypical cells and lipoblasts. **B:** Dedifferentiated areas of the tumor contain more spindled cells.

or within septae that divide the tumor into lobules. Atypical stromal cells are also present. The tumors may contain focal necrotic areas. The diagnosis rests on finding atypical lipoblasts with cytologic features of malignancy (Fig. 19.53).

Pleomorphic liposarcomas contain disorganized sheets of pleomorphic, malignant lipoblasts. The cells have extreme nuclear hyperchromasia and pleomorphism with numerous monstrocellular forms. Some tumors contain dedifferentiated areas. Histologically, dedifferentiated liposarcomas consist of mixtures of areas of well-differentiated, sclerosing liposarcoma or pleomorphic liposarcoma admixed with areas of morphologically high-grade, nonlipogenic sarcoma.

Lipoleiomyosarcomas arise in the retroperitoneum and secondarily involve the bowel. Lipoleiomyosarcomas show typical well-differentiated liposarcoma with multifocal gradual transitions into smooth muscle areas. The smooth muscle areas exhibit low cellularity, mild to moderate nuclear atypia, and low mitotic activity. The areas seem to arise from or blend with the vascular smooth muscle cells within the tumors (149).

AGGRESSIVE MESENTERIC FIBROMATOSIS (DESMOID TUMORS)

Aggressive mesenteric fibromatosis (AMF) is a neoplastic, monoclonal myofibroblastic proliferation that is prone to aggressive local recurrences, but it does not metastasize

(150). Despite its rarity, AMF is the most common mesenteric tumor (151). The lesions arise de novo, secondary to trauma, or in association with familial adenomatous polyposis (FAP), Gardner syndrome (152), or Crohn disease (153). Patients range in age from 8 to 72 years (154), with a mean of 34 to 46.2 years. In FAP patients, desmoid tumors arise in the surgical bed of the previously resected bowel. They also arise in the mesoappendix. Estrogens may play a role in the genesis of some lesions (155). Deep fibromatoses have somatic *β-catenin* or *adenomatous polyposis coli (APC)* gene mutations leading to nuclear accumulations of *β*-catenin (156). In contrast, superficial fibromatoses lack these mutations (157). The *APC* mutations tend to occur at or beyond codon 125 (see Chapter 13).

AMF affects the intestines and stomach and may extend into the liver, retroperitoneum and pancreas. It presents as a slow-growing tumor that causes obstruction, ischemia, intestinal fistulae, or ureteral obstruction. Tumor behavior varies from that of a benign neoplasm to a deeply invasive tumor characterized by the presence of numerous recurrences. Many regard these locally aggressive tumors as low-grade fibrosarcomas. Patients usually die from obstruction, as large bulky tumor masses compress the bowel loops or infiltrate the bowel wall. The lesions appear as localized, firm, irregular, poorly defined mesenteric masses (Fig. 13.13). These lesions may be quite large, measuring up to 10 cm in diameter. Their cut surfaces have a tan-gray whorled

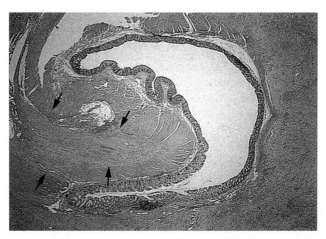

FIG. 19.54. Whole mount demonstrating colonic luminal compression by surrounding mesenteric fibromatosis. The areas of fibromatosis appear somewhat bluer than the native muscle and are outlined by the *arrows*. The fingerlike extension on the left-hand side of the photograph (*arrows*) pushes into the bowel lumen, compromising its size.

homogeneous fibrous appearance without hemorrhage, necrosis, or cyst formation, differentiating the lesions from GISTs. Occasional foci of myxoid degeneration are present.

AMF consists of a variably cellular (usually low to moderate cellularity) proliferation of uniform, bland plump spindle or stellate cells with thin, tapering eosinophilic cytoplasm and elongated, delicate nuclei without significant mitotic activity or necrosis. Occasionally, the cells have more abundant cytoplasm with a rounded or stellate shape and plump nuclei. The nuclei contain evenly dispersed chromatin and small central nucleoli. Mitotic activity is usually less than three mitoses per 50 hpf. In a small percentage of tumors, mitoses can be focally increased (as high as 11 mitoses/50 hpf) in cells that are larger and plumper. Atypical mitoses and cytologic atypia are absent.

The cells are arranged in long, sweeping fascicles, sometimes with a focal storiform pattern. Delicate collagen fibrils, which in some cases can become quite dense and even acquire a keloidal appearance, surround the tumor cells. The amount of collagen is generally greater than that seen in GISTs. Fingerlike projections of the lesion extend into the mesenteric fat and bowel wall (Fig. 19.54) and the cells irregularly infiltrate the muscularis propria. However, they rarely infiltrate the mucosa. Dilated thin-walled veins are common, sometimes accompanied by extravasated red cells and hemosiderin deposits suggesting areas of Kaposi sarcoma. Scattered inflammatory cells and myxoid features may be present (158).

The differential diagnosis of fibromatosis includes inflammatory lesions, low-grade fibrosarcoma, inflammatory myofibroblastic tumor, sclerosing mesenteritis, GIST, and neurofibroma. The lack of an inflammatory component, except possibly in areas of ulceration, mitigates against an inflammatory condition. Distinguishing between AMF and

GIST is important for two reasons. The diagnostic criteria for malignancy in GISTs do not apply to AMF, which, although focally mitotically active, consists of benign tumors without metastatic capability. Further, it is important to distinguish between the two lesions because of the therapeutic implications. The presence of homogeneously distributed wavy spindle cells lacking atypia associated with abundant, sometimes keloidal collagen accompanied by thick-walled arteries and dilated thin-walled veins and an infiltrating pattern of growth characterize AMF. AMF does not show the cystic changes, necrosis, nuclear palisading, or skeinoid fibers seen in GISTs (158).

The confusion between GISTs and AMF is compounded by CD117 immunostaining. CD117 positivity, a key criterion for the diagnosis of a GIST, is present in many desmoid tumors depending on the antibody used to stain the tumors (154,158). The antibody produced by DAKO is positive, whereas that produced by Santa Cruz biotechnology is negative (154). β-Catenin nuclear positivity is present in AMF and negative in GISTs (156,157). CD34 immunostains can be helpful since many GISTs are CD34+ and AMF is negative. Features that may be used to distinguish between these two lesions are listed in Table 19.12.

AMF can consist of locally aggressive lesions that recur but do not metastasize. Surgical excision with negative margins represents adequate treatment. However, local recurrences frequently occur as the result of incomplete resection because the tumor commonly extends beyond the obvious gross limits of the tumor margins. It infiltrates with numerous fingerlike extensions, which, if not removed, become the source of subsequent recurrences. Patients with FAP have much more aggressive lesions than those without FAP in that the risk of recurrence, the presence of multiple lesions, and the death rate due to the disease is significantly greater relative to non-FAP patients (159).

Radiation therapy may be effective in controlling primary and recurrent lesions (160). Sometimes it is combined with hyperthermia. Recent attention has focused on the use of chemotherapy. One study demonstrated long-term regression of desmoid tumors treated with combined endocrine therapy using goserelin acetate, tamoxifen, medroxyprogesterone acetate, and interferon-γ (161). It is conceivable that imatinib methylate may be effective in treating these tumors, since there have been reports of responses to treatment with this drug in desmoids that express either PDGFRA or c-kit (162). Nonsteroidal anti-inflammatory drugs may also be effective.

INFLAMMATORY MYOFIBROBLASTIC TUMORS (INFLAMMATORY PSEUDOTUMORS)

Inflammatory myofibroblastic tumors (IMTs; also known as inflammatory pseudotumors and inflammatory fibrosarcoma) are uncommon mesenchymal lesions typified by

TABLE 19.12   Gastrointestinal Stromal Tumor (GIST) Versus Aggressive Mesenteric Fibromatosis (AMF)

	GIST	AMF
Location	Primarily bowel wall	Primarily mesentery or retroperitoneum
Histology	Spindle epithelial cells	Monotonous spindle cells
	Necrosis and hemorrhage frequent	No necrosis or hemorrhage
Mitoses	Variable	Usually <3/50 hpf although up to 11/50 hpf
IHC	Vimentin+ (100%), CD34+ (63%), SMA+ (75%), desmin+ (8%), S100+ (16%), CD117+	Weak staining for SMA 75% CD117+ (see text)
Outcome	Related to tumor size, mitotic activity	Generally good outcome May have recurrences
Gross	Expanded multilobular lesion Focal area of cysts Liquefactive necrosis	Firm, gray-tan masses Infiltrating margins
Stroma	Myxoid; hyalinized Skeinoid fiber prominent	Collagenous with fine collagen fibroids No skeinoid fibers

hpf, high-powered field; IHC, immunohistochemistry.

proliferations of spindle cells admixed with lymphocytes and plasma cells. Once thought to be reactive, these lesions are now considered to be neoplastic (163). Therefore, the terminology of these lesions has shifted from inflammatory myofibrohistiocytic proliferations or pseudosarcomatous myofibroblastic proliferations to inflammatory myofibroblastic tumors. Many believe that this tumor derives from myofibroblastic cells. However, it may represent a proliferative lesion of fibroblastic reticulum cells (164).

The tumors develop in patients of diverse ages and race. Many affected patients are children with a mean age of approximately 10 years (165). The tumors have been described in patients with HIV infection (166) and chronic granulomatous disease (167). The etiology of this lesion is unclear; some postulate that it may be related to EBV infections. Others have found human herpesvirus-8 (HHV-8) viral sequences in the tumor cells (168).

IMTs often show clonal aberrations involving chromosome 2p23, the site of the human *ALK* gene (169–171). *ALK* rearrangements and/or *ALK1* and p80 immunoreactivity are reported in 33% to 67% of the tumors (163). The rearrangements result in the constitutive activation and overexpression of the *ALK* kinase domain (171). Fusion oncogenes have been identified in a small proportion of IMTs with *ALK* rearrangements (170). *ALK* rearrangements can be identified by fluorescence in situ hybridization (FISH).

Patients commonly present with abdominal pain, an abdominal mass, and, occasionally, diarrhea or intestinal obstruction (165). Some patients have prominent systemic manifestations, including fever, night sweats, weight loss, and malaise. Abnormal laboratory tests may include elevated erythrocyte sedimentation rates, thrombocytosis, and hypergammaglobulinemia. These often resolve when the lesion is removed.

IMTs have been described in the intestines, rectum, appendix, gastroesophageal junction, and mesentery, where they present as well-circumscribed, lobular, multinodular, or whorled firm masses with a white-tan or yellow colored fleshy or myxoid appearance. Secondary changes include hemorrhage, necrosis, calcification, and ossification. The lesions range in size from 0.4 to 36 cm. Those arising in the mesentery and abdomen tend to be large. The lesions may be sessile or polypoid; some are pedunculated and some are large and ulcerated, mimicking GISTs.

Most IMTs are ill-defined myofibroblastic submucosal lesions that may infiltrate the muscularis propria. The lesions show wide variability in their histologic features and cellularity. IMTs contain a mixture of inflammatory cells (lymphocytes, plasma cells, and eosinophils) and spindle-shaped myofibroblasts. The stroma can be edematous, myxoid, fibrotic, or hyalinized. Lymphoid follicles may be present. A small number of neutrophils are present in approximately half of the cases. The proportion of spindle cells to inflammatory cells varies in different areas.

Three major histologic patterns are identified: A fibromyxoid/vascular pattern, a proliferating pattern, and a sclerosing pattern (165). The fibromyxoid pattern represents the early stage of the lesion; the sclerosing form is the late stage. The fibromyxoid/vascular pattern resembles inflammatory fibroid polyps and predominates in approximately 24% of cases. It is characterized by widely separated stellate or spindle cells and a myxoid edematous or loose delicate fibrous stroma with a more or less rich vascular network and inflammatory cells, somewhat resembling nodular fasciitis. In the proliferating pattern, compact proliferations of spindle-shaped cells are arranged in a storiform or fascicular growth pattern. Mitoses can be seen and rare tumors contain cells with mild cytologic atypia. On occasion, there are spindle or oval atypical cells with vesicular nuclei and prominent nucleoli resembling ganglion cells or Reed-Sternberg cells (228). Mitoses are generally scanty (zero to two mitoses per 10 hpf), but there can be as many as 15 mitoses/10 hpf (228). Both the spindle cells and the large ganglionlike cells overexpress the *ALK* protein.

The differential diagnosis of gastrointestinal IMTs includes GISTs, smooth muscle tumors, follicular dendritic cell tumors, fibrohistiocytic sarcomas, desmoid tumors, sclerosing mesenteritis, inflammatory fibroid polyps, Hodgkin and non-Hodgkin lymphoma, and metastatic carcinoma. The lesions are positive with antibodies to smooth muscle actin (86%), muscle-specific actin (82%), desmin (41%), cytokeratin (26%), vimentin, calponin, factor XIIIA, ALK, CD68, and CD117 (172). The lesion may be positive for EBV by in situ hybridization and immunohistochemistry for LMP1, but polymerase chain reaction (PCR)-amplified EBV DNA sequences are not present.

Some patients have an adverse outcome, whereas others have a favorable prognosis, but there are no clear-cut factors that distinguish between the two different clinical outcomes. Intra-abdominal and retroperitoneal tumors are more likely to be aggressive than similar tumors arising elsewhere (172). Approximately one quarter of IMTs recur locally, and rare examples undergo malignant transformation and metastasize. High cellularity and increased numbers of mitoses associate with an unfavorable outcome (173). All IMTs with an adverse outcome show the proliferative histologic pattern (165). In most IMTs with a favorable prognosis, mitoses range from zero to two per 50 hpf; four patients had seven mitoses per 50 hpf. Mitoses range from one to seven per 50 hpf in cases with an adverse prognosis. Cellular atypia is found in 60% of IMTs with a favorable prognosis and 100% of those with an adverse outcome. Cellularity is high in many patients with a favorable prognosis. In patients who die of their disease, high cellularity is present and is characterized by prominent atypical bizarre-shaped cells intermixed with rounded cells rather than the spindle cell proliferation, marked nuclear pleomorphism, and infiltrating borders (165,173). Necrosis may be present.

The major therapy for IMTs is surgical resection with re-excision of recurrent tumors.

MALIGNANT FIBROUS HISTIOCYTOMAS

Malignant fibrous histiocytoma (MFH), the most common soft tissue sarcoma, may also originate in the GI tract. It can arise throughout the gut (Fig. 19.55) (174–176). MFHs may also arise outside of the gastrointestinal tract, extending or metastasizing into it. MFHs arise spontaneously or they may complicate previous radiotherapy. Patients range in age from 17 to 74; most patients are males. Patients present with intussusception, obstruction, or other primary gastrointestinal complaints.

MFHs appear as single or multiple, sessile or pedunculated masses. Histologically, the tumors show a mixture of pleomorphic spindled cells with atypical nuclei and rounded histiocytes arranged in a storiform pattern. The round histiocytes have eccentrically placed nuclei and abundant eosinophilic vacuolated cytoplasm. Fibroblasts, inflammatory cells, and histiocytes may be accompanied by xanthoma cells. Some tumors exhibit a prominent hemangiopericytomalike pattern. Bizarre pleomorphic giant cells may be seen. The tumors may contain multiple hyperchromatic nuclei and prominent nucleoli. Mitoses are usually abundant and atypical. Pleomorphic MFHs may or may not exhibit the classic storiform pattern. Extratumoral vascular invasion may be evident at the time of diagnosis. The tumors tend to involve all layers of the gastrointestinal wall. Inflammatory MFHs may also develop in the GI tract (176).

BENIGN VASCULAR TUMORS

Solitary or multiple benign vascular tumors arise in the intestinal tract. These lesions include (a) multiple phlebectasias, (b) cavernous hemangiomas (diffuse or polypoid), (c) capillary hemangiomas, and (d) angiomatoses. When multiple, angiomas associate with similar neoplasms in other organs, including the liver, and skin (177). Gastrointestinal hemangiomas are classified according to the size of the vessel affected into capillary, cavernous, or mixed lesions. Gastrointestinal hemangiomas have been reported in patients from 2 months to 79 years of age, and no definite sex predilection is identified. They usually present in young persons, often in the 3rd decade of life (178). Benign vascular tumors are more common in the small intestine than in the rest of the gut (177). Esophageal and small intestinal hemangiomas tend to be smaller when they become symptomatic than gastric hemangiomas. Intestinal bleeding, with or without anemia, is the most common presenting symptom. The bleeding may be massive and may lead to death. Larger intestinal lesions produce intussusceptions. Large mesenteric cavernous hemangiomas may weigh up to 5 kg and diffusely involve the small intestine (177). With large lesions such as this, it is impossible to tell whether the site of origin is in the small bowel or the mesentery.

Capillary Hemangiomas

Capillary hemangiomas are usually solitary with a predilection for involving the small intestine, appendix, and perianal skin (236). They generally arise from submucosal vessels, and often have a thin fibrous capsule. They tend to enlarge toward the lumen, presenting as bluish polypoid masses. Alternatively, they appear as localized; smooth; blue, red, wine- or plum-colored; submucosal deformities or ill-defined nodular masses. The cut surfaces appear thickened with numerous dark red nodules. They measure from several millimeters to 11 cm in diameter.

The hemangiomas consist of a proliferation of densely packed small capillaries without interanastomosing vascular channels (Fig. 19.56). The vascular channels are lined by a

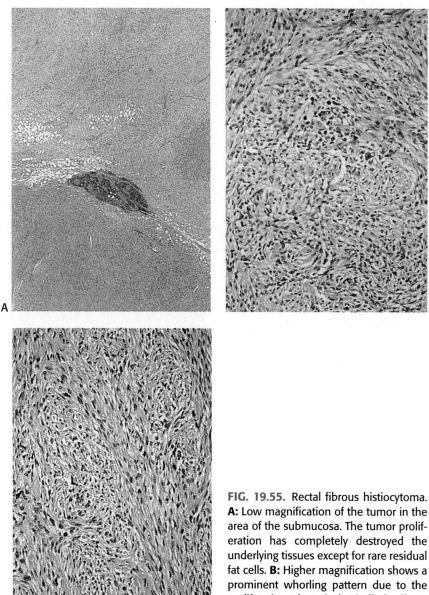

FIG. 19.55. Rectal fibrous histiocytoma. **A:** Low magnification of the tumor in the area of the submucosa. The tumor proliferation has completely destroyed the underlying tissues except for rare residual fat cells. **B:** Higher magnification shows a prominent whorling pattern due to the proliferation of atypical spindled cells. **C:** The long fascicles of spindled cells in a storiform arrangement are obvious.

single layer of well-differentiated endothelial cells. Venous hemangiomas contain thick-walled vessels and smooth muscle cells. Hemangioendotheliomas are capillary hemangiomas with many layers of endothelial cells, often obliterating the vascular lumens. Cross sections of capillary–cavernous hemangiomas show solid areas of hyperplastic endothelial cells and semi-obliterated vascular spaces that alternate with large blood-filled sinuses lined by a single layer of endothelial cells. Connective tissue septa with moderate amounts of muscle and elastic tissue support the vascular spaces (177).

Cavernous Hemangiomas

Cavernous hemangiomas generally arise in the large or small intestine (Figs. 19.57 and 19.58). The esophagus is the least common site of origin (179). Cavernous hemangiomas are bluish purple, soft, and compressible lesions arising from larger submucosal arteries and veins. They diffusely infiltrate large segments of the bowel wall, adjacent soft tissues, or other organs (177). The serosa often demonstrates an irregular varicose vascular network (177).

Four types of cavernous hemangioma exist: (a) multiple phlebectasia type, (b) simple polypoid type, (c) diffuse expansile type, and (d) multiple diffuse expansive type. Cavernous hemangiomas often measure <5 mm. Most lesions remain confined to the submucosa, where they rarely exceed 1 cm in diameter. *Cavernous hemangiomas of the multiple phlebectasia type* consist of multiple small discrete lesions found in any gastrointestinal segment. As many as 50 separate tumors may exist in a 20-cm length of the small

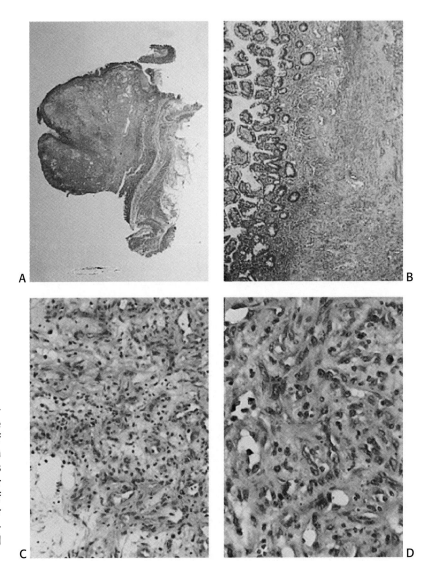

FIG. 19.56. Capillary hemangioma with features of granuloma pyogenicum. **A:** Whole mount section demonstrating the presence of a large polypoid mass. **B:** Higher magnification shows that the small intestinal tumor consists of a proliferation of small capillaries. **C:** Higher magnification demonstrating the presence of capillaries and inflammatory cells. **D:** Higher magnification showing the presence of a proliferation of large numbers of capillary-sized vessels.

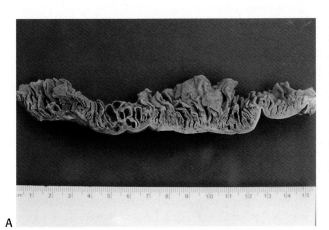

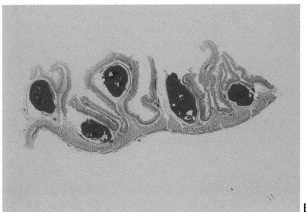

FIG. 19.57. Cavernous hemangioma of the small bowel. **A:** Gross appearance showing the widened intestinal folds. **B:** Low-power view shows multiple large blood filled spaces. (Pictures courtesy of Dr. YZ. Hui, Peoples Hospital, Beijing Medical University, Beijing, China.)

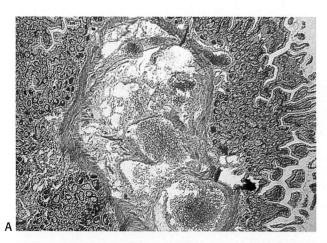 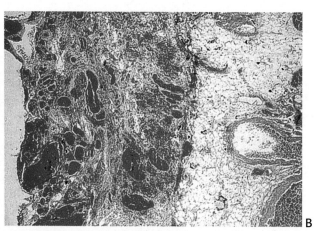

FIG. 19.58. Small intestinal angiomatosis. **A:** Low-power view of small intestinal angiomatosis extensively involving the submucosa. **B:** Near-confluent irregular collection of blood vessels characteristic of angiomatosis.

intestine. The lesions are easily overlooked during pathologic examination since the vessels collapse when they are no longer filled with blood. *Cavernous hemangiomas of the simple polypoid type* consist of single isolated cavernous lesions associated with the submucosal vascular plexus (Fig. 19.59). When they enlarge, they prolapse into the GI lumen causing ulceration, hemorrhage, and intestinal obstruction. These lesions are less common than the phlebectasia type. *Cavernous hemangiomas of the diffuse expansile type* exhibit great variability in size and shape. Many tumors involve up to 20 to 30 cm of the GI tract in one contiguous segment. Grossly, they produce soft, compressible, nodular, dark purple, submucosal elevations. The periphery of these tumors often shows numerous dilated tortuous vessels as well as an abundance of smooth muscle and fibrous connective tissue stroma, suggesting that normal vessels may become incorporated into the tumors. *Cavernous hemangiomas of the multiple diffuse expansile type* may occur simultaneously in separate organs throughout the body, including the skin.

Cavernous hemangiomas consist of large blood-filled spaces or sinuses lined by single or multiple endothelial layers. The supporting stroma contains scant connective tissue septa with variable numbers of smooth muscle fibers. Growth occurs at the tumor periphery by angioblastic proliferation, dilation of the capillary spaces, and fusion of intervascular connective tissue walls to form septa. Degenerative and sclerosing changes include the presence of thrombi in the cavernous spaces, overgrowth of fibrous tissue, hyalinization, edema, and focal calcification (177).

Angiomatoses

The *Klippel-Trenaunay syndrome* consists of a triad of congenital anomalies: (a) port wine stain hemangiomas (naevus flammeus), (b) varicose veins, and (c) hypertrophy of the soft tissue and bone with an overgrowth of the ipsilateral limb. Visceral complications are common and may cause life-threatening complications. Patients may present with recurrent intestinal bleeding. Cavernous hemangiomas and venous fibromuscular dysplasias are the most prominent and consistent vascular lesions other than the cavernous hemangioma, which are present, but they are not specific for this syndrome. The dysplastic veins may also have deformed and insufficient or absent valves (180).

Osler-Weber-Rendu disease is widespread among various ethnic groups and ranges in frequency from about 1 in 2,000 to 40,000 depending on the geographic location. Mutations in the endothelial cell surface protein endoglin leads to the disease (181). The three requisites for establishing the diagnosis include (a) a history of repeated hemorrhages; (b) telangiectasias of the mucous membranes, viscera (liver, genitourinary tract, GI tract), and skin; and (c) a familial occurrence (182). Epistaxis in early childhood or young adulthood is often the first manifestation of the disease. The vascular tumors increase in number and variety with age, leading to the later appearance of angiomatous lesions on the skin, face, and mucous membranes. These lesions bleed spontaneously or following trauma, and can cause severe anemia. A significant difference exists in the age of onset of epistaxis (median 11 years) and of GI bleeding (mean 55.5 years) (183).

Hemangiomas develop anywhere in the GI tract, but are most common in the stomach and duodenum (184). There are two major types of mucosal lesions: Stellate or spindle angiomata and nodular or plaquelike angiomas. Stellate angiomata consist of a flat or raised punctiform central area, from which radiate easily visible vessels that appear bluish red and fade on pressure. Nodular angiomata are sometimes surrounded by a pale halo, appear as solid tumors that are bluish red, and lack the "spider legs" of the stellate type. The angiomas measure 1 to 3 mm in diameter and are not obliterated by pressure. Microscopically, the lesions consist of multiple, thin, dilated venules and capillaries lined by a single layer of benign endothelial cells.

The *blue rubber bleb nevus syndrome* (BRBNS) consists of cutaneous and GI tract cavernous hemangiomas. The term describes cutaneous bluish lesions that look and feel like rubber nipples. Most cases are sporadic, although an autosomal

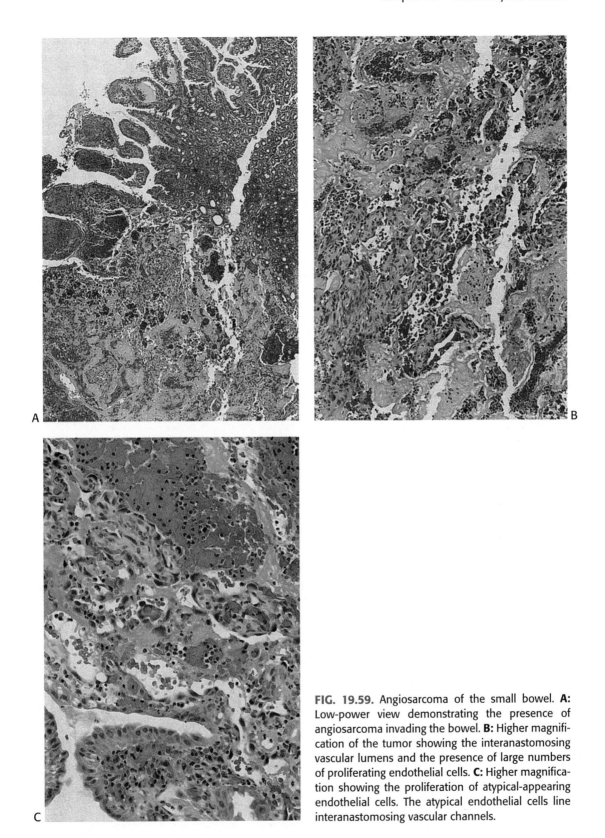

FIG. 19.59. Angiosarcoma of the small bowel. **A:** Low-power view demonstrating the presence of angiosarcoma invading the bowel. **B:** Higher magnification of the tumor showing the interanastomosing vascular lumens and the presence of large numbers of proliferating endothelial cells. **C:** Higher magnification showing the proliferation of atypical-appearing endothelial cells. The atypical endothelial cells line interanastomosing vascular channels.

dominant pattern of inheritance has been suggested in some instances. GI involvement usually affects the small intestine, although lesions develop in the esophagus, stomach, colon, rectum and anus, mesentery, and peritoneum (184). The condition is present from birth or early childhood. Lesions then increase in both size and number with age. Complications include gastrointestinal bleeding, consumptive coagulopathies, chronic anemia, intussusception, and orthopedic complications (183). Resection may be required if the patient becomes severely symptomatic.

Hemangiomas accompanied by multiple enchondromas characterize *Maffucci syndrome* (185). Large diffuse hemangiomas cause a coagulopathy due to platelet sequestration and consumption in the hemangioma and clotting within the neoplastic vascular network. The triad of thrombocytopenia, hemangiomas, and a consumptive coagulopathy constitutes *Kasabach-Merritt syndrome* (186). The hemangiomas consist of localized giant vascular lesions. The consumptive coagulopathy causes a disturbance in the thrombohemolytic balance that leads to acute bleeding or predisposes the patient to thrombosis. Resection cures patients with a coagulopathy.

Angiosarcomas

GI angiosarcomas are very rare (177). The gut may be affected by either primary or secondary lesions (187). Angiosarcomas typically complicate longstanding lymphedema, radiation (188), or foreign bodies (189). The latency period following radiation ranges from 37 months to 50 years (190). Clinical symptoms include intestinal bleeding, anemia, abdominal pain, perforation, acute abdomen, and intestinal obstruction (187). Primary tumors arise in the stomach, small intestine, rectum, esophagus, retroperitoneum, and appendix, with the small intestine being the most common site (187). The tumors tend to be multicentric in origin and extensively invade the bowel wall. They present as polypoid, macular, or purplish lesions with poorly defined margins and prominent submucosal or serosal hemorrhagic nodules. They may appear edematous and ulcerated.

Angiosarcomas consist of a network of irregular interanastomosing delicate vascular channels lined by abnormal plump endothelial cells with large hyperchromatic nuclei (Figs. 19.59 and 19.60). The vascular spaces contain intraluminal tufts or papillary projections of neoplastic endothelium. Some channels contain erythrocytes, whereas others are devoid of red blood cells. This pattern may be obscured by solid sheets of spindled, epithelioid, or undifferentiated cells, making the diagnosis difficult, particularly if the typical anastomosing vascular spaces are absent. *Epithelioid angiosarcoma*s contain sheets of large plump polygonal endothelial cells with little vascular architectural differentiation. Such tumors may be mistaken for other sarcomas, lymphomas, malignant melanomas, mesotheliomas, or poorly differentiated carcinomas (Fig. 19.60).

The typical immunohistologic profile of angiosarcoma includes positivity for CD34, CD31, vimentin, factor VIII, UAE1, and cytokeratins AE1/AE3, CAM5.2, CK-7, CK-8, and CK-19. Cytokeratin-20 is characteristically negative. Rare cases may be focally positive for EMA. Cytokeratin staining is variable and ranges from focal to extensive (187), making the differential diagnosis challenging. Epithelioid angiosarcomas may be diffusely and strongly positive for cytokeratins and only show subtle signs of vascular differentiation, creating a potential diagnostic confusion with primary or metastatic carcinoma. For this reason, the tumors should always be stained with several vascular markers. However, there may be staining with only one marker such as CD31, suggesting that angiosarcomas show different levels of differentiation and individual expression patterns of the various endothelial cell markers (191). More than half of angiosarcomas express c-kit, but these tumors lack *KIT* mutations (192).

Florid vascular proliferations developing secondary to intussusception and mucosal prolapse may show features that overlap with angiosarcoma and are in the differential diagnosis of this lesion. The latter is a vascular proliferation due to repeated mucosal trauma and ischemia (193). The benign histologic features help distinguish the lesion from angiosarcoma.

Angiosarcomas often disseminate by the time they are detected, leading to the diffuse seeding of the liver, omentum, and peritoneum with multiple red hemorrhagic-appearing nodules. Many patients die of their disease between 1 and 33 months after diagnosis.

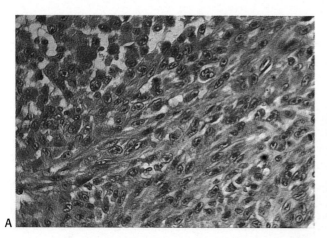
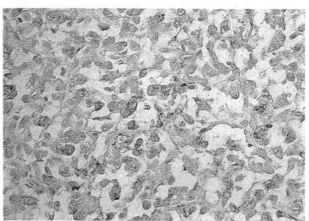

FIG. 19.60. Epithelioid angiosarcoma. **A:** Histologic features of an angiosarcoma without prominent vascular channels. **B:** Factor VIII–related antigen is positive in the majority of tumor cells.

TABLE 19.13 Variants of Kaposi Sarcoma

Type	Risk Group	Gastrointestinal Involvement
Classic	Elderly men of Eastern European or Mediterranean origin	80% of patients
Endemic	African adults and children	Rare
Immunosuppression related	Organ transplant patients	50% of patients
AIDS associated	HIV-infected persons	Common

Kaposi Sarcoma

Incidence/Epidemiology

Four distinct clinical and epidemiologic forms of Kaposi sarcoma (KS) are recognized (Table 19.13). The *classic indolent variant* primarily affects elderly men of Eastern European or Mediterranean origin with a male:female ratio of 15:1. *Endemic African KS* is common in equatorial Africa affecting HIV-negative children and middle-aged adults. *AIDS-associated KS,* the most aggressive form of KS, often causes patient death. Risk factors for tumor development include the number of sexual partners, use of nitrite inhalants, and receptive anal intercourse. Men most likely to develop KS engage in oral–anal contact with multiple partners. The average age at diagnosis is 30 to 40 years (194). This disorder was highly prevalent early in the AIDS epidemic, but there was a marked reduction in its incidence between 1994 and 2003 following the introduction of highly active antiretroviral therapy (HAART) (195). Organ transplant recipients and patients receiving immunosuppression for other disorders develop the *iatrogenic form of KS.* The median interval from organ transplantation to the diagnosis of KS is 29 to 31 months, and as in other forms, men are more commonly affected than women.

Pathogenesis

Whether KS represents a clonal neoplastic process or a polyclonal hyperplastic or inflammatory proliferative disorder is controversial (196). Factors favoring a dysregulated inflammatory response include the following: (a) in early KS, the number of spindle cells is low compared with the surrounding inflammatory cells; (b) KS cells in culture require exogenous growth factors, and when implanted into nude mice induce an inflammatory angiogenic reaction but do not induce tumors as would be expected of neoplastic cells (197); (c) regression of KS can happen spontaneously or when the immunosuppression is relieved; (d) KS lesions are multifocal (198); and (e) cytogenetic abnormalities are rare and inconsistent (196). However, X chromosome inactivation within a single lesion and a comparison of multiple lesions from single patients support a clonal origin in a subset of advanced cases (199). More recent studies have shown varying monoclonality, oligoclonality, and polyclonality from lesions of various patients (200). One possibility for these results is that KS starts as a hyperplastic polyclonal lesion that gives rise to a clonal cell population only under specific circumstances, with HHV-8 infection preceding the clonal expansion and sarcoma development (198). The pathogenesis of KS may therefore involve a complex interaction of viral infection, genetic factors, and immunosuppression.

Since HIV-infected persons have a disproportionate incidence of KS among homosexual or bisexual men, a sexually transmitted cofactor, in addition to the background of HIV infection, has been thought to be responsible for the development of KS. Today, we know that HHV-8 plays a major role in the development of all forms of KS (201). The virus is sexually transmitted and viral sequences are present in both endothelial cells and spindle cells (202). HHV-8 latently infects endothelial cells as well as peripheral blood monocytes and B lymphocytes in KS (203). HHV-8 escapes human leukocyte antigen (HLA) class I–restricted antigen presentation to cytotoxic T lymphocytes by increasing endocytosis of major histocompatibility class (MHC) class I chains from the cell surface, thereby enabling latent infection and immune escape in primary and chronic infections (198). Viral oncogenesis and cytokine-induced growth, as well as some immunocompromised states, contribute to KS development. Several virally encoded genes (*bcl2, interleukin 6, cyclin D, G-protein–coupled receptor, and interferon regulatory factor*) provide key functions related to vascular proliferation, inhibition of apoptosis, and survival. Growth promotion of KS is further stimulated by various proinflammatory cytokines and growth factors such as tumor necrosis factor-α, interleukin 6, basic fibroblast growth factor, and vascular endothelial growth factor. These result in a hyperplastic polyclonal spindle cell lesion derived from lymphoid endothelia. HHV-8 induces the expression of both angiogenic and invasion factors including vascular endothelial growth factor and matrix metalloproteinases, allowing the tumors to progress and grow (204).

The development of antibodies to the HHV-8 latency-associated nuclear antigen (LANA) is considered the hallmark of latent HHV-8 infection. Seropositivity for antibodies to LANA is found in >85% of KS patients (205) and the presence of LANA antibodies in HIV-infected patients strongly associates with the risk of developing KS (206).

Clinical Course

The clinical course varies with the type of KS that is present. Gastrointestinal mucosal lesions usually follow the appearance of skin lesions, but not always. Classic KS usually has an indolent course as does the endemic form of the disease in adults. This contrasts with an aggressive course in children with endemic KS. Iatrogenic KS has an indolent or aggressive course depending in part on the degree of immunosuppression that is present. AIDS patients have a high incidence of GI and visceral involvement. The clinical course of AIDS-related KS varies from a slowly progressive disease evolving over many years to a rapidly fulminant progression evolving over weeks to months. Three factors associate with a shortened survival: The presence of systemic symptoms (fever, drenching night sweats, and weight loss), CD4 lymphocyte counts <300/mm³, and a history of opportunistic infection (207). In the absence of these factors, the median survival approximates 31 months. The presence of a coexisting opportunistic infection associates with a median survival of only 7 months. Mortality increases significantly in patients with GI involvement, perhaps because the extent of visceral involvement parallels the severity of immunosuppression and thus parallels susceptibility to life-threatening infections.

The location of nonvisceral Kaposi sarcoma, in skin versus lymph nodes, does not predict the likelihood of GI Kaposi sarcoma, and the absence of skin or lymph node Kaposi sarcoma does not exclude the possibility of GI involvement. Patients with extensive cutaneous lesions are likely to have GI involvement, but we have seen GI involvement in the absence of cutaneous disease. GI KS often remains silent because the nodular lesions have room to expand into the bowel lumen before becoming symptomatic. Symptoms include dysphagia and odynophagia resulting from oropharyngeal and esophageal lesions. Abdominal pain, melena, hemorrhage, obstruction, fever, diarrhea, intussusception, weight loss, hematemesis, perforation, peritonitis, mesenteric pseudocyst, protein-losing enteropathy, malabsorption, and an ulcerative colitis–like syndrome with toxic megacolon complicate intestinal lesions. Appendiceal lesions cause acute appendicitis.

Pathologic Features

KS lesions develop anywhere in the GI tract (Figs. 19.61 to 19.63). The size and number of lesions vary with the disease stage. The lesion begins in mucosal and submucosal locations, eventually producing discolored intraluminal nodular growths. Small lesions may be invisible grossly. The disease presents as a single focus or patchy studding of the bowel with innumerable irregular nodules varying in size from a few millimeters that are easily overlooked to raised, reddish lesions measuring up to 4 cm in size. Luminal KS lesions show three distinct growth patterns: Maculopapular (often hemorrhagic) lesions, polypoid lesions, and umbilicated nodular lesions. They appear reddish, gray-white, violaceous brown, or blue, and nipplelike, depending on the relative amounts of vascular and spindle cell components and associated reactive fibrosis. The lesions do not blanch and are not usually painful or tender.

The histologic features of KS are similar in all of the epidemiologic types. Early-stage lesions resemble granulation tissue; late-stage lesions can resemble angiosarcomas or fibrosarcomas. Variable inflammatory infiltrates containing lymphocytes, plasma cells, macrophages, and histiocytes surround early lesions, suggesting the presence of granulation

A, B
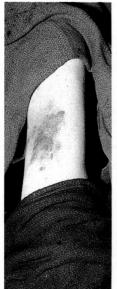 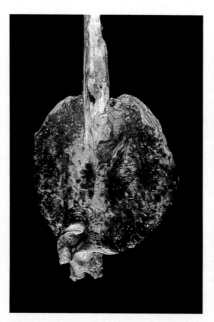 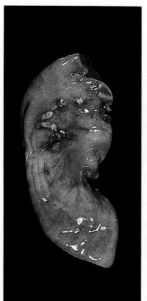 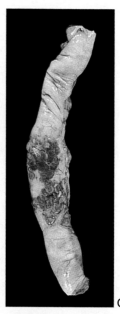
C, D

FIG. 19.61. Disseminated Kaposi sarcoma in an AIDS patient. **A:** Skin changes of Kaposi sarcoma seen on the upper arm of a patient with disseminated disease. **B:** Gastric mucosa showing the presence of numerous violaceous nodules within the gastric mucosa. All of these histologically were Kaposi sarcoma. **C, D:** Portions of small intestine showing the presence of serosal implants of Kaposi sarcoma.

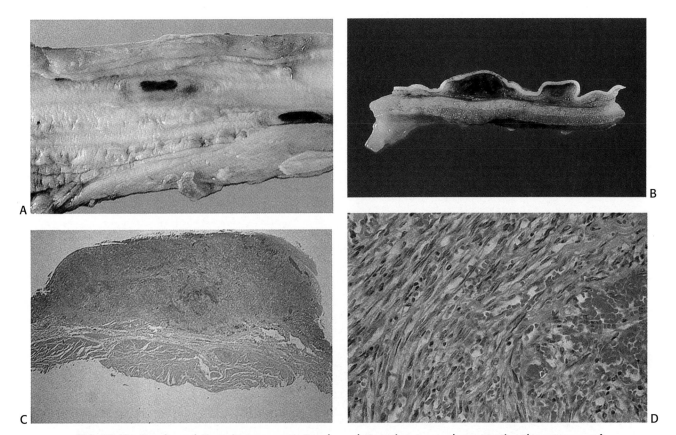

FIG. 19.62. Esophageal Kaposi sarcoma. **A:** Esophageal Kaposi sarcoma demonstrating the presence of plaquelike lesions. **B:** Cross section through several of these lesions showing the presence of submucosal lesions covered by the white epithelium of the esophagus. The Kaposi sarcoma expands the submucosa. **C:** Histologic features of small intestinal plaquelike lesion expanding the submucosa. **D:** Histologic features of the lesion shown in C showing characteristic spindle-shaped cells with red blood cells percolating between them.

tissue. The inflammation is usually less in AIDS-associated KS than in classic KS. Some lesions appear as nothing more than a mild mucosal expansion of spindled cells without much atypia, resembling a hyperplastic muscularis mucosae or fibromuscular obliteration of the lamina propria.

As the lesions progress from early to later stages, one sees loss of vascular spaces and an increase in the number of spindle cells. Nodular spindle cell areas blend with more angiomatous areas. Interwoven bundles of spindle cells extend in various directions throughout the tissues. Although nuclear atypia and mitotic figures may be present, they are rarely prominent. Mature lesions consist of proliferations of interweaving spindle-shaped cells that tend to form vascular spaces within a network of reticulin and collagen fibers. Dilated, thin-walled, anastomosing vascular spaces usually intermingle with spindle cells. Flat to plump endothelial cells line the vascular spaces. The endothelial cells may protrude into the vascular lumens, but they are not atypical and therefore differ from the endothelium seen in angiosarcomas. Extravasated erythrocytes (Fig. 19.63) percolate through the lesion and hemosiderin deposits are present in the surrounding tissue. Clues to the diagnosis, especially in early lesions,

include an appropriate clinical history, knowledge of the endoscopic findings, recognition of nuclear crowding and hyperchromasia in the spindled cells, recognition that the slits and spaces contain red blood cells and are thus vascular spaces, and the tendency for KS cells to overrun or obliterate the muscularis mucosae. The lesions may be surprisingly subtle and easily missed, even by experienced pathologists. Early lesions can be distinguished from granulation tissue by the presence of angulated disorganized vascular channels. The lining cells of well-developed vascular structures are usually positive with vascular markers. The spindle cells are consistently positive for CD34 and commonly positive for CD31 but are factor VIII negative. All cases, regardless of the epidemiologic subgroup, are positive for HHV-8.

Distinguishing KS from other benign or malignant vascular tumors as well as other nonvascular spindle cell neoplasms can be challenging. The differential diagnosis includes angiosarcoma, spindle cell hemangioma, leiomyomas, pyogenic granuloma, and spindle cell melanoma. LANA expression is a highly sensitive and specific marker of KS and helps to correctly identify the lesion in difficult cases (208).

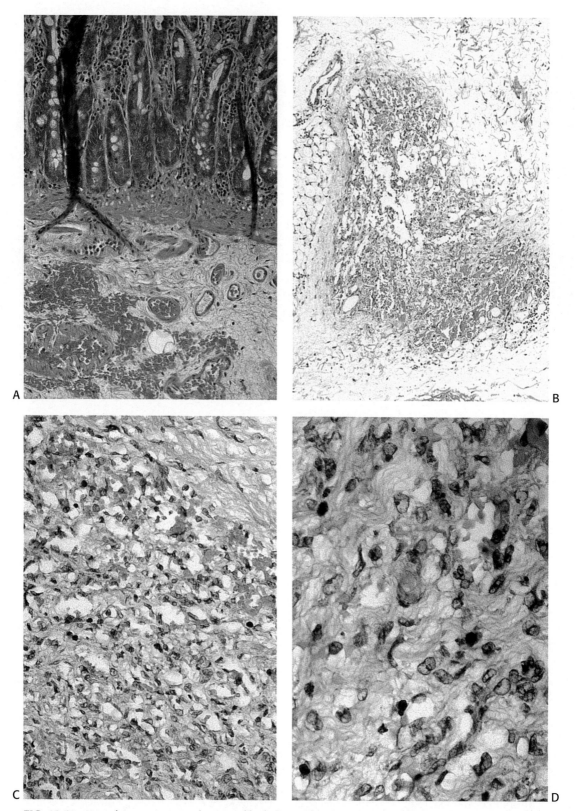

FIG. 19.63. Kaposi sarcoma. **A:** Angiomatouslike lesion within the submucosa demonstrating widely dilated vascular spaces in the absence of a spindle cell proliferation. **B:** Another lesion demonstrating more compact cellular proliferations and loss of some of the angiomatous regions. **C:** Higher magnification shows the presence of a sclerotic tumor with slitlike spaces. **D:** Higher magnification shows the cytologic atypia and eosinophilic globules.

Treatment

GI involvement in AIDS patients associates with a poor prognosis. Patients with classic KS with a single lesion are typically cured by local excision. In immunocompetent patients with multiple lesions, observation may be appropriate and some lesions may regress or show little progression over time. In patients with disease limited to a single region, radiation therapy may be appropriate. In patients with extensive or recurrent disease, some combination of surgery, chemotherapy, and/or radiation therapy may be appropriate. Patients with HIV-associated KS may benefit from HAART. Patients may also receive a combination of radiation therapy, chemotherapy, and biologic agents (209).

Lymphangioma

Lymphangiomas are less common than hemangiomas. They develop in patients ranging in age from 3.5 to 78 years (210). In Europeans and Americans, a 2:1 female:male ratio exists. This ratio reverses in the Japanese (211). Symptoms vary depending on location and size. Large polypoid lesions cause obstruction or intussusception. Esophageal lymphangiomas may cause dysphagia. In contrast, most intestinal lymphangiomas remain asymptomatic and are discovered incidentally. Some patients develop protein-losing enteropathy (212), hypogammaglobulinemia, and T-cell lymphopenia (213) or potassium loss that is cured by lesional resection (214). Rectal lesions cause pain or bleeding. These lesions may enlarge due to continuing engorgement with chyle and localized secondary inflammation rather than proliferation of the neoplastic cells (210).

Generally, lymphangiomas are solitary, but multiple lesions do occur. The term *lymphangiomatosis* describes the presence of multiple lymphangiomas. Gastrointestinal lymphangiomas occur most frequently in the colon, followed by the duodenum and stomach. Esophageal lesions are rare. When extensive, the lesions may involve the small intestine, large intestine, appendix, mesentery, gallbladder, and biliary tree (213). Lymphangiomas can be recognized by their pale translucent cystic appearance and their deformation under pressure. They appear as a pink, tan, or yellow, oval or spherical lesion with a smooth mucosal surface, often with a broad base (Fig. 19.64). Small lymphangiomas may be grossly invisible or they appear as intramucosal, intramural, intraluminal, sessile, or pedunculated lesions, ranging in size from 1.5 to 23 cm (average size 2.8 cm). Larger tumors may circumferentially involve an intestinal segment. An abrupt transition occurs between the lesion and adjacent normal tissues. When cut, lymphangiomas have a multicystic cut surface that exudes clear yellowish or milky fluid.

Lymphangiomas are characterized by a localized proliferation of dilated lymphatics lined by benign endothelial cells. In their simplest form, one sees an ill-defined, multilobulated mass composed of dilated, variably sized endothelial-lined lymph vessels with a cellular fibrous connective tissue stroma or sometimes a loose myxoid stroma (Figs. 19.65 and 19.66). The lymphatic channels connect the tumor to the adjacent lymphatic system. Cellular variants contain prominent endothelial and stromal cells that almost obliterate the vascular lumina. Occasionally, frayed smooth muscle fibers course through the connective tissue. In contrast to hemangiomas, lymphangiomas do not contain blood within the vascular spaces and they do not express factor VIII–related antigen unless one uses proteolytic digestion before immunostaining, in which case some lesions may become positive. They are positive for D2-40 and Lyve-1.

Multifocal Lymphangioendotheliomatosis with Thrombocytopenia

Multifocal lymphangioendotheliomatosis with thrombocytopenia is a newly recognized congenital clinicopathologic entity in which there are extensive venous and lymphatic malformations. Patients with GI involvement usually have multifocal involvement, including the skin and gut, and there is occasional involvement of other sites. The lesions resemble the acquired lesions recently classified as benign lymphangioendothelioma, which consists of small vessels

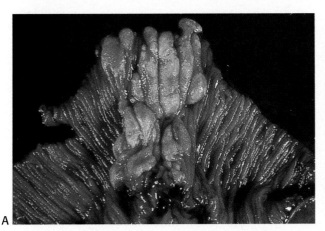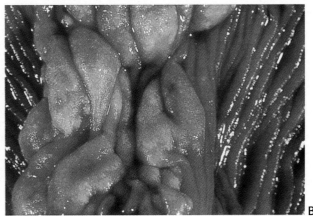

FIG. 19.64. Lymphangioma. **A:** Gross photograph of a lobulated lymphangioma. **B:** Higher magnification.

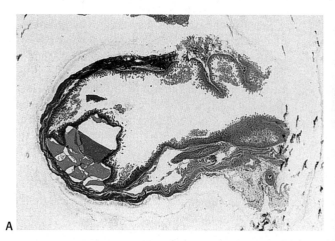

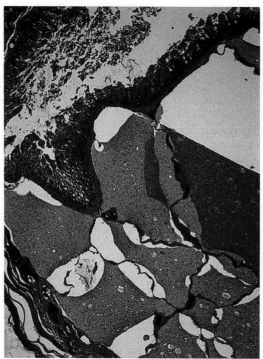

FIG. 19.65. Small intestinal lymphangioma. **A:** Whole mount section showing a localized submucosal cystic mass containing pink material. **B:** Higher magnification illustrating the presence of numerous vascular spaces containing lymph.

lined by a single layer of endothelial cells rimmed by loosely arranged stroma. The perivascular stroma can be myxoid with scattered hemosiderin deposits that have chronic fluctuating levels of thrombocytopenia. The tumor vessels are immunoreactive for Lyve-1 (215).

Hemangiolymphangioma

Some tumors have features of both a lymphangioma and a hemangioma (216) with an interanastomosing meshwork of lymphatics and blood vessels. The lymphatics contain a fine

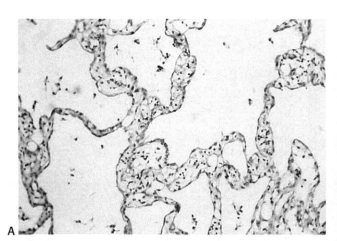

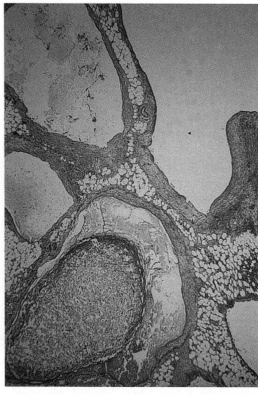

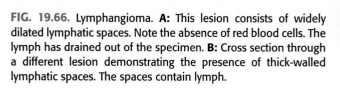

FIG. 19.66. Lymphangioma. **A:** This lesion consists of widely dilated lymphatic spaces. Note the absence of red blood cells. The lymph has drained out of the specimen. **B:** Cross section through a different lesion demonstrating the presence of thick-walled lymphatic spaces. The spaces contain lymph.

eosinophilic precipitate consistent with lymph and valvelike structures surrounded by regular nodular smooth muscle coats. Other areas of the tumor resemble lymphangiomyoma with a prominent muscular component. One may identify muscular arteries and veins filled with calcified thrombi. Such a lesion can be designated as a hemangiolymphangioma with focal smooth muscle proliferation.

Glomus Tumors

Patients range in age from 19 to 90 years with a median age of 55 years (217), usually affecting females. The clinical manifestations of the tumors resemble those produced by any gastrointestinal mass. Glomus tumors develop in the gastric (218), intestinal (217), and esophageal submucosa. They present as whitish, intramural, circumscribed polypoid, sometimes ulcerated masses, measuring 1.7 to 7.0 cm in diameter. A rare patient developed multiple gastric and perigastric glomus tumors (219). There is also a unique report of a massive gastric glomus tumor that filled the abdominal cavity; it was present for decades (220).

Most tumors consist of multiple cellular nodules separated by strands of smooth muscle cells. Dilated veins without glomus tumor elements are often present among the lobules and in the tumor periphery. Some tumors have a solid pattern with inconspicuous vessels; others have a predominantly trabecular pattern with a hyalinized stromal pattern. The tumor cells have sharply defined cell membranes and centrally located, round uniform nuclei with delicate chromatin and inconspicuous nucleoli (Fig. 19.67) (217). Focal oncocytic changes, prominent clear cell features, or mild nuclear atypia may be present. Thrombosis may lead to the formation of phleboliths. Foci of hyaline and myxoid change may be present, particularly in the center of the tumor (217). Vascular invasion and focal atypia are relatively common but mitotic activity is low (one to four mitoses per 50 hpf) and the mitoses are not atypical. Focal signet ring cell morphology can be present. Some tumors consist of multiple nodules

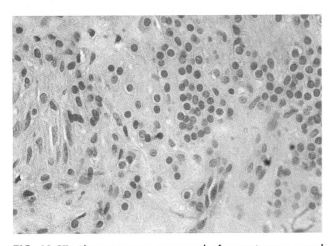

FIG. 19.67. Glomus tumor composed of monotonous round cells, sometimes in a perivascular location.

set in a desmoplastic stroma representing *the infiltrative variant of glomus tumor*. Histologically, these lesions somewhat resemble desmoplastic small round cell tumors or even carcinoid tumors. Osseous metaplasia may also be present.

Glomus tumors may be diagnosed by endoscopic ultrasound-guided needle aspiration biopsy. The specimens demonstrate cohesive clusters of uniform, small, round to polygonal cells with ill-defined cytoplasmic borders and scanty amphophilic cytoplasm. The nuclei are round with smooth nuclear membranes and evenly distributed dusty chromatin. Small, short, spindled, normal-appearing endothelial cells intermingle with the epithelioid cells.

The differential diagnosis of glomus tumors includes GISTs, gangliocytic paragangliomas, hemangiopericytomas, carcinoid tumors, and lymphomas. Glomus tumors are positive for α-smooth muscle actin, HHF-35, H-caldesmon, and calponin, and nearly all have a netlike pericellular laminin and collagen IV positivity (217). The tumors are negative for desmin, S100, CD34, CD117, and cytokeratin. The tumors may show focal synaptophysin positivity, but chromogranin is negative. The tumors lack GIST-specific *KIT* mutations.

Overall, glomus tumors have an excellent prognosis, but there is a small unpredictable potential for malignant behavior, usually in the face of very low mitotic activity, particularly if vascular invasion is present (217).

HEMANGIOPERICYTOMA

Hemangiopericytomas affect all age groups, but they occur most commonly in the 5th and 6th decades without a sexual predilection. These tumors develop throughout the gut, with the small bowel representing the most common site of origin (221). Obstruction, intussusception, and bleeding are some of the more common presenting features. These rare tumors arise from pericytes surrounding small blood vessels, and they affect all layers of the bowel wall (221) and its mesentery. The tumors diffusely infiltrate the bowel wall, ranging in size from microscopic lesions to tumors weighing >1 kg. They appear as grayish pink, sessile, polypoid, or nodular lesions traversed by coarse fibrous trabeculae extending into the muscularis propria. Hemangiopericytomas contain abundant, uniformly distributed, branching blood vessels lined by flattened endothelium. Pericytes compress the vascular lumina into slitlike spaces. Oval to round pericytes surround the vessels with a reticulin band separating the two; reticulin stains show that the cellular proliferations lie outside the endothelial lining. Fifty-three to ninety percent of tumors are malignant (221,222), but no single histologic criterion exists that reliably differentiates benign from malignant tumors. Factors considered to be important include increased cellularity, hyperchromasia, prominent mitotic activity, necrosis, and hemorrhage.

The differential diagnosis of hemangiopericytomas includes vascular smooth muscle tumors, fibrous histiocytomas, and glomus tumors, but immunostains serve to distinguish among these entities. The tumors also exhibit a characteristic reticulin staining pattern. A complicating factor regarding hemangiopericytomas is the fact that many tumor types may exhibit hemangiopericytomatous histologic patterns and thus these tumors need to be adequately worked up for these other tumor types before diagnosing a primary gastrointestinal hemangiopericytoma.

PERIVASCULAR TUMORS

Epithelioid Cell Tumor ("PEComa")

PEComas are mesenchymal neoplasms characterized by perivascular epithelioid cell (PEC) differentiation and myomelanocytic marker expression. They are related to angiomyolipomas and lymphangioleiomyomatosis. These tumors may be benign and malignant. PEComas develop exclusively in young women; some patients have tuberous sclerosis (223). The tumors arise in the small bowel, cecum, and perirectal area (224) as well as outside the gut, extending into it (225).

Benign PEComas consist of sheets and packets of large polygonal cells with glycogen-rich clear or eosinophilic cytoplasm. Focally, the tumors demonstrate papillarylike configurations or pseudoglandular or spindle cell areas. There are often prominent nucleoli with mild to moderate nuclear pleomorphism. Mitotic figures are rare. Multinucleated giant cells may be present in some tumors. The tumors are traversed by a delicate vasculature, mimicking clear cell carcinoma (223). Abundant brown, Fontana-Masson–positive pigment is evident in a fraction of the neoplastic cells.

Malignant PEComas resemble their benign counterparts, but in addition there are prominent areas of coagulative necrosis and lymphovascular invasion. Mitotic activity is variable and can be low or extremely brisk. The tumor cells exhibit moderate nuclear atypia with focally prominent large nucleoli (226). Tumor emboli are often seen in the lymphovascular spaces at the periphery of the tumors. The tumor may metastasize to the regional lymph nodes, liver, lungs, and bone.

PEComas do not express epithelial markers but express the melanocytic markers HMB45 and Melan-A. The spindle cells express myogenic markers, staining strongly for smooth muscle actin and moderately for muscle-specific actin. There may be membrane staining with CD10, moderate focal estrogen receptor expression (225), and positivity for microphthalmia transcription factor and calponin. Desmin, keratins, S100, CD34, progesterone receptor, chromogranin, EMA, and CEA are negative (225). CD117 can be expressed in some cells, but *KIT* mutations are absent (225).

PEComas may be divided into benign, borderline, and malignant tumors (227). Recurrence and/or metastasis strongly associate with a tumor size >8 cm and mitotic activity greater than one mitosis per 50 hpf and necrosis.

Small PEComas without any worrisome histologic features are likely to be benign. PEComas with only nuclear pleomorphism or large PEComas without worrisome histologic features may be classified as borderline lesions (227). Therapy consists of resection.

Lymphangioleiomyomatosis

Lymphangioleiomyomatosis (LAM) is a rare disorder occurring nearly exclusively in premenopausal women. The disease is usually sporadic, but it often affects patients with tuberous sclerosis (227) or MEN-1. The disorder is characterized by multiple tumor nodules that may exceed 3 cm in diameter and may contain multiple large cysts filled with yellow-tan chylous fluid. LAM is not primarily a gastrointestinal tumor, but it can secondarily involve the serosal surfaces of the appendix and intestines in women with widespread disease. LAM is characterized by proliferations of short spindled smooth muscle cells arranged in fascicular, trabecular, and papillary patterns. The spindle cell areas may associate with more cellular areas composed of plump epithelioid cells arranged around dilated branching endothelial-lined channels. Irregular smooth muscle proliferations possessing irregularly shaped, slightly enlarged nuclei can also be seen in the walls of the lymphatics that merge with the smooth muscle of the venous wall. This lymphangiomatous component does not involve the circumference of the lymphatic vessel uniformly and is more readily identified in the pericolonic fat (Fig. 19.68). Immunohistochemical studies show strong reactivity for α-smooth muscle actin and smooth muscle myosin heavy chain. There is weak to moderate reactivity for desmin. HMB45, estrogen receptor, and progesterone receptor may also be positive, particularly in the epithelioid cells (227).

ANGIOMYOLIPOMAS

Angiomyolipomas are clonal neoplastic lesions with hamartomalike features that occur sporadically or as part of the tuberous sclerosis complex (228). These lesions show a female predominance. They may develop primarily in the bowel (229), usually in the large bowel, or they may extend into the bowel from the kidney. Colonic lesions present as small mucosal polyps. Angiomyolipomas are believed to arise from multipotential perivascular epithelioid cells and share the expression of HMB45 with the other perivascular-type lesions.

These well-circumscribed tumors contain a variable admixture of thick-walled blood vessels, bundles of smooth muscle, and mature adipose tissue. The spindle cells preferentially surround blood vessels, from which they appear to fan out. Tumors with characteristic features are easy to diagnose. However, the range of morphologic appearances is quite broad; they are variously described as pleomorphic, epithelioid (230), atypical, and carcinomalike (231). Some

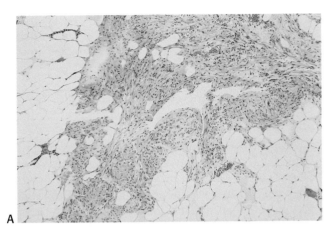
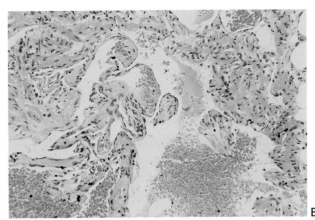

FIG. 19.68. Lymphangiomyoma. **A:** A spindle cell proliferation is present in the mesocolon. **B:** Higher magnification discloses the intermingling of smooth muscle cells, blood vessels, and lymphatic spaces.

colonic tumors have an atypical epithelioid appearance with a predominance of smooth muscle and ganglionlike cells, bizarre nuclear forms, and intranuclear inclusions (228). These tumors may show considerable pleomorphism, a feature that may lead to misdiagnosis, particularly in extrarenal lesions. The most distinctive component of the tumor is an HMB45-positive epithelioid smooth muscle cell, similar to that seen in lymphangiomyoma/lymphangiomyomatosis and PEComa (228). The tumors also express MELAN-A and microphthalmia transcription factor (232,233).

The differential diagnosis of gastrointestinal angiomyolipoma includes epithelioid variants of smooth muscle tumors, PEComas, and metastatic tumors. A clue to the diagnosis may come from a disproportionate degree of cytologic atypia in relation to other tumor features (mitotic rate, lack of necrosis, and circumscription) (227). Angiomyolipomas with signet ring features may resemble GISTs with signet ring features but angiomyolipomas are CD117 or CD34 negative and HMB45 positive. The differential diagnosis also includes metastatic melanoma. The lack of MELAN-A and S100 staining in the spindle and epithelioid cells rules out this possibility. However, the presence of pigment does not exclude a diagnosis of angiomyolipoma because melanin or melaninlike pigment may occur in these tumors. HMB45 and vimentin positivity is common to both lesions.

INTRA-ABDOMINAL DESMOPLASTIC SMALL ROUND CELL TUMORS

Desmoplastic small round cell tumors (DSRCTs) are rare, typically involving the peritoneum of children and young adults with a mean age of 10 and a strong male predilection (male:female ratio of 4:1) (234). A diagnostic chromosomal translocation (11;22)(p13q12) creates a fusion of the WT1 (Wilms tumor) gene on chromosome 11 with the EWS (Ewing sarcoma gene) on chromosome 22 (235). The chimeric protein produced by the translocation can be

detected immunohistochemically using an antibody raised against the carboxy terminal of WT1.

Patients present with abdominal distension, pain, a palpable abdominal mass, weight loss, ascites, or signs of intestinal obstruction or umbilical hernia (236). Lesions identified at the time of colonoscopy appear as diffuse white elevated lesions resembling aphthous erosions. Unusually high serum CA125 levels may be present (237). Variably sized but usually large intra-abdominal masses associate with smaller peritoneal implants of a similar appearance. The tumors can be >40 cm in diameter.

The tumor is characterized by sharply circumscribed nests or clusters of small round undifferentiated cells surrounded by a desmoplastic stroma. The cell nests vary in size and shape and glandlike spaces may be present. There may also be peripheral palisading of basaloid cells, central necrosis, and calcification. One may see uniform-appearing spindle cells with eosinophilic or clear cytoplasm, signet ring cells, and cells with marked nuclear pleomorphism. These cells are typically uniform with scanty cytoplasm and indistinct cell borders. The cells may contain cytoplasmic inclusions and an eccentric nucleus, imparting a rhabdoid appearance. The tumor cells are PAS positive. Mitotic figures and single cell necrosis are common (238).

Immunohistochemically, the tumors are positive for low-molecular-weight cytokeratin, EMA, vimentin, and CD57. They are variably positive for desmin in a dotlike pattern (238). Most tumors have nuclear reactivity for the C-terminal region of the Wilms tumor protein (238). WT1 immunoreactivity is not seen in Ewing sarcoma/primitive neuroectodermal tumors (PNETs) or neuroblastomas, making it a useful marker to separate DSRCTs from other small round blue cell tumors (239). DSRCTs are also focally positive for NSE, CD99, actin, PGP9.5, and S100 protein (240). Rare cases are cytokeratin negative, but the correct diagnosis can be established by utilizing molecular techniques to demonstrate the diagnostic translocation (241).

Patients with DSRCTs are typically treated by debulking procedures and postoperative chemotherapy and irradiation.

This tumor is highly aggressive and >90% of patients die from tumor progression within 3 to 46 months of their initial diagnosis (235). Tumor regression has been noted during multiagent chemotherapy, but prolonged survival is rare.

OTHER RARE MESENCHYMAL TUMORS

PNETs and *Ewing sarcomas* are usually grouped together as a single disease because of their characteristic diagnostic cytogenetic abnormality, usually a t(11;22), that results in EWS-FLI-1 gene fusion, creating an EWS/FLI fusion protein (242). This group of tumors typically affects younger patients (children and adolescents). Patients with gastrointestinal lesions present with obstruction or intussusception (243,244).

Both Ewing sarcomas and PNET are small, round blue cell tumors that lack obvious histologic differentiation. The tumors grow in a sheetlike, vaguely lobular growth pattern, with a well-developed capillary vasculature and a uniform population of round cells approximately two times the size of an endothelial cell. PNETs exhibit a mild to moderate degree of spindle cell growth and occasionally poorly formed rosettes. The cells possess a small amount of clear to lightly eosinophilic cytoplasm, regular nuclear contours, finely dispersed chromatin, and inapparent or small nucleoli. Geographic necrosis and individual degenerating cells (so-called dark cells) are frequently present. One often sees transmural involvement of the bowel wall with focal extension into adjacent organs. PAS staining shows the presence of occasional cytoplasmic PAS-positive granules. Rare mitoses are seen. The tumor cells of Ewing sarcomas/PNETs sometimes express morphologic and immunophenotypic evidence of neural differentiation, and it is now generally accepted that PNET is the more differentiated spectrum of Ewing sarcoma.

The tumors are positive for CD99 and FLI-1 (245), with FLI-1 positivity being present in approximately 70% of cases. FLI-1 is also routinely positive in lymphoblastic lymphomas and other non-Hodgkin lymphomas and, occasionally, in neuroblastoma, Merkel cell carcinoma, and melanoma (245). CD117 expression is found in many Ewing family–like tumors (246). The tumors also show diffuse cytoplasmic activity for vimentin and a focal paranuclear dot pattern of cytoplasmic cytokeratin immunoreactivity. As many as 25% of morphologically typical Ewing family tumors are positive with the broad-spectrum cytokeratin monoclonal cocktail AE1/AE3 (245). Because PNETs and Ewing tumors lack specific histologic features, cytogenetic and molecular demonstration of the t(11;22)(EWS-FLI-1) or variant translocations have emerged as the gold standard for diagnosing the Ewing family of tumors (245).

Primary gastrointestinal *synovial sarcomas* are rare, usually developing in adolescents. They arise in the stomach, esophagus, or small intestinal mesentery (246,247,248). Synovial sarcomas also metastasize to the GI tract. These tumors are typically biphasic and exhibit the classic features of synovial sarcomas arising elsewhere. These tumors are positive for cytokeratin and EMA and the diagnosis is confirmed by demonstrating the (X;18) chromosomal translocation. CD117 immunoreactivity may be present in these lesions, allowing synovial sarcomas to be confused with GISTs. However, the presence of the characteristic synovial sarcoma translocation allows one to distinguish between these two tumors.

Both *chondromas* and *osteochondromas* develop in the esophagus (249). They presumably develop in the submucosal glands and they likely resemble pulmonary hamartomas rather than being true neoplasms (250). These arise in the cervical esophagus and contain osseous and cartilaginous tissues along with fibrous tissue, adipose tissue, and glands (250).

Rhabdomyomas develop in the esophagus (251), colon (252), and anorectum (253). Rare *rhabdomyosarcomas* arise in the esophagus, stomach, duodenum, ileum, ampulla of Vater, and anal and perianal regions (254–257). Patients range in age from 3 to 59 years. Anal and perianal tumors resemble either embryonal (botryoid) or alveolar rhabdomyosarcomas. The tumors range in size from 1 to 20 cm with a median diameter of 4 cm. They may appear as infiltrative lesions or may form intraluminal polyps with infiltrating margins. The tumors are characterized by the presence of strap cells with eosinophilic cytoplasm lying in a myxoid matrix.

Alveolar soft part sarcomas (ASPSs) may be primary or secondary in the gut (258,259). The tumor affects adolescents and young adults with a predilection for affecting females (260). The tumors show a unique transcript, ASTL-TFE3, that creates a new fusion protein (261). Grossly, GI ASPSs appear as well-circumscribed "glittery yellow" nodules (Fig. 19.69). The tumor shows a characteristic alveolar whorled arrangement. The uniform-appearing tumor cells are polygonal with abundant eosinophilic granular cytoplasm and indistinct cell borders (Fig. 19.70). The cells contain 1 to 20 large, round, eosinophilic nuclei arranged in a horseshoe pattern. Vascular invasion is common. Mitoses are rare. Numerous diastase-resistant, PAS-positive granules and crystals are present.

Extraordinarily *giant cell tumors* arise in the GI tract (262). Colonic lesions may present as a long, irregular, stiff homogeneous grayish white stricture with areas of yellowish and brownish discoloration. Histologically, the tumor replaces the mucosa and muscular coat. It contains multinucleated giant cells similar to those described for giant cell tumors arising in other sites (262).

Rare primary *clear cell sarcomas* develop in the intestines and stomach (263–265) in patients ranging in age from 13 to 57 years. The tumors measure up to 7 cm in diameter and present as any other mass lesion. They center in the bowel wall with extension both into the mucosa and serosa. The neoplastic polygonal cells have either a clear or densely eosinophilic cytoplasm with centrally located, round to oval nuclei with irregular contours. They appear normochromatic

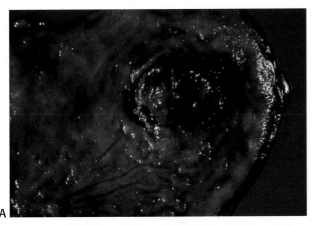

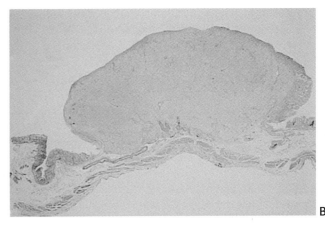

FIG. 19.69. Primary alveolar soft part sarcoma of stomach. **A:** Gross photograph demonstrating the presence of a polypoid nodule in the wall of the stomach. **B:** Tumor arising from the muscular layer of the bowel wall. (Case courtesy of Dr. Yagihashi, Department of Pathology, Hirosaki University School of Medicine, Hirosaki, Japan.)

or slightly hyperchromatic. Mitotic activity is generally high. Necrosis is scanty and generally limited to areas adjacent to ulcerations. Scattered osteoclastlike multinucleated giant cells are present. They are sometimes grouped focally so that some regions of the tumor contain many whereas others contain none (266). The tumor may exhibit a solid growth pattern with a tendency to form tumor nests. In other areas, perivascular pseudopapillae and alveolar formations may be seen.

These tumors frequently contain melanin. They are diffusely positive for S100 and often stain with HMB45, Melan

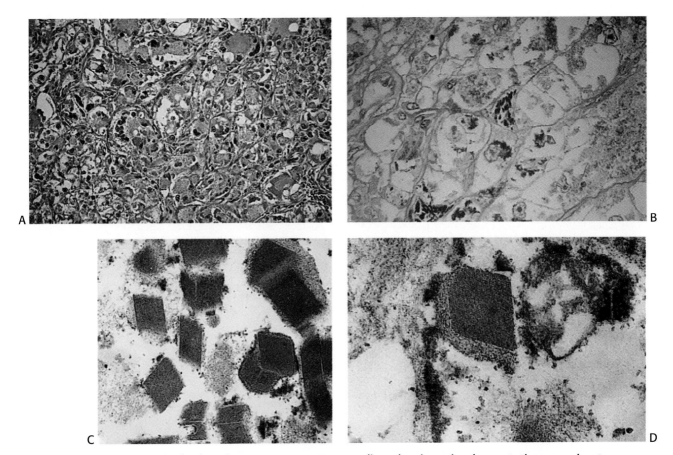

FIG. 19.70. Gastric alveolar soft part sarcoma. **A:** Hematoxylin and eosin section demonstrating a prominent alveolar arrangement. Multinucleated giant cell formation is frequently present. Occasional spherical inclusion bodies are also identified. **B:** Crystalline inclusion bodies present in the cytoplasm of the tumor cells. These are periodic acid–Schiff positive. **C:** Electron micrograph demonstrating the presence of the crystalline bodies. **D:** Higher magnification of the crystalline bodies present in this tumor.

A, tyrosinase, and other melanoma markers. They are also positive for microphthalmia transcription factor (MITF) (267). The tumor cells are negative for CD117, CD34, CD3, CD45, EMA, and usually cytokeratin. However, rarely, the tumors show aberrant cytokeratin expression. The differential diagnosis includes GISTs. The negativity for CD117, CD34, and PDGFRA effectively rule out this diagnosis. The histologic features, combined with the positivity for melanocytic markers, also raise the possibility of metastatic melanoma. However, clear cell sarcoma can be identified by the presence of the characteristic t(12;22)(q13;q12) translocation involving EWS and ATF-1 (267). The tumors are often aggressive, but they can have a variable course. The tumors metastasize to regional lymph nodes, the liver, and intra-abdominal sites. Prognosis is better if the tumor is small and superficial.

Elastofibromas may develop within the gastrointestinal tract, having been reported in the stomach, colon, rectum, and greater omentum (268,269). Patients range in age from 58 to 76. The cut surface of the lesion appears as a gray-white thickened submucosal layer with a rubbery elastic consistency. Gastric elastofibromas present more like mass lesions than those arising in the colon and rectum. The thickened areas contain abundant acellular collagen fibers containing numerous elastinophilic thick serrated fibers and globules.

REFERENCES

1. Kindblom LG, Remotti HE, Aldenborg F, et al: Gastro-intestinal pacemaker cell tumor (GIPACT): gastrointestinal stromal tumors show phenotypic characteristics of the interstitial cells of Cajal. *Am J Pathol* 1998;152:1259.
2. Miettinen M, Sarlomo-Rikala M, Lasota J: Gastrointestinal stromal tumors: recent advances in understanding of their biology. *Hum Pathol* 1999;30:1213.
3. Miettinen M, Lasota J, Sobin LH: Gastrointestinal stromal tumors of the stomach in children and young adults. A clinicopathologic, immunohistochemical and molecular genetic study of 44 cases with long-term follow-up and review of the literature. *Am J Surg Pathol* 2005;29:1373.
4. Bates AW, Feakins RM, Scheimberg I: Congenital gastrointestinal stromal tumour is morphologically indistinguishable from the adult form, but does not express CD117 and carries a favorable prognosis. *Histopathology* 2000;37:316.
5. Carney JA, Swee RG: Carney complex. *Am J Surg Pathol* 2002;26:393.
6. Hirota S, Nishida T, Isozaki K, et al: Familial gastrointestinal stromal tumors associated with dysphagia and novel type germline mutation of KIT gene. *Gastroenterology* 2002;122:1493.
7. Miettinen M, Fetsch JF, Sobin LH, Lasota J: Gastrointestinal stromal tumors in patients with neurofibromatosis 1. A clinicopathologic and molecular genetic study of 45 cases. *Am J Surg Pathol* 2006;30:90.
8. Miettinen M, Sobin LH, Lasota J: Gastrointestinal stromal tumors of the stomach: a clinicopathologic, immunohistochemical, and molecular genetic study of 1765 cases with long-term follow-up. *Am J Surg Pathol* 2005;29:52.
9. Robinson TL, Sircar K, Hewlett BR, et al: Gastrointestinal stromal tumors may originate from a subset of CD34-positive interstitial cells of Cajal. *Am J Pathol* 2000;156:1157.
10. Torihashi S, Nishi K, Tokutomi Y, et al: Blockade of kit signaling induces transdifferentiation of interstitial cells of Cajal to a smooth muscle phenotype. *Gastroenterology* 1999;117:140.
11. Heinrich MC, Rubin BP, Longley BJ, et al: Biology and genetic aspects of gastrointestinal stromal tumors: KIT activation and cytogenetic alterations. *Hum Pathol* 2002;33:484.
12. Corless CL, McGreevey L, Haley A, et al: KIT mutations are common in incidental gastrointestinal stromal tumors one centimeter or less in size. *Am J Pathol* 2002;160:1567.
13. Prakash S, Sarran L, Socci N, et al: Gastrointestinal stromal tumors in children and young adults: a clinicopathologic, molecular, and genomic study of 15 cases and review of the literature. *J Pediatr Hematol Oncol* 2005;27:179.
14. Lasota J, Wozniak A, Sarlomo-Rikala M, et al: Mutations in exons 9 and 13 of KIT gene are rare events in gastrointestinal stromal tumors. A study of 200 cases. *Am J Pathol* 2000;157:1091.
15. Andersson J, Sjogren H, Meis-Kindblom JM, et al: The complexity of KIT gene mutations and chromosome rearrangements and their clinical correlation in gastrointestinal stromal (pacemaker cell) tumors. *Am J Pathol* 2002;160:15.
16. Corless CL, Fletcher JA, Heinrich MC: Biology of gastrointestinal stromal tumors. *J Clin Oncol* 2004;22:3813.
17. Penzel R, Aulmann S, Mock M, et al: The location of KIT and PDGFRA gene mutations in gastrointestinal stromal tumors is site and phenotype associated. *J Clin Pathol* 2005;58:634.
18. Hartmann K, Wardelmann E, Yongsheng MA, et al: Novel germline mutation of *KIT* associated with familial gastrointestinal stromal tumors and mastocytosis. *Gastroenterology* 2005;129:1042.
19. Kato H, Nakamura M, Orito E, et al: A case of gastrointestinal stromal tumor with internal tandem duplication in the 3'-terminal of the KIT juxtamembrane domain. *Dig Dis Sci* 2005;50:70.
20. Vu HA, Xinh PT, Kikushima M, et al: A recurrent duodenal gastrointestinal stromal tumor with a frameshift mutation resulting in a stop codon in KIT exon 13. *Genes Chromosomes Cancer* 2005;42:179.
21. Heinrich MC, Corless CL, Duensing A, et al: PDGFRA activating mutations in gastrointestinal stromal tumors. *Science* 2003;299:708.
22. Yantiss RK, Rosenberg AE, Sarran L, et al: Multiple gastrointestinal stromal tumors in type I neurofibromatosis: a pathologic and molecular study. *Mod Pathol* 2005;18:475.
23. Nemoto H, Tate G, Schirinzi A, et al: Novel NF1 gene mutation in a Japanese patient with neurofibromatosis type 1 and a gastrointestinal stromal tumor. *J Gastroenterol* 2006;41:378.
24. Perry CG, Young WF, McWhinney SR, et al: Functioning paraganglioma and gastrointestinal stromal tumor of jejunum in three women. *Am J Surg Pathol* 2006;30:42.
25. Chen H, Hirota S, Isozaki K, et al: Polyclonal nature of diffuse proliferation of interstitial cells of Cajal in patients with familial and multiple gastrointestinal stromal tumours. *Gut* 2002;51:793.
26. Fletcher CD, Berman JJ, Corless C, et al: Diagnosis of gastrointestinal stromal tumors: a consensus approach. *Hum Pathol* 2002;33:459.
27. Lee JR, Joshi V, Griffin JW Jr, et al: Gastrointestinal autonomic nerve tumor: immunohistochemical and molecular identity with gastrointestinal stromal tumor. *Am J Surg Pathol* 2001;25:979.
28. Carney JA, Sheps SG, Go VLW, et al: The triad of gastric leiomyosarcoma, functioning extra-adrenal paraganglioma and pulmonary chondroma. *N Engl J Med* 1977;296:1517.
29. Suster S, Fletcher CD: Gastrointestinal stromal tumors with prominent signet-ring cell features. *Mod Pathol* 1996;9:609.
30. Richmond JA, Mount SL, Schwartz JE: Gastrointestinal stromal tumor of the stomach with rhabdoid phenotype: immunohistochemical, ultrastructural and immunoelectron microscopic evaluation. *Ultrastruct Pathol* 2004;28:65.
31. Suarez-Vilela D, Izquierdo-Garcia FM: Cytotoxic T-lymphocyte-rich, gastrointestinal stromal tumour. *Histopathology* 2003;43:398.
32. Miettinen M, Sarlomo-Rikala M, Sobin LH, et al: Esophageal stromal tumors: a clinicopathologic, immunohistochemical, and molecular genetic study of 17 cases and comparison with esophageal leiomyomas and leiomyosarcomas. *Am J Surg Pathol* 2000;24:211.
33. Miettinen M, El-Rifai W, Sobin L, et al: Evaluation of malignancy and prognosis of gastrointestinal stromal tumors: a review. *Hum Pathol* 2002;33:478.
34. Trupiano JK, Stewart RE, Misick C, et al: Gastric stromal tumors: a clinicopathologic study of 77 cases with correlation of features with nonaggressive and aggressive clinical behaviors. *Am J Surg Pathol* 2002;26:705.
35. Tworek JA, Appelman HD, Singleton TP, et al: Stromal tumors of the jejunum and ileum. *Mod Pathol* 1997;10:200.
36. Goldblum JR, Appelman HD: Stromal tumors of the duodenum: a histologic and immunohistochemical study of 20 cases. *Am J Surg Pathol* 1995;19:71.

37. Brainard JA, Goldblum JR: Stromal tumors of the jejunum and ileum: a clinicopathologic study of 39 cases. *Am J Surg Pathol* 1997;21:407.

38. Miettinen M, Makhlouf H, Sobin LH, Lasota J: Gastrointestinal stromal tumors of the jejunum and ileum. A clinicopathologic, immunohistochemical and molecular genetic study of 906 cases before Imatinib with long-term follow-up. *Am J Surg Pathol* 2006;30:477.

39. Miettinen M, Sobin LH: Gastrointestinal stromal tumors in the appendix: a clinicopathologic and immunohistochemical study of four cases. *Am J Surg Pathol* 2001;25:1433.

40. Miettinen M, Sarlomo-Rikala M, Sobin LH, et al: Gastrointestinal stromal tumors and leiomyosarcomas in the colon: a clinicopathologic, immunohistochemical, and molecular genetic study of 44 cases. *Am J Surg Pathol* 2000;24:1339.

41. Miettinen M, Furlong M, Sarlomo-Rikala M, et al: Gastrointestinal stromal tumors, intramural leiomyomas, and leiomyosarcomas in the rectum and anus: a clinicopathologic, immunohistochemical, and molecular genetic study of 144 cases. *Am J Surg Pathol* 2001;25:1121.

42. Tworek JA, Goldblum JR, Weiss SW, et al: Stromal tumors of the anorectum: a clinicopathologic study of 22 cases. *Am J Surg Pathol* 1999;23:946.

43. Loughery MB, Mitchell C, Mann GB, et al: Gastrointestinal stromal tumor treated with neoadjuvant Imatinib. *J Clin Pathol* 2005;58;779.

44. Abdulkader I, Cameselle-Teijeiro J, Forteza J: Pathological changes related to imatinib treatment in a patient with a metastatic gastrointestinal stromal tumour. *Histopathology* 2005;46:470.

45. Pauwels P, Debiec-Rychter M, Stul M, et al: Changing phenotype of gastrointestinal stromal tumours under imatinib mesylate treatment: a potential diagnostic pitfall. *Histopathology* 2005;47:41.

46. Miettinen M, Lasota J: Gastrointestinal stromal tumors—definition, clinical, histological, immunohistochemical, and molecular genetic features and differential diagnosis. *Virchows Arch* 2001;438:1.

47. Dorfman DM, Bui MM, Tubbs RR, et al: The CD117 immunohistochemistry tissue microarray survey for quality assurance and interlaboratory comparison: a College of American Pathologists Cell Markers Committee study. *Arch Pathol Lab Med* 2006;130:779.

48. Yamaguchi U, Hasegawa T, Masuda T, et al: Differential diagnosis of gastrointestinal stromal tumor and other spindle cell tumors in the gastrointestinal tract based on immunohistochemical analysis. *Virchows Arch* 2004;445:142.

49. Wang L, Vargas H, French SW: Cellular origin of gastrointestinal stromal tumors: a study of 27 cases. *Arch Pathol Lab Med* 2000;124:1471.

50. Sarlomo-Rikala M, Tsujimura T, Lendahl U, et al: Patterns of nestin and other intermediate filament expression distinguish between gastrointestinal stromal tumors, leiomyomas and schwannomas. *APMIS* 2002;110:499.

51. West RB, Corless CL, Chen X, et al: The novel marker, DOG1, is expressed ubiquitously in gastrointestinal stromal tumors irrespective of KIT or PDGFRA mutation status. *Am J Pathol* 2004;165:107.

52. Kim, K-M, Kang DW, Moon WS, et al: PKCθ expression in gastrointestinal stromal tumor. *Mod Pathol* 2006;19:1480.

53. Emory TS, Sobin LH, Lukes L, et al: Prognosis of gastrointestinal smooth-muscle (stromal) tumors: dependence on anatomic site. *Am J Surg Pathol* 1999;23:82.

54. Appelman HD, Lewin K: Mesenchymal tumors and tumor-like proliferations of the stomach. In: *Tumors of the Esophagus and Stomach*, AFIP Fascicle, Third Series. Washington, DC: AFIP, 1996.

55. Evans HL: Smooth muscle tumors of the gastrointestinal tract. A study of 56 cases followed for a minimum of 10 years. *Cancer* 1985;56:2242.

56. Lasota J, Sarlomo-Rikala M, Miettinen M: Mutations in exon 11 of c-Kit occur preferentially in malignant versus benign gastrointestinal stromal tumors and do not occur in leiomyomas or leiomyosarcomas. *Am J Pathol* 1999;154:53.

57. Taniguchi M, Nishida T, Hirota S, et al: Effect of c-kit mutation on prognosis of gastrointestinal stromal tumors. *Cancer Res* 1999;59:4297.

58. Rubin BP, Singer S, Tsao C, et al: KIT activation is a ubiquitous feature of gastrointestinal stromal tumors. *Cancer Res* 2001;61:8118.

59. Andersson J, Bumming P, Meis-Kindblom JM, et al: Gastrointestinal stromal tumors with KIT exon 11 deletions are associated with poor prognosis. *Gastroenterology* 2006;130:1573.

60. Lasota J, Dansonka-Mieszkowska A, Sobin LH, et al: A great majority of GISTs with PDGFRA mutations represent gastric tumors of low or no malignant potential. *Lab Invest* 2004;84:874.

61. DeMatteo RP, Lewis JJ, Leung D, et al: Two hundred gastrointestinal stromal tumors: recurrence patterns and prognostic factors for survival. *Ann Surg* 2000;231:51.

62. Irving JA, Lerwill MF, Young RH: Gastrointestinal stromal tumors metastatic to the ovary. A report of five cases. *Am J Surg Pathol* 2005;29:920.

63. Tuveson DA, Willis NA, Jacks T, et al: STI571 inactivation of the gastrointestinal stromal tumor c-KIT oncoprotein: biological and clinical implications. *Oncogene* 2001;20:5054.

64. Joensuu H, Fletcher C, Dimitrijevic S, et al: Management of malignant gastrointestinal stromal tumours. *Lancet Oncol* 2002;3:655.

65. Debiec-Rychter M, Cools J, Dumez H, et al: Mechanisms of resistance to imatinib mesylate in gastrointestinal stromal tumors and activity of the PKC412 inhibitor against imatinib-resistant mutants. *Gastroenterology* 2005;128:270.

66. Tamborini E, Bonadiman L, Greco A, et al: A new mutation in the KIT ATP pocket causes acquired resistance to imatinib in a gastrointestinal stromal tumor patient. *Gastroenterology* 2004;127:294.

67. Frost MJ, Ferrao PT, Hughes TP, et al: Juxtamembrane mutant V560GKit is more sensitive to imatinib (STI571) compared with wild-type c-kit whereas the kinase domain mutant D816VKit is resistant. *Mol Cancer Ther* 2002;1:1115.

68. Chen LL, Trent JC, Wu EF, et al: A missense mutation in KIT kinase domain 1 correlates with imatinib resistance in gastrointestinal stromal tumors. *Cancer Res* 2004;64:5913.

69. Antonescu CR, Sommer G, Sarran L, et al: Association of KIT exon 9 mutations with nongastric primary site and aggressive behavior: KIT mutation analysis and clinical correlates of 120 gastrointestinal stromal tumors. *Clin Cancer Res* 2003;9:3329.

70. Andrejauskas-Buchdunger E, Regenass U: Differential inhibition of the epidermal growth factor-, platelet-derived growth factor-, and protein kinase C-mediated signal transduction pathways by the staurosporine derivative CGP 41251. *Cancer Res* 1992;52:5353.

71. Takubo K, Nakagawa H, Tsuchiya S, et al: Seedling leiomyoma of the esophagus and esophagogastric junction zone. *Hum Pathol* 1981;12:1006.

72. Vortmeyer AO, Lubensky IA, Skarulis M, et al: Multiple endocrine neoplasia type 1: atypical presentation, clinical course and genetic analysis of multiple tumors. *Mod Pathol* 1999;12:919.

73. Matsukuma S, Takeo H, Ohara I, et al: Endoscopically resected colorectal leiomyomas often containing eosinophilic globules. *Histopathology* 2004;45:302.

74. Deyrup AT, Lee VK, Hill CE, et al: Epstein-Barr-Virus-associated smooth muscle tumors are distinctive mesenchymal tumors reflecting multiple infection events. *Am J Surg Pathol* 2006;30:75.

75. Billings SD, Folpe AL, Weiss SW: Do leiomyomas of deep soft tissue exist? An analysis of highly differentiated smooth muscle tumors of deep soft tissue supporting two subtypes. *Am J Surg Pathol* 2001;25:113.

76. Sloper JC: Idiopathic diffuse muscular hypertrophy of the lower oesophagus. *Thorax* 1954;9:136.

77. McKeeby JL, Li X, Zhuang Z, et al: Multiple leiomyomas of the esophagus, lung, and uterus in multiple endocrine neoplasia type 1. *Am J Pathol* 2001;159:1121.

78. Goh SG, Ho JM, Chuah KL, et al: Leiomyomatosis-like lymphangioleiomyomatosis of the colon in a female with tuberous sclerosis. *Mod Pathol* 2001;14:1141.

79. Siegler RW, Rothstein RI, Beecham JB, et al: Gastro-esophageal-vulvar leiomyomatosis presenting over the course of 20 years. *Arch Pathol Lab Med* 1996;120:1141.

80. Lonsdale RN, Roberts PF, Vaughan R, et al: Familial oesophageal leiomyomatosis and nephropathy. *Histopathology* 1992;20:127.

81. Zhou J, Mochizuki T, Smeets H, et al: Deletion of the paired a5(IV) and a6(IV) collagen genes in inherited smooth muscle tumors. *Science* 1993;261:1167.

82. Povey S, Burley MW, Attwood J, et al: Two loci for tuberous sclerosis: one on 9q34 and one on 16p13. *Ann Hum Genet* 1994;58:107.

83. Guillem P, Delcambre F, Cohen-Solal L, et al: Diffuse esophageal leiomyomatosis with perirectal involvement mimicking Hirschsprung disease. *Gastroenterology* 2001;120:216.

84. Freni SC, Keeman JN: Leiomyomatosis of the colon. *Cancer* 1977;39:263.

85. Tavassoli FA, Norris HJ: Peritoneal leiomyomatosis (leiomyomatosis peritonealis disseminata): a clinicopathologic study of 20 cases with ultrastructural observations. *Int J Gynecol Pathol* 1982;1:59.

86. Kaplan C, Benirschke K, Johnson KC: Leiomyomatosis peritonealis disseminata with endometrium. *Obstet Gynecol* 1980;55:119.

87. Akkersdijk GJ, Flu PK, Giard RW, et al: Malignant leiomyomatosis peritonealis disseminata. *Am J Obstet Gynecol* 1990;163:591.

88. Miettinen M, Kopczynski J, Makhlouf HR, et al: Gastrointestinal stromal tumors, intramural leiomyomas, and leiomyosarcomas in the duodenum: a clinicopathologic, immunohistochemical, and molecular genetic study of 167 cases. *Am J Surg Pathol* 2003;7:625.

89. Hou YY, Tan YS, Xu JF, et al: Schwannoma of the gastrointestinal tract: a clinicopathological, immunohistochemical and ultrastructural study of 33 cases. *Histopathology* 2006;48:536.

90. Mulvihill JJ, Parry DM, Sherman JL, et al: NIH conference: neurofibromatosis 1 (Recklinghausen disease) and neurofibromatosis 2 (bilateral acoustic neurofibromatosis). An update. *Ann Intern Med* 1990;113:39.

91. Kwon MS, Lee SS, Ahn GH: Schwannomas of the gastrointestinal tract: clinicopathological features of 12 cases including a case of esophageal tumor compared with those of gastrointestinal stromal tumors and leiomyomas of the gastrointestinal tract. *Pathol Res Pract* 2002;198:605.

92. Daimaru Y, Kido H, Hashimoto H, et al: Benign schwannoma of the gastrointestinal tract: a clinicopathologic and immunohistochemical study. *Hum Pathol* 1988;19:257.

93. Lewin MR, Dilworth HP, Abu AK, et al: Mucosal benign epithelioid nerve sheath tumors. *Am J Surg Pathol* 2005;29:1310.

94. Nabeya Y, Watanabe Y, Tohnosu N, et al: Diffuse schwannoma involving the entire large bowel with huge extramural development: report of a case. *Surg Today* 1999;29:637.

95. Miettinen M, Shekitka KM, Sobin LH: Schwannomas in the colon and rectum: a clinicopathologic and immunohistochemical study of 20 cases. *Am J Surg Pathol* 2001;25:846.

96. Murase K, Hino A, Ozeki Y, et al: Malignant schwannoma of the esophagus with lymph node metastasis: literature review of schwannoma of the esophagus. *J Gastroenterol* 2001;36:772.

97. Hornick JL, Fletcher CD: Intestinal perineuromas: clinicopathologic definition of a new anatomic subset in a series of 10 cases. *Am J Surg Pathol* 2005;29:859.

98. Xu GF, O'Connell P, Viskochil D, et al: The neurofibromatosis type 1 gene encodes a protein related to GAP. *Cell* 1990;62:599.

99. Menon AG, Anderson KM, Riccardi VM, et al: Chromosome 17p deletions and p53 gene mutations associated with the formation of malignant neurofibrosarcomas in von Recklinghausen neurofibromatosis. *Proc Natl Acad Sci USA* 1990;87:5435.

100. Berner JM, Sorlie T, Mertens F, et al: Chromosome band 9p21 is frequently altered in malignant peripheral nerve sheath tumors: studies of CDKN2A and other genes of the pRB pathway. *Genes Chromosomes Cancer* 1999;26:151.

101. Wang Q, Lasset C, Desseigne F, et al: Neurofibromatosis and early onset of cancers in hMLH1-deficient children. *Cancer Res* 1999;59:294.

102. Gallinger S, Aronson M, Shayan K, et al: Gastrointestinal cancer and neurofibromatosis type 1 features in children with a germline homozygous MLH1 mutation. *Gastroenterology* 2004;126:576.

103. Riccardi VM: Von Recklinghausen's neurofibromatosis. *N Engl J Med* 1981;305:1617.

104. Westenend PJ, Smedts F, de Jong MCJW, et al: A 4-year-old boy with neurofibromatosis and severe renovascular hypertension due to renal arterial dysplasia. *Am J Surg Pathol* 1994;18:512.

105. Behranwala KA, Spalding D, Wotherspoon A, et al: Small bowel gastrointestinal stromal tumours and ampullary cancer in Type 1 neurofibromatosis. *World J Surg Oncol* 2004;2:1.

106. Shekitka KM, Sobin LH: Ganglioneuromas of the gastrointestinal tract. Relation to Von Recklinghausen disease and other multiple tumor syndromes. *Am J Surg Pathol* 1994;18:250.

107. Dahl EV, Waugh JM, Dahlin DC: Gastrointestinal ganglioneuromas. *Am J Pathol* 1957;33:953.

108. Weidner N, Flanders DJ, Mitros FA: Mucosal ganglioneuromatosis associated with multiple colonic polyps. *Am J Surg Pathol* 1984;8:779.

109. Haggitt RC, Reid BJ: Hereditary gastrointestinal polyposis syndromes. *Am J Surg Pathol* 1986;10:871.

110. Devroede G, Limieux B, Masse S, et al: Colonic hamartomas in tuberous sclerosis. *Gastroenterology* 1988;94:182.

111. Carney JA, Go VL, Sizemore GW, et al: Alimentary-tract ganglioneuromatosis: a major component of the syndrome of multiple endocrine neoplasia, type 2b. *N Engl J Med* 1976;295:1287.

112. D'Amore ES, Manivel JC, Pettinato G, et al: Intestinal ganglioneuromatosis: mucosal and transmural types: a clinicopathologic and immunohistochemical study of six cases. *Hum Pathol* 1991;22:276.

113. Mendelsohn G, Diamond MP: Familial ganglioneuromatous polyposis of the large bowel—report of a family with associated juvenile polyposis. *Am J Surg Pathol* 1984;8:515.

114. Santoro M, Carlomagno F, Romano A, et al: Activation of RET as a dominant transforming gene by germline mutations of MEN2A and MEN2B. *Science* 1995;267:381.

115. Hegstrom JL, Kircher T: Alimentary tract ganglioneuromatosis-lipomatosis, adrenal myolipomas, pancreatic telangiectasias, and multinodular thyroid goiter. *Am J Clin Pathol* 1985;83:744.

116. Lashner BA, Riddell RH, Winans CS: Ganglioneuromatosis of the colon and extensive glycogenic acanthosis in Cowden's disease. *Dig Dis Sci* 1986;31:213.

117. Demos TC, Blonder J, Schey WL, et al: Multiple endocrine neoplasia (MEN) syndrome type IIB: gastrointestinal manifestations. *Am J Roentgenol* 1983;140:73.

118. Rescorla RJ, Vane DW, Fitzgerald JF, et al: Vasoactive intestinal polypeptide-secreting ganglioneuromatosis affecting the entire colon and rectum. *J Pediatr Surg* 1988;23:635.

119. Feinstat T, Tesluk H, Schuffler MD, et al: Megacolon and neurofibromatosis: a neuronal intestinal dysplasia. *Gastroenterology* 1984;86:1573.

120. Harries K, Nunn T, Shah V, et al: First reported case of esophageal paraganglioma. A review of the literature of gastrointestinal tract paraganglioma including gangliocytic paraganglioma. *Dis Esophagus* 2004;17:191.

121. Westbrook KC, Bridger WM, Williams GD: Malignant non-chromaffin paraganglioma of the stomach. *Am J Surg* 1972;124:407.

122. Kheir SM, Halpern NB: Paraganglioma of the duodenum in association with congenital neurofibromatosis. *Cancer* 1984;53:2491.

123. Skoldberg F, Grimelius L, Woodward ER, et al: A family with hereditary extraadrenal paragangliomas without evidence for mutations in the von Hippel-Lindau disease or ret genes. *Clin Endocrinol* 1998;48:11.

124. Baysal BE, Ferrell RE, Willett-Brozik JE, et al: Mutations in SDHD, a mitochondrial complex II gene in hereditary paraganglioma. *Science* 2000;287:848.

125. Mariman ECM, van Beersum SEC, Cremers CWRJ, et al: Fine mapping of a putatively imprinted gene for familial non-chromaffin paragangliomas to chromosome 11q13.1 evidence for genetic heterogeneity. *Hum Genet* 1995;95:56.

126. Niemann S, Muller U: Mutations in SDHC cause autosomal dominant paraganglioma type 3. *Nat Genet* 2000;26:268.

127. Mulligan LM, Kwok JB, Healey CS, et al: Germline mutations of the RET protooncogene in multiple endocrine neoplasia type 2A. *Nature* 1993;363:458.

128. Latif F, Tory K, Gnarra J, et al: Identification of the von Hippel-Lindau tumor suppressor gene. *Science* 1993;260:1317.

129. Horenstein MG, Hitchcock TA, Tucker JA: Dual CD117 expression in gastrointestinal stromal tumor (GIST) and paraganglioma of Carney triad: a case report. *Int J Surg Pathol* 2005;13:87.

130. Pipeleers-Marichal M, Goossens A, De Waele B, et al: Granular cell tumour of the appendix in a patient irradiated for a rectal carcinoma. *Virchows Arch A Pathol Anat* 1990;417:177.

131. Sailors JL, French SW: The unique simultaneous occurrence of granular cell tumor, gastrointestinal stromal tumor, and gastric adenocarcinoma. *Arch Pathol Lab Med* 2005;129:121.

132. Vinco A, Vettoretto N, Cervi E, et al: Association of multiple granular cell tumors and squamous carcinoma of the esophagus: case report and review of the literature. *Dis Esophagus* 2001;14:262.

133. Marinho A, Moura A, Baptista M, et al: Granular cell tumour and leiomyomatosis of the esophagus—a non-coincidental association? *Pathol Res Pract* 1996;192:492.

134. Johnston J, Helwig EB: Granular cell tumors of the gastrointestinal tract and perianal region: a study of 74 cases. *Dig Dis Sci* 1981;26:807.

135. David O, Jakate S: Multifocal granular cell tumor of the esophagus and proximal stomach with infiltrative pattern: a case report and review of the literature. *Arch Pathol Lab Med* 1999;123:967.

136. O'Donovan DG, Kell P: Malignant granular cell tumour with intraperitoneal dissemination. *Histopathology* 1989;14:417.

137. Buley ID, Gatter KC, Kelly PMA, et al: Granular cell tumours revisited. An immunohistological and ultra-structural study. *Histopathology* 1988;12:263.

138. Parfitt JR, Mclean CA, Joseph MG, et al: Granular cell tumors of the gastrointestinal tract: expression of nestin and clinicopathologic evaluation of 11 patients. *Histopathology* 2006;48:424.

139. Mazur MT, Shultz JJ, Myers JL: Granular cell tumor. Immunohistochemical analysis of 21 benign tumors and one malignant tumor. *Arch Pathol Lab Med* 1990;114:692.

140. Tzilinis A, Fessenden JM, Ressler KM, et al: Transanal resection of a colonic lipoma, mimicking rectal prolapse. *Curr Surg* 2003;60:313.

141. Snover DC: Atypical lipomas of the colon: report of two cases with pseudomalignant features. *Dis Colon Rectum* 1984;27:485.

142. Kato K, Matsuda M, Onodera K, et al: Angiolipoma of the colon with right lower quadrant abdominal pain. *Dig Surg* 1999;16:441.

143. Mohl W, Fischinger J, Moser C, et al: Duodenal angiolipoma: endoscopic diagnosis and therapy. *Z Gastroenterol* 2004;42:1381.

144. McGregor DH, Kerley SW, McGregor MS: Gastric angiolipoma with chronic hemorrhage and severe anemia. *Am J Med Sci* 1993;305:229.

145. Ramirez JM, Ortego J, Deus J, et al: Lipomatous polyposis of the colon. *Br J Surg* 1993;80:349.

146. Santos-Briz A, Garcia JP, Gonzalez C, et al: Lipomatous polyposis of the colon. *Histopathology* 2001;38:81.

147. Amato G, Martella A, Ferraraccio F, et al: Well differentiated "lipoma-like" liposarcoma of the sigmoid mesocolon and multiple lipomatosis of the rectosigmoid colon. Report of a case. *Hepatogastroenterology* 1998;45:2151.

148. Panagopoulos I, Hoglund M, Mertens F, et al: Fusion of the EWS and CHOP genes in myxoid liposarcoma. *Oncogene* 1996;12:489.

149. Vartanian RK, O'Connell JX, Holden JK, et al: Primary jejunal well-differentiated liposarcoma (atypical lipomatous tumor) with leiomyosarcomatous dedifferentiation. *Int J Surg Pathol* 1996;4:29.

150. Middleton SB, Frayling IM, Phillips RK: Desmoids in familial adenomatous polyposis are monoclonal proliferations. *Br J Cancer* 2000;82: 827.

151. Weiss S, Goldblum JR: *Enzinger and Weiss's Soft Tissue Tumors.* 4th ed. St. Louis: Mosby, 2001, pp 309–346.

152. Burke AP, Sobin LH, Shekitka KM, et al: Intraabdominal fibromatosis. A pathologic analysis of 130 tumors with comparison of clinical subgroups. *Am J Surg Pathol* 1990;14:335.

153. Slater G, Greenstein AJ: Mesenteric fibromatosis in Crohn's disease. *J Clin Gastroenterol* 1996;22:147.

154. Yantiss RK, Spiro IJ, Compton CC, et al: Gastrointestinal stromal tumor versus intra-abdominal fibromatosis of the bowel wall: a clinically important differential diagnosis. *Am J Surg Pathol* 2000;24:947.

155. Wilcken N, Tattersall MH: Endocrine therapy for desmoid tumors. *Cancer* 1991;68:1384.

156. Montgomery E, Torbenson MS, Kaushal M, et al: Beta-catenin immunohistochemistry separates mesenteric fibromatosis from gastrointestinal stromal tumor and sclerosing mesenteritis. *Am J Surg Pathol* 2002;26:1296.

157. Montgomery E, Lee JH, Abraham SC, et al: Superficial fibromatoses are genetically distinct from deep fibromatoses. *Mod Pathol* 2001;14:695.

158. Rodriguez JA, Guarda LA, Rosai J: Mesenteric fibromatosis with involvement of the gastrointestinal tract. A GIST simulator: a study of 25 cases. *Am J Clin Pathol* 2004;121:93.

159. Lynch HT, Fitzgibbons R Jr, Chong S, et al: Use of doxorubicin and dacarbazine for the management of unresectable intra-abdominal desmoid tumors in Gardner's syndrome. *Dis Colon Rectum* 1994;37:260.

160. Goy BW, Lee SP, Eilber F, et al: The role of adjuvant radiotherapy in the treatment of resectable desmoid tumors. *Int J Radiat Oncol Biol Phys* 1997;39:659.

161. Bauernhofer T, Stoger H, Schmid M, et al: Sequential treatment of recurrent mesenteric desmoid tumor. *Cancer* 1996;77:1061.

162. Mace J, Sybil Biermann J, Sondak V, et al: Response of extraabdominal desmoid tumors to therapy with imatinib mesylate. *Cancer* 2002;95: 2373.

163. Cook JR, Dehner LP, Collins MH, et al: Anaplastic lymphoma kinase (ALK) expression in the inflammatory myofibroblastic tumor: a comparative immunohistochemical study. *Am J Surg Pathol* 2001;25:1364.

164. Nonaka D, Birbe R, Rosai J: So-called inflammatory myofibroblastic tumour: a proliferative lesion of fibroblastic reticulum cells? *Histopathology* 2005;46:604.

165. Coffin CM, Watterson J, Priest JR, et al: Extrapulmonary inflammatory myofibroblastic tumor (inflammatory pseudotumor). A clinicopathologic and immunohistochemical study of 84 cases. *Am J Surg Pathol* 1995;19:859.

166. Aboulafia DM: Inflammatory pseudotumor causing small bowel obstruction and mimicking lymphoma in a patient with AIDS: clinical improvement after initiation of thalidomide treatment. *Clin Infect Dis* 2000;30:826.

167. Purdy DJ, Levine EJ, Forsthoefel KJ, et al: Periampullary pseudotumor secondary to granulomatous disease. *Am J Gastroenterol* 1994;89:2087.

168. Gomez-Roman JJ, Sanchez-Velasco P, Ocejo-Vinyals G, et al: Human herpesvirus-8 genes are expressed in pulmonary inflammatory myofibroblastic tumor (inflammatory pseudotumor). *Am J Surg Pathol* 2001;25:624.

169. Coffin CM, Patel A, Perkins S, et al: ALK1 and p80 expression and chromosomal rearrangements involving 2p23 in inflammatory myofibroblastic tumor. *Mod Pathol* 2001;14:569.

170. Lawrence B, Perez-Atayde A, Hibbard MK, et al: TPM3-ALK and TPM4-ALK oncogenes in inflammatory myofibroblastic tumors. *Am J Pathol* 2000;157:377.

171. Debelenko LV, Arthur DC, Pack SD, et al: Identification of CARS-ALK fusion in primary and metastatic lesions of an inflammatory myofibroblastic tumor. *Lab Invest* 2003;83:1255.

172. Meis-Kindblom JM, Kjellstrom C, Kindblom LG: Inflammatory fibrosarcoma: update, reappraisal, and perspective on its place in the spectrum of inflammatory myofibroblastic tumors. *Semin Diagn Pathol* 1998;15:133.

173. Makhlouf HR, Sobin LH: Inflammatory myofibroblastic tumors (inflammatory pseudotumors) of the gastrointestinal tract: how closely are they related to inflammatory fibroid polyps? *Hum Pathol* 2002;33:307.

174. Aagaard MT, Kristensen IB, Lund O, et al: Primary malignant non-epithelial tumours of the thoracic oesophagus and cardia in a 25-year surgical material. *Scand J Gastroenterol* 1990;25:876.

175. Jiao YF, Nakamura S, Sugai T, et al: p53 gene mutation and MDM2 overexpression in a case of primary malignant fibrous histiocytoma of the jejunum. *APMIS* 2002;110:165.

176. Murata I, Makiyama K, Miyazaki K, et al: A case of inflammatory malignant fibrous histiocytoma of the colon. *Gastroenterol Jpn* 1993;28:554.

177. Gentry R, Dockery MB, Clagett, OT: Vascular malformations and vascular tumors of the gastrointestinal tract. *Int Abstr Surg* 1949;88:281.

178. Garvin PJ, Herrmann V, Kaminski DL, et al: Benign and malignant tumors of the small intestine. *Curr Probl Cancer* 1979;3:1.

179. Ruiz AR Jr, Ginsberg AL: Giant mesenteric hemangioma with small intestinal involvement: an unusual cause of recurrent gastrointestinal bleed and review of gastrointestinal hemangiomas. *Dig Dis Sci* 1999; 44:2545.

180. Lie JT: Pathology of angiodysplasia in Klippel-Trenaunay syndrome. *Pathol Res Pract* 1988;183:747.

181. Bourdeau A, Cymerman U, Paquet ME, et al: Endoglin expression is reduced in normal vessels but still detectable in arteriovenous malformations of patients with hereditary hemorrhagic telangiectasia type 1. *Am J Pathol* 2000;156:911.

182. Smith CR, Bartholomew LG, Cain JC: Hereditary hemorrhagic telangiectasia and gastrointestinal hemorrhage. *Gastroenterology* 1963;44:1.

183. Cynamon HA, Milov DE, Andres JM: Multiple telangiectasias of the colon in childhood. *J Pediatrics* 1988;112:928.

184. Vase P, Grove O: Gastrointestinal lesions in hereditary hemorrhagic telangiectasia. *Gastroenterology* 1986;91:1079.

185. Hall BD: Intestinal hemangiomas and Maffucci's syndrome. *Arch Dermatol* 1972;105:608.

186. Blix S, Aas K: Giant hemangioma, thrombocytopenia, fibrinogenemia and fibrinolytic activity. *Acta Med Scand* 1961;169:63.

187. Allison KH, Yoder BJ, Bronner MP, et al: Angiosarcoma involving the gastrointestinal tract: a series of primary and metastatic cases. *Am J Surg Pathol* 2004;28:298.

188. Wolov RB, Sato N, Azumi N, et al: Intra-abdominal "angiosarcomatosis" report of two cases after pelvic irradiation. *Cancer* 1991;67:2275.

189. Ben-Izhak O, Kerner H, Brenner B, et al: Angiosarcoma of the colon developing in a capsule of a foreign body. *Am J Clin Pathol* 1992;97:416.

190. Nanus DM, Kelsen D, Clark DGC: Radiation-induced angiosarcoma. *Cancer* 1987;60:777.

191. Mori S, Itoyama S, Mohri N, et al: Cellular characteristics of neoplastic angioendotheliosis. An immunohistological marker study of 6 cases. *Virch Arch A Pathol Anat Histopathol* 1985;407:167.

192. Miettinen M, Sarlomo-Rikala M, Lasota J: KIT expression in angiosarcomas and fetal endothelial cells: lack of mutations of exon 11 and exon 17 of c-kit. *Mod Pathol* 2000;13:536.

193. Bavikatty NR, Goldblum JR, Abdul-Karim FW, et al: Florid vascular proliferation of the colon related to intussusception and mucosal prolapse: potential diagnostic confusion with angiosarcoma. *Mod Pathol* 2001;14:1114.

194. Biggar RJ, Horn J, Lubin JH, et al: Cancer trends in a population at risk of acquired immunodeficiency syndrome. *J Natl Cancer Inst* 1985;74:793.

195. Mocroft A, Kirk O, Clumeck N, et al: The changing pattern of Kaposi sarcoma in patients with HIV, 1994-2003. *Cancer* 2004;100:2644.

196. Ensoli B, Barillari G, Buonaguro L, Gallo RC: Molecular mechanisms in the pathogenesis of AIDS-associated Kaposi's sarcoma. *Adv Exp Med Biol* 1991;303:27.

197. Salahuddin SZ, Nakamura S, Biberfeld P, et al: Angiogenic properties of Kaposi's sarcoma-derived cells after long-term culture in vitro. *Science* 1988;242:430.

198. Hengge UR, Ruzicka T, Tyring SK, et al: Update on Kaposi's sarcoma and other HHV8 associated diseases. Part 2: pathogenesis, Castleman's disease and pleural effusion lymphoma. *Lancet Infect Dis* 2002;2:344.

199. Rabkin CS, Janz S, Lash A, et al: Monoclonal origin of multicentric Kaposi's sarcoma lesion. *N Engl J Med* 1997;336:988.

200. Gill PS, Tsai YC, Rao AP, et al: Evidence for multicolonality in multicentric Kaposi's sarcoma. *Proc Natl Acad Sci USA* 1998;95:8257.

201. Ambroziak JA, Blackbourn DJ, Herndier BG, et al: Herpes-like sequences in HIV-infected and uninfected Kaposi's sarcoma patients. *Science* 1995;268:582.

202. Cohen J: Is a new virus the cause of KS? *Science* 1994;268:1803.

203. Boshoff C, Schultz TF, Kennedy MM, et al: Kaposi's sarcoma-associated herpesvirus infects endothelial and spindle cells. *Nat Med* 1995;1:1274.

204. Wang L, Wakisaka N, Tomlinson CC, et al: The Kaposi sarcoma-associated herpesvirus (KSH/HHV-8) K1 protein induces expression of angiogenic and invasion factors. *Cancer Res* 2004;64:2774.

205. Simpson GR, Schultz TF, Whitby D, et al: Prevalence of Kaposi's sarcoma associated herpesvirus infection measured by antibodies to recombinant capsid protein and latent immunofluorescent antigen. *Lancet* 1996;348:1133.

206. Martin JN, Ganem DE, Osmond DH, et al: Sexual transmission and the natural history of human herpesvirus 8 infection. *N Engl J Med* 1998;338:948.

207. Levine AM: AIDS-related malignancies: the emerging epidemic. *J Natl Cancer Inst* 1993;85:1382.

208. Patel RV, Goldblum JR, His ED: Immunohistochemical detection of human herpes virus-8 latent nuclear antigen-1 is useful in the diagnosis of Kaposi sarcoma. *Mod Pathol* 2004;17:456.

209. Antman K, Chang Y: Kaposi's sarcoma. *New Engl J Med* 2000;342:1027.

210. Mahle C, Schwartz M, Popek E, et al: Intra-abdominal lymphangiomas in children and adults. Assessment of proliferative activity. *Arch Pathol Lab Med* 1997;121:1055.

211. Kuroda Y, Katoh H, Ohsato K: Cystic lymphangioma of the colon: report of a case and review of the literature. *Dis Colon Rectum* 1984;27:679.

212. Zilko PJ, Laurence BH, Sheiner H, et al: Cystic lymphangioma of colon causing protein losing enteropathy. *Am J Dig Dis* 1975;20:1076.

213. Amadori G, Micciolo R, Poletti A: A case of intra-abdominal multiple lymphangiomas in an adult in whom the immunological evaluation supported the diagnosis. *Eur J Gastroenterol Hepatol* 1999;11:347.

214. Schaefer JW, Griffin WO, Dublier LD: Colonic lymphangiectasis associated with a potassium depletion syndrome. *Gastroenterology* 1968;55:515.

215. North PE, Kahn T, Cordisco MR, et al: Multifocal lymphangioendotheliomatosis with thrombocytopenia: a newly recognized clinicopathological entity. *Arch Dermatol* 2004;140:599.

216. Farley TJ, Klionsky N: Mixed hemangioma and cystic lymphangioma of the esophagus in a child. *J Pediatr Gastroenterol Nutr* 1992;15:178.

217. Miettinen M, Paal E, Lasota J, et al: Gastrointestinal glomus tumors: a clinicopathologic, immunohistochemical, and molecular genetic study of 32 cases. *Am J Surg Pathol* 2002;26:301.

218. Hamilton LW, Phil M, Shelbourne JD, et al: A glomus tumor of the jejunum masquerading as a carcinoid tumor. *Hum Pathol* 1982;113:859.

219. Haque S, Modlin IM, West AB: Multiple glomus tumors of the stomach with intravascular spread. *Am J Surg Pathol* 1992;16:291.

220. Warner KE, Haidak GL: Massive glomus tumor of the stomach: 20-year follow-up and autopsy findings. *Am J Gastroenterol* 1984;79:253.

221. Binder SC, Wolfe HJ, Deterling RA Jr: Intra-abdominal hemangiopericytoma: report of four cases and review of the literature. *Arch Surg* 1973;107:536.

222. McMaster MJ, Soule EH, Ivins JC: Hemangiopericytoma: a clinicopathologic study and long-term follow up of 60 patients. *Cancer* 1975;36:2232.

223. Bonetti F, Martignoni G, Colato C, et al: Abdominopelvic sarcoma of perivascular epithelioid cells. Report of four cases in young women, one with tuberous sclerosis. *Mod Pathol* 2001;14:563.

224. Birkhaeuser F, Ackermann C, Flueckiger T, et al: First description of a PEComa (perivascular epithelioid cell tumor) of the colon: report of a case and review of the literature. *Dis Colon Rectum* 2004;47:1734.

225. Evert M, Wardelmann E, Nestler G, et al: Abdominopelvic perivascular epithelioid cell sarcoma (malignant PEComa) mimicking gastrointestinal stromal tumour of the rectum. *Histopathology* 2005;46:115.

226. Hornick JL, Fletchler CDM: PEComa: what do we know so far? *Histopathology* 2006;48:75.

227. Folpe AL, Mentzel T, Lehr H-A, et al: Perivascular epithelioid cell neoplasms of soft tissue and gynecologic origin. *Am J Surg Pathol* 2005;29:1558.

228. Bonetti F, Pea M, Martignoni G, et al: The perivascular epithelioid cell and related lesions. *Adv Anat Pathol* 1997;4:343.

229. Maluf H, Dieckgraefe B: Angiomyolipoma of the large intestine: report of a case. *Mod Pathol* 1999;12:1132.

230. Martignoni G, Pea M, Bonetti F, et al: Carcinoma-like monotypic epithelioid angiomyolipoma in patients without evidence of tuberous sclerosis: a clinicopathologic and genetic study. *Am J Surg Pathol* 1998;22:663.

231. Tsui WM, Colombari R, Portmann BC, et al: Hepatic angiomyolipoma: a clinicopathologic study of 30 cases and delineation of unusual morphologic variants. *Am J Surg Pathol* 1999;23:34.

232. Jungbluth AA, Busam KJ, Gerald WL, et al: A103: an anti-melan a monoclonal antibody for the detection of malignant melanoma in paraffin-embedded tissues. *Am J Surg Pathol* 1998;22:595.

233. Zavala-pompa A, Folpe AL, Jimenez RE, et al: Immunohistochemical study of microphthalmia transcription factor and tyrosinase in angiomyolipoma of the kidney, renal cell carcinoma and renal and retroperitoneal sarcomas: comparative evaluation with traditional markers. *Am J Surg Pathol* 2001;25:65.

234. Dorsey BV, Benjamin LE, Rauscher F 3rd, et al: Intra-abdominal desmoplastic small round-cell tumor: expansion of the pathologic profile. *Mod Pathol* 1996;9:703.

235. Gerald WL, Ladanyi M, de Alava E, et al: Clinical, pathologic, and molecular spectrum of tumors associated with t(11;22)(p13;q12): desmoplastic small round-cell tumor and its variants. *J Clin Oncol* 1998;16:3028.

236. Lae ME, Roche PC, Jin L, et al: Desmoplastic small round cell tumor: a clinicopathologic, immunohistochemical, and molecular study of 32 tumors. *Am J Surg Pathol* 2002;26:823.

237. Ordonez NG, Sahin AA: CA 125 production in desmoplastic small round cell tumor: report of a case with elevated serum levels and prominent signet ring morphology. *Hum Pathol* 1998;29:294.

238. Ordonez NG: Desmoplastic small round cell tumor: II: an ultrastructural and immunohistochemical study with emphasis on new immunohistochemical markers. *Am J Surg Pathol* 1998;22:1314.

239. Barnoud R, Sabourin JC, Pasquier D, et al: Immunohistochemical expression of WT1 by desmoplastic small round cell tumor: a comparative study with other small round cell tumors. *Am J Surg Pathol* 2000;24:830.

240. Norton J, Monaghan P, Carter RL: Intra-abdominal desmoplastic small cell tumour with divergent differentiation. *Histopathology* 1991;19:560.

241. Trupiano JK, Machen SK, Barr FG, et al: Cytokeratin-negative desmoplastic small round cell tumor: a report of two cases emphasizing the utility of reverse transcriptase-polymerase chain reaction. *Mod Pathol* 1999;12:849.

242. Hu-Lieskovan S, Zhang J, Wu L, et al: EWS-FLI1 fusion protein up-regulates critical genes in neural crest development and is responsible for the observed phenotype of Ewing's family of tumors. *Cancer Res* 2005;65:4633.

243. Folpe AL, Goldblum JR, Rubin BP, et al: Morphologic and immunophenotypic diversity in Ewing family tumors: a study of 66 genetically confirmed cases. *Am J Surg Pathol* 2005;29:1025.

244. Shek TW, Chan GC, Khong PL, et al: Ewing sarcoma of the small intestine. *J Pediatr Hematol Oncol* 2001;23:530.

245. Folpe AL, Hill CE, Parham DM, et al: Immunohistochemical detection of FLI-1 protein expression: a study of 132 round cell tumors with emphasis on CD99-positive mimics of Ewing's sarcoma/primitive neuroectodermal tumor. *Am J Surg Pathol* 2000;24:1657.

246. Gonzalez I, Andreu EJ, Panizo A, et al: Imatinib inhibits proliferation of Ewing tumor cells mediated by the stem cell factor/KIT receptor pathway, and sensitizes cells to vincristine and doxorubicin-induced apoptosis. *Clin Cancer Res* 2004;10:751.

247. Anton-Pacheco J, Cano I, Cuadros J, et al: Synovial sarcoma of the esophagus. *J Pediatr Surg* 1996;31:1703.

248. Helliwell TR, Raraty M, Morris AI, et al: Biphasic synovial sarcoma in the small intestinal mesentery. *Cancer* 1995;75:2862.

249. Mahour GH, Harrison EG Jr: Osteochondroma (tracheobronchial choristoma) of the esophagus. Report of a case. *Cancer* 1967;20:1489.

250. Saitoh Y, Inomata Y, Tadaki N, et al: Pedunculated intraluminal osteochrondromatous hamartoma of the esophagus. *J Otolaryngol* 1990;19:339.

251. Pai GK, Pai PK, Kamath SM: Adult rhabdomyoma of the esophagus. *J Pediatr Surg* 1987;22:991.

252. Yang AH, Chen WY, Chiang H: Malignant rhabdoid tumour of colon. *Histopathology* 1994;24:89.

253. Lapner PC, Chou S, Jimenez C: Perianal fetal rhabdomyoma: case report. *Pediatr Surg Int* 1997;12:544.

254. Willen R, Lillo-Gil R, Willen H, et al: Embryonal rhabdomyosarcoma of the oesophagus. Case report. *Acta Chir Scand* 1989;155:59.

255. Fox KR, Moussa SM, Mitre RJ, et al: Clinical and pathologic features of primary gastric rhabdomyosarcoma. *Cancer* 1990;66:772.

256. Caty MG, Oldham KT, Prochownik EV: Embryonal rhabdomyosarcoma of the ampulla of Vater with long-term survival following pancreaticoduodenectomy. *J Pediatr Surg* 1990;25:1256.

257. Mihara S, Yano H, Matsumoto H, et al: Perianal alveolar rhabdomyosarcoma in a child: report of a long-term survival case. *Dis Colon Rectum* 1983;26:728.

258. Yagihashi S, Yagihashi N, Hase Y, et al: Primary alveolar soft-part sarcoma of stomach. *Am J Surg Pathol* 1991;15:399.

259. Zilber S, Brouland JP, Voisin MC, et al: Colonic metastases of alveolar soft-part sarcoma: a case report and review of the literature. *Ann Diagn Pathol* 2003;7:306.

260. Bu X, Bernstein L: A proposed explanation for female predominance in alveolar soft part sarcoma. Noninactivation of X; autosome translocation fusion gene? *Cancer* 2005;103:1245.

261. Ladanyi M, Lui MY, Antonescu CR, et al: The der(17)t(X;17) (p11;q25) of human alveolar soft part sarcoma fuses the TFE3 transcription factor gene to ASPL, a novel gene at 17q25. *Oncogene* 2001;20:48.

262. Eshun-Wilson K: Malignant giant-cell tumour of the colon. *Acta Pathol Microbiol Scand* 1973;81:137.

263. Achten R, Debiec-Rychter M, De Wever I, et al: An unusual case of clear cell sarcoma arising in the jejunum highlights the diagnostic value of molecular genetic techniques in establishing a correct diagnosis. *Histopathology* 2005;46:472.

264. Fukuda T, Kakihara T, Baba K, et al: Clear cell sarcoma arising in the transverse colon. *Pathol Int* 2000;50:412.

265. Pauwels P, Debiec-Rychter M, Sciot R, et al: Clear cell sarcoma of the stomach. *Histopathology* 2002;41:526.

266. Zambrano E, Reyes-Mugica M, Franchi A, et al: An osteoclast-rich tumor of the gastrointestinal tract with features resembling clear cell sarcoma of soft parts: reports of 6 cases of a GIST simulator. *Int J Surg Pathol* 2003;12:75.

267. Antonescu CR, Tschernyavsky SJ, Woodruff JM, et al: Molecular diagnosis of clear cell sarcoma. Detection of EWS-ATF1 and MITF-M transcripts and histopathological and ultrastructural analysis of 1 case. *J Mol Diagn* 2002;4:44.

268. Saint-Paul MC, Musso S, Cardot-Leccia N, et al: Elastofibroma of the stomach. *Pathol Res Pract* 2003;199:637.

269. Goldblum JR, Beals T, Weiss SW: Elastofibromatous change of the rectum. A lesion mimicking amyloidosis. *Am J Surg Pathol* 1992;16:793.

Note: Page numbers followed by f indicate figure; those followed by t indicate table.